TEXTBOOK OF

Medical-Surgical Nursing

LILLIAN SHOLTIS BRUNNER,
R.N., M.S.N., Sc.D., F.A.A.N.

Consultant in Nursing, Schools of Nursing:
Presbyterian-University of Pennsylvania Medical
Center, Philadelphia, Pennsylvania, and Bryn
Mawr Hospital, Bryn Mawr, Pennsylvania,
formerly Assistant Professor of Surgical Nursing,
Yale University School of Nursing

DORIS SMITH SUDDARTH,
R.N., B.S.N.E., M.S.N.

Consultant in Health Occupations, Job Corps
Health Office, U.S. Department of Labor;
formerly Coordinator of the Curriculum,
Alexandria Hospital School of Nursing,
Alexandria, Virginia

TEXTBOOK OF

Medical-Surgical Nursing

Fourth Edition

J. B. Lippincott Company • Philadelphia • Toronto

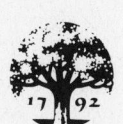

Fourth Edition

Copyright © 1980, 1975, 1970, 1964 by J. B. Lippincott
Company

Distributed in Great Britain by Harper & Row, Ltd.

ISBN 0-397-54238-0

Printed in the United States of America

3 5 7 9 8 6 4

Library of Congress Cataloging in Publication Data

Brunner, Lillian Sholtis.
    Textbook of medical-surgical nursing.

    Bibliography: p.
    Includes index.
    1. Nursing. 2. Surgical nursing. I. Suddarth,
Doris Smith, joint author. II. Title. II. Title:
Medical-surgical nursing. [DNLM: 1. Nursing care.
2. Surgical nursing. WY150 B897t]
RT41.B86   1980   610.73   79-27506
ISBN 0-397-54238-0

PREFACE

In the decade of the eighties, the only certainty for nursing and other health professions will be the certainty of change. The nurse will face unprecedented challenges and opportunities. Shifting attitudes, inflationary pressures, cost consciousness, a revolution of rising expectations and research advances will influence health care. The nurse should be assertive in reaching for excellence in nursing theory and practice even while moving in new and unfamiliar directions. The spirit of inquiry and an understanding of the human mind and body are basic to the care of the client/patient in any environment.

To alleviate the effects of the patient's health problems in the medical-surgical setting, the nurse has to have a knowledge of normal physiology and how it is altered by disease, and an understanding of principles and rationale of management, nursing interventions and strategies. This core of knowledge is fundamental to patient assessment, which requires a perceptive and educated mind. Analysis of clinical evidence, the basic material with which the nurse works, is based on an understanding of the patient's problems.

Therefore, the authors continue to present the theoretical principles and concepts of medical-surgical nursing from both a biological and a clinical point of view. The common clinical problems are presented in a logical framework to encourage decision making and competence in patient care. Every condition has been reviewed, updated and amplified to reflect the results of ongoing research in health and illness care.

The revised first unit presents a broad view of nursing in today's world. Several conceptual models in nursing currently in use as a framework for nursing curricula are presented as examples of contemporary models in nursing. It is not the intent of the authors to suggest that any of these be adopted since a conceptual framework must be agreed upon by the individual faculty in light of their philosophy. Nursing and the health care delivery system and the roles of the nurse as practitioner, leader and researcher are reviewed. The nursing process, termed the essence of nursing, is detailed in a separate chapter.

Since the American public is beginning to realize the necessity of accepting greater individual responsibility for health, nurses along with other health educators are becoming sensitive to their roles as teachers. A new chapter, Patient Education/Health Teaching, includes the nature of teaching and learning and the nursing process in patient teaching. Patient education is also emphasized in the discussion of major clinical conditions.

There are two new chapters in Unit Three, Biophysical and Psychosocial Concepts Related to Health and Illness. Recognizing that improved nutrition will promote wellness and help cut the nation's health care costs, Chapter 9, Nutritional Considerations in Health Care has been added. It includes nutritional assessment and counseling in health and disease. The nutritional support of patients with cancer, renal disease, diabetes, gastrointestinal and cardiovascular diseases has been expanded. The rationale of the nutritional support is discussed from the point of view of biochemical changes that take place in disease necessitating dietary modifications.

A major advance has developed through the understanding of the immune nature of disease. Chapter 10, The Immune System and Immunopathology, will aid in learning how the body's immune system normally functions and its relationship to disease, specific treatment and ultimate prognosis.

In response to reader requests, Chapter 19, Intraoperative Nursing Management, has been written to give the framework of perioperative techniques and management to enable the nurse to supply supportive therapy before, during and after the operation.

Because of almost daily developments in the field of cancer research, Chapter 16, Diagnostic Radiology, Radiotherapy and Nuclear Medicine is offered to guide the nurse through the intricacies of the physics of radiation, its biological aspects, clinical application and nursing support. A section on radiopharmaceuticals, the techniques involved, and results to be expected from nuclear medicine procedures has been added.

A physiological overview precedes each clinical section. The prevention of illness and health maintenance are stressed. Risk factors have been identified whenever feasible to help sharpen assessment and case-finding skills.

The chapters have been reorganized to take cognizance of changes in the nursing curricula, advances made in biomedical research and to promote the acquisition of ever changing and increasing knowledge. Nursing is a uniquely human skill and the techniques of nursing are included where appropriate along with the management of emotional, psychosocial and behavioral aspects of patient care.

A serious attempt has been made to avoid the use of the pronouns *she/her* in referring to the nurse. However, this has been difficult. The nurse authors recognize and respect our male nurse colleagues as equal partners in providing the best care to all humans. Another hard decision involved references to the patient. Single gender pronouns are used to maintain the clarity and flow of the text. Any apparent discrimination is truly unintentional.

Because the art is long, the subject matter vast, and the value of human life immeasurable, the study of nursing is the task of a lifetime. We offer this revised volume in the hope that it will increase understanding and clinical expertise as the nurse engages in the most challenging and rewarding task—that of caring for patients.

LSB and DSS

CONTRIBUTORS

ABASS ALAVI, M.D.
Assistant Professor of Nuclear Medicine, Hospital of the University of Pennsylvania, Philadelphia
Chapter 16: Nuclear Medicine

JANE B. ALAVI, M.D.
Hematology-Oncology Section, Hospital of the University of Pennsylvania, Philadelphia
Chapter 32: Assessment and Management of Patients with Hematologic Disorders

PETER H. ARGER, M.D.
Associate Professor of Radiology, Hospital of the University of Pennsylvania, Philadelphia
Chapter 16: Diagnostic Radiology

PATRICIA J. BALDWIN, R.N., D.N.SC.
formerly Assistant Professor and Chairman of Cardiovascular Nursing, The Catholic University of America, Washington, D.C.
Chapter 28: Management of the Patient in the Cardiac Care Unit

BRENDA G. BARE, R.N., M.S.N.
Acting Curriculum Coordinator, Alexandria Hospital, Alexandria, Virginia
Chapter 1: Nursing in Today's World: Concepts and Implementation
Chapter 2: The Nursing Process
Chapter 3: Patient Teaching/Health Education

HERBERT H. BUTLER, M.D.
Emergency Department Physician, Underwood-Memorial Hospital, Woodbury, New Jersey
Chapter 27: Electrocardiograms and Heart Arrhythmias

EDWARD D. CRANDALL, M.D.
Associate Professor of Medicine, UCLA School of Medicine, Los Angeles, California
Physiology and selected sections on Pathophysiology

JAMES F. ELAM, PH.D.
Clinical Biochemist, Pathology Department, Alexandria Hospital, Alexandria, Virginia
Appendix: Diagnostic Studies and Their Meanings

ARON B. FISHER, M.D.
Associate Professor of Medicine and Physiology, University of Pennsylvania School of Medicine, Philadelphia
Physiology and selected sections on Pathophysiology

RONALD J. GLASSER, M.D.
Pediatric Nephrology, Department of Pediatrics, University of Minnesota, Minneapolis
Chapter 10: The Immune System and Immunopathology

CAMILLUS J. R. JOHNPULLE, M.B.B.S.
Medical Staff, Department of Anesthesia, St. Mary's Hospital, West Palm Beach, Florida
Chapter 24: Respiratory Intensive Care Nursing

SILVIA PRODAN LANGE, R.N., M.N.
Clinical Specialist, Department of Psychological and Social Medicine, Presbyterian Hospital of Pacific Medical Center, San Francisco, California
Chapter 11: Illness as a Human Experience

THOMAS E. MACNAMARA, M.B., CH.B.
Professor and Chairman, Department of Anesthesia, Georgetown University School of Medicine, Washington, D. C.
Chapter 24: Respiratory Intensive Care Nursing

MARGO McCAFFERY, R.N., M.S.
Consultant in the Nursing Care of Patients with Pain, Santa Monica, California; Assistant Clinical Professor, Nursing, University of California, Los Angeles
Chapter 14: The Person Experiencing Pain

RUTH MROZEK, R.N., M.N.
Clinical Specialist in Nursing, Pittsburgh, Pennsylvania
Chapter 6: Documentation of Nursing Practice

CHARLES B. MULHERN, M.D.
Assistant Professor, Radiation Therapy, Hospital of the University of Pennsylvania, Philadelphia, Pennsylvania
Chapter 16: Diagnostic Radiology

THOMAS E. PIEMME, M.D.
Director, Office of Continuing Medical Education, George Washington University, Washington, D.C.
Chapter 4: Clinical Interviewing
Chapter 5: Physical Assessment

MELVYN P. RICHTER, M.D.
Assistant Professor Radiation Therapy, Hospital of the University of Pennsylvania, Philadelphia
Chapter 16: Radiotherapy
Chapter 45: Radiotherapy: Management of Patients with Gynecologic Disorders

MONA B. SHEVLIN, PH.D.
Assistant Professor of Counseling and Guidance, School of Education, The Catholic University of America, Washington, D.C.; Director of the Counseling Center for Greater Washington
Chapter 13: Developmental Concepts of the Life Cycle

H. MILLARD SMITH, M.D., PH.D.
formerly Director of Clinical Pharmacology, Schering Corporation; Associate Professor of Physiology, University of Arkansas; Associate Professor of Physiology, Loma Linda University
Chapter 7: Homeostatic Mechanisms and Pathophysiologic Processes
Chapter 15: Cell Cycle in Oncology: Nursing the Patient with Cancer

BEATRICE K. SPARLING, R.N., M.S.N.
Cardiovascular Clinical Nursing Specialist; Assistant Professor, Nursing Program, Division of Health Technology, Northern Virginia Community College, Annandale, Virginia
Chapter 29: Management of the Cardiovascular Surgery Patient

SALLY GALBRAITH THOMAS, R.N., PH.D., F.A.A.N.
Assistant Professor of Nursing, School of Nursing, University of California, Los Angeles
Psychosocial Problems faced by the Patient with Breast Cancer, in Chapter 46: Management of the Patient with Breast Disorders

EILEEN STRELING TURNER, R.N., M.S.N.
Clinical Director, Hong Kong Adventist Hospital, Hong Kong
Chapter 29: Management of the Cardiovascular Surgery Patient

KYRIAKE V. VALASSI, PH.D.
Professor of Nutritional Biochemistry, School of Nursing, The Catholic University of America, Washington, D.C.
Chapter 9: Nutritional Considerations in Health Care

ACKNOWLEDGMENTS

Nursing shares an intricate colleague-relationship with other disciplines and benefits by the mutual exchange of this knowledge and expertise. The authors express special appreciation to the following persons:

LUCY JO ATKINSON, R.N., M.S., Director of Educational Services, Ethicon, Inc., Somerville, New Jersey

MARJORIE H. BAER, R.N., B.A., M.N., Assistant Director, School of Nursing, The Bryn Mawr Hospital, Bryn Mawr, Pennsylvania

JULIA W. BALZER, R.N., M.N., Consultant, Clinical Specialist, Psychiatric-Mental Health Nursing; Northern Virginia Mental Health Institute, Falls Church, Virginia

ELIZABETH W. BAYLEY, R.N., M.S.N., M.S., Clinical Specialist in Burn Nursing, Department of Nursing, Crozer-Chester Medical Center, Chester, Pennsylvania

STEPHEN J. BEDNAR, M.D., Assistant Professor of Medicine, Georgetown University Medical Center, Washington, D.C.

JUDITH S. BOYD, R.N., B.A., formerly Director of Nursing Services, National Orthopedic and Rehabilitation Hospital, Arlington, Virginia

FRANK P. BROOKS, M.D. Sc.D. (Med.), Professor of Medicine and Physiology, School of Medicine, University of Pennsylvania

CONNIE J. DELANEY, R.N., M.A., Instructor in Nursing, Luther College, Department of Nursing, Decorah, Iowa

ROBERT DiBIANCO, M.D., Chief of Noninvasive Cardiac Laboratories, Veterans Administration Hospital, Washington, D.C.

JOHN C. DONALDSON, CDR., M.C., U.S.N., Assistant Head, Pulmonary Branch, National Naval Medical Center, Bethesda, Maryland

E. ANNE DOTSKA, R.N., M.A. Ed., Instructor in Nursing, Bryn Mawr Hospital School of Nursing, Bryn Mawr, Pennsylvania

KATHLEEN A. EGAN, R.P.T., Department of Physical Medicine, Crozer-Chester Medical Center, Upland, Chester, Pennsylvania

MERVYN L. ELGART, M.D., Professor and Chairman, Department of Dermatology, George Washington University Medical Center, Washington, D.C.

THOMAS G. FRAZIER, M.D., F.A.C.S., Assistant Surgeon, Bryn Mawr Hospital; Instructor in Surgery, Thomas Jefferson University, Philadelphia, Pennsylvania

BARBARA GASTELL, M.D., M.P.H., Expert, National Institute on Aging, National Institutes of Health, Bethesda, Maryland

LEE GIGLIOTTI, R.N., M.S.N., Assistant Clinical Professor of Nursing, University of Pennsylvania; Director, Oncology Nursing, Hospital of the University of Pennsylvania, Philadelphia, Pennsylvania

CECIL P. GREENE, A.M., BRIT.I.R.E., C.L.T., C.C.E., Clinical Engineer, Clinical Engineering Services, Stafford, Virginia

GEORGE W. GREGORY, CDR., M.C., U.S.N., Department of Cardiovascular and Thoracic Surgery, National Naval Medical Center, Bethesda, Maryland

MAUREEN HARRIS, Ph.D., Program Director, National Diabetes Data Group, National Institutes of Health, Bethesda, Maryland

PATRICIA ROBERTSON HERCULES, R.N., M.S., Assistant Professor in Nursing, Houston Baptist University, Houston, Texas

LOIS M. HOSKINS, R.N., M.S.N., Ph.D., Assistant Professor of Nursing, The Catholic University of America, Washington, D.C.

JAMES R. HOWE, M.D., Clinical Instructor, Neurosurgery, George Washington University Medical Center, Washington, D.C.

PAMELA F. HUMPHREY, R.P.T., Washington Adventist Hospital, Takoma Park, Maryland

RUTH H. KIRKMAN, R.N., M.S., Director of Nursing, Crozer-Chester Medical Center, Upland, Chester, Pennsylvania

LOUIS J. LaBORWIT, Ph.D., Chief Speech Pathologist, Department of Physical Medicine and Rehabilitation, Georgetown University Hospital, Washington, D.C.

STEPHEN M. LEVIN, M.D., Assistant Clinical Professor of Orthopedic Surgery, Howard University, Washington, D.C.

JONI MAGEE, M.D., Instructor, Obstetrics and Gynecology, Thomas Jefferson University; Attending Physician, Booth Maternity Center and Methodist Hospital, Philadelphia, Pennsylvania

ERNEST L. McKENNA, JR., M.D., Clinical Professor of Otolaryngology, Thomas Jefferson University, Philadelphia, Pennsylvania

HARRY C. MILLER, M.D., Professor and Chairman, Department of Urology, George Washington University Medical Center, Washington, D.C.

M. BARRY MOSKOWITZ, D.M.D., Clinical Associate in Restorative Dentistry, School of Dental Medicine, University of Pennsylvania, Philadelphia, Pennsylvania

JOHN H. MOYER, M.D., D.Sc., Professor of Medicine and Director of Regional Affairs, Temple University School of Medicine, Philadelphia; Senior Vice-President and Director, Professional and Educational Affairs, Conemaugh Valley Memorial Hospital, Johnstown, Pennsylvania

DAVID NAIDE, M.D., Associate Professor of Medicine; Chief, Vascular Section, Hahnemann Medical College and Hospital; Chief, Vascular Clinic, Graduate Hospital, Philadelphia, Pennsylvania

PHILIP R. NAST, M.D., Attending Gastroenterologist, Bryn Mawr Hospital, Bryn Mawr, Pennsylvania; Associate Professor Gastroenterology, School of Medicine, University of Pennsylvania, Philadelphia, Pennsylvania

HENRY J. NEALIS, M.D., Ophthalmologist, Bryn Mawr Hospital, Bryn Mawr, Pennsylvania

A. E. PARRISH, M.D., Director, Division of Renal Diseases, George Washington University Medical Center, Washington, D.C.

DONALD M. PORETZ, M.D., Chief, Infectious Diseases, Fairfax Hospital, Falls Church, Virginia

JAMES W. PREUSS, M.D., Clinical Instructor, Neurosurgery, Georgetown University Medical Center, Washington, D.C.

BASIL M. RIFKIND, M.D., F.R.C.P., Chief, Lipid Metabolism Branch; Project Officer, Lipid Research Clinics Program; Division of Heart and Vascular Diseases, National Institutes of Health, Bethesda, Maryland

ROGER D. SOLOWAY, M.D., Gastroenterology, Hospital of the University of Pennsylvania; Associate Professor of Medicine, School of Medicine, University of Pennsylvania, Philadelphia, Pennsylvania

BARRY E. STIMMEL, R.P.T., Washington Adventist Hospital, Takoma Park, Maryland

LEROY D. VANDAM, M.D., Professor of Anaesthesia, Harvard Medical School; Anesthesiologist-in-Chief, Peter Bent Brigham Hospital, Boston, Massachusetts

NANCY S. WEXLER, Ph.D., Psychologist, Neurological Disorders Program, National Institute for Neurological and Communicative Disorders and Stroke, National Institutes of Health, Bethesda, Maryland

ARTWORK

The authors are particularly indebted to *Neil O. Hardy* for his ingenious interpretation of the authors' art requests and for the consistency of outstanding quality in his unique art style.

Artists:
Shirley Baty, William Burke, Nancy Lou Gahan, Timothy Hengst, E. Thompson Thayer

Photography:
Glenn Dalby

LIBRARY/RESEARCH

ALBERT M. BERKOWITZ, Chief of Reference Services Division, and the Reference Staff, National Library of Medicine, Bethesda, Maryland

JEAN CROSIER, References Services Division, National Library of Medicine

LESLIE D. GUNDRY, Chief Medical Librarian, Bryn Mawr Hospital and School of Nursing, Bryn Mawr, Pennsylvania

ALICE MACKOV, Reference (Head), Scott Memorial Library, Thomas Jefferson University, Philadelphia, Pennsylvania

ALEXANDER G. KULCHAR, Medical Librarian, Bryn Mawr Hospital and School of Nursing, Bryn Mawr, Pennsylvania

JACQUELINE VAN DE KAMP, References Services Division, National Library of Medicine

The authors express appreciation to

DIANA INTENZO, editor, for her continued expert overall supervision, knowledgeable guidance, and personal interest. Her commitment to excellence is deeply appreciated.

JEANNE WALLACE, copy editor, for her continued meticulous attention to detail, concern for meeting time schedules, and especially for her gracious and calming personality.

MARY MURPHY, secretary, for her efficiency and speed in providing materials, and for her quiet, warm and pleasant manner.

DAVID T. MILLER, Vice-President, for his constant support, expectation of the best, and global awareness of trends.

the many others of the Lippincott/Harper team who have been our loyal friends and supporters.

LSB DSS

CONTENTS

Unit Three   Biophysical and Psychosocial Concepts Related to Health and Illness

Unit Four   Concepts and Challenges in Patient Management

Unit Five   Perioperative Management of the Surgical Patient

Unit Six   Problems Affecting Oxygen-Carbon Dioxide Exchange and Respiration

Unit Seven Cardiovascular, Circulatory, and Hematologic Problems

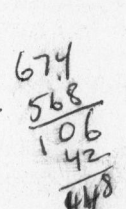

Unit Eight   Digestive and Gastrointestinal Problems

Unit Nine   Metabolic and Endocrine Problems

Unit Ten   Renal and Urinary Problems

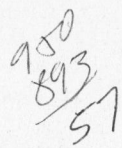

Unit Eleven   Sexual and Reproductive Problems

Unit Twelve   Integumentary Problems and Disorders of Protective Function

Unit Thirteen   Sensorineural Problems

Unit Fourteen   Musculoskeletal and Locomotion Problems

Unit Fifteen Other Acute Problems

Health
Maintenance
and Health Needs

UNIT ONE

1

NURSING IN TODAY'S WORLD: Concepts and Implementation

NURSING DEFINED

Since the era of modern nursing began, nursing leaders have attempted to define nursing in such a way as to articulate clearly the roles and functions of the nurse. Included in these definitions are: the services provided by the nurse, the setting within which the profession of nursing functions, the characteristics of the person who is the recipient of nursing care, and those attributes that distinguish nursing from other service-oriented disciplines in the health care delivery system. While definitions of nursing have evolved over the years, a universally accepted definition does not exist.

Since the time of Florence Nightingale, who wrote in 1858 that the real goal of nursing was "to put the patient in the best condition for nature to act upon him," nursing leaders have defined nursing as both an art and a science. In the earlier years, they tended to emphasize the nursing services that are directed toward the care of the sick. More recently, they have stressed the maintenance and promotion of health as well as the prevention of illness.

One of the classic definitions of nursing, as formulated by Virginia Henderson (1966), delineates the unique function of the nurse as follows:

> to assist the individual, sick or well, in the performance of those activities contributing to health or its recovery (or to peaceful death) that he would perform unaided if he had the necessary strength, will or knowledge. And to do this in such a way as to help him gain independence as rapidly as possible.[*]

[*]Henderson, V.: The Nature of Nursing. New York, The Macmillan Company, 1966.

Review of the literature since the time of Henderson's definition of nursing reveals a multitude of attempts at further defining the unique function of the nurse — unique with regard to the functions of other health care disciplines. Most of these formulations have attempted to define nursing as a profession directed toward meeting both the health and illness needs of "man," who is viewed holistically as having physical as well as emotional, psychological, intellectual, social, and spiritual needs. One such definition of nursing is that presented by Yura and Walsh (1978).

> Nursing is an encounter with a client and his family in which the nurse observes, supports, communicates, ministers, and teaches; she contributes to the maintenance of optimum health, and provides care during illness until the client is able to assume responsibility for the fulfillment of his own basic human needs; when necessary, she provides compassionate assistance with dying.[†]

Because of the diversity of definitions of nursing that exist in the literature, individual nurses and groups of nurses are left with the choice of subscribing to one of these definitions, of combining components of several definitions, or of developing their own. Whatever the choice, the selected definition should reflect a view of man as an integrated whole — a bio-psycho-social being. With such a view, the holistic concept of health is then seen as including physical, emotional, psychological, intellectual, social, and spiritual aspects of human functioning that are interrelated, interdependent, and of equal importance.

[†]Yura, H., and Walsh, W. B.: The Nursing Process, 3rd edition. Appleton-Century-Crofts, 1978.

- Nursing then can be defined as a service-oriented health profession that is directed toward meeting the health and illness needs of the individual relative to all aspects of his or her functioning capacity.
- The goal of nursing can be defined as the promotion, maintenance, and restoration of health with concern for the biological and psychosocial factors of health and illness, and with respect for the needs and rights of the person to whom nursing care is rendered.

CONCEPTUAL MODELS IN NURSING

If nurses are to accomplish the goals of nursing as defined by nursing leaders, nursing must have a body of theoretical knowledge upon which to base its practice. "Theory building" in nursing is still in its infancy. In the past, nursing has utilized theories from various biopsychosocial sciences. Only within the past several decades have nurses made concerted efforts toward identifying a circumscribed body of knowledge that is unique to nursing and that can serve as the theoretical basis for the practice of nursing. Such a theoretical basis, when more fully developed, will consist of scientifically derived general principles that will serve to describe, explain, and predict the practice of nursing. Nursing theories will provide a guide for viewing nursing holistically and for determining the probable results of nursing actions in advance of their implementation. However, only as theories of nursing evolve and mature and as they are tested and retested will a general theory of nursing develop.

Much of the progress that has been accomplished in the pursuit of a scientific theory of nursing has been in the areas of concept formalization and model construction. Because nursing is a practice-oriented discipline, concepts of nursing have been evolving over the years. However, it has only been within recent years that nurses have attempted to articulate these concepts, to propose that they be utilized as the framework for nursing practice, and to test and validate them. Many concepts which have their foundations in the biopsychosocial sciences have been found to be particularly applicable to nursing and to serve as useful components of frameworks for nursing practice.

Several of the broad concepts which have been utilized extensively as frameworks for nursing curricula and for nursing practice throughout the country include (1) the wellness-illness continuum, (2) developmental processes throughout the life cycle, and (3) stress-adaptation.

The *wellness-illness continuum* provides a means by which the nurse focuses on the patient's positive health attributes and characteristics within the dimensions of his illness or potential illness situation. With such a focus, the nurse then assists the patient to utilize his attributes in attaining and maintaining the highest level of wellness that is possible within his physical and psychosocial limitations.

The *developmental processes* approach to nursing provides a frame of reference that emphasizes the complexity of variables that are involved in each of the developmental stages of the life cycle. Such a framework provides direction for the nurse in assisting the patient to accomplish his developmental tasks as they are affected by his state of health and wellness.

The *stress-adaptation framework* emphasizes the role of the nurse in assessing the patient's behavioral responses to the demands of his internal and external environment. Nursing goals are then directed toward assisting the patient to strive toward adaptive behavior that promotes health and prevents illness.

These broad concepts and other related concepts, while serving as useful frameworks for nursing practice, are not in and of themselves unique to nursing. Therefore, nursing leaders have attempted to develop more fully concepts that are inherent within nursing itself and to construct models that describe the relationships between these concepts and their subconcepts. Three such conceptual models of nursing are the *life processes model* developed by Rogers (1970), the *self-care model* as advocated by Orem (1971), and the *adaptation model* as formulated by Roy (1974).

These are certainly not the only conceptual models of nursing that have been developed, nor is it the intent of the authors to suggest that nurses should subscribe to any one of these models, forsaking other models that may also serve as valuable frameworks for the practice of nursing. However, it is the intent of the authors to present these models as *examples* of contemporary models of nursing, with the hope that they will generate interest, enthusiasm, and inquiry into the present status and future potential of conceptual frameworks of nursing and the state of theory building in nursing.

The Life Processes Model

The life processes model of nursing focuses on the wholeness of the human organism in the person who is the recipient of nursing care. It is Rogers's belief that the purpose of the scientific body of knowledge of nursing is to describe, explain, and make predictions about mankind. Such knowledge leads to the evolution of theories that serve to guide nursing practice. Rogers identified fundamental human attributes which constitute the following basic assumptions upon which nursing science is built:

1. Man is a unified whole possessing his own integrity and manifesting characteristics that are more than and different from the sum of his parts.
2. Man and the environment are continuously exchanging matter and energy with one another.

3. The life process evolves irreversibly and unidirectionally along the space-time continuum.
4. Pattern and organization identify man and reflect his innovative wholeness.
5. Man is characterized by the capacity for abstraction and imagery, language and thought, sensation and emotion.

The qualities of the life processes as described in these assumptions include: wholeness, openness, unidirectionality, pattern and organization, sentience and thought. The underlying principles describe man as a dynamic entity who interacts mutually and simultaneously with his environment. The changes which occur during this interaction are irreversible, nonrepeatable, and rhythmical, increasing in complexity and proceeding by the continual repatterning of man and his environment.

- With such a view of man, the goal of nursing becomes that of promoting the person's interaction with his environment in such a way that the maximum state of health that is possible is realized by the utilization of the individual's own energies and potential.

This holistic concept of human functioning serves as the basis for making predictions about nursing intervention. Data gathered for making nursing diagnoses are derived from the total pattern of events that have influenced the extent to which man is achieving his maximum health potential. These data then serve as the basis for the establishment of short-term and long-term health goals for the individual, his family, and society, and for the implementation of nursing actions directed toward the achievement of these goals. These nursing actions are aimed at helping the individual to repattern his relationship with himself and his environment so that his maximum health potential can be attained. Such a conceptual model of nursing as proposed by Rogers contributes to the pursuit of a scientific theory of nursing. Testing, retesting, and validation of the model will no doubt serve to further the science of nursing.

The Self-Care Model

Orem has developed a concept of nursing that places emphasis on the person's need for self-care—those activities which an individual practices for the purpose of maintaining life, health, and well-being. It is the concern of nursing to provide for and manage the person's self-care actions in an attempt to promote life and health and to assist him to recover from disease and injury or to cope with their effects. The need for nursing exists when an adult is unable to satisfactorily meet his self-care demands, or when a parent is unable to meet these demands for his child.

- Nursing is responsible for assisting the person to overcome those circumstances which interfere with self-care and which cause self-care limitations and deficits.

There are two broad categories of self-care demands: universal self-care demands and health-deviation self-care demands. *Universal self-care demands* are those that are required of all individuals in order to maintain integrated human functioning. *Health-deviation self-care demands* are those that occur as a result of disease, injury, disfigurement, or disability and require that changes be made in the person's routine of self-care depending upon the nature and extent of the demands. Self-care activity is deliberate action. It is goal-directed, self-initiated, and self-directed, and is affected by the person's values and goals.

Orem identifies three systems of nursing activities which are designed to meet the individual's self-care requirements according to the extent to which self-care action is disrupted: the wholly compensatory system, the partly compensatory system, and the supportive-educative system. The *wholly compensatory system* is utilized when the individual is unable to assume an active role in his care and the nurse assists him by acting for and doing for him. The *partly compensatory system* is utilized when the nurse and the individual participate in accomplishing therapeutic self-care actions. The major responsibility for the performance of these actions may be assumed by the nurse or by the individual, depending upon his physical or medically prescribed limitations, his knowledge and skills, and his psychological readiness to accomplish such activities. The *supportive-educative system* is utilized when the individual is capable of performing, or learning to perform, those measures which are necessary to accomplish his self-care demands, but for which he needs assistance in the form of support, guidance, and teaching.

Thus, as the health status of the individual changes, his needs for nursing activity may demand a change in the nursing system that is appropriate to meet his needs. Such a conceptual model of nursing can serve as a framework for guiding and directing nursing care. However, further validation of the concept is necessary for the continuation of nursing's pursuit of a sound theoretical base.

The Adaptation Model

The adaptation model of nursing developed by Roy is a systems model that incorporates interactionist concepts. Adaptation is defined as the process of change, a universal phenomenon of man. Within the model, man is viewed as a biopsychosocial being who is in constant interaction with his environment—an interaction that requires man to make continual adaptations. The capacity for adaptation depends upon the stimuli to which he is exposed and the level of his adaptation. The adaptive level is determined by the effect of three classes of stimuli: focal stimuli, or those stimuli with which the person is immediately confronted; contextual stimuli, which include all other stimuli that are present; and residual stimuli, or stimuli that the person has experienced in the past, such as beliefs, attitudes and traits. Humans have four modes of adaptation: physiologic, self-concept, role function, and interdependence relations. Thus, adaptive or positive responses to stimuli serve to maintain the total integrity of the individual.

- The role of nursing is that of promoting adaptation in all four modes during health and illness through utilization of the four components of the nursing process: assessing, planning, implementing, and evaluating.

During the assessment phase of the nursing process, the individual's position on the health-illness continuum is identified and the effectiveness of his ability to cope with the stimuli with which he is confronted is evaluated. The planning phase of the nursing process involves the establishment of goals for changing maladaptive behavior to adaptive behavior. Then, the nursing process is completed by the implementation and evaluation of a plan of nursing action directed toward promoting adaptation. The adaptation model of nursing has recently been put into operation by several schools of nursing. However, it continues to require further validation as a framework for the practice of nursing.

Overview

These are but three of the available models of nursing which can serve as frameworks for nursing practice. Educators throughout the country are utilizing these models, adapting them to meet their own individual needs, following other models of nursing, or developing new models. A curriculum based upon a conceptual model provides the student and the graduate with a framework for nursing practice within which the nurse can function while providing nursing care and can be guided in furthering her nursing education experiences. It is the hope of the authors that students and graduates who utilize any of the various nursing models can appropriately incorporate into their own frameworks of nursing practice the information about health, illness, and specific disease entities included in this book. Only with an acute appreciation for the physiological as well as the psychosocial needs of the individual who has a right to health but who experiences the threat of illness can practitioners of nursing fulfill the expectations that are centered in them by society and by the nursing profession.

NURSING AND THE HEALTH CARE DELIVERY SYSTEM

HEALTH DEFINED

The nursing profession exists to meet the health needs of the people. Hence, as health needs change so must health care. Unprecedented changes have occurred in the structure of our society, in life styles, and in scientific and

technological advances. These changes have altered the pattern of disease and the traditional therapeutic approaches as well as the concept of health care and the expectations which society has of the health professions. Today health is considered more than a basic human right; it has become a matter of public concern, national priority, and political action.

Our health system has traditionally been an illness system. However, the current trend is to emphasize health and its promotion. Health has been defined by the World Health Organization as a "state of complete physical, mental, and social well being and not merely the absence of disease and infirmity."* However, such a definition of health does not allow for any variation in the degrees of wellness or of illness. The concept of a health-illness continuum (as first described by Dunn [1961]) has markedly affected the purposes of the health professions. By viewing health and illness on a graduated continuum, a person is seen as having neither complete health nor complete illness. Instead a person's state of health is ever changing and has the potential for ranging from high-level wellness to extremely poor health with imminent death. Thus, a person is viewed as simultaneously possessing degrees of both health and illness. A person who has a chronic illness cannot meet the expectations of health as defined by the WHO definition of health. However, according to the health-illness continuum, the person with a chronic illness can attain a high level of wellness if he is successful in meeting his health potential within the limits of his chronic illness.

Continued emphasis on health and on the potential for health has resulted in the promotion of massive health programs as well as rehabilitative programs. With the shift in emphasis from cure to prevention and health maintenance, a wide range of techniques have come into use, including multiphasic screening, disease detection, examination for "wellness," environmental and mental health programs, accident prevention, and nutrition and health education. Special efforts are being made in this regard to reach and motivate members of various socioeconomic groups concerning life style and health practices. The main thrust is to design a health care delivery system so that the goals of comprehensive health care can be available to all the people at a tolerable cost. Of course, this type of health care has broad political and sociological implications as organizers, consumers, politicians, and health care providers become involved in the planning.

CONCEPT OF PROMOTION OF WELLNESS AND HEALTH MAINTENANCE

Health workers need to gain a vision of the concept of wellness, of what society could accomplish if it were

*Preamble of the Constitution of the World Health Organization.

a leader may be rather subtle. She may serve primarily as the patient's advocate, anticipating and meeting the needs which he is unable to meet for himself. She must not only be acutely aware of the patient's needs but able to communicate his needs to other health care professionals involved in his care and to coordinate the efforts of all of these persons in an effort to promote goal achievement.

Outside the hospital setting the persons served by nurses are more independent and more capable of making decisions about their health and the health behaviors they will strive to achieve. For this reason, the leadership role of the nurse in such a setting may be less subtle than in the hospital setting. The leadership skills utilized by the nurse are the same as those used within the hospital setting, but they must be adapted to the environmental variables that affect the patient population, specifically those varibles that affect their health needs and how they can be met. Environmental variables such as cultural values, attitudes, resources, and the influence of community leaders are just a few of the factors which must be considered by the nurse when attempting to effect changes in the health behaviors of persons within a community.

Research Role

The research role of the nurse is a role which has not been fully accepted and utilized by nurses in general. Instead, this role has been left to academicians, nurse scientists, graduate nursing students, and researchers from other disciplines. It has only been recently that nurses in general have recognized the acute need for nursing research. Likewise, nurses have just begun to appreciate the significant contributions that can be made to nursing research by nurses without advanced degrees.

The primary task of nursing research is to develop nursing theories that will serve as the scientific basis for the practice of nursing. Further studies are needed to determine the actual effects of nursing intervention and nursing care. Without such research efforts the science of nursing will not grow, and a scientifically based rationale for making changes in nursing practice will not be generated.

It is the responsibility of all nurses to become involved in nursing research—to accept their research role. Nurses who have preparation in research methodology can use their research knowledge and skills to initiate and implement timely studies of nursing. This is not to say that nurses who do not initiate and implement studies of nursing do not play a significant role in nursing research. Every nurse has valuable contributions to make to nursing research and a responsibility to make these contributions. All nurses must constantly be on the alert for nursing problems and important questions about the practice of nursing which can serve as the basis for the articulation of researchable problem areas. Those nurses

directly involved in giving patient care are often in the best position to identify such problems and questions. Their clinical insights are invaluable. Nurses also have a responsibility to become actively involved in ongoing research studies. This participation may involve facilitating the data collection process or it may involve the actual collection of data. Their interpretation of the study to other health care professionals or to patients and their families is often of invaluable assistance to the nurse who is conducting the study.

Above all, nurses must use research findings in their nursing practice. Research for the sake of research is meaningless. Only with the utilization of research findings in clinical nursing practice will the science of nursing be furthered. Research findings can only be substantiated through utilization and validation. Nurses must be continually aware of studies that are directly related to their own area of clinical practice. The findings of these studies must then be employed in an attempt to improve patient care and to validate the findings themselves. The attitude of every health care agency and every nursing unit within such an agency should be one of interest in the progress of nursing research and enthusiasm in the implementation of research findings. It must also be remembered that communication of research findings is imperative. When findings of studies are not made available to other nurses, the impact of the findings on nursing practice is diminished.

Thus, research is an inherent part of nursing. The future of nursing science depends upon the active involvement of nurses in the implementation and utilization of nursing research. Nurses must cultivate their curiosity about nursing practice and their belief in the worth of the practice of nursing by accepting their research role and responsibility. Only with the questioning mind of nurses can nursing research be generated. The scientific basis of nursing depends upon the research efforts of all nurses, practitioners and researchers alike.

THE PATIENT/CLIENT: CONSUMER AND RECIPIENT OF HEALTH CARE

The term "patient," which is derived from the Latin verb meaning *to suffer,* has traditionally been used to describe those persons who are recipients of nursing care. The connotation commonly attached to the word is one of dependence. For this reason many nurses prefer to use the term "client," which is derived from the Latin verb meaning *to lean* and which connotes alliance and interdependence. For the purposes of this book the term "patient" will be utilized throughout, but with appreciation for each nurse's prerogative to choose the term that seems most suitable.

THE PATIENT'S PROBLEMS

The central figure in health care services is, of course, the patient. Although the patient reports to the hospital or health facility with a health problem or problems (increasing numbers of patients have multiple disease disorders), he also comes as an individual, a member of a family, and a citizen of the community. Undoubtedly, he is laden with a number of personal concerns that have been amplified and compounded by illness. Confronting him, perhaps, are problems that he feels are inescapable and insurmountable; problems that demand a solution but are incapable of solution; problems for which he feels solely responsible and which he is reluctant to share. He may be wholly absorbed in problems that are of minor consequence while dismissing others that truly are of paramount importance relative to his illness. One of the nurse's important functions is to help him to sort out his problems, reduce them to their essentials, place them in proper perspective, and cope with them effectively.

Troublesome Symptoms as Problems

From the standpoint of the symptomatic patient, the most important problem confronting him is his major symptom. If he is gasping for breath, his most pressing need is to be relieved of his respiratory distress. Dyspnea is his primary problem. To evaluate this symptom and alleviate it effectively, the nurse must understand correctly the pathologic physiology underlying the patient's dyspnea. Is it caused by pulmonary congestion? by pneumonia? by pleurisy? or by asthma? Does the patient have respiratory obstruction? Should he be placed in an orthopneic position? or in low Fowler's position? or should he lie flat? Should he be receiving oxygen? Is he in need of tracheal suction? Is endotracheal intubation likely to be required? Should a sedative be administered, or is sedative medication strictly contraindicated in this patient? Close scrutiny of the patient might convince the nurse that his breathing, although abnormally rapid and deep, is not attended by discomfort and does not involve undue effort. In other words, this particular patient is not dyspneic but hyperpneic. Hyperpnea is a different symptom altogether, and the problems it entails are quite different from those of dyspnea. Is this a case of hysterical hyperventilation? or diabetic acidosis? or has this patient been poisoned? On the appropriate answers to these and a host of other pertinent questions may hinge the correctness of diagnosis, the effectiveness of nursing intervention, and, in many instances, the very survival of the patient.

Every step in the care of the patient represents a team effort, and a key member of the health team charged with this responsibility is the professional nurse. Among the most important of her contributions to this joint effort are her clinical observations. To what extent these observations are significant, informative, and helpful depends on how well the nurse knows and understands symptoms. Confronted with a symptom, the nurse must be able to recognize it as a deviation from the normal. She should also be aware of the patterns of illness in the community and the characteristics of the population being served. Table 1-1 specifies the leading causes of

TABLE 1-1.   DEATH RATES FOR 15 LEADING CAUSES OF DEATH: UNITED STATES, 1976

RANK[1]	CAUSE OF DEATH	DEATH RATE (PER 100,000 POPULATION)	PERCENT OF TOTAL DEATHS
	All causes	889.6	100.0
1	Diseases of heart	337.2	38.0
2	Malignant neoplasms, including neoplasms of lymphatic and hematopoietic tissues ...	175.8	19.8
3	Cerebrovascular diseases	87.9	10.0
4	Accidents	46.9	5.3
—	Motor vehicle accidents	21.9	—
—	All other accidents	25.0	—
5	Influenza and pneumonia	28.8	3.2
6	Diabetes mellitus	16.1	1.8
7	Cirrhosis of liver	14.7	1.6
8	Arteriosclerosis	13.7	1.5
9	Suicide	12.5	1.4
10	Certain causes of mortality in early infancy	11.6	1.3
11	Bronchitis, emphysema, and asthma	11.4	1.3
12	Homicide	9.1	1.0
13	Congenital anomalies	6.1	0.7
14	Nephritis and nephrosis	4.0	0.4
15	Peptic ulcer	3.0	0.3
—	All other causes	110.9	12.5

[1]Rank based on number of deaths.
From "Final Mortality Statistics, 1976." *Monthly Vital Statistics Report.* National Center for Health Statistics.

death in the U.S., and hence indicates the most common clinical problems that will be encountered in nursing practice.

THE PATIENT'S BASIC NEEDS

Certain basic needs are common to all human beings and demand satisfaction accordingly. Such needs are dealt with on the basis of priority, meaning that certain needs are more pressing than others. However, once an essential need is met, a person moves to a need on a higher level. Approaching needs according to priority reflects Maslow's hierarchy of needs, in which human needs may be ranked as follows: physiologic needs, safety needs, the need to belong, the need for recognition, esteem, and affection, the need to create, the need for knowledge and comprehension, and aesthetic needs.*

Physiologic Needs

These needs predominate in the motivation of human behavior and drive the mechanisms that maintain *homeostasis* — the constancy of the internal environment of an organism (see Chapter 7). They involve the regulation of respiratory, nutritive, and excretory functions, as well as maintenance of the water content of tissues, adjustments of body temperature, and the operation of numerous protective mechanisms. These needs are powerful; unless satisfied, they dominate the conscious mind. For example, if a patient is obliged to restrict his fluid intake for therapeutic reasons, thirst will absorb his thoughts. He may discuss nothing but drinking, complain incessantly of thirst, and repeatedly question his nurse and physician as to when fluids will be forthcoming. During this period he is not likely to be too concerned about the aesthetic features of his environment. As soon as his thirst is quenched he becomes aware of other needs; now he may be disturbed by the absence of privacy.

Safety Needs

If the physiologic needs are satisfied, the concern for safety emerges. The normal adult is able to protect himself and usually does not feel endangered. He is relatively "safe" from death. His job is "safe." His insurance program and his savings account furnish a sense of economic security.

Illness naturally poses a threat. The sick person may be apprehensive in response to the many different persons with unfamiliar functions who enter his room. Diagnostic tests and therapeutic procedures may contribute to his fears. He wants to feel safe and secure. Although he may not express his feelings in these terms, he wants the health team to be aware of his insecurity. To help protect the patient from danger the nurse must know the nature

*Maslow, A. H.: Motivation and Personality, New York, Harper, 1954.

of his illness and be cognizant of any possible complications. If complications should occur, she should be able to provide intelligent care. The nurse's role in promoting the psychological safety of the patient is discussed in Chapter 11.

Need for Affection and Recognition

Once the patient's physiologic and safety needs have been satisfied, his need for affection will become apparent. Every individual, sick or well, desires the companionship and recognition of others. A sick person wants and needs his family or, in their absence, friends. Thus any signs of friendliness are usually appreciated. The wise nurse is constantly aware of this need and of its importance in relation to the patient's morale. One way to achieve this end is to help the family members to feel that they have a definite contribution to make to the patient's recovery. The nurse will seek relevant information from them concerning his habits, preferences, and antipathies, and will be guided by this information to whatever extent may be possible.

Man is by nature a social being, abhorring isolation. Illness removes him from his relatively convivial world and transplants him into a strange environment, an environment that is entirely unsought and unfamiliar, one in which he feels incompetent and alone. Previously an actively contributing member of society, he now must accept a position of dependency. This patient needs to preserve his self-esteem. He needs to be recognized as an individual, a distinct personality. The professional nurse, imbued with the concept of the individual worth and the dignity of man, sees to it that this need is fulfilled. She takes time to listen to the patient. To the extent that he desires it and opportunity permits, she joins him in conversation. She exhibits interest in all matters that seem important to him — her attentiveness, thoughtfulness, and kindliness conveying the conviction that he is held in esteem and affection, and that his needs and problems are recognized.

The Creative Impulses

Once the patient's physiologic needs have been compensated and he is feeling secure, esteemed, and wanted, his creative impulses may now emerge. During the course of a short hospital stay this need is not likely to be frustrated. However, the patient with a protracted illness must be assured an opportunity to express himself creatively and to be, or at least feel, useful.

The Need to Know and Understand

This need is a strong drive. The intelligent person seeks information, organizes it, analyzes it, and searches for its meaning. In general, patients want to know what is in store for them and they are thwarted by explanations that are too brief or vague. Many have studied and know a surprising amount about the bodily functions. However, while some of their information may be factual some of it is likely to be erroneous, and correction or clarification is usually necessary. Their instruction is the responsibility of the nurse, and the teaching of patients is one of the most responsible functions of her profession. To teach correctly and effectively the nurse must have a thorough knowledge of the subject, be skilled in communication, and be cognizant of the basic mechanisms of learning. The explanations, while simple for the sake of comprehension, at the same time must be meaningful if they are to be accepted.

Much of the instruction will refer to specific tests or treatments that are in prospect and will describe the technical steps involved, the sensations likely to be experienced and the aftereffects to be anticipated, as well as what the patient can do to facilitate the procedure, minimize his discomfort, and reduce complications. Of course, when discussing anything with the patient the nurse must take into consideration his physical and emotional status, his intelligence, his experience as a patient, and his awareness of the situation, as well as the urgency of his need to know and understand. She also must consider the possible implications of her intended remarks and guard with equal care against inaccuracies on her part and misunderstandings on the part of the patient.

Aesthetic Needs

These needs vary in importance from individual to individual, but for all patients the most salutary environment is one that is orderly and one in which there is beauty. The patient with highly developed aesthetic sensibilities will be distressed by unpleasant sights, sounds, odors, and disarray. He may crave flowers, books, or music — amenities which, when supplied, add immeasurably to his well-being.

Summary

In concluding this discussion, it may be pointed out that most of the needs of the average individual, ill or well, can be satisfied only in part. Moreover, the nurse whose responsibility and privilege it is to help the patient meet his problems must recognize the fact that some problems can be neither eliminated nor solved. In relation to the patient with such a problem the nurse's role is to help him to make a mature, objective, and compensatory adjustment to its continued existence or to its imperfect solution, if this solution is the best that can be achieved.

APPROACH TO THE PATIENT

As nursing searches for ways of fulfilling patient needs, it has devised various methods of approaching the patient. During the 1950s and 1960s the concept of team nursing came to the fore. In recent years, however, some questions have been raised concerning the effectiveness of team nursing, and a different approach in the form of primary nursing has been advocated and implemented in many hospital settings. Although primary nursing is now becoming the predominantly favorite means of organizing patient care, team nursing is still found in many health care institutions.

The Nursing Team

Team nursing, as the term implies, refers to the care of patients by an organized group of nursing personnel, rather than by an individual nurse. The team is led by a qualified nurse who interprets and coordinates the plans for care. The needs and nursing requirements of each patient are assessed and a plan of care is developed on a collaborative and cooperative basis and implemented by the team. Decisions are made concerning what types of skills will be required and who can best provide the care.

Comprising the team are professional nurses, nursing students, practical nurses, and nursing assistants. To each of these individuals specific responsibilities are delegated that are in keeping with his or her educational background and experience.

The *team leader* is responsible for planning and evaluating the care of each patient. She delegates responsibilities to the personnel working with her and guides and supports the activities of every team member. The functions of the *professional nurse* are determined largely by the needs of the patient and the nature of his problems. She undertakes the care of patients whose conditions are complex, requiring judicious decisions, experienced health teaching, or advanced nursing skills. In addition, she assists the other team members in the care of their patients.

The *nursing student* participates to an extent commensurate with her education and in a manner that should prove of mutual benefit to her and to the patients whose care she is assigned.

The role of the *practical nurse* is dictated by her educational background, clinical experience, and individual competence, and by the needs of the team. The nursing assistants perform the functions for which they are trained. Each member has a distinctive contribution to make to the patient's care and to the smooth functioning of the team.

The *team conference* serves as a "clearinghouse" for the exchange of information concerning each patient. Such a conference is scheduled daily and usually is held as soon as possible after the completion of the major portion of the patient's care. The team leader inscribes pertinent notations on the nursing care plan, revising the latter according to the suggestions offered and the solutions proposed at the conference. Thus, the patient benefits promptly and directly from the combined observations, the cumulative knowledge, and the joint problem-solving ability of the several team members, all of whom are operating in concert to provide nursing care of the highest possible quality.

Primary Nursing

Primary nursing, not to be confused with primary health care, which deals with first-contact general health care, refers to comprehensive care that is provided with continuity. Individualized total care is provided to the patient by the same nurse from the time of the patient's admission until his discharge. This type of nursing care eliminates the fragmented care that has typified team nursing and serves to accomplish a goal for which nurses have recognized a need for years: it allows the nurse to once again give direct patient care rather than manage and supervise the functions of others who care for the patient. In essence it allows the nurse the opportunity to implement her practitioner role and her leadership role within the framework of rendering direct patient care.

The focus of primary nursing is the patient. The primary nurse accepts total responsibility for quality nursing care for the patient. This nursing care is directed toward meeting his total, individualized nursing needs — his biopsychosocial needs. The primary nurse is responsible and accountable for involving the patient and his family directly in all facets of his care. The primary nurse has autonomy that allows her to make decisions with the patient and his family concerning his care. Thus, the primary nurse is a facilitator of family-centered as well as patient-centered nursing care. All communications with other members of the health team regarding the patient and his health care are made by the primary nurse. This allows the nurse to provide for continuity of care and to promote collaborative efforts directed toward the assurance of quality care. It provides the other health care professionals with the opportunity to communicate directly with the nurse who is responsible for the patient's care.

Ideally the number of patients for whom the nurse is the primary nurse is limited to three or four. However, this number may range from one to ten depending upon the extent of the nursing needs of the patients. The nurse meets the patient as soon as possible after his admission to the health care facility. This allows her to begin to establish a relationship with the patient which will continue until discharge and, in some cases, after discharge. It allows the patient to identify with the nurse who will be responsible for his care on a continuous basis. Each day that the primary nurse works, she cares for the patient. She is aware of problems and needs as they arise, and she assumes the responsibility for securing the means to solve the problems and to meet the needs. Prior to the patient's discharge to another health care facility or to his home, the primary nurse assumes the responsibility for making the appropriate referrals and for assuring that all relevant information is provided to those persons who will be involved in his care. Throughout the entire admission the nurse continually strives to involve the patient's family in his care and in the preparations that are made for his discharge.

During the times when the primary nurse is not scheduled to work she is assisted by an associate nurse, or co-nurse. This associate nurse implements the nursing care plan and provides feedback to the primary nurse that is invaluable in evaluation of the care plan. However, it remains the responsibility of the primary nurse to make sure that the patient's needs are met and that continuity of care is not lost when she is not present to render the care herself.

Within the concept of primary nursing, the head nurse functions as a consultant for the primary nurses and she strives toward providing opportunities for these nurses to continually improve their clinical expertise. The head nurse initiates the nurse-patient relationship by assigning the primary nurse to her designated patients. This is done with knowledge of the primary nurse's capabilities and her particular areas of nursing expertise. The head nurse then serves as a resource person for the primary nurse when she is confronted with patient problems or needs which she is unable to resolve. Periodic evaluation of the primary nurse's performance is the responsibility of the head nurse. Frequent interaction with the primary nurse and her patients gives the head nurse much information that can be used positively in assisting the primary nurse to utilize her capabilities to their utmost and to make strides toward overcoming her limitations. The head nurse also functions as a primary nurse for a small group of patients. By assuming such responsibility she is allowed to utilize her clinical expertise in giving direct patient care and to serve as a role model for her primary nurses.

Practical nurses, nursing assistants, and nursing students assist within the primary nursing framework. The responsibility for maintaining continuity of total individualized nursing care remains with the primary nurse. However, when direct patient care is not given by the primary nurse, other members of the health team assume this responsibility. They implement the plan of care developed by the primary nurse and consult with the primary nurse when changes in the plan of care seem warranted. In such instances the primary nurse serves as a valuable consultant and teacher for associate nurses and other personnel. Nursing care conferences provide a means for the exchange of information. In these conferences the quality of care rendered to the patient is the focus, and continuity of individualized total patient care is the goal.

SUMMARY

Throughout this chapter, the evolution of the profession of nursing has been explored. Many references have been made to the significance of nurses as members of the health team. Over the years nurses have striven to change their role from one of subservience to other members of the health team, particularly the physician, to one that is collegial. As nursing practitioners and researchers make advances in the area of concept formalization and theory building, the unique competencies of the profession of nursing become more clearly articulated. It becomes increasingly more evident that nursing provides certain health care services that are unique to this profession. However, nursing continues to recognize the importance of collaboration with other health care disciplines in meeting all of the health care needs of patients. The diagram prepared by Engel (1977) (see Fig. 1-1) which depicts the task-oriented relationships between nurses and physicians in terms of equivalent, superior, and unique competencies suggests that nursing is realizing its goal of attaining a collegial relationship with physicians.

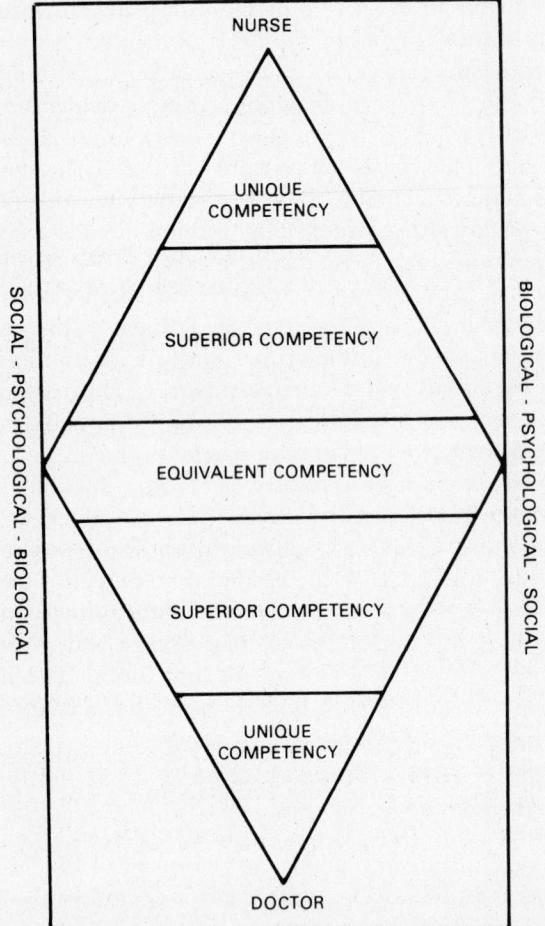

Figure 1-1.   Task-oriented relationships between doctors and nurses in the care of patients in terms of the relative competencies of each. The area of equivalent competency applies to tasks for which either a doctor or nurse would be qualified. Superior competency implies that both doctor and nurse have a measure of competency to perform a particular task or exercise a particular judgment, but that education and experience renders one superior to the other. Unique competency refers to activities which only members of one discipline or subdiscipline are qualified to carry out. In any particular situation the health professional most qualified available at that moment is the one to assume responsibility. For the same problem, under certain circumstances this may prove to be a nurse, under different circumstances, a physician, depending on individual qualifications and availability. (From Engel, G. L.: The biopsychosocial model and the education of health professions. Annals of the New York Academy of Sciences, vol. 310, 1978.)

BIBLIOGRAPHY

BOOKS

Chaska, N. L. (Ed.): The Nursing Profession. Views Through the Mist. New York, McGraw-Hill, 1978.

DiVincenti, M.: Administering Nursing Service. Boston, Little, Brown, 1977.

Dunn, H. L.: High-Level Wellness. Arlington, Va., R. W. Beatty, 1961.

Henderson, V.: The Nature of Nursing. New York, Macmillan, 1966.

King, I. M.: Toward a Theory for Nursing. New York, John Wiley and Sons, 1971.

Maslow, A. H.: Motivation and Personality. New York, Harper and Brothers, 1954.

Murray, R. and Zentner, J.: Nursing Concepts for Health Promotion. Englewood Cliffs, N.J., Prentice-Hall, 1975.

Nightingale, F.: Notes on Nursing: What It Is, and What It Is Not. New York, D. Appleton, 1860.

Orem, D. E.: Nursing: Concepts of Practice. New York, McGraw-Hill, 1971.

Rogers, M. E.: An Introduction to the Theoretical Basis of Nursing. Philadelphia, F. A. Davis, 1970.

Roy, C.: Introduction to Nursing: An Adaptation Model. N.J., Prentice-Hall, 1976.

————: The Roy Adaptation Model. *In* Riehl, J. P., and Roy, C.: Conceptual Models for Nursing Practice. New York, Appleton-Century-Crofts, 1974.

Theory Development: What, Why, How? NLN Publication #15-1708, 1978.

Yura, H., Ozimek, D., and Walsh, M. B.: Nursing Leadership: Theory and Process. New York, Appleton-Century-Crofts, 1976.

ARTICLES

Theories and Concepts of Nursing

Bush, H. A.: Models for nursing. Advances in Nursing Science, *1*:13-21, January 1979.

Carper, B. A.: Fundamental patterns of knowing in nursing. Adv. in Nurs. Sci., *1*:13-23, Oct. 1978.

Chater, S. S.: A conceptual framework for curriculum development. Nurs. Outlook, *23*:428-433, July 1975.

Chinn, P. L., and Jacobs, M. K.: A model for theory development in nursing. Adv. in Nurs. Sci., *1*:1-11, Oct. 1978.

Donaldson, S. K., and Crowley, D. M.: The discipline of nursing. Nurs. Outlook, *26*:113-120, Feb. 1978.

Fawcett, J.: The relationship between theory and research: a double helix. Adv. in Nurs. Sci., *1*:49-62, Oct. 1978.

Fenner, K.: Developing a conceptual framework. Nurs. Outlook, *27*:122-126, Feb. 1979.

Hardy, M. E.: Perspectives on nursing theory. Adv. in Nurs. Sci., *1*:37-48, Oct. 1978.

Henderson, V.: The concept of nursing. J. Adv. Nurs., *3*:113-130, Mar. 1978.

Jacobs, M. K., and Huether, S. E.: Nursing science: the theory-practice linkage. Adv. in Nurs. Sci., *1*:63-73, Oct. 1978.

Kritek, P. B.: The generation and classification of nursing diagnoses: toward a theory of nursing. Image, *10*:33-40, June 1978.

Peterson, C. J.: Questions frequently asked about the development of a conceptual framework. J. Nurs. Ed., *76*:22-32, Apr. 1977.

Reilly, D. E.: Why a conceptual framework? Nurs. Outlook, *23*:566-569, Sept. 1975.

Stillman, M. J.: Territoriality and personal space. AJN, *78*:1670-1672, Oct. 1978.

Health, Health Belief Model, Sick Role Behavior

Becker, M. H.: The health belief model and sick role behavior. Health Ed. Monographs, *2*:409-419, Winter 1974.

Becker, M. H., Drachman, R. H., and Kirscht, J. P.: A new approach to explaining sick-role behavior in low-income populations. AJPH, *64*:205-216, Mar. 1974.

Hoffman, C. A.: The house of medicine. JAMA, *221*:483-485, July 31, 1972.

Parsons, T.: Definitions of health and illness in the light of American values and social structure. *In* Jaco, E. J.: Patients, Physicians and Illness. New York, Free Press, 1972.

Roles of Nurses

Disch, J. M.: The clinical nurse specialist in a large peer group. J. Nurs. Admin., *8*:17-20, Dec. 1978.

Engel, G. L.: The biopsychosocial model and the education of health professionals. Ann. N. Y. Acad. Sci., *310*:169-181, June, 1978.

Friss, L.: What do nurses do? J. Nurs. Admin., *7*:24-28, Oct. 1977.

Haase, P. T.: Pathways to practice. Part I. AJN, *76*:806-809, May 1976.

————: Pathways to practice. Part II. AJN, *76*:950-954, June 1976.

Henry, O. M.: Progress of the nurse practitioner movement. Nurse Practitioner, *3*:4, May-June 1978.

Lieb, R.: Power, powerlessness and potential — nurses' role within the health care delivery system. Image, *10*:75-82, Oct. 1978.

Roy, C., and Obloy, M.: The practitioner movement — toward a science of nursing. AJN, *78*:1698-1702, Oct. 1978.

Nursing Leadership

Cutter, M. J.: Nursing leadership and management: an historical perspective. Nurs. Admin. Quart., *1*:7-19, Fall 1976.

Zorn, J. M.: Nursing leadership for the 70's & 80's. J. Nurs. Admin., 7:33-35. Oct. 1977.

Nursing Research

Ashley, J. A.: Foundations for scholarship: historical research in nursing. Adv. in Nurs. Sci., *1*:25-36, Oct. 1978.

Conway, M. E.: Clinical research: instrument for change. J. Nurs. Admin., *8*:27-32, Dec. 1978.

deTornyay, R.: Nursing research — the road ahead. Nurs. Research, *26*:404-407, Nov.-Dec. 1977.

Dimond, M., and Slothower, K.: Research in nursing administration: a neglected issue. Nurs. Admin. Quart., *2*:1-8, Summer 1978.

Jacox, A., and Prescott, P.: Determining a study's relevance for clinical practice. AJN, *78*:1882-1889, Nov. 1978.

Kinney, M. R., and Jackson, B. S.: Exploratory nursing research for prescribing patient care. Heart & Lung, 7:295-298, Mar.-Apr. 1978.

Primary Nursing

Brown, B.: The autonomous nurse and primary nursing. Nurs. Admin. Quart., *1*:31-36, Fall 1976.

Ciske, K. L.: Misconceptions about staffing and patient assignment in primary nursing. Nurs. Admin. Quart., *1*:61-68, Winter 1977.

Dahlen, A. L.: With primary nursing we have it all together. AJN, *78*:426-428, Mar. 1978.

McCarthy, D., and Schifalacqua, M. M.: Primary nursing: its implementation and six month outcome. J. Nurs. Admin., 7:29-32, May 1978.

Olsen, A.: Change takes time. Nurs. Admin. Quart., *1*:51-59, Winter 1977.

Smith, C. C.: Primary nursing care — a substantive nursing care delivery system. Nurs. Admin. Quart., *1*:1-8, Winter 1977.

The Evanston story: primary nursing comes alive. Nurs. Admin. Quart., *1*:9-50, Winter 1977.

2

THE NURSING PROCESS

The nursing process has been accepted as the essence of nursing. It is a deliberate, problem-solving approach to meeting the health care and nursing needs of patients. Although the steps of the nursing process have been delineated in various ways by many nursing leaders, the commonalities found in all definitions are: assessment, planning, implementation, and evaluation. These fundamental components can be utilized to define the nursing process as follows:

1. Systematic assessment of the patient's problems for the purpose of establishing nursing diagnoses
2. Development of a plan of care to solve the problems
3. Implementation of the plan of care or supervision of the implementation of the plan of care by others
4. Evaluation of the effectiveness of the plan of care in resolving the assessed problems

- *Thus, the nursing process is a data-collection, decision-making process that incorporates evaluation and subsequent modification as feedback mechanisms that promote the ultimate resolution of the patient's nursing problems.*

Division of the nursing process into four distinct components or steps serves to emphasize the critical nursing actions that must be accomplished when the nurse assumes responsibility for resolving the patient's nursing problems. However, the nurse must remember that the process as a whole is cyclic, the steps being interrelated, interdependent, and recurrent (Fig. 2-1).

ASSESSMENT

The assessment component of the nursing process begins with the nurse's first encounter with the patient. It involves the systematic collection of data about the pa-

tient's nursing needs and the utilization of this data to formulate nursing diagnoses.

- *The nursing diagnoses then become the basis for the nursing care plan.*

Sensitive and continuous nursing assessment is essential in order to maintain an awareness of the patient's needs and the effectiveness of the nursing care that he receives.

History Taking

Assessment of the patient's nursing needs is accomplished by means of the nursing history and the physical examination of the patient. The nursing history is carried out for the purpose of determining the patient's state of wellness or illness and is best accomplished as part of a planned interview.

The interview is a dialogue between the patient and the nurse and is a very personal experience. Interviewing is an art that requires wisdom, judgment, tact, and experience. It involves the sensitive direction of a conversation with a patient in order to obtain information about him. The nurse's approach to the patient will largely determine the amount and quality of information that is received. Achieving a relationship of mutual trust and respect requires the ability to communicate a sincere interest in the patient. The patient should be made as comfortable as possible and afforded privacy for the interview.

The principles involved in interviewing a patient are:

1. Listening and questioning
2. Observing and interpreting
3. Synthesizing
4. Incorporating what is learned into a plan of care

18

To learn about a patient one must talk little and listen a lot. Listen to the patient with "hearing ears." What is he saying? Because an ill person is so suggestible, do not put words in his mouth. Let him tell his story in his own way. Although many topics may be brought up, look for the main area of concern. Give the patient time, without interruptions, to tell why he is seeking help. Be attentive not only to his verbal expression but also to his nonverbal behavior, which may be exhibited in such subtle forms as gestures, posture, and facial expressions. Anxiety is present in almost every patient; it may be well concealed but it is there. Anticipate the patient's anxieties and try to relieve them during the interview. All inquiries should be relevant. The patient has the right to expect something from each interview. He should especially be made to feel that he is being understood.

The use of a nursing history guide may help the nurse to obtain pertinent information and to facilitate the course of the interview. A variety of nursing history guides have been developed by individual nurses and committees of nurses. Many health care agencies have developed guides that are specifically directed toward obtaining the information that is most essential for their particular patients. Guides that are standard for a particular health care agency tend to reflect the agency's specific philosophy and concept of man, nursing, and health. These nursing history guides are just that — guides. They are designed to guide the interview but must be adapted to the individual responses, problems, and needs of the patient. As the nurse gains expertise in conducting a nursing history she should strive toward developing her own format, one that allows for adaptability and flexibility while still obtaining the essential information. This essential information must reflect an assessment of the total patient with regard to his basic human needs and his state of wellness or illness. A variety of models can serve as the framework for the assessment of basic needs. Maslow's Hierarachy of Needs and Erikson's Eight Ages of Man are two examples of frameworks which provide bases for the assessment of the total needs of the client — his physical, psychological, emotional, intellectual, social, and spiritual needs. The questions in the chart on page 20 are offered as guidelines for interviewing, but the questions actually asked are determined by the reaction of the individual patient.

In some instances it may be appropriate for the patient to fill out the nursing history form. If this technique of history taking is utilized, it remains the responsibility of the nurse to verify and clarify the information provided by the patient and to seek any additional information that

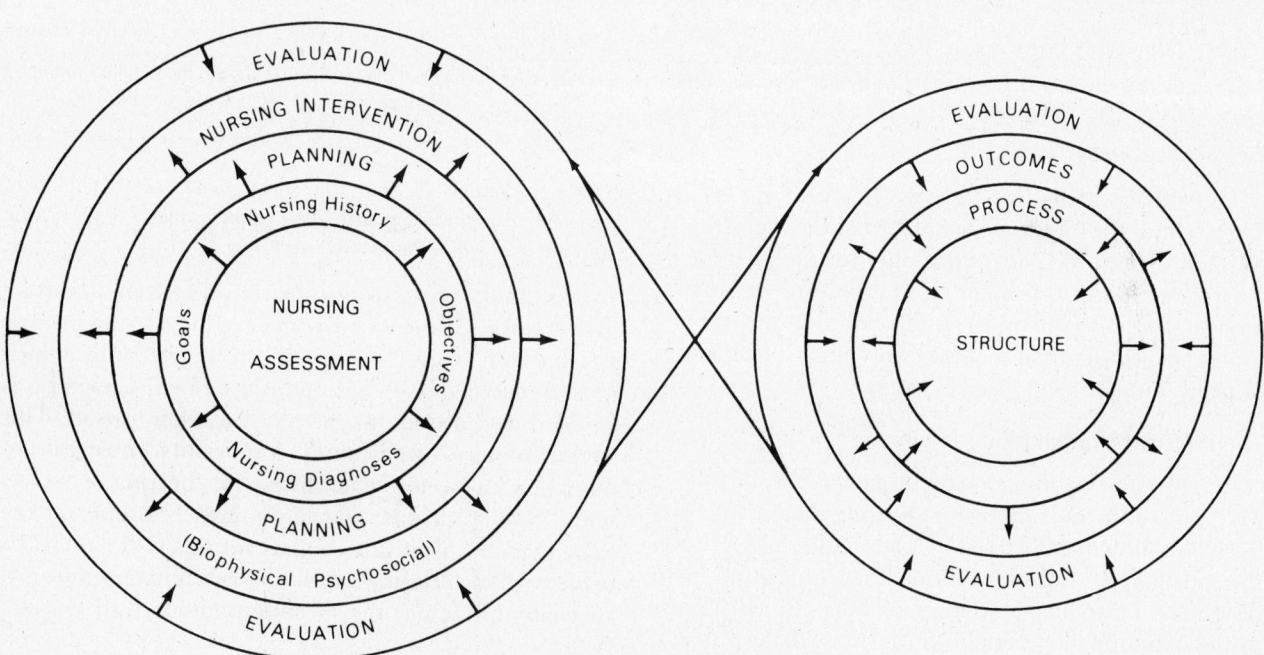

NURSING PROCESS

Figure 2-1. The nursing process is depicted schematically in the circle on the left. Starting from the innermost circle, nursing assessment, the process moves outward through the taking of the nursing history, the making of nursing diagnoses, the setting of goals and objectives, planning, and actual nursing intervention, and arrives at the ongoing process of evaluation. To show the consistent role of evaluation, the right circle indicates a gearlike activity: (1) structure—the organizational pattern within which the nursing process takes place and which involves personnel, environment, and facilities; (2) process—the providing of care, including the interaction which takes place between the patient recipient and the care provider; and (3) the final outcome—the condition of the patient/client following this process.

GUIDELINES FOR INTERVIEWING PATIENTS

Guiding Principle: At the beginning of the interview, focus on what is most troublesome to the patient—what are his symptoms or complaints? Why is he seeking help now?

What brought you to the hospital?

What is causing you the most discomfort?

When did the complaints appear?

Describe your life situation at the time of the onset of your illness.

Do you believe you are getting better or worse? (the directional trend: improvement or deterioration)

What do you think made you sick?

What do you do for yourself at home when you are sick?

How has this illness affected your way of life? For how long?

What factors aggravate or help your condition?

Are you taking any medications?

Do you have any allergies? (food, drugs)

Do you have any elimination (bowel or urinary) problems?

What is your greatest concern?

Are you being informed about tests and treatment?

Guiding Principle: Learn about the patient's background and experience in order to determine his needs.*

Where is your home?

Do you have a family?

What family member do you usually turn to for help?

What type of work do you do? or, if someone else is the provider, what type of work does he do?

Has your illness interfered with your work?

What activities, hobbies, and forms of recreation do you enjoy?

Guiding Principle: Ascertain what can be done to support the patient and help him make the best use of his resources. What are his defects? Limitations? Strengths?

What are your food preferences? Dislikes?

What are your sleeping habits?

    Regular retiring time?

      Do you like a night light?

      How many pillows do you use?

Do you have any limitations of seeing? hearing? walking?

What personal preferences do you have?

    Sleep late?

    Ice or tapwater to drink?

Would it be helpful to have a family member or friend stay with you?

What annoys you most about being in the hospital?

What do you miss the most in the hospital?

How long do you think you will stay?

What could the nursing staff do that would be most helpful to you?

*Social, cultural, educational levels, and the patient's readiness to learn can be assessed throughout the interview. Clues to the patient's financial status are obtained from his belongings, room, data on the chart, etc.

---

is necessary to identify the patient's nursing needs. Throughout the interview the nurse has the opportunity to interact with the patient not only for the purpose of data collection but also for the purpose of conveying interest, support, and understanding to the patient. For a more detailed discussion of the concepts and techniques of clinical interviewing, see Chapter 4.

The Physical Examination

The physical examination of the patient may be carried out prior to the nursing history, during the nursing history, or following the nursing history, depending upon the patient's physical and emotional state, his response to his illness and to hospitalization, and the immediate priorities of his illness situation. The purpose of the physical examination is to elicit those parameters of physical functioning which indicate that a nursing need exists. The examination is designed to determine the patient's physical alterations and limitations and also to determine his assets which may serve to complement his limitations.

- *To accomplish the purposes of the physical examination the nurse must be skilled in the techniques of inspection, palpation, percussion,* *and auscultation; she must also have a sound basic knowledge of anatomy and physiology and of the symptomatology of the disease process with which the patient presents.*

Because the physical examination is such an important part of the assessment component of the nursing process and because it involves specific technical skills which must be learned and continuously refined, Chapter 5 is devoted to the study of the physical examination. This chapter requires careful study, for the nurse must learn to observe with "seeing" eyes, hear with "hearing" ears, feel with "feeling" hands, and interpret the findings of the examination. Significant observations that should be made with each clinical condition appear in the appropriate chapter in which the specific condition is discussed.

Other Components of the Data Base

Following the nursing history and the physical examination, the nurse seeks additional relevant information from the patient's family and/or significant others, from other members of the health team, and from the patient's health record or chart. Depending upon the patient's immediate illness needs, this information may have been obtained prior to the nursing history and the physical examination. Whatever the sequence of events, the nurse utilizes all available sources of pertinent data to complete the nursing assessment. It is paramount that she study the patient's health record to determine the problem that caused the patient to seek help.

A tentative medical diagnosis has usually been formulated by the physician upon the patient's admission to the hospital. It is absolutely essential to understand the pathophysiological processes underlying this diagnosis. "Therapeutic conversation" is no substitute for knowing the effects of altered physiology, rationale of treatment, and potential complications. This knowledge helps the nurse to anticipate problems that may evolve, to formulate a nursing approach to their solution, and to participate with other members of the health team in providing coordinated health care.

Nursing Diagnosis

The assessment component of the nursing process is concluded with the formulation of the nursing diagnoses. As soon as possible after the completion of the nursing history and the physical examination the nurse organizes, analyzes, synthesizes, and summarizes the data collected and determines the patient's need for nursing care.

• *Those health problems that have the potential for resolution by means of nursing actions are identified as nursing diagnoses.*

Nursing, unlike medicine, does not yet have a standard taxonomy of diagnostic labels which convey the same meaning to all nurses. Until recently the nursing literature has revealed little substantive content regarding the classification of nursing diagnoses. The National Conferences on the Classification of Nursing Diagnoses held in the mid-1970s have provided an impetus for the identification and classification of nursing diagnoses according to symptomatology. The diagnostic categories identified by the conference groups are gaining general acceptance by nurses but require further validation and expansion. Nurses and nursing students alike who are assuming the practitioner role of nursing have a unique opportunity to utilize the presently defined nursing diagnoses and to develop additional diagnoses which describe those health problems that are amenable to nursing care.

When developing the nursing diagnoses for a particular patient, the nurse must first identify the commonalities among the assessment data collected. These commonalities lead to the categorization of related data that reveal the existence of a problem and the need for nursing intervention. *The patient's nursing problem is then defined as the nursing diagnosis.*

It must be remembered that nursing diagnoses are *not* medical diagnoses; they are *not* medical treatments prescribed by the physician; they are *not* diagnostic studies; they are *not* the equipment utilized to implement medical therapy; and they are *not* the problems that the nurse experiences while caring for the patient. They *are* the patient's health problems that have the potential for resolution by means of nursing actions. Nursing diagnoses that are succinctly stated in terms of the specific problems of the patient will guide the nurse in the development of the nursing care plan.

In order to give additional meaning to the diagnosis, the characteristics and the etiology of the problem must be identified and included as a part of the diagnosis. Consider this clinical example:

> Assessment of a patient with a medical diagnosis of diabetes mellitus reveals that the patient does not comply with his dietary regimen. He has the financial means necessary for purchasing the foods included in his diet, he has the home facilities required for preparing his foods, and he expresses a sincere desire to comply with his diet. However, he does not have an understanding of the food exchange system that is necessary for meal planning.

For this patient, the nursing diagnosis of "noncompliance" would give little guidance to the nurse in establishing a plan of care to meet the patient's needs. However, a more specific diagnosis of "noncompliance with dietary regimen related to lack of understanding of the diabetic exchange system" provides the nurse with information regarding the characteristics and cause of the problem. With such a diagnosis, the nurse is then ready to plan nursing care measures directed toward resolution of the problem.

PLANNING

Once the nursing diagnoses have been identified, the planning component of the nursing process follows. This phase involves:

1. The assignment of priorities to the nursing diagnoses
2. The specification of short-term, intermediate, and long-term goals of nursing action
3. The identification of specific nursing actions appropriate for attaining the goals
4. The documentation of the nursing diagnoses, goals, nursing actions (nursing orders), and expected outcomes on the nursing care plan

Also, during this phase of the nursing process it is the responsibility of the nurse to communicate to the appropriate persons any assessment data indicative of health needs that can best be met by other members of the health team.

Setting Priorities

The assignment of priorities to the nursing diagnoses should be a joint effort by the nurse and the patient and/or his family members. Any disagreement about the priorities should be resolved in a way that is mutually acceptable. Consideration must be given to the urgency of the problems, the most critical problems receiving the highest priorities. Maslow's hierarchy of needs provides a useful framework for the determination of priority problems. The use of this hierarchy requires that high priorities be given to physical needs. Subsequent to the resolution of physical needs, priorities are reassigned according to the urgency of needs at other levels of the hierarchy (see page 13).

Establishing Goals for Nursing Action

After the priorities of the nursing diagnoses have been established, the short-term, intermediate, and long-term goals and the nursing actions appropriate for attainment of the goals are identified. The patient and/or his family should be included in the establishment of the short-term, intermediate, and long-term goals of the nursing actions. The short-term goals are those which are of immediate concern and which can be reached in a short period of time. The intermediate and long-term goals require a longer period of time for their accomplishment and usually involve prevention of complications and further health problems, health education, and rehabilitation. For example, goals for an uncontrolled diabetic patient with a nursing diagnosis of "noncompliance with dietary regimen related to lack of understanding of the diabetic exchange system" may be stated as follows:

Short-term goal: oral intake and tolerance of 1,500 calorie diabetic diet spaced in three meals and one snack

Intermediate goal: planning of meals for one week based on diabetic exchange system

Long-term goal: compliance with prescribed diabetic diet

The patient and/or his family should be included whenever possible in the decisions about the nursing actions to meet the goals. Involvement of the patient and his family in the planning of nursing actions promotes their cooperation in the implementation of nursing care. The identification of appropriate nursing actions and their related goals depends upon the nurse's recognition of the strengths and potential of the patient and/or his family, her understanding of the pathophysiological alterations which he experiences, and her sensitivity to his emotional, psychological, and intellectual response to his illness state. Likewise, the nurse's knowledge of nursing, her clinical experience, and her awareness of available supporting resources influence the validity of the nursing actions which she identifies as appropriate for resolving the patient's problems.

Establishing Expected Outcomes

Expected outcomes of the nursing actions should be stated in terms of the patient's behaviors, and they should be realistic and measurable. Standard outcome criteria established by the health care agency for the target population applicable to the patient should be utilized whenever possible. However, it may be necessary to adapt these outcome criteria so that they are realistic in terms of the specific patient's potential for resolution of his problems. The critical time period within which the outcomes should be demonstrated by the patient are also identified.

- The outcomes which define the expected behavior of the patient will serve as the basis for evaluation of the effectiveness of the nursing actions.
- The critical time periods provide a time frame for determining the effectiveness of the nursing actions and the existence of a need for additional or altered nursing care.

Team Planning

Ideally, the accomplishment of all aspects of the planning phase of the nursing process is a group effort. The nurse collaborates with other members of the nursing team, with the patient and his family, and with appropriate resource persons from the health care agency and community agencies.

In planning with other members of the nursing team, the nurse recognizes that each team member has a role that is supported and respected. Of course, the physician initiates the medical regimen and is a valuable counselor, teacher, and resource person. A nurse clinical-specialist, when available, can make a significant contribution.

Because the plan revolves around a patient, he should have a part in it. The ultimate goal is to help the patient help himself. This means the patient is accepted as a worthy individual and his right to self-determination is respected. Since the plan is oriented in terms of the patient's goals and capabilities, he has every right to express his feelings and voice his opinions about his care. He should be kept informed about his current health status (when feasible), any change in plans, the roles of health care personnel, and the resources available to him.

It is also important to remember that the patient is part of a family. The family members have needs that arise from the patient's illness. They may be included in the planning by questioning them about the patient's reactions and informing them about the nursing care plan and the expected results of treatment. The family may also make pertinent observations and offer effective suggestions.

Another aspect of care planning takes into account the fact that the patient comes from the community. Community agencies have an interest in the patient and are involved in planning. This means that the nurse must be aware of the community services that may be offered a patient following discharge from the hospital. These agencies can be informed of the goal to be reached and decisions can then be made regarding the type of services that will be needed. Many communities have a directory listing all community resources available. These include community health and visiting nursing services, home-making services, meals on wheels, social and recreational services, etc. A knowledge of these resources and the method of referral is of inestimable value in helping to cope with long-term health needs.

Formulating the Nursing Care Plan

The entire planning phase of the nursing process culminates in the formulation of the patient's nursing care plan by the professional nurse. The nursing care plan serves to communicate the following information to all members of the nursing team:

1. The nursing diagnoses and their priorities
2. The goals of the nursing actions
3. The nursing actions which are expressed in the form of nursing orders
4. The outcome criteria which identify the expected behavioral outcomes for the patient
5. The critical time period within which the outcome must be met

The information incorporated into the nursing care plan should be written in a concise, systematic manner that facilitates its use by all nursing personnel. Space must be provided in the care plan for documentation of the patient's response to the nursing actions—the outcomes. It must be remembered that the care plan is subject to change as the patient's problems change, as the priorities of the problems shift, as resolution of problems occurs, and as additional information about the patient's state of health is collected. As the nursing actions are implemented, the patient's responses are evaluated and documented, and the care plan is changed accordingly. A well developed, continuously updated nursing care plan is the patient's greatest assurance that his nursing problems will be solved and that his basic needs will be met. (A sample nursing care plan appears on pages 24-25.)

IMPLEMENTATION

The implementation phase of the nursing process follows the formulation of the nursing care plan. Implementation refers to carrying out the proposed plan of care. The nurse assumes responsibility for the implementation but includes the patient and his family and other members of the nursing team and the health team as appropriate. The activities of all persons involved in implementation are coordinated by the nurse.

- The nursing care plan serves as the basis for implementation.
- The short-term, intermediate, and long-term goals are utilized as a focus for the implementation of the designed nursing actions.
- While implementing nursing care, the nurse continually assesses the patient and his response to the nursing care.

- Alterations are made in the care plan as the patient's condition, problems, and responses change and as reassignment of priorities is required.

Implementation includes all of the nursing actions that are directed toward resolution of the patient's nursing problems and meeting his health needs. Some of these needs have already been discussed (page 22). Needs specific to certain conditions are presented in the chapter in which the particular condition is discussed.

General Categories of Nursing Action

Included among nursing actions are hygienic care; promotion of physical and psychological comfort; support of respiratory and elimination functions; facilitation of the ingestion of food, fluids, and nutrients; environmental management; health teaching; promotion of a therapeutic relationship; and a host of therapeutic nursing activities. The nurse utilizes judgment in the selection of nursing actions that are based on physiologic fact.

This knowledge of physiology must be constantly sought, integrated, and applied. Consider this clinical example:

A patient with bronchiectasis is exhausted from repeated episodes of unproductive coughing. Traditionally the doctor would be notified and a medication for cough given. The more self-directing nurse, using nursing abilities based on an understanding of altered pathophysiology, will listen to the patient's lungs with a stethoscope, locate the area of congestion, position him for drainage, and then assist him to assume the posture which will help him cough up the mucus. Of course the physician is notified and his medical regimen for the patient is followed.

- *All nursing actions are patient-focused and goal-directed. They are based on scientific principles and are implemented with compassion, surety, and a willingness to understand.*

Delegating Nursing Action

The nurse may delegate certain specific actions to other members of the nursing team. When delegating, the nurse must know the capabilities and limitations of the members of the nursing team, select the most appropriate person to implement the actions, and supervise the performance of the actions. The nursing team member should be provided with all of the information that she needs to effectively perform the actions in such a way that the patient remains the focus of the actions at all times.

Many members of the nursing team and the health team may become involved in the patient's care. In order to provide for coordination and continuity of care, information about the patient's response to his care and any changes that must be made in the plan of care must be communicated verbally and in writing to the appropriate persons. Continual updating of the care plan is of paramount importance in assuring coordination and continuity.

EXAMPLE OF A NURSING CARE PLAN

Mrs. Jane Rollins, a 56-year-old housewife, was admitted to the nursing unit from the diabetic clinic. She had been diagnosed as having diabetes mellitus five years ago and had been controlled with 15 Units of Lente Insulin daily and a 1,500 calorie ADA diet. Her clinic record revealed that she had been examined in the clinic every six months and that her fasting blood sugar ranged between 130-140 mg./100 ml., with no glucosuria or acetonuria. Her weight was stable at 61.2-63.5 kg. (135-140 lbs.). Five days prior to admission she developed flu-like symptoms which did not subside with rest, fluids, and aspirin. She presented with the following signs and symptoms: T 38.4 C. (101.2 F.), P 96, R 24, BP 136/84, nausea, anorexia, malaise, dry skin and mucous membranes, and 4+ glucosuria. The admission blood sugar was 355 mg./100 ml. Mrs. Rollins reported that she had discontinued her insulin therapy three days prior to admission when she experienced loss of appetite. The physician's orders upon admission included: sliding scale regular insulin therapy, 1,800 calorie ADA diet, and daily FBS.

Nursing Diagnosis: Hyperglycemia related to discontinuation of insulin
therapy and increased metabolism

Goals—Short-term: State of hydration restored
Tolerance for oral fluids (1,800 calories/day)
Urine free of sugar and acetone

Intermediate: Resumes daily self-administration of Lente Insulin

Long-term: Complies with insulin administration regimen.

Nursing Orders	Outcome Criteria	Critical Time*	Outcome
Continue assessment of state of glycemia: diabetic urines q.4 hr. check daily FBS	Urine free of glucose and acetone (or no greater than 1+ glucose)	48 hrs.	Urine free of glucose and acetone 24 hrs. after admission.
observe for hyperglycemia: weakness, polydipsia, polyuria, dry skin and mucous membranes, anorexia, decreased mental acuity, acetone breath	FBS returns to range of 130-140 mg.	48 hrs.	FBS 138 mg. 36 hrs. after admission. (Lente Insulin resumed 3 days after admission.)
observe for hypoglycemia: nervousness, weakness, sweating, headache, impaired vision, hunger, irritability	Free from symptoms of hyperglycemia	48 hrs.	Appetite improved, skin less dry, mucous membranes moist; no further symptoms of hyperglycemia.
	Free from symptoms of hypoglycemia	48 hrs.	No symptoms during first 48 hrs.
Continue assessment of state of hydration: I & O q. 8 hrs. observe skin turgor and texture observe texture of mucous membranes of eyes and mouth Vital signs q. 4 hrs.	Intake of minimum of 2,000 ml./day Intake equals output, +200 ml./day	24 hrs. 48 hrs.	1st 24 hrs.: intake: 2,500 ml. output: 1,800 ml. 2nd 24 hrs.: intake: 2,300 ml. output: 2,050 ml.
	Skin elastic; free from excessive dryness or moisture	24 hrs.	Tissue turgor good, skin less dry within 24 hrs.
	Mucous membranes moist	24 hrs.	Mucous membranes of eyes and mouth moist within 24 hrs.
	Temperature, pulse, and respirations within normal limits	48 hrs.	1st 24 hrs.: T: 37.6°-38.3° C. (99.8°-101° F.) 2nd 24 hrs.: T: 36.7°-37.2° C. (98°-99° F.) P: 70-84/minute R: 14-20/minute, normal depth

*These times have not been standardized but are individualized according to the patient's needs.

Nursing Orders	Outcome Criteria	Critical Time*	Outcome
Encourage intake of foods and fluids desired, within restrictions of 1,800 calorie ADA diet	Tolerates intake of 1,800 calorie ADA diet	48 hrs.	Tolerated 1,800 calorie full liquid diet within 24 hrs. Tolerated standard 1,800 calorie ADA diet within 48 hrs.
Encourage self-care: testing of urine a.c. and h.s.	Tests urine for glucose and acetone a.c. and h.s.	3 days	Testing done a.c. 2nd h.s. beginning 48 hrs. after admission
	Demonstrates proper technique of urine testing	3 days	Procedure performed accurately
administration of insulin	Administers insulin daily, a.c. breakfast	3 days	Resumed self-administration of insulin 48 hrs. after admission
	Demonstrates proper technique of insulin administration with rotation of sites and recording of type, amount, and time of administration	3 days	Procedure performed correctly Identified proper sites and significance of rotation; recorded type, amount, time of administration
Diabetic teaching about compliance with insulin regimen	(see teaching plan)		

*These times have not been standardized but are individualized according to the patient's needs.

Recording Outcomes

The implementation phase of the nursing process is concluded when the nursing actions have been completed and when the patient's responses to the actions have been recorded. Recordings should be made concisely, precisely, and objectively. The recordings should:

- be related to the nursing diagnoses
- describe the nursing actions and the patient's responses to the actions, and
- include any additional pertinent data.

Only with accurate recording can evaluation be carried out. Documentation of information provides the basis for the measurement of the patient's behavioral response to the nursing actions—his accomplishment of the defined outcome criteria.

EVALUATION

Evaluation is the final component of the nursing process and is directed toward determining the patient's response to the nursing actions and the extent to which the goals have been achieved. The nursing care plan provides the basis for evaluation, the nursing diagnoses, goals, nursing actions, and outcome criteria provide the specific guidelines that dictate the focus of the evaluation.

Evaluation will answer the following questions:

- Were the nursing diagnoses accurate?
- Did the patient meet the outcome criteria?
- Did the patient meet the criteria within the critical time period?
- Have the patient's nursing problems been resolved?
- Have the patient's nursing needs been met?
- Should the nursing actions be retained, altered, or discontinued?
- Have new problems evolved for which nursing actions have not been planned or implemented?
- What factors influenced the achievement or lack of achievement of the goals?
- Do priorities need to be reassigned?
- Should changes be made in the goals and outcome criteria?

Objective data that answer these questions must be collected from all available sources (i.e., patient, family and/or significant others, nursing and other health team members). This data should be available in the patient's record and should be substantiated by direct observation of the patient.

Quality Assurance

Evaluation has traditionally been the most neglected component of the nursing process. However, during the past decade the increased emphasis placed on professional accountability and the advent of quality assurance programs have tended to focus much attention on evaluation.

- The concept of quality assurance refers to the accountability of the health professions to society for the quality, quantity, and costs of the health services provided.

STEPS OF THE NURSING PROCESS

ASSESSING

1. Conduct the nursing history.
2. Perform the physical examination.
3. Interview the patient's family and/or significant others.
4. Study the health record.
5. Formulate the nursing diagnoses.
   a. Organize, analyze, synthesize, and summarize the collected data.
   b. Identify the patient's nursing problems.
   c. Identify the defining characteristics of the nursing problems.
   d. Identify the etiology of the nursing problems.
   e. State nursing diagnoses concisely and precisely.

PLANNING

1. Assign priority to the nursing diagnoses.
2. Specify the goals.
   a. Develop short-term, intermediate, and long-term goals.
   b. State the goals in realistic and measurable terms.
3. Identify nursing actions appropriate for goal attainment.
4. Establish outcome criteria.
   a. Make sure that the outcomes are realistic and measurable.
   b. Identify critical times for the attainment of outcomes.
5. Develop the written nursing care plan.
   a. Include nursing diagnoses, goals, nursing actions, and outcome criteria.
   b. Write all entries precisely, concisely, and systematically.
   c. Keep the plan current and flexible to meet the patient's changing problems and needs.
6. Involve the patient, his family and/or significant others, nursing team members, and other health team members in all aspects of planning.

IMPLEMENTING

1. Put the nursing care plan into action.
2. Coordinate the activities of the patient, his family and/or significant others, nursing team members, and other health team members.
3. Record the patient's responses to the nursing actions.

EVALUATING

1. Collect objective data.
2. Compare the patient's behavioral outcomes to the outcome criteria. Determine the extent to which the goals were achieved.
3. Include the patient, his family and/or significant others, nursing team members, and other health team members in the evaluation.
4. Identify alterations that need to be made in the nursing diagnoses, goals, nursing actions, and outcome criteria.
5. Continue all steps of the nursing process: assessing, planning, implementing, evaluating.

The priority of the health professions for the establishment of quality assurance programs was stimulated by the enactment of the Social Security Amendments of 1972 which provided for the creation of PSROs as a system for evaluating the quality of health care delivered. PSROs are based on the concept of peer review, which allows the specific profession to establish its own norms, standards, and criteria for review and to carry out the review process. Nursing, as a nonphysician health care profession, has accepted its responsibility for implementation of peer review and thus for accountability for the quality of the nursing care provided. Nurses have recognized their accountability to their patients, their employing institutions, their colleagues and subordinates, other members of the health care team, and the nursing profession.

Quality assurance programs in nursing are viewed as evaluation systems composed of three dimensions: structure, process, and outcome.

The *structural dimension* focuses on the organization within which nursing care is provided.

The *process dimension* focuses on the actual performance of the tasks, functions, and activities of nursing care.

The *outcome dimension* focuses on patient welfare, the end results of the care provided to the patient.

Evaluation of structure, process, and outcome are all important and are interrelated, each influencing the other. However, outcomes which provide clinical evidence of the results of care are the ultimate validators of the care rendered. Outcomes focus the attention of the practitioner on the response of the patient to the care that he received.

Outcome Criteria

Goals for accountability and quality assurance in nursing are being realized. The American Nurses' Association has developed basic standards that provide a general model for nursing practice by which the quality of nursing practice may be evaluated. Record-keeping has been revised to provide a problem-oriented approach to documentation of data. The Problem-Oriented Medical Record (POMR) focuses attention on the patient and his problems and allows for the systematic documentation of data by various health team members. The use of outcome criteria as validators of the nursing process has become an accepted trend. Nurses in various health care settings have developed outcome criteria for specific patient populations. Likewise, the American Nurses' Association has developed outcome criteria which have served as guidelines and as prototypes for criteria utilized in various health care agencies. The nursing audit has become an accepted method for comparing results of the actual nursing performance with the established criteria. Nursing audit may involve concurrent review or retrospective review of the patient's record. While the patient is in a health care agency there can be a concurrent review of the patient's record by a nursing group to evaluate whether or not quality care has been given. This provides the opportunity to make changes. There can be a retrospective review of the patient's record (after he leaves the health care agency) which provides another method of evaluation. However, this method of evaluation does not provide an opportunity to make changes for the specific patient who is evaluated.

All methods utilized to accomplish the evaluation component of the nursing process are directly related to the nursing care plan. Evaluation of the patient's response to nursing actions is accomplished by comparing the patient's behavioral outcomes with the established outcome criteria. This information then serves as a basis for modification of the nursing care plan.

Evaluation should include self-assessment by the nurse. This can be done through courses of study, programmed learning, study of cause and effect, etc. The nurse in reviewing the care plans should decide how many correct decisions were made in nursing assessment, planning, and implementation, as compared with ineffective decisions, and how effective the nursing care is, as measured by valid outcome criteria.

However, it is not enough to evaluate only the effectiveness of the nursing care. An important phase of evaluation is "What should be done to improve the nursing care?" Other nursing actions may have to be tried. Goals may have to be redesigned. Priorities may have to be reassigned. Outcome criteria may have to be made more realistic. There must be a continuous and thorough scrutiny of the care provided. Then changes are made, plans altered, and a course of action initiated that will be most supportive to the patient.

Thus the steps of the nursing process are cyclic and recurrent. Each step is ongoing and is related to all other steps. Continuous evaluation provides the means for maintaining the viability of the entire nursing process and for demonstrating accountability for the quality of nursing care rendered.

For an overall view of the steps of the nursing process see the summary chart on page 26.

BIBLIOGRAPHY

BOOKS

American Nurses' Association: Guidelines for Review of Nursing Care at the Local Level. Washington, D.C., U.S. Government Printing Office, 1976.

Campbell, C.: Nursing Diagnosis and Intervention in Nursing Practice. New York, John Wiley and Sons, 1978.

Erikson, E. H.: Childhood and Society. New York, W. W. Norton, 1963.

Gebbie, K. M., ed.: Summary of The Second National Conference: Classification of Nursing Diagnoses. St. Louis, Clearinghouse-National Group for Classification of Nursing Diagnosis, 1976.

Little, D. E., and Carnevali, D. L.: Nursing Care Planning. Philadelphia, J. B. Lippincott, 1976.

Mayers, M. G.: A Systematic Approach to the Nursing Care Plan. New York, Appleton-Century-Crofts, 1976.

Mayers, M. G., Norby, R. B., and Watson, A. B.: Quality Assurance for Patient Care: Nursing Perspectives. New York, Appleton-Century-Crofts, 1976.

Phaneuf, M. C.: The Nursing Audit. Self-regulation in Nursing Practice. New York, Appleton-Century-Crofts, 1976.

Yura, H., and Walsh, M. B.: Human Needs and the Nursing Process. New York, Appleton-Century-Crofts, 1978.

———: The Nursing Process. New York, Appleton-Century-Crofts, 1978.

ARTICLES

Barba, M., Bennett, B., and Shaw, W. J.: The evaluation of patient care through use of ANA's standards of nursing practice. Supervisor Nurse, *9*:42-54, Jan. 1978.

Block, D.: Criteria, standards, norms — crucial terms in quality assurance. J. Nurs. Admin., 7:20-30, Sept. 1977.

———: Evaluation of nursing care in terms of process and outcome: issues in research and quality assurance. Nurs. Research, *24*:256-263, July-Aug. 1975.

Chow, R. K.: Assuring the quality of care: a personal perspective — from tailoring to outcome measurement. Nurs. Leadership, *1*:11-22, Sept. 1978.

Gordon, M.: Nursing diagnosis and the diagnostic process. A. J. N., *76*:1298-1300, Aug. 1976.

Henderson, B.: Nursing diagnosis: theory and practice. Adv. in Nurs. Sci., *1*:75-83, Oct. 1978.

Hover, J., and Zimmer, M. J.: Nursing quality assurance: the Wisconsin system. Nurs. Outlook, *26*:242-248, Apr. 1978.

Hushower, G., Gamberg, D., and Smith, N.: The nursing process in discharge planning. Supervisor Nurse, *9*:55-58, Sept. 1978.

Kritek, P. B.: The generation and classification of nursing diagnoses: toward a theory of nursing. Image, *10*:33-40, June 1978.

Langford, T.: Establishing a nursing contract. Nurs. Outlook, *26*:386-388, June 1978.

Laros, J.: Deriving outcome criteria from a conceptual model. Nurs. Outlook, *25*:333-336, May 1977.

Mundinger, M. O., and Jauron, G. D.: Developing a nursing diagnosis. Nurs. Outlook, *23*:94-98, Feb. 1975.

Roy, C.: A diagnostic classification system for nursing. Nurs. Outlook, *23*:90-94, Feb. 1975.

———: The impact of nursing diagnosis: AORN J., *21*:1023-1030, May 1975.

Schmidt, A., and Deets, C.: Responsibility for audit criteria. AORN J., *27*:657-662, Mar. 1978.

Snyder, P. J.: Goal setting. Supervisor Nurse, *9*:61-64, Sept. 1978.

Vengroski, S. M., and Saarmann, L.: Peer review in quality assurance. AJN, *78*:2094-2096, Dec. 1978.

3

PATIENT EDUCATION/HEALTH TEACHING

HEALTH EDUCATION TODAY

Perhaps one of the greatest challenges facing members of the nursing profession today is that of meeting the health education needs of the American public. In this respect nurses are becoming increasingly sensitive to and conscious of their role as teachers. Health education is considered to be an independent function of nursing practice and a primary responsibility of the nursing profession.

- Health education is an essential component of nursing care and is directed toward promotion, maintenance, and restoration of health and adaptation to residual effects of illness.

The emphasis that has been placed on the need for health education during recent years perhaps stems in part from the belief of many health care leaders that the American public has the right to expect and receive comprehensive health care, including health education. It also reflects the emergence of a better informed American public who are asking more significant questions about health, health care, and the services offered by the health care delivery system. Because of the emphasis that the American culture places on health and the responsibility of each individual for the maintenance and promotion of his own health, it is the obligation of the members of the health care delivery system and, specifically, of nurses, to make health education available to the American public.

One of the largest groups of people in need of health education today are those persons with chronic illnesses. The number of people in this category is continually rising. It is the belief of many health care leaders that persons with chronic illness are entitled to as much health care information as they can handle in order that they may actively participate in and assume the responsibility for much of their own care. Health education can aid the individual in adapting to his illness, in cooperating with his prescribed therapy, and in learning to solve problems when confronted with new situations. Health education can prevent rehospitalization for the same condition, a frequent result when a person does not understand how to care for his chronic condition.

- The goal of health education is teaching people to live life to its healthiest—that is, to strive toward achieving one's maximum health potential.

Every contact that a nurse has with a patient should be considered an opportunity for patient teaching. It is the patient's right to decide whether or not he will learn, but it is the nurse's responsibility to present him with the information that he needs in order to make the decision and to motivate him to appreciate the need for learning.

COMPLIANCE

Inherent within the area of patient teaching is the concern for the promotion of the patient's compliance with his therapeutic regimen. Many patients are given the responsibility for managing their own care at home. The patient's responsibility may include taking medications, adhering to a diet, restricting his activities, observing himself for signs and symptoms of illness, carrying out specific hygienic measures, seeking periodic evaluation of his health status, and attending to a host of other therapeutic and preventive measures. The fact that many patients do not comply with their prescribed regimens cannot be ignored or minimized. The rates of patient compliance with therapeutic and preventive regimens are generally very low, especially when the regimens are complex or of long duration. The characteristics of noncompliant patients and their reasons for not complying with their prescribed therapy have been the subjects of many studies. For the most part, the findings of these studies have been inconclusive. No one factor has been found to be the predominant cause of noncompliance. Instead, it seems that a wide range of variables interacting with one another influence the degree of compliance. The influencing factors include:

- demographic variables such as age, sex, race, socioeconomic status, and education
- illness variables, such as the severity of the illness and the relief of symptoms afforded by the therapy
- psychosocial variables such as intelligence, attitudes toward health professionals, and acceptance or denial of illness

Knowledge alone concerning health and health promotion and illness and illness prevention has not been found to be a sufficient stimulus to motivate total compliance. However, it has been found that some degree of compliance in some patients is obviously enhanced by the use of teaching programs and by methods directed toward stimulating motivation to comply. The problem of noncompliance with therapeutic regimens is a substantial one that needs to be remedied in order to assist patients to adequately participate in self-care and to successfully achieve their maximum health potential.

The role of the nurse in teaching and directing patients toward compliance behavior is a significant one. It is the responsibility of the nurse to assess all variables that may have an effect upon the patient's compliance behavior and to use this information when developing and implementing the patient's teaching plan.

THE NATURE OF TEACHING AND LEARNING

When learning is defined as the acquiring of knowledge, attitudes, or skills, and teaching is defined as helping another person to learn, it becomes evident that the teaching-learning process is an active one. It requires the active involvement of both the teacher and the learner in the effort to reach the desired outcome—change in behavior. The teacher does not give knowledge to the learner but instead serves as a facilitator of learning. In general, there is a lack of knowledge about how learning occurs and is affected by teaching. No single theory of learning suffices to explain how learning occurs. However, some specific principles of learning and some guidelines for teaching have been identified.

Learning Readiness

There are many variables, both internal and external, that affect the learner and the learning situation. One of the most significant of these factors is the learner's readiness to learn—his physical, emotional, and experiential readiness to learn.

Physical readiness is of vital importance because until a patient is physically capable of learning, attempts at teaching and learning may be both futile and frustrating. A patient who is experiencing acute pain is unable to focus his attention away from the pain long enough to concentrate on learning. Likewise, a patient who is short of breath will concentrate his energies on breathing rather than on learning.

- Utilizing Maslow's hierarchy of needs is helpful in considering the concept of physical readiness for learning.

Emotional readiness involves the patient's motivation to learn. Until the person has begun to accept his illness or to accept the fact that illness is a threat to him, he will not be motivated to learn. If his therapeutic regimen is not acceptable to him or is in conflict with his life style, he may consciously avoid learning. Until he recognizes the need to learn and his own ability to learn, teaching efforts may be thwarted. However, it is not always wise to wait for the patient to become emotionally ready to learn—this time may never come unless efforts are made by the nurse to stimulate the patient's motivation to learn. Illness and the threat of illness are usually accompanied by anxiety and stress. The nurse who recognizes the patient's reactions to his illness or threatened illness can use simple explanations and instructions to alleviate his anxieties and to further motivate him to learn. It must be remembered that since learning involves changes in behavior it normally produces mild anxiety. Such anxiety is often a useful motivating factor.

- Emotional readiness can be promoted by creating a warm, accepting, positive atmosphere and by establishing realistic learning goals with the patient so that he can realize success and a feeling of accomplishment which in themselves are motivators of learning.

Feedback about progress also serves to motivate learning. Such feedback should be presented in the form of positive reinforcement when the patient is successful and constructive criticism when he is unsuccessful.

Experiential readiness to learn refers to the patient's past experiences that enable him to learn what is being taught. Previous educational experiences and life experiences in general are significant determinants of the patient's approach to learning. A person who has had little or no formal education may not be able to understand the instructional materials presented to him—although this is not always true. The person who has experienced difficulty in learning in the past may be hesitant to make new attempts to learn. Many behaviors required for meeting one's maximum health potential require a rather extensive background of knowledge, physical skills, and attitudes. If the person does not have this background upon which to build, learning may be very difficult and very slow for him. For example, until a patient understands the basics of normal nutrition he may not be able to understand the restrictions of a special diet. Also, a person who is not future-oriented will be unable to appreciate many aspects of preventive health teaching. And a person who does not view the desired learning as meaningful to himself and his life style will reject teaching efforts.

Thus, experiential readiness is closely related to emotional readiness, since motivation tends to be stimulated by one's appreciation for the need to learn and by those learning tasks that are familiar, interesting, and meaningful.

- Prior to initiating a teaching-learning program the nurse must assess the patient's physical and emotional readiness to learn as well as his level of attainment of those behaviors that are prerequisites to learning what is being taught. This information then becomes the basis for the goals to be established, goals which in themselves can motivate the patient to learn.
- Involvement of the patient in the establishment of goals that are mutually acceptable to him and to the nurse serves the purpose of encouraging the patient to be actively involved in the learning process and to share the responsibility for his learning progress.

The Learning Atmosphere

Although a teacher is not always necessary, most patients who are attempting to learn new or altered health behaviors will need the services of a nurse-teacher at least part of the time. The interpersonal interaction between the patient and the nurse who is attempting to meet the patient's learning needs may be formal or informal depending upon the method and techniques of teaching that are found to be most appropriate for the individual patient.

The nurse facilitates learning by manipulating those external variables that affect the patient's learning. For example, the physical environment should be such that it is conducive to learning. That is, the room temperature, lighting, noise levels, and the like should be appropriate to the learning situation. Also, the time selected for teaching should be suited to the patient's needs. Scheduling a teaching session at a time of day when the patient is fatigued, when he is anticipating diagnostic or therapeutic procedures about which he is anxious, or when he has visitors does not provide a conducive learning environment. Timing of teaching may also be determined by visits of the family members, if they are to be included in the teaching plan.

Teaching Techniques

The nurse also facilitates learning by selecting teaching techniques and methods that are most appropriate to meet the individual patient's needs.

The lecture or explanation method of teaching is commonly used but should always be accompanied by discussion. The discussion is important, since it affords the patient an opportunity to express his feelings and concerns, to ask questions, and to receive clarification of any misinformation or misunderstandings that he may have.

Group teaching is appropriate for some patients because it allows them not only to receive the information that is needed but also to experience security through being a member of a group. Patients with similar problems or learning needs have the opportunity to identify with each other and thus to gain moral support and encouragement. However, it must be remembered that all patients do not relate well in groups and therefore may not benefit from such experiences.

Demonstration and practice are often essential ingredients of the patient's teaching program, especially when skills are to be learned. The nurse first demonstrates the skill to the patient and then allows him ample opportunity to practice the skill. When special equipment is necessary to perform the skill, such as insulin syringes, colostomy bags, dressings, and the like, it is important that the nurse provide the patient with the same equipment that he will be using after he leaves the hospital. Learning to perform a skill with one kind of equipment and then having to change to a different kind of equipment is more than can be expected of most patients.

Teaching aids are available to supplement the abilities of the nurse to help the patient to learn. These include books, pamphlets, pictures, films, slides, tapes, and models. Such teaching aids are invaluable when utilized appropriately. It is the responsibility of the nurse to carefully review all such aids before presenting them to patients in order to be sure that they are designed to meet the individual patient's learning needs.

Reinforcement and follow-up are also important factors to consider, since learning takes time. The patient must be allowed ample time to learn and to have his learning reinforced. A single teaching session is never adequate. Follow-up sessions are imperative in order to promote the patient's confidence in his ability to follow through with what he has learned. Such sessions also give the nurse the opportunity to evaluate the patient's progress and to plan for additional teaching sessions as required. It is also important to realize that the patient may not be able to transfer what he has learned in the hospital to his home setting. Thus, arrangements for follow-up after discharge are often essential for assuring that the full benefits of the hospital teaching program have been realized.

THE NURSING PROCESS IN PATIENT TEACHING

The teaching-learning process is an integral part of the nursing process. With a focus on learning and with regard for the principles of teaching and learning, the steps of the nursing process — assessment, planning, implementation, and evaluation — are utilized for the purpose of meeting the teaching and learning needs of the patient and his family.

Assessment

Assessment in the teaching-learning process is comparable to that component of the nursing process. It is directed toward the systematic collection of data about the patient's learning needs and his readiness to learn. All internal and external variables that affect the patient's readiness to learn are assessed. A learning assessment guide may be helpful in obtaining pertinent information about the patient's need to learn and his readiness to learn. Some of the learning assessment guides available are very general and are directed toward the assessment of general health information. Others are specific to common medication regimens or disease processes. An example is the *Diabetes Mellitus Assessment Guides* published by the American Diabetes Association, North Carolina affiliate, Inc. These assessment guides are designed for the assessment of the diabetic's learning needs with regard to all aspects of the diabetic regimen. Such guides serve to facilitate the asessment but must be adapted to the individual responses, problems, and needs of the patient. As soon as possible after completing the assessment, the nurse organizes, analyzes, synthesizes, and summarizes the data collected and determines the patient's need for teaching. Nursing diagnoses that specifically relate to the patient's learning needs are then succinctly stated and serve to guide the nurse in the development of the teaching plan.

Planning

Once the nursing diagnoses related to the patient's need for learning have been identified, the planning component of the teaching-learning process follows. This plan follows the same sequence utilized in the nursing process:

1. Assigning priorities to the diagnoses
2. Specifying the short-term, intermediate, and long-term goals of learning
3. Identifying specific teaching actions appropriate for attaining the goals
4. Documenting the diagnoses, goals, teaching actions (teaching orders), and expected outcomes on the teaching plan

As in the nursing process, the assignment of priorities to the diagnoses should be a joint effort by the nurse and the patient and/or his family members. Consideration must be given to the urgency of the patient's learning needs, the most critical needs receiving the highest priority.

After the priorities of the diagnoses have been established, the short-term, intermediate, and long-term goals and the teaching actions appropriate for attaining the goals are identified. Studies have indicated that teaching is most effective when the patient's goals and the nurse's goals are in agreement. Goal-directed learning should begin with the establishment of goals that are appropriate to the situation and that are realistic in terms of the patient's ability to achieve them. Goals should be individualized according to the needs of the patient, specifically the needs perceived by the patient, and must be acceptable to the nurse, the patient, and the family. Involving the patient and his family in goal establishment and subsequent planning of teaching actions promotes their cooperation in the implementation of the teaching plan.

Expected outcomes of the teaching actions are stated in terms of the patient's behaviors. Every effort is made to develop outcome criteria that are realistic and measurable. The critical time period within which the outcomes should be demonstrated by the patient are also identified. The outcome criteria and the critical time periods will serve as a basis for evaluation of the effectiveness of the teaching actions.

During the planning phase, the nurse gives consideration to the sequence in which the subject matter will be presented to the patient when each of the nursing actions is implemented. An outline is often helpful for arranging subject matter and for ensuring that all necessary information is included. Also during this time, the nurse selects and secures the appropriate teaching aids to be used in implementing the nursing actions.

The entire planning phase of the teaching-learning process is concluded with the formulation of the patient's teaching plan by the nurse. This teaching plan communicates the following information to all members of the nursing team:

1. The nursing diagnoses that specifically relate to the patient's learning needs and the priorities of these diagnoses
2. The goals of the teaching actions
3. The teaching actions, which are expressed in the form of teaching orders
4. The outcome criteria, which identify the expected behavioral outcomes for the patient
5. The critical time period within which the outcome must be met
6. The patient's behavioral responses (must be documented on the teaching plan)

The same rules that apply to writing and revising the nursing care plan apply to the teaching plan. (A sample

EXAMPLE OF A TEACHING PLAN
(For background information see nursing care plan example, page 24.)

Assessment of Mrs. Rollins' teaching and learning needs revealed the following:

basic knowledge about diabetes mellitus and the relationship between insulin, diet and activity
inadequate understanding of the relationship between hyperglycemia and physical and emotional stress
accurate administration of Lente Insulin 15U daily with acceptable rotation of injection sites and record keeping
acceptable practices of urine testing
inadequate knowledge of causes, signs, and symptoms of hyperglycemia and hypoglycemia
compliance with 1800 calorie ADA diet
acceptable practices of foot care and general hygiene

Nursing Diagnosis: Potential noncompliance with insulin administration regimen related to inadequate understanding of hyperglycemia and hypoglycemia
Goals—Short-term: Daily self-administration of Lente Insulin utilizing proper technique, rotation of sites, and record keeping
Intermediate: Describes effect of physical and emotional stress on diabetic control
Long-term: Consults diabetic clinic when confronted with symptomatology indicative of need for alteration of insulin dosage

TEACHING ORDERS	OUTCOME CRITERIA	CRITICAL TIME	OUTCOME
Reinforce knowledge regarding principles and practices of insulin administration.	Explains in her own words the necessity for and the action of insulin	3 days	Related explanation accurately
	Demonstrates proper technique of administration of insulin	3 days	Procedure performed accurately 3 days after admission; identified
	Records type, amount, and time of insulin injection	3 days	proper sites and significance of rotation; rotates between both
	Explains in her own words the rationale for rotating insulin injections	3 days	thighs and abdomen; skin of thighs and abdomen free of lipodystrophies; recorded type,
	Rotates insulin injection sites	3 days	amount and time of administration
Explain and discuss the following topics:	Identifies causes of hypoglycemia	5 days	Identified causes and symptoms accurately
causes of hypoglycemia	Identifies symptoms of hypoglycemia	5 days	
symptoms of hypoglycemia relationship between insulin, diet, activity, and stress with relation to hypoglycemic reactions	Explains in her own words the relationship between insulin, diet, activity, and stress with relation to hypoglycemic reactions	5 days	Related explanation accurately
immediate and delayed management of hypoglycemic reactions	States time of day when hypoglycemic reaction is most apt to occur	5 days	Related time accurately
	Describes immediate and delayed management of hypoglycemic reactions	5 days	Described management accurately
	Carries sugar on person at all times	5 days	Carries 2 packages of sugar in purse
Explain and discuss the following topics:	Identifies causes of hyperglycemia	5 days	Identified causes and symptoms accurately
causes of hyperglycemia symptoms of hyperglycemia	Identifies symptoms of hyperglycemia	5 days	
relationship between insulin, diet, activity, and stress with relation to hyperglycemia management of hyperglycemia	Explains in her own words the relationship between insulin, diet, activity, and stress with relation to hyperglycemia	5 days	Related explanation accurately

TEACHING ORDERS	OUTCOME CRITERIA	CRITICAL TIME	OUTCOME
	Describes the management of hyperglycemia	5 days	Described management accurately; continues to remain hesitant about reporting symptoms of hyperglycemia, including glucosuria, to diabetic clinic nurse
	Explains importance of reporting persistently positive urine tests for glucose and acetone	5 days	
Notify diabetic clinic nurse of patient's need for reinforcement of teaching regarding hypoglycemia and hyperglycemia after discharge from hospital (referral sent to diabetic clinic nurse on 1/8/80)	During next clinic visit, explains to clinic nurse the causes and symptoms of hypoglycemia and hyperglycemia; the relationship between insulin, diet, activity, and stress with relation to hypoglycemia and hyperglycemia; the management of hyperglycemia and hypoglycemia	first clinic visit after discharge	
	Seeks assistance from diabetic clinic nurse when confronted with symptoms of hyperglycemia or hypoglycemia	after discharge	

teaching plan appears on pages 32-33. Note that it is not different from but is simply a continuation of the nursing care plan.)

Implementation

The implementation phase of the teaching-learning process follows the formulation of the teaching plan. The patient, his family, and other members of the nursing team and the health team are included in the implementation. The activities of all of these persons are coordinated by the nurse, and the teaching plan serves as the basis for implementation.

- It is important to remain flexible during the implementation phase of the teaching-learning process and to continuously assess the patient's responses to the teaching actions and to make alterations in the teaching plan as necessary.

It is highly desirable that the nurse utilize her creativity to the fullest to promote and sustain the patient's motivation to learn; she should anticipate teaching needs that may arise after the patient's discharge from the hospital that are not foreseen by the patient while he is still in the hospital. Then, and only then, can she assist the patient in transferring knowledge from the hospital to his home. The implementation phase is concluded when the teaching actions have been completed and when the patient's responses to the actions have been recorded. This record serves as the basis for the evaluation of the patient's accomplishment of the defined outcome criteria.

Evaluation

Evaluation is the final component of the teaching-learning process and is directed toward the determination of the patient's response to the teaching actions and the extent to which the goals have been achieved. Evaluation for the teaching-learning process will answer the same question as that used for the nursing process but with specific regard to teaching and learning. An important phase in evaluation remains "What should be done to improve the teaching?" Answers to this question will dictate changes that must be made in the teaching plan.

It should never be assumed that an individual has learned because he has been taught. Learning does not automatically follow teaching. A variety of measurement techniques can be used to measure changes in behavior that give evidence of learning. These include direct observation of behavior, using rating scales, checklists, or anecdotal notes to document the behaviors, and indirect measures such as oral questioning and written tests. Measurement of actual behavior (direct measurement) is the most accurate and appropriate technique in many patient teaching situations. However, it should be supplemented with indirect measurements whenever possible. When more than one measurement technique is employed, the reliability of the resultant data is enhanced since each individual measurement technique carries with it a potential source of error.

The use of measurement techniques is only the beginning of evaluation. It is followed by the interpretation of the data and the making of value judgments about learning and teaching. Such evaluation should be done periodically throughout the teaching-learning program, at its conclusion, and at varying periods subsequent to the program. Evaluation of learning after hospitalization is highly desirable but is not always feasible in terms of time, economics, and nursing personnel required for such evaluation. However, coordination of efforts and sharing of information between hospital-based and community-based nursing personnel serves to facilitate such post-hospital evaluation.

• It should always be remembered that evaluation is not the end step in the teaching-learning process. The information gathered during evaluation should be utilized to redirect teaching actions with the goal of improving the patient's responses and outcomes that result from the teaching actions.

As in the nursing process, the steps of the teaching-learning process are cyclic and recurrent. Each step is ongoing and is related to all other steps. Continuous evaluation provides the means of maintaining the viability of the entire teaching-learning process and for demonstrating accountability for the quality of the teaching provided.

The guide which follows is intended to assist in the nurse's utilization of the teaching-learning process.

A GUIDE TO PATIENT TEACHING

ASSESSING

1. Assess the patient's readiness for health education.
   a. What are his health beliefs and behaviors?
   b. What psychosocial adaptation is he making?
   c. Is he ready to learn?
      Is he able to learn these behaviors?
      What additional information about him is needed?
      What are his expectations?
2. Formulate the nursing diagnoses that relate to the patient's learning needs.
   a. Organize, analyze, synthesize and summarize the collected data.
   b. Identify the patient's learning problems, their characteristics, and etiology.
   c. State nursing diagnoses concisely and precisely.

PLANNING

1. Assign priority to the nursing diagnoses that relate to the patient's learning needs.
2. Specify the short-term, intermediate, and long-term nurse-patient established learning goals.
3. Identify teaching actions appropriate for goal attainment.
4. Establish outcome criteria.
5. Develop the written teaching plan.
   a. Include diagnoses, goals, teaching actions, and outcome criteria.
   b. Put the information to be taught in logical sequence.
   c. Write down the key points.
   d. Select appropriate teaching aids.
   e. Keep the plan current and flexible to meet the patient's changing learning needs.

6. Involve the patient, his family and/or significant others, nursing team members, and other health team members in all aspects of planning.

IMPLEMENTING

1. Put the teaching plan into action.
2. Know the material to be presented.
3. Use language the patient can understand.
4. Use appropriate teaching aids.
5. Use the same equipment that the patient will utilize after discharge.
6. Encourage the patient to actively participate in learning.
7. Record the patient's responses to the teaching actions.

EVALUATING

1. Collect objective data.
   a. Observe the patient.
   b. Ask questions to determine if he understands.
   c. Use rating scales, checklists, anecdotal notes, and written tests when appropriate.
2. Compare the patient's behavioral outcomes to the outcome criteria. Determine the extent to which the goals were achieved.
3. Include the patient, his family and/or significant others, nursing team members, and other health team members in the evaluation.
4. Identify alterations that need to be made in the teaching plan.
5. Make referrals to appropriate sources or agencies for reinforcement of learning after discharge.
6. Continue all steps of the teaching process: assessing, planning, implementing, evaluating.

BIBLIOGRAPHY

BOOKS

Redman, B. K.: The Process of Patient Teaching in Nursing. St. Louis, C. V. Mosby, 1976.

Zander, K. S., Bower, K. A., Foster, S. D., Towson, M. C., Wermuth, M. R., and Woldum, K. M.: Practical Manual for Patient-Teaching. St. Louis, C. V. Mosby, 1978.

ARTICLES

General

del Bueno, D. J.: Patient education: planning for success. J. Nurs. Admin., 7:3-7, June 1978.

Dziurbejko, M. M., and Lardin, J. C. Including the family in preoperative teaching. AJN, 78:1892-1894, Nov. 1978.

Levin, L. S.: Patient education and self-care: how do they differ? Nurs. Outlook, 26:170-175, Mar. 1978.

Mayer, G. G., and Peterson, C. W.: Theoretical framework for coronary care. Nursing education. AJN, 78:1208-1211, July 1978.

Murray, R., and Zentner, J.: Guidelines for more effective health teaching. Nursing '76, 6:44-53, Feb. 1976.

Redman, B. K.: Curriculum in patient education. AJN, 78:1363-1366, Aug. 1978.

Compliance with Therapeutic Regimens

Carpenter, J. O., and Davis, L. J.: Medical recommendations — followed or ignored? Factors influencing compliance in arthritis. Arch. Phys. Med. & Rehab., 57:241-246, May 1976.

Connelly, C.E.: Patient compliance: a review of the research with implications for psychiatric-mental health nursing. J. Psychiat. Nurs., 16:15-18, Oct. 1978.

Given, C. W., Given, B. A., and Simoni, L.E.: The association of knowledge and perception of medications with compliance and health states among hypertensive patients: a prospective study. Res. in Nurs. & Health, 2:76-84, July 1978.

How can you improve patient compliance? Nursing '78, 8:40-47, May 1978.

Komaroff, A. L.: The practitioner and the compliant patient. AJPH, 66:833-835, Sept. 1976.

Romankiewicz, J. A., Gotz, V., Capelli, A., and Carlin, H. S.: To improve patient adherence to drug regimens: an interdisciplinary approach. AJN, 78:1216-1219, July 1978.

Rosenstock, I. M.: Patients' compliance with health regimens. JAMA, 234:402-403, Oct. 1975.

Steckel, S. B., and Swain, M. A.: Contracting with patients to improve compliance. Hospitals, J.A.H.A., 51:81-84, Dec. 1, 1977.

Zifferblatt, S. M.: Increasing patient compliance through the applied analysis of behavior. Preventive Med., 4:173-182, June 1975.

Health
Assessment
of the
Client/Patient

UNIT TWO

4

CLINICAL INTERVIEWING

No more important facet of the nurse–patient relationship exists than the clinical interview. It is through this device that the quality of the relationship is established, that information sufficient to provide a thorough assessment of the patient's problem is obtained, and that help is begun. Behaviors appropriate to the interview, and the techniques required to elicit cogent information, are not intrinsic to our social lives. These behaviors and techniques must be learned. No skill of the health professional requires more careful development than the skill of appropriate clinical interviewing.

THE ROLE OF THE NURSE

The role of the nurse in the provision of health care is a dynamically changing one. The scope of nursing now includes not only those functions for which the nurse has traditionally been prepared but a breadth of activities once reserved for physicians and other members of the health care team. *Nurse clinicians* and *nurse practitioners* are taught to employ skills that include gathering the patient data base and performing the physical examination. The concept that only the physician may diagnose and treat has become outmoded. Indeed, the concept should have been regarded as nonsense many years ago. Even in the traditional mode, the nurse who detected that the patient had fever, and responded appropriately, was "diagnosing" and "treating."

The concept of the health team is a relatively recent one. Intrinsic to the concept is an interdependence of health professionals, including physicians, nurses, physician's assistants, social workers, and others, each maximizing his or her skills in contributing to the resolution of patient problems. Common to all members of the health professions must be the capacity to interview the patient within the frameworks associated with each of their roles on the team.

The domain of the nurse may be restricted to a nursing assessment alone (see Chapter 6) or may be expanded to include the acquisition of the data base. Irrespective of the role of the nurse on the team, the team concept implies a knowledge by the nurse of the expected functions of all other members of the team. Thus, the nurse must be thoroughly familiar with the content of the data base and the system in which it is acquired.

Critical to the knowledge necessary to provide an optimum contribution to the team is an awareness of (1) the attributes of the skilled interviewer, (2) the content of the data base that emerges from the interview efforts of all the members of the team, and (3) the techniques of interviewing that not only provide maximum relevant information but also carry the health team toward the resolution of the patient's problem.

ATTRIBUTES OF THE INTERVIEWER

- The first responsibility of the interviewer upon initial contact with the patient is to put the patient at ease and provide for his comfort.

The nurse should introduce herself to the patient, defining her role on the health team, if appropriate, and explaining what she is about to do and why it is important. The setting of the interview should be conducive to open communication without anxiety. Thus the nurse should insure privacy for the interview. If visitors are present, they should be asked to leave, firmly but politely, since a patient may find it difficult to communicate when visitors (even close relatives) are in the room. Distractions caused by radios or television sets also should be excluded from the environment.

The interview must be conducted with due consideration for the patient's comfort and self-respect. Before beginning, the nurse should see that the patient is comfortable. If the interview is taking place in a hospital room, the nurse may ask the patient if he would like another pillow or would prefer to be seated in a chair rather than in bed. The patient who is short of breath will be made more comfortable if allowed to sit rather than lie down. If the patient is in pain or in urgent need of going to the bathroom, his discomfort should be attended to before the interview is allowed to continue. It is unnerving to both patient and interviewer if the patient feels the urge to use the toilet facilities either before or during the interview. Frequently the patient will convey this need by nonverbal behavior that clearly says "I have to go to the bathroom." If such is the case, he should be given the opportunity.

- The interviewer should permit the patient to express himself fully.

Whether the interview is relatively directive or non-directive, the patient should not be interrupted in his response to questions. The patient's own questions and verbalized anxieties should be responded to. Moreover, the patient should be encouraged to ask questions. A frequent response by the patient to a question in a sensitive area might be, "Why do you need to know that?" The importance of the interviewer's question can usually be expressed in a context that will make it entirely understandable and acceptable to the patient. In the event that it is not, the interviewer might pursue another line of questioning and return to the sensitive area when trust has been established.

- The interviewer must take pains to reassure the patient and convey an understanding of the nature and intensity of the problem.

Properly done, such reassurance moves the interviewer from the inquiring to the therapeutic mode. The interviewer must also convey understanding of and respect for the patient's beliefs and attitudes. This must be done in spite of the fact that such beliefs and attitudes may be sharply at variance with those held by the interviewer. There is no place in the interview for a comment such as "You don't really believe that, do you?" If the patient does not believe it, it is unlikely that he would state it candidly to a health professional conducting an interview. A nonjudgmental attitude is especially necessary when dealing with matters related to human sexuality, drug and alcohol abuse, and racial and ethnic matters.

Since the interviewer may elicit a wide variety of attitudes and experiences related to human sexual behavior, it is important to remember that one person's perversion may be part of another's life style.

- The interviewer must take into account the patient's cultural background.

Cultural attitudes about family relations and the role of women should be accepted at face value, as should attitudes toward pain, illness, and hospitalization. These beliefs and attitudes may be derived from personal experiences that are different from experiences common to those who have spent several generations in the English-speaking world.

- The interviewer should be aware of her or his own feelings and attitudes.

Patient behavior that the nurse might find offensive in herself, her family, or her friends may arouse hostility, anger, anxiety, or even, at times, revulsion. The true professional cannot allow this to be conveyed to the patient. Quite unconsciously, the interviewer might convey irritation, boredom, or disbelief. Similarly, the interviewer may be acutely uncomfortable when dealing with certain kinds of illnesses, because of his or her own fears or because he or she finds it difficult to relate to the personality associated with the illness. For example, the nurse may find herself irritated by the passive dependence commonly associated with asthma and bowel disorders. Or her own ethical and moral sense may make it difficult for her to relate to the alcoholic and the drug-dependent patient. It is a frequent failing of health professionals to view self-inflicted illness with disdain, hostility, and anger. The situation is compounded when the patient is acutely intoxicated and may return hostility for hostility. The first step in dealing effectively with such patients is to understand the inner compulsions that cause the interviewer to reject the patient.

- The interviewer should be attuned to nonverbal communication and should learn to recognize gestures that convey defensiveness, hostility, confidence, impatience, etc.

The nurse should learn to respond to body language the same way she responds to the spoken word. Since much has been written about body language, a quick perusal of an illustrated book on this subject will be highly rewarding to anyone involved in professional-client relationships. Frequently, the body language and the patient's verbal expression are at variance. Often this is obvious—as when the patient describes a seemingly happy event, yet appears to be on the verge of tears. The interviewer might respond to such inconsistencies by drawing them to the patient's attention.

- The interviewer should communicate in a manner that is consistent with the patient's level of understanding.

This is especially true in regard to the patient's educational background. The nurse is a highly intelligent person selected from the population for advanced education by virtue of capacities and opportunities not possessed by a large segment of the population. Her use of the English language is sophisticated, and she also possesses a health care vocabulary that is foreign to the majority of the population. Questions must be phrased in such a way that they are well understood by the patient, and counseling must be done using as few technical terms as possible. If the patient does not understand the language being used, it is unlikely that he will interrupt for clarification, largely out of fear tht he will appear ignorant. Careful questioning may reveal the level of the patient's understanding of an issue that has just been discussed.

A second factor influencing the patient's level of understanding is cultural background. The Puerto Rican mother, for example, has a different perception of personal health than does a mother born and raised in an American suburb. Pregnancy is not something for which she would seek care and attention until labor begins. Thus she would not understand the need for prenatal care as advocated by health professionals. Nor would a woman from a culture in which obesity is a way of life and admired by males understand the need for diet and weight control. Similarly, Oriental women, not accustomed to complaining of pain, even when severe, would not appreciate the advantages of taking analgesics. All such differences in outlook must be taken into account when dealing with members of other cultures.

Even differences in the life experiences of those who are well educated and from the same cultural background must be considered. An only child of an urban or suburban family may be ill-equipped to deal with the problems of being a mother, in contrast to a woman from a rural society who is reared in a family of eight or ten children. In large families, older children participate in rearing the young.

- The interviewer should terminate the interview in an appropriate manner that will ensure that the patient has understood the major points discussed.

The nurse should inquire whether the patient has any questions and should search for any lack of understanding that may have derived from the interview. Showing concern for the patient's insights will help provide a bridge for future encounters. It might also be appropriate to spell out the objectives to be accomplished in subsequent interactions.

CONTENT OF THE INTERVIEW

When the patient is seen for the first time by the health team (except in the emergency care situation) the first requisite is to obtain a *data base*. The nurse may be respon-sible for all or part of the data base, but clearly she must be familiar with all of its facets and the role to be played by other members of the team in acquiring the requisite information. The data base contains the following components:

1. Patient profile (introductory identifying data)
2. Informant
3. Chief complaint
4. History of present illness
5. Past medical history
6. Review of systems
7. Family history
8. Patient profile (amplification of 1)
9. Physical examination
10. Radiologic and laboratory information
11. Problem formulation, assessment, and plan

Patient Profile (Introductory Identifying Data)

The introductory identifying information helps to put much of the history in context. Certainly this information must include the age and sex of the patient, marital status, race, and occupation. Some people prefer a full patient profile at this juncture, but most believe a full profile to be inappropriate until such time as the interviewer has obtained the trust and confidence of the patient. Moreover, a patient in pain, or with an equally urgent problem for which he seeks attention, is unlikely to put a great deal of confidence in an interviewer who is more concerned with the details of his marital status than with quickly addressing the problem for which the patient seeks help.

The Informant

The informant may not always be the patient, as is the case if the patient is a child or an elderly person, or is unconscious, in a coma, or suffering a severe psychiatric disturbance. The interviewer should assess the reliability of the informant and the usefulness of the information provided. For example, hysterical or depressed patients are unlikely to provide a reliable data base, while patients who abuse drugs and alcohol are likely to use denial as part of their operating mechanism. It is reasonable for the interviewer to make such judgments (based on the context of the entire interview) and to incorporate them in the record.

Chief Complaint

The chief complaint is that issue which brings the patient to seek help. Frequently the patient appears without complaint, seeking an ongoing relationship with a health team or requesting a "check-up." If this is the case, it should be noted in lieu of a chief complaint. Once the patient has expressed his complaint, his exact words should be transposed to the record in quotation marks.

However, a statement such as, "Doctor Smith sent me," is not a chief complaint. Although such information can be included as part of the introductory patient profile, the patient should be asked why he sought Dr. Smith's attention and this reason should be entered as the chief complaint.

Frequently the patient will have more than one problem and, therefore, more than one complaint. These should be listed in terms of the patient's priorities and then explored through the present illness as separate entities, if they represent separate problems, or as a single present illness if they are multiple manifestations of one cohesive problem.

History of Present Illness

Of all the facets of the data base, the history of the present illness is the most difficult to elicit. It is relatively easy to extract the facts related to a past medical history or to a review of systems, and certainly a wide range of health professionals are taught to deal with the social and emotional facets of the data base. The techniques of the physical examination may be taught to anyone who has a modest knowledge of anatomy and physiology. However, cogent exploration of the facts related to a present illness requires substantial knowledge of the pathophysiology and natural history of disease. If one does not know, for example, the manifestations of acute pericarditis, it is difficult to subtly extract information which will allow the diagnosis to be made. Moreover, the history of any illness is the single most important factor in enabling the health professional to arrive at a diagnosis. The physical examination is helpful but usually reveals manifestations that are an expected consequence of the story that has unfolded. Occasionally laboratory and radiologic information can be singularly helpful; only rarely do they establish the diagnosis. On the other hand, judicious selection of laboratory and radiologic inquiry demands a careful history.

The "present illness" may well be but one episode in a sequence that is contained within a single disease process. An episode of insulin shock, for example, is only one of an ordered series of occurrences that define the natural history of diabetes. In such an instance, the entire course of the diabetic illness must be unfolded in order to put the current complaint in context. Although the episode of insulin shock gains prominence in the delineation of the story, the description of it must be obtained in the context of the natural history of the disease and communicated to the record in a similar manner. Dates of onset of the various manifestations of a complicated illness are critical to the analysis of the problem. They must be obtained and set down in an orderly fashion. The chronology should include factors which have precipitated changes in the course of the illness, medical interventions, and dates of hospitalization, surgical procedures, etc.

Specific symptoms such as pain, headache, fever, change in bowel habits, discharge from an orifice, etc. must be delineated in detail. Critical to the analysis of symptoms are location, quality, severity, and duration of the complaint. The interviewer must pursue the persistence and/or intermittence of the symptom, those factors which aggravate or alleviate it, and any associated manifestations of which the patient may be aware. Information about this last point is most difficult to obtain, since the patient will frequently not associate two events that are in fact related to a common problem. Clarity emerges as a result of the care with which the development of symptoms is explored.

Past Medical History

The interviewer should obtain and record in chronological order all significant past illnesses, injuries, and operations, including dates, duration, complications, and facts related to hospitalization. To the extent that a particular hospitalization or major medical intervention is related to the present illness, it need not be repeated; rather, reference to the history of the present illness may be indicated. Careful exploration of the past medical history will include medications prescribed and taken, immunizations, and evidence of allergies to drugs or other substances.

Review of Systems

Part of the data base should include a complete inventory of major body organ systems in terms of the presence or absence of symptoms past or present. Illnesses that have been previously described under the history of the present illness or under the past medical history need not be repeated. Reference may be made to the appropriate location of relevant information. The system review should include an overview of general health as well as symptoms related to the skin, eyes, ears, nose, mouth, cardiovascular system, pulmonary system, gastrointestinal system, endocrine system, and genitourinary and reproductive systems. There is an increasing tendency among health professionals to codify the past medical history and review of systems in a formal checklist that may be kept as part of the medical record. Many of these are commercially available and others are prepared by health teams in a manner appropriate to team function. One asset of the "checklist" process is that it is easily audited and less subject to error than is relying on the interviewer to obtain information relevant to each organ system. On the whole it is an encouraging development and one which will gain increased usage.

Family History

Details with respect to the state of health of all first-order relatives should be obtained. First-order relatives include parents, brothers and sisters, and children. The interviewer should seek information regarding specific inherited or communicable diseases not only among first-order but also among second-order relatives. Thus, it is important to know if grandparents or cousins have had diabetes, tuberculosis, hypertension, and cancer. One should attempt to determine which members of the family constellation are living with the patient, and the state of health of each.

Patient Profile

The patient profile obtained at this stage of the interview is an amplification of the identifying information that was sought at the beginning of the interview. Critical to an analysis of the patient's problem, his capacity to deal with that problem, and the health team's capacity to provide assistance, is knowledge of the patient's family origin, issues surrounding the patient's growth and development, and the patient's current life situation. With respect to the last item, it is important to inquire about the quality of intimate relationships, about the occupation, education, religion, goals, and aspirations of the patient, and about the patient's past responses to stressful situations. It is important to know what the illness means to the patient in order to put in context the patient's capacity to deal with that illness. It is important to know what kind of emotional and physical support exists within the patient's home and social environment. That support will inevitably be called upon by the health team in the event of serious illness. In terms of the quality of intimate relationships, one should seek information regarding the patient's capacity for sexual expression and the degree to which he gains satisfaction and gratification from his relationships. The issue of sexuality is vital to every patient, but is rarely raised by the patient if the health professional does not express an openness and willingness to deal with sexual matters.

The Remainder of the Data Base

The physical examination is treated in Chapter 5 of this text. Problem formulation, assessment, and the plan for the management of patient problems are included in the discussion of the problem-oriented record in Chapter 6. It should not be forgotten, however, that they are an integral part of the data base that is needed to evaluate the patient initially and to complete the framework around which care is provided on a continuing basis.

TECHNIQUES OF THE INTERVIEW

Whatever the purpose of the interview, and whatever content is to be obtained by the nurse, some general principles applicable to all professional-client relationships should be understood.

ASSURING TRUST AND CONFIDENCE. Accuracy of information and the capacity to provide help and assistance to the patient are functions of the degree to which trust and confidence have been achieved by the interviewer. The patient who seeks health care for a specific problem is almost invariably anxious. He does not really understand the significance of his symptoms. Compounding this are fears related to potential disruption of the patient's life style, and perhaps apprehension regarding the costs of medical care. Given this set of circumstances, the patient feels helpless, for he perceives that the outcome with respect to both his health and his economic well-being lies in the hands of others. At the same time the health team may well be inundated with numerous other patients with other problems, many of which are grave, and all of which are time-consuming. It is understandable that the team will therefore seek information efficiently and attempt to resolve problems firmly. In such a setting it is easy to slip into an ambience wherein the health professionals become authority figures and the patient's dependence is unnecessarily heightened. Respect for the patient as an individual deteriorates.

ENCOURAGING SPONTANEITY. The goal of the clinical interview is to obtain all of the facts that will influence both the diagnosis and the therapeutic approach. However, in pursuing this objective, one must constantly strive to assert the least amount of authority necessary to obtain information in the time allotted. This can best be achieved in an atmosphere that encourages spontaneity on the part of the patient. Optimal spontaneous behavior can be a function of both the physical setting and the behavior of the interviewer.

It is the interviewer's role to facilitate spontaneous behavior and the unrestricted recitation of the problem as the patient perceives it. We have spoken earlier of the importance of nonverbal communication on the part of the patient. There is also a role for nonverbal communication on the part of the nurse. The nurse may actively encourage the patient to elaborate, or to continue, by nodding her head or by repeating the last few words if the patient appears hesitant. A puzzled look will encourage the patient to clarify apparent inconsistencies in the story. Questions should be open-ended. "How can we help you?" "Tell me about it." "How did it feel?" are all appropriate questions. "Was it a sharp pain?" "Did it happen only on weekdays?" are inappropriate questions. Such questions presume the answer. Although one certainly wishes to obtain that information, it should be sought in a more open-ended way. One will find the patient attempting to "help" the nurse by providing the answer that she wishes to hear.

EXPRESSING UNDERSTANDING. Silence is not undesirable in the interview situation. The patient may be emotionally overcome or may be attempting to formulate an accurate description of events. Such silences should not be intruded upon by the interviewer. Nor should tearful episodes be interrupted. One should resist the urge to tell the patient that matters are going to be all right or to provide similar verbal reassurances. Things may not be all right, and the reassurance may appear false. Moreover, one has much to learn by inquiring why the patient became fearful. Reassurance can be conveyed by nonverbal communication. Open-ended statements such as "You look sad" or "You seem frightened" will encourage the patient to elaborate upon his feelings and at the same time convey the interviewer's understanding and empathy.

ASKING SUITABLE QUESTIONS. Ultimately, in order to refine the details that are important to the analysis of symptoms, one must resort to some degree of direct questioning. Such questions should provide the patient with options for his response. "Does the pain have any relationship to meals?" gives the patient the option of answering yes or no. "Does the pain come before the meal, during the meal, or after the meal?" again gives the patient the opportunity to select from among several options. This more direct line of questioning should be deferred until later in the interview, when the patient has had an opportunity to express himself as fully as possible and his urge to "help" the interviewer has been submerged by a well developed sense of trust and confidence.

It is not to be presumed that the approach to every patient will be the same. Clearly, the nurse will have to be more directive with the garrulous patient and will have to encourage the patient who is more taciturn or who is depressed. The sophistication that allows modulation of the interview technique comes only with experience.

SUMMARY. In summary we might comment that interviewing skill has always been necessary for the nurse as a means of fulfilling her responsibility. The nurse is, however, currently being asked to expand her role and to apply the interview skill over a wider range of activities. In order to fulfill the broader role to which the nurse must address herself she will have to cultivate the attributes of attitude and behavior necessary for the skilled interviewer and refine the techniques that promote optimum communication.

NURSING HISTORY
*Nursing Assessment and Data Base**

Purpose: To obtain pertinent information from a newly admitted patient in order to initiate a nursing care plan including outcome criteria.

I. GENERAL PATIENT/CLIENT DATA BASE

A. Identification
  1. Name: Age: Sex: Race: Adm. Date:
  2. Marital Status: Education: Household Size:
  3. Occupation: Work Patterns:
  4. Appearance at First Sight
     Physical:
     Emotional:
  5. Significant Cultural Factors:
  6. Financial Status (relating to care):
B. General Health History
  1. Medical Diagnosis
     Primary:
     Secondary:

2. Family History	Living	Age at Death	Cause of Death
Father:			
Mother:			
Siblings:			

  3. Health Practices: Recreational, religious, and nutritional
     a. Smoking: Amount
     b. Alcohol: Amount
     c. Exercise: Type and frequency
     d. Recreational and diversional activities:
     e. Nutrition: Quality, special habits, idiosyncrasies, preferences
     f. Religious beliefs: Impact on health

---

*This tool is only a guide. More or fewer points of inquiry may be required.

I. GENERAL PATIENT/CLIENT DATA BASE (CONTINUED)

    4. Health Resources Utilized

	Yes	How Often		Yes	How Often
Family physician:			Dentist:		
Specialist:			Podiatrist:		
Community Nursing:			Psychiatrist:		

    5. Allergies:

        How Managed

      Food

      Drug

      Other

    6. Medications:

Name	Dosage	Purpose	Frequency

II. SPECIFIC HEALTH-ILLNESS DATA BASE—PSYCHOSOCIAL ASSESSMENT

  A1. Perception of Illness and Hospitalization:

    1. What brought you to the hospital?

    2. What is your understanding of the cause and possible treatment of your illness?

    3. How do you feel about your illness?

    4. What are your expectations?

    5. What is the role of your family, friends, etc.?

    6. Adequacy of post-hospital care

  A2. Nursing Awareness and Evaluation

    1. Pertinent physical and psychosocial needs expressed by patient/client

    2. General level of understanding and ability to communicate

  B. Coping Mechanisms:

    1. What previous illnesses have you had? Hospitalizations?
       How were these managed? Adverse recollections?

    2. Do you have concerns about this admission?

    3. What resources can you tap to help you? (Family, religion, etc.)

    4. What other stressful experiences have you had? How did you handle these?

  C. Comfort and Safety Measures:

    1. Discomforts? Causes:

    2. Measures to promote comfort and safety

  D. Relations with Others: Psychosocial Needs

    1. Does the person (family or significant others) closest to you know that you are in the hospital?

    2. Can we contact anyone for you?

      3. Self-Concept (body image)

        a. Family role   c. Body function

        b. Job role   d. Sexual function

      4. Self-Esteem (belonging)

        a. Family   c. Co-workers

        b. Friends   d. Others

      5. Dependence-Independence-Interdependence

        a. Family   c. Co-workers

        b. Friends   d. Others

      6. Esthetic Practices

        a. Hospital unit   b. Home care

III. ASSESSMENT OF PHYSIOLOGICAL FUNCTIONS

  A. Sensory: Stimuli-Response

    Mental Status:

      Alert   Depressed

      Confused   Irritable

      Disoriented   Dizzy, lightheaded

    Vision: Hearing:

      Glasses, contact lenses   Each ear

      Headaches, blurred vision   Aids

      Diagnostic test results   Diagnostic test results

III. ASSESSMENT OF PHYSIOLOGICAL FUNCTIONS (CONTINUED)

A. Sensory: Stimuli-Response (Continued)
   Communication:
      Speaks clearly   Relates well to others
      Understands language   Eye contact

B. Neurologic
   Levels of consciousness   Vertigo, syncope
   Muscle tone, paralysis   Pupillary reactions
   Memory, orientation   Cranial nerve deficiencies:
   Seizures, tremors   Taste, hearing, etc.
   Gait   Diagnostic test results

C. Integument
   Skin condition—general   Feet: Nails
      Folds: axillary, groin, etc.   Between toes
   Diaphoresis   Corns, calluses
   Hair

D. Respiratory
   Respirations: Cough: character, sputum
      Rate and character   Skin color
      Breath sounds   Respiratory aids
      Chest expansion   Diagnostic test results

E. Cardiovascular
   Blood pressure   Edema and positional color of lower
   Pulses and nature   extremities
   Color and temperature of extremities   Complaints of dizziness, restlessness, etc.
   Supportive aids: Diagnostic test results
      Oxygen, pacemaker, etc.

F. Gastrointestinal
   1. Nutritional   Dentures
      Nature of diet, quality of meals   Fluid-drinking habits and preferences
      Appetite, anorexia, flatulence   Discomforts: nausea, vomiting, pain
      Food preferences, dislikes   Surgically created diversions
                                    Diagnostic test results

   2. Elimination
      Defecation patterns, stool   Hemorrhoids
         characteristics
      Constipation, diarrhea

G. Urinary
   Voiding patterns   Urinary diversions
   Nocturia, frequency, pain, etc. Diagnostic test results

H. Reproductive
   Male: Female:
      Genital infections   Menstrual history
      Prostate problems   Pregnancies
      Impotence   Menopausal age
      Sexual activity   Vaginal discharge
                                       Last Pap test

I. Musculoskeletal
   Ability to work   Range of motion
   Nature of muscle tone   Supportive aids or prosthesis
   Spinal deviations: scoliosis, lordosis

BIBLIOGRAPHY

BOOKS

Conn, H. F., et al.: Family Practice. *In* Froehlich, R. E., and Verby, J. E., eds.: Interviewing Techniques. Philadelphia, W. B. Saunders, 1973.

Enclow, A. J.: Interviewing and Patient Care. New York, Oxford University Press, 1972.

Froehlich, R. E., and Bishop, F. M.: Clinical Interviewing Skills. 3rd ed. St. Louis, C. V. Mosby, 1977.

Prior, J. A., and Silberstein, J. S.: Physical Diagnosis: The History and Examination of the Patient. St. Louis, C. V. Mosby, 1977.

Raus, E. E., and Raus, M. M.: Manual of History Taking, Physical Examination and Record Keeping, Philadelphia, J. B. Lippincott, 1974.

ARTICLES

Eggland, E. T.: How to take a meaningful nursing history. Nursing '77, 7:22–30, July, 1977.

Porter, A., et al.: Patient needs on admission, AJN, 77:112–113, Jan. 1977.

5
PHYSICAL ASSESSMENT

The basic tools of the physical examination are the human senses of vision, hearing, touch, and smell. These human tools may be augmented by special man-made tools (e.g., the stethoscope, the ophthalmoscope) to permit better definition of visual and acoustic details, but these man-made tools should be recognized for what they are: extensions of the human senses. One may hear it implied that some of these tools are sophisticated devices that require divine knowledge for their use; in fact, they are simple instruments that anyone can learn to use, and use well. Sophistication comes with the interpretation of what is being seen and heard.

THE PROCESSES OF PHYSICAL EXAMINATION

Four fundamental processes are employed in the examination of the patient: *inspection, palpation, percussion,* and *auscultation.*

Inspection

The first fundamental process is inspection. The power to observe is one that must be cultivated. General inspection is carried out at the first moment of contact with the patient. The examiner introduces herself to the patient, perhaps shakes hands with him, and exchanges the first words of communication. Many impressions register in this exchange, and numerous valuable observations can be made. The patient is old or young (how old? — how young? — appropriate to his/her stated age?); the patient is thin or fat; the patient is anxious, or perhaps

depressed; the patient is normal in body habitus or perhaps deformed in some way (what way? — how different from expected normal?).

Two commonly used phrases are too frequently used as excuses for insufficient attention to the details of observation. *"The patient looks sick."* In what way does the patient look sick? Is he pale; is his skin clammy; is the patient grimacing in pain; is the patient dyspneic; is the skin jaundiced or cyanotic; does the patient have edema? What specific physical features or behavioral manifestations convey that he is "sick"? *"The patient appears chronically ill."* In what way does the patient appear chronically ill? Does he appear to have lost weight? Patients who lose weight secondary to malignancy or other muscle-wasting disease appear different from those who are merely thin. The distribution of their weight loss takes a different form. Does the skin have the appearance of chronic illness? That is, is it pale, or does it give the appearance of dehydration or loss of subcutaneous tissue? These are important observations that health professionals frequently fail to note on the record.

Among general observations that should be noted in the initial examination of the patient are posture and stature, body movements, nutrition, speech pattern, and body temperature.

POSTURE AND STATURE. The posture that a patient assumes can often reveal much about his illness. Patients with the dyspnea of cardiac disease prefer to sit and may complain of "smothering" if forced to lie down for even brief periods of time. Persons with emphysema not only sit upright, but assume a posture that is quite characteristic. They thrust their arms forward and laterally onto the edge of the bed ("tripod position") in order to place accessory muscles of respiration at an optimum mechanical advantage for respiratory assistance. Patients with abdominal pain due to peritonitis prefer to lie perfectly still. Even slight jarring of the bed by the examiner will incite agonizing accentuation of pain. On the other hand, patients with abdominal pain due to renal or biliary colic are exceedingly restless. They may writhe in bed or even rise to pace the room. Patients with meningeal irritation associated with headache cannot flex the head or the legs without aggravating their pain.

BODY MOVEMENTS. Abnormalities of body movement may be of two general kinds: generalized discontinuity of voluntary or involuntary movement, or asymmetry of movement. In the former category are included tremors of a wide variety, some of which may occur at rest (Parkinson's disease), while others are incited only on voluntary movement (cerebellar ataxia). Other tremors may exist both during rest and activity (delirium tremens of the alcoholic, thyrotoxicosis). Some voluntary or involuntary movements are fine, others quite coarse. At the extreme are the convulsive movements of epilepsy or tetanus and the gross choreiform movements of patients with rheumatic fever or Huntington's disease.

Asymmetry of movement is seen in patients with disease of the central nervous system (CNS), principally in those who have had cerebral vascular accidents. The patient may manifest drooping of one side of the face and/or be incapable of normal movement of the right or left upper and lower extremities. Strength is impaired on the involved side, and the patient walks with a foot-dragging gait.

NUTRITION. States of nutrition are important to note. Obesity may be generalized as a function of excessive intake of calories or may be specifically localized to the trunk in patients with endocrine disorders (Cushing's disease) or those who have been taking steroid drugs for long periods of time. Loss of weight may be generalized as a function of caloric deprivation or may be reflected more strikingly in loss of muscle mass in patients whose diseases interfere with protein building.

SPEECH PATTERN. Speech may be slurred owing to central nervous system disease or because of incapacity to articulate due to damage to cranial nerves. Damage to the recurrent laryngeal nerve will produce hoarseness, as will those diseases which produce edema or swelling of the vocal cords. Speech may be halting or interrupted in flow in some CNS disorders (multiple sclerosis).

BODY TEMPERATURE. The recording of body temperature is a part of every physical examination. Fever is an increase in body temperature above normal. Normal for most persons is an average of 37.0°C. (98.6°F.). It should be recognized that there is some variation from 37.0°C. (98.6°F.) that is still within the range of normal. Some persons are quite normal at 36.6°C. (98°F.), and others at 37.3°C. (99°F.). Children playing hard during summer months quite regularly run temperatures as high as 37.7°C. (100°F.), and occasionally higher, but this should subside quite promptly, with rest. Moreover, it should be recognized that there is a normal diurnal variation of a degree or two in body temperature throughout the day. Most persons achieve their low early in the morning. Body temperature rises during the day to 37.3°C. (99°F.) or 37.5°C. (99.5°F.) and then subsides through the night.

Palpation

Palpation is a vital part of the physical examination. Many structures of the body, although not visible, are assessable by the hand and may, in a way, be "felt." Examples include blood vessels, lymph nodes, the thyroid, the organs of the abdomen and pelvis, and the rectum.

Sounds generated within the body, if within specified frequency ranges, also may be "felt." Thus, certain murmurs generated in the heart or within blood vessels (thrills) may be detected. Thrills create a sensation to the hand much like the purring of a cat. Voice sounds are transmitted along the bronchi to the periphery of the lung. These may be perceived by touch and will be altered by certain disease states within the lung. The phenomenon is called *tactile fremitus* and is useful in assessing diseases of the chest.

Percussion

The technique of percussion translates the application of physical force into sound. It is a most difficult art to perfect, but one capable of yielding much information about disease processes in the chest and abdomen. The principle is to set the chest wall or abdominal wall into vibration by striking it with a firm object. The sound produced is reflective of the structure of underlying thoracic or abdominal contents.

The procedure (for right-handed persons; hands should be reversed if the examiner is left-handed) is conducted as follows (Fig. 5-1): Place the distal phalanx of the left middle finger firmly against the chest wall. The other fingers should be held away from the chest wall, since any pressure they might exert against the thorax would tend to mute or dampen the sound produced. The right hand now becomes the striking object. The middle finger of the right hand is used to strike the terminal phalanx of the middle finger of the left hand just behind the nail bed. If done sharply, a brief resonant tone will be produced. The motion of the right hand should be dominantly a wrist action. The forearm itself should be held steady. The clarity of the sound produced is dependent on the brevity of the action. The intensity is a function of the force used.

The vibration of the chest wall or abdominal wall incited by percussion reflects the nature of thoracic or

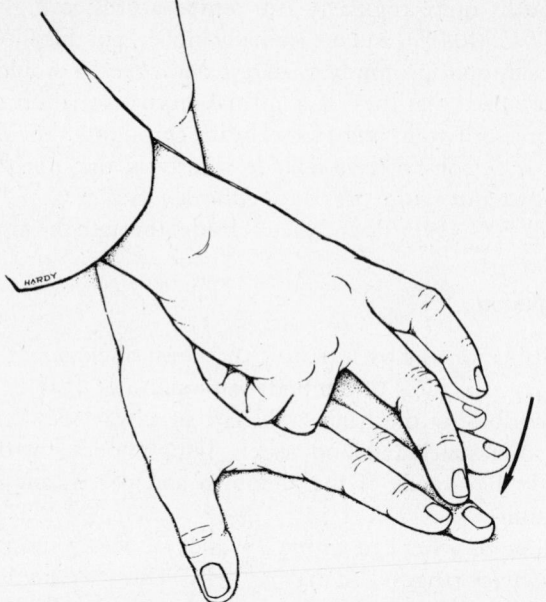

Figure 5-1. Percussion technique. The middle finger of the right hand strikes the terminal phalanx of the middle finger of the left hand. Care should be taken that only the terminal part of the middle finger of the left hand is in contact with the area to be percussed. The middle finger of the right hand should be held rigidly. It is properly a wrist action, and the intensity and clarity of the note will be a function of the quickness with which it is performed.

abdominal contents to a depth of 4 to 6 cm (Fig. 5-2). Definition of structures deeper than this must be left to other methods. One must become familiar with the range of normal tones produced by percussion of the chest wall. The tone is obviously influenced by the thickness of the wall as well as the nature of underlying structures. The range of tone produced in normal persons is called *normal resonance*. Persons with emphysema and overinflated lung tissue produce a tone that is lower in frequency and longer in duration than normal resonance. This is called *hyperresonance*. Air trapped in an enclosed structure under tension (tension pneumothorax, obstructed bowel, etc.) will produce a high frequency drumlike sound that is appropriately called *tympany*. Consolidation or increase in density of normal air-containing lung tissue produces a shorter, higher pitched sound that is termed *dull*. The presence of a large nonresonant mass, such as fluid, in the chest or abdomen, will almost totally impede any motion of the chest or abdominal wall. The sound produced is said to be *flat*.

Percussion gives one the capacity to assess such normal anatomical details as the degree to which the diaphragm descends during inspiration. The sound over lung tissue is normally resonant; the sound over apposing diaphragm is dull. One may percuss the border of the heart. One may determine the level of pleural effusion or the location of pneumonic consolidation or atelectasis of a lobe of the lung. Further application of the technique will be discussed under examination of the thorax and abdomen.

Auscultation

Sound is produced within the body either by the movement of air through hollow structures or by the forces set up by the movement of columns of fluid that set solid structures in motion. Examples of acoustical phenomena of clinical importance include the movement of air through the trachea and bronchi (breath sounds), the movement of air past functioning vocal cords (spoken voice), the movement of air through the intestines (bowel sounds), the movement of blood through vascular structures that provide critical resistance to flow (murmurs), and the impedance to flowing blood provided by closed valves and the heart wall (heart sounds). Physiological sounds may be normal (e.g., first and second heart sounds) or pathological (e.g., murmurs in diastole produced in the heart, or rales in the lung). Some normal sounds may be distorted by pathology of structures through which the sound must travel (e.g., changes in the character of breath sounds as they travel through the consolidated lung of lobar pneumonia).

Sound produced within the body, if of sufficient amplitude, will set in vibration all structures between the origin of the sound and the body surface. Sound vibration emanating from the body surface may be captured directly by the examiner's ear or, more appropriately, by the stethoscope, an instrument devised as an extension of the human ear.

Although the stethoscope does not have the capacity to amplify sound, it does channel it, thereby making physiologic sound more readily available for our critical evaluation. Two end-pieces are available for the stethoscope—the *bell* and the *diaphragm*. Many stethoscopes come with both pieces built into a single head. Alternating between the pieces becomes a matter of turning the head of the stethoscope or flipping a switch. The bell is better suited for the transmission of very low frequency sounds; the diaphragm is more appropriately constructed for the reception of high frequency sounds. The ear pieces of the stethoscope should fit snugly into the ear canals, and the tubing should not be more than 20 cm. in length. Dual tubing transmits sound more faithfully than single tubing.

Sound produced by the body has the features of sound produced in any other manner. That is, it is characterized by intensity, frequency, and quality. The intensity, or loudness, associated with physiologic sound is low. Rarely may sounds of the body, except for speech, be heard without direct application of the ear or the stethoscope to the body surface. With respect to frequency, or pitch, it may be said that physiologic sound is in reality

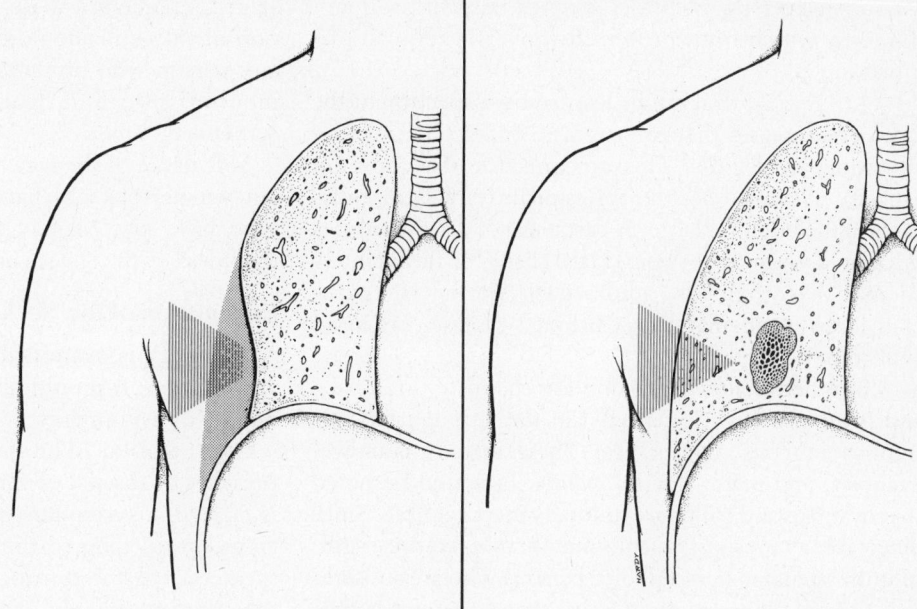

Figure 5-2. This figure illustrates graphically the fact that masses more than 6 cm. from the surface of the chest wall will not impair normal resonance over the lung. An effusion under the pleural surface produces dullness, whereas a tumor mass near the hilum of the lung cannot be detected.

"noise," in that most sounds consist of a frequency spectrum as opposed to single frequency sounds that we associate with music or the tuning fork. The frequency spectrum may be quite low, yielding a rumbling noise, or comparatively high, producing a harsh or blowing sound. The third feature of sound is quality. This relates to overtones and is the characteristic of sound that allows one to differentiate sound produced by the piano from that produced by the violin. This has little relevance, however, for physiologic sound.

The fundamental processes of inspection, palpation, percussion, and auscultation will now be discussed with respect to the various organ-systems and parts of the body to which they may be applied.

EXAMINATION OF THE HEAD AND NECK

In examining the head and the sensory organs contained within it, inspection is the principal process employed. Palpation is used to some extent and auscultation to a very limited degree.

Examination of the Head

HEAD SIZE.   The head is inspected for its size and shape. A grossly small head is called *microcephaly* and is always associated with mental retardation. Enlargement of the head may occur for one of several common reasons. In infancy, when the fontanelles are open and increased intracranial pressure allows separation of the bony components of the calvarium, an enlarged head may be due to

hydrocephalus secondary to stenosis of the aqueduct or to overproduction of cerebrospinal fluid. Enlargement of the head in adult life is less common but may be seen in overproduction of growth hormone, an entity known as *acromegaly*. This disease is associated with broadening of the nose and marked enlargement of the jaw, the hands, and the feet. Enlargement of the frontal part of the skull may also be seen in *Paget's disease* of the bone. This is associated with bowing of the legs and other skeletal deformities.

HAIR AND SCALP.   The hair and scalp should be examined routinely. The most common abnormality to be encountered is *seborrhea*, commonly known as dandruff. Baldness is common in men, rare in women. It is almost universally congenital, even when occurring at a young age. A history of male baldness on either side of the family predisposes any young person to early loss of hair. Interestingly, baldness is frequently associated with excessive body hair.

Any serious illness, especially one associated with protein loss and negative nitrogen balance, may be associated with transient hair loss (*alopecia*). It should be understood that a certain percentage of the hairs of the head are lost from their follicles daily. In the event that protein building is interrupted, sustained growth of the hair is aborted, and more vulnerable hairs are lost at an earlier stage of their growth. These may then fall out prematurely. The process is restored to normal once protein again becomes available for tissue synthesis.

One of the more common causes of hair loss that is seen today is that induced by antineoplastic and chemotherapeutic drugs. The treatment of cancer and the leukemias is almost invariably associated with alopecia.

This is in keeping with the effect of the drugs on any tissue in which high protein turnover is requisite to function.

FACE. A great deal can be learned by inspection of the face. The diseases that present with characteristic facial alteration are legion. This accounts for the common capacity of trained health professionals to recognize diseases in the public at large. A partial list of disease entities associated with stereotypical facial change includes myxedema, thyrotoxicosis, acromegaly, scleroderma, discoid lupus erythematosus, Cushing's disease, carcinoid syndrome, and mongolism.

A number of alterations in body chemistry are easily, and most observably, reflected in the face and its contiguous mucous membranes. These include jaundice, cyanosis, and pallor due to anemia. It should be noted that cyanosis and pallor are mutually incompatible. Since detectable cyanosis in mucous membranes requires 5 gm. of unoxygenated hemoglobin, persons who are substantially anemic (possession of fewer than 10 gm. of hemoglobin per 100 ml. of blood) cannot appear cyanotic except in extreme oxygen deprivation. On the other hand, persons who are polycythemic easily display cyanosis.

SOFT TISSUE. Auscultation of the head and palpation of soft tissue around the head are occasionally useful. Cerebrovascular accidents may result from arteriovenous malformations within the skull; more frequently they result from stenotic lesions of the cerebral vasculature. Murmurs may be produced in the skull in either circumstance. Frequently these are easily heard, and auscultation of the skull should be a part of the examination of any person who presents with hemiparesis or with the meningismus and headache associated with intracerebral bleeding.

Soft tissue of the face takes on a characteristic consistency in persons who have Cushing's disease and in those who have myxedema. This is reflected in a palpable thickness of the cheeks and jowls.

Examination of the Neck

The neck is examined by inspection, palpation, and auscultation. It should first be observed for any obvious masses or asymmetry.

LYMPH NODES. The neck should be palpated for the presence or absence of abnormal lymphadenopathy. This is done in a systematic manner beginning with the occiput, proceeding to the posterior triangle of the neck (posterior to the sternocleidomastoid muscle), then to the anterior triangle of the neck (forward of the sternocleidomastoid muscle), and concluding in the supraclavicular area. Lymph nodes should be noted for their location, size, consistency, mobility, and the presence or absence of tenderness. Inflamed nodes may be moderately enlarged and are commonly tender but usually movable. The nodes of tuberculosis may become fixed to deep structures or to the skin. The nodes of malignancy are often quite hard, tend to coalesce or "mat," and are frequently fixed to subcutaneous tissue.

TRACHEA. The position and mobility of the trachea is noted. The trachea should be in the midline as it enters the thoracic inlet behind the sternum. Deviation of the trachea may result from pressure of a mediastinal mass or from major pathology within the thorax affecting the lung. A large pneumothorax or pleural effusion will deviate the trachea to the contralateral side. Substantial atelectasis of the lung will draw the trachea toward the side of the lesion. Mediastinal inflammation and aneurysm formation may fix the trachea to cardiovascular structures so that it tugs with each cardiac contraction.

THYROID. The thyroid gland should be palpated routinely (Fig. 5-3). The isthmus of the thyroid may be located within a centimeter of the cricoid cartilage. The two lobes are then found on either side of the trachea extending under the sternocleidomastoid muscle. The thyroid is most effectively palpated from the rear with both hands circumscribing the patient's neck. The patient's head is turned gently to the left as the fingers explore the extent of the thyroid beneath the left sternocleidomastoid muscle, then turned gently to the right as the process is repeated on the opposite side. The thyroid is noted for enlargement, symmetry, and consistency, if enlarged. The gland of thyrotoxicosis due to diffuse hyperplasia is quite soft. Malignancy within the gland is perceived as hard nodularity. All nodules of the

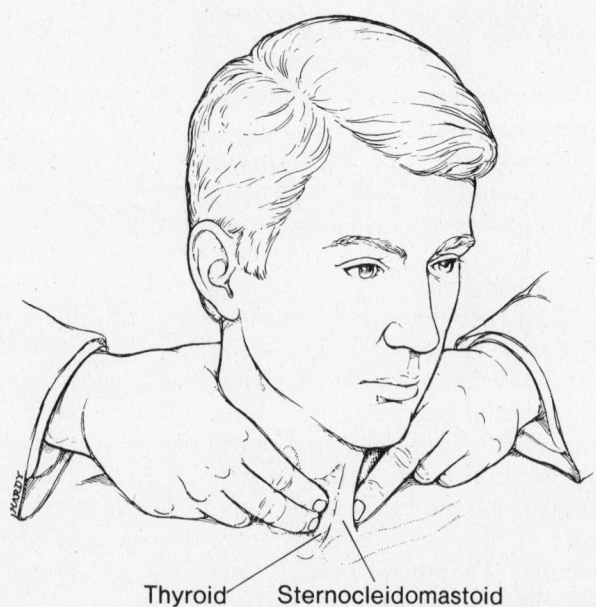

Thyroid   Sternocleidomastoid

Figure 5-3. Technique for palpation of the thyroid gland. The isthmus of the thyroid may be felt in the midline approximately 1 cm. below the cricoid cartilage. The gland is felt laterally beneath the tendinous insertion of the sternocleidomastoid muscle.

thyroid are not malignant, however, but should be noted since they must be evaluated by the physician.

VEINS. A discussion of the veins of the neck is included under the consideration of the cardiovascular system. The veins are normally visible, though not pulsatile, while the patient is lying down. They should collapse at about 30 degrees of elevation. Persistence of distended neck veins as the patient sits implies an increase in central venous pressure or obstruction to superior vena caval emptying into the right atrium. Carotid pulsation may be readily apparent in the neck, especially in disease states associated with high cardiac output. Occasionally, superficial neck veins may be seen, and the neck may be observed to pulsate with each systole. There may well be some doubt about whether the pulsations are venous (a- or v-waves associated with cardiac insufficiency) or arterial and quite innocent. Simple compression of the vein as it emerges from behind the clavicle should resolve the dilemma. If the pulsations disappear upon finger pressure, they must be assumed to be venous. If they do not, they are probably arterial.

ARTERIES. The stethoscope is placed over the carotid arteries in the examination of every patient, especially those over 40. Systolic murmurs may reflect narrowing of the carotid arteries or may be transmitted into the carotid arteries by a stenotic aortic valve. A hum or continuous murmur of torrential blood flow may be heard over the enlarged thyroid gland in active thyrotoxicosis.

Examination of the Eye

Examination of the eye is an exceedingly critical facet of the physical examination, not only because of the importance of the function of the eye to the well-being of the patient, but also because the eye is reflective of many facets of the general state of health. The retina, which may be viewed with the ophthalmoscope, is the only site in the human body where a vascular bed may be examined directly. Diseases such as hypertension and diabetes, both exceedingly common in the population, produce changes that are readily observable. The pupil may be said to be a window to the human microcirculation.

VISUAL ACUITY. Visual acuity may easily be tested in any physician's office and may be assessed by the nurse. Formal testing of visual acuity should be a part of the data base of every patient.

Testing of visual acuity is accomplished by means of an eye chart placed 6 meters (20 feet) from the patient. If space is lacking, an inverted eye chart may be placed directly behind the patient's head, and a mirror placed 3 meters (10 feet) from the patient. The patient is instructed to cover one eye with a card, to keep both eyes open, and to read each line of the chart until he is no longer able to distinguish the details for a given size of print. If the patient wears glasses, his acuity should be assessed with and without corrective lenses.

Illiteracy may be circumvented by the use of charts that display the letter "E" in four different positions. This enables one to assess the vision of children as young as 5 years of age.

Visual acuity is expressed in a ratio that relates what the patient *should* see at 20 feet to what the patient *can* see at 20 feet. Acuity of 20/50 means that the patient can see at 20 feet what he should see at 50 feet; 20/200, the boundary of legal blindness, indicates that the patient can see at 20 feet what he should be able to see at 200 feet. Such patients can only discern with accuracy the large letter at the top of the chart. The patient whose visual acuity is less than 20/20 when corrected by his or her own glasses should be referred to an ophthalmologist.

Near vision is not usually tested in routine office practice. Patients who have complaints of difficulty reading at close range should be referred to an ophthalmologist. This is common after the age of 40 when the lens may become rigid and incapable of accommodating its shape to close-range vision. This condition is known as *presbyopia*. For such patients bifocals are available to help correct close- and far-range vision through separate lenses contained within one pair of glasses.

EXTERNAL EVALUATION OF THE EYE. The eye is protected by a layer of epithelium that runs continuously from the palpebral junction behind the lids and is then reflected over the anterior surface of the globe, stopping at the cornea. The junction of the conjunctiva and the cornea is called the *limbus*.

Examination of the conjunctiva may reveal plethora or hyperemia of the circulation due to generalized hyperemia or to local inflammation or irritation. *Petechiae* caused by capillary hemorrhaging are more apparent on mucous membranes than on the skin. They often appear on the conjunctival surface of the eye. Jaundice, cyanosis, and pallor may be detected by inspecting the conjunctiva and the sclera beneath.

The cornea should be inspected for opacities and for superficial abrasions. Since the cornea is transparent, the latter may be difficult to detect even though quite extensive. Abrasions may be made more apparent by the instillation of fluorescein dye onto the corneal surface. This is not a routine procedure and should not be conducted by the nurse unless she is specially trained in this technique.

The pupils should be round, regular, equal in diameter, and equivalently reactive to light. Although a small percentage of the population may have unequal pupils that may be considered normal, the phenomenon is sufficiently unusual that it should lead to thorough examination in order to ascertain that the inequality is not due to central nervous system disease. When confronted with light, the normal pupil promptly constricts in a regular concentric fashion. The unstimulated opposite pupil will constrict as well. Constriction of the stimulated pupil is called the *direct light reflex,* whereas constriction of the opposite pupil is termed *consensual light reflex*. Exploration of this phenomenon will allow one to separate damage to the optic nerve from blindness due to more central disease. Direct light stimulation of the nerve-damaged eye will result in neither a direct nor a consensual light reflex. Stimulation of the uninvolved eye will, however, result in consensual constriction of the pupil of the damaged eye, since the consensual reflex is not dependent upon transmission through the optic nerve. Rather, it is a ganglion function of the autonomic nervous system. The pupil that is capable of constricting in response to the light is also capable of constricting in response to accommodation. If the patient is asked to focus upon a finger or other object held 30–45 cm. (12 to 18 inches) from the eye and then abruptly focus on a distant wall, the pupil will be seen to change in size as a function of the change in accommodation. Autonomic disease due to central nervous system syphilis or to diabetes may result in a pupil that is incapable of responding to light but retains its capacity to respond to accommodation. Such a pupil is known as an *Argyll Robertson pupil*.

The iris may be inspected for the presence of *synechiae,* white ridges of scar tissue around its rim, that are remnants of old, healed iritis.

OCULAR TENSION. An increase in intraocular tension is the cardinal manifestation of glaucoma, a disease responsible for more than one fifth of the blindness seen in the United States. Experienced observers are capable of assessing ocular tension by applying finger pressure over the sclera of the closed eye, but this method is highly inaccurate and should not be relied upon. Rather, skill in the use of the tonometer should be attained and employed as part of the examination for routine health maintenance. The tonometer is an instrument that allows the pressure of ocular fluid behind the cornea to be balanced by a sequence of small weights until the resultant forces are equal. At this point a needle in the instrument swings freely to indicate that balance has been attained. The cornea is anesthetized with a Pontocaine derivative. The palpebral fissure is held open with the thumb and forefinger while the tonometer is placed directly on the corneal surface (Fig. 51-10). No risk of injury to the cornea exists when the procedure is done gently and by experienced hands.

ASSESSMENT OF EXTRAOCULAR MUSCLES. Synergistic action of six small muscles attached to each eye, enervated by three of the cranial nerves, results in parallel gaze. Although the mechanism by which this takes place is highly complex, and analysis of abnormality requires the physician, assessment can be done by the nurse. Deviation of either eye to the temporal side of the head is called an *exotropia;* deviation to the nasal side is called *esotropia*. These conditions are known respectively to the lay public

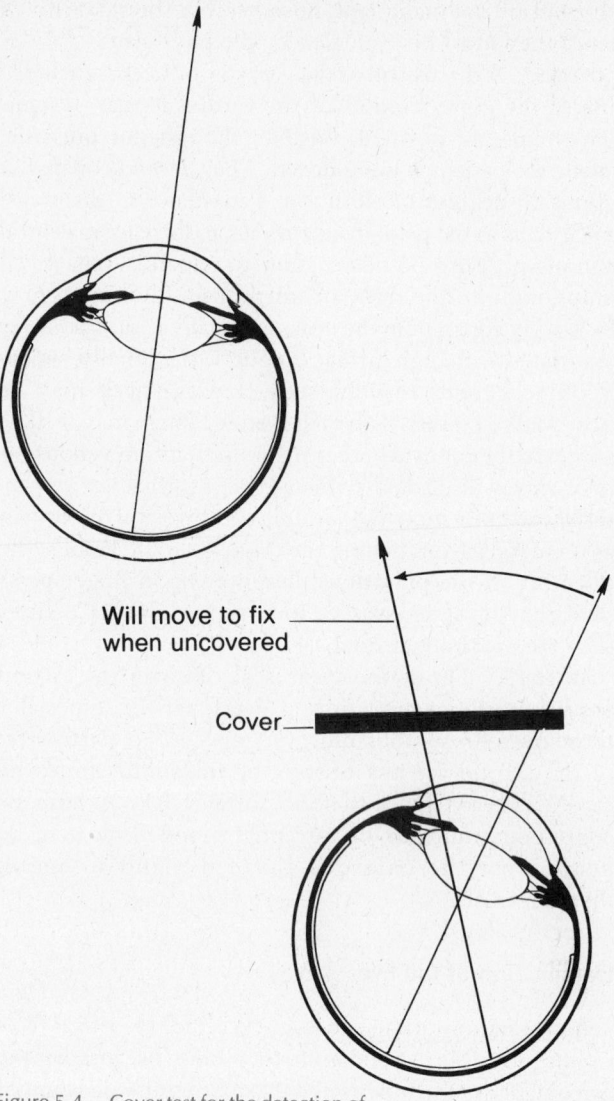

Will move to fix when uncovered

Cover

Figure 5-4. Cover test for the detection of esophoria.

as "wall-eye" and "cross-eye." The muscles of the eye are able to compensate involuntarily for up to 15 degrees of malalignment of the two eyes. This is not accomplished without effort, however, and persons with 10 to 15 degrees of malalignment may suffer headache when reading extensively and may note double vision when tired or inebriated.

Parallel alignment of the eyes may be easily detected by shining a light directly into the face while the patient is staring at the light source. The light should be reflected from the pupils of both eyes identically. Central positioning of the light reflex from one pupil associated with asymmetry in the other indicates disturbance in parallax vision. In spite of normal alignment of both eyes when they function together, the tendency of either eye to drift to the nasal or temporal side (and the necessity to involuntarily compensate for this with effort) may be assessed by the *cover test* (Fig. 5-4). One eye is covered by a card or by the hand of the examiner, and the patient is asked to focus the free eye on a stationary object. He is instructed to keep the covered eye open. The card or hand is abruptly removed from the covered eye, and it is this eye to which the examiner devotes his attention. If the eye, when uncovered, has drifted to the temporal side, it will snap back into alignment when the cover is removed. Conversely, if it has drifted to the nasal side, the reverse phenomenon will occur. The tendency of an eye to drift, when covered, to the temporal side is called an *exophoria;* a tendency of an eye to drift to the nasal side is called an *esophoria* (Fig. 5-4).

Integrity of the nervous control of the muscles of the eye may be assessed by directing the patient to move his eyes in the six cardinal positions of gaze (Fig. 5-5) while following an object. The object should be moved laterally to either side along the horizontal axis and then along two oblique axes, each of which makes a 60-degree angle with the horizontal. Each of the cardinal positions of gaze represents the function of one of the six extraocular muscles attached to each eye. If *diplopia,* or double vision, develops during the transition to any one of the cardinal positions of gaze, the examiner has an indication that one or more of the extraocular muscles are failing to function properly.

When extraocular movements are checked, the eye should be observed for *nystagmus*. Nystagmus is an irregular jerking movement of the eyes in the process of transferring gaze to a lateral position. Nystagmus has two components: a quick component in one or the other direction, and a slower subsequent component that brings the eye back to the intended position. A number of conditions cause nystagmus, many of which are benign, whereas others may reflect severe pathology.

ASSESSMENT OF FIELD OF VISION. Although the visual field may be assessed with a high degree of precision by an ophthalmologist, it may be readily assessed in the office or at the bedside of the patient, when the examiner is concerned with gross disturbance of the visual field. Such a circumstance may arise, for example, in assessing the patient with a cerebrovascular accident. Such patients commonly lose one quarter or one half of the visual fields of both eyes. While focusing on an object held directly in front of the eye, the patient should be able to perceive a second object within 60 degrees to the nasal side, 90 degrees to the temporal side, 50 degrees superiorly, and 70 degrees inferiorly to the line of vision. A simple and reliable method of testing the fullness of the visual field is to have both the examiner and the patient focus on an object held midway between them on a direct line as each stares toward the other's eye. The examiner may then take another object (or a finger) and move it along a plane halfway between the examiner and the patient. It should appear in the patient's field of vision at the same time as it appears in the examiner's field of vision. Lack of perception within one half of the visual field, common in stroke, is called *hemianopia*.

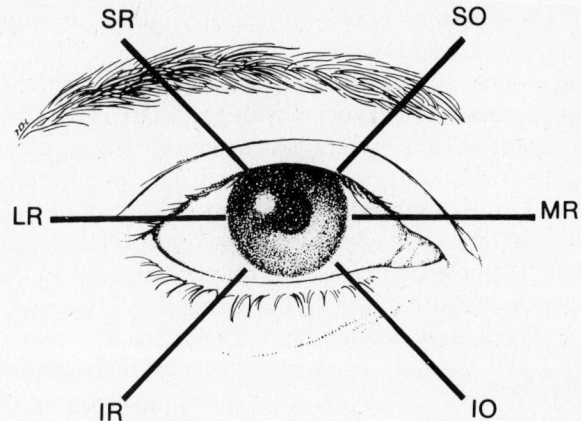

Figure 5-5. Cardinal positions of gaze.

OPHTHALMOSCOPY. The nurse can easily become proficient in the use of the ophthalmoscope. The ophthalmoscope is an instrument that projects light through a prism and bends the light at 90 degrees, allowing the observer to view the retina through a lens in such a way that the line of vision is parallel to the bent ray of light (Fig. 5-6). A number of lenses are available and are arranged on a wheel so that they may be chosen by rotating the wheel with the index finger without interrupting the inspection. The standard ophthalmoscope contains an array of gadgetry that includes grids, slits, filters, and the like—none of which are particularly use-

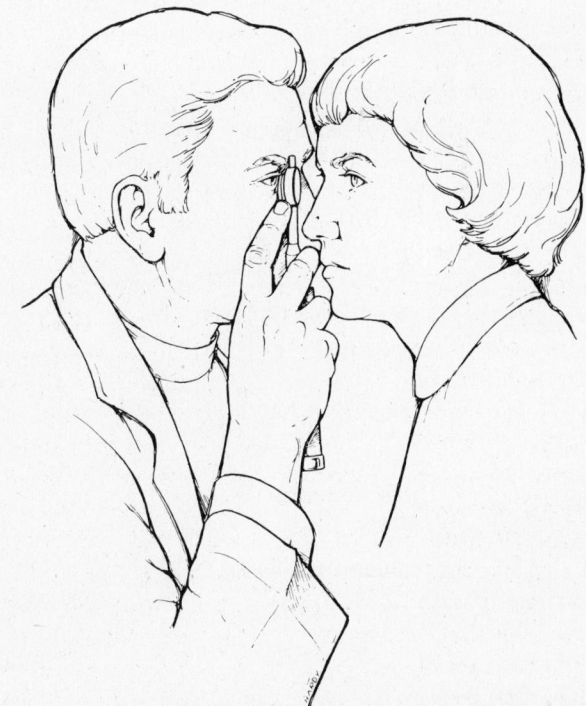

Figure 5-6. Technique for the proper use of the ophthalmoscope. The right eye of the examiner looks into the patient's right eye. The index finger is used to adjust the lens for proper focus.

ful. The small unfiltered aperture is appropriate and most useful for standard ophthalmoscopy.

In order to avoid a confrontation of noses, the right eye of the patient is examined with the right eye of the examiner, the left eye of the patient with the left eye of the examiner. The room is darkened so that the pupil will be dilated. Alternatively, dilatation can be accomplished with a drop of phenylephrine (Neo-Synephrine) in patients in whom there is no suspicion of glaucoma. The patient is instructed to hold the eyes still and focus on a real or imaginary distant object. The ophthalmoscope is gripped firmly in the hand, with the index finger resting on the lens wheel. The head of the ophthalmoscope is braced within the angle made by the brow and the nose. The lens chosen for initial inspection should be the one labeled zero unless the examiner is knowingly correcting his or her own defect in visual acuity. If the examiner wears glasses, it is better to remove the glasses and become familiar with which lens is analogous to zero for the examiner with 20/20 vision. Provided the patient has 20/20 vision, the zero lens should enable the examiner to obtain a precise focus on the retina. If the retina is out of focus, the lens wheel is rotated until it is brought into focus. The choice of a lens labeled with a red numeral implies that one is focusing further away than normal; the choice of a lens labeled with a black numeral implies that one is focusing nearer to the examiner. The examiner will choose lenses among the red series for patients who are *hyperopic,* and lenses in the black series for patients who are *myopic*.

With the room in darkness, the patient appropriately gazing into the distance, and the ophthalmoscope appropriately positioned within the cradle of the brow and nose, the examiner may now approach the patient. He stands within 0.7 meters (2 feet) of the patient and focuses the light directly on the pupil. If this has been done appropriately, the pupil will glow red. This is known as the *red reflex*. The examiner should then approach the patient until their foreheads touch. At this point, provided the proper lens has been selected, the retina should be in focus, and the venules and arterioles that course through the retina are readily apparent (Fig. 5-7). In scanning the surface of the retina it is important that the examiner hold the scope firmly and move his head rather than the instrument. Proficiency in the use of the ophthalmoscope can be readily attained with a little practice.

The examiner should first focus on the optic disc. In the event that the disc is not in view when the retina is first visualized, the veins that are within the field of vision should be followed down their tributaries toward the disc from which the arterioles emerge and the venules enter. This is analogous to following the limbs of a tree until one sees the trunk. The optic disc is examined for size, shape, color, and the sharpness of its margin. The disc is circular and pearly white in color. The margin is sharp and occasionally surrounded by a rim of dark pigment. One must become familiar with what is regarded as a normal size. In the center of the disc there is frequently a small physiologic cup into which the central

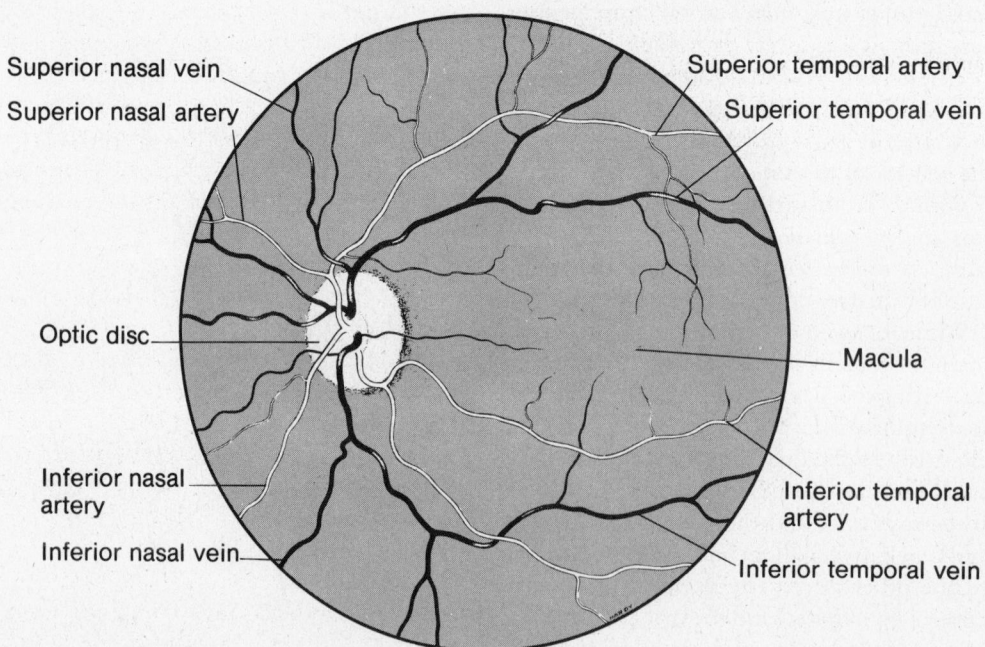

Superior nasal vein

Superior nasal artery

Optic disc

Inferior nasal artery

Inferior nasal vein

Superior temporal artery

Superior temporal vein

Macula

Inferior temporal artery

Inferior temporal vein

Figure 5-7. Display of the retina as seen through the ophthalmoscope. The ophthalmoscope is capable of visualizing only a portion of the retina at any one time. It is best to identify the disc, ascertain the sharpness of disc margins, and then follow each of the vessels that emerge from the disc at least three disc diameters along their course. The macular area should then be identified for any lesion that may be present.

vein of the retina recedes. To accurately focus on the base of this cup one may have to choose another lens in the direction of the red sequence. A deep cup is seen in glaucoma. Edema of the optic disc with concomitant blurring of the disc margin is seen with increases in cerebrospinal fluid pressure. The disc becomes pink, and accurate focus may require shifting to a lens in the direction of the black sequence. This is termed *papilledema*. *Optic atrophy* is characterized by extreme pallor of the disc and reduction of its size.

The remainder of the retina is now examined. Abnormalities may be precisely located for other observers by using a standard nomenclature that makes reference to an imaginary clock face, and by referring to the diameter of the disc to delineate distance. Thus a hemorrhage may be noted to be one half of the disc diameter in size, located two disc diameters away from the disc margin at two o'clock. Any observer should be able to replicate this finding.

The examiner should now follow each of the major vessels from the margin of the disc. The arterioles are lighter in color and narrower than the venules. Under normal circumstances the vein is 30 to 50 percent broader than the artery. It should be understood that the walls of the vessels are essentially transparent and that what is being observed is the blood column itself. Thus, the color difference should be readily understood, since oxygen has been removed at the level of the capillary bed.

The venules may be dilated in a number of clinical circumstances. These include conditions which increase cerebrospinal fluid pressure, with consequent compression of the central retinal vein as it runs through the optic nerve, and conditions which increase the viscosity of blood, interfering with flow. Prominent among the latter are polycythemia and sickle cell disease.

The arterioles are narrowed in hypertension. Moreover, they indent the vein at points of crossing—a phenomenon known as *nicking*. It may seem paradoxical that although the arteriole appears narrower in hypertension, it impresses upon the vein in a manner that impedes venous blood flow. It should be remembered, however, that one is examining only the blood column and that the wall of the artery in hypertension is, in fact, thicker than normal so that the external diameter of the vessel, invisible to the eye, is wider than usual. Another phenomenon associated with hypertension is a widening of the normal *light reflex,* the narrow linear streak of light that reflects from the surface of the arteriole.

Advanced hypertension is associated with hemorrhages and exudates. Hemorrhaging within the retina may be superficial or deep. Superficial hemorrhages will obscure the vessels that lie beneath them, whereas deep hemorrhages will appear much darker and do not interfere with the capacity to observe the vessels that course through the substance of the retina. This distinction is important since there are different implications for hemorrhages depending upon their location.

Exudates are of two classes, commonly referred to as *soft* and *hard*. Soft exudates result from microinfarcts of the retina. They are fluffy, appear quickly, and may totally resolve in a matter of weeks. Hard exudates result from venous stasis. They are sharply delineated, usually quite small, and, once formed, remain as permanent abnormalities within the retinal substance.

Severe sustained hypertension may be associated with an increase in cerebrospinal fluid pressure and may be accompanied by papilledema.

The changes of hypertension may be graded in severity. Grade I changes include simple narrowing, increased tortuosity of the arterioles, and an increase in the arteriolar light reflex. Grade II changes are similar, with the addition of arteriovenous nicking. Grade III changes include the presence of hemorrhages and exudates. Grade IV hypertensive retinopathy is accompanied by papilledema.

The changes associated with diabetes are quite distinctive and include such phenomena as the development of capillary microaneurysms and the formation of arteriovenous malformations near the disc. This latter phenomenon is called *neovascularization*. For a proper appreciation of these changes, audiovisual presentations of retinal photographs should be consulted. They are readily available in most libraries.

Although all of the techniques which have been discussed for the examination of the eye will not be performed on every patient, they are all quite simple and may be readily mastered by the nurse examiner. Routinely one should inspect the conjunctiva, the cornea, and the pupil and assess extraocular motion. Ophthalmoscopic examination should be a part of every reasonably complete physical examination. Although visual acuity should be part of the data base, it need not be assessed more often than once every year or two except in elderly individuals.

Examination of the Ear

The ear can easily be examined with an otoscope and should be checked as part of the routine physical examination.

EARDRUM. Proper inspection of the tympanic membrane requires that the ear canal be free of cerumen. If the membrane cannot be well visualized, wax may be removed with a cerumen scoop, or the ear canal may be gently irrigated with warm tap water. In the event that firmly adherent cerumen is present, a small amount of mineral oil or an analogous commercial preparation may have to be instilled within the ear canal and the patient instructed to return for subsequent removal of the wax and inspection of the ear. This should not be negated, since earwax is a common cause of hearing deficit in the population.

The tip of the otoscope is gently placed within the external auditory canal. Better visualization will be achieved if the examiner gently applies traction to the ear in a superior-posterior direction (Fig. 5-8). The tympanic membrane should then be brought into view. Since the floor of the canal is not flat but convex, the inferior border of the drum, and the anterior portion as well, may be hidden from view. This should not, however, prevent reasonable assessment of the tympanic membrane. The membrane is pearly gray and reflects light from the otoscope just inferior to its epicenter (Fig. 5-9). In middle ear infection the drum may bulge, or an air fluid level may be seen lying behind it. Abnormalities should be dealt with by the physician.

LEVEL OF HEARING. Hearing may be effectively screened by assessing the patient's capacity to interpret a whispered voice or the ticking of a watch. Hearing loss may be of one of two types. The first type is a conductive deficit due to disease of the tympanic membrane or middle ear that inhibits the transmission of sound to the inner ear where it is converted to a neural impulse. The second type of loss is a nerve deficit involving damage to the eighth cranial nerve or to its connections with the central nervous system. These may be distinguished through the use of a tuning fork specifically selected for frequencies within the conversational voice range. The best frequency to apply to an assessment of hearing is 512 cps.

When the tuning fork is made to vibrate and is placed on the vertex of the skull, it will normally be heard equally in the two ears. If there is a conductive deficit in one ear, the sound will be heard better in the deficient ear. This is because the inner ear is protected, or masked, from extraneous sound that might reach it through the normal pathway. That is, there is no competition for conducted sound. In nerve deafness, conducted sound will be appreciated only in the better ear. This phenomenon is referred to as the *Weber test*.

If the tuning fork is placed on the bony prominence of the temporal bone behind the ear in normal persons it will be heard clearly initially but will gradually die out. When the sound is no longer conducted through bone, the examiner then takes the vibrating prongs and places them 2 cm. (1 inch) from the opening of the external auditory canal. Sound will again be heard and will eventually die out. Thus, under normal circumstances, air conduction is better than bone conduction. In conductive hearing loss, however, bone conduction exceeds air conduction. That is, once bone conduction through the temporal bone has died out, the patient is unable to hear the fork through the usual conductive mechanism. In contra-

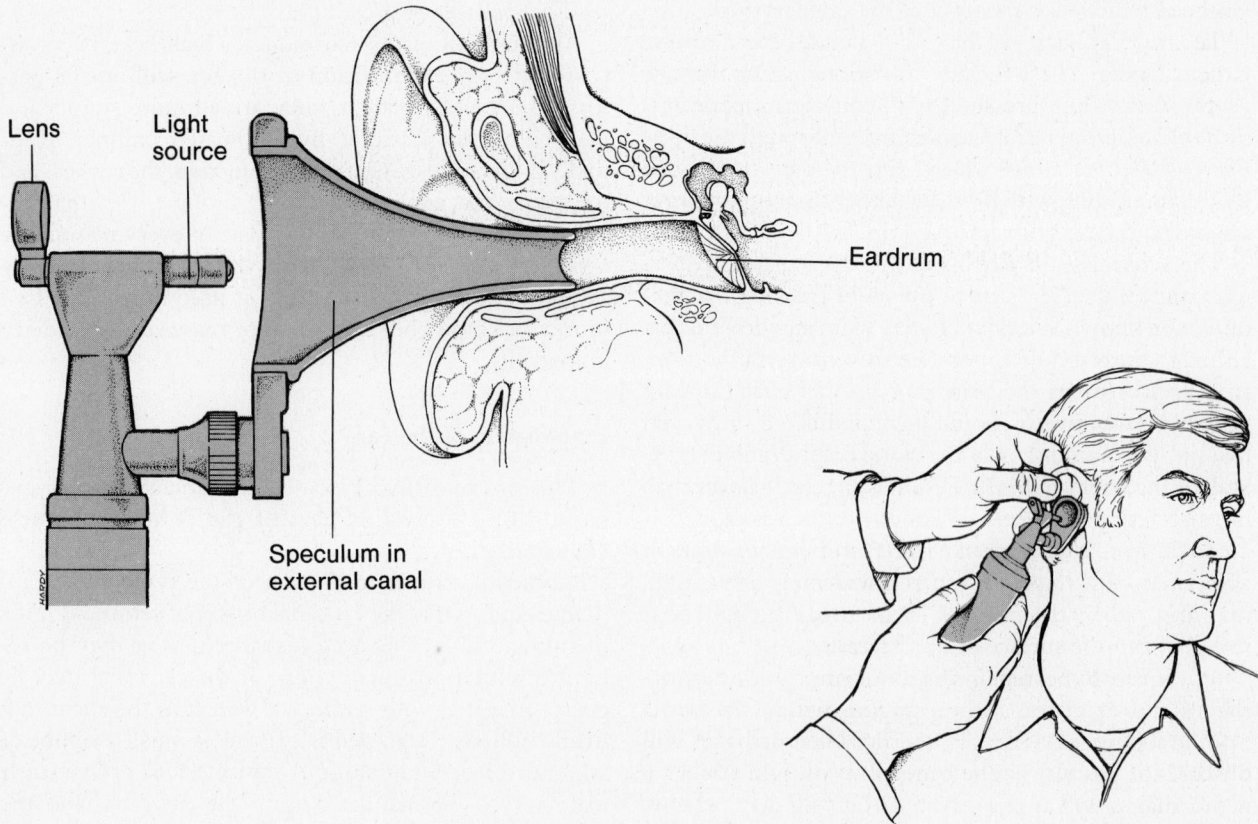

Lens

Light source

Eardrum

Speculum in external canal

Figure 5-8. Technique for using the otoscope.

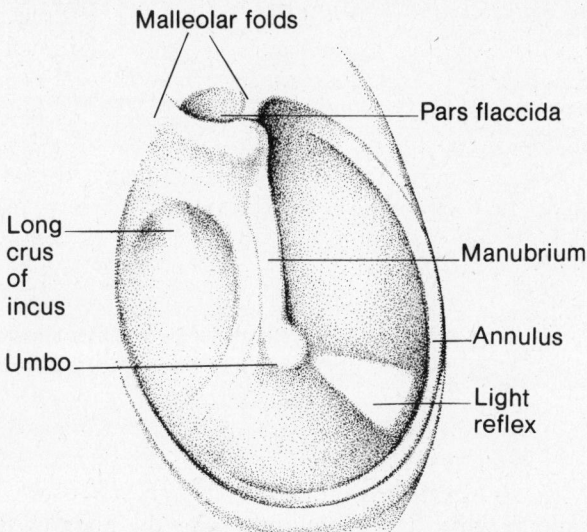

Figure 5-9. Display of the eardrum as it would be visualized through the otoscope.

distinction, nerve deafness permits sound to be conducted by air better than by bone, although both are conducted poorly, and all sound may be perceived to be distant and faint. This is known as the *Rinne test*. Use of the Weber and Rinne tests in concert enables one to distinguish conductive loss from nerve loss when hearing is impaired. These tests are not necessarily a part of the usual physical examination, but will be useful if the patient reports hearing deficit or if the examiner detects an inability of the patient to perceive such sounds as a ticking watch or a whispered voice.

Examination of the Mouth

The nursing assessment of a patient with a mouth or neck problem can be accomplished by interrogation and the use of simple equipment: a good light, 4″ x 4″ gauze squares, tongue depressor, finger cots, and a pair of sterile gloves.

At the outset, ask the patient if he has noticed any irritation or change in the mouth, throat, or voice. Inquire if he uses tobacco or smokes a pipe and how much alcohol he drinks, if any.

The mouth should be examined carefully for mucosal lesions and for adequacy of dental care. The tongue should be well papillated and the floor of the mouth and buccal mucosa free of lesions. The pharynx and the tonsillar fossae should be examined for increased vascularity and for the presence of abnormal lymph tissue. Purulent material within tonsillar crypts should be cultured, especially if the office visit is occasioned by sore throat.

Sit in front of the patient so that his mouth is below your eye level. Adjust the spotlight and the head lamp for proper lighting. Inspect the patient's mouth from front to back, using a laryngeal mirror, gloves, or finger cots if need be. The mirror shoud be dipped in warm water and then dried so as to prevent fogging.

With each thumb on the outer cheek and the two index fingers in the mouth, fold the upper lip up and out and the lower lip down so that it is possible to visually inspect both gutters along the upper and lower jaws. With the thumb on the outer cheek and the index finger at the mouth corner, push the cheek in so that the mucous membrane inside the mouth can be seen. Determine if it is moist and glistening or dry or if there is any inflammation, keratosis, or unilateral abnormality.

Ask the patient to stick out his tongue and move it up, down, and from side to side. Any limitation of movement may indicate a tumor. Wrap a piece of gauze around the tip of the tongue and then pull it gently forward and to one side. Using a tongue depressor in the other hand, push the middle of the tongue up so that a good view of the floor of the mouth is possible (Fig. 5-10A). Repeat on other side. Use care so that the sensitive lingual frenum is not injured. Inspect the posterior tongue with a mirror; also check the roof of the mouth, and the hard and soft palates. Palpate all surfaces and record any area of roughness, induration, or granularity. Examine the gums and teeth, and check the undersurface of the chin (Fig. 5-10B).

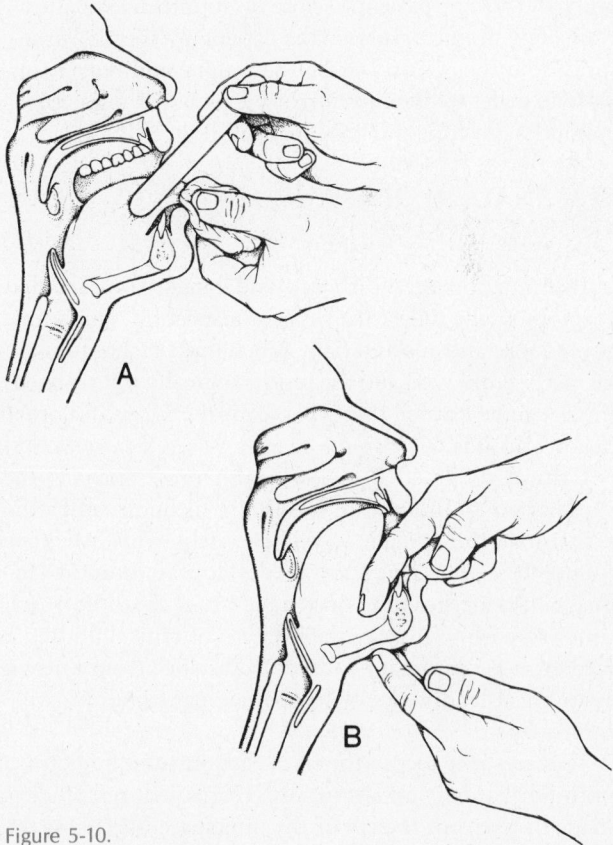

Figure 5-10.

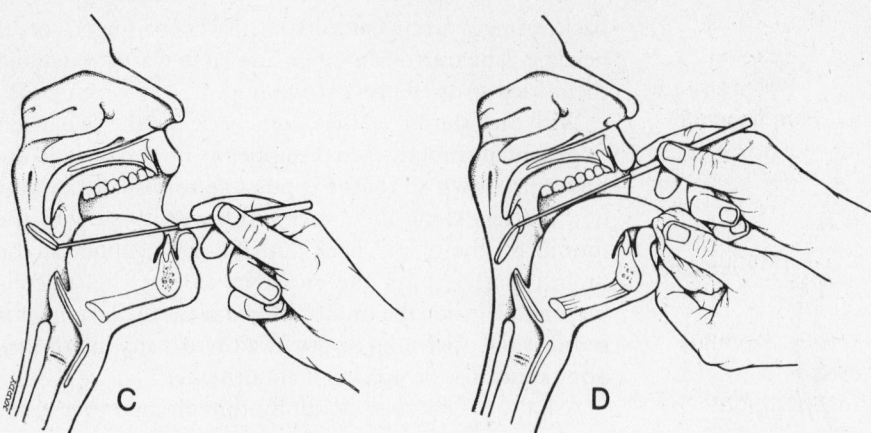

Figure 5-10—*Continued*. Nursing assessment of the patient's mouth. *A.* Observe the floor of the mouth. *B.* Examine underneath surface of chin. *C.* View the tonsillar-pharyngeal area. *D.* Inspect the larynx.

To inspect the tonsillar-pharyngeal area, have the patient relax his tongue. Place the mirror or tongue blade as far back on the tongue as possible without touching the soft palate (Fig. 5-10C); press downward. This causes a reflex retraction of the uvula and a contraction of the muscles of the oropharynx, permitting a good view of the tonsillar fossae and posterior pharyngeal wall.

LARYNX. If the patient is hoarse or gives a history of voice changes, the larynx should be carefully inspected with a laryngeal mirror. Some patients may require a nonreactive topical anesthetic spray of the oral pharynx in order to tolerate the mirror examination. Spray sparingly and ask the patient to close his mouth and swallow; wait a few minutes. Inform the patient not to spit out the spray solution. Gently grasp the tongue and pull it forward in order to obtain a mirror view of the tongue base, epiglottis, larynx, and nasopharynx (Fig. 5-10D).

EXAMINATION OF THE THORAX AND LUNGS

Examination of the thorax and lungs is an art that employs to the fullest the skills of inspection, palpation, percussion, and auscultation. When these techniques are properly employed and the results logically interrelated, much can be learned that will escape the x-ray and other diagnostic aids.

Critical to practice in the health professions is the capacity to communicate to others, through either the written or the spoken word, precisely what we have found. It is thus necessary to develop a common language. It is inefficient to draw a picture of the thorax each time we wish to display the location of critical findings. Rather, it is customary to refer to distance from known anatomical landmarks or from imaginary lines in common usage.

With respect to the thorax, location may be defined both horizontally and vertically. Horizontal reference is made in terms of the rib or the interspace overlying the examiner's findings (Fig. 5-11). On the anterior surface, identifying the specific rib is facilitated by locating the

angle at which the manubrium joins the body of the sternum in the midline. The second rib joins the sternum at this prominent landmark. Other ribs may be identified by counting down from the second rib. The interspaces are referred to in terms of the rib immediately above the interspace. Thus, the fifth intercostal space is the space below the fifth rib. It is in this interspace that the male nipple and the impulse of the heart may be seen in normal persons.

Location of ribs on the posterior surface of the thorax is more difficult. The first step is to identify the spinous process. This may be accomplished by finding the most prominent of the spinous processes, the seventh cervical vertebra (*vertebra prominens*). When the neck is slightly

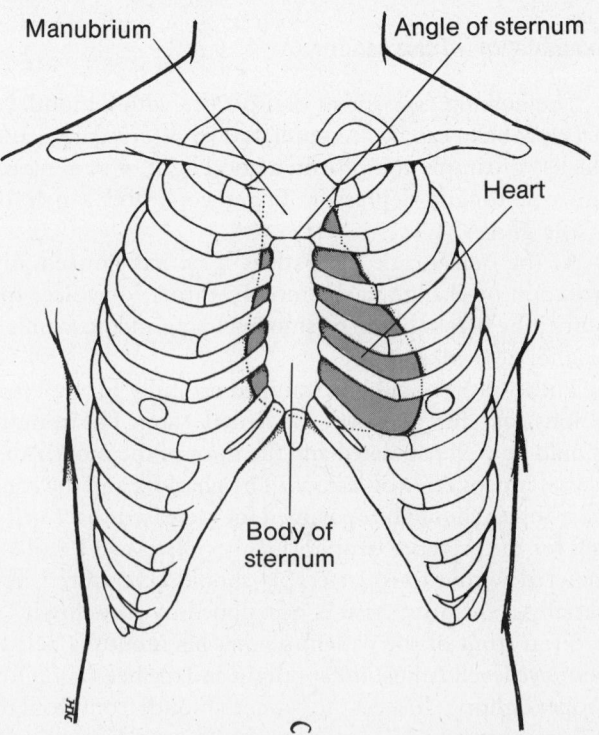

Figure 5-11. Topography of the anterior thorax.

flexed the seventh cervical spinous process stands out. Others may then be identified by counting down.

To identify thoracic findings in terms of vertical location, reference is made to several imaginary lines (Fig. 5-12). The *midsternal line* is drawn down through the center of the sternum. The *midclavicular line* is an imaginary line drawn from the middle of the clavicle. The point of maximum impulse of the heart most generally lies along this line. When the arm is abducted from the body at 90 degrees, imaginary vertical lines may be drawn from the anterior axillary fold, from the middle of the axilla, and from the posterior axillary fold. These lines are called respectively the *anterior axillary line,* the *midaxillary line,* and the *posterior axillary line*. A line drawn vertically through the superior and inferior poles of the scapula is called the *scapular line,* and a line drawn down the center of the vertebral column is called the *vertebral line*.

It should now be apparent that the examiner can easily be understood when referring to a sound heart in the sixth left intercostal space at the anterior axillary line. Similarly, one may describe an area of dullness extending from the vertebral to the scapular line between the seventh and tenth ribs on the right without equivocation or confusion.

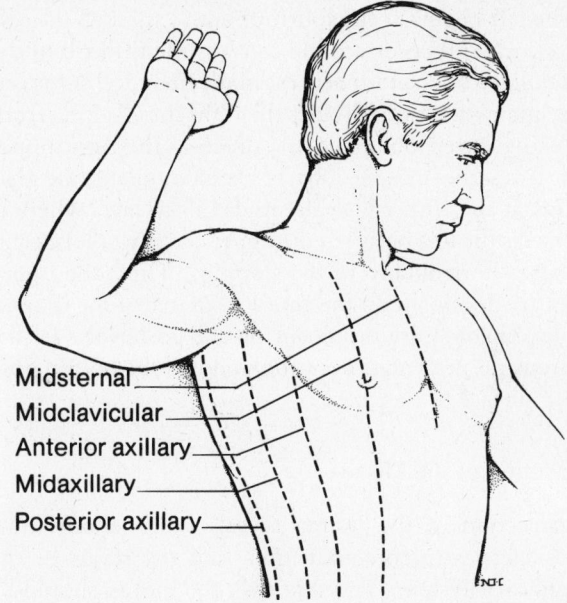

Midsternal
Midclavicular
Anterior axillary
Midaxillary
Posterior axillary

Figure 5-12. Imaginary "longitudinal lines" that permit verbal reference to the location of abnormalities over the chest wall.

Topographically, the lobes of the lung may be located on the surface of the chest wall in the following manner (Fig. 5-13). The line between the upper and lower lobes

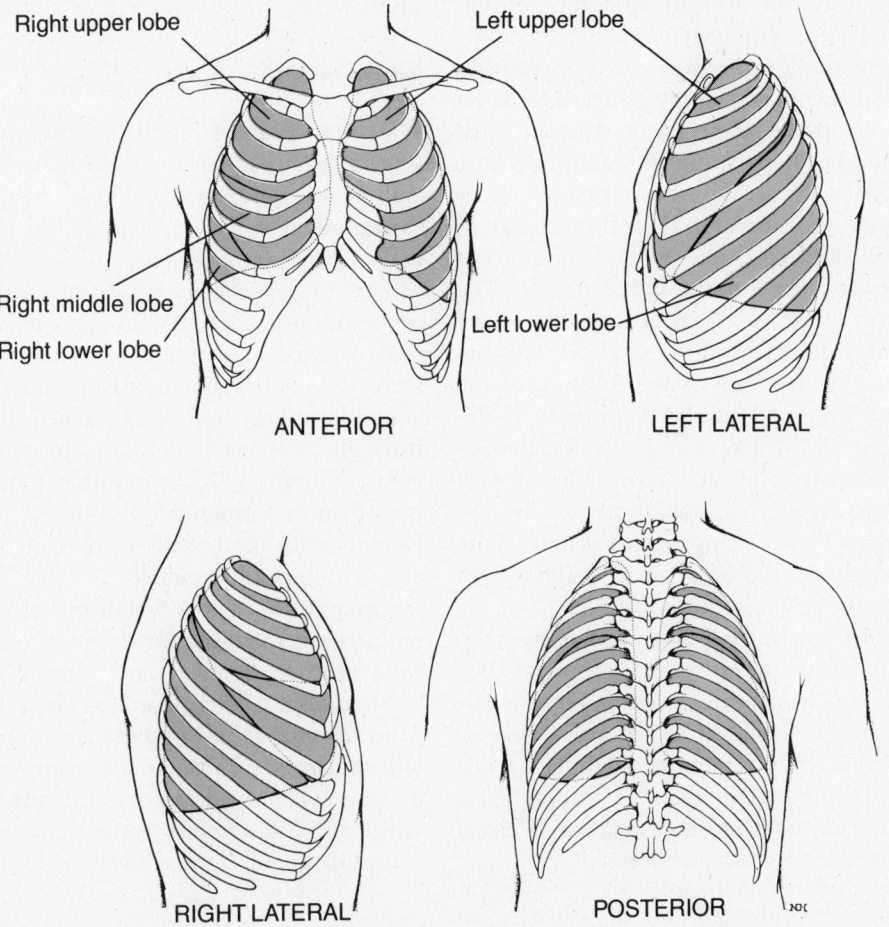

Right upper lobe

Left upper lobe

Right middle lobe

Right lower lobe

Left lower lobe

ANTERIOR

LEFT LATERAL

RIGHT LATERAL

POSTERIOR

Figure 5-13. Topographical relationship of the ribs to the lobes of the lung.

on the left begins at the fourth thoracic spinous process posteriorly, proceeds around to cross the fifth rib in the midaxillary line, and meets the sixth rib at the sternum. This line on the right divides the right middle lobe from the right lower lobe. The line dividing the right upper lobe from the middle lobe is an incomplete one that begins at the fifth rib in the midaxillary line, where it intersects the line between the upper and lower lobes and traverses horizontally to the sternum. Thus, the upper lobes are dominant on the anterior surface of the thorax; the lower lobes are dominant on the posterior surface. There is no presentation of the middle lobe on the posterior surface of the chest.

Inspection of the Thorax

Inspection of the thorax reveals much about musculoskeletal structure, nutrition, and the status of the respiratory system. The skin over the thorax should be observed for color and turgor and for evidence of loss of subcutaneous tissue. The musculature of the thorax may reflect recent weight loss. Asymmetry, if present, should be noted.

BREATHING PATTERNS. Noting the manner in which the patient breathes is of particular importance. Normally the ribs articulate with the spine at a 45-degree angle. The act of breathing elevates the ribs, thrusting the sternum forward and up. The interspaces widen, and the angle that the ribs make with the spine more nearly approaches a 60-degree angle. Patients with emphysema have excessive residual volume; that is, they cannot expel the usual volume of air from the lungs during expiration. Because of the large residual volume, the ribs make a less acute angle with the spine, and the sternum is thrust forward excessively, even during expiration. This has the effect of *increasing the anteroposterior diameter* of the thorax. The ribs are, moreover, more widely spaced, and the interspaces tend to bulge on expiration. As a result of overinflation of the lungs, not only is the capacity of the thorax to expand limited, but the diaphragm is depressed, limiting vertical filling. Consequently, the patient must bring into play accessory muscles of respiration such as the sternocleidomastoids. The appearance of the patient with emphysema is thus quite characteristic and allows the observer to diagnose the disease easily, even from a distance.

Observation of the rate and depth of respiration is also important. An increase in the rate of respiration is called *tachypnea;* an increase in depth is called *hyperpnea*. An increase in both rate and depth is referred to as *hyperventilation*. At the extreme of hyperventilation is the marked increase in rate and depth (both to their maximum) that is associated with the severe acidosis of diabetic or renal origin, and that is called *Kussmaul* respiration.

The inspiratory phase of respiration is the only one requiring energy in normal physiology. Expiration is passive. Inspiration occupies the first third of the respiratory cycle, expiration the latter two thirds. With more rapid breathing, inspiration and expiration will be more nearly equal.

In thin persons it is quite normal to note a slight retraction of the intercostal spaces during quiet breathing. Bulging during expiration implies obstruction of expiratory air flow, as in emphysema. Marked retraction of inspiration, most especially if asymmetrical, implies blockage of a branch of the respiratory tree. Asymmetrical bulging of the interspaces, on one side or the other, is created by an increase in pressure within the hemithorax. This may be a result of air trapped under pressure within the pleural cavity where it does not belong (pneumothorax), or the pressure of fluid within the pleural space (pleural effusion).

The severe pain associated with pleurisy causes intercostal muscle spasm and a "lag" in respiration on the involved side.

Certain patterns of respiration are characteristic of specific disease states. Although the nurse need not recognize the specific pattern nor be acquainted with the association of a certain pattern with a disease state, she should be able to describe abnormal patterns of rhythmicity.

Palpation of the Thorax

TACTILE FREMITUS. Sound generated by the larynx travels distally along the bronchial tree to set the chest wall in resonant motion. This is especially true of consonant sounds. The capacity to feel sound on the chest wall is called *tactile fremitus*.

There is a wide variation in normal fremitus. It is obviously influenced by the thickness of the chest wall, most especially if that thickness is muscular, although the increase in subcutaneous tissue associated with obesity has some influence. Lower pitched sounds travel better through the normal lung and incite the chest wall to greater vibration. Thus, fremitus is more pronounced in men than in women because of the deeper male voice. Patients with the hoarse voice of myxedema will have augmented tactile fremitus.

The physics of sound transmission through the lung requires explanation. Air does not conduct sound well; solid substance (tissue) does, provided that it has elasticity and is not conglomerated into a nonresonant mass. Thus, an increase in solid tissue per unit volume of lung will enhance fremitus. An increase in air per unit volume of lung will impede sound. Patients with emphysema will exhibit almost no tactile fremitus. A patient with consolidation of a lobe of the lung due to pneumonia will have an increase in tactile fremitus over the distribution of the projection of that lobe on the surface of the chest wall. Air in the pleural space will not conduct sound. Compression of the lung by an external mass, or force, results in an increase in solid lung tissue per unit volume as air is forced out of the lung. The result will be a segmental increase in tactile fremitus. Such a circumstance is called *compression atelectasis*. Obstruction of a bronchus also results in atelectasis as air trapped in the obstructed portion of the lung is gradually resorbed. This is called *obstructive atelectasis*. Obstructive atelectasis, in contradistinction to compression atelectasis, will not transmit sound since the bronchus through which the sound must travel is blocked. Fluid within the pleural cavity represents too large a mass to respond to transmitted sound and will not vibrate. Thus, the chest wall over a pleural effusion displays no tactile fremitus. Occasionally a *pleural friction rub,* the sound created by the rubbing together of the two pleural surfaces when they are diseased, can be felt during respiration.

PROCEDURE. Palpation of the chest wall may be done either with the tips of the fingers or with the forward part of the palm (Fig. 5-14). Touch should be applied lightly. The patient is instructed to speak in a clear voice some phrase dominated by consonants. Traditionally the phrase used is "ninety-nine." The patient repeats this as the examiner palpates over the surface of the thorax.

POSITION OF TRACHEA. A critical item of palpation with respect to the thorax is the position of the trachea. Although more appropriately felt when examining the neck, it is discussed here because of its importance in diagnosing chest disease. A large pleural effusion or a pneumothorax under tension will displace the trachea to the *contralateral* side (side opposite to the lesion). Obstruction of a bronchus with resorption of air from the affected lung tissue will displace the trachea to the *ipsilateral* side (side of involvement). Deviation of the trachea may best be appreciated in the suprasternal notch between the heads of the sternocleidomastoid muscles.

Percussion of the Thorax

Percussion of the thorax can be highly informative. It gives the examiner the opportunity to determine the location and size of the heart within the thorax, to ascertain the magnitude of descent of the diaphragm during maximum inspiration, and to detect a spectrum of disease processes within the thorax.

SIZE OF THE HEART. For the sake of efficiency the border of the heart is percussed at the same time that the examiner percusses the thorax over the lung for the assessment of pulmonary pathology. Only the left border of the heart may be located this way in normal man. It extends to the midclavicular line in the fifth intercostal space. The right border lies under the right margin of the sternum, but the sternum is a sounding board and does not permit

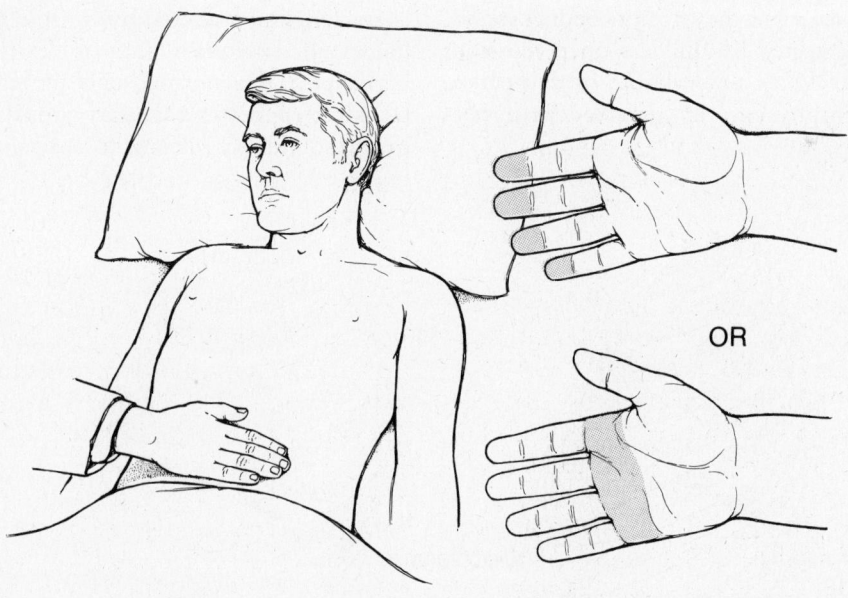

OR

Figure 5-14.   The technique of palpation. The most sensitive area of the hand for an individual might be either the fingertips or the palmar surface over the heads of the metacarpal bones. The sensitive area of the hand may be used to detect fremitus, thrills, or temperature differences over the surface of the body.

definition of the border. Enlargement of the heart to either the left or right may easily be noted. In many persons who have very thick chests, or are obese, or have emphysema, the heart may lie sufficiently far beneath the thoracic surface that not even its left border can be noted unless the heart is enlarged.

POSITION OF THE DIAPHRAGM. The normal resonance of the lung stops at the diaphragm, where it becomes dull. Quite obviously the position of the diaphragm will be different during inspiration than it is during expiration. It is convenient to have the patient take a deep inspiration and hold it while the maximum descent of the diaphragm is determined, usually along the scapular lines bilaterally. The patient is then instructed to expire fully and hold it while the diaphragmatic level is again assessed (Fig. 5-15).

Maximum excursion of the diaphragm may amount to as much as 8 or 10 cm. (3 or 4 inches) in healthy tall young adult males. For most persons it is usually 5 to 7 cm. (2 to 2¾ inches). Less than 4 cm. (1½ inches) of excursion of the diaphragm is abnormal. The diaphragm will be seen to be 2 cm. (¾ inch) or so higher on the right than on the left. This is because of the spatial relationships of the heart and the liver above and below the left and right segments of the diaphragm respectively.

INDICATION OF DISEASE. Dullness over the lung is a function of increased density of the lung, and will be seen in those circumstances that lead to an increased transmission of sound, i.e., consolidation and compression atelectasis. On the other hand, pleural effusion and obstructive atelectasis, while they do not conduct sound, are, nevertheless, detected by dullness on percussion. Pneumothorax produces a tympanic, or drumlike, sound, whereas emphysema is perceived as hyperresonant.

Auscultation of the Thorax

Auscultation is useful in assessing the sound of breathing through the bronchial tree and in evaluating the quality of the *spoken voice*.

BREATH SOUNDS. The sound of normal breathing that is detected on the chest wall is generated by the rate at which air flows through the higher passages of the bronchial tree. Since inspiration is shorter than expiration, it is logical that air flows at a higher rate of speed during inspiration. Thus it should not be surprising that inspiratory sound is louder than expiratory sound. Indeed, the sound generated during expiration occurs only during the first few seconds of the expiratory phase, if at all. Duration of inspiratory sound exceeds that of expiration by a ratio of approximately 2 to 1, a reversal of the actual time spent in expiration versus inspiration. The interval between the end of expiratory sound and the beginning of inspiration is usually silent.

The normal breath sounds described above represent *vesicular breathing*. It is heard throughout the lung except directly over the major bronchi where expiratory sound is as prominent as inspiratory sound, although of higher pitch (Fig. 5-16). Breath sounds heard over the major bronchi are referred to as *bronchial* or *bronchovesicular* sounds.

The sound generated by breathing, like tactile fremitus, is greater when transmitted through lung tissue where there is an increase in the amount of solid tissue per unit volume of lung. The quality of the sound is quite characteristically altered by consolidation. The sound is louder; the expiratory phase is clearly heard, and it is of higher pitch than normal, since the higher frequencies are transmitted better through consolidated lung. Such breath sounds are referred to as *tubular breathing,* or *bron-*

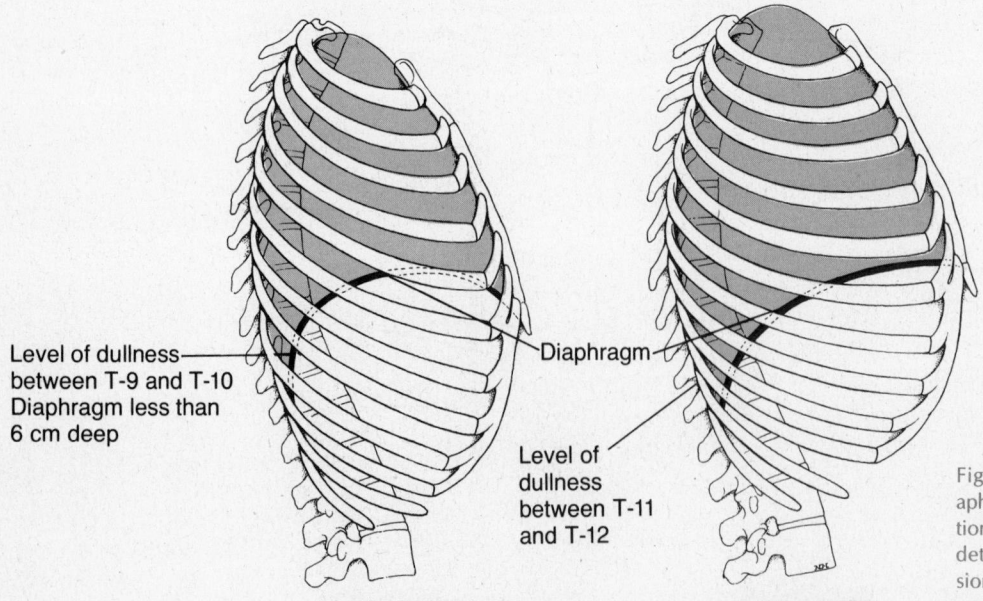

Level of dullness between T-9 and T-10 Diaphragm less than 6 cm deep

Diaphragm

Level of dullness between T-11 and T-12

EXPIRATION

INSPIRATION

Figure 5-15. Position of the diaphragm on inspiration and expiration. Movement of the diaphragm is detectable by percussion. Excursion in the normal person should amount to 5-8 cm.

chial breathing, since the sound resembles that heard over the major bronchi in normal physiology.

For reasons that are entirely analogous to those mentioned with respect to tactile fremitus, bronchial breathing is characteristic of both consolidated lung and compression atelectasis. No breath sounds are heard over a pleural effusion, over a pneumothorax, or over a lung that is atelectatic secondary to an obstructed bronchus.

The breath sounds of the patient with emphysema deserve comment. They are faint, often completely absent. When heard, the expiratory phase is prolonged and may exhibit a high-pitched whistling tone called *wheezing*. This same sound is also heard in asthma and, indeed, in any process associated with marked bronchoconstriction.

SPOKEN VOICE. The examiner must become familiar with the sound of the normal spoken voice. Characteristically the voice sounds as though it is coming through a tunnel. Syllables are not distinguishable. Only the lower pitched sounds are heard. This normal *vocal resonance* is substantially altered by consolidation of pulmonary tissue. The sound is increased in intensity and sharpened in clarity. These characteristics produce a quality of spoken voice termed *bronchophony*. More striking is the change in advanced consolidation. Syllables become clearly distinguishable, and the voice assumes a bleating quality called *egophony*. Spoken voice is usually tested by having the patient repeat the phrase "ninety-nine" while the examiner listens. Egophony is best appreciated by having the patient repeat the letter "e." The distortion produced by consolidation transforms the sound into a clearly heard "a" rather than "e."

Bronchophony and egophony have precisely the same connotation as bronchial breathing and an increase in tactile fremitus. Where one is detected, so should the others be. Admittedly, change in tactile fremitus is more subtle and might be missed, given a lesser degree of consolidation. Bronchial breathing and bronchophony should present the examiner with little difficulty.

A very subtle finding, heard only in the presence of rather dense consolidation is the phenomenon of *whispered pectoriloquy*. Transmission of high frequency components of sound is so enhanced that even whispered words are heard, a circumstance not noted in normal physiology. The implication is the same as that of *egophony*.

ABNORMAL BREATH SOUNDS. In diseases involving the bronchial tree and the alveoli in such a way that fluid or mucus obstructs air flow, certain sounds, termed *adventitious sounds,* may be heard. Sounds heard in inspiration are called *rales* (Fig. 5-17). Rales sound much like the crackling of tissue paper or the rubbing of hairs together at the end of the stethoscope. *Fine rales* are heard at the end of inspiration and are produced in the alveoli. *Medium rales* are produced in middle-to-late inspiration and emanate from bronchioles and very small bronchi. *Coarse*

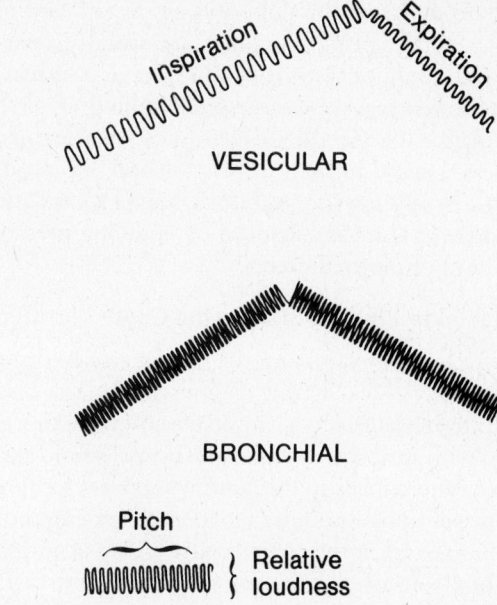

Figure 5-16. Bronchial breathing differs from vesicular breathing in that higher frequencies are transmitted, the sounds are of greater intensity, and the expiratory phase is prolonged beyond normal.

rales have a gross moist sound. They are produced in medium bronchi and are heard in early-to-middle inspiration. Another class of sounds, termed *rhonchi,* are

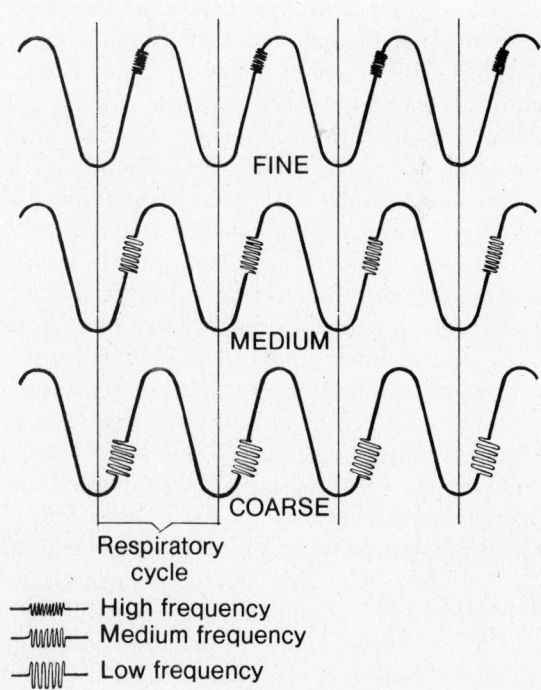

Figure 5-17. Rales may be distinguished by their quality and their position in the respiratory cycle. Fine rales are of higher frequency and occur near the end of inspiration. Coarse rales are of lower frequency, are louder, and occur in midinspiration.

generated from larger bronchi and are heard in both inspiration and expiration. They are usually coarse sounds, although occasionally they have a musical quality and often may be cleared by coughing.

Inflammation of pleural surfaces induces a leathery, rough sound, heard in both inspiration and expiration. The sound is called a *friction rub*. It seems to be quite "close" to the ear and is enhanced by applying pressure with the head of the stethoscope.

Interpretation of Physical Signs in the Chest

The processes of examining the thorax and the information that is yielded permit diagnosis of major chest disease. Extreme lateral hyperresonance over the thorax, combined with an absence of transmission of sound and a deviation of the trachea to the contralateral side, implies the presence of a pneumothorax, that is, the presence of a large amount of air in the pleural space. A lag in respiration on one side of the thorax combined with a flat percussion note and an absence of transmitted sound implies pleural effusion. Figure 5-18 summarizes in pictorial form the major lesions of the thorax that are accessible to analytic diagnosis.

As the reader has by now surmised, the finesse with which one can examine the chest for the presence or absence of disease is intricate and time-consuming. A question naturally arises: are all of the potential physical signs to be elicited in all patients? This is not feasible, nor is it desirable. Application of the tools of physical examination should always be selective. Respiration should be observed in every patient. Palpation of the chest wall for the presence and normalcy of tactile fremitus is easily accomplished. Percussion of the descent of the diaphragm is simple and yields a great deal of information. Likewise, auscultation of the chest walls for normal transmission of breath sounds over each lobe is simple and rewarding. On the other hand, an attempt to elicit egophony or whispered pectoriloquy is useless and unnecessarily time-consuming unless some facets of the history or some prior observation on physical examination leads one to pursue the inquiry in a more intricate manner. The examiner should seek to avoid the automatism that leads to uniform examination of all patients. The patient with neurological disease deserves a more detailed examination of the nervous system than the patient with chest disease, and vice versa, unless disease of the two systems coexists.

The above statement is not meant to imply that examination of patients should be superficial; rather, it should be thoughtful. The attempt to elicit physical findings should be based upon all the information available at the time the examination is conducted. This same principle will apply to the examination of other organ systems.

EXAMINATION OF THE BREAST

Breast examination should be conducted during any general physical or gynecologic examination, or whenever the patient presents with suspicion, complaint, or fear of breast disease.

The patient should be stripped to the waist and, initially, should be sitting in a comfortable position facing the examiner with her hands in her lap. The breasts should be inspected for symmetry. Elevation, deformity, or dependency of either breast is cause for suspicion. The nipples, although variable from patient to patient, should have a similar appearance. Retraction of the nipple or evident discharge is abnormal. Bulging or retraction of any portion of the breast should be noted. The breast should be observed for redness, or for "orange-peel" appearance of the skin. The latter is due to lymphatic blockage by tumor cells creating edema and pitting of the skin.

Lymph nodes in both the supraclavicular and axillary areas are examined by palpation. To examine axillary lymph nodes the patient's arm should be gently abducted from the thorax by the examiner's hand. The patient's right elbow may be grasped with the examiner's right hand, the forearm supported on the examiner's forearm. The left hand is then free to palpate the axilla noting the presence or absence of nodes which may be lying against the thoracic wall. The procedure should be reversed for the examination of the left axilla. Lymph nodes should be noted for size, number, mobility, and consistency. The arm is put through a full range of motion in order to uncover any nodes or mass lesions that may be hidden under the pectoralis muscle or under subcutaneous fat.

The patient should now lie comfortably on the examining table. When the right breast is examined, the right shoulder may be elevated on a small pillow in order to balance the breasts on the chest wall. Otherwise, a mass may be missed in the thick tissue if the breast is allowed to fall to the side. The same procedure is followed for the examination of the opposite breast. The breast is palpated gently and in an orderly fashion beginning at 12 o'clock and proceeding clockwise over the entire surface in smaller concentric circles. When the medial half of the breast is palpated, the arm may be actively or passively moved above the head in order to tense the pectoralis muscles and provide a flatter surface. When the lateral half of the breast is palpated, the arm is brought back to the patient's side. The examiner may do this by simple manipulation of a relaxed elbow. A prolongation or "tail" of breast tissue may extend toward the axilla along the pectoralis tendon toward its insertion. This may be mistaken for pathology. If it is bilaterally symmetrical, it is normal.

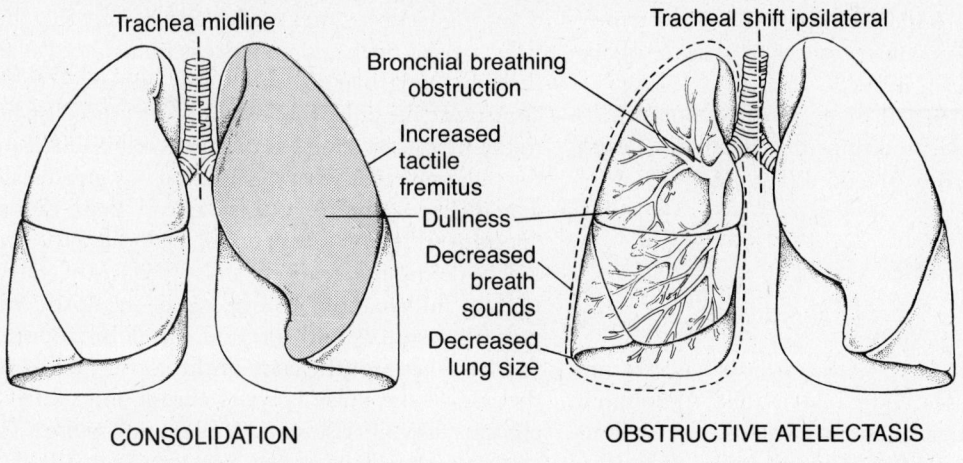

CONSOLIDATION

- Trachea midline
- Bronchial breathing obstruction
- Increased tactile fremitus
- Dullness

OBSTRUCTIVE ATELECTASIS

- Tracheal shift ipsilateral
- Decreased breath sounds
- Decreased lung size

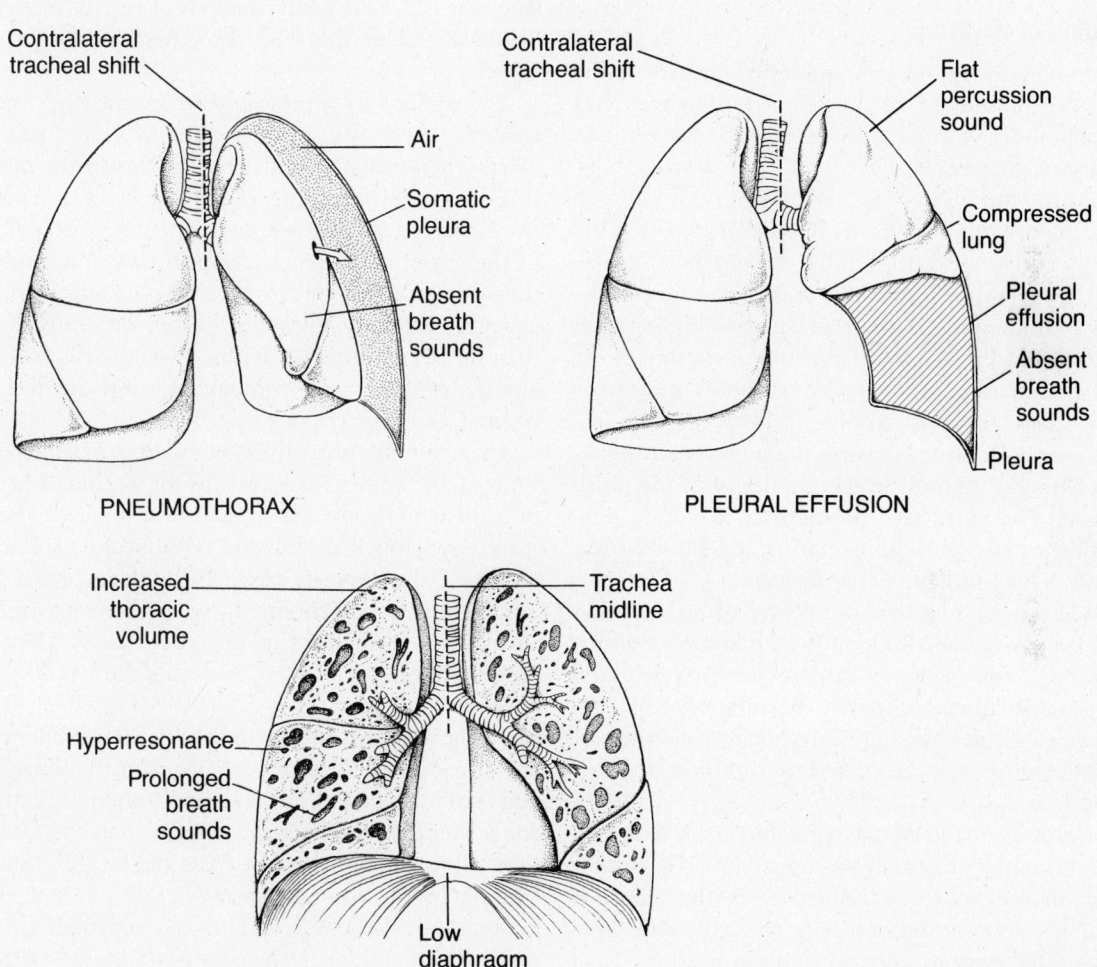

PNEUMOTHORAX

- Contralateral tracheal shift
- Air
- Somatic pleura
- Absent breath sounds

PLEURAL EFFUSION

- Contralateral tracheal shift
- Flat percussion sound
- Compressed lung
- Pleural effusion
- Absent breath sounds
- Pleura

EMPHYSEMA

- Increased thoracic volume
- Trachea midline
- Hyperresonance
- Prolonged breath sounds
- Low diaphragm

Figure 5-18. Pathophysiology of five contrasting conditions that may be revealed by physical diagnosis of the chest.

67

Lastly, the areola around the nipple should be gently compressed to determine the presence or absence of abnormal secretion.

The patient is instructed in performing breast self-examination, a simple procedure that facilitates health maintenance if uniformly practiced (Fig. 46-1).

EXAMINATION OF THE CARDIOVASCULAR SYSTEM

For convenience, all facets of the cardiovascular examination will be discussed under one heading, although it must be recognized that different portions of the examination will be done at different times during the evaluation of the patient because it is more convenient to do so.

Examination of the Pulse

In examining the pulse one is interested not only in the obvious information to be determined from rate and rhythm, but in the configuration of the pulse wave and in the quality of the vessel itself.

The normal pulse rate may vary from a low of 50 in healthy, athletic young adults to rates well in excess of 100 following exercise or during times of excitement. Anxiety will frequently elevate the pulse rate during the physical examination. If the rate appears higher than expected, it may be well to reassess it near the end of the physical examination at a time when the examiner has established better rapport with the patient.

Equally important in assessing the pulse is noting its rhythm. Minor variations in the regularity of the pulse are normal. The pulse rate, particularly in young persons, will speed up during inspiration and slow during expiration. This is called *sinus arrhythmia*.

An understanding of the complexity of arrhythmias that may be encountered during the examination requires a sophisticated knowledge of cardiac electrophysiology, a knowledge usually possessed by the nurse who specializes in cardiovascular nursing. Nurses can, nevertheless, frequently describe the disordered rhythm in terms that are helpful.

An arrhythmia may be quite regular in its presentation or totally irregular. Examples of "regular" arrhythmias are those in which, for example, every third beat is dropped, or every second beat appears earlier than normal so that the heartbeats appear to occur in pairs. Total irregularity of the pulse is much more common than regular irregularity. An "irregularly irregular" pulse is called *atrial fibrillation*. Atrial fibrillation is very common in serious heart disease and is created by chaotic contraction of the atrium. Hundreds of contractions of the atrium occur in the course of a minute, but no more than 160 to 170 of these will get through the AV node to result in ventricular contraction. Some of the ventricular con-

tractions occur so quickly after one another that the aortic valve fails to open and no pulse is transmitted at all, even though ventricular excitation has occurred. In this circumstance the pulse that might be measured by listening to the first heart sound at the apex will be different from the pulse rate that will be perceived in some distal vessel. The difference between this "apical" pulse rate and the "peripheral" pulse rate is called a *pulse deficit*.

The configuration of the pulse frequently conveys important information. In stenosis of the aortic valve the pulse pressure is narrow, and the pulse appears to be feeble. When insufficiency of the aortic valve is present, the rise of the pulse wave is abrupt and its fall is precipitous, giving rise to a "collapsing" pulse. The true configuration of the pulse is best appreciated by palpating over the carotid artery rather than the distal radial artery, since the dramatic characteristics of the pulse wave may be distorted or damped by transmission to smaller vessels.

The quality of the peripheral vasculature is of vital concern, especially in older patients. The pulse rate is usually determined by placing the tips of the index and middle finger over the radial artery. Once rate and rhythm have been determined, one can assess the quality of the vessel itself. Does it appear to be thickened? Is it tortuous? Can calcium be palpated along its wall? In order to properly assess the vessel, one must do more than simply compress it. It is necessary to slide the fingers along the vessel and compare it with the feel of the normal vascular tree.

The examiner must always be alert to occluded vessels. One of the carotid vessels may be occluded in elderly persons who have extensive vascular disease. The occlusion may happen slowly and without the production of "stroke," the opposite vessel being adequate to provide ample flow to the brain. Lower extremity vessels are most often influenced by atherosclerosis. The femoral vessels should be assessed, as should the *dorsalis pedis* and the *posterior tibial* arteries of the feet (Fig. 31-2). It should be recognized that in approximately 10 percent of people the dorsalis pedis arteries are not palpable. However, in such circumstances both are usually absent together, and the posterior tibial arteries are more than adequate, since they alone supply the feet. Absence of pulsation of all vessels in the lower extremities is characteristic of coarctation of the aorta. This is a common congenital anomaly of children, one that is associated with severe hypertension, and one that is corrected by surgery. Palpation of femoral arteries is a mandatory part of the examination of every patient, regardless of age.

Examination of Blood Pressure

Blood pressure occurs as a cyclic phenomenon and is measured in millimeters of mercury. The peak of the cycle is called the *systolic pressure;* the low point of the cycle is called the *diastolic pressure*. Blood pressure is usually expressed as the ratio of the systolic over the diastolic pressure, with normal values measuring 120/80 mm. Hg.

The difference between systolic and diastolic pressure is called the *pulse pressure*. Normally this amounts to 40 mm. Hg. An increase in blood pressure is called *hypertension;* a decrease is called *hypotension*. The systolic pressure may be elevated alone (*systolic hypertension*) and of necessity results in a widening of the pulse pressure. This happens in atherosclerosis (hardening of the arteries) and in thyrotoxicosis. Elevation of the diastolic pressure is always associated with elevation of the systolic pressure, and the circumstance represents true hypertension. An increase of the diastolic pressure to 95 mm. Hg gives rise to concern, particularly in younger patients; an increase in excess of 95 mm. Hg in the diastolic pressure constitutes true hypertension and requires investigation and control.

The blood pressure is measured by the use of the sphygmomanometer and the stethoscope. The sphygmomanometer consists of an inflatable cuff and a pressure gauge that communicates with the hollow portion of the cuff. The device is calibrated in such a manner that the pressure that is read from the manometer is quite comparable to the pressure in millimeters of mercury that is being transmitted to the brachial artery. The cuff is wrapped around the upper arm tightly and is inflated by a bulb. Pressure on the cuff is increased until the radial pulse disappears. The disappearance of the radial pulse signifies that systolic blood pressure has been exceeded and the brachial artery is occluded. Since the manometer reads the pressure to which the brachial artery is exposed, this must be in excess of 120 mm. Hg. If one now slowly

lowers the pressure within the cuff by deflating the bulb, there will come a point at which a pulse will again become discernible in the radial artery. This is the systolic blood presure. At the same time, a sound is produced within the brachial artery just below the cuff and is audible with the stethoscope. This sound (*Korotkoff sound*) coincides with each pulse beat and will continue to emanate from the brachial artery until the pressure in the cuff has been reduced below diastolic pressure. At that point, the sound ceases. In actual practice, the sound more often becomes muffled (changes character) as diastolic pressure is reached and then disappears at 10 to 20 mm. Hg below normal diastolic pressure. One is interested in the point at which the sound becomes muffled. If there is any doubt, the blood pressure may be recorded as a tripartite pressure (120/80/60) to imply that the sound became muffled at 80 mm. Hg and disappeared at 60 mm. Hg.

Accurate recording of the blood pressure depends upon attention to several critical details. The cuff must be firmly wrapped around the arm. It should not be too loose. The stethoscope has to be placed directly over the brachial artery, just below the crease of the elbow, the point at which the brachial artery emerges from the two heads of the biceps muscle. The cuff must be appropriate to the size of the arm. If the cuff is too large for the arm, as in a child, one will underestimate the magnitude of pressure; that is, the pressure obtained will be substantially below true pressure. If the arm is excessively large, as it is in many obese persons, one will overestimate the level of pressure; that is, the patient will appear to be hypertensive when the pressure is, in fact, normal (Fig. 5-19). Special cuffs are manufactured for obese persons and for children.

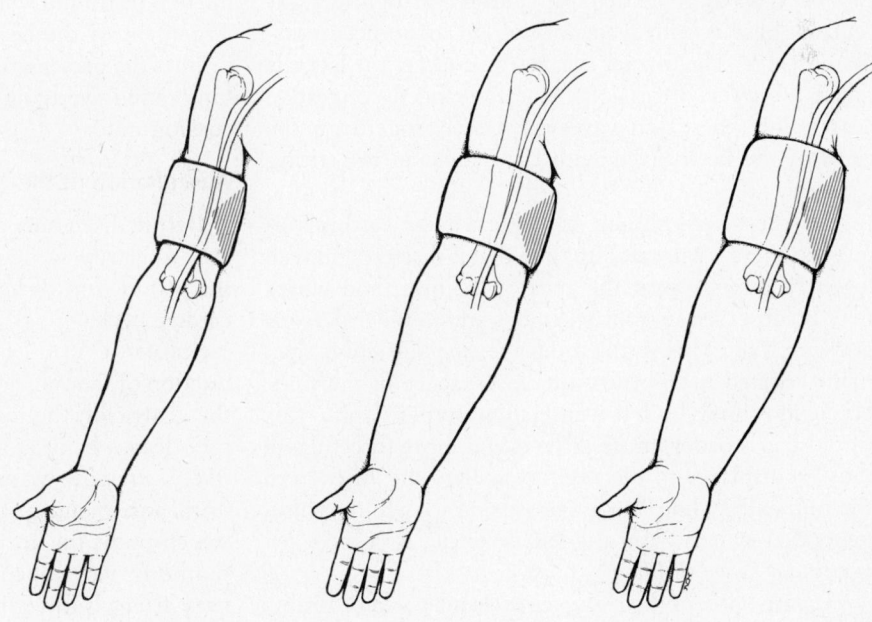

Figure 5-19. Illustration of blood pressure cuff transmission to the brachial artery. Panel to the left represents the normal transmission as it would occur in a normal sized arm. The center panel demonstrates that with obesity the usual size cuff will not transmit faithfully to the brachial artery without excessive generation of pressure, providing a falsely elevated reading. The panel to the right illustrates the use of a wider ("obesity") cuff in order to obtain accurate readings from persons who are overweight.

The measurement of blood pressure is an exercise that a nurse is expected to be able to perform well and reliably. Proper measurement takes practice. Pressure in hypertensive persons should be measured while the patient is lying down, sitting, and then standing. It should be measured in both the right and the left arm. Unless there is disease of the vasculature, a difference of no more than 5 mm. Hg should be found.

Blood pressure can also be measured in the lower extremities. However, an extra wide cuff should be used, and the results interpreted with some skepticism. The measurement has little practical utility.

Inspection of the Heart

Inspection with respect to the cardiovascular system involves two important observations. First the venous system is inspected and any venous pulsations observed; second the *precordium* (surface of the thorax overlying the heart) is inspected for abnormal pulsation.

It is especially important to observe the external jugular veins in the neck. These are frequently distended while the patient lies supine on the examining table or in the bed. As the patient is elevated, however, the distention of the veins will disappear. They are not normally apparent once the angle that the patient makes with the examining table exeeds 30 degrees. Obvious distention of the veins with the patient at 45 to 90 degrees (sitting up) implies an abnormal increase in the volume of the venous system secondary to the retention of fluid or obstruction to flow in the superior vena cava. The former circumstance is much more common and is associated with congestive heart failure.

When the neck veins are distended, they easily conduct pulsations that emanate from the heart. They may conduct a wave associated with contraction of the atrium and/or a wave generated by contraction of the right ventricle that is conveyed through an incompetent tricuspid valve. The former is called an *a-wave;* the latter is called a *v-wave*. Occasionally, in advanced congestive heart failure, these two waves may be seen together in the veins of the neck, even with the patient in the sitting position.

The chest wall should be observed for cardiac impulses. There is a normal impulse that is discrete and well localized directly over the apex of the heart and which may be observed in young persons and in older persons who are thin. This is called the apex *impulse* and is normally located in the fifth intercostal space in the midclavicular line. In left ventricular hypertrophy this impulse is broader, more diffuse, and more forceful and may be displaced to the anterior axillary line or even to the midaxillary line. Such a broad and forceful impulse, generated as it is from the left ventricle, is called a *left ventricular heave* or *lift*.

Hypertrophy of the right ventricle may also be visibly discernible on the chest walls. When apparent, it is located just to the left of the sternum and is broad, diffuse, and forceful. It is usually centered in the third or fourth intercostal space near the sternal junction. When present, it is called a *right ventricular heave* or *lift*.

Palpation of the Heart

The apex impulse, as well as left and right ventricular heaves, may easily be palpated. The apex impulse will be palpated as a discrete thrust in its normal location. Left and right ventricular heaves will appear to "lift" the hand from the chest wall itself. This merely tends to confirm the observation previously made on inspection.

The sounds of the heart may frequently be palpated on the chest wall. This is true of the first and second heart sounds when they are increased in intensity and usually implies pathology within the heart, since an increase in intensity of sufficient magnitude to be apparent to the hand bespeaks an intensity born of increased pressure within a chamber.

Murmurs, when they are exceptionally loud, may also be palpated and are felt by the fingers or palm as a "purring" sensation. This phenomenon is called a *thrill* and is always indicative of significant pathology within the heart. Thrills also may be palpated over vessels when there is significant substantial obstruction to blood flow and will occur over the carotid arteries in the presence of narrowing (or stenosis) of the aortic valve.

Percussion of the Heart

Percussion of the heart was described earlier in the discussion of percussion of the thoracic wall and is mentioned here as a part of the examination of the cardiovascular system. By practicing percussion, the examiner will become familiar with the border of the normal heart and will be able to easily identify any enlargement of the heart. An absence of cardiac dullness implies the presence of emphysema, where air trapped in lung tissue overlying the heart obscures the normal percussion note.

Auscultation of the Heart

Before discussing auscultation of the heart, it is necessary to clarify some physical principles as they relate to the production of heart sounds. Let us first review the cardiac cycle.

CARDIAC CYCLE. The cardiac cycle begins with contraction of the ventricles. As pressure is generated within the ventricles, the mitral and tricuspid valves close, and their leaves balloon into the left and right atria, respectively. Pressure within the ventricles continues to rise until aortic and pulmonic pressures are exceeded, at which point the aortic and pulmonic valves open. The pulmonic valve opens first, since pressure in the pulmonary artery is lower than that in the aorta. The period of time between closure of the atrial ventricular valves and the opening of the semilunar valves is called *isometric ventricular contraction*. Opening of the semilunar valves (aortic and pulmonic valves) is the point at which *systole* begins. Systole continues until ventricular energy is spent, aortic and pulmonic pressures exceed pressures within the ventricle, and the semilunar valves close. The aortic valve closes first under normal circumstances, since aortic pressure exceeds pulmonic pressure. Pressure in the ventricle then falls precipitously until it dips below the pressure within the atria, at which time the mitral and tricuspid valves open, and diastole begins. The period of time between the closure of the semilunar valves and the opening of the atrioventricular valves is called *isometric ventricular relaxation*. Once the mitral and tricuspid valves have opened, the ventricles begin to fill. This phase of the cardiac cycle is called *diastole*. Filling is at first rapid, ultimately approaching a plateau. Near the end of diastole the atria contract against the partially filled ventricle and augment the volume of the ventricular cavities by an additional 10 percent of volume. Almost immediately thereafter, the mitral and tricuspid valves rebound to a closed position, the ventricles promptly contract, ballooning the valves back into the atrium, and the cycle begins again.

HEART SOUNDS. Closure of the valves gives rise to "heart sounds" which may be heard on the chest wall. These are called the *transient heart sounds*. In normal physiology the periods of systole and diastole are silent. Pathology of the ventricle, however, can give rise to transient sounds in systole and diastole that are called *gallops, snaps,* or *clicks*. Significant pathological narrowing of the valve orifices at times when they should be open or residual gapping of valves at times when they should be closed gives rise to prolonged sounds which are called *murmurs*. Proper interpretation of normal and abnormal sounds over the precordium is a sophisticated and challenging process, but one with which the nurse can become familiar.

Auscultatory Valve Areas. Events occurring at each of the four valves are uniquely reflected at specific locations on the chest wall (Fig. 5-20). These locations do not correspond to the anatomical location of the valve within the chest. Rather, they are reflective of the patterns of radiation of heart sounds toward the chest wall. Sound in vessels through which blood is flowing is always reflected downstream. Events of the mitral valve are usually best heard in the fifth intercostal space at the midclavicular line. This is called the *mitral valve area*. Events occurring at the tricuspid valve are best heard in the fourth intercostal space just to the left of the sternum. This is called the *tricuspid valve area*. The *aortic valve area* is located in the second intercostal space to the right of the sternum, and the *pulmonic valve area* is located in the second intercostal space to the left of the sternum. When

cardiac pathology is indicated, it is wise to listen to each valve area in turn with both the bell and the diaphragm. Thus, there are a minimum of eight specific maneuvers that must be undertaken.

Timing of the events in the cardiac cycle is vital. Occasionally, when the sounds are prominent and both systole and diastole are filled with murmurs, it is possible to get lost in the cycle. It is helpful to palpate the carotid artery, thus identifying systole and assessing all else accordingly. One additional note may be helpful. In advanced cardiac pathology it may be necessary to identify as many as four or five different sounds within a single cardiac cycle. If a patient has a tachycardia, this implies that one must identify, describe, and evaluate bits of information that are occurring as often as 500 times per minute. It is useful to separate the cycle and concentrate on selected facets of it rather than attempt to interpret the entire cycle at first hearing. One should first identify the first heart sound and concentrate on it, excluding all other information. One should then listen to the second heart sound, again excluding all other facets of the cycle. One may then focus attention on the systolic interval, and finally on the diastolic interval. Once the characteristics of each phase of the cycle have been determined, the relationship of one to another and the synthesis of events within the cycle may then be summarized. This is entirely analogous to the assessment of a piece of music or a painting. One perceives an overview, analyzes the component parts, and then summarizes the net effect of what he has seen or heard.

Transient Heart Sounds. The *first heart sound* is created by the simultaneous closure of the mitral and tricuspid valves. Although heard over the entire precordium, it is best heard in the mitral area. It is increased in

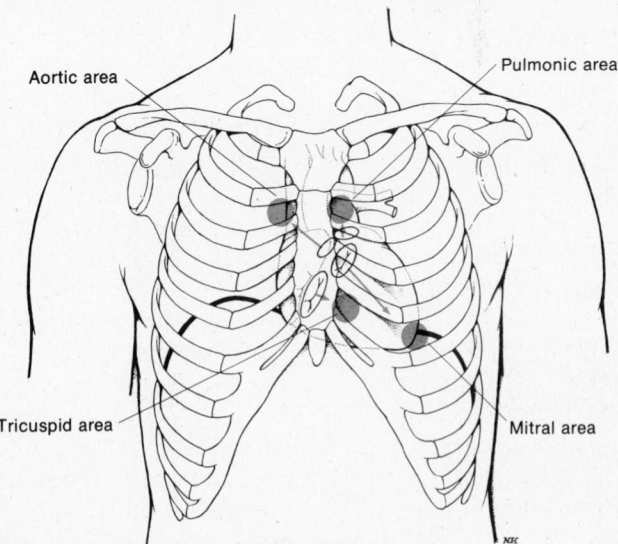

Figure 5-20. Topographical anatomy of the heart as it projects upon the thoracic wall.

intensity when the valve leaflets are made rigid by calcium in rheumatic heart disease and in any circumstance in which ventricular contraction intervenes at a time when the valve is caught wide open. The latter circumstance will occur, for example, when a premature ventricular contraction interrupts the normal cardiac cycle. The first heart sound varies in intensity from beat to beat when atrial contraction is not synchronous with ventricular contraction. This is because the valve may be closed or partially closed on one beat and quite widely patent on the subsequent one as a function of irregular atrial activity. The first heart sound is easily identifiable and serves as the point of reference for the remainder of the cardiac cycle (Fig. 5-21).

The *second heart sound* is produced by the closure of the aortic and pulmonic valves. It is quite usual for these valves to close separately, the aortic valve first, followed by the pulmonic valve, and for the resultant sounds to be clearly distinguished as a "split" second sound. It is even more usual for this split to be accentuated on inspiration and to disappear on expiration as a function of respiratory influence on right ventricular ejection (augmenting it on inspiration, inhibiting it on expiration). The aortic com-

ponent of the second sound is heard clearly in both the aortic and pulmonic areas and is heard less clearly at the apex. The pulmonic component of the second sound, if present, may only be heard over the pulmonic area. Thus, one may hear a "single" second heart sound in the aortic area and a split second heart sound in the pulmonic area. Hypertension of either the systemic or pulmonary systems will increase the intensity of the respective component of the second sound. Narrowing of either valve orifice, as a function of either congenital or rheumatic heart disease, will decrease the intensity of the sound generated by the respective valve. A congenital septal defect between the two atria (*atrial septal defect*) is of particular interest because it delays pulmonic valve closure until quite late and gives rise to a very wide split in the second heart sound. Moreover, this split does not change with respiration. This sign is absolutely diagnostic of an atrial septal defect.

Gallop Sounds. Impedance to diastolic filling of the ventricle in certain disease states may give rise to transient vibrations in diastole that are much akin to, although usually softer than, the first and second heart sounds. Heart sounds then come in triplets and have the acoustical

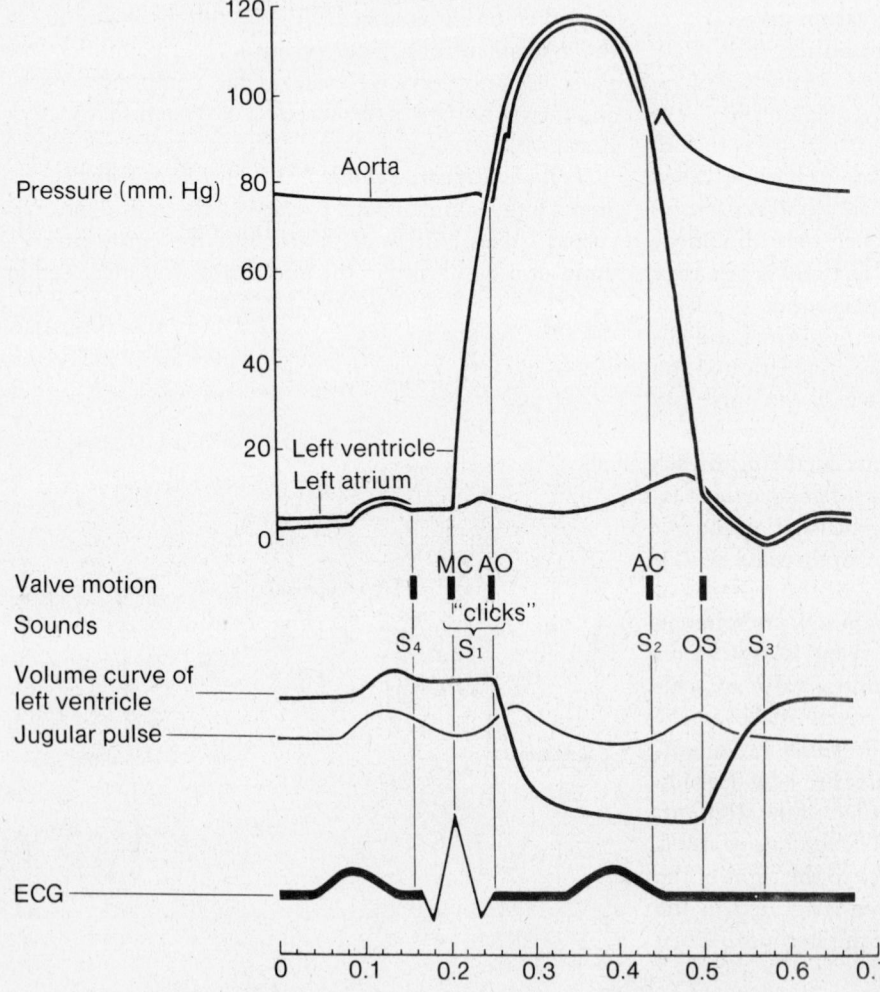

Figure 5-21. Events in the cardiac cycle. Three pressure curves are displayed: aortic, ventricular, and left atrial. In addition, the jugular venous pulse with its a-wave and v-wave, and the volume curve of the left ventricle are displayed. Electrocardiographic events precede the mechanical events by the indicated periods of time. Valve closure and opening are indicated, as is the relationship of the cardiac sounds to these events.

effect of a galloping horse; they are therefore called *gallops*. This may occur early in diastole during the rapid-filling phase of the cardiac cycle, or it may occur at the time of atrial contraction. A gallop sound occurring during rapid ventricular filling is called a *third heart sound* or protodiastolic gallop. Such a sound is heard in patients who have myocardial disease or in those who are in congestive heart failure and whose ventricles fail to eject all of their blood during systole. The protodiastolic gallop is a cardinal sign of heart failure.

Gallop sounds which are heard during atrial contraction are called *fourth heart sounds* or *presystolic gallops*. They are often heard when the ventricle is hypertrophied, although not to the point of failure. Such a circumstance might occur in aortic stenosis or in hypertension. Indeed, a presystolic gallop is an expected finding in hypertension with diastolic pressures of 100 mm. Hg. On rare occasions all four heart sounds may be heard within a single cardiac cycle, giving rise to what is called a *quadruple rhythm*.

It should be noted that gallop sounds are very low frequency sounds and may only be heard with the bell of the stethoscope placed very lightly against the chest. They are heard best at the apex, although occasionally when emanating from the right ventricle they may be heard to the left of the sternum.

Snaps and Clicks.   Stenosis of the mitral valve due to rheumatic heart disease gives rise to an unusual sound very early in diastole that is high-pitched and best heard along the left sternal border. The sound is caused by high pressure in the left atrium abruptly displacing a rigid mitral valve. The sound is called an *opening snap*. It occurs too long after the second sound to be mistaken for a split second sound and too early in diastole to be mistaken for a gallop. It is almost always associated with the murmur of mitral stenosis and is very specific for that disease.

In an analogous manner stenosis of the aortic valve gives rise to a short, high-pitched sound immediately after the first heart sound that is called an *ejection click*. This is due to very high pressure within the ventricle displacing a rigid and calcified aortic valve.

Murmurs.   Murmurs are created by the turbulent flow of blood past a critically narrowed valve, by the regurgitant flow of blood through a valve that has failed to close properly, or by the flow of blood through a congenital defect within the wall of the ventricle or between the aorta and the pulmonary artery. Murmurs are characterized and consequently identified by several characteristics, including timing in the cardiac cycle, location on the chest wall, intensity, pitch, quality, and pattern of radiation.

The *timing* of the murmur in the cardiac cycle is vital. First of all the observer must determine whether the murmur is occurring in systole or in diastole. Does it begin simultaneously with the first heart sound, or is there some delay between the sound and the beginning of a systolic murmur? Does the murmur run up to (or through) the second heart sound, or is there again delay between the end of the murmur and the occurrence of the second heart sound? Are diastolic murmurs continuous, or do they die out in mid or late diastole?

Location of the murmur is highly critical. The diastolic murmur of *mitral stenosis* is heard only at the apex (mitral area) and may indeed be confined to only a few centimeters of the chest wall. The murmurs of *aortic and pulmonic stenosis,* although usually widely heard, are nevertheless best heard over their respective valve areas. The murmur of *aortic insufficiency* is best heard along the left sternal border between the third and fourth interspace. (The murmur of *aortic insufficiency* may not be heard at all in the aortic area. This is because the "forward" direction of blood flow for regurgitation at the aortic valve is in the reverse direction, and the point has previously been made that murmurs radiate "downstream." For this reason the fourth intercostal space just to the left of the sternum is frequently called the *secondary aortic area*.)

The *intensity* of murmurs is conventionally graded from I through VI. The student will have difficulty hearing a grade I murmur. A grade II cardiac murmur should be easily perceived. Murmurs of grades IV or louder are usually associated with thrills that may be palpated on the surface of the chest wall. A grade VI murmur can often be heard with the stethoscope off the chest. A murmur may vary in intensity from its inception to its conclusion. This is very characteristic of certain valvular disorders. The murmur of aortic stenosis, for example, begins sometime after the first heart sound, increases in intensity to midsystole, and then decreases in intensity, stopping prior to the second heart sound. The sound configuration is referred to as "diamond" in shape, and the murmur is referred to as an *ejection murmur* (Fig. 5-22). The midsystolic increase in intensity is characteristic of murmurs that result from ejection through either the aortic or the pulmonic valve. The murmur of mitral insufficiency and

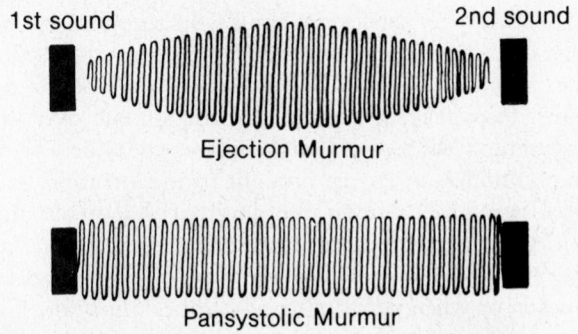

1st sound   2nd sound

Ejection Murmur

Pansystolic Murmur

Figure 5-22.   Differentiation between ejection murmurs generated at the pulmonic and aortic valves and pansystolic murmurs generated at the mitral and tricuspid valves. Ejection murmurs begin after the first sound, peak in midsystole, and generally conclude before the second sound. Pansystolic murmurs are of equivalent intensity throughout systole, beginning with the first sound and ending with the second sound.

the murmur of a ventricular septal defect are, on the other hand, constant in intensity throughout systole. Moreover, they begin simultaneously with the first heart sound and end simultaneously with the second heart sound. These murmurs are referred to as *holosystolic* or *pansystolic*.

The next important quality of a murmur is its *pitch*. The murmur of mitral stenosis is a low, rumbling sound, often heard only with the bell placed lightly on the chest wall. By contrast, the murmur of aortic insufficiency is a very high-pitched murmur, occasionally "whistling" in character, heard best with the diaphragm. Other murmurs, especially the murmur of aortic stenosis, contain the full spectrum of sound frequency, a characteristic that makes the murmur appear to be very harsh in quality.

The last feature of concern is *radiation* of the murmur. The murmur of mitral insufficiency, best heard at the apex (mitral area), radiates into the axilla. This, of course, reflects the "downstream" nature of its transmission. The murmur of aortic stenosis will, for analogous reasons, radiate into the carotid arteries in the neck. The murmur of pulmonic stenosis, which may sound identical to that of aortic stenosis, will not radiate into the neck; rather, it may radiate into the left shoulder or into the back.

FRICTION RUB. In serious pericarditis, a harsh grating sound can be heard both in systole and diastole and is called a *friction rub*. It is caused by the abrasion of the pericardial surfaces during the cardiac cycle. This may be confused with a murmur; care should be taken to identify the sound when appropriate and to distinguish it from murmurs that may be heard in both systole and diastole.

Interpretation of Cardiac Sounds

The interpretation of cardiac sounds is a difficult art to acquire. It requires intimate knowledge of cardiac physiology and the pathophysiology of cardiac diseases. However, there are different levels of performance at which the nurse may be expected to function — levels at which auscultation of the heart may be part of her role. The first level of function is simply the recognition that what one is hearing is not normal. There may be a third heart sound; there may be a murmur in systole or diastole; there may be a pericardial friction rub over the midsternum; the second heart sound may be widely split. These findings are to be brought to the attention of a physician and acted upon accordingly. This level of function is useful in screening. It is the kind of activity that one engages in when doing school physicals on normal children or when performing physical examinations for insurance companies.

The second level of function employs pattern recognition. The nurse correctly observes the findings and is capable of recognizing the constellation of sounds and its diagnostic significance, if the constellation is a common one. This is the role into which the nurse practitioner has recently been placed. The nurse practitioner can and should be capable of recognizing mitral stenosis, an atrial septal defect, aortic insufficiency, etc.

At its most sophisticated level cardiac diagnosis can be interpretive. Nurses properly trained can differentiate among arrhythmias and respond accordingly. They can determine the significance of the appearance and disappearance of gallops during treatment of patients who have had myocardial infarctions or are in heart failure. This is the role into which the coronary care nurse and the cardiovascular nurse specialist have been cast. They function with a team of professionals for whom the fine details of cardiovascular diagnosis have become highly tuned, shared skills.

It might be useful to delineate the characteristic features of the most common cardiac abnormalities, leaving the less common ones to the interested nurse who should consult appropriate textbooks. One might note that the description of the constellation of findings in common cardiovascular conditions is analogous to describing the opening bars of a symphony in words. A symphony has to be heard to be appreciated. Several excellent and highly useful recordings of characteristic heart sounds are available. These should be obtained and listened to until one is secure in recognizing the patterns.

Mitral stenosis results from the fusion, thickening, and calcification of the cusps of the mitral valve as a result of rheumatic heart disease. The first heart sound is increased in intensity. Systole is silent. The second heart sound is followed by a high-pitched opening snap best heard along the left sternal border. Coincidentally with the opening snap there begins a low-pitched rumbling murmur that may die out in late diastole or continue throughout the diastolic period, becoming accentuated during atrial contraction at the end of diastole and culminating in the loud first heart sound. The murmur of mitral stenosis is low in intensity, never exceeding grade III.

The mitral valve may be sufficiently damaged during repeated attacks of rheumatic fever that the cusps do not completely close during systole. The valve then becomes incompetent, leading to *mitral insufficiency*. The murmur of mitral insufficiency begins coincidentally with the first heart sound, and it maintains a constant intensity throughout systole, culminating in the second heart sound. Occasionally, mitral stenosis and mitral insufficiency coexist, giving rise to the features of both.

Aortic stenosis implies fusion of the cusps of the aortic valve. This may be congenital in origin or may be the result of rheumatic fever. In the latter instance the valve is rigid and calcified. The murmur of aortic stenosis, as was noted earlier, begins shortly after the first heart sound, peaks in midsystole, and comes to an end before the second heart sound. In advanced aortic stenosis no second heart sound is heard. Aortic stenosis must be distinguished from *pulmonic stenosis;* the murmurs are similar, but the murmur of pulmonic stenosis will not radiate into the carotid arteries.

Aortic insufficiency is caused by the failure of the cusps of the aortic valve to completely close during diastole. This may be due to disease of the valves secondary to rheumatic fever or may be the result of dilatation of the aortic valve ring secondary to syphilis. The first heart sound is normal. Systole is silent. The second heart sound is prominent and is followed by a high-pitched decrescendo murmur that dies out in late diastole. Occasionally aortic stenosis and insufficiency will coexist, and the features of both are seen in the same patient.

As is the case with examination of the chest, physical examination of the cardiovascular system is complex and may be time-consuming. One may ask what constitutes a competent and sufficiently thorough examination. In the absence of cardiac symptoms one should certainly assess the blood pressure and the pulse rate. Blood pressure may indeed be the most important observation that we make in the examination of any patient, since hypertension is exceedingly common in the population and amenable to adequate control. Inspection of the anterior thorax is easily accomplished, and an apex impulse, if present, should be noted. It is unusual for healthy adults over the age of 30 to exhibit an apex impulse, and its presence may be a clue to underlying cardiac hypertrophy. Percussion of the cardiac border in normal persons is not usually rewarding and only yields valuable information when cardiac hypertrophy is anticipated. The heart should be listened to with care in the four principal areas. Any variation from normal mandates more intensive investigation.

EXAMINATION OF THE ABDOMEN

Examination of the abdomen calls for a departure from the usual ordered process of inspection, palpation, percusssion, and auscultation. Palpation of a painful abdomen can incite paroxysms of colic or inhibit early bowel sounds in a resolving peritonitis. Thus, physical manipulation of the abdomen is deferred until last. The order then is: inspection, auscultation, percussion, and palpation.

Topography of the Abdomen

The abdomen is conventionally divided into four quadrants by a vertical midline and a horizontal line through the navel (Fig. 5-23). Thus, the liver lies in the

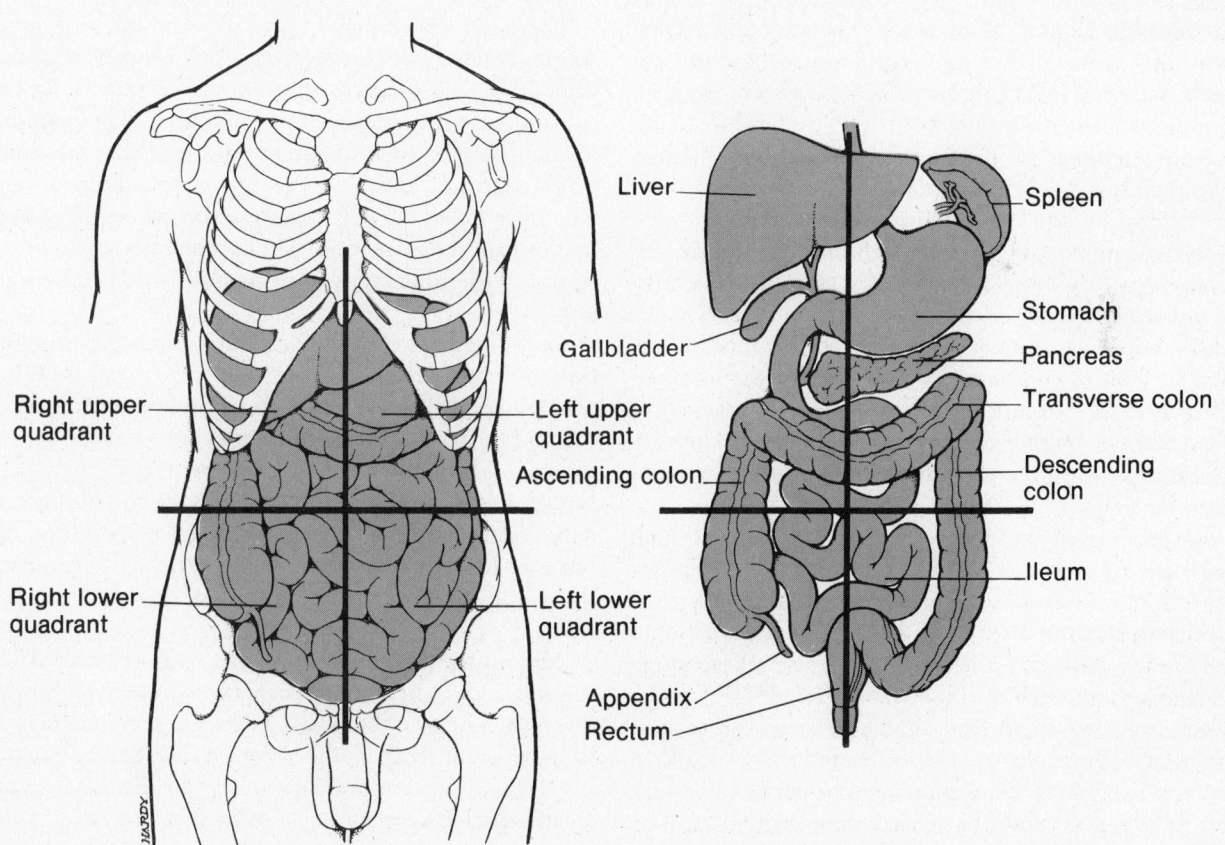

Figure 5-23. Topography of the abdomen as it is related to the location of the abdominal viscera.

right upper quadrant, the spleen in the left upper quadrant, the appendix and cecum in the right lower quadrant, and the sigmoid colon in the left lower quadrant. The midportion of the abdomen above the umbilicus is referred to as the epigastrium, and the midportion of the abdomen below the umbilicus is referred to as the hypogastrium. The antrum of the stomach, the pylorus, and the first third of the duodenum lie in the epigastrium. The bladder lies in the hypogastrium.

Inspection of the Abdomen

SKIN. Inspection of the abdomen begins with an observation of the skin, which can offer clues to the patient's state of health and past history. For example, the skin over the abdomen will provide early evidence of jaundice. With appropriate lighting, jaundice may be as easily discerned on the trunk as it is in the sclerae. Abdominal skin can also reflect the state of hydration of the patient. If the skin "tents" after the abdominal wall is pinched, the patient may be dehydrated. The skin should also be observed for scars of previous surgery. Frequently patients will neglect to tell the examiner about an appendectomy in the distant past or other surgical procedures that may have occurred in childhood. Such scars should be explained and noted.

HERNIAS. Hernias may be quite visible. Many patients, especially children, have evident umbilical hernias that have no clinical significance. The abdominal contents may herniate through an old scar where muscle layers separated following surgery. Such a hernia may be demonstrated by having the patient lift his head from the bed, thus tensing the abdominal musculature while increasing intra-abdominal pressure. A small bulge reveals the hernia. Inguinal and femoral hernias may also be observed. Inguinal hernias, though rare in women, are exceedingly common in men. They may protrude into the scrotum and often contain bowel and occasionally other abdominal organs. Femoral hernias, more common in women, occasionally bulge below the inguinal ligament. Failure to observe a hernia does not necessarily mean that one is not present. Frequently inguinal hernias decompress when the patient lies down, only to emerge when he stands.

ASCITES. Tense ascites (peritoneal cavity filled with fluid) is readily noted on observation. However, lesser degrees of ascites may be less apparent and may thus make it difficult to distinguish between moderate ascites and obesity. However, the tendency of the flanks to bulge with ascites represents a subtle but real difference between ascites and obesity. In the presence of ascites, superficial veins may appear in the abdominal wall. In rare instances such veins are related to portal hypertension in which anastomotic veins develop around the umbilicus, and resemble a multilegged hydra, a rather startling phenomenon referred to as a *caput medusa*. Much

more commonly, especially in patients who have long-standing ascites from whatever etiology, longitudinal veins will appear on both sides of the abdomen. These have nothing to do with portal hypertension. Rather, they reflect an attempt to decompress the inferior vena cava through superficial epigastric veins into the superior vena cava. They are the result of the compression of the inferior vena cava by the mass of the fluid.

PERISTALTIC WAVES. In patients who have bowel obstruction, most especially those who are thin, one may see peristaltic waves of activity crossing the abdomen. This is diagnostic of obstruction.

PAIN. Patients with abdominal pain should be observed closely. The patient with pain due to peritonitis will lie quite still and will find that any movement, active or passive, exacerbates the pain and is unbearable. The patient will frequently draw his knees up into a fetal position and lie on his side in a vain attempt to achieve a position of comfort. The patient with abdominal pain that is colicky in nature due to biliary disease, bowel obstruction, or urinary tract disease is more likely to be restless, writhing in the bed and frequently alternating between a sitting and lying position; he may even occasionally pace the floor.

Auscultation of the Abdomen

There is a wide range of intensity and pitch of bowel sounds that may be considered normal. Therefore, attention should be focused only on the extremes. At one extreme is a total absence of bowel sounds. The examiner should listen in each quadrant for more than a minute before stating definitively that bowel sounds are absent. The absence of bowel sounds accompanies peritoneal irritation or inflammation. The combination of no bowel sounds with other signs of peritonitis is termed *paralytic ileus*.

At the other extreme are the high-pitched, "tinkling" bowel sounds of gastrointestinal obstruction. When obstructed, the bowel fills with air, and peristaltic movement of the tensely distended bowel produces the characteristic high-pitched sound. Both peritonitis (ileus) and bowel obstruction are associated with the absence of defecation and/or the passing of gas. Therefore, the capacity to have a bowel movement virtually eliminates the possibility that either peritonitis or bowel obstruction exists.

Abdominal murmurs associated with obstructed vessels may also be heard. In patients who have hypertension due to renal artery stenosis, a systolic murmur may be heard over the flank on the involved side. Severe narrowing of the lower abdominal aorta or the iliac arteries due to atherosclerosis may be associated with systolic murmurs as well. Usually these will radiate into the femoral vessels and are easily heard there.

Percussion of the Abdomen

SIZE OF ABDOMINAL ORGANS. Percussion of the abdomen helps delineate the size of abdominal organs such as the liver, spleen, and bladder. The tone produced by percussion over the liver is dull. The upper border of this dullness is usually at the sixth or seventh rib in the midclavicular line on the right, whereas the lower border is at the costal margin. The total span of liver dullness in the midclavicular line ranges from 8 cm. (3 inches) in small persons to 12 cm. (4¾ inches) in large, muscular men. A liver span in excess of 12 cm. implies hepatic enlargement.

Although the spleen lies just under the left costal margin it usually cannot be felt, nor can it be percussed. Occasionally, when the spleen is moderately enlarged, as in infectious mononucleosis, it may be percussed, although not palpated.

The bladder is often percussable in the hypogastrium. This is useful in differentiating "overflow" incontinence of a distended and obstructed bladder from incontinence due to autonomic neuropathy. The nurse may frequently use percusssion of the abdomen as a guide in determining whether or not a patient needs to be catheterized.

ASSESSMENT OF ASCITES. Percussion is exceedingly useful in the assessment of ascites. When the patient lies on his back, fluid is dependent, and the bowel floats on the surface. If one begins at the midline and percusses laterally one can detect a sharp difference between the hyperresonance of the floating bowel and the dull or flat sound that emerges at the fluid level. If the patient is then turned on his side, the bowel will again float to the top, and the fluid will flow into the dependent flank. If one then again percusses the abdomen, one finds that the fluid level has shifted toward the umbilicus. This phenomenon is called *shifting dullness* and is absolutely diagnostic of ascites.

Another test for ascites is the demonstration of a *fluid wave*. If the examiner places the palm of his hand against one flank, and taps the opposite flank, the impact of the tap will be felt by the hand. One caution should be exerted. The subcutaneous tissue of obese persons may transmit a fluid wave that might falsely be interpreted as showing evidence of ascites. Subcutaneous transmission may be precluded, however, by having the patient place the edge of his hand firmly against the midline of the abdomen to interrupt superficial wave transmission.

Palpation of the Abdomen

Palpation of the abdomen should be approached gently, especially in those patients who have abdominal pain. Furthermore, one begins palpation as far away from the site of pain as possible, moving circumferentially and palpating the painful area last. If the painful area is palpated first, muscle guarding will be induced, preventing the examiner from gaining useful information elsewhere in the abdomen.

PAIN. The first concern is tenderness. Tenderness is usually most exquisite over the area where the patient complains of pain, but it may be elicited elsewhere as well. Quite often palpation of another part of the abdomen will result in pain perceived in the quadrant in which the disease process is located. For example, palpation anywhere in the abdomen of the patient with appendicitis will elicit pain in the right lower quadrant. Pain, especially the pain of peritonitis, is almost always associated with muscle guarding, even to the point of rigidity. This is an involuntary process and cannot be controlled by the patient. The absence of muscle guarding in the presence of pain provoked by palpation should alert the examiner to the possibility of malingering. This is a useful observation in identifying patients who achieve primary or secondary gain from their illness.

Occasionally pain is not elicited on direct palpation, but may emerge when the hand is abruptly removed from the abdomen. This phenomenon is called *rebound tenderness* and is highly suggestive of peritoneal irritation. Of even greater diagnostic significance is *referred rebound tenderness* in which the abrupt withdrawal of the hand from the abdomen results in rebound tenderness referred to the site of the disease. An example of this is again noted in appendicitis. One may well be able to palpate the left lower quadrant to a reasonable depth without eliciting pain, but the abrupt withdrawal of the hand results in the perception of severe pain in the right lower quadrant.

ABDOMINAL ORGANS. The examiner should next attempt to palpate body organs. The liver may be palpable in the right upper quadrant, the spleen in the left upper quadrant. A palpable liver may not necessarily represent enlargement, although the inference is usually justified (Fig. 5-24). An example of a normal palpable liver is that which occurs in the patient with emphysema whose diaphragm is depressed, forcing the liver below the right costal margin. A palpable spleen is considered by most observers to be indicative of splenic enlargement and disease. The normal kidney may be palpable in thin persons with pliable abdominal walls. However, this is unusual and probably not worth eliciting unless disease of the kidney is suspected.

The liver and spleen may be distinguished from other masses by their motion on diaphragmatic excursion. A deep inspiration will cause either or both to descend several centimeters. The failure of a palpable mass to descend implies that it is not attached to the diaphragm but lies behind the peritoneum.

Palpable organs should be characterized by the examiner. Of concern is their size, their consistency, whether or not they are tender, and whether they are regular or irregular in outline. If the liver is enlarged, the degree to which it descends below the right costal margin should be recorded in order to provide some impression of its total dimension. The liver of cirrhosis is small and hard in

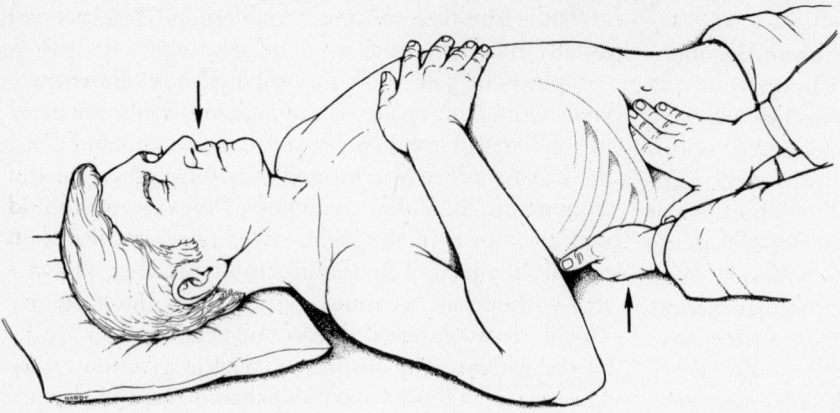

Figure 5-24. Technique for palpation of the liver. As the patient inhales, a palpable liver edge will descend to meet the index finger of the right hand.

consistency, while the liver of acute viral hepatitis is quite soft, and the edge is easily moved by the hand. The spleen likewise may be very firm, as in Hodgkin's disease, or quite soft, as in infectious mononucleosis. (The spleen may be ruptured by vigorous palpation in infectious mononucleosis.) Tenderness of the liver implies recent acute enlargement with consequent stretching of the liver capsule. The absence of tenderness implies that the enlargement is chronic. The liver of viral hepatitis is tender; the liver of alcoholic hepatitis demonstrates no tenderness. The examiner should determine whether the liver edge is sharp and smooth or whether it is blunt. He should determine whether the enlarged liver is nodular or whether its surface is smooth. The nodules of portal cirrhosis are too small to be felt through the abdominal

wall, but the nodules of metastatic malignancy are frequently easily palpable, providing a high index of suspicion of the disease being dealt with. The kidneys of polycystic disease are large, and cyst masses are easily palpable. Although rare, the disease is usually discovered by careful physical examination.

The abdomen should be carefully and systematically palpated for masses that do not represent body organs. The examiner should begin in one quadrant and proceed circumferentially and in narrowing concentric circles. Masses felt should be characterized with respect to size, consistency, presence or absence of tenderness, and whether or not they seem uniform and smooth or multinodular.

HERNIAS. Although many hernias are evident, others, especially those through the inguinal ring, appear only intermittently and with increases in intra-abdominal pressure. The indirect inguinal hernia follows the course of the spermatic cord through the abdominal musculature. One is able to palpate the external inguinal ring and to determine whether it is normal or whether it is widely patent, permitting descent of intra-abdominal contents into a hernial sac. The technique (Fig. 5-25) is as follows:

The male patient may be examined in either a standing or a recumbent position. The examiner should identify the spermatic cord as it disappears under the skin, subcutaneous tissue, and fascia of the anterior abdominal wall. The finger is placed beside the spermatic cord at the very base of the scrotum, catching a small part of the scrotal fold as the finger ascends. The finger should then be advanced under the skin and subcutaneous tissue of the abdominal wall, following the spermatic cord, until the cord is felt to enter the ring of the external oblique muscle. One will feel a small depression that should admit no more than the pad of a fingertip under normal circumstances. This is the inguinal ring. In the presence of a hernia one may be able to pass the finger through the external oblique muscle toward the internal inguinal ring. In the event that the ring is found to be larger than normal, the examiner should ask the patient to bear

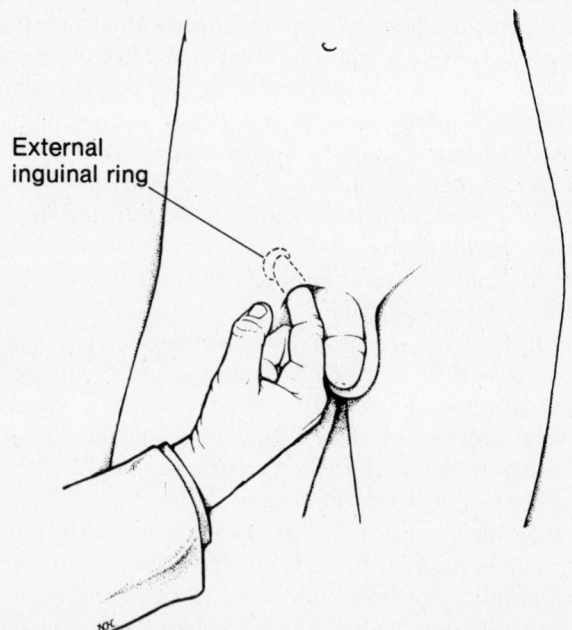

External inguinal ring

Figure 5-25. Technique for the detection of an indirect inguinal hernia. The spermatic cord lies under the index finger and enters the abdomen at the external inguinal ring.

down as though he is having a bowel movement (Valsalva maneuver). If a hernia exists, the examiner will feel a sac of peritoneum with or without omentum or bowel emerging through the external inguinal ring to meet the finger.

Interpretation of the Abdominal Examination

The routine physical examination should include inspection of the abdominal wall for scars of previous surgery and other obvious abnormalities. It should also include attempted palpation of normal body organs (especially liver and spleen) and careful palpation for abnormal masses. Symptoms or signs that refer to the abdomen indicate more thorough examination, as was the case with the examination of the chest and of the cardiovascular system.

THE RECTAL EXAMINATION

The rectal examination is an essential part of the physical assessment of all patients over 40 and should be incorporated as a part of the periodic assessment, probably every year or so, of all patients. The examination may be done in one of several positions (Fig. 5-26). In hospitalized patients who are confined to bed, it is most conveniently performed in the left lateral position with the patient lying on the left side, his right knee drawn up to the level of his chest. In the office the examination may be done with the patient bending over the examining table. Female patients are most conveniently examined in a dorsolithotomy position at the same time that the pelvic examination is being conducted. Further discussion of the examination of the female patient will be deferred until the section on examination of the genital system (see page 80).

ANAL CANAL.   The examiner should first note the anus, observing whether external hemorrhoidal tags are present and whether the anus is free of fissures and fistuli. The index finger of the gloved hand should be lubricated and inserted slowly into the anal canal. The examiner should note whether good sphincter tone is present, and then should slowly advance the index finger along the anal canal and into the rectum. Internal hemorrhoids are not palpable unless they are thrombosed.

PROSTATE.   The plum-sized normal prostate usually has a median raphe (indentation) and is felt on the ventral surface of the rectal wall. On either side of the prostate the rectal folds fall away. The finger should be swept around the rectal mucosa, observing for masses or polyps. Fecal material which may be mistaken for polypoid masses may be differentiated by sweeping them away from the rectal mucosa. The prostate should be carefully palpated for enlargement or for stony hard masses within its resilient body. Hard masses within the prostate usually represent malignancy.

FECES.   When the finger is withdrawn, fecal material will usually cling to the glove. This material should be examined by appropriate solutions for content that may represent blood within the stool.

EXAMINATION OF THE GENITALIA

Genital examination is a part of the complete physical examination in all circumstances. Most health professionals understand this basic principle when examining female patients, especially since the advent of the highly

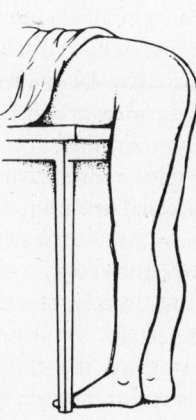

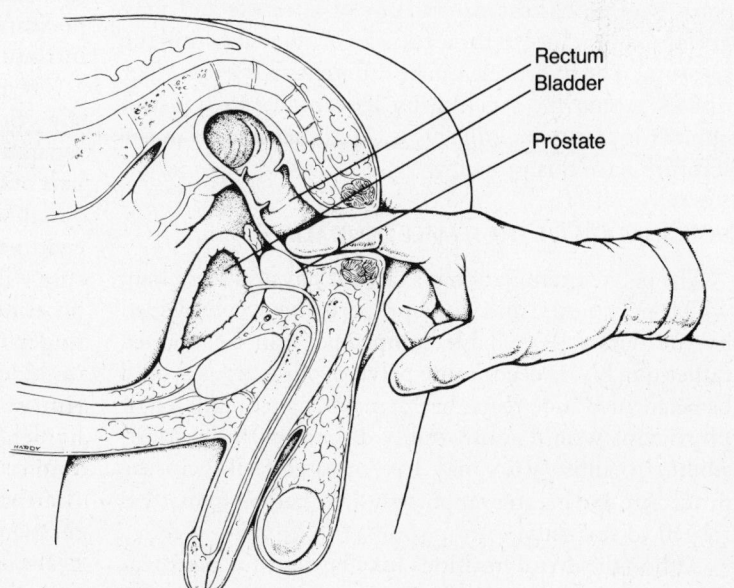

Rectum
Bladder

Prostate

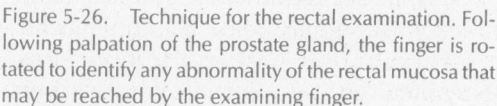

Figure 5-26.   Technique for the rectal examination. Following palpation of the prostate gland, the finger is rotated to identify any abnormality of the rectal mucosa that may be reached by the examining finger.

efficacious Papanicolaou smear for cancer of the cervix. Too frequently, however, they fail to give the male genitalia the same careful attention.

EXAMINATION OF THE MALE GENITALIA

The penis of the male may be observed for the location of the urethral opening and for any lesions along the skin of the shaft. An abnormal location of the urethral opening along the dorsal midline of the shaft is called *epispadias;* an abnormal urethral opening along the ventral surface of the shaft is called *hypospadias*. The examiner should observe whether or not the penis has been circumcised. If uncircumcised, the foreskin should be retracted back from the glans penis. Inability of the foreskin to be retracted over the glans is called *phimosis*. Occasionally, inflammation of the foreskin in a retracted position does not allow the foreskin to be drawn forward over the glans. This circumstance is called *paraphimosis*. The glans of the uncircumcised penis should be palpated, especially in older individuals, to determine if any part of it has a firmer consistency than the remainder. This is indicative of carcinoma of the glans penis. Carcinoma of the circumcised penis does not occur.

The scrotum and its contents also should be examined. Normal testes are of firm consistency and measure 6 to 8 cm. (2½ to 3 inches) in their longest polar length. Testes of less than 4 cm. (1½ inches) in polar length are atrophied or represent abnormal development (Klinefelter's syndrome). The testicles should be palpated for firm masses within their substance. Other masses within the scrotum include the *varicocele* and the *hydrocele*. The varicocele represents enlargement of the pampiniform plexus of veins that surrounds the spermatic cord and feels like a "bag of worms." The hydrocele is a collection of fluid within a peritoneal remnant lying along the spermatic cord. It often has the consistency of a testicle and may give the appearance of three testicles contained within the scrotum. The hydrocele can be differentiated from other masses within the scrotum by its capacity to transmit light. It is said to *transilluminate*. No other masses in the scrotum have this property.

EXAMINATION OF THE FEMALE GENITALIA

The pelvic examination is a facet of physical asessment which may easily, and quite properly, be accomplished by the nurse. Reasonable competency can be attained rather quickly. Indeed, more pelvic examinations would be performed and greater health maintenance rendered, if physicians would comfortably discharge this responsibility to those who may have greater facility in the procedure and greater rapport with the patient in matters related to sexuality.

Although several positions may be used for performing the pelvic examination, the dorsolithotomy position is preferred and is more amenable to office practice. If the examiner is required to perform the pelvic assessment in the hospital on a patient who is too ill to be placed on a table equipped with stirrups, the *Sims' position* may be used. In the Sims' position the patient lies on her left side with her left arm behind her and her right leg bent at a 90-degree angle. The right labia may be retracted for adequate access to the vagina.

The patient should be instructed to void prior to the pelvic examination. The urine may be retained, if a urine specimen is part of the total assessment procedure. The patient should then be placed on the table in stirrups and encouraged to relax so that her buttocks are presented at the edge of the examination table and her thighs spread as widely apart as possible. The patient should be appropriately draped to avoid embarrassment should other members of the health team enter the room.

The left hand should be gloved so that the right hand is free to use appropriate instruments. (Left-handed persons should reverse this instruction.) When the patient is prepared, the *labia majora* and *minora* should be examined. The epidermal tissue of the labia majora, with its hair follicles characteristic of skin, fades to the pink mucous membrane of the vaginal introitus. In the nulliparous woman the labia minora should come together at the opening of the vagina. In women who have borne children, the labia minora may gape and vaginal tissue may protrude. The patient should be asked to bear down. Birth damage to the anterior vaginal wall may have resulted in incompetency of musculature so that a bulge representing bladder intrusion into the submucosa of the anterior vaginal wall may be seen. This is called a *cystocele*. Analogously, such trauma may have affected the posterior vaginal wall so that a bulge representing the cavity of the rectum may protrude, presenting as a *rectocele*. The cervix or the uterus itself may descend under pressure through the vaginal canal and present itself at the introitus. This is termed *prolapse* of the uterus.

The introitus should be free of hair follicles and free of superficial mucosal lesions. The labia minora may be separated by the fingers of the gloved hand and the lower part of the vagina palpated. In virginal women a *hymen* of variable thickness may be felt circumferentially within a centimeter or two of the vaginal opening. The hymeneal ring will usually permit the admission of two fingers, but occasionally is sufficiently restricting so that only one finger may enter the vagina. Rarely, the hymen totally occludes the vaginal entrance. In nonvirginal women a rim of scar tissue representing the remnants of the hymeneal ring may be felt circumferentially around the vagina near its opening. The greater vestibular glands (Bartholin's glands) lie between the labia minora and the remnants of the hymeneal ring. These glands frequently become infected in gonococcal disease. Patients may occasionally present with an abscess of one of these glands.

Speculum Examination

Three sizes of the bivalved Graves' speculum are available. The speculum may be warmed with running tap water to make it less uncomfortable when it is inserted. It should not be lubricated, since lubrication with commercial jellies may interfere with the examination of the cervical cytology. Two setscrews may be seen on the speculum. One is along the handle and holds the two valves of the speculum together. This one should be tightened. The setscrew that holds the thumb-rest in place should be loosened. The speculum should be grasped in the right hand with the thumb against the back of the thumb-rest in order to keep the tips of the valves closed. The speculum should be rotated slightly counterclockwise, and the vaginal orifice held open by the thumb and the forefinger of the gloved left hand. The speculum should be gently inserted into the posterior portion of the introitus and slowly advanced to the top of the vagina (Fig. 5-27). The tip of the speculum may then be elevated and the speculum rotated to a transverse position. The speculum is then slowly opened and should reveal the cervix of the uterus. The cervix having been brought into view, the setscrew of the thumb-rest may be tightened to hold the speculum open.

The cervical os should first be cultured. This is particularly important if any purulent material appears at its opening. Many authorities now advocate routine culture for gonococcus in light of the evidence that the disease is now ubiquitous in the population, afflicting all age groups and all socioeconomic strata. Gonococcal disease is silent in more than one third of the women afflicted by it. Culture may be done with a cotton-tip applicator and immediately placed in an appropriate medium for transmission to the laboratory.

The next procedure is the scraping of the cervix for cancer cytology by the *Papanicolaou* method with a wooden spatula specially constructed for the purpose.

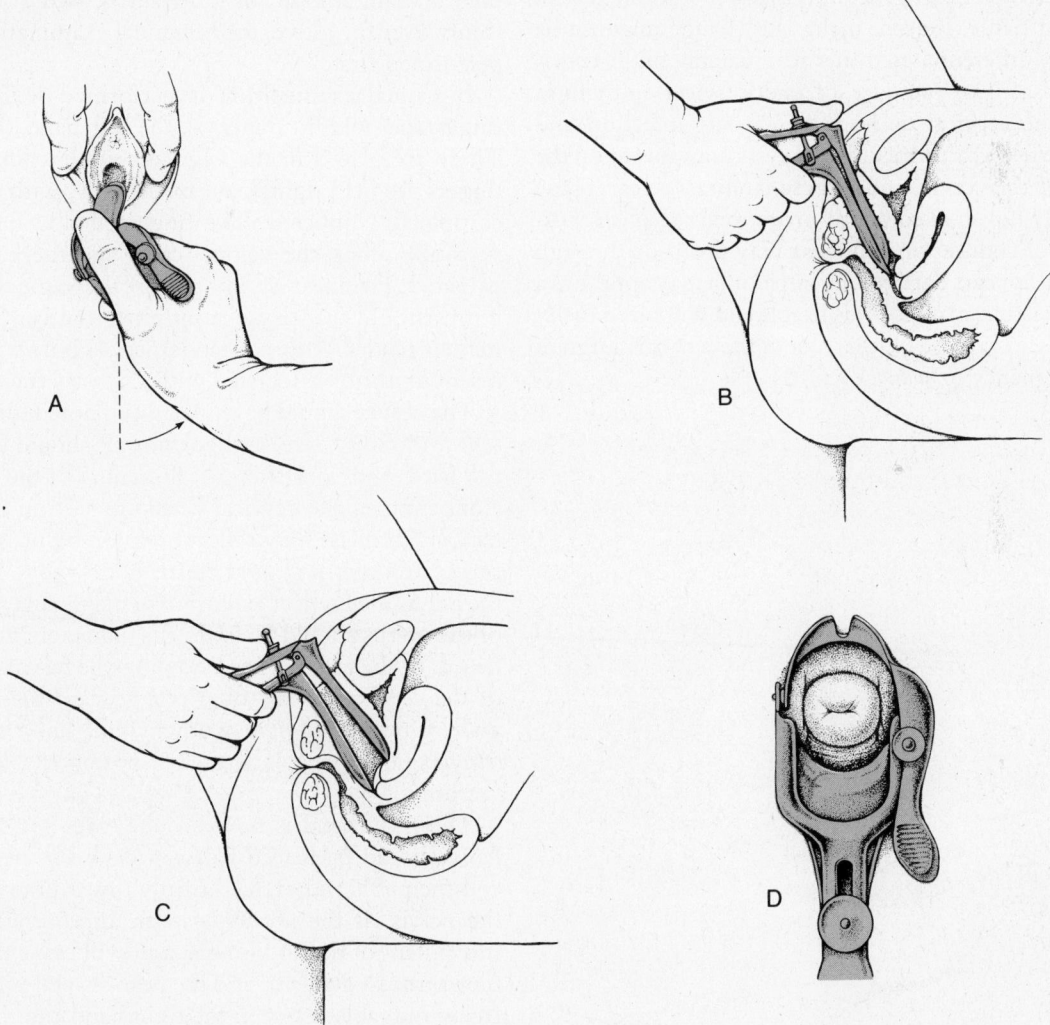

Figure 5-27. Technique for speculum examination of the vagina and cervix.

The tip of the spatula should be placed in the cervical os and the spatula rotated 360 degrees firmly but non-traumatically (Fig. 44-4). Cellular material clinging to the spatula should then be smeared on a glass slide, and the slide promptly placed in fixative solution or sprayed with commercially available fixative material. It should then be transmitted to the laboratory along with culture material that may have been extracted from the cervical os.

The cervix should now be inspected. In nulliparous women, the cervical os will be 2 to 3 mm. in diameter and smooth. Women who have borne children may have a laceration, usually transverse, frequently giving the cervical os a "fishmouth" appearance. Moreover, epithelium from the endocervical canal may have grown out onto the surface of the cervix, appearing as beefy red surface epithelium circumferentially arranged around the os. This is commonly called a *cervical erosion*. Although not always differentiable from a cervical carcinoma, the cervical erosion is, in general, less sharply outlined than malignant tissue. Indeed, malignant change may not be obviously differentiated from the remainder of the cervical mucosa. The presence of endocervical epithelium around the cervical os leads to chronic infection and discharge from the orifice. Small cysts may appear on the surface of the cervix under these circumstances. These are usually bluish in color and are termed *nabothian cysts*. A polyp of endocervical mucosa may protrude through the os and appears dark red. A carcinoma may appear as a cauliflower-like growth. It is friable and will bleed easily when traumatized. A bluish color of the cervix is a sign of early pregnancy (*Chadwick's sign*).

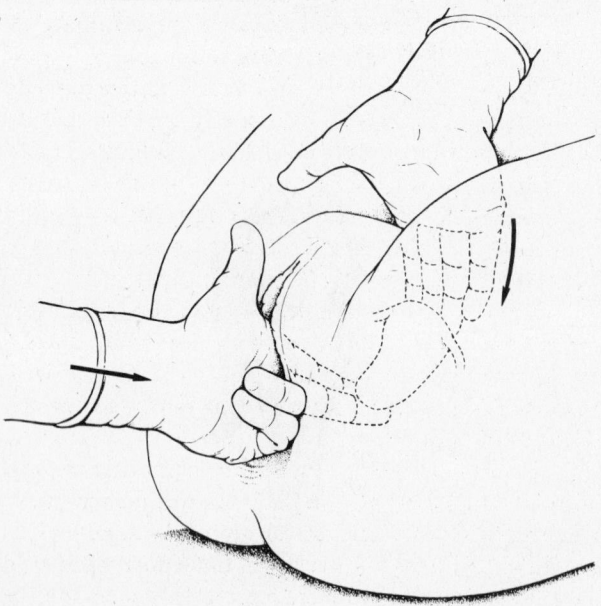

Figure 5-28. Technique for the bimanual examination of the pelvis in the female.

The vagina may be examined as the speculum is withdrawn. It is smooth in young girls and becomes more thickened after puberty, with many rugae and much redundancy in the epithelium. Vaginal discharge may be present. Discharge due to bacteria is yellow and has a purulent appearance. Discharge due to Trichomonas is thin and watery, often yellow, and occasionally frothy. Discharge due to Monilia is thick and white and may have a cheesy appearance. As the speculum is withdrawn, the patient is again instructed to bear down. If the speculum is rotated, a cystocele or rectocele may well bulge into the vaginal canal.

Bimanual Examination

Some physicians prefer to perform the bimanual examination before the speculum examination. On the other hand, the bimanual examination requires lubrication of the gloved left hand, which may interfere with cytologic examination of the cervical smear. However, if only a small amount of lubricant is used and is spread thinly over the glove, the bimanual examination may be performed first.

Bimanual examination is performed with the forefinger and middle finger of the left hand (Fig. 5-28). These are placed in the vaginal orifice while the other fingers are held tightly out of the way, with the thumb completely adducted. The fingers should be advanced vertically along the vaginal canal and the vaginal wall palpated. Firmness of any part of the vaginal wall may represent old scar tissue from birth trauma. Such tissue may be tender. Anterior tenderness or burning may represent urethritis associated with a urinary tract infection.

The cervix should be palpated and noted for its consistency, mobility, size, and position. It should be firm but not hard, and uniformly so. Softening of the cervix and elongation of the cervical canal are seen in early pregnancy. Hardness may reflect invasion by neoplasia. The cervix and uterus should be freely movable. Fixation in the pelvis may reflect extension of malignancy. The body of the uterus should be twice the diameter and twice the length of the cervix. The body may be felt on either side of the cervix curving anteriorly toward the abdominal wall. One out of five women will, however, have a *retroflexed* uterus which curves posteriorly toward the sacrum.

The right hand is now brought into play. The right hand should be placed halfway between the umbilicus and the pubis and pressed firmly toward the opening of the pelvis. If the uterus is in an appropriate position, movement of the abdominal wall will cause the body of the uterus to descend, and the pear-shaped organ will be freely movable between the right hand and the examining fingers of the left hand. A reasonably accurate impression can be gained of the size, mobility, and regularity of contour of the uterus.

The right and left parametria should now be palpated. The tube and ovary are contained within these structures. The fingers of the left hand are moved first to one side, then to the other, while the right hand is moved correspondingly to either side of the abdominal wall. The adnexae should be trapped beween the two examining hands and should be palpated for obvious mass, tenderness of adnexal tissue, and mobility of the parametrial contents.

RECTOABDOMINAL EXAMINATION

Examination of the rectum is, of course, a normal part of the physical examination and can be done immediately after the pelvic examination. It may be useful in selected instances to use the rectal approach to palpate the pelvic contents. Examples include young virginal women whose vaginas may not admit the examining fingers, women whose vaginas have been foreshortened by surgery and/or irradiation, and those who are suspected of having abnormal tissue present in the parametria. The parametria wing back posteriorly from the uterus and are more accurately palpable from the rectal approach. The gloved finger of the left hand may be inserted into the rectum and the right hand used to compress the abdominal wall in a manner analogous to the bimanual examination of the vagina. The uterus should be easily palpable, and the adnexal structures, which include the ovary and the fallopian tube, may be palpated by moving the finger to the left and right of the cervix.

Upon withdrawal of the finger from the rectum, fecal material clinging to the glove may be smeared and stained appropriately for blood and iron products as in any rectal examination.

THE NEUROLOGICAL EXAMINATION

Although the neurological examination may be limited in most instances to a simple screening, it is necessary for the examiner to be able to conduct a reasonably thorough neurological assessment if the history or other physical findings warrant it. In capable hands, the neurological examination is a sophisticated and subtle process, comprising a large number of tests of highly specialized function that allow the knowledgeable clinician to localize neurological disease and assess the probabilities of cause. Unlike respiratory, cardiac, or abdominal diseases, neurological disease does not remain hidden and is not likely to be asymptomatic. On the contrary, a neoplastic or vascular lesion no larger than a pencil eraser can wreak havoc with the central nervous system if located in a critical area. Tumors of the brain are fatal not because they metastasize but because, in a tightly confined space, they interfere with critical function.

As in other facets of the physical assessment, the neurological examination follows a logical sequence and should be pursued from higher levels of cortical function through to a determination of the integrity of peripheral nerves.

Much of the patient's neurological function can be assessed during the examiner's effort to obtain a history and during the routine of the earlier parts of the physical examination. One can learn much about speech patterns, mental status, gait, stance, motor power, and coordination. The simple act of shaking a patient's hand as he enters the room conveys an enormous amount of information to the alert observer. Certain neurologic illnesses present in characteristic ways. The appearance of the patient with Parkinson's disease is immediately evident upon inspection. This syndrome carries with it a masklike facial appearance, a characteristic tremor, and a unique gait. Similarly, one may easily recognize the patient with Huntington's disease, hemiparesis, tabes dorsalis, and many other characteristic neurologic syndromes.

Mental Status

Higher intellectual function should be tested in the event that any doubt exists about the patient's intellectual competence. Often patients in a toxic state, or those who have destruction of frontal cortex, may appear superficially normal until or unless one or more tests of integrative capacity are performed. First, the examiner should determine whether the patient is oriented to time, place, and person. Does the patient know what day it is, what year it is, or who is the president of the United States? Is the patient aware of where he is? Is the patient aware of who you are, and of his purpose for being in the room? Is the capacity for immediate memory intact? A person with an average I.Q. should be able to repeat seven digits without faltering and should be able to recite five digits backwards. The examiner might ask the patient to count backwards from 100, or to subtract 7 from 100, then 7 from that, then 7 from that, etc. The capacity to interpret well-known proverbs is a test of even higher intellectual function. Does the patient know what is meant by "The early bird catches the worm"?

It is important to determine thought content, but this usually emerges in the course of the interview. Preoccupation with death or morbid events, evidence of hallucinations, paranoid ideation, are all important and can be diagnostically critical.

The examiner may now look at more specific areas of higher cortical function. *Agnosia* is the inability to interpret or recognize objects seen through the special senses. The individual may see a pen but not know what it is called or what to do with it. He may even be able to describe it but not to interpret its function. The patient may experience auditory or tactile agnosia, as well as visual agnosia. Each of the dysfunctions implicates a different part of the cortex.

The impairment to understanding or using speech is called *aphasia*. Right-handed persons usually have a dominant left cerebral hemisphere, and vice versa. A mass lesion or infarction of the dominant hemisphere will result in varying degrees of aphasia. There are a wide variety of expressions of aphasia that reflect lesions that may be located in the frontal, parietal, or temporal cortex. While a knowledge of the anatomical relationships required for proper analysis is not necessary, the examiner should be able to elicit a speech abnormality. In a *motor aphasia,* the patient is unable to articulate well. He may delete pronouns and other small words in his sentence structure. He may use incorrect words, and in the extreme, this takes on the characteristic of jargon speech. This latter phenomenon is termed *paraphasia*. Some patients, on seeing a familiar object, are unable to name it, although they have no difficulty understanding the purpose or function of the object. Other patients are incapable of reading, although they may use speech correctly. This is termed *dyslexia*. Aphasia should be differentiated from *dysarthria*. Dysarthria is the loss of the capacity to articulate and may be a function of cranial nerve damage rather than central or cortical dysfunction.

Interpretation of neurological abnormalities is a highly sophisticated and technical process. It is the obligation of the examiner to record and report what is found. Analysis, and the conclusions that may be drawn from these findings, will usually depend upon extensive knowledge of neuroanatomy, neurophysiology, and neuropathology.

Examination of the Cranial Nerves

There are 12 pairs of cranial nerves that emerge from the undersurface of the brain. They are designated by the Roman numerals I to XII according to the order of their placement.

The cranial nerves may be tested in order, as follows:

CRANIAL NERVE I (OLFACTORY NERVE). Sense of smell may be assessed through the use of a nonirritating substance. The patient is asked to close his eyes and identify tobacco, the mint odor of lifesavers, soap, etc. Substances such as ammonia are astringent and are identified by the irritation they produce rather than by their odor. On the other hand, the claim of inability to identify the odor of a noxious substance such as ammonia may be helpful in identifying the hysteric and distinguishing that individual from the person who has a true loss of the sense of smell.

CRANIAL NERVES II (OPTIC NERVE), III (OCULOMOTOR NERVE), IV (TROCHLEAR NERVE, AND VI (ABDUCENS NERVE). The function and method of assessing these nerves has been covered under the discussion of the eye, and may be referred to for review. (See page 54.)

CRANIAL NERVE V (TRIGEMINAL NERVE). The trigeminal nerve supplies motor fibers to the muscles of the jaw and sensation to the entire face and cornea. Adequate function of the motor component may be determined by having the patient clench his jaw and move it from side to side against a resisting hand. The sensory component of the trigeminal nerve is represented in three branches. The first emerges above the orbit; the second emerges through the maxilla; and the third emerges through the mandible. Competence may be assessed by determining the patient's sensitivity to pinprick over the distribution of all three branches. A wisp of cotton touched against the temporal surface of the cornea should elicit a blink if sensation is intact. This is termed the *corneal reflex*.

CRANIAL NERVE VII (FACIAL NERVE). The facial nerve provides motor fibers to all of the muscles of the face and accounts for taste on the anterior two thirds of the tongue. Integrity of the facial nerve may be assessed by asking the patient to make facial grimaces, including showing the teeth and wrinkling the forehead. When paralyzed, the affected side of the face will appear smooth, without wrinkles or expression. One should pay particular attention to the forehead. Since forehead musculature is supplied from fibers deriving from both sides of the cortex, cortical damage accompanying a stroke will not interfere with the capacity to wrinkle the forehead, even though the remainder of the face may have lost its capacity for function. On the other hand, direct injury of the facial nerve will result in uniform loss of function over the entire side of the face, including the forehead. A common but subtle sign of facial malfunction is the loss of normal creasing of the affected side of the face, accompanied by a slight droop of the mouth. Asymmetry of the face should lead one to examine carefully facial nerve function.

Taste is provided to the anterior third of the tongue by sensory fibers that accompany the facial nerves. Taste may be assessed by the patient's capacity to discriminate among sweet, salty, bitter, and sour substances.

CRANIAL NERVE VIII (ACOUSTIC NERVE). The auditory component of the function of the acoustic nerve is discussed earlier, under examination of the ear. Deafness may derive either from a conduction defect in the middle ear or from a neurologic deficit in the inner ear or along the course of the acoustic nerve. The Weber and Rinne tests will distinguish between these two sources of hearing difficulty. These should be reviewed from the earlier discussion.

The vestibular branch of the acoustic nerve innervates the semicircular canals and provides sensory input for the maintenance of balance. Abnormalities of the vestibular portion of the acoustic nerve will be reflected in *nystagmus*. Instruct the patient to look to the side. If nystagmus is present, the patient will have difficulty maintaining deviation of the eye. The eye will tend to drift toward the center and then snap back toward the deviated position. More sophisticated testing of the vestibular component of the acoustic nerve is accomplished by irrigating the ear canal with ice water. In this instance, integrity of the vestibular component of the eighth nerve will result in vertigo and nystagmus. Its absence indicates abnormality.

CRANIAL NERVE IX (GLOSSOPHARYNGEAL NERVE). The ninth nerve is responsible for taste in the posterior portion of the tongue and, in conjunction with the tenth nerve, results in coordinated pharyngeal contraction. The absence of a gag reflex may be attributed to damage of the ninth nerve, although this is a normal finding in many persons.

CRANIAL NERVE X (VAGUS NERVE). Although the vagus nerve plays an enormous role in autonomic function, it is difficult to assess its competence by physical examination. If one or the other vagus nerve is damaged, however, the uvula will be seen to deviate toward the normal side when the patient is asked to make a sound with his mouth open. If the patient can swallow normally and speak clearly, the vagus nerve is almost certainly intact.

CRANIAL NERVE XI (SPINAL ACCESSORY NERVE). The spinal accessory nerve innervates the sternocleidomastoid and trapezius muscles. The patient may be asked to raise his shoulder against resistance and turn his head against opposing pressure exerted by the examiner's hand.

CRANIAL NERVE XII (HYPOGLOSSAL NERVE). The hypoglossal nerve innervates motor function of the tongue. Damage to this nerve will result in deviation of the tongue toward the involved side when the patient is asked to protrude his tongue. Atrophy of the tongue is seen early in lesions of the twelfth nerve.

Examination of the Motor System

The motor system is quite complex, and the end result of motor function is a synthesis of the integrity of the corticospinal tracts, the extrapyramidal system, and cerebellar function. A motor impulse traverses two neurons. The *upper motor neuron* begins in the cortex of the opposite side of the brain, descends through the internal capsule, crosses to the opposite side in the brain stem, descends through the corticospinal tract, and synapses with the *lower motor neuron* in the cord. The lower motor neuron receives the impulse in the posterior part of the cord and runs to the myoneural junction. The other two systems, the extrapyramidal system and the cerebellar system, act as modifiers. When abnormality exists, it is the function of the examination to discern whether the problem lies with the upper motor neuron, the lower motor neuron, the extrapyramidal system, or the cerebellar system.

One begins by testing muscle strength. This is best accomplished by ascertaining the patient's ability to flex or extend his extremity against resistance. The function of an individual muscle or group of muscles is evaluated by placing the muscle at a disadvantage. The quadriceps, for example, is a powerful muscle responsible for straightening the leg. Once the leg is straightened, it is exceedingly difficult for the examiner to flex the knee. On the other hand, if the knee is flexed, and the patient is asked to straighten the leg against resistance, a more subtle disability can be brought out. It is critically important to compare the two sides if one is looking for minor degrees of disability.

Some authorities have advocated the use of a five-point scale for strength of motor power. A five would indicate full power of contraction; a four would indicate fair, but not full, strength; a three would imply just sufficient strength to overcome the force of gravity; a two indicates the ability to move but not to overcome the force of gravity; a one indicates minimal contractile power; a zero implies no contraction whatsoever.

Assessment of motor power can be as restricted or detailed as the examiner wishes. One may quickly test the strength of the proximal muscles of the upper and lower extremities, comparing the two. The motor capacity of the finer muscles that control the function of the hand and of the foot can then be assessed. Weakness may result from a lesion within the brain or spinal cord, or from disease of the peripheral nerves. Disease of the brain or spinal cord is referred to as an *upper motor neuron lesion;* disease of the peripheral nerve is referred to as a *lower motor neuron lesion*. Upper motor neuron lesions result in spastic paralysis and are accompanied by rigidity and hyperactive reflexes. Usually, under these circumstances, fine movements are lost while more gross function of powerful proximal muscles is preserved. Lower motor neuron lesions are associated with flaccidity of muscle groups, atrophy of muscles, and marked decrease in or absence of reflex activity.

Extrapyramidal disease (Parkinson's disease, for example) results in rigidity, even though motor power is intact. This can best be tested by alternately flexing and extending a limb in order to demonstrate rigidity of the muscle groups that control the action of that limb. In the instance of Parkinson's disease, there is a "jerking" quality to the rigidity that is referred to as *cogwheeling*. Other features of extrapyramidal disease include the loss of those associated movements that give the body its fluid gait. The face takes on the appearance of a plastic mask. In addition, there are spontaneous tremors that are characterized by being present when the patient is at rest.

Cerebellar influence on the motor system is reflected in discoordination and tremor. The discoordination is referred to as *ataxia*. This is expressed in an incapacity to perform rapid alternating movements, and an inability to carry out coordinated movements such as placing the finger on the nose or running the heel down the anterior surface of the tibia. More gross ataxic movements include *athetoid* movements, which are writhing and dance-like, and *choreic* movements, which are quick, erratic, and spontaneous, so that the patient appears to be lurching from position to position. Involuntary movements of muscles or muscle groups that are abrupt are called *myoclonus*. Tremor due to cerebellar disease does not occur at rest, but occurs during action as the patient is about to touch or lift an object. This is called an *action tremor*.

Examination of the Reflexes (Fig. 5-29)

The motor reflexes are involuntary contractions of muscles or muscle groups in response to abrupt stretching near the site of the muscle's insertion. The tendon is struck directly with a reflex hammer, or indirectly by striking the examiner's thumb, which is placed firmly against the tendon. In testing the reflexes, we are examining involuntary reflex arcs that depend upon the presence of afferent stretch receptors, spinal synapses, efferent motor fibers, and a variety of modifying influences from higher levels. Common reflexes that may be tested include the biceps, the brachioradialis, the triceps, the quadriceps, and the gastrocnemius. Wide variation in reflex response may be considered normal. However, it is more important that the reflexes be symmetrically equivalent. When the comparison is made, both sides should be equivalently relaxed and each tendon struck with equal force. The absence of reflexes is significant, although ankle jerks (gastrocnemius reflex) might well be absent in older people.

The *biceps reflex* is elicited by striking the biceps tendon of the flexed elbow. The examiner should support the forearm with one arm, while placing the thumb against the tendon and striking the thumb with the reflex hammer. The *triceps reflex* is elicited by striking the triceps tendon just above the elbow. The *patellar reflex* is brought out by striking the patellar tendon of the flexed and relaxed knee. The *Achilles reflex (ankle jerk)* is elicited by striking the stretched Achilles tendon.

When reflexes are exceedingly hyperactive, a phenomenon called *clonus* may be elicited. If the foot is abruptly dorsiflexed, it may "chatter" for two or three beats before it settles into a position of rest. Occasionally in central nervous system disease, this activity will persist, and the foot will not come to rest while the tendon is being stretched but will persist in repetitive activity. The unsustained clonus associated with normal but hyperactive reflexes is not considered pathological. Sustained clonus always indicates the presence of nervous system disease.

Certain superficial reflexes may be elicited by scratching the skin of the abdominal wall or the inside of the thigh in men. The former results in involuntary contraction of the abdominal muscles, and the latter results in retraction of the scrotum. Although interesting phenomena, they have little clinical significance.

A well-known reflex, indicative of central nervous system disease afflicting the corticospinal tracts, is the *Babinski sign*. If the lateral aspect of the sole of the foot is stroked in normal persons, the toes will contract and be drawn tightly together. In persons with central disease of the motor system, the toes will fan out and be drawn back. This is normal in newborn infants but represents serious pathology in the adult. There are a variety of described reflexes which convey similar information. Many of them are interesting, but not particularly informative.

Sensory Examination

The sensory system is even more complex than the motor system, since sensory modalities are carried in different tracts, located in different portions of the cord. It is well to remember that the sensory examination is largely subjective and requires the cooperation of the patient. It is common for patients who are malingering or hysterical to report absence of sensation, when in fact this is not so. It would be well for the examiner to become familiar with dermatomes that represent the distribution of the peripheral nerves that ramify from the spinal cord. Most sensory deficits result from peripheral neuropathy and will follow anatomic dermatomes. Exceptions to this include major destructive lesions of the brain, loss of sensation which may affect an entire side of the body, and the neuropathies associated with alcoholism which occur in a glove and stocking distribution.

Pain and temperature sensation are carried together in the lateral part of the cord. Thus, it is not necessary to test for temperature sense in most circumstances. Pain may be assessed by determining the patient's sensitivity to pinprick. The pin must be applied with equal intensity at all times and the two sides tested symmetrically.

The fibers for *touch* may be tested by having the patient close his eyes while the examiner touches him with a wisp of cotton and has him indicate where he has been touched.

Vibration and proprioception (the subjective sense of joint position) are carried together in the posterior part of the cord. Vibration may be evaluated through the use of a low frequency (128 or 256 CPS) tuning fork. The handle of the vibrating fork should be placed against a bony prominence and the patient asked whether or not he feels a buzz. He should signal the examiner when the buzz ceases. Position sense may be determined by asking the patient to close his eyes and indicate, as the toes are moved, in which direction movement has taken place. Vibration and position sense will be lost together, frequently in circumstances where all others remain intact.

Having tested peripheral sensation, one must now ask the question, whether *integration of sensation* in the brain is being carried out properly. This may be done by testing two-point discrimination. That is, if the patient is

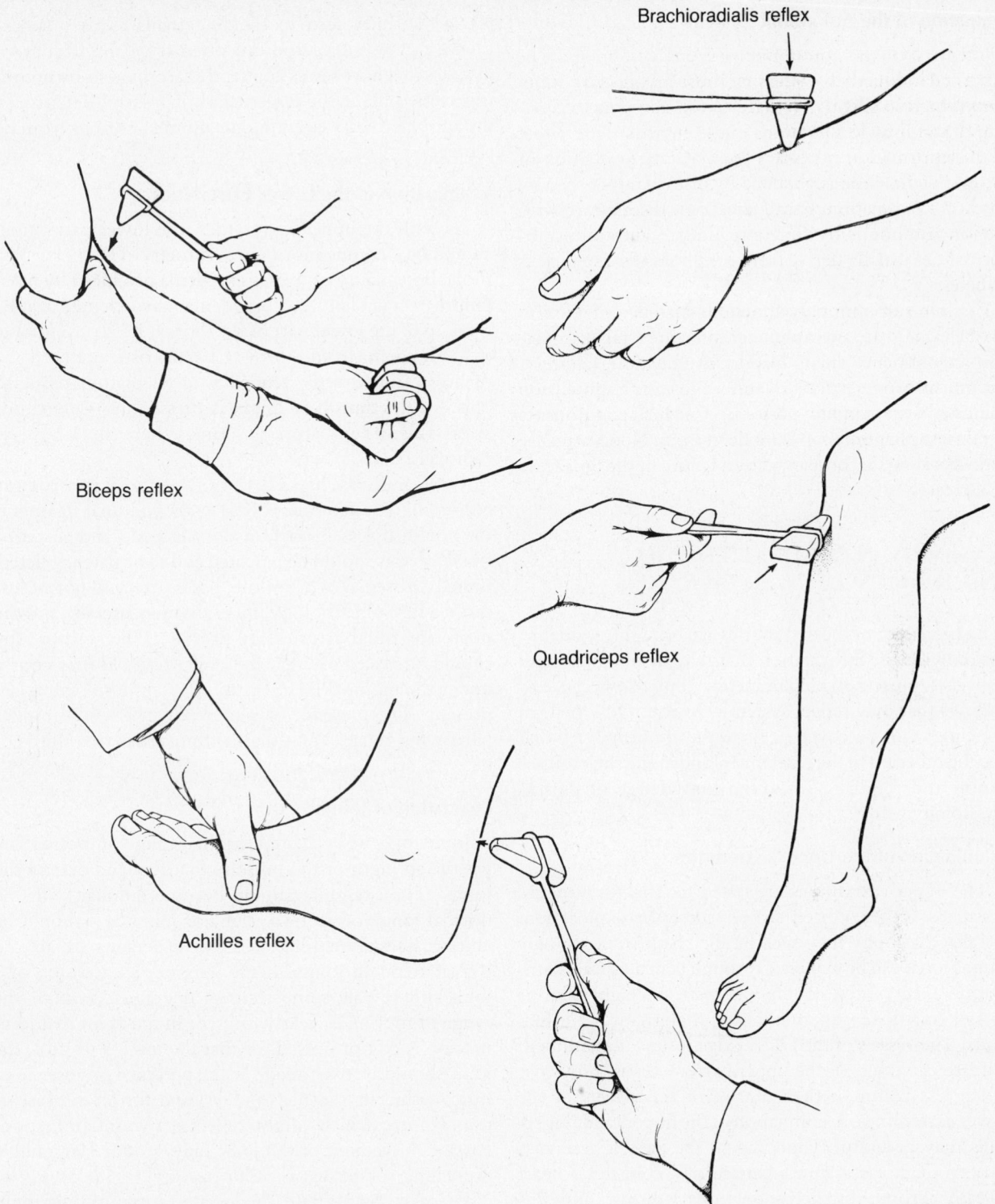

Brachioradialis reflex

Biceps reflex

Quadriceps reflex

Achilles reflex

Figure 5-29. Proper technique for the elicitation of the major tendon reflexes. The tendon is struck directly with the reflex hammer. Normal reflexes are symmetrical.

touched with two sharp objects simultaneously, are they perceived as two, or as one? If a patient is touched simultaneously on opposite sides of the body, he should normally recognize that he has been touched in two places. If he recognizes only one, the one not recognized is said to demonstrate *extinction*. A good test of higher cortical sensory ability is that of *stereognosis*. The patient should be instructed to close his eyes and identify a variety of objects (keys, coins, etc.) which are placed in his hand by the examiner.

Evaluation of the Autonomic System

Integrity of the autonomic nervous system may be evaluated indirectly by assessing those involuntary functions which so silently, yet effectively, allow us to function through wide alterations in the environment. Most of the information necessary for accurate evaluation of autonomic function is obtained by history rather than by physical examination. Focal neurologic disease rarely results in autonomic dysfunction. Rather, autonomic abnormalities usually derive from metabolic disease such as diabetes.

Possible autonomic dysfunctions include: a failure to sweat, inadequate anal sphincter tone on rectal examination, incontinence due to bladder dysfunction, failure of erection and/or ejaculation, and orthostatic hypotension (fainting in the standing position). Cardinal components of this last phenomenon are a decrease in blood pressure upon standing, accompanied by a failure of the pulse rate to increase.

EXAMINATION OF THE EXTREMITIES AND THE MUSCULOSKELETAL SYSTEM

Examination of the extremities can be highly valuable, not only for the information that may be obtained with respect to musculoskeletal function, but also because of findings that may reflect systemic disease. Only general principles will be covered, since the abnormalities that may be reflected in the extremities and in the skeleton are legion and require substantial knowledge of pathophysiology.

Examination of the Upper Extremities

The upper extremities are noted for their symmetry. Localized or generalized atrophy deserves exploration. Localized atrophy may well be the result of neurologic damage that can be explored through neurological examination. Generalized atrophy may reflect weight loss due to systemic disease — metabolic, malignant, or infectious. The vessels of the upper extremities are examined. Disease of vessels of the upper extremities is, however, much less common than disease of the vessels of the lower extremities. Examination of the fingers and fingernails may be useful. Clubbing of the nails is seen in a variety of diseases, most particularly congenital heart disease, chronic obstructive pulmonary disease, and cancer of the lung. Fingernails grow rapidly, replicating themselves in 4 to 6 months. The growth of the fingernail requires the capacity to synthesize body protein. Chronic disease or acute disease which interferes for a period of time with protein building may transiently halt the growth of the fingernail. This may then be reflected in transverse lines seen in the fingernails as they subsequently grow out. One can often trace the history of diseases that have remissions and exacerbations by noting transverse lines in the fingernails much as one determines the age of a tree by counting the number of rings from its center.

Examination of the Lower Extremities

As with the upper extremities, the lower extremities should be examined for their symmetry. The most common abnormality of the legs is edema produced by heart failure or renal failure. This edema may extend variably, even up to the lower part of the thorax. It is conventional to grade edema from 1 to 4+. Characteristic of the edema of heart failure is the tendency of edematous tissue to "pit." If the thumb or finger is pressed into edematous skin, the indentation remains when the finger is removed.

Vascular disease of the lower extremities is exceedingly common. The femoral vessels at the inguinal ligament, the popliteal vessels, and the dorsalis pedis and posterior tibial arteries should be palpated and their patency determined. Absence of a dorsalis pedis artery is not necessarily a sign of pathology if it is absent bilaterally and the posterior tibial arteries are present. The stethoscope should be placed over the femoral arteries as they course under the inguinal ligament to ascertain if murmurs are present. The presence of a murmur in a vessel implies narrowing to an extent that compromises two thirds of its cross sectional area.

Evaluation of Joints

Joints may be evaluated for their range of motion and for the strength of the muscles that flex and extend the joints. The examiner should become familiar with the normal range of motion of major joints and should be able to assess functional loss. Most persons are able to hyperextend all joints. If the maximum extension of a joint still reveals some residual degree of flexion, the range of motion is clearly limited. In the event that joint motion is compromised, or that the joint is painful, the joint should be examined for the presence or absence of fluid within its capsule (*effusion*) and for an increase in temperature which might reflect active inflammation. Passive movement of the joint may produce an audible crunching sound that is called *crepitus*.

Diseased joints and the tissues surrounding them should be examined for nodule formation. Rheumatoid arthritis, gout, osteoarthritis, and rheumatic fever, all produce characteristic nodules that are diagnostic of the disease. The nodules of rheumatoid arthritis are soft and occur within and along tendons that provide extensor function to the joints. The nodules of gout are hard and lie within and immediately adjacent to the joint capsule itself. Frequently they rupture, exuding uric acid crystals onto the skin surface. The nodules of osteoarthritis represent bony overgrowth that has resulted from destruction of the cartilaginous surface of bone within the joint capsule.

Atrophy of muscle will result from disuse as effectively as it will from neurological damage. Thus, the muscles which provide function to a diseased joint will atrophy when the joint is kept passive to avoid the pain which may arise from moving it. This is dramatically seen in rheumatoid arthritis of the knees, in which the quadriceps muscle may atrophy in a very dramatic way. Often the size of a diseased joint is exaggerated by the atrophy of muscles proximal and distal to that joint.

Examination of the Spine

The normal curvature of the spine is convex through the thoracic portion and concave through the cervical and lumbar portions. The concavity of the lumbar spine is referred to as *lumbar lordosis* and is normal. Excessive curvature of the thoracic spine is called *kyphosis*. Deviation of the spine to the left or right is termed *scoliosis*. Kyphosis and scoliosis may result from damage to the paraspinal musculature in poliomyelitis or from disease of the vertebral column such as that which may be seen in tuberculosis.

Back pain is an exceedingly common patient presentation. It is often difficult to determine whether back pain results from an organic lesion or is a functional abnormality without organic cause. Organic lumbar pain produces a triad of physical findings that are characteristic: (1) a straightening of the lumbar spine due to a loss of the normal lumbar lordosis, (2) paraspinal muscle spasm which causes tenderness when palpated, and (3) an inability to flex the spine so that, when the patient is asked to touch his toes, he bends from the hips rather than the waist.

THE EXAMINATION IN REVIEW

Although in this chapter we have approached the physical examination by discussing each organ system as a separate unit (i.e., respiratory system examination, neurological examination, etc.), the actual sequence of assessment is usually determined by efficiency and patient comfort. All relevant organ systems are tested in the process, but not necessarily in the sequence described. For example, when the face is examined it is appropriate at the same time to check for facial asymmetry and, thus, for the integrity of cranial nerve VII; one does not return to this point later, as part of a "neurological" examination. Were we not to combine systems in this manner, the patient would be put through a sequence of sitting up, lying down, sitting up, etc. that would be—to say the least—exhausting.

Moreover, the point should be emphasized that the "complete" physical examination is not a "routine." Many of the elements that we have discussed fall in the category of "sub-routines," which would be selectively addressed to the patient as a function of his or her particular problem. If, for example, a healthy 20-year-old college student reports for an examination in order to satisfy a requirement to play basketball, and reports no history of neurological abnormality, the requirements for an adequate survey of the neurological system are minimal. Conversely, a complaint of transient numbness and diplopia should elicit from the examiner a quite complete neurological investigation. In the same vein, a person with pleuritic chest pain should receive a much more intensive examination of the chest than the person with, for instance, leg cramps.

BIBLIOGRAPHY

BOOKS

Bates, B.: A Guide to Physical Examination, 2nd ed. Philadelphia, J. B. Lippincott, 1979.
Bouchier, I. A. D., and Morris, J. S.: Clinical Skills: A System of Clinical Examination. Philadelphia, W. B. Saunders, 1976.
Delp, M., and Manning, R. T.: Major's Physical Diagnosis, 8th ed. Philadelphia, W. B. Saunders, 1975.
DeGowin, E. L., and DeGowin, R. L.: Bedside Diagnostic Examination, 3rd ed. New York, Macmillan, 1976.
Friedman, H. H., and Papper, S.: Problem-oriented Medical Diagnosis. Boston, Little, Brown, 1975.
Gillies, D. A., and Alyn, I. B.: Patient Assessment and Management by the Nurse Practitioner. Philadelphia, W. B. Saunders, 1976.
Hobson, L. B.: Examination of the Patient: A Text for Nursing and Allied Health Personnel. New York, McGraw-Hill, 1975.
Judge, R. D., and Zuidema, G. D.: Methods of Clinical Examination, 3rd ed. Boston, Little, Brown, 1974.
Malasanos, L., et al.: Health Assessment. St. Louis, C. V. Mosby, 1977.
Prior, J. A., and Silberstein, J. S.: Physical Diagnosis: The History and Examination of the Patient, 5th ed. St. Louis, C. V. Mosby, 1977.
Sana, J. M., and Judge, A. D.: Physical Appraisal Methods in Nursing Practice.
Sherman, J. L., and Fields, S. K.: Guide to Patient Evaluation, 3rd ed. Flushing, N.Y., Medical Examination Pub. Co., 1978.

ARTICLES

Jarvis, C. M.: Perfecting physical assessment, Part 1. Nursing '77, 7:28-37, May, 1977; Part 2, Nursing '77, 7:38-45, June, 1977; Part 3, Nursing '77, 7:44-53, July, 1977.

Keane, A.: The assessment of physical health, Chap. 4 (pages 54-84) in Kintzel, K. C., ed.: Advanced Concepts in Clinical Nursing, 2nd ed. Philadelphia, J. B. Lippincott, 1977.

Penta, F. B., and Penta, M. Q.: Physical examination simulators. Nurs. Digest, 3:40-42, Mar./Apr. 1975.

Stright, P. A., and Soukip, S. M.: How to hear it right: evaluating and choosing a stethoscope. AJN, 77:477, Sept. 1977.

Warren, J. V.: Ten tips to help you make better use of your stethoscope. Med. Opinion 3:31-37, Nov. 1974.

Wong, D. M.: Providing experience in physical assessment for students in basic programs. AJN, 75:974-975, June 1975.

6

DOCUMENTATION OF NURSING PRACTICE: Problem-Oriented Recording

The problem-oriented health record system was devised by Lawrence Weed, M.D. over ten years ago. Since then, many health care delivery systems have incorporated it into their practice settings and many others have adapted it by modifying various components of the system. Dr. Weed's purpose in developing this system of documentation for the patient's health record was to promote a systematic method of organizing all the information needed to accurately diagnose illness and treat patients.

- The problem-oriented system uses the scientific method of problem solving to provide an organized approach to documenting the handling of a patient's problems.

The overall intent of the problem-oriented method of charting is to change the record from a source-oriented document to an integrated patient problem-oriented record that follows the format of a book. The health record starts with a preface or introduction of the patient (Data Base), proceeds to a table of contents (Patient Problem List), develops the succeeding chapters based on the Problem List (Patient Progress Notes) and finally reaches a conclusion (Discharge Summary).

THE PURPOSES OF PATIENT HEALTH RECORDS

The chief purposes of the health record are to provide a means of communication between the members of the health team participating in patient care and to facilitate coordinated planning and continuity of care. The record fulfills other functions as well: it serves as the business and legal record for the hospital and for the professional staff responsible for the care of patients; it serves as a basis for evaluating the quality of care as well as for reviewing the effective utilization of patient care health practices; and it provides data useful in research, education, and short- and long-range planning.

Nursing care has not always been documented in consistent fashion. The focus in charting has frequently been on recording nursing interventions such as tasks and routines. These functions are only one component of nursing practice and often represent areas that nurses have delegated to the nonprofessional members of the nursing team. This type of charting effectively demonstrates the traditionally dependent role of nursing practice — which has consisted in following the licensed physician's and dentist's orders for medications and treatments. The areas which reflect the independent functions of nursing practice, such as prevention, health maintenance, restorative nursing measures, and the psychosocial responses of the patient, as well as discharge planning and patient-family teaching have not been readily documented on the patient's health record. A retrospective review of nurses' charting in any setting illustrates the generalizations nurses have used when charting — for instance, "Good day, up in chair," "Slept well," "No complaints," etc. Very little evidence of patient progress or the effectiveness of the patient care plan was documented.

Today the major frame of reference, or philosophy, of nursing practice is based on the "nursing process," which includes the professional nurse's role in assessing, planning, implementing, and evaluating the patient care given by nurses. This frame of reference for nursing practice, which is analogous to the problem-oriented system of recording, thus makes the nursing process concept attainable and operational in everyday practice.

Although the problem-oriented system does not in itself improve care, it does provide nursing with a tool for documenting nursing practice that is based on scientific method rather than intuition. It also forces the nurse back to the patient's bedside, which enables her to record most effectively all of the parameters she has considered in assessing the patient.

COMPONENTS OF THE PROBLEM-ORIENTED SYSTEM

The problem-oriented system consists of four components: (1) the data base, (2) the problem list, (3) patient care plans, and (4) progress notes for follow-up on each problem and plan, along with a discharge or transfer summary.

Data Base

The data base is a compilation of all of the data obtained on each patient at the time of entry into the health care system. It consists of a complete health history, physical examination, nursing assessment, patient profiles from other sources such as social worker, pharmacist, nutritionist, dentist, physical therapist, respiratory therapist, relevant laboratory and radiologic data, and any other data or profiles from other members of the health team involved in the patient's care. The form and content of the data base should be predetermined and the specified data should be collected for all patients within the institution. Although many disciplines may participate in collecting different parts of the patient data base, all of the baseline information should be placed together in the same section of the health record.

- The data base should not remain source-oriented, as in the traditional record; nor should the same information be recorded by each discipline. Only new information or additional history or observations should be noted.

When all disciplines are not using the problem-oriented system it is not always possible to achieve an integrated data base. In this case the nursing department should determine what information is needed about all patients and should seek to avoid duplication of the physician's notes as much as possible.

The nursing assessment, interview, and history or profile of the patient should be obtained on admission or shortly thereafter by the nurse or the nonprofessionals on the nursing team. The general admission information, which serves as the baseline data for nursing, consists of such items as height, weight, temperature, pulse, respiration, and blood pressure. In addition, the patient's diet at home may be included, as well as any assistive devices or prostheses such as dentures, canes etc., that the patient has brought with him or that he uses to maintain his independence. Other possible entries include the patient's orientation to his environment; for instance, bed controls, intercom system, bathroom facilities, etc.

The remainder of the nursing assessment or patient's data base must be collected by the professional nurse and could include the patient/family assessment factors found on page 96.

Experience with the problem-oriented system and the nursing process has shown that definite time limits need to be established by the organization so that the patient's problems may be identified as quickly after admission as possible. Many organizations set 8 to 24 hours as the time limit.

After collaborating with the patient in describing the problems he perceives, discussing any additional problems identified from the information given, and selecting only relevant data, the nurse is now ready to record the information on the patient's health record. This information can then be inserted in the section with the physician's history and physical examination; however, if the record is still source-oriented, the data base will be the first sheet in the nursing section and should not be removed or thinned from the record during the patient's stay. The patient's data base for nursing now becomes the introduction or preface to all future patient interactions or responses to treatment.

Patient Problem List

The patient problem list becomes the first page of the health record. It serves as the "Table of Contents" for patient information. Generally, if all professionals are using the problem-oriented system, the primary or responsible physician assumes the responsibility of formulating the patient's problems from the data base.

- For clarification, a patient problem is defined as anything that relates to the patient, endangers his health, requires specific management, and concerns any member of the health team.
- These problems are numbered and are used by all concerned for making plans and writing titled and numbered patient progress notes.

Patient problems are classified according to field of interest and level of understanding and thus fall into the following categories:

Medical Problems

   Diagnosis: (e.g., adenocarcinoma of the fundus of the uterus)

   Physiologic Finding: (e.g., blood in the vagina)

   Symptom or Physical Finding: (e.g., spotting or postmenopausal bleeding)

   Abnormal Laboratory Finding: (e.g., positive PAP smear)

Social Problems:
  (e.g., teenage son with drug problem)
Demographic/Environmental Problems (i.e., health hazard)
  (e.g., smoked two packs of cigarettes a day for 20 years; takes unopposed estrogens)
Psychiatric Problems:
  Diagnosis: (e.g., acute psychotic depression)
  Behavioral Manifestations: (e.g., denial of spotting for six months)
Past Problems (i.e., from all categories)
  (e.g., history of appendectomy, 1948)

The patient's problems are also classified by status. Active or inactive and resolved problems should all be listed on the "Master Problem List." The problem list must be modified as the patient changes and as more information is gained. A problem is modified by inserting an arrow with the date above it, followed by the updated or new diagnosis or by the word "dropped" or "resolved." The problem may be updated as follows:

1-7-80 Postmenopausal bleeding
1-8 Total hysterectomy with bilateral salpingo-oophorectomy
→
1-8 Adenocarcinoma of fundus of the uterus
→

Minor problems or episodes may be labeled "temporary problems" in the progress notes (e.g., patient incident, such as a fall, or a headache after a spinal tap). When a second progress note is written it is usually easy to decide whether the incident should be transferred to the problem list and given a permanent number, or dropped.

If all professionals are not using the problem-oriented system, the same nurse who collected the data base will initiate the patient-problem list. (See page 92.) The problem is always stated at the nurse's current level of understanding. The nurse is able to list chronic medical problems, past problems, symptoms, physical findings, and abnormal laboratory findings as well as social, demographic, or behavioral problems. The nurse does not make a medical diagnosis, but as more information is available from the diagnostic studies and the physician's physical examination, the nurse does update the problem list.

• The most important fact to remember is that if all disciplines are using the system as originally intended, there should be only one patient-problem list. If each discipline begins to develop its own patient-problem list, the record becomes totally confused.

Patient Care Plans

Patient care plans are initiated for each problem that is identified and are keyed by number to the problem list. This is the next step in the scientific method of solving problems, and when a well conceived plan is written initially, all that is necessary for long periods of time in

the progress notes is a record of the data on observations of the patient in response to the diagnostic or therapeutic treatment ordered. In many institutions, to facilitate following the plan of care, a card file called a Kardex is used. This does not substitute for documenting the plan in the progress notes, unless the Kardex is considered a permanent part of the health record. More and more institutions are moving toward making the Kardex care plan a permanent part of the record and are recording it in ink rather than in pencil. The Kardex care plan involves all of the professional members of the health team, as required by the patient's problems, so that all members are working together toward the same goal and all of their efforts are congruent.

The plan for each problem should contain three essential components:

1. Directives for the need to collect more data.
   (The physician will consider the "rule-outs" or the "possibles," each of which should always be coupled with an action.)
      Example: R/O kidney disease; schedule IVP for Wednesday.
   (Nursing will consider the need for more information.)
      Example: Monitor intake and output x 72 hours.
2. Directives for management or treatment of the problem.
   (The physician will prescribe specific modalities.)
      Example: Aldomet 250 mg. p.o., q.i.d.
   (Nursing will order specific nursing measures to be taken.)
      Example: B.P., lying and standing q.i.d.
3. Directives for teaching the patient and one or more family members about his problem, its treatment, and what is expected of him in managing the problem and maintaining an optimum level of health.
   (The physician will document what the patient has been told about his illness and what is being planned for him or his family.)
      Example: Patient told that this problem should not interfere with occupation and he should be able to return to work in three weeks.
   (The nurse will document whether the patient and his family can repeat or verbalize any instructions given to them.)
      Example: Attended group classes on 3-10; able to answer all questions regarding diet, activity, and medications he will be taking when he returns home.

Whether or not nurses are the only ones implementing the system, they can use the above components in developing their patient care plans. The nurse will need to develop the skill of stating her plans in the form of specific directives in the progress notes, so that they can eventually be transcribed by the unit clerk to the Kardex.

Patient Progress Notes

The progress notes are written in a format which not only relates them clearly and unmistakably to the problem but also utilizes the scientific method of problem solving on a day-by-day basis (see page 99). Progress notes are written in a narrative form using the acronym "SOAPIE."

S: Subjective data (symptoms that the patient describes)

O: Objective data (signs that the professional observes)

A: Assessment (the professional's conclusion about the subjective and objective data)

P: Plan (immediate or future, including patient education)

I: Intervention (nursing action done to, for, or with the patient)

E: Evaluation (patient outcome of nursing process)

Flow sheets are used to follow or monitor a problem that does not lend itself to a single note or requires that multiple parameters be observed and recorded more often than every six hours or four times a day; or they may be used for the documentation of nursing and patient activities such as treatments, daily care, etc.

• The Progress Notes are the most critical part of the problem-oriented system. They are the mechanism which provides a minute-by-minute ongoing assessment of the patient's problem. The progress notes can detect faulty understanding and poor decisions made by the health care provider. They do not improve care, but they can identify inadequate logic in seconds. Progress notes provide the feedback on problem identification and the plans formulated. If all professionals are recording on integrated progress notes the patient has a greater chance of receiving continuity of care.

The progress notes always begin with the date, time, and problem number and title, and they continue using the following format:

SUBJECTIVE DATA: The subjective or symptomatic data are obtained from the patient's or family's point of view. When recording subjective data consider the following: onset (date, time, type), intensity, quality, location, radiation, number of episodes, time of day of episodes, sources of relief (rest, position, medication), precipitating factors, factors that make the problem worse, other associated symptoms existing at the same time, overall course, the degree to which the symptoms have affected the patient's life style, etc.

OBJECTIVE DATA: These include actual clinical observations or laboratory findings appropriate to the problem. When recording objective data always include the following: location, size, shape, color, temperature, moisture, consistency. Also note presence or absence of swelling, movement, weakness, associated pain with movement or touch. Many nurses record their nursing actions in this section; others add their immediate interventions to the plan component of the progress notes.

ASSESSMENT: This is the portion of the progress notes which deals directly with the subjective and objective data just collected and which presents the health care provider's conclusion based on that information. If both are consistent with the problem statement, little needs to be said here. One way of considering assessment in relation to patient progress or regress will be a comparison with the previous documentation using such terms as "improved," "worse," or "deteriorating," or "same" or "stable." If the problem is a new one, then the subjective and objective data should support a new assessment of what is going on with the patient. If the problem statement and the subjective and objective data are not consistent, then one can quickly assess the logic or accuracy of the information recorded.

Assessment occurs when the provider records his thinking and conclusions at his level of understanding.

PLAN: The original or initial plan, if well thought out and developed, will continue to be followed or will be modified as new information is obtained. The plan will always consider the three areas described earlier: the need for more information, management, and treatment, and patient and family education.

INTERVENTION AND EVALUATION: Nurses use the same problem-oriented procedure to document their practice. However, there are two components that many nurses have added in order to comply with the requirements of the nursing process and of some regulatory agencies for documenting nursing practice. These components are labeled *I*, for the nursing intervention which was carried out immediately (e.g., raise the head of the bed, notify the physician, etc.), and *E*, for evaluation of the nursing intervention (was it effective or ineffective?) as documented according to patient outcomes. Sometimes the evaluation will appear in the next progress note because more time is needed to observe the patient's response to the nursing intervention.

One can see that when the plan is incorporated in the patient progress notes, it readily becomes a permanent part of the legal record and the Kardex system reverts to being a tool to facilitate the implementation of the plan.

Discharge or Transfer Summary

The last portion of the record should be a summary of each problem, using the "SOAP" format. The summary should include:

• the cause of the problem
• the status of each problem
• the intervention or management used to handle the problem
• the future plans for following the problem at home, in the office, clinic, or extended care facility
• agency referrals made
• instructions and verification of the patient's or family's knowledge of the problem and their responsibility in dealing with it.

This summary is vital to the next set of health care providers. It is often done by the physician and includes the contributions made by all of the other health professionals. Even if the physician does include the health team approach in his summary, the nursing and other disciplines involved should include in their discharge summaries the specific goals with which their professions were directly involved.

The transfer summary is most appropriate when the patient is progressing from one level of care to another. An example of this would be the transfer from an intensive care unit to a general patient unit.

SUMMARY

The problem–oriented system makes it possible to document health care practice using the scientific method. It will eventually lend itself to computerization, but at present it can easily be recorded manually. The total concept, when implemented, improves communication among all health professionals. The system promotes the continuing education of each individual member of the health team; the systematic gathering, recording, and assessment of data, the development and implementation of plans, and the evaluation of results constitute an effective learning process. Above all, the system provides a more meaningful way of reviewing the patient's profile by focusing on the patient and all of the factors that affect his recovery or return to optimum health.

The problem–oriented system is important to nursing practice because it makes the nursing process operational and has the potential of contributing to nursing research by helping to define and evaluate nursing practice.

REMINDERS TO CONSIDER BEFORE WRITING PROBLEM-ORIENTED PROGRESS NOTES

1. Have the patient's problem list in front of you or open to the problem list on the patient's health record.
2. Think about your patient in light of each problem listed in the active column. Are there any new problems to be added or considered as a result of your observations or interactions with the patient today?
3. Read the immediately previous notes so that you will not unnecessarily repeat information already recorded and so that you will be aware of plans which are in progress.
4. Decide which are the most important problems for you to discuss; always consider life-threatening or major problems first (e.g., although a myocardial infarction may be a very threatening problem, if it is relatively stable or has recently been discussed, the patient's acute anxiety may be a more pertinent topic; it may have a significant impact on his survival).
5. A follow-up note on data-base information or on your plans identified in previous notes may be appropriate if the data is now available, or you might want to comment on the effectiveness or ineffectiveness of your plan (e.g., vital signs, weight, response to treatment or nursing measures, etc.).
6. Always begin your note with the date, time, problem number, and title. List the subjective or objective data using the factors suggested in this chapter. Record both follow-up data and any new information you have gathered.

7. Write an assessment for each problem considered, stating your thoughts at the level at which you actually understand the information. If you want to write about specific observations or responses to medications or treatments with which you have had little experience, look them up first—you may find valuable information that will help all members of the health team or you might learn that your idea does not logically follow from the data you have available.
8. Review the plan for each problem listed, or initiate a new plan if you have identified a new problem. Always consider the following three factors:
   a. The need for more information: such as specific observations which might help clarify the problem.
   b. Nursing intervention: such as specific nursing measures you can order or initiate to resolve the problem (e.g., have patient turn, cough, and take deep breaths every hour for 24 hours).
   c. Patient or family teaching: what you have told or plan to tell the patient and his family about this problem to increase their understanding of the management.
9. Write a progress note when there is something pertinent to say, such as when there has been a change. Some days several notes for the day or for the shift, may be indicated, whereas on other days *no* notes will be appropriate for some problems.

SOME DON'TS WHEN RECORDING ON THE PROGRESS NOTES

DON'T include comments on nonproblem items (e.g., bed baths, h.s. care given, doing well, etc.)

DON'T write about things that have already been discussed unless you disagree with the data listed or the conclusions drawn. Be sure to defend your position with exact literature references if you do disagree.

DON'T include comments on normal physiologic functions unless they are pertinent to a particular problem (e.g., the daily bowel movements should be kept on a routine care flow sheet unless you are discussing a patient who has diarrhea or who has a previously identified problem such as constipation).

DON'T use the progress notes to record routine tests done or care given (e.g., these can be checked off on the Kardex care plan or considered recorded when the laboratory or x-ray reports come back.

NURSING ASSESSMENT

White, Susan   11322.1
Dr. Stone   198-74-0360
MTS   1/21/80
59677 25 8-9-49 F.S. Cath.
176 Hollow St. Pgh 15215
HSA 6605-00   198-74-0360
Unemployed R.N.
Parents-Teresa 412-264-7657

NURSING DATA BASE

GENERAL ADMISSION INFORMATION

DATE: 1/21/80   TIME: 1:00 pm.

BASELINE DATA: Height: 163cm. Weight: 49.5 Kg Temp.: 37.6°c Pulse: 120   Resp.: 22   BP: Ra: 106/70 La: 110/74

PROSTHESES OR ASSISTIVE DEVICES: None

DIET AT HOME: General-when eating

ALLERGIES: "Compazine"   SIGNATURE: R. Jones, R.N.

PATIENT/FAMILY ASSESSMENT

REASON FOR HOSPITALIZATION OR ADMITTING PROBLEM: Nausea, vomiting. lower abdominal pain with cramping, diarrhea-small amounts of green liquid stool 3-4x day.

DURATION OF THIS PROBLEM: 2 weeks without a normal B.M., poor appetite and weaker past week.

OBSERVATION OF PATIENT'S CONDITION: Very ill young lady with Cushingoid appearance
Gastrointestinal status: Distended abdomen, mild epigastric tenderness
Neurological status: Alert and oriented to time, place, and person; no loss of sensation
Respiratory status: No difficulty at this time, R.22
Skin condition: Skin-clear, no petechiae on body; gums-oral mucosa look clear.

CONCURRENT CONDITIONS: "Hodgkins Disease since 1975." Dx 7/75 of Hodgkin's Stage IV B.

PREVIOUS EXPERIENCE WITH HOSPITALIZATIONS: 6th admission here. Rx 8/75 with Exploratory Lap with Splenectomy; 10/76 Radiation Therapy with 4000 Rads to all nodes. 8/77 chemotherapy
MEDICATION: Prednisone 30mg q.d. with Maalox. Darvon 65mg. Dalmane 30mg. HS PRN.

REACTION TO ALLERGIES: "Compazine makes me hyperactive"

PATTERNS:
HYGIENE: "Usually shower when I feel good"
REST/SLEEP: 6-7 hours/night, retires 11-12 midnight, arises 6-7 a.m.
MEALS/DIET: General. but appetite poor past 2 wks; has been eating soup, cereals, eggs
ACTIVITY STATUS: Independent in ADL; OOB as tolerated.
ELIMINATION—BOWEL: Diarrhea 3-4x day-"maybe I am impacted from Vincristine"
       BLADDER: 4-5x day, q.s. no recent change, "occ. nocturia if I can't sleep"
MENSTRUAL HISTORY: Lmp 1/25/78 No change recently.

HEALTH HAZARD APPRAISAL: BSE q month, To M.D. office q. month, no smoking or alcohol

LIFE STYLE: Prior to 7/75 worked as R.N. in ICU at local hospital. Since 1976 worked only 1 mo. Lives with parents. "Mother fusses over me."

TYPICAL DAY PROFILE: "Up at 7 a.m., bkft with parents, watch T.V., nap, lunch. Sew or knit, frequent vistors. "Boyfriend hasn't given up on me." "Now what!" Anxious and
MENTAL/EMOTIONAL STATUS: "was doing well until this happened!" teary-eyed. Depressed and angry during interview.

SAFETY APPRAISAL: No problem unless she gets weaker and is unable to get OOB s help.

DISCHARGE PLANNING: Anticipated LOS 1-2 wks if present problem is resolved s̄ surgery and if chemotherapy is completed. Will have to return to clinic each month. Reinforce patient and family as to what to watch for after discharge, if no further relapse.

INFORMANT: Patient, old charts, physician.

SIGNATURE:

Based on form used by Presbyterian-University Hospital Nursing Service Department, Pittsburgh, Pa.

NAME: Susan White

PATIENT CARE PLAN A

ALLERGIES: Idiosyncrasy to Compazine

Date Ordered	#	Medications	Dosage	Rte.	Time Symbol	Time - Hours	To Be Disc.	Date Ordered	Specimens and Cultures	INIT.	Date To Be Done	Date Ordered	Diagnostic Procedures	Date To Be Done
1/21	2	Decadron	1mg.	I.V.	q6h	12-6-12-6		1/21	Urine R+m	RJ		1/21	Chest X-Ray	7/21
1/21	2	Prednisone	10mg.	P.O	q6h	10-4-10-4						1/21	ECG	7/21
1/21	2	maalox	30ml.									1/21	Flat Plate Abd.	7/21
									Standing Blood Work					
1/25	2	Thorazine	25mg.	IM	1/2hr	1/2hr ā Chemo Rx						1/21	Consults — Surg. C-RS	
1/25	1	Darvon	65mg.	PO	q4h	PRN							Dr. C. Watson	Date Seen 1/21
1/24	1	Talwin	50mg.	IM	q4h	PRN								
1/22	4	Oxaine	5 ml.	PO	PRN	Leave at bedside								
1/21	4	Peppermint H2O	8 ml.	PO	PRN									
1/21	3	Valium	5mg.	IM	q6h	PRN			Routine Blood Work					
1/21	1	Codeine Sulph.	30mg.	IM	q4h	PRN						1/21	CBC & Diff	1/21
												1/21	Retic. Platelets	1/21

Based on form used by Presbyterian-University Hospital Nursing Service Department, Pittsburgh, Pa.

PATIENT CARE PLAN B

Patient Profile

White, Susan   1132a.1
Dr. Stone   1   198-74-0360
M+S   2   1-21-80
56977   a5   8-9-55 F3 Cath
176 Hollow St.   Pgh. 15215
HSA 6605-00 198-74-0360
Unemployed R.N.
Parents-Teresa   412-264-7657

DATE—DIET:	DATE—ACTIVITY STATUS:	DATE—CARE CATEGORY
/a liquids as tol.	1/a1 Bed rest c̄ BRP as tol.	1/a1 Partial → Self
	PROSTHESES: None	HT. 163 cm WT. 49.5 kg.
DATE—OPERATION:	SAFETY APPRAISAL: Instruct to seek assistance when getting up c̄ I.V.	TPRq 4h. while awake B/Pq
		Assessment Done by 1/a1 Ruth Jones

#	PATIENT PROBLEM LIST	#	Date	Treatments and Nursing Directives	Time
1.	Abdominal Pain 1/a1 partial intestinal obstruction	1 1a	1/a1 1/a1	Intake and Output NG tube to intermittent low suction; cont. irrigation 30 ml NSS	7-3-11 8-10-12 etc
	a. Nausea and vomiting	1a	1/a1	Mouth care c̄ baking soda/water pik q4h/ PRN p̄c meals	8-1a-4-8 etc
	b. Abdominal cramping	1b	1/a1	Check for bowel sounds q4h	8-1a-4-8 etc
	c. Diarrhea	1c	1/a1	Observe color, consistency q record on Flow Sheet	
2.	Hodgkins IVB	a	1/a1	Check for constipation due to chemotherapy side effects daily	
3.	Adaptation to illness	a	1/a1	Weigh daily Observe skin for petechiae and pruritus	7:30 A.M.
	a. Depression			Give premedication ½ hr. before chemotherapy	
	b. Anger			Urine reductions q.i.d. x 48 hrs., then 1x daily	7-11-4-9
4.	Esophagitis	3a	1/a1	Accept her behavior; let her know you understand	
5.	Cushingoid appearance			She will talk if she trusts you. Pretends sleep when unable to talk	
6.	Allergy or idiosyncrasy to Compazine	3b	1/a1	Easily recognized-refuses Rx, meds, pulls out NG tube. Knows diagnosis. Answer	
7.	1975- Exp. Lap. with Splenectomy			- Sometimes more frightened (because she is an R.N.)	
				honestly and keep her informed of Rx, tests, Plans,	
#	DISCHARGE PLANNING:	4	1/a4	Give oxaine 15 min āc - avoid acidic juices or drinks	
1	Reinstruct about changes in bowel habits - develop regime q discharge	5	1/a1	Concerned over body image. Very attractive c̄ Prednisone, Boy-	
2	Support patient (ex: concerns over diagnosis) by listening to her. Work with parents to support end-stage disease at home or in hospital. Sacraments of the sick 1/24/80			friend still visits - Provide privacy. Help her to look attractive when it is known he is coming. Assess parents response to her body image change. Explain drug effects.	

Tent. Disch.	Name	Attending Physician	Intern	Room
2 weeks	Susan White	Dr. Stone	Smiley	1132a.1

NURSES' PROGRESS NOTES

DATE	TIME	PROBLEM	PROGRESS NOTES
1/22/	7-12N	#1 Partial Intestinal Obstruction	S: pain and cramping in abdomen is less today.
			O: Abdomen softer, sluggish peristalsis. N-G tube draining small amount (50-100 ml.) clear yellow liquid. No diarrhea or formed stool.
			A: fecal impaction may be beginning to move
			P: If peristalsis improves, remove N-G tube and start on liquids.
			I: Notified Dr. Smiley. S.S. enema ordered and given.
			E: Enema effectual for return of yellow liquid with many small pieces of hard brown stool.
1/23/	7-12N	#1 Partial Intestinal Obstruction	S: Requesting more to eat than sips of water.
			O: Active bowel sounds, abdomen soft, small formed B.M.
			A: Obstruction resolved. Impaction broken up.
			P: Begin bowel regime to keep stool soft and formed. Instruct patient in importance of having B.M. every day because of constipating effect of chemotherapy.
			I: Dr. Smiley notified. N-G tube removed. Started on liquids as tolerated.
			E: Tolerated liquid lunch; will add more full liquids to evening meal.

Each Progress Note consists of the number and title of problem as stated on the Problem List and any or all of the following components:

S — Subjective Data (Symptoms)
O — Objective Data (Measurable Signs)
A — Assessment (Conclusion)
P — Plan — Immediate or Future
I — Intervention — Nursing Action
E — Evaluation — Effectiveness of Intervention

Based on form used by Presbyterian-University Hospital Nursing Service Department, Pittsburgh, Pa.

SPECIAL CARE
FLOW SHEET

Define parameters as need for each patient.

NOS._____PROBLEMS_____

DATE 12 pm._____to 12 pm._____

TIME	Blood Pressure	Pulse	Respirations	Temperature	Central Venous Pressure	Urine Volume	Specific Gravity								REMARKS

Based on form used by Presbyterian-University Hospital Nursing Service Department, Pittsburgh, Pa.

DISCHARGE SUMMARY

DATE	REMARKS

2/3/80

#1 Partial Intestinal Obstruction
S: "No discomfort. BM's are soft and moving regularly."
O: Soft abdomen. No diarrhea.
A: Obstruction due to impaction relieved through scheduled bowel regulation program.
P: Continue daily pericolace; reemphasize to patient the importance of keeping her stool soft and moving daily because of side effect of medication, Vincristine. To notify M.D. if laxative needed.

#2 Hodgkins IV B
S: Understands diagnosis of Hodgkins IV B
O:
A: End stage of disease progressing
P: Worked with parents to accept progression of disease and the minimal response to chemotherapy. Taught them what to expect such as edema, ascites, further weakness, etc. To avoid bruising, since platelets are up.

2/3/80

#3 Adaptation to Illness

S: Still angry about having disease; has not been able to accept condition.
O: Lashes out at parents, crying, very frightened of going home.
A: Still needs much support to begin to accept living one day at a time.
P: Referred her to Visiting Nurse Association in Pittsburgh for Patient/Family Support.

#4 Esophagitis
S: No complaints of heartburn any longer.
A: Problem resolved at this time.
P: Given prescription for Oxaine and instructed to take it if heartburn recurs.

#5 Cushingoid Appearance
S: Concerned over physical appearance and what it will do to her relationship with boyfriend and family.
O: Moon-shaped face, slight hump on back, beginning to look more and more Cushingoid. Urine reduction negative.
A: Steroid dose (Prednisone) will continue to be given, so Patient/Family need to be aware of sign and symptoms of diabetes.
P: Continue to encourage her fix herself up with makeup and set her hair, etc. Instructed family in observation of signs and symptoms of diabetes, such as polyuria, polydipsia and polyphagia. Taught her to check urine at least once a day. Instructed family to make as few comments as possible about physical appearance.

2/3/80

Discharged home with parents,

R. Smith. R.N.

BIBLIOGRAPHY

BOOKS

Accreditation Manual for Hospitals. Chicago, Joint Commission on Accreditation of Hospitals, Feb. 1978.

Bailey, J., and Claus, K.: Decision Making in Nursing: Tools for Change. St. Louis, C. V. Mosby, 1975.

Easton, R.: Problem-Oriented Medical Record Concepts. New York, Appleton-Century-Crofts, 1974.

Gebbie, K., and Lavin, M., eds.: Classification of Nursing Diagnoses: Proceedings of the First National Conference, St. Louis, C. V. Mosby, 1975.

Little, D., and Carnevali, D.: Nursing Care Planning, 2nd ed. Philadelphia, J. B. Lippincott, 1976.

Vaughn-Wrobel, B., and Henderson, B.: The Problem-Oriented System in Nursing: A Workbook, St. Louis, C. V. Mosby, 1976.

Walker, H. K., et al., eds.: Applying the Problem-Oriented System. New York, Medcom Press, 1973.

Walker, J. B., et al., eds.: Dynamics of Problem-Oriented Approaches: Patient Care and Documentation. Philadelphia, J. B. Lippincott, 1976.

Weed, L: Medical Records, Medical Education and Patient Care. Cleveland, Case Western Reserve University Press, 1968.

Yura, H., and Walsh, M. B.: The Nursing Process: Assessing, Planning, Implementing and Evaluating, 3rd ed. New York, Appleton-Century-Crofts, 1978.

ARTICLES

Ansley, B.: Patient-oriented recording, Nursing '75, 5:52-53, Aug. 1975.

Atwood, J., and Yarnall, S. R., eds.: Symposium on the problem-oriented record. Nurs. Clin. N. Am., 9:entire issue, June 1974.

Bertucci, M., et al: Comparative study of progress notes using problem-oriented and traditional methods of charting. Nurs. Research, 23:351-354, July-Aug. 1974.

Eggland, E. T.: How to take a meaningful nursing history. Nursing '77, 7:22-30, July, 1977.

Mitchell, P. H.: A systematic nursing progress record: The problem-oriented approach. Nurs. Forum, 12:(2) 187-210, 1973.

Porter, A., et al.: Patient needs on admission. AJN, 77:112-113, Jan. 1977.

Rieder, K., and Wood, M.: Problem-orientation: an experimental study to test its heuristic value. Nurs. Research, 27:25-29, Jan.-Feb. 1978.

VanMeter, M. J., and Scott, L. K.: An experience with problem-oriented nursing notes. J. Neurosurg. Nurs., 7:42-56, July 1975.

Woody, M., and Mallison, M.: The problem-oriented system for patient-centered care. AJN, 73:1168-1175, July 1973.

Biophysical and Psychosocial Concepts Related to Health and Illness

UNIT THREE

7

HOMEOSTATIC MECHANISMS AND PATHOPHYSIOLOGIC PROCESSES: The Internal Environment

The great French physiologist Claude Bernard laid down a major biological principle when he wrote: "The condition for a free life is the constancy of the internal environment." The "internal environment" is the fluid that bathes the cells of the body, as contrasted with the external environment that surrounds man as a whole organism. As long as this fluid, a water solution of gases, ions, and nutrients, is relatively constant in composition and temperature, the cell can carry on its functions, despite the fact that man lives in an external environment hostile to the existence of the cell. Because the cell is thus protected, humans are not confined, as is the amoeba, to a pond sufficiently rich in oxygen and nutrients, but are free to move in the external world to the extent that inventive ingenuity permits. In short, the range and variety of activities and choices available to humans depend upon both the functional integrity of the cell and the stability of the internal environment.

A PHYSIOLOGIC DEFINITION OF DISEASE

For the purposes of this chapter, *disease* is defined as any process or event that promotes a change in the internal environment that results in loss of cell function and thus limits man's freedom to act in the external world. To the nurse, disease is displayed as a changing state or shifting pattern of patient response that is the result of disease processes on the one hand and bodily defenses and therapeutic responses on the other. Disease described in the context of physiology or pathophysiology is most useful as the nurse attempts to answer two questions: What is the current status of the patient? and What is the response of the patient to therapy?

The physiologic definition given above is used for two reasons: (1) Many serious illnesses provoke and evoke change in the internal environment; and (2) most therapy is directed toward the restoration of a normal internal environment. For instance, the patient with advanced emphysema who is cyanotic, acidotic, fighting for every breath, and able to climb only a few stairs without rest has his freedom of choice severely restricted because his oxidative energy supply for cell function is limited. The decreased pulmonary gas exchange results in a loss of the rapid respiratory mechanism for neutralizing hydrogen ions and in retention of carbon dioxide, producing a respiratory acidosis in addition to the metabolic acidosis of hypoxemia and a change in blood pH. Since the structure of most body proteins is pH-dependent, such a change in pH results in a change of structure and cell functions, especially of the cell wall. This patient is seriously ill because his internal environment is altered.

The chronic smoker with mild to moderate bronchitis and bronchoconstriction is not ill while carrying on sedentary activity, but if he must run to the bus stop, the reduction in ventilatory function would force a slackened pace. This means that his freedom of choice of action is restricted and his health compromised. A patient who has had a coronary occlusion is confined to bed lest the output of the heart be insufficient to maintain adequate transport of gases in the blood or adequate blood pressure. Recovery is associated with increasing activity (freedom of choice) without breathlessness, fatigue, or an unusually rapid or erratic heart rate.

On the other hand, a woman awaiting surgery for carcinoma of the uterus who has a stable pulse, normal blood pressure, and quiet respiration and who is eating well and able to care for herself is, in terms of homeostasis, far less ill than an emphysematous man who is cyanotic and dyspneic with lungs full of rhonchi and who has bleeding hemorrhoids.

The physiologic viewpoint, then, is useful for minute-to-minute (intensive care) or hour-to-hour care of the patient. The resulting nursing action will be commensurate with the patient's need, and the objective will be to preserve the entire organism as well as treat the disease.

MECHANISMS FOR MAINTAINING HOMEOSTASIS

The bodily state associated with a stable internal environment is called *homeostasis*. The machinery and method for obtaining homeostasis are discussed next.

The *internal environment* is the intracellular or interstitial fluid bathing each cell, a water solution of inorganic salts and organic substances filtered from the plasma through the capillary wall. Its composition is similar to that of plasma without protein. However, the interstitial fluid of the brain (cerebrospinal fluid) is produced by active cellular processes and differs somewhat from interstitial fluid derived from blood plasma (Table 7-1).

Although the composition of the internal environment may vary locally from tissue to tissue because of differences in cellular activity and metabolism, its average composition is relatively constant, a consequence of the free exchange of substances back and forth between blood and interstitial fluid. Blood, in turn, is continuously being "mixed," as it is collected and redistributed in the blood vessels of the body and lungs.

Various exchanges take place between the external and internal environments: respiratory gases, foodstuffs, water, and heat. These exchanges are effected by the lungs, kidneys, gastrointestinal tract, and skin, and the activity of these organs varies to compensate for cellular activity ranging from rest to extreme exercise. The circulatory system acts as the middleman between the variable organ and the stable fluid. For instance, carbon dioxide, one end product of energy production in the cell, when dissolved in water forms a weak acid capable of changing the internal environment as it diffuses out of the cell and into the bloodstream. However, the CO_2 is buffered by the acid-neutralizing capacity of the blood and is transported to the lungs for elimination into an external environment that is low in CO_2 content.

ROLE OF THE KIDNEYS. Even more dramatic is the role of the kidney, which removes certain chemicals dissolved in the blood by filtration and by renal tubular excretion. It then returns most of the filtered chemicals to the blood and eliminates excess or unwanted substances by way of the urine.

Table 7-2 illustrates the overall activity of the kidney; several consequences of renal function are apparent. About 170 L. of kidney filtrate are formed per 24 hours by the recirculation of about 3 L. of plasma per minute through the kidney, thus providing for a continuous adjustment of the composition of the blood. Some substances important to cell function (such as glucose) are almost totally reabsorbed, while other substances produced or eaten in excess of need (e.g., potassium) are excreted in amounts sufficient to avoid accumulation. Thus, the kidney is capable of a wide variety and range of activities. A small change in renal function results in a major deviation in the internal environment, or depar-

TABLE 7-1.   COMPOSITION* OF SERUM, INTERCELLULAR FLUID, CEREBROSPINAL FLUID, AND INTRACELLULAR FLUID OF MUSCLE CELLS

	SERUM	INTER-CELLULAR FLUID	CEREBRO-SPINAL FLUID	INTRA-CELLULAR† FLUID
Na	138	140	141	10
K	4	4	3	150
Ca	7	7	2.5	—
Mg	—	—	—	40
Cl	102	114	127	15-20
HCO$_3$	26	29	18	10
PO$_4$,SO$_4$	3	3	1.5	150
Protein	15	—	—	40

*mEq./L. These substances are frequently reported in terms of mg./100 ml.
†Skeletal muscle.
Note: Only ions are considered, including the ionic equivalency of protein, which is a charged molecule at bodily pH values.

TABLE 7-2*   THE KIDNEY AS A HOMEOSTATIC ORGAN

SUBSTANCE	AMOUNT FILTERED PER 24 HOURS	AMOUNT EXCRETED PER 24 HOURS	PERCENT REABSORBED
Water	170 L.	1.5 L.	99%
Glucose	170 gm.	0 gm.	100%
Sodium	560 gm.	5 gm.	99%
Potassium	29 gm.	2.7 gm.	90%
Urea	51 gm.	30.0 gm.	60%
Ammonia†	—	1.0 mg.	0%

*The examples given are typical of a healthy man at rest and do not show the range possible in disease, exercise, or water excess or deprivation.
†Secreted after formation by the renal tubules.

ture from homeostasis. Were the kidney to excrete 10 percent instead of 1 percent of the filtrate water, a person would spend much of his time drinking and eliminating water. Diabetes insipidus, produced by a deficiency of antidiuretic hormone of the neurohypophysis is such a disease state.

SODIUM BALANCE. Now let us put the action of the kidney into the scheme of sodium balance to illustrate in simple form the interacting shifts and flow of materials in and through the body, at the same time noting that the balance is maintained (Fig. 7-1).

Depending on the diet, about 2 to 10 grams of sodium a day are absorbed via the intestines, and a corresponding amount is excreted into the urine or perspiration, if conditions of heat regulation so require. The kidney acts as the adjusting organ, filtering out of the blood about 600 grams of sodium and returning about 99 percent to the blood over a 24-hour period. The excreted sodium thus is only a minor fraction of the sodium processed by the kidney, and the kidney operates well within its enormous reserve capacity. The net flow is unidirectional, open-ended, and variable. This is the overall balance.

In contrast to the net flow for the entire body, sodium is transferred in and out of different compartments of the body continuously but with no net loss. Some shifts are generally in *equilibrium* from moment to moment; that is

to say, inward flow is equal to outward flow as in the case of exchange between plasma and interstitial fluid. Some shifts are transient, such as the temporary net inflow of sodium into a nerve cell during the formation and progress of the nerve impulse over the nerve, an event corrected by the outward pumping of sodium by the nerve metabolic processes in less than a few seconds of time. By contrast, during digestion large volumes of digestive juice rich in sodium are secreted into the intestines and are then reabsorbed over a few hours time. Renal compensation for this large but temporary shift outside the body fluid compartment is achieved by decreased sodium and water excretion during the period of digestion.

Thus the flow and exchange of sodium within the body go on continuously, leading to temporary shifts and imbalances; but over a period of hours or days there is a stable state, in which the concentration of sodium in the internal environment remains steady.

This relative constancy of composition is the result of a *dynamic* type of equilibrium, the stability achieved by continuous small reciprocal exchanges of chemical substances between cell, interstitial fluid, and blood everywhere throughout the body, along with a continuous, variable action of the organs of homeostasis. Stability is achieved by continuous controlled cellular activity.

This situation is analogous to that of two equally

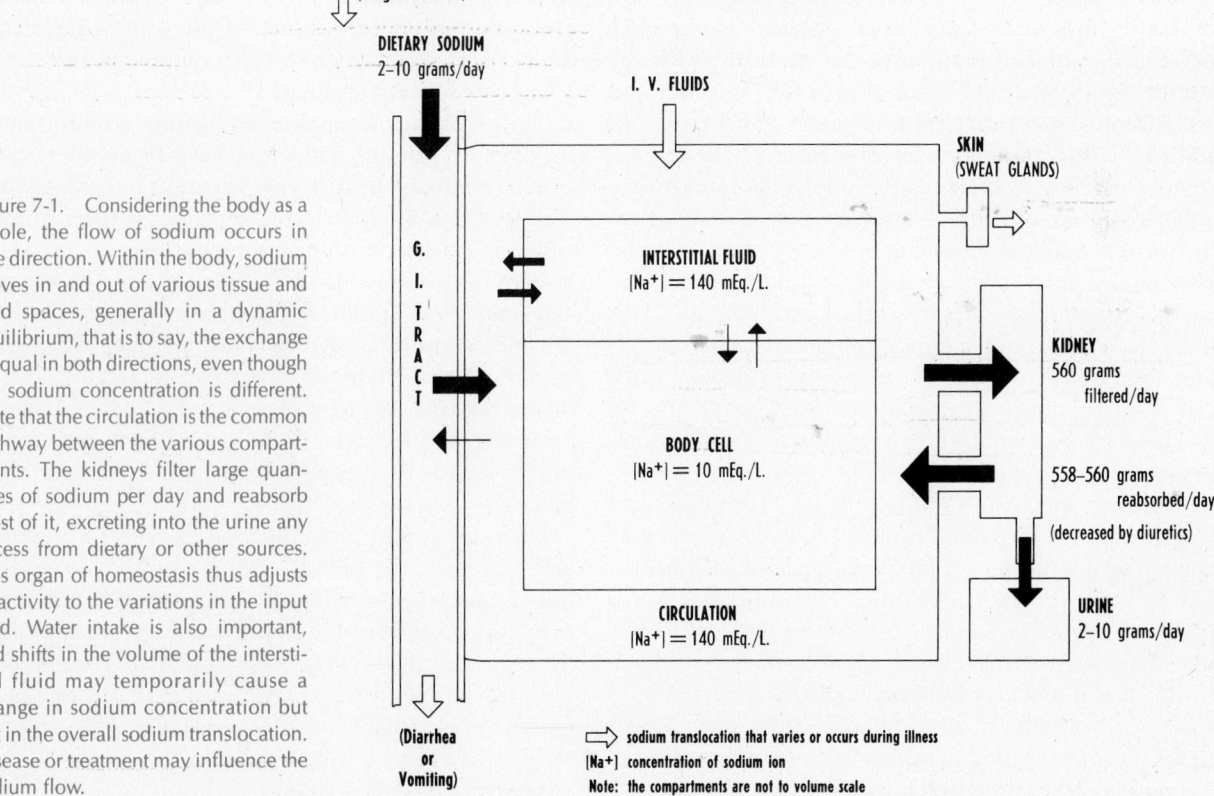

DYNAMICS OF SODIUM TRANSLOCATION

Figure 7-1. Considering the body as a whole, the flow of sodium occurs in one direction. Within the body, sodium moves in and out of various tissue and fluid spaces, generally in a dynamic equilibrium, that is to say, the exchange is equal in both directions, even though the sodium concentration is different. Note that the circulation is the common pathway between the various compartments. The kidneys filter large quantities of sodium per day and reabsorb most of it, excreting into the urine any excess from dietary or other sources. This organ of homeostasis thus adjusts its activity to the variations in the input load. Water intake is also important, and shifts in the volume of the interstitial fluid may temporarily cause a change in sodium concentration but not in the overall sodium translocation. Disease or treatment may influence the sodium flow.

(Drugs with Na+)

DIETARY SODIUM
2–10 grams/day

I. V. FLUIDS

SKIN
(SWEAT GLANDS)

G.
I.
T
R
A
C
T

INTERSTITIAL FLUID
[Na+] = 140 mEq./L.

KIDNEY
560 grams
filtered/day

BODY CELL
[Na+] = 10 mEq./L.

558–560 grams
reabsorbed/day
(decreased by diuretics)

CIRCULATION
[Na+] = 140 mEq./L.

URINE
2–10 grams/day

(Diarrhea or Vomiting)

⇨ sodium translocation that varies or occurs during illness
[Na+] concentration of sodium ion
Note: the compartments are not to volume scale

skilled and powerful wrestlers who have brought one another to a standstill, equilibrium being achieved by continuous small and opposing shifts in muscular activity.

It is important to grasp the concept that the patient lying in bed has within his system a continuous ongoing process of change so balanced and regulated that the whole organism appears stable, and that disease is expressed by the appearance of an unstable state, sometimes by the minute (respiratory distress), the hour (diabetes), or months (cancer).

OTHER ORGANS OF HOMEOSTASIS. The other organs of homeostasis have analogous abilities and the capacity for wide changes in function to provide for continuous adjustment in the composition of the blood. Diseases of the organs of homeostasis (heart, lungs, kidney, liver, gastrointestinal tract, skin) are serious because they change the internal environment. As a consequence, cellular activity in general is altered, diminished, or halted. For this reason, then, examination of blood to determine the status of the interstitial fluid and examination of the heart, lungs, liver, and kidney to determine the status of the organs of homeostasis constitute the crux of all diagnostic procedures and allow an estimate of prognosis.

Approximately 70 percent of the lungs, kidney, liver, or heart muscle can be surgically removed or damaged before homeostasis during body rest is altered. The enormous *physiologic reserve* of function allows a wide variation in total body activity, ranging from sleep to Olympic competition.

STEADY STATE AS AN OPEN-ENDED SYSTEM. Though the end-function of the organs of homeostasis is to keep the internal environment constant, they act on molecules and use energy sources that are not reused or recycled but enter and leave the body in a one-way flow pattern termed *open-ended*. For example, in the adult, each day about 2,000 ml. of water, 2,500 kilocalories of energy in the form of food, and varying quantities of oxygen and various ions enter the body and leave as urine containing various molecules in solution, or heat, or CO_2, etc. This flow of materials and energy through the body is necessary for two reasons: (1) the molecular structure of the cell is continuously degraded, removed, and replaced; and (2) the cells manufacture new substances such as fat, glycogen, or hormones, or perform such energy-consuming mechanical functions as shortening and lengthening the muscles. From day to day a person may appear to be the same, but this apparent stability or steady state actually is dynamic. The molecules of the body are being exchanged for identical molecules at an unceasing but variable rate. If a wall contained a million bricks, and if each day 100 original bricks were removed from various parts of the wall and replaced, in 10,000 days the entire wall would have been entirely replaced. Yet on any one day the wall functioned as a wall and with little apparent change. Entirely analogous is the situation

of the body's cellular structure. For this reason the patient is analyzed for "balance," or intake-output, of water, minerals, and energy because alteration of the flow of energy or materials means a loss of the steady state. Disease frequently causes an unsteady state with gradual but inexorable loss of cell integrity and a change in homeostasis. Vomiting, gastrointestinal obstruction, diarrhea, or pneumonia causes a decreased input or increased output of material and energy. For this reason therapy often is directed toward maintaining the open-ended steady state: intravenous fluids with glucose and salts, diuretics, oxygen, and so forth. Any analysis of disease must include an estimate of the disruption of the open-ended steady state, since in many cases cellular or organ malfunction that is trivial in terms of cellular integrity, such as viral enteritis, may be rapidly fatal in an infant because of water and salt loss.

HORMONES AS HOMEOSTATIC REGULATORS. The function of the organs of homeostasis is regulated by means of hormones and/or the activity of the nervous system. Insulin and the regulation of blood sugar via the liver; parathyroid hormone and the regulation of blood calcium and phosphorus via the kidney; neural control of the respiratory muscles regulating the rate and depth of respiration and thus of gas exchange; neural control of the rate and force of cardiac contraction—all are examples of *regulation of homeostasis*. Obviously, deficiency or excessive action of hormones or of the nervous system must result in disease. A blow on the head may cause sufficient neuronal injury to cause muscular paralysis, preventing respiratory muscles from contracting so that the victim is unable by himself to supply the needs of his open-ended energy system.

The regulating organ receives continuous information about the results of regulation by way of the nervous system or the bloodstream, a situation termed *feedback*. The feedback then alters the function of the regulator, enhancing or diminishing its activity. For instance, the level of sugar in the blood flowing through the pancreas determines the amount of insulin released from the islet cells of the pancreas. After a meal the blood sugar rises because of the intestinal absorption of glucose. Insulin then is released to enhance absorption of glucose into the body cells and to promote the formation of glycogen in the liver, thus correcting the postprandial rise in blood glucose.

During exercise, when glucose is metabolized and tends to leave the blood, insulin secretion is reduced, glycogen storage is reduced, and epinephrine is released to aid the breakdown of glycogen to glucose in the liver by a process called glycogenolysis, with release from the liver to the bloodstream. Meanwhile the mean blood glucose level remains relatively unchanged because production and use are balanced.

Feedback is called *positive* if the substance regulated enhances the action of the regulator, and *negative* if it decreases the action of the regulator. An example of negative feedback is the ingestion of an excessive amount of water, which reduces the release of antidiuretic hormone from the neurohypophysis, with the result that less renal tubular absorption of water occurs until the excess water is voided as urine.

Disease may be a consequence of abnormal regulation of homeostasis. Examples are diabetes insipidus due to deficiency of antidiuretic hormone; paroxysmal atrial tachycardia following excess sympathetic nervous system stimulation; and renal edema due to excessive aldosterone, a hormone of the adrenal cortex which decreases the loss of sodium by way of the kidney.

COMPENSATION.   Finally, the role of *compensation* must be discussed. The organs of homeostasis or their regulators are capable of a wide range of activity. Witness the range of the volume of air breathed: 0.3 to 150 L./minute; or of the heart rate: 40-150 beats/minute; or urinary volume and concentration. These organs, if healthy, can increase their activity in the presence of disease processes which continuously tend to change the internal environment. Consider now an example.

The thyroid hormone controls the rate of energy metabolism, as generally measured by oxygen consumption or heat exchange, through an iodine-containing hormone, thyroxine, produced by its cells. If the food is deficient in iodine the continuous loss of iodine to the open-ended system is halted by means of a compensatory enlargement or hypertrophy of the thyroid cells which capture with great efficiency all iodine from the food or previously released thyroxine. The enlarged thyroid is called a goiter, and what is termed a disease is actually compensation to provide for homeostasis. The enlargement is due to the release of thyroid-stimulating hormone (TSH) from the anterior pituitary, a consequence of decreased circulating thyroid hormone (positive feedback).

Disease also follows loss of compensation. If a person rises suddenly from a sitting or lying position, the venous return to the heart is reduced because about 1 liter of blood is temporarily pooled in the legs. A fall in blood pressure is avoided by a compensatory increase in heart output. Ordinarily, however, the adjustment is rapid, the change in heart rate is small, and the blood pressure is steady. After squatting for a few minutes and then rapidly standing, even the young may experience transient dizziness because of the decreased cardiac output, loss of blood pressure, and decreased perfusion of the brain. The dizziness occurs because some brain cells have no energy reserve, and hence adequate blood pressure and flow to the brain to provide oxygen and glucose homeostasis are of the utmost importance. In the treatment of hypertension, drugs which block or diminish the activity of the sympathetic nervous system, such as reserpine or guanethidine, interfere with the vascular and cardiac compensation to change in posture, and orthostatic hy-

potension follows. Getting out of a chair in such instances becomes a study in slow motion and a search for a support to prevent falling.

SUMMARY.   To summarize briefly, homeostasis in an open-ended system results from the varying activities of organs of homeostasis regulated by hormonal, humoral, and neural mechanisms often via a positive or negative feedback, circulation being the common mediator. The equilibrium achieved is a dynamic steady state.

Disease results when any of these interacting and interrelated organs and phenomena are altered by (1) a change in the organ cells themselves by infection, trauma, or degeneration, (2) a change in formation, release, or action of the regulators, or (3) over- or under-compensatory action of the organs for changes elsewhere.

Nursing Implications

Now, to put these concepts to practical use, the nurse will combine observation and assessment of the patient with a review of the patient's record and will make two decisions:

1. What is the current status of the patient?
2. Is the clinical trend toward or away from health and a steady state?

A set of questions and the sources for the answers leading to these two decisions are presented as follows:

Question 1:   Is the patient in dynamic balance?
   Sources: a. Heat balance: body temperature
                b. Water balance: water intake and output, daily body weight
                c. Calorie balance: recorded food intake, long-term body weight
                d. Nitrogen balance: recorded food intake

Examples: If the patient has a fever and a limited calorie intake of 2 or 3 liters of intravenous infusions of glucose in water, then he is most likely suffering from a negative calorie and protein balance, which is a serious situation in the young and lethal in aged patients, who are already depleted of bodily nutritional stores. If the patient is on bed rest, this automatically means a negative calcium balance. If he is vomiting and has diarrhea, the result may be a negative mineral and water balance. An elderly patient with an adequate intake of water by vein not approximately equaled by urine volume must be perspiring, dehydrated, or edematous, since there is an apparent positive water balance.

Question 2:   Is the patient in a homeostatic state as determined by analysis of blood and urine?
    Sources: a. Electrolytes
                 b. Creatinine or BUN
                 c. Blood sugar
                 d. Blood gases, pH

Examples: The nurse should scan the record to obtain the current status and to determine if there has been a change. Obviously, a rising BUN indicates a serious immediate threat more than does a stable elevated BUN in known chronic renal disease, for the latter state may last for years.

Question 3: Are the principal organs of homeostasis functioning with good reserve?

Sources:
    a. Circulation: blood pressure, pulse, ECG, hemoglobin, hematocrit
    b. Lungs: rate and depth of respiration, respiratory distress, cyanosis, chest film, auscultation for estimate of ventilation
    c. Liver: size, blood enzymes, bilirubin
    d. Kidneys: output, specific gravity, urinalysis, BUN, creatinine clearance

Question 4: Does the patient have any reserve in terms of willed activity?

Sources:
    a. State of consciousness and intellectual activity
    b. Motor function: bed rest, bathroom privileges, feeding activity

This list shows that no special tools are needed to arrive at some estimate of the patient's functional state. Systematic nursing assessment will alert to a change in functional state and to the need for prompt and further observation. These questions ask nothing about disease and pathology but about *function* (physiology).

BRIEF SURVEY OF OTHER MECHANISMS OF DISEASE

Developmental defects are not an uncommon cause of disease. Overt anatomic defects such as imperforate anus or cardiac abnormalities make homeostasis impossible or else attainable only by restricted activity. Other defects, more subtle in expression, are molecular or cellular in scope and are often a result of genetic abnormality. Examples are: clotting defects such as hemophilia; anemia in sickle-cell disease; and enzyme defects such as phenylketonuria.

Allergic and autoimmune diseases (i.e., diseases associated with the development of antibodies and abnormal proteins in the body) are disruptive to homeostasis.

One of the allergic diseases, asthma, produces readily demonstrable changes in homeostasis. Because of constriction of bronchial muscle, resistance to air flow is increased, ventilation of the lungs is decreased, and exchange of respiratory gases is altered. Carbon dioxide accumulates, oxygen supply is insufficient, and respiratory acidosis, hypoxemia, and reduced reserves for energy from oxidative sources result. By marked muscular effort the severe asthmatic may obtain sufficient oxygen to support life under conditions of reduced activity while the kidney excretes acid to compensate for the acidosis.

Diseases of metabolism and the endocrine glands may best be considered in their relationship to homeostasis. Abnormalities of growth or of the sex hormones do not usually alter homeostasis; alterations are confined to specific tissues not vital to survival. Metabolic diseases involving blood vessels, such as atherosclerosis, are most serious when the blood vessels of the organs of homeostasis are involved.

Deficiency of calories, protein, or other essential nutrient elements is a common cause of human misery and a serious one because man exists in an open-ended system. Many diseases cause malnutrition: diarrhea, malabsorption syndromes, intestinal obstruction; but poverty, ignorance, poor health habits, and faulty dentition or ill-fitting dentures are frequent causes. In the United States, obesity caused by calorie excess is the most common nutritional defect. Although not usually classified as a disease, obesity is associated with an increased incidence of heart and arterial disease and a shorter life span. In fact, most acute illnesses are laid on a foundation of chronic disease either fully compensated by physiological means or ignored until the acute episode.

Altered regulation of cell growth and reproduction is also an important cause of disease and in this class may be placed growths, benign or malignant, of any tissue. Generally, in these instances, death comes from malnutrition or interference with the organs or regulators of homeostasis.

Diseases of striated muscles, the skeleton, the sense organs, the motor control of skeletal muscles, and the skin (save for sweating and heat regulation) may not disturb homeostatic mechanisms, but may change our relation to the external environment. Since the bulk of man's thought and activity is directed to the external environment, such diseases are serious tragedies. The victim of stroke may linger on for years, his mechanism for homeostasis intact; yet he is restricted in choice and freedom because still-living muscle cells are not stimulated and coordinated to permit purposeful movement.

Infection, parasitic infestation, trauma, and poisoning come from without. There are bodily defenses for these: white cells, blood clotting, fibrous tissue repair, vomiting. Generally, cause and effect can be traced in these instances.

Finally, to be mentioned but not discussed is the *interaction between the mind and the body*. Anxiety, depression, and neurotic behavior with attendant physical symptoms are major contributors to the discomfort of modern man, though life is not threatened and homeostasis generally is secure. Pain, though not a disease, may seriously influence behavior and restrict activity, thus providing a diseaselike state.

Mental disease is not discussed because the pathogenesis is largely unknown, although in some instances evidence points to biochemical changes at the cellular level as one basis for such disease.

STRESS: PHYSIOLOGIC REACTION TO INJURY AND DISEASE

Local Response and Defenses

Cell injury can be caused by a variety of factors (infections, heat, cold, chemicals, mechanical injury, etc.). Each of these causes provokes a local response to the injury as a result of the release of chemical substances from the damaged cells: histamine, lysosomes, and kinins. These chemical substances have the following effects:

1. Dilatation of capillaries and arterioles with a resultant increase in local blood flow
2. Increased permeability of the capillaries with a translocation of protein and water from the blood to tissue space and a resultant swelling and local accumulation of hormones, antibodies, and nutrients
3. Stimulation of nerve endings by kinins with a resulting sensation of pain and flow of information to the central nervous system (protective reflexes, generalized bodily responses to the local injury)
4. Migration of white blood cells to the injured area by means of chemical attraction (polymorphonuclear cells migrate to sites of bacterial invasion where their action results in the formation of pus; monocytes and lymphocytes are attracted in cases of viral invasion; and eosinophils come into play in allergic injury by antigens)

The external signs of this complex response to injury are swelling (edema, wheal formation in allergy), redness, pain, and loss of function. The process is basically the same for each response; variations depend on the cell injured, the resistance of the host to injury, and the nature of the cause of injury. Thus the body has a predetermined ready response to a mosquito bite or to myocardial death following coronary artery occlusion.

Generalized Stress Responses and Defenses

Other predetermined ready defenses against disease involve organ activity at a distance from the site of the disease. First, the ordinary activity of the organs of homeostasis may be augmented: increased cardiac output with fever and attendant increase in metabolic activity; increased respiratory volume for the same reason. Second, the activity of the pituitary and adrenal endocrine glands and the sympathetic nervous system is augmented and integrated into a pattern of response to protect the entire organism against disease and to integrate the homeostatic response so that it is commensurate with bodily defense requirements.

The action of the homeostatic organs adjusts, via the control system, to the needs of the entire body, depending on the activity undertaken, whether it be sleeping or running a marathon. Bodily response can be affected by numerous factors: (1) disease can disrupt cellular activity or structure and damage the control system; (2) the external environment can be hostile (cold, heat, starvation); (3) emotional control can be lost (anger, depression, grief); or (4) the need for physical activity can become greatly increased (chopping wood, running up stairs). In such situations, a condition of *stress* occurs. Stress relates to marked demands on the organs of homeostasis, such as those that occur when disease causes a reduction in the actual physiological reserve or when muscular effort exhausts potential reserves without benefit of training or conditioning. (Running is less stressful to the athlete than to the once-a-month jogger, and pneumonia is less stressful to the young man than to the older heavy smoker suffering from chronic obstructive pulmonary disease.)

However, the homeostatic balances generally do not succumb to stress, because of the stress "team" that is called into play — the adrenal gland and the sympathetic nervous system, which superimpose a set of controls and responses on practically every cell.

ADRENAL GLAND AND CORTISOL.   The adrenal gland, derived from two germ layers, releases two different kinds of hormones and is controlled in turn by two different types of mechanisms. The medulla, derived from ectoderm, releases epinephrine and is under the control of the sympathetic nervous system. The cortex, derived from mesoderm, releases the hormones cortisol and aldosterone.

Cortisol release is regulated by the adenohypophysis, through its hormone adrenocorticotrophin (ACTH), in conjunction with a negative feedback as part of the control. Aldosterone, a regulator of salt and water excretion by the kidneys, is guided by the renin-angiotensin system of the kidney.

Stress (due to injury, emotional instability, disease, social changes) acting by way of the central nervous system causes the neurohypophysis to release a hormone called ACTH-releasing factor, which in turn stimulates the adrenal cortex to produce the hormone cortisol. Cortisol has a universal effect, influencing practically every cell in the body and producing the following important results:

1. Conversion of bodily protein to glucose (gluconeogenesis), which allows energy sources to be mobilized, but at the expense of body proteins, especially muscle and skin
2. Inhibition of protein synthesis so that antibodies are not formed; hence antigen-antibody reactions are diminished and tissue transplants are not rejected, though at the price of delayed wound healing
3. Stabilization of lysosomes, which prevents cellular self-digestion in inflammatory states but reduces the destruction of bacteria

Cortisol thus maintains the blood sugar in fasting states (sleep, postsurgical state, vomiting) and reduces inflammatory responses (swelling, fever, pus, etc.) and bodily defenses against disease. Therefore, cortisol is used to fight uncontrolled inflammation which in itself is a disease, as in septic shock, rheumatoid arthritis, excessive fibrosis and scarring, and excessive mucus in the small bronchi.

Other effects of cortisol are (1) decrease in the number of circulating eosinophils, (2) increase in the number of circulating lymphocytes, (3) inhibition of fibroblast formation, and (4) decrease in the rate of epithelialization of the skin.

SYMPATHETIC NERVOUS SYSTEM. Walter Cannon pointed out the role of the sympathetic nervous system in protecting the body against external events that threaten homeostasis, especially hunger, cold, trauma, and sudden environmental changes. Some of the same responses may occur in states of fear and rage. They are:

1. Activation of a liver enzyme, phosphorylase, to promote glycogenolysis
2. Increase in the rate of strength of contraction of the heart to maintain blood pressure
3. Constriction of the blood vessels of the skin to reduce heat loss and skin hemorrhage
4. Increase in the clotting ability of the blood
5. Dilatation of skeletal muscle arterioles and constriction of splanchnic vessels to redistribute blood
6. Inhibition of the intestinal wall muscle
7. Dilatation of bronchial muscle to provide easier air flow

All of the above reactions protect against external hazards. In addition, fatigue is postponed and energy sources are mobilized. Thus, the sympathetic nervous system is a defense system against external threat and can be considered a general homeostatic mechanism and one that acts rapidly (within seconds); whereas the hypothalamic-pituitary-adrenocortical system is slower, taking minutes to hours to achieve its obvious effects.

The substance released by both the adrenal gland and the sympathetic nervous system is a hormone, and thus every cell is potentially regulated by alteration in permeability, stimulation or suppression of function, or stimulation of enzyme activity.

GENERAL ADAPTATION SYNDROME. Hans Selye has emphasized the stereotyped nonspecific reactions of the hypothalamic-pituitary-adrenocortical system to any kind of stress. The general gross responses are: enlargement of the adrenal cortex, shrinkage of the thymus gland, stomach ulceration (stress ulcers), decreased circulation of eosinophils, and loss of body weight (protein catabolism) — all end results of the effects of corticol. The entire process and the results Selye termed the "general adaptation syndrome," meaning adaptation to stress. In turn, the general syndrome is divided into three phases, depending on the duration and degree of the stress: (1) the *alarm reaction,* during which the chemicals released by the local tissues in response to injury stimulate the central nervous system, via the limbic system and the hypothalamus, to initiate the rapidly acting sympathetic nervous system responses and the slower pituitary-adrenal responses; (2) the *stage of resistance* to stress, dominated by the pituitary-adrenal hormones, in which tissue responses are sustained but the inflammatory local responses are not permitted to be exuberant; and (3) if the stress goes on, the *stage of exhaustion,* when the bodily defenses are insufficient to cope with the ongoing disease process. This descriptive analysis provides a framework for thinking about disease and disease processes.

Emotional stress — anger, frustration, and anxiety — provoke not a triple local response but an increased release of cortisol and sustained excessive sympathetic nervous system activity (tachycardia, pallor, sweaty palms and skin). Thus the general response systems, which are designed to protect the body from stress, now produce effects that are diseaselike, so that a disease of adaptation results. Another example is essential hypertension characterized by excessive salt and water retention, the effect of inappropriate aldosterone secretion and/or sustained vasoconstriction of the arterioles via the sympathetic nervous system. Therapy is directed to dietary salt restriction, diuretics, and/or sympathetic nervous system blocking agents or drugs acting directly to relax the smooth muscle of arterioles.

SUMMARY

Disease is a dynamic, ever changing expression of the balance between cell damage or abnormal cell activity and the body's defense mechanisms or compensations. It becomes serious when a major organ of homeostasis is extensively damaged or when it is functioning maximally. Once the internal environment is substantially altered, then all cells are damaged or die. Death is generally defined as cessation of the activity of the heart and lungs, the principal organs of homeostasis. More recently, the absence of cerebral function as measured by the electroencephalograph is now considered an indication of death, and so a regulator of homeostasis is included in the definition of death.

REPRESENTATIVE PATHOPHYSIOLOGIC PROCESSES

The aim of the rest of this chapter is to present the pathogenesis of several diseases as examples of the principles discussed. Flow diagrams indicate major events in the development of disease and for clarity are divided into *antecedent* events that may be considered the prime cause of disease, and *action* events that show the interrelation of disease and bodily response. In the latter case, cause and effect are displayed for the major facets of the disease. Regretably, arrows and words but dimly portray the shifts in the patient's condition, moment by moment or day by day in acute illness, or week by week in chronic illness. The influence of normal or abnormal physiological cycles, of social adjustments between patient and hospital personnel or family, of unknown or expressed anxiety and concern, and of the patient's total life experience on the development and course of disease, is well recognized by the health team. These variables cannot be inserted into a flow diagram—yet, they may be major factors governing the course of the disease.

Four diseases are discussed and the major characteristics of each are pointed out. Pollinosis (seasonal allergic rhinitis due to pollens) is associated with an abnormal defense mechanism, that of defense against foreign protein. Sickle cell anemia is an example of the effect of a genetic defect, in this case in the formation of hemoglobin. The disease is caused by a small change in the structure of a molecule. Addison's disease, caused by decreased function of the adrenal cortex, is an example of loss of regulation of a part of the internal environment, principally sodium and water, and carbohydrate metabolism. Left-sided heart failure shows the effect of the abnormal function of an organ of homeostasis.

Seasonal Allergic Rhinitis Due to Pollens (Pollinosis) (Flow Diagram I)

Typically, allergies are characterized by a marked cellular response to trivial challenge and represent an exaggerated immune reaction. The protein structure of the body is, in part, unique to the organism and is a product of genetic inheritance. Invasion by a foreign protein, called an antigen (through bacteria, blood transfusion, gastrointestinal absorption of protein), provokes the formation of a body protein called an antibody, which is able to combine with the antigen and render it incapable of injuring cells. The antibodies may circulate in the bloodstream as globulin or may be fixed in the tissues.

The lymphocyte that "stores" the information about a previous invasion by foreign protein or other antigenic substance is in many cases maintained throughout the lifetime of the individual, and hence when the antigen reappears, specific antibodies can be formed quickly by the conversion of the specific lymphocytes to plasma cells that actually produce the immune globulins. In multiple myeloma, a disease associated with hyperplasia of the plasma cells in bone marrow, large quantities of immune globulins or of fragments of immune globulins are produced.

The use of vaccines against common infectious diseases involves the deliberate introduction of foreign protein into the body, in order to stimulate antibody formation. Following vaccination against tetanus, the effective levels of antibody may be available for years, and the concentration or titer is readily increased by a so-called booster dose.

In seasonal allergic rhinitis, antibodies of immunoglobulin class E (IgE) coating the mucosa of the nose

PATHOPHYSIOLOGY OF POLLINOSIS
(Flow Diagram I)

Antecedents

Inherited tendency to abnormal immune response (atopy)
Entry of antigen protein substance (pollen)

↓

Lymphocytes transformed into plasma cells

↓

Formation of circulating protein antibodies (immunoglobulins) by immune cells (probably lymphocytes) that not only *immunize* but *sensitize* (skin-sensitizing antibodies or reagin)

Attachment of "skin sensitizing" antibodies to nasal mucosa

Action

Pollen released into air	contact with sensitized mucosa	

→ antigen antibody reaction with cell injury

release of histamine other substances (kinins)

↓

sympathetic nervous system activity	diminishes these responses	1. capillary dilatation (congestion) 2. tissue fluid transudation (nasal discharge, sneezing) 3. stimulation of mucus production 4. stimulation of naked nerve endings ——→ itching

Addenda

Repeated antigen challenge leads to desensitization (mechanisms unknown)

and conjunctiva and specific for a given pollen (antigen) combine with the pollen. As a result, cell injury occurs, as is indicated by copious secretions, edema of the mucosa, sneezing because of the secretions, and local itching. When the offending pollen is blown away, the allergic condition ceases.

Cell stimulation is due in part to the release of histamine and other as yet poorly identified substances. Therapy takes four major lines:

1. Hyposensitization by repeated injections of the offending pollens in low concentration
2. Administration of antihistamine; that is, substances protecting cells against the effects of histamine
3. Removal of offending pollens (by air conditioning)
4. Suppression of the immune response by means of corticosteroids

Sickle Cell Anemia (Flow Diagram II)

Sickle cell anemia is the result of the physical deformity of red cells following altered aggregation of hemoglobin molecules within the cell. The complex protein molecule referred to as S hemoglobin differs from the normal hemoglobin molecule by the introduction of a single amino acid, valine, instead of glutamic acid. The cause of this chronic inherited defect is a fault in the desoxyribonucleic acid of the gene controlling production of the

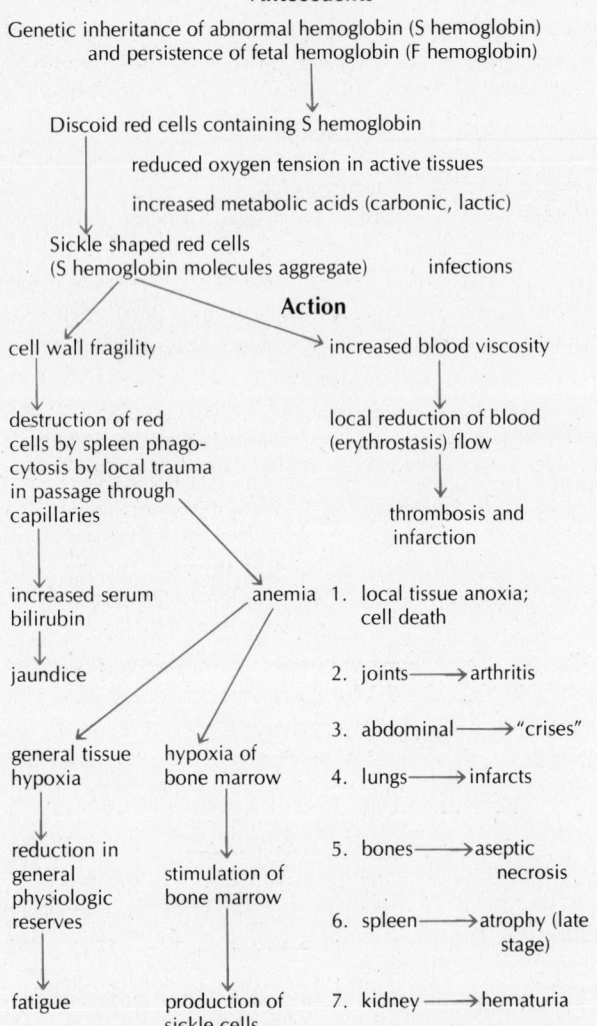

PATHOPHYSIOLOGY OF SICKLE CELL ANEMIA
(Flow Diagram II)

Antecedents

Genetic inheritance of abnormal hemoglobin (S hemoglobin) and persistence of fetal hemoglobin (F hemoglobin)

Discoid red cells containing S hemoglobin

reduced oxygen tension in active tissues

increased metabolic acids (carbonic, lactic)

Sickle shaped red cells
(S hemoglobin molecules aggregate)   infections

Action

cell wall fragility   increased blood viscosity

destruction of red cells by spleen phago-cytosis by local trauma in passage through capillaries   local reduction of blood (erythrostasis) flow

thrombosis and infarction

increased serum bilirubin   anemia   1. local tissue anoxia; cell death

jaundice   2. joints──→arthritis

                           3. abdominal──→"crises"

general tissue hypoxia   hypoxia of bone marrow   4. lungs──→infarcts

                           5. bones──→aseptic necrosis

reduction in general physiologic reserves   stimulation of bone marrow   6. spleen──→atrophy (late stage)

fatigue   production of sickle cells   7. kidney──→hematuria

Compensation

1. Decreased oxygen is the stimulus for red cell production in the bone marrow, which produces red cells sufficient to correct the anemia and attendant hypoxia. This is an example of positive feedback. The compensation produces further pathology in the bone vessels.
2. The greater the amount of F hemoglobin in the cells the less the sickling effect.
3. Local vessel dilatation following tissue injury and an inflammatory reaction are present. The white cells and other sources of proteolytic enzymes remove dead cells; fibrous tissue replacement occurs.

abnormal S hemoglobin in the bone marrow. Since the sickle cell is resistant to invasion by the parasite of malaria, this latter disease may promote the survival of the genetic trait by natural selection.

In the capillaries serving actively metabolizing cells, the normal reduction in oxygen and the production of acids such as carbonic and lactic acids cause the S hemoglobin to aggregate, and the coin-shaped red cell is distorted into a sickle shape. The abnormal cells do not readily slip and squeeze through the capillaries, and a logjam of red cells causes local stasis of blood flow with attendant cell damage due to hypoxia and altered local internal environment. In the general circulation, the red cells generally maintain the normal anatomic shape.

The severity of the disease depends on the number of abnormal cells and on local tissue factors governing blood flow at the arteriole-capillary-venule level. Ordinarily the course of the disease is chronic, with exacerbations associated with infection or other disease. Though not life-threatening, sickle cell anemia does restrict the freedom of its victim to participate in a wide range of life's activities.

Adrenal Cortical Insufficiency (Addison's Disease) (Flow Diagram III)

Certain disease states can cause the partial loss of adrenal cortical tissue. This loss leads to major changes in the internal environment because the hormone aldosterone, which normally controls the absorption of sodium by the kidney, is deficient, so that sodium is excreted in increased amounts. Sodium is the chief ion of the extracellular fluid from the standpoint of total concentration and of its key position in regulation of water volume and thus blood volume. Since the ionic concentrations of the internal environment must be kept relatively stable, retention of sodium ions by the kidney is always associated with water retention and expansion of the fluid volume; and to a greater or lesser degree, sodium loss is usually associated with water loss, contraction of the fluid volume, and, thus, dehydration. Where sodium goes, water usually follows.

Loss of sodium and water is associated with decreased blood perfusion of the kidney and an increase of blood urea nitrogen, so-called prerenal azotemia.

The normal functional integrity of the cell wall in part depends upon the concentration of the sodium and potassium ions on the inside (high potassium) and outside (high sodium) of the cell. An important consequence of this asymmetrical distribution of ions is the creation of an ion-battery with an excess positive electrical charge on the outer surface and a corresponding excess negative charge on the inside. Migration of these ions across the cell surface follows cell stimulation, and charged-particle migration causes an electric current which serves to initiate biochemical activities of the cell such as contraction of

PATHOPHYSIOLOGY OF ADRENAL CORTICAL INSUFFICIENCY
(Addison's Disease)
(Flow Diagram III)
Antecedents

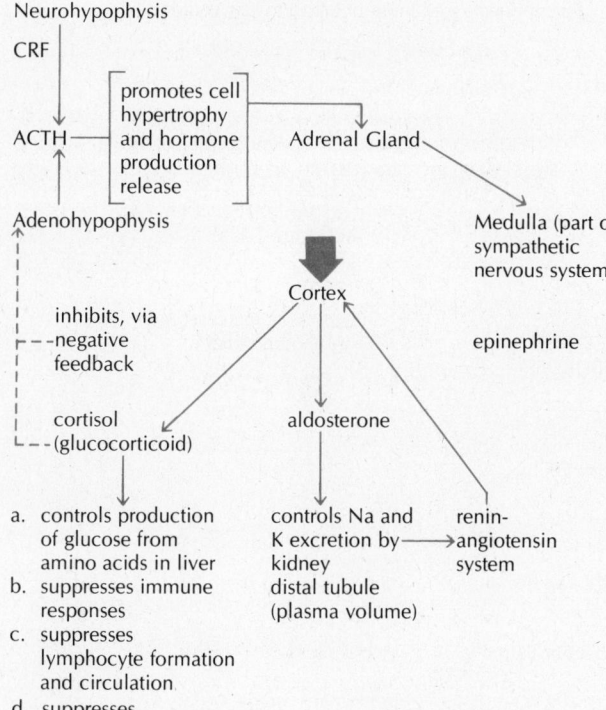

Neurohypophysis

CRF

ACTH ⟶ promotes cell hypertrophy and hormone production release ⟶ Adrenal Gland

Adenohypophysis

Medulla (part of sympathetic nervous system)

Cortex

epinephrine

inhibits, via negative feedback

cortisol (glucocorticoid)

aldosterone

a. controls production of glucose from amino acids in liver
b. suppresses immune responses
c. suppresses lymphocyte formation and circulation
d. suppresses eosinophil circulation

controls Na and K excretion by kidney distal tubule (plasma volume)

renin-angiotensin system

Action
(via the cyclic AMP System)

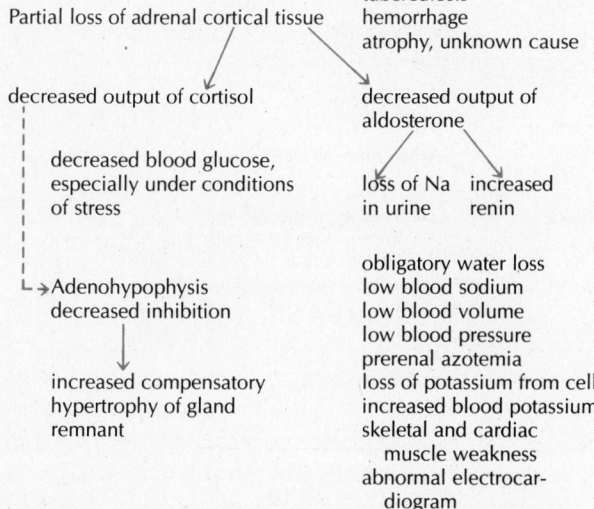

Partial loss of adrenal cortical tissue

tuberculosis
hemorrhage
atrophy, unknown cause

decreased output of cortisol

decreased output of aldosterone

decreased blood glucose, especially under conditions of stress

loss of Na in urine

increased renin

Adenohypophysis decreased inhibition

increased compensatory hypertrophy of gland remnant

obligatory water loss
low blood sodium
low blood volume
low blood pressure
prerenal azotemia
loss of potassium from cell
increased blood potassium
skeletal and cardiac muscle weakness
abnormal electrocardiogram

Compensation

1. hypertrophy of gland remnant by adenohypophysis via release of ACTH
2. salt "craving," a desire of unknown mechanism, leads to intake of salt

muscle protein and release of enzymes. The electrocardiogram is a graphic registration of the complex electrical fluctuations passing over heart muscle as the excited cell membranes allow small reversible migrations of sodium and potassium ions into and out of the cell. In Addison's disease, sodium loss is followed by the loss of potassium from the cell into the extracellular fluid. The increased potassium concentration in the extracellular fluid produced during exacerbations of the disease causes an abnormal electrocardiogram. A further consequence of the sodium and potassium shifts is muscle weakness, both skeletal and cardiac.

The adrenal cortex produces a second hormone, cortisol, as was noted earlier. Cortisol and its metabolites control the formation of glucose from amino acids in the liver, a process called *gluconeogenesis*. By this metabolic mechanism, glucose can be formed from noncarbohydrate stores and during periods of stress or starvation glucose homeostasis can be maintained. Because Addison's disease curtails cortisol production, the patient tends to have a low blood sugar and does not tolerate fasting.

Lymphocytosis occurs because the normal suppressive action of cortisol on the lymphocyte is absent or diminished. Because enhanced adrenal cortical activity is part of the bodily response to stress of any type, such as cold, heat, starvation, infection, and injury, the Addisonian does not tolerate stress, and major illness may rapidly become lethal. As in all endocrine disorders, the clinical picture varies with the degree of hormonal deficit.

Compensation is achieved by hypertrophy of the remaining cells of the adrenal cortex through the stimulus of adrenocorticotrophin hormone (ACTH) of the adenohypophysis released now from the inhibition of normally circulating levels of cortisol. Salt "hunger" leads to an appetite for salt which relieves the most serious aspect of this disease. Replacement therapy provides cure in the same sense that insulin provides a cure for diabetes mellitus.

A partial Addison's disease can be produced by giving exogenous cortisol or a chemical congener (prednisone, etc.) to treat disease. True to the negative feedback arrangement, the adenohypophysis no longer produces ACTH, and the adrenal cortex atrophies. If the exogenous hormone is abruptly withdrawn, then there is insufficient adrenal gland tissue to produce the necessary daily requirements of cortisol. Aldosterone secretion, under the control of the renin-angiotensin system is not involved.

Note: Hyperpigmentation occurs in Addison's disease, but the mechanism is not understood. Enhanced activity of a melanocyte-stimulating hormone of the neurohypophysis has been advanced as an explanation.

Chronic Heart Failure Due to Mitral Stenosis (Flow Diagram IV)

Ordinarily, failure of the muscle of each heart chamber to pump out the incoming blood is a slowly developing process, though sudden demands on the heart may lead to acute failure. All organs, and in particular those of homeostasis, depend upon adequate blood flow for cell function; and their cell function in turn changes or normalizes the concentration of selected substances in the blood. Therefore, partial loss of the pumping action of the heart can lead to rapid and dangerous alterations of the internal environment. Symptoms arise from every organ and tissue. Left-sided failure is usually a way-station in the course of total right- and left-heart failure.

Because, in left-sided failure due to mitral stenosis, blood cannot readily flow from the left atrium to the left ventricle, the lung serves as a reservoir for blood, and pulmonary edema follows. Dyspnea, first on exertion and then as a paroxysmal nocturnal event, is the most important symptom. Hypoxemia is the consequence, and all tissues may function only to the limit allowed by reduced oxygen pressure. Poor perfusion of the myocardium by way of the coronary arteries leads to a still less efficient pump.

Because renal blood flow and pressure are reduced, sodium retention occurs, with retention of water as a consequence, leading to an expansion of blood and interstitial fluid volume. This increased circulating fluid is likewise stored in the lung, and another vicious cycle is set up.

Cardiac compensatory activity occurs. Stretching of the chamber wall by the blood left behind after a contraction of a chamber, combined with the normal incoming flow, results in a more forceful contraction of the atrium and a greater flow of blood past the narrowed valve orifice of mitral stenosis. Since no valves exist in the great pulmonary veins, the enhanced filling and contraction pressure is transmitted back to the lungs. Normally the pulmonary arterial and venous pressures are too low to cause filtration of water through the capillary to the alveoli. However, with enhanced venous pressures, edema fluid further accumulates and dyspnea follows. As the pulmonary venous pressure rises, the right ventricle must contract more forcibly to provide for a forward flow of blood. If the right ventricle fails, then right-heart failure, with enhanced central venous pressure, generalized edema, and liver and gastrointestinal congestion, occurs.

An abnormal rhythm, atrial fibrillation, frequently occurs and the atrium ceases to act as a pump at all. Stasis of flow of blood in the atrium may be sufficient to allow blood clotting, thrombus formation, and ultimately an embolus.

Although cardiac muscle and renal compensation may

PATHOPHYSIOLOGY OF LEFT-SIDED HEART FAILURE
(Flow Diagram IV)

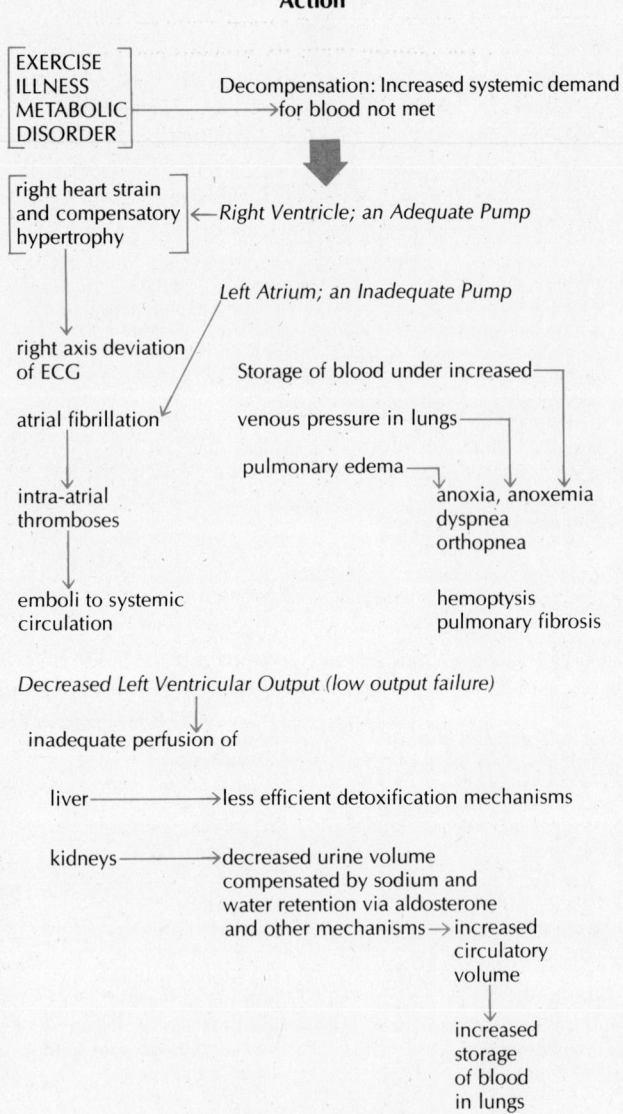

Antecedents

MITRAL STENOSIS FOLLOWING RHEUMATIC FEVER

Decreased Input of Blood to Left Ventricle

Decreased Left Ventricular Output

Diminished Perfusion of Systems Organs

INTERIM COMPENSATION: Hypertrophy of Atrial Muscle with Increased Atrial Output, Increased Contraction Force of Right Ventricle

Action

EXERCISE / ILLNESS / METABOLIC DISORDER — Decompensation: Increased systemic demand for blood not met

right heart strain and compensatory hypertrophy ← *Right Ventricle; an Adequate Pump*

Left Atrium; an Inadequate Pump

right axis deviation of ECG

atrial fibrillation

Storage of blood under increased venous pressure in lungs

pulmonary edema

intra-atrial thromboses

anoxia, anoxemia dyspnea orthopnea

emboli to systemic circulation

hemoptysis pulmonary fibrosis

Decreased Left Ventricular Output (low output failure)

inadequate perfusion of

liver————→less efficient detoxification mechanisms

kidneys————→decreased urine volume compensated by sodium and water retention via aldosterone and other mechanisms→increased circulatory volume ↓ increased storage of blood in lungs

brain————→decreased cerebral blood flow cerebral edema, anoxia Cheyne-Stokes respiration fatigue, personality change

skin————→compensation by vasoconstriction

provide temporary improvement, the only effective compensation is a reduction in tissue activity, and this must necessarily be of skeletal muscle. Rest, reduced muscle activity, is essential to a mode of living that will make the fewest demands on the heart. An upright position to permit drainage of edema fluid to the lowest parts of the lung and body will relieve the dyspnea.

BIBLIOGRAPHY

BOOKS

Brobeck, J. R., ed.: Best and Taylor's Physiological Basis of Medical Practice, 10th ed. Baltimore, Williams and Wilkins, 1979.

Cannon, W. B.: Bodily Changes in Pain, Hunger, Fear and Rage, 2nd ed. New York, Appleton-Century-Crofts, 1929.

Grollman, S.: The Human Body. Its Structure and Physiology. New York, Macmillan, 1978.

Guyton, A. C.: Basic Human Physiology: Normal Function and Mechanisms of Disease, 2nd ed. Philadelphia, W. B. Saunders, 1977.

_____: Textbook of Medical Physiology, 5th ed. Philadelphia, W. B. Saunders, 1976.

Luciano, D. S., Vander, A. J., and Sherman, J. H.: Human Function and Structure. New York, McGraw-Hill, 1978.

Miller, F. N.: Peery and Miller's Pathology, 3rd ed. Boston, Little, Brown, 1978.

Ross, G.: Essentials of Human Physiology. Chicago, Year Book Publishers, 1978.

Schottelius, B. A., and Schottelius, D. D.: Textbook of Physiology, 18th ed. St. Louis, C. V. Mosby, 1978.

Selye, H.: The Stress of Life, rev. ed. New York, McGraw-Hill, 1976.

Strand, F. L.: Physiology. New York, Macmillan, 1978.

ARTICLES

Frain, M., and Valiga, T. M.: The multiple dimensions of stress. Topics in Clin. Nsg., 1:43-52, Apr. 1979.

Marcinek, M. B.: Stress in the surgical patient. AJN, 77:1809-1811, Nov. 1977.

Shaw, S. E.: Health education for the public: Stress and stress management. Topics in Clin. Nsg., 1:53-57, Apr. 1979.

Stephenson, C. A.: The stress response. Stress in critically ill patients. AJN, 77:1806-1808, Nov. 1977.

Sutterley, D. C.: Stress and health: A survey of self-regulation modalities, Topics in Clin. Nsg., 1:1-21, Apr. 1979.

8

FLUIDS AND ELECTROLYTES: Balance and Disturbances

BODY FLUIDS

Since water makes up such a large percentage of the total body mass (approximately 60 percent), it is hard to imagine life without it. Indeed water provides the necessary medium in which most of the reactions of the body can occur. Total body water is distributed in the blood, the interstitial fluid surrounding the cells, and the water inside the cells. A variety of inorganic chemicals, including the electrolytes, and a number of organic compounds, including proteins and nutrients, are dissolved in the body water. The amount of water in the body represents the balance between water intake and water excretion. Relatively small disturbances in the body water balance can cause symptoms; the loss of 25 percent of the body water is generally fatal. Disturbances in the electrolyte composition of the body water can have marked effects upon body function. An important factor in the management of many disease processes is the correction of abnormalities of body water content and electrolyte composition.

BODY FLUID COMPARTMENTS

The total body water is distributed among various body compartments, as is indicated in Figure 8-1. Approximately 66 percent of the total body water (40 per-

118

cent of body weight) is contained within the cells and is referred to as the intracellular fluid. Approximately 25 percent of the total body water (15 percent of body weight) is contained around the cells and is referred to as the interstitial fluid. Most of the remainder (approximately 8 percent) of the body water (5 percent of body weight) forms the blood plasma. In addition, there are small amounts of water in specialized compartments within the body such as the cerebrospinal fluid, joint fluid, pericardial fluid, and pleural fluid. All of the body fluid that is not contained within cells is referred to as *extracellular fluid*.

ELECTROLYTES AND NONELECTROLYTES

Body water contains a variety of dissolved substances, including organic molecules such as proteins and lipids, and inorganic substances such as dissolved salts and dissolved gases. An important group of compounds are the blood electrolytes. Electrolytes are charged particles, or ions, that result from the dissociation of dissolved molecules. For example, salt (NaCl) when dissolved in water dissociates into a sodium ion, Na^+, and a chloride ion, Cl^-. Positively charged ions are called cations and include sodium (Na^+), potassium (K^+), calcium (Ca^{++}), and magnesium (Mg^{++}). Negatively charged electrolytes are called anions and include chloride (Cl^-), bicarbonate

(HCO_3^-), sulfate ($SO_4^=$), and phosphate ($PO_4^\equiv$). Some organic molecules such as the amino acids can also ionize when dissolved in water. In any solution, the total number of cations and the total number of anions must be equal.

The average electrolyte composition of the vascular, interstitial fluid, and intracellular fluid compartments is shown in Table 8-1. Generally, the units of electrolyte concentration are expressed in either millimoles (mmol.) per liter or milliequivalents (mEq.) per liter. One millimole of an ion is equal to its molecular weight in milligrams. For example, 23 milligrams of sodium (molecular weight 23) equals 1 millimole of sodium; if this amount is present in 1 liter of solution, the concentration is 1 millimole per liter. One milliequivalent is equal to the molecular weight in milligrams divided by the valence of the ion. The valence of an ion is a measure of its net electrical charge. Since the valence of the sodium ion is 1, a solution containing 1 millimole of sodium per liter also has a concentration of 1 milliequivalent per liter. However, a solution containing calcium in a concentration of 1 millimole per liter has 2 milliequivalents per liter since the valence of calcium is 2.

There are marked differences in the concentrations of various ions between intracellular fluid on the one hand and blood plasma and interstitial fluid on the other (see Table 8-1). The composition of blood plasma and interstitial fluid is similar with respect to ions, since the capillary wall is permeable to these small molecules which equilibrate between the two compartments. However, the capillary wall is relatively impermeable to plasma proteins because of their large size. As a result, the protein component of interstitial fluid is much smaller than that of plasma. Cell membranes are relatively impermeable to most ions and, therefore, the ionic concentrations in the intracellular fluid are markedly different from those in the interstitial compartment.

Two ions of particular importance are sodium and potassium. Intracellular sodium concentration is very low and intracellular potassium concentration is very high compared with the concentrations in the extracellular fluid. These differences are due to the property of cell membranes known as *active transport,* a process in which sodium is actively extruded from cells in exchange for potassium. The high intracellular potassium concentration is an important factor in normal protein synthesis and metabolism and also in allowing excitable cells such as nerve and muscle cells to transmit electrical impulses. Calcium is present in very low concentration in intracellular fluid, probably due to intracellular compartmentalization and active extrusion of calcium from the cell interior. Chloride and bicarbonate ion concentrations are also low within the cell. On the other hand, magnesium and phosphate ions that are bound to large molecules are present in concentrations that are much higher inside the cells than in the interstitial fluid.

The maintenance of these differences between intracellular and extracellular fluid is important for normal cell function.

EXTERNAL EXCHANGES OF FLUIDS AND ELECTROLYTES

The fluid within the body is in a dynamic state since there is constant fluid intake and constant fluid excretion. The total body fluid at any time represents the balance between intake and output. Normally, intake occurs by absorption through the gastrointestinal tract after the ingestion of water or other fluids. In addition, the metabolism of foodstuffs by the body liberates small amounts of water. Through the sensation of thirst, the volume of fluid intake is normally closely matched to the volume of fluids lost from the body. In the hospitalized patient, intravenous administration can also be utilized to replace fluid losses.

Fluid is lost from the body primarily through the normal excretory routes of urine and feces. Additional water is lost from the skin through evaporation and through the lungs during respiration; these are called *insensible losses*. In a normal individual, the amount of fluid ingested and eliminated per day is approximately 2,000 ml. This is typically accounted for by approximately 1,300 ml. in the urine, 200 ml. in the feces, and 500 ml. in insensible losses. A mechanism for variable water loss from the body is sweating. The loss of water through sweating can be as high as one liter per hour in hot, humid weather.

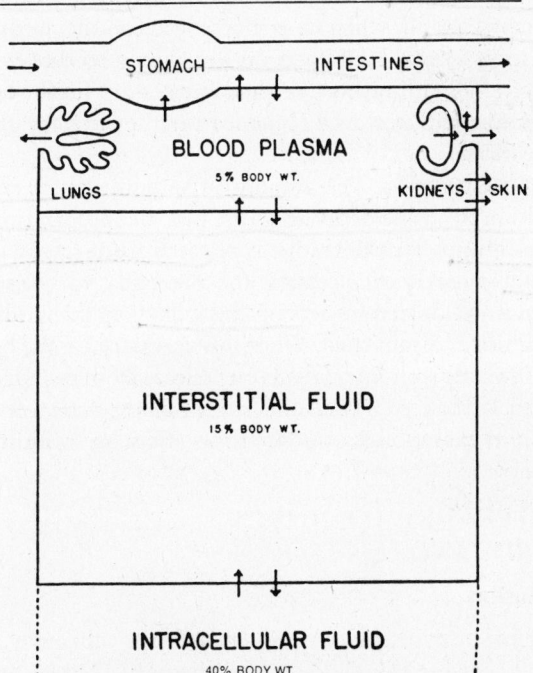

Figure 8-1. Schematic diagram of the distribution of body fluid among the intracellular, interstitial and blood plasma compartments.

TABLE 8-1.   COMPOSITION OF THE BODY FLUIDS. CONCENTRATIONS ARE EXPRESSED IN MILLIEQUIVALENTS PER LITER

SUBSTANCE	BLOOD PLASMA	INTER-STITIAL FLUID	INTRA-CELLULAR FLUID
Sodium	146.0	141.0	9
Potassium	4.4	4.1	145
Calcium	4.0	3.8	0
Magnesium	3.0	2.7	40
Total cations (+)	157.4	151.6	194
Chloride	106.0	114.0	6
Bicarbonate	28.0	30.0	11
Phosphate	2.1	2.0	90
Sulfate	1.1	1.2	20
Protein	17.0	1.0	67
Organic acids	3.2	3.4	0
Total anions (−)	157.4	151.6	194

In order to maintain constant conditions in the body, the intake of each of the electrolytes must equal its excretion. For example, the elimination of sodium in the urine, through the skin with perspiration, and in the gastrointestinal tract with the feces must equal the intake of sodium by mouth or by vein. Similar balances must hold for all of the other ions listed in Table 8-1.

REGULATION OF ELIMINATION OF FLUIDS AND ELECTROLYTES

ADH.   The amount of water that is eliminated in the urine depends on the blood concentration of antidiuretic hormone (ADH). This hormone is released from the pituitary gland when it is necessary for the body to conserve water. ADH acts on the kidney so that water excretion is diminished. When it is necessary for the body to eliminate water, ADH release from the pituitary gland is reduced.

ALDOSTERONE.   The amount of sodium that is eliminated in the urine depends on the blood concentration of aldosterone. This hormone is released from the adrenal gland when it is necessary for the body to conserve sodium. Aldosterone acts on the kidney so that sodium excretion is diminished. When it is necessary for the body to eliminate sodium, aldosterone release from the adrenal gland is reduced. The influence of aldosterone on potassium excretion is opposite to its effect on sodium.

INTERNAL EXCHANGES OF FLUIDS AND ELECTROLYTES

Diffusion

Substances dissolved in water, such as electrolytes, can move between two fluid compartments by the process of diffusion. *Diffusion* is defined as the tendency of particles to move from regions of high concentration to regions of low concentration. Cell membranes contain specialized proteins that can enhance the rate of transfer of some substances into or out of the cell. This process is called *facilitated diffusion*. Both nonfacilitated and facilitated diffusion are passive processes, i.e., no energy input is required. Most particles equilibrate across capillary walls by passive diffusion.

Osmosis

Water diffusion occurs across most capillary and cell membranes in order to achieve an equal water concentration on both sides of the membrane. The tendency of water to diffuse from one compartment to another depends on its *osmolality* which is defined as the total concentration of particles dissolved in a liter (actually a kilogram) of water. When a compound such as sodium chloride is dissolved in water, it dissociates into a cation (sodium) and an anion (chloride). Therefore, if a solution contains 150 millimoles per liter of sodium chloride, it would contain 150 milliequivalents per liter of sodium and 150 milliequivalents per liter of chloride. This solution has an osmolality of 300 milliosmols per liter.

Certain substances, when placed in aqueous solution, do not dissociate as do the electrolytes. These substances remain as single, uncharged particles. Examples of such substances that are physiologically important include glucose, urea, and other organic compounds. These nonelectrolytes contribute to the osmolality of the fluid but do not contribute to the total cation or anion concentration of the solution.

The osmolality of normal human plasma, interstitial fluid, and intracellular fluid is approximately 300 milliosmols/liter. The reason that osmolality of all body fluid compartments is equal is that water moves easily across membranes if small differences in osmolality arise. This movement of water, called *osmosis*, restores the condition of equal osmolality on both sides of the membrane.

Active Transport

In most cells, sodium is actively extruded from the intracellular fluid into the extracellular fluid. Potassium is transported in the opposite direction. These ion movements are equal to and are in the reverse direction from those that are constantly occurring by passive diffusion. They are examples of active transport, a process that requires biological energy. In the case of sodium and potassium, the active transport process is called the "Sodium–Potassium pump." The energy utilized for active transport is produced by metabolic processes occurring in every cell of the body. It is stored in the form of a chemical called adenosine triphosphate (ATP) and is liberated for use by the action of an enzyme called adenosine triphosphatase (ATPase).

REGULATION OF BODY FLUID pH

Hydrochloric acid (HCl), when dissolved in water, is dissociated into the cation hydrogen (H^+) and the anion chloride (Cl^-). The concentration of hydrogen ions in solution determines the acidity or pH of the solution. pH is defined as the negative logarithm of the hydrogen ion concentration. For example, if a solution contains 10^{-7} mol/liter of H^+, its pH is 7.0.

The pH of blood is normally at 7.4. This corresponds to a hydrogen ion concentration of approximately 4×10^{-8} mol/liter. Intracellular fluid is slightly more acid than blood, having a pH in the range of 6.6 to 7.2. The range of blood pH compatible with life is 6.8 to 7.8.

The pH of the extracellular fluid is regulated by its content of CO_2 and bicarbonate. These two compounds can be interconverted as shown by the following chemical reaction:

$$CO_2 + H_2O \longleftrightarrow H_2CO_3 \longleftrightarrow H^+ + HCO^-_3$$

Carbon dioxide (CO_2) reacts reversibly with water to form carbonic acid (H_2CO_3), which then dissociates into hydrogen ions (H^+) and bicarbonate ions (HCO^-_3). Because of this interaction, the pH is determined by the ratio of carbonic acid (HCO^-_3) to carbon dioxide (CO_2). At pH 7.4, the ratio of the concentrations of HCO^-_3 and CO_2 is 20:1 (Fig. 8-2). The ratio is normally maintained very close to this value by the actions of the kidney and the lungs, which excrete bicarbonate ions and carbon dioxide, respectively. Both the lung and kidney can greatly vary their excretion rates and thereby control the bicarbonate to CO_2 ratio and body fluid pH.

The lung and the kidney require minutes and hours, respectively, to compensate for changes in body fluid pH. The initial line of defense against change in pH is the chemical buffers of the body. *Buffers* are substances capable of binding hydrogen ions. They prevent large changes in pH when acids or alkali are actually added to the body fluids. The most important buffers from a physiological standpoint are the body proteins. Other compounds such as phosphates and ammonia contribute to total body buffering.

GAINS AND LOSSES IN BODY FLUIDS

Water and electrolytes are gained and lost by the body in various ways. Water alone is gained by drinking distilled water and by the oxidation of foodstuffs and body tissues. If the water contains electrolytes, as in the case of well water, softened water, mineral water, or most city water, then both water and electrolytes are gained. Electrolytes are also obtained from food. Hospitalized patients are often given water and electrolytes by way of nasogastric tube, intravenous needle, or rectal tube.

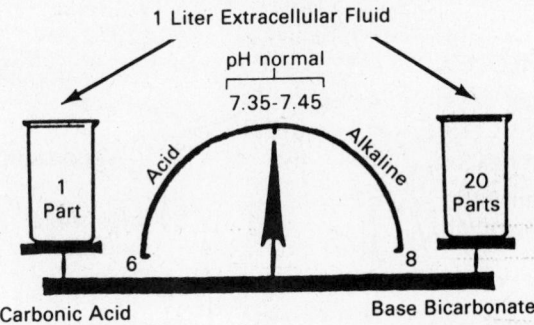

NORMAL ACID-BASE BALANCE

Figure 8-2. Acid-base balance is normal when pH is between 7.35 and 7.45. If the pH drops below 7.35, acidosis (acidemia) is present; if the pH is above 7.45, alkalosis (alkalemia) is present. In extracellular fluid, there is approximately 1 part of dissolved carbon dioxide to 20 parts of bicarbonate. (Adapted from Thorek, P.: Illustrated Preoperative and Postoperative Care. J. B. Lippincott.)

The body loses water and electrolytes normally through the skin in perspiration, through the kidneys in urine, in bowel movements, and from other minor sources such as saliva and tears (Fig. 8-3). Additional water is lost through the skin in insensible perspiration, which continues night and day, and through the lungs in breathing.

• In illness or injury, abnormal losses can occur through burn or wound exudate, hemorrhage, vomiting and diarrhea (Fig. 8-4).

• Postoperatively, fluids and electrolytes are commonly lost through gastric, intestinal, or biliary drainage procedures.

• Effusions of fluid can occur into various body cavities including the pleural and peritoneal spaces.

The general state of fluid balance in the healthy adult can readily be assessed by comparing the volume of fluid ingested by mouth with the volume of urine. The difference between intake and output in the normal person reflects the insensible losses from the body. Abnormal differences between intake and output of water and electrolytes result in body fluid imbalances.

• Accurate intake-output records aid tremendously in assessing the state of fluid balance in the hospitalized patient.

WATER AND ELECTROLYTE IMBALANCES

Imbalances are generally defined in terms of changes in the extracellular fluid, since this compartment is most easily sampled by analysis of the blood. Imbalances include changes in the volume of the extracellular fluid, in the composition of its major electrolytes, and in its acid-base status. Imbalances can exist alone or in combination and are generally associated with one or more disease states.

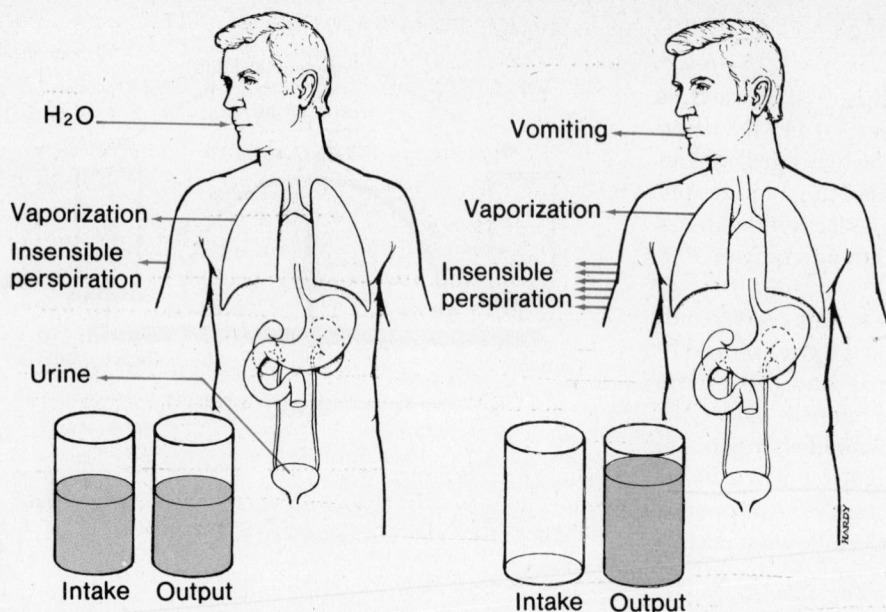

H₂O

Vaporization

Insensible
perspiration

Urine

Intake   Output

Vomiting

Vaporization

Insensible
perspiration

Intake   Output

Figure 8-3. *(Left)* Normal fluid balance. Water is taken in as such. Water is lost by vaporization from the lungs and the skin (insensible loss) and in the urine. The small amount normally lost in the feces is not indicated. The amount lost as sensible perspiration is highly variable and is not indicated. Daily intake and output are equal. *(Right)* Output exceeds intake. Water is lost by vomiting. No water is taken in either as such or in food. The only source is the water of oxidation produced in the cells as the body tissues are consumed. Water is also lost by vaporization, while the insensible loss from the skin is increased, due to the elevation of the body temperature or to hot weather. Little or no urine is formed. The variable loss by sensible perspiration is not shown.

CHANGES IN VOLUME OF EXTRACELLULAR FLUID

Extracellular Fluid Volume Deficit

Extracellular fluid volume deficit represents a loss of water from the extracellular space. Generally, electrolytes are also lost. This imbalance is called *hypovolemia*. The patient with extracellular fluid volume deficit usually has a history that includes one or more of the following: decreased water intake, vomiting, diarrhea, a systemic infection, fistulous drainage, intestinal obstruction, or severe burn. In addition, fluid can be sequestered within the body cavities and thereby remain inaccessible to the blood volume. The most common example is peritonitis, which may occur following intestinal perforation or acute pancreatitis.

The symptoms and signs of this imbalance can include dry skin and mucous membranes, thirst, oliguria (low urinary output of 100–400 ml./24 hours) or anuria (reduced urinary output of 100 ml. or less/24 hours), acute weight loss (in excess of 5 percent in the child or adult, 10 percent in the infant), lassitude, a drop in body temperature, decreased blood pressure, and rapid pulse (tachycardia). The laboratory findings reveal an increase in the red cell count, packed cell volume, and hemoglobin concentration of the blood.

Extracellular Fluid Volume Excess

This imbalance represents an excess in the volume of the extracellular fluid caused by an increase of water in the extracellular space. Generally, electrolytes are retained as well. This imbalance is called *hypervolemia fluid volume overload*. Volume overload may be caused by congestive heart failure, excessive ingestion of sodium chloride or electrolyte mixtures, administration of adrenocortical hormones (especially for long periods), hyperaldosteronism, or renal disease. A patient with extracellular fluid volume excess may have been given excessive quantities of an isotonic solution of sodium chloride intravenously. Symptoms exhibited include puffy eyelids, shortness of breath, edema, moist rales in lungs, and acute weight gain. A decrease is shown in the red cell count, the packed cell volume, and the hemoglobin concentration of the blood.

CHANGES IN COMPOSITION OF EXTRACELLULAR FLUID

Sodium Deficit

Sodium deficit of extracellular fluid represents a loss of sodium in excess of extracellular water loss or extracellular water gain in excess of sodium gain. The primary mechanism may be decreased intake or increased output of sodium or increased intake or decreased output of water. This imbalance is called *hyponatremia*. In the patient with sodium deficit, there is frequently a history of excessive sweating with ingestion of plain water, surgical drainage with administration of hypotonic fluids, or administration of a potent diuretic. These syndromes are associated with excessive sodium loss. Sodium deficit associated with increased intake of water is seen with parenteral infusion of an electrolyte-free solution and repeated administration of water enemas. Sodium deficit due to increased intake of water also results from drowning in fresh water. In some diseases, the normal control system for water balance is disturbed and antidiuretic hormone (ADH) is released in excessive amounts. This results in water retention in excess of salt retention and leads to hyponatremia.

Symptoms of hyponatremia include lethargy, confusion, and coma. If the condition develops rapidly, convulsions may occur as well. The symptoms are due to swelling of the cells of the brain as water moves from extracellular to intracellular fluid compartments by means of osmotic forces. If the etiology of the hyponatremia is excessive sodium loss from the body, total body water and blood volume are likely to be decreased as well. Consequently, manifestations of hypovolemia including hypotension, rapid, thready pulse, and cold, clammy skin can occur. The normal range of serum sodium concentration is 135 to 145 mEq/L. Symptoms of hyponatremia generally do not occur until the serum sodium concentration is decreased to less than 125 mEq/L.

Sodium Excess

Sodium excess in the extracellular fluid is called *hypernatremia*. In the patient with sodium excess, there is frequently a history of normal salt intake in the presence of decreased water intake, excessive ingestion of sodium chloride without increased ingestion of water, or drowning in salt water. These syndromes represent sodium gain in excess of water gain. Hypernatremia also occurs if water is lost from the body in excess of salt. This occurs with high fever (insensible losses from skin and lungs), profuse watery diarrhea, excessive sweating, loss from skin with burns, or in the disease diabetes insipidus (lack of normal ADH output from the pituitary gland) in which excessive urinary loss of water occurs.

With hypernatremia, mental symptoms including dullness and stupor are common because of dehydration of the cells of the brain. The symptoms of both hyponatremia and hypernatremia are similar, since they are caused in each case by disordered function of the brain secondary to water shifts between intracellular and extracellular fluid compartments. If the etiology of the hypernatremia is excessive water loss, symptoms and signs include intense thirst, oliguria, dry mucous membranes, and other manifestations of dehydration.

Potassium Deficit

Potassium deficit, known as *hypokalemia,* is caused by either a deficient intake or excessive loss of potassium from the body. It is seen most frequently in patients taking diuretics that result in excessive potassium loss

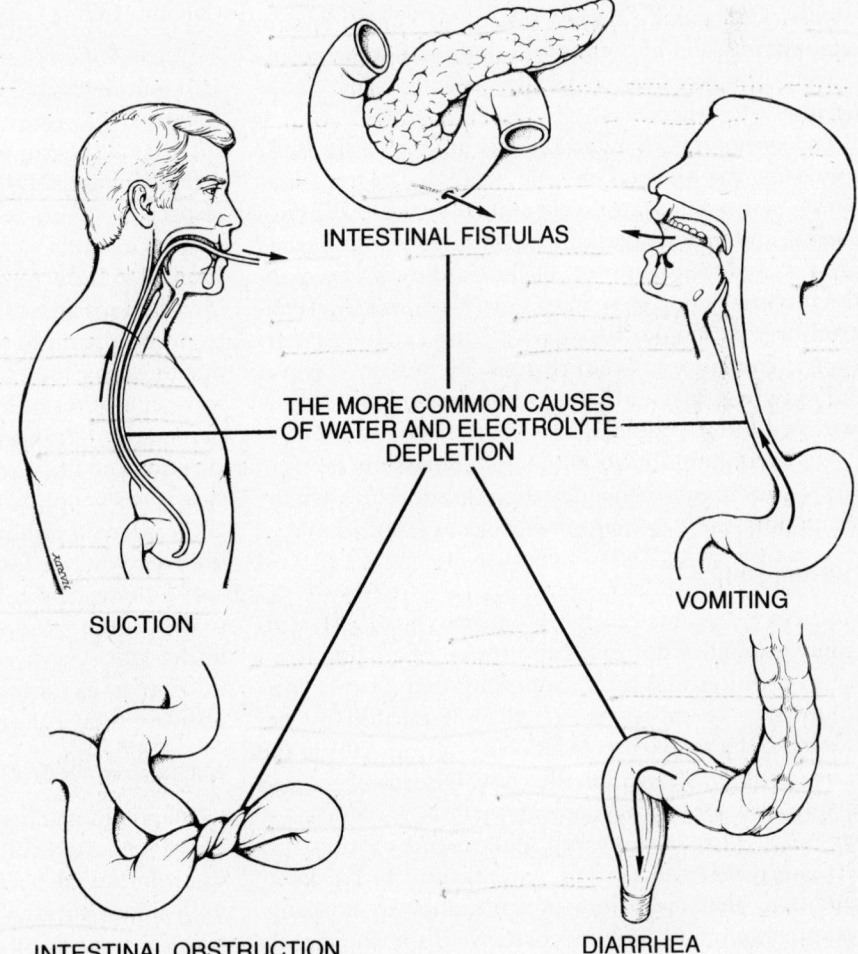

Figure 8-4. Causes of water and electrolyte depletion.

with the urine. Another common cause is loss of potassium from the gastrointestinal tract with vomiting or diarrhea. The condition may occur from the prolonged parenteral administration of solutions low in potassium, from the loss of potassium through fistulas of the small intestine or colon, and from the metabolic changes that occur during diabetic acidosis.

In the early stages of potassium deficit, symptoms are nonspecific. The patient has malaise or "just does not feel well." As the deficit becomes more severe, symptoms relating to the muscular system appear. In the *skeletal muscles,* there is generalized weakness and a decrease in or absence of reflexes; in severe cases, total paralysis may occur. Weakness of the *respiratory muscles* may cause shallow respiration. Gaseous distention of the gastrointestinal tract due to paralytic ileus may occur. Serious cardiac arrhythmias are common, especially in patients receiving digitalis. The electrocardiogram shows characteristic changes.

The normal value for serum potassium concentration is 3.5 to 5 mEq/L. Potassium concentration below 3.0 mEq/L. may lead to serious consequences.

Potassium Excess

Potassium excess in extracellular fluid is called *hyperkalemia.* One usually finds a history of kidney failure, excessive infusion of potassium solutions, adrenal insufficiency, or massive tissue damage, as with burns, crushing injuries, or hemolysis.

The symptoms of hyperkalemia are primarily those involving the skeletal muscles and the heart. Neuromuscular manifestations are similar to those of hypokalemia and include weakness, paresthesias, diminished reflexes, and respiratory paralysis. Cardiovascular manifestations include a slow heart rate (bradycardia), hypotension, ventricular fibrillation, and cardiac arrest. Typical electrocardiogram changes are peaked T waves and slow conduction through the ventricular muscle (widened QRS complex).

Mild symptoms occur with serum potassium levels of 5 to 7 mEq/L. Severe manifestations may occur when the serum potassium concentration exceeds 7 mEq/L.

Calcium Deficit

Calcium deficit is called *hypocalcemia.* It is most commonly a result of decreased absorption of calcium from the gastrointestinal tract. Superimposed on this condition may be excessive excretion of calcium by the kidneys or excessive precipitation of calcium salts in the bones or other sites within the body. Disorders that lead to impaired absorption include vitamin D deficiency, pancreatic insufficiency and other forms of intestinal malabsorption, and chronic renal failure. In the latter condition, there is failure of the kidney to normally activate vitamin D. In hypoparathyroidism, the regula-

tory system for calcium is disordered. As a consequence, there is decreased absorption from the gastrointestinal tract, decreased resorption of calcium from bone, and increased excretion in the urine. The most common cause for hypoparathyroidism is inadvertent surgical removal of the parathyroid glands during thyroid surgery. Severe magnesium deficit can also cause hypoparathyroidism, owing to depression of parathyroid gland function. Hypocalcemia can result from massive blood transfusions when formation of a complex occurs between calcium and the citrate added as an anticoagulant to blood during storage. In patients with decreased serum albumin, the total serum calcium is decreased, but this may not represent a true hypocalcemia since the biologically active free (unbound) serum calcium is normal.

Symptoms of hypocalcemia include tingling of the ends of fingers, tetany, abdominal cramps, muscle cramps, carpopedal spasms, and convulsions. The electrocardiogram shows a prolonged Q-T interval.

Normal serum calcium concentration is 8.8 to 10.4 mg./100 ml. or 4.4 to 5.2 mEq/L. The level of depressed serum calcium that results in symptoms is highly variable in different individuals.

Calcium Excess

Calcium excess, or *hypercalcemia,* is most often associated with increased absorption of calcium from the gastrointestinal tract or increased resorption of bone. Increased gastrointestinal absorption occurs with increased vitamin D intake, ingestion of excess calcium (especially when taken in conjunction with antacids), adrenal insufficiency in which there is increased production of vitamin D, and sarcoidosis in which there is increased sensitivity to the effects of vitamin D. Increased resorption from bone may occur with bony destruction due to cancer metastases, multiple myeloma, prolonged immobilization of the patient, and thyrotoxicosis. Hyperparathyroidism results in both increased calcium absorption and increased calcium resorption. Symptoms of this imbalance include hypotonicity of the muscles, anorexia, nausea, abdominal pain, constipation, polyuria with dehydration, and mental changes including psychoses, dullness, and coma. Chronic hypercalcemia can lead to deposition of calcium salts in many tissues, especially in the kidney, where kidney stones result. The plasma calcium is characteristically above 5.8 mEq/L. in the presence of symptoms.

Magnesium Deficit

Magnesium deficit, or *hypomagnesemia,* is usually associated with decreased absorption of magnesium from the gastrointestinal tract. It is most commonly associated with malabsorption syndromes or chronic alcoholism. Clinical conditions that may lead to malabsorption of magnesium include diseases of the small intestine, surgical removal of portions of the intestine, or enterostomy. Magnesium deficit may also occur after prolonged parenteral administration of magnesium-free solutions. Magnesium deficit is not common, and usually occurs in combination with other electrolyte abnormalities. It is difficult to distinguish the symptoms and signs of hypomagnesemia from those of hypokalemia or hypocalcemia. The major signs and symptoms of hypomagnesemia include weakness, tremors, personality changes, vertigo, convulsions, confusion, and hyperactive reflexes. The serum magnesium level is normally between 1.4 and 2.0 mEq/L. Severe symptoms usually do not occur unless the serum concentration of magnesium is 0.8 mEq/L. or less.

Magnesium Excess

Magnesium excess, or *hypermagnesemia,* is seen only in patients to whom exogenous magnesium has been administered. The hypermagnesemia in most patients is mild and asymptomatic. Severe hypermagnesemia is seen in patients with renal failure who are given exogenous magnesium. Symptoms of hypermagnesemia include hypotension, nausea, vomiting, drowsiness, hyperreflexia, and muscular weakness. Symptoms do not usually occur until the serum magnesium level rises to 3 to 5 mEq/L. or higher.

Phosphate Deficit and Excess

Phosphorus in the form of phosphate ions is usually present in the normal serum in a concentration ranging from 0.8 to 1.5 mEq/L. Serum phosphorous may be elevated (hyperphosphatemia) in renal failure and hypoparathyroidism. Symptoms are usually not present in hyperphosphatemia. However, when high levels are maintained for long periods of time, calcium phosphates may abnormally deposit in various sites in the body. A low serum phosphate level, called *hypophosphatemia,* is usually due to hyperparathyroidism. Acute changes may be unaccompanied by symptoms. However, persistent hypophosphatemia may be associated with anorexia, dizziness, bone pain, muscular weakness, and a wobbling gait.

ACID-BASE DISTURBANCES

When the concentration of hydrogen ions increases (pH decreases) and the extracellular fluid becomes acid, the patient is said to have *acidosis.* When the concentration of hydrogen ions decreases (pH increases) and the extracellular fluid becomes alkaline, or basic, the patient has *alkalosis.* Any condition that increases the carbon dioxide or decreases the bicarbonate ion concentrations leads to an increased hydrogen ion (H^+) concentration (acidosis). Any condition that increases bicarbonate ion con-

centrations or decreases carbon dioxide concentrations leads to decreased hydrogen ion concentration (alkalosis). Hydrogen ion balance can be altered by two types of disturbances — metabolic and respiratory. Metabolic disturbances affect primarily the bicarbonate ion concentration, and respiratory disturbances affect primarily the carbon dioxide concentration of body fluids.

Primary Bicarbonate Deficit (Metabolic Acidosis)

A primary deficit in the bicarbonate ion concentration of the extracellular fluid is called *metabolic acidosis* (Fig. 8-5). This imbalance is often associated with diabetic ketosis and renal failure. It may also occur with starvation, severe diarrhea, or the ingestion of certain poisons such as methyl alcohol, ethylene glycol, paraldehyde, and salicylate.

Symptoms and signs of metabolic acidosis are stupor, deep rapid breathing (Kussmaul respirations), weakness, and, if the imbalance is severe, unconsciousness. Laboratory findings show a urine pH below 6.0, plasma bicar-

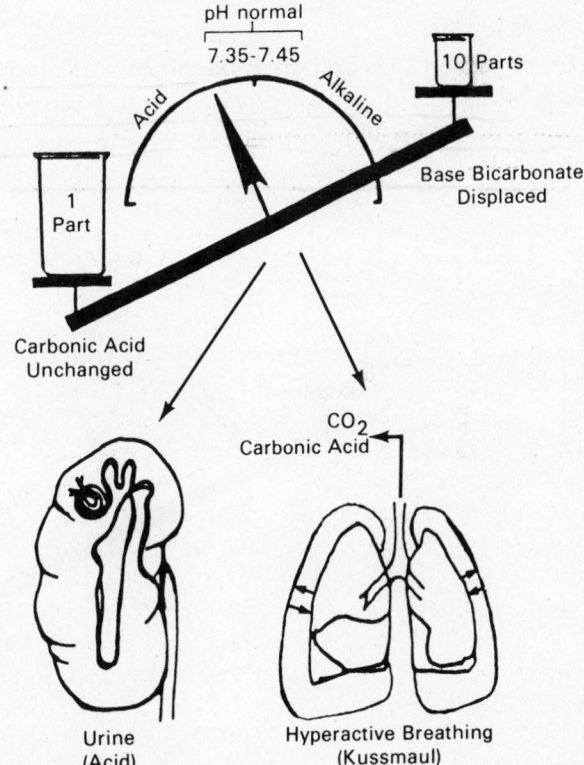

METABOLIC ACIDOSIS

Figure 8-5. Metabolic acidosis (bicarbonate deficit). In this condition serum bicarbonate levels are low and the pH of the extracellular fluid drops below 7.35. The normal CO_2-HCO_3^- ratio of 1 to 20 is now changed to 0.7 to 10. The lungs attempt to compensate by hyperventilation, thus blowing off excess carbon dioxide. The kidneys attempt to compensate by excreting hydrogen ions (acid) and conserving bicarbonate. The urine becomes acid. (Adapted from Thorek, P.: Illustrated Preoperative and Postoperative Care. J. B. Lippincott.)

bonate below 25 mEq/L. in adults and below 20 mEq/L. in children, and a plasma pH below 7.35. Blood carbon dioxide tension (PCO_2) is usually low (below 30 mm. Hg) due to hyperventilation.

Primary Bicarbonate Excess (Metabolic Alkalosis)

A primary excess of bicarbonate ion, called *metabolic alkalosis,* may result from loss of hydrogen ion from the body. This can be understood by reference to the following equation:

$$CO_2 + H_2O \longleftrightarrow H_2CO_3 \longleftrightarrow H^+ + HCO^-_3$$

Metabolic alkalosis is most commonly seen with vomiting or nasogastric suction in which hydrogen-ion-containing digestive juice is lost from the body. Metabolic alkalosis also occurs following excessive ingestion of sodium bicarbonate or other alkali (Fig. 8-6).

The symptoms and signs of metabolic alkalosis include hypertonicity of the muscles, tetany, and depressed respiration. Laboratory findings include a urine pH of 7.0, plasma bicarbonate above 29 mEq/L. in adults and above 25 mEq/L. in children, a plasma pH above 7.45, and a plasma potassium below 4 mEq/L. Blood carbon dioxide partial pressure (PCO_2) is usually slightly elevated (44 to 48 mm. Hg).

Primary Carbon Dioxide Deficit (Respiratory Alkalosis)

Any condition that results in an increased rate and depth of breathing with the resultant excessive elimination of carbon dioxide will cause an increase in blood pH and *respiratory alkalosis*. This condition is seen with oxygen lack, fever, anxiety, intentional overbreathing, and early in salicylate intoxication. The symptoms include tetany, convulsions, and unconsciousness. Laboratory findings include a urine pH above 7.0, PCO_2 less than 35 mm. Hg, and a plasma pH above 7.45. Plasma bicarbonate is only moderately lowered below its normal value (25 mEq/L).

Primary Carbon Dioxide Excess (Respiratory Acidosis)

Primary carbon dioxide excess, called *respiratory acidosis*, is brought on by any condition that impairs the elimination of carbon dioxide by the lung. It occurs most commonly with emphysema, obstruction of the breathing passages, and overdose with morphine, barbiturate, or other sedatives. It can also occur as a result of breathing excessive carbon dioxide. Symptoms of respiratory acidosis include headache, disorientation, weakness, and lethargy. Laboratory findings reveal a urine pH below 6.0, plasma pH below 7.35, and a PCO_2 greater than 45 mm. Hg. Plasma bicarbonate is elevated if the condition is chronic.

Diagnosing Acid-Base Imbalance

One can learn whether a patient has acidosis or alkalosis simply by determining the plasma pH, which can be done directly by a pH meter. Either heparinized arterial blood or "arterialized" blood from a warmed ear lobe or fingertip can be used.

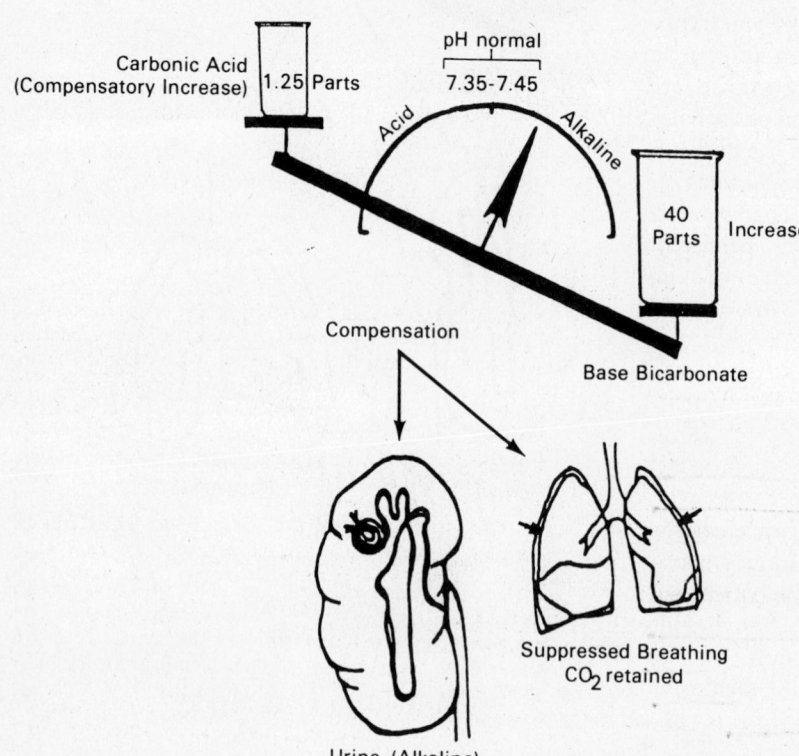

METABOLIC ALKALOSIS

Carbonic Acid (Compensatory Increase) 1.25 Parts

pH normal 7.35-7.45

Acid   Alkaline

40 Parts   Increased

Compensation

Base Bicarbonate

Suppressed Breathing CO_2 retained

Urine (Alkaline)

Figure 8-6. Metabolic alkalosis (bicarbonate excess). In this condition the serum bicarbonate concentration is increased and the pH is increased above 7.45. The normal CO_2-HCO_3^- ratio of 1 to 20 is changed to 1.25 to 40. The lungs compensate by retaining carbon dioxide by hypoventilation. The kidneys compensate by retaining hydrogen ions and excreting bicarbonate ions; the urine becomes alkaline. (Adapted from Thorek, P.: Illustrated Preoperative and Postoperative Care. J. B. Lippincott.)

Although the plasma pH answers the basic question, whether the patient is in acidosis or alkalosis, it does not tell us whether the condition is a result of metabolic acidosis or alkalosis, respiratory acidosis or alkalosis and/or renal or pulmonary compensatory mechanisms. This crucial question can be answered only by careful analysis of history, physical examination, and all laboratory findings including PCO_2 and bicarbonate.*

The PCO_2 is measured by a PCO_2 meter. Normal PCO_2 values range from 36 to 44 mm. Hg for arterial blood.

Plasma bicarbonate cannot be measured directly, so it is measured indirectly via the CO_2 content. Do not be misled by the names of this test: *it is not done to determine the plasma CO_2 but, rather, the plasma bicarbonate*. In this test, sulfuric acid is added to the test plasma so that the bicarbonate ion forms gaseous CO_2, which is then measured. The CO_2 gas dissolved in the plasma is measured along with the CO_2 freed from the bicarbonate. The total measurement, therefore, represents both the CO_2 released from bicarbonate and the CO_2 gas dissolved in the plasma. Their sum represents the CO_2 *content,* which normally ranges from 24 to 33 mEq/L. In the normal individual, the CO_2 content largely reflects bicarbonate with a small (<5%) contribution from dissolved CO_2.

The CO_2 content, bicarbonate, pH, and PCO_2 all can be determined if any two of the values are known. Figure 8-7 provides a summary of the changes in direction of pH, bicarbonate, and PCO_2 in acid–base disturbances.

Protein Deficit

The concentration of proteins in the blood can be decreased due either to decreased production or increased loss in the urine or feces. This condition, often involving only the serum albumin, is called *hypoproteinemia.* The disease most commonly associated with decreased albumin production is cirrhosis of the liver. The diseases most commonly associated with increased loss of albumin are the chronic kidney diseases that constitute the nephrotic syndrome. Less common causes of chronic

Imbalance	pH	Bicarbonate	pCO₂
Respiratory acidosis	↓	↑	⬆
Respiratory alkalosis	↑	↓	⬇
Metabolic acidosis	↓	⬇	↓
Metabolic alkalosis	↑	⬆	↑

Figure 8-7. Summary of changes in direction of blood gas values in acid-base disturbances. The heavy arrows indicate the primary abnormality.

protein loss are a wide variety of gastrointestinal conditions that result in increased excretion in the feces. The normal serum albumin is 3.5 to 5.5 g./100 ml. Severe albumin deficit is characterized by a serum albumin concentration less than 2.0 g./100 ml.

The major sign of hypoproteinemia is the formation of generalized edema. This represents a shift of fluid from the vascular space to the interstitial fluid compartment. It occurs because the osmotic pressure in the intravascular space is reduced when hypoproteinemia is present (see Vascular Physiology). If the loss of fluid from the vascular space is severe, the symptoms and signs of hypovolemia may occur.

THERAPY

The physician keeps three goals in mind in planning day-to-day treatment for the patient with an actual or potential body fluid disturbance:

1. Repairing preexisting deficits of water and electrolytes
2. Providing water and electrolytes to meet the maintenance needs of the patient

---

*Diagnosis is even more difficult when one is dealing with a mixed disturbance resulting from several primary and compensatory processes affecting the same blood gas values. For example, how can one differentiate between a metabolic acid-base disturbance with respiratory compensation and a metabolic acid-base disturbance combined with a respiratory acid-base disturbance? Nomograms are helpful, but they cannot tell the whole story. It is absolutely essential to have clinical information concerning the specific patient. McCurdy presents a "system for diagnosing clinical acid-base disorders [that is] easy to use and avoids most of the pitfalls of quick decisions based only on fluid gas values and nomograms":

1. Study the history for processes that may lead to simple acid-base disorders.
2. Note the findings on physical examination that suggest an acid-base imbalance.
3. Check the routine electrolytes for
    a. plasma bicarbonate
    b. unspecified anions (To calculate the unspecified, or undetermined, anions, including anionic proteins, phosphates, sul-

fates, and organic acids, subtract the sum of bicarbonate and chloride from the serum sodium concentration; this undetermined, or unspecified anion fraction, also described as the anion gap or delta, is normally less than 12-14 mEq/L. If the total is higher than 14, metabolic acidosis is present.)
    c. plasma potassium, which usually moves opposite to arterial pH.
4. Examine other laboratory data for disease processes associated with acid-base disturbances.
5. Explain the blood gas values. If a change in PCO_2 or HCO^-_3 is attributed to compensatory mechanisms rather than to an additional primary acid-base disturbance, be sure it is within physiologically possible limits. The procedure for making this determination is explained clearly in the splendid article by McCurdy†

†McCurdy, D. K.: Mixed metabolic and respiratory acid-base disturbances: diagnosis and treatment. Chest, *62*:35S-44S, Aug. 1972 Supplement.

TYPES OF WATER AND ELECTROLYTE IMBALANCES

	CAUSES	SYMPTOMS	LABORATORY FINDINGS
EXTRACELLULAR FLUID VOLUME DEFICIT (Hypovolemia)	Decreased water intake Vomiting Diarrhea Systemic infection Fistulous drainage Intestinal obstruction Sequestered fluid in body cavities	Dry skin Dry mucous membrane Thirst Oliguria Anuria Acute weight loss Lassitude Drop in body temperature Decreased blood pressure Tachycardia	Increase in red cell count Packed cell volume Hemoglobin concentration
EXTRACELLULAR FLUID EXCESS (Hypervolemia)	Congestive heart failure Excessive ingestion of sodium chloride or electrolyte mixtures Long-term administration of adrenocortical hormones Hyperaldosteronism Renal diseases Excessive quantities of isotonic solutions intravenously	Puffy eyelids Shortness of breath Moist rales in lungs Acute weight gain	Decrease in red cell count Packed cell volume Hemoglobin concentration
SODIUM DEFICIT (Hyponatremia)	Excessive sweating with ingestion of plain water Surgical drainage with administration of hypotonic fluids Administration of potent diuretic Excessive release of antidiuretic hormone	Lethargy Confusion Coma Possibly convulsions Possibly hypotension, rapid thready pulse, and cold clammy skin	Serum sodium concentration is decreased to less than 125 mEq/L.
SODIUM EXCESS (Hypernatremia)	History of normal salt intake in presence of decreased water intake. High fever Profuse watery diarrhea Excessive sweating Loss (fluid) from skin with burns Polyuria (diabetes insipidus)	Stupor Intense thirst Oliguria Dry mucous membrane Dehydration	Serum sodium is greater than 145 mEq/L.
POTASSIUM DEFICIT (Hypokalemia)	Deficient intake of potassium Excessive loss of potassium Diuretic Vomiting—diarrhea Prolonged parenteral administration of solution low in potassium Loss of potassium through fistulas	"Just does not feel well" Generalized weakness Decrease or absence of reflexes Total paralysis may occur Shallow respiration Gaseous distention of gastrointestinal tract Cardiac arrhythmias	Serum potassium below 3.0 mEq/L.
POTASSIUM EXCESS (Hyperkalemia)	History of kidney failure Excessive infusion of potassium solutions Adrenal insufficiency Massive tissue damage	Muscle weakness Paresthesias Diminished reflexes Respiratory paralysis Bradycardia Hypotension Ventricular fibrillation Cardiac arrest	Mild symptoms when serum potassium is 5 to 7 mEq/L. Severe manifestations when serum potassium exceeds 7 mEq/L.
CALCIUM DEFICIT (Hypocalcemia)	Absorption of calcium from gastrointestinal tract Excessive secretion of calcium by kidneys	Tingling of fingertips Tetany Abdominal cramps Muscle cramps	Normal serum calcium concentration is 4.4 to 5.2 mEq/L. For hypocalcemia, depressed calcium is highly variable

128

TYPES OF WATER AND ELECTROLYTE IMBALANCES (CONTINUED)

	CAUSES	SYMPTOMS	LABORATORY FINDINGS
CALCIUM DEFICIT (Hypocalcemia)	Excess precipitation of calcium salts Vitamin D deficiency Pancreatic insufficiency Intestinal malabsorption Chronic renal failure Massive blood transfusion	Carpopedal spasms Convulsions Prolonged Q-T interval on electrocardiogram	
CALCIUM EXCESS (Hypercalcemia)	Increased absorption of calcium from gastrointestinal tract Increased vitamin D intake Ingestion of excess calcium (antacids) Adrenal insufficiency with increased production of vitamin D Sarcoidosis Cancer metastasis Prolonged immobilization Thyrotoxicosis	Hypotonicity of muscles Anorexia Nausea Abdominal pain Constipation Polyuria with dehydration Psychosis Coma	Plasma calcium about 5.8 mEq/L.
MAGNESIUM DEFICIT (Hypomagnesemia)	Decreased absorption of magnesium from the gastrointestinal tract. Malabsorption syndromes Chronic alcoholism	Weakness Tremors Personality changes Vertigo Convulsions Confusion Hyperactive reflexes	Serum magnesium level is 0.8 mEq/L. or less
MAGNESIUM EXCESS (Hypermagnesemia)	Renal failure (patients who are given exogenous magnesium)	Hypotension Nausea Vomiting Drowsiness Hyperreflexia Muscular weakness	Serum magnesium rises to 3 to 5 mEq/L. or higher

3. Replacing water and electrolytes lost through vomiting, diarrhea, tubular drainage, wound or burn drainage, diuresis, etc.

There are many different methods for achieving these goals, but rather than describe them all, we shall present one simple method that has worked well in practice and that will give the nurse a basic understanding of the principles involved in fluid therapy. This method was developed by Butler and his co-workers at the Massachusetts General Hospital and has been used with great success in many parts of the world.

Testing Renal Function

Because various types of solutions, particularly those containing potassium, can be hazardous if renal function is not adequate, an important step in fluid therapy is the determination of the status of the kidneys. If any of the following criteria exist *in the absence of coexisting nonrenal diseases,* a therapeutic test for functional renal depression may be carried out:

- specific gravity of the urine above 1.030
- less than three voidings in 24 hours
- no urine in the bladder

For the therapeutic test, an initial hydrating solution is administered. Such a solution might be 5 percent glucose in water with 3 grams of sodium chloride added per liter (0.3% NaCl). The solution is administered at a rate of approximately 5 to 10 ml./m.^{2} body surface/minute for 45 minutes. If the urinary suppression is due to volume deficit, the therapeutic test will reestablish urinary flow. If the kidneys begin to function, the initial hydrating solution is discontinued, and therapy is started with appropriate solutions for fluid and electrolyte maintenance. If urinary flow is not restored, the rate of infusion is reduced to 2 ml./m.^{2} body surface/minute and continued for another hour. If urination has not occurred at the end of this period, the physician assumes that he is dealing with primary renal disease rather than with functional renal depression caused by loss of extracellular fluid. Thus, he focuses his attention on correcting the renal problem.

Administering Fluid Therapy

Assuming the patient's kidneys have been shown to be functional, the physician can proceed with therapy to repair preexisting deficits and to provide water and electrolytes for maintenance. To accomplish these goals, a single solution of the type devised by Butler, modified as needed to treat specific imbalances, may be used. Maintenance requirements can be met by the administration of 1,500 ml. of a Butler-type solution*/m.² body surface/day. If the patient has a moderate preexisting deficit, this can be corrected and the maintenance needs met by giving 2,400 ml./m.² body surface/day. If the patient has a severe preexisting deficit, then one can correct the deficit and provide maintenance by giving 3,000 ml./m.² body surface/day.

The Butler-type solution is administered intravenously, orally, or by nasogastric tube, but not subcutaneously. When the solution is given intravenously, the usual rate of administration is 3 ml./m.² body surface/minute.

For correcting continuing abnormal losses, as in vomiting or severe diarrhea, replacement solutions with a composition resembling that of the body fluid being lost are added to the daily fluid ration. For example, if the patient loses gastric juice, a gastric replacement solution is administered intravenously. Such abnormal losses are usually replaced on a volume-for-volume basis. A typical rate of administration for replacement solutions is 3 ml./m.² body surface/minute.

This simple plan of therapy can be used for treating body fluid disturbances that occur as a result of differences between intake and output, such as the following:

- fluid volume deficit of extracellular fluid
- sodium excess of extracellular fluid
- potassium deficit of extracellular fluid
- primary bicarbonate deficit of extracellular fluid
- primary bicarbonate excess of extracellular fluid

The other fluid and electrolyte imbalances require therapy specifically tailored to the imbalance, as will be described in the discussion which follows.

*The solution of the type devised by Butler is formulated so that when one uses it to meet the patient's fluid volume requirement, it supplies electrolytes in quantities balanced between the minimal needs and maximal tolerances of the patient. Hence, it is sometimes called a *balanced solution,* as by Snively and Sweeney. The Butler-type solution is hypotonic with respect to electrolytes, being only 1/3 to 1/2 as concentrated as plasma. Therefore, it provides free water to form urine and to carry out metabolic functions. It contains carbohydrate to reduce tissue destruction, counteract ketosis, and spare protein. What the Butler-type solution really does is to use the body's homeostatic mechanisms, which selectively retain the electrolytes that are required and reject those that are not. When used properly, it has a great margin of safety.

Fluid Volume Excess

The object of therapy in this imbalance is to reduce the extracellular fluid volume to normal without altering the electrolyte concentration of the fluid. This is usually accomplished by the administration of diuretics.

Sodium Deficit

In treating sodium deficit, the goal is to restore the sodium level of the extracellular fluid to normal without causing a fluid volume excess or deficit. If the extracellular fluid volume is already excessive, the imbalance is corrected by restricting fluids. If fluid volume is normal or low, isotonic sodium chloride is administered. Occasionally a 3 percent solution of sodium chloride may be required to rapidly correct a sodium deficit.

Potassium Excess

When the kidneys are functional, an uncomplicated potassium excess can be treated simply by avoiding additional potassium, either orally or parenterally. If the kidneys are impaired, however, several methods of removing excessive potassium from the extracellular fluid can be used. These methods include the administration of insulin and dextrose intravenously or the use of ion exchange resins orally or per rectum. Peritoneal dialysis or hemodialysis may be necessary when potassium excess is accompanied by severe kidney disease.

Calcium Deficit

In acute calcium deficit, a 10 percent solution of calcium gluconate diluted with isotonic solution of sodium chloride should be administered intravenously. This is particularly important if tetany or convulsions have occurred.

Calcium Excess

Treatment of calcium excess should be directed at correcting the underlying condition. For emergencies, the patient can be treated with forced diuresis (to increase renal calcium excretion), adrenal corticosteroids (to decrease intestinal calcium uptake), or mithramycin (to decrease calcium resorption from bone). Chronic calcium excess is sometimes treated by oral administration of phosphate. If other imbalances are also being treated, calcium-free solutions should be used.

Protein Deficit

Protein deficit is corrected by the administration of high-protein foods, high-protein supplements, or amino acids, with provision of generous quantities of calories. In recent years, intravenous hyperalimentation has become available.

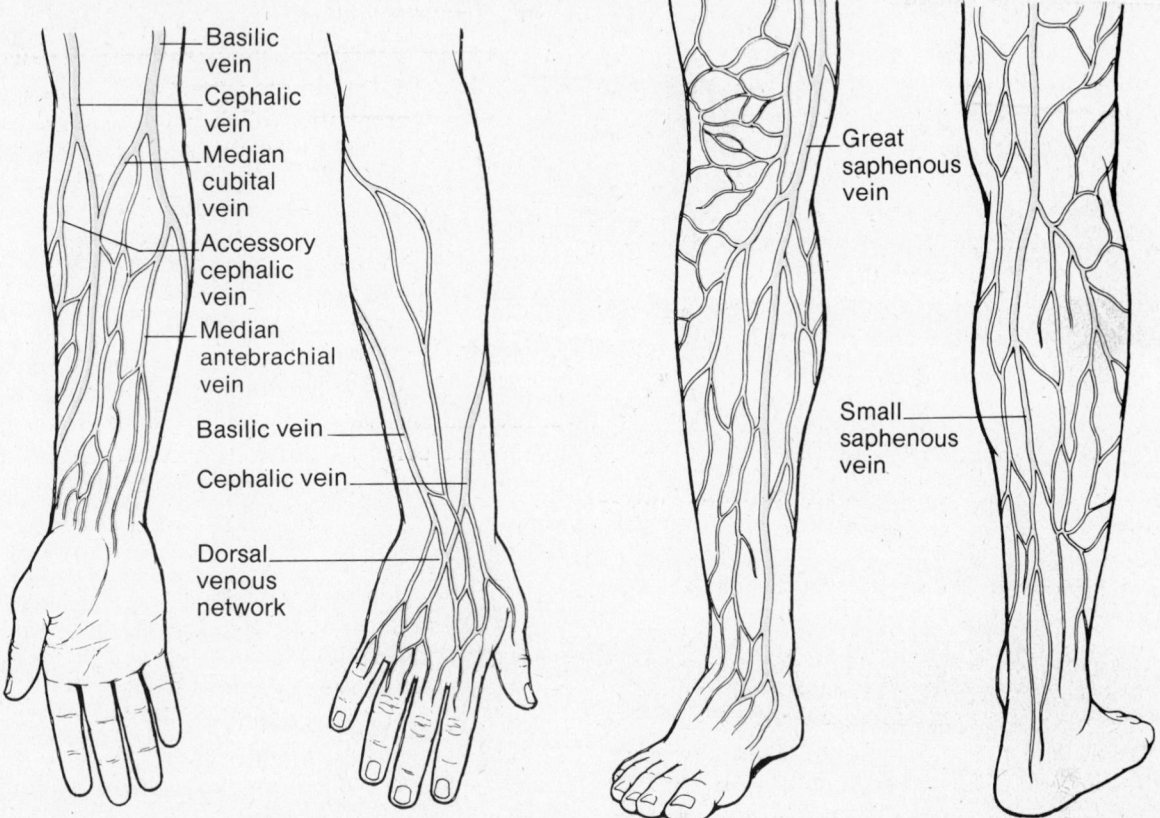

Figure 8-8. Sites of election for the insertion of intravenous needles for the parenteral administration of fluids or blood transfusion.

Primary Carbon Dioxide Imbalance

These imbalances are due to alterations in the respiratory status of the patient and should be treated by correcting the primary abnormality. Their treatment does not necessarily require fluid therapy.

Solutions Available

Solutions used vary greatly from hospital to hospital, and the nurse should become familiar with those used in the local hospital. This can be done by talking with physicians and by reading the literature provided by the hospital's pharmaceutical supplier.

With respect to IV push medications, observe carefully the manufacturer's instructions as to the proper diluent. The objective is to promote maximal stability of the ingredients after mixing. In some instances, the diluent may be sterile water (e.g., Betalin Complex); in others, the diluent may be 5 percent dextrose in water (e.g., Leritine). Incompatibilities should be carefully avoided by meticulously following manufacturer's instructions.

METHODS OF ADMINISTRATION

Because the nurse plays a major role in the administration of parenteral fluids, it is imperative that the basic principles of safe administration be understood. (The Guidelines on page 136 give a step-by-step summary of nursing action in administering an intravenous infusion in an arm vein.)

INTRAVENOUS ROUTE

An excellent route for the quick administration of water and electrolytes, medications, and nutrients is through the veins, or intravenously. (See page 720, parenteral nutrition.) Fluids administered intravenously pass directly into the extracellular fluid, and the body homeostatic mechanisms act rapidly to prevent the infusion from producing abnormal changes in the volume or electrolyte concentration of extracellular fluid. When nutrients are needed in a hurry, the intravenous route is essential. Provided due care is exercised, relatively large volumes of fluids can be safely administered by this route.

Choice of Veins

The veins in and around the cubital fossa (antecubital, basilic, and cephalic veins) are the most common sites for venipuncture because they are large and easily accessible (Fig. 8-8). They can accommodate large needles, large volumes of fluids, and all but the most irritating intravenous solutions. Other commonly used veins include

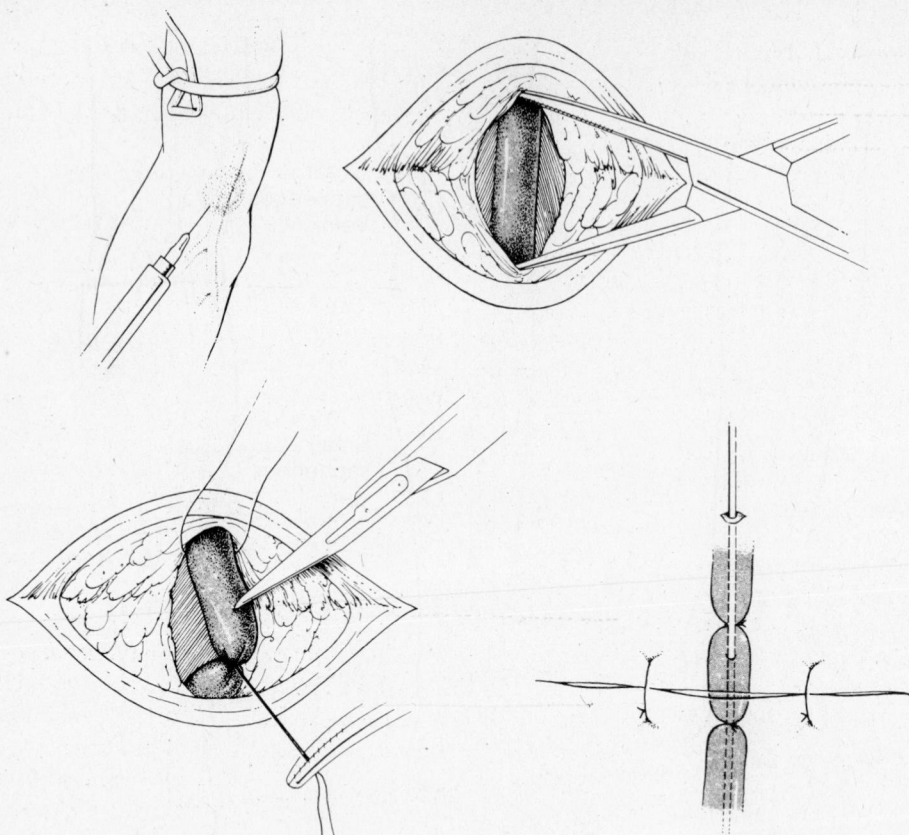

Figure 8-9. Cutdown technique. A cutdown is a surgical procedure and must be done with appropriate precautions—but if you observe these, it can be relatively simple. After preparing the skin over the chosen site, infiltrate a local anesthetic *(top, left)*. Then make a transverse incision and gently dissect the subcutaneous tissue down to the vein *(top, right)* and free it from the medial antebrachial nerve. Pass sutures under the vein at both ends of the freed segment, tie the vein off distally, and pull slightly on the distal suture to raise the vein *(bottom, left)*. Then make a puncture wound in the skin about an inch to an inch and a half distal to the transverse incision and pass the catheter subcutaneously up to the incision *(bottom, right)*. Puncture the vein and thread the catheter in, tie the vein over the catheter, and close the incision. The tunneling technique reduces the risk of infection from skin bacteria. (From Wilson, R. F.: Securing the lifeline. Emergency Medicine, *10*:1978)

veins in the forearm (basilic and cephalic veins), veins in the radial area of the wrist, veins in the hand (metacarpal and dorsal venous plexus), femoral and saphenous veins in the thigh, veins in the foot (dorsal venous plexus, medial and lateral marginal veins), and scalp veins in infants and in the aged.

The selection of a vein depends upon a number of factors, including availability of sites (depends upon condition of veins), size of needle to be used, type of fluids to be infused, volume, rate, and length of infusion, degree of mobility desired, and the skill of the operator. The more distal sites are used first, leaving the larger vessel sites for emergency use or for times when small vessel sites are inaccessible.

Choice of Needle/Catheter

Fluids are introduced into the vein through a steel needle, a plastic needle, a plastic catheter threaded through a metal needle, or a plastic catheter introduced by means of a cutdown (minor surgical procedure). Steel needles are usually used for short-term infusions. The size of the needle to be used depends upon the vein and the type of solution. Nineteen or 20-gauge, (2.5 to 4 cm. [1 to 1½ inch]) needles are the most commonly used; an 18-gauge needle is indicated for blood administration—the smaller the gauge number, the larger the internal diameter of the needle.

Long lines are catheters threaded through a metal needle inserted into the antecubital, subclavian, internal jugular, or external jugular veins. These are usually threaded into the superior vena cava or right atrium to measure central venous pressure or to administer drugs which would cause sclerosing in smaller veins. Once the catheter is in place, the needle is withdrawn and its point covered with a needle guard to prevent injury (see p. 728 for special procedure and precautions).

Catheters about 20 cm. (8 inches) in length are used in the antecubital fossa. Shorter plastic catheters, 5 to 7½ cm. (2 to 3 inches) are inserted by being threaded over a steel needle; the needle is then withdrawn leaving the catheter in place and permitting freer mobility of the patient.

The shortest indwelling line is the "butterfly," which is a steel needle with plastic wing handles (scalp-vein).

A cutdown, which involves insertion of a catheter through a slit in the vein, is used when veins are hard to find and long-term fluid therapy is anticipated (Fig. 8-9). Obese patients, infants, or those in or almost in shock frequently require cutdowns.

Patient Education

Although intravenous therapy is common, the patient needs to know what it is all about, what the limitations or restrictions are, and how the proper functioning of the infusion can be monitored. The patient can report significant changes in the flow rate and the emptying of a bag or flask, and any deviations from proper functioning at the infusion site, such as tenderness, erythema, puffiness, leakage, or accidental trauma.

Patient Comfort Measures

1. Include the patient in decision-making; if there are no contraindications to using any extremity for an infusion, find out if the patient has a preference.
2. For an initial infusion, the most distal good site is used first. Subsequently, if fibrosis or vein injury occurs, it does not affect the proximal sites, which are used next.
3. Restrict movement of the site by supporting the area with a padded armboard or padding. Place the extremity in a comfortable natural position.
4. Use hypoallergenic tape so that skin irritation is minimized.
5. Tell the patient what restrictions of movement are required and what range of motion is permitted.
6. Let the patient participate in care by monitoring the infusion and reporting any untoward developments.
7. Place the call device and any equipment for personal needs within reach of the patient's free arm.
8. In transporting a patient, be conscious of anything that could bump or disturb the infusion components.

Preparation of the Vein

Before venipuncture, it is necessary to distend the vein. This can usually be accomplished by applying a tourniquet. The tourniquet should be applied lightly and should restrict only outflow. Sometimes it may be necessary to distend the vein by other methods, such as placing the part in a dependent position for several minutes or warming the entire extremity by applying warm towels, immersing it in warm water, or using an electric hair dryer or an electric blanket.

Preparation of Infusion Site

If a large gauge needle is to be used, a small amount of 1 percent procaine should be injected before the needle is inserted. This should only be done at the request of the physician; the patient should be queried about a possible allergy to procaine before the injection is given. The injection site should be scrubbed with an iodine preparation followed by an alcohol wipe before the needle is inserted. Sometimes the area is cleaned with a detergent-germicide or other antiseptics prior to wiping with alcohol.

To Prevent Bubbles in Intravenous Tubing

Often the reservoir is hung on the IV pole, the clamp is opened, and fluid is permitted to flow *downward* through the tubing. As fluid flows rapidly in rivulets, air rises upward, competing for the same space. These actions, together with surface tension effects, cause bubbles. However, research by Hanneman has shown that a safer

method is to allow fluid to flow *upward*, so that a continuous column of air is displaced by a solid column of fluid (Fig. 8-10). In this method, no mixing or bypassing of air can occur.

The steps of this method are carried out as follows:

- Step 1. Partially fill drip chamber (by squeezing burette or chamber itself).
- Step 2. Using the right index finger as a guide, form a "U"-shaped loop with the tubing at the base of the drip chamber. With the left hand, open the flow valve slightly to allow liquid to rise to the level of the drip chamber (Fig. 8-11, left).
- Step 3. Reposition tubing so that the level of liquid in the tubing is again lower than the liquid level in the drip chamber so that the liquid continues to flow upward (Fig. 8-11, right).
- Step 4. Repeat Step 3 until liquid reaches end of tubing. Then arrange tubing in the usual position for attachment to the needle or catheter.

Insertion of Needle

In most cases, the bevel of the needle should be facing upward during insertion. However, when a large needle is introduced into a small vein, it may be necessary for the bevel to face downward to prevent the needle from piercing the posterior wall of the vein when the tourniquet is removed. The needle should pierce the skin to one side of and about 1-2 cm. (½ to 1 inch) below the point where the needle will enter the vein. The needle should enter the skin at a 45-degree angle; after the skin is pierced, the angle is decreased. The free hand is used to palpate the vein while the needle is being introduced. After the needle enters the vein, it should be inserted very slowly. It is threaded into the lumen approximately 1.25-2 cm. (½ to ¾ of an inch). The tourniquet is released. Frequently, a thin stream of blood is seen in the tubing when the needle enters the vein.

Securing the Needle and Initiating Fluid Flow

Next, in order to anchor the needle comfortably and safely, a cotton ball or small gauze pad is placed under the hub of the needle and fixed in place with adhesive tape.

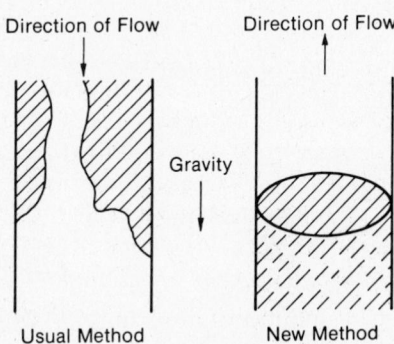

Figure 8-10. Comparison of usual IV filling method (downflow) vs. new method (upflow).

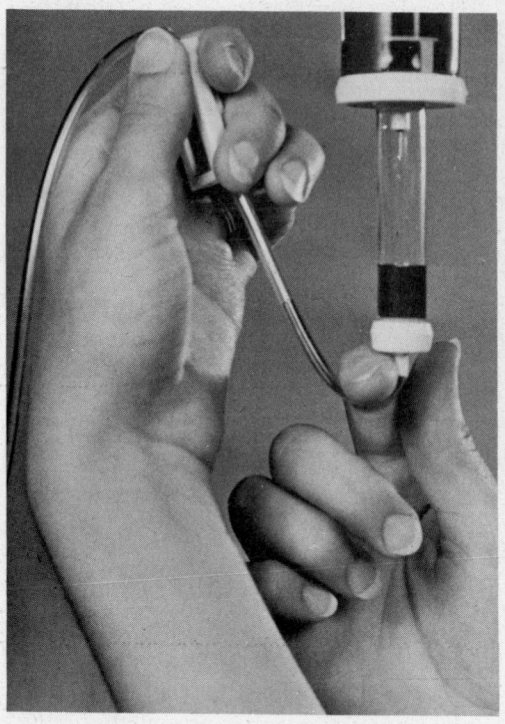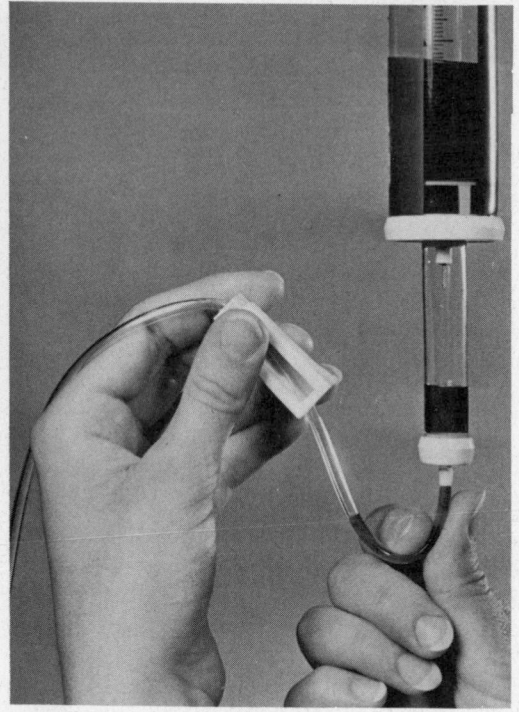

Figure 8-11 *(left)*. Steps 1 and 2 of upflow method; *(right)*, step 3 of upflow method. From Hannemann, R. E., et al.: Preventing bubbles in intravenous tubing, JAMA, 236:2488-89, Nov. 29, 1976.

Another strip of tape should be placed over the needle to help hold it steady. A loop should be made in the tubing and taped in place to allow some slack and to minimize pull on the needle when the patient moves.

When the needle is secured in place, the fluid is then started and the prescribed flow rate established.

Determining Flow Rate

There are several ways of determining the flow rate. When flow rate is calculated for a particular patient, it is necessary to check the manufacturer's directions. (Calculators are available from manufacturers of parenteral solutions.)

Example:
*Method:**

Step 1
$$\frac{\text{Total Amounts of Solution}}{\text{Number of Hours}} = \text{Number of ml./hr.}$$

Step 2
$$\frac{\text{ml./hr.}}{60} = \text{Number of ml./min.}$$

Step 3
ml./min. × number of drops/ml.
    = number of drops/min.

*Scherer, J. C.: Introductory Clinical Pharmacology, Philadelphia, J. B. Lippincott, 1975, p. 101.

Sample Calculation:
The orders are: 1,000 ml. (amount of IV solution)
                8 hours (time the solution is to be infused)
The drop factor delivered by the solution set is 15 gtts./min.

Step 1
$$\frac{1,000}{8} = 125 \text{ ml./hr.}$$

Step 2
$$\frac{125 \text{ ml./hr.}}{60} = 2.08 \text{ ml./min.}$$

Step 3
15 × 2.08 = 31.20 (rounded off to 30 or 31 gtts./min.)

Following the calculation, a "time-tape" can be placed on the infusion flask or bag to indicate the amount of solution the patient is to receive each hour and the number of drops per minute.

Factors affecting flow rate:

• Position of the needle in the vein. If the bevel is against the wall of the vein, it will restrict fluid flow.
• Height of the flask or bag. If elevated, flow of solution is increased.
• Patency of tubing and needle. Check for kinks and blood clots.

INFUSION PUMPS. These are automatic devices designed to control IV flow rates with greater precision than the traditional gravity flow. Many pumps are equipped with alarms or lights to alert the attendant that the solution source is almost empty, that air is in the tubing, or that the infusion is infiltrating.

Infusion pumps determine flow rate capability and the type of disposable administration set required. They move fluid by compressing intravenous tubing (peristaltic pump) or by forcing fluid through a cylinder (piston and cylinder pump).

There are many models available, all with advantages and disadvantages. Most are costly, require storage space, and take time to learn how to operate. Ideally, the infusion pump should:

1. Operate accurately and have separate alarms for detecting the following:
   a. end of infusion
   b. presence of air bubbles
   c. a change in rate flow
   d. infiltration
   e. occlusion
   f. mechanical failure (low battery power)
2. switch to a battery source should electrical power go off
3. be easy to use, safe, and quiet
4. be compact and inexpensive

Heparin Lock

Heparin lock is similar to a winged (clamp vein) needle with tubing about 8.75 cm. (3½ inches) long capped by a resealable rubber adapter plug. It is used for intermittent administration of such medications as antibiotics, chemotherapeutic agents, steroids, and heparin. The advantages are that it avoids repeated venipuncture (or intramuscular or subcutaneous injections) provides freedom of movement for the patient, and may be functional without an intravenous fluid drop (which could contribute to vascular overload and electrolyte imbalance). The heparin lock can be used immediately for intravenous infusion by removing the plug and attaching the flushed IV set.

After a medication is given through the heparin lock, heparin is immediately flushed to prevent clot formation. The prescribed amount of heparin is drawn into a syringe, the adapter is scrubbed with alcohol, and the heparin needle is inserted. After a gentle pull-back on the plunger to ensure the position of the needle, the heparin is gently instilled while the needle is withdrawn. Note that some medications are incompatible with heparin; for these, normal saline should be the flush solution.

Strict asepsis is required while the heparin lock is in place. It is discontinued if no longer needed; keeping it in place "just in case" incurs an unjustified risk of phlebitis, infiltration, and discomfort. The heparin lock should be changed every 72 hours and the date recorded on the tape. Swelling, pain, redness, or undue discomfort justify its withdrawal and discontinuance.

COMPLICATIONS OF THERAPY

The use of intravenous infusions should be initiated only when necessary, because the possibility of complications is significant. The shorter the lines, both external and internal, the better. Steel needles are preferable to plastic catheters except where the secureness of the line is of concern. (The incidence of infections and problems is lower when steel needles are used, but this may be related to shortened time of use.)

Infection

Meticulous attention to the principles of asepsis will prevent the high incidence of infection.

- The flask or bag should be carefully examined for evidence of contamination of the fluid, such as cloudiness, stringy elements, discoloration, cracks, or puncture sites. (If there is a question, do not use the solution; report the problem.)
- Proper handwashing should be carried out before and after every patient contact to minimize a source of contamination. (Note that contaminated hand lotion may be a source of infection.)
- Adequate cleansing of the infusion site is necessary to remove dirt and dead skin so that such particles are not carried into the vein during skin puncture.
- If an emergency intravenous infusion is begun under questionable conditions, it should be replaced as soon as practical.
- Aseptic technique relates to all parts of the infusion system. Sterile disposable gloves are worn in assembling, flushing, and initiating the infusion.
  The best skin preparations include iodine-based solutions, followed by alcohol wipes. (If the patient is allergic to iodine, then alcohol or an effective skin antiseptic is used.)
- Before a dressing and tape are applied after the line is functioning, antibiotic ointment may be applied to the needle insertion site. (The effectiveness of this practice continues to be studied because of the alterations in skin flora resulting from the antibiotics and the possibility of candidal infections.)
- The catheter/cannula is anchored securely and the insertion site is covered with a sterile dressing.
- All connecting links in the system and any infusion into the system to administer medications are potential entry routes for contaminants (Fig. 8-12).
- The date the infusion was started should be recorded and the set changed completely at least every 12 hours; certainly the system should not be left in place longer than 24 hours. (The incidence of infection rises with the length of time the set is in place.)

Pyrogenic Reactions

Pyrogens, foreign proteins that can cause a febrile reaction, are sometimes present in the infusion solution or in the administration setup. The symptoms of a pyrogenic reaction usually begin about 30 minutes after the start of the infusion and include an abrupt temperature elevation (from 37.8° to 41.1° C., or 100° to 106° F.) accompanied by severe chills, backache, headache, general malaise, nausea, and vomiting. Vascular collapse

GUIDELINES TO ADMINISTERING AN INTRAVENOUS INFUSION IN AN ARM VEIN

PREPARATION OF THE PATIENT

Nursing Action	Rationale
1. Place patient in bed in semi-Fowler position.	1. Is comfortable for patient. Permits arm to be placed in flexed, comfortable position.
2. Inform patient of the procedure and its purpose.	2. Solicits patient's understanding and cooperation.
3. Remove sleeve of patient's garment.	3. Permits removal of gown or pajama top if necessary during infusion without cutting sleeve.
4. Position (but do not tighten) tourniquet under lower end of upper arm (5 cm. above joint.)	4. Immobilizes arm while needle or catheter is in vein; prevents dislodging of needle and vein injury.
5. Place padded splint under arm; fix arm to splint by bandaging firmly.	5. Prevents constriction of nerves or blood vessels.
6. Connect intravenous materials; hang fluid receptacle after checking label for proper solution.	6. Intravenous fluids are medications. Verify labels!
7. Allow fluid to flow through the system; tighten the clamp; lay sterile needle in or on sterile surface until arm is prepared.	7. Eliminates air bubbles (these could cause air emboli).

PROCEDURE

1. Tighten tourniquet, with latter proximal to infusion site. Ends of tourniquet should be on side of arm opposite to infusion site.	1. Distends veins for better visualization. Prevents contamination of injection area by tubing ends.
2. Request patient to open and close his fist. Palpate and note suitable vein for injection.	2. Contraction of lower arm muscles forces blood into veins, thereby distending them further.
3. Cleanse skin thoroughly, using an antiseptic (of room temperature) on a cotton ball; apply friction in a circular motion outward from injection site.	3. Removes skin pathogens and sebum that might otherwise be drawn into the subcutaneous tissue or vein as the needle is advanced. Avoid application of cold antiseptic solution, particularly if patient has very small veins, since cold application would further constrict the vessels.
4. Use thumb to apply tension down on tissue and vein about 5 cm. (2 inches) distal to injection site.	4. Aids in anchoring vein as needle is introduced.
5. Hold the needle at a 45-degree angle alongside the wall of the vein in the direction and near the intended site of injection; pierce skin.	5. This angle permits greatest ease and accuracy in entering the vein.
6. Decrease angle of needle until it is nearly parallel with the skin and slightly to one side of the vein; apply pressure in same direction to puncture and enter the vein.	
7. If there is a backflow of blood through the needle, the vein has been entered; advance the needle slowly about 2.5 cm. (1 inch) while lifting the vein.	7. Prevents the needle from becoming dislodged from the vein and puncturing the posterior wall of the vein.
8. Release tourniquet.	8. Permits infusion solution to enter circulatory system.
9. Release clamp on infusion tubing and relax skin tension.	9. Allows flow of solution and prevents blood from clotting in the needle.
10. Slip a sterile gauze square (3″ x 3″) under the needle (double if necessary) to anchor it in the proper position.	10. Prevents needle orifice from pressing against vein wall and prevents needle from piercing vein wall.
11. Anchor needle in position, using adhesive strips; fasten a loop of tubing to prevent pull on needle.	11. Effective taping allows some mobility for the patient and retains safe inflow of solution.
12. Regulate flow rate of infusion.	12. Proper monitoring of solution will prevent overloading of circulatory system.

DISCONTINUATION OF INFUSION

1. Gently loosen adhesive taping and fixation near injection site.
2. Place a sterile gauze square over needle or cannula where it enters vein; withdraw needle (or cannula) and exert pressure at site. If bleeding persists, apply a gauze square or Band-Aid.
3. Remove adhesive marks with solvent.
4. Record:
    a. Nature of therapy and time given
    b. Type of solution and rate of flow
    c. Total amount of solution
    d. Any problems
    e. Patient's reaction

with hypotension and cyanosis may occur if the reaction is severe. The severity of the reaction depends upon the amount of pyrogens infused, the rate of flow, and the patient's susceptibility.

- If symptoms of pyrogenic reactions occur, the infusion should be stopped at once and the physician notified.

Also, the nurse should check the patient's vital signs. The solution should be saved so that it can be cultured if necessary.

Commercially prepared solutions and administration sets are pyrogen-free, but contaminants can enter these solutions after the seal is broken.

- Solutions not used immediately after the seal is broken should be discarded.
- Solutions should be discarded if there is any evidence of cloudiness in a solution that is normally clear.

A contaminated needle as the source of a pyrogenic reaction is easily overlooked.

- Any hypodermic needle that is to be reused must be properly cleaned and sterilized.

The only safe alternative is to use disposable needles exclusively. Special care must be taken when adding medications to the infusion fluid to avoid introducing organisms into the solution.

Local Infiltration (Extravasation)

The dislodging of a needle and the local infiltration of solution into the subcutaneous tissues are fairly common, especially when a small, thin-walled vein is used and the patient is active. Edema at the site of injection, failure to get blood return into the tubing when the bottle is lowered below the needle, discomfort in the area of injection (the degree of discomfort depends on the type of solution), and a significant decrease in the rate of infusion or a complete stop in the flow of the fluid are indications of infiltration.

Some solutions, such as hypertonic carbohydrate solutions, solutions with a pH varying greatly from that of the body (such as protein hydrolysates, sixth molar sodium lactate, or ammonium chloride), and potassium solutions, often cause great pain if they infiltrate the subcutaneous tissues. The local irritation may cause tissue slough, especially when norepinephrine (Levophed) is the offending solution.

- When infiltration is apparent, the infusion should be immediately discontinued.

Circulatory Overload

Administration of excessive intravenous fluids may overload the circulatory system and cause increased venous pressure, venous distention, increased blood pressure, coughing, shortness of breath, increased respiratory rate, and pulmonary edema with severe dyspnea and cyanosis. Patients with cardiac decompensation are particularly prone to circulatory overload.

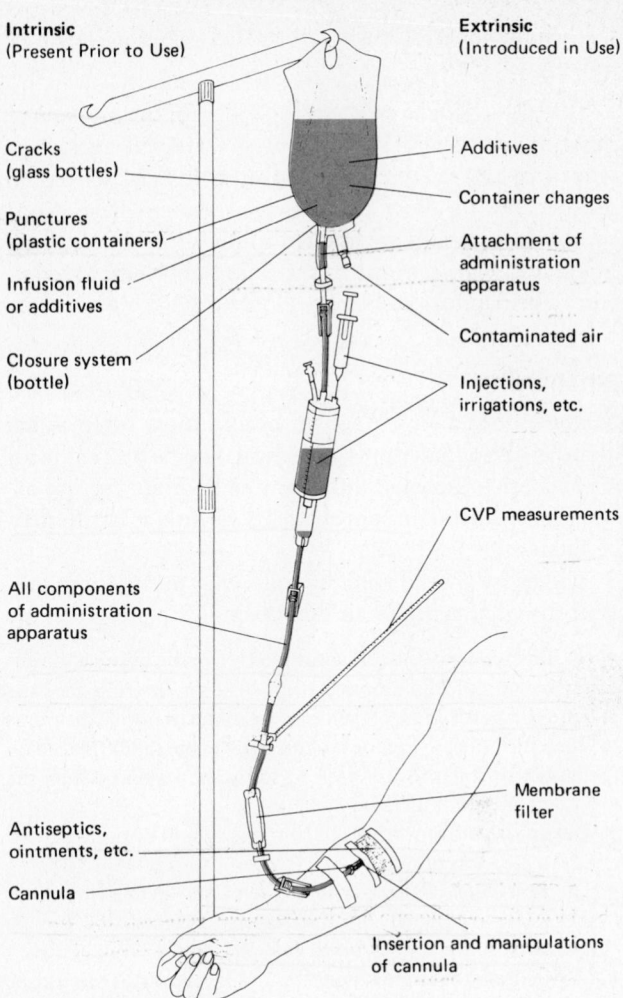

Figure 8-12. Potential mechanisms for contamination of IV infusion systems. (Drawing by N. L. Gahan from Maki, D. G.: Preventing infection in intravenous therapy. Hospital Practice, 1976)

- If the patient displays signs of circulatory overload, the infusion should be stopped and the physician notified immediately.
- The patient can be raised to a sitting position to aid breathing.

Thrombophlebitis

Thrombophlebitis is a condition associated with clot formation in an inflamed vein. It may be induced chemically or mechanically. Some degree of venous irritation occurs with all intravenous infusions, but it is usually of significance only in infusions kept going in the same site for longer than 12 hours. Thrombophlebitis is indicated by pain along the course of the vein and redness and edema at the injection site. If the condition is severe, systemic reactions to the infection may occur (tachycardia, fever, and general malaise).

Irritating solutions, such as alcohol, can help cause thrombophlebitis. Hypertonic solutions are often associated with venous irritation; carbohydrate solutions in excess of 10 percent almost always produce this reaction. Solutions with an alkaline or acid pH are more frequently associated with thrombophlebitis than are solutions that approximate body pH.

- When thrombophlebitis is detected, the infusion should be stopped.

The physician may change the order for the infusion to prevent more veins from being irritated and consequently unavailable. The infusion is best started in another site to allow the damaged vein to heal. Cold compresses usually are applied to the thrombophlebitic site. Later, warm, moist compresses can be employed to relieve discomfort and to promote healing.

Air Embolism

Even though air embolism occurs most often when blood is given under pressure, the danger is present in all intravenous infusions. Small amounts of air are not always harmful; but in some patients, as little as 10 ml. may be fatal.

The nurse should take the following measures to prevent the occurrence of air embolism:

- An infusion should be discontinued *before* the bottle and tubing are completely emptied to prevent air entering the vein from the bottle. The patient may be asked to notify the nurse when the infusion is about to run out. A tape can be placed on the side of the infusion flask to show the level at which the patient should notify the nurse.
- The needle and any other attachments should be tightly fitted to the infusion tubing.
- The first bottle to empty in a Y-type set (parallel hookup) should be completely clamped off so that air will not be drawn from the empty bottle into the vein.
- Instructions for use of blood pumping apparatus should be carefully followed when blood or any other fluid is given under pressure.
- The extremity receiving the infusion should not be elevated above the level of the heart since this results in venous collapse and negative venous pressure. Negative pressure in the vein receiving the infusion draws in large amounts of air if there are any defects in the apparatus.
- The clamp used to regulate fluid flow rate should be kept at a low level—preferably no higher than the level of the heart, certainly no higher than 4 to 11 cm. above the heart. Venous pressure normally causes a column of water to rise 4 to 11 cm. above the level of the heart. If the flow regulating clamp is placed above this height, a negative pressure will result in the tubing below. The negative pressure can be great enough to draw in sizable amounts of air if there are any defects in the apparatus.
- Permitting the infusion tubing to drop below the level of the extremity may help prevent air from entering the vein if the infusion flask empties unobserved.

Air embolism is manifested by sudden vascular collapse, with symptoms of cyanosis, hypotension, weak rapid pulse, venous pressure rise, and loss of consciousness.

- If an air embolism occurs, the administration tubing should be clamped immediately.

- The patient should be turned on his left side in the head-down, feet-up position so that air in the right ventricle floats away from the pulmonary air flow tract.
- Oxygen should be administered.

Speed Shock

Speed shock, a systemic reaction, may occur as a result of too rapid administration of solutions containing drugs. The drug floods the bloodstream, and toxic concentrations are supplied to organs that have a rich blood supply, such as the heart and the brain. Syncope and shock may occur.

- The flow rate should be checked often and reduced if untoward symptoms (which vary with the offending drug) develop.

BIBLIOGRAPHY

BOOKS

Collins, R.D.: Illustrated Manual of Fluid and Electrolyte Disorders. Philadelphia, J. B. Lippincott, 1976.

Goldberger, E.: A Primer of Water, Electrolyte and Acid-base Syndromes, 5th ed. Philadelphia, Lea and Febiger, 1975.

Metheny, N. A., and Snively, W. D., Jr.: Nurses' Handbook of Fluid Balance, 3rd ed. Philadelphia, J. B. Lippincott, 1979.

Plumer, A.: Principles and Practice of Intravenous Therapy. Boston, Little, Brown, 1975.

ARTICLES

Fluids and Electrolytes

Adlard, J. M., and George, J. M.: Hyponatremia. Heart & Lung, 7:587-593, Aug. 1978.

Cohen, S., et al.: Metabolic acid-base disorders, Part 1, Chemistry and Physiology. (Programmed Instruction) AJN, 77:P.I., 1-32, Oct. 1977.

———: Metabolic acid-base disorders, Part 2, Physiological Abnormalities and Nursing Actions. AJN, 78:1-20, Jan. 1978.

Coniglione, T. C.: Treatment of hypercalcemia and hyperkalemia, Med. Times, 106:69-75, July 1978.

Dutcher, I. E., and Hardenburg, H. C., Jr.: Water and Electrolyte Imbalance. Chap. 10 in Meltzer, et al.: Concepts and Practices in Intensive Care for Nurse Specialists, 2nd ed. Bowie, Md., The Charles Press, 1976, pp. 341-385.

Elbaum, N.: Detecting and correcting magnesium imbalance, Nursing '77, 7:34-38, Aug. 1977.

Grant, M. M., and Kubo, M. M.: Assessing a patient's hydration status. AJN, 75:1306-1311, Aug. 1975.

Lee, C. A., et al.: What to do when acid-base problems hang in the balance. Nursing '75, 5:32-37, Aug. 1975.

Macleod, S. M.: The rational uses of potassium supplements. Postgrad. Med., 57:123-128, Feb. 1975.

Metheny, N. A.: Water and electrolyte balance in the postoperative patient. Nurs. Clin. N. Am., 10:49-57, Mar. 1975.

Metheny, N. A., and Snively, W. D., Jr.: Perioperative fluids and electrolytes. AJN, *78*:840-845, May 1978.

Myers, F. J., and Pennock, B. E.: The acid-base map—an additional tool for dealing with a difficult problem. Med. Times, *106*:38-42, July 1978.

O'Dorisio, T. M.: Hypercalcemic crisis. Heart & Lung, *7*:425-434, May-June, 1978.

Papper, S.: Metabolic acidosis—diagnosis and treatment. Med. Times, *106*:83-88, July 1978.

Schwartz, A. B.: Therapy of hypokalemia. Am. Fam. Physic., *13*:148-149, Apr. 1976.

Snively, W. D., Jr., and Beshear, D. R.: Water and electrolytes in health and disease. Chap. 16 in Kintzel, K. C.: Advanced Concepts in Clinical Nursing. Philadelphia, J. B. Lippincott, 1977.

Twombly, M.: The shift into third space. Nursing '78, *8*:34-41, June 1978.

Yusuf, M., et al.: Calcium chloride and severe thrombosis of an extremity. Conn. Med., *42*:89-90, Feb. 1978.

Methods of Intravenous Infusion

Arnold, T. R., and Hepler, C. D.: Bacterial contamination of intravenous fluids opened in unsterile air. Am. J. Hosp. Pharmacy, *28*:614-619, Aug. 1971.

Beaumont, E.: The new infusion pumps, Nursing '77, 7:31-35, July 1977.

Bodnar, A., and D'Agostino, J.: IV therapy. Part I, Infection control. J. Pract. Nurs., *27*:18-21, Aug. 1977; Part II, *27*:24-27, Sept. 1977.

Egan, A.: Perfecting piggy-back techniques. Nursing '74, *4*:27-33, Jan. 1974.

Gump, D. W.: Bugs along the lifeline. Emerg. Med., *10*:57-65, Apr. 1978.

Hannemann, R. E., et al.: Preventing bubbles in intravenous tubing. JAMA, *236*:2488-2489, Nov. 29, 1976.

Hanson, R. L.: Heparin-lock or keep open IV? AJN, *76*:1102-1103, July 1976.

Harrison, M. J., and Healy, T. E. J.: Intravenous administration sets: The effect of flushing and filtration on particulate contamination. Brit. J. Anesthesia, *46*:59-65, Jan. 1974.

Lang, S. H., et al.: Reducing discomforts from IM injections. AJN., *76*:800-801, May 1976.

Maki, D. G.: Lifelines gone bad. Emerg. Med., *10*:71-94, Apr. 1978.

Michael, S. L.: Home IV therapy. AJN., *78*:1223-1226, July 1978.

"Plastic containers for intravenous solutions." Med. Letter, *17*:43-44, May 9, 1975.

Ungvarski, P. J.: Parenteral therapy. AJN., *76*:1974-1977, Dec. 1976.

Weiss, Y., and Nissan, S.: A method for reducing the incidence of infusion phlebitis. Surg., Gyn., & Obstet., *141*:73-74, July 1975.

Wilson, J. A.: Infection control in injection therapy. Heart & Lung, *5*:430-436, June 1976.

Wilson, R. F.: Securing the lifeline. Emerg. Med., *10*:43-51, Apr. 1978.

Woodside, W., et al.: Intravenous fluids as vehicles of infection. The Pharm. J., *215*:606, Dec. 20 and 27, 1975.

9
NUTRITIONAL CONSIDERATIONS IN HEALTH CARE

NUTRITIONAL CARE

Nutrition is a critical factor in the promotion of health, in the prevention of disease, and in recovery and rehabilitation from illness or injury. In health programs today, many disciplines work together to deliver comprehensive services.

Nutritional care (the application of the science of nutrition to the health care of people) is an integral part of nursing practice. The nurse's helping relationship with the patient or client is multifaceted and varies with the clinical setting. For instance, in primary health care facilities such as prenatal clinics and health maintenance organizations, the purpose of health care is prevention, and attention is focused on the maintenance of health and the prevention of disease. On the other hand, in community hospitals and other medical centers crisis intervention or restoration of health may be stressed, whereas in extended care facilities, the goals of care are frequently geared to rehabilitation.

The dimensions of clinical nutrition are well expressed by the American Dietetic Association in the following definition:

> Clinical nutrition is that branch of the health sciences having to do with diagnosis, treatment and prevention of human disease caused by deficiency, excess or metabolic imbalance of dietary nutrients.*

*ADA Guidelines for dietary counseling. J. Am. Diet. Assoc.: 66:571-575, June 1975.

The practice of clinical dietetics is a health service designed to help people maintain or reestablish a positive state of health. This can be accomplished by providing individualized professional guidance to assist a person in adjusting his daily food consumption to meet his health needs.

The Nurse's Role in Nutrition

As a member of the health care team, the nurse should possess a body of knowledge that can serve as a basis for sharing responsibility in nutritional care counseling. Included in this knowledge base is an understanding of the biological, behavioral, and natural sciences as they relate to nutritional health care.

In the clinical area, specific nursing activities related to nutritional care may include the following:

- To observe, record, and report the patient's response to diet by recording food and fluid intake and to make appropriate substitutions of food where needed in consultation with the dietition and the physician.
- To assist the patient at mealtime if necessary, by providing a pleasant atmosphere that is conducive to eating and by helping the handicapped patient to make adjustments in self-feeding.
- To interpret the prescribed diet to the patient by supplying information relating the modifications of diet to the illness.
- To maintain lines of communication with the physician and the dietitian regarding the patient's expressed dietary needs and to obtain a diet prescription if necessary.
- To plan for home care by arranging counseling sessions for the patient and family members and by suggesting agencies

for outside assistance or providing appropriate literature, if available, regarding the details of the diet.

Regardless of diagnosis, the patient should receive a nutritionally adequate diet in order to maintain tissue and body function. Such a diet will speed recovery and build up resistance to infection. Although meeting the patient's nutritional needs requires coordinated effort on the part of the medical, nursing, and dietary staff, the nurse is the member of the health team who spends considerable time in providing direct services to the patient and establishing a good rapport with him. Therefore, the nurse is in a position to help the patient accept his modified diet.

THE IMPORTANCE OF NUTRITION

The quality of nutritional intake has direct effect on physical and mental function. Proper nutrition is conducive to mental efficiency and concentration. On the other hand, nutritional inadequacy during the growth period may result in permanent changes in the size and chemical composition of the brain. All nutrients are involved in maintaining a healthy body: carbohydrates (glucose) are the chief energy source utilized by the cells; protein is needed for muscle building and for enzyme function in oxidizing glucose; vitamins are necessary for numerous body functions, as is evidenced by the wide range of symptoms related to various vitamin deficiencies (Table 9-1).

Primary and Secondary Nutritional Deficiency

Nutritional deficiency may result from the lack of one or more nutrients in the diet. This type of deficiency is termed *primary*. Underlying reasons for dietary lack may be poor food habits, poverty, ignorance of proper nutritional practices, poor selection of food, lack of food supply and lack of facilities for preserving and storing food.

Even if the diet is adequate in quantity and quality, other factors may interfere with the utilization of nutrients. This type of deficiency is termed *secondary* or conditioned.

The following factors may contribute to secondary nutritional deficiency:
1. Factors that interfere with ingestion: gastrointestinal disturbances, loss of teeth, anorexia, diarrhea
2. Factors that interfere with absorption: achlorhydria, gastrointestinal surgery, biliary disease, frequent use of mineral oil, parasitism
3. Factors that interfere with utilization: liver disease, diabetes mellitus, hypothyroidism, malignancy, alcoholism, antimetabolite and sulfa therapy
4. Factors that increase nutritive requirements: fever, hyperthyroidism, burns, growth, pregnancy, lactation
5. Factors that increase excretion: polyuria, excessive perspiration, diuretic therapy
6. Factors that increase nutrient destruction: lead poisoning, achlorhydria, sulfonamide therapy, frequent use of alkalizers

TABLE 9-1. VITAMIN DEFICIENCY SYMPTOMS IN MAN

Vitamin A Retinol	Night blindness; keratinization of epithelial tissues; xerophthalmia; faulty bone and tooth development
Vitamin D Calciferol	Rickets in children; delayed dentition; osteomalacia in adults
Vitamin E a-tocopherol	Hemolysis of red blood cells; mild anemia; protection of unsaturated fatty acids
Vitamin K	Prolonged clotting time; hemorrhagic disease in newborn infants; bleeding tendencies in biliary disease or surgical procedures
Thiamin	Poor appetite, atony of the gastrointestinal tract, deficient hydrochloric acid. Mental depression; apathy; beriberi; fatigue; neuritis; paralysis; edema; cardiac failure
Riboflavin	Cracks at corners of lips (cheilosis); scaly desquamation around mouth; glossitis; eye irritation; photophobia; corneal vascularization
Niacin Nicotinamide Nicotinic acid	Dermatitis (particularly areas exposed to light); neuritis; confusion; scaly skin; pellagra
Pyridoxine (B_6)	Nervous irritability, convulsions; dermatitis; anemia
Folic acid Folacin	Megaloblastic anemia; diarrhea; gastrointestinal disturbances
Vitamin B_{12} Cobalamin	Pernicious anemia due to genetic lack of intrinsic factor; neurologic degeneration; lack or deficiency in vegetarians (strict)
Vitamin C Ascorbic acid	Scurvy: red, swollen, bleeding gums; poor wound healing, capillary fragility; subcutaneous hemorrhage

If no intervention takes place, the effects of nutritional deficiency may become progressive, leading to depletion of body nutrient reserves, anatomical lesions, and chemical and functional changes.

Certain signs and symptoms that suggest possible nutritional deficiency are easy to note because they are specific. However, there are physical signs which have no relation to poor diet and which must be carefully distinguished from nutritional deficiencies. Some of the physical signs may be the result of other factors such as poor hygiene or exposure to the sun or, possibly, systemic disorders. A physical sign that suggests a nutritional abnormality should be considered a clue rather than a diagnosis and as such should be pursued further. For example, certain signs that may appear to indicate nutritional deficiency may actually reflect other conditions, such as endocrine disorders, infectious disease, or disorders affecting digestion and absorption capacity or excretion or storage of nutrients in the body.

NUTRITIONAL ASSESSMENT AND COUNSELING

Assessment of nutritional status can be determined by one or more of the following methods:

- Medical and clinical examination
- Anthropometric measurements
- Biochemical tests
- Dietary intake

Clinical Examination

The state of nutrition is easily reflected in a person's appearance. Although the most obvious physical sign of good nutrition is a normal body weight with respect to height, body frame, and age, other tissues can serve as indicators of nutritional status; these include the hair, skin, teeth, gums, mucous membranes, mouth and tongue, skeletal muscles, abdomen, lower extremities, and thyroid gland (Table 9–2).

ANTHROPOMETRIC MEASUREMENTS. The most common anthropometric measurements include height, weight, and the circumferences of the triceps, subscapular area, and the arm. When anthropometric measurements are gathered as part of data collection, standardized equipment and procedures are used, as well as standard measurement guides. Although such measurements focus on undernutrition, they will also detect obesity. (See Table 9–8 for skinfold thickness and arm and muscle circumference, and Table 9–3 for ideal adult weight.)

Biochemical Assessment

Biochemical assessment reflects both the tissue level of a given nutrient and any abnormality of metabolism in the utilization of nutrients. These determinations are made from blood studies (serum protein, serum albumin and globulin, hemoglobin, serum vitamin A, carotene, and vitamin C), and urine studies (creatinine, thiamin, riboflavin, niacin, and iodine). Some of these tests, while reflecting recent intake of the elements detected, can also identify suboptimum levels when there are no clinical symptoms of deficiency. (Table 9–9 provides a suggested guide for the interpretation of blood data.)

TABLE 9-2. PHYSICAL SIGNS INDICATIVE OF NUTRITIONAL STATUS

BODY AREA	SIGNS OF GOOD NUTRITION	SIGNS OF POOR NUTRITION
Hair	Shiny, lustrous; firm, healthy scalp	Dull and dry, brittle, depigmented, easily plucked
Face	Skin color uniform; healthy appearance	Skin dark over cheeks and under eyes, skin flaky, face swollen
Eyes	Bright, clear, moist	Eye membranes pale, dry (xerophthalmia); Bitot's spots, increased vascularity, cornea soft (keratomalacia)
Lips	Good color (pink), smooth	Swollen and puffy (cheilosis), angular lesion at corners of mouth (angular fissures)
Tongue	Deep red in appearance, surface papillae present	Smooth appearance, swollen, beefy red, sores, atrophic papillae
Teeth	Straight, no crowding, no cavities, bright	Cavities, mottled appearance (fluorosis), malpositioned
Gums	Firm, good pink color	Spongy, bleed easily, marginal redness, recession
Glands	No enlargement of the thyroid	Thyroid enlargement (simple goiter)
Skin	Smooth, good color, moist	Rough, dry, flaky, swollen, pale, pigmented; lack of fat under skin
Nails	Firm, pink	Spoon shaped, ridged
Skeleton	Good posture, no malformation	Poor posture, beading of ribs, bowed legs or knock knees
Muscles	Well developed, firm	Flaccid, poor tone, wasted, underdeveloped
Extremities	No tenderness	Weak and tender; presence of edema
Abdomen	Flat	Swollen
Nervous system	Normal reflexes	Decrease in or loss of ankle and knee reflexes

Assessment of Food Intake

The appraisal of food intake considers quantity and quality of diet and also frequency of consumption of certain food items, in order to determine current or customary intake of nutrients. Commonly used methods of determining individual consumption include the food record and intake estimation by recall. These methods are discussed with the patient and explained during the taking of the diet history.

The *food record* is used most often in nutritional status studies. The person is asked to keep a record of food actually consumed over a period of time, varying from three to seven days. Some instructions are given for accuracy in estimating and describing the specific foods consumed. This method appears to be fairly accurate, depending on the subject's integrity and ability to estimate quantity of food.

The *24-hour recall* method is, as the name implies, recall of food intake over a 24-hour period. The subject is asked by the interviewer to recall all food eaten during the previous day and to estimate the quantities of the food consumed. Information obtained by this method is not always representative of usual intake. For this reason, at the end of the interview the subject is asked if the previous day's food intake was a typical one. To obtain supplementary information regarding the typical diet, the interviewer should also ask how frequently foods from certain food groups are eaten.

The dietary and biochemical data for most nutrients provide more information than the clinical examination. The clinical examination is not sensitive enough to detect subclinical deficiencies unless such deficiencies become so advanced that overt signs develop. A low dietary intake of nutrients over a period of time may lead to low biochemical levels and, without nutritional intervention, may result in characteristic and observable signs and symptoms.

Evaluation of the Dietary Information

Once the dietary information has been obtained, the diet must be evaluated for its nutritive value. The first method is to use accceptable food composition tables, like those issued by the Department of Agriculture. The diet is then calculated in terms of grams and milligrams of specific nutrients. The total nutritive value is then compared with the Recommended Dietary Allowances (RDA) (Table 9-4), and the nutritional evaluation is expressed in terms of percentage of adequacy for each nutrient.

A second method of evaluation is to compare the diet data with recommendations based on foods selected from various food groups for various age levels, such as the "Basic Four Food Groups," or "The Guide to Good Eating" (Table 9-5).

TABLE 9-3. IDEAL WEIGHTS DERIVED FROM
LIFE INSURANCE STATISTICS
Desirable weights for women aged 25 and over

HEIGHT WITH SHOES 2-INCH HEELS FEET	INCHES	SMALL FRAME	MEDIUM FRAME	LARGE FRAME
4	10	92- 98	96-107	104-119
4	11	94-101	98-110	106-122
5	0	96-104	101-113	109-125
5	1	99-107	104-116	112-128
5	2	102-110	107-119	115-131
5	3	105-113	110-122	118-134
5	4	108-116	113-126	121-138
5	5	111-119	116-130	125-142
5	6	114-123	120-135	129-146
5	7	118-127	124-139	133-150
5	8	122-131	128-143	137-154
5	9	126-135	132-147	141-158
5	10	130-140	136-151	145-163
5	11	134-144	140-155	149-163
6	0	138-148	144-159	153-173

For nude weight, deduct 2 to 4 lbs.
Prepared by Metropolitan Life Insurance Company.

Desirable weights for men aged 25 and over

HEIGHT WITH SHOES 1-INCH HEELS FEET	INCHES	SMALL FRAME	MEDIUM FRAME	LARGE FRAME
5	2	112-120	118-129	126-141
5	3	115-123	121-133	129-144
5	4	118-126	124-136	132-148
5	5	121-129	127-139	135-152
5	6	124-133	130-143	138-156
5	7	128-137	134-147	142-161
5	8	132-141	138-152	147-166
5	9	136-145	142-156	151-170
5	10	140-150	146-160	155-174
5	11	144-154	150-165	159-179
6	0	148-158	154-170	164-184
6	1	152-162	158-175	168-189
6	2	156-167	162-180	173-194
6	3	160-171	167-185	178-199
6	4	164-175	172-190	182-204

For nude weight, deduct 5 to 7 lbs.
Prepared by Metropolitan Life Insurance Company.

The choice of a method for dietary evaluation depends on the purpose of the assessment. If the health counselor is interested in knowing about intake of specific nutrients such as vitamin A, iron, or calcium, then the food record method would be the one to use. The food intake would be analyzed by consulting an official publication listing foods according to composition and nutrient content. This analysis would then be compared with the Recommended Daily Allowances (Table 9-4) and the nutrient intake evaluated in terms of percentage of adequacy in reference to that standard.

If the purpose of the assessment is to obtain information for diet instruction, then a more appropriate method of data collection would be the 24-hour recall question-

TABLE 9-4. RECOMMENDED DAILY DIETARY ALLOWANCES

Revised 1973 by the Food and Nutrition Board, National Academy of Sciences-National Research Council.
Designed for the maintenance of good nutrition of practically all healthy people in the United States.*

	AGE YEARS	WEIGHT (KG)	WEIGHT (LBS)	HEIGHT (CM)	HEIGHT (IN)	ENERGY (KCAL)	PROTEIN (G)	VITAMIN A ACTIVITY (RE)	VITAMIN A ACTIVITY (IU)	VITAMIN D (IU)	VITAMIN E ACTIVITY (IU)	ASCORBIC ACID (MG)	FOLACIN (MCG)	NIACIN (MG)	RIBOFLAVIN (MG)	THIAMIN (MG)	VITAMIN B6 (MG)	VITAMIN B12 (MCG)	CALCIUM (MG)	PHOSPHORUS (MG)	IODINE (MCG)	IRON (MG)	MAGNESIUM (MG)	ZINC (MG)
Infants	0.0-0.5	6	14	60	24	kg x 117	kg x 2.2	420	1,400	400	4	35	50	5	0.4	0.3	0.3	0.3	360	240	35	10	60	3
	0.5-1.0	9	20	71	28	kg x 108	kg x 2.0	400	2,000	400	5	35	50	8	0.6	0.5	0.4	0.3	540	400	45	15	70	5
Children	1-3	13	28	86	34	1,300	23	400	2,000	400	7	40	100	9	0.8	0.7	0.6	1.0	800	800	60	15	150	10
	4-6	20	44	110	44	1,800	30	500	2,500	400	9	40	200	12	1.1	0.9	0.9	1.5	800	800	80	10	200	10
	7-10	30	66	135	54	2,400	36	700	3,500	400	10	40	300	16	1.2	1.2	1.2	2.0	800	800	110	10	250	10
Males	11-14	44	97	158	63	2,800	44	1,000	5,000	400	12	45	400	18	1.5	1.4	1.6	3.0	1,200	1,200	130	18	350	15
	15-18	61	134	172	69	3,000	54	1,000	5,000	400	15	45	400	20	1.8	1.5	2.0	3.0	1,200	1,200	150	18	400	15
	19-22	67	147	172	69	3,000	54	1,000	5,000	400	15	45	400	20	1.8	1.5	2.0	3.0	800	800	140	10	350	15
	23-50	70	154	172	69	2,700	56	1,000	5,000		15	45	400	18	1.6	1.4	2.0	3.0	800	800	130	10	350	15
	51+	70	154	172	69	2,400	56	1,000	5,000		15	45	400	16	1.5	1.2	2.0	3.0	800	800	110	10	350	15
Females	11-14	44	97	155	62	2,400	44	800	4,000	400	12	45	400	16	1.3	1.2	1.6	3.0	1,200	1,200	115	18	300	15
	15-18	54	119	162	65	2,100	48	800	4,000	400	12	45	400	14	1.4	1.1	2.0	3.0	1,200	1,200	115	18	300	15
	19-22	58	128	162	65	2,100	46	800	4,000	400	12	45	400	14	1.4	1.1	2.0	3.0	800	800	100	18	300	15
	23-50	58	128	162	65	2,000	46	800	4,000		12	45	400	13	1.2	1.0	2.0	3.0	800	800	100	18	300	15
	51+	58	128	162	65	1,800	46	800	4,000		12	45	400	12	1.1	1.0	2.0	3.0	800	800	80	10	300	15
Pregnant						+300	+30	1,000	5,000	400	15	60	800	+2	+0.3	+0.3	2.5	4.0	1,200	1,200	125	18	450	20
Lactating						+500	+20	1,200	6,000	400	15	80	600	+4	+0.5	+0.3	2.5	4.0	1,200	1,200	150	18+	450	25

*The allowances are intended to provide for individual variations among most normal persons as they live in the United States under usual environmental stresses. Diets should be based on a variety of common foods in order to provide other nutrients for which human requirements have been less well defined.

naire. The frequency with which certain foods are consumed can then be compared with the "Basic Four" food groups as a reference for dietary adequacy or excess.

Additional available information, obtained during the interview, should include: methods of preparing food, sources available for food (donated foods, food stamps), food buying practices, vitamin and mineral supplements, and income range.

Conducting the Interview

As was indicated in the chapter on Interviewing Techniques, it is important that the interviewer establish a rapport with the patient in order to promote respect and trust. The success of the interviewer in eliciting pertinent information for dietary assessment depends on the quality of communication established at the outset.

In the initial stages of the interview, the interviewer should introduce and explain the purpose of the interview. The rest of the session should be conducted in a nondirective and exploratory way, allowing the respondent to express his feelings and thoughts. At the same time, the respondent should be encouraged to respond specifically to the questions asked.

The manner in which a question is asked will influence the extent to which the respondent will cooperate. To this end, the interviewer should accept a reply to a question without expressing disapproval, either directly by comment or indirectly by facial expression. For example, if the respondent says, "We eat rattlesnake meat as an appetizer," the reviewer should not express amazement or disgust by making faces or saying anything negative.

Sometimes a series of questions is necessary in order to elicit the information needed. Consider the following exchange:

> Interviewer: "What time did you get out of bed yesterday?"
> Respondent: "I got up at six o'clock in the morning to prepare breakfast for my husband and I had a cup of coffee with him."
> Interviewer: "Did you put anything in your coffee?"
> Respondent: "Only a teaspoon of sugar, nothing else."
> Interviewer: "Did you have anything else with your coffee?"
> Respondent: "No, not at that time. I had breakfast later, around eight o'clock in the morning."

When attempting to elicit information about the kind and quantity of food eaten at a particular time, the interviewer should not ask a suggestive question such as "Did you put sugar or cream in your coffee?" Also, assumptions should not be made about the size of servings. Instead, questions should be phrased so that quantities

TABLE 9-5. BASIC FOUR FOOD GROUPS THE DAILY GUIDE TO GOOD EATING

FOOD GROUPS	RECOMMENDED AMOUNTS	
Milk Group (8-ounce cups)	Children under 9	2 to 3 cups
	Children 9-12	3 to 4 cups
milk, cottage cheese	Adolescents	4 or more cups
	Adults	2 or more cups
ice cream, yogurt	Pregnant women	3 or more cups
	Nursing mothers	4 or more cups
Meat Group (2-3 ounce serving) (cooked, without bone) lean beef, veal, pork, lamb, poultry, fish	2 servings total	
Alternatives: dried beans, peas, lentils (1 cup cooked, serving) peanut butter (4 tablespoons serving) eggs (2)		
Vegetables, Fruits (½ cup serving, 1 piece fruit)	4 servings total	
Dark green or yellow	1 serving vitamin A rich	
Citrus fruit or vegetable	1 serving vitamin C rich—or 2 servings of a fair source	
Other vegetables and fruits	2 or more servings	
Breads and Cereals bread, rolls, biscuits, muffins (1 slice or small piece) ready to eat cereals (1 ounce serving) cooked cereal, cornmeal, grits macaroni, noodles, rice, spaghetti (½ to ¾ cup cooked, serving)	4 servings total	
Miscellaneous Group cream, bacon, butter, margarine, shortening, oil, salad dressing, olives, jam, jelly, sugar, candy, cake, pie, carbonated beverages, relishes, alcoholic beverages, snack foods, pretzels, potato chips, etc.	Provide mostly calories for the day's total intake	

are more clearly determined. For example, to help determine indirectly the size of one hamburger eaten, the following question may be asked: "How many hamburgers were prepared out of the pound of ground meat you said you bought?" Another approach to determining quantities is to use food models of known sizes in estimating portions of meat, cake, or pie or to record quantities in common measurements such as cups, spoonfuls, etc. (or according to size of containers, when discussing intake of bottled beverages).

In recording a particular combination dish such as "Spanish rice" or "stew," ask for the ingredients in the recipe, recording the largest quantities first. Note whether the ingredients were raw or cooked and the number of servings provided by the recipe. When the client has finished listing the foods for the recall questionnaire, it may be helpful to read the list of foods back and ask if anything was forgotten, such as fruit, cake, candy, between-meal snacks, or cocktails.

Assessing Food Consumption

An example of a 24-hour recall form is detailed in Table 9-6. This sample contains dietary information about Mrs. Brown, a 25-year-old housewife, indicating the different kinds of food she consumed, the times during the day when she consumed them and the quantities she consumed, as measured in household units. An assess-

ment of the adequacy of this diet, using the "Basic Four" food groups as a reference standard, is shown in Table 9-7. The chart indicates that Mrs. Brown's diet is adequate with respect to the bread and cereal group and foods rich in vitamin A, low in food sources of calcium and vitamin C, and only slightly lacking in servings of protein foods.

On the other hand, Mrs. Brown's 24-hour recall record shows an excessive intake of high-calorie foods from the miscellaneous food group. This food consumption practice is reflected in her weight, which is 19 percent over acceptable normal standards — enough to characterize her as obese.

TABLE 9-6. 24-HOUR RECALL QUESTIONNAIRE FOR ADULTS

NAME *MRS. BROWN*   DATE OF RECALL *3/4*   DAY OF RECALL *TUESDAY*
AGE *25 YEARS*   MALE _____   FEMALE ✔   OCCUPATION *HOUSEWIFE*
HEIGHT (INS.) *64*   WEIGHT (lbs.) *138*   IDEAL WEIGHT (lbs.) *116*   % OF IDEAL *119%*

INGESTION PERIOD	KINDS OF FOODS AND DESCRIPTION	AMOUNT IN HOUSEHOLD UNITS	FREQUENCY OF CONSUMPTION OF VARIOUS FOODS	TIMES PER DAY-WEEK-MONTH ×D	×W	×M
6:00 A.M.	coffee	1 cup	milk, whole		4	
	sugar	1 tsp	milk, skim			
	cream	2 tbsp	yogurt		3	
			cheese		3	
			ice cream		5	
8:00 A.M.	cornflakes	1 cup	beef		4	
	milk, whole	½ cup	pork			1
			lamb			1
12:00 NOON	sandwich		fish		1	
	bread, white	2 slices	poultry		3	
	peanut butter	2 tbsp	eggs		5	
	apple	1 small	cream	3		
	coffee	1 cup	butter		3	
	sugar	1 tsp	margarine	3		
	cream	2 tbsp	oil	1		
			salad dressings	1		
3:00 P.M.	Coca-Cola, regular	1 (12-ounce can)	vegetables			
	Almond Joy bar	1½ ounces	green—yellow	1		
			citrus fruits		3	
6:30 P.M.	fried filet of sole	3 ounces	legumes			
	green beans	½ cup	beans		1	
	boiled potato	1 medium	chick peas			1
	lettuce salad	1 cup	lentils			
	french dressing	2 tbsp	potatoes	1		
	muffin	1 small	breads	3		
	coffee	1 cup	pastas		4	
	sugar	1 tsp	rice			
	cream	2 tbsp	cakes	1		
			pies		4	
10:30 P.M.	chocolate cake (8″ diam.)	1/16 cake	candy bars	1		
	Coca-Cola, regular	1 (12-ounce can)	jams—jellies		5	
			sugar	3		
			alcoholic bev.			
			carbonated bev.	3		
			coffee, tea	3		
			snack foods	1		
			vitamin suppl.			
			mineral suppl.			

Planning for Nutritional Care

A plan of action for nutritional care should be based on the results of the dietary assessment and the client's profile. Using the example given previously in Table 9-7, the goal for the nutritional care of Mrs. Brown involves helping her to state clearly and set specific objectives for achieving her goal of weight reduction.

Two main objectives derived from the nutritional assessment are:
• Appropriate food selection for a balanced diet
• Appropriate food intake for weight control

To help the client understand why a good diet is necessary to maintain health the nutritional plan should include a discussion of the nutrient contributions from each of the "Basic Four" food groups and their recommended levels. Specifically, in Mrs. Brown's case, it would be desirable to increase consumption of foods from the milk group and add citrus fruits, in order to achieve an adequate intake of calcium and vitamin C respectively.

Discussing the specific foods in the miscellaneous group that contribute mainly "empty calories" helps to ensure the effectiveness of a weight control plan. The frequent consumption of such foods eventually contributes to overweight.

The initial planning sessions based on clearly defined objectives will help in nutritional counseling and, later, in evaluating progress.

Dietary Counseling Based on Client Needs

Once the dietary evaluation is complete, it is important to discuss the results with the client. The positive aspects of the diet should be stressed and suggestions made for improving intake of foods from the "Basic Four" daily guide.

In the case of Mrs. Brown, to achieve the set objectives, it would be important to involve her in the planning for her diet by assigning her certain activities:

1. Plan meals for a week using as a guide the "Basic Four" food groups for nutritional adequacy.
2. Learn to make appropriate choices from food exchanges considering size of servings within the prescribed calorie levels for weight reduction.
3. Develop skill in planning low calorie snacks using fruit and low calorie food.

The instructions should be stated clearly and simply, in terms adapted to the client's educational background. The nutritional counseling may be initiated by the dietitian, while the nurse, as a team member of the health group, can supplement the client's knowledge and offer motivation to follow the prescribed diet.

Various teaching methods can be used to achieve the learning objectives. If programmed instruction is avail-

TABLE 9-7. DIETARY ADEQUACY OF FOOD INTAKE OF A 25-YEAR-OLD HOUSEWIFE, USING THE BASIC FOUR FOOD GROUPS AS A REFERENCE STANDARD*

BASIC FOUR GROUP AND MISCELLANEOUS FOODS	DIETARY ADEQUACY
Milk Group	−1½ cups
Meat Group	−½ serving
Vegetables, Vitamin A rich	OK
Fruits, Vitamin C rich	−1 serving Vitamin C rich
Bread-Cereal Group	OK
Miscellaneous Foods	Additional: Sugar Cream Coca-Cola Salad Dressing Chocolate Cake Candy Bar

*Dietary information derived from Table 9-6, the 24-hour recall questionnaire

able, this teaching technique can provide general nutritional knowledge as part of counseling, while allowing the client to learn at his own pace. If group instruction is used, it can offer an opportunity for several people to share their experiences of a common problem such as weight reduction and thereby provide encouragement and a positive outlook for following the dietary program. Individual instruction can then be used to deal with any specific problems the client may have. Such teaching should be coupled with written instructions for an individualized plan such as a dietary list and charts for plotting the rate of weight loss relevant to the individual client. Additional available literature in the form of leaflets and pamphlets would be very helpful during counseling.

In summary, the nurse plays an important role in providing individualized professional guidance to the person who must adjust daily food consumption to meet health needs. She may consult with a dietitian or a nutritionist or may refer the client to them. When functioning in a primary health care setting in the community, the nurse should be aware that the client is autonomous and has the power to accept or reject the plan of care. Therefore, it is extremely important to develop skills which will gain the client's cooperation in focusing on the objectives of the plan and carrying out the prescribed regimen.

Evaluating the Counseling Process

The success of nutritional counseling is evaluated in terms of desirable changes in the client's behavior relevant to the objectives of the plan of care. For example, if the client demonstrates knowledge and skill in planning an adequate diet, then this accomplishment can be used as one of the points in the evaluation. If Mrs. Brown substitutes fruit for candy bars as snacks in her daily diet, this is an indication that the counseling sessions have been successful. Other criteria may include the quality and quantity of the nutritional knowledge gained by the client as indicated by tests given before and after counseling. Or, the actual loss of weight demonstrated on a weight reduction chart may reflect how successfully this objective has been attained.

Evaluation also leads to reassessment, replanning or reteaching as the client's situation either changes or shows no improvement. In the latter instance, it would be necessary to revise the plans to reinforce the learning or develop alternative ways of dealing with the situation. Inherent in this approach is an understanding that behavioral changes are made slowly and that the client, as a human being, has rights, values, and an individual life style.

At the same time that the client's progress is being evaluated, the nurse counselor is evaluating her own effectiveness in accordance with standards of competent professional practice.

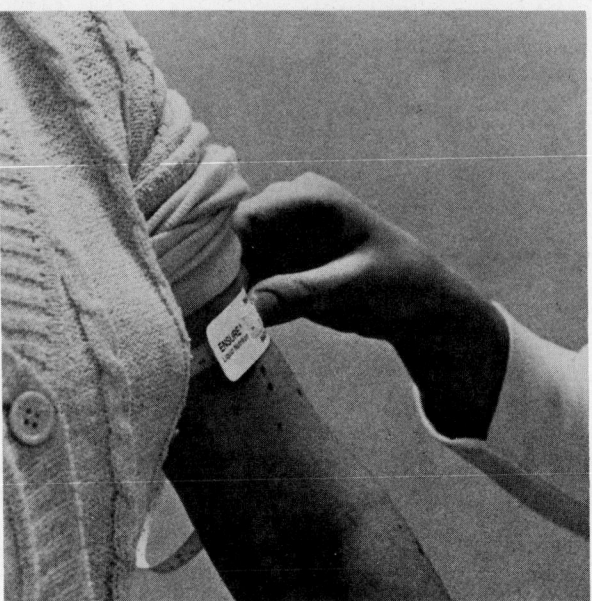

Figure 9-2. Measurement of arm muscle circumference. (Photo by Doug Herdman/Kettering Medical Center)

NUTRITION IN DISEASE

Many disease conditions produce metabolic alterations that result in *negative nitrogen balance*. When these conditions are coupled with anorexia they can lead to malnutrition. It is known that malnutrition interferes with wound healing, increases susceptibility to infection, and contributes to prolonged bed confinement in the hospital population.

Butterworth cites several examples of nutritional neglect in hospitals. He points out that iatrogenic malnutrition has become a significant factor in determining the outcome of illness in many patients.

Among the undesirable practices affecting the nutritional health of hospital patients are:
- prolonged use of glucose and saline IV therapy
- withholding of meals because of diagnostic tests
- use of tube feedings in inadequate amounts and of uncertain composition
- failure to recognize increased nutritional needs resulting from injury or illness

Many drugs also influence the nutritional status of patients. Some of these medications may have a specific appetite-depressant effect, may irritate the mucosa, or may cause nausea and vomiting. Others may influence bacterial flora in the intestine or directly affect nutrient absorption, so that secondary malnutrition results.

The body in starvation may convert protein to glucose for energy; the result is persistent loss of muscle tissue. One sensitive indicator of the body's gain or loss of protein is its *nitrogen balance*. An adult is said to be in *nitrogen equilibrium* when the nitrogen intake (from food) equals the nitrogen output (in urine, feces, and perspiration); it is a sign of health. A positive nitrogen balance exists when nitrogen intake exceeds nitrogen output and indicates tissue growth, such as occurs during pregnancy, childhood, recovery from surgery, and rebuilding of wasted tissue. Negative nitrogen balance indicates that tissue is breaking down faster than it is being replaced. It can be brought about by fever, surgery, burns, and other debilitating diseases as well as by starvation. For instance,

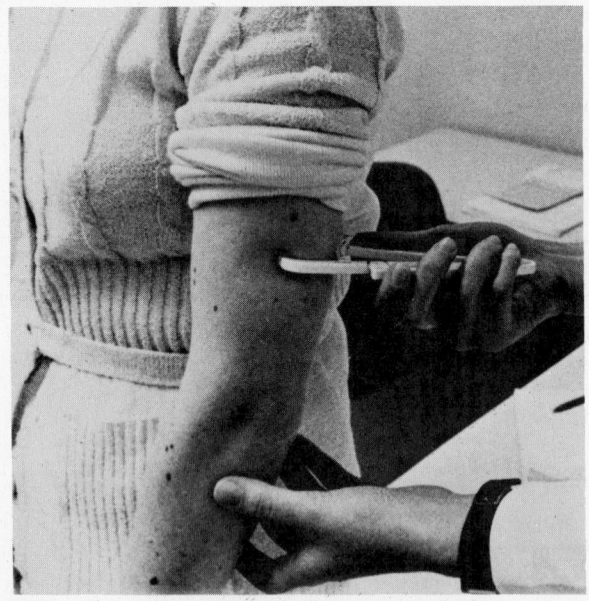

Figure 9-1. Skinfold calipers for measurement of skinfold thickness. (Photo by Doug Herdman/Kettering Medical Center)

each gram of nitrogen loss in excess of intake represents the depletion of 6.25 grams of protein or 25 grams of muscle tissue. Therefore, a negative nitrogen balance of 10 grams per day for 10 days could mean the wasting of 2.5 kilograms (5.5 pounds) of muscle tissue.

Nutritional Assessment of the Hospitalized Patient

If the hospital has a metabolic nutrition support unit, it is managed by a physician working with a specially trained team consisting of a pharmacist, a nurse clinician, and a dietitian. Nutritional assessment of the hospitalized patient includes the following parameters:

1. Anthropometric measurements
   Weight/height
   Triceps skinfold thickness
   Midarm and arm muscle circumferences
2. Biochemical measurements
   Albumin
   Transferrin
   Total lymphocyte count
   Creatinine/height index
   Urinary tests (sodium, potassium, urea, creatinine)

Weight loss is an extremely important measurement since it reflects inadequate calorie intake. In the semi-starved patient, weight loss indicates an increased loss of protein from the body cell mass. With respect to *anthropometric measurements* for protein calorie malnutrition, the best available indicators are triceps skinfold thickness (Fig. 9-1), which indicates fat stores, and muscle circumference (Fig. 9-2), which indicates the state of muscle protein (Table 9-8).

Lower serum albumin and *transferrin* levels are useful measures of visceral protein deficits in adults and are expressed as percentages of normal values (Table 9-9).

Both are indicators of the degree of malnutrition. Serial measurements of these are used to assess the results of nutritional therapy.

Reduced amounts of *leukocytes* in hospitalized patients who become acutely malnourished as a result of stress and low-calorie feeding are associated with impairment of cellular immunity.

Information about *electrolyte balance* provides an assessment of kidney function as a metabolic response to infused electrolytes. The creatinine/height index calculated over a 24-hour period assesses the metabolically active tissue and indicates the degree of protein depletion, comparing expected body mass for height and actual body cell mass.

Diagnostic Categories of Malnutrition

After the data for nutritional assessment have been collected, determination of the category of malnutrition which applies to the individual patient becomes the first consideration in order to plan an effective regimen for nutritional support of the hospitalized patient. Table 9-10 indicates nutritional status classification.

Not every patient with an eating problem can be considered a candidate for special nutritional therapy, but the nurse should be on the alert for any secondary nutritional problems which may be dealt with through the nursing care plan. An example of how the nurse can deal with such problems within the framework of the health care team and the Problem Oriented Medical Record system is found on page 151.

Total Parenteral Nutrition

Sometimes patients are so weak that eating sufficient food to meet their needs is impossible, and parenteral and enteral nutrition are required.

TABLE 9-8.   ANTHROPOMETRIC MEASUREMENTS
STANDARD VALUES AT VARIOUS DEFICIENCY LEVELS

		TRICEPS SKINFOLD (ADULT)			
	(mm.) STANDARD	90% STANDARD	80% STANDARD	70% STANDARD	60% STANDARD
Male	12.5	11.3	10.0	8.8	7.5
Female	16.5	14.9	13.2	11.6	9.9
		ARM CIRCUMFERENCE (ADULT)			
	(cm.) STANDARD	90% STANDARD	80% STANDARD	70% STANDARD	60% STANDARD
Male	29.3	26.3	23.4	20.5	17.6
Female	28.5	25.7	22.8	20.0	17.1
		MUSCLE CIRCUMFERENCE (ADULT)			
	(cm.) STANDARD	90% STANDARD	80% STANDARD	70% STANDARD	60% STANDARD
Male	25.3	22.8	20.2	17.7	15.2
Female	23.2	20.9	18.6	16.2	13.9

Adapted from: C. E. Butterworth, G. L. Blackburn, Hospital malnutrition. Nutrition Today, 10(2):11-12, Mar./Apr. 1975.

TABLE 9-9.   SUGGESTED GUIDE TO INTERPRETATION OF BLOOD DATA*

	DEFICIENT	LOW	ACCEPTABLE	HIGH
Total plasma protein: gm/100 ml	< 6.0	6.0 -6.4	6.5 -6.9	≥7.0
Serum albumin (electrophoretic method): gm/100 ml	< 2.80	2.80-3.51	3.52-4.24	≥4.25
Serum globulin (percent of serum protein):				
Alpha₁		....	4-7	
Alpha₂		....	9-11	
Beta		....	11-15	
Gamma		....	12-16	
Hemoglobin, gm/100 ml:				
Men	<12.0	12.0 -13.9	14.0-14.9	≥15.0
Women (nonpregnant, nonlactating; ≥13 years)	<10.0	10.0 -10.9	11.0-14.4	≥14.5
Children (3-12 years)	<10.0	10.0 -10.9	11.0-12.4	≥12.5
Hematocrit (PCV), percent:				
Men	<36	36-41	42-44	≥45
Women (nonpregnant, nonlactating; ≥13 years)	<30	30-37	38-42	≥43
Children (3-12 years)	<30.0	30.0 -33.9	34.0-36.9	≥37.0
Plasma ascorbic acid: mg/100 ml	< 0.10	0.10-0.19	0.20-0.39	≥0.40
Plasma vitamin A: μg/100 ml	<10	10-19	20-49	≥50
Plasma carotene: μg/100 ml	₃	20-39	40-99	≥100
Red cell riboflavin: μg/100 ml-red blood cells	<10.0	10.0 -14.9	15.0-19.9	≥20

*Except for the particulates in blood, serum levels of nutrients in children do not differ appreciably beyond infancy from those of adults. Similarly, with the exception of hemoglobin and hematocrit, the serum levels of blood constituents in women of child-bearing age are comparable to those of males.
From: Interdepartmental Committee on Nutrition for National Defense. Manual for Nutrition Surveys, 2nd ed.

Total parenteral nutrition (TPN) is indicated when the oral route is unavailable due to surgery or obstruction, when oral intake is inadequate, and when peripheral infusion of nutrients cannot meet the patient's needs.

The clinical situations for which TPN may be indicated can be summarized as follows; they include circumstances in which:

- The patient is *unable* to ingest any food orally or by tube (major burns, esophageal and gastric carcinoma).
- The patient can and does ingest food (orally or by tube) but *not enough* to maintain an anabolic state (radiation enteritis, malabsorption syndromes, Crohn's disease).
- The patient is able to ingest food orally but *refuses* to do so (e.g., the geriatric postoperative patient, the adolescent with anorexia nervosa, and the psychiatric patient in prolonged depression).
- The patient *should not be fed* orally or by tube feeding (such as those with acute pancreatitis, high enterocutaneous fistula, chronic diarrhea).

TABLE 9-10.   NUTRITIONAL STATUS CLASSIFICATION

STANDARDS		MILD	MODERATE	SEVERE
Albumin	gm%	3.5-3.0	<3.0-2.5	<2.5
Transferrin	mg%	200-180	<180-160	<160
Lymphocyte count		1,800-1,500	<1,500-900	<900
Triceps Skinfold	% deficit			
Mid-arm Circum.	% deficit	>5-15%	>15-30%	>30%
Arm Muscle Circum.	% deficit			

Adapted from: M. V. Kaminski, A. L. Winborn. Nutritional Assessment Guide. Midwest Nutrition, Education and Research Foundation Inc., 1978.

- A patient who is emaciated may require more energy sources as well as electrolytes, vitamins, and minerals. Because of protein wasting this patient requires a greater supply of protein than he did while in the healthy state. He also may have an impaired metabolism, so that infusion of metabolic end products for oxidation and synthesis is required.

The duration of TPN treatment for any given patient must be determined individually and cannot be prescribed in advance. It depends on the extent and nature of injury or disease, the healing rate, and the previous degree of nitrogen balance.

The TPN mixture for each patient is prescribed by the physician, who is guided by the initial assessment report; he adjusts it as often as necessary to suit the therapeutic regimen and the patient's condition.

Nutritional Requirements in Parenteral Nutrition

Calorie requirements for maintenance are estimated to be 30 to 35 cal./kg./day, with a nitrogen-calorie ratio of 1:300. For anabolic nutrition the calorie level is approximately 40 to 45 cal./kg./day, with a nitrogen-calorie ratio of 1:200. This level appears to be adequate for most patients.

Glucose, which is the most physiological sugar, is given to patients on TPN in solution concentrations of 20 to 40 percent. Such a concentration is necessary in order to supply the daily requirement of about 3,000 calories without fat. For fat-intake needs, *Intralipid*, a fat emulsion, has been approved by FDA and has been used successfully in parenteral nutrition. It contains essential fatty acids. It has been given in about 1.5 to 2.5 mg./kg. units to patients receiving 2,500 to 3,500 calories. It must

APPLYING POMR TO A NUTRITIONAL PROBLEM

Date: 4/26/80

Problem: Difficulty in mastication and swallowing due to radiation treatment in the pharyngeal area.

S: Mr. R., an elderly male, refuses to eat. He complains of difficulty in masticating and swallowing, and of tasteless food. After one or two bites he pushes away the tray. He prefers to take a few sips of milk now and then. He feels weak and responds indifferently to his nurse's encouragement to eat.

O: The patient's height is 158 cm. (5'6"), his weight on admission was 58 kg. (128 lbs.). His present weight is 52 kg. (114 lbs.). Serum albumin is 2.5 gm./100 ml. Hemoglobin is 11 gm./100 ml. and hematocrit 36%. The prescribed hospital diet is 1,800 calories.

A: The radiation treatment has caused soreness and dryness of the mouth and has resulted in "mouth blindness," or lack of taste. Further, inability to accept food has caused a progressive weight loss. The mild degree of malnutrition that has developed has contributed to his weakness and affected his morale.

P: In an attempt to minimize mouth soreness and dryness, discuss and demonstrate mouth care to the patient and suggest, in consultation with the physician, suitable preparations available for relief of mouth dryness, especially during periods of eating. Subsequently, consult with the dietitian for more acceptable foods for the patient, such as creamy dishes and dishes with gravy, to facilitate swallowing. To improve appetite, substitute foods with aroma to compensate for loss of taste and to stimulate appetite. Between meals provide high-calorie, high-protein beverages taken in small sips, such as milkshakes or other commercial preparations to increase nutritional intake. Socialize frequently with patient to encourage verbalization of feelings and involve him in the selection of his menu. Continue to encourage other forms of interaction to keep his morale high.

---

be pointed out that the needs and disease states of the individual patient must be taken into consideration when fat is included in parenteral nutrition.

Nitrogen estimation for nitrogen equilibrium is approximately 8 gm./day (1 g. nitrogen is approximately 6.25 g. protein; therefore 8 x 6.25 = 50 gm. protein per day.) The positive nitrogen balance in most patients can be achieved with 12 to 13 gm./day of nitrogen (12-13 x 6.25 = 75-81 gm. protein). For patients with burns or sepsis the amount of protein might be further increased to achieve nitrogen balance. The sources of nitrogen for parenteral nutrition are protein hydrolysates, crystalline amino acids, or whole blood and serum albumin. For TPN, amino acid mixtures are used, in which case the eight essential amino acids should be present in adequate amounts and in proper balance for maintenance needs and protein synthesis.

Vitamins are needed for proper metabolism of amino acids, fats, and carbohydrates. Vitamins in parenteral nutrition are given on the basis of assumptions made from oral requirements previously established. Usually an injection of 1.4 ml. of multivitamin is added to 1 liter of amino acid-glucose solution, and these are given with the solution to patients.

Electrolytes and inorganic trace minerals are also important nutrients. Sodium deficit decreases protein utilization, and potassium is needed for better glucose infusion. Calcium is required for bone mineralization and normal function of the parathyroid gland. Other inorganic elements such as phosphorous, chloride, acetate, and others are also included according to the patient's needs.

These solutions are mixed and prepared in the hospital pharmacy under a laminar-flow hood using aseptic techniques to maintain sterility.

Most of the solutions currently used for TPN in the United States are hyperosmotic. The basic nutrient solution is about six times more concentrated than blood. The route of administration of such concentrated solutions should be via the right subclavian vein or external jugular vein. In that region high blood flow permits rapid dilution that minimizes the undesirable effects of phlebitis and thrombosis.

Nursing Roles

Nursing roles in parenteral therapy may be described as follows:

- The hyperalimentation nurse clinician participates in nutritional assessments, follows the patient's progress, and monitors for possible complications.
- The nurse coordinator is trained to assist in catheter insertion and in the safe delivery of solutions.

These are the new challenges for nurses working with multidisciplinary teams in a nutritional support service; their participation in education, research, and service in this relatively new modality will help to reduce morbidity and mortality in hospitalized patients.

BIBLIOGRAPHY

BOOKS

Exchange Lists for Meal Planning, rev. ed. New York, American Diabetes Association, 1976.

Interdepartmental Committee on Nutrition for National Defense: Manual for Nutrition Surveys, 2nd. ed. Bethesda, Md., National Institutes of Health, 1963, p. 250.

Lagua, R. T., Claudio, V. S., and Thiele, V. F.: Nutrition and Diet Therapy; Reference Dictionary, 2nd. ed. St. Louis, C. V. Mosby, 1974.

Meng, H. C.: Parenteral nutrition. *In* H. A. Schneider, C. E. Anderson, and D. B. Coursin, eds.: Nutritional Support of Medical Practice. Hagerstown, Md., Harper and Row, 1977.

Munro, H. N.: Protein hydrolysates and amino acids. *In* P. L. White, M. E. Nagy, and D. C. Fletcher, eds.: Total Parenteral Nutrition. Acton, Mass., Publishing Sciences Group, 1974, pp. 59-79.

Weed, L. L.: Medical Records, Medical Education and Patient Care. Cleveland, The Press of Case Western Reserve University, 1970.

Wilson, E. D., Fisher, K. H., and Fuqua, M. E.: Principles of Nutrition, 3rd ed. New York, J. Wiley, 1975.

ARTICLES

ADA guidelines for diet counseling. J. Am. Diet. Assoc., *66*:571-575, June 1975.

Bistrian, B. R., et al.: Cellular immunity in semistarved states in hospitalized adults. Am. J. Clin. Nutr., *28*:1148-1155, Oct. 1975.

Bollet, A. J., and Owens, S.: Evaluation of nutritional status of selected hospitalized patients. Am. J. Clin. Nutr., *26*:931-938, Sept. 1973.

Butterworth, C. E., Jr.: The skeleton in the hospital closet. Nutr. Today, *9*:4-8, Mar.-Apr. 1974.

————: The dimensions of clinical nutrition. Am. J. Clin. Nutr., *28*:943-945, Sept. 1975.

———— and Blackburn, G. L.: Hospital malnutrition. Nutr. Today, *10*:8-18, Mar.-Apr. 1975.

Christaki, G., ed.: Nutritional assessment in health programs. Am. J. Pub. Health Supplement, *63*:18-21, Nov. 1973.

Dudrick, S. J., et al.: Can intravenous feeding as the sole means of nutrition support growth in the child and restore weight loss in an adult? Ann. Surg., *169*:974-984, June 1969.

Newton, M. E., Beal, M. E., and Strauss, A. L.: Nutritional aspects of nursing care. Nurs. Res. *16*:46-49, Winter 1967.

Viteri, F. E., and Alvarado, J.: The creatinine height index: its use in the estimation of the degree of protein depletion and repletion in protein calorie malnourished children. Pediatrics *46*:696, Nov. 1970.

Woody, M., and Mallison, M.: The problem-oriented system for patient-centered care. AJN, *73*:1168-1175, July 1973.

10

THE IMMUNE SYSTEM AND IMMUNOPATHOLOGY

There are a large number of medical conditions called collagen diseases that are in reality immunological disorders. Included in this category are such diseases as dermatomyositis, polyarteritis nodosa, scleroderma, rheumatic fever, rheumatoid arthritis, systemic lupus erythematosus, mixed connective disease, and rheumatoid arteritis.

Much, if not all, of the confusion concerning these diseases lies in the old-fashioned terminology used in identifying them. Terms such as "collagen," "rheumatoid," and "arteritis" are solely descriptive in nature and refer only to the major tissues affected in the diseases; they offer little by way of explanation. Yet, all of these conditions can be understood by realizing that first and foremost they are diseases caused by the body's own immune system.

"Immunity" refers to the body's specific protective response to an invading foreign agent or organism. However, pathological developments within this system lead to certain disease manifestations. Therefore, the term "immunopathology" is used to describe the study of diseases caused by the immune reaction—that protective response which the body initiates but which paradoxically turns on the body and causes tissue damage and disease. However, to understand immunopathology we must first understand how the body's immune system normally functions.

THE IMMUNE SYSTEM

General Immune Responses

When the body is attacked by bacteria or viruses, it has three means of defending itself—the phagocytic immune response, the humoral or antibody immune response, and the cellular immune response.

The first line of defense, the *phagocytic immune response*, involves the white blood cells (granulocytes and macrophages) which actually have the ability to ingest foreign particles. These cells can move to the point of attack to engulf and destroy the foreign agents.

The second protective response, the *humoral or antibody response*, begins with the lymphocyte cells which can transform themselves into plasma cells that manufacture antibodies. It is the antibodies, which are highly specific proteins, that are transported in the bloodstream and have the ability to disable the invaders.

A third mechanism of defense, the *cellular immune response*, also involves the lymphocytes which, besides transforming themselves into plasma cells, can also turn into special killer T cells that can attack the microbes themselves.

Of the three modes of immune response, the formation of antibodies constitutes the major protective device employed by the immune system.

Antigens and Antibodies

The part of the attacking organism that is responsible for stimulating the production of an antibody is called an *antigen*. In strict molecular terms, an antigen is a small patch of proteins on the outer surface of the microorganism. A single bacterium, even a single large molecule such as a toxin (diphtheria or tetanus toxin), may have several such antigens or "markers" on its surface and can therefore induce the body to produce a number of different antibodies. Once an antibody is produced, it is released into the bloodstream and carried to the attacking organism where it combines with the antigen on its surface, coupling with it like a complementary piece of a jigsaw puzzle (Fig. 10-1).

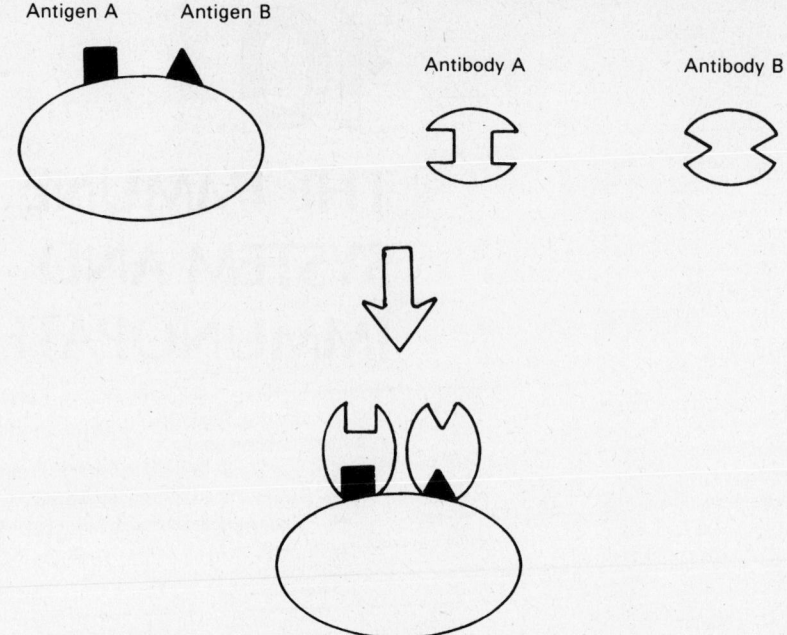

Figure 10-1.   Antigens A and B cause the production of specific antibodies A and B, which couple with corresponding antigens.

Stages of the Immune System Response

There are four well-defined stages in an immune response: recognition, proliferation, response, and the effector stage.

Recognition

The basis of any immune reaction is first and foremost recognition. It is our immune system's ability to recognize antigens on materials as "foreign," or "non-self," that is the initiating event in the mounting of any immune reaction. The body must first recognize invaders as "foreign" before it can react to them.

SURVEILLANCE BY LYMPH NODES AND LYMPHOCYTES.   The body accomplishes its surveillance in two ways. First, instead of being localized centrally in one large organ far away from the obvious points of microbial attack such as the skin, mouth, eyes and throat, the immune system is widely dispersed — distributed close to all of the body's surfaces, internal as well as external, in the form of tiny organs called lymph nodes. Second, a steady succession of sentries in the form of small lymphocytes is continuously being discharged from lymph nodes into the bloodstream where they patrol the tissues and vessels that drain the areas served by that node. Basically, it is the lymphocytes and lymph nodes that make up our immune system.

LYMPHOCYTES.   There are two kinds of lymphocytes, those in the lymph nodes themselves and those that circulate. Figure 10-2 shows the path taken by the recirculating lymphocytes. Taken in aggregate, the total number of lymphocytes in the body add up to a mass of cells of impressive size. Radioactive labeling of circulating lymphocytes has shown that these cells have no particular fate but simply recirculate from the blood to lymph nodes — and from their lymph nodes back into the bloodstream again in a never-ending series of patrols. Rather astonishingly, these circulating lymphocytes can survive for decades. Some of these small, hardy cells maintain their solitary circuits for the lifetime of the person.

The exact way in which circulating lymphocytes recognize antigens on foreign surfaces is not known. At present the accepted theory is that recognition depends upon specific receptor sites on the surface of the lymphocytes. It appears that macrophages, a type of granulocyte found in the tissues of the body, play an important though as yet undefined role in helping these circulating lymphocytes to process the antigens. Foreign materials enter the body and a circulating lymphocyte comes into physical contact with the surfaces of these materials. Upon contact, the lymphocyte, with the help of macrophages, either removes the antigen from the surface or in some way picks up an imprint of its structure. For example, during a streptococcal throat infection, the streptococcal organism gains access to the mucous membranes of the throat, and a circulating lymphocyte moving through the tissues of the neck bumps up against the organism. The lymphocyte familiar with the surface markers on the cells of its own body recognizes the antigens on the microbe as being different (non-self) and the streptococcus as being antigenic (foreign). This triggers the second phase, the immune response — proliferation.

Proliferation Stage

The circulating lymphocyte containing the antigenic message returns to the nearest lymph node. Once in the node, these "sensitized" lymphocytes stimulate certain of the dormant lymphocytes residing there first to enlarge, divide, and proliferate, and finally to differentiate into antibody-producing plasma cells. Swelling of the lymph nodes in the neck in conjunction with a sore throat is one example of the immune response.

The Response Stage

In the response stage, the changed lymphocytes will function in either a humoral or cellular fashion.

HUMORAL. The production of antibodies to a specific antigen is called a humoral response, humoral referring to the fact that the antibodies are released into the bloodstream and so reside in the plasma or fluid fraction of the blood, one of the classical four "humours" of the body. (An explanation of antibody function can be found on page 157.)

CELLULAR. The exact mechanism of the cellular response is not yet known. It is thought that the returning sensitized lymphocytes probably migrate to areas of the lymph node (other than those areas containing lymphocytes programmed to become plasma cells) where they stimulate the residing lymphocytes to become cells that upon being released back into the circulation will attack microbes personally rather than through the production of antibodies (Fig. 10-3).

These transformed lymphocytes have been given the descriptive name *killer T cells.* The *T* stands for the fact that during the embryologic development of the immune system, these lymphocytes spent some time in the thymus of the developing fetus, during which time they were genetically programmed to become (under the di-

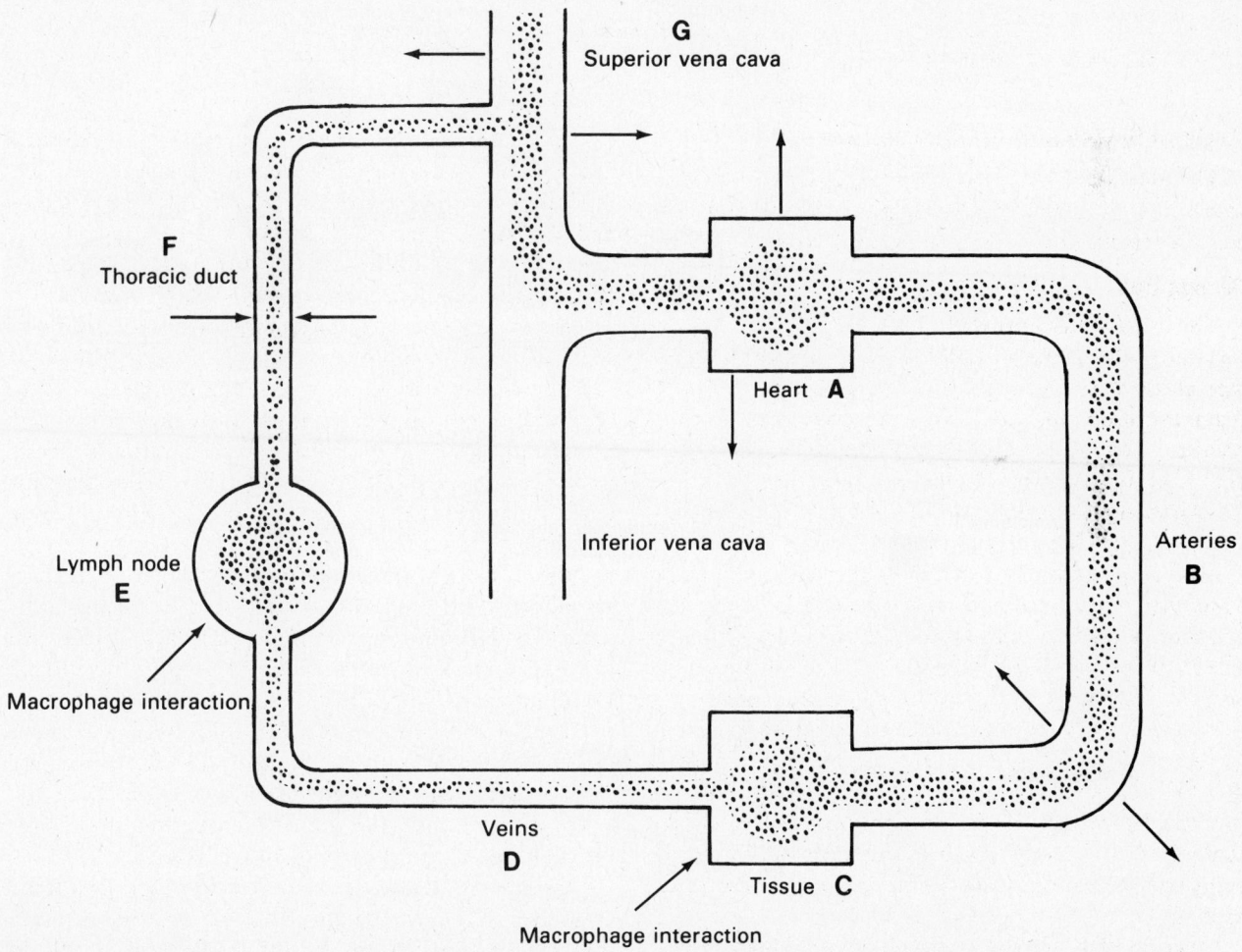

Figure 10-2.   Recirculation of small lymphocytes is depicted schematically. For convenience, we shall begin the lymphocyte circuit in the heart *A.* From *A,* the lymphocytes tumble into the aorta and from the aorta into arteries *B* and eventually out into the tissues of the body *C.* Cells then enter the veins *D* and from there move into the nearest lymph node *E.* The cells moving through the lymph node leave the node via the lymphatic drainage, eventually entering the thoracic duct *F,* through which they enter *G,* the superior vena cava, via the large veins of the neck. The superior vena cava then takes the cells back to the heart to begin another circuit that will take the circulating lymphocyte to another part of the body.

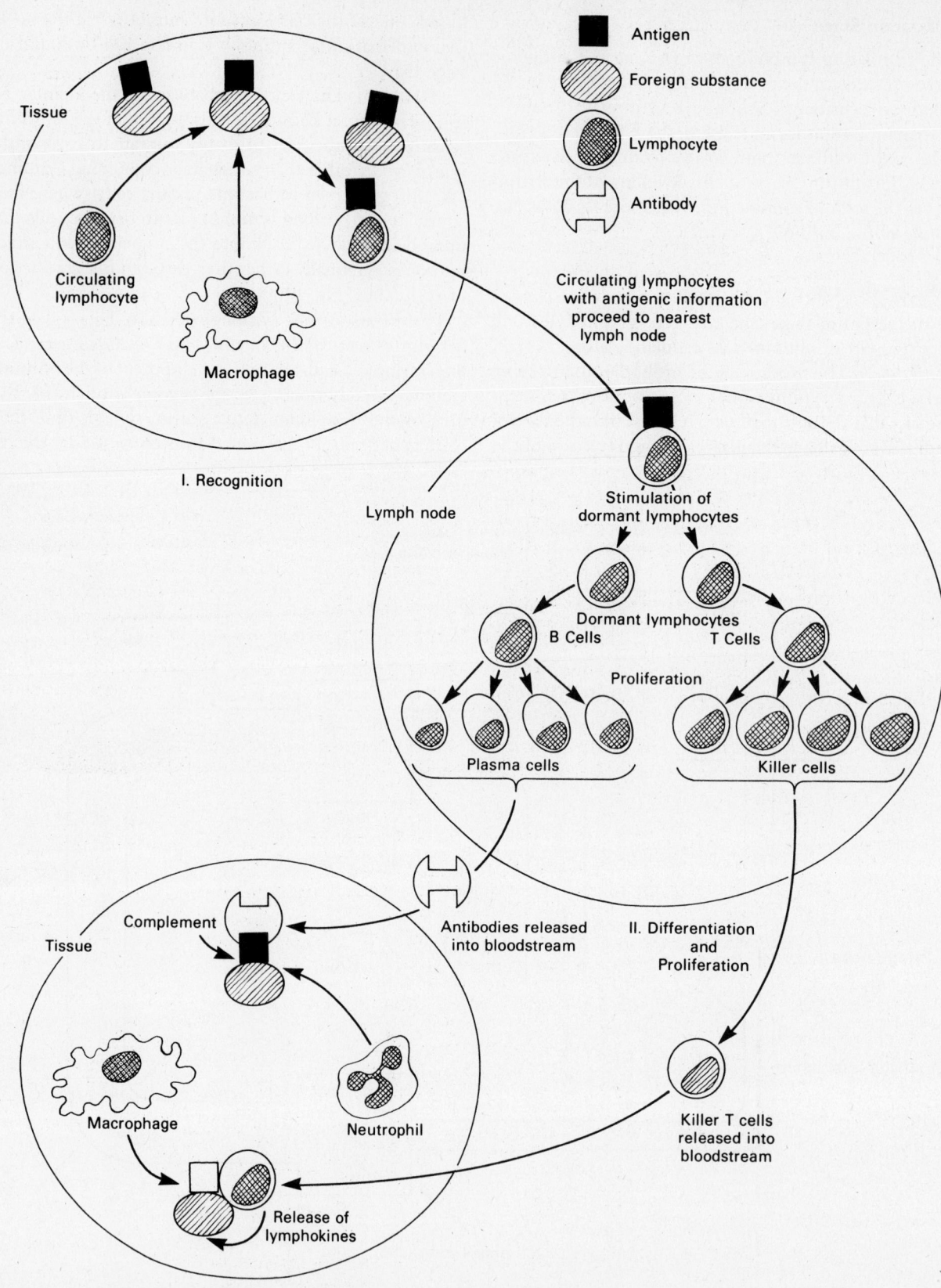

Figure 10-3. Cellular response.

rection of an antigenically sensitized circulating lymphocyte) killer T cells rather than plasma cells. Viral rather than bacterial antigens induce a cellular response. This response is manifested by the increasing number of lymphocytes seen in the blood smears of people with viral illnesses, for instance, in the lymphocytosis occurring in infectious mononucleosis.

Most immune reactions to antigens involve both humoral and cellular responses, though usually one predominates. During transplantation rejections, the cellular reaction predominates, whereas in the bacterial pneumonias and sepsis it is the humoral response that plays the dominant protective role (Table 10-1).

The Effector Stage

In the effector stage the antibody of the humoral response or the killer T cell of the cellular response reaches and couples with the antigen on the surface of the foreign object. The coupling initiates a series of events that in the majority of instances results in the total destruction of the invading microbes or the complete neutralization of the toxin. The events involve an interplay of antibodies, complement, and action by the killer T cells.

ANTIBODIES. To understand how the production of antibodies can protect the body we must understand what an antibody looks like and how it works. Figure 10-4 is a schematic representation of an antibody molecule. The various parts have been designated as the Fab fragments and the Fc end.

It is important here to define the "Ig" designation of antibodies. *Ig* refers to the term immunoglobulin. Early

TABLE 10-1. COMPARISON OF CELLULAR AND HUMORAL IMMUNOLOGIC RESPONSE

CELL MEDIATED IMMUNE RESPONSES	HUMORAL MEDIATED IMMUNE RESPONSES
Transplant rejection	Bacterial phagocytosis and lysis
Delayed hypersensitivity-tuberculin reaction	Viral and toxin neutralization
Contact dermatitis	Anaphylaxis
Graft-vs.-host reactions	Allergic hay fever and asthma
Tumor surveillance and/or destruction	Immune complex disease
Intracellular infections	

in the study of the types and kinds of proteins circulating in blood, machines were developed that could separate blood proteins by the electronic changes on their surfaces. Antibodies were found to be contained in a class of circulating proteins migrating through the electronic field at a rate different from those of the other blood proteins, such as hemoglobins or the clotting factors.

These antibody proteins, defined solely by how they migrated through the charged field, were listed as globulins because of other physical and chemical properties that showed they belonged to the general class of proteins called globulins. They were also given the name immunoglobulins, since they were globulins involved in the immune response. We now know that the body produces five different kinds of globulin antibodies arbitrarily designated as IgA, IgM, IgG, IgD, and IgE, each type differing in size and amino acid composition (Table

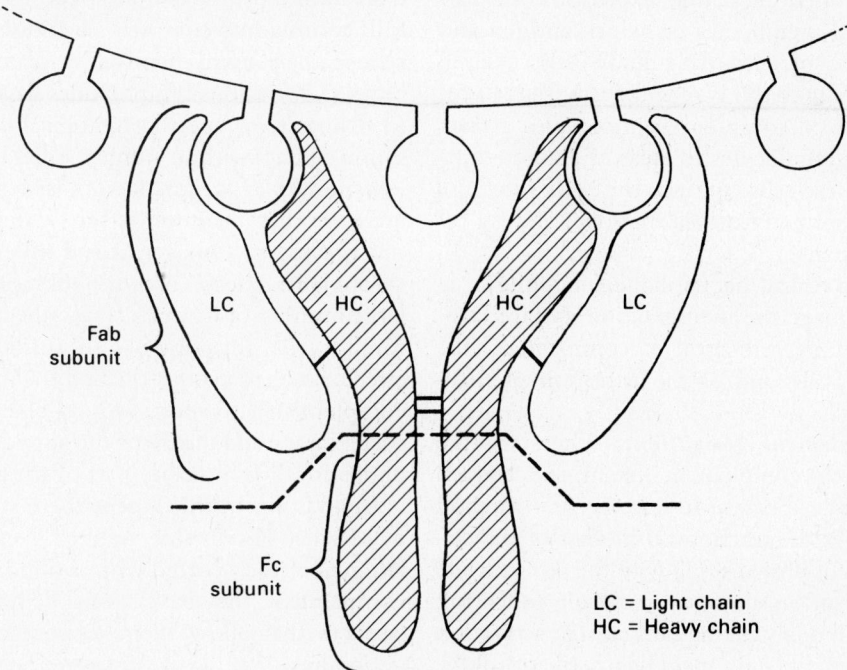

Fab subunit

Fc subunit

LC   HC   HC   LC

LC = Light chain
HC = Heavy chain

Figure 10-4. Antibody molecule.

TABLE 10-2. CLASSES OF IMMUNOGLOBULINS

PROTEIN		SPECIES	AMINO ACID CHAIN LENGTH	PROTEIN MOLECULAR WEIGHTS
IgG (IgG_1, IgG_2, IgG_3, IgG_4)	Δ	Human	450	150,000
IgA (IgA_1, IgA_2)	$\square$	Human	470	58,000
IgM		Human	575	950,000
IgD		Human	—	175,000
IgE		Human	550	77,000

Δ Subclasses of IgG molecules
$\square$ Subclasses of IgA molecules

10-2). The most common antibodies, however, are those of the IgG class. Each antibody molecule made against a particular antigen has a slightly different configuration from those of the amino acids making up its Fab (antigen binding) fragments, so that each Fab fragment fits specifically onto the antigen it was made against (Figure 10-4) and onto no other antigen. The Fab part of the molecule can be considered to be the "recognition" end of the antibody. Once the Fab segments couple with its antigen, the Fc fragment through a change in the antibody's configuration, becomes available to the circulation; i.e., it becomes exposed to the blood passing by, and this exposure allows it to interact with the first of a series of 20 circulating proteins, called the complement system.

COMPLEMENT. The term "complement" refers to a number of circulating plasma proteins made in the liver that can be activated when an antibody couples with its antigen. Once activated, these unique proteins cause alterations of the cell membranes on which antigen and antibody complex form, permitting fluid to enter the cell and leading eventually to cell lysis and death (Fig. 10-5). In addition, activated complement molecules attract macrophages and granulocytes to areas of antigen-antibody reactions. These cells continue the body's defense by devouring the antibody-coated microbes and by releasing bacterial agents.

It is important to realize that antibodies coupling to an antigen do not damage the membrane or surface. Destruction is caused by activation of complement, the arrival of killer T cells and/or the attraction of macrophages.

Classical Complement Activation. There are two ways of activating the complement system; one, termed the classical pathway, because it was the first method discovered, involves the reaction of the first of the circulating complement proteins (C_1) with the receptor site of the Fc portion of an antibody molecule following coupling of the antibody with the antigen. The activation of the first complement component then activates all the other components in the sequence in which the other components were discovered, namely C_1, C_4, C_2, C_3, C_5, up to C_9 respectively. According to the order of reaction, the C components are designated as follows: $C_{1\text{ qrs}}$, C_4, C_2, C_3, C_5, C_6, C_7, C_8, and C_9. C_4 is the second reactant in sequence, rather than C_2, the first four complement components having been numbered before their reaction sequence was known.*

Alternate Pathway of Complement Activation. The alternative method of complement activation occurs without the formation of antigen-antibody complexes. This alternate pathway can be initiated by bacterial products, thus bypassing the requirement for antibody production and/or antigen-antibody coupling. Whatever the method of activation, however, once activated the complement can and does destroy cells.

This destruction is not only therapeutic but lifesaving, if the cell attacked by the complement system is a true foreign invader such as a streptococcus or staphylococcus. However, if that cell is in reality part of the person — a cell of his brain or liver, the tissue lining his blood vessels, or the cells of a donor organ — the result can be devastating disease and even death. The result of the immune response — the implacableness of its attack on any material read as foreign, the deadliness of the struggle — is obvious in the pus (the remains of microbes, granulocytes, and macrophages, circulating and killer T-cell lymphocytes, plasma proteins, complement, and antibodies) that accumulates in wound infections and abscesses.

KILLER T CELLS AND K CELLS. It is not only the complement system that can destroy foreign cells but also sensitized lymphocytes and killer T cells. Cellular rather than humoral destruction is carried out when killer T cells coming into contact with antigenically foreign cells release their own chemical mediators called lymphokines. The various lymphokines have been given names to denote their specific biological effects (Table 10-3). Upon contact with an antigen, killer lymphocytes release low molecular weight factors which attract, hold, and activate other uncommitted circulating lymphocytes and macrophages. One sensitized killer lymphocyte can, through its release of lymphokines, quickly recruit a large number of other cells into the area of antigenically foreign cells, amassing in a short time a large number of effector cells to protect the body. Unfortunately, as with complement activation, such cellular activation can cause tissue injury and disease if the supposedly "foreign" cell under attack is in reality part of the person.

In addition to the T cells there are effector lymphocytes called K cells that, unlike killer T cells, only attack antigens already coated with antibody. Like molecules of complement, they have special Fc receptor sites on their surfaces that allow them to couple to the Fc end of antibodies.

*Austen, K. F., et al.: Nomenclature of complements. Int. Arch. Allerg., *37*:661, 1970.

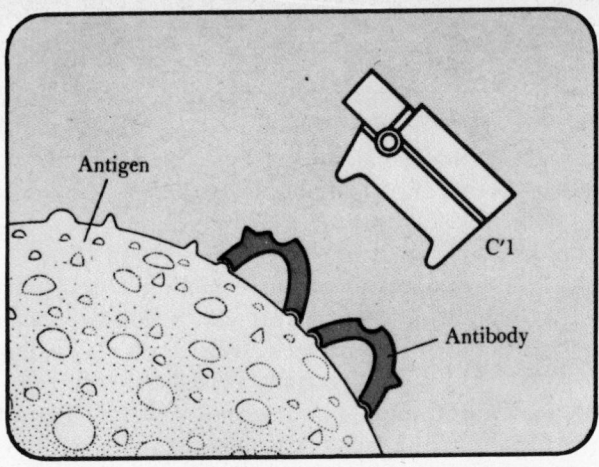

Initiating the sequence is the combination of antigen and complement-fixing antibody. It is hypothesized that under certain conditions, complement binding sites are then exposed.

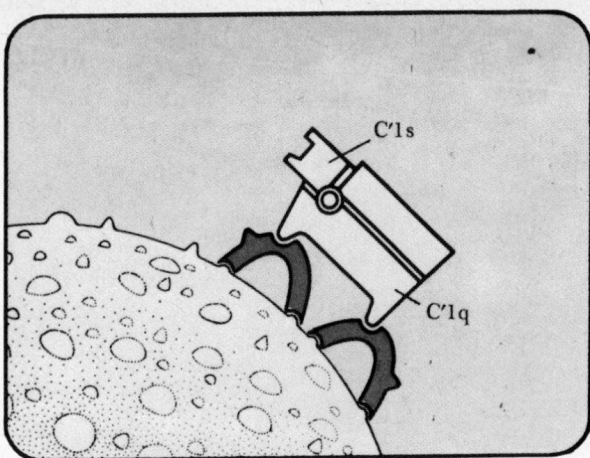

C'1 combines with these sites, with C'1q (a gamma globulin) attaching to the antibody. Enzymatic site (at C'1s) capable of acting with next component is converted to its active form.

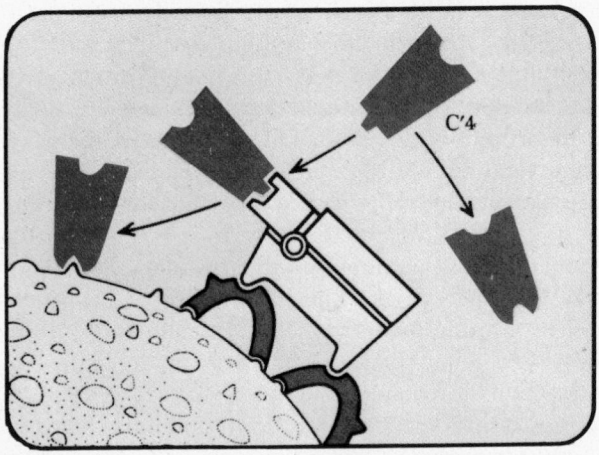

Next in order of appearance is C'4, which is acted upon by C'1s, exposing site for binding C'4 to the surface of the antigen or to the antibody. If unbound, C'4 cannot function in hemolysis.

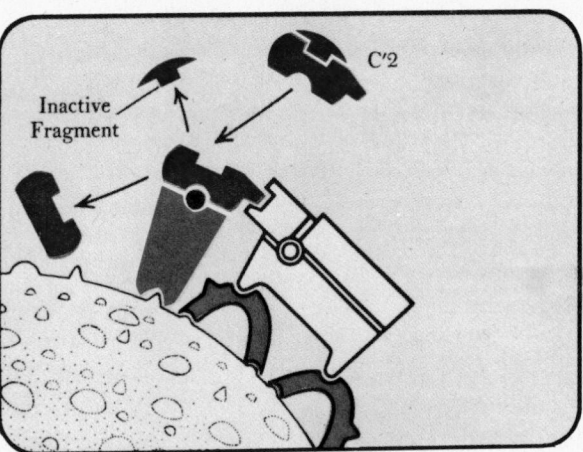

C'2 also interacts with C'1. An inactive fragment is cleaved out, preparing activated C'4-C'2 complex to act on next component. Magnesium is needed for integrity of this complex.

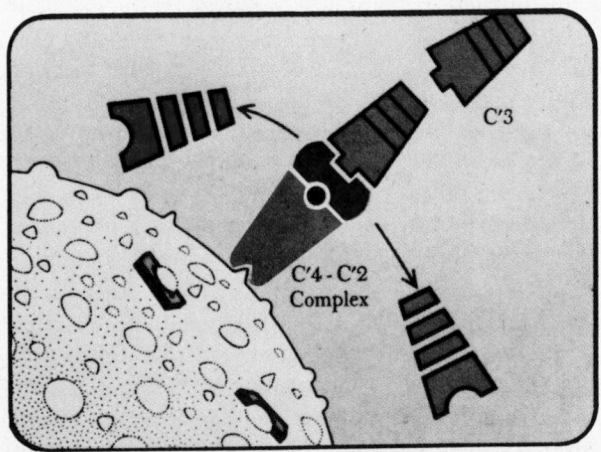

If C'3 appears during the few minutes the C'4-C'2 complex is active, it may be cleaved into at least four parts, one of which may become bound to the surface of the cell.

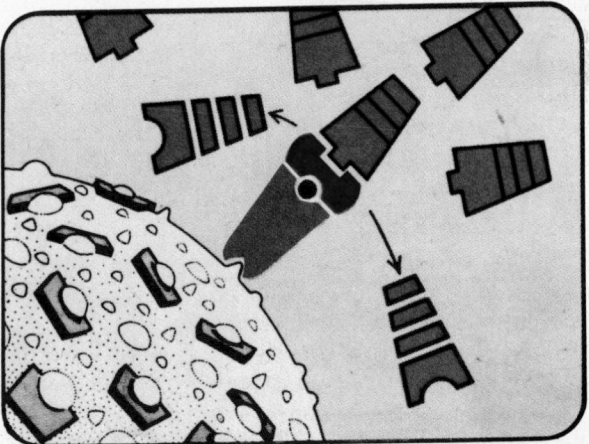

Each C4-C'2 complex can apparently mobilize hundreds of C'3 molecules, thus providing tremendous amplification of immunologic functions served by C'3 and perhaps later C' components.

Figure 10-5.   The complement sequence of activation. C'1, the first component of complement, is made up of 3 subunits called C'1q, C'1s, and C'1r. Activation mechanisms are explained under each individual panel. (Drawings by Irving Geis from Gewurz, H.: The immunologic role of complement. *Hospital Practice*, Vol. 2, No. 9, Sept. 1967, and Good, R. A., and Fisher, D. W., eds.: Immunobiology. Sinauer Associates, Inc., Sunderland, Mass. Reprinted with permission.)

TABLE 10-3. LYMPHOCYTES AND THEIR EFFECTS

LYMPHOKINE	EFFECT
Permeability factor	Increases vascular permeability, allowing white cells into area
Interferon	Interferes with viral growth, stopping the spread of viral infection
Migration inhibitory factor	Suppresses movement of macrophages, keeping macrophage in area of foreign cells
Skin reactive factor	Induces inflammatory response
Cytotoxic factor	Kills certain antigenic cells
Macrophage chemotatic factor	Attracts macrophages into the area
Lymphocyte blastogenic factor	Stimulates more lymphocytes, recruiting additional lymphocytes into the area
Macrophage aggregation factor	Causes clumping of macrophages and lymphocytes
Macrophage activation factor	Causes macrophages to adhere to surfaces more readily
Proliferation inhibitor factor	Inhibits growth of certain antigenic cells
Cytophilic antibody	A factor that binds to an Fc receptor on macrophages that permits them to bind to antigens

BASIS OF IMMUNOPATHOLOGY

The difference between the protective nature of the immune response and its disease-causing potential starts with recognition of what is foreign and what is not. If the antigen is truly foreign we are protected; if not, autoimmune (self-immunized) disease is caused. Antibody-antigen interactions can cause bodily damage in six ways:

1. by antibodies binding to and neutralizing normally biologically active molecules (neutralization)
2. by antibodies destroying normal cells (cytotoxicity)
3. by the deposition of the antibody antigen complexes in tissues and the activation of complement as well as the attraction of granulocytes and K cells to the area of the immune complexes (toxic complex)
4. by the destruction of tissues by sensitized lymphoid cells, killer T cells, due to direct infiltration of the tissues by the lymphoid cells (delayed hypersensitivity)
5. the accumulation of large masses of cells in an area where the antigen is not easily removed or destroyed (granulomatous reactions)
6. the combining of an antigen with an antibody, i.e., most cell destruction, causing the immediate release of pharmacologic agents (anaphylactoid reactions)

We are now aware that a large number of diseases result from just such events.

Nowhere though, has the understanding of immune mechanisms been more productive in deciphering the secrets of disease than in the condition known as *systemic lupus erythematosus* (SLE). The unraveling of the cause of this once baffling condition serves as the model for the basic understanding of all immune mediated diseases.

Systemic Lupus Erythematosus (SLE)

The first recognition of this condition as a distinct entity occurred in 1892. In that year a noted German physician described two types of the disease: an acute, relatively benign form, entailing a facial rash, often preceded by an arthritis; and a second, more malignant form, again with a facial rash, but also with seizures, pneumonia, and often death within two weeks of the appearance of the rash. In 1904, Sir William Osler, an English clinician, reaffirmed the German observations but for the first time emphasized the widespread organ involvement in both types of the disease.

In 1924, Drs. Liebman and Sachs described pathologically unique lesions on the heart valves of patients with SLE. In 1935, Boehr pointed out the kidney destruction in this condition. In 1948, Dr. Hargrove of the Mayo Clinic reported a strange cell circulating in the blood of SLE patients. He called these cells, which he found only in the blood of patients with systemic lupus erythematosus, LE (lupus erythematosus) cells.

In 1955, Moore and Lutz reported that SLE patients had a unique antibody circulating in their blood. However, what that antibody was made against remained unknown.

Shortly after the report of Moore and Lutz, Elliot and Mathieson proved that SLE patients had decreased levels of complement in the circulation. In addition, the LE cells of Hargrove were found to be granulocytes that had ingested circulating antibody. In 1957, the antibody in the serum of these patients was found to be made against DNA, and in 1966, the presence of the antigen DNA itself was found in the blood of SLE patients. Recently, autopsy and biopsy studies using new immunofluorescent techniques have shown antibodies, complement, and in some cases, DNA, to be physically deposited in the diseased kidneys, skin, brains, hearts, and joints of SLE patients.

It is now known that SLE patients make antibodies against their own DNA as well as against other parts of their cells. In addition, the whole seemingly unrelated array of multisystem organ involvement is explained by one cause, namely the deposition of these antigen antibody complexes throughout the body. The immune system of a patient with SLE mounts an immune response against constituents of his own cells and the antigen-antibody complexes resulting from that response cause widespread disease.

For all the precision and effectiveness of our immune system, it is in reality a mindless police force that, once set in motion, will attack any antigen recognized correctly or incorrectly as foreign until it or the antigen is destroyed or neutralized. In SLE we know that the antigens are parts of the patient's own cells, most specifically the patient's own DNA. Two explanations of how this occurs have been offered. They have relevance to all other autoimmune diseases as well.

Mechanisms of Autoimmune Reactions

The first explanation states that SLE is in reality a virus-induced disease. It is postulated that a person with SLE is infected with an as yet unknown virus. The virus gets into the patient's cell, damages the cell, and releases the DNA into the systemic circulation where the body's circulating lymphocytes reads the released DNA as "foreign." Since normally DNA is kept sequestered inside the nuclei of a person's cells and thus away from patroling lymphocytes, when this molecule is released into the bloodstream it is read as foreign and antibodies are made against it. It should be noted here that antibodies can fix to antigens on cell surfaces or to antigens floating free in the bloodstream. In either case, the antigen-antibody complexes bind and activate complement. If this reaction occurs in the circulation, the complexes carried along in the circulation are then deposited in the walls of small vessels all over the body. Once these complexes are deposited, complement is activated, damaging the vessels in which the complexes are deposited and destroying them, much as innocent bystanders can be injured by a shell that accidentally goes off.

The second theory holds that an individual with SLE has a genetically defective immune system that leads to abnormal antibody production against a wide variety of antigens, including the person's own host molecules. To support this theory there are cases of drug-induced SLE. Drugs, including Dilantin used in treating epilepsy, isoniazid in tuberculosis, hydralazine in hypertension, and procainamide in cardiac arrhythmia, cause some people to produce antibodies against their own tissues, mimicking all the signs and symptoms of naturally occurring SLE. This misidentification of host molecules as foreign occurs through the physical binding of the drugs to the patient's own molecules, which chemically changes them so that the patient's genetically aberrant immune system reads these altered molecules as foreign.

The Autoimmune Diseases

SLE fulfills the criteria for an autoimmune disease: (1) the presence of abnormal antibodies in these patients' serum, (2) the low complement levels, and (3) the deposition of immune complexes and complement in their diseased organs—all of which point to this condition's being the result of an autoimmune process. The precise mechanisms involved in many of the other conditions now thought to be of autoimmune origin have not been as clearly worked out as they have been for SLE, though the immune nature of these conditions is obvious (Table 10-4). The nature of the offending antigens might remain obscure; yet, it is clear in the majority of autoimmune diseases that the inciting event may be one of the following:

1. The release of sequestered antigens by tissue damage caused either by a virus or a toxin
2. The altering of host molecules through some chemical or physical means
3. The cross-reactivity of an antibody made against a foreign antigen with a molecular constituent of normal tissue

As immunologic methodologies and techniques improve, the various mechanisms of injury as well as the antigens involved in these autoimmune diseases will become as well defined as they have been for systemic lupus erythematosus.

Treatment

Two types of drugs have been employed as treatment regimens in the immune mediated diseases. In general, both types interfere with immune responses either by suppressing lymphocyte interactions and/or proliferation, or through disrupting antibody production.

STEROIDS. Although the precise actions of steroids on the immune response have yet to be completely worked out, it is known that steroids enter cells and interfere with cellular functions. In the case of lymphocytes, there is inhibition of growth and sometimes even cell death. In addition, steroids have been shown to interfere with

TABLE 10-4. PRESUMPTIVE EVIDENCE FOR THE IMMUNE NATURE OF "COLLAGEN" DISEASE

DISEASE	EVIDENCE FOR INVOLVEMENT OF IMMUNE MECHANISMS
Polyarteritis	Complexes of hepatitis viruses and immunoglobulin found in the vessels of one half of the reported cases
Systemic lupus erythematosus	Circulating antinuclear antibodies
Rheumatoid arthritis	Presence of rheumatoid factor, a circulating IgM antibody to the patient's own immunoglobulins; decreases levels of complement in affected joints
Scleroderma	Circulating antibodies to components of cell nuclei
Dermatomyositis	Experimental production of a similar disease in animals by immunization with muscle tissue
Mixed connective tissue disease	High titers of circulating antibody to components of cell nuclei
Rheumatic fever	Circulating antibodies cross-reacting specifically with antigens in streptococci and heart muscle.

humoral responses, by inhibiting the production of antibodies, and with cellular responses, by affecting killer T-cell differentiations. Steroids are also thought to interfere with the liberation and/or action of mediators such as the lysozymal enzyme released by macrophages and the lymphokines of killer T cells; thus steroids influence tissue damage and inflammation in this way rather than by specifically interrupting the immune response itself.

IMMUNOSUPPRESSIVE MEDICATIONS. The alkylating agent cyclophosphamide (Cytoxan) and the purine analogue azathioprine (Imuran) are both drugs that interfere with DNA replication.

These medications disturb the fundamental mechanisms concerned with cell growth and differentiation and therefore interfere with rapidly proliferating tissues. Since the immunological system, when mounting an immune response, is composed at all levels of cells undergoing rapid growth and differentiations, the immunosuppressive medications are particularly effective in blunting or stopping the mounting of an immune response.

SUMMARY

Immune mechanisms serve to protect the body from foreign invaders as well as to neutralize circulating toxins. It is clear that these same immune mechanisms can account for a large number of human diseases. The understanding of the immune nature of disease has provided a major advance in medicine, allowing physicians and nurses to better understand the nature of disease, its specific treatments, and ultimate prognosis.

BIBLIOGRAPHY

BOOKS

Anderson, W. A. D., and Kissane, J. M., eds.: Pathology, 7th ed. St. Louis, C. V. Mosby, 1977.

Glasser, R. J.: The Body is the Hero. New York, Random House, 1976.

Good, R. A., and Fisher, D. W., eds. Immunobiology, 5th ed. Sunderland, Mass., Sinauer Associates, 1973.

Goodman, L. S., and Gilman, A.: The Pharmacological Basis of Therapeutics, 5th ed. New York, Macmillan, 1975.

Ropes, M. W.: Systemic Lupus Erythematosus. Cambridge, Mass., Harvard University Press, 1976.

Weiser, R. S., et al.: Fundamentals of Immunology for Students of Medicine and Related Sciences. Philadelphia, Lea and Febiger, 1971.

ARTICLES

Antibodies yield their secrets and display therapeutic versatility. JAMA Medical News, 235:583-590, Feb. 8, 1976.

Balow, J. E., et al.: Immunosuppressive effects of glucocorticosteroids: Differential effects of acute vs. chronic administration on cell mediated immunology. J. Immunol., 114:1072-1076, Mar. 1975.

Capra, J. D., and Edmundson, A. B.: The antibody combining site. Scient. American, 236:50-59, Jan. 1977.

Croft, C. L.: BCG administration and nursing implications. AJN, 79:315-319, Feb. 1979.

Dharan, M.: Immunoglobulin abnormalities, AJN, 76:1626-1628, Oct. 1976.

Dodd, M. J.: Theoretical bases of immunotherapy. AJN, 79:309-314, Feb. 1979.

Donley, D. L.: Nursing the patient who is immunosuppressed. AJN, 76:1619-1625, Oct. 1976.

Good, R. A.: Harnessing the immunity system: From potential to reality. CA — A Cancer J. for Clinicians, 25:178-186, July-Aug. 1975.

Hurd, E. R., and Giuliano, V. J.: Effect of cyclophosphamide on B and T lymphocytes in patients with connective tissue disease. Arthritis & Rheumatism, 18:67-75, Jan.-Feb. 1975.

Isler, C.: Newest treatment for cancer: Immunotherapy. RN, 39:35-38, Apr. 1976; and 39:29-31, May 1976.

McKhann, C. F., and Yarlott, M. A.: Tumor immunology. CA — A Cancer J. for Clinicians, 25:187-197, July/Aug. 1975.

Nysather, J. O., et al.: The immune system: Its development and functions. AJN, 76:1614-1616, Oct. 1976.

Schern, P. S., and Winokor, S. H.: Immunosuppressive and cytotoxic chemotherapy. Long term complications. Ann. Int. Med., 82:84-95, 1975.

Sell, S.: Immunopathology. Teaching monograph, Am. J. Pathol., 90:215-279, Jan. 1978.

Sinkovics, J. G.: Clinical immunotherapy for tumors. Postgrad. Med., 59:110-116, Feb. 1976.

Smith, R. D.: Defense against cancer. The Sciences, 16:21-26, Jan./Feb. 1976.

Sullivan, B. P.: Patient responses to BCG therapy for malignant melanoma. AJN, 79:320-324, Feb. 1979.

Yu, D. T. Y., et al.: Human lymphocyte subpopulation. Effect of corticosteroids. J. Clin. Invest., 53:565-571, 1974.

11

ILLNESS AS A HUMAN EXPERIENCE

ASPECTS OF COMMUNICATION

The experience of illness precipitates many stressful feelings and reactions, for example, anxiety, anger, denial, shame, guilt, and uncertainty. The diagnostic tests, the medical treatment, the prognosis, the body changes, the reactions of family and friends, the experience of hospitalization, and the projected changes in life style—all take part in a person's adaptation to the new situation. Usually, a sick person is exceptionally sensitive and vulnerable. His whole life has been changed at least temporarily, and he often struggles with the resurgence of past experiences as he copes with the present reality and the anticipated future. The nurse is a central figure in the patient's immediate life. Through sensitive understanding and intelligent action she can provide many opportunities for the patient to maintain his basic security, self-esteem, and integrity.

The basic nurse-patient relationship takes into account the physician, the family, other patients, the rest of the health team, and society at large. The relationship is established and maintained by the communication process—a complex, dynamic exchange of verbal and nonverbal messages.

Communication is based on mutually intelligible symbols. To be understood, a person must have a knowledge of himself and his needs, an ability to speak the language and express himself clearly, and a familiarity with the usual conventions of the situation. To understand others, he must be able to observe and evaluate behavior. To make oneself understandable and to understand others is vital to the establishment of relationships. The patient whose English is inept or who speaks a foreign language, or whose ability to express himself is markedly impaired through physical or psychological causes, poses a challenge to the nurse.

The process of communication may be considered to consist of four segments: (1) *I* (2) *am communicating something* (3) *to you* (4) *in this situation.* Breakdowns in communication can be pinpointed by identifying the segment in which the interference is taking place.

The sender of the message, the *I,* is affected by such factors as age, sex, socioeconomic status, marital status, occupation, intelligence, physical condition (especially as related to the nervous system and the organs of communication), personality, and current emotional status.

The message, *am communicating something,* consists of both verbal and nonverbal elements that may be complementary or incongruous. The patient who says, "Oh, I'm fine. Nothing is the matter," while restlessly moving about, wringing his hands and sighing, frequently illustrates the latter.

The receiver of the communication, *to you,* is influenced by the same factors as the sender with respect to behavior. The ability to hear or "read" a patient's behavior depends largely upon the ability to listen openly and sensitively. The presence of stereotypes, misconceptions, and anxiety may prevent the nurse from correctly identifying the message from a particular patient.

The context of the communication, *in this situation,* refers to the sociocultural status of the patient, the context of illness, the social order of the hospital, and immediate environmental aspects. The importance of understanding the cultural background and the values of

163

patients has gained recognition in all areas of nursing. When patients enter the hospital world, they may be overwhelmed and bewildered by the change in their status and role. The nurse plays a vital part in orienting patients to their new position. She also needs to acquaint them with the scope of her professional services. Many people do not know that the nurse is prepared and eager to help them with a wide variety of health needs. In addition to performing the traditional services related to physical needs, she offers help as a health teacher, a rehabilitation worker, a communications link with other professional services, and, in some instances, a psychotherapeutic counselor.

A person in the first stages of adapting to illness, who is taking the defensive measure of denying his illness, does not seek or welcome accurate information about his condition or treatment. A nurse who attempts to do effective health teaching will find her efforts of little avail at this time. The behavior of the patient, the questions he asks or avoids, and his reactions to the changes in his health status all give clues to his readiness and his needs. In turn, the patient is also very sensitive to the reactions of the medical and nursing staff and seeks to interpret nonverbal messages with regard to his prognosis, especially when it is not favorable.

Developing skill in listening to and talking with patients is a continuous process that improves with experience. The nurse communicates with patients in order to identify their health needs, to clarify misconceptions, and to help them verbalize their fears and reactions to their situations. Anxiety can be lessened or channeled through sharing it with another person. The nurse concerns herself with the impact of illness in the patient's life situation. At the same time, she must be aware of the right of the patient to privacy about his life and recognize that her purpose in talking with him is to help him.

The expressive function of the nurse involves helping the patient to maintain equilibrium and motivation and supporting his attempts to cope with the experience of illness and treatment, by providing direct gratifications that reduce his tension level and help him to adapt to the process. The provision of physical comfort and support is combined with such interpersonal activities as explaining, reassuring, understanding, protecting, and simply being with the patient. When a patient is acutely ill, communication generally takes place on a primitive, chiefly nonverbal level. A touch, a soft but reassuring tone of voice, and the presence of the nurse may convey to the patient that he is not alone and that he is being cared for. When it is anticipated that a patient will experience a direct interference with communication patterns as a result of treatment, it is vital to set up a system of communication in advance. One patient reported: "The worst part about my laryngectomy was that I couldn't tell anyone what I needed—but the magic slate helped."

An important part of the development of interpersonal and communication tools is the nurse's understanding of herself, her characteristic interpersonal needs, and her usual patterns of communication. As she becomes more aware of her own needs, she is better able to identify those of her patients and to know when her own perceptions and reactions are preventing her from accurately assessing the situation. This is particularly true when the patient's behavior is frustrating, puzzling, hostile, or demanding. The nurse must be able to evaluate her own responses so that she does not retaliate with anger or rejection. The situations that lead to feelings of helplessness and hopelessness must be talked about and shared so that the nurse can maintain her own equilibrium and give optimal nursing care to patients with incurable, repulsive, or terminal conditions. The nurse's awareness of her own need for approval and recognition plays an important part in her reactions to patient behavior and to the behavior of her co-workers, her supervisors, and the medical staff.

BASIC EMOTIONAL NEEDS

Everyone has the same basic emotional needs. These have been categorized by some authorities as love, trust, autonomy or self-control, self-esteem, identity, and productivity. Another list includes the desire for recognition, new experiences, security, and response—the giving and receiving of personal appreciation, love, and affection. The foregoing needs are summarized as: (1) inclusion, (2) control, and (3) affection. The nonrealization of a need leads to undesirable consequences. The discrepancy between the need and its fulfillment results in feelings that are labeled *anxiety*.

The *need for inclusion* is defined behaviorally as the need to establish and maintain satisfactory relationships with people with respect to association and interaction. It refers to the establishment and maintenance of a feeling of mutual interest in others. The need for inclusion is the need to feel that the self is significant and worthwhile. Inclusion behavior refers to association between individuals and is indicated by such words as "associate," "interact," "belong," "join," and "communicate." Lack of inclusion is connoted by words such as "excluded," "ignored," "withdrawn," "aloof," or "isolated." The need to be included is shown by the desire to attract attention and interest. The "demanding" patient who frequently signals and monopolizes the staff with extensive conversation may simply be indicating strong needs for inclusion. The nurse who feels personally slighted when a patient ignores her attempts at polite conversation or treats her like a servant rather than a professional person may be demonstrating her own inclusion needs.

The desire for prestige and status is a part of inclusion

needs; the individual needs people to pay attention to him, know who he is, and distinguish him from others. Identity is closely related to inclusion. One is known as a distinct individual, who therefore deserves attention. The height of inclusion is to be understood, which implies that someone is interested enough to seek and discover a person's particular characteristics, likes, and dislikes.

When a person enters a hospital situation, his first crisis involves inclusion needs. Will the staff know who he is? Will he be treated like a person and not just another case — "Room 111" or "the new cardiac"? Many routines of hospital admission strip the patient of his outward signs of prestige and status. His clothes and belongings, even his dentures, may be taken away. He receives a uniform, and often humiliating, hospital gown. He may be bombarded by a series of questions relating to the most intimate details of his life. He is expected to join the patient "group" but may be given little explanation or few guidelines about what to do. When it is necessary to place a patient in isolation, attention should be given to his inclusion needs — the nurse becomes a vital link in satisfying them.

Other ways to help a patient with his inclusion needs include giving him a thorough and considerate orientation to his physical surroundings. The nurse can inquire about any questions the patient has, what he expects from his treatment, and how he expects her to help him. She can give him some guidelines about the scope of her professional responsibility, explaining that she will be available to help him in a variety of ways and that she will maintain her interest in him as an individual.

The patient who is withdrawn and avoids association with others may have unmet inclusion needs. He may not talk to his roommates or the nurse and may spend long periods sleeping or with the curtains pulled. A certain amount of regression and isolation is often a necessary part of adaptation to illness and recovery, but extremes over a period of time are significant. Underneath an apparent indifference to others may lie a basic anxiety in relation to people. The patient's worst fear may be that others will ignore him and show no interest in him, although he disguises his fear with a lack of interest in others and a seeming independence. Patients who feel abandoned and isolated from their families and friends, who believe that they are so changed now as to be unacceptable, or who feel rejected and ignored by the medical and nursing staff, may give up the struggle. On the other hand, such patients may get lifesaving reassurance and support from the nurse who continues to include them in the human race and communicates her recognition of their individuality and worth.

Part of the decision of where to place a patient is based on his need for inclusion. Will he do better in a room with three other people? How close to the nursing station should he be? Patients who are together for long periods of time, such as in an orthopedic ward or a rehabilitation facility, demonstrate a particularly wide variety of inclusion needs.

The second major need is *control*. This is the need to establish and maintain a satisfactory relation to others with regard to power, decision-making, and authority. It has to do with the feeling of mutual respect for the competence and responsibility of oneself and others. Control needs are suggested by such words as "dominance," "influence," "boss," "rebellion," "submission," "leader," "noncooperation," and "follower." Control represents assumption of power over others and therefore over one's own future, whereas *being* controlled means giving up responsibility for oneself.

When a person comes to a hospital, he struggles with his need for control. In addition to the problems of inclusion, he may find other people making decisions for him that he would ordinarily make for himself — when to get up, what to eat, and when to go to the toilet. The rules of the hospital may take away his usual decision-making capacity. An extreme example of control behavior is the person who completely gives up or abdicates his own responsibility. He is a clinging, helpless patient who seeks direction from everyone about what to do and how to do it. This reinforces his conviction that he is incompetent, irresponsible, and powerless. Behind these beliefs often lie anxiety, hostility, and a lack of trust in others as well as oneself. Helping the patient to assume responsibility early for making decisions about his own care are nursing actions that help to increase a sense of self-control and responsibility.

The other extreme in control behavior is reflected in actions of constant rebellion and domination. Although the patient's overt behavior may be that of a strong, competent, responsible person, his underlying feelings may be those of uncertainty in his own power. He takes every opportunity to disprove these fears and therefore has a great deal of difficulty in accepting the need for dependency in such matters as bed rest or following "doctor's orders." Nurses also need to examine their own needs for power and control in relation to patients, coworkers, and physicians.

The third major need is that of *affection*. This represents the need to establish with another person a give-and-take relationship based on mutual liking. Affection is suggested by such words as "love," "like," "emotionally close," "personal," "friendship," "intimacy." Lack of affection is connoted by "hate," "dislike," and "emotionally distant." The need for affection is usually met by family members, spouses, and close friends. When a person is separated from these sources by illness or hospitalization, he may not have the need satisfied. Being emotionally close to another generally results in confiding to that person one's innermost anxieties, wishes, and feelings. In the hospital setting, the patient may turn to the nurse to share these things, especially if the family member is unavailable or too anxious to listen. One difference between a social and a professional relationship is that the former implies mutuality of need-satisfaction, the latter, that the patient's needs are the focus without the nurse's burdening him with her own problems. However, the need for affection in both patient and nurse must be considered, particularly when the relationship continues over a period of time.

Aspects of inclusion, control, and affection behavior are overlapping and continuous. Inclusion is primarily related to the formation of a relationship, whereas control and affection are demonstrated within the relationship. Inclusion is related to feeling "in" or "out," control to "top" or "bottom," and affection to "remote" or "close." Generally, a person establishes an equilibrium between himself and other people in these three different areas. Sickness with hospitalization disturbs this equilibrium, giving rise to a wide variety of new stresses.

ANXIETY

Anxiety is a normal reaction to stress and threat. It is an emotional reaction to the perception of danger, real or imagined, that is experienced physiologically, psychologically, and behaviorally. Anxiety and fear are often used synonymously; however, fear generally refers to a specific threat, anxiety to a nonspecific one. A person experiencing anxiety may feel uneasy and apprehensive, and may have a vague sense of dread. Feelings of helplessness and inadequacy may be present along with a sense of alienation and insecurity. The intensity of these feelings may range from mild to severe enough to cause panic, and the intensity may be increased or diminished by interpersonal means.

Anxiety is caused by a threat to the functioning of the organism—either to physical survival or to the integrity of the psychosocial self (self-image). Often, the threat affects both of these areas: a person who is anxious because of acute pain may also be anxious in response to his feelings about his levels of courage and dependency. Illness and hospitalization include the following anxiety-precipitating threats: general threat to life, health, and body integrity; exposure and embarrassment; discomfort from pain, cold, fatigue, and changes in diet; deprivation of sexual satisfaction; restriction of movement; isolation; interruption or loss of one's means of livelihood; precipitation of a financial crisis; dislike, rejection, or ridicule from others as the result of the condition; inconsistent and unpredictable behavior of the authority figures on whom one's welfare depends; frustration of goals and expectations; confusion and uncertainty about the present and the future; separation from family and friends.

Physiologic reactions to anxiety are primarily reactions of the autonomic nervous system and are defensive in nature. They include increases in pulse and respiratory rates, shifts in blood pressure and temperature, relaxation of the smooth muscles in the bladder and bowel, cold, clammy skin, increased perspiration, dilated pupils, and dry mouth. The bodily responses to mild anxiety initially promote learning and the ability to function, but as the reaction increases in severity, learning decreases, perception is reduced or distorted, and the ability to concentrate is greatly diminished. Nurses must be able to evaluate the level of anxiety in a patient so that they can be effective in reducing it. An extremely anxious person is suffering and is very uncomfortable. He has difficulty giving or receiving information of any kind. As far as health matters are concerned, he learns little and magnifies or distorts what he hears.

Characteristic manifestations of anxiety reflect a person's individuality. They include withdrawal, muteness, hyperactivity, swearing, talking and joking excessively, striking out verbally or physically, fantasizing, complaining, and crying. The specific means of coping with anxiety, whether successful or not, varies with individuals and with the situation. One disadvantage of enforced immobility and isolation is that a person who is used to active approaches in handling anxiety is deprived of his usual means of coping and so must develop alternative channels.

Nursing intervention in anxiety includes four aspects:

1. Recognition by the nurse that the patient is anxious. She is aware of situations that can potentially precipitate anxiety and is alerted to physiologic, emotional, and behavioral clues.
2. The nurse verbally encourages the patient to recognize and express his feelings of anxiety.
3. If the source of the anxiety is external, such as poor orientation to the ward or disturbing noises and sights, the nurse may take steps to change these conditions or, if this is impossible, help the patient to understand and cope with his reactions. She encourages the patient to share his immediate experience by open-ended statements such as "Tell me what happened" or "What was going on?" Patients often need help in describing their reactions and thoughts. To ask initially "Why are you anxious?" may or may not result in the information. The person may be too afraid or unsure to tell you, he may not know why he is anxious, or he may resent the inquisition.
4. The nurse helps the patient to cope with what is now a specific threat. He may be helped to reevaluate the situation and his reaction to it. Many times just the sharing of a feeling reduces its intensity. The nurse asks the patient what he usually does to handle anxious feelings and helps him to use similar or other means. The physical presence of the nurse may help, as well as the appropriate use of touch, physical care, and tone of voice.

The apprehension of patients recovering from surgery may be demonstrated by their anxiety about whether the operation was a success and whether they will survive the bewildering, painful, often uncertain postoperative period. The expert physical nursing care given in the recovery room or intensive care unit must take into consideration the patient's fears resulting from isolation, the weird noises and equipment attached to all parts of the body, the blinking, beeping monitor signaling the body's functioning, and the periods of disorientation and loss of physical and emotional control. In this tense situation the nurse must be constantly aware of her own behavioral manifestations of anxiety.

Illness and its treatment precipitate anxiety. For many people, early conflicts are revived. There is often a great deal of uncertainty about the future. The nurse sometimes may be powerless to decrease the patient's anxiety at all, but she can avoid adding to it. For some patients, the thought of getting well and leaving the hospital produces anxiety. The nurse can be helpful to these people by encouraging them to mobilize their strengths and by encouraging decision-making and the reacquisition of responsibility.

Nursing in almost all areas is a profession that deals continually with anxiety. The intimate association with life, death, and all the stages in between arouse within the nurse conscious and unconscious fears about her own vulnerability. Recognition, achievement, and attention are all important to her; she must be able to say that she did all that was possible. There are emotional "high risk" situations in nursing, such as the intensive care unit and the emergency room, in which the nurse's understanding and management of her own anxiety as well as that of patients and their families is vital.

BODY IMAGE

The concept of body image is useful in understanding the many complex reactions of people to changes in health status. Body image may be considered as the total, constantly changing and evolving perception of one's physical self as separate and distinct from all others. This perception is based on inner sensations and functionings as well as on information derived from the external environment. Society prescribes norms of physical appearance and behavior. The perception of body image operates on both conscious and unconscious levels.

Integration of experiences regarding the use of the body takes place over a long period of time. The formative years of childhood are particularly significant in laying down the basic body image and its relation to the personality. While a child is being held, fondled, fed, played with, and toilet-trained, he gradually accumulates related concepts pertaining to his ability to use his physical body, his degree of pride, and his sense of identity. Through sensory impressions, mobility, and touch he experiences pleasure, pain, shame, failure, or pride of accomplishment, as he tests out his boundaries and abilities. As the small child becomes aware of his separation from others, he grows increasingly conscious of his own body, its relation to others, and his ability to control his muscles in the acts of locomotion, bowel and bladder retention and release, motor coordination, and speech. During this period, he begins to master these abilities, and thus acquires pride and self-esteem. If he is not able to gain this mastery, because of loss of self-control and parental overcontrol, he may develop basic attitudes which lead him to regard his body as inadequate, worthless, and shameful. Illness, with enforced dependency and lack of body control, reactivates in persons of all ages many of these early conflicts and perceptions of body image. Feeling ashamed of a disfigurement or deformity stems from early feelings of smallness, weakness, and ugliness as compared to others. The prominent sociocultural values of youth, physical attractiveness, health, and wholeness are incorporated early and reinforced throughout life.

Threats to the body image, and hence to self-esteem, are recognizable in many nursing situations. Feelings of shame, inadequacy, and guilt may be precipitated, depending on the patient's definition of the situation. Violation of modesty and invasion of privacy cause anxiety and embarrassment. Exposure of the body during physical examinations and such treatments as enemas and catheterizations may be upsetting, even though expected as part of the therapeutic regimen. The disturbance in usual elimination processes and the need for using a bedpan or talking about bowel and bladder habits threatens self-esteem. This is a major problem for people requiring the type of surgery that produces such drastic changes as a colostomy or ileostomy.

Major changes in the body image are brought about by amputation of any part or by surgery on the face, hands, and reproductive organs—areas particularly related to identity and self-esteem. Other parts of the body may have unconscious symbolic meanings for a person, and so he may react in an unexpected way to relatively minor, external changes.

Besides the sudden changes in body structure and functioning that occur through accident or surgical intervention, subtle changes occur in progressive diseases such as arthritis, obesity, and multiple sclerosis. Even normal changes in the body, such as occur in puberty and pregnancy, pose a problem of altering the body image. During adolescence there is a sensitive, often painful awareness of the body and its many changes. Complexion, weight, and development of primary and secondary sexual characteristics are closely linked to feelings of worth and sexual desirability.

Changes in the body image may result from such side effects of medication as development of a moon face, changes in the secondary sex characteristics, and growth of facial hair. The reaction of the body to radiation treatment may further threaten the body image, as may changes in skin color, such as occurs in jaundice.

Changes in medical technology require that nurses meet the challenge of new and different approaches to helping people. A person with chronic kidney damage extends his body image to include the "artificial kidney." Organ transplants are another development that raises questions about body image. What does it mean to a person to have another person's heart beating in his chest? What would it be like to have parts of your own body live on after you are clinically dead?

The first step in understanding the concept of body image is to become more aware of one's own attitude toward health, illness, mutilation, disfigurement, and changes in body functioning. Anxiety, revulsion, disgust, and pity are often automatic responses to abnormal body appearance and functioning. To help patients who have these conditions, nurses must come to grips with their own feelings. A patient has a right to expect that nurses will be knowledgeable about his condition, will be impartial toward it, will be willing to help him, and will be concerned about him. A patient often uses the nurse's reactions as a test of whether he is still a worthwhile person in spite of his altered appearance or functioning.

The nurse needs to learn what alteration in the body can mean to the individual patient and what adjustments it will require. Both the patient and his family should be considered, because ideally the adjustment that takes place is mutual. In formulating the nursing care plan for a particular patient, it is useful to include the ability of the family to help the patient cope with changes, orientation to reality, specific problems in coping and methods of coping, and nursing care. The nurse needs to determine how she can support the family and the steps she will take in response to the patient's positive moves. She can anticipate grief, mourning, and anger as reactions to changes in body appearance and functioning. The need for hope and steps toward full rehabilitation must be supported.

Even after the patient has begun to alter his body image and feels worthwhile and accepted in the hospital setting, he is faced with adjusting to society. Many conditions of altered appearance and functioning are stigmatizing. Because of their close proximity to illness, nurses may lose sight of the fact that being disfigured or incapacitated still evokes negative responses and rejection by most of the population. Any such stigma implies that the person is not quite normal—that he is a disabled person, rather than a person having a specific disability. The tendency to stereotype denies the person's individuality. A person with an obvious physical disability has a major problem in handling tensions in interpersonal situations. He may be subjected to curiosity and stares. He may be asked intrusive questions about his condition or treated as if he were completely helpless.

If the condition is not readily visible, learning to exercise information control may help one to avoid being stigmatized. For instance, wearing a prosthesis for a mastectomy can keep one's radical surgery from becoming common knowledge. Talking about one's health status, body functioning, and difficulties in adjustment are appropriate with health personnel and close family and friends. With other people, excessive dwelling on these topics may lead to rejection and ostracism.

A person making necessary adjustments to alterations in his body is often faced with physical and social insecurity. A physically normal person has a general idea of how high the bus steps are and is able to read from a menu. However, the person with a physical impairment may have to make constant and vigilant adaptations to his physical world. The person who uses a wheelchair must find a restroom large enough for him to maneuver in; one with diabetes must calculate his allowed intake at a cocktail party; a man with crutches may find a revolving door almost impossible to manage. Adaptation requires energy, ingenuity, and persistence. Sometimes an individual limits his living space and activities in order to provide more predictable situations. Although this arrangement may be safer, it also limits a person's full participation in life.

Reactions of others toward a person with a disability are ambiguous and conflicting. Acceptance and rejection, sympathy and pity, trust and fear, curiosity and revulsion, valuation and devaluation face him in countless interpersonal situations. He is often unsure of where he stands, particularly with strangers. He is also often unsure of himself, because the process of adaptation and self-acceptance is a shifting one.

STAGES IN ADAPTATION TO ILLNESS

The transition from health to illness is a complex and highly individualized experience. The two main tasks to be faced by anyone with a developing condition are: (1) to modify his body image, his concept of himself, and his relation to people and work; and (2) to readjust to the realistic limitations and adaptations of the condition. These two tasks begin to take place within a setting in which the person is being treated for his physical disturbance.

In the cycle of health and illness, most people go through three stages: (1) the transition from health to illness, (2) the period of "accepted" illness, and (3) convalescence. The duration and quality of the experience an individual has in these stages vary with his personality, the specific disorder, and the changes made in his life.

FIRST STAGE. The development of symptoms usually is accompanied by unpleasant sensations, loss of vigor and stamina, and a decrease in ability to function. Certain symptoms such as chest pain, indigestion, or headache may increase in frequency and intensity. Anxiety is often present and the person handles it with his usual coping devices. To ward off the prospect of sickness, one person may plunge into activity, keeping late hours with extra work and social activities. Another may become passive and withdrawn, hoping that the vague symptoms will go away. A person may put off going to the doctor for fear of the diagnosis, which may be particularly threatening if a familiar disease such as cancer is suspected. Anxiety, guilt, shame, and denial are prominent during this initial period. If the symptoms persist, the person may be impelled to seek medical attention. He may have distinctly ambivalent feelings toward examinations and diagnostic tests, of which cancelled or missed appointments are often indices. Some patients go from doctor to doctor, hoping to find out "what is really the matter" or seeking evidence that a previous diagnosis was inaccurate.

If a person experiences a serious injury or a sudden catastrophe such as a heart attack or a cerebral vascular accident, he is instantly shifted from health to illness. His immediate concern is that help will not arrive in time, or that the strangers he is suddenly so dependent upon are not competent. If he is unconscious, his family may experience similar fears. This apprehension may be expressed through excessive demands, refusal to cooperate or accept the proposed treatment, and suspicion of the motives and methods of those trying to help. To offset this type of reaction, it is helpful to obtain information about close relatives and contact the person's own physician, if possible. Calm explanation of the necessary procedures and technical skill in carrying them out will convey to the patient that he is being cared for adequately.

When a patient is experiencing shock, disbelief, and denial of his condition, the nurse can help by listening to him. In a noncritical way, she does not support the denial but accepts the patient's need to cope with his situation in this way at the present time. She establishes herself as a helpful professional person who wants to understand the patient and his current dilemma. She orients him to his immediate environment and answers his questions.

SECOND STAGE. The second stage is a shift to the period of accepted illness. The patient recognizes and admits that he is sick and in need of help from others, specifically from the medical and nursing staff. Temporarily, he withdraws interest and concern from his usual adult responsibilities and applies himself to the task of getting well. He becomes preoccupied with himself, his symptoms, and treatment. Interest in current events and even concern about family and friends may be quite limited. The patient becomes self-centered, and shows increased dependency and preoccupation with somatic concerns. His behavior is often described as regressive, since it represents a return to earlier forms of acting, feeling, and participating with others. A certain amount of regression is considered necessary, so that the person can allow himself to rest in bed, eat a specified diet, and just let his body heal. People who normally resist being dependent may find this very difficult. They may be so frightened

that they continue to deny their condition in part or refuse to follow prescribed treatment. They push themselves beyond their physical limits and leave treatment before it is indicated. Other dependency problems evolve when a person receives so much gratification from this state that he attempts to continue it indefinitely; the term "hospitalitis" refers to this situation.

Nursing students are often concerned that the patient will become too dependent on them. There must be a realistic evaluation of the stage of illness, the patient's needs for dependency, and his need for a trusting, caring person. Nurses who care for the same patients over a long period of time should evaluate their own needs for dependency and for having people dependent on them. The nurse can help a patient to move through the stages of illness.

During the stage of accepted illness, the patient may express anger, guilt, and resentment. He may be very critical of his care and medical management, attacking the very people on whom he so depends. The most helpful nursing approach is to view this reaction as the patient's way of dealing with his situation and to try to understand how he feels. The nurse should encourage the patient to express his feelings, without passing judgment, moralizing, or arguing. She assumes responsibility for his care, but should be alert to individual differences and provide opportunities for him to make decisions and assume responsibility whenever indicated. As the patient becomes more assured of the nurse's availability, interest, and competence, he is less anxious and more willing to relinquish his dependence on her. During this period, the patient may be experiencing an acute sense of loss, of which the clinical picture is often depression with sadness, hopelessness, and anger. He may be mourning the loss of his state of health and vigor, the loss of a body part or function, or the changes in his job or family. He may be mourning his own death in advance.

THIRD STAGE. The third stage in adaptation is called the convalescent period or the period of restitution. The return of health and physical strength often precedes the patient's feeling and acting "well." Just as a lag usually occurs in the initial stage between the appearance of physical symptoms and the emotional acceptance of illness, a reverse lag occurs at the other end. Getting well implies giving up a dependent, regressive position and resuming adult responsibilities and normal relations with others. Although some people are reluctant to give up the patient role, most are motivated toward health but are afraid or hesitant to try out new skills. This is particularly true if the illness and treatment require major changes in work and family relations. The nurse can help the patient in this stage by assuming a role analogous to that of an adequate parent of a teenager. The nurse gradually relaxes protection and offers guidance, advice, and encouragement to progress. She quietly retires to the sidelines, ready to reassure the patient but encouraging him to experiment with new skills; she steps in only when gross errors in judgment occur. The patient senses the confidence of the nurse and is reassured by it, especially when ideal or perfect results are not expected.

During this stage the nurse can stimulate the patient to renew his interest in the world, to communicate better with his family, and to make plans for the future. For example, groups of people with similar conditions, such as colostomies or laryngectomies, have formed clubs in the local community. These club members may be called upon to talk to the patient both pre- and postoperatively in order to convey hope and to give realistic, firsthand information on coping with their common disability. At first, the patient may be overwhelmed by anxiety or grief and unable to use this service to full advantage. As he recovers, he may be reminded and encouraged to avail himself of this help. It is important, however, to keep in mind individual differences, since some people prefer not to affiliate themselves with a group of this type. The connotation of being "different," of having a stigmatizing condition, may be too painful to accept.

The stages of transition from health to illness and back to health are most clearly defined when a person has an acute, discrete condition that responds favorably to treatment. A similar series of steps takes place in adapting to a chronic condition, as identified by Crate. She describes the stages as disbelief, developing awareness, reorganization, resolution, and identity changes. In a successful adaptation to a chronic illness, the person can comfortably or resignedly regard himself as having a specific condition. He acknowledges and copes with the necessary changes in his life imposed by the condition. Although he may have gone through periods of despair, anger, and self-depreciation, he is able to regard himself as a worthwhile person who happens to be dependent. The nurse needs to be aware of the changes in feelings during the adaptation, to recognize deviations from the usual patterns, and to help the patient move forward through the process. Adaptation to chronic illness is a lengthy and continuous process. The extent of adaptation required depends on the type of illness, the degree of disability, and the patient's unique personality. Some chronic illnesses are relatively stable, with few changes; others have acute remissions and slow degeneration; others are terminal. Throughout, the nurse is in a position to provide skilled nursing care along with compassion, concern, and intelligent approaches to help guide the patient and his family in their struggle.

ANGER AND HOSTILITY

In addition to anxiety, expressions of anger are common in nursing situations. Conflict and frustration often precipitate aggression, a complex reaction of feelings and behavior that varies in intensity, duration, and expression. Words such as "irritated," "sullen," "unfriendly," "hostile," "assertive," "belligerent," "defiant," "uncooperative," "resentful," "enraged," "furious," and "indignant" describe various forms of aggressiveness. Anger, the general term for this emotion, is one way of handling anxiety, particularly in response to real or perceived threat, insult, or injury. To be a patient means to be sick, helpless, controlled by others, and assaulted—however therapeutically—by needles, catheters, enemas, and surgical procedures. Being told to wait for medication angers many patients who are in pain. Being awakened in the middle of the night to cough and take deep breaths taxes anyone's patience. Hospital rules such as lights out and restrictions on visitors may arouse feelings of anger. When a patient is new to the hospital or clinic, he is often uncertain and anxious about his diagnosis, treatment, and prognosis; as a defense he may flare up at the nurse or withdraw in sullen noncommunicativeness. Expressions of anger may decrease markedly as the element of the unknown is reduced and the patient becomes more familiar with his surroundings, the personnel, and the treatment program. On the other hand, anger may increase if the threat grows and the patient's needs are not met adequately.

A person who has been angry, unhappy, and chronically dissatisfied with himself and others brings this behavior with him to the clinical setting. He may be argumentative, demanding, unappreciative, sarcastic and unwilling to go along with nursing care. Extreme overfriendliness, ingratiation, and refusal to make any decision concerning one's care are also expressions of aggression. Occasionally, a patient is aggressive to the point of violence—throwing his dinner tray, shouting, cursing, doing or threatening to do physical harm. Nonverbal expressions of anger—glaring eyes, clenched fist, a sneer—can be nearly as eloquent.

The usual social responses to anger are counterattack, withdrawal or avoidance of the situation. A nurse's initial reaction to an angry patient is to treat him as she would in social circumstances. Many times this is not appropriate from the therapeutic standpoint. The professional nursing responsibility is to try to help this person even with and in spite of his anger. The nurse does this by first recognizing her own responses to angry behavior. It is not unusual for a nurse to experience feelings of irritation and annoyance. She may be frightened, embarrassed, and hurt. When a patient lashes out at her verbally, she may feel inadequate and guilty even if she has acted appropriately. She may feel helpless or immobilized to the extent that she dreads caring for the patient and begins to avoid him whenever possible. This kind of behavior may heighten the patient's frustration by leaving him isolated, helpless, and unable to depend on the nursing staff to meet his physical and emotional needs. Thus a vicious circle is established.

Aggressive behavior that is ascribable to a toxic condition is acceptable; the patient can be excused because he was delirious or "not in his right mind." The continuously hostile patient who is fully conscious and in control is much harder to understand and deal with. The expression of anger in the clinical situation may reflect the person's best manner of coping with threats that surround him. Anger may be an attempt to relieve feelings of helplessness and dependency. In other situations, anger may indicate part of the grief process or emergence from apathy and depression. A patient's anger may vanish when someone helps him to identify what is frustrating or threatening him and to take steps toward successfully dealing with the threat.

It is not unusual for people to displace feelings of anger—that is, to express them toward someone or something other than the original frustrator. When one believes oneself to be in a vulnerable position, it may not be safe to express dissatisfaction and anger directly. Therefore, one takes it out on somebody less likely to retaliate or less vitally important to one's emotional and physical well-being. A patient may be very angry with his physician but afraid to complain for fear that he will receive less attention. Instead, he bawls out the nurse and later insists that she contact his doctor. Or, the nurse and the doctor may have a covert misunderstanding; she finds herself snapping at the aides and being irritable with the patients. Generally, direct expressions of anger are not socially acceptable, and outbursts may be followed by guilt, shame, and profuse apologies. Moreover, there exist cultural and socioeconomic differences in the expression of anger, and the nurse may find herself bewildered, insulted, and overwhelmed by behavior considered normal and expected by another individual.

Therapeutic responses to angry patients are based on the attempt to understand the person and his situation. The nurse is aware of her own reaction to the patient and attempts to help him sort out the issues involved. She enables the patient to maintain his dignity, pride, and self-esteem. She sets limits on his behavior so that he does not hurt himself or others and helps him to find more appropriate means of expressing his feelings. Although she may feel angry or frightened in reaction to the behavior, she uses her feelings for further problem solving rather than giving way to retaliation or withdrawal. Helpful questions in arriving at a nursing care plan for patients who are angry and hostile include the following: When does the patient get angry and how does he show it? Does his anger interfere with his receiving the care he needs? Why does his behavior bother me? How do I react? Does he get angry with other people too? Is there someone who does get along with him? What does that person do that is different? Does the patient's hostility serve a useful purpose? How much of this behavior reflects his usual way of reacting to people? How much is

he willing to change? What realistic goals shall we work toward? Are there any other resources—doctor, family, psychiatric nursing consultant, psychiatrist, occupational therapist, or other patients—that we could call in? If the patient stops expressing anger, will he develop more destructive patterns?

Learning to work therapeutically with angry, hostile patients is a challenging and rewarding part of nursing. Patients who disguise temporary fear and shame with anger appreciate the nurse who stands by them in the crisis without condemnation, rejection, or retaliation. Patients who have made a lifelong adjustment by means of hostile attack are also grateful, although they may never express it directly, to the nurse who refuses to be alienated and who applies herself to understanding and caring for him.

BEHAVIOR MODIFICATION

People react to illness and hospitalization with many different kinds of behaviors, some of which are maladaptive and destructive. In such situations, the nurse can help the patient to adjust his behavior by means of *behavior modification,* which is the systematic application of learning theory in order to change undesired, disruptive, and maladaptive patterns of behavior.

Behavior that is learned and continued is behavior that is reinforced—rewarded. There is a system of rewards and punishments (even if not acknowledged) in all social systems, including the hospital. Patients bring their learned behavior patterns with them and react to the new interpersonal environment accordingly.

The patient's behavior may be regarded as maladaptive and destructive if he experiences incontinence for no obvious physiologic reason, creates eating disturbances, displays temper outbursts, refuses to participate in treatment, has crying jags, complains continually of pain problems, and makes incessant demands. Behavior modification may be of help with such patients, as well as with sick children, patients with chronic conditions, or those undergoing long-term hospitalization.

If the patient's behavior tags him as "difficult," the nurse should study him to identify (1) what constitutes his maladaptive behavior and how it interferes with his care, progress, and rehabilitation, (2) how and by whom his behavior is reinforced, and (3) how the environment, the sequence of behaviors, and their reinforcers can be changed so that the behavior changes. At the same time, the nurse should examine her own behavior to see if she is playing a part in continuing the unsatisfactory situation. Nursing behavior can influence a patient's behavior in either a positive or negative direction. Positive reinforcers include spending time with the patient, paying attention to him, smiling at him, showing interest in discussing certain subjects with him, providing food, granting privileges such as watching TV, staying up late, and going out on pass, giving backrubs, contacting the physician, and administering p.r.n. medications. Negative behavior may be triggered by frowning at the patient, failing to respond to him, and ignoring him.

GRIEF AND MOURNING

Grief is a complex of emotional responses to the anticipated or actual loss of someone or something valued. The loss may be that of a relative or friend, a part of the body, a job, health, or life. Feelings of anxiety, helplessness, hopelessness, guilt, anger, depression, remorse, sadness, and loneliness are part of grief. Mourning refers to the processes that follow the loss and ultimately result in overcoming the grief. There are many cultural factors involved in the specific way in which grief and mourning take place, from the extremes of stoic acceptance to elaborate and ritualistic weeping, keening, and public display.

The intensity of grief and mourning depends on the significance and extent of the loss to the person. It is generally greater if the loss, especially through death, comes suddenly. If the survivor has been particularly dependent upon the deceased person, or if in any way he was responsible for the death, grief is intensified. A person who is very sensitive to separation as a result of early separations may be deeply affected. Ambivalence (mixed feelings) is present in all significant relationships. If the ambivalence is marked, grief may be particularly intense. Guilt and irrational ideas about the causation of the death may prevent a person from facing himself and mourning effectively.

The stages of mourning are similar to the stages of adaptation to illness—shock and disbelief, awareness, and restitution. Upon recognition of a loss, people often experience a sinking feeling, tightness in the throat, loss of appetite, fatigue, tension, and acute anxiety. The sensorium is altered, and there is a feeling of unreality and distance from people. There is a preoccupation with the deceased or lost object and a state of readiness for its return. Feelings of guilt may be present, and there may be soul-searching and remorse about things that could have been done differently. The grieving person's relationships with other people lack warmth and are characterized by irritation and the desire not to be bothered. He is likely to slow up activities, neglect personal care, and be restlessly, purposelessly active. He may develop symptoms similar to those of the deceased one. Sometimes the shock of the loss is accepted intellectually and the person goes through the motions of making arrangements and caring for others. His emotional reaction is cut off in his attempt to protect himself from the pain of the loss.

In the stage of developing awareness, the person experiences pain, anguish, emptiness, and acute sadness. Crying or the desire to cry is common and often elicits support from others. Many people cannot allow themselves to cry in public and need privacy to handle their grief.

In the stage of restitution, the physical reality of the loss is emphasized. In the case of death, the funeral makes this fact unavoidable. In the case of an amputation, the sight of the stump and the first attempt of using a prosthesis underline the reality. The mourner begins a long process of coping with the absence of the loved person or object. There may be repetitive talk about the person or object and there is a tendency to idealize them, so that only pleasant memories are reinforced. Gradually, this assists in the task of achieving emotional detachment. As dependence on the lost object decreases, the person begins to develop new interests and invests his energy in other people. He is able to remember the relationship more realistically, with its good and bad aspects, and can talk about it without emotional dependence on the memory of the relationship.

Nursing intervention to help patients handle their feelings with the experience of grief and mourning includes anticipating reactions to loss, supporting the patient's usual coping mechanisms, and allowing the patient to express feelings when he wishes. The nurse provides privacy and availability when needed. When a body part or function is lost, the nurse designs specific nursing care and manipulates the environment to prevent additional loss of self-esteem. To maintain resources and give complete care, the nurse includes the family in the plan of care. The presence and willingness of the nurse to participate in the painful experiences that accompany grief help to prevent feelings of total abandonment. By being aware of the usual patterns of grief and mourning, the nurse is able to recognize maladaptive patterns and help evaluate the need for other types of therapeutic intervention, such as psychotherapy.

DENIAL

A common response to a shift in health status is denial. When symptoms of illness threaten a person, he may avoid facing his fear of them by unconsciously denying their existence or their significance. Denial is an ego-defense mechanism that protects the person from recognizing painful and disturbing aspects of reality. It serves to diminish anxiety. However, an increase in the number and intensity of symptoms may force a person to abandon the denial.

Denial may possibly underlie the behavior of patients who do not follow treatment regimens and who miss appointments or transfer to another doctor. Inappropriate cheerfulness or lack of concern about symptoms of the illness may indicate denial. If anxiety, depression, and anger are not expressed in situations in which they could be expected, the patient may be protecting himself by denial. The ignoring of certain aspects of reality may indicate denial, as in the case of a coronary patient who experiences substernal pain and attributes it to indigestion. Obese patients who explain their trouble as "glandular" and deviate from their reducing diets also demonstrate this behavior. Denial may prevent a person from seeking help or it may interfere with his treatment program. However, it is also a means of maintaining psychological equilibrium. When the stress and anxiety decrease, so does the need for denial. Denial mechanisms may be operating in members of the patient's family as they try to protect themselves from recognizing the severity of the condition. Even when the possibility of imminent death is discussed, the family may deny that this is possible and act (or fail to act) accordingly.

In dealing with denial of illness as a nursing problem, the nurse assesses the extent to which the denial is harmful and in which ways it is beneficial. The necessary nursing judgments and intervention can then be based on this assessment. Generally, the defense of denial is not challenged directly, because such an action tends to reinforce the denial or leaves the person without adequate ego protection. The nurse does not support or encourage the denial. The nurse is available so that when the patient is able to relinquish his denial, he can be helped to cope with the onset of reality. Sometimes a person appears to use denial defenses, although he is consciously acting in such a manner in order to protect the feelings of his family. This may happen when the patient is aware that he will die soon but perceives that his family would be more comfortable if he continued the mutual deception. If the nurse conveys interest in and concern for this patient, he may choose to talk about his feelings, thus lessening his isolation.

Denial is a coping mechanism that nurses use to handle their own painful feelings about illness, radical surgery, and death. A nurse may find this defense necessary in order to continue functioning in some areas over a long period of time. If the nurse can talk about these feelings with other nurses and develop more realistic ways of dealing with the stresses, she may be better equipped to help patients cope with their use of denial.

PSYCHOSOMATIC INTERACTIONS

Knowledge about the relationship between emotions and physical reactions is increasing. This is a highly complex and little understood matter that the mass media have simplified to the point where the terms "psychosomatic," "neurotic," "imaginary," "faking," "malingering," "pyschogenic," and "somatopsychic" are used loosely and produce much confusion.

Anxiety is experienced as both emotional and physiologic reactions. Many people seek treatment for symptoms that are due to chronic, continued anxiety. The anxiety may represent a reaction to reality factors in the present, such as a job or a marriage, or to long-standing conflicts over sexuality, dependency, aggression, and other factors.

Anxiety reactions in which the symptoms center around one organ system are described in the nomenclature as *psychophysiologic reactions* having autonomic and visceral responses (e.g., "psychophysiologic reaction, cardiovascular," if the symptoms are predominantly cardiac in nature). Any organ system can be affected. When actual structural changes do occur, the condition is described as a *psychosomatic illness* that has resulted from a combination of emotional and physiologic factors. Common conditions that are generally considered to involve psychosomatic factors are: peptic ulcer, chronic ulcerative colitis, hyperthyroidism, bronchial asthma, essential hypertension, and neurodermatitis. The frequency and severity of these illnesses point to the need for greater understanding of the relationship between mind and body.

Another manifestation of underlying emotional conflict that expresses itself in physical symptoms is *hypochondriasis*. A hypochondriacal patient may be totally absorbed in his body and its functioning, and presents endless complaints and reports. A person uses this means in attempting to meet long-standing dependency needs. The nurse must evaluate her reactions to such a patient's complaints and demands. Frustration and anger are common responses to this type of patient. The hardworking nurse often resents someone who avoids adult responsibility so easily. Expressing this anger directly to the patient is not helpful, since he is struggling to maintain some kind of equilibrium. Not recognizing her own anger could result in the nurse's avoiding the patient and not caring for his realistic needs. If the nurse goes overboard and attempts to meet all of the patient's unsatisfied dependency needs, she soon finds that the patient is insatiable—a bottomless pit. Finding a reasonable middle ground is a challenge in working with these patients. Very little is known about successful nursing approaches to hypochondriacal patients. Excessive preoccupation with one's body, accompanied by unusual ideation, may be a sign of more severe emotional disorders, such as psychotic depression or schizophrenia. Through proper assessment of needs and evaluation of behavior, the nurse may help plan for more appropriate treatment.

Another group of physical reactions that have an emotional basis are *conversion reactions*. Conversion is an ego defense mechanism in which anxiety is eliminated or reduced by the production of a physical symptom. This symptom may be directly related to the emotional conflict; the hand that would strike out is paralyzed; the eyes that would look at the forbidden become blind. In most instances the conflict and the symbolic meaning of the symptom are complex, disguised, and difficult to unravel. These patients come into a medical-surgical setting for differential diagnosis. A conversion reaction may possibly develop after an organic illness has occurred, which tends to prolong the secondary gains of dependency and security.

Generally, the symptoms of conversion reactions simulate disturbances in the voluntary nervous system or in the organs of the special senses. Disturbances of sensation and motion are the most common. Sensation changes include anesthesia, paresthesia, and pain. Loss of hearing and sight are much more common than loss of the other special senses. Disturbances of motion include paralysis, usually of the limbs or speech mechanism, and uncontrolled movements such as tics and nonorganic convulsions. If the symptom is diagnosed as a conversion reaction, the treatment is generally best directed by a psychiatrist. The nurse can help greatly by accurately observing the patient's behavior, including his reaction to other people. She must keep in mind that symptom formation in a person with a conversion reaction occurs on an unconscious level—the patient is not faking, nor are his symptoms imaginary. This is his way of coping with situations at the present time; with professional help he may be able to find more adequate ways of doing so.

Disturbances in orientation occur frequently in patients on medical-surgical services. Acute brain syndrome, which may be a reaction to anesthesia, infection, surgical or metabolic disturbances, overdose of drugs or alcohol, or assault of the brain as in head injury, often produce delirium. *Delirium* is a state of altered consciousness or awareness manifested by disorientation and confusion. It is induced by interference with the metabolic processes of the brain and is generally acute in onset and reversible. The first signs are restlessness, anxiety, and suspicion, which quickly mount to agitation, excitement, and confusion. The patient often begins to hallucinate and experience delusions. These distortions of reality are extremely frightening, and the desperate behavior of the person experiencing them necessitates skilled nursing action. Patients recovering from cardiac surgery, in particular, often become delirious. It is necessary to reduce the terror and extreme anxiety of these patients not only for emotional reasons, but also to prevent overloading the body with more stress.

Nursing care for a delirious patient includes continual reorientation, a calm voice, and adequate lighting through the night. If possible, the same nurses should attend the patient much of the time, since they repeatedly demonstrate by familiar words and action that he is safe and cared for. It often helps to tell the patient that you know he is very frightened, but that the things he is experiencing are a reaction to his illness that will go away. Hallucinations caused by organic processes are often vivid and threatening. Along with visual hallucinations, the patient may experience tactile hallucinations in which he feels he is being touched or bugs are crawling on him.

Acute brain syndrome is treated by alleviating the causative agents, and the nurse must be aware that proper hydration, nutrition, and medication are directed toward this end. Restraints may be necessary to keep the patient in bed, but they may also frighten and irritate him. The nurse must be aware of his distortion of reality and poor judgment in order to protect him from injuring himself or others. Patients have walked out of unprotected windows while delirious.

Following an episode of delirium, a person may experience anxiety and shame over his behavior when not in full control. He may fear that he has acted inappropriately, hurt someone, or said vulgar or obscene things. He may be afraid of having told confidences and secrets about himself. If the patient gives evidence of such concern, the nurse can encourage him to talk about his fears and then reassure him that his behavior was understandable in the situation and that his confidence will not be betrayed. This is a potentially shameful situation in which the rights, dignity, and privacy of the patient must be protected.

Chronic brain syndrome may result from damage to brain tissue sustained by the causes of acute brain syndrome, or from long-term infections such as syphilis, heavy mental intoxication, circulatory disturbances such as cerebral arteriosclerosis, convulsive disorders, disturbances of growth, metabolism, or nutrition, intracranial neoplasm, prenatal factors, and diseases of unknown etiology such as multiple sclerosis. The behavior common to people with these conditions is described as *dementia,* and it represents chronic, irreversible brain damage with deterioration of intellectual capacities due to structural changes. Both delirium and dementia are characterized by loss of abilities—defects in memory, orientation (of time, place, and person), and judgment. In planning nursing care and long-term treatment, the individual's strengths must be evaluated along with his limitations. Environmental manipulation and simplification may help him to live his life to the fullest.

DYING AND DEATH

To give maximal help to the dying patient and his family, nurses need to examine their own feelings about death and to understand better the reactions of other people toward death. Each person dies in his individual style, just as he lives in his own style. One of the major problems in understanding death is that, in our culture, it has been a taboo topic. Death is a strange and foreign experience to most people, even more so now that many people die in hospitals and nursing homes rather than in their own homes. Many nursing students come into contact with death for the first time in their medical-surgical clinical experience.

For most people, even the thought of death is frightening, and when one is in robust health, it seems almost impossible. Regardless of one's religious beliefs, it is difficult to imagine oneself as no longer existing in the world. Nurses are deeply committed to life and health. The dying patient is in direct opposition to that commitment. Sometimes the medical and nursing staff react to a dying patient as if their failure of skill or care is responsible for the impending death. It helps to realize that, although nothing can be done to reverse the ultimate process, the dying person can be helped in his last human contacts.

It is generally accepted that it is the physician's responsibility to decide what information to give the patient about his diagnosis and prognosis. It is important that the physician and nurse share information that will help determine what is most beneficial for the patient. The nurse, through observations and interactions, can assess the patient's and the family's understanding of the disease and their intellectual and emotional patterns, including their coping abilities. The nurse is then more sensitive to the verbal and nonverbal cues of the patient and his family and can determine how to help them most in this time of great need. An understanding of the emotional reactions of the patient facing death is important for the nurse.

Stages of Dying

People face death in many ways. According to studies done by Kübler-Ross, the emotional responses of a person facing death can be traced through five stages: denial and isolation, anger, bargaining, depression, and acceptance. These five stages do not always occur in sequence. They may be mixed or they may be experienced as overlapping phases. At times a patient seems to move back and forth through the stages.

DENIAL AND ISOLATION. Recognition and acceptance of the fact that death is to be faced shortly is difficult; the common reaction is to insulate oneself until other defenses are marshalled. Denial permits hope to exist. Often the patient may be ready to accept the fact that he is going to die but his family continues to express denial. This in turn delays the time when the patient can communicate his concerns. Denial and isolation are short-lived because the patient begins to think about unfinished business; there are personal affairs to be straightened out, children to consider, and financial arrangements to be made.

ANGER. The next emotional expression is anger. "Why me?" is the question put forth. It does not require an answer, but the patient is helped if the nurse is present to offer support and to listen. Behavior of the patient during this stage is difficult because nothing that is done for him seems to please him. The nurse can expect this expression of anger and, rather than take it personally, should try to determine what is causing it. The patient must be allowed to express his anger, his sense of helplessness, and his outrage, for when his feelings have been vented, he will be able to move more rapidly into the stage of bargaining.

BARGAINING. Bargaining is a phase of coping during which the dying person attempts to negotiate a trade. Usually it involves a deal with God, the physician, or the nurse. "If I can live long enough to attend my son's wedding, I'll be ready to die." If at all possible the patient should be granted his request.

DEPRESSION. The fourth stage is depression; at this time the full impact of the inevitable is apparent to the patient. His defense mechanisms are no longer effective and his sadness and anguish are expressed. By crying he also elicits the support of loved ones or the nurse. The resolution of this phase leads quietly into the last stages of acceptance.

ACCEPTANCE. This is a time of peace and contentment. The patient seems to be desirous of time alone with his thoughts. Quiet visiting with minimal verbalization is most supportive. It appears to be a time for the patient to review his past and contemplate the unknown future.

Summary

Although an underlying principle in all areas of nursing is that the person is an individual who should be treated with respect and dignity, studies have shown that the social value placed upon a person determines how he is treated when dying. Such factors as age, color, socioeconomic status, attractiveness, and former accomplishments greatly affect a patient's treatment, and thus the intensity of his experience of abandonment, isolation, and loneliness while he is dying. Many times, the nurse caring for the dying patient becomes his most important link with life. The nurse is the one who can make him as physically comfortable as possible, and also is in a privileged position to help him and his family with one of the most difficult and painful parts of life—leaving it. The nurse stays with him to the end and tries to comfort the family left behind.

It is an emotional strain to attend people who are dying. Nurses assigned to areas in which death frequently occurs must be able to share their feelings and reactions with each other. It is also desirable that these nurses move periodically to other wards in which the recovery rate is high, in order to recharge their hope.

BIBLIOGRAPHY

BOOKS

Aguilera, D. C., and Messick, J. M.: Crisis Intervention: Theory and Methodology, 3rd ed. St. Louis, C. V. Mosby, 1978.

Barton, D., ed.: Dying and Death, a Clinical Guide for Caregivers. Baltimore, Williams and Wilkins, 1977.

Carlson, C. E., ed.: Behavioral Concepts and Nursing Interventions. Phila., W. B. Saunders, 1978.

Epstein C.: Nursing the Dying Patient: Learning Processes for Interaction. Reston, Va., Reston Pub. Co., 1975.

Kübler-Ross, E.: On Death and Dying. New York, Macmillan, 1969.

Garfield, C. A.: Pyschosocial Care of the Dying Patient. New York, McGraw-Hill, 1978.

Howard, J., and Strauss, A.: Humanizing Health Care. New York, John Wiley and Sons, 1975.

Lipp, M. R.: Respectful Treatment: The Human Side of Medical Care. Hagerstown, Md., Harper and Row, 1977.

Lowery, B.: Some psychological concepts of health-related behavior. *In* Kintzel, K. C., ed.: Advanced Concepts in Clinical Nursing, 2nd ed. Philadelphia, J. B. Lippincott, 1977, Chap. 3, pp. 37-53.

Robinson, L.: Liaison Nursing, Psychological Approach to Total Care. Philadelphia, F. A. Davis, 1974.

Schwartz, L. H., and Schwartz, J. L.: The Psychodynamics of Patient Care. Englewood Cliffs, N. J., Prentice-Hall, 1972.

Sell, I. L.: Dying and Death, an Annotated Bibliography. New York, Tiresias Press, 1977.

Strain, S.: Psychological Care of the Medically Ill. New York, Appleton-Century-Crofts, 1975.

ARTICLES

Bandman, E. L., and Bandman, B.: The nurse's role in protecting the patient's right to live or die. Adv. in Nurs. Sci., 1:21-35, Apr. 1979.

Boyajian, A.: Fighting despair. AJN, 78:76-77, Jan. 1978.

Carper, B. A.: The ethics of caring. Adv. in Nurs. Sci., 1:11-19, Apr. 1979.

Curtin, L. L.: The nurse as advocate: A philosophical foundation for nursing. Adv. in Nurs. Sci, 1:1-10, Apr. 1979.

Forsyth, G. L.: Exploration of empathy in nurse-client interaction. Adv. in Nurs. Sci., 1:53-61, Jan. 1979.

Frain, M., and Valiga, T. M.: The multiple dimensions of stress. Topics in Clin. Nurs., 1:43-52, Apr. 1979.

Hazzard, M. E., and Thorndal, M. L.: Patient anxiety: Teaching students to intervene effectively. Nurse Educator, 4:19-21, Jan.-Feb. 1979.

Jean Johnson researches stress reduction. AJN, 78:128-129, Jan. 1978.

Lemandri, B. J., and Boyle, D. W.: Instilling hope. AJN, 78:79-80, Jan. 1978.

Moritz, D. A.: Understanding anger. AJN, 78:81-83, Jan. 1978.

Programmed Instruction: Helping Depressed Patients in General Nursing Practice. AJN, 77:P.I. 1-32, June 1977.

Shaw, S. E.: Health education for the public: Stress and stress management. Topics in Clin. Nurs., 1:53-57, Apr. 1979.

Shubin, S.: R_x for stress — your stress. Nursing '79, 9:52-55, Jan. 1979.

Snyder, J. C., and Wilson, M. F.: Elements of psychological assessment. AJN, 77:235-239, Feb. 1977.

Sutterly, D. C.: Stress and health: A survey of self-regulation modalities. Topics in Clin. Nurs., 1:1-21, Apr. 1979.

Swanson, D. W., et al.: Results of behavior modification in the treatment of chronic pain. Psychosomat. Med., 41:55-61, Feb. 1979.

Concepts and Challenges in Patient Management

UNIT FOUR

12

PRINCIPLES
AND PRACTICES
OF REHABILITATION

PHILOSOPHY OF REHABILITATION

It is never how high one rises that determines one's merit, but rather how far one has come, considering his difficulties.
— ARCHIBALD RUTLEDGE

Rehabilitation is a dynamic, active program which enables an ill and disabled person to achieve his greatest possible level of physical, psychological, mental, social, and economic efficiency. How close he comes to achieving this goal determines the degree to which he becomes a socially and economically independent member of society. Rehabilitation has been called the third phase of medicine, the first being prevention, the second diagnosis and treatment, the third convalescence and rehabilitation. Modern rehabilitation is a process whereby a patient adjusts to a handicap by learning how to integrate all of his resources and to concentrate more on existing abilities than on the permanent disabilities with which he must live. Genuine adjustment is in great part an inner process, because it involves reorientation of the patient's values.

The first comprehensive program in rehabilitation was started in 1947 at the Bellevue Hospital in New York City by Dr. Howard Rusk. Since then, programs have been developed in most medical centers. Many health facilities have elaborate departments; however, a successful program can be carried out even in a small hospital and with a minimum of personnel and equipment. A positive point of view plus dedication, patience, and willingness to move through the many stages from inactivity to activity must be demonstrated by the patient and all those who work with him in achieving this goal.

Rehabilitation concerns not only the individual; it also concerns the nation. Early in 1962 the Department of Health, Education and Welfare launched a new approach in public welfare that stressed "services instead of support, rehabilitation instead of relief." The promotion of rehabilitation services and the family-centered approach are receiving particular emphasis. The Social and Rehabilitation Service (SRS) created in 1967 within the Department of Health, Education and Welfare combines the programs of Welfare Administration, the Vocational Rehabilitation Administration, the Medicaid program and the Mental Retardation Division of the Public Health Service.

The federal funds to support state agency services can provide up to 80 percent of the costs, thereby offering an incentive to the individual states to provide more rehabilitation services for the handicapped. The economic advantage of such an emphasis is readily apparent; instead of an individual receiving welfare aid, there is a person who will be rehabilitated into employment. Instead of being dependent on society, he will contribute to it. The effect on the individual is to change him from a hopeless dependent to an active, self-sufficient citizen. But it is even more important that the person is helped to develop a satisfying way of life that preserves the uniqueness of his individuality. He gains inner strength from his own resources that makes it possible for him to partake of the joys and meet the problems of life in a meaningful way.

The trend in rehabilitation is to include not only the physically, mentally, and emotionally handicapped, (including those suffering from cancer), but also to take in the aged and those who are disadvantaged from problems of poverty or social deprivation.

In the hospital setting, the patient and his problems are evaluated and a program is set up to enable him to achieve self-sufficiency up to the level of his capabilities and desires. His abilities are stressed, rather than his disabilities. Since each patient has a different level of capability, the program is individualized. The ultimate goal is to obtain optimal function in his daily routine—i.e., the activities of daily living. Rehabilitation goals must be realistic, taking into consideration the patient's ability (the most important factor) and then his disability. Through such a program the patient is motivated and helped to attain social interdependence and greater economic security.

THE REHABILITATION TEAM

Rehabilitation is a creative process that requires a team of people working together and contributing specialized services. The team members represent a variety of disciplines, each health professional making a unique contribution. They meet in group sessions at frequent intervals to evaluate the patient's progress and make the necessary program changes.

The *rehabilitation nurse* is responsible for developing a patient care plan directed toward defined patient goals and for coordinating the actions of other team members toward these goals. Additional goals include the prevention of complications and the restoration and maintenance of optimal physical and psychosocial health. The nurse establishes a sustained and supporting relationship with the patient and applies nursing assessment and intervention in skin care, positioning, transfer techniques, bladder and bowel management, nutrition, psychosocial support, and patient education. In accordance with the ANA Standards of Rehabilitation Nursing Practice, the functions of rehabilitation nursing may be listed as follows:

- Collecting data on the health status of the patient
- Developing a nursing diagnosis (identifying the problems, limitations, and methods of adaptation to health problems)
- Developing goals for nursing care (the end state toward which nursing action is directed)
- Prescribing action to meet the goals (priority setting, alternative interventions, etc.)
- Implementing the nursing care plan
- Evaluating the nursing care plan in terms of stated goals
- Reassessing and reordering priorities and setting new goals; revising the plan of care*

*Adapted from the American Nurses' Association Division of Medical-Surgical Nursing Practice and the Association of Rehabilitation Nurses: Standards of Rehabilitation Nursing Practice. Kansas City, ANA, 1977.

The *physician* has the responsibility of making the diagnosis so that therapy can be directed toward realistic goals; part of this responsibility includes directing the patient's therapeutic program.

The *physiatrist* is a physician-specialist in physical medicine and rehabilitation with responsibility for testing the patient's physical functioning, determining the potential functional goal, and supervising the rehabilitation program.

The *physical therapist* teaches and supervises the patient through a prescribed exercise program designed to strengthen weak muscles and prevent deformities. The physical therapist also teaches new ways of locomotion, transportation, and daily activities.

The *psychologist* assesses the patient's motivation, values, and attitudes toward the disability and also works with the family to help them cope with the problems that have arisen as a result of the patient's condition.

The *occupational therapist* develops skills to assist the patient in adapting to home and work situations. Practical projects are devised to improve the patient's coordination and maintain his interest.

The *social worker* investigates the patient's background and socioeconomic status and assists the patient and his family in adjusting to the home and social environment.

The *vocational counselor* tests the patient to determine his interests and aptitudes so that vocational training can be instituted. He also helps plan job modifications and advises the patient of employment opportunities.

The *rehabilitation engineer* uses technology in designing and constructing devices that help severely and multiply-handicapped persons to function despite their disabilities.

The importance of rehabilitation is often underestimated. Approximately 14 percent of the population of the United States have some limitation of activity. Many older people (whose numbers are increasing) have disabling conditions requiring rehabilitation services. Every patient, regardless of his problem or diagnosis, has the right to rehabilitation services. Thus, rehabilitation is a large and growing area of nursing responsibility.

Rehabilitation is an integral part of nursing and *should begin with the initial contact with the patient*. Every major illness carries with it the threat of disability. If the patient is hospitalized with a burn and develops a contracture deformity, his recovery time will be greatly delayed. Disabilities are not static but tend to become worse, and some complications of inactivity can give the patient more pain and discomfort than the initial injury or disease.

Though not all hospitals have departments of physical medicine and rehabilitation, *the principles of rehabilitation are basic to the care of all patients,* and the pages that follow point out how the nurse applies them. Other aspects of rehabilitation are discussed under the appropriate clinical conditions throughout the book.

PSYCHOLOGICAL IMPLICATIONS OF A DISABILITY

A physical disability often has a deep psychological significance to the patient. It has a direct impact on the patient's body image and can cause a state of conflict. Physically, a part of his body has deteriorated. He may have the shattering realization that he can do less than he did formerly. His shape and posture may have changed, as may his state of mind. Even his position in society may be altered, as well as his social interaction with others. He perceives himself as a second-class citizen, a devalued person. In short, he feels that he is different.

Disability may mean hardship or even tragedy to the individual, depending on his occupation, cultural background, and social status, and on the support he receives from or provides for his family.

A person usually goes through a series of emotional reactions to a newly acquired disability. The first reaction may be confusion, disorganization, and denial. The patient is in a state of conflict and has to cope with problems of forced dependence, loss of self-esteem, and feelings that his personal and family integrity are threatened. The patient may refuse to accept his new limitations and at times has an unjustified overconfidence in speedy recovery. His false hopes lead him to hear only what he wants to hear. He is likely to be self-centered and even childlike in his demands. The mechanism of denial may be useful up to a certain point, but eventually the reality of the situation must be accepted.

The patient may progress to a stage of depression and grief in which he appears to mourn for his lost function or missing body part. (Depression may also be caused by sensory deprivation and restricted environmental stimulation.) There may be behavioral changes, particularly regression. This stage of grief appears to be a necessary phase in adapting to the disability. Mourning is part of the process of working through all the meanings of the loss. Therefore, the patient should not merely be encouraged blithely to "cheer up." Such an approach can evoke extreme hostility and provoke behavior which will result in a "problem patient." The nurse, simply because of her understanding and her ready-to-act presence, can transmit a feeling of caring.

Following the stage of depression and grief, there is generally a period of adaptation and adjustment. In time, the patient becomes more familiar with his condition and is able to tolerate it better. As he revises his body image and modifies his former picture of himself, he redirects his energies toward coping with his physical functioning.

He is able to accept a degree of dependency and not resent being "waited upon." He begins to realize that hopelessness is futile and knows that he must adapt to the permanent aspects of the disability while relentlessly pursuing victory over temporary weaknesses.

The acceptance of the limitations imposed by the disability and the total investment of the patient in his rehabilitation program is basic to adjustment. It is from this point in rehabilitation that the patient begins to look ahead and to develop realistic goals for his future.

At the same time it is important to realize that not every patient will progress in orderly fashion through the stages of grieving. Many frequently fluctuate between acceptance and grief, so that angry outbursts and depression may continue long after the usual period of mourning has supposedly passed. Each new situation (going home, starting vocational rehabilitation, entering a new relationship) reminds the patient anew of his limitations, of his changed body image and the reality of the permanence of his situation. Thus, even though the disabled person makes progress and increases his independence, he must continually deal with the grief process and the need to grow throughout his life.

At the other end of the spectrum are those patients who do not accept their disability but instead waste emotional energy in rebelling futilely against unalterable damage. Or, there are those patients who ignore the disability and refuse to put forth any effort to adapt for everyday life. Still others may overreact and build a false reputation for being "cheerful and courageous." Although "ignoring" may seem healthy, often it includes a total rejection of the disability, which keeps the patient from doing the small things that will be helpful to him. These patients may require assistance from either a psychologist or a psychiatrist.

In general, the nurse's responsibility is to assess the patient's reaction to his disability and work with him, always emphasizing his assets, and at the same time listening to him, encouraging him, and sharing in his satisfactions and triumphs as he progresses in his program. It is through the support and inspiration of the members of the rehabilitation team that the patient becomes all that he is capable of being.

SEXUALITY AND THE DISABLED

There is a growing recognition of the sexual concerns and problems of the handicapped. This involves not only sexual activity per se but also the individual's concept of his masculinity or her femininity and the way he or she reacts to others and is perceived by them. Sexual matters are considered to be in the very private realm, and the patient is apt to be reticent about discussing his feelings. The professional person is focusing so intently on the rehabilitation of the patient, i.e., helping him to gain independence, that there is a tendency to forget that sexuality is part of the patient's personality. Recognizing and dealing with sexual concerns is basic in establishing feelings of self-worth, which are so essential to total rehabilitation. Professional personnel, family members, and the community must deal with the reality that handicapped persons are sexual beings.

The relationships of the handicapped individual concerning love, sex, marriage, and reproduction must be based on the capacity of the individual and the couple to give and receive love and to share intimacies and satisfaction. The reader is referred to the bibliography at the end of the chapter for additional reading on this subject.

PRINCIPLES AND PRACTICES OF REHABILITATION NURSING

The most common complications that threaten a patient with a prolonged illness or disability are contractures, pressure sores, and bladder and bowel problems.

Contractures result when muscles are not used or put through their full range of motion. The contracture is actually a shortening of the muscle which leads to deformity. These deformities may be prevented if the causal conditions are understood properly and preventive measures are instituted early.

When tissues do not receive adequate nourishment, circulation, and exercise, they tend to deteriorate and to atrophy. Initiating deliberate and proper measures can combat and prevent tissue damage and pressure sores.

Bladder and bowel difficulties may result from disease, injury, or shock. In many patients, refunctioning can be accomplished through individualized teaching and persistent attention to the establishment of regular function.

The major responsibilities of the nurse in rehabilitation are: (1) to prevent deformities and complications, (2) to motivate, to teach, and to support the patient (and his family when necessary) during the daily activities of living which include self-care, and (3) to refer the patient for proper follow-up care and supervision. Each of these categories will now be discussed in detail.

PREVENTION OF DEFORMITIES AND COMPLICATIONS

Deformities and complications of illness or injury often can be prevented by proper positioning in bed, frequent changes of position, passive mobilization (range of motion exercises), and active exercise.

POSITIONING

Unless contraindicated, the patient should be turned frequently. The reasons for changing body position are:

- to prevent contractures
- to stimulate circulation and to help prevent thrombophlebitis, pressure sores, and edema of the extremities
- to promote lung expansion
- to promote drainage of respiratory secretions
- to relieve pressure on a body area

The most common positions that the patient assumes in bed are the dorsal, or supine, the side-lying, or lateral, and the prone positions. The essential principles of body alignment necessary for maintaining these positions follow.

DORSAL OR SUPINE POSITION

1. The head is in line with the spine, both laterally and anteroposteriorly.
2. The trunk is positioned so that flexion of the hips is minimized.
3. The arms are flexed at the elbow with the hands resting against the lateral abdomen.
4. The legs are extended with a small, firm support under the popliteal area.
5. The heels are suspended in a space between the mattress and the footboard.
6. The toes are pointed straight up.
7. Trochanter rolls are placed under the greater trochanters in the hip joint areas.

SIDE-LYING OR LATERAL POSITION

1. The head is in line with the spine.
2. The body is in alignment and is not twisted.
3. The uppermost hip joint is slightly forward and supported in a position of slight abduction by a pillow.
4. A pillow supports the arm, which is flexed at both the elbow and the shoulder joints.

PRONE POSITION (ON ABDOMEN)

1. The head is turned laterally and is in alignment with the rest of the body.
2. The arms are abducted and externally rotated at the shoulder joint; the elbows are flexed.
3. A small flat support is placed under the pelvis, extending from the level of the umbilicus to the upper third of the thigh.
4. The lower extremities remain in a neutral position.
5. The toes are suspended over the edge of the mattress.

THERAPEUTIC EXERCISES

Exercise involves the function of muscles, nerves, bones, and joints as well as the cardiovascular and respiratory systems. *Return to function is dependent upon the strength of the musculature that controls the joints.* Therapeutic exercises are prescribed by the physician and performed with the assistance and guidance of a physical therapist and/or nurse.

The overall objectives are to develop and retrain deficient muscles, to restore as much normal movement as possible, in order to prevent deformity, and to stimulate the functions of various organs and body systems.

Exercise is also valuable in helping to restore the motivation and well-being of the patient. It can help to lift the mind from pessimism and depression to optimism and good humor. The patient should have a clear understanding of what the exercise is to accomplish.

Exercise, when correctly done, assists in (1) maintaining and building muscle strength, (2) maintaining joint function, (3) preventing deformity, (4) stimulating circulation, and (5) building tolerance and endurance. There are five types of exercise: passive, active assistive, active, resistive, and isometric. The description, purpose, and action of each of these exercises are summarized in Table 12-1.

Range of Motion Exercises

Each joint of the body has a normal range of motion. In many musculoskeletal and neurological conditions the joints may lose their normal range, stiffen, and produce a permanent disability. If the range of motion is limited, the functions of the joint and of the muscle that moves the joint are impaired. In order to prevent painful deformities, range of motion activities are carried out when permitted, to either maintain or increase the maximal motion of a joint and to prevent deterioration.

These exercises should begin as soon as the patient's clinical condition allows. The range of motion exercises are planned for the individual to accommodate the wide variation in the degrees of motion that persons of varying body build and age groups can attain.

TABLE 12-1. THERAPEUTIC EXERCISES

EXERCISE	DESCRIPTION	PURPOSES	ACTION
Passive	An exercise carried out by the therapist or the nurse without assistance from the patient.	To retain as much joint range of motion as possible; to maintain circulation.	Stabilize the proximal joint and support the distal part. Move the joint smoothly, slowly, and gently through its full range of motion. Avoid producing pain.
Active assistive	An exercise carried out by the patient with the assistance of the therapist or the nurse.	To encourage normal muscle function.	Support the distal part and encourage the patient to take the joint actively through its range of motion. Give no more assistance than is necessary to accomplish the action. Short periods of activity should be followed by adequate rest periods.
Active	An exercise accomplished by the patient without assistance. Activities include turning from side to side, from back to abdomen, and moving up and down in bed.	To increase muscle strength.	Active exercise when possible should be done against gravity. The joint is moved through full range of motion without assistance. (Make sure that the patient does not substitute another joint movement for the one intended.)
Resistive	An active exercise carried out by the patient working against resistance produced by either manual or mechanical means.	To provide resistance in order to increase muscle power.	The patient moves the joint through its range of motion while the therapist resists slightly at first and then with progressively increasing resistance. Sandbags and weights can be used and are applied at the distal point of the involved joint. The movements should be done smoothly.
Isometric or Muscle setting	Alternately contracting and relaxing a muscle while keeping the part in a fixed position. This exercise is performed by the patient.	To maintain strength when a joint is immobilized.	Contract or tighten the muscle as much as possible without moving the joint; hold for several seconds, then "let go" and relax. Breathe deeply.

DEFINITIONS

Abduction—movement away from the midline of the body

Adduction—movement toward the midline of the body

Flexion—bending of a joint so that the angle of the joint diminishes

Extension—the return movement from flexion; the joint angle is increased

Inversion—movement that turns the sole of the foot inward

Eversion—movement that turns the sole of the foot outward

Dorsiflexion—movement that flexes or bends the foot toward the leg

Plantar flexion—movement that flexes or bends the foot in the direction of the sole

Pronation—rotation of the forearm so that the palm of the hand is down

Supination—rotation of the forearm so that the palm of the hand is up

Rotation—turning or movement of a part around its axis
Internal: turning inward, toward the center
External: turning outward, away from the center

TECHNIQUE

The patient must be in a comfortable position, lying supine with his arms to the side and his knees extended. Good body posture is to be maintained in each position assumed during the exercise. The bed should be high enough to permit the nurse to reach effectively the part to be exercised. Unless prescribed otherwise, a joint should be moved through its range of motion from 3 to 10 times, at least once a day. The extremity is held at the joint and the joint is moved smoothly, slowly, and gently through its range. If the joint is painful, as in arthritis, the extremity may be supported in the muscular area. A joint should not be moved beyond its free range of motion. Therefore, the motion should be stopped at the point of pain. When muscle spasm is present, the joint should be moved slowly and to the point of resistance. Then a gentle, steady pressure is exerted until the muscle relaxes.

When range of motion exercises are performed, consideration must be given to the bones above and below the joint to be moved. For example, when the elbow is taken through its range of motion, the humerus must be stabilized while the radius and the ulna are moved through their range of motion in the elbow joint. (Refer to Table 12-2 and Fig. 12-1 for joint motion and a pictorial review of range of motion exercises.)

Deterrents to Exercise

FEAR AND PAIN. The ability of a patient to follow a pattern of exercises may be thwarted by *fear* and *pain*. These produce increased tension and may result in muscle spasm and tightness of joint ligaments. If fear and pain are not relieved, they may lead to stiffness of joints, limitation in range of motion, muscle contractures, and poorly coordinated muscle activity. For example: *pain* in the chest, as observed in chest and breast surgery, cardiac pain, or burns of the thorax, frequently causes many patients to hold the arm close to the body, resting it on the chest or abdominal wall with the elbow flexed. If permitted to continue for prolonged periods of time, this practice may result in tightness of the ligaments around the shoulder and elbow joints; and spasm of the large pectoral muscles and biceps may lead to adaptive shortening, tightening, and contractures of these muscles. The weight of the arm on the chest and/or the abdomen restricts the expansive motion of the chest wall and muscles of respiration, which leads to inadequate ventilation.

Fear (as observed in patients who have had cardiac, chest, or breast surgery, infections in the lungs, and burns of the chest wall) often causes these patients to assume protective positions that are restrictive in nature and prevent proper physiologic alignment.

PREVENTING EXTERNAL ROTATION OF THE HIP

Patients who are in bed for periods of time may develop external rotation deformity of the hip. The hip is a ball-and-socket joint and has a tendency to rotate outward when the patient lies on his back. A trochanter roll extending from the crest of the ilium to the midthigh will prevent this deformity (Fig. 12-2). With correct placement, the trochanter roll serves as a mechanical wedge under the projection of the greater trochanter.

PREVENTING FOOTDROP (PLANTAR FLEXION)

Footdrop is a deformity in which the foot is plantar flexed (the ankle bends in the direction of the sole of the foot). If the condition continues without correction, the patient cannot hold the foot in a normal position and will walk on his toes without touching the ground with the heel of his foot. The deformity is caused by contracture of both the gastrocnemius and the soleus muscles. It may also be produced by loss of flexibility of the Achilles tendon.

- Prolonged bed rest, lack of exercise, incorrect positioning in bed, and the weight of the bedding forcing the toes into plantar flexion are factors that contribute to footdrop.

To prevent this crippling deformity, a footboard or pillows are used to keep the feet at right angles to the legs when the patient is in a supine position. The feet are positioned so that both plantar surfaces are firmly against the footboard or pillows. The patient is encouraged to flex and then to extend (curl and stretch) his feet and toes frequently. The ankles should be moved clockwise and counterclockwise in a rotary motion several times each hour.

TABLE 12-2. RANGE OF MOTION

SHOULDER

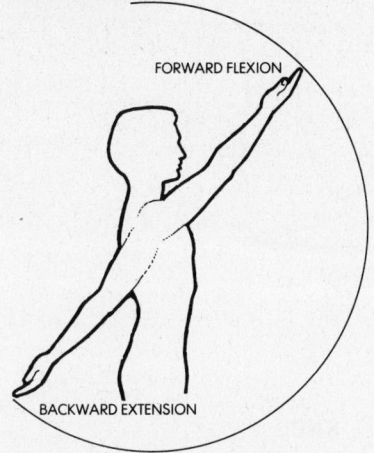

FORWARD FLEXION

BACKWARD EXTENSION

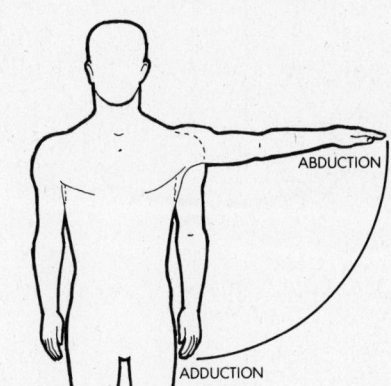

ABDUCTION

ADDUCTION

ELBOW

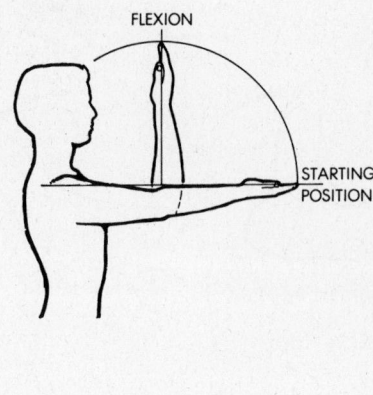

FLEXION

STARTING POSITION

FOREARM

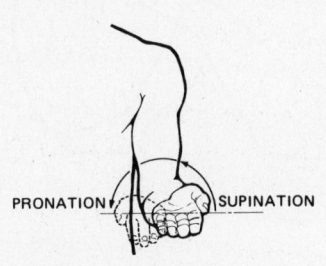

PRONATION   SUPINATION

WRIST

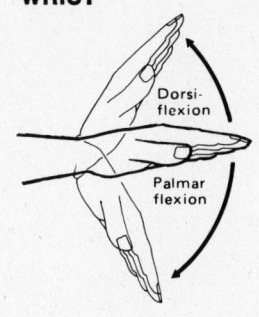

Dorsi-flexion

Palmar flexion

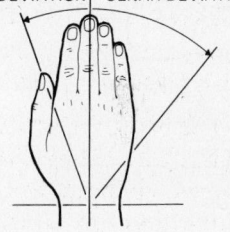

RADIAL DEVIATION   ULNAR DEVIATION

THUMB

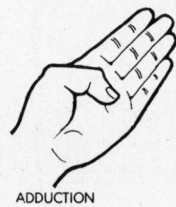

ADDUCTION

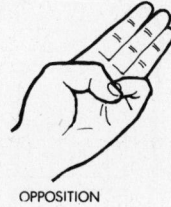

OPPOSITION

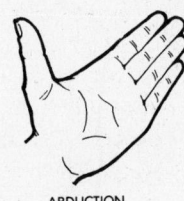

ABDUCTION

FINGERS

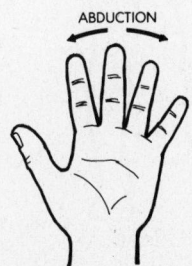

ABDUCTION

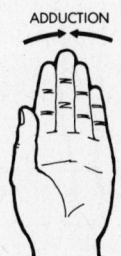

ADDUCTION

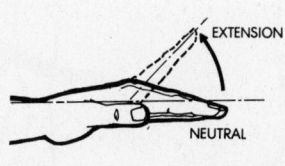

EXTENSION

NEUTRAL

185

TABLE 12-2.   RANGE OF MOTION *(Continued)*

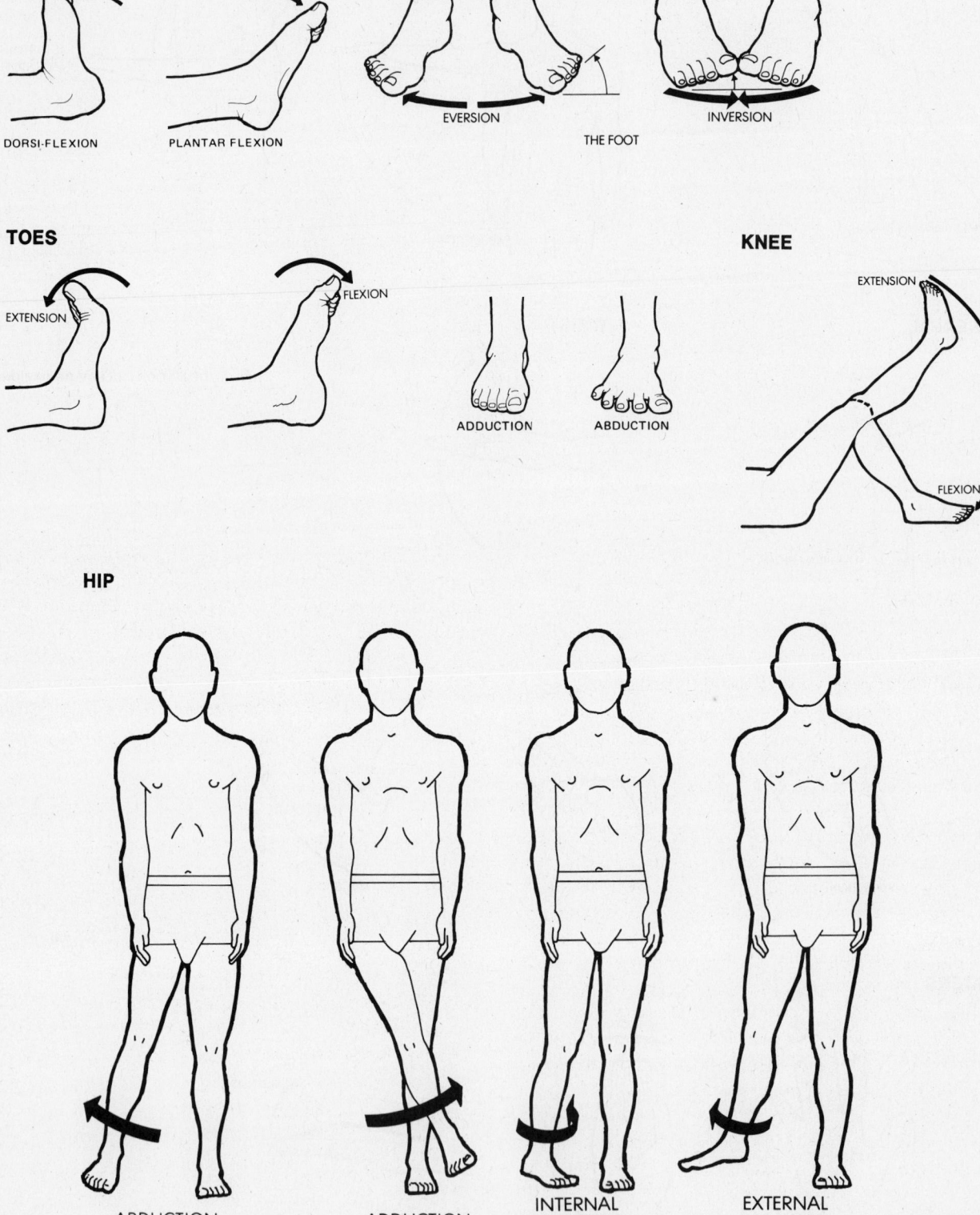

ANKLE

DORSI-FLEXION

PLANTAR FLEXION

FOOT

EVERSION

THE FOOT

INVERSION

TOES

EXTENSION

FLEXION

ADDUCTION

ABDUCTION

KNEE

EXTENSION

FLEXION

HIP

ABDUCTION

ADDUCTION

INTERNAL ROTATION

EXTERNAL ROTATION

TABLE 12-2.   RANGE OF MOTION *(Continued)*

CERVICAL SPINE

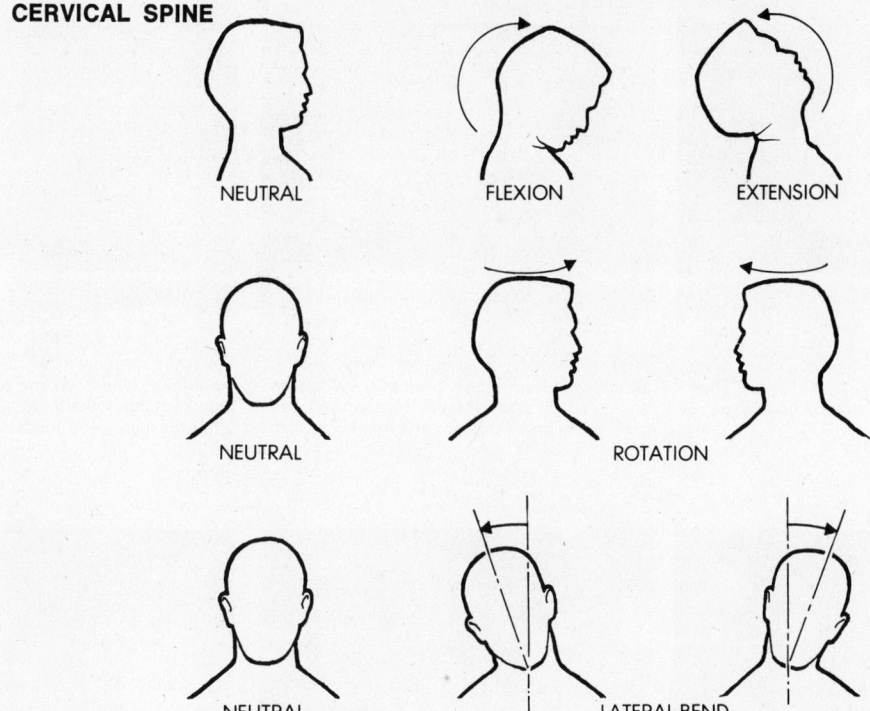

NEUTRAL   FLEXION   EXTENSION

NEUTRAL   ROTATION

NEUTRAL   LATERAL BEND

PREVENTING AND TREATING PRESSURE SORES

Pathogenesis

Pressure sores (bedsores, decubitus ulcers) are localized areas of infarcted soft tissues produced by pressure. Pressure is exerted on the skin and subcutaneous tissues by the object on which they rest, such as the mattress, chair seat, cast, etc. There is compression of the small nutrient vessels of the skin and underlying tissues, which results in tissue anoxia or ischemia. The cutaneous tissues become broken or destroyed, leading to progressive destruction of underlying soft tissue. Once the skin breaks, an ulcer may form which may be painful and very slow to heal. Invasion by a profusion of microorganisms (streptococci, staphylococci, *Pseudomonas aeruginosa, Escherichia coli, Proteus* species) and secondary infections is difficult to avoid. There emanates from the lesion an obnoxious-smelling discharge which is the product of bacterial invasion and tissue breakdown. The lesion, if large enough, permits a continuous loss of serum which may deplete the circulating blood and the entire body of essential protein constituents. Also, when the ulcer is infected, it may extend deep into the fascia, muscle, and bone, and multiple large sinus tracts may radiate from it. Thus, systemic infection can easily develop, especially from bloodstream invasion by gram-negative bacilli.

Other factors contribute to the development of pressure sores. (See chart below.) Anemia, whether caused by hemorrhage, nutritional deficiency, or infection, decreases the body's oxygen carrying ability and predisposes to ulcer formation. Patients with nutritional deficiencies have negative nitrogen, phosphorus, sulfur, and calcium balances, which will produce wasting of tissue and loss of weight.

**RISK FACTORS
FOR DEVELOPMENT OF PRESSURE SORES**

Prolonged pressure

Immobility, compromised mobility

Loss of protective reflexes, motor or sensory deficit/loss

Shearing forces, friction, trauma

Malnutrition, hypoproteinemia, vitamin deficiencies, anemia

Skin dryness, excessive skin moisture, maceration

Edema, poor skin perfusion

Infection

Advancing age

Equipment: traction, casts, restraints, improper bedding and seats

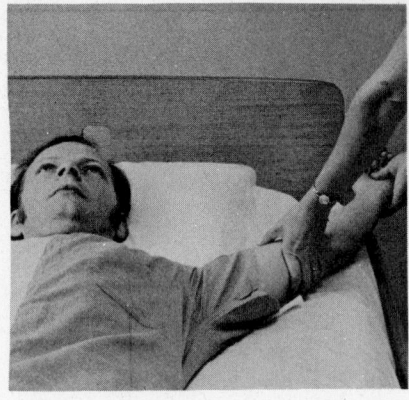

Abduction of shoulder. Move arm from side of body to above the head. Then return arm to side of body or neutral position (adduction).

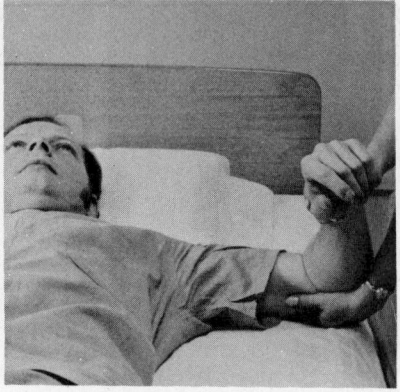

Internal rotation of shoulder. With arm at shoulder height, elbow bent at a 90-degree angle, palm toward feet—turn upper arm until palm and forearm face backward.

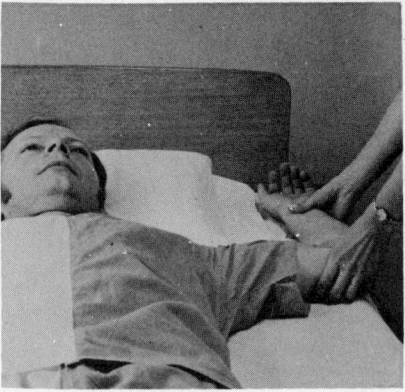

External rotation of shoulder. With arm at shoulder height, elbow bent at 90-degree angle, palm toward feet—turn upper arm until the palm and forearm face forward.

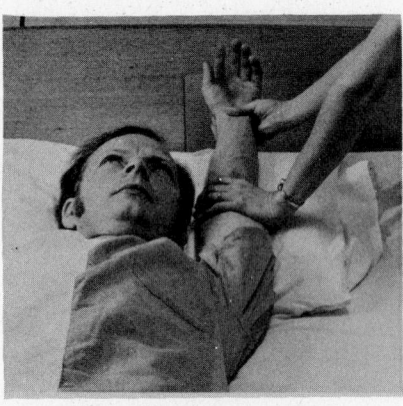

Forward flexion of shoulder. Move arm forward and upward until it is alongside of head.

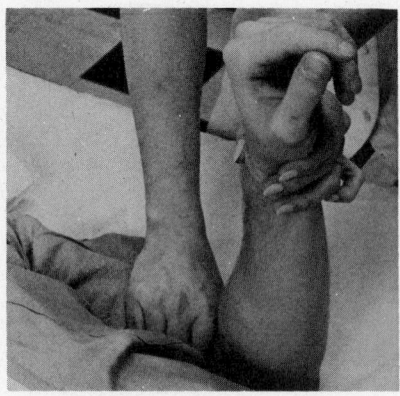

Pronation of forearm. With elbow at waist, arm bent at 90-degree angle—turn hand so that palm is facing down.

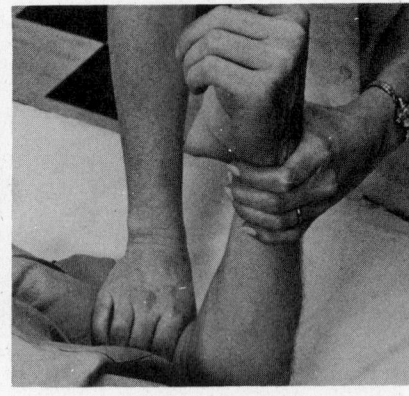

Supination of forearm. With elbow at waist, arm bent at 90-degree angle, turn hand so that palm is facing up.

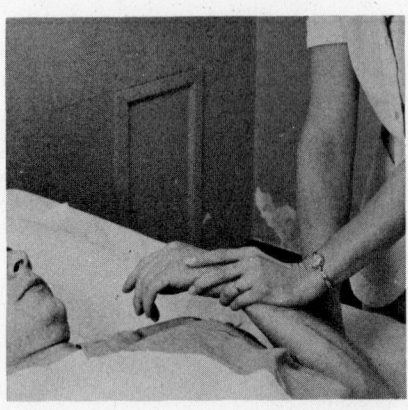

Flexion of elbow. Bend elbow, bringing forearm and hand toward shoulder. Then return forearm and hand to neutral position (arm straight).

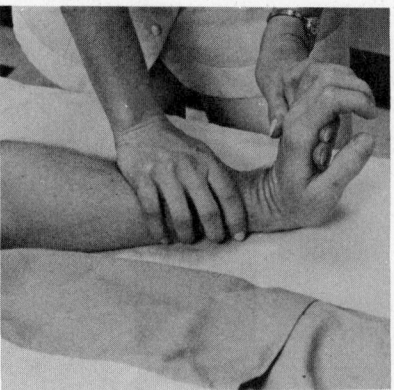

Wrist extension.

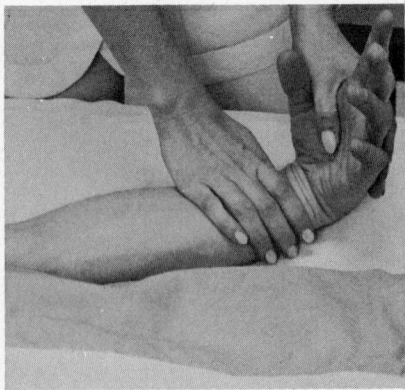

Flexion of wrist. Bend wrist so that palm is toward forearm. Straighten to a neutral position.

Figure 12-1.   Range of motion exercises.

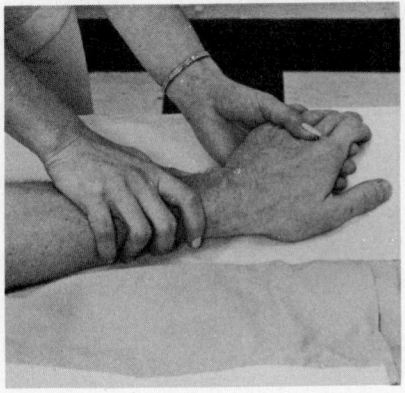
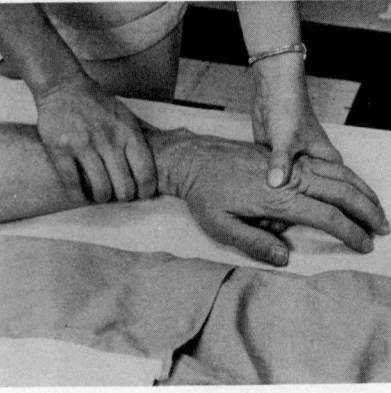
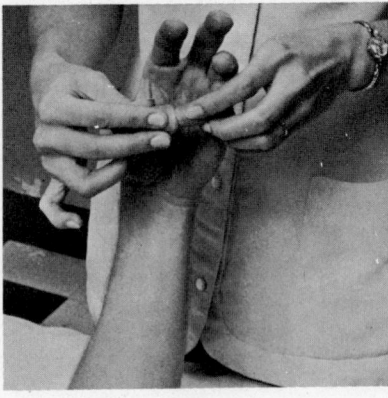

Ulnar deviation. Move hand sideways so that the side of hand on which little finger is located moves toward forearm.

Radial deviation. Move hand sideways so that side of hand on which thumb is located moves toward forearm.

Thumb opposition. Move thumb out and around to touch little finger.

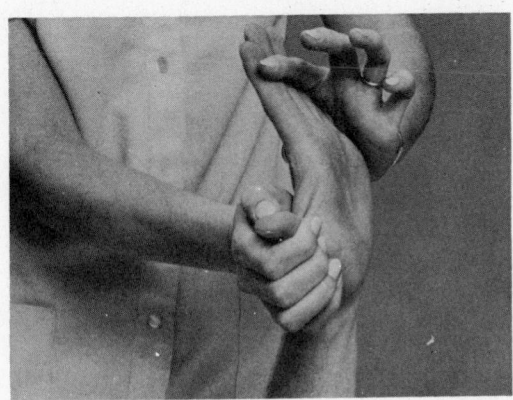
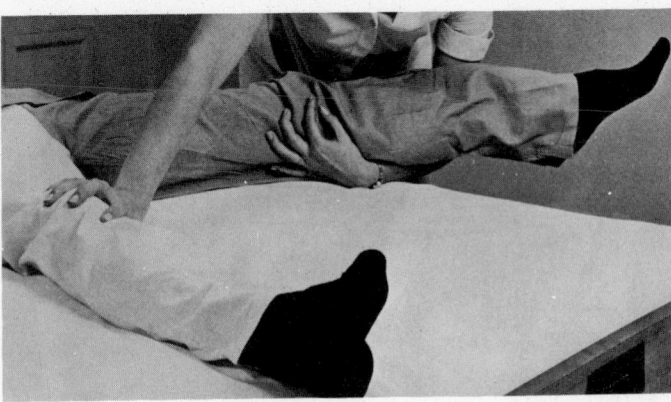

Extension of fingers.

Abduction-adduction of hip. Move leg outward from the body as far as possible. Return leg from abducted position to neutral position and across the leg as far as possible.

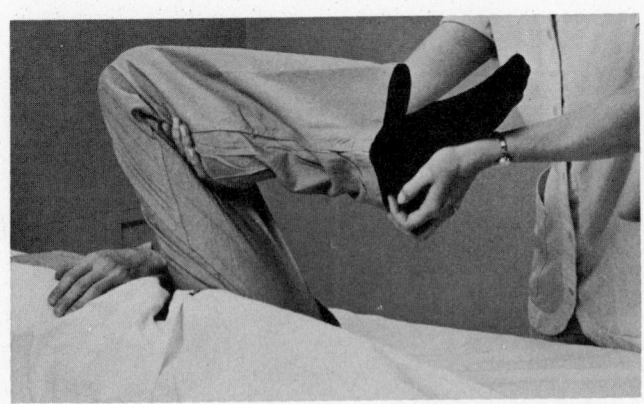
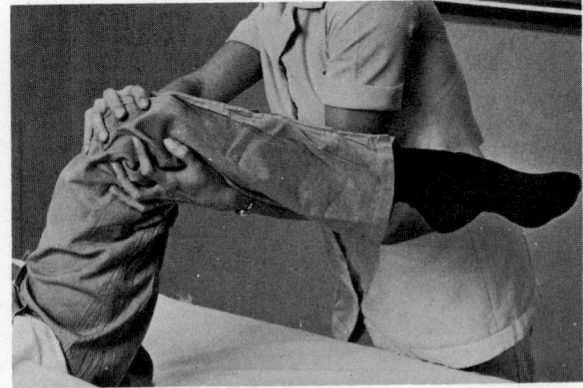

Flexion of hip and flexion of knee. Bend hip by moving the leg forward as far as possible. Return leg from the flexed position to the neutral position.

Internal-external rotation of hip. Turn leg in an inward motion so that toes point in. Turn leg in an outward motion so that toes point out.

Figure 12-1.   Range of motion exercises *(Continued)*.

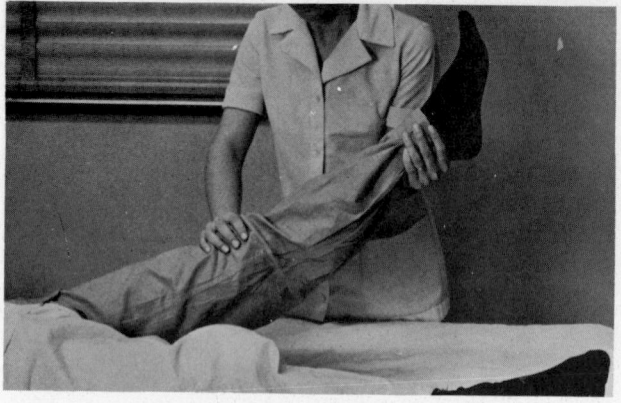

To stretch hamstring muscles, straighten leg and raise.

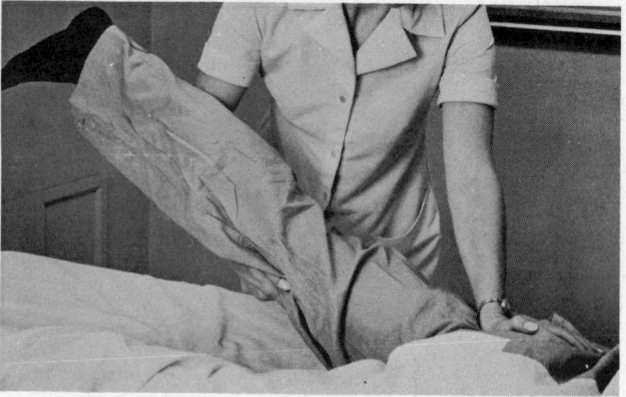

Hyperextension of hip. Place the patient in a prone position and move leg backward from the body as far as possible.

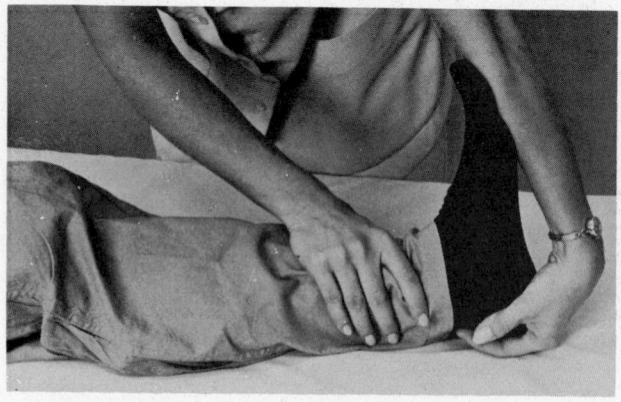

Dorsiflexion of foot. Move foot up and toward the leg. Then move foot down and away from the leg (plantar flexion).

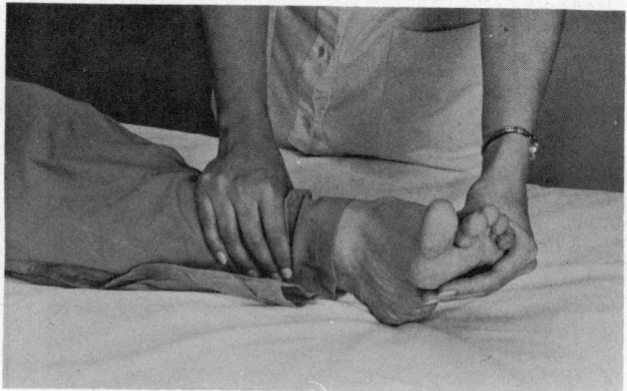

Inversion and eversion of foot. Move foot so that sole is facing outward (eversion). Then move foot so that sole is facing inward (inversion).

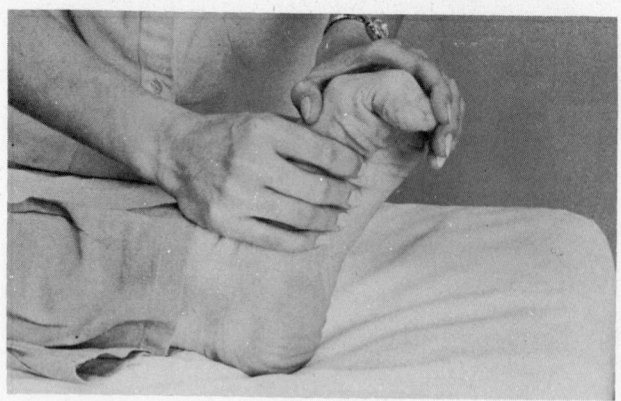

Flexion of toes. Bend the toes toward the ball of foot.

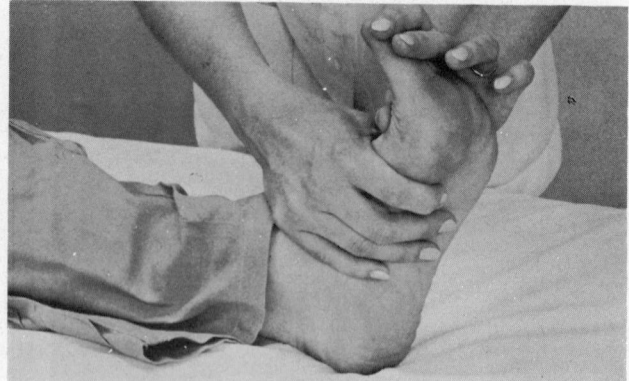

Extension of toes. Straighten toes and pull them toward the leg as far as possible.

Figure 12-1.　Range of motion exercises *(Continued)*.

Other metabolic disorders can also contribute to low protein levels. Persons with malabsorption syndrome may develop protein deficiency and severe anemia because of failure to absorb folic acid. Diabetic persons may have a poor quality of tissue which is easily injured. Many persons have hidden vitamin C deficiencies. In all of these conditions there is evidence of protein depletion (in the form of low serum albumin) that can lead to a pressure sore when illness supervenes.

Motor paralysis with associated muscular atrophy causes reduction of padding between the overlying skin and the underlying bone, and leads to pressure sores. Paralyzed patients tend to lie in one position, with the body weight concentrated on small areas of skin. This high pressure collapses blood vessels and impedes blood flow causing a pressure sore to form in a very short time. If the patient has suffered sensory loss he will not be aware of pain and pressure and will not be aware that the skin is breaking down.

Shearing force is created by the interplay of two other forces: gravitational forces that pull the patient's body towards the foot of the bed, and resting forces created by friction taking place on the skin surface. Shearing forces, by pulling on tissues, stretch and injure tissues and blood vessels. This type of shearing force is applied when the patient is pulled up in bed, is allowed to slump in bed or a chair, or moves up in bed by digging his heels or elbows into the mattress. To prevent this, the patient should be lifted, not dragged up, in bed or on a chair.

Other causes of pressure sores are edema, which impairs circulation and interferes with the supply of nutrients to the cells, and moisture and friction, which irritate the skin and make it less resistant to injury. Physiological change in the skin, especially in older patients, because of reduced production of sebum, is another factor.

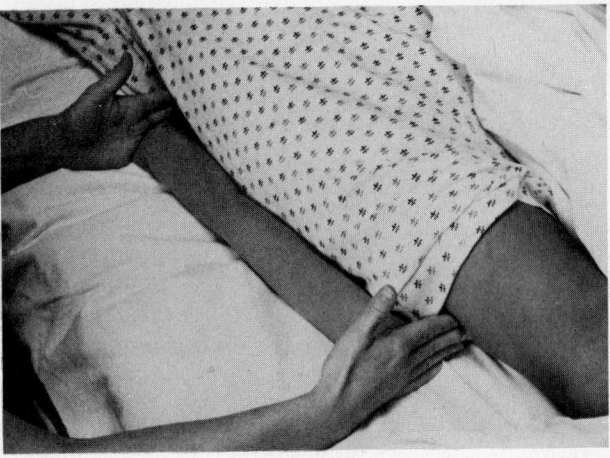

Figure 12-2. Placement of trochanter roll. (From Farrell, J.: Illustrated Guide to Orthopedic Nursing. J. B. Lippincott, 1977)

In summary, the basic causes of pressure sores are pressure (Fig. 12-3), blocking of blood flow, and lack of normal movement.

Signs and Symptoms of Pressure Sores

The first sign of a potential pressure sore is the appearance of erythema (redness) of the skin, which will blanch on pressure. The redness progresses to a dusky, cyanotic blue-gray appearance which is the result of skin capillary occlusion and subcutaneous weakening. Blistering and a break in the skin occur, and the early stages of necrosis follow. This process may involve deeper soft tissues, bursae, muscles, tendons, and even bone and/or joints. If the ulcer is long-standing and has repeatedly broken down and healed, secondary induration (hardening of tissue) develops and the blood supply to the area is compromised by underlying scar tissue. Deep pockets of infection are often present. These may be covered by a dark crust which also impedes healing.

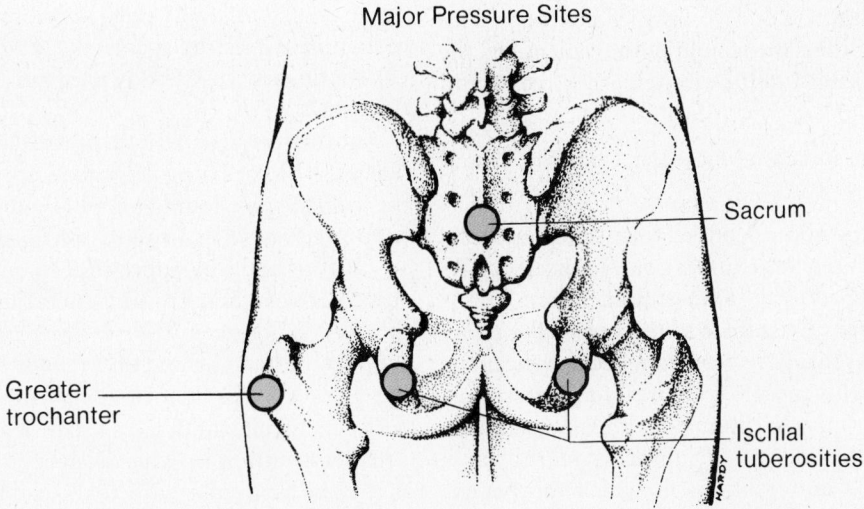

Major Pressure Sites

Sacrum

Greater trochanter

Ischial tuberosities

Figure 12-3. Areas of major pressure sites where pressure sores can develop.

NURSING ASSESSMENT

- Inspect each pressure site for erythema.
  Press on the area. Look for blanching.
  Note how long hyperemia persists following removal of pressure.
- Palpate for warmth.
  Is skin temperature increased?
- Inspect for dry skin, moist skin, break in the skin.
- Palpate peripheral pulses to evaluate circulatory status.
- Check patient's record for hematocrit, hemoglobin and serum albumin levels.

Prevention of Pressure Sores

The prevention of pressure sores is one of the most important considerations in the nursing management of patients. Pressure sores develop with alarming rapidity — within 2 to 4 hours at sites where there is unrelieved pressure. They are a serious complication that may occur in any patient. Their presence greatly prolongs the patient's convalescence and imposes a tremendous physical and economic burden.

The best treatment of pressure sores is prevention. If one bears in mind that the weight-bearing prominences are covered only by skin and small amounts of subcutaneous fat, it is easily seen that the majority of pressure sores are located at such sites: the sacrum, greater trochanter, and ischial tuberosities, especially in persons who sit for prolonged periods (Fig. 12-3). Other bony promontories that are susceptible to pressure sore development are the knees, malleoli, heels, and elbows.

The principles that underlie the nursing management are:
- to relieve or remove pressure
- to stimulate the circulation
- to keep the skin clean and in a healthy condition

RELIEF OF PRESSURE. The patient needs frequent changes of position and the avoidance of positions that result in excessive pressure. Such measures will prevent prolonged blocking of blood flow which interferes with skin nutrition. Shifting the weight of the patient lets the blood flow back and helps tissue to recover from pressure.

- Thus the patient should be turned at 1-hour or 2-hour intervals.

He should be positioned on all four sides (laterally, prone, dorsally) in sequence unless contraindicated. The skin should be inspected at each position change.

One way to avoid pressure is to use one of the many mechanical devices that have been designed as a means of providing support for specific body areas or for distributing pressure uniformly. An alternating pressure pad mattress covered with 2.5 cm. (1″) thick foam rubber is especially valuable in conditions in which the patient cannot turn. The alternating inflation and deflation of the pad produces constriction followed by dilatation of the superficial blood vessels of the skin. By such action, pressure on any one part is reduced and the blood supply is increased.

For patients susceptible to pressure on bony prominences there is a variety of pads and supportive devices available that can be placed on top of the mattress. The gel-type flotation pad reduces pressure because the material is similar in consistency to human adipose tissue and "gives" with the patient's weight. Soft, moisture-absorbing padding is also useful since the softness and resilience of padding allows for even distribution of pressure and the dissipation and absorption of moisture, while providing for freedom from wrinkles and friction. Bony prominences may be protected by inserting pieces of gel pads, sheepskin padding, or soft foam rubber beneath the sacrum, the trochanters, heels, elbows, scapulae, and the back of the head when there is pressure on these sites. The patient should not be placed on a poorly ventilated mattress that is covered with plastic or some other impermeable material.

The use of the flotation mattress, or water bed, for treatment of pressure sores has been advocated. As the patient's body sinks into the fluid, additional surface becomes available for weight bearing, thereby further decreasing body weight per unit area. (Pascal's law states that the weight of the body floating on a fluid system is evenly distributed over the entire supporting surface.) Thus the body weight is lightened and there is less pressure on the body parts. However, shearing forces can be built up on the water bed as the patient's body is suspended on the plastic covering over the surface of the water. The Rehabilitation Engineering Center at Rancho Los Amigos Hospital developed a multifluidic unresisting displacement (MUD) bed, sometimes called a high density fluid support system (HDF). The patient is floated on a bed of high density fluid, a mixture of bentonite clay and barites. Since this fluid is twice as dense as water there is equal distribution of pressure and reduction of pressure against the total body surface as the patient floats with his body partly in and partly out of the fluid mixture.

Another way to relieve pressure over bony prominences is the bridging technique accomplished through the correct positioning of pillows. Just as a bridge is supported on pillars to allow traffic to move underneath, so can the body be supported by pillows to allow for space between bony prominences and the mattress. For the feet and extremities, a footboard or pillows will support the bedding and thus reduce pressure. To protect the heels 2.5 cm. (1″) of foam rubber may be placed between a well laundered soft sheet and the mattress.

Patients sitting in wheelchairs for prolonged periods should be protected with foam-padded seatboards that are cut out posteriorly over ischial areas. This is useful since the weight of the body is usually spread over a smaller area of skin when the patient is sitting in a chair. The patient should be reminded to shift his weight frequently and raise himself up for a few seconds every half hour while sitting in a chair (Fig. 12-4).

STIMULATION OF CIRCULATION. Since the stimulation of circulation relieves tissue ischemia, the forerunner of pressure sores, the patient is encouraged to keep active. Active and passive exercises increase muscular, skin, and vascular tone. The patient should be ambulated whenever possible since the level of mobility is an important criterion for prognosis and treatment. (Activity also stimulates the metabolic processes and helps to improve morale.) Frequent skin massage with lotion is useful as another means of stimulating the blood flow in the skin. A gentle circular motion is used around bony prominences and other vulnerable areas. If an abrasion is discovered, massage should be directed in ever-widening circles away from the lesion. Again, turning aids the circulation. The use of a rocking bed and a tilt table also aids in stimulating circulation.

SKIN CARE AND GENERAL HYGIENE. Maceration of the skin by continuous moisture must be prevented by meticulous hygienic measures. The skin should be washed with a mild soap and water and blotted dry with a soft towel. The skin then is lubricated with an emollient lotion or a thin layer of silicone cream to keep it soft and pliable. It is desirable that the patient assist in caring for his skin. He should be encouraged to inspect it at frequent intervals for evidence of pressure. He should be taught to use a mirror and inspect posterior areas, if he is paraplegic or has other neuromuscular disorders. He should massage and stroke lightly around bony prominences since this promotes venous return, reduces edema, and increases vascular tone. Foreign bodies should be kept out of the bed because they serve to irritate the skin. Foundation sheets should be tightly stretched to prevent wrinkles.

The patient's nutritional status must be adequate and a positive nitrogen balance maintained. Pressure sores develop more quickly and are more resistant to treatment in patients suffering from nutritional disorders. A high protein diet with protein supplements may be helpful. Iron preparations and whole blood transfusions may be necessary since the hemoglobin level is a critical criterion for the development of pressure sores. Vitamin C is necessary for healing and tissue vitality.

Treatment

If a pressure sore develops, the objectives of treatment are to continue preventive measures on a more vigorous level (remove the pressure), encourage restoration of circulation and cellular function, and prevent necrosis of deeper structures. The metabolic processes are stimulated by keeping the patient as active as possible. Blood flow may be improved by gentle massage of the adjacent

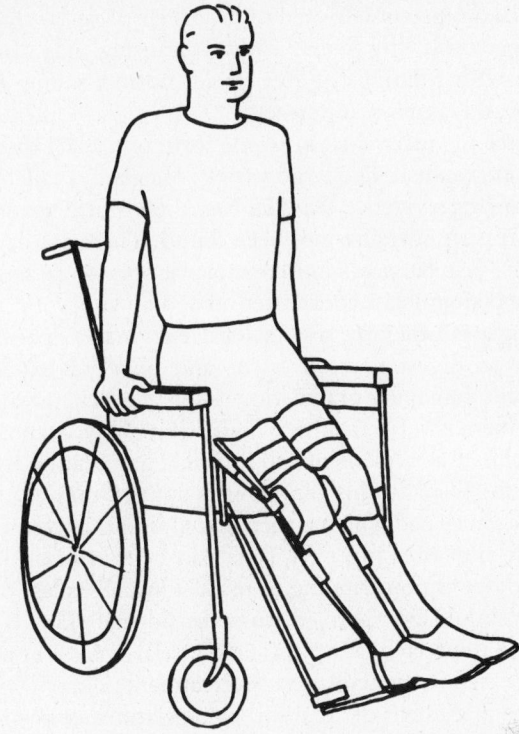

Figure 12-4. Wheelchair push-up to prevent ischial pressure sores. These push-ups should become an automatic routine (every 30 minutes) for the person with paraplegia. He should stay up, out of contact with the seat, for 60 seconds. (From Hirschberg, G. G., Lewis, L., and Vaughan, P.: Rehabilitation. Philadelphia, J. B. Lippincott, 1976)

area. The patient is placed on a high-protein, high-vitamin diet to promote healing. These wounds leak body fluids and protein, placing the patient in a catabolic state and predisposing to the serious problem of secondary infection.

Patients who have pressure sores are usually malnourished and tend to have hypoproteinemia and vitamin deficiencies. Protein deficiency must be corrected in order to heal a pressure sore, and carbohydrates are necessary to "spare" proteins and provide an energy source. Extra protein is added to the diet and the regular diet may have to be supplemented with tube feedings. Wound healing is also dependent on collagen. In turn, ascorbic acid (vitamin C) is necessary for collagen formation. Therefore, patients with pressure sores require additional vitamin C. Supplemental zinc is a stimulant to wound healing in those patients who suffer from a zinc deficiency.

The ulcer must be cleansed daily to clear up sepsis and stimulate the regeneration of epithelium. The ulcer(s) is debrided of necrotic material because devitalized tissue promotes the development of infection and impedes healing. Dead bone must also be removed. Debridement may be done by surgical dissection or electrocautery. Cultures are obtained of the material deep in the ulcer to ascertain whether anaerobes are present. If anaerobes are found, oxygen is delivered to the deeper areas by hydrogen peroxide irrigations. Topical cleansing may also be done with solutions of acetic acid, normal saline, half-strength Dakin's solution, etc.

After the ulcer is clean, some form of topical therapy may be applied. The large variety of agents available is convincing evidence that the best therapeutic modality for pressure sores has not been found. There are drying agents, skin barriers, antiseptic plastic sprays, an aerosol spray containing a corticosteroid and an antibiotic, etc. Collagenase therapy uses a local enzymatic debriding agent to digest necrotic tissue and purulent exudates without damaging granulation tissue. This chemical debridement is very effective when used with hydrotherapy to facilitate debridement and promote granulation tissue growth. Usually this ointment is applied directly to a sterile gauze pad which is then placed over the wound. A plastic film dressing or a Telfa pad held in place with paper tape is nonirritating to most skin. All excess ointment should be removed from the normal skin. If the wound is infected, a topical antibacterial agent is applied before enzymatic (collagenase) treatment.

The placement of an absorbable gelatin sponge at the base of the ulcer (changed daily) has also been successful. This pad is a synthetic material with a physical consistency similar to that of human fat tissue. It provides a layer of "artificial fat" over a bony prominence.

Physical therapy modalities such as air, sunlight, whirlpool baths, ultraviolet irradiation and ultrasound have also been used successfully. Oxygen applied directly on the ulcer (hyperbaric oxygen therapy) has been employed to direct more oxygen to the tissues, hasten metabolic processes, and reduce healing time.

Surgical intervention is necessary when the ulcer does not respond to conventional treatment. Incision and drainage are carried out if the ulcer is not draining properly. Skin grafts may be necessary. Sometimes the ulcer, scar tissue, underlying bursa, and bone must be removed before healing will take place.

SUPPORTING THE PATIENT IN DAILY SELF-CARE

ACTIVITIES OF DAILY LIVING

Activities of daily living (ADL) are those self-care activities which must be accomplished each day in order for the patient to maintain some degree of independence and participate in society. ADL include personal hygiene, dressing, eating, toileting, getting in and out of bed (transfers), using a wheelchair, ambulating (when possible), and performing manual tasks. The goal for the patient is to care for himself in his daily routine without depending on others. The role of the nurse is to teach, support, and supervise the patient while he performs these activities.

An Activities of Daily Living program is started as soon as the rehabilitation process starts. The longer a muscle is in disuse, the weaker and more atrophied it becomes. The patient must learn that he will lose what he does not use.

In order to effectively teach a person methods of self-care he must be motivated. "I would rather do it myself" is a good concept for the patient to develop. The nurse teaches and guides, but the patient must do the work. Since there are individual differences in all persons, self-care techniques need to be flexible and adapted to the patient's needs and mode of living. It is important to remember that there is usually more than one way to accomplish self-care. Since many patients do not perform these commonplace activities easily, a great deal of common sense and a little ingenuity are frequently called for. Often a simple maneuver requires concentration and the exertion of considerable effort.

By using an "Activities of Daily Living (ADL) Sheet" (Fig. 12-5) to evaluate the ability of a patient to perform certain activities, it is possible to determine his limitations. Another advantage of such a guide is that it shows the patient how he is progressing from one time to the next; this may be a valuable morale booster. When a patient's progress can be demonstrated, there is a tendency for such evidence to be a source of motivation. Also the ADL sheet keeps the staff informed of the activities that the patient can perform independently and those that will require assistance.

Before initiating an ADL program, the nurse must understand the patient's medical condition, his functional capacity, and his therapeutic goal as well as the details of his care. It is also wise to learn about the patient's family background and educational level in order to know how much support the family can give.

TEACHING THE ACTIVITIES OF DAILY LIVING

Since there are many ways to teach a task, the following is offered as a guide:

1. Ascertain what methods can be used to accomplish the task. (Example: There are several ways of putting on a given garment.)
2. Determine what the patient can do by watching him perform.
3. Ascertain the motions necessary for the accomplishment of the activity.
4. Encourage the patient to exercise the muscles necessary to perform the motions involved in the activity.
5. Select activities that encourage gross functional movements of the upper and lower extremities (e.g., bathing, holding larger objects).
6. Gradually include activities that use finer motions, (e.g., buttoning clothes, eating with a spoon).
7. Increase the period of activity as rapidly as the patient can tolerate.

ACTIVITIES OF DAILY LIVING (ADL) SHEET

EVALUATION OF THE PATIENT'S FUNCTIONING

	Total Assistance	Partial Assistance	Independent

Prescribed Activities:

Range of Motion

Positioning

Use of Tilt Table

  Degree

  How long

Exercises

  Breathing

  Balancing

  Crutch Training

  Parallel Bars

  Steps

Other Information:

Appliances or Prosthesis

Ambulation

Time Permitted Up

Bladder/Bowel Program

Bathing/Grooming Schedule

Speech Problems

Activities Being Learned

Name:

Diagnosis:

Doctor:

Functional Capabilities:

1. Flexes neck

2. Raises hand to head

3. Raises hand behind head

4. Reaches out at shoulder level to side (laterally)

5. Pronates/supinates forearm

6. Grasps objects

7. Begins grasp ability

8. Closes fist

9. Opens fist

10. Flexes and extends knee joint

11. Touches floor while seated

12. Crosses leg over opposite knee while sitting (with or without help of hands)

13. Transfers from sitting to standing (with or without holding to support)

14. Walks

Figure 12-5.   On the actual chart there is sufficient space left under each item for notes.

8. Perform and practice the activity in a real-life situation.
9. Encourage the patient to perform every activity up to his maximal capabilities within the framework of his disability.
10. Support the patient by giving justifiable praise for effort put forth and for acts accomplished.

The ADL Sheet is an information sheet for those who are taking care of the patient. The data on it serve to inform each member of the rehabilitation team what activities the patient can perform. It also serves as an index of progress. For example, after it has been determined that the patient can bathe himself, this information is noted on the ADL Sheet. The nurse who is responsible for the patient reviews this sheet at morning care time and notes what the patient is capable of doing and what activities he is learning. Thus the patient does not regress, because all members of the rehabilitation team are working toward the same goal.

The ADL Sheet in Figure 12-5 is a guide to the assessment of the functions of the patient. These activities are key goals. If the patient can sit up and raise his hands to his head, he probably can begin to bathe himself. By asking the patient to perform certain motions the nurse can determine what activities he will be able to do.

ADAPTIVE EQUIPMENT (SELF-HELP DEVICES). If the patient has difficulty in performing the activity, an adaptation will have to be made. Often a new method can be learned. If the patient cannot quite reach his head, perhaps he will be able to touch his head by leaning forward. Or, if the method cannot be changed, adaptive equipment (self-help devices) may be used—such as those devised by adding a long handle to a comb, "building up" the handle of a spoon, or making similar modifications. Equipment such as an automatic toothbrush has been found to improve the oral hygiene of those having limited movements of the hands, wrists, and arms. Be alert to "gadgets" coming on the market that may be useful to the handicapped. There are mobility aids and systems for the paralyzed and cerebral palsied, educational aids, occupational and vocational tools, personal aids, and writing, typewriting, and communication aids that have been designed and are in use.

ASSISTING THE PATIENT WITH AMBULATION

The Use of the Tilt Table

Weight-bearing on the long bones is essential for normal physiologic functioning. In order to prevent complications of inactivity, the upright position with weight-bearing on the long bones is desirable at the earliest possible time. This position prevents decalcification of the bones, thus aiding in the maintenance of normal acid-base balance and the prevention of renal calculi; it also stimulates circulation to the lower extremities.

Some disabilities, such as spinal cord injuries, orthostatic hypotension, brain damage, and those re-

quiring extended periods in the recumbent positions, prevent patients from assuming an upright position by the usual methods. In such instances a tilt table can be of tremendous use. A tilt table is a board or table that can be tilted gradually from a horizontal to a vertical position, permitting the patient to assume an upright position. It helps the patient with his weight-bearing activities and standing balance, prevents disuse syndrome, and conditions the vascular system. Before the patient is placed on a table, a compression leotard or a snug-fitting abdominal binder and elastic bandages are applied from the toes to the groin. Compression on the abdomen prevents pooling of blood in the splanchnic area and subsequent postural hypotension and inadequate cerebral circulation. Compression applied to the legs restricts the vascular walls of the blood vessels and prevents blood from pooling in the legs and edema from developing.

Tilting the patient from a supine to an upright position causes a decrease in the systolic blood pressure. For this reason a blood pressure cuff is applied before the table is tilted. The table should be tilted gradually, and someone should stay with the patient throughout this process. If the patient feels dizzy and his blood pressure drops, return him to a flat position. Observe for pallor, diaphoresis, tachycardia, and nausea. These are the signs and symptoms of insufficient cerebral circulation. The tilt of the table is increased by 5- to 10-degree increments. The angle of the tilt is determined by the patient's tolerance and the desired amount of weight-bearing. Be careful that the patient does not stand too long, especially if he cannot move his extremities. Prolonged standing may cause pressure ulceration on the bottom of the feet. The feet should be protected with a pair of properly fitted shoes.

Transfer Activities

A transfer is the movement of the patient from one piece of furniture or equipment to another; i.e., from bed to chair or bed to wheelchair.

As soon as the patient is permitted out of bed, transfer activities are started. While still confined to his bed, it is important that the patient practice "push-up" exercises to strengthen the arm and shoulder extensors. It is desirable that the patient be able to raise and move his body in different directions by means of these push-up exercises. A simple, effective procedure follows:

1. Have the patient sit upright in bed.
2. Place a book under each hand.
3. Instruct the patient to push down on the book and thus raise his body weight.

Since the nurse is so frequently concerned with getting weak and incapacitated patients out of bed, it is important to be familiar with the techniques of moving the

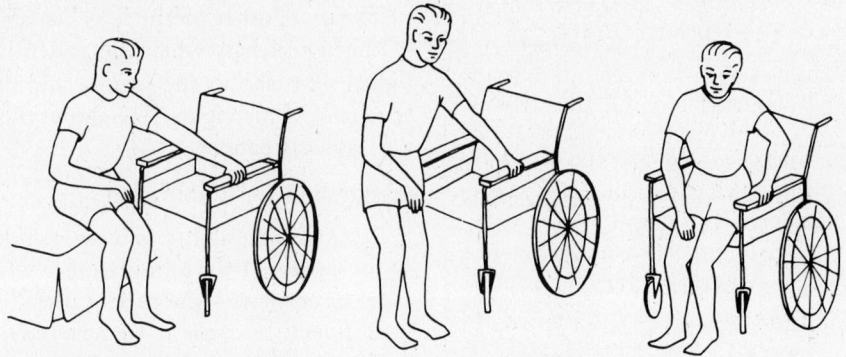

A. Weight-bearing transfer from bed to chair. The patient stands up, pivots until his back is opposite the new seat and sits down.

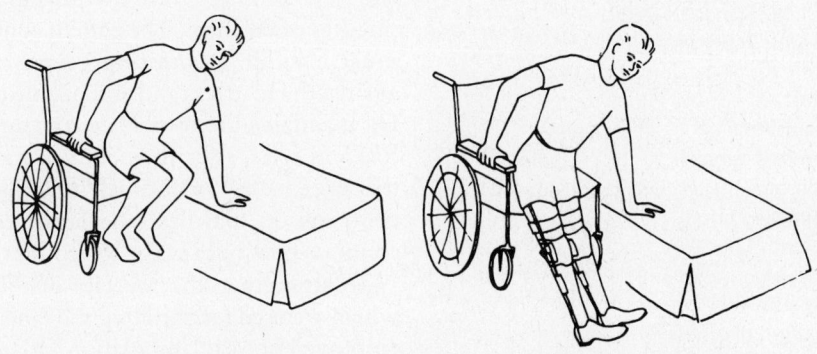

B. (*Left*) Non-weight-bearing transfer from chair to bed. (*Right*) With legs braced.

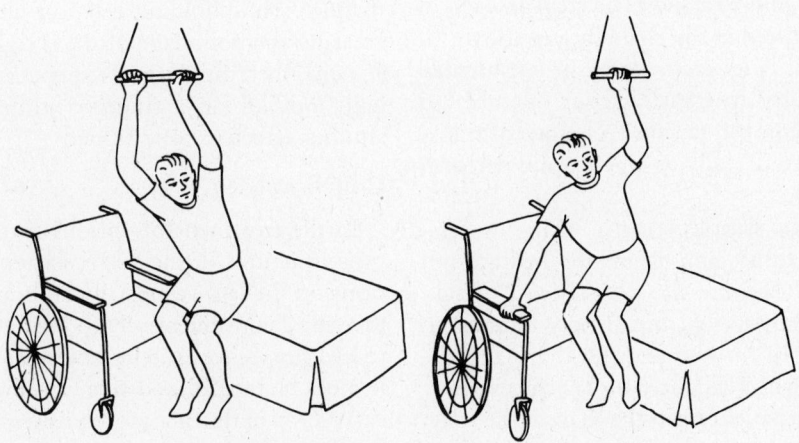

C. (*Left*). Non-weight-bearing transfer, pull-up method.
(*Right*). Non-weight-bearing transfer, combined method.

Figure 12-6. Methods of transferring the patient from the bed to a wheelchair. The wheelchair is in a locked position. (From Hirschberg, Lewis, and Vaughan: Rehabilitation. Philadelphia, J. B. Lippincott, 1976)

ASSISTING THE PATIENT OUT OF BED

Technique for moving the patient to the edge of the bed:
- Move head and shoulders of patient toward the edge of the bed.
- Move feet and legs to the edge of the bed (The patient is now in a crescent position that gives good range of motion to the lateral trunk muscles.)
- Place both arms well under patient's hips. (Before the next maneuver you should tighten [set] the muscles of your back and abdomen.)
- Straighten your back while moving the patient toward you.

Technique for sitting patient on the edge of the bed:
- Place arm and hand under shoulders of the patient.
- Instruct the patient to push his elbow into the bed while you lift his shoulders with one arm and swing his legs over the edge of the bed with the other. (Gravity pulls the legs downward, which aids in raising the patient's trunk.)

Technique for assisting patient to stand:
- Place patient's feet well under him.
- Face the patient while firmly grasping each side of his rib cage with your hands.
- Push your knee against one knee of the patient.
- Rock the patient forward as he comes to a standing position. (Your knee is pushed against the patient's knee as he comes to the standing position.)
- Ensure that the patient's knees are "locked" (full extension) while he is standing. (Locking the knees of the patient is a safety measure for those who are weak or have been in bed for a period of time.)
- Give the patient *enough time* to balance himself.
- Pivot the patient to position him to sit in the chair.

patient to the edge of the bed, sitting him on the edge of the bed and assisting him to stand. The steps in each of these maneuvers are listed in the chart shown above.

Before the patient is taught to transfer, he is evaluated to determine his ability to transfer from one area to another. The nurse demonstrates the technique of transfer and the patient then is ready to practice and perform this activity (Fig. 12-6).

USE OF A TRANSFER OR SLIDING BOARD. If the muscles that the patient uses to lift himself off the bed are not strong enough to overcome the resistance of body weight, a polished light-weight board may be used to bridge the gap between the bed and the chair, and the patient slides across on it. This board (or bench) also may be used to transfer the patient from the chair to the toilet or the bathtub.

- Place one side of the transfer board under the patient's buttocks and the other side on the surface to which the transfer is being made, i.e., the chair.
- Instruct him to push up with his hands to shift the buttocks and then to slide across the board to the other surface.

There are other methods of transferring from the bed to the wheelchair when the patient is unable to stand. Figure 12-6 shows the weight and non-weight-bearing transfers, while Figure 12-7 shows the vertical transfer of a paraplegic patient.

Preparation for Ambulation

Regaining the ability to walk is a prime morale builder. To be prepared for ambulation—whether with braces, cane, or crutches—the patient must be strengthened and conditioned. *Exercise is the foundation of preparation.* By performing mat and parallel-bar exercises, the patient develops balance and coordination and strengthens his muscles. The following are preconditioning exercises that the nurse can teach and supervise.

To strengthen the muscles needed for ambulation, *quadriceps setting* is used. The quadriceps muscles are also guardians of the knee joint. Strengthening of these muscles acts as a deterrent to flexion contractures or instability of the knee. The patient contracts the quadriceps muscle while attempting to push the popliteal area against the mattress and at the same time raising the heel. He maintains the muscle contracture until the count of five and relaxes for the count of five. He should repeat this exercise 10 to 15 times hourly. In *gluteal setting,* he contracts or "pinches" the buttocks together until the count of five, relaxes for the count of five, and repeats.

To strengthen the muscles of the upper extremities, which are used for handling the cane, crutches, or walker employed in early ambulation, *sit-ups* are helpful. While in a sitting position, the patient raises his body from the chair by pushing his hands against the chair seat (or mattress). He also should be encouraged to do *push-ups* while in a prone position. Teach him to *raise his arms* above his head and lower them in a slow, rhythmical manner while holding traction weights—gradually increasing the poundage of the weights. He can *strengthen his hands* by crumpling newspaper and squeezing a rubber ball. *Pull-ups* on a trapeze, while lifting the body, is another effective conditioner.

Crutch-walking

In the treatment of various forms of arthritis and of most fractures of the lower extremity, and after operations on the leg—especially after amputation—crutches provide a convenient method for getting from one place to another. Since crutch-walking is not an inherited skill, it must be taught, and this learning process must begin early. One of the first prerequisites is to develop power in the shoulder girdle and upper extremities which will bear the patient's weight while he is crutch-walking. One way to strengthen these muscles is to use parallel bars in preparation for crutch-walking.

The following muscle groups are important for crutch-walking:

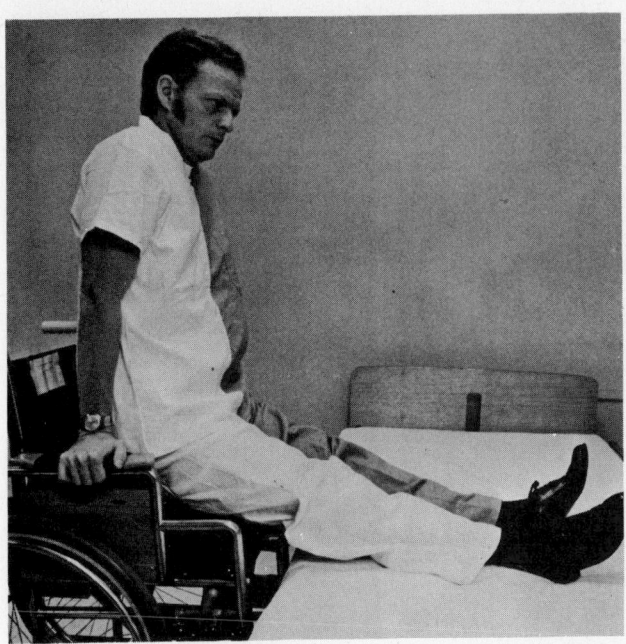 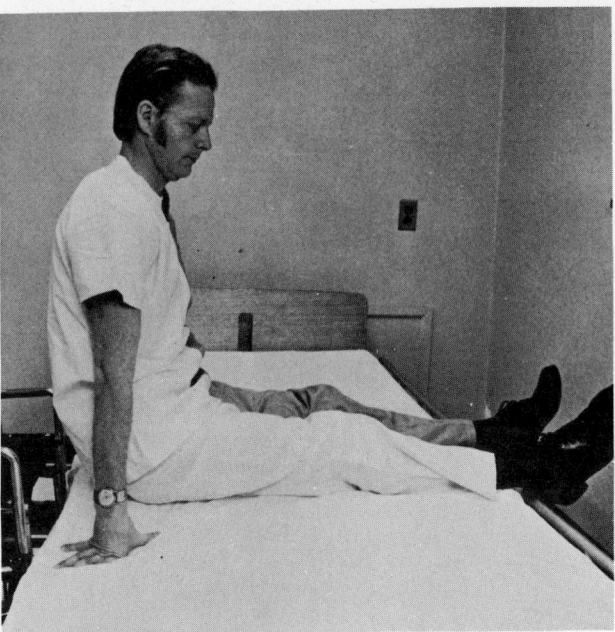

Figure 12-7.   Vertical transfer of a paraplegic patient. The wheelchair is placed facing the bed with the wheels locked and the pedals in the "down" position. The patient pushes up on his hands and arms and slides his body forward onto the bed. This is a non-weight-bearing transfer in which the patient is able to transfer on the same level. With conditioning and practice, this transfer can be done to a higher or lower level by the push-up method.

1. Arm flexors — to move the crutches forward
2. Forearm flexors — to hold the crutch at the correct angle
3. Finger and thumb flexors — to grip the crutches
4. Wrists and dorsiflexors — to keep hands on the hand pieces
5. Shoulder girdle depressors and downward rotators — to support the body on the crutches when the body is raised from the floor

Of equal importance is psychological preparation, which can be developed long before the physical need is present. The individual needs of each patient must be considered and the methods of approach directed to them. The patient's age, his interests, and his future intentions, as well as his prognosis, are essential factors.

MEASUREMENT FOR CRUTCHES.   Adjustable crutches are practical because the disease may cause changes in the muscles and the joints, or because the patient may improve and progress to a different crutch base and gait.

To measure a standing patient for crutches, measure 3.75–5.0 cm. (1½ to 2 inches) from the axillary fold to a position on the floor 10 cm. (4 inches) in front of the patient and 15 cm. (6 inches) to the side of his toes. (This is merely an approximate measure. It is desirable to have a 2-finger width insertion between the axillary fold and the armpiece.)

If the patient has to be measured while lying down, measure from the anterior fold of the axilla to the sole of the foot, and then add 5 cm. (2 inches). Another method is to determine the height of the patient and subtract 40 cm. (16 inches).

The hand piece should allow 20 to 30 degrees of flexion at the elbow. The wrist should be extended and the hand dorsiflexed. The patient should wear shoes that fit well and have firm soles. The crutches should be fitted with large rubber suction tips before measuring.

The maintenance of an erect posture is essential to crutch-walking. Before trying to use crutches, the patient should learn to stand by a chair on the unaffected leg in order to achieve balance. The nurse explains and demonstrates to the patient how he should manipulate his crutches before he attempts to do so.

CRUTCH STANCE.   The *tripod position* is the basic crutch stance. The crutches rest approximately 20–25 cm. (8 to 10 inches) in front and to the side of the patient's toes. This gives the strongest and most balanced support. Since, to provide stability, a greater height requires a broader base, a taller patient needs a wider base and a shorter patient a narrower base.

The patient must be taught to support his weight on the hand piece (Fig. 12-8). If the weight is borne on the axilla, the pressure of the crutch can damage the brachial plexus nerves and produce "crutch paralysis." A foam rubber pad on the underarm piece will relieve pressure on the upper arm and the thoracic cage.

Ability to shift body weight is the next step. The crutch gait selected depends on the nature of the patient's disability. The nurse must know how much (if any) weight can be placed on the affected side and whether the crutches are being used for balance and support.

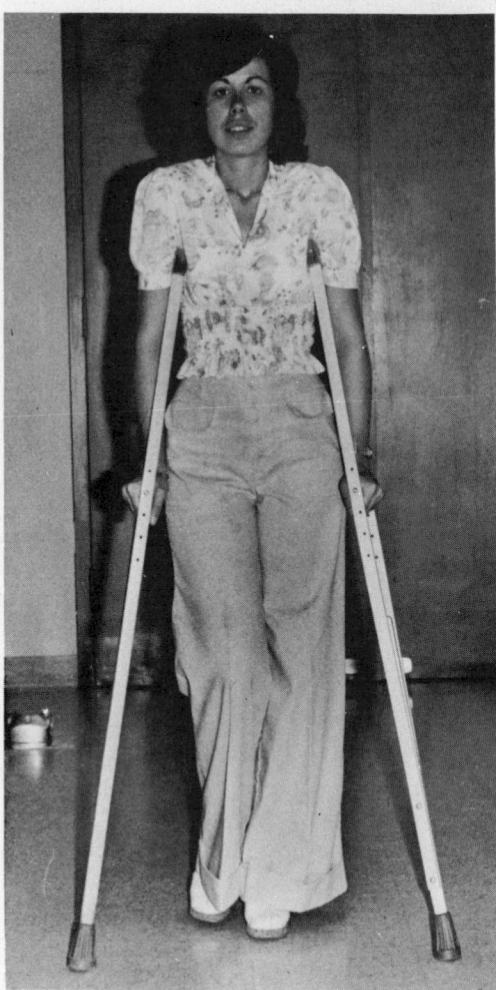

Figure 12-8. The tripod position for the basic crutch stance. Note that the patient's weight is borne not in the axilla but on the palm of the hand. (Courtesy, National Orthopedic and Rehabilitation Hospital.)

CRUTCH GAITS. The selection of the crutch gait depends on the type and severity of the disability and on the patient's physical condition, arm and trunk strength, and body balance. The patient should be taught two gaits so that he may change from one to another. Shifting crutch gaits relieves fatigue since each gait requires the use of a different combination of muscles. (If a muscle is forced to contract steadily without relaxing, the circulation of the blood to the part is reduced.) A faster gait can be used for making speed, whereas a slower one is used in crowded places.

All gaits begin in the tripod position. The more common gaits are the 4-point, the 2-point, the 3-point, and the swinging-to and swinging-through gaits. The sequence of movements for each of these gaits is listed in the chart which follows.

The patient should not practice crutch-walking for too long, especially if he has been in bed for a prolonged period. Such signs as sweating or shortness of breath

GAITS FOR CRUTCH-WALKING

4-POINT GAIT

This gait can be used when supported weight bearing is permitted for both legs. It is safe and gives maximal balance because there are always three points of contact with the floor; thus it is slow because it requires constant shifting of weight.

Sequence:
1. right crutch
2. left foot
3. left crutch
4. right foot

2-POINT GAIT

This gait is faster, since there are only two points of contact with the floor at one time.

Sequence:
1. Advance right crutch and left foot.
2. Simultaneously shift weight and advance left crutch and right foot.

THE 3-POINT GAIT

This is a faster gait but requires more strength and balance. The patient must be able to support his entire body weight on his arms.

Sequence:
1. Advance the weaker leg and both crutches simultaneously.
2. Advance the stronger lower extremity.

THE SWINGING-TO AND SWINGING-THROUGH GAITS

These gaits are more advanced.
Swinging-to Gait:
Sequence:
1. Bear weight on good leg.
2. Place crutches at an equal distance ahead of you.
3. Swing to a position that is even with the crutches.
4. Weight is shifted to the palm of the hands and back to the good leg.

Swinging-through Gait:
Sequence:
1. Lift both legs off the ground simultaneously and swing forward while pushing up on the crutches.
2. Advance crutches forward.
3. Lift and swing body beyond the crutches.

should be indications that the lesson on crutches should be stopped and the patient permitted to rest or go back to bed.

OTHER CRUTCH MANEUVERING TECHNIQUES. Before a patient is sent home on crutches, it is important to ascertain whether or not he can dress himself, get in and out of chairs, on and off the toilet, in and out of doors, up and down stairs and ramps, and in and out of a car, taxi, or public conveyance.

The following procedures should be taught to the patient.

TO GO DOWN STAIRS:

Walk forward as far as possible on the step. Advance crutches to the lower step. The weaker leg is advanced first and then the stronger one. In this way the stronger extremity shares the work of raising and lowering the body weight with the patient's arms.

TO GO UP STAIRS:

Advance the stronger leg first up to the next step. Then advance the crutches and the weaker extremity. (Strong leg goes up first and comes down last.) A memory device for the patient is "up with the good; down with the bad."

TO SIT IN A CHAIR:

Grasp the crutches at the hand pieces for control and bend forward slightly while assuming a sitting position.

TO STAND UP:

Place one or both feet in a wide stance under the chair or as close to the chair as possible. Grasp the hand pieces of the crutches (one in each hand or both hand pieces in one hand). Push down on the hand pieces while raising the body to a standing position.

Ambulation with a Cane

A cane is used to help the patient walk with greater balance and support. It also relieves the pressure on weight-bearing joints. To fit the patient for a cane, have him flex his elbow at a 30 degree angle and hold the cane 15 cm. (6 inches) lateral to the base of his fifth toe. Adjust the cane so that the handle is approximately level with the greater trochanter. An adjustable aluminum cane fitted with a gently flaring tip that has flexible and concentric rings gives optimum stability and enables the patient to walk with greater speed and less fatigue.

CANE-FOOT SEQUENCE:

1. Hold the cane fairly close to the body to prevent leaning.
2. Hold the cane on the unaffected (good) side.
3. Advance the cane at the same time the affected leg is moved.

To go up and down stairs:

1. Step up on the unaffected extremity.
2. Then place the cane and affected extremity up on the step.
3. Reverse this procedure for descending steps. (Strong leg goes up first and comes down last).

ASSISTING WITH PROSTHETIC AND ORTHOTIC APPLIANCES

A *prosthesis* is an artificial replacement for a missing portion of the body. An *orthosis* (commonly known as a brace) is an orthopedic device or appliance used to provide support and alignment, prevent or correct defor-

mities, and improve the function of the body. A prosthetist or an orthotist fits these appliances only by prescription of the physician.*

Preprosthetic Care

The nurse performs an essential function in the preprosthetic phase of the patient's care by helping him to develop an attitude of realistic hopefulness and by preventing deformities so that the time between the healing of the tissues and the fitting of the prosthesis is kept to a minimum. In the amputation of an extremity, the physical therapist (or the nurse) is responsible for bandaging the stump correctly, so that proper shrinkage and shaping of the stump occurs and the patient can be fitted more effectively with a prosthesis (see pages 1315-1316).

Braces

A *brace* is a support that protects weakened muscles, prevents and corrects deformities, immobilizes and protects a diseased or injured joint, protects painful, inflamed or healing tissue, and aids in the control of involuntary muscle movements. Thus braces are supportive, corrective, and protective as well as dynamic (with springs, cables and elastic bands) and preventive.

Clinical indications for bracing include pain, weakness, or paralysis of a part of the body. The patient is fitted for a brace according to the prescription of the physician. In recent years, synthetics, particularly thermoplastics, have been used in braces. They are functional, lighter, and more cosmetically acceptable to the patient. Velcro straps are also gaining increasing usage.

In caring for a patient wearing a brace, the nurse has the major responsibility of encouraging him to continue under the supervision of a competent therapist or orthotist until he can wear the appliance with ease. It is also important to encourage the patient to wear the brace as directed and check to see that it is not applied too tightly and that no skin problems or pressure sores are developing from the brace.

The following are the main points to emphasize in teaching the patient to care for braces:

1. Place the brace on a table or the floor, or prop it against the wall when it is not in use; hanging may cause distortion of its position.
2. Twisting of the brace may occur with use; check alignment frequently. Look down the full length of the brace. The joints should coincide with the body joints.
3. Before putting a brace on, check carefully for worn areas,

---

*Specific prostheses are described later in this book, when the clinical conditions calling for them are discussed, e.g., limb prostheses for the amputee and a breast prosthesis for the patient who has had a radical mastectomy. Information concerning prosthetic and orthopedic appliances may be obtained also from The American Orthotic and Prosthetic Association, 1440 N Street, N.W., Washington, D.C. 20005.

missing or loose screws, and the condition of straps and buckles.

4. Pressure areas may occur if metal or plastic rubs the skin. Check the skin for reddened areas immediately after removing the brace.
5. Keep the heels and soles of the shoes in good condition.
6. Clean and dry the brace, when necessary, at night.
7. To clean the plastic parts:
   a. Wipe the plastic parts with a damp cloth.
   b. Do not oil plastic surfaces and joints.
8. To clean the metal parts:
   a. Remove rust or corrosion spots with steel wool.
   b. Clean dirt out of metal joints and locks with a pipe cleaner dipped in a solvent.
   c. Clean the metal parts with a solvent.
   d. Apply a light coat of paste wax to the metal parts to prevent rust.
   e. Put oil in metal joints with an eyedropper or toothpick.
9. Have the brace checked periodically.

HELPING TO OVERCOME ELIMINATION PROBLEMS

Urinary and bowel incontinence are frequent problems in the disabled patient. Bladder and bowel control are important functions of the body and are influenced by prescribed social behavior. Incontinence may curtail a person's independence and limit his sense of social acceptance. Patients with various medical and surgical conditions have to be trained to regain control of these functions.

Bladder Training

Incontinence should not be regarded as inevitable in any patient, since bladder training is an available alternative in most instances. This facet of care (bladder training) is a part of nursing function.

True incontinence may be caused by obvious urologic problems or by congenital or acquired neurologic disease. Neurologic incontinence and its management are discussed on pages 914–916.

For patients with incontinence from other causes, the key to successful urinary control is:

- sufficient fluid intake (2,500 ml. daily)
- establishment of regular times to void, i.e., a habit pattern

A schedule is set up with definite times indicated for the patient to try to empty his bladder using either the bedpan or the toilet. The interval between voidings in the early phase of the training period is fairly short (1½ to 2 hours), but as the patient's bladder capacity increases, the interval is lengthened. A suggested procedure is to give a measured amount of fluid every 2 hours. After drinking, the patient waits for 30 minutes and then attempts to void. He gradually lengthens the period between voiding times. (It is best to give larger amounts of fluid during the day and to withhold fluids after 5 P.M.)

The patient is encouraged to hold his urine until the specified voiding time. Usually, there is a relationship between drinking, eating, exercising, and voiding, and the alert patient soon can determine his own intake schedule. Have the patient keep a written voiding schedule which will give a continuous record of the time and amounts of fluid ingested and the time and amount of each voiding. Regularity is the key to success. To assist in the act of voiding the patient should either stand or sit with the thighs flexed and the feet and the back supported. Increasing intra-abdominal pressure by massage over the bladder or by leaning forward while sitting will help to initiate evacuation of the bladder.

For the confused elderly patient, watch and determine when he is incontinent and take him to the bathroom before involuntary voiding occurs. Create an environment which keeps sensory monotony to a minimum. Orient the patient to time and place. Extend his social environment beyond the confines of his room and try to increase the number of his social contacts. An alarm clock may be set at regular intervals throughout the day and several times during the night to remind the patient to void. The patient must approve of the program and have a sincere desire to establish control. It may take several weeks to accomplish this end; patience and persistence on the part of both nurse and patient plus expressions of approval for even slight gains are necessary. It is also important to encourage the patient to continue with self-care and the exercise and occupational therapy programs—boredom and frustration can lead to incontinence. Have the patient wear his own clothing, since this enhances his self-esteem and dignity and is a strong deterrent to regressive behavior. The use of a diaper at any time is discouraged, because its psychological effect is one of regression rather than progression.

Bowel Training

The objectives of a bowel training program are to develop regular bowel habits and to prevent fecal incontinence, impaction, and irregularity.

- The first essential step in bowel training that requires reflex assistance is the establishment of regularity.

Any attempts at evacuation should be made within 15 minutes of the same time daily. An active aid to bowel evacuation is the stimulation of peristalsis and the gastrocolic and duodenocolic reflexes. Therefore, the patient should establish his bowel evacuation time after a regularly scheduled meal. One of the best times is after breakfast. However, if the patient has a previously established habit pattern, it should be followed.

Physical activity is another helpful aid to peristaltic activity and bowel movement. Unless contraindicated by other existing conditions, the diet should include adequate roughage and a fluid intake between 2,000 and

4,000 ml. daily. Prune juice or fig juice (120 ml.) taken 30 minutes before a meal once daily is helpful when constipation is a problem.

The reflex habit should be established by regularity early in the course of the patient's illness. It may be aided by mechanical means. About 30 minutes before the scheduled bowel time, a glycerine suppository is inserted into the rectum in order to stimulate the anorectal reflex. After the scheduled interval, the patient is encouraged to attempt to have a bowel movement. If at all possible he should assume the normal position for defecation. Instruct him to bear down and to contract his abdominal muscles. If need be, he can lean forward to increase intra-abdominal pressure. The patient may be taught to apply pressure to the abdominal wall to assist with defecation.

After this routine is well established, mechanical stimulation with the suppository probably will not be necessary, and in a few weeks the patient will be having regular daily bowel movements.

PROMOTING CONTINUITY OF PATIENT CARE

The objective of a referral system is to maintain continuity of care when the patient is transferred from the health care facility to his home or an extended care facility. It is ideal to begin formulating a plan for discharge when the patient is first admitted to the hospital. The patient's functional potential is estimated by the rehabilitation team, and discharge plans are made with this in mind.

Frequently the community health nurse is the case finder whose astute observations make the rehabilitation services possible for the patient. By visiting the patient in the hospital, the community health nurse is able to see what adjustments will have to be made in the home. It may be necessary to help the family select, improvise, or borrow needed equipment from another agency. Plan with the patient ways and methods of coping with problems that may arise. Prior to discharge, the patient may experience "separation anxiety" as he realizes that he is leaving the protected environment of the hospital. Give him increased support and encouragement to ease him through this phase.

The family will need to know as much about the patient's condition and care as possible so that they will not fear his return home. Their attitude toward the patient, his disability, and his return home, should be assessed. After the patient comes home, the community health nurse makes sure that he does not "lose ground" and that he is able to maintain the independence that he gained in the hospital.

Not all families can be expected to carry on the arduous programs of exercise and physical training that a patient

may need. The family may require family therapy to allow them to discuss and explore their feelings and attitudes (rejection, aversion, avoidance) toward the disabled family member.

The Activities of Daily Living Sheet is sent home with the patient so that the community nurse knows exactly what activities the patient can perform. The nurse continues to reinforce the teaching that has been done and helps the patient to achieve attainable goals. The degree to which he adapts to his home and community environment depends on the confidence and self-esteem developed during his rehabilitation program and on the acceptance and reactions of his family, employer, and community members.

If the patient is transferred to an extended care facility, his ADL Sheet goes with him to orient the staff to activities that he can perform independently.

The Rehabilitation Services Administration provides services whereby disabled persons or those disadvantaged by advanced age or other conditions obtain the help they need to engage in gainful employment. These services are provided by state agencies and include diagnostic, medical, surgical, psychiatric, and hospital services, and assistance in securing prosthetic appliances. There is a counseling, training, placement, and follow-up service available to help the patient to select and attain a vocational objective.

A selected list of agencies and organizations, both governmental and private, that work with or for patients needing rehabilitation services is listed on page 205.

BIBLIOGRAPHY

BOOKS

American Academy of Orthopaedic Surgeons: Atlas of Orthotics: Biomechanical Principles and Applications. St. Louis, C. V. Mosby, 1975.

American Nurses Association Division on Medical-Surgical Nursing Practice and the Association of Rehabilitation Practice: Standards of Rehabilitation Nursing Practice. Kansas City, ANA, 1977.

Basmajian, J. V., ed.: Therapeutic Exercise, 3rd ed., Baltimore, Williams and Wilkins, 1978.

Bender, M., et al.: Teaching the Moderately and Severely Handicapped. Baltimore, University Park Press, 1976.

Bonner, C. D.: Homburger and Bonner's Medical Care and Rehabilitation of the Aged and Chronically Ill. Boston, Little, Brown, 1974.

Boroch, R. M.: Elements of Rehabilitation in Nursing. St. Louis, C. V. Mosby, 1976.

Cash, J. E., ed.: A Textbook of Medical Conditions for Physiotherapists. Philadelphia, J. B. Lippincott, 1976.

Christopherson, V. A., Coulter, P. P., and Wolanin, M. O.: Rehabilitation Nursing: Perspectives and Applications. New York, McGraw-Hill, 1974.

Cobb, A. B.: Medical and Psychological Aspects of Disability. Springfield, Charles C Thomas, 1973.

Daniels, L., and Worthingham, C.: Therapeutic Exercise for Body Alignment and Function, 2nd ed., Philadelphia, W. B. Saunders, 1977.

Garrett, J. F., and Levine, E. S.: Rehabilitation Practices with the Physically Disabled. New York. Columbia University Press, 1973.

Gilbert, A.: You Can Do It From A Wheelchair. New Rochelle, N.Y., Arlington House Publishers, 1973.

Goldenson, R. M., Dunham, J. R., and Dunham, C. S.: Disability and Rehabilitation Handbook. N.Y., McGraw-Hill, 1978.

Hardy, R. E., ed., et al.: Severe Disabilities. Springfield, Charles C Thomas, 1974.

Hirschberg, G. G., Lewis, L., and Vaughan, P.: Rehabilitation: A Manual for the Disabled and Elderly, 2nd ed. Philadelphia, J. B. Lippincott, 1976.

Hollis, M.: Practical Exercise Therapy. Philadelphia, J. B. Lippincott, 1976.

Ince, L. P.: Behavior Modification in Rehabilitation Medicine. Springfield, Charles C Thomas, 1976.

————: The Rehabilitation Medicine Services. Springfield, Charles C Thomas, 1974.

Kenedi, R. M., and Cowden, J. M., eds. Bed Sore Biomechanics. London, Macmillan Press Ltd., 1975.

Laurie, G.: Housing and Home Services for the Disabled. Hagerstown, Md., Harper and Row, 1977.

Levitan, S. A., and Taggart, R.: Jobs for the Disabled. Baltimore, Johns Hopkins University Press, 1977.

Marinelli, R. P., and Dell-Orto, A. E.: The Psychological and Social Impact of Physical Disability. New York, Springer, 1977.

May, E. E., et al.: Independent Living for the Handicapped and the Elderly. Boston, Houghton Mifflin, 1974.

Meislin, J.: Rehabilitation Medicine and Psychiatry. Springfield, Charles C Thomas, 1976.

Murdoch, G., ed.: The Advance in Orthotics. Baltimore, Williams and Wilkins, 1976.

Nichols, P. J. R.: Rehabilitation Medicine: The Management of Physical Disabilities. London, Butterworth, 1976.

Perske, R., et al.: Mealtimes for Severely and Profoundly Handicapped Persons. Baltimore, University Park Press, 1977.

Robinault, I. P., ed.: Functional Aids for the Multiply Handicapped. Hagerstown, Md., Harper and Row. 1973.

Rosen, M., Clark, G. R., and Kivitz, M. S.: Habilitation of the Handicapped. Baltimore, University Park Press, 1977.

Rusalem, H., and Milikin, D., eds.: Contemporary Rehabilitation. New York, New York University Press, 1976.

Rusk, H. A.: Rehabilitation Medicine. St. Louis, C. V. Mosby, 1977.

Shestack, R.: Handbook of Physical Therapy, 3rd ed. New York, Springer, 1977.

Shivers, J. S., et al.: Therapeutic and Adapted Recreational Services. Philadelphia, Lea and Febiger, 1975.

Sister Kenny Institute Staff: Introduction to Bowel and Bladder Care. Minneapolis, Sister Kenny Institute, 1975.

Sister Kenny Institute Staff: Nursing Care of the Skin, rev. ed. Minneapolis, Sister Kenny Institute, 1975.

Sister Kenny Institute Staff: Wheelchair Selection: More than Choosing a Chair with Wheels, rev. ed. Minneapolis, Sister Kenny Institute, 1977.

Sorenson, L., et al.: Ambulation Guide for Nurses. Minneapolis, Sister Kenny Institute, 1974.

Stryker, R.: Rehabilitative Aspects of Acute and Chronic Nursing Care, 2nd ed. Philadelphia, W. B. Saunders, 1977.

Stubbins, J., ed.: Social and Psychological Aspects of Disability. Baltimore, University Park Press, 1977.

Valletutti, P. J., and Christoplos, F., eds.: Interdisciplinary Approaches to Human Services. Baltimore, University Park Press, 1977.

Washburn, K. B.: Physical Medicine and Rehabilitation: A Practitioner's Guide. New York, Medical Examination Pub. Co., 1976.

ARTICLES

Principles and Philosophy of Rehabilitation

Garrett, J. F.: Professionalism in rehabilitation in the 1980's. Arch. Phys. Med. Rehabil., 57:93-97, March, 1976.

Hein, E., and Leavitt, M.: Providing emotional support to patients. Nursing '77, 7:39-41, May 1977.

Kowalsky, E. L.: Grief: A lost life-style. AJN, 78:418-420, Mar. 1978.

Niles, B.: The nurse makes rehabilitation really happen. Occup. Health & Safety, 46:14-16, May-June, 1977.

Rusk, H. A.: Rehabilitation knowledge in search of understanding. Arch. Phys. Med. Rehabil., 59:156-160, Apr. 1978.

Sink, J.: Trends in rehabilitation. J. Rehabil., 43:36-40, Jan.-Apr. 1977.

Steger, H. G.: Understanding the psychologic factors in rehabilitation. Geriatrics, 31:68-73, May, 1976.

Wilke, H. H.: Creating the caring community. Arch. Phys. Med. Rehabil., 58:97-100, Mar. 1977.

Pressure Sores

Barton, A. A.: Prevention of pressure sores. Nurs. Times, 73:1593-1595, Oct. 13, 1977.

Berger, E. M., and DeGregories, P.: Decubitus ulcers. An ounce of prevention. Phys. Ther., 56:1374-1375, Dec. 1976.

El-Toraei, I., and Chung, B.: The management of pressure sores. J. Dermatol. Surg. Oncol., 3:507-511, Sept.-Oct., 1977.

Fulghum, D. D.: Ascorbic acid revisited. Arch. Der., 113:91-92, Jan. 1977.

Gruis, M. L., and Innes, B.: Assessment: Essential to prevent pressure sores. AJN, 76:1762-1764, Nov. 1976.

Jungreis, S. W.: Exercises for expediting mobility in bedridden patients. Nursing '77, 7:47-51, Aug. 1977.

Kavchak-Keyes, M. A.: Four proven steps for preventing decubitus ulcers. Nursing '77, 7:58-61, Sept. 1977.

Stewart, P., and Wharton, G. W.: Bridging: An effective and practical method of preventive skin care for the immobilized person. South. Med. J., 69:1469-1473, Nov. 1976.

Tepperman, P. S., et al.: Pressure sores: Prevention and step-up management. Postgrad. Med., 62:83-89, Sept. 1977.

Wilson, R.: The MUD bed and its implications for nursing care. Nurs. Clin. N. Am., 11:725-730, Dec. 1976.

Rehabilitation Practices

Alves, R., and Martin, T. A.: An overview of orthotics and prosthetics. ONA J., *4*:231-235, Sept. 1977.

Ford, J. R., and Duckworth, B.: Moving a dependent patient safely, comfortably: Part I, positioning. Nursing '76, *6*:27-36, Jan. 1976.

Foss, G.: Breaking the architectural barrier with crutches, wheelchairs and walkers. Nursing '73, *3*:16-31, Oct. 1973.

Gordon, M.: Assessing activity tolerance. AJN, *76*:72-75, Jan. 1976.

Habeeb, M. C., and Kallstrom, M. D.: Bowel program for institutionalized adults. AJN, *76*:606-608, Apr. 1976.

Hirschberg, G. G., Lewis, L., and Vaughan, P.: Promoting patient mobility. Nursing '77, *7*:42-47, May 1977.

Jefcoate, R.: Electronic technology for disabled people. Rehabil. Lit., *38*:110-115, Apr. 1977.

Long, B. C., and Buergin, P. S.: The pivot transfer. AJN, *77*:980-982, June 1977.

Perry, J., ed.: Upper extremity orthotics. Phys. Ther., *58*:264-320, Mar. 1978.

Sexuality and the Disabled

BOOKS

Barnard, M. U., Clancy, B. J., and Krantz, K. E., eds.: Human Sexuality for Health Professionals. Philadelphia, W. B. Saunders, 1978.

Beach, F. A., ed.: Human Sexuality in Four Perspectives. Baltimore, Johns Hopkins University Press, 1977.

Browning, M. H., and Lewis, E. P., eds.: Human Sexuality: Nursing Implications. New York, American Journal of Nursing Company, 1973.

Dunham, C. S.: Social-sexual relationships. *In* Goldenson, R. M., et al., eds: Disability and Rehabilitation Handbook, pp. 28-35. New York, McGraw-Hill, 1978.

Green, R., ed.: Human Sexuality: A Health Practitioner's Text. Baltimore, Williams and Wilkins, 1975.

Greengross, W.: Entitled to Love: The Sexual and Emotional Needs of the Handicapped. London, Malaby Press, 1976.

Heslinga, K., Schellen, A., and Verkuyla, A.: Not Made of Stone: The Sexual Problems of Handicapped People. Springfield, Charles C Thomas, 1974.

Robinault, I. P.: Sex, Society and the Disabled. Hagerstown, Md., Harper and Row, 1978.

Woods, N. F.: Human Sexuality in Health and Illness. St. Louis, C. V. Mosby, 1975.

ARTICLES

Berkman, A. H., Weissman, R., and Frielich, M. H.: Sexual adjustment of spinal cord injured veterans living in the community. Arch. Phys. Med. Rehab., *59*:29-33, Jan. 1978.

Finch, E.: Sexuality and the disabled. Canad. Nurse, *73*:19-20, Jan. 1977.

Griffin, E. R., Tomko, M. A., and Timms, R. J.: Sexual function in spinal-cord injured patients: Rev. Arch. Phys. Med. Rehab. *54*:539-543, Dec. 1973.

Krozy, R.: Becoming comfortable with sexual assessment. AJN, *78*:1036-1038, June 1978.

MacRae, I., and Henderson, G.: Sexuality and irreversible health limitations. Nurs. Clin. N. Am. *10*:587-597, Sept. 1975.

Paradowski, W.: Socialization patterns and sexual problems of the institutionalized chronically ill and physically disabled. Arch. Phys. Med. Rehab. *58*:53-59, Feb. 1977.

Rosenbaum, M.: Sexuality and the physically disabled: The role of the professional. Bull. N. Y. Acad. Med. *54*:501-509, May 1978.

Vemireddi, N. K.: Sexual counseling for chronically disabled patients. Geriatrics, *33*:65-69, July 1978.

Zalar, M.: Human sexuality — a component of total patient care. Nurs. Dig. *3*:40-43, Nov.-Dec. 1975.

AGENCIES

Governmental

Department of Health, Education, and Welfare, Washington, D.C. 20201.:

Office of Education: Bureau of Education for the Handicapped.

Office of Human Development: Architectural and Transportation Barriers Compliance Board; Clearinghouse on the Handicapped; Developmental Disabilities Office; National Clearinghouse on Aging; President's Committee on Mental Retardation; Rehabilitation Services Administration; Public Services Administration.

Social Security Administration.

Department of Housing and Urban Development (HUD), Washington, D.C. 20410.:

Elderly and Handicapped Policy Office.

Department of Labor, Washington, D.C. 20201.:

President's Committee on Employment of the Handicapped.

Veterans Administration, Washington, D.C. 20420.

Voluntary Organizations

Consult Directory of National Information Sources on Handicapping Conditions and Related Services. (Prepared by Clearinghouse on the Handicapped, Office for Handicapped Individuals, Office of Human Development, U.S. Department of Health, Education, and Welfare.) *This directory contains abstracts and addresses of 270 organizations offering services, information and resources to handicapped individuals.*

Obtained from: Superintendent of Documents, Government Printing Office, Washington, D.C. 20420.

Geriatrics, i.e., care of the aged, has come to deserve specific emphasis in the nursing curriculum. This specialty has as its prime concern the health and the well-being of a large and important segment of the patient population, and it deals with problems of therapy and rehabilitation that are inherently and uniquely complex. Thus, the whole field of gerontology, the study of the aging process and its effects on older persons, becomes more important with each passing day.

Aging is a normal process of time-related change that occurs throughout life. It involves all aspects of the organism and is largely characterized by a decline in functional efficiency and decreased capacity to compensate and recover from stress. It does not necessarily occur in an interrelated or synchronous manner, but it does involve physiological, psychological, and social changes that interact to influence behavior and adaptation. Old age is a normal part of human development and is the final phase of the life cycle. Aging is not something that happens to the other person but is a unique and highly personal experience that affects everyone who lives long enough. Successful adaptation to the aging process probably correlates with the person's previous ability to cope and adapt to change. Other influences include environmental factors, education, and sociocultural determinants as well as the health status of the entire body.

In the past, society tended to shrug off the problems of the aged, possibly because the signs of aging are visible and may stimulate anxiety in younger persons concerning their own mortality. Also, there has been some reluctance to invest too much time and effort in the aged because they are at the end of their life span. However, as the debilitating effects of disease, disability, and various social problems are reduced and eliminated, it becomes a challenge to visualize those normal developmental processes that continue into old age: creativity, life experience, perspective, and judgment.

As a result of current research and observation, new concepts have developed with respect to the quantity and quality of human life. The current generation is described as the generation of the "active elderly." Scientific progress points to projections of greater life expectancies and to a vastly improved quality of life in the years to come. This *quality* of a person's life should be the special concern of those in the helping professions: physicians, psychiatrists, psychologists, social workers, clergymen, and nurses.

DEVELOPMENTAL CONCEPTS OF THE LIFE CYCLE

Mature Adulthood

Adulthood is not a period of stability and certainty but one of change. The changes that occur during this stage of life have no absolute chronological or sequential order, although certain events are biologically, psychologically, and socially determined or expected. The impact of the change, which often includes new sets of relationships, new expectations, and altered or modified self-evaluation, inevitably involves the adult in transitions or turning points. The events of adult life entail either role gains or role losses. For example, getting married, having a child, obtaining a job, and receiving a promotion are usually perceived as role gains; getting divorced, being chronically ill, retiring from work, going through menopause, and being widowed are perceived as role losses.

The main themes of adulthood include *stress, stocktaking,* and *shifts in time perspective* and *locus of control.*

Major stresses are caused by events that upset the sequence and rhythm of the life cycles—as when the death of a parent occurs during a person's childhood rather than in middle age; when marriage does not come at its desired or appropriate time; when the birth of a child occurs too early or too late; when occupational achievement is delayed; when grandparenthood, retirement, major illness, or widowhood occur in an atypical time frame.

The primary source of stress for middle-aged men is their work. For middle-aged women, stress is related to their concern for their husbands' work and health and with events in the lives of their children.

Although adults of any age may go through the process of reassessment, the "stock-taking" of middle age is characterized by a focus on the inner self, a concern with self-development, and a reexamination and reevaluation of competency. The period of "middlescence" often causes people to see their children as capable of getting more enjoyment from sex, love, and life in general than they can; and at the same time they are aware that their children view them as being on the decline. For some middle-aged people, the position of being "caught between two generations" intensifies a sense of loss and fear of aging and reconfirms the feeling that they are no longer masters of their fates and their environment.

People inclined toward this view may be described as having an external *locus of control,* so that they feel like puppets on a string, controlled by other people or by impersonal social forces or fate. On the other hand, people with an internal locus of control perceive themselves as having power over their own destiny. These are the middle-aged people who view middle adulthood as a period of maximum capacity which underscores their ability to handle a highly complex environment and more challenging self goals. In these people, stock-taking produces a renewed sense of self as they triumph over difficulties and develop new coping skills. For others, however, it is a time of feeling trapped, anxious, or panicked by life events. Many of these people become immobilized, are unable to act, and sink into deep depression.

One of the most startling events in middle age is a shift in time perspective; one starts thinking in terms of the time left to live, rather than the time lived since birth. This awareness of mortality appears to be somewhat more important to men than to women. Men become more conscious of their loss of strength and vitality, more preoccupied with their health, and more fearful that time is running out. Women become more concerned with the health of the significant people in their lives, particularly their spouses. Women may "rehearse for widowhood." However, like men, women become overwhelmingly aware that they have little time left. The shift in time perspective brings a confrontation with death, which now becomes a personal reality rather than something that happens to other people.

An awareness that life in middle age is not progressing as smoothly as expected may lead middle-aged adults to believe that they are abnormal. They often do not realize that other adults experience self-doubt, lost hopes, and feelings of inadequacy. One of the most important services rendered by members of the helping professions is to assure those people who are struggling with the "crisis" of middle age and aging that they are not alone and that what they feel is within the range of normal experience.

Developmental Theories and Themes of Aging

Certain theoretical models of human development help to point out important turning points during the late years of the life cycle. The theories concerning the life cycle incorporate the social, psychological, and biological factors of developmental growth and relate them to age to identify milestones and time development.

The theories of Buhler, Jung, and Erikson, which are considered to be three of the most prominent theories of adult development, have as a common theme the goal of personal resolution in the second half of life.

Buhler's theories were based on a collection of 400 biographies and autobiographies collected in the 1930s in Vienna; she developed a methodology for analyzing these biographies to reveal an orderly progression of phases based on changes in events, attitudes, and accomplishments during the life cycle.

Buhler perceived the period between 45 and 65 as the period of self-assessment of the results of striving for goals determined in early life stages. The period from 65 on is one of awareness of the experience of fulfillment or failure, and the remaining years are spent in either a continuance of previous activities or a return to the need-satisfying orientations of childhood. The conclusion from Buhler's studies is that the individual's assessment of whether he did or did not reach fulfillment was a more critical factor in how well he adjusted to old age than biological decline and insecurity. A person's own sense of having realized his goals and reached a sense of fulfillment may be the crucial final result of lifelong goal-setting and striving.

Jung saw no clear sense of meaning or purpose in old age in our society. He stated that although many people reach old age with unsatisfied demands, it is "fatal" for such persons to look back. It is essential that they have a goal in the future, in order to live the second half of life with as much purpose as the first. Jung suggested that in the second half of life the individual direct his attention inward, so that through an intensive inner exploration he may find a meaning and totality in life that makes the acceptance of death possible.

Erikson developed the concept of the eight ages of man, each representing crucial turning points in the life span that stretches from birth to death. Erikson's theory was more fully explored by Peck in an attempt to define more precisely the crucial issues of middle age and old age. According to this expanded theory, the years between 40 and 50 challenge those values which a person places on physical power in favor of the values placed on wisdom. People who cling to their waning physical powers become more and more depressed, but persons who shift to using their mental abilities as a primary resource appear to age more successfully. At this point in their lives, if men and women redefine themselves as individuals and companions, with less stress on the sexual element, then interpersonal relationships may take on a greater depth of understanding and enhance their marital union. People in their forties must make a shift in emotional openness. They must reach out to possible friends to supplant the loss of children leaving home, parents dying, and/or old friends leaving and/or dying.

As persons move along the life span, toward old age, there are three central issues to challenge them. First, to develop varied interests so that when they retire or when their children leave home they can engage in meaningful activities that offer a sense of satisfaction. Also, older people need to find comfort in human relations to transcend the illness and pain of their fragile bodies. Finally, the old person must be able to find a gratifying meaning for life in the future potential of his family, his ideas, his creations, or future generations, in general.

The theorists view the first part of life as growth and expansion, and the latter part of life as inner withdrawal and contraction. The tasks of later life involve finding meaning and wholeness in life and considerations about oncoming death. It would appear that a person's own sense of having realized, or not realized, chosen goals will be more critical in determining how successfully he adapts to aging than biological decline and personal insecurity.

Kinds of Aging

BIOLOGICAL AGING. Aging occurs with such changes as whitening of the hair, wrinkling of the skin and decline in eye focus and high-register hearing. The most serious change for most people is their heightened vulnerability to and lessened ability to recuperate from various illnesses. Biological aging, for each individual, depends on a combination of factors, including genetic inheritance, finances, and good health. However, biological aging is secondary to other problems in its impact on most people.

PSYCHOLOGICAL AGING. Psychological aging refers to a role which the individual assigns to himself as he reaches a certain chronological age. The two major threats felt by the older person are the deterioration of his concept of self, which results in loss of self-esteem, and extensive and continual grief over frequently occurring losses. People spend their lives attempting to enhance their self-concepts while simultaneously attempting to deter actions by themselves and others that would erode this concept.

The plight of the aged in a youth-oriented society continues to receive attention, and the process of gerontological counseling is now recognized as a specialized form of helping. Individually designed adaptive responses are the helping person's most effective tools.

Older persons are not (as sterotyping would lead us to believe) incapable, inactive, and deficient in intellect and sexual function. They do not spend their time complaining, reminiscing, talking of illnesses, and attending funerals.

The older person should be encouraged to see himself as in a dynamic period of growth, rather than in a period of rapid deterioration. Perceiving self with an ongoing continuous potential permits the older person to reflect, not ruminate, on the past, while continuing to cultivate a hopeful vision for the future.

The sense of psychological loss intensifies as the older person ages and vitality decreases, while vulnerability increases. Many older people become enraged at the helplessness they feel in the face of seemingly uncontrollable events, including the apparent attempts of other people to crush their individuality.

The older person, for the most part, wishes to be treated as a person of worth and dignity. He does not wish to be tolerated, indulged, patronized, or perceived as a pet. People working with and caring for the elderly should not consider them "cute little old ladies" or "dear little old men." Listening attentively, focusing the patients' attention on the here and now, and discussing with them their plans for the future will underscore the feeling that they are being related to as people, each unique and distinct from the other.

SOCIOGENIC AGING. Society imposes roles on people as they reach a certain chronological age. Older persons are seen by many people in our society as either *nonpeople* or *expendable people,* merely because they have lived longer. One of the major difficulties for older people is that their perceptions of themselves reflect the way society has viewed them and the manner in which they themselves have internalized these roles.

A significant amount of current research indicates that a large proportion of mental and attitudinal changes in old people do not arise from biological effects but rather from societal prescribed role definitions. Older people have been told by our society that they are supposed to be physically, socially, sexually, and intellectually infirm — slow in comprehending events going on around them and rigid in their ways of thinking and behaving.

Our society devalues people once they leave the ranks of the "employed." Yet society automatically retires a worker at the magical age of 70 years. Because educational institutions historically have prepared people to fill work-oriented roles, society tends to classify the elderly as "nonpeople" when they reach retirement. Society also seems to take the attitude that older people should run away and hide until they die. It is important to note that the combination of psychological and sociogenic aging causes more debilitation than biological aging for many people.

PROFILE OF THE AGING AMERICAN

The age "65" generally is thought of as the beginning of old age, but this figure has been rather arbitrarily selected for social (retirement) and legislative (Social Security) purposes. Some specialists in the field of gerontology refer to the "young old" as those in the 65 to 74 age group while the term "old old" is reserved for those over 75.

At present, over 11 percent of the population in the United States is over 65 years of age, and demographic projections suggest that the elderly may constitute about 13 to 21 percent of the population by the year 2030 (Fig. 13-1). People over age 65 are the fastest growing age group in this country and their numbers are expected to continue growing into the twenty-first century at a faster pace than the rest of the population. The projected life span average from birth for the female is 75.3 years and for the male, 67.6 years. Each day, there is a net increase of more than 1,400 persons of age 65 and over, and the number of older persons in the United States is already larger than the population of 22 states. The older a person is, the greater the probability of his living longer. The forces producing this phenomenon include medical advances that have reduced maternal and infant mortality and have enabled more people to live to old age.

The elderly population has become older. An analysis of the statistics reveals that those over 75 are the fastest growing segment of the senior citizen group. Although the numbers of people 60 years old and over have increased nearly 7 times since 1900, the 75-and-over age group has experienced a tenfold increase, and the 85-plus group has grown by about 17 times.

There are more older women among elderly people in general due to the longer life span of women. Most women are usually younger than their husbands and often outlive them by several years. Widows constitute 23 percent of women 60 to 64 years of age, whereas among those 70 to 75 years and older, the figure jumps to 70 percent. Most elderly widows live alone, one fourth of their number subsisting on incomes below the Federal government's poverty index.

Medical advances also have made an impact on blacks and other nonwhite races. Life expectancy in these groups has nearly doubled. The nonwhite elderly population is expected to grow about 300 percent by 2035, thereby increasing this proportion of the elderly population from one tenth to one sixth.

The popular picture of old people as frail, institutionalized beings is grossly misleading. Over 95 percent of older Americans live in the normal community, not in institutions, and an increasing number of these elderly people live alone. According to the latest statistics, the proportion of those living alone has increased from one sixth of all noninstitutionalized elderly persons in 1960 to one fourth. Again, this trend is most noticeable among elderly women and has resulted mainly because of the increased numbers of widows and the availability of greater financial security (supplemental Social Security income) and more and better coverage under private pension plans and health care support programs (Medicare).

Impact and Implications for Health Care

Persons in the 75-year-old and older group require additional resources to handle some of the unique physical and emotional problems which occur more frequently in this age group as a result of chronic disease and impairment. Members of the "old–old" group have more problems than do the "young old." Persons 75 and older spend an average of four and a half times as many days in short-stay hospitals as the national average and 70 percent more than persons who are 65 to 74 years of age. Three fourths of all nursing home residents are 75 or older and over one third are 85 and older. Thus there is greater

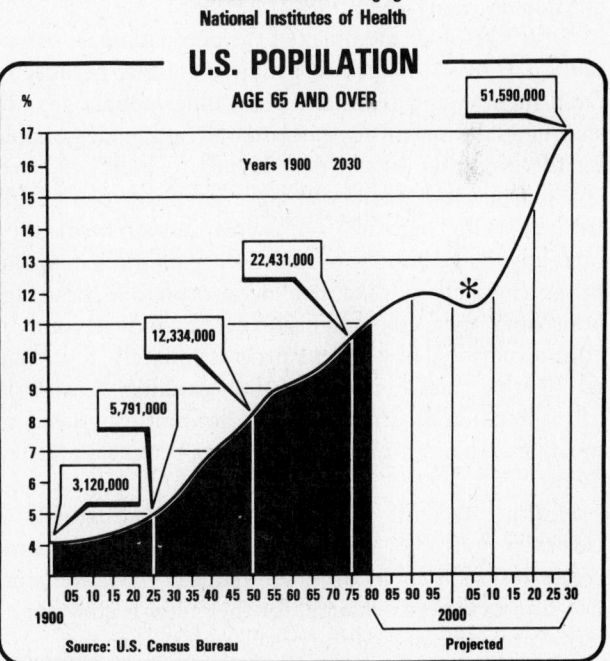

* Decrease due to lowered birth rate during depression of 1930's.

Figure 13-1.   Age Gauge—chart shows the percentage of the American population 65 and older from 1900; with predictions for 1980 to 2030. (National Institute on Aging, National Institutes of Health.)

demand for health practitioners, facilities, and supportive services for those over 75.

The social and economic backgrounds of many members of the "old-old" group differ from those of elderly citizens in the "young-old" group. Many were immigrants who had little formal education and worked throughout their lives for relatively low salaries. In the future more older persons will have been born in this country, will be much better educated, will have worked at higher paying occupations and will benefit from a variety of economic and retirement plans. And they will be more accustomed to regarding social services and supports as rights. The changing needs of the nation's population will have a definite impact on the health care professions.

Economic Factors Affecting Older People

Level of income undoubtedly affects quality of living as well as health. Currently, one of every nine couples in which the husband is over 65 receives an income of less than $4,000. At the other end of the income scale, one of every five elderly couples has an income of $15,000 or more. However, the income of elderly persons living alone or with nonrelatives falls toward the lower income scale, two of every five having incomes under $3,000. About 15 percent of persons over 65 have incomes below the poverty level. Among elderly whites, one of every eight (13 percent) is poor, but about one third (35 percent) of elderly blacks and elderly persons of other races are considered poor.

Thus, the older members of the population are essentially part of a low-income group, primarily because of fixed income and inflation. Most older people are not sharing in the increasing standard of living made possible by the economy which they helped to build. In part, compulsory retirement plans prevent most old people from working regularly, and when they do work they earn less than younger people. Older consumers spend proportionately more of their incomes on food, housing, household operation, and health care than their younger counterparts. They spend proportionately less than younger persons on transportation, clothing, household furnishings, and recreation. It is not that they need so much less; they simply cannot afford a better standard of living.

Health care costs are a large item in the budgets of elderly people. Not only do their health care needs increase just as their incomes are reduced by retirement, but also their needs change, for they now require long-term care as a result of the prevalence of chronic conditions, diseases, and impairments. Currently the health care costs of the elderly account for about 30 percent of the nation's spending for health services.

Current population trends, marked by an increasing number of older people, call for major adjustments in our socioeconomic planning.

Housing for the Aged

About 82 percent of elderly family heads own their homes, while 18 percent rent. Among elderly persons living alone, 59 percent own their homes and 41 percent rent. One sixth (16%) of elderly persons in rental housing live in public or government subsidized private housing.

Since a place to live is a basic human need, and since it is desirable that older people live independently as long as possible, there is a growing trend toward providing housing especially designed for older Americans. The Housing Assistance Administration of the Department of Housing and Urban Development is providing housing units for the older members of the population. The buildings are planned and designed to prevent accidents; they are easy to maintain, modest in size, and within walking distance of varied facilities. The Rent Supplement Program allows older citizens with low incomes to live in decent housing by providing them with rent supplements. This is of special interest to community health nurses as well as allied health workers who are engaged in helping the aged solve their problems.

Since elderly people have a difficult time adapting to a changing environment, it is helpful if their dwelling can be adapted to their needs. For people in their seventies, such safety measures as adequate illumination, nonslip flooring, and grab bars in strategic places are especially important. Single-level living quarters may also be desirable. The very old may also need facilities offering group dining and nursing and medical services.

PHYSIOLOGIC CHANGES THAT OCCUR WITH AGE

The process of aging varies with each individual, since hereditary and environmental factors influence longevity. Intensive and systematic study of aging, both experimentally and clinically, has revealed certain facts about the aging process. Aging occurs on all levels of bodily function: cellular, organic, and systemic. At least in laboratory settings, it appears that cells have a definite life span; they do not divide indefinitely but demonstrate a decreasing capacity for cellular division with age. Also, the cells of elderly persons may not perform as well as those of the young. Some of the research at the cellular level indicates that body cells may age and die because they lack the ability to repair damage that they sustain as a result of their own metabolic processes or as a result of adverse environmental effects.

Grossly speaking, *loss of cells and loss of physiologic reserve make up the dominant processes of aging.* This loss of reserve capacity may occur in many organ systems because of a gradual loss of functional units, a gradual impairment of the remaining units, decreased coordination of functional units, or a combination of these factors.

There are wide differences in aging; different organ systems are affected at different rates, even in the same individual. However, the overall effect of aging is seen in altered body functions—usually in the direction of deterioration.

Changes in Homeostasis

Homeostasis is the body's ability to maintain a stable internal environment (see Chapter 7). The complex mechanism of homeostasis regulates fluid and electrolyte balance, blood pressure, temperature, and food intake. Man is dependent upon the functional integrity of the cell and the stability of the internal environment. If the homeostatic mechanisms are functioning properly, the body is able to adapt or react to stress. However, with aging these mechanisms become less efficient and reserve power is lost. The body usually can function adequately at rest and during short periods of moderate activity, but when external stresses such as trauma or infection occur, there is little or no reserve capacity. This in turn makes the person more vulnerable to disease. Breakdown of bodily function can follow. Recovery is also affected, since more time is required for the body to return to normal after illness. Thus, to cope with these physiological changes the older person must make adjustments in living by reducing the level of activity.

Changes in the Nervous System

The nervous system is extremely vulnerable to the aging process, as is seen in the progressive loss of cells that occurs with advancing years. There are approximately half as many brain cells in the frontal area of the brain at age 80 as at 40, with a resulting decrease in brain weight. (However, the reserve capacity of the brain generally can compensate for this deficiency.) The steady loss of neurons begins surprisingly early in life and affects both the brain and spinal cord. There is progressive atrophy of the convolutions (gyri) of the brain surface and consequent widening and deepening of the spaces (sulci) between the convolutions. There is also a decrease in the blood flow to the brain. Both the physiological changes in the brain and the reduced blood supply may be related to personality changes sometimes encountered in the elderly. This may account for the fact that as we grow older there is a tendency to become slightly forgetful (particularly short-term memory), to respond more slowly, to awaken earlier in the morning, and, perhaps, to become more inflexible. More time is frequently needed for decision making. However, there is generally little decline in intelligence test scores up to age 75 although there is a decline in speed of response. Tests have shown that persons with advanced education and ability usually show little or no intellectual deterioration with age as long as there is no time pressure. Many older people remain creative late into life.

Changes in the Special Senses

The aging process produces varying degrees of impairment in hearing, vision, smell, taste, and pain perception, as well as diminished sensations of touch and a slowing of reflexes.

A decrease in the sense of smell and in the number of taste buds at times contributes to a loss of appetite; diminished sensitivity to thirst needs can lead to dehydration and confused behavior as a result of fluid imbalance.

Hearing impairment, which usually is first noticed in the higher frequencies, can result in impairment of speech discrimination and a loss of the full sense of background noises. Since sensory stimulation helps to maintain orientation to one's surroundings, these losses in sensory perception can contribute to the withdrawal and social isolation of some patients.

Vision is affected by a decrease in visual acuity (ability to discriminate fine detail) and accommodation to glare and by a marked diminution of night vision and the peripheral field of vision. This can be particularly frustrating, because reading and television viewing are favorite activities of many older persons who are unable to engage in more strenuous pursuits. The implications for nursing are many; it is necessary to provide increased illumination without glare, use night lights, and employ caution in moving elderly patients from lighted rooms to darkened rooms so as to allow time for adjustment from day to night vision. The major ophthalmological problems in older people include presbyopia (difficulty in seeing clearly at close range), lacrimal disturbances, cataract, macular degeneration, glaucoma, diabetic retinopathy, and retinal detachment. Newer methods of diagnostic instrumentation and medical and surgical therapy have improved the opportunities for visual rehabilitation.

PAIN PERCEPTION AND TEMPERATURE REGULATION. Perception of some types of pain decreases, and referral of pain from one part of the body to another seems to become more common with advancing age. In fact, the elderly can be free of pain in some acute disorders such as myocardial infarction, pneumonia, appendicitis, and peritonitis.

The temperature-regulating mechanisms are less reliable and the heat-generating activities are reduced. In the presence of infection the aged person may show a *decrease* or little change in body temperature rather than a definite elevation. Therefore, one must watch for changes in facial appearance and small increases in respiratory rate as possible signs of infection in the aging person.

Cardiovascular Changes

In older people, the heart is able to pump effectively under normal circumstances, but because it lacks much of its physiological reserve, it reacts poorly to sudden stress such as blood loss, excessive parenteral fluids, or sudden effort. When normal homeostasis is upset, congestive heart failure, arrhythmias, and myocardial ischemia may develop.

The signs of arteriosclerosis become clinically recognizable when it has reached an advanced stage in the elderly. The arteries of old people show progressive chemical and anatomical changes, with an increase in cholesterol, other lipids, and calcium. The elastic fibers progressively straighten, fray, split, and fragment. Poor circulation due to hardening of the arteries is a cause of many of the ills of the aged. Although blood pressure in the aged may fluctuate, arterial hypertension is indicated when *persistent* elevations of both systolic and diastolic values are present.

Respiratory Changes

Most of the changes that occur in pulmonary function in the aged result from loss of elastic tissue surrounding the alveoli and alveolar ducts and from changes in the anteroposterior diameter of the chest due to rib and vertebral calcification. There are also changes in the tissues of the lung and a decline in its functional capacity, size, and structure, as well as weakening of the respiratory muscles. Vital capacity becomes reduced while there is a concurrent increase in residual volume. Changes in the pulmonary vasculature also occur. However, ventilation usually remains adequate to meet the demands of ordinary activity. Normally, elderly people should be free from chronic respiratory symptoms and infection, as long as their health status is normal.

Changes in Kidney Function

Kidney function declines with age because of a reduction in the number of glomeruli and diminished filtration and tubular function. The blood flow to the kidney is reduced as a result of decreased cardiac output and increased peripheral resistance. Because of these changes, the kidney becomes a less effective waste disposal system and loses its efficiency in homeostatic control. However, its initial reserve capacity is so great that under normal circumstances it continues to function adequately throughout life.

Metabolic Changes

As the body ages, the basal metabolic rate slows and the quantity of oxygen used by the tissues is reduced. As metabolic processes change, the glucose tolerance curve tends toward that of the diabetic. If normal standards for glucose tolerance tests were applied to the aged, 50 percent of this population would be classified as diabetics. Therefore, the usefulness of conventionally interpreted glucose tolerance tests for the aged is in doubt, except for those with long-standing diabetes. Special tables to aid in interpreting glucose tolerance tests in older patients are available.

GASTROINTESTINAL CHANGES. In some older persons, gastrointestinal function is impeded by a combination of factors, including loss of teeth or inadequately fitting dentures, an impaired swallowing mechanism, or diminishing gastric and enzyme secretions. Absorption of nutrients and minerals may also be lessened and gastrointestinal motility reduced. One chronic complaint frequently encountered in the elderly is constipation, but the usual causes are lack of fiber and bulk and poor bowel habits rather than a "sluggish bowel."

Musculoskeletal Changes

Generally there is a slow and steady atrophy of muscle which results in muscle wasting, particularly of the trunk and extremities. With loss of muscle power there is a decrease in strength, endurance, and agility. Bones gradually lose calcium and become more porous and lighter. Because bones become more brittle, falls are especially dangerous in the elderly. Ligaments calcify and ossify and joints become stiffened from erosions of cartilaginous joint surfaces. Changes in the lining of joint cavities can produce degenerative changes. Such changes contribute to reduction in height and sometimes to a stooped posture and a limited ability to "get around." However, many disabilities occurring from muscular insufficiency can be prevented and corrected. Lifelong exercise programs can help to minimize age-related musculoskeletal changes. Since lack of activity aggravates disability from musculoskeletal changes, the aged need to be encouraged to be physically active within the level of their ability and to maintain optimum nutrition, particularly with respect to an adequate intake of protein, calcium, and vitamins.

Skin and Connective Tissue Changes

The skin is among the first structures to show the most obvious changes associated with aging. As a person ages there is loss of subcutaneous supporting tissue and resultant thinning of the skin. With the loss of subcutaneous fat, the skin assumes the characteristic appearance of aging—folds, lines, wrinkles, and slackness. Thinning and loss of the hair occur, as well as variations in pigmentation of the skin and hair. Purpura and ecchymoses may appear because of the greater fragility of the dermal and subcutaneous vessels and loss of subcutaneous tissues supporting the skin capillaries. Minor trauma can easily cause bruising.

The dermis becomes relatively dehydrated and loses strength and elasticity. The skin in general is prone to excess dryness and itching. The diminished capillary bed and atrophying glands are one cause of the elderly person's inability to cope with cold, heat, and soap.

As a protective measure, older people should avoid overexposure to the sun, which tends to accelerate aging of the skin and increases the tendency to skin cancer. Older people should also protect themselves against minor trauma since the skin gradually loses its ability to heal, particularly in diabetics and those with impaired circulation due to atherosclerosis in the lower extremities.

Reproductive Changes and Changes in Sexual Activity

Physiologic changes occurring with the menopause can have impact on sexual function and activity in older women. Atrophy of the vaginal canal and diminished vaginal secretions can lead to local irritation, bleeding, and pain with sexual activity. This problem is treatable. In older men, there may be diminished and delayed ability to achieve a full penile erection and a reduction in the frequency of ejaculation. These physiological changes are frequently associated with psychological changes.

Although there may be an overall decline in sexual activity with advancing age, substantial numbers of older people continue to desire and engage in sexual activity. Sexual desires and capabilities, though modified, may remain sufficiently intact to function in late life. Studies have suggested that continued sexual activity in the aged is dependent upon previous sexual behavior and experience and the availability of a partner. The fact that the majority of aged women are widows may have something to do with the seeming decline in sexual interest in older women.

PREVENTIVE CARE AND HEALTH MAINTENANCE FOR THE AGED

Preventive health care in the elderly is most important because people in this age group have less resilience and suffer more deleterious consequences from any breakdown in homeostasis. Preventive care in the elderly means maintaining health and function, detecting disease at an early stage, and preventing the deterioration of an existing condition.

People who care for and about the aged must have a positive feeling about the health potential of these elderly patients. (One has to be "tough" to reach old age.) Older persons must be educated about health conservation. Of course, the ideal practice would be to detect disease and provide remedial care in the pregeriatric years in order to prevent disabling diseases. Nurse practitioners who have special abilities, education, and interest in geriatrics are making great strides in promoting the health care of the elderly.

Health Appraisal

Elderly persons as a whole are less likely to present themselves for physical examination because they may be inclined to overlook serious symptoms as mere signs of "old age." In addition, lack of mobility and money, a decreased sensitivity to some types of pain, and depression are factors leading to self-neglect.

Varied health assessment techniques can be implemented to help detect and identify elderly people at risk. One such assessment approach uses an automatic medical screening program. The medical history is combined with certain physiological parameters to obtain a health profile. This system uses automated procedures, computer analyses, and read-out results to obtain health information. With this method the state of wellness is assessed and the probability of the presence of one or more diseases and patterns of change is identified. This is correlated with the findings from the physical examination. In part because the natural history of disease is altered in old age, many physical problems do not become obvious until they are considerably advanced.

Many authorities believe that a comprehensive annual physical examination, including blood examinations, urinalysis, and stool test, should be carried out annually. Of special importance is the ECG which shows heart abnormalities often unappreciated by the elderly patient. Equally important is a chest x-ray which can provide evidence of congestive heart failure, chronic lung disease, tuberculosis, cancer, the size of the heart, and changes in large blood vessels and bony structures of the chest. Pulmonary function tests are used to evaluate the effects of such diseases as emphysema. The Papanicolaou smear is important in elderly women to detect cancer of the cervix, as is the tonometer test for glaucoma. It is wise to monitor the weight of older people since subtle weight losses can herald the presence of cancer. Hearing and vision should be tested and corrected, as sensory deprivation can cause a downhill course.

Assessment of health habits is necessary as a basis for health counseling. Positive measures for maintaining health include weight control, exercise, proper nutrition, avoidance of cigarette smoking and the promotion of accident prevention. All of these appear to contribute to longevity and improved quality of life.

Nutritional Support

Dietary inadequacies in the elderly result from such factors as poor nutritional habits, economic constraints, and underlying disease conditions. Nutrition can have a tremendous impact on health maintenance and disease prevention as well as on the treatment of disease. In general the nutritional requirements of the elderly appear to be similar to those of other mature adults except that calorie intake should generally be reduced. The calorie requirement decreases about one third because lean body mass, metabolic rate, and physical activity decline with age. The calorie intake is adjusted on an individual basis to maintain normal weight and to prevent overweight and underweight. However there is some evidence that the overall mortality rate is lowest among elderly people who are mildly or moderately overweight.

Older people are vulnerable to low nutrient intake. Dietary studies show that calcium, thiamine, ascorbic acid, and vitamin A are the nutrients most commonly lacking in the diets of the aged.

With aging there is a decrease in the amount of body protein, which largely reflects the decrease in skeletal muscle mass. Some researchers recommend that the protein content of the diet should be more than 10 percent (and possibly 12 to 14 percent) of the calorie total. Though total body protein breakdown and synthesis decrease with age and one might expect that the protein needs of the elderly would be reduced, there is not enough information concerning the amino acid requirements of the elderly. Physical and psychological stress may result in negative nitrogen balance. Problems of malabsorption and metabolic changes may reduce the efficiency of utilization of nitrogen. For these reasons the amount of protein should be individually assessed. One gram of protein per kilogram of ideal weight has been recommended as a desirable standard for protein intake for older people.

There is some disagreement over what constitutes an appropriate intake of vitamins for the elderly. The few studies available do not suggest that higher requirements exist in the aged, but the elderly may respond to vitamin supplementation because their vitamin intake is generally low.

Among the minerals, calcium intake especially may have to be supplemented. The high incidence of osteoporosis in older women seems to be age-related.

The addition of a moderate amount of fiber to the diet may alleviate the constipation and flatulence that are common complaints in this age group.

Other factors contributing to nutritional deficiencies are social isolation, lack of interest in cooking and eating, and problems in food shopping. Weak and shaky hands can make some types of cooking hazardous. Eating is a social occasion and many of life's enjoyable moments are associated with food. When the social element is removed and the person lives alone, there is a temptation to stop eating regular meals. Many depend to an undesirable extent on foods and snacks that are inexpensive and can be prepared with the least effort. Persons living at poverty levels cannot afford to buy the protective foods that are needed. Therefore, the proportion of carbohydrates in the diet may be excessively high, as in the "tea-toast" regimen, and the protein consumption far below the minimum requirements.

Loss of interest in food is also prompted by physiological changes such as decreased production of saliva and an inability to chew properly because of poorly fitting dentures or the loss of teeth. By the age of 75, 66 percent of Americans have lost their teeth. People with poorly fitting dentures or no teeth at all tend to eat soft foods, particularly starches and sweets.

Other reasons for loss of appetite in many older people include the loss of taste buds (up to 50 percent) and a diminished ability to smell. Difficulty in swallowing is also seen.

Appetite can be improved by beginning the meal with appetite stimulants such as fruit juices and soups made from meat extract. Frequent nutritious small feedings can also help to increase food intake in the anorectic patient. When counseling the patient on diet modifications and working out a dietary regimen related to a specific disorder, the nurse should consider the patient's lifelong food habits. The mere fact that the patient is old does not necessarily mean that food must be soft and bland. It is important that the food be served attractively and be as palatable as possible.

The benefit of eating in a social setting is important to physical and mental well-being. Therefore, the patient should be encouraged to eat with others, attend church dinners and "pot-luck" occasions, and share hostess duties with others. The federal government is subsidizing a program to provide meals for the elderly in a social setting. The nurse can direct persons to these centers for senior citizens that serve hot lunches. "Meals on Wheels" is primarily for the homebound.

Exercise

Activity is one key to the prevention of premature aging. Many of the health problems of the aged arise from a lack of conditioning and a diminished response to stress. Inactivity is a serious threat to the aged and weakness or stiffness of major postural muscles ultimately causes problems in mobility. Exercise maintains muscular tone throughout the body and is effective in the prevention of and rehabilitation following cardiovascular disease. Exercise training improves functional capabilities, increases vitality, and has psychological benefits. However, there is no evidence that it increases life expectancy.

The goal of physical training for the aged is to extend their active, productive years. A systematic program of exercise that emphasizes the relaxation and stretching of tight muscles as well as the strengthening of weak muscles constitutes a helpful reconditioning plan. Usually the older person should start with relaxation exercises and then progress to limbering exercises before undertaking the strengthening exercises. For older people, the exercise is not repeated more than 2 to 3 times to avoid stiffening of joints. The program is gradually increased in intensity. An individualized and supervised program can be applied to the bedridden as well as the ambulatory patient.

The President's Council on Physical Fitness and Sports and the Administration on Aging have published an exercise program for older Americans titled "The Fitness

Challenge in the Later Years"* which presents graded exercise programs that give a balanced workout, utilizing all major muscle groups.

Accident Prevention

About 24,000 persons 65 years old and over die each year from accidental injuries. Nurses are all too familiar with the frail aged person who is admitted to the hospital with a fractured hip that leads to prolonged incapacity, pressure sores, indwelling catheter, depression, and death. For the elderly person, a fall can literally be the "beginning of the end." National Safety Council figures show that persons over 65 account for 31 percent of hospital days due to injury, 23 percent of all accidental deaths, and 18 percent of all patients hospitalized for accidents. For persons over 65 who are hospitalized for accidental injuries, the average stay is 13.5 days, whereas the average is 8.0 days for other age groups.

Most accidents involving older people occur in the home, and falls are the most common type of accidents. The following suggestions may help older persons to avoid accidents.

1. All stairs should have handrails.
2. Grab bars should be installed next to the bathtub, the shower, and the toilet.
3. Shoes should fit, and the laces must be tied securely; loose slippers are a hazard.
4. Personal belongings and other frequently used items should be stored at a level that is between the hip and the eyes, in order to avoid climbing or bending.
5. Older pedestrians must be reminded to be cautious, since their hearing and vision are often impaired.

Plans should be made to deal with emergencies for those living alone and for the handicapped. A buddy system in which telephone contact is made daily is useful, since elderly persons are prone to "drop attacks" and may lie on the floor unattended for long periods of time. Emergency numbers should be written in large letters and placed in a conspicuous place and/or tape recorded for persons with visual impairment.

HEALTH PROBLEMS OF THE AGED

DISEASE AND AGING

As was indicated earlier, the aged are particularly vulnerable to disease because of such factors as their decreased physiological reserve, a less flexible homeostatic mechanism, and lessened defense mechanisms of the body. Chronic diseases have been called "the companions

*Dept. of Health, Education and Welfare. Publication No. OHDS-75.

of the aged," and most persons over 65 are affected by at least one chronic disease. The major disorders of old age include heart disease, malignancy, cerebrovascular disease (mainly senile dementia and stroke), influenza, and pneumonia. Coronary heart disease is the most frequently seen cardiac condition. Cancer of the alimentary tract, especially of the colon, is also common. Sometimes cancers progress more slowly in the aged.

Disease in the aged does not always present with classic signs and symptoms. The usual clinical manifestations may be absent, attenuated, or disguised, and atypical signs and symptoms may be present. Complaints may be overlooked and attributed to aging and senility. Although older people have reduced physiologic reserve, some of the diseases of the aged are curable, or preventable, and the progress of others can be slowed. It is necessary to distinguish disease caused by physical insults and time-related changes from those caused by the effects of socioeconomic adversities and personal crises.

Many of the disabilities associated with old age develop as a result of degenerative vascular disease, namely arteriosclerosis. Multiple small thromboses of the arteries in the cerebral cortex are responsible for the mental deterioration of some so-called "senile" patients. When such occlusions occur, the patient may no longer be able to integrate thoughts or observations, and may lose the ability to recall recent events, becoming increasingly irritable, and exhibiting signs which in many respects seem to represent a reversion to childhood. The patient may also become less responsive to the environment. On the other hand, an older person may suffer immediate death or serious disability if a sudden occlusion develops in a large arteriosclerotic artery in the brain or if a cerebral hemorrhage occurs. Another complication of arteriosclerosis is occlusive vascular disease of the lower extremities, resulting in intermittent claudication and, possibly, gangrene, which can sometimes necessitate amputation of one or both extremities.

Arteriosclerosis is apt to involve the coronary arteries of the heart and those supplying the kidney. Therefore the elderly patient is unusually subject to cardiac disorders such as angina, acute coronary insufficiency, acute myocardial infarction, arrhythmia, and heart failure which may seriously limit the capacity for physical exertion and can produce transient ischemic episodes and falls. The impairment of kidney function brings with it the ultimate prospect of chronic renal failure.

Gastrointestinal disturbances commonly occur in the older age groups because of neoplastic disease, reduction of the blood supply to the gastrointestinal tract, neuromuscular degenerative changes, alterations of the intestinal linings, and loss of secretions. If impaired peristalsis of the esophagus occurs (due to diminished muscle and nerve function) swallowing will become difficult and may possibly lead to aspiration pneumonia.

- Because of swallowing difficulties that can occur with age, it is necessary to elevate the head of the bed while feeding an elderly patient who cannot sit up.

Abdominal emergencies, such as internal bleeding or intestinal obstruction, do not always occur with classic symptoms in the elderly. Fainting may signal occult gastrointestinal bleeding. An intestinal obstruction may be silent but is always a serious event. In general, gastrointestinal disturbances create problems in nutritional management and symptomatic therapy.

A respiratory infection in the older person is an *acute emergency* and is complicated by the patient's inability to cough up secretions because of a lack of sufficient expulsive power. Patients with chronic obstructive pulmonary disease often develop respiratory complications following illness, surgery, or trauma.

- Confusion is often the first sign of respiratory infection in the elderly.
- Sedatives or tranquilizers should be given with caution because they make the patient vulnerable to ventilatory failure and suppress the cough reflex.
- Elderly patients with even "minor" respiratory infections require vigorous treatment.

Other frequently occurring disorders in the aged include atrophic and ulcerative lesions of the skin and mucous membranes and enlargement of the prostate gland with urinary obstruction. Description of these and other degenerative disorders are included in the appropriate sections of this text.

Falls in the Elderly

Persons aged 65 or older account for 23 percent of all accidental deaths in the United States, and falls lead the list of major causes. For an aging person, a fall may be a frightening experience that can lead to immobilization and possibly to pneumonia and complete loss of the ability to walk. Falls by the elderly may result from age-related physiologic decline in postural control (particularly swaying) and deterioration of the central nervous system or from lightheadedness, postural hypotension, heart block, and arrhythmias. Many times falls occur when an elderly person hurries in response to the need to void or defecate.

Special danger arises from osteoporosis, a condition in which the bones lose calcium and thus become thin and brittle. This condition renders an elderly person susceptible to major fractures. (Hip fracture, Colles' fracture, and compression fractures of the spine are common in older people.) The joints are very often affected by degenerative (hypertrophic) arthritis, causing pain and limiting the motion of the back and of the weight-bearing joints. The eroded joint can "give in," causing the patient to fall.

- A fracture should be suspected in any elderly person who falls.

To reduce the frequency of falls among hospitalized older people, the following measures have been recommended:*

1. Implementing a treatment and rehabilitation program
2. Assessing patient dexterity and carrying out frequent monitoring during the first week of hospitalization, the time period when many falls occur
3. Placing the incapacitated or hemiplegic patient in a wheelchair equipped with a seat belt, pillow and stable-mounted table
4. Keeping corridors free of furniture and service equipment
5. Having patient wear nonskid shoes
6. Stabilizing bed tables; placing them in easy reach and immobilizing them when in use
7. Using low beds with low bedrails for confused and restless bed patients
8. Using stable chairs with arms and a seat height suitable for rising and sitting
9. Instructing patients to arise slowly when experiencing a sudden need to void or defecate
10. Using a television camera for continued monitoring of areas where there are restless bed patients, etc., for the recognition and prevention of dangerous situations.

MENTAL HEALTH OF THE AGED

The basic psychological needs of all people include respect, security, and self-esteem, as well as a need to feel appreciated and valued by others. These psychological needs are threatened during times of stress and crisis. For the aged, illness makes it more difficult to fulfill these needs. Even in the absence of serious illness, the elderly person is vulnerable to emotional and mental stress because of the sense of loss that can come from the death of friends and family members as well as from retirement, somatic changes, and failing health and mental faculties. Failure to adapt during any time of the life cycle can result in physical and emotional illness.

Although most people maintain their intellectual competence, the incidence of psychiatric and cognitive disorders increases with age; some of these are residuals of lifelong conflicts that never were resolved. Of the elderly living in the community, an estimated 15 to 25 percent have moderate to severe psychiatric impairment. More than half of those living in nursing homes suffer from senile dementia. Many display signs of regression or turn to alcohol or drugs in reaction to pain, grief, and despondency. Other mental disorders that make their appearance late in life include depression, senile dementia, and persistent paranoid state. Psychiatric symptoms in

---

*Sehested, P., and Severin-Nielsen, T. Falls by hospitalized elderly patients: Causes, prevention. Geriatrics, *32*:101-108, Apr. 1977.

the elderly may also be the result of metabolic, toxic, infectious, cardiopulmonary, or drug-induced disorders. Even a sudden environmental change or hospitalization can produce confusion in a previously alert elderly person or can convert a mildly confused patient into a psychotic one. Unfortunately, psychiatric problems are often overlooked and mental changes are mistakenly regarded as part of the aging process.

Depression

Depression is the most common emotional disorder in the aged; approximately one million older Americans suffer from this affective disorder. (Depression may also be attributable to biochemical or endogenous factors.) Depression and grief are common in the aged since losses are inevitable. The accumulation of many losses—losses of people, of things, and of hope—may deplete the individual's inner resources and the ability to cope. Depression resulting from losses can easily be overlooked and may be mistaken for physical or organic mental illness. The patient may exhibit anger, denial, withdrawal, or other maladaptive responses that move him further away from reality. He may become overly helpless or dependent. Physical complaints may serve to mask true feelings. Depression in the aged is usually manifested by feelings of apathy, quietness, and emptiness that may be mistaken for "senile" changes. In any depression, especially when associated with guilt, there is a risk of suicide. Suicide in old age is allied to physical disease, social isolation, and grief and is more prevalent among males, especially white males in their eighties.

TREATMENT. There is a natural tendency for depressive illness to improve. The treatment of depression should be as vigorous in the aged as in the young. Antidepressant drugs are usually prescribed with smaller starting doses and smaller dosage increments. In depressions resulting mainly from losses, the therapeutic approach is one of empathy; offering a sympathetic ear and understanding heart can help the patient to see that depression is the outcome of human problems. Sometimes treatment focuses on assisting the patient to complete the grieving process. Referral to community resources such as the community mental health service can be very beneficial. But services cannot substitute for emotional ties with people. The presence of a confidant and personal contacts serve to increase the confidence and self-esteem of the patient. The seriously depressed patient may require hospitalization, especially if there are suicidal tendencies.

Senile Dementia (Chronic Organic Brain Syndrome)

The term *dementia* refers to signs and symptoms of intellectual dysfunction due to differing etiologies and varying pathophysiologic mechanisms that can occur alone and in combination. It is believed to result from diffuse impairment of brain tissue. The most common long-term disorders of cognitive functioning (attention, learning, memory) in the elderly are seen in senile dementia (often called Alzheimer's disease). Other conditions resulting in dementia include Pick's disease and Jakob-Creutzfeldt disease.

Senile dementia generally refers to a disturbance of mental status or mental deterioration occurring after the age of 65, but a similar or identical condition may also begin earlier in life. There are neuropathologic changes associated with changes in the patient's cognitive function, which may include loss of neurons, neurofibrillary tangles, granulovascular changes, and neuritic (senile) plaques in the brain. The patient usually experiences gradual deterioration of memory, which at first may be minor and almost imperceptible and is often overlooked and mistakenly thought to be the result of physical illness or emotional upset. Gradually there is impairment of intellectual function and judgment, disorientation, and shallow and/or labile affect. Behavioral changes such as irritability, anger, restlessness, agitation, and depression are sometimes seen and may be a reaction to senile dementia or the result of loss of cerebral function. In time the individual's ability to carry out self-care activities, to relate to others, and to cope with environmental situations is affected. Varying patterns in the sequence of changes and in the rate of change occur from patient to patient.

Senile dementia is devastating to the human personality and is a source of anguish and frustration to the patient and loved ones. Senile dementia and related disorders are associated with a high mortality rate and significantly shortened life expectancy. It is perhaps the fifth greatest killer in the United States, since death can result from pneumonia, "benign neglect," and the effects of multiple medications which contribute to cardiovascular and neurological problems, malnutrition, and dehydration.

Management of the Dementias

The goal of treatment is to relieve some of the psychosocial stresses and to improve the general health of the patient. Unfortunately there is no treatment to halt the progressive deterioration of brain function. Patients with mild or moderate involvement may be well aware of their intellectual deficiencies and react to their personality loss with anxiety. Drug therapy (antianxiety agents; antidepressants) may be prescribed to handle behavioral disturbances and to improve the patient's subjective feelings. Medication can improve sleeping patterns.

The patient requires understanding support from family and health care personnel. Negative feelings and rejection can precipitate more anxiety, depression, and bizarre behavior and further accentuate feelings of insecurity and worthlessness and loss of self-esteem.

A major objective is to keep the patient functioning as

long as possible. A greater sense of security can be promoted with an orderly and rather ritualistic existence. Memory aids (lists of daily activities, labeled items) may help in day-to-day living, with emphasis placed on "now." Senile behavior is neither endorsed nor encouraged. Caring persons can help the patient to continue social contacts as long as possible. When the problems become too difficult for the family to manage, the patient may be placed in an extended care facility. The nursing approach to the confused patient is summarized on page 219, and the reader is referred to a psychiatric nursing textbook for other appropriate nursing interventions. The community services and facilities that may be helpful are listed in the chart that appears below.

Acute Brain Syndrome (Delirium or Acute Confusional States)

Acute brain syndrome is a temporary psychiatric state caused by a physiologic or an anatomical insult to brain tissue. The disorders have a relatively sudden onset and are potentially reversible. They are associated with acute physical illness or physiological disturbances, cardiac and circulatory problems, neurologic conditions, cerebrovascular disorders, dehydration, electrolyte imbalance, alcohol or drug toxicity, and a wide variety of infections. A reduction of cognitive function and delirium are usually present.

- An underlying physical cause should be suspected in any patient who has *sudden* changes in intellectual function.

COMMUNITY SERVICES AND FACILITIES OF BENEFIT TO PATIENTS WITH CHRONIC BRAIN SYNDROME

Recreational and social therapy
Occupational and physical therapy
Friendly visitors
Visiting nurses
Home health aides
Homemakers
Companions
Social workers
Clergymen
Protective and legal services
Programs (VISTA, Senior Aide, SCORE, Peace Corps, Foster Grandparents, Greenthumb, etc.)
Voluntary agencies
Departments of welfare and public assistance
Information and referral services
Screening and evaluation centers
Foster home care
Community mental health centers
Day care and day hospitals
Community senior citizens centers

(From Plutzky, M.: Principles of psychiatric management of chronic brain syndrome. Geriatrics, 29:124, 1974. Reproduced with permission of the author from Geriatrics, Volume 29, Number 8, Page 124. Copyright The New York Times Media Company, Inc.)

In the management of acute brain syndrome the basic disease must be treated or the etiologic toxic agent must be removed. Specific treatment is aimed at alleviating or curing the condition that underlies the confusion: antimicrobials for infection; removal of drugs; correction of fluid, electrolyte, and metabolic imbalances; removal of fecal impaction; correction of heart failure; treatment of stroke. Appropriate medication such as the phenothiazines, which exert much of their calming action on the lower brain centers, may be administered. The nursing approaches which may be beneficial to the confused elderly patient are found on page 219.

MANAGEMENT OF THE ELDERLY PATIENT

Geriatric nursing is a growing challenge in today's world. As more and more elderly people become part of the nurse's clientele, all of the nurse's scientific and humanistic resources are tapped. Not only are there multiple medical problems and nursing needs that must be managed simultaneously, but psychological and socioeconomic problems must be attended to as well. In general, an elderly patient requires 20 percent more time in nursing care and general assistance than a younger patient. When one approaches a frail, older person with multiple diseases that require several modes of treatment, more than the usual degree of assessment, clinical judgment, and nursing proficiency is required. Gerontologic nursing requires an understanding of the human condition enhanced by compassion, patience, and respect. At the same time great rewards can be gained by interacting with and learning from people who have accumulated a lifetime of experience by successfully adapting to and coping with major social, economic, and personal crises. The underlying principle in approaching the elderly patient is to recognize and respect the individuality and uniqueness of the person.

NURSING ASSESSMENT

With a view to understanding the total person, the nurse assessess the patient and seeks information for developing a nursing care plan; she then initiates the plan and evaluates its effectiveness. Knowing the patient's early history can help in developing nursing interventions and prevention strategies. One of the best ways of gathering data is taking the history and then engaging in conversation with the patient. The goal is to answer the question: *What are the assets and limitations of this patient?*

The nurse should be seated near the patient in order to maintain eye contact and should speak slowly and clearly in simple sentences. Hearing the life history is a process that takes time. The older patient usually has a slower response time, so the nursing interview should be slow

NURSING APPROACH TO THE "CONFUSED" OLD PERSON

A. Changes in mental status may be the first sign of illness in the elderly.
  1. Expect an underlying physical cause in any patient who has *sudden* changes in intellectual functioning.
  2. Confusion and disorientation may be first sign of infection (e.g., pneumonia), cardiac failure, coronary occlusion, electrolyte imbalance, stroke, dehydration, anemia, malignancy.

B. Aging is not synonymous with senility — senile dementia is a *degenerative* disease of the elderly.

C. Determine when and how the confusion developed.
  1. When was the patient last clear mentally?
    a. Are there any other symptoms? urinary frequency? cough? pain?
    b. What medications are being taken? (Ask to see them.)
  2. Assess the patient.

Physical Status	**Mental Status**
a. Observe respirations and pulse; take temperature.	a. Where are you now?
b. Check the state of hydration — tongue, tissue turgor.	b. What is today's date? day of month? year?
c. Examine for peripheral edema.	c. How old are you?
d. Look for alterations in color.	d. When is your birthday?
e. Check for evidence of injury.	e. Where do you live?

D. A new environment may bring on confused or "senile" behavior without physiological causes.
  1. Be optimistic about this turn of events; act on the assumption that this behavior is temporary.
  2. Accept the person as he is, without judgment or criticism.
  3. Maintain eye contact.
  4. Pay attention to what the patient is saying—often a person who is considered confused is only transiently so and much of what he is saying makes sense.
  5. Pick out "meaningful" comments and continue talking with him.
  6. Explain the patient's situation to him repeatedly.
  7. Make short frequent contacts.
  8. Call the person by name each time a contact is made; touch the patient when you speak to him.
    a. Talk directly to him.
    b. Answer questions in simple, short sentences.
  9. Show the person your name tag.
  10. Convey a therapeutic attitude—listening, smiling, talking, and touching.

E. Provide sufficient sensory input that is recognized as friendly.
  1. Keep the patient oriented with respect to time and place.
    a. Remind him of time, date, and place each morning and whenever necessary.
    b. Keep a calendar and clock, both with easily readable numbers, within his range of vision.
  2. Encourge family to bring in pictures, family album, etc., since familiar objects promote a sense of continuity, aid memory, and provide security and comfort.
  3. Use pictures, music, color, indoor gardens, etc., to enhance the environment.
  4. Read newspaper headlines. Discuss current events.
  5. Take the patient outdoors.
  6. Give the patient something to occupy his hands and mind.
  7. Keep the room well lighted to reduce confusion and fear; use nightlights to reduce risk of "sundowning" (worsening of a condition at night).
  8. Maintain a calm environment. Remove unduly stressful stimuli.
  9. Arrange for visits from others to counteract isolation.
    a. Have family sit by bed so that patient can see and touch them.
    b. Utilize services of a volunteer if no family is available.

F. Respect the patient's territorial rights.
  1. Do not move his personal belongings.
  2. Avoid changing rooms.
  3. Have the patient's personal belongings where he can see and use them.

G. Encourage the patient to assume a *well* and *active* role.
  1. Encourage him to dress in clean, attractive clothing *daily*—the wearing of nightwear confuses the concept of day and night (suggest up-to-date clothing as gifts).
  2. See that he wears shoes—not slippers.
  3. Encourage the patient to *walk* and not use the wheelchair, which limits his enviornment.

NURSING APPROACH TO THE "CONFUSED" OLD PERSON (CONTINUED)

    4. Encourage the patient to eat at a table and not at the bedside.
    5. See that he wears his glasses, hearing aid, dentures, or other prostheses.
    6. Be sure he is drinking adequate fluids.
  H. Attempt to alleviate the patient's anxiety and restlessness.
    1. Try "laying on of hands"—touching, stroking, hugging; many aged persons have no one to touch them.
    2. Use warm baths, warm milk, back massage, and understanding and compassion as therapeutic modalities.
    3. Give the patient gentle and constant reassurance.
  I. Avoid endorsing senile behavior.
    1. Do not agree with confused statements.
    2. Avoid letting the patient "ramble." Direct him back to reality.
    3. Be consistent. Each member of the health care team should know the nursing objectives and use the same approach.
    4. Schedule the patient's daily activities and adhere to the schedule to promote security.

---

and relaxed. In addition to the patient's responses, non-verbal clues such as facial expression and posture ("body language") should be noted. Touching the patient can be reassuring.

The following list of questions is offered as a guide in the nursing assessment of elderly patients.

Physiological Assessment

How does the patient describe the activities of a "typical" day?

How effective is the patient at self-care?

How much physical capacity does the patient have?

How much muscle strength and coordination does the patient have?

How well does the patient see and hear?

What are the patient's usual eating, sleeping, elimination, and activity patterns? What constitutes a "normal" bowel movement?

What will the patient have to do to regain or maintain functioning ability?

Socioeconomic Assessment

What is the patient's background? early history?

How many person-to-person contacts does the patient have in a day?

What is the family structure?

What family members are living?

Who visits the patient?

What is the patient's religion?

What are the patient's living arrangements?

Are the patient's activities limited because of transportation problems? high-crime environment?

Is the patient economically self-sufficient?

How much independence does the patient possess?

Does the patient participate in any phase of community life?

How can the environment be adjusted to maintain independence?

Psychological Assessment

Is the patient alert and optimistic in outlook?

What does the patient identify as his major concerns and problems?

What are the patient's attitudes toward aging?

What are the patient's attitudes toward himself/herself? Is there a feeling of being needed? useful?

What psychological defenses does the patient use?

What are the patient's activities, interests, and hobbies?

What ego strengths did the patient use in the past?

What are the patient's plans and hopes?

All of these factors affect the patient's reaction to illness and hospitalization. The more the nurse knows about the patient the more effective is the care given. Since the older patient has more complicated problems and less flexibility for solving them, the nurse may be the only one to whom the patient can turn for help to identify, face, and solve the problems.

PSYCHOSOCIAL CONSIDERATIONS

A newly admitted patient should be made to feel welcome and at home and should be introduced to nearby patients if circumstances allow. At this early meeting, the nurse can observe any incapacities such as difficulty in hearing, tremor of an extremity, problems in mobility, etc. In elderly patients more than in younger patients, a sudden change from accustomed surroundings to the impersonal routine of a hospital can produce a feeling of insecurity and emotional stress. The understanding nurse can do much to help the patient over this hump of transition between home and institution. Placing the patient near another patient provides an opportunity to talk to someone and helps in making the necessary adjustments to the hospital environment. Touching the patient's hand or shoulder when giving explanations is especially helpful in promoting acceptance, relaxation, and confidence. Many older people have lost all of their social contacts, and the nurse may be the only "caring" person.

Sometimes the transition to a new environment may bring on temporary states of anxiety, confusion, regression, and disorientation. Senile behavior may be exhibited without physiological cause. The patient may be misjudged as being senile when the real cause is fear, depression, and a feeling of hopeless inadequacy. When symptoms and behavior of senility occur, such as confusion, incontinence, etc., act on the assumption that they are temporary. The nursing approach should be a positive one, conveying the idea that the problem can be altered.

In order to reduce psychic stress, changes should be kept to a minimum. The same personnel should care for the patient whenever possible. The environment should be kept simple and predictable, and a few of the patient's possessions should be kept in plain sight. *Normal routine* should be written on the nursing care plan and adhered to so as to provide reassurance. Since it is sometimes difficult for the elderly to recall names and places and recent events, especially in an anxiety-provoking situation such as hospitalization, the nurse should identify herself by name with each contact. To minimize the confusion that often occurs with hospitalization, the patient's family and friends are encouraged to maintain contact and visit frequently.

Like everyone else, older persons respond to suggestions. It is helpful to remind the patient of past successes and to note that each period of life also has its unique problems, benefits, and gratifications. Accepting the patient as he is gives him the assurance that there are caring persons who will help when needed. The demonstration of respect and friendship will do much to enhance self-esteem and mobilize personal resources for self-help.

The elderly fear loneliness and dependency with all of their attendant pains and anguish. As soon as the patient enters the hospital, references and plans should be made concerning discharge from the hospital. This dispels much of the ever present fear of invalidism, dependency, and death. *All nursing activities are directed toward restoration of the ability for self-care.*

The successful nurse early recognizes differences in older people. Some may be old and physically frail but mentally alert and fresh in spirit. Very readily one may detect an inherent sense of humor, a philosophical frame of mind, or a thwarted and depressed personality. Often the patient's temperament will direct the course of progress. Keen observation of these manifestations will present a challenge to the nurse in developing the plan of care.

A fixed routine provides a sense of security for some elderly persons. To know that a certain activity takes place at a certain time provides a schedule which can be anticipated and planned for. The nurse can further convey a feeling of acceptance by remembering the patient's desires and idiosyncrasies even when they seem trivial.

Before procedures or examinations are done or the siderails put into place, explanations should be offered in order to eliminate fears and tensions. Since older people object to being hurried, sufficient time should be allowed in preparing for a treatment. Every effort should be made to help the older patient feel confidence in those responsible for giving care.

DRUG THERAPY FOR THE ELDERLY

Elderly people use more drugs than any other age group, averaging more than 13 prescriptions and renewals a year. One of every four prescriptions is dispensed to a person over 65. Small wonder that the aged are apt to have more adverse drug reactions and interactions than younger people. One study reported that 59 percent of the elderly outpatient population with chronic illness made errors in self-administration of prescribed medications and 25 percent committed potentially serious errors.

Physiological Considerations

There is great variability in the absorption, distribution, metabolism, and excretion of drugs in older patients due in part to a reduced capacity of the liver and kidneys to metabolize and excrete the drugs and to lowered levels of circulatory and nervous system efficiency in coping with the effect of certain drugs. Many drugs and their metabolites are excreted by the kidney. However, in the elderly patient, both glomerular and tubular functions are reduced.

- Those administering medications to the elderly must be aware of the commonly used drugs which are primarily removed from the body by renal excretion. An estimate of renal function should be made before such drugs are given.
- At the same time, it is important to realize that decline in cardiac output may decrease the delivery rate to the target organ or storage tissue.
- Changes in the gastrointestinal system may also affect drug therapy. In some elderly patients, a reduced number of mucosal cells and a slowing of gastric motility can prevent the drug from reaching therapeutic plasma and tissue concentrations, and delayed gastric emptying has undesirable effects on drugs which are acid-labile or are metabolized by the stomach mucosa. Alterations in intestinal motility and activity thus change the drug's contact time with the absorptive surface of the mucosa.
- As a result of a slowing metabolism, the drug levels may increase in the tissues and plasma, leading to a prolongation of drug action.

Because some or all of the organ systems may be marginally operational, older patients are apt to show paradoxical or unusual responses to drugs and to develop toxic reactions and their complications. In addition, the elderly have multiple medical problems requiring multiple drug treatment. Table 13-1 lists examples of diseases which may affect drug responses through pharmacokinetic alterations.

Nutritional Considerations

In any drug regimen for the elderly, one must bear in mind that drugs are capable of altering the patient's nutritional status, which may already be compromised by a marginal diet and chronic disease and its treatment. Drugs can depress the appetite, cause nausea, irritate the stomach, and decrease absorption of nutrients, in addition to altering the electrolyte balance and carbohydrate and fat metabolism. A few examples of drugs that are capable of altering the nutritional status are the antacids (producing thiamine deficiency), cathartics (diminished absorption), corticosteroids (lower serum calcium by reducing its absorption), aspirin (associated with folate deficiency), and phenothiazines and tricyclic depressants (increased food intake and weight gain).

Possible Drug Side Effects

The drugs commonly used by elderly persons are capable of producing potentially serious problems.

- Since sedatives and hypnotics can lead to confusion, delusion, hallucinations, falls, habituation, agitation, and possibly noisy behavior, such drugs should be given in smaller doses. Caution should also be taken when opiates are administered since they act as respiratory depressants.
- Before a prescribed opiate is given, the respiratory rate should be counted; if the rate drops below 10 per minute, the drug should be withheld. Because of the addicting nature of these drugs, no opiate should be given for longer than 72 hours unless specifically prescribed.
- The side effects of commonly used pain relievers must be taken into account when older patients are concerned. Although salicylates are well tolerated, they can produce salicylism, electrolyte depletion, and possibly serious bleeding from prolonged prothrombin time. Phenacetin, a frequently used over-the-counter pain reliever, may be nephrotoxic and habit-forming.
- If tranquilizers are used for older patients, it is important to note that some (the phenothiazines) can cause hypotension, cerebral depression, and worsening of the agitated state. The minor tranquilizers meprobamate and chlordiazepoxide are useful in alleviating symptoms of anxiety in the ambulatory patient and in calming agitation. However, these drugs have a narrow therapeutic range, so that they may worsen the agitation and produce uninhibited aggressive states in some patients.
- Central nervous system stimulants may be prescribed with the hope of relieving depression, apathy, and lethargy. However, these drugs are given in small dosages since they have a tendency to exaggerate confusion and accentuate paranoia in some patients who have chronic brain disorder. The tricyclic antidepressants may cause cardiac tachyarrhythmias and conduction disturbances.

- Since the heart conduction system, in general, is less effective in older patients, even small doses of digitalis can cause arrhythmias and gastrointestinal and mental symptoms that develop without warning. Digitalis is also not as well tolerated because of less effective kidney function, a decrease in myocardial potassium, and reduction in body weight. As a result, supplementary potassium and careful dosage maintenance are required.
- Digoxin has a potentially fatal myocardial impact. Diuretics are commonly prescribed for heart failure and can produce debilitating volume and electrolyte depletion.

In teaching the patient about the medication regimen, speak slowly and clearly, since he may have a hearing, seeing, and/or memory loss. Tell the patient what each medication is used for and what its side effects are. Then write out the drug regimen.

The patient often feels that unless a drug has been prescribed, adequate treatment has not been given. As with other age groups, this type of thinking must be corrected. Reinforce the concept that health maintenance includes proper nutrition, a daily program of activity and periodic health checkups. Drugs are no substitute for caring persons and sound health practices. Patient compliance will be improved when the drug regimen is kept as simple as possible and when the patient is made a partner in the drug-taking regimen.

The patient should not be "fed" medication, but should be encouraged to take it himself. It is also a good idea to give the patient a sip of water before a pill or capsule is swallowed to prevent it from sticking in the throat. Finally, if a patient has a history of suicide threats or attempts, the nurse must be sure that the medication (pill or capsule) is actually swallowed and not retained between the cheeks and the gums or teeth.

GENERAL NURSING INTERVENTIONS

Temperature Regulation

As a person ages, the body becomes less efficient in temperature regulation. In general, older people cannot tolerate a cold environment and are very susceptible to hypothermia. The nursing approach is to palpate the skin for warmth, particularly the extremities, and to make sure that the environmental temperature is adequate. Extra blankets may be added for warmth. Conversely, older persons with cardiovascular disease are prone to develop heat stroke. Efforts are directed to maintain heat and humidity at comfortable levels by fans, air conditioning, and humidifiers or dehumidifiers during hot weather.

Hygienic Care

With aging the skin becomes thin and inelastic, predisposing the elderly patient to pressure sores. Pressure is the underlying cause of all pressure sores, and because the

TABLE 13-1.   EXAMPLES OF DISEASES OR CONDITIONS WHICH MAY AFFECT
DRUG RESPONSE THROUGH PHARMACOKINETIC ALTERATIONS*

DISEASE/CONDITION	EFFECT
Absorption Pyloric stenosis Gastric ulcer Vagotomy (surgical or chemical) Diabetic gastroparesis Severe malabsorption syndrome Achlorhydria	A decreased gastric emptying rate may result in failure to achieve adequate drug concentrations. Drug absorption may be decreased. The absorption of certain basic drugs which require a low gastric pH for complete dissolution may be reduced.
Distribution Congestive heart failure Hypoalbuminemia Amputations	Drugs may be inadequately distributed to other parts of body exposing the regional priorities systems, i.e., heart and brain, to excessive drug concentrations (e.g., lidocaine, procainamide, theophylline). For highly albumin-bound drugs, low serum albumin concentrations may lead to clinical toxicity if the concentration of unbound pharmacologically active drug in the plasma remains increased (e.g., prednisone, phenytoin, phenylbutazone). Failure to take into account the lost muscle mass in the amputee may lead to toxicity with drugs that preferentially distribute into lean body tissue (e.g., digoxin, gentamicin, kanamycin).
Renal Excretion Kidney dysfunction Congestive heart failure	Drugs which are largely excreted unchanged in the urine can accumulate to toxic levels if no precautions are taken to reduce the dose and/or administer less frequently. Since the relative degree of glomerular and tubular dysfunction will often vary with the cause of nephropathy, the frequently observed linear relationship between creatinine and drug clearances may not apply for drugs which are primarily secreted by the tubules. A significant reduction in cardiac output can result in large decreases in renal blood flow and, to a lesser extent, glomerular filtration rate. Maintenance doses of drugs which are excreted via the kidney may have to be reduced.
Drug Metabolism *Liver Disease*—because the pathophysiology of acute and chronic liver disease is very different, it is evident that their effect on drug metabolism may also differ. Acute liver disease—there is primarily hepatocellular necrosis with subsequent decreased activity of drug metabolizing enzymes. Hepatic blood flow is generally regarded as normal, and serum albumin concentration is usually unchanged. Chronic liver disease—there is often replacement of functional tissue by fibrosis, reduced liver blood flow, and decreased serum albumin concentrations. The activity of the drug metabolizing enzymes may be normal or decreased depending upon the degree of compensatory hepatocellular hyperplasia.	The capacity to metabolize drugs may be significantly impaired during an acute bout of hepatitis (viral). Furthermore, there is no correlation between conventional liver function tests and the prolongation of drug half-life. Complete recovery from viral hepatitis is usually followed by a corresponding recovery of drug metabolizing capability. The capacity to metabolize drugs may be significantly impaired in chronic liver disease. However, much variability in drug metabolism rates may be seen because of the heterogeneity of the disease. Again there is often no relationship between drug metabolizing ability and the common biochemical tests of liver function. In any form of liver disease, the administration of drugs whose major means of elimination is by hepatic metabolism dictates that frequent clinical and laboratory asessments are necessary for adjusting dosage regimens.
Congestive Heart Failure	In patients with a low cardiac output, proportional, reductions in liver blood flow can be anticipated. Furthermore, in right-sided heart failure, the increased right auricular pressure is readily transmitted to the hepatic veins resulting in liver congestion with possible centrizonal liver cell necrosis. Dosage regimens for drugs which are cleared from the plasma principally by hepatic metabolism may have to be decreased.

*(From William Reichel: Clinical Aspects of Aging. Baltimore, Williams and Wilkins, 1978.)

older patient is sometimes content to lie in bed without moving, the nurse must encourage the patient to turn and move frequently and to engage in graduated activity. (The prevention of pressure sores is discussed on page 187.)

In the aged there is reduction of sebum, sweat, and the water binding capacity of the skin, resulting in a tendency of the skin surface to crack. Rather than avoid bathing, the patient should be advised to lubricate the skin with an ointment (Aquaphor®) that traps the moisture. At the same time, special attention must be given to the removal of soapy water from the skin. The danger of residual soap and consequent lysis of the skin is greatest between the toes and fingers and in areas where there are folds. Bathing in hot water and using detergent soaps or bubble baths are to be avoided, since these substances aggravate dryness. Senile pruritus is a result of atrophic changes in the epidermis and dermal appendages. The management of pruritus is discussed on page 1048.

Foot Care

For elderly people, foot care is essential in order to maintain mobility and physical well-being, and independence. Common foot disorders of this age group include calluses, bunions, toenail problems, corns, and fungus infections. The feet of older people have survived a lifetime of use, misuse, and trauma. As musculoskeletal problems develop, biomechanical changes occur. All of these are compounded by diabetes, edema, and peripheral vascular ischemia, which increase the patient's susceptibility to infection.

Patient assessment includes attention to possible foot problems as indicated by the patient's complaints and to any signs of abnormality that may suggest possible underlying systemic disorders. The skin is one of the first structures to show degeneration changes associated with aging. The following are offered as guidelines for assessing the lower extremities and feet:

- Is the skin of the extremities thin and shiny?
- Is there loss of hair on the toes? on the front of the legs?
- Are there complaints of pain? paresthesia?
    Is pain intensified at night? relieved by walking?
    Is there pain on rest?
- Is there brownish pigmentation? skin erosion? rubor?
- Is the skin mottled?
- Is the extremity cool?
- Does the patient complain of numbness? tingling? burning?
- Are the pulses weak, decreased, or absent?

CARE OF THE TOENAILS. Thickened and deformed toenails in the elderly occur as a result of vascular insufficiency, nutritional changes, and trauma to the nail matrix. Before the toenails are trimmed, the feet should be soaked in tepid water for 10 or 15 minutes. Soaking softens the nail plate, loosens subungual debris, decreases the possibility of bacterial infection, and helps to relax the patient. The feet are dried by blotting them with a towel instead of wiping them vigorously, since friction can injure skin that is delicate, atrophic, or ischemic.

- Sit facing the patient. (The patient's feet should be placed on a footrest.)
- Observe the nails, skin temperature, texture, and color and look especially for breaks in the skin and signs of infection, redness, and edema.
- Locate the nail and differentiate the nail from the nail bed; a curette can be used for this. (The growth pattern of some nail plates is altered so that it is frequently difficult to distinguish the nail plate from the nail bed.)
- Apply antiseptic solution to the areas around the toenails before cutting the nails. Frequently, the nails are so thick that thinning is required before cutting is possible. This is accomplished by rubbing an emery board across the nail surface.
- To cut the toenails, use only the tip of sterile nail nippers, starting at one corner and taking small "bites" across the entire nail plate. Follow the contour of the nail plate. Little or no force should be necessary.
- Cut the nail so that it rests freely and without pressure on the nail bed. It should be cut even with the end of the toe and the edges should be smoothed with an emery board.
- Use a curette to carefully debride around and under the nail plate. Debriding removes subungual debris which may be causing discomfort.
- Apply an antiseptic to the nail plates and toes that have been treated, in order to prevent infection.
- Avoid cutting nails if force is required, if a toe is exuding purulent material or is gangrenous, or if a subungual neoplasm is suspected.
- The feet of the diabetic patient should be treated with special care, preferably by a podiatrist.

Oral and Dental Care

Loss of teeth in the aged usually occurs from degeneration of the periodontal structures: gingivae, alveolar bone, and periodontal membrane. Half of the elderly have no natural teeth. Although a good percentage of these people have dentures, many do not wear them or wear them infrequently for a variety of reasons, including traumatic ulcers and the need for refitting or replacement. Many mistakenly believe that there is no need for dental consultation after the teeth have been removed and replaced by dentures.

Dry mouth, abnormal taste, and burning sensations (from atrophy of taste buds, dehydration, reduced salivary flow, iron and vitamin B complex deficiencies, and low estrogen levels) are common complaints. All of these may result in poor eating habits, which further produce degeneration of oral tissues.

The components of dental care for the aging patient (gerodontics) include: eating a proper diet, maintaining healthy oral and denture-bearing structures, being motivated to seek proper care, and having adequate dental services available. The objectives of dental care are to preserve the remaining teeth and to carry out reconstructive procedures, modifying and adding to existing appliances and designing and fitting partial or complete sets of dentures. If an elderly person has not worn dentures for a long time, it may be wise not to secure dentures but to make sure that the diet has all of the proper nutrients, since adequate nutrition is fundamental to the health of the oral structures.

Receding gums and denture movement accentuate the spaces between the teeth. Tooth brushing will not remove retained food particles, and toothpicks and dental floss will be required. An electric toothbrush or Water Pic® is helpful in carrying out an effective oral hygiene program, especially in patients who have tremors, paralysis, or other physical impairments. Persons with decreased salivary flow resulting in cracked lips and fissures of the tongue should be encouraged to drink more water and to use soothing mouthwashes. Unfortunately not too much can be done to correct the problem, since the salivary glands may have undergone regressive changes.

The dentures should be regarded as prostheses. The person with dentures requires a nonabrasive denture cleaning paste and denture brush. Particles of food that harbor bacteria or yeast can become lodged in the mouth area that is covered by the dentures. Dentures should be stored in fresh water at night.

For the patient who is confined to bed, mouth care should be supervised by the nurse. By carefully evaluating the condition of the mouth, the nurse is able to meet the patient's nutritional needs more effectively, to request dental attention when necessary, and to prevent infections. Any areas of chronic irritation, ulceration, whitening, and thickening should be referred for evaluation by the dentist.

Elimination Problems

Many elderly people become very concerned about bowel elimination and have problems with constipation because of altered gastrointestinal motility, decreased mucus secretion, and changes in muscle tone and elasticity of the colon, as well as changes in diet.

Problems of constipation and bowel incontinence often can be reduced through systematic habit training. While the patient is in the hospital, a bedside commode is easier to use and is more acceptable than a bedpan. Indwelling catheters should not be used to treat urinary incontinence; evidence shows that catheterization is a means of introducing organisms into the urinary tract. The cause of urinary incontinence should be determined. If no pathological problem can be found, fear, social withdrawal, and loneliness may be factors.

• Experience in long-term care facilities has shown that systematic bladder and bowel training programs, combined with exercises, ambulation, and social activities, can produce significant decreases in the frequency of incontinence.

Sensory Impairments

Approximately 30 percent of all older persons have hearing loss, which is understandably the most difficult sensory loss for the elderly. Perhaps only one ear is involved or only certain ranges of sound may not be detectable. Whatever the difficulty, simple gestures and signals by the nurse may be understood clearly. Most patients who have diminished hearing are reluctant to call attention to it; therefore, it is up to the nurse to take the initiative in discovering this or any other handicap. The nursing approach to the individual with a hearing loss is discussed on page 1153.

Further, *visual impairment* may predispose the patient to accidents. Grab rails in the bathroom should be available, and all rooms should be well lighted, especially the path from bed to bathroom at night. The bed should be equipped with side rails to remind the patient to remain in bed at night. Side rails can also be held onto when raising to a sitting position and when turning over in bed.

Appearance

An attractive appearance is a great morale booster; to look well implies that one feels well. Since older people at times neglect their appearance, they need to be encouraged to look their best.

Both men and women enjoy nice clothes or a bit of color to brighten their appearance. Even some conservative men seem to like bright-colored pajamas. A small flower on the lapel of a man's bathrobe will brighten his spirits. A shave and a haircut do for a man what lipstick does for most women. Almost everyone finds the fragrance of certain dusting powders and colognes refreshing. This has special appeal when the scent is in keeping with the individual's personality. Surely the nurse will be able to find at least one thing that will help immeasurably to cheer an older patient.

Physical Activity/Rehabilitation

The goal of rehabilitation of the elderly patient is to reestablish self-care and, if possible, to improve ambulatory capacity. An exercise program in accordance with the patient's exercise tolerance is necessary to achieve this goal.

Walking activities should be encouraged as soon as the patient is able. Instruction in the proper use of aids such as a walker, crutches, or a cane, must be given to the patient, as well as reasons for why it is important to maintain proper body posture and how to achieve it.

The dangers of prolonged bed rest, even prolonged sitting, are numerous and should be avoided even when the patient objects to a change. The rocking chair is more helpful than a straight or an overstuffed chair, since it enables all but the most feeble to exercise with dignity at any time. Use of the calf and forearm muscles encourages venous return and increases cardiac output. Pulmonary ventilation is increased and hypostatic pulmonary congestion is discouraged. From the psychological point of view, rocking is socially acceptable; in such a chair, one can participate in home activities and be an integral part of the family.

Recreation

In the words of Piersol and Bortz, "The society which fosters research to save human life cannot escape responsibility for the life thus extended. It is for science not only to add years to life, but more important, to add life to the years."

Recreation is more than just having fun; it is fundamental to physical and mental well-being. No matter how old or disabled one becomes, the desire for the dignity that comes only through purposeful activity is never lost.

As soon as the patient is capable of participating in any type of group activity or is willing to undertake some project on an individual basis, such activity should be planned. The nurse can enlist the help of other personnel, such as occupational therapists, and volunteer aides, and of members of the family, in organizing activities designed to occupy the patient's time pleasantly, maintain his enthusiasm, and keep him in possession of his faculties and aware of his own personal worth. If a project is successful in this respect, one of the most important goals in the therapeutic process will have been accomplished.

No plan for rehabilitation will be successful unless it is continued beyond the walls of the hospital. Continuity of care can be planned with the community health nurse and other community agencies as well as the patient's own family. In many instances, the geriatric patient does not have a family that he can return to. Real adjustments may have to be made. The smoother the transfer, the more graceful will be the resumption of normal living for the elderly.

The Family

The idea that older people are rejected by their families is an exaggeration. Old people are not usually ignored by their familes nor estranged from their children. Many live within a day's journey of a family member. The cooperation of the family should be enlisted as early as possible in the management of the patient in order to assure convalescent care and protection against possible complications and further recurrences of the disease. Providing information on aging is helpful to families in promoting understanding, support, and improved relationships with older family members.

A developmental crisis occurs when the mental or physical health of an aged parent begins to decline. The inability of the parent to live independently places new demands on adult children who are faced with making a critical decision at this turning point in their own lives. As the shift in roles occurs, there may be feelings of guilt and anger, unresolved conflicts, financial strain, and social pressures. The nurse must recognize and understand that the family is likely to have ambivalent feelings about caring for the parent. Alternative options that the family may consider are provision of support services such as homemaker services, Meals on Wheels, visits by the community health nurse, and more frequent contacts by the family to assist the patient to continue living in the present setting. If the patient cannot continue to be independent, an extended care facility or retirement home may be the answer. Or the children may have the parent live with one of them, although potential areas of conflict may arise with respect to lack of space and privacy, entertainment of friends (both of adult children and parents), expenses, recreation, vacation, child rearing, and management of household tasks. Such conflicts should be anticipated, identified, and discussed, and steps should be taken to resolve such problems at an early date. The nurse can assist in providing the therapeutic climate in which the family can ventilate their feelings, reduce anxiety and guilt, explore options, and establish priorities.

THE ELDERLY PATIENT UNDERGOING SURGERY

Surgery imposes physical and psychological stress, but because of advances in evaluation techniques, surgical procedures, anesthetic techniques, and monitoring capabilities, older patients tolerate elective surgery surprisingly well. The principle to be kept in mind during preoperative evaluation, surgery, and postoperative care is that the aged patient has *less physiological reserve* (the ability of an organ to return to normal after a disturbance in its equilibrium) than younger patients. The special requirements for optimum results following surgery on an elderly patient include: (1) skillful preoperative evaluation and treatment; (2) experienced and careful anesthesia and surgery; and (3) meticulous and competent postoperative management. The hazards of surgery for the aged are proportional to the number and severity of coexisting diseases and the nature and duration of the operative procedure.

Psychological Considerations

Confidence will be strengthened if the geriatric patient fully realizes that the contemplated operation is less hazardous than the disease it is expected to remedy. Years of living have a tendency to broaden the patient's ability to adjust to crises. On the other hand, one must not assume that the patient is unconcerned or values life less than a younger patient. In old age one is more conscious of the shortness of the remaining years. The patient may re-

SUMMARY OF THE PRINCIPLES UNDERLYING THE NURSING MANAGEMENT OF THE ELDERLY PATIENT

1. Growth and adaptation continue to occur when the individual's strengths and potential are recognized and reinforced.
2. Nursing care must be individualized, taking into consideration the patient's past experiences, needs, and individual goals.
3. Realistic and attainable goals, which are understood by the patient, are set to help establish a sense of accomplishment and purpose.
   a. Engage in mutual goal setting when possible; preserve a reason for living.
   b. Keep communicating to the patient the planned goals of care.
   c. Support the patient's belief in his/her own inner resources.
4. The patient should be an active participant in the plan of care.
   a. Learn something about the patient before the initial encounter; find out the patient's strengths.
   b. Consult the patient's preferences.
   c. Concentrate on what the patient can do.
   d. Ask the patient's opinions.
   e. Encourage the patient to make choices and decisions.
   f. Avoid making decisions for the patient; this promotes low self-esteem, dependency, and depression.
   g. Support the patient during periods of anxiety. Direct attention to the gains being made.
   h. Urge the patient to remain active.
5. Nursing activities should be done *with* the patient rather than *for* the patient.
6. Necessary modifications and compromises imposed by the physiological limits of aging must be reflected in the medical and nursing management of the patient.
7. The individuality of the patient should be encouraged—to preserve identity and sense of control.
   a. Encourage the patient to have and use personal possessions that help to bridge the gap between past and present.
   b. Respect the patient's right to self-direction.
   c. Give the patient *time* to express his or her feelings.
   d. Help the patient to retain the social graces.
   e. Help the patient to cope with thoughts of death.
8. Elderly persons should be kept in the mainstream of life to prevent physical, emotional, and mental deterioration.
   a. Avoid removing the element of challenge. Encourage contact with others.
   b. Work out a "buddy system" to prevent loneliness and isolation.
   c. Stimulate mental acuity and sensory input.
   d. Encourage physical activity.
   e. Share your world with the patient.
   f. Remember the patient's preferences; accept his or her idiosyncracies.
   g. Provide opportunities for the patient to do some tasks of daily living (water plants; wash own stockings).
   h. Provide meaningful diversional activity.
   i. Give the patient something to look forward to.
9. The patient's potentialities should be utilized.
   a. Select activities that are in keeping with lifelong interests.
   b. Do not attempt to alter lifelong character and behavior patterns.
   c. Give the patient time to listen, to learn, and to adapt.
   d. Help the patient to learn new ways to maintain independence.

quire repeated explanation, clarification, and positive reassurance. The objective is to secure the patient's *active* cooperation; if this is to be achieved, a kindly, considerate approach is basic. The psychological preparation consists of giving simple and straightforward information about what can be expected before and after surgery.

Preoperative Assessment

A careful preoperative evaluation is done in order to assess the patient's physical status and his ability to adapt to operative stress and to correct, as far as possible, existing defects. All medication that the patient is taking should be brought into the hospital and reviewed, since some drugs interact with anesthetic agents and can produce dangerous side effects.

Specific instructions are given in deep breathing and movement of the extremities, and the reasons why these actions are to the patient's advantage are presented.

Preparation for surgery demands a meticulous evaluation of the cardiovascular, respiratory, and renal systems as well as the nutritional and hydration status of the patient. Although the patient may be admitted for one specific problem, frequently there are several degenerative diseases affecting vital systems. Ideally, all deficiencies should be corrected before the patient is taken to the operating room; in reality, some compromises are necessary. After data gathering and assessment are completed, the anesthesia plan, surgical procedure, and postoperative activities are discussed by appropriate members of the health team.

Cardiovascular Function. Cardiovascular diseases are the most common abnormalities in the elderly surgical patient. The status of the heart's pumping action and the adequacy of the blood vessels are determined and baseline electrocardiograms are obtained. An effort is made to determine the level of the patient's normal activity and then to evaluate cardiovascular reserve. The cardiovascular response to stress may be assessed before and after exercise.

In the presence of atherosclerosis, the heart, brain, and kidneys are very sensitive to the further reduction of perfusion and oxygenation that anesthesia may produce.

The ECG will demonstrate evidences of hypertrophy and conduction abnormalities. Cardiac arrhythmias can often be controlled and congestive heart failure improved, but other manifestations of arteriosclerosis are altered very little by preoperative treatment. Coronary artery disease is considered the most serious heart disease of this age group; its presence increases the operative risk. Medical treatment of anginal symptoms should precede surgery.

The presence of arrhythmias, congestive heart failure, coronary insufficiency, and severe diastolic hypertension increases the mortality rate. If the patient is in congestive heart failure, careful adjustment of digitalis levels, administration of diuretics (with care taken not to dehydrate the patient), sodium restriction, and bed rest are indicated before surgery. As with other patients, tranquilizing drugs, reserpine, propranolol, and monoamine-oxidase inhibitors are preferably discontinued 10 days before the operation. (Under stress these agents may produce alterations in cardiovascular responses.) If the patient is hypertensive the blood pressure is controlled before elective surgery and, if possible, is maintained below 160/100 mm. Hg.

Peripheral Vascular Assessment. Varying degrees of arterial insufficiency and tissue ischemia are present in the aged. Easy fatigability and numbness of an extremity on exercise, with relief on rest, are common. The peripheral pulses, including the temporal, carotid, brachial, radial, femoral, popliteal, dorsalis pedis, and posterior tibial pulses, should be evaluated and appropriate ones marked before surgery.

Making sure that the patient avoids positions that permit venous stasis or pressure on the blood vessels is a nursing responsibility. Thus the patient should be instructed to avoid crossing his legs while sitting. The head and foot of the bed must not be elevated at the same time since this position encourages venous stagnation in the pelvic veins. Elastic stockings, if worn throughout the hospital stay, help to keep venous blood in the deeper circulation. Sitting in a chair with the feet hanging down should be discouraged. Since activity improves circulation, the patient should be ambulated as much as possible.

Respiratory Assessment. Although there is some degree of impaired pulmonary function in all postoperative patients, the elderly are at special risk for pulmonary complications because of changes in the lungs and chest due to aging. The lungs of the elderly lose some of their elastic recoil, and chest compliance is reduced. There is a progressive decrease in vital capacity.

Preoperative assessment includes history, physical examination, chest x-ray, pulmonary function studies, and arterial blood gas analysis. Graded stress testing is directed toward eliciting stress responses. If dyspnea develops it must be determined whether shortness of breath is the result of a cardiac problem, underlying pulmonary disease, or both.

While caring for the patient, look at the nature and quality of respirations, shortness of breath, coughing and sputum production, and smoking habits. Infection, abnormal states of hydration, and retained secretions are risk factors which respond to therapy before surgery.

• After the operation, the nursing actions are directed towards ensuring adequate hydration, checking for evidence of retained secretions by means of auscultation of the chest, promoting frequent deep breathing and coughing to prevent pulmonary complications, and encouraging early ambulation.

Renal Function Assessment. Disorders of renal function and urinary disturbances are common in the elderly. Between the ages of 50 and 80 the average urea clearance declines 50 percent. A serum creatinine test and blood urea nitrogen test are done preoperatively to identify renal impairment so that suitable measures can be taken to prevent renal failure. Other tests are done as indicated. In the male, urethral stricture and urethritis, and prostatic hyperplasia and prostatitis are frequently observed urinary problems. It is wise to have the elderly male practice using the urinal while lying in bed in the preoperative period since voiding during the postoperative period may be a real problem.

Fluid, Electrolyte, and Nutritional Management. Electrolyte and fluid deficits should be restored before surgery is undertaken. Serum potassium levels are evaluated since a low potassium level increases susceptibility to possible ventricular arrhythmias and digitalis intoxication. When an older patient is given a transfusion, the central venous pressure should be monitored. The urinary output also serves as a guide in the correction of dehydration states.

The patient may suffer from nutritional deficiency resulting from chronic illness, socioeconomic factors, and poor dietary habits. The goal of nutritional support is to supply the necessary calories and protein to meet metabolic demands and prevent nitrogen loss. Supportive feedings, including oral, hyperalimentation, and tube feedings are given as necessary. The patient's weight, fluid, and electrolyte balance as well as renal and hepatic functions are monitored.

Preoperative Medication

The purposes of preoperative medications are to calm the patient and to depress secretions. Since drug sensitivity is usually increased in elderly individuals, a conservative approach is used and smaller dosages generally are given. Preoperative medication may not be given at all to the acutely ill or debilitated patient. The preoperative medication may be given to the aged patient earlier on the morning of surgery, because of delayed absorption.

Anesthesia

The anesthesia chosen depends on the patient's physiologic status, the length of the operation, and the experience and preference of the anesthesiologist. The arterial partial pressure of oxygen may be temporarily lowered during induction, intubation, and extubation, causing arrhythmias in the elderly. All inhalational anesthetics are potential respiratory and myocardial depressants.

Regional anesthesia, especially spinal anesthesia, is useful for patients undergoing transurethral resection, inguinal herniorrhaphy, orthopedic procedures, and for poor risk patients who would poorly tolerate inhalation anesthesia. It must be remembered, that even though the blood vessels of the elderly patient may be quite inelastic, a profound drop in blood pressure may occur.

If the drop in blood pressure is sudden and prolonged it may lead to circulatory insufficiency. This in turn may cause cerebral ischemia, thrombosis, followed by embolism, infarction, and anoxemia. To maintain blood pressure at a normal level is of utmost importance in these patients.

It is well to remember that excessive or over-rapid infusions may cause pulmonary edema.

Postoperative Management

The immediate postoperative care is the same as that for any patient, but additional support is given to any impaired function of the cardiovascular, pulmonary, and renal systems.

- Since the possibility of shock is greater in the older patient, it is necessary to monitor the pulse, respiratory rate, blood pressure, and urinary output (and central venous pressure and blood gas determinations if indicated) and to watch for deviation from baseline readings.

Transfer of the patient from the operating room table to the bed is done *slowly* and carefully while monitoring the effects of this action upon the blood pressure and assessing for evidence of hypoxia. Special attention is given to keeping the patient warm, since body temperature in the elderly is labile. Position should be changed frequently not only for comfort, since lying in one position can be painful, but also to avoid pulmonary and circulatory complications.

Prevention of Complications

Since the patient has a lesser margin of reserve, it is important that complications be prevented, for one postoperative complication can lead to another. The system that is most defective usually fails first. The aged cannot tolerate prolonged periods of stress.

Shock. Shock causes death more frequently among patients over 60 than among younger patients. An older person cannot tolerate a reduction of blood volume or hypotension for even a short period of time, especially since the heart and blood vessels do not constrict as readily. An added problem for the patient who has sclerotic and narrowed arteries and develops hypotension from shock is a serious reduction in the perfusion of coronary or cerebral vessels. Therefore, the blood pressure must be maintained as close as possible to the patient's normal blood pressure. The urinary output, an indication of adequate blood volume and perfusion, should be between 15 to 25 ml. per hour.

In treating shock with fluid replacement, it is important to monitor the patient's central venous pressure to prevent overloading of the circulation, which places an unnecessary burden on the heart.

For the treatment of shock, see pages 364–370.

Postoperative Respiratory Complications. The most frequent respiratory complication of the aged is pneumonia. Decreased lung expansion, weakness, relative fixity of the rib cage, and drug depression of cough reflexes contribute to such complications.

- Measures to prevent respiratory complications include frequent turning, early ambulation, use of small doses of analgesia, removal of tracheobronchial secretions, and breathing exercises.

Yawning is an effective way to prevent or correct atelectasis. Taking a deep breath and holding it as long as possible helps to increase ventilation. If the tracheobronchial tree cannot be cleared by suction and aspiration, a tracheostomy may be necessary.

Hydration. Hydration and replacement of electrolyte losses following surgery are the same as for any surgical patient. Substantial amounts of potassium are lost immediately after the operation from fever, acidosis, or breakdown of tissue. Certain considerations should be noted when parenteral infusions are given to elderly patients.

- After the first few postoperative hours, the patient's head and shoulders are raised during replacement therapy in order to reduce the pressure in the pulmonary circuit and avoid pulmonary edema.
- Since an older person's heart and circulatory system cannot stand overloading, infusions and transfusions are given slowly. If there is any question, central venous pressure monitoring will reveal circulatory overloading.
- Usually the older patient needs to be encouraged to drink enough fluids. An output of one liter or more indicates that intake is sufficient. Obviously, the recording of intake and output is important.

Gastrointestinal Distention and Ileus. Gastrointestinal distention and ileus (cessation of intestinal motor action) is encountered following extensive trauma and intra-abdominal operations as well as in systemic and abdominal disease states. Retroperitoneal hemorrhage, intra-abdominal hemorrhage, lack of muscle tone of the large bowel, and fecal impaction can produce ileus, as can the use of narcotics which can reduce peristalsis. A common cause of postoperative distention is retention of swallowed air in the gastrointestinal tract.

- To prevent postoperative distention, a nasogastric tube may be introduced into the gastric lumen. Management of ileus usually requires decompression by intubation into the small bowel. Keep in mind that an indwelling nasogastric tube in an older patient can cause erosion and perforation of the esophagus and can prevent bronchial secretions from being raised. In addition, nasogastric suction is not well tolerated in the elderly.

In older people, the sluggish peristalsis in the colon sometimes results in incomplete evacuation and therefore in retention of fecal material in the sigmoid colon and the rectum. The absorption of fluid produces a hard fecal mass which is irritating to the intestine and often produces frequent small stools, a sort of pseudodiarrhea. Digital examination reveals a hard mass of fecal material in the rectum. When the mass is broken up by the finger and by enemas, the symptoms are relieved.

Management of Postoperative Pain. Postoperative pain relief may be achieved with fairly small amounts of narcotic drugs, such as codeine. The side effects of narcotics — depressed ventilation and diminished circulation — are dangerous. Enough drug should be given to reduce the pain but not enough to make it difficult for the patient to perform the required exercises. Moving about is much more desirable than being in a prolonged stuporous condition from oversedation. A certain degree of relaxation can also be achieved with reassurance.

Exercise and Ambulation. Activity in bed as well as out of bed is essential to recovery.

- Bed exercises include turning from side to side, flexing and extending the legs and the arms, deep breathing, and deliberate coughing.
- In getting out of bed, the patient should turn to his operated side and bend his knees upward. As he swings his feet over the side of the bed, the nurse can assist him to a sitting position.
- Sitting positions that promote venous stasis in the lower extremities are to be avoided. *Ambulation means that the patient walks, not sits in a chair.*

Patients with preexisting cardiovascular and pulmonary conditions should be watched carefully, because overexertion may cause a breakdown of these functions. As the period out of bed is gradually increased, the stability of the vital signs serves as a measure of the patient's reaction to exercise and ambulation activities.

Convalescence

Convalescence in the elderly may be difficult because strength is regained slowly. Above all, the older patient needs a great deal of patience. Some authorities advocate that one day be allowed for each decade of one's age for convalescence from acute illness. Patients often find this difficult to accept.

Every attempt should be made to maintain an interest in people and to prevent psychological withdrawal. A major concern for the patient and the family is how care will be provided following discharge from the hospital. Of course, this challenge should be addressed by all concerned upon admission. The patient may be fearful of returning home alone, yet the children may not have room to accommodate another person in the house. If the patient must remain alone, there is a problem of increased isolation due to lessened activity following surgery.

The older patient must be encouraged to become proficient in self-care in order to become self-sufficient as quickly as possible. Thus, the nurse must refrain from becoming overly protective when caring for an elderly patient, at the same time providing necessary emotional support as plans are made for the future.

BIBLIOGRAPHY

BOOKS

General

Aiken, L.: After Life. Philadelphia, W. B. Saunders, 1978.

Barton, D., ed.: Dying and Death. A Clinical Guide for Caregivers. Baltimore, Williams and Wilkins, 1977.

Behnke, J. A., Finch, C. E., and Moment, G. B., eds.: The Biology of Aging. New York, Plenum Press, 1978.

Bell, B. D.: Contemporary Social Gerontology. Springfield, Charles C Thomas, 1976.

Bellak, L., and Karasu, T. B., eds.: Geriatric Psychiatry. New York, Grune and Stratton, 1976.

Birren, J. E., and Schaie, K. W., eds.: Handbook of the Psychology of Aging. New York, Van Nostrand Reinhold, 1977.

Brickner, P. W.: Home Health Care for the Aged. New York, Appleton-Century-Crofts, 1978.

Brocklehurst, J., ed.: Textbook of Geriatric Medicine and Gerontology. Edinburgh, Churchill Livingstone, 1978.

Burnside, I. M.: Nursing and the Aged. New York, McGraw-Hill, 1976.

Burnside, I. M., Ebersole, P., and Monea, H. E.: Psychosocial Caring Throughout the Life Span. New York, McGraw-Hill, 1979.

Busse, E. W., and Pfeiffer, E.: Behavior and Adaptation in Late Life, 2nd ed. Boston, Little, Brown, 1977.

Butler, R. N., and Lewis, M. I.: Aging and Mental Health, 2nd ed. St. Louis, C. V. Mosby, 1977.

Cape, R.: Aging: Its Complex Management. Hagerstown, Md., Harper and Row, 1978.

Davis, R. H.: Aging: Prospects and Issues. Los Angeles, University of Southern California Press, 1976.

Edington, D. W., and Edgerton, V. R.: The Biology of Physical Activity. Boston, Houghton Mifflin, 1976.

Eliopoulos, C.: Gerontological Nursing Practice. Hagerstown, Md., Harper and Row, 1979.

Eisdorfer, C., and Friedel, R. O., eds.: Cognitive and Emotional Disturbance in the Elderly. Chicago, Year Book Medical Publishers, 1977.

Epstein, C.: Learning to Care for the Aged. Reston, Va., Reston Publishing Co., 1977.

Finch, C. E., and Hayflick, L.: Handbook of the Biology of Aging. New York, Van Nostrand Reinhold, 1977.

Herzog, B. R.: Aging and Income: Programs and Prospects for the Elderly. New York, Human Sciences Press, 1978.

Jarvik, L. F., and Kratz, H., eds.: Aging into the 21st Century. New York, Gardner Press, 1978.

Katzman, R., Terry, R. D., and Bick, K. L.: Alzheimer's Disease: Senile Dementia and Related Disorders. New York, Raven Press, 1978.

Kayne, R. C.: Drugs and the Elderly. Los Angeles, University of Southern California Press, 1978.

Moss, F. E., Jr., and Halamandaris, J. D.: Too Old, Too Sick, Too Bad. Germantown, Aspen Systems Corp., 1977.

Nandy, K.: The Aging Brain and Senile Dementia. New York, Plenum Press, 1977.

Reichel, W., ed.: Clinical Aspects of Aging. Baltimore, Williams and Wilkins, 1978.

Reichel, W., and Schechter, M., eds.: The Geriatric Patient. New York, Hospital Practice Pub. Co., 1978.

Rockstein, M., and Sussman, M. L.: Nutrition, Longevity and Aging. New York, Academic Press, 1976.

Rosenfeld, A. H.: New Views on Older Lives. Washington, D.C., U. S. Gov't. Printing Office, 1978.

Schneider, E. L.: The Aging Reproductive System. New York, Raven Press, 1978.

Siegel, J. H., and Chodoff, P.: The Aged and High Risk Surgical Patient: Medical, Surgical and Anesthetic Management. New York, Grune and Stratton, 1976.

Shephard, R. J.: Physical Activity and Aging. Chicago, Year Book Medical Pub., 1978.

Smith, W. L., and Kinsbourne, B. M.: Aging and Dementia. New York, Spectrum Publications, 1977.

Strain, J. J.: Psychological Interventions in Medical Practice. New York, Appleton-Century-Crofts, 1978.

Storandt, M., Siegler, I. C., and Elias, M. F.: The Clinical Psychology of Aging. New York, Plenum Press, 1978.

Verwoerdt, A.: Clinical Geropsychiatry. Baltimore, Williams and Wilkins, 1976.

Willington, F. L.: Incontinence in the Elderly. New York, Academic Press, 1976.

Watson, W. H., and Maxwell, R. J.: Human Aging and Dying. New York, St. Martin's Press, 1976.

Weiner, M. B., Brok, A. J., and Snadowsky, A. M.: Working with the Aged. Englewood Cliffs, N. J., Prentice Hall, 1978.

Zinberg, N. E., and Kaufman, I., eds.: Normal Psychology of the Aging Process. New York, International Universities Press, 1978.

Developmental Concepts

Barrow, G. M., and Smith, P. A.: Aging, Ageism and Society. New York, West Publishing Co., 1979.

Gutmann, D.: Female ego styles and generational conflict. *In* Bardwick, J., et al., eds.: Feminine Personality and Conflict. Monterey, Calif., Brooks/Cole, 1970.

Kimmel, D. C.: Adulthood and Aging. New York, John Wiley and Sons, 1974.

Lowenthal, M. F.: Some potentialities of a life-cycle approach to the study of retirement. *In* Carp, F. M., ed.: Retirement. New York, Behavioral Publications, 1972.

Neugarten, B. L.: The awareness of middle age. *In* Neugarten, B. L., ed.: Middle Age and Aging. Chicago, University of Chicago Press, 1968.

———: Adult personality: Toward a psychology of the life cycle. *In* Neugarten, B. L., ed.: Middle Age and Aging. Chicago, University of Chicago Press, 1968.

———: Adaptation and the life cycle. *In* Schlossberg, N. K., and Entine, A. D., eds.: Counseling Adults. Monterey, Calif., Brooks/Cole, 1977.

Sorenson, R. C.: Adolescent Sexuality in Contemporary America: Personal Values and Sexual Behavior — Ages 13-19. New York, World Publishing Co., 1973.

Troll, L. E.: Early and Middle Adulthood: The Best is Yet to Be — Maybe. Monterey Calif., Brooks/Cole, 1975.

ARTICLES

Care of the Aged

Campbell, J. C.: Detecting and correcting pulmonary risk factors before operation. Geriat., 32:54-57, May 1977.

Combs, K. L.: Preventive care in the elderly. AJN, 78:1339-1341, Aug. 1978.

Friedman, S. A., and Steinheber, F. U., eds.: Symposium on geriatric medicine. Med. Clin. N. Am., 60:1059-1332 (entire volume), Nov. 1976.

Glover, B. H.: Sex counseling of the elderly. Hosp. Pract., 12:101-113, June 1977.

Griggs, W.: Sex and the elderly. AJN, 78:1352-1354, Aug. 1978.

Kraus, H.: Reconditioning aging muscles. Geriat., 33:93-96, June 1978.

Lore, A.: Supporting the hospitalized elderly person. AJN, 79:496-499, Mar. 1979.

Malinchak, A. A., and Wright, D.: Older Americans and crime: The scope of elderly victimization. Aging: 281-282:10-16, Mar.-Apr. 1978.

McGreehan, D. M., and Warburton, S. W.: How to help families cope with caring for elderly members. Geriat., 33:99-106, June 1978.

Mead, W. F.: The aging heart. Am. Fam. Phys., 18:73-80, Aug. 1978.

Reichel, W.: Multiple problems in the elderly. Hosp. Pract., 11:103-108, Mar. 1976.

Schwartz, D. R.: Public health nursing's responsibilities for care of the aged. Bull. N. Y. Acad. Med., 54:555-560, June 1978.

Sehested, P., and Severin-Nielsen, T.: Falls by hospitalized elderly patients; causes, prevention. Geriat., 32:101-108, Apr. 1977.

Tarara, E. L., and Spittel, J. A.: Clues to systemic diseases from examination of the foot in geriatric patients. J. Am. Podiatry Assoc., 68:387-394, June 1978.

Drugs and the Elderly

Cooper, J. W.: Drug therapy in the elderly: Is it all it could be? Drugs, 18:25-26, July 1978.

Gordon, F. S.: Geriatric medications: Tailoring cardiovascular therapy to the patient. RN, 41:54-61, Mar. 1978.

Gotz, B. E., and Gotz, V. P.: Drugs and the elderly. AJN, *78*:1347-1351, Aug. 1978.

Korcok, M.: Drugs and the elderly. Can. Med. Assoc. J., *118*:1320, 1325-1326, 20 May, 1978.

Mental Health

Burnside, I. M.: Eulogy for Ms. Hogue. AJN, *78*:624-629, Apr. 1978.

Comfort, A.: The myth of senility. Postgrad. Med., *65*:130-142, Mar. 1979.

Glickman, L., and Friedman, S. A.: Changes in behavior, mood or thinking. Med. Clin. N. Am., *60*:1297-1313, Nov. 1976.

Jacobson, S. B.: Geriatric psychiatry today. Bull. N. Y. Acad. Med., *54*:568-572, June 1978.

Mooney, C. M.: Psychologic problems of the aged. J. Am. Geriat. Soc., *26*:268-273, June 1978.

Salzman, C., and Shader, R. I.: Depression in the elderly. I. Relationship between depression, psychologic defense mechanisms and physical illness. J. Am. Geriat. Soc., *26*:253-260, June 1978.

Nutrition

Albanese, A. A., ed.: Nutrition of the elderly. (Symposium). Postgrad. Med., *63*:117-172, Mar. 1978.

Bozian, M. W.: Nutrition for the aged or aged nutrition. Nurs. Clin. N. Am., *11*:169-177, Mar. 1976.

Fulmer, T. T.: If elderly patients can't chew. AJN, *77*:1615, Oct. 1977.

Harper, A. E.: Recommended dietary allowances for the elderly. Geriat. *33*:73-78, May 1978.

Templeton, C. L.: Nutrition counseling needs in a geriatric population. Geriat., *33*:59-66, Apr. 1978.

Psychological Support

Blazer, D.: Techniques for communicating with your elderly patient. Geriat., *33*:79-84, Nov. 1978.

Burnside, I. M.: Listen to the aged. AJN, *75*:1800-1803, 1822, Oct. 1975.

Cohen, G. D.: Approach to the geriatric patient. Med. Clin. N. Am., *61*:855-866, July 1977.

Coleman, C. A., Jr.: Gymnasium for the mind. Geriat., *33*:97-100, Apr. 1978.

Hayter, J.: Positive aspects of aging. J. Gerontolog. Nurs., *2*:19-23, Jan.-Feb. 1976.

Hogstel, M. O.: How do the elderly view their world? AJN, *78*:1335-1336, Aug. 1978.

McIver, V.: Freedom to be: A new approach to quality care for the aged. Can. Nurse, *74*:19-26, Mar. 1978.

Rowe, D.: Aging—a jewel in the mosaic of life. J. Am. Diet. Assoc., *72*:478-486, May 1978.

Psychosocial Aspects: Developmental Concepts

Gould, R.: The phases of adult life: A study in developmental psychology. Am. J. Psychiat., *129*:521-531, Nov. 1972.

Lowenthal, M. F., and Weiss, L.: Intimacy and crises in adulthood. Counseling Psychol., *6*(1):10-15, 1976.

Neugarten, B. L.: Adaptation and the life cycle. Counseling Psychol., *6*(1):16-20, 1976.

Neugarten, B. L., and Gannon, D.: Attitudes of middle-aged persons toward growing older. Geriat., *14*:21-24, Jan. 1959.

Neugarten, B. L., and Kraines, R. J.: Menopausal symptoms in women of various ages. Psychosomat. Med., *27*:266-273, May-June 1965.

Neugarten, B. L., Moore, J. W., and Lowe, J. C.: Age norms, age constraints, and adult socialization. Am. J. Sociol., *70*:710-717, May 1965.

Rotter, J.: Generalized expectancies for internal versus external control of reinforcement. Psycholog. Monographs, *80*:(whole No. 609) 1966.

AGENCIES

Governmental

Administration on Aging, 330 Independence Ave., S.W., Washington, D.C. 20201

Center for Studies of the Mental Health of the Aging, National Institute of Mental Health, Parklawn Building, 5600 Fishers Lane, Rockville, Md. 20857

National Institute on Aging, National Institutes of Health, Bethesda, Md. 20205

Federal Advisory Groups

Counselor to the President on Aging, The White House, Room 425, Executive Office Building, Washington, D.C. 20503

Federal Council on Aging, 330 Independence Ave. H.E.W. North #4260, Washington, D.C. 20201

National Advisory Council on Aging, Building 31, Room 5C-07, National Institutes of Health, Bethesda, Md. 20205

Voluntary

Aging Research Institute, 342 Madison Ave., New York, N.Y. 10017

Alzheimer's Disease Society, 32 Broadway, New York, N.Y. 10004

American Association of Homes for the Aging, 1050 17th St., N.W., Washington, D.C. 20036

American Association of Retired Persons, 1909 K St. N.W., Washington, D.C. 20049

American Geriatrics Society, 10 Columbus Circle, New York, N.Y. 10019

American Podiatry Association, 20 Chevy Chase Circle, N.W., Washington, D.C. 20015

Gerontological Society, 1 Dupont Circle, Suite 520, Washington, D.C. 20036

Gray Panthers, 3625 Chestnut St., Philadelphia, Pa. 19104

National Council on the Aging, 1828 L St., N.W., Washington, D.C. 20036

National Council of Senior Citizens, 1511 K St., N.W., Washington, D.C. 20005

National Geriatrics Society, 212 West Wisconsin Ave., Milwaukee, Wis. 53203

National Safety Council, 444 North Michigan Ave., Chicago, Ill. 60611

14

THE PERSON EXPERIENCING PAIN

Pain disables and distresses more people than any single disease entity. It is probably the most common and compelling reason why a person seeks medical assistance. Most of the medical-surgical problems included in this book are associated with pain, resulting either from the disease process, diagnostic tests, or therapeutic procedures.

Ironically, little is known about pain. Most experts consider it a mysterious phenomenon that defies precise definition. At the very least it appears to have three components: (1) a stimulus, physical or mental; (2) a bodily sensation of hurting; and (3) the reaction of the person experiencing it.

The nurse spends more time with the patient with pain than any other member of the health team and therefore has the opportunity to make a significant contribution toward increasing the patient's comfort and relieving pain. The physician must seek to verify the patient's complaint of pain by establishing the cause and treating it. The nurse, in addition to assisting the physician with this goal, also makes a major contribution to palliative pain relief—relief of pain that does not necessarily involve curing the cause of the pain.

In actual clinical practice, when direct care is given to a patient with pain, it is virtually essential that the nurse adopt the patient's point of view about his pain. Unless he is a malingerer, who consciously lies, the patient does not doubt that he has pain. A cardinal rule in the care of patients with pain is that all pain is real, regardless of its cause—even when the cause remains unknown. Therefore, the nurse's verification of pain is based simply upon the patient's indication that it exists.

Within this context, *the nursing definition of pain may be stated as whatever bodily hurt the patient says he has, existing whenever he says it does.* This definition encompasses three important points that are ultimately relevant to assessment, intervention, and evaluation.

First, the nurse believes the patient. It is important to avoid making the erroneous judgment that the patient does not have pain because no cause can be found or because the pain is not of physical origin. Although some painful sensations are initiated by or sustained by the mental or psychological state of the individual, the patient actually feels a sensation of pain. He is not merely thinking or imagining that he has pain.

Secondly, what the patient "says" about his pain need not be only verbal statements that it exists. Indeed, some patients cannot or will not verbalize. Therefore, the nurse is responsible for eliciting information from the patient and for observing the many nonverbal behaviors that indicate the presence of the pain sensation and all that the patient experiences in relation to his pain.

Thirdly, the nurse realizes that pain is an experience to which the patient responds as a total human being. Consequently, effective management of pain requires knowledge of physiological, psychological, and cultural aspects of the individual patient.

NURSING ASSESSMENT

Assessment of the patient experiencing pain involves:

- recognizing whether the pain is acute or chronic
- identifying the phases of the experience
- observing the patient's behavioral responses
- identifying the factors that influence the pain and the patient's response to it

A thorough assessment is of the utmost importance. To help the patient with his pain, the nurse must know that pain is occurring and how it is affecting the patient. This is not always obvious. There may be a language barrier, or the patient may try to hide his pain because he fears the diagnosis or the treatment. Or, the patient may exhibit minimal responses to pain and, therefore, may appear not to experience pain.

DIFFERENCES BETWEEN ACUTE AND CHRONIC PAIN

The differences between acute and chronic pain have implications for both assessment and treatment. Differences in cause and duration provide a helpful framework for examining the main differences in the effects that pain has upon the patient and the possible variations in the ways pain can be treated.

ACUTE PAIN. Acute pain, which is a very common daily occurence, is usually defined as an episode of pain that lasts from a split second to about six months. Classically, organic disease or injury is present, although healing may also be accompanied by acute pain. As the healing process progresses, the pain subsides and gradually disappears.

Injuries or diseases that cause acute pain may require treatment or may heal spontaneously. For example, a prick of the finger may heal rapidly, the pain subsiding quickly, perhaps within a few minutes. On the other hand, a streptococcal throat infection will require more direct treatment, such as the administration of antibiotics. In the case of a more drastic condition such as appendicitis, surgery may be necessary. In these cases, the pain decreases with healing of the disease or surgical trauma.

CHRONIC PAIN. Chronic pain is defined simply as pain that lasts for six months or longer. Six months is a rather arbitrary period of time for differentiating between acute and chronic pain. An episode of pain may assume the characteristics of chronic pain long before six months has elapsed, or some types of pain may remain primarily acute in nature for longer than six months. Nevertheless, after six months, the majority of pain experiences are characterized by some of the major symptoms associated with chronic pain.

There are at least three main varieties of chronic pain: limited pain, intermittent pain, and persistent pain.

Limited pain is pain that is expected to end eventually. Examples of this type of pain include pain from slowly healing injuries such as burns or torn nerves and muscles. Although torn muscles and nerves may take months to heal, particularly if the patient does not take care to prevent added injury, one can expect that healing will take place and pain will diminish. The situation for the patient with severe burns is even more exacting since he may experience repeated, almost continuous episodes of pain for up to 18 months or longer while the burns heal and reconstructive surgeries are performed. Although 18 months is a rather long time, the pain is not expected to last indefinitely.

With *intermittent pain,* the patient has fairly well defined episodes of pain interspersed with pain-free intervals. However, these episodes may recur rather frequently over a period of years. Hence, this is a type of chronic pain. Physical pathology may exist which accounts for the pain, or the cause may be elusive. Examples of intermittent chronic pain are migraine headache, sickle cell crisis, and back pain that flares up for a few weeks several times a year.

Persistent pain is more or less constant. This type of pain is often called chronic benign pain. The use of the word benign is misleading because it suggests pain of mild intensity and of minimal importance to the patient. Certainly this is not the case. Nonetheless, the word benign has been chosen to help differentiate this type of pain from that caused by malignancy. Cancer pain may last several years, but ultimately its duration is limited due to the underlying pathology. Chronic benign pain lasts indefinitely, perhaps 20 or 30 years, but the underlying pathology is not a direct threat to life. The cause of the pain may be unknown, or, if known, it may not respond to currently available treatment. The most common example of chronic benign pain is low back pain.

PHASES OF THE PAIN EXPERIENCE

The patient may experience any or all of the three phases of a pain experience:

1. the anticipation of pain
2. the sensation of pain
3. the aftermath of pain.

Each of these phases must be assessed because each requires nursing intervention, not just the phase during which pain is sensed. Even the patient who has relatively persistent and chronic pain may experience modified forms of these phases as the pain waxes and wanes in intensity.

The anticipation of pain is sometimes more difficult for the patient to bear than the actual sensation of pain. In addition, what happens, or fails to happen, during the anticipation phase profoundly affects the patient's response to the sensation of pain.

Of the three phases, the most frequently overlooked is probably the aftermath. However, close observation may reveal any number of behavioral responses indicating such feelings as fear, embarrassment, or guilt. These feelings may last from hours to months following the cessation of the pain sensation.

BEHAVIORAL RESPONSES

The patient's responses during any of the three phases of pain experience may be any one or a combination of a large number of possible reactions. These may include physiological manifestations, verbal statements, vocal behaviors, facial expressions, body movements, physical contact with others, or alterations in response to the surrounding environment. These behaviors vary greatly from one person to another and may differ within the same person from one time to the next.

When the nurse observes the patient's behavioral response, the purpose is to identify the following:

1. The phase of pain the patient is experiencing, i.e., anticipation, sensation, or aftermath.
2. The severity of the patient's pain. Whenever possible, it is helpful if the nurse asks the patient to rate his discomfort or the degree to which his discomfort bothers him by some scale such as none, slight, moderate, severe, or very severe.
3. The patient's tolerance for this particular painful sensation. Pain tolerance may be defined as the maximum intensity or duration of pain the person is willing to endure.
4. Characteristics of the painful sensation. These include location (see Fig. 14-1 for areas to which pain in various organs may be referred), duration, rhythmicity (periods of waxing and waning of the intensity or existence of pain), and the quality (e.g., pricking, burning, aching).
5. Effects of pain upon activities of daily living, e.g., sleep, appetite, concentration, interactions with others, and physical movement. (Acute pain is usually associated with anxiety, chronic pain with depression.)
6. What the patient believes will help him with his pain. Many patients have definite ideas about what will increase or decrease the intensity of their pain or what will make it more tolerable.
7. The patient's concerns about his pain. This may include a wide variety of items, such as financial burdens, prognosis, interference with role performance, and body image changes.

Assessing the Harmful Effects of Pain

Special emphasis should be placed upon assessing the harmful effects of pain. Frequently the initial effect of a painful sensation is that of a helpful warning signal. Pain warns us that injury has occurred and that efforts must be taken to treat the injury or prevent further injury. After this initial warning signal, the existence of pain becomes a distressing and often harmful experience. Prolonged or chronic pain may prevent rehabilitation from an illness, or the pain itself may become a disability. Prolonged pain may result eventually in depression, perpetual fatigue due to inability to sleep well, weight gain, problems with

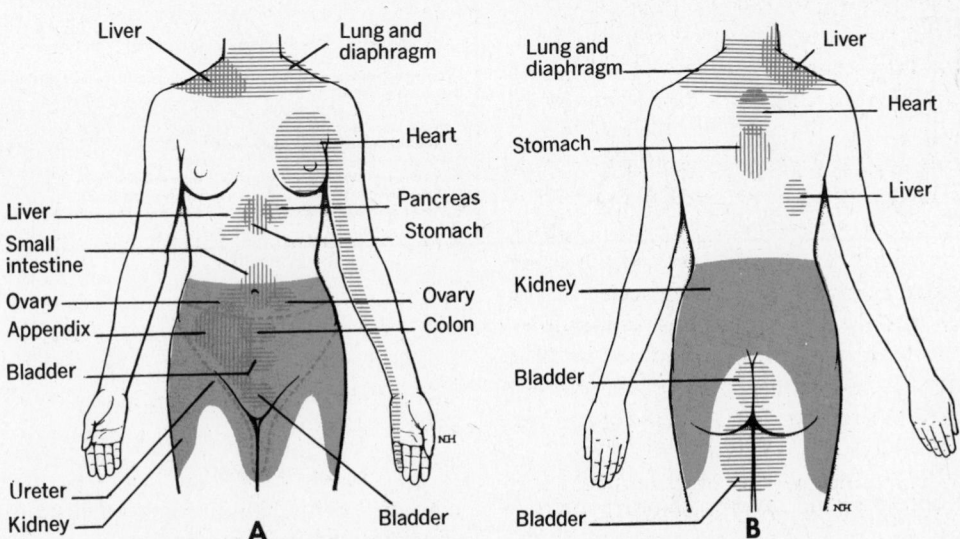

Figure 14-1. Referred pain. *A* anterior view; *B* posterior view. (From Chaffee and Greisheimer: Basic Physiology and Anatomy, 3rd ed. Philadelphia, J. B. Lippincott.)

McGill-Melzack
PAIN QUESTIONNAIRE

Patient's name _____ Age _____
File No. _____ Date _____
Clinical category (e.g. cardiac, neurological, etc.): _____

Diagnosis: _____
_____

Analgesic (if already administered):
1. Type _____
2. Dosage _____
3. Time given in relation to this test _____
Patient's intelligence: circle number that represents best estimate
1 (low)   2   3   4   5 (high)

••

This questionnaire has been designed to tell us more about your pain. Four major questions we ask are:
1. Where is your pain?
2. What does it feel like?
3. How does it change with time?
4. How strong is it?

It is important that you tell us how your pain feels now. Please follow the instructions at the beginning of each part.

_____
© R. Melzack, Oct. 1970

Part 1. Where is Your Pain?

Please mark, on the drawings below, the areas where you feel pain. Put E if external, or I if internal, near the areas which you mark. Put EI if both external and internal.

Part 2. What Does Your Pain Feel Like?

Some of the words below describe your present pain. Circle ONLY those words that best describe it. Leave out any category that is not suitable. Use only a single word in each appropriate category—the one that applies best.

1	6	11	16
Flickering	Tugging	Tiring	Annoying
Quivering	Pulling	Exhausting	Troublesome
Pulsing	Wrenching		Miserable
Throbbing			Intense
Beating	**7**	**12**	Unbearable
Pounding	Hot	Sickening	
	Burning	Suffocating	**17**
2	Scalding		Spreading
Jumping	Searing		Radiating
Flashing			Penetrating
Shooting	**8**	**13**	Piercing
	Tingling	Fearful	
3	Itchy	Frightful	**18**
Pricking	Smarting	Terrifying	Tight
Boring	Stinging		Numb
Drilling			Drawing
Stabbing	**9**		Squeezing
Lancinating	Dull	**14**	Tearing
	Sore	Punishing	
4	Hurting	Gruelling	**19**
Sharp	Aching	Cruel	Cool
Cutting	Heavy	Vicious	Cold
Lacerating		Killing	Freezing
	10		
5	Tender		**20**
Pinching	Taut	**15**	Nagging
Pressing	Rasping	Wretched	Nauseating
Gnawing	Splitting	Blinding	Agonizing
Cramping			Dreadful
Crushing			Torturing

Part 3. How Does Your Pain Change With Time?

1. Which word or words would you use to describe the pattern of your pain?

1	2	3
Continuous	Rhythmic	Brief
Steady	Periodic	Momentary
Constant	Intermittent	Transient

2. What kind of things relieve your pain?

3. What kind of things increase your pain?

Part 4. How Strong Is Your Pain?

People agree that the following 5 words represent pain of increasing intensity. They are:

1	2	3	4	5
Mild	Discomforting	Distressing	Horrible	Excruciating

To answer each question below, write the number of the most appropriate word in the space beside the question.

1. Which word describes your pain right now? _____
2. Which word describes it at its worst? _____
3. Which word describes it when it is least? _____
4. Which word describes the worst toothache you ever had? _____
5. Which word describes the worst headache you ever had? _____
6. Which word describes the worst stomach-ache you ever had? _____

Figure 14-2. McGill-Melzack Pain Questionnaire. The first time the patient completes this questionnaire, the nurse should read the instructions out loud to the patient to make sure that they are fully understood. Otherwise errors tend to occur. It is especially important for the patient to understand that he is to choose only one item from a word list, that he need not choose a word from every subclass, and that he is to describe his pain as it exists at that moment, not previous pain. Initially the questionnaire usually requires 15 to 20 minutes. If the patient uses it often, eventually he may be able to complete it in 5 to 10 minutes. (From: Melzack, R.: The McGill pain questionnaire: Major properties and scoring methods. Pain, *1*:277-299, 1975, pages 280-281.)

concentration, job loss, and divorce or other interpersonal problems.

Acute pain may result in problems that retard recovery from the acute illness associated with the pain. Acute pain may disturb the amount and quality of sleep, decrease appetite, reduce fluid intake, and cause nausea and vomiting. For years the value of rest and nutrition have been recognized as important factors in recovery from

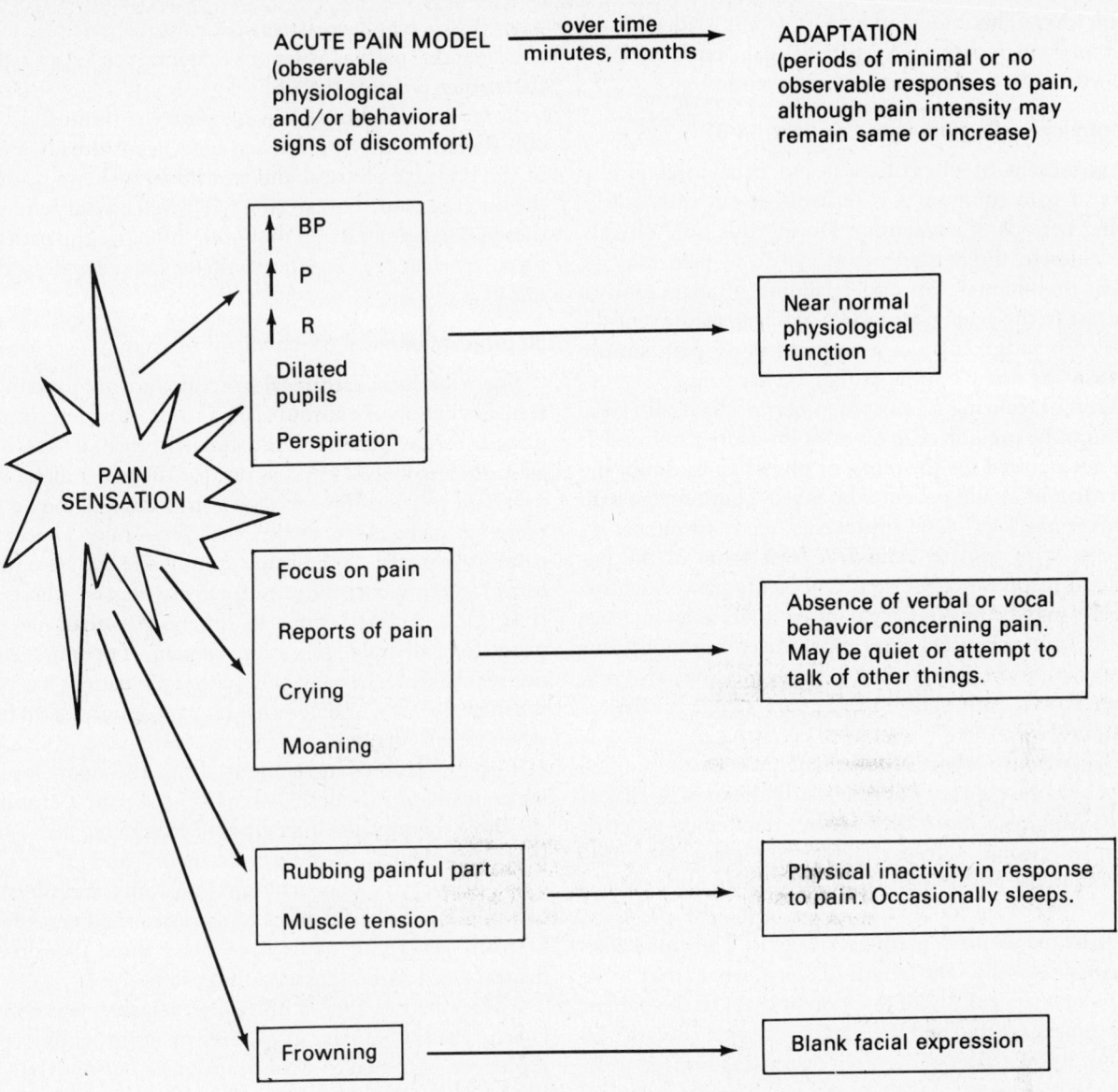

ACUTE PAIN MODEL
(observable
physiological
and/or behavioral
signs of discomfort)

over time
minutes, months

ADAPTATION
(periods of minimal or no
observable responses to pain,
although pain intensity may
remain same or increase)

PAIN SENSATION

BP
P
R
Dilated pupils
Perspiration

Near normal physiological function

Focus on pain
Reports of pain
Crying
Moaning

Absence of verbal or vocal behavior concerning pain. May be quiet or attempt to talk of other things.

Rubbing painful part
Muscle tension

Physical inactivity in response to pain. Occasionally sleeps.

Frowning

Blank facial expression

Figure 14-3. Examples of adaptation of responses to pain.

illness. When pain interferes with sleep and nutritional intake, the patient is deprived of his natural resources for getting well. In addition, the nausea, vomiting, or decreased fluid intake is a potential threat to fluid and electrolyte balance.

Assessing the existence of pain, its nature, and the distressing and harmful effects requires that the nurse ask specific questions and make careful observations. Global questions are not sufficient. For many reasons, patients tend to give incomplete and inaccurate reports of their pain experience unless the nurse asks for details.

Assessment Tools

The McGill-Melzack Pain Questionnaire (Figure 14-2) may be especially helpful in assessing pain in some pa-

tients. It provides a method of obtaining information about the location, intensity, quality, and pattern of the patient's pain, and about factors that relieve or increase the pain. For patients with chronic pain it may be used on a regular basis, e.g., daily, weekly, or before and after pain-relieving treatments. Portions of the questionnaire may be adapted for use for patients with acute pain. For the patient who has difficulty localizing pain or who gropes for words to describe the pain, the questionnaire may be a welcome aid for communicating with the health team.

Repeated observations of the same patient's responses to pain often reveal certain behaviors that the patient tends to exhibit repeatedly in response to the pain experience. The patient's responses, particularly any pattern of responses, should be reported to other members of the health team. This information helps others to identify the existence and qualities of the patient's pain experience and also assists them with plans for intervention.

Adaptation of Responses to Pain (Fig. 14-3)

Assessment of physiological and behavioral indications of pain sometimes is difficult, if not impossible, during periods of adaptation. During this time observable clues to the existence and nature of pain may be absent or minimal. An understanding of adaptation in contrast to the acute pain model will help to prevent the erroneous judgment that a patient has no pain simply because "he doesn't act as though he has pain."

Without realizing it, most members of the health team appear to be prejudiced in favor of the acute pain model. It is not unusual for the nurse or physician to doubt the statement of a calm patient who says, "I have severe pain in my right leg." One mistakenly tends to expect *all* patients with pain to exhibit at least some of the behavioral responses associated with acute pain. Such responses may be physiological in that there is an increase in pulse and respiratory rates and the occurrence of pallor and perspiration. The patient in acute pain may also cry, moan, frown, immobilize a body part, clench his fist, or withdraw.

The responses a particular patient makes to the sudden onset of acute pain are not necessarily the ones he makes when pain lasts more than a few minutes or when it becomes chronic. Obviously the body is unable to sustain an intense physiological reaction to pain for weeks or years, or even several hours.

Other behavioral manifestations of pain may also change drastically. The fatigue of being in pain may leave the patient too exhausted to moan or cry. Or, the patient may appear relaxed and involved in activities because he has become a master of the art of distracting himself from pain. It is unfortunate when the patient who has succeeded in minimizing the effect of chronic pain upon his life is then doubted by others. His is a bitter victory.

Regardless of the type of adjustment made by the patient with chronic pain, pain over an extended period of time often produces behaviors typical of a disability. To some extent the patient usually is unable to continue the activities and interpersonal relationships he engaged in before pain began. This may range from merely having to curtail his participation in some vigorous sport to being unable to take care of his personal needs, such as undressing.

Preexisting Factors Influencing the Pain Experience

All aspects of the patient's pain experience are subject to the influence of a large number of factors. These factors may increase or decrease the perceived intensity of pain, increase or decrease the patient's tolerance for pain, and elicit one particular set of behavioral responses rather than other possible reactions.

Some are situational, arising from the immediate circumstances. Others, discussed here, were already a part of the patient's physical and emotional makeup prior to the onset of pain. This section will dwell on only a few of these preexisting factors that both influence the patient's pain experience *and* interfere with the nurse's understanding of it.

Neurophysiological Mechanisms of Pain

Specific neuroanatomical structures are involved in the transformation of a stimulus into a sensation perceived as painful by the patient. Unfortunately this fact tends to leave the erroneous impression that there is a direct and invariant relationship between a stimulus and the occurrence of pain. As a result, the nurse may expect all patients exposed to the same stimulus (e.g., appendectomy) to experience the same intensity of pain. This is *not* true. Comparable lesions in different patients do not produce comparable sensations of pain. If the nurse does not realize this, she may believe that the patient has pain when he does not or that he has no pain or only slight pain when he is actually experiencing severe pain.

There is lack of agreement about the neurological mechanisms that underlie a sensation of pain. Currently the three theories most frequently considered are (1) the specificity theory, (2) the pattern theory, and (3) the gate control theory. The neurological anatomy and physiology possibly involved in the transmission and perception of pain, according to each of these three theories, is diagrammed and discussed in Figure 14-4.

These theories are not mutually exclusive, and none is considered entirely accurate or comprehensive. However, each makes a contribution to our understanding of what causes a person to perceive pain following a specific stimulus.

The gate control theory provides a particularly helpful basis for beginning to appreciate the individuality of the pain experience. It suggests that the existence and intensity of pain is dependent upon various neurological activities that include the transmission of signals from the cortex and thalamus. These structures send signals that involve the individual's memories and feelings along with cultural influences.

Cultural Influences

Early in childhood a person begins to learn what those around him expect and accept with respect to painful experiences. For example, the person may learn that an injury sustained while he is engaging in a sport is not expected to hurt as much as a comparable injury caused

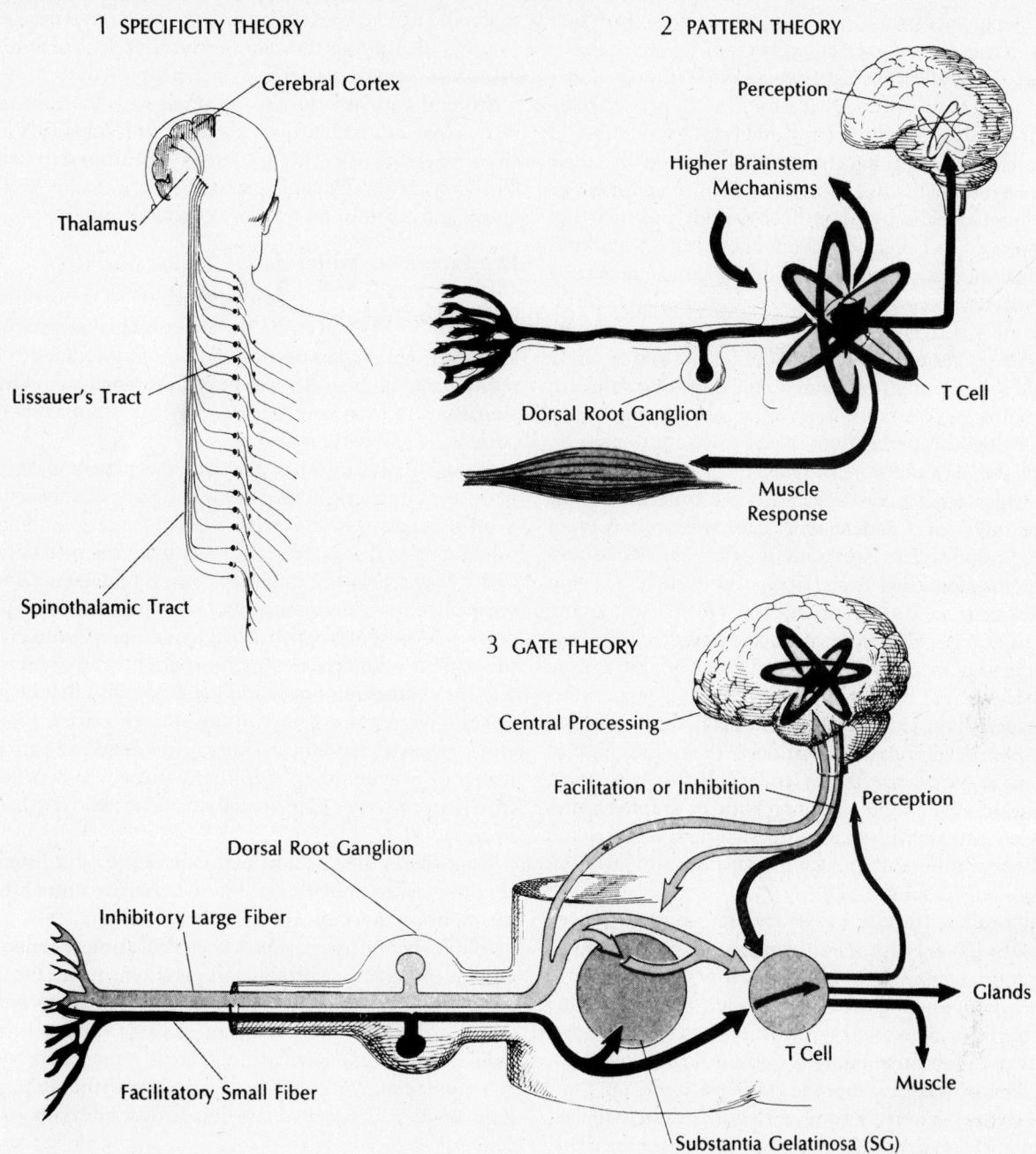

1 SPECIFICITY THEORY

Cerebral Cortex

Thalamus

Lissauer's Tract

Spinothalamic Tract

2 PATTERN THEORY

Perception

Higher Brainstem Mechanisms

Dorsal Root Ganglion

T Cell

Muscle Response

3 GATE THEORY

Central Processing

Facilitation or Inhibition

Perception

Dorsal Root Ganglion

Inhibitory Large Fiber

Glands

T Cell

Muscle

Facilitatory Small Fiber

Substantia Gelatinosa (SG)

Figure 14-4. Three theories of pain transmission and perception are schematized above. The earliest was the Specificity Theory (1), which held that pain stimuli enter the spinal cord through spinal nerves and synapse ipsilaterally, then rise several levels in Lissauer's tract. They then cross the cord and ascend to the thalamus where they synapse again and rise to the cerebral cortex where pain is perceived. (2) The Pattern Theory postulates stimuli entering from nerves through dorsal root ganglia into the spinal cord. The so-called T cell is in the lateral horn of the spinal cord. It sets up a response, part of which results in an impulse to higher brain-stem mechanisms. These, in turn, modulate the response by action on the T cell, which fires and sends impulses to brain, causing perception, and to striated muscle, facilitating response. (3) The Gate Theory depends on concept of two "parallel" fibers, both with cell bodies in the dorsal root ganglia. The large fiber has basically an inhibitory effect on pain perception, the small fiber basically a facilitatory effect. The large fiber acts upon the substantia gelatinosa (SG) and stimulates it. Such stimulation will prevent firing of the T cell, which is necessary for pain perception. The small fiber can overcome or modify the large fiber's influence on the SG, and/or it can directly stimulate the T cell to fire. The large fiber may also act directly on the brain's central processing mechanisms, although the pathways of this action have not been defined. Impulses may be either inhibitory or facilitatory. If the latter, the result will be firing of the T cell, producing pain perception and endocrine and muscle responses. (From: Hospital Practice, Special Report: Recent Studies on the Nature and Management of Acute Pain, Jan. 1976. Reprinted with permission.)

by an unexpected accident. Or, he may simply learn that the latter warrants a greater expression of pain than the former. From all of his experiences with stimuli he begins to learn from others what stimuli are supposed to be painful and what kind of behavioral responses he should make. The people in his culture teach him this by their behavior toward him. They may ignore, punish, or praise him, depending upon his behavior and their beliefs. Since these beliefs vary from one culture to another, it is apparent that patients reporting the same intensity of pain will not necessarily respond to it in the same ways.

The individual is in the process of learning the culture's expectations about pain throughout his life and is rarely affected by consistent exposure to the opposing values of other cultures. Consequently a person tends to grow up believing that his perceptions of and reactions to pain are the only correct and normal ones.

Consider what may happen when a nurse from one culture cares for a patient with pain who comes from another culture. The expectations of the nurse's culture may include avoiding expressions of pain such as crying and moaning, seeking immediate relief from pain, giving efficient descriptions of the pain, and having confidence in the health professions. This nurse may tend to ignore or be skeptical of the patient whose cultural experiences have taught him to moan and complain about pain, to refuse pain relief measures that do not cure the cause of the pain, to use adjectives like "unbearable" in describing his pain, and to be somewhat distrustful of the physician's ability. A patient with still another cultural background may behave differently, or he may behave similarly but for different reasons.

Many other attitudes and behaviors—a patient's preference for having visitors or being alone, or his attitude toward his diagnosis—may vary from one culture to another. Recognizing the values of one's own culture and learning how these values differ from those of other cultures helps immeasurably in overcoming the tendency to evaluate behavior on the basis of one's personal cultural expectations. A nurse with this outlook will have a greater understanding of what the patient is experiencing. Assessment is far more accurate when it takes into account the wide range of possible attitudes and behavioral responses, and interventions for pain relief are more effective when the nurse is able to respond to the patient's particular beliefs and values.

One word of caution to the nurse who embarks upon further study of the expectations which different cultures have in relation to painful experiences. Because of the research design, much of the written material on this fascinating subject tends to identify certain characteristics according to particular sociocultural groups. This may mislead the nurse by seeming to suggest that a patient can be stereotyped according to his cultural membership. Each patient's personal experiences vary too much for

this to be true. It is more productive to use this information for identifying those questions that the nurse must ask about every patient. For example, determining whether a patient wants to be alone with his pain, and why, is far more helpful in planning individualized care than identifying the patient's membership in a sociocultural group and then assuming that his preferences will correspond to those of that group.

Past Experience with Pain

It is tempting and seemingly logical to expect that a person who has had multiple or prolonged experiences with pain will be less anxious and more tolerant of pain than a person who has not experienced much pain. Occasionally this may be observed, but for the majority of patients, the reverse is true.

Probably the more experience the patient has with pain, the more frightened he will be about subsequent painful events. He may also tend to be less willing to tolerate pain, that is, to want relief from the pain sooner and at lower levels of intensity. This is understandable if we realize that, unfortunately, most patients with pain receive unsatisfactory pain relief from time to time. Thus the patient with repeated pain experiences may learn to fear the escalation of pain and the possibility that he will not receive relief. Further, quite simply, once a patient experiences severe pain, he knows just how bad pain can become. On the other hand, the patient who has never experienced severe pain actually does not know what to be afraid of!

Sometimes the effect of past experience with pain is a result of an accumulation of many separate painful events throughout the patient's life. For other patients, past painful experiences may have been more or less constant, as in prolonged or chronic and persistent pain. The patient who feels pain for months or years may suffer additional effects from this type of past experience with pain. Notably the patient's personality may undergo a change. He may become quite irritable, withdrawn, and depressed, and others may find him unpleasant to be around.

The undesirable effects that may result from past experiences point up the need for the nurse to be attentive to all of the patient's experiences with pain. If the patient's pain is regularly relieved, promptly and adequately, perhaps he will be less fearful of future pain and more able to tolerate it.

NURSING MANAGEMENT

Basic Care Plan

Once information about the patient is organized, it provides a basis for designing individualized nursing care. *First the nurse plans to alter factors that influence the nature of the pain sensation and factors that increase the intensity of the patient's behavioral responses to the pain experience.* Of course, some influencing factors cannot or should not be altered. For example, if one factor that causes a painful sensation is pressure from an inoperable malignancy, then it may be impossible to alter this factor. The malignancy simply cannot be removed. However, in some cases positioning, drug therapy, or radiation may decrease the pressure. An example of a factor that both should not and essentially cannot be altered is the influence of the patient's cultural expectations upon his behavioral responses to pain.

Since it may not be possible or desirable to alter some of the patient's responses to his pain experience, *the second part of the nurse's plan of care includes determining appropriate responses to the patient's behaviors and attitudes regarding pain*. For example, the patient's cultural and personal experiences may have taught him that the preferred and natural response to pain experiences is not to share his feelings and sensations with anyone. Another patient may feel quite the opposite, wanting to describe his feelings and pain in detail. Appropriate and helpful nursing approaches to these two patients will differ markedly.

After examining what can be done to assist the particular patient with his pain experience, *the third phase of the nurse's plan is to select appropriate goals for nursing intervention.* Whenever possible these goals are shared with the patient. For a few patients the goal may be total elimination of the painful sensation. For most patients this is rarely realistic. Other goals may include a decrease in intensity, duration, or frequency of pain; a decrease in the extent to which pain bothers the patient; or a decrease in the patient's anxiety during the anticipation, presence, or aftermath of pain.

Principles Related to Pain Relief

GATE CONTROL THEORY. Just as no one really knows how a sensation of pain is produced, no one knows exactly why certain nursing activities may relieve pain. However, the gate control theory (previously mentioned as a possible explanation of the neurophysiological mechanism underlying the pain sensation; see page 238.) is very useful in understanding and devising measures that may relieve pain. In fact, the gate control theory seems to be far more helpful to the clinical practitioner as a conceptual model than it is for the neurophysiologist, who is concerned with studying the neuroanatomy and physiology of pain.

As the name suggests, the gate control theory proposes that there are gating mechanisms in the nervous system that can determine the flow of pain impulses up to the level of consciousness (the thalamus and cerebral cortex). Conceptually, if the gate is open, pain impulses reach the level of awareness. If the gate is closed, pain impulses are stopped and are not felt consciously. If the gate is partially closed, not all pain impulses reach the level of awareness and the intensity of the pain sensation is thus reduced.

The gate control theory stipulates three broad categories of activity that can influence the opening and closing of the gate to the flow of pain impulses.

The following is a brief discussion of these three categories, along with mention of the pain relief measures that can be derived from them.

1. *Activity in the large and small diameter nerve fibers.* Most pain impulses probably travel along the small diameter nerve fibers. Activity in the large diameter nerve fibers may "close the gate" to impulses that travel along the small diameter fibers. For the purposes of intervention it is fortunate that the skin contains a multitude of large diameter nerve fibers. Thus, various forms of cutaneous stimulation may be used to decrease the intensity of pain.
2. *Impulses from the brain stem.* In the brain stem the reticular formation monitors and regulates sensory input. If the patient is subjected to some form of sensory restriction, such as monotony, facilitative impulses may reach the gate from the brain stem, increasing pain by opening the gate to the transmission of pain impulses. However, inhibitory impulses may be sent from the brain stem to the gate if the patient receives sufficient or maximum sensory input. Intervention that takes advantage of this concept includes deliberate distraction strategies, guided imagery, and the avoidance of a monotonous environment for the patient with pain.
3. *Impulses from the cerebral cortex and thalamus.* Processes related to thoughts, emotions, and past experiences are subserved in part by neural activity in these structures. Therefore, an individual's own unique memories, feelings, and level of comprehension may influence whether or not pain impulses are transmitted beyond the gating mechanism to the level of awareness. Some of the cerebral activity is a result of past experience and some is generated by the present situation. In a general sense this can be referred to as the presence or absence of anxiety about pain.

Managing Anxiety Related to Pain

It is well known that anxiety may have a profound influence upon the sensation of pain. For that reason, whether or not anxiety is desirable and what should be done about it will be considered in some detail in the following discussion of the three phases of the pain experience—anticipation, sensation of pain, and aftermath.

ANTICIPATION PHASE. During the anticipation phase of the pain experience, it is desirable for the patient to have a moderate amount of anxiety about the impending pain so that he will be motivated to find methods of coping with it. This degree of anxiety is manifested by the patient's worrying about his anticipated pain some of the time but not all of the time. Usually this anxiety can be produced by informing the patient about when his pain will occur, where it will occur, how intense it will be, and how long it will last. The nurse then channels this anxiety into helping the patient learn a variety of pain relief measures (See pages 243-247).

During the anticipatory phase of pain, teaching the patient about the nature of the impending painful experience and what he can do to obtain relief usually minimizes the anxiety he will have when he actually feels the pain sensation. With this approach, the patient knows that he can do something about the pain when it occurs. Hence, anticipation of pain is less likely to increase anxiety as much as it would if the patient had no knowledge of what to do about the pain. Learning about pain relief measures probably gives the patient a sense of control over sensations of pain. This control seems to affect the patient's appraisal of the threat of pain—he views pain as less threatening.

One of two extremes of reaction sometimes occurs when a patient is taught about a future painful event: intense anxiety or no anxiety. The nurse may employ desensitization, a form of behavior therapy, as a method of presenting information to the highly anxious patient.

To use desensitization the nurse first constructs a hierarchy of stimuli that are frightening to the patient. She then provides a relaxing and pleasurable environment for the patient, begins talking with him about the least frightening stimulus, and progresses up the hierarchy until the patient shows signs of anxiety. At this point she reverts to a less frightening stimulus. This process is repeated at intervals until the patient's anxiety about the most frightening stimulus decreases to a moderate level.

Other anxiety-reducing techniques that may also be effective involve administering tranquilizing drugs, focusing the patient's attention on one specific problem, or eliminating a source of anxiety, for instance, by helping an anxious relative to become less anxious. In some instances it may be necessary to postpone a painful event until the patient's anxiety can be decreased.

The person who shows little or no anxiety about impending pain may simply know from his past experiences that he has a high tolerance for pain. But some patients who show low anxiety or no anxiety are denying the fact that they may have pain. When pain actually occurs, these patients tend to be quite anxious and to have considerable difficulty in coping with pain. What can be done to assist these patients prior to the painful event is largely unknown. We do not yet know with certainty whether it is better to continue to give them information or to give them no information. When giving the patient specific information about pain does not produce seemingly appropriate anxiety, further information probably should be brief, essential, and general. Emphasis should be placed upon pain relief measures.

Preferably, when the nurse suspects that the patient's lack of anxiety reflects an effort to deny information he receives about pain, she explores with the patient whether he wants more information about either pain or its relief. At this point in our knowledge, it appears that his decision should be respected. However, the patient should be closely observed for a marked increase in anxiety as the time approaches for the painful event to occur. The previous suggestions regarding interactions with patients with moderate and severe anxiety can then be employed, depending upon the level of anxiety noted.

At times the nurse may be tempted not to tell a patient that he may experience pain or that the pain may be much greater than he seems to think. She may reason that such knowledge will make him anxious. Indeed, she may be correct. The prospect of pain usually arouses some anxiety in the patient. The nurse must appreciate the necessity of this anxiety and help the patient to use it in a constructive manner—learning about pain relief. If the patient is to learn ways of increasing his ability to cope with pain, he must first know that pain may occur. Failure to forewarn the patient of pain is probably a mistake *unless* one of the following conditions exists: (1) previous experience shows that forewarning this patient produces such a high level of uncontrollable anxiety that the patient is unable to take positive steps toward learning to handle his pain; (2) the patient specifically requests that he not be forewarned, and this request has been thoroughly explored with the patient; or (3) previous experience shows that teaching this patient about pain and its relief damages his coping mechanism of denial and that he has no other effective mechanism for coping with stress.

What the nurse tells the patient about the pain relief measures available and their effectiveness may also be relevant to the anxiety component of the patient's pain experience. The nurse may prevent an increase in anxiety by explaining briefly to the patient the general type of pain relief he can expect from each pain relief measure. For example, if the patient expects distraction or morphine to eliminate his pain totally, his anxiety may increase when this does not happen. These pain relief measures along with many others do not usually eliminate the sensation of pain and may not even reduce its intensity. Instead, they tend to increase the patient's tolerance for pain or render pain much less bothersome to the patient.

THE SENSATION OF PAIN. During the time when pain sensations are felt by the patient, it is desirable to reduce the patient's anxiety to as low a level as possible. When the patient is anxious about his pain there is a tendency for him to perceive a greater intensity of pain or to be less tolerant of the pain. This in turn produces greater anxiety. Thus a spiraling process is initiated in which the patient becomes more anxious and experiences greater pain or becomes progressively less tolerant of pain.

Obviously it is extremely important to interrupt this process as soon as possible. Low levels of anxiety or pain are easier to reduce or control than are higher levels. *Consequently, pain relief measures should be utilized before pain becomes severe.* Many patients have the impression that they should not employ pain relief measures until pain approaches or exceeds the maximum level they are able to tolerate. It is advisable to explain to all patients that pain relief or pain control is more successful if they employ pain relief measures before pain becomes unbearable.

Anxiety during the anticipatory and sensation phases of the pain experience may be managed effectively by nursing activities related to establishing a relationship with the patient with pain and by patient teaching (see below). Almost all nursing interventions for pain relief contribute in some way toward utilizing anxiety or decreasing anxiety.

AFTERMATH. During the aftermath phase of pain, when the pain sensation subsides, it is hoped that the patient's anxiety also will subside. When this does not happen, certain techniques that help the patient to assimilate the pain experience are useful nursing interventions (see page 244).

For many patients the experience of pain continues after the sensation of pain ceases or subsides. Some patients continue to fear pain simply because they do not know that there is no longer any danger that pain will occur. Conveying to the patient that the source of noxious stimuli has been removed or decreased helps prevent him from anxiously expecting pain to continue or to occur again shortly.

Most patients do not seem simply to forget about a painful experience as soon as pain is no longer felt or anticipated. The patient may be disturbed about his behavioral responses to the pain experience or he may be concerned about how others view his responses. He may have unclear and somewhat frightening ideas about the cause of his pain or the treatment for it. His general sense of personal safety and control may be shaken by his having felt more intense pain than he had ever imagined was possible. The patient who is relieved of chronic pain actually may experience an identity crisis, fearing what he will be like without his pain. In the aftermath phase the patient also may suddenly begin trembling or perspiring. He may have nausea, vomiting, or chills. Some patients have nightmares about a painful experience for weeks and months after it is over. Obviously the care of the patient with pain, especially the management of anxiety, extends beyond the anticipation and sensation phases of pain.

NONINVASIVE PAIN RELIEF MEASURES

Perhaps because of the lack of either knowledge or time, many patients and health team members tend to regard analgesics as the major method of pain relief. However, there are many nursing activities that can be used to assist the patient with his pain experience. Table 14-1 outlines various categories of such nursing activities, including:

- Establishing a relationship with the patient
- Teaching the patient about pain and its relief
- Using the patient-group situation
- Managing other people who come in contact with the patient
- Using cutaneous stimulation
- Providing distraction from pain
- Promoting relaxation
- Using guided imagery
- Administering pharmacological agents
- Decreasing noxious stimuli
- Utilizing the assistance of other professionals
- Being with the patient
- Conveying to the patient that the source of noxious stimuli has been removed or decreased
- Assisting with the assimilation of the painful experience

The purpose of the table is merely to introduce the nurse to the variety of nursing activities that may be used to help patients with their pain experiences. This brief synopsis is *not* intended to provide a basis of knowledge sufficient to prepare the nurse to use all of these measures in the actual care of patients. For help in acquiring this knowledge the nurse is referred to the reference at the bottom of the table. Through reading and practice the nurse easily may learn to use these activities with patients.

Some of the noninvasive nursing activities listed in Table 14-1 will be discussed here in more detail. "Noninvasive" simply means that no physical or bodily intrusion is involved. Although noninvasive pain relief measures are not necessarily a substitute for analgesics, for brief episodes of pain lasting only seconds or minutes, a noninvasive technique may be all that is necessary or appropriate. In other instances, especially when there is severe pain that lasts for hours or days, the use of some noninvasive techniques along with medications may be the most effective way to relieve pain.

Relationship and Teaching

The two pain relief measures basic to all others are the nurse-patient relationship and patient teaching about pain and its relief. These activities may actually produce pain relief in the absence of any other pain relief measures. Certainly each may enhance the effectiveness of all other pain relief measures used with the patient. Certain aspects of the relationship and teaching serve to reduce the patient's anxiety about pain, and, as was indicated earlier, reducing anxiety commonly results in pain relief, either by decreasing the intensity of pain or by rendering the pain more tolerable to the patient.

Trust is also an extremely important aspect of the nurse-patient relationship. Conveying to the patient that his complaints about pain are believed can help reduce his anxiety. Some patients spend considerable time and en-

TABLE 14-1.   NURSING ACTIVITIES TO ASSIST THE PATIENT WITH HIS PAIN EXPERIENCE*

CATEGORY OF NURSING ACTIVITY	EXPLANATION	EXAMPLE OF NURSING ACTIVITY
1. Establishing a relationship with the patient with pain	Interacting with the patient as a total person, believing what he says he experiences, and respecting his reactions and attitudes regarding pain (see text).	Telling the patient you believe what he says about his pain experience.
2. Teaching the patient about pain and its relief	Using a variety of the patient's sensory modalities for the purpose of conveying to him information about his pain experience (see text).	Explaining the quality and location of impending pain by applying pressure and pulling the skin in the area where the patient will have an incision.
3. Using the patient-group situation	Using the principles of small group functioning to teach the patient and his family about the patient's pain experience.	The nurse, two female patients with arthritis, and their husbands discussing modifications in home-making activities following discharge from the hospital.
4. Managing other people who come in contact with the patient	Assisting other people to reach their maximum potential for helping the patient with his pain experience.	Talking alone with a patient's wife who shows marked anxiety in the presence of her husband when he complains of his undiagnosed abdominal pain.
5. Using cutaneous stimulation	Using various qualities, locations, durations, and intensities of stimuli in contact with the skin (see text).	Applying a hand-held vibrator to the scalp and back of the neck to relieve headache.
6. Providing distraction from pain	Obtaining the patient's response to and participation in stimuli through the major sensory modalities (see text).	Helping the patient to use "he-who" breathing during a painful dressing change.
7. Promoting relaxation	Using a variety of techniques to assist the patient to avoid fatigue and to achieve skeletal muscle relaxation.	Helping the patient learn to use slow, rhythmic breathing.
8. Using guided imagery	Assisting the patient to imagine a pleasant event as a substitute for the pain experience or to imagine a means of ridding his body of the pain (see text).	Helping the patient imagine that he is ridding himself of pain as he exhales slowly.
9. Administering pharmacological agents	Giving to the patient and explaining the effects of medications with pain-relieving potential; assisting the physician in determining the patient's need for analgesics (see text).	Administering analgesics on a preventive basis.
10. Decreasing noxious stimuli	Using a variety of techniques to reduce the transmission of pain signals to the cortex of the brain.	Splinting an abdominal incision during coughing and deep breathing.
11. Utilizing the assistance of professionals	Assisting the patient, his family, and his physician to identify the need for additional help in dealing with pain; assisting the patient and his family to obtain this help and to utilize it to their best advantage.	Suggesting to the patient that his clergyman may be able to counsel him about his concern (reduce his anxiety) that his pain is punishment for a sin.
12. Being with the patient	Identifying and responding to the patient who would benefit from the mere presence of the nurse or someone else.	Getting a hospital volunteer to sit at the bedside of the patient who does not want to be alone with his pain experience.
13. Conveying that the source of noxious stimuli has been removed or decreased	Conveying to the patient, when appropriate, that something has been done to diminish or eliminate a cause of his pain (see text).	Telling the patient that the needle for his lumbar puncture has just been removed and all that remains is to cleanse his back.
14. Assisting with the assimilation of the painful experience	Identifying the patient's need for and assisting him with the intellectual and emotional incorporation of a painful experience (see text).	Discussing with the patient what sensations he felt and what he was thinking while experiencing his myocardial infarction on the previous day.

*This table is adapted from McCaffery, M.: Nursing Management of the Patient with Pain, 2nd ed. Philadelphia, J. B. Lippincott, 1979.

ergy trying to convince others that they have pain. Perhaps their pain is doubted because no cause can be found for it, or because their behavior is not "typical" for what the health team expects. To say to a patient, "I know you have pain (or discomfort), I only want to understand it better," often will set the patient's mind at rest. Occasionally a patient who has feared that no one will believe him will become tearful with gratitude and relief when he knows that he can trust the nurse and that she believes him.

As quickly as possible upon encountering a patient with pain, the nurse must convey to the patient that she cares about helping him to obtain pain relief. Often the patient does not know where to turn for help in relieving the pain. Indeed, sociologists have noted that seldom is anyone on the health team explicitly held responsible for providing pain relief. However, when the nurse says very simply, "Let me know when you begin to hurt so I can help you do something about it," she quickly conveys to the patient that she cares and in some way assumes responsibility for helping with his pain.

The nurse also provides vital information, via patient teaching, about how pain can be controlled. The patient needs to know, for example, that pain should be reported in the early stages before it becomes severe. Too often the patient waits as long as he can endure the pain before reporting it. At that point the pain may be intense and his anxiety may be very high. It is much easier to prevent severe pain and panic than to relieve them once they exist.

Cutaneous Stimulation

According to the gate control theory, stimulation of large diameter nerve fibers in the skin may reduce the intensity of pain. This can be accomplished in an almost infinite variety of ways. In devising methods of cutaneous stimulation for pain relief, the nurse considers which quality of stimulation is to be used and the location, duration, and intensity of stimulation. Unfortunately, the approach is one of trial and error, but common sense often is an effective guide.

Various qualities of cutaneous stimulation are easily available at low cost. Some may require a physician's order or may be contraindicated, but usually some type of stimulation will be permissible. Different types of skin sensations may be elicited when the following measures are applied: pressure, vibration, heat, cold, bathing, lotion, menthol cream, and transcutaneous electric nerve stimulation (TENS). Although TENS is not as readily available as the other measures, it has proven to be very helpful in both acute and chronic pain relief, and its use is becoming more widespread. It consists of a battery operated unit with electrodes that are applied to the skin to produce a tingling, vibrating, or buzzing sensation in the area of pain.

When cutaneous stimulation is employed, it is applied to different areas of the body. While in some instances, stimulating the skin on or near the site of pain is suitable, in other instances such direct stimulation over the pain site must be avoided because it elicits more pain. If stimulation of the skin near the painful site is ineffective or painful, trigger points may be used. These areas are usually located at some distance from the pain site and cause pain when stimulated. The technique is to apply stimulation at first to the area near the trigger point, and then to work gradually toward the trigger point in an effort to eradicate it.

The intensity of stimulation is generally moderate. Mild stimulation tends to be ticklish or annoying, whereas intense stimulation may cause pain.

In general, the duration of cutaneous stimulation and the intervals between applications of it vary considerably. Some patients experience pain relief for hours or days following cutaneous stimulation. Others obtain relief only while stimulation is being applied. For these patients, use of a menthol cream or a TENS unit is an efficient means of providing continuous stimulation. It takes only a few minutes to apply, but the stimulation lasts for hours. The TENS unit may be worn 24 hours a day.

Oddly enough, the side of the body opposite the painful area may be stimulated for pain relief. For example, the pain of "tennis elbow" on the left side may be relieved better by applying menthol cream to the right elbow rather than the left. This is especially helpful to remember when the site of pain is difficult to stimulate directly, such as when a thick cast has been applied over a painful area or when the entire limb is injured or burned.

Distraction

Distraction, or focusing the patient's attention away from his painful sensations, may be an effective method of pain relief. In some instances it may decrease the perceived intensity of pain, but usually it renders the pain less bothersome to the patient and increases his tolerance for pain. These results are understandable when one considers that pain exists only in the sense that the person is aware of it. In other words, the totally unconscious person does not feel pain. Pain tends to draw attention to itself; but if the conscious person is made less aware of pain or pays less attention to it, he naturally will be less bothered by pain and more tolerant of it.

There are many degrees and types of distraction, ranging from the maintenance of normal and typical levels of sensory input in the environment to the use of highly complicated physical and mental activity. The mere avoidance of sensory restriction is a mild form of distraction.

Sensory restriction may occur when one of the patient's modalities is deprived of stimuli (e.g., bilateral eye patches), when there is a reduction in the patterning and meaningful organization of input (e.g., sounds of cardiac monitors and suction machines), or when there is a lack of variation in stimuli (i.e., boredom). Any of these situations can affect the patient's pain experience. The patient may react with an increased sensitivity to painful stimuli, a decreased tolerance for pain, or an increase in the number of mild discomforts. When the environmental stimuli are deficient in amount, patterning, or variation, the person's centrally regulated thresholds for sensation tend to be lowered. This apparently allows the person to utilize more of the available input. Consequently he is more sensitive to input such as pain.

If the patient with pain is experiencing some form of sensory restriction, pain relief may result when the nurse provides compensating environmental stimuli. This is a very mild form of distraction that focuses the patient's attention away from his painful sensations. The nurse simply is arranging an environment that is more "normal" for the patient. The distraction may merely involve minimizing strange noises, making brief but frequent visits to the patient, bringing him a snack, and/or teaching him physical exercises appropriate to his condition. The latter is a particularly effective method of reducing the effects of sensory restriction.

More deliberate and intense forms of sensory input may be necessary to distract the patient from brief episodes of increased pain, such as bone marrow aspiration or wound debridement, or longer periods of moderate to severe intensities of pain. Some patients are able to utilize distraction for hours.

The value of distraction techniques for pain relief sometimes is misunderstood by the health team. A common misconception is that the patient who can be distracted from his pain does not have as much pain as he seems to want others to believe. However, distraction is a powerful method of pain relief. Doubting the patient's pain because he uses distraction effectively may produce the unfortunate result of causing the patient to stop using the distraction.

The effectiveness of distraction depends upon the degree to which the patient makes an effort to receive and create sensory input other than pain. As a general rule, pain relief is increased in direct relation to the patient's active participation, the number of sensory modalities used, and the patient's interest in the stimuli. Therefore, seeing, hearing, and keeping a box score of a baseball game will distract the patient from his pain more than would only one or two of these activities. Involving the sensory modalities of seeing, hearing, and movement is more effective than using only one or two modalities. If the patient prefers baseball to football, stimuli related to baseball will distract him from pain more than stimuli associated with football.

Increasing the complexity of the distractor as pain increases will work, however, only up to a certain level of pain intensity. With severe pain, the patient is unable to concentrate well enough to engage in highly complicated mental or physical activities.

Many patients devise their own distraction strategies. The patient may hum, mentally calculate math problems, or choose an absorbing television program. The nurse may support these efforts and assist the patient to elaborate upon them.

Under conditions of brief, severe pain, it may be necessary to teach the patient a distraction strategy. A technique that may be taught quickly, even to patients who are debilitated, fatigued, sedated, or in severe pain, is to combine rhythmic rubbing with visual concentration. The patient is asked to open his eyes, stare at a specific spot on the wall or ceiling, and rub a part of his body. The rubbing may be done initially by the nurse. Then the nurse may take the patient's hand and guide him in doing the rubbing. Rubbing with a firm, circular motion on bare skin seems to be effective. The rubbing and staring involve a steady source of sensory input through visual and tactile-kinesthetic modalities along with a focus of rhythm. Sensory input through several modalities combined with rhythm are common characteristics of successful distraction techniques.

A more complicated but highly effective distraction method is "he-who" rhythmic breathing. Ideally the patient is instructed in this technique prior to the onset of or increase in pain. It is also helpful if the nurse demonstrates the method and does it along with the patient. The patient is asked to breathe shallowly. He can be helped to identify this level of breathing by asking him to open his mouth, breathe in, and note when a cool sensation is felt about mid-throat. Then he whispers "he." He inhales shallowly again, then whispers "who." This is repeated again and again. The rate begins slowly and may accelerate as the pain increases in intensity. The patient automatically exhales when he whispers the words. Therefore, there is seldom any need to mention exhalation.

If "he-who" breathing is used for more than a few minutes it is possible that the patient will develop hyperventilation. This need not be a serious problem if the patient is instructed to report the first signs of hyperventilation, i.e., numbness or tingling in the fingertips or around the mouth. The cause of hyperventilation often is forceful exhalation or too rapid a rate of breathing. These can be corrected and the patient can continue to use the distraction.

Relaxation

Skeletal muscle relaxation may reduce the intensity of pain or increase pain tolerance. More often, however, it is combined with other pain relief measures such as pharmacological agents and cutaneous stimulation to enhance their effectiveness. Many people learn relaxation techniques for the purpose of dealing with life stresses. Community agencies offer adult education programs in transcendental meditation, yoga, hypnosis, music therapy, and a variety of other potentially relaxing activities. If a patient already knows a technique for relaxing, the nurse may need only suggest that he use it in the presence of pain or to prevent an increase in pain.

Almost all patients with chronic pain need to learn some method of relaxing and to employ it on a regular basis several times a day. In most patients, chronic pain causes fatigue and muscle tension. Regular periods of relaxation are needed to combat this. Sometimes muscle tension contributes directly to increasing pain.

A simple relaxation technique for patients with acute or chronic pain consists of abdominal breathing at slow, rhythmic rate. The patient may close his eyes and picture the air entering and leaving his lungs as he performs this activity. About six to nine breaths per minute is a slow and comfortable rate. The patient maintains a constant rhythm by counting silently and slowly to himself as he inhales ("in, 1, 2") and as he exhales ("out, 1, 2, 3"). When the nurse is teaching this technique to the patient it is helpful to count out loud for him at first. Initially the patient may benefit from keeping his eyes open and watching the nurse breathe in coordination with him.

Slow rhythmic breathing may also be used as a distraction technique. It may not be relaxing to the patient until he has practiced it and has become skillful in using it.

Guided Imagery

Therapeutic guided imagery may be defined as the use of one's imagination in an especially designed manner to achieve a specific positive effect. In this instance the effects desired are relaxation and pain relief. Imagery of various types is capable of altering body functions over which we seem to have no direct or conscious control. Most people have experienced this in the form of increased cardiac rate (pounding heart) and/or perspiration when a distressing mental image comes to mind just before falling asleep. Although images of this sort seem to provoke a stress response, certain other images seem to evoke relaxation responses or pain relief. A considerable amount of the nurse's time usually is required to teach and explain the technique of guided imagery. The patient, too, must invest time and energy in practicing it. For these reasons guided imagery most often is taught to patients with chronic pain, although it is effective with acute pain as well. To learn to use guided imagery the patient must be able to concentrate, use his imagination, and follow directions. Therefore, this technique is not appropriate for the patient with brain damage. Also it is not advisable to try to teach it when the patient is fatigued, sedated, or in severe pain.

One simple form of therapeutic guided imagery for relaxation and pain relief consists of combining the slow rhythmic breathing described as a relaxation technique with a mental image of relaxation and comfort. With eyes closed, the patient imagines that each time he exhales slowly he is breathing out muscle tension and discomfort, leaving behind a relaxed and comfortable body. Another variation involves suggesting that the patient imagine a ball of healing energy, like a white light, either on his chest or in his lungs. Each time he inhales he can imagine that the air sends the ball of healing energy to the area of discomfort. Each time he exhales, he can imagine that the ball floats away from his body, carrying with it the pain and tension. It enters the body again immediately, in a purified state, and can be circulated to the area of discomfort again.

Usually the patient is asked to practice guided imagery for about five minutes, three times a day. Several days of practice may elapse before the patient finds that he can reduce the intensity of pain through this technique. Pain relief can continue for hours after the imagery is used. Most patients begin to experience the relaxing effects of guided imagery the first time they try it.

MEDICATIONS FOR PAIN RELIEF

Whether pain is acute or chronic, certain guidelines are useful when medications are indicated for the relief of pain. Usually medications are most effective when a preventive approach is used and when the dose and interval between doses is individualized to meet the patient's needs.

Preventive Approach

Using a preventive approach to pain relief means that medications (analgesics in particular) are given before the pain occurs, if it can be predicted, or at least before it reaches a severe intensity. If the patient's pain is expected to occur daily for a great portion of the 24-hour period, a regular schedule may be indicated, rather than the usual p.r.n. method.

A preventive approach has many advantages. It usually takes a smaller dose to alleviate mild pain or prevent the occurrence of pain than it does to relieve severe pain. Thus, a preventive approach may result in a lower total 24-hour dose. This helps prevent tolerance to analgesics and decreases the severity of side effects such as sedation and constipation. Further, pain relief can be more complete with a preventive approach. For example, there need not be any peaks of severe pain and the patient spends less time in pain. On a p.r.n. approach to pain relief, the patient must experience pain, obtain his analgesic, and wait for it to take effect. Within a 24-hour period this may result in his spending a total of several hours in pain.

It is also felt that the better pain control achieved with a preventive approach will reduce the likelihood of the patient's craving the drug. Some health team members seem to feel that the frugal use of narcotics will help prevent addiction in the patient with acute pain. However, there is no basis for this belief. Certainly a patient who is in pain and has his analgesic withheld is more likely to crave the medication than the patient whose pain is relieved before it becomes distressing to him.

Individualized Doses

Individualizing the dose and the interval between doses is necessary because patients metabolize and absorb medications at different rates, and because adjustments are required for varying intensities of pain. It should not be at all surprising that a certain dosage of a narcotic given at specified intervals would be effective for one patient but totally inappropriate for another. However, too often analgesics, especially narcotics, are ordered and given in a very standardized and inflexible manner. The nurse must remember that there are no magic numbers for milligrams or for hours between doses. For example, when a patient metabolizes 100 mg. of meperidine IM in two hours, it should be understood that this is a well documented physiological phenomenon, not a drug abuse problem.

Drug Preferences

With both acute and chronic pain it is wise to utilize aspirin or acetaminophen (e.g., Tylenol, Datril) to the extent possible. Those drugs provide non-narcotic analgesia without the unpleasant sedation and constipation that so often accompany narcotics. Furthermore, when narcotics are necessary it is logical to give these non-narcotic analgesics concurrently, because their effects decrease the dosage of narcotic needed. Also, aspirin and acetaminophen produce analgesia by action at the peripheral nervous system level, whereas narcotics act at the central nervous system level.

For the patient who has chronic pain, whether it is of malignant or benign origin, the use of tricyclic antidepressants may be considered. Usually they are not appropriate for acute pain. However, patients with chronic pain almost always are depressed. These drugs have an antidepressant effect after about 14 days. Since they have a sedative effect and the total daily dose may be given at bedtime, they assist with sleep disturbances. Recently it has been discovered that tricyclic antidepressants probably have an analgesic effect after 10 days of regular administration. Thus, the patient may benefit from a certain level of non-narcotic analgesia.

If narcotics are necessary for chronic pain, priority should be given to the oral route of administration. Currently the drug of choice is methadone. It is less expensive than most other narcotics and it appears to be capable of dealing with severe pain if necessary. A 20 mg. dose of methadone, taken by mouth, is approximately equal in analgesic effect to 10 mg. of morphine sulfate IM. It is reliably absorbed from the gastrointestinal tract, and it has a longer duration of action than most narcotics. It seems to cause less nausea, vomiting, and sedation. For patients with cancer pain, Brompton's mixture (a liquid given orally and containing a variety of drugs plus either heroin or morphine), is frequently given. But, those who have worked with both Brompton's mixture and methadone now consider methadone superior. However, successful results can be obtained with either drug, if used properly.

Proper use, as was mentioned previously, involves a preventive approach. Drugs such as methadone and Brompton's mixture are rarely very effective if they are given on a p.r.n. basis. Almost always they are given on a regular schedule around the clock for prolonged pain, particularly cancer pain. The patient is awakened at night for his scheduled dose if it can be predicted that pain will awaken the patient or will be out of control by morning.

SPECIAL FACILITIES*

Over the last decade many pain clinics have been established in the United States to help patients with chronic pain. They tend to utilize a multidisciplinary approach and to offer a variety of perspectives on the relief of pain. Therapy may include biofeedback, acupuncture, nerve blocks, hypnosis, autogenic training, group therapy, medication, physical therapy, nutritional counseling, and many others. Not all pain centers offer the same approaches to pain relief. Some clinics or centers treat the patient on an outpatient basis, whereas others admit the patient to a pain control unit (PCU).

When the patient is not able to obtain satisfactory pain relief, the physician may refer him to a pain center for evaluation and treatment. Unfortunately there are not nearly enough pain centers to care for all the patients with chronic pain. The waiting lists at such clinics often are quite long.

Hospice settings have been developed in some areas to give care and symptomatic relief to the dying patient. Pain control is one of their primary goals. Again, there are not enough of these agencies to care for all of the patients who need them.

*For information on how to obtain *Pain Clinic Directory, 1977,* listing the locations of and services offered by pain clinics throughout the world, write: Committee on Pain Therapy & Acupuncture, American Society of Anesthesiologists, 515 Busse Hwy., Park Ridge, Ill. 60068.

For assistance in locating hospice programs that are being developed or providing service in your area (directory being prepared), write Public Information Dept., Hospice, 765 Prospect St., New Haven, Conn. 06511.

EVALUATION OF THE EFFECTIVENESS OF PAIN RELIEF MEASURES

To determine objectively the effectiveness of nursing activities designed to help the patient with his pain experience, the patient's behavioral responses prior to intervention are compared with those which follow intervention. After the nurse intervenes, she once again assesses the patient's behavioral responses, much as she did in her initial assessment. This assessment is repeated at appropriate intervals following the intervention.

• Care should be taken not to equate sedation with pain relief.

The *comparison* of these assessments reveals the effectiveness of the pain relief measures. This provides a basis for continuing or modifying nursing intervention.

GUIDELINES TO NURSING MANAGEMENT OF THE PATIENT WITH PAIN

I. Assess the patient's behavioral responses to the pain experience.
  1. Identify whether the pain is acute or chronic.
  2. Identify the phase or phases (anticipation, presence, aftermath) the patient experiences.
  3. During each phase of the pain experience observe all of the patient's behavioral responses, using the following as a guide:
    a. Physiological manifestations
    b. Verbal statements
    c. Vocal behaviors
    d. Facial expressions
    e. Body movements
    f. Physical contact with others
    g. Alterations in response to the surrounding environment
    h. Adaptation of physiological and/or behavioral responses
  4. Use the patient's behavioral responses to determine the following:
    a. Severity of pain
    b. Tolerance for pain
    c. Characteristics such as location, duration, rhythmicity, and quality
    d. Harmful effects of pain upon recovery
    e. What the patient believes will help him with his pain
    f. The patient's concerns about his pain
    g. Any pattern in the patient's behaviors, i.e., behaviors the patient tends to exhibit repeatedly
II. Assess factors that influence each of the following:
  1. The presence of each phase of the pain experience
  2. The nature of the painful sensation(s)
  3. The patient's behavioral responses, including his concerns and beliefs
III. Organize the most pertinent findings of the assessment of the patient.
  1. Identify the phases of the patient's pain experience and the nature of the pain sensation(s) and identify those factors that influence the existence of the phases of the pain experience and the nature of the pain sensation(s).

2. Describe the patient's behavioral responses to each phase of the pain experience and identify those factors that help to explain why the patient behaves as he does.
IV. Plan and implement nursing intervention to assist the patient with his pain experience.
  1. Identify realistic goals for nursing intervention.
  2. Use the following categories of nursing activities as a guide to selecting and implementing nursing measures that will alter factors that influence the patient's experiences and behaviors during each phase of his pain and that are appropriate responses to the patient's behaviors:
    a. Establishing a relationship with the patient with pain
    b. Teaching the patient about pain and its relief
    c. Using the patient-group situation
    d. Managing other people who come in contact with the patient
    e. Using cutaneous stimulation
    f. Providing distraction from pain
    g. Promoting relaxation
    h. Using guided imagery
    i. Administering pharmacological agents
    j. Decreasing noxious stimuli
    k. Utilizing the assistance of other professionals
    l. Being with the patient
    m. Conveying that the source of noxious stimuli has been removed or decreased
    n. Assisting with assimilation of the painful experience
  3. Select a variety of nursing activities, remembering that establishing a relationship with the patient with pain and teaching him about pain are basic to the effectiveness of all other pain relief measures.
V. Evaluate the effectiveness of nursing intervention.
  1. Compare the patient's behavioral responses prior to intervention with his responses following intervention.
  2. Modify nursing intervention in accordance with the results of the evaluation and the patient's changing status.

BIBLIOGRAPHY

BOOKS

Bonica, J. J., and Albe-Fessard, D. G., eds.: Advances in Pain Research and Therapy, vol. 1. New York, Raven Press, 1976.

Crue, B. L., Jr., ed.: Pain Research and Treatment. New York, Academic Press, 1975.

Donavan, M. J., and Pierce, S. G.: Cancer Care Nursing. New York, Appleton-Century-Crofts, 1976.

Fagerhaugh, S. Y., and Strauss, A.: Politics of Pain Management: Staff-Patient Interaction. Menlo Park, Calif., 1977.

Fordyce, W. E.: Behavioral Methods for Chronic Pain and Illness. St. Louis, C. V. Mosby, 1976.

Jacox, A. K., ed.: Pain: A Source Book for Nurses and Other Professionals. Boston, Little, Brown, 1977.

Kroger, W. S., and Fezler, W. D.: Hypnosis and Behavior Modification: Imagery Conditioning. Philadelphia, J. B. Lippincott, 1976.

McCaffery, M.: Nursing Management of the Patient with Pain, 2nd ed. Philadelphia, J. B. Lippincott, 1979.

Melzack, R.: The Puzzle of Pain. New York, Basic Books, 1973.

Sternbach, R. A.: Pain, A Psychophysiological Analysis. New York, Academic Press, 1968.

————: Pain Patients: Traits and Treatment. New York, Academic Press, 1974.

Zborowski, M.: People in Pain. San Francisco, Jossey-Bass, 1969.

ARTICLES

Barrins, P. C.: What nurses need to know about hypnosis. RN, *38*:37-54, Jan. 1975.

Benson, M. K. D.: Surgical management. Nurs. Mirror, *144*:49-53, Jan. 13, 1977.

Blackwell, A. K., and Blackwell, W.: Relieving gas pains. AJN, *75*:66-67, Jan. 1975.

Breedon, S., and Kondo, C.: Using biofeedback to reduce tension. AJN, *75*:2010-2012, Nov. 1975.

Copley, I. J.: No matter what you call it, it's still pain to the patient. RN, *41*:64, Feb. 1978.

Coxhead, C. E.: Physiotherapy in low back pain. Nurs. Mirror, *144*:57-59, Jan. 13, 1977.

Craven, J., and Wald, F. S.: Hospice care for dying patients. AJN, *75*:1816-1822, Oct. 1975.

Davis, A. J.: Teaching your patients to use electricity to ward off pain. RN, *41*:43-45, Feb. 1978.

Davitz, L. J., and Davitz, J. R.: How nurses view patient suffering. RN, *38*:69-74, Oct. 1975.

Davitz, L. J., Sameshima, Y., and Davitz, J. R.: Suffering as viewed in six different cultures. AJN, *76*:1296-1297, Aug. 1976.

Dell, D. D., and Snyder, J. A.: Marijuana: pro and con. AJN, *77*:630-635, Apr. 1977.

Everall, M.: Cold Therapy. Nurs. Times, *72*:144-145, Jan. 29, 1976.

Fagerhaugh, S. Y.: Pain expression and control on a burn care unit. Nurs. Outlook, *22*:645-650, Oct. 1974.

Harris, C. M.-T.: The mechanics of lifting. Nurs. Mirror, *144*:60-61, Jan. 13, 1977.

Hassid, P.: Focus . . . on the behavioral responses. AJN, *76*:1244, Aug. 1976.

Holdcroft, A.: Analgesia and anesthesia. Nurs. Times, *141*:60-63, July 3, 1975.

Hogan, L., and Beland, T.: Cervical spine syndrome. AJN, *76*:1104-1107, July 1976.

Isler, C.: New approach to intractable pain. RN, *38*:17-21, Jan. 1975.

Iveson-Iveson, J.: Aspirin reincarnated. Nurs. Mirror, *142*:39, Mar. 18, 1976.

Jacox, A. K.: Assessing pain. AJN, *79*:895-900, May 1979.

Johnson, J. E., and Rice, V. H.: Sensory and distress components of pain. Nurs. Res., *23*:203-209, May-June 1974.

Johnson, M.: Pain: How do you know it's there and what do you do?. Nursing '76, *6*:48-50, Sept. 1976.

Kerrane, T. A.: The Brompton Cocktail. Nurs. Mirror, *140*:59, May 1, 1975.

Maher, R. M.: Cancer pain in relation to nursing. Nurs. Times, *71*:344-349, Feb. 27, 1975.

Marks, R. M., and Sachar, E. J.: Undertreatment of medical inpatients with narcotic analgesics. Ann. Int. Med. *78*:173-181. Feb. 1973.

McCaffery, M.: Current misconceptions about the relief of acute pain. *In* Crue, B. L., Jr., ed.: Chronic Pain—Further Observations from City of Hope. Spectrum Publications, Jamaica, N. Y., 1979.

————: Dorsal column stimulation. Nursing '75, *5*:54-55, Aug. 1975.

————, and Hart, L. L.: Undertreatment of acute pain with narcotics. AJN, *76*:1586-1591, Oct. 1976.

————: Technique to help a patient relax. AJN, *77*:795, May 1977.

Munley, M. J., and Keane, M. C., eds.: Impressions of pain: A nursing diagnosis. Nurs. Clin. N. Am., *12*:609-668, Dec. 1977.

Naish, J.: Discomfort after food. Nurs. Times, *71*:2060-2062, Dec. 25, 1975.

O'Brien, E. A.: Nursing care following back surgery. Nurs. Mirror, *144*:54-56, Jan. 13, 1977.

O'Dell, A. J.: Hot packs for morning joint stiffness. AJN, *75*:986-987, June 1975.

Ostrow, L. S.: New hope for patients with trigeminal neuralgia. AJN, *76*:1301-1303, Aug. 1976.

Ostrowski, M. J., and Dodd, V. A.: Transcutaneous nerve stimulation for relief of pain in advanced malignant disease. Nurs. Times, *73*:1233-1238, Aug. 11, 1977.

Pace, J. B.: Helping patients overcome the disabling effects of chronic pain. Nursing '77, 7:38-43, July 1977.

————: Commonly overlooked pain syndromes responsive to simple therapy. Postgrad. Med., *58*:107-113, Oct. 1975.

Paige, R. L., and Looney, J. F.: Hospice care for the adult. AJN, *77*:1812-1815, Nov. 1977.

Plein, J. B.: Perspectives on aspirin, part 1: Aspirin as an analgesic. Nurse Practitioner, *1*:34-36, Mar.-Apr. 1976.

Rose-Neil, S.: Acupuncture. Nurs. Times, *72*:687-689, May 6, 1976.

Ryan, B. J.: Biofeedback training: The voluntary control of mind over body and mind. Nurs. Forum, *1*:48-55, 1975.

Saunders, C.: Control of pain in terminal cancer. Nurs. Times, *72*:1133-1135, July 22, 1976.

Smith, S. E.: How drugs act—10: Drugs and pain. Nurs. Times, *71*:1379-1380, Aug. 28, 1975.

————: How drugs act—20: Drugs and anaesthesia. Nurs. Times, *71*:1780-1781, Nov. 6, 1975.

Stewart, E.: To lessen pain: Relaxation and rhythmic breathing. AJN, *76*:958-959, June 1976.

Thomas, B. J.: Headache. RN, *38*:20-23, Oct. 1975.

Troup, J. D. G.: The causes, prevention, and treatment of low back pain. Nurs. Mirror, *144*:46-49, Jan. 13, 1977.

Twedt, B.: Control of pain in orthopedic patients. RN, *38*:39-41, Apr. 1975.

Wiener, C. L.: Pain assessment on an orthopedic ward. Nurs. Outlook, *23*:508-516, Aug. 1975.

Wilson, R. L.: An introduction to yoga. AJN, *76*:261-263, Feb. 1976.

Wing, D. M.: A different approach to IM injections. AJN, *76*:1239-1240, Aug. 1976.

15

ONCOLOGY: NURSING THE PATIENT WITH CANCER

Cancer should be regarded as a disease process that begins when abnormal cells are derived from normal body cells by some poorly understood mechanism of change. As the disease progresses, these abnormal cells proliferate, still within a local area. However, a stage is then reached in which the cells acquire invasive characteristics and changes occur in surrounding tissues. The cells infiltrate these tissues and gain access to lymph and blood vessels whence they are transported to form metastases (cancer spread) in other parts of the body.

Although the disease process can be described in the general terms used above, it should be noted that cancer is not a single disease with one cause; rather it is a group of distinct diseases with different causes, manifestations, treatments, and prognoses.

In order to understand the pathophysiology of cancer, let us take a brief look at the structure and function of the normal cell and relate these phenomena to the aberrant behavior of the cancer cell.

CELL STRUCTURE, GROWTH, AND FUNCTION: NORMAL AND MALIGNANT

The basic unit of independent life is the cell, from which the organism as a whole is formed. The living cell is capable of fulfilling the following functions: (1) separation from the rest of the universe by a boundary (the cell membrane) that can selectively allow the flow of salts, water, nutrients, and various chemical compounds in and out of the cell; (2) conversion of energy in chemical bonds to useful work, such as contraction of protein molecules, formation of secretions, synthesis of compounds, transportation of molecules (various portions of the cell); (3) chemical synthesis or degradation of molecules (generally enzymatic processes); (4) reproduction; (5) cellular control, development, and differentiation (genes of the nucleus); and (6) defense against changes in environment or forces that threaten cellular integrity. Like the cell, the entire human body has mechanisms for each of these six functions, except that specialization of function, and control systems are more highly developed. Yet all of this must spring from the information present in code form in the nucleic acids of the cell nucleus—and that from a single cell, the fertilized egg. The variations of the basic ideas of cell biology are rich and complex, and what follows is but a faint indication of the whole.

A summary of cell substructures and their functions may be found on page 252.

Control of Cellular Biochemical Events: Role of Nucleic Acids

The control and direction of chemical events provide order and continuity in the life of the cell. Proteins are the bricks of the cellular house, or the catalysts, organizers, and controllers of chemical reactions. They are formed by the combined action of nucleic acids in the nucleus (DNA) and in the cytoplasm (RNA) on amino acids. All of the information needed for the biochemical life of the cell in space and in time is found in the genes of the chromosomes, and this information is transformed into protein molecules.

251

CELL STRUCTURE AND FUNCTION

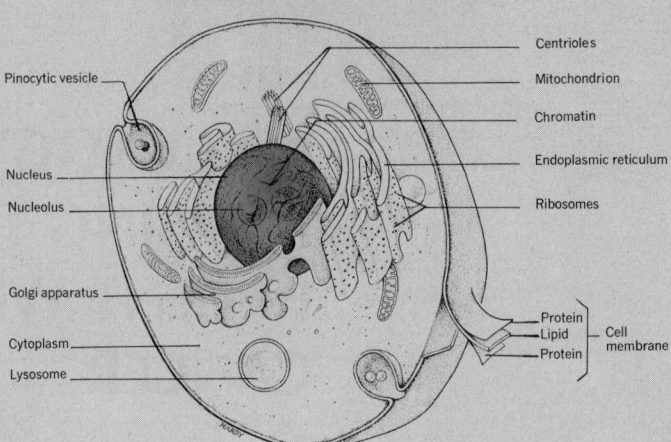

CELL MEMBRANE

A mosaic of lipids and globular proteins that acts as a boundary between the cell and the environment. It also provides for two-way transport of chemical substances by the following means:

1. diffusion from an area of high concentration to one of low concentration
2. specific "carrier proteins" or enzymes that pick up the transported molecules at specific points and move them through the membrane
3. "carrier proteins" that utilize chemical energy to transport molecules against a chemical gradient (potassium into the cell, sodium out of the cell)
4. infoldings of the cell that engulf substances, creating pockets that then reopen inward or outward (pinocytosis)

The cell membranes also act as "recognizers" of foreign substances by means of immunoglobulins that cast the cell and combine with antigens to initiate the series of chemical responses called antigen-antibody reactions which are important to immunity.

MITOCHONDRION

The mitochondrion is an organelle ("little organ") with enzymes arranged on shelves (cristae) formed from covering membrane. It functions as a means for transferring chemical energy in hydrogen bonds in foodstuffs to adenosine triphosphate (ATP), a common source of energy for cell activities such as transport of molecules, contraction of protein molecules (muscle), and synthesis of chemical compounds. The hydrogen combines with oxygen to form water, and the carbon from which the hydrogen is taken is finally converted into carbon dioxide. The ATP as it releases its energy is converted into *adenosine monophosphate* (AMP), which is ready to again accept hydrogen bond energy to form ATP. Mitochondria, then, capture chemical energy to do chemical work by means of oxidative metabolism.

ENDOPLASMIC RETICULUM

A variable network of tubular or vesicular (bubble-shaped) protein structures that are the sites of synthesis of various molecules needed by the cells. Smooth, or agranular, endoplasmic reticulum is involved in lipid synthesis (especially triglycerides), conjugation of bile pigments, conversion of glycogen to glucose (glycogenolysis), and drug detoxification. Granular endoplasmic reticulum is studded with ribosomes composed of ribonucleic acids, and is important in protein synthesis.

GOLGI APPARATUS

A variable structure, loosely organized; probably another form of the endoplasmic reticulum associated with the forma-tion of secretory molecules (usually arranged in granules), such as the digestive enzymes of the pancreas and the small bowel that are released from the cell. Other digestive enzymes remain in the cell as packets surrounded by a layer of lipoprotein. The function of these packets, called lysosomes, is to digest foreign substances (bacteria) in the cell, or the cell itself in case of cell death (cytolysis).

STRUCTURES SPECIALIZED FOR A PARTICULAR CELL

microtubules   Protein structures of cilia or sperm that provide motion

myofibrils   Protein structures that shorten and lengthen, as in muscle

CENTRIOLES

A complex of short rods forming a hollow cylinder, generally found near the nucleus. During cell division these migrate to opposite sides of the nucleus and act as a center for the formation and organization of microtubules that make up the spindle and aster of the metaphase portion of mitosis. They may also produce cilia and flagella.

NUCLEUS

A cell organelle containing deoxyribonucleic acid (DNA), and separated from the cytoplasm by a membrane derived from endoplasmic reticulum. Because of its intense staining properties, DNA is called *chromatin*, and may be dispersed or formed into knots, or, during cell division, organized into rodlike units called *chromosomes*, which in turn have subunits called *genes*. Genes control the synthesis of protein in cells according to the information contained in the DNA strands. Thus the nucleus contains the data bank and control system which direct the unfolding biochemical events that constitute the life of the cell.

NUCLEOLUS

A substructure of the nucleus, present in variable numbers, which contains fibrous structures and ribonucleic acid, a component in the sequences of chemical events that originate in the nucleus and end with the formation of protein in the cytoplasm.

PRODUCTS OF CELL ACTIVITY

Lipid droplets formed in the cell or, in the case of the intestine, absorbed. Granules, probably enzymes, or histamine in macrophages, etc. Glycogen, or cell starch. Small filaments.

WATER AND SOLUBLE SUBSTANCES

Sodium, potassium, urea, glucose, protein molecules, anions, in great numbers.

The answers to a few basic questions will shed some light on the process: What is deoxyribonucleic acid (DNA)? In what sense is it an information data bank? How is a readout (formation of protein) of the information accomplished? DNA is formed from three molecules: phosphate, a five-carbon sugar called deoxyribose, and a variety of purines and pyrimidines (called bases). These are arranged in long strands, the elements being repeated along the strands (Fig. 15-1). The backbone of each strand consists of phosphate sugar linkage. The strands occur in pairs and are twisted together to the right in corkscrew fashion to form a helix. The bases are the purines adenine and guanine and the pyrimidines thymine and cytosine, which are arranged in specific sequences and pairs. The specific arrangement of the bases constitutes the code for the formation of proteins.

Most of the information concerning the role of DNA in heredity and in protein synthesis comes from the study of the DNA strands (prokaryocytes) in viruses and bacteria, in which each chromosome is a single circular strand of DNA with a molecular weight of about a million. Probably this information is true for the human complex chromosomes with strands whose molecular weight approaches a billion. The following discussion refers to prokaryocyte material.

Three bases (a triplet) constitute the unit of the code system (codon). Twenty amino acids are coded, and each has more than one triplet; three codons are used to determine the length of the protein chain and to signal the start or stop of the protein synthesis. DNA must express its code through ribonucleic acid (RNA) contained in the nucleoli and in the cytoplasm. RNA, like DNA, is a helix made up of a sugar, phosphate, and bases, except that the 5-carbon sugar is ribose and the pyrimidine uracil is used instead of thymine. In addition, RNA is a single rather than a double strand. RNA occurs in three forms: messenger RNA, ribosome RNA, and transfer RNA, each with its own function.

A skeleton of the theory of protein synthesis goes something like this:

A DNA helix partially untwists, exposing a section called a gene, which controls the formation for a specific protein. Molecules of ribose, phosphate, and particular bases line up against corresponding units in the DNA, and an enzyme RNA polymerase joins these units together to form messenger RNA. Messenger RNA, now carrying the code, moves to the cytoplasm where it attaches to ribosome RNA. This attachment permits the messenger RNA to accept alignment of amino acids in the sequence determined by the code. The amino acids are brought to the ribosome RNA by transfer RNA that is specific for the amino acid. When all the amino acids are lined up, enzymes join them together, and the protein chain is formed. Thousands of forms of messenger RNA occur, about 60 of transfer RNA, and a few of ribosome RNA.

Twisting and untwisting of DNA, length of sequence, signals to start and to stop synthesis are factors involved in the process. DNA can also reproduce itself via the enzyme DNA polymerase.

During cell reproduction, either for growth or replacement, the DNA is duplicated; the DNA strands are untwisted, replicated, and parcelled into two groups, each containing identical genetic material, the latter process being called *mitosis*. The result is two cells with identical structure and heredity, each cell containing the DNA structure possessed originally by the fertilized ovum. Sex cells (ova or spermatozoa), when dividing, parcel out only one half of the genetic material to each of the resulting cells (reduction division, or meiosis). Fertilization of the ovum restores the full complement of DNA (46 chromosomes) but they are of differing heredity, since genetic material from two separate individuals is combined.

The fascinating subject of change in heredity, whether by the combination of DNA from two differing individuals (the usual method), by change in DNA itself (mutation), or by differing expressions of genetic potentiality (dominant or recessive inheritance) cannot be discussed here. These variations permit the recognition of the indi-

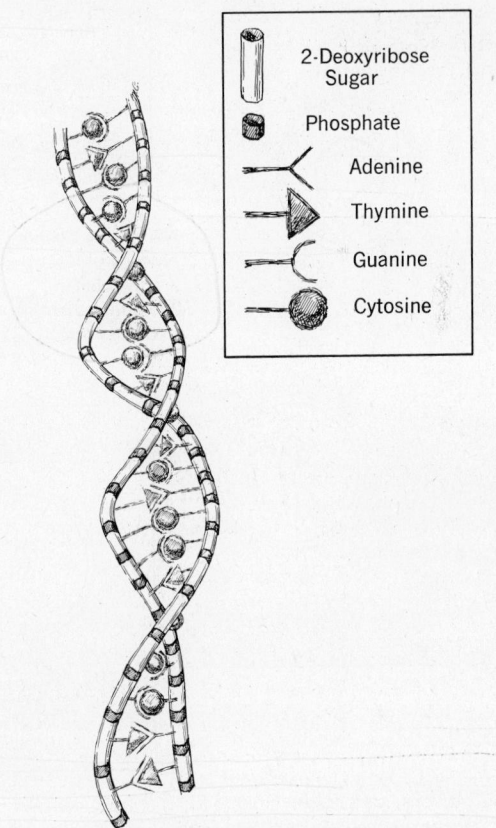

2-Deoxyribose Sugar

Phosphate

Adenine

Thymine

Guanine

Cytosine

Figure 15-1. Schematic representation of the spiral ladder arrangement of repeating nucleotide units found in the DNA molecule. It is thought that anywhere from 500 to 1,000 of these rungs make up a single gene, and that there are over 1,000 genes in a single chromosome. (From Chaffee and Greisheimer: Basic Physiology and Anatomy. J. B. Lippincott, 1974.)

vidual in such details as hair color, sex, body build, and height, or, more subtly, in such manifestations as abnormal lipid transport proteins (hyperlipidemia), some forms of anemia (thalassemia or sickle cell anemia) or of intelligence (mongolism), or absence of enzymes (various heritable metabolic disorders). Thus the variable heredity derived from the union of sex cells may be expressed as disease or as physical and mental superiority.

The Cell Cycle

The completed division of a cell is called a *cell cycle*. Cells in tissues are divided into three populations: (1) continuously dividing cells (bone marrow stem cells, crypt cells of the small intestine), (2) nondividing cells (neurons), (3) resting cells (liver, thyroid gland) that are

capable, when appropriately stimulated, of reproducing. The reference event in the cell cycle is *mitosis*, when the chromosomes are dividing into two portions and are pulled by contracting microtubules (asters) into daughter cells; the cycle extends from mid-mitosis to mid-mitosis of the daughter cells. With respect to DNA, the cycle is marked by two events: the unseen synthesis of DNA (S period of time), and the seen mitosis; the remaining periods are resting periods as far as DNA replication or distribution is concerned. These phases may be identified as follows: S (DNA synthesis), G_0 (resting phase), G_1 (early protein synthesis), G_2 (RNA synthesis and expanded protein synthesis) and M (metaphase). In cells of the human colon, the time of S is 25 hours; of G_1, 15 hours; of G_2, 3 hours; and of M, 1 hour.

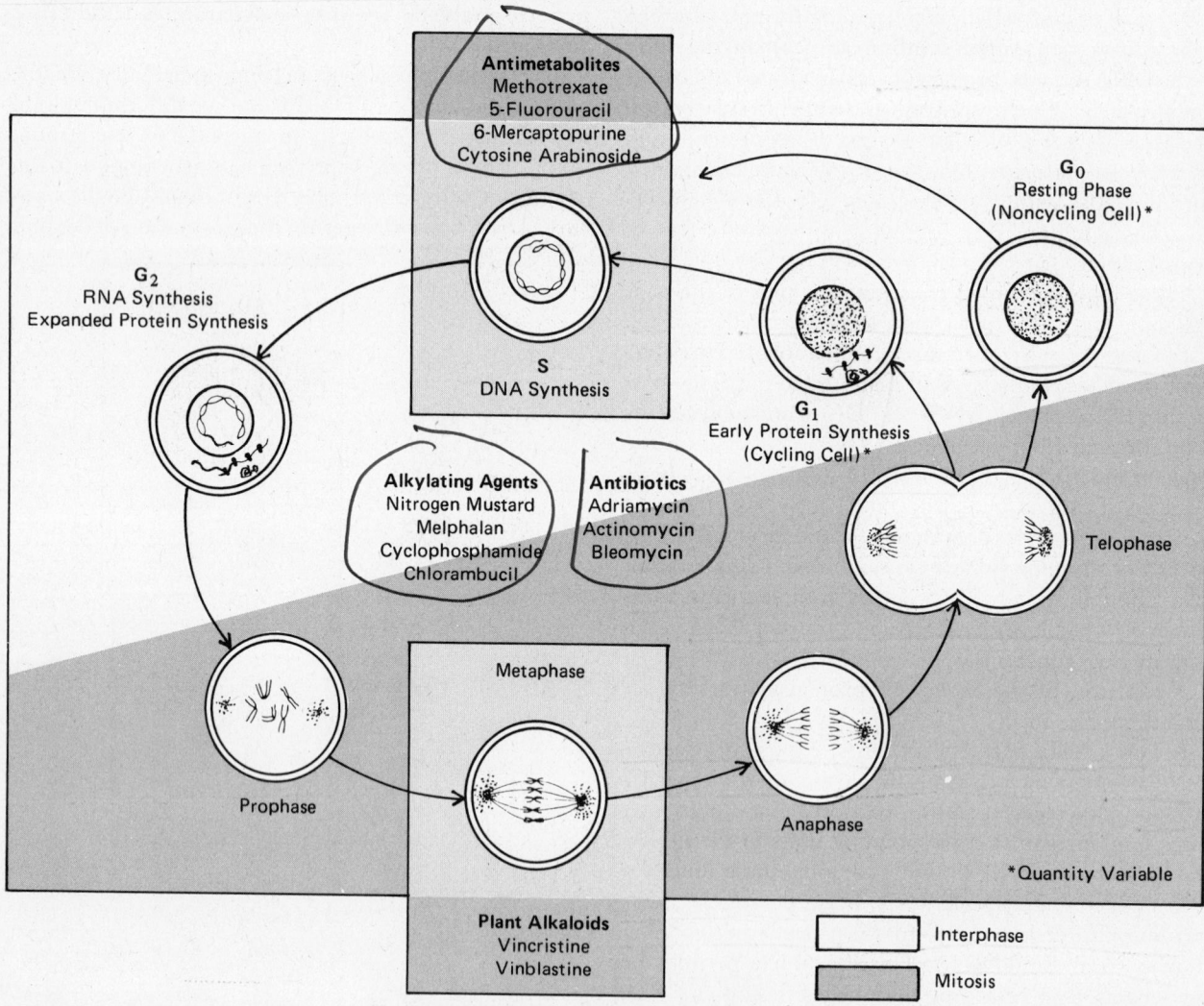

Figure 15-2. Drugs listed in Table 15-1 in terms of their marrow-suppressive properties and chronology of associated nadirs are identified in the schematic diagram above in terms of where, during the cell cycle, they exert their distinctive tumor-killing effect. Actually, all the drugs are active during the entire cycle, but the antimetabolites are particularly effective during the period when a large proportion of tumor cells are in the S phase; similarly the plant alkaloids are relatively most effective during metaphase. Neither of these drug classes is as effective (on a relative dose basis) as the alkylating agents during the resting phase (G_0). No effort has been made in the diagram to indicate the relative time spent by the cell in each phase of the cycle. (Drawing by N. L. Gahan from Lokich, J. J.: Managing chemotherapy—induced bone marrow suppression in cancer. Hospital Practice, *11*:63, Aug. 1976)

Cancer, DNA, and the Cell Cycle

There is a relationship between cancer, DNA, and the cell cycle. Cancer may be considered an unfortunate change in replication structure or control (mutation). Several possible mechanisms have been studied: (1) incorporation of viral DNA into the genetic structure; (2) changes in DNA repair mechanisms; (3) changes in DNA structure caused by radiation, drugs, metabolic diseases, or recurrent cell injury. These cells with altered DNA enter the active cell cycle and, released from physiologic controls, reproduce endlessly.

Principle of Cancer Therapy

The aim of cancer therapy is to destroy all of the cancer cells, while avoiding normal cell damage. The cell in active division, particularly during DNA synthesis or replication, is most sensitive to the toxic effect of chemicals and radiation (x-ray beam, radioactive isotopes, or radium). Development of antitumor drugs has been directed toward either DNA structure or synthesis, or toward protein synthesis, because a change in either will prevent cell duplication.

Figure 15-2 pictures the distribution of various cancer chemotherapeutic agents according to position of maximum effect in the cell cycle. During chemotherapy, any normal cells in the S portion of the cycle (DNA synthesis) are vulnerable, along with the cancer cells. If large numbers of cancer cells are in the S phase, and but few normal cells, then chemotherapy may result in satisfactory tumor destruction. Agents directed toward RNA and protein synthesis (antibiotics and alkylating agents) are nonspecific in that all cells are active in these chemical activities. Obviously, the normally continuously dividing cells (bone marrow stem cells, gastrointestinal cells) are exceptionally sensitive to the action of anticancer agents, and thus the side effects of anemia, diminished white cell count, and diarrhea are explained. Table 15-1 lists the various types of anticancer agents and their relationship to side effects, marrow suppression in particular. When serious white cell depression occurs, the patient then is liable to invasion by bacteria and viruses, and hence to life-threatening infection.

One of the main thrusts of current research is the search for chemical agents that synchronize cancer cell division so that all are in the S phase; then, antitumor treatment would be maximally effective. The need to localize anticancer drugs to the tumor as much as possible is obvious.

The unfolding of the DNA-protein synthesis story and the framework of the cell cycle have yielded a good theoretical basis for the development of new agents, particularly those that focus on single anatomical targets or chemical events.

TABLE 15-1.   INCIDENCE AND CHRONOLOGY OF MARROW SUPPRESSION BY CANCER CHEMOTHERAPEUTIC AGENTS

DRUG CLASS	EXAMPLES	MARROW SUPPRESSION	NADIR DAY	SIGNIFICANT MARROW SUPPRESSION	OTHER DOSE-LIMITING TOXICITY
I. Alkylating Agents	Nitrogen mustard Melphalan Cyclophosphamide (CTX) Chlorambucil	Yes	6-8	4-10 days	Nausea and vomiting Cystitis (CTX)
II. Antimetabolites	Methotrexate	Yes	6-9	4-12 days	Stomatitis, renal and hepatic abnormalities
	5-Fluorouracil 6-Mercaptopurine Cytosine arabinoside				
III. Antibiotics	Adriamycin (AD) Actinomycin	Yes	10-14	4-7 days	AD-cardiac toxicity[2] BLM-pulmonary toxicity,[2] dermatitis, fever
	Bleomycin (BLM)[1]	No	—	—	
IV. Natural Products (Plant Alkaloids)	Vinblastine Vincristine[1]	Yes No	4-7 —	3-10 days —	Neurotoxicity
V. Other Compounds	DTIC (Dacarbazine)[1]	Occasional	—	—	Nausea and vomiting, flu syndrome
	Steroids[1]	No	—	—	
					STZ-nephrotoxicity
	Nitrosoureas-BCNU, CCNU, MeCCNU[2]	Yes	20-25	10-40 days	
	Streptozotocin (STZ)[1]	No	—	—	

1 Nonmarrow suppressive at therapeutic doses
2 Maximum cumulative dose limited
(From Lokich, J. J.: Managing chemotherapy—induced bone marrow suppression in cancer. Hospital Practice, *11*:63, Aug. 1976)

CANCER PREVENTION AND CONTROL

The greatest opportunity for achieving cancer cure exists in the early stage of the disease. A localized tumor is easier to treat than the systemic spread of a malignancy; small tumors are more amenable to eradication than large cancers. These facts constitute the rationale for early detection.

Cancer prevention and control can be accomplished by persistently concentrating on several approaches:

1. Promoting research
2. Providing education
3. Eliminating or controlling risk factors and agents that may cause cancer
4. Diagnosing cancer in its earliest stages when curative treatment is possible

CANCER RESEARCH

The National Cancer Act of 1971 has spurred research in the struggling effort to learn the cause and accomplish the cure of cancer. Increased funds have established special cancer centers at research hospitals across the nation and have helped to finance new cancer-control plans and wider testing of anticancer drugs. A National Cancer Plan has been developed which consists of two parts: (1) the Strategic Plan and (2) the Operational Plan. The goal of the strategic plan is to develop the means of reducing the incidence of morbidity and mortality due to cancer in humans. To achieve this, seven objectives have been identified:

1. Reduce the effectiveness of external agents in producing cancer.
2. Modify individuals to minimize their cancer risk.
3. Prevent normal cells from becoming precancerous.
4. Prevent precancerous cells from becoming malignant and cancer-spreading.
5. Accurately assess the risks for both individuals and population groups of developing cancer, and assess the present extent and course of cancer.
6. Develop cancer cures.
7. Improve the rehabilitation of cancer patients.

CAUSATIVE FACTORS

Cancer prevention requires knowledge about causative factors and the measures which can be taken to avoid exposure to them. Causative factors may be grouped under four headings: physical, chemical, genetic, and viral.

Physical Causes

Physical factors associated with cancer include exposure to radiation and physical trauma.

RADIATION. The main types of radiation covered under this heading are actinic radiation, ultraviolet radiation, and radiation from diagnostic and nuclear devices.

Actinic Radiation. Undesirable effects of actinic radiation result from excessive exposure to sunlight, which causes squamous and basal-cell carcinoma of the skin. Since such lesions affect areas of exposed skin such as the face and hands, these areas need to be protected, especially in people with light coloring, since fair skins are affected more readily than dark skins.

Ultraviolet Radiation. Excessive exposure to this type of radiation also is to be avoided; protection is provided by suitable clothing and barrier creams.

Radiation from Radium, X-rays, and Explosion of Nuclear Devices. It is advisable to reduce to an absolute minimum the total amount of this type of radiation. Radiodiagnostic examinations should be made only when there is definite need, and radiotherapy should not be used for noncancerous lesions. When persons are exposed to radiation occupational hazards, a radiological protection service should be instituted. (See Chapter 16).

TISSUE INJURY. Injuries to tissue (apart from radiation) may be a causative cancer factor. There is evidence that physical injury may contribute to the subsequent development of certain cancers including bone sarcoma and sarcoma of soft tissues, testis, and skin.

Chemical Carcinogens

Through the years, various chemical compounds have been linked to cancer, including aromatic polycyclic hydrocarbons (coal tar), aromatic amines, aminostilbenes, urethane, and such metals as nickel, iron, beryllium, chromium, arsenic, asbestos, azo dyes, nitroso-amines, and lactones. Other chemical carcinogens include agricultural insecticides, herbicides, fertilizers, and preservatives.

FOOD AND CANCER. Although nitrites are used as food additives in many countries, they are thought to react with amines to form carcinogens. Legislative controls are necessary to reduce or limit the use of such carcinogenic compounds in food processing.

INDUSTRIAL ENVIRONMENTS. In certain "dirty" industries, conditions exist that seem to be conducive to the development of cancer. This is particularly apparent in chemical plants and asbestos processing companies where the incidence of lung, liver, and bladder cancer is higher than in clean industries.

PHARMACEUTICAL PRODUCTS. Certain cancers are seen today in patients who received certain medications, such as arsenical preparations, 20 years ago. Stilbestrol, a medication given to selected pregnant women approximately 20 years ago has been under study as a carcinogen because, upon reaching puberty, some of the female offspring of the women who received this drug have developed vaginal adenosis, a precursor of vaginal carcinoma.

SMOKING AND CANCER. Cigarette smoking has not only been implicated as a cause of lung cancer but also has been associated with cancer of the mouth, pharynx, esophagus, proximal end of the stomach, and urinary bladder. Smoking less may help an individual to increase his chances of not getting cancer.

Genetic Factors

Although more knowledge is being gained about the genetic aspects of cancer, not enough is known at present to include it as a part of active cancer prevention. However, there seems to be a genetic predisposition or familial tendency toward acquiring cancer. Persons whose immediate family members have cancer of the breast, stomach, colon, uterus, or lung are more likely to develop a similar cancer.

Viral Causes

Since viruses are known to cause certain tumors in animals, there has been a resurgence of interest in attempting to identify viruses as a cause of some human cancers. If it is possible to prove that humans can be affected by oncogenic viruses, it could lead to the development of immunotherapy and protective vaccination with significant implications for prevention.

THE NURSE AND THE CANCER PATIENT

The nurse is a very important member of any cancer care team. In the hospital, the skill of the nurse is a necessary adjunct to that of the surgeon, the radiologist, and the internist. At home, the patient who is being treated for cancer may be cared for by the community health nurse. In industry, the nurse is effective in the detection and care of illness of employees and often is concerned about the health of their families as well. In all ramifications of the health field, the nurse contributes knowledge and expertise in case-finding, assessment, treatment, referral, rehabilitation, and advanced care of persons who have cancer.

The hope of cure in malignant disease depends on treatment of the malignancy before it has spread beyond the localized stage. This means that treatment should be given as soon as possible after the malignancy is recognized, but it must also be understood that in some patients diagnosis may be made after the tumor has spread, making it impossible to cure the patient by our present methods of therapy.

Rapid progress is being made in the education of the public about the dangerous consequences of untreated tumors. The nurse is one of the most effective agents in the dissemination of such information. Not infrequently patients or their friends will question the nurse concerning "a lump that has formed" or a rapid loss of weight with increasing "indigestion."

To answer such questions it is important to know what symptoms and signs suggest malignant disease: (see also Table 15-2).

C — Change in bowel or bladder habits
A — A sore that does not heal
U — Unusual bleeding or discharge
T — Thickening or lump in breast or elsewhere
I — Indigestion or difficulty in swallowing
O — Obvious change in wart or mole
N — Nagging cough or hoarseness

If these symptoms occur in a person past middle age, they are especially suggestive, because cancer occurs most frequently at that time of life. Knowing that only early treatment can cure, the nurse should urge an immediate examination by a physician. The diagnosis is confirmed by the use of biopsy, cytologic test, endoscopy, roentgenogram, scan, ultrasound, or blood tests.

Role of the Nurse

The responsibility of the nurse begins in the early stages of cancer detection and progresses through the following roles:

- supporting the patient undergoing diagnostic procedures
- recognizing the psychological and spiritual needs of the patient
- meeting the fluid and nutritional needs of the patient
- assisting in carrying out treatments for the malignancy itself
- assisting in the rehabilitation and convalescence of the patient
- assisting in the follow-up of all treated patients
- aiding in the collection of data for research

In caring for the patient with a malignant tumor, the nurse finds that the health care team is rarely limited to the surgeon, the patient and the nurse, but often includes the medical oncologist, radiotherapist, medical social worker, nutritionist, occupational and physical therapists, psychiatrist, and clergyman. Over and above this, one cannot overlook the fact that the patient's family plays a significant role.

CLASSIFICATION OF CYSTS AND TUMORS

Cysts

A *cyst* is an abnormal collection of fluid within a definite sac or wall. Cysts may form in several different ways. When the outlet to a gland becomes blocked and the gland continues to secrete, a *retention cyst* is formed.

TABLE 15-2.   CANCER SITES: SYMPTOMS AND RISK FACTORS

	LUNG	ESOPHAGUS	STOMACH	COLON	BREAST	UTERUS (Endometrium)	CERVIX
Symptoms	Chronic cough Dyspnea Hemoptysis	Hoarseness Cough Dyspnea Hemoptysis	Progressive loss of appetite Blood in stool Vomiting Gastric fullness	Change in bowel habits Blood in stool	Change in size, texture, shape Mass Nipple discharge Abnormal nipple inversion	Abnormal vaginal bleeding Persistent vaginal discharge	Abnormal vaginal bleeding Persistent vaginal discharge Postcoital pain or bleeding
Moderate Risk (2-3 times)	Smoking 5-9 cigarettes per day or Family history (parents, siblings)	Heavy alcohol consumption (more than three 2-oz. 80-proof drinks a day or the equivalent in wine or beer) or smoking one pack of cigarettes	Family history (parents, siblings) or Frequent consumption of dried or smoked fish, pickled vegetables	Family history (parents, siblings) or High-fat, high-protein diet Polyps	Family history (mother, sisters) or Possibly high-fat diet or Menopause after age 52 or Obesity or Having first child after age 30 or Having no children	Family history (sisters, mother) or Early menses or Menopause after age 52 or Moderately overweight or Childlessness or Medium doses of estrogen medication or Obesity, hypertension, diabetes	Many sexual partners or Early sexual intercourse (before age 18) Early age at first pregnancy
Great Risk (4 times greater)	Family history and smoking 1-9 cigarettes per day or Smoking 10 or more cigarettes per day or Exposure to air pollution, metal dusts, asbestos	Smoking pack of cigarettes or more *and* heavy alcohol consumption	A combination of stomach cancer risk factors or Pernicious anemia, gastritis, or diabetes	Ulcerative colitis or Familial polyposis or A combination of two colon cancer factors	Two or more breast cancer risk factors	Obesity or A combination of two or more of the other uterine cancer risk factors or High-dose, long-term estrogen therapy	First intercourse before age 18 and many sexual partners or Familial incidence Multiple diseases, Type II herpes virus

(Adapted from Whelan, E. M., and Cole, P.: Cancer News, 1978; published by the American Cancer Society, Inc., with permission.)

Remnants of fetal organs secrete a fluid which can form cysts (called *epidermoid cysts*), often of considerable size, especially when springing from the pelvic organs of the female. An extravasation of blood in the tissues may become surrounded by a definite wall and form an *extravasation cyst*.

Cysts may be formed by parasites, especially the *Taenia echinococcus (Echinococcus granulosus)* or dog tapeworm. These cysts, spoken of as *hydatid cysts*, often are of considerable size and usually are found in the liver.

TREATMENT.   Cysts of several types should be removed when possible, because occasionally they change into malignant growths. They often become infected, at which time incision and drainage are necessary.

Tumors

A tumor is a new growth of tissue (neoplasm) in which the multiplication of cells is progressive and uncontrolled. According to gross appearance, a tumor may be described as *exophytic*, that is, growing away from the surface, *verrucous*, growing along the surface, or *infiltrative*, invading the tissue right from the beginning.

Benign or Nonmalignant Tumors

Some tumors are surrounded by a definite capsule and remain localized in the tissue from which they spring. They disturb their host only by exerting pressure on the surrounding structures or by robbing the normal tissues of their blood supply. These tumors usually grow rather slowly, and once removed they do not tend to recur. Such tumors are spoken of as *benign or nonmalignant*.

Malignant Tumors

Other neoplasms are not surrounded by a capsule, but grow by invasion into the tissues surrounding them; these are *malignant tumors*. Such tumors invade the blood vessels or the lymphatics and extend rapidly along these open channels. Often the tumor cells are broken off and carried by the blood and the lymph to other parts of the body, where they set up a secondary growth.

Secondary growths are looked for at the nearest lymph filter, the lymph nodes. Here cells are caught and may begin to form an independent tumor like the parent or primary growth. Thus, in every patient with cancer of the breast, the axilla is examined carefully for enlarged lymph nodes, because it is known that the lymph flow from the breast is through the axillary lymph nodes.

Tumor cells that invade the blood vessels are carried to organs where the venous blood passes through a capillary bed; thus we see secondary tumors appearing in the lung from a cancer of the breast or in the liver when the cells are carried by the portal venous system from a tumor in the abdomen. This property of tumors is called *metastasis*, and the new or secondary growth is called a *metastatic growth*. The cells of these secondary tumors grow rapidly and under the microscope resemble the rapidly growing cells found in the embryo. They invade the surrounding tissues in such a manner that it is nearly impossible to remove all the tumor cells and, therefore, they tend to recur after the main body of the tumor has been removed.

TABLE 15-3.   COMPARISON OF BENIGN AND MALIGNANT CELLS

	BENIGN	MALIGNANT
Cell type	Adult	Young
Mitotic action	Slight	Usually considerable
Parent resemblance; morphology	Close resemblance to tissue of origin	Cells tend to be anaplastic—less differentiated than normal cells from which they derive
Encapsulation	Often present	Never present
Growth rate	Slow expansion	Rapid infiltration
Spread	Never occurs; remains localized	Forms secondary growths by metastasis through both lymph and blood stream
Recurrence	Does not tend to recur when removed	Tends to recur when removed, because of infiltration
Tissue destruction	Harms the host only by pressure of growth on surrounding structures	Causes loss of weight and strength, anemia, cachexia, and eventually death.

TABLE 15-4.   THE TNM SYSTEM

T—Primary Tumor
N—Regional Lymph Nodes
M—Distant Metastasis

This classification is extended by the following designations:
Tumor:

    TO—No tumor clinically
    TIS—Carcinoma *in situ*
    T1, T2, T3, T4—Ascending degrees of increase in tumor size and involvement

Nodes:

    NO—No regional lymph node involvement assessed clinically
    NX—Regional lymph nodes cannot be assessed clinically
    N1, N2, N3, N4—Ascending degrees of nodal involvement

Metastasis:

    MO—No evidence of distant metastasis
    M1, M2, M3, M4—Ascending degrees of metastatic involvement of the host

TNM assignments may be grouped into a small number of clinical stages. Stage-grouping by site is recommended on the basis of field trials.

American Cancer Society

The rapid growth of the tumor and its secondary growths saps the vitality of its host, with the result that there is a rapid loss of weight and strength. These tumors bleed easily, producing a loss of the red cells in the blood—an anemia. The patient finally becomes thin, pale, and weak, a shadow of his former self. This condition is spoken of as *cachexia*. The course of the disease frequently ends in death.

Since a tumor that is at first benign may take on malignant characteristics, it is well to remove all tumors as soon as they are discovered in most instances. For a comparison of the characteristics of benign and malignant tumors see Table 15-3.

TNM SYSTEM. The TNM system is a method of categorizing the primary lesion and extent of involvement, in the clinical assessment of malignant disease. Specific criteria modify this system according to the anatomical site. An explanation of the TNM designations and system is given in Table 15-4.

Subdivisions on Basis of Tissue

Neoplasms are subdivided further according to the kind of tissue of which they are formed (Table 15-5). In embryonic life there are three divisions of tissue from which all others are formed: (1) endoderm, (2) mesoderm, and (3) ectoderm.

Endoderm is the tissue from which the lining membranes (mucosa) of the respiratory tract, the gastrointestinal tract, and the genitourinary tract are formed.

Mesoderm is the tissue from which muscles, bones, fascia, and connective tissue are formed.

Ectoderm is the tissue from which come the skin cells and the cells composing hair follicles, sweat glands, and the entire nervous system.

TABLE 15-5. CLASSIFICATION OF TUMOR CELLS

ORIGIN OF CELL	BENIGN	MALIGNANT
Epithelium:	Papilloma	Cancer—carcinoma
Skin epithelium	Wart (verruca)	
Gland epithelium	Polyp	Basal cell carcinoma
	Adenoma	Adenocarcinoma
Endothelial Tissue:		Endothelioma
Blood vessels	Hemangioma	Hemangiosarcoma
	Glomus tumor	Hemangioendothelioma
	Hemangiopericytoma	Malignant hemangiopericytoma
Lymph vessels	Lymphangioma	Lymphangiosarcoma
Lymphoid tissue		Lymphosarcoma
Connective Tissue:		
Fibrous tissue	Fibroma	Fibrosarcoma
Adipose tissue	Lipoma	Liposarcoma
Cartilage	Chondroma	Chondrosarcoma
	Osteochondroma	Primary
	Chondroblastoma	Secondary
	Enchondroma	
Bone	Osteoma	Osteosarcoma
	Osteoid osteoma	
	Osteoblastoma	
Marrow elements:		
Hematopoietic cells		Plasma cell myeloma
		Ewing's sarcoma
		Reticulum cell sarcoma
Muscle tissue:	Myoma	Myosarcoma
Smooth muscle	Leiomyoma	Leiomyosarcoma
Striated muscle	Rhabdomyoma	Rhabdomyosarcoma
Nerve tissue:		
Nerve fibers	Neuroma	Neurogenic sarcoma
Ganglion cells	Ganglioneuroma	Neuroblastoma
Glial cells	Glioma*	Glioblastoma
Meninges	Meningioma	
Pigmented neoplasm	Nevus—mole	Malignant melanoma
Notochord		Chordoma
Uncertain origin	Giant cell tumor	Giant cell tumor
		Adamantinoma

*Many classify glioma as malignant

COMPLEX TISSUES. Some tumors, thought to result from embryologic maldevelopment, contain more than one of the embryonal tissues. Tumors containing two of the tissues, called *teratomas* or *dermoids*, are not infrequently seen in operations on the ovary or the testicle. They may contain bone, teeth, and muscle—all of which arise from the mesoderm—and hair, skin, and subcutaneous glands, all of which develop from the ectoderm.

New growths often are composed of more than one tissue and are named accordingly—fibroadenoma, fibrolipoma, osteosarcoma, and so forth.

INCIDENCE OF VARIOUS MALIGNANCIES

The importance of malignant growth to the nursing and the medical professions can be understood if some of the facts concerning its incidence are reviewed. It is estimated that in the United States malignancy annually exacts a toll of at least 395,000 lives (Fig. 15-3), ranking second as the principle cause of death, being exceeded only by heart disease (Table 15-6). More than one out of six deaths that occur in adults are caused by malignancy. It is estimated that more than 128,000 cancer patients might have been saved in 1979, for example, had they recognized early symptoms and sought prompt treatment. At present only one in three cancer victims is saved, although one in two could be saved if diagnosed early enough and given better treatment. Cancer affects men and women of all ages and of all races (Fig. 15-4). No organ of the body is exempt (Table 15-7).

DESIGN OF CANCER THERAPY

Malignant neoplasms usually lead to certain death if untreated, and benign tumors may become malignant without warning. Therefore, it must be realized that the patient who is the host of tumors of any kind is the potential victim of a fatal disease.

Surgery is the most frequently used and most effective method available today for the treatment of cancer. *Radiotherapy* (see Chapter 16) is another frequently used modality of treatment; its objective is to destroy malig-

TABLE 15-6. MORTALITY FOR LEADING CAUSES OF DEATH: UNITED STATES, 1976

RANK	CAUSE OF DEATH	NUMBER OF DEATHS	DEATH RATE PER 100,000 POPULATION	PERCENT OF TOTAL DEATHS
	All Causes	**1,909,440**	**889.5**	**100.0**
1	Diseases of Heart	723,729	337.1	37.9
2	Cancer	377,312	175.8	19.8
3	Stroke	188,623	87.9	9.9
4	Accidents	100,761	46.9	5.2
5	Influenza & Pneumonia	61,666	28.7	3.2
6	Diabetes Mellitus	34,508	16.1	1.8
7	Cirrhosis of Liver	31,453	14.7	1.6
8	Arteriosclerosis	29,366	13.7	1.5

Source: Vital Statistics of the United States.
Prepared by: Research Department, American Cancer Society, 1978.

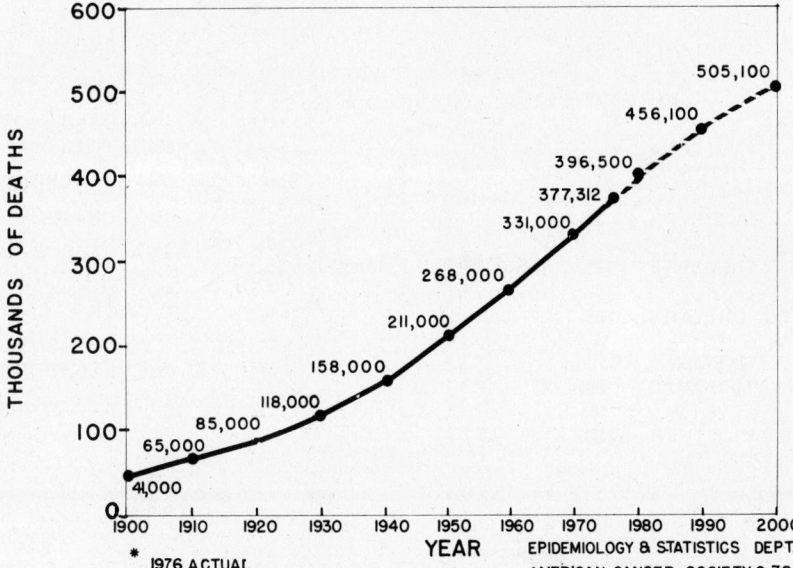

FORECAST OF CANCER DEATHS
(IF PRESENT TRENDS CONTINUE)

Figure 15-3. Forecast of cancer deaths. Note that the solid line through 1976 tells the actual number of deaths from cancer, whereas the dotted line is a statistician's prediction for the years to come—if present rates continue. It is hoped that some more effective means will be found to prevent deaths from cancer. (American Cancer Society)

nant cells with minimum damage to surrounding normal tissue. This form of therapy has been particularly effective in treating seminoma of the testis, retinoblastoma in children, early Hodgkin's disease, and squamous cancer of the cervix and nasopharynx.

If the tumor is limited in its location, surgery and/or radiotherapy may be curative; when this is not the case, these treatment modalities are effective in preparing the patient for chemotherapy and immunotherapy.

Chemotherapy has become more popular and widespread since World War II when it became apparent that chemicals could destroy or significantly inhibit cancer cells without unreasonable toxic effects. There are at least 40 clinically effective chemotherapeutic agents. By this form of therapy alone, significant cure rates have been realized for patients with choriocarcinoma and Burkitt's lymphoma. A significant number of patients can achieve normal life expectancies with drug therapy for the following forms of cancer: lymphocytic leukemia, Hodgkin's disease, Ewing's tumor, Wilms' tumor, testicular tumors, retinoblastoma, histiocytic lymphomas, and embryonal rhabdomyosarcoma.

Endocrinotherapy is a form of management involving the manipulation of hormonal concentrations as they affect tumors of hormone-dependent organs—i.e., breast and prostate. The chief advantage of this form of treatment is that it is physiologic and relatively nontoxic.

Immunotherapy is the newest therapeutic modality for cancer. It is still largely investigative, but it is showing promise and is of great interest.

Adjuvant therapy is the term applied to the combined use of more than one form of therapy. For example, in surgical adjuvant therapy, surgery becomes only one step in a multidisciplinary approach that may also include chemotherapy, immunotherapy, and/or radiation therapy.

SURGERY FOR CANCER

Surgical removal of the entire cancer is regarded as the best method of treatment. However, surgical procedures may be carried out with a variety of objectives in mind in which the emphasis may be mainly diagnostic, prophylactic, curative, reconstructive, or palliative. Or, the chief goal may be the relief of pain.

DIAGNOSTIC. Diagnostic surgery usually is performed to obtain a *biopsy*, the excision of a piece of tissue from a suspicious growth. This tissue is examined under the microscope by a pathologist, who prepares the tissue as a frozen section (rapid) or a paraffin section (permanent). By freezing the tissue first and then slicing it for examination under the microscope, the pathologist is able to quickly examine and report the nature of the cells. The embedding of tissue in paraffin takes longer, but the slice of tissue offers a clearer view of cells and the specimen can be kept for a period of time. Diagnostic surgery may also take the form of a laparotomy, which allows the surgeon to visually determine the extensiveness of cancer spread and the probability of removal. Endoscopy in its various forms can also be performed, allowing for visual and biopsy determinations. Staging to determine the extensiveness of the invasion of cancer can also be done surgically.

1979 ESTIMATED CANCER INCIDENCE BY SITE AND SEX†

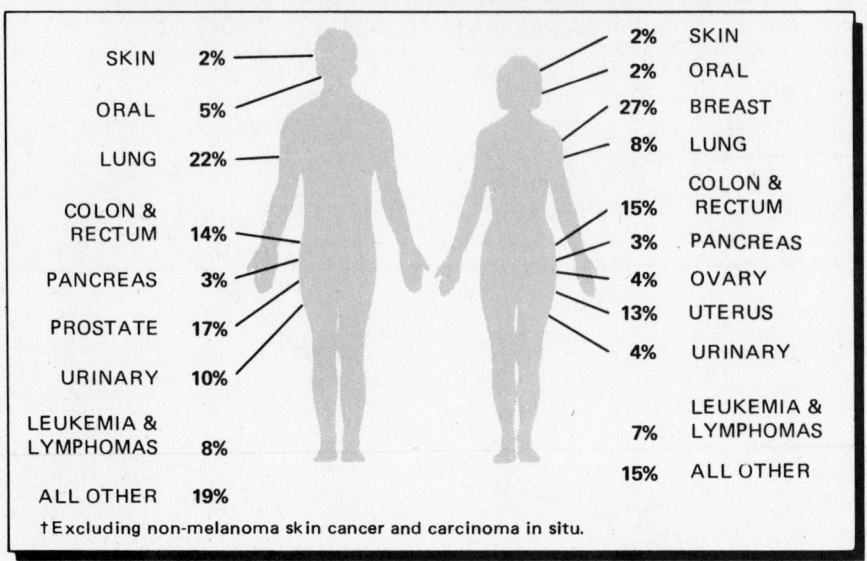

†Excluding non-melanoma skin cancer and carcinoma in situ.

1979 ESTIMATED CANCER DEATHS BY SITE AND SEX

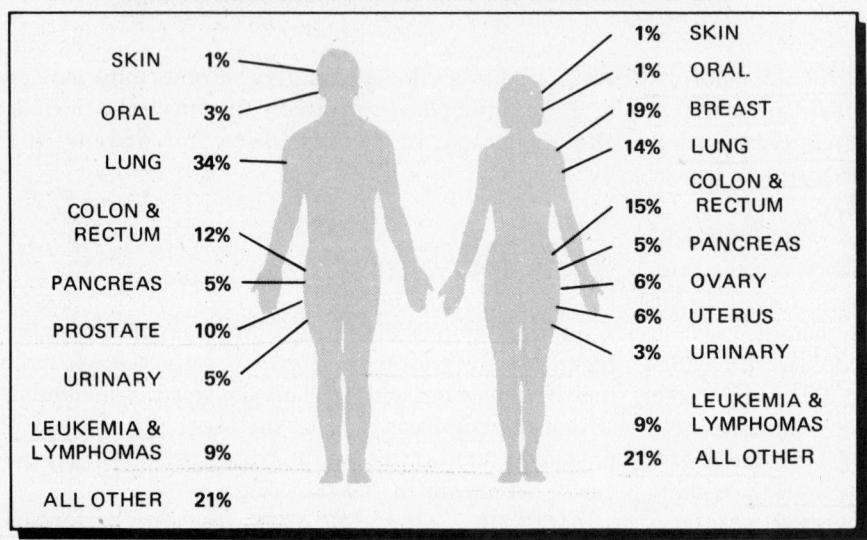

Figure 15-4. Cancer incidence and death by site and sex. (Courtesy, American Cancer Society)

PROPHYLACTIC. Prophylactic surgery involves the removal of lesions which are apt to develop into cancer if they are left in the body. An example is the removal of small tumors (polyps) that often grow in the colon. These may be detected by roentgenograms or sigmoidoscopy.

CURATIVE. The purpose of surgery is to remove the entire tumor with the least disturbance of function. When the tumor is excised along with the lymphatic channels that drain the area near the tumor, the procedure is referred to as "total" or "en bloc" surgery. If the cancer has metastasized, surgery is no longer curative.

RADICAL. On occasion, when the cancer has spread, it may be necessary to perform an amputation of an extremity or even a hemipelvectomy, which includes removal of a section of the pelvis as well as the leg. Extensive internal cancer may require a pelvic exenteration, the removal of several affected organs in the lower abdomen. These procedures are considered mutilating and disfiguring and are only performed with due consideration of the patient's ability to accept the losses in exchange for life. Psychological problems are commonly encountered and must be given priority in the general care of the patient.

RECONSTRUCTIVE. This type of surgery may follow curative or radical surgery and is carried out in an attempt to produce a better return of function and/or a better cosmetic effect. It may be done in one operation or in stages.

PALLIATIVE. Palliative surgery is performed as an at-

TABLE 15-7.   LEADING CANCER SITES, 1979*

SITE	ESTIMATED NEW CASES 1979	ESTIMATED DEATHS 1979	WARNING SIGNAL IF YOU HAVE ONE, SEE YOUR DOCTOR	SAFEGUARDS	COMMENT
Breast	107,000	35,000	Lump or thickening in the breast, or unusual discharge from nipple.	Regular checkup. Monthly breast self-exam.	The leading cause of cancer death in women.
Colon and Rectum	112,000	52,000	Change in bowel habits; bleeding.	Regular checkup, including digital, occult blood and proctoscopic exams, especially after age 40.	Because of accuracy of available tests, is potentially a highly curable disease.
Lung	112,000	98,000	Persistent cough, or lingering respiratory ailment.	80% of lung cancer would be prevented if no one smoked cigarettes.	The leading cause of cancer death among men and rising mortality among women.
Oral (including Pharynx)	24,000	9,000	Sore that does not heal. Difficulty in swallowing.	Regular checkup.	Many more lives should be saved because the mouth is easily accessible to visual examination by physicians and dentists.
Skin	14,000†	6,000	Sore that does not heal, or change in wart or mole.	Regular checkup, avoidance of overexposure to sun.	Skin cancer is readily detected by observation, and diagnosed by simple biopsy.
Uterus	53,000‡	11,000	Unusual bleeding or discharge.	Regular checkup, including pelvic examination with PAP test.	Uterine cancer mortality has declined 70% during the last 40 years with wider application of the PAP test. Postmenopausal women with abnormal bleeding should be checked.
Kidney and Bladder	51,000	18,000	Urinary difficulty. Bleeding—in which case consult doctor at once.	Regular checkup with urinalysis.	Protective measures for workers in high-risk industries are helping to eliminate one of the important causes of these cancers.
Larynx	10,000	3,500	Hoarseness—difficulty in swallowing.	Regular checkup, including laryngoscopy.	Readily curable if caught early.
Prostate	64,000	21,000	Urinary difficulty.	Regular checkup, including palpation.	Occurs mainly in men over 60, the disease can be detected by palpation at regular checkup.
Stomach	23,000	14,000	Indigestion.	Regular checkup.	An 80% decline in mortality in 50 years, for reasons yet unknown.
Leukemia	22,000	15,000	Leukemia is a cancer of blood-forming tissues and is characterized by the abnormal production of immature white blood cells. Acute lymphocytic leukemia strikes mainly children and is treated by drugs which have extended life from a few months to as much as ten years. Chronic leukemia strikes usually after age 25 and progresses less rapidly.		
Lymphomas	39,000	20,000	These cancers arise in the lymph system and include Hodgkin's disease and lymphosarcoma. Some patients with lymphatic cancers can lead normal lives for many years. Five-year survival rate for Hodgkin's disease increased from 25% to 54% in 20 years.		

*All figures rounded to nearest 1,000.   †Estimate new cases of non-melanoma skin cancer over 300,000.

‡If carcinoma in situ is included, cases total over 98,000.
INCIDENCE ESTIMATES ARE BASED ON RATES FROM N.C.I. SEER PROGRAM 1973-76.

(American Cancer Society)

tempt to relieve the complications of cancer, such as ulcerations, obstruction of the gastrointestinal tract, pain produced by extension of the tumor to surrounding nerves, and bleeding and nutritional loss from the extensive tumor growth. Therefore, palliative surgery may give the patient improved health and comfort for a longer period of time than would otherwise be the case. Thus, in bleeding or obstructing tumors of the stomach or bowel, usually the tumor is resected in spite of the fact that the patient may have metastatic extension to the liver.

RELIEF OF PAIN.   In addition to attempts to remove the complications of tumors, other measures are sometimes employed specifically to relieve pain. These include radiation therapy; operations on nerves, the spinal cord, or the brain to divide the pathways that carry pain sensation; the use of hormones in the case of tumors that are affected by hormone stimulation, such as those in the breast or the testes; and the removal of hormone-producing glands such as the pituitary, the adrenal, the ovary, and the testis. None of these procedures can produce a cure for the cancer, but they may relieve pain and in some patients may produce a regression of the tumor for a time.

CHEMOTHERAPY FOR CANCER

The hope for a cancer cure by means of chemical agents (chemotherapy) depends on understanding and making use of the biochemical and metabolic differences between normal and neoplastic cells that allow tumor cells to be destroyed while healthy tissue remains intact. *In general it can be said that as yet no drugs have been discovered that can cure malignant tumors.* Some of the drugs produce a regression of the tumor or its metastases, and the use of chemotherapeutic agents at the time of surgery may reduce or slow up the appearance of secondary growths. In some patients, pain and other symptoms are relieved for a time.

Chemotherapeutic agents are used as the primary treatment for patients with leukemia and choriocarcinoma. Life expectancy can be extended in patients with Hodgkin's disease, other types of lymphomas, Ewing's tumor, Wilms' tumor, embryonal rhabdomyosarcoma, testicular tumors, and retinoblastoma. In such patients, there may be a remission but never a cure. In solid tumors the mass may become smaller and surface ulcerations may heal for a time. In some treatment regimens, two or more drugs may be used together or in sequence. Chemotherapy may be used as adjuvant therapy to surgery to prevent recurrence of some cancers.

The *rationale* for administering these drugs is based on their ability to destroy young, rapidly multiplying cells; the cells comprising malignant tumors possess these characteristics. It is believed that these drugs interfere with the manufacture of nucleic acids that are necessary for the building of genetic structures in cells. As a result, cellular growth and reproduction are inhibited.

However, there also are normal cells in the body that have short life spans and compensate for this by rapid cell proliferation. The majority of these normal, rapidly reproducing cells are located in the bone marrow, the lining of the gastrointestinal tract, and the hair follicles. Unfortunately, the drugs cannot differentiate between rapidly dividing cells that are normal and those that are abnormal. As a result of their effects on normal susceptible cells, toxic signs and symptoms may occur that constitute a major challenge to the nurse.

Chemotherapeutic agents are prescribed after several determinations are made: (1) What is the nature of the tumor? (2) Is this therapy to be used as an adjuvant to some other method of cancer treatment or is it considered after other methods have failed? (3) How effective is each drug for this particular patient? (4) What is the appropriate dosage in relation to the patient's weight and height, in view of the narrow margin between therapeutic dose and toxic level? (5) How much time should be allowed between series of dosages so that normal tissue can recover from toxic effects? (6) What are the side effects, particularly the extent of damage to bone marrow which reduces the number of white cells, red cells, and platelets? (7) Has liver function been affected, since these drugs are metabolized in the liver? (8) Has kidney function been affected, since chemotherapeutic agents are excreted via the kidneys? (9) What other agents can be used simultaneously or sequentially to produce maximum effectiveness?

Specific Agents Used in Cancer Chemotherapy

1. **POLYFUNCTIONAL ALKYLATING AGENTS.** Nitrogen mustards and the polysaccharides are examples of cytotoxic, poisonous agents. These poisons destroy both normal and tumor cells. It is believed that cells in mitosis (rapidly dividing tumor cells) are more sensitive to toxicity than normal adult cells, and that tumors of well-differentiated cells are less sensitive to toxicity than those of less well-differentiated cells in some tumors. By acting with deoxyribonucleic acid in the nucleus, these agents hinder cell growth and division. The chief disadvantage of most of these drugs is their destructive effect on bone marrow, one of the body's chief sources of new blood cells. Other manifestations are nausea, vomiting, stomatitis, and diarrhea.

2. **ANTIMETABOLITES.** The antimetabolites include folic acid and purine antagonists, which are synthetic substances similar to those that nourish the normal cell during its growth and development. However, they differ enough in their chemical composition so that, although the drugs are taken into the cell substance, they cannot be used by the cell. Thus, they deceive the cell and act as a monkey wrench in the cellular machinery. The signs and symptoms indicating evidence of toxicity are similar to those of the alkylating agents.

3. **STEROID COMPOUNDS, ACTH, AND CASTRATION.** Alteration of the endocrine environment is a major approach in the chemotherapy of certain types of neoplastic disease: namely, tumors arising in organs usually under hormonal influence, such as the prostate (castration) and the breast (androgen and estrogen therapy). The patient receiving this form of therapy will need to be observed for signs of toxicity such as fluid retention, hirsutism, nausea, and vomiting. Oophorectomy, adrenalectomy, and pituitarectomy represent similar forms of therapy.

4. **ANTIBIOTICS.** Drugs such as adriamycin, bleomycin, dactinomycin, and mithramycin are being used in cancer chemotherapy. A newcomer is mitomycin C, which demonstrates significant effectiveness in gastrointestinal cancer when used with 5-fluorouracil and arabinosylcytosine.

TABLE 15-8 NEOPLASTIC DISEASES THAT RESPOND TO CHEMOTHERAPY

TYPE OF CANCER	USEFUL DRUGS [C]* [A]†	PERCENT RESPONSE RATE	SURVIVAL OF RESPONDERS (PERCENT)
PROLONGED SURVIVAL OR CURE			
Gestational trophoblastic tumors	Methotrexate, Dactinomycin, Vinblastine	70	Cured
Burkitt's tumor	Cyclophosphamide	50	Cured
Testicular tumors:			
Seminoma	Cyclophosphamide, Radiotherapy	90-95	50-60 Cured
Other	Chlorambucil, Methotrexate, Bleomycin, Dactinomycin, Mithramycin, cis-Platinum (II) diammine dichloride, Vinblastine, [C] [A]	90-95	(15-30 prolonged remission)
Wilms' tumor	Dactinomycin with surgery & radiotherapy, Vincristine [C] [A]	30-40 / 80-90	Cured (advanced stage) / Cured (early stage)
Neuroblastoma	Cyclophosphamide, Adriamycin, Procarbazine, Vincristine [C]	>50 / 5-80	(advanced stage) long-term survival depending on stage
Acute lymphoblastic leukemia	6-Mercaptopurine, Methotrexate, Daunorubicin, Prednisone, L-Asparaginase, 1,3-bis (β-Chloroethyl)-1-nitrosourea, Vincristine [C]	90	70 beyond 5 years
Lymphosarcoma (children)	Same as acute lymphoblastic leukemia [C]	>90	Definite increase
Hodgkin's disease Stages 11B, 111B & IV	Nitrogen mustard (Mustargen), Adriamycin, Bleomycin, Prednisone, 5-(3, 3-Dimethyl-1-triazene)-imidazole-4-carboxamide, Procarbazine, Vincristine, Vinblastine [C]	70	40 beyond 5 years
PALLIATION AND PROLONGATION OF LIFE			
Prostate carcinoma	Estrogens, castration	70	Some increase
Breast carcinoma	Alkylating agents, 5-Fluorouracil, Methotrexate, Adriamycin, Androgens, Estrogens, Prednisone, Nafoxidine, Tamoxifen, Vincristine [C] [A]	60-80	Increase
Acute myeloblastic leukemia	Arabinosylcytosine & 6-Thioguanine, Daunorubicin, Prednisone [C]	65	Increase
Chronic lymphocytic leukemia	Alkylating agents, Prednisone	50	Probable increase
Lymphosarcoma (adults)	Alkylating agents, Nitrosoureas, Prednisone [C]	50	Probable increase
Osteogenic sarcoma	Methotrexate-Citrovorum factor (calcium leucovorin), Adriamycin [C] [A]	20	Increase (advanced stage) / Marked increase with adjuvant Rx (early stage)
PALLIATION WITH UNCERTAIN PROLONGATION OF LIFE			
Chronic granulocytic leukemia	Alkylating agents, 6-Mercaptopurine, Hydroxyurea	90	good control during most of course
Multiple myeloma	Alkylating agents, Prednisone, 1,3-bis (β-Chloroethyl)-1-nitrosourea, Vincristine [C]	60	
Ovary	Alkylating agents, cis-Platinum (II) diammine dichloride	30-40	
Endometrium	Progestins	25	

*[C] Combination chemotherapy shown to be effective
†[A] Adjuvant chemotherapy shown to be effective
(Source: Krakoff, I. H.: Cancer chemotherapeutic agents. CA—A Cancer J. for Clinicians, 24, May-June 1977, American Cancer Society. Also personal communication with Dr. Krakoff.)

TABLE 15-8. (continued)

TYPE OF CANCER	USEFUL DRUGS [C]* [A]†	PERCENT RESPONSE RATE	SURVIVAL OF RESPONDERS (PERCENT)
UNCERTAIN PALLIATION			
Lung	Alkylating agents	30-40	brief responses
Head and neck	Alkylating agents, Methotrexate-Citrovorum factor (calcium leucovorin), Bleomycin, cis-Platinum (II) diammine dichloride	20-30	brief responses
Large bowel	Arabinosylcytosine, 5-Fluorouracil, Mitomycin C 1-(β-Chloroethyl)-3-(4-methylcyclohexyl)-1-nitrosourea [C]	30-50	
Stomach	Arabinosylcytosine, 5-Fluorouracil, Mitomycin C [C]	30	
Pancreas	5-Fluorouracil (islet cell: Streptozotocin)	<10 (80—in treatment of hypoglycemia)	
Liver	5-Fluorouracil	<10	
Cervix	Alkylating agents, Bleomycin	20	
Melanoma	Alkylating agents, 5-(3,3-Dimethyl-1-triazene)-imidazole-4-carboxamide, Vinblastine	20	
Adrenal cortex	o,p'-Dichlorodiphenyldichloroethane	Relief of Cushingoid syndrome	
Soft tissue sarcoma	Methotrexate-Citrovorum factor (calcium leucovorin), Adriamycin	20	
LOCAL CHEMOTHERAPY			
Intracavitary injection for recurrent effusion	Alkylating agents, 5-Fluorouracil, Quinacrine	50—effusions controlled	
Intrathecal injection for meningeal leukemia	Arabinosylcytosine, Methotrexate	80—improvement for 2 months	
Extracorporeal perfusion for cancer of extremities	Alkylating agents	Irregular and uncertain	
Continuous infusion for cancer of head and neck, liver and pelvis	5-Fluorouracil, Methotrexate-Citrovorum factor (calcium leucovorin)	Irregular and uncertain	

5. MISCELLANEOUS. Plant alkaloids, vinblastine (Velban) and vincristine (Oncovin) are derived from the flowering herb, periwinkle. Toxic manifestations of vinblastine (used in Hodgkin's disease) are nausea, vomiting, leukopenia, and epilation. Vincristine given to children with acute leukemia may produce side effects of leukopenia and neuromuscular disturbances.

Methods of Administration

The cancer chemotherapeutic drugs may be given orally, intravenously or intramuscularly into the systemic circulation, or intra-arterially, depending on the drug and the carcinoma. In addition, efforts may be made to introduce high concentrations of the drug into the tumor area by injection into its vascular supply. These efforts require complicated techniques that usually are carried out in specialized clinics.

Perfusion and Regional Infusion

Perfusion technique allows the administration of large doses of extremely toxic drugs to an isolated extremity, organ, or region of the body. Such a dose could not be tolerated by the entire body.

PATIENT PREPARATION. On admission and preoperatively the patient is weighed, because the amounts of chemotherapeutic drug and heparin given are calculated on the basis of kilograms of body weight. Blood, urine, and x-ray studies are also done. Preparation of the patient for surgery includes answering his many questions. It is the physician's responsibility to inform the patient of what can be expected of this therapy, including side effects, so that informed consent may be obtained.

PROCEDURE. In the operating room, the tumor-bearing area is excluded from the general circulation for a set period of time, and a prescribed amount of drug is perfused into the isolated area. A catheter is placed in the desired artery under aseptic conditions and is then attached to intravenous tubing and the perfusion bag. The perfusion is controlled by an infusion pump or an arterial pressure cuff. During the procedure, tourniquets and/or ligatures are used in an effort to prevent seepage of the drug into the systemic circulation. Obviously, it is easier to prevent leakage into the systemic circulation when an extremity is involved, than when the torso is perfused.

For percutaneous introduction of the catheter into a

TABLE 15-9.   SPECIFIC AGENTS USED IN CANCER CHEMOTHERAPY

AGENTS	PRINCIPAL ROUTE OF ADMINIS- TRATION	USUAL DOSE	ACUTE TOXIC SIGNS	MAJOR TOXIC MANIFESTATIONS
POLYFUNCTIONAL ALKYLATING AGENTS				
Methylbis (β-Chloroethyl) Amine (HCL HN2, Mustargen)	I.V.	0.4 mg./kg. single or divided doses	Nausea and vomiting	Therapeutic doses moderately depress peripheral blood cell count; excessive doses cause severe bone marrow depression with leukopenia, thrombocy- topenia and bleeding. Maximum toxicity may occur two or three weeks after last dose. Dosage, therefore, must be carefully controlled. Alopecia and hemorrhagic cystitis occur occasionally with cyclophosphamide.
Chlorambucil (Leukeran)	Oral	0.1-0.2 mg./kg./day 6-12 mg./day	None	
Melphalan (Alkeran)	Oral	0.1 mg./kg./day x 7 2-4 mg./day maintenance	None	
Cyclophosphamide (Endoxan, Cytoxan)	I.V.	3.5-5.0 mg./kg./day x 10 (40-60 mg./kg. single dose)	Nausea and vomiting	
	Oral	50-200 mg./day		
Triethylenethio- phosphoramide (TSPA, Thio-TEPA)	I.V.	0.8-1.0 mg./kg. or 0.2 mg./kg./day x 4.5	None	
Busulfan (Myleran)	Oral	2-6 mg./day	None	
ANTIMETABOLITES				
Methotrexate (Methotrexate)	Oral I.V. I.V.	2.5-5.0 mg./day 25-50 mg. 1 2x weekly 200 mg.-10 gm. with CF rescue	None	Oral and digestive tract ulcerations; bone marrow depression with leukopenia, thrombocytopenia and bleeding. Toxicity enhanced by impaired kidney function.
6-Mercaptopurine (6-MP, Purinethol)	Oral	2.5 mg./kg./day	None	Therapeutic doses usually well tolerated, excessive doses cause bone marrow depression.
6-Thioguanine (6-TG, Thioguan)	Oral	2.0 mg./kg./day		
5-Fluorouracil (5-FU, Fluorouracil)	I.V.	12 mg./kg./day x 3 Smaller dose, 1.2 x weekly for maintenance	None	Stomatitis, nausea, GI injury, bone marrow depression.
Arabinosylcytosine (Ara-C. Cytosar)	I.V.	1.0-3.0 mg./kg./day x 10-20	Nausea and vomiting	Bone marrow depression, megaloblastosis, leukopenia, thrombocytopenia.
ANTIBIOTICS				
Adriamycin	I.V.	50-75 mg./m.², in single or divided doses every 3 weeks	Nausea and vomiting	Stomatitis, GI disturbances, alopecia, bone marrow depression. Cardiac toxicity at cumulative doses over 500 mg./m.²
Bleomycin (Blenoxane)	I.V. S.C.	0.25 mg./kg./day x 5.7 Maintenance 1.0-2.0 mg./day	Nausea and vomiting, chills, fever	Mucocutaneous ulcerations alopecia, pulmonary fibrosis in approximately 5% patients.
Dactinomycin (Cosmegan)	I.V.	0.01 mg./kg./day x 5 or 0.04 mg./kg. weekly	Nausea and vomiting	Stomatitis, GI disturbances, alopecia, bone marrow depression.
Daunorubicin**	I.V.	0.8-1.0 mg./kg./day x 3.6 Total doses never to exceed 25 mg./kg.	Nausea and vomiting, fever	Bone marrow depression with leukopenia and thrombocytopenia, alopecia, stomatitis; cardiac toxicity at cumulative doses over 25 mg./kg.

**Available for experimental use only.

Source: Krakoff, I. H.: Cancer chemotherapeutic agents. CA—A Cancer Journal for Clinicians, Vol. 27, No. 3, May/June 1977.

(continued)

TABLE 15-9. (continued)

AGENTS	PRINCIPAL ROUTE OF ADMINIS- TRATION	USUAL DOSE	ACUTE TOXIC SIGNS	MAJOR TOXIC MANIFESTATIONS
ANTIBIOTICS (CONTINUED)				
Mithramycin	I.V.	25 micrograms/kg. every other day x 3-4	Nausea and vomiting	Bone marrow depression particularly thrombocytopenia, bleeding, hypocalcemia, hepatic toxicity at large doses.
Mitomycin C (Mutamycin)	I.V.	0.06 mg./kg. 2x weekly	Nausea and vomiting	Bone marrow depression.
STEROID COMPOUNDS				
Androgen				
Testosterone propionate	I.M.	50-100 mg. 3x weekly	None	Fluid retention, masculinization.
Fluoxymesterone (Halotestin)	Oral	10-20 mg./day		
Estrogen				
Diethylstilbestrol	Oral	Breast: 1-5 mg., 3/day Prostate: 1 mg./day	Occasional nausea and vomiting	Fluid retention, feminization.
Ethinyl estradiol (Estinyl)	Oral	Breast: 0.1-1.0 mg., 3/day Prostate: 0.1 mg./day		Uterine bleeding.
Progestin				
Hydroxyprogesterone caproate (Delalutin)	I.M.	1 gm. 2x weekly	None	
6-Methylhydroxyprogesterone (Provera)	Oral I.M.	100-200 mg./day 200-600 mg. 2x weekly		
Adrenal Cortical Compounds				
Cortisone acetate	Oral	20-100 mg./day	None	
Prednisone (Meticorten)	Oral	15-100 mg./day		Fluid retention, hypertension, diabetes, increased susceptibility to infection.
Dexamethasone (Decadron)	Oral	0.5-4.0 mg./day		
Methylprednisolone sodium succinate (Solu-Medrol)	I.M. I.V.	10-125 mg./day		
Hydrocortisone sodium succinate (Solu-Cortef)	I.V.	100-500 mg./day		
MISCELLANEOUS DRUGS				
L-Asparaginase**	I.V.	200-1,000 IU/kg. 3-7x weekly for 28 days	Nausea and vomiting, fever, hypersensitivity reactions	Anorexia, weight loss. Somnolence lethargy, confusion. Hypoproteinemia (including albumin and fibrinogen). Hypolipidemia and (?) hyperlipidemia, abnormal liver function tests, fatty metamorphosis of the liver. Pancreatitis (rare). Azotemia. Granulocytopenia, lymphopenia, and thrombocytopenia (usually mild and transient).
1,3-bis (β-Chloroethyl)- 1-nitrosourea (BCNU)**	I.V.	100 mg./m.^{2} every 6 weeks	Nausea and vomiting	Bone marrow depression with leukopenia and thrombocytopenia.
1, (β-Chloroethyl)-3- (4-methylcyclohexyl)- 1-nitrosourea (MeCCNU)**	Oral	120-150 mg./m.^{2} every 6 weeks		
Streptozotocin**	I.V.	1 gm./day	Nausea and vomiting	Skin eruptions, diarrhea, mental depression, muscle tremors.

TABLE 15-9. (continued)

AGENTS	PRINCIPAL ROUTE OF ADMINIS-TRATION	USUAL DOSE	ACUTE TOXIC SIGNS	MAJOR TOXIC MANIFESTATIONS
MISCELLANEOUS DRUGS (CONTINUED)				
o.p. DDD (Mitotane)	Oral	2-10 gm./day	Nausea and vomiting	
Dimethyl imidazole triazeno carboxamide (DTIC)	I.V.	2-4 mg./kg./day x 10	Nausea and vomiting	Bone marrow depression.
Hydroxyurea (Hydrea)	Oral	20-40 mg./kg./day	None	Bone marrow depression.
Nafoxidine**	Oral	60 mg. 3/day	None	Dermatitis.
Tamoxifen**	Oral	2-12 mg./m.² 2/day	None	Mild bone marrow depression.
cis-Platinum (II) diammine dichloride	I.V.	1 mg./kg. every 3 weeks 3 mg./kg. every 3 weeks with mannitol diuresis	Nausea and vomiting	Bone marrow depression, renal tubular damage, deafness.
Procarbazine (Matulane)	Oral	50-300 mg./day	Nausea and vomiting	Bone marrow depression with leukopenia and thrombocytopenia, mental depression.
Quinacrine	Intrapleural	100-200 mg./day x 5	Local pain, fever	
Vinblastine (Velban)	I.V.	0.1-0.2 mg./kg. weekly	Nausea and vomiting	Alopecia, areflexia, bone marrow depression.
Vincristine (Oncovin)	I.V.	0.015-0.05 mg./kg. weekly	None	Areflexia, muscular weakness, peripheral neuritis, paralytic ileus, mild bone marrow depression.

**Available for experimental use only.

major artery, it is necessary to use fluoroscopic guidance. This method has the chief advantage of not requiring major surgery, and it can be repeated at intervals. The vessels usually perfused for a lesion in the lower extremity are the iliac, femoral, and popliteal arteries and veins. For upper extremity perfusion, the axillary artery and vein are injected, whereas the abdominal aorta and the vena cava are used in pelvic perfusion (Figs. 15-5 and 15-6).

In patients requiring liver perfusion, a Teflon catheter is placed in the hepatic artery and attached to a portable pump. Such therapy can continue for the desired number of days even after the patient leaves the hospital. In this instance, a self-contained pump is worn beneath the clothing, as a hearing aid would be.

Regional infusions may be used for head and neck cancer, gastric tumors, or cancer of the liver. Usually this procedure is reserved for patients who have had maximum radiation therapy and all the surgery possible. The same side effects that may occur with systemic chemotherapy may also occur with regional perfusion, since some of the medication does seep into the general circulation.

NURSING MANAGEMENT. The treatment plan should be explained to the patient, with the realization that this patient has probably already experienced many forms of therapy for the malignancy. Thus there is a need for support, understanding, and reinforcement of hope.

Following the administration of the chemotherapeutic agent, blood tests are done frequently to check on bone marrow depression. Tissue in the local area is observed frequently for any reaction such as erythema, mild edema, blistering, and petechiae. Any noticeable change is documented, with a full description. Pain usually is not a problem, but if it is present, it may indicate severe injury to normal tissue.

The patient should be encouraged to attend to mouth hygiene. If mouth ulcers, mucositis, tissue sloughing, and swallowing problems develop, special mouth care is given by the nurse.

A tracheostomy set is kept nearby in the event of respiratory difficulties. Oropharyngeal secretions may have to be aspirated. An accurate record of intake and output is kept and a high-calorie diet is offered. If mouth lesions and swallowing problems occur, the diet is modified so that the patient may continue to receive adequate

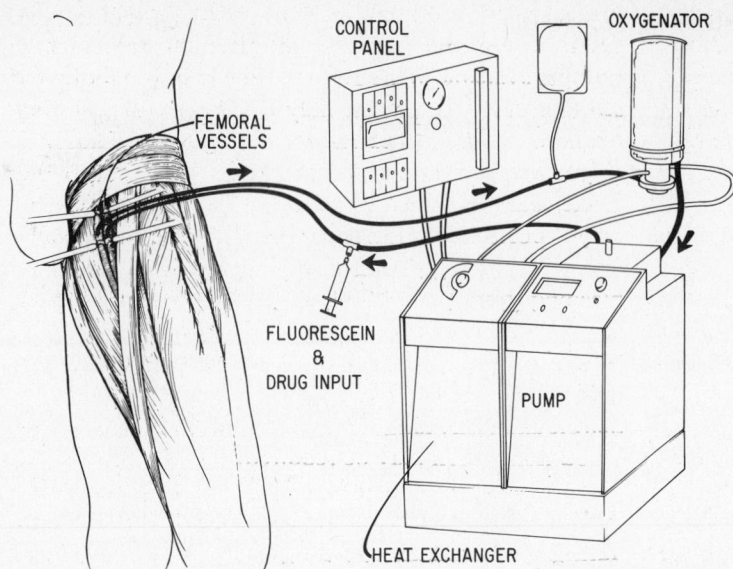

Figure 15-5. This diagram shows equipment used in the operating room to perfuse a lower extremity. The appropriate vessels are exposed, the patient is systemically heparinized and the vessels are cannulated. Tubing is connected to a pump oxygenator. The extremity is placed on bypass after the tourniquet is applied above the cannula insertion site. Whole blood initiates the process of priming the pump and starting the infusion. Arrows indicate the direction of drug input and fluorescein. The dye, fluorescein, is used to demonstrate extent of perfusion when the extremity is viewed in the dark using a Wood's lamp. (Illustration courtesy Peter R. Jochimsen, M.D.)

nutriments in softer form (baby foods may be convenient). Nasogastric feedings may be needed if mouth problems interfere with proper diet maintenance.

If the infusion has to be discontinued temporarily because white blood cell or platelet counts fall below a certain level, the patency of the tubing is maintained by flushing with heparinized solution.

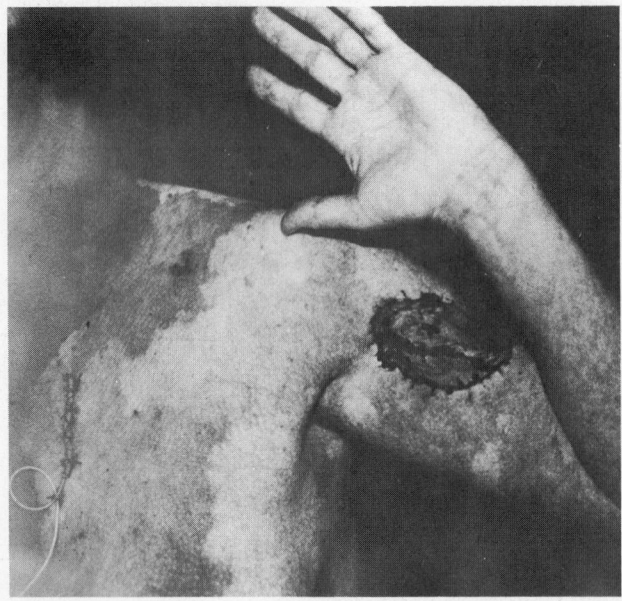

Figure 15-6. Note on the left that an arterial line is placed in the thyrocervical trunk in such a fashion that a chemotherapeutic drug may be given to the left upper extremity. This photograph was taken in the dark after fluorescein (which was injected into the arterial line) was injected. The light areas demonstrate the areas being infused by the drug, whereas the darker areas show that no drug is present. This patient had an excision on the upper arm for recurrent malignant melanoma. (Illustration courtesy Peter R. Jochimsen, M.D.)

The patient who has had an aortic perfusion should be observed for signs of malaise, nausea, vomiting, rising temperature, blood pressure, and pulse (note signs indicative of a hypotensive reaction). Fluids are given intravenously for the first 48 hours; the patient's total intake and output are recorded accurately. The patient is turned frequently, because pressure areas develop easily. These patients require emotional support; for those having surgery, the principles of effective postoperative care are followed.

Nursing Care of Patients Receiving Chemotherapeutic Agents

ANTICIPATORY NURSING. Knowledge of the expected drug action and the signs of toxicity enables the nurse to assess the patient's reactions to the chemotherapeutic agents. It is understood that these signs may occur in different intensities in different patients and that they may vary with different drugs. The evaluation of the therapeutic effectiveness of a drug requires an understanding not only of drug action but of anticipated effect. It is important to know whether these effects will be immediate or delayed. The nurse will initiate those activities which will prevent or minimize adverse reactions wherever possible.

SAFER DRUG ADMINISTRATION. When the drug used is a chemical that may cause tissue damage if extravasated, it is desirable to use discrimination in selecting a vein for administration of the chemotherapeutic agent and extreme caution while administering it. The area chosen should be one which will allow the needle to be secured safely, so that it will not be easily dislodged if the extremity is moved. Some advocate using larger vessels in preference to smaller veins in order to minimize the chemical irritation of the interior surface of the vein.

When injecting the medication directly into a vein is contraindicated, an infusion may be used prior to administering the drug, or a Y-tube (or side arm of IV tubing) may be used. It is advisable to avoid administering the drug into an extremity which has had other pathology, such as lymph node dissection, hematoma, scarring, or sclerosis.

When an infusion is started, the "butterfly" needle is preferred (page 132). A single puncture of the skin and vessel is desirable, since repeated punctures may initiate a hematoma or further traumatize the area.

While the chemotherapeutic agent is being administered, the patient should be observed and instructed to report and describe any discomforts. If problems occur, it may be necessary to terminate the procedure and restart the medication at another site.

Extravasation (escape of infusion fluids into the tissues) may occur even if the aforementioned precautions are followed. The local signs include a reddened, mottled, and/or swollen area. The result may be tissue breakdown, possible necrosis, and pain.

To promote comfort and slow down tissue metabolism, ice compresses may be applied immediately. The next day, heat may be applied to assist in removing dead cells. If necrosis does not occur, there still may be pain for a few days due to phlebitis. However, should necrosis occur, an early consultation with a plastic surgeon may be recommended.

When extravasation occurs with Mustargen, the specific antidote, sodium thiosulfate, should be injected immediately into the area.

TOXIC REACTIONS. The multiplicity of toxic reactions that can occur may interfere with the patient's basic needs for food, oxygen, fluid, and body protection as well as with psychosocial needs, especially those relating to the acceptance of a change in self-image and body concept. The ingenuity of the nurse will sometimes be taxed in coping with the variety and complexity of the nursing problems encountered while striving to meet the needs of the patient.

Since virtually all drugs used in cancer chemotherapy can be harmful to the fetus if taken during pregnancy, it may be advisable to warn women of childbearing age to avoid conception while they are being treated with these agents.

SIDE EFFECTS. Because certain cells are more vulnerable to the chemotherapeutic agents than others, a common *triad of symptoms* related to the gastrointestinal tract may occur: *stomatitis, nausea and vomiting,* and *diarrhea.* As a result, the patient's nutritional status may be jeopardized, fluid and electrolyte balance may be affected, and various feelings of discomfort may occur during certain intervals of the chemotherapy cycle.

The bone marrow depression caused by these drugs presents another triad of clinical manifestations. All cells produced by the bone marrow, namely, leukocytes, erythrocytes, and platelets, are affected, reducing the number available in the body to cope with metabolic and stress needs. The patient may develop *anemia, bleeding tendencies,* and *decreased resistance to infection.* Thus it is important to observe for evidence of infection since a low white count often occurs with anticancer drugs. Laboratory reports are followed to note whether the platelet count is low, suggesting that the patient is in danger of bleeding (gums, nosebleed, etc.). Urine and stool specimens are checked for evidence of bleeding.

When red cells are depressed, there is a possibility that anemia may develop, causing the patient to become lethargic and easily fatigued. If the anemia becomes severe, blood transfusion may be required.

It is well to note that bone marrow suppression is a cyclical phenomenon which occurs at a predictable time during the chemotherapy program. Levels of the bone marrow elements should return to normal before the next cycle of chemotherapy is commenced.

Hyperuricemia can occur because of the breakdown of large numbers of tumor cells following use of alkylating agents and antimetabolites; allopurinol can sometimes prevent this. See Table 15-9 for specific side effects.

NUTRITION. The patient's nutritional state may be endangered because of nausea, vomiting, and anorexia. Electrolyte depletion and loss of necessary nutrients may disturb cellular function at a time when the patient's metabolic requirements are urgent. Various dietary supports may be provided. By catering to individual preferences and providing snacks, supplements, and frequent small feedings, the nurse can encourage the patient to maintain an adequate dietary intake. A frequent check of weight may reveal changes due to impaired nutrition.

MOUTH CARE. The patient receiving chemotherapeutic drugs may experience signs and symptoms that are pronounced. Commonplace nursing care does not always suffice. For example, if the patient develops inflammation of the oral mucosa, how does the nurse modify the manner in which oral hygiene is given so that the oral cavity does not become a breeding place for bacteria and the inflamed mucosa is not injured to a greater degree? Frequent cleaning of the mouth with soft, nonabrasive materials, followed by a soothing coating of the mucosa, would be pleasant to the patient and would reduce irritation. Rinsing the mouth with warm saline at 4-hour intervals is also helpful. Lemon juice and mineral oil or glycerine are not recommended since these substances have a tendency to coat organisms rather than remove them; they also decrease saliva and change the pH of the mouth.

When a patient is discharged while he still has mouth problems, it is important that the nurse help set up a pattern of care for good oral hygiene so that complications may be minimized.

Since stomatitis is a side effect of therapy, the nurse should promote measures to prevent further oral discomfort. The patient should be counseled against eating spicy food that could aggravate an already painful mouth. Ill-fitting dentures should be adjusted to prevent irritation. Alcoholic beverages will need to be diluted and smoking discouraged to reduce the severity of oral symptoms. One way of bypassing the discomfort of eating with a painful mouth is to suggest that the patient use a mouthwash or a rinse of lidocaine (Xylocaine) at mealtime to anesthetize the oral mucosa.

SKIN CONDITION. Because antineoplastic medications disturb cell growth and thus interfere with wound healing it is important to examine the skin for lesions and breaks and to assess general muscle tone and skin turgor.

PSYCHOSOCIAL NEEDS. Perhaps the greatest psychosocial need arising from the use of chemotherapeutic agents is the patient's need to regain an acceptable self-concept and body image. As a result of the effect of these drugs on the hair follicles, the patient may develop alopecia. With the loss of hair, patients may become so depressed that they refuse to interact with others and may even have difficulty looking at themselves. The nurse can be very helpful in these instances by stressing the temporary aspect of the problem and the fact that there will be regrowth of hair. A wig may be the answer for the female patient. In place of a wig, attractive scarves and roller caps can be used to deemphasize this problem. For men, attractive hairpieces are available.

Learning about the effects of various antineoplastic drugs will enable the nurse to recognize that certain patient reactions such as depression, malaise, euphoria, etc., may be due to the medications. The patient may feel somewhat reassured to know that such feelings are not psychotic and that they may disappear once the drug treatment is terminated.

ATTITUDE. Some amount of toxicity is expected for a portion of the chemotherapy cycle. It must be remembered that the goal of chemotherapy is to maximize the potential benefits of the drugs and minimize the toxicity. Therefore, it is imperative to sort out one's own feelings toward this mode of therapy and the discomforts it causes. The personal attitude conveyed to the patient and family is of the utmost importance and will affect the caliber of nursing care that the nurse will be capable of giving.

It is hoped that the patient may experience a decrease in pain, an eventual increase in the feeling of well-being, a more hopeful attitude, and, ultimately, prolongation of life. The nurse should continually exert conscious efforts to broaden personal perspectives in order to act more effectively through attitude as well as through knowledge and skill to administer quality nursing care to patients receiving drugs for the treatment of cancer.

Reverse Isolation Unit

The care of a patient whose immune defenses have been reduced by chemotherapy presents a nursing challenge. Such a patient requires strict aseptic precautions, physical barrier isolation, and antibiotic prophylaxis. At the National Institutes of Health, a laminar air-flow room (LAFR) module has been developed (Fig. 15-8) for

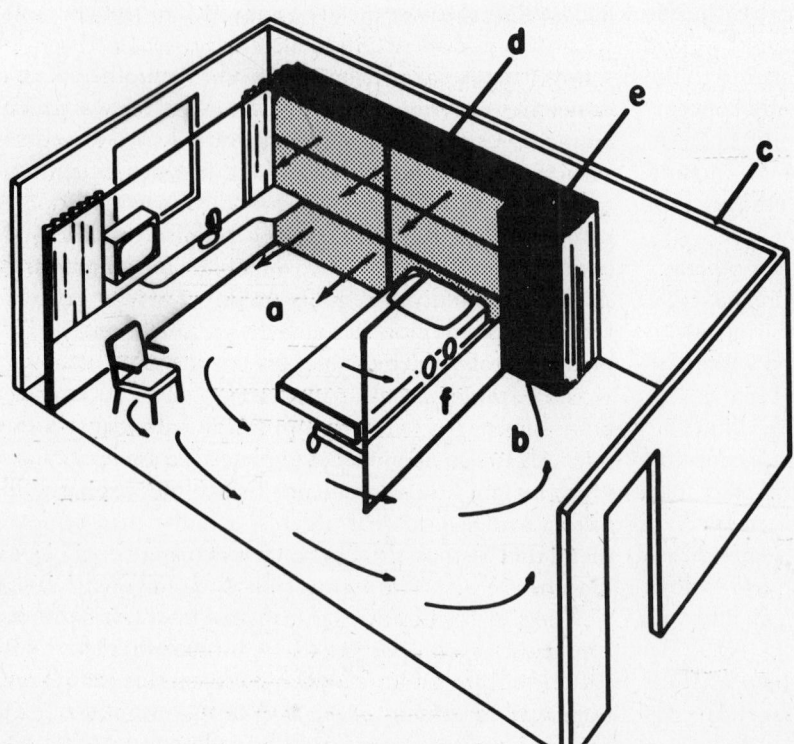

Figure 15-7. The floor plan of the LAFR shows the isolation area as a room within a larger room. Arrows at (a) indicate the influx of 99.9% sterile air entering in horizontal lines moving with uniform velocity. Circulation pattern is in one direction only. The air-filtering cycle begins with air at (b) that is drawn into the filter just outside the module to remove lint and dust. The air continues through a bank of filters (d and e). (c) is the outer wall of the large room. Note at (f) the two portholes through which the hands of the nurse, physician, or physical therapist work as they contact the patient from the outside of the plastic screen. (Courtesy, National Institutes of Health)

the purpose of providing reverse-isolation for the infection-prone patient who is undergoing intensive intravenous chemotherapy. A barrier is set up within which the patient is free from contact with exogenous organisms, and the possibility of infection is thus reduced.*

The continuous air flow (100 feet per minute) prevents airborne organisms from moving against the flow of air toward the patient. The nurse or visitor may stand outside the isolation area (b in Fig. 15-7) and not infect the patient. Personnel who enter the unit must wear a sterile gown, cap, mask, gloves, and shoe covers. This unit allows the patient more freedom and a more normal environment than the previously limiting "life island."

IMMUNOTHERAPY FOR CANCER

In the field of immunology, several breakthroughs have occurred in recent years, giving impetus to renewed research to determine the clinical potential for treating cancer. Evidence indicates that host immunity is an important factor in resistance to cancer. Recent studies show that the thymus gland is essential for developing host resistance and that it is particularly essential in certain immunologic phenomena, including immunity to tumor growth.

The thymus, a large lymphoid organ in the upper anterior mediastinum, produces a hormone, thymosin. This hormone appears to play a role in the differentiation of certain thymus-dependent cells (T cells). It is believed that thymus-dependent T cells protect man from daily neoplastic insults not only by identifying cancer cells but also by eliminating them.

Present research attempts are directed toward challenging the body's defense mechanisms with foreign microorganisms, the objective being to stimulate the immune response (particularly T cells) to release macrophages and phagocytes and thereby kill the tumor.

There is much about the complex field of immunology that is unknown; however, researchers are optimistic about the potential for treating cancer. The chief problem has been the small number of patients tested and the lack of controls.

PSYCHOLOGICAL ASPECTS OF NURSING THE CANCER PATIENT

The Optimistic Psychosocial Approach

Because there are so many kinds of cancer (over 100), the diagnosis of cancer need not indicate a fatal outcome. Many forms of cancer are curable; many others achieve "cure" status if they are treated early.

*For more detailed information, see Seidler, F. M.: Innovative approaches in cancer nursing management. Proceedings of the National Conference on Cancer Nursing, American Cancer Society, 1974, pp. 18-24.

It is generally held, in the field of oncology, that the patient has a right to know the diagnosis and participate in all decisions relative to his care. However, there are numerous factors to be considered in this regard as will be discussed in the next section.

The manner in which a patient accepts the information that he has cancer often depends on his philosophy of life and his views of life and death. The greatest support may be spiritual consolation. Therefore, the nurse should arrange to have available those spiritual resources that are most likely to meet the patient's individual needs.

Once the diagnosis of cancer has been established, a very effective and comfortable way of accepting the illness is to live wholly for the present. Projecting thoughts to the future adds doubts and fears; planning and living each day as it comes can provide a sense of achievement. The patient from this point of reference realizes he is still here and acquires a feeling of extension of life. The opposite is true if the reference point is projected to a year from now, for his future then seems shortened and limited. Even dividing one's time into blocks of days walled in by visits to the doctor can be helpful. These units of time are quantities that can be appreciated and coped with by the patient.

It is hoped that the prospect of a breakthrough in treatment is closer with each passing day. Countless hours spent in study and analysis are added daily to hundreds of thousands of dollars spent on research. Tomorrow could be the day when significant contributions will be made in the treatment of many kinds of cancer.

In modern cancer therapy the possibility exists that extensive surgery and irradiation therapy may produce changes that are disfiguring or multilating and not easily borne by the patient. The problems thus created may be almost overwhelming. They begin before operation, when the question is raised as to how much the patient should be told about the details of his disease and his operation; they must be handled differently for each patient.

Since surgery or other treatments for cancer interrupt the patient's life style, it is important to assist him in adapting to a change in his mode of living. How he adapts depends upon the values he places on his behavior, his self-image, and his attitudes toward particular body parts and social and sexual interaction. Cancer and cancer treatment can seriously disrupt the patient's adaptive process, resulting in depression until new methods of coping with an altered life style are found and coping skills developed.

The adaptation that has to be made must begin in the preoperative period. To this end, the patient participates in the plan of treatment so that, in a sense, he has a real part in all that is done for, by, and with him. Patients are particularly in need of support and reassurance in order to establish confidence in the skill of the surgeon and the hospital environment. When the patient approaches surgery with a sense of hopefulness and expectation, excellent results can be anticipated from a psychological point of view. If, however, surgery is approached with the conviction that the operation is going to be painful, disfiguring, and mutilating, it is almost to be expected that depression and a marked sense of weakness will become apparent postoperatively. The postoperative symptoms of depression may take the form of sleep disturbance, loss of appetite, and other manifestations that may persist for an indefinite period. In their depression, patients may think that the attitudes of nurses, physicians, and attendants show hostility.

A patient who has not taken part in the planning process may experience feelings of dejection accompanied by a sense of helplessness. Such anxiety often makes the patient turn to other people for help, advice, consolation, and reassurance. This state is usually temporary, and the nurse, who is closest to the patient, can be of invaluable aid during this period of rehabilitation. Kindness, warmth, and understanding provide the security the patient needs.

The nurse, of all health personnel, has the most sustained and intimate contact with the patient during hospitalization and thus is the person to whom the patient turns most often for understanding and support during the early postoperative period. If the nurse is able to meet these needs, not only will the pressure and the anxiety be alleviated, but also the patient's perception of the hospital experience will be modified.

In summary, the psychology of the cancer patient is the psychology of a person who is facing a fundamental struggle with security and self-value. Such problems can be met best by working with professional persons. The nurse is in a very advantageous position to aid the patient in efforts to overcome depression and anxiety and to resume normal function after surgery.

Gravity of Prognosis

What is in the mind of a patient suffering from a fatal disease? What are his hopes and fears? How nearly does he suspect intuitively the truth of the situation, and, if he knows the truth, by what psychological mechanisms is he saved from despair? How specifically and in what detail should he be informed regarding his illness and its probable outcome? If he demands an accurate appraisal of his status and a true estimate as to the prognosis, ought not this be supplied? What is his family to be told? What are the responsibilities of the nurse with respect to the transmission of diagnostic and prognostic information to the patient's family?

These and similar questions regularly confront physicians and nurses responsible for the care of the seriously ill. Some of them may be answered without equivocation, with a reasonable degree of certainty and without important reservations, while others, depending on the personal philosophy of the physician, on the family, and on the status of a particular patient, may be answered in generalizations which, although basically valid, are open to a variety of interpretations.

First, with respect to the nurse-patient and the nurse-family relationship, it may be stated that whatever information is to be supplied concerning the diagnosis, whether or not it has been definitely established, never should be volunteered to the patient or his family by the nurse, except as planned in mutual discussions with the patient's physician. By the same token, whatever prognostications are offered by the nurse should be as specific as the physician's, and no more. Finally, any remarks of the nurse's that have a bearing on the possible implications of the diagnosis, prognosis, or treatment should be made advisedly, in the light of the physician's known views and intentions. This admonition deserves considerable emphasis, for nothing is more destructive of confidence and morale than an impression of inconsistency, and nothing is more threatening to therapeutic success than confusion and distrust in the mind of the patient. Obviously, all of the statements and actions of the nurse should be calculated to convey a sense of truthfulness and even guarded optimism; no matter how grave the situation or depressing the outlook, the nurse can lend a great deal of encouragement without exceeding either the bounds of reality or professional responsibilities.

Normally, protective psychological mechanisms operate in patients with lethal disease, apparently to excellent effect, for many such patients do not become acutely anxious or profoundly depressed, even when it is seemingly obvious that a fatal outcome is imminent. The precise nature of these mechanisms presumably differs according to the individual and the situation. A conversion of the patient's will to live to a complete acceptance of the idea of death, even a desire for death, may be one aspect of this process of psychological adaptation in patients with prolonged and painful illnesses, although in most instances there is no sign of a death wish. On the contrary, the evidence suggests that the desire to live persists with great tenacity, ideas of death apparently being altogether excluded from awareness.

It is not often that the physician or the nurse must decide how much of the tragic truth to tell; they seldom are asked. An occasional patient does persist in his direct questioning, apparently with logical reason, perhaps related to his business plans or obligations to his family. Under these circumstances some physicians may feel justified in offering a complete evaluation of the case in detail and stating their conclusions in definite terms. The usual experience, i.e., a frank discussion, does not often result in total decompensation, and should always be accompanied by compassionate support.

Members of the patient's family and those of his associates who require explicit information, of course, must be made aware of the complete situation, and at least one member of the immediate family should be advised from the outset regarding all possible developments. If this is done, candid discussions concerning prognoses with the victims of hopeless disease are rarely justified. Optimism is to be strengthened, not destroyed, if the humane objective of patient care is to be served completely.

Esthetic Factors

Facial tumors are often unsightly, causing the patient to feel very sensitive about his appearance. Such lesions should be covered, if possible, and other features of the patient accented to detract attention from the tumor site. This can be done by careful grooming, attractive garments, etc. Bright lights in a room should be replaced by softer lights, inasmuch as shades of light and dark can tone down unsightly areas. The nurse can use her ingenuity in helping this individual to bear his burden more easily.

One of the most unpleasant features of cancer in exposed areas on the body is the foul odor that appears sooner or later as a result of the sloughing of tissues. Every effort should be made to keep the patient and his room clean. Dressings should be changed frequently, removed quickly from the patient's room, and deposited in a metal-covered container until they are sent to the incinerator. Bedclothes and the patient's clothing should be changed when soiled. The use of absorbent pads may help when drainage is present. The room should be ventilated properly.

If deodorants are necessary, several of the essential oils, such as oil of geranium, oil of eucalyptus, or oil of orange, may be used. Neutroleum alpha is lasting and not unpleasant when 1 or 2 drops are applied to the dressing or the bedclothing. Powdered charcoal in the dressing or potassium permanganate solution 1:2,000 as an irrigation often helps. Activated zinc peroxide is also effective in cleansing and deodorizing these wounds. Commercially prepared products can be disseminated from a bottle with a wick, by spray, or by means of an electric deodorizer to absorb odors. These are quite successful.

The nurse should try to maintain a rational psychological approach toward death. Often, the nurse is the person to whom the patient turns when he wants to talk about himself, his fears, his hopes, etc. To be able to listen and to offer encouragement are extremely important assets. Many times a patient demonstrates hostility and rebellion. The nurse, by remaining tolerant, offers the patient understanding in spite of his unpleasant actions. This approach will eventually uncover the reasons for the patient's outbursts and will help him to resolve his feelings. (See Psychological Aspects of Nursing the Cancer Patient, page 273.)

Occupational and Recreational Therapy

Statistics reveal that the home is best suited for the care of the cancer patient for several reasons. The environment is familiar, and friends and family are at hand. Many times, the patient can perform some household duties, and this promotes feelings of usefulness. It is also easier to pursue hobbies, such as caring for tropical fish, developing a miniature garden, etc. In addition, the financial burden on the family is reduced. At the same time, the family has the responsibility for the patient's care and knows what is happening to him, which often is not the case when he is in an institution.

For the patient who does not have a home, the next best available environment should be sought. The nurse with sympathetic understanding can help the patient to make contact with the proper agencies for the adjustment of any social and economic problems.

For an overall view of caring for the patient with advanced cancer see the guidelines on page 276.

The Hospice

The concept of the hospice originated in Great Britain but is growing in popularity in this country. The underlying purpose of the hospice is to provide a unit that serves only terminally ill patients, whether it be near or apart from a general hospital. Rooms are decorated in pleasant colors and furnished in a homelike manner. The philosophy of care is designed to promote comfort, and time is provided by those in attendance to talk to and listen to the patient and his family. Pain medications are given in pleasant-tasting concoctions, and special requests are honored if possible.

Each patient decides, with the support of the staff and his clergyman, whether he wishes to be at home or in the hospice. If he prefers his home, a member of the staff will visit the home daily to support and comfort him and his family. If he elects the hospice, he is never left alone when members of the family are not with him. Hospice care does not terminate with the patient's death. Support for the family is continued through a bereavement program.

NURSING CARE OF THE PATIENT WITH ADVANCED CANCER

Some authorities claim that the most important aspect of the care of the terminal patient is good nursing management. Frequent changes of bed linen, cleanliness, and keeping the patient warm are all comfort measures that can relieve a great deal of pain. During this care probably the most common emergency that the nurse should anticipate is hemorrhage, due to erosion of blood vessels by the malignancy itself, secondary necrosis, or the sloughing of tissue following irradiation. In some instances, the nurse can control bleeding by digital pressure. In cases of hemorrhage that cannot be controlled by local measures, the patient should be kept quiet in the recumbent position and the physician notified. The nurse should have the necessary equipment available for treating shock and hemorrhage (see pages 364, 371).

Ambulation

The patient is kept ambulatory as long as possible; however, the nurse must recognize when it is undesirable for him to get out of bed. In this instance, simple exercises or passive range of motion may be indicated.

Pain

Medications are used to control pain so that it is not a persistent and continuous symptom. This means finding an analgesic in a dose suitable to relieve pain, and then giving the analgesic on a regular schedule (not p.r.n.) so that pain does not reemerge. The same criterion applies to the administration of sedatives, antidepressants, and tranquilizers.

THE PATIENT WITH ADVANCED CARCINOMA
Objectives and Principles of Medical, Surgical and Nursing Management

A. To control the carcinogenic growth
  1. Prepare the patient for surgery, radiotherapy, and/or chemotherapy and/or immunotherapy.
    a. Assist with diagnostic tests to determine if metastasis has occurred.
    b. Combat local and systemic infections.
    c. Correct existing anemia and electrolyte imbalance.
    d. Give the patient psychological support.
      (1) Explain the treatment to help patient mobilize his intellectual functions and defenses to cope with the anticipated stress.
      (2) Offer reassurance and support.
      (3) Listen to and support the patient as he displays his anxieties.
  2. Assist with the treatment as prescribed.
    a. Surgical treatment
    b. Radiotherapy
    c. Chemotherapy
    d. Immunotherapy

B. To recognize the possibility of complications contributing to the patient's discomfort and illness and to initiate preventive and treatment measures
  1. Radiation sickness
    a. Administer vitamin B as prescribed.
    b. Give sedatives, antihistamines, and antiemetic drugs.
    c. Offer small, frequent feedings of high caloric, high protein foods.
    d. Increase fluid intake.
    e. Report patient's reactions.
  2. Diarrhea
    a. Give low residue or bland diet.
    b. Use anodyne suppositories.
    c. Instill oil enemas to soothe rectal mucosa.
    d. Give antidiarrhea medications as prescribed.
  3. Skin reaction
    a. Observe the skin for erythema.
    b. Apply oil or bland cream to radiation site.
    c. Protect skin from sunlight, heat, trauma, and tight clothing.
    d. Avoid irritation with soap and water.
    e. Observe for telangiectasis (a permanent, weblike dilatation of capillaries and small arteries).

  4. Bone marrow depression
    a. Report results of laboratory evaluation.
    b. Observe for evidences of bleeding.
    c. Protect the patient from infection.
    d. Offer medicated mouthwashes to soothe oral mucosa.
  5. Infection
    a. Take temperature at regular intervals since fever in patients with cancer usually indicates infection.
    b. Observe patient with hematologic malignancies and those receiving chemotherapy for symptoms of infection due to granulocytopenia, lymphopenia.
    c. Give antibiotics as ordered; most infections in cancer patients are caused by gram negative bacilli.
    d. Give fever sponges and apply cold compresses to head, encourage fluids, administer antipyretic drugs to promote comfort.
  6. Hemorrhage
    a. Evaluate patient with terminal cancer for possibility of
      (1) Thrombocytopenia
      (2) Defects in platelet function
      (3) Necrosis and sloughing of tumor
      (4) Ulceration or invasion and rupture of vessels
    b. Give platelet transfusion or whole blood transfusions as indicated.
    c. Administer anticoagulants (heparin) as indicated.
  7. Anemia
    a. Evaluate patient for weakness and symptoms of anemia due to
      (1) Blood loss
      (2) Hemolysis
      (3) Myelophthisis (wasting of spinal cord)
      (4) Inadequate erythropoiesis
    b. Prepare patient for transfusion of whole blood or packed cells to maintain hemoglobin above 8 gm.
  8. Malnutrition
    a. Assess patient for body wasting and anorexia.
    b. Correct electrolyte imbalance.
    c. Utilize vitamin supplements.
    d. Administer infusions of protein hydrolysates, glucose, and vitamins as directed.

C. To relieve the patient's pain
1. Develop an understanding of the patient's emotional makeup, his relation to his family, and the projected emotional climate at home.
2. Evaluate the quality, intensity, and duration of pain as well as the patient's response to pain.
3. Establish the specific source of pain, since all of the patient's symptoms are not necessarily caused by cancer.
4. Promote the general comfort of the patient (i.e., turning, moving, ambulating).
5. Determine the physical resources available at home.
6. Administer agents to relieve pain when indicated.
   a. Use specific drugs for the relief of nausea and vomiting.
   b. Give ataractic agents for the relief of fear and apprehension.
   c. Utilize hot and cold compresses if indicated.
   d. Give sedative and hypnotic drugs to induce sleep.
   e. Apply local anesthetics if the situation warrants.
   f. Administer muscle relaxant drugs and antispasmodics; use non-narcotic drugs when possible; use the smallest amount of narcotic possible.
   g. Give analgesic drugs for more intense pain.
   h. Use tranquilizers to provide a sense of well-being.
7. Assist with surgical treatment for the relief of pain.
   a. Prepare for alcohol injections to block nerve pathways for sensory benefit.
   b. Prepare patient for treatment of accessible painful nodule(s).
      (1) Excision
      (2) Injection with alkylating agent
      (3) Anesthetic infiltration or neurosurgical interruption of sensory supply
   c. Prepare for localized radiotherapy for deep lesions.
   d. Prepare for presacral neurectomy when visceral pain is predominant.
   e. Prepare for cordotomy when pain is intractable.
8. Assure patient that severe pain will be alleviated.
9. See Chapter 9 for additional therapeutic and psychosocial concepts of pain control.

D. To control malodor
1. Remove the odor at its source.
2. Encourage good personal hygiene.
3. Give normal saline irrigations (if indicated) to external lesions.
4. Administer prescribed vaginal irrigations when discharging vaginal lesions are present.
5. Keep perineal area shaved if malodorous discharge is present.
6. Change perineal pads frequently; remove and wrap in paper and place in covered container *outside* the patient's room.

E. To control the bleeding
1. Observe for increasing pulse rate.
2. Observe for amount and color of blood.
3. Apply digital pressure if site is accessible.
4. Utilize vaginal or rectal packing as indicated.
5. Prepare patient for cauterization and ligation of exposed vessels if indicated.

F. To care for bladder frequency and incontinence
1. Initiate a bladder control program.
2. Keep an accurate intake and output record.
3. Give meticulous skin care to perineal area.
4. Watch for formation of a vesicovaginal or rectovaginal fistula.
5. Insert an indwelling catheter if all other measures fail.

G. To prevent constipation
1. Encourage fluids and regular meals.
2. Place patient on prune juice and glycerine suppository regimen.

H. To reduce edema due to blocking of lymphatic vessels
1. Encourage motion and exercise.
2. Elevate edematous extremity.
3. Utilize nursing measures to prevent pressure sores.
   a. Relieve the pressure.
   b. Encourage circulation to the part.
   c. Put extremities through range of motion exercises.

I. To assist the patient to cope with his situation
1. Help the patient to feel that he is understood.
2. Help the patient to work out his feelings.
3. Accept the psychological defense mechanisms used by him.
4. Recognize that the patient's loss of resources leads to helplessness, fear, and anger.
5. Encourage the patient to talk about his *feelings* and his situation.
6. Develop a supportive relationship with the patient.
7. Utilize all measures to keep the patient's ego intact.
   a. Encourage him to make decisions and choices.
   b. Answer his questions.
   c. Listen to him.
   d. Provide a daily schedule for the patient, including short daily rest periods.
   e. Encourage him to keep active and to have interesting pursuits.
8. Help restore patient's self-esteem and purpose by offering help when needed and accepting irrational expectations and hostility.
9. Demonstrate concern for a suffering human by giving expert care and contributing something to his welfare.

J. To maintain the patient at optimal physical and emotional condition
1. Give a high caloric, high protein diet (gavage feedings if indicated).
2. Keep caloric intake up with between-meal feedings.
3. Give supplementary vitamins and hematinics.
4. Administer blood transfusions as prescribed.
5. Encourage regular rest periods and arrange for periods in the outdoors.
6. Keep the patient as active as possible to build up endurance and avoid debilitation.
7. Support the patient during his anxiety and stress.
8. Maintain a cheerful and optimistic attitude.
9. Encourage verbalization.
10. Do little "extras" for the patient.
11. Include the family in the patient's care.

BIBLIOGRAPHY
BOOKS
Cancer

Baserga, R., ed.: The Cell Cycle and Cancer. New York, Marcel Dekker, Inc. 1971.

Becker, F. F., ed.: Cancer. New York, Plenum Press, 1977.

Belonado, A. A., and Stahl, D. A.: Cancer Nursing. Garden City, N.Y. Med. Examination Pub., 1978.

Berkley, G. E.: Cancer: How to Prevent It and How to Help Your Doctor Fight It. Englewood Cliffs, N. J., Prentice-Hall, 1978.

Bloom, W., and Fawcett, D. W.: A Textbook of Histology, 10th ed. Philadelphia, W. B. Saunders, 1975.

Cullen, J. W., ed., et al.: Cancer: The Behavioral Dimensions. New York, Raven Press, 1976.

del Regato, J. A., and Spjut, H. J.: Cancer, 5th ed. St. Louis, C. V. Mosby, 1977.

Donovan, M. I., and Pierce, S. G.: Cancer Care Nursing. New York, Appleton-Century-Crofts, 1976.

Earl, A. M., et al.: The Nurse as a Care Giver for the Terminal Patient and His Family. New York, Columbia University Press, 1976.

Glasser, R. J.: The Greatest Battle. New York, Random House, 1976.

Greenspan, E. M.: Clinical Cancer Chemotherapy. New York, Raven Press, 1975.

Hall, T. C.: The cellular mechanisms of cancer chemotherapy. *In* Cancer Chemotherapy: Fundamental Concepts and Recent Advances. Yearbook Medical Pub. Inc., Chicago, 1975, pp. 295-309.

Hardy, R. E., and Cull, J. G.: Counseling and Rehabilitating the Cancer Patient. Springfield, Charles C Thomas, 1975.

Kruse, L. C., et al.: Cancer: Pathophysiology, Etiology, Management. St. Louis, C. V. Mosby, 1979.

Lehninger, A.: Biochemistry, 2nd ed. New York, Worth, 1975.

Nealon, T. F.: Management of the Patient with Cancer. Philadelphia, W. B. Saunders, 1976.

New York Academy of Sciences: Cancer and the Worker. New York, N. Y. Academy of Sciences, 1977.

Nursing '77: Helping Cancer Patients—Effectively. Horsham, Pa., Intermed Communications, 1977.

Paterson, B. H., and Kellogg, C. J.: Current Practice in Oncologic Nursing. St. Louis, C. V. Mosby, 1976.

Siegenthaler, W., and Luthy, R.: Current Chemotherapy. Washington, D. C., American Society for Microbiology, 1978.

Southern, C. M., and Friedman, H., eds.: International Conference on Immunotherapy of Cancer. New York, N. Y. Academy of Sciences, 1976.

Whelan, E.: Preventing Cancer. New York, W. W. Norton, 1978.

Winick, M., ed.: Nutrition and Cancer. New York, J. Wiley and Sons, 1977.

ARTICLES
General

Barber, J.: Hypnosis as a psychological technique in the management of cancer pain. Cancer Nurs., *1*:361-363, Oct. 1978.

Bonica, J. J.: Cancer pain: a major national health problem. Cancer Nurs., *1*:313-316, Aug. 1978.

Belt, R. J., et al.: Incidence of hemorrhagic complications in patients with cancer. JAMA, *239*:2571-2574, June 16, 1978.

Blot, W. J.: Geography of cancer. Cancer News, *32*:18-22, Winter 1977.

Burkhalter, P. K.: Cancer quackery. AJN, 77:451-453, Mar. 1977.

Carrol, R. M.: BCG immunotherapy by the tine technique: The nurse's role. Cancer Nurs., *1*:241-246, June, 1978.

Copeland, E. M., III: Intravenous hyperalimentation as an adjunct to cancer patient management. CA—A Cancer J. for Clinicians, *28*:322-330, Nov./Dec. 1978.

Craytor, J. K., et al.: Assessing learning needs of nurses who care for persons with cancer. Cancer Nurs., *1*:211-220, June 1978.

Croft, C. L.: BCG administration and nursing implications. AJN, *79*:315-319, Feb. 1979.

Damadian, R.: Nuclear magnetic resonance: A noninvasive approach to cancer. Hosp. Pract., *12*:63-70, July 1977.

Dodd, M. J.: Theoretical bases of immunotherapy (BCG in cancer therapy). AJN, *79*:310-314, Feb. 1979.

Dreizen, S., et al.: Oral complications of cancer radiotherapy. Postgrad. Med., *61*:85-92, Feb. 1977.

Fitzwater, J.: Nursing protocols for reducing sepsis rates in cancer patients. Surg. Team, *5*:34-43, May/June 1976.

Halman, M., and Suttinger, J.: Family-centered care for cancer patients. Nursing '78, *8*:42-43, Mar. 1978.

Isler, C.: Delivering total care—everywhere. RN, *41*:59-62, Apr. 1978.

————: Approaching the final days. RN, *41*:63-65, Apr. 1978.

James, V.: Caring for the cancer patient. Nursing '77, 7:30-33, Aug. 1977.

Kastenbaum, B. K., and Spector, R. E.: What should a nurse tell a cancer patient? AJN, *78*:640-641, Apr. 1978.

Kennedy, P. S., and Luedke, D. W.: Adenocarcinoma of unknown origin. Postgrad. Med., *65*:151-160, Jan. 1979.

Kennedy, T. J., et al.: Carcinomatous change in old scars. Am. Fam. Physic., *16*:106-107, July 1977.

Lande, S.: A gift of hope. AJN, 77:639-640, Apr. 1977.

Miaskowski, C.: The Bromptom cocktail. Cancer Nurs., *1*:451-455, Dec. 1978.

Miller, M. W., and Nygren, C.: Living with cancer—coping behaviors. Cancer Nurs., *1*:297-302, Aug. 1978.

Miller, S. A.: Oncology nurse and chemotherapy. AJN, 77:989-993, June 1977.

Mundinger, M. O.: Nursing diagnosis for cancer patients. Cancer Nurs., *1*:221-226, June 1978.

Murawski, B. J., et al.: Social support in health and illness; the concept and its measurement. Cancer Nurs., *1*:365-371, Oct. 1978.

Newell, G. R., and Golumbic, N.: What you can do to protect yourself against cancer. AORN J., *25*:909-923, Apr. 1977.

Oberst, M. T.: Cancer cachexia. Cancer Nurs., *1*:402, Oct. 1978.

Park, D.: Basic cancer concepts. (Programmed Instruction). Cancer Nurs., *1*:65-80, Feb. 1978.

Parsons, J., ed.: Needs of the cancer patient. (entire issue) Nurs. Digest, *5*:No. 2, 1977.

Pastan, I.: Cyclic AMP. Scient. American, *227*:97-105, Aug. 1972.

Paulen, A.: Caring for the patient who's "well." RN, *41*:56-58, Apr. 1978.

Pomerance, W.: The cancer-screening dilemma. Postgrad. Med., *64*:43-50, Aug. 1978.

Ridgway, H. B.: Skin signs of internal malignancy. Am. Fam. Physic., *17*:123-129, Mar. 1978.

Rowlingson, J. C.: Management of cancer pain. Cancer Nurs., *1*:317-318, Aug. 1978.

Shubin, S.: Cancer widows. Nursing '78, *8*:56-60, Apr. 1978.

Simon, M. A. S.: No one should face cancer alone — not even a nurse. RN, *41*:79-86, Mar. 1978.

Smith, D. S., and Chamorro, T. P.: Nursing care of patients undergoing combination chemotherapy and radiotherapy. Cancer Nurs., *1*:129-134, Apr. 1978.

Sugarbaker, E. V., et al.: Interdisciplinary cancer therapy: Adjuvant therapy. Curr. Prob. in Surg., *14*:1-69, June 1977.

Sullivan, B. P.: Patient responses to BCG therapy for malignant melanoma. AJN, *79*:320-324, Feb. 1979.

"The future of cancer control." New Eng. J. Med., *298*:567-568, Mar. 9, 1978.

Theologides, A.: Weight loss in cancer patients. CA — A Cancer J. for Physic., *27*:207-208, July/Aug. 1977.

Valassi, K.: Nutritional management of cancer patients in a variety of therapeutic regimens. Arch. Phys. Med. & Rehab., *58*:393-397, Sept. 1977.

Valentine, A. S.: Caring for the young adult with cancer. Cancer Nurs., *1*:385-389, Oct. 1978.

Van Scoy-Mosher, C.: The oncology nurse in independent professional practice. Cancer Nurs., *1*:21-28, Feb. 1978.

Welch, D.: Assessing psychosocial needs involved in cancer patient care during treatment. Oncology Nurs. Forum, *6*:12-18, Jan. 1979.

"What's new in cancer control?" AJN, *76*:962, June 1976.

Whelan, E. M.: What is your cancer risk? Med. Times, *105*:96-103, Dec. 1977.

White, L. N., et al.: Screening of cancer by nurses. Cancer Nurs., *1*:15-20, Feb. 1978.

Winters, W. D.: Viruses and cancer. AJN, *78*:249-253, Feb. 1978.

Chemotherapy

Becker, F. F.: Chemotherapy. *In* Cancer. New York, Plenum Press, 1977, Chap. 5.

Burns, N.: Cancer chemotherapy: A systemic approach. Nursing '78, *8*:56-63, Feb. 1978.

Bruya, M. A., and Madeira, N. P.: Stomatitis after chemotherapy. AJN, *75*:1349-1352, Aug. 1975.

Carter, J.: Role of the oncology nurse in regional infusion chemotherapy. AORN J., *25*:662-668, Mar. 1977.

DiPalma, J. R.: Cancer chemotherapy. RN, *39*:85-88, Apr. 1976.

————: Laetrile: When a drug is not a drug. Am. Fam. Physic., *15*:186-187, Jan. 1977.

Dreizen, S., et al.: Cutaneous complications of cancer chemotherapy. Postgrad. Med., *58*:150-158, Nov. 1975.

Einhorn, L. H.: Cancer chemotherapy. Am. Fam. Physic., *15*:186-190, Mar. 1977.

Gullo, S.: Chemotherapy, what to do about special side effects. RN, *40*:30-32, Apr. 1977.

Gutterman, J. U., et al.: Chemoimmunotherapy of human solid tumors. Med. Clin. N. Am., *60*:441-462, May 1976.

Harris, J. G.: Nausea, vomiting and cancer treatment. CA — A Cancer J. for Physic., *28*:194-201, July/Aug. 1978.

Herbst, S. F.: A new approach to parenteral drug administration. AJN, *75*:1345, Aug. 1975.

Hess, C. M.: Intra-arterial chemotherapy: Making it safer and more successful. Nursing '74, *4*:30-34, May 1974.

Hubbard, S., and Devita, V.: Chemotherapy research nurse. AJN, *76*:560-565, Apr. 1976.

Levine, M. E.: Cancer chemotherapy — a nursing model. Nurs. Clin. N. Am., *13*:271-280, June 1978.

Livingston, R. B.: Chemotherapy of solid tumors. Postgrad. Med., *59*:121-125, Feb. 1976.

Lokich, J. J.: Managing chemotherapy — induced bone marrow suppression in cancer. Hosp. Pract., *11*:61-67, Aug. 1976.

Marino, E. B., and LeBlanc, D. H.: Cancer chemotherapy. Nursing '75, *5*:22-33, Nov. 1975.

McMullen, K.: When the patient is on bleomycin therapy. AJN, *75*:964-966, June 1975.

Morrow, M.: Nursing management of the adolescent (The effect of cancer chemotherapy on psychosocial development). Nurs. Clin. N. Am., *13*:319-336, June 1978.

Morton, D. L., et al.: BCG immunotherapy as a systemic adjunct to surgery in malignant melanoma. Med. Clin. N. Am., *60*:431-439, May 1976.

Nirenberg, A.: High-dose methotrexate. AJN, *76*:1776-1780, Nov. 1976.

Pilapil, F., and Studva, K. V.: Cancer chemotherapy (Programmed Instruction). Cancer Nursing. *1*:153-164, Apr. 1978; 260-271, June 1978; 409-420, Oct. 1978.

Rosner, F.: Is chemotherapy carcinogenic? CA — A Cancer J. for Clinicians, *28*:57-58, Jan./Feb. 1978.

Van Scoy-Mosher, M. B.: Chemotherapy: A manual for patients and their families, Cancer Nurs., *1*:234-240, June 1978.

Wallace, S., and Goldstein, H. M.: Intravascular occlusive therapy. Postgrad. Med. *59*:141-146, Feb. 1976.

Zia, P. K.: Cyclophosphamide. Cancer Nurs., *1*:83-85, Feb. 1978.

Zubrod, G. C.: Treatment of the patient with cancer by chemotherapy. *In* Nealon, T. F.: Management of the Patient with Cancer, Phila., W. B. Saunders, 1976, Chap. 3.

BOOKLET

Mourad, L. A., and Donahue, M. P.: Guide to the Administration of I.V. Chemotherapeutic Agents. Columbus, Ohio, OSU Comprehensive Cancer Center (1580 Cannon Drive, Columbus, Ohio 43210), 11 pages, $ 0.30.

Perfusion and Regional Infusion

Carter, J.: Role of the oncology nurse in regional infusion chemotherapy. AORN J., *25*:662-668, Mar. 1977.

Hess, C. M.: Intra-arterial chemotherapy: Making it safer and more successful. Nursing '74, *4*:30-34, May 1974.

Hobbs, B., and Ness, S.: Rationale for and long-term care of indwelling arterial infusion systems. Oncol. Nurs. Forum, *4*:6-7, Oct. 1977.

Jochimsen, P. R., and Lawton, R. L.: Aggressive regional therapy of melanoma involving the extremity. J. Iowa Med. Soc., *67*:315-319, Aug. 1977.

AGENCIES

American Cancer Society
777 Third Avenue
New York, N.Y. 10017

16

DIAGNOSTIC RADIOLOGY, RADIOTHERAPY, AND NUCLEAR MEDICINE

Generally, radiation is used in medicine in three ways—for diagnosis, therapy, and research. For any of these, the available radiation sources can be listed simply as roentgenographic and fluoroscopic machines (x-rays), natural and artificial radioactive isotopes, and the high energy particle machines.

Radiation is effective in destroying cancer cells and preventing their spread. In the individual whose malignancy has spread to such an extent that other forms of treatment are ineffective, radiation may be used as a palliative measure to keep the patient comfortable.

Instruction concerning the nature of radiation is essential in order to reduce fears and to promote the safety of all persons who come in contact with it.

THE PHYSICS OF RADIATION

Radioactivity

Everything in our universe, including man, has been subjected to radiation since the universe was formed. This ever present radiation, called natural background, is a normal part of nature's balance and presents no hazard to ordinary living. Scientists discovered x-rays in 1895 and one year later identified radioactivity. Ever since, significant progress has been made in the field of radiation physics.

The elements of the nucleus of an atom achieve stability because of the effect of neutrons on protons. However, in the heavier elements, this becomes increasingly difficult, and such atoms are said to be unstable. In order to become more stable, nuclei give up energy in the form of rays or particles—alpha (α), beta (β), and gamma (γ). Such disintegration is referred to as radioactivity. The relation of physics and radioactivity to therapy is diagrammed in Figure 16-1.

Radioisotopes

The atoms of each chemical element have the same number of protons, so that each atom of the element has the same physical and chemical properties. However, a different form of the same chemical element, called an isotope, may exist. An *isotope* is an element whose nucleus contains a constant number of protons but has a differing number of neutrons, which has the effect of changing its weight. To indicate an isotope, the total number of neutrons and protons is appended, e.g., in cobalt-59 (^{59}Co), the isotope of cobalt has a total of 59 protons and neutrons. The optimal ratio between protons and neutrons in a chemical element is one that is stable—^{59}Co is an example. By using nuclear reactors and high speed particle accelerators, it is possible to bombard a stable isotope such as ^{59}Co with additional neutrons. When ^{59}Co absorbs an extra neutron, an unstable or radioactive isotope is formed, ^{60}Co. This isotope has valuable medical uses.

Most radioisotopes emit *particulate radiation* (small fragments of the nucleus having mass and size) and *electromagnetic radiation* ("rays" that have no mass). The basic radiation type is presented by *alpha* and *beta* particles, which are actually parts of radioactive atoms; these break away and travel at high speeds and with great energies.

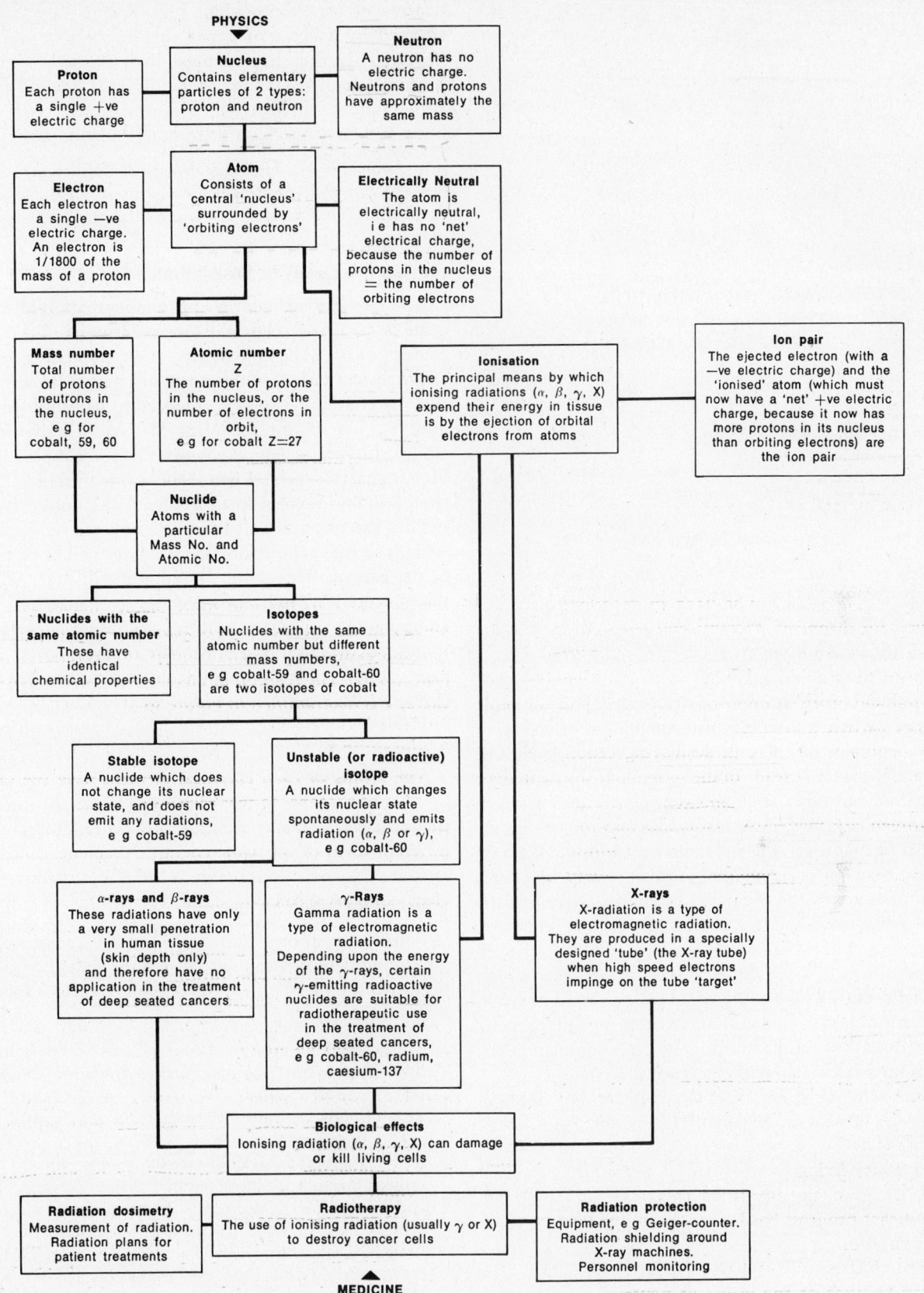

Figure 16-1. An outline of basic physics of radiation and its relation to medicine. (From Mould, R. F.: Physics and radiotherapy. Nurs. Times, March 1974.)

UNITS TO MEASURE AMOUNT OF ACTIVITY	
Curie (Ci)	the basic measure or unit to measure the amount of activity in a radioactive sample
Millicurie (mCi)	one thousandth of a curie
Microcurie (μ)	one millionth of a curie
Picocurie (pCi)	one trillionth of a curie

UNITS TO MEASURE AMOUNT OF RADIATION TO WHICH A GIVEN SUBSTANCE IS EXPOSED OR ABSORBED	
Roentgen (R)	a standard unit of *exposure* (applicable to x-ray and gamma rays)
Milliroentgen (mR)	one thousandth of a roentgen
Rad	a unit to measure absorbed dose (1 rad—amount of radiation required to deposit 100 ergs of energy per gram of irradiated material)
Rem	a unit of measure of radiation dose equivalent which takes into account the relative biological effectiveness ("roentgen equivalent man")

X-ray is a good example of electromagnetic radiation, one of the basic types. It is made up of rays, or waves, of very high electric energy traveling at very high speeds. When electromagnetic radiation arises from natural or artificially created radioactive isotopes, instead of an x-ray machine, it is called *gamma radiation.*

All four of these types of radiation (α, β, γ, X) act on living tissue by ionization or, in other words, by alteration of atoms in the chemical systems of the cell. If the level of radiation and its resulting intracellular ionization is low enough, no irreversible damage is done to the cell or organism as a whole. However, if the level is high enough, the cell may be altered or even destroyed. When such ionization occurs in the cells of the gonads, genetic mutations may result. Radiation effect is cumulative; the ionization that occurs in cells is not reversible.

The different kinds of rays are capable of different

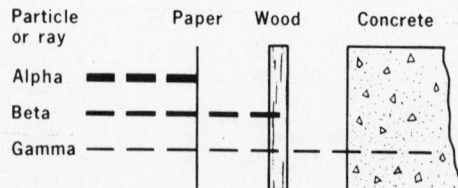

Figure 16-2. Relative penetration of alpha, beta and gamma radiation. (U.S. Atomic Energy Commission)

degrees of penetration (Fig. 16-2). Alpha rays can be stopped by a sheet of paper, and most beta rays are hindered by a thin sheet of metal. In tissue, beta rays have a range of up to 15 mm. Gamma rays are the most penetrating of the three; they can penetrate the human body and can cause hazards to others near the patient.

• To summarize, the amount of damage or destruction to tissue varies with the type of radiation, the dosage and intensity of radiation, and the nature of the site to be irradiated.

Radioactive Decay or Disintegration

The rate at which atoms emit their radiation (disintegrate or decay) varies from isotope to isotope. The decay rate or *half-life* is the time (hours, days, months, or years) required for one half of the atoms of a particular radioactive material to decay or be reduced to half of its initial activity. For example, iodine-131, has a half-life of slightly more than 8 days, whereas radium-226 has a half-life of over 1600 years. When a radioactive agent is administered in an unsealed form to a patient, another factor besides the physical half-life of the radioactive element will play a role in how long radioactivity will be retained in the patient. This is the "biological half-life," which depends on how the body handles injected material. The combination of physical and biological half-lives determines the overall effective half-life of the isotope. Isotopes of longer life are implanted in the patient in sealed containers and then removed for use at another time. An example of this is cobalt-60, which has a half-life of about 5 years.

BIOLOGICAL ASPECTS AND CLINICAL APPLICATION

Effect of Radiation on Tissue

Ionizing radiation is harmful to living tissue; therefore good judgment is required to weigh the benefit of radiation exposure versus the risk of tissue damage. Factors that influence such risk are:

1. The dose rate—a prescribed dose causes less tissue destruction if given in small amounts over a long period of time than when given all at once.
2. Area of body exposure—the larger the area exposed, the greater the effect.
3. Cell susceptibility—rapidly dividing cells with no specialized function are more sensitive than nondividing cells and highly differentiated cells (e.g., lymphocytes and germ cells are more sensitive than nerve or muscle cells).
4. Biological variability—some individuals are more susceptible to radiation than others; e.g., the healthy person is more responsive than the malnourished. Noteworthy also is that those skin cells which are more radioresistant are cured of cancer when sufficient radiation is used.

The fact that the injury extends to all components of the exposed tissue and affects most severely the cells that are growing fastest, i.e., those engaged in tissue regeneration and repair, accounts for the slow healing and extensive scarring that are characteristic of radiation damage.

The *skin* is especially vulnerable to radiation injury by virtue of its exposed location. Healing is likely to be protracted and permanent changes caused by radiation are unusually extensive.

Bone marrow is one of the most radiosensitive of normal tissues, and damage to the marrow is potentially the most lethal of the complications of excessive irradiation. Interruption of marrow function results, in 7 to 8 days, in a fall in circulating platelets to thrombocytopenic levels, giving rise to a hemorrhagic diathesis for which a platelet transfusion may be given. Agranulocytosis develops in about 2 days, causing a heightened susceptibility to bacterial infection that may prove to be as hazardous as thrombocytopenia. Fortunately, antibiotic therapy affords some protection against sepsis in these patients.

Radiation cataracts have been described after excessive exposure of the *eyes* to neutron or x-radiation, and diffuse, incapacitating fibrosis of the *lungs* may follow injudicious irradiation of the thorax. Damage to the *fetus in utero*, with production of congenital malformations, is apt to occur as a result of irradiation during the period from the second to the sixth week of gestation.

SHORT-TERM EFFECTS. If a person has had a major portion of the body exposed to large doses of radiation (over 100 rems) in a short period of time, the symptoms of radiation syndrome will be apparent (see Table 16-1). This is manifested in four stages: (1) prodromal—nausea, vomiting, and malaise; (2) latent—symptoms subside; (3) illness—general malaise, epilation, hemorrhage (purpura, petechiae, nosebleeds, etc.), pallor, diarrhea, inflammation of mouth and throat; and (4) recovery or death.

LONG-TERM EFFECTS. The long-term effects of radiation are an area of public health concern because of the possible involvement of large numbers of people who may be exposed to low levels of radiation over a long period of time. The classic example is the experience of the women employed in the early 1920s to paint watch and clock dials

TABLE 16-1. SUMMARY OF CLINICAL EFFECTS OF ACUTE IONIZING RADIATION DOSES*

RANGE	0 to 100 rems Subclinical range	100 to 1,000 rems Therapeutic range			Over 1,000 rems Lethal range	
		100 to 200 rems	200 to 600 rems	600 to 1,000 rems	1,000 to 5,000 rems	Over 5,000 rems
		Clinical surveillance	Therapy effective	Therapy promising	Therapy palliative	
INCIDENCE OF VOMITING	None	100 rems: 5% 200 rems: 50%	300 rems: 100%	100%	100%	
DELAY TIME	—	3 hours	2 hours	1 hour	30 minutes	
LEADING ORGAN	None	Hematopoietic tissue			Gastrointestinal tract	Central nervous system
CHARACTERISTIC SIGNS	None	Moderate leukopenia	Severe leukopenia, purpura, hemorrhage, infection, epilation above 300 rems		Diarrhea, fever, disturbance of electrolyte balance	Convulsions, tremor, ataxia, lethargy
CRITICAL PERIOD POST-EXPOSURE	—	—	4 to 6 weeks		5 to 14 days	1 to 48 hours
THERAPY	Reassurance	Reassurance, hematologic surveillance	Blood transfusion, antibiotics	Consider bone marrow transplantation	Maintenance of electrolyte balance	Sedatives
PROGNOSIS	Excellent	Excellent	Good	Guarded	Hopeless	
CONVALESCENT PERIOD	None	Several weeks	1 to 12 months	Long	—	
INCIDENCE OF DEATH	None	None	0 to 80% (variable)	80 to 100% (variable)	90 to 100%	
DEATH OCCURS WITHIN	—	—	2 months		2 weeks	2 days
CAUSES OF DEATH	—	—	Hemorrhage, infection		Circulatory collapse	Respiratory, failure, brain edema

*U.S. Dept. of Defense: The Effects of Nuclear Weapons, p. 591, Washington, D. C., Supt. of Documents.

with luminizing (radium–containing) paints. Years later, bone sarcomas resulted from the carcinogenic effect of the radium. Another example is the Hiroshima survivors who continue to show the effects of low levels of radiation.

When the gonads are exposed to radiation, the long-term effects may not be apparent in the individual but may appear in his progeny. Genetic mutations can be transmitted to subsequent generations. Among the most serious of the late consequences of irradiation damage is the increased susceptibility to malignant metaplasia and the development of cancer at sites of earlier irradiation. Evidence cited in support of this relationship refers to the increased incidence of carcinoma of skin, bone, and lung after latent periods of 20 years and longer following irradiation of those sites. Further support has been adduced from the relatively high incidence of carcinoma of the thyroid 7 years and longer following low-dosage irradiation of the thymus in childhood, and from the increased incidence of leukemia following total body irradiation at any age.

Evidence for long-range damage from irradiation in the form of gene mutations in exposed germ plasm is derived almost entirely from observations on insects and small animals and is based on analogy. Statistical arguments and analogies aside, the potential capacity of radiation to produce gene mutations can scarcely be discounted; the existence of the threat cannot be denied. Accordingly, precautions against unnecessary or excessive exposure to radiation are appropriate, and every available safeguard against radiation damage is definitely indicated.

RADIATION DETECTION, CONTROL, AND PRECAUTIONS

Radiation Detection and Control

Although radiations are very powerful, they cannot be directly seen, heard, smelled, tasted, felt, or in any other way detected by ordinary human senses. However, their characteristic ability to ionize matter through which they pass makes it possible to detect and measure them. Instruments have been developed which record the number of rays or particles of radiation that pass through the detecting unit in a given period of time. These instruments, such as Geiger counters, detect radioactivity and measure its general strength.

Radiation has the additional property of affecting the emulsion of photographic film as light does in a camera. Film badges can be worn while working with or near radiation. When the film from the badge, is developed, the extent of exposure can be determined. This knowledge of total radiation exposure is very important.

Within certain limits, cells live quite well while being constantly exposed—there is always a low continuous radiation background. At the other extreme, too much radiation exposure can cause physical damage and death.

In this country, and in much of the world, laws require that radiation sources and devices be used only by persons who are trained in their theory and operation and who agree to abide by specified standards and limits. Such standards, if properly observed, should enable anyone to work with or near radiation throughout his life without noticeable physical damage, shortening of life expectancy, or genetic harm to future generations. Detailed specific dosage and exposure limits need not concern the nurse who is not working directly in a radiology department, so long as the precautions are carefully followed as outlined by the hospital radiologist for any particular patient involving radiation. Exposure ordinarily will be only occasional and, assuming proper precautions, very slight. However, for patients being treated by means of nuclear medicine, the precautions are more exacting, as is indicated in the charts on pages 300–302.

Prevention of Radiation Damage

Improvements in equipment for diagnostic radiology are clearly desirable and are constantly in progress. Policies have been recommended, more rigid than those of the past, regarding the extent to which diagnostic x-ray examinations should be carried out and the frequency with which they should be repeated. Examinations for possible pregnancy or for purposes of pelvimetry, for example, are discouraged, as are all x-ray studies that are undertaken in the absence of disease. Perhaps the most important aspect of any program that might be designed for the prevention of radiation damage concerns the education of practitioners who work with radiologic apparatus but are untrained in radiology.

Finally, it should be emphasized that the benefits of radiation therapy should never be denied to a patient with a radiosensitive neoplasm because of considerations regarding long-range radiologic safety. As a result of intensive publicity regarding the dangers of radioactive fallout and the complications of radiation damage in general, anxiety over the potential complications of radiotherapy, including x-ray irradiation and the use of radioisotopes, is prevalent among the uninformed public. The nurse is very likely to be in a position to allay such fears in the minds of many patients for whom irradiation has been recommended but who are inclined to refuse it on the grounds of its inherent risks.

Roentgenologic Precautions

The safety of the patient, the therapist, the nurse, the x-ray technician, and any other personnel who might be present during radiography, fluoroscopy, or radiotherapy demands strict observance of certain precautions, including the following:

- No one should be in the room with a patient who is undergoing x-ray therapy or roentgenography.
- The fluoroscopic equipment and technique should be such as to prevent the leakage of radiation.
- Each individual in the fluroscopic room should protect himself from scattered radiation by wearing a lead apron and, if indicated, lead-impregnated gloves.
- Complete protection of the patient's gonads during radiography and x-ray therapy should be assured by means of appropriate lead shielding.
- The symbol indicating the presence of radioactive material should be displayed in a prominent place as a means of warning all personnel of the need for caution (Fig. 16-3).

The nurse should be familiar with these stipulations and their purpose so that they may be clearly explained to the patient.

When a patient is receiving x-ray therapy, he ought to know why he seems to be left alone when receiving treatment and that a technician is always nearby and can see him through a window or via TV monitoring. Also, the patient should know that there is an intercommunication system that allows him to talk to the technician. It is well to remember that external radiation will never cause any patient to become radioactive himself. He cannot possibly present any radiation hazard to himself, other patients, or the nurse.

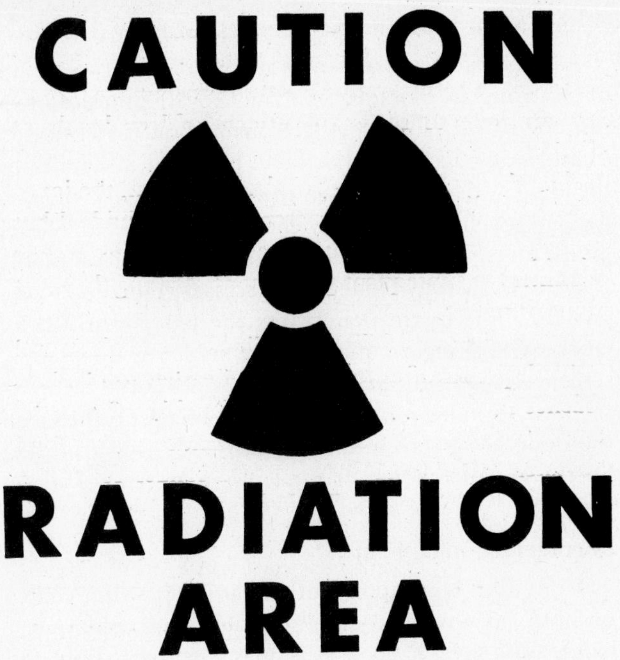

DIAGNOSTIC RADIOLOGY

Diagnostic radiology has assumed an ever increasing role in the overall management of patients. Disease or injury often causes alterations in the function and structure of tissue which may be detected roentgenographically. Therefore, evaluation of the patient frequently requires a roentgenographic examination.

Basic procedures that are employed in various x-ray studies are of immediate concern to the nurse. In certain examinations the nurse is a direct participant and can influence the success or failure of the examination by the manner in which certain preliminary preparative measures are carried out. For example, the nurse can prepare the patient by allaying any suspected fears and by making sure that the patient receives the proper medication at the proper time prior to the examination. The nurse's familiarity with diagnostic roentgenology in general and her appreciation of the objectives of specific tests are essential to understanding patients and their problems.

It is important to understand not only the diagnostic capabilities of the roentgenographic examination, but also the exposure factors and economic considerations

CAUTION

RADIATION AREA

Figure 16-3. Radioactive material warning symbol.

involved. A major goal of modern radiology is to minimize exposure of the population to diagnostic radiation. Employing proper safeguards in the use of radiation equipment is one means of accomplishing this end.

Certain basic considerations should be discussed concerning radiation dose and its beneficial and potentially harmful effects. Frequently patients ask the nurse questions such as "Am I getting too much x-ray?" In general, diagnostic doses of radiation are relatively insignificant, although exposure of the gonads must be considered. Although a single exposure during one examination on one patient is little cause for concern, continued or cumulative radiation exposure can be hazardous and can have far-reaching implications if the exposure occurs during the reproductive years. Certainly, the scientific data gathered from animal experiments support the basis for this concern. The logical conclusion, therefore, is to minimize exposure to radiation whenever possible and to consider all untoward effects. For example, in view of the known fact that the fetus is extremely sensitive to radiation, it may be wise, when doing a nonemergency roentgenographic workup on a female patient of childbearing age, to carry out the procedure during the patient's menstrual period to assure that the patient is not pregnant.

In the final analysis, responsible medical judgment must balance the potential benefits versus the potential risks of any roentgenologic examination. Any examination done unnecessarily should be considered as "too much x-ray"—yet no examination important to the diagnostic or therapeutic management of the patient should be withheld.

Nature of the X-ray Image—Concept of X-ray (Fig. 16-4)

As was noted earlier, x-rays are one part of a spectrum of electromagnetic radiation. The rays are produced in a cathode ray tube in which electrons are boiled off a heated filament and accelerated across a potential difference to the anode, the target. When the electrons strike the target, energy, including x-ray energy, is produced. The x-ray beam is passed from the target through a collimator (Fig. 16-4), thereby reducing unnecessary radiation to the patient. The beam penetrates the patient and then emerges, striking the film cassette holder or fluroscopic screen. A roentgenographic image is produced on an x-ray film. (Similarly, in fluroscopy the image produced on the fluorescing screen during fluroscopy is transmitted by the use of mirrors or a television screen for direct vision.)

Roentgenographic Film

X-ray film is composed of a clear plastic base, coated on both sides with an emulsion layer containing silver halide. The silver halide emulsion is sensitive to light and x-rays. During exposure of the film to x-rays and during the process and development procedure, there is a physicochemical alteration of the silver halide emulsion. The blackening of the film producing the intelligible image is caused by the effects on the silver halide of the amounts of radiant energy that reach the film through the object examined.

Differential Absorption

The amount of radiant energy reaching the film cassette is in large part affected by the differential absorption characteristics of tissue. Basically there are four radiographic densities: air, fat, soft tissue, and bone. Absorption is dependent in turn, upon the tissue density and volume irradiated. A given thickness of bone will absorb more than the same thickness of muscle (soft tissue), and a given thickness of fat will absorb more than a similar volume of air. It is this characteristic that allows demarcation of anatomical structures within the body.

In order to achieve the necessary degree of inequality in density where no such inequality exists (as is the case with vessels in soft tissue or with the lumen of the bowel), it may be necessary to introduce either an artificial high-density "contrast medium" or a natural low-density contrast agent, such as air. This will delineate the lumen of any tube or hollow viscus containing the contrast agent, thereby improving radiographic contrast and diagnostic capability. The roentgenographic study of the gastrointestinal tract, the gallbladder, the bronchi, the kidneys, the spinal canal, the genitourinary tract and blood vessels, etc., depend in each case on the ingestion or the injection of an appropriate contrast agent.

TOMOGRAPHY. Another type of radiographic examination is tomography, also known as body section radiography, planigraphy, or laminography. These terms all refer to a method of radiographic examination in which it is possible to examine a single layer or plane of tissue by blurring out the planes of tissue both above and below the area of interest. This is accomplished by simultaneous motion of the x-ray tube and film cassette in geometric relation to the plane to be examined. Geometrically, the plane of focus represents the fulcrum of the motion of the tube and film, i.e., the only area not in motion, with respect to the tube and film. This procedure is frequently

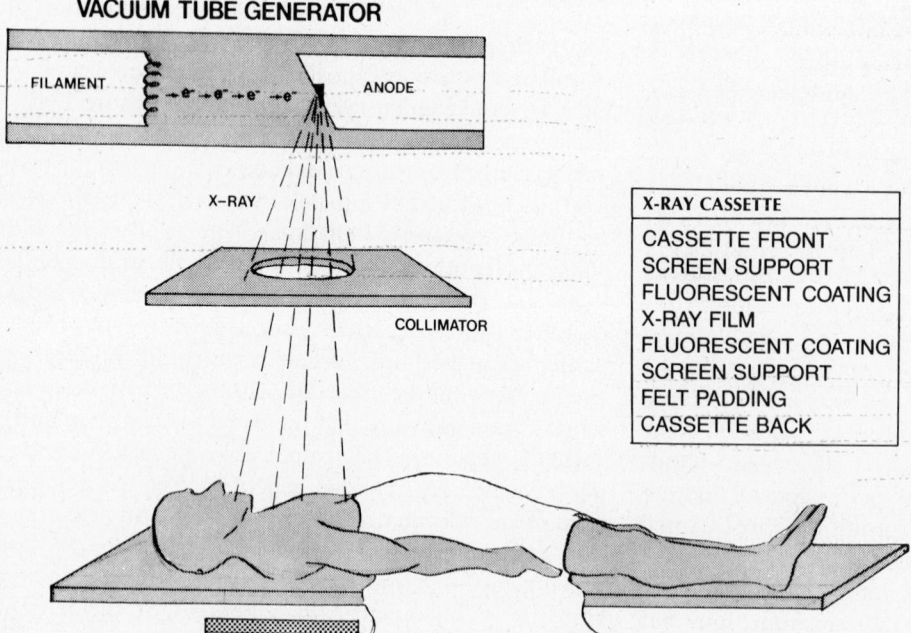

VACUUM TUBE GENERATOR

FILAMENT → e⁻ → e⁻ → e⁻ → e⁻   ANODE

X-RAY

COLLIMATOR

X-RAY CASSETTE

CASSETTE FRONT
SCREEN SUPPORT
FLUORESCENT COATING
X-RAY FILM
FLUORESCENT COATING
SCREEN SUPPORT
FELT PADDING
CASSETTE BACK

X-RAY CASSETTE

Figure 16-4. Production of x-ray and roentgenogram. Insert shows makeup of typical film cassette.

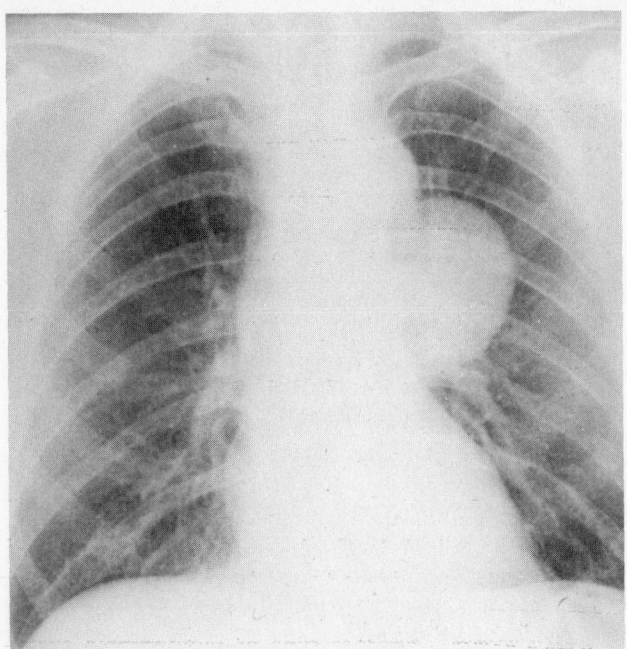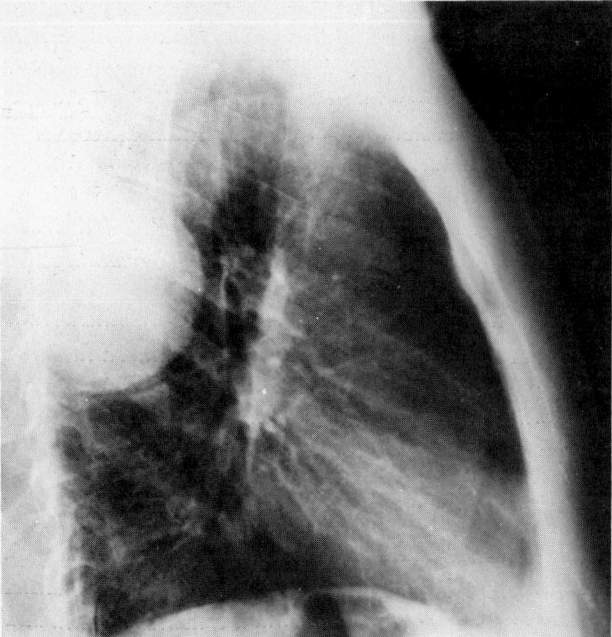

Figure 16-5. PA (posteroanterior) and lateral roentgenograms demonstrate large mass in posterior left chest representing "cannonball" metastasis from primary liposarcoma arising in left thigh.

helpful in blurring out any overlying, confusing edges. Multiple views of a body region focused at successively deeper layers visualize clearly some structures that would otherwise be obscured. For example, a tumor partially obstructing a bronchial lumen or an area of bone destruction in the vertebral column may be more clearly visualized by this technique.

Roentgenographic Examination of the Chest (Fig. 16-5)

The chest roentgenographic examination is extremely important in diagnosing pulmonary disease and in evaluating abnormalities of the mediastinum, including the heart and the bony thorax. The chest roentgenogram is not only helpful in the workup of the patient at the time of the examination, but also serves as a normal baseline or as a record of the stage or progression of disease. Even though chest radiography may frequently demonstrate lesions not detectable by other means, it is not meant to supplant clinical history and physical examination.

Routine examination of the chest basically includes posteroanterior (PA) and lateral projections (Fig. 16-5). These are usually taken with the tube-film at a distance of 6 feet. It is desirable to have the patient inhale deeply or moderately at the time of examination in order to reduce distortion and allow for magnification of the image.

A wealth of information is obtainable from a chest roentgenogram. Since direct measurement of thoracic structures may be obtained, the lung and pulmonary vessels can be well visualized as can the trachea and proximal bronchi by virtue of their air-containing lumen. The heart and its chambers can be clearly seen, especially when barium is present in the esophagus allowing the posterior surface of the heart to be outlined. While soft tissue and osseous thorax can be noted, mediastinal structures may not be seen as distinct entities because of a lack of inherent contrast within the mediastinum. However, a pathologic process such as neoplasm or bronchogenic cyst may be visualized by virtue of the displacement of normal structures from their usual location.

Special views, including oblique or apical lordotic positions, may be obtained to further evaluate a suspected abnormality. Chest tomography can help outline detailed anatomy of the lung and its vascular structures or demonstrate a cavity in a tuberculous parenchymal lesion. Fluoroscopy is occasionally helpful in evaluating the chest, particularly in differentiating vascular from nonvascular structures and in assessing diaphragmatic motion or the location of a lesion. Fluoroscopic controls can also be used in bronchography in which the bronchial tree is studied by introducing opaque material into the desired bronchus or bronchi. This is usually done to detail the anatomy of the bronchial tree and to outline the extent of known disease, such as bronchiectasis, or to determine the presence of suspected disease, such as lung tumor.

Roentgenographic Examination of the Abdomen

Abdominal x-rays are most frequently taken in the anteroposterior position. Frequently, this view (often referred to as a "scout roentgenogram") is accompanied

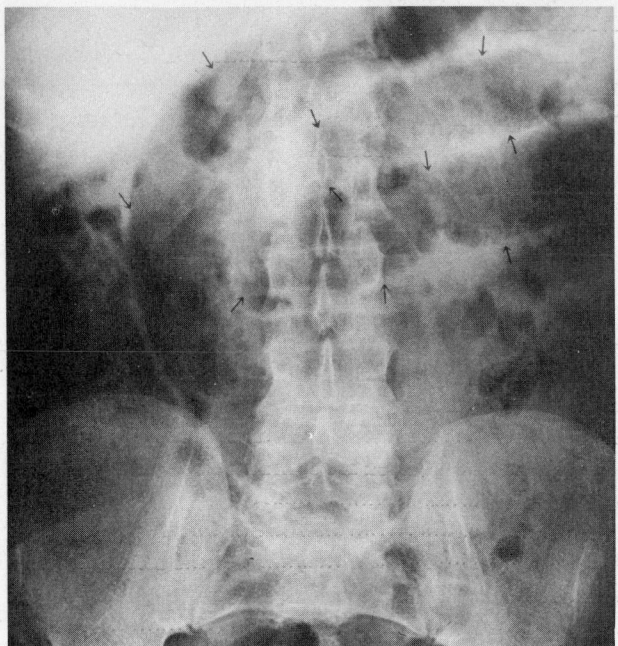
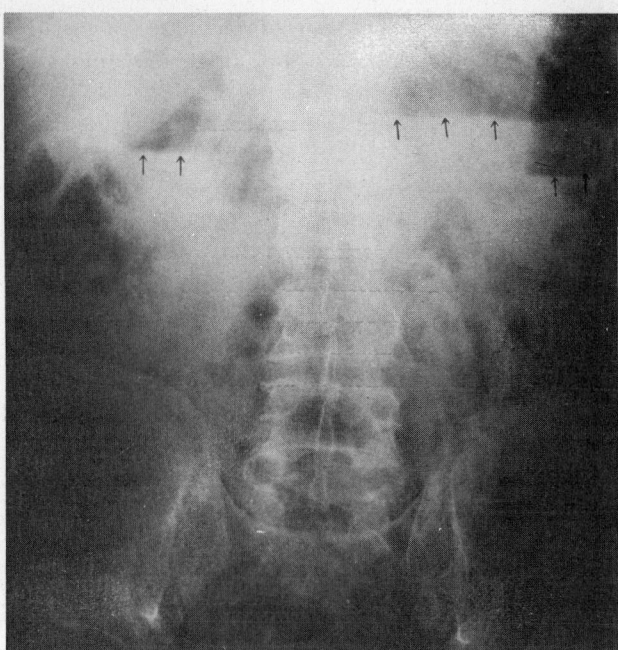

Figure 16-6. Supine and erect roentgenograms of abdomen demonstrate multiple dilated air-fluid filled loops of small bowel consistent with the diagnosis of small bowel obstruction. Arrows indicate loops.

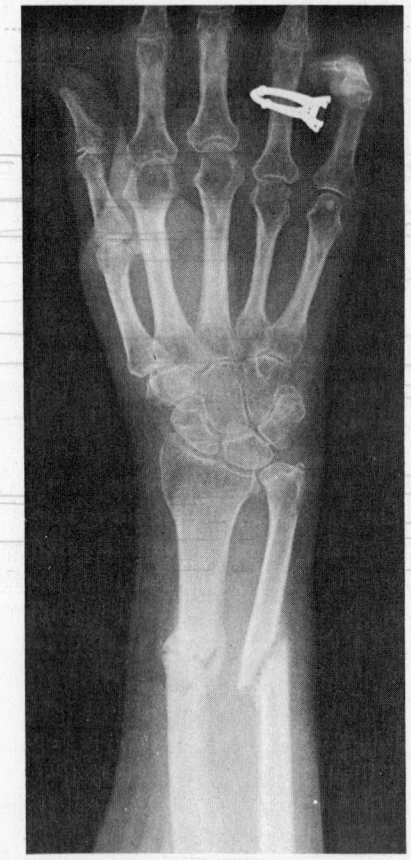

Figure 16-7. AP roentgenogram of left forearm demonstrating healing fractures of distal radius and ulna. (Note ring on third finger.)

by an erect anteroposterior view of the abdomen (Fig. 16-6). In certain situations in which the patient cannot stand, a special view, such as the decubitus view, is obtained. This view is taken with the patient lying on his side with the film cassette placed behind and the x-ray beam directed through the body on a horizontal plane. Another possible view is the direct lateral view, which is used in certain instances, such as in suspected cases of calcified abdominal aortic aneurysm.

A variety of conditions can be ascertained through abdominal x-ray, including bowel obstruction, collection of intra-abdominal fluids (such as ascites or abscess) calculi of the gallbladder or urinary tract, and other pathologic intra-abdominal calcifications. Abdominal organs viewed include the liver, kidney, and spleen. The pancreas, on the other hand, is a difficult organ to visualize by routine roentgenogram. Therefore, pancreatic pathology is usually detected only by displacement of normal structures.

Contrast agents are particularly useful in evaluating the function and anatomical detail within the lumen of abdominal structures in the biliary system and in the gastrointestinal and genitourinary tracts. For example, opaque contrast material can help to outline nonopaque gallstones or diagnose a nonfunctioning gallbladder. An ulcer will be seen as a persistent collection of contrast material. The bowel wall surrounding the ulcer may also be visualized indicating the benign or malignant nature of the ulcer.

The examination of the retroperitoneum, particularly

the pancreas, has always been a difficult area to visualize roentgenographically because of the lack of natural contrast substances, either air or fat. Ultrasound and computed body tomography have been particularly helpful in this difficult area.

Skeletal Roentgenograms (Fig. 16-7)

Skeletal problems, particularly fractures, are well visualized roentgenographically, as is the process of fracture healing. However, the soft tissues of the joints, including cartilage, are not visualized normally without the use of a contrast medium, which is injected into the joint to outline these structures. This latter technique is called *arthrography.*

Roentgenograms of the skeleton may be helpful in establishing or excluding the diagnosis of nutritional and endocrine disorders that are complicated by derangements of protein metabolism or calcium and phosphorus deposition. Abnormal radiolucency of the bones indicating demineralization of the skeleton is a characteristic, for example, of rickets, hyperparathyroidism, and myelomatosis. The various types of arthritis often demonstrate roentgenographic changes sufficiently characteristic to allow differentiation. Paget's disease (a congenital disorder) and osteoporosis appear as regions of increased bone density. Furthermore, chronic lead intoxication or hypervitaminosis A may be established by skeletal roentgenograms. Lymphomas and metastasizing carcinomas or sarcomas may often manifest themselves in the skeletal system in the form of osteolytic or osteoblastic lesions. The most common sites of metastatic disease within the skeleton are those areas with active bone marrow and, therefore, relatively high blood perfusion, including the skull, pelvis, and vertebrae.

Computerized Tomography

The detail and inner structure of an object can be mathematically reconstructed from the information obtained from numerous projections taken from multiple angles. This technique has been used in astronomy, electron microscopy, and computerized tomography.

In computerized tomography (CT) two processes are involved: (1) various views are taken in a single plane, and (2) the data acquired are computed and presented as a recognizable cross-sectional image.

The image results from an x-ray beam passing through the body at many angles. Readings of the attenuation of the x-ray beam are recorded by detectors and stored in the computer. This data is then computed (reconstructed) into the image by using complex mathematical equations. The gray scale or brightness of each portion of the cross-sectional image is related to its degree of x-ray absorption. The image is displayed on an oscilloscope or a television monitor and can be permanently recorded on x-ray or polaroid film.

Machines are currently available which can literally scan "head to toe." Scan time ranges from 2 to 18 seconds.

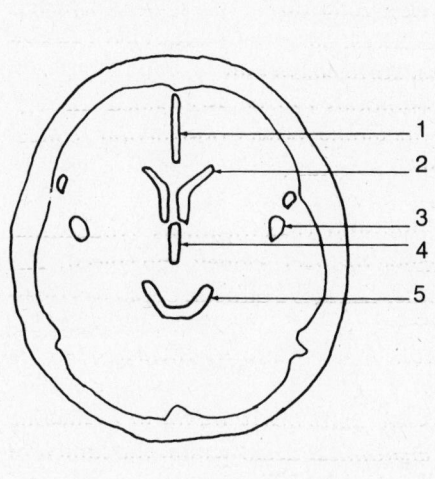 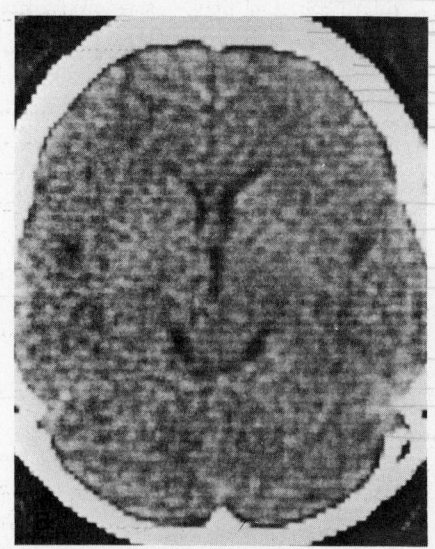 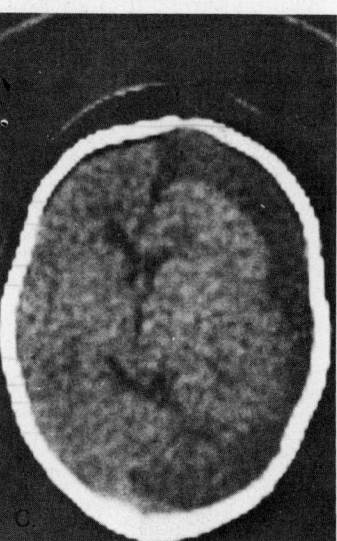

Figure 16-8. CT scans. (Figures courtesy Robert A. Zimmerman, M.D., Hospital of the University of Pennsylvania)

A. Line drawing of *B*. 1—interhemispheric fissure between frontal lobes of brain; 2—frontal horns; 3—temporal horn; 4—third ventricle; 5—fourth ventricle.

B. CT of brain through level of frontal horns. See *A* for detailed anatomy.

C. CT of brain following head trauma. Note radiolucent area (blacker area) surrounding the brain on the right. This represents a chronic subdural hygroma from previous bleeding after trauma. Note the shift of the midline of the brain to the left. The ventricular system is dilated (compare with *B*).

For head scans, spine and extremity scans, and most chest scans, no preparation is necessary. Since intravenous contrast material may be used to enhance a questionable area, knowledge of allergic reactions to contrast materials used in previous studies is quite important.

Body scans require that the gastrointestinal tract be clear of content, including any trace of barium. Therefore, laxatives may have to be given prior to the examination.

• For abdominal body scanning, the patient should be NPO after midnight prior to the day of the examination.

Since the patient will likely receive oral gastrografin, intravenous contrast media, and intravenous glucagon, it is again important to know the allergic history of the patient and whether the patient is diabetic.

Head scans are used in the evaluation of most cranial problems including brain tumors, intracranial hemorrhage and ischemic disease, infection, hydrocephalus, demyelinating diseases, congenital abnormalities, cervical spinal cord lesions and various eye, ear, nose, and throat diseases. Figure 16-8 shows the contrast between a normal CT of the head and one taken of a patient who has suffered severe head trauma.

Scanning can be done on nearly any part of the body including the lungs and pleura, mediastinum, liver, gallbladder and biliary tree, pancreas, spleen, urinary tract and adrenals, retroperitoneum, pelvis, and extremities. Figure 16-9 shows a pancreatic pseudocyst demonstrated by CT.

Computerized tomography has already had a profound effect on the practice of medicine and will probably have an even greater effect in the future. It is hoped that it will decrease the number of tests, reduce hospital inpatient time, replace more invasive modalities, and decrease the need both for exploratory surgery and, possibly, for hospitalization.

Diagnostic Ultrasound

Ultrasound (high frequency sound above the hearing range) has become established as a diagnostic modality with a wide variety of uses in clinical medicine. The high frequency sound is generated by a transducer (crystal) and converted into a molecular beam which then enters the body. A small percentage of the beam is reflected back to the transducer from tissue interfaces of different densities. The greater the difference in the tissue densities at the interface, the greater the amount of sound reflected back to the transducer.

The reflected sound wave bounces back to the transducer, which records how long it took to come back and how much of the original sound wave came back. By timing the wave, an accurate depth measurement can be made.

As the transducer is drawn over the skin surface, it generates a two-dimensional cross-sectional image of that part of the body. The echoes come from various tissue interfaces both outside and inside the underlying organs. The depth recording and the intensity recording of these echoes produce a cross-sectional image showing the outlines and internal structures of organs based on their sound reflection properties.

Because fluid is homogeneous, there are no internal echoes in fluid. Ultrasound, therefore, is a very sensitive instrument for distinguishing solid from cystic structures.

Because of the great differences that exist between the density of soft tissue and that of air or bone interfaces,

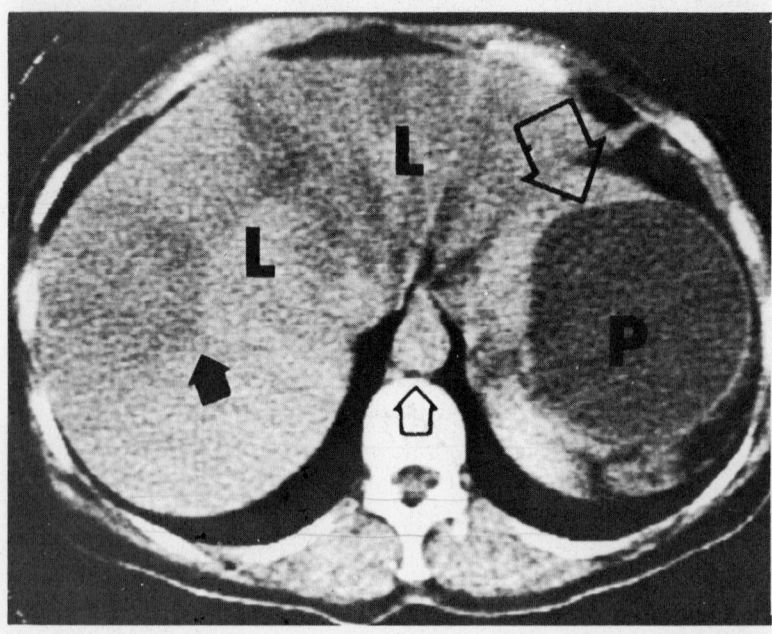

Figure 16-9. CT of body demonstrating pancreatic pseudocyst. Note well circumscribed radiolucent (blacker) pseudocyst (P) on the patient's left (scans of the body are viewed from the patient's feet). Solid black arrow points to radiolucent areas in the liver (L) which are fatty infiltrations due to cirrhosis. Outlined arrow placed on the lumbar vertebral body points to the upper abdominal aorta.

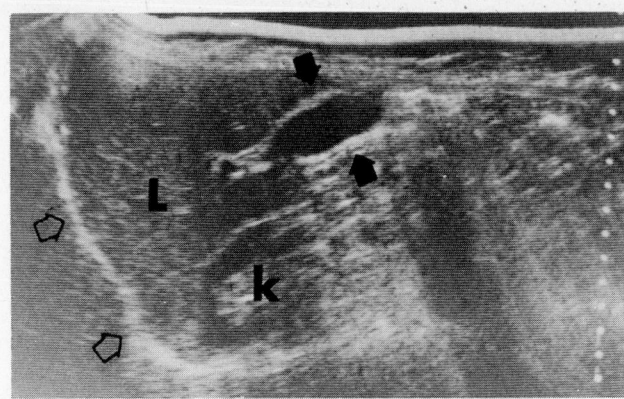

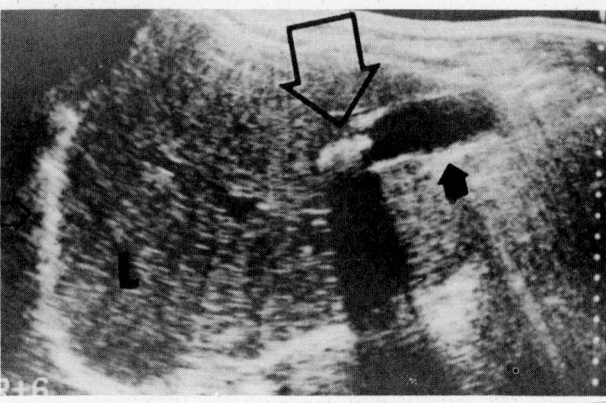

Figure 16-10. A. Ultrasound scan of normal gallbladder. Longitudinal (sagittal) section to the right of the midline. Tubular echo-free area (solid black arrows) is normal gallbladder in its usual relationship to the liver (L) and right kidney (K). Outlined arrows point to the dense echoes of the right diaphragm.

B. Gallstones. Longitudinal (sagittal) section to the right of the midline. Note the gallbladder (solid black arrow), with dense echoes and acoustic shadowing in the superior aspect (large outlined arrow) indicating presence of gallstones. Liver (L) and right diaphragm (small outlined arrow) are also seen.

ultrasound does not penetrate air or bone. Barium also reflects the sound wave. This is why ultrasound has little application in chest studies and why preparation of the patient is important in abdominal work.

- When ultrasound of the abdomen is scheduled, the patient should be in a fasting state and possibly prepped with an anti-gas agent such as simethicone.
- Ultrasound should be done before any contemplated barium studies such as UGI or BE (upper GI or barium enema).
- Good hydration is important since sound is transmitted best in well hydrated patients.

Ultrasound has wide application including brain, thyroid, neck, heart, chest for pleural effusions, liver, gallbladder and ducts, pancreas, retroperitoneum, aorta, and kidney and pelvis.

Figure 16-10 illustrates a normal gallbladder and one with stones demonstrated by the use of ultrasound.

Because experiments to date indicate that it causes no detectable tissue damage, ultrasound is widely used for pregnancy evaluation. Location of the placenta, gestational age, and some abnormalities may be demonstrated.

RADIATION THERAPY

Principles and Purpose of Radiation Therapy

Radiation therapy is the use of *ionizing radiation* for the treatment of patients with malignant tumors. The ionizing radiations are electromagnetic waves that are generated by radioisotopes: cobalt, radium, and cesium — and by electromechanical devices such as linear accelerators and betatrons. Charged particles may also be used, and machines are now available for the medical application of neutron, proton, and pi meson beams. X-ray treatments

may be delivered by *external beam* (cobalt machine, linear accelerator) (Fig. 16-11), by *intracavitary* means (within a cavity, i.e., intrauterine and vaginal), or by *interstitial* means (within tissue, i.e., radioactive implants). Frequently, combinations of external and internal treatments are used in an attempt to cure local or regional disease or to palliate symptoms and signs of advanced disease such as pain, bleeding, and obstruction.

A common characteristic of all malignant cells is their capacity for unlimited proliferation. The rate at which this occurs varies with the tumor type. Ionizing radiation

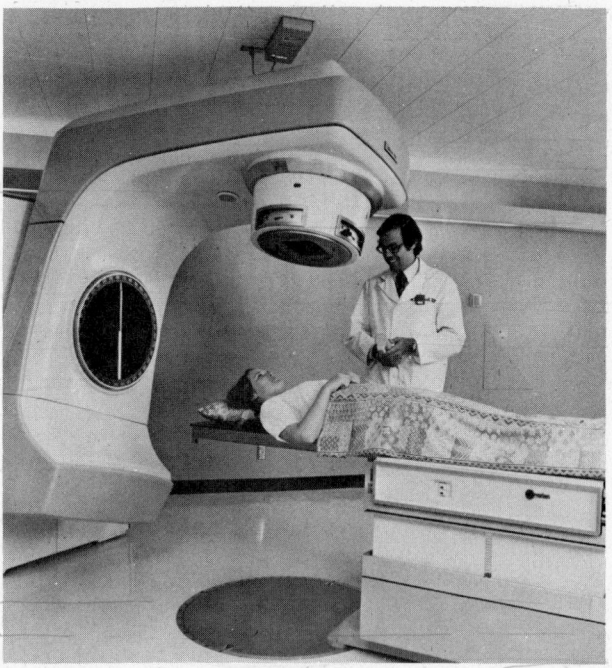

Figure 16-11. Clinac 6X™, 6-million electron volt (MeV) linear accelator for radiotherapy. (Courtesy Varian)

interferes nonspecifically with cellular division, and if enough lethal radiation damage has been deposited within the cell, the cell will be unable to reproduce itself successfully. However, cell death may not occur immediately but may be delayed for a number of cellular divisions extending from hours to months. Malignant cells probably have the same capacity to repair radiation damage as do normal cells but they cannot repopulate as rapidly. This difference makes possible the x-ray eradication of tumors. The radiation therapist attempts to increase the therapeutic ratio between normal tissue tolerance and tumor kill by a variety of means.

While tumors cause problems by replacing normal tissues, malignant tumors have the additional ability to *metastasize* by disseminating through the bloodstream and the lymphatic system. Knowledge of the potential pattern of spread of a specific tumor enables the radiation therapist and other members of the cancer treatment team to plan specific therapy. If radiation treatments are elected, the radiation therapist will design treatment portals to encompass these sites. Different doses will be utilized depending on the type of tumor treated and the extent of gross and microscopic disease.

Radiation therapy may be used in conjunction with surgery, either preoperatively or postoperatively, with or without chemotherapy. In preoperative radiation, the objectives are (1) to reduce the possibility of local recurrence by destroying the peripheral, better oxygenated malignant cells which will not be extirpated by surgery, (2) to reduce tumor bulk and volume, thereby facilitating surgery, and (3) possibly to decrease the likelihood of metastatic spread at the time of surgery. Postoperative irradiation may be used when there is residual tumor or a high likelihood of local recurrence. Such irradiation may include the original tumor volume and adjacent lymph-node-bearing areas. The timing of the irradiation in relation to surgery, either before or after, may not be crucial.

In modern radiation therapy, a *treatment simulator* is utilized to determine the *treatment portals,* that is, the specific area of treatment. A simulator not only has the same mechanical characteristics and beam geometry of the treatment unit but also can take high quality diagnostic x-ray films utilizing fluoroscopic guidance. From these planning films, a formal treatment plan is developed by the radiation therapist in conjunction with a radiation physicist and a radiation dosimetrist. In this fashion, exact measurements can be made and exact doses can be determined for the target volume.

Initiation of Therapy

Once dosage has been determined, the patient begins the course of radiation therapy, which may be brief or protracted. Small lesions, such as superficial skin cancers, may be treated for cure by very rapidly utilizing high radiation doses over a brief period. Extensive deep-seated lesions, however, will require a radiation program extending over weeks or months. This is called *fractionation* (the daily repeated dose), and it is utilized by the radiation therapist to allow the normal tissues to repopulate themselves. The traditional radiotherapy program is given Monday through Friday, 5 days a week with daily fraction sizes varying usually from 150 to 300 rad tumor dose. The *rad* is a unit of absorbed dose in tissue corresponding to 100 ergs per gram of tissue. During the course of therapy, the radiation therapist and the nurse regularly monitor the patient's tolerance of the program and the response of the disease.

Delivering high doses of irradiation to deep-seated tumors while shielding critical structures such as the spinal cord, heart, kidneys, and bowel has accounted in large part for the recent progress in cancer management. Such diseases as Hodgkin's disease, cervical and uterine cancer, seminomas and pediatric tumors such as Wilm's disease, and rhabdomyosarcoma have a high likelihood of cure with radiation alone or radiation in combination with surgery and chemotherapy. High energy treatment machines (*supervoltage*) deposit their maximum dose deep within tissue, thereby reducing to a minimum the severe skin reactions seen with low energy equipment (*orthovoltage*) used in the past. Orthovoltage deposits its maximum energy in the skin and subcutaneous tissues, limiting the total dose that can be delivered to a deep-seated tumor and is therefore no longer used in curative radiotherapy. Another advance, collimation of the beam, limits the unwanted scatter to normal uninvolved tissues and thus increases the patient's tolerance of the radiation treatment.

Side Effects of Radiation Therapy

The side effects of the treatment depend greatly on the volumes of normal tissue that must of necessity be included in the radiation field. With early, confined disease, the radiation may be restricted to the tumor and a small amount of normal neighboring tissue. In this situation radiation side effects may be minimal. With more advanced disease, large volumes are treated and side effects increase proportionately. Daily dose and total dose also play a role here; as each increases, the acute and chronic reactions may increase.

NURSING SUPPORT

Physical and Psychological Preparation

The nurse, as a key member of the cancer management team, helps to prepare the patient for the emotional stress of radiation treatment by anticipating and relieving common apprehensions and managing common side effects. For the patient who has a malignancy, radiation therapy may be misinterpreted as representing terminal care. The nurse should be aware of this apprehension and direct the assessment and nursing plan accordingly, recognizing that radiation therapy is often curative and frequently capable of extending the quality of meaningful life. The nurse and physician should confer about how the purpose of the treatment may best be explained to the patient and the family.

There are certain similarities between a diagnostic x-ray study and an x-ray therapy session. For one thing, the patient must remain still and in some instances must be immobilized with external devices to prevent movement. The treatment period is relatively brief—2 to 3 minutes—and the patient feels no special sensation during treatment. During the actual treatment, all personnel leave the room to avoid exposure to the radiation. Being left alone in a room with huge radiation equipment may frighten the patient unless reassurance and explanation are given by the nurse prior to the session. It is equally important to reassure the patient that the treatment will not make him radioactive unless radioactive material has been taken internally or placed in body cavities or tissues (e.g., intrauterine radium in uterine and cervical malignancy).

It may be necessary for the radiation therapist to mark the exact area of treatment on the skin. Pen markings or, preferably, permanent inconspicuous dots may be placed at the edges and center of the treatment area. Such marks should be preserved and care taken to see that they are not washed off by the patient or nurse unless permission is given by the radiotherapist.

Occasionally the treatment course may be altered from the initial plan. Such a change may prove discouraging to the patient. Again, the nurse will be crucial here in helping the patient and the family to understand the reasons for the change.

Skin Reactions

The skin in areas that are being treated may become tender and reddened. Advise the patient not to apply ointments, lotions, cosmetics or powders to these sites since they may increase the irritation. Likewise, discourage vigorous drying or the use of tight-fitting garments. The region should be kept dry and open to the air as much as possible. *Cornstarch* acts as an excellent drying agent and does not increase the radiation reaction. Even long after a course of radiation therapy, the patient should be cautioned against undue irritation to the area from friction and excessive exposure to sunlight.

Systemic Reactions

Individual responses to radiation therapy vary. The side effects one encounters depend on the nature and extent of the illness and the area of treatment. The patient should be encouraged to report all symptoms to the medical team. Most physical reactions to radiation are

TABLE 16-2. DIETARY SUPPORT OF COMMON COMPLICATIONS OF RADIOTHERAPY

REGION	COMPLICATIONS	NUTRITIONAL SUPPORT
Head-neck, oropharyngeal	Teeth susceptible to deterioration	Serve foods steaming, to impart aroma.
	Postradiation mouth blindness: loss of taste for sweet-bitter-salt-sour	Serve meals with sauces or gravies to facilitate mastication and swallowing.
	Mouth very dry Mastication, swallowing very difficult	Serve meals appealing in color, form, texture to overcome anorexia.
	Anorexia, nausea, vomiting	Serve fragrant foods and beverages to compensate for loss of taste.
Intestinal	Early symptoms: Acute or subacute enteritis, diarrhea, abdominal pain, distention, nausea, vomiting	High calorie, high protein, low fat intake B_{12} supplementation
		If food tolerated: low residue diet small frequent feedings ample amount of fluids
	Later symptoms: Intestinal stenosis, fibrosis Edema, loss of weight Loss of fluids and electrolytes	If stenosis and fibrosis: tube feedings

(Valassi, K.: Nutritional management of cancer patients in a variety of therapeutic regimens, Arch. Phys. Med. & Rehabil. *58*: Sept. 1977)

temporary and can be alleviated by nursing care and medication.

Adequate *nutrition* is essential during the course of treatment. Since patients frequently experience anorexia (loss of appetite), food and vitamin supplements are needed. Persons undergoing treatment to the head and neck region and chest may experience pharyngitis or esophagitis. For these patients, soft or pureed foods and high-calorie liquids are beneficial. Hyperalimentation may be required on a temporary basis to maintain the patient in positive nitrogen balance. (See Table 16-2: Dietary Support of Common Complications of Radiotherapy.)

Thick, tenacious sputum, loss of taste, and *dry mouth* are frequent side effects (often long-lasting) when the upper aerodigestive tract is irradiated. Frequent irrigation of the oral cavity with a dilute saline or bicarbonate solution, particularly after meals, is recommended.

Nausea and *vomiting* are usually experienced only by patients undergoing large volume irradiation to the thorax and upper midabdomen. It is rarely experienced by those whose radiation portals are away from these sites. Antiemetics such as phenothiazine compounds, the careful selection of fluids and foods palatable to the patient, frequent small meals, and the constant reassurance of the nursing team may greatly improve this condition.

Diarrhea and *abdominal cramping* may be experienced by patients receiving pelvic and lower abdominal irradiation. Maintaining fluid balance, using a low fiber diet, and judiciously administering antispasmodic drugs may greatly alleviate this side effect.

Increased *urinary frequency, urgency,* and *dysuria* are symptoms of acute radiation cystitis which may be experienced by persons undergoing pelvic irradiation. After infection has been excluded, antispasmodics and local urinary tract anesthetics are usually beneficial.

Weakness and fatigue often result from a protracted course of radiation therapy. This fatigue may be temporary, lasting from a few weeks to months. During this period normal activity should be interspersed with time for rest and relaxation. The nurse can often help the patient through these difficult days by showing an understanding of why the patient feels discouraged and listless.

Hair loss due to irradiation is only produced within the treated area and nowhere else. Should the scalp not be in the portal, balding will not occur. Hair loss may not be permanent and hair may begin to grow back within 3 months of the completion of the program.

In summary, the nurse is a crucial part of the cancer management team. Knowledge of the realities of the treatment program will help to allay the fears and apprehensions of the patient, and nursing support will facilitate the patient's progress through therapy. The better the communication between the radiation therapist, nurse, and patient, the more successful will be the outcome of the treatment program.

NUCLEAR MEDICINE

BASIC CONCEPTS

During the past 10 to 15 years nuclear medicine has progressed from a minor subspecialty under the jurisdiction of other branches of medicine to a separate specialty with its own training program and specialty board. This rapid growth has occurred mainly because of the development of improved imaging devices and better radiopharmaceuticals. Nuclear medicine procedures are simple to perform, their adverse effects on the patient are relatively slight, and they yield valuable information not attainable by any other means. All medical personnel dealing directly with patients should have at least a limited acquaintance with radiopharmaceuticals, the instruments involved, and the results to be expected from nuclear medicine procedures. Although this section will deal mainly with imaging techniques employed in nuclear medicine, there will be a brief discussion of nonimaging in-vivo examinations, therapeutic uses of radioactive isotopes, and radiation precautions.

Radiopharmaceuticals

The radiopharmaceutical contains a radionuclide (radioactive element) which is used either to localize an organ or a system in the body for a diagnostic purpose, or to irradiate an organ or a system for therapeutic purposes. Radiopharmaceuticals are also used in studies which are performed on body constituents in a test tube. Because these agents are used only in very minute quantities, no pharmacological response is noted with these chemicals. The radioactive atom disintegrates and in so doing emits energy of two types: either particulate radiation, such as alpha or beta particles, or electromagnetic radiation, such as gamma or x-rays. The electromagnetic radiation is employed in diagnostic tests, whereas particulate radiation is utilized for internal therapy.

The majority of radionuclides utilized clinically are obtained from nuclear reactors or cyclotrons. Radionuclides with very short half-lives (less than 2 hours) have limited use because of rapid decay of activity. Radionuclides with very long half-lives (months), because of both significant radiation exposure to the patient and environmental hazards, have been replaced by relatively short half-life radionuclides.

In the majority of cases, the radionuclide is only a part of the pharmaceutical, serving as the "tag" to make measurement or detection possible. In these instances the chemical and biological behavior of the material labeled determines its use in the procedure. Mechanisms of localization include the following: active transport (thyroid scanning with radioiodine), phagocytosis (liver scanning with tagged colloidal particles), sequestration (spleen scanning with red blood cells), capillary blockage (lung scanning with labeled macroaggregated albumin), simple or exchange diffusion (bone scanning), and compartmental localization (cardiac scanning with tagged human serum albumin).

Of all the radionuclides available to nuclear medicine laboratories, 99m-technetium (99mTc) is most commonly used in the practice of nuclear medicine today, replacing Iodine 131 in many radiopharmaceutical preparations. Preference for 99m-technetium is based upon short half-life (6 hours), lack of particle emission, reasonable cost, and ease of availability. It should be pointed out that before any ^{131}I-tagged agent is used, the patient's thyroid should be blocked by administering 10 drops of Lugol's solution several hours before the agent is given, and it is advisable to continue this once daily for a couple of days (except in thyroid studies).

Instrumentation

Basically two types of instruments are used in nuclear medicine laboratories.

1. Instruments used in performing in-vitro tests, in which radiopharmaceuticals are added to a sample of the patient's

blood constituents or urine, etc., to determine the amount of specific substance present.

2. Instruments employed in performing in-vivo tests, in which a radiation detection device is used to measure radioactivity in different organs from outside the patient.

The scintillation counter is the detector most widely employed in everyday clinical nuclear medicine in both types of instruments. The instruments currently available for in-vivo procedures include three major categories: (1) stationary probes, (2) scanners, and (3) cameras.

Using modern instruments and new radiopharmaceuticals, most nuclear medicine procedures require 20 to 45 minutes to be completed.

SPECIFIC TISSUE SCANNING

The Thyroid

Because of the early availability of radioiodine, the thyroid gland was one of the first organs studied with radionuclides. A large number of thyroid tests (both in-vivo and in-vitro) are now available to the clinician.

THYROID UPTAKE STUDIES

This test is based on the ability of the thyroid gland to trap and retain iodine. External detection systems can be employed to determine the percentage uptake of iodine at a specific time. Most laboratories ask patients to fast overnight.

Prior to performing the procedure, medical personnel should question the patient concerning:

1. Any previous studies with radiographic iodinated contrast media, topical application of iodine-containing compounds, oral ingestion of iodides and medications which contain iodine. All of these agents increase the body's iodide pool and hence decrease tracer uptake in the thyroid gland.
2. Prior use of antithyroid drugs (propylthiouracil and methimazole), which interfere with thyroid function.
3. Administration of thyroid preparations such as thyroid extracts and synthetic thyroid preparations, which again interfere with entrapment of the administered tracer dose.

In most laboratories the uptake of iodine at 2 and 24 hours is routinely measured and expressed as percentage thyroidal uptake compared with total administered dose. This test is more reliable in hyperthyroidism than hypothyroidism and should be used in combination with other tests of thyroid function to provide an accurate diagnosis of many diseases of the thyroid.

THYROID SCANNING

The thyroid gland traps and retains the iodine for a sufficient period of time to allow excellent pictures of the gland to be obtained by scintillation techniques. Iodine-131 was the first radiopharmaceutical used to scan the thyroid gland. However, in recent years it has been replaced in many laboratories by 99m-Tc pertechnetate, which is trapped like iodine but not organified into the thyroid hormones. As with thyroid-uptake determination, antithyroid medications, exogenous iodine, or certain drugs may prevent satisfactory concentration of radioiodine and 99m-Tc by the thyroid gland. Recently, ^{123}I has become available as a preferable agent for thyroid studies. This radionuclide does not emit beta rays, hence is superior to ^{131}I for diagnostic studies. This agent will be used widely in the near future.

The normal thyroid gland varies in shape. In the majority of individuals, the two lobes of the thyroid gland are attached in the middle by a bridge of activity called the isthmus. Abnormal scans usually exhibit change in thyroidal size, shape, and position as well as function. Hyperfunctioning areas are generally referred to as "hot" nodules, whereas hypofunctioning areas are called "cold" nodules. The scan is helpful in the evaluation of thyroid nodules, carcinomas, and masses in the tongue, neck, and mediastinum.

The Respiratory System

Since the introduction of the perfusion lung scan in 1963, lung scanning has been used very extensively in the examination of patients with pulmonary disease, especially pulmonary embolism. Perfusion lung scan is performed by IV injection of particles larger than 10 microns in size. These particles are trapped in the arterioles or capillaries of the lung in the first pass and remain there for several hours. This allows a satisfactory study to be obtained very shortly after the introduction of these particles and up to a couple of hours later.

Two commonly used agents for perfusion lung scanning are 99m-Tc and ^{131}I MAA or microspheres. When ^{131}I MAA is used, Lugol's solution must be given to the patient several hours prior to the scanning to reduce radiation to the thyroid gland.

A chest x-ray should be obtained immediately before or after lung scan for comparison. Scans in pulmonary embolism will reveal areas of absent perfusion, which appear normal on the corresponding chest x-ray. In patients with abnormal chest x-rays due to pneumonia, tuberculosis, and other pulmonary diseases, perfusion lung scans will reveal defects which should not be misinterpreted as pulmonary embolism. Repeating lung scans 7 to 10 days after the initial diagnosis of pulmonary embolism is of importance in the follow-up of these patients, since most of these clots start to resolve after they have lodged in pulmonary arteries. Patients with emphysema will also show areas of defect on perfusion lung scans. However, most of these patients have normal chest x-rays, and it is necessary to obtain another radioisotopic study using Xenon-133 (^{133}Xe) to further substantiate this diagnosis. The latter study involves inhalation of ^{133}Xe which has been introduced into a closed system such as a respirometer. In this study, areas of emphysema will be seen as regions of poor ventilation. In contrast, in patients with pulmonary embolism, ventilation to the areas of embolism is intact.

Myocardial Scanning

In recent years the application of radioisotopic techniques has significantly improved our capabilities in the evaluation of patients with cardiovascular disorders. After intravenous injection of ^{99m}Tc pertechnetate or ^{99m}Tc-tagged albumin, transit of activity through the major venous sytem, right heart, lung, left heart, and aorta and its branches can be evaluated. With a similar technique the left to right shunt can be detected and quantified noninvasively. If sufficient time (5 to 10 minutes) is allowed to elapse after intravenous injection of agents such as ^{99m}Tc albumin or ^{99m}Tc-tagged red blood cells, the activity will equilibrate throughout the vascular system and blood pool images can be obtained. This test has been used in the past to detect pericardial effusion and placental localization. However, most recent *ultrasonic* techniques appear to be superior in the evaluation of these disorders. With the aid of an electrocardiograph attached to a scintillation camera, it is possible to obtain an image of the blood pool of the heart at the end of systole and diastole (gated cardiac blood pool studies). From these images one can observe the cardiac wall motion in normal and pathologic states. Also, ejection fraction (percent of blood ejected with each cardial cycle) during cardiac contraction can be calculated from this information. With the aid of newer computer programs, the cardiac cycle has been divided into multiple intervals, and images obtained in these intervals can provide cinematographic visualization of cardiac chambers from systole to diastole.

Although it is possible to evaluate the myocardium indirectly by blood pool imaging, the introduction of myocardial imaging agents enables one to visualize abnormalities in the myocardium. One of the early radionuclides used for myocardial scanning was potassium 43. This agent in recent years has been replaced by thallium 201, which has better physical characteristics for modern instruments. These agents are injected intravenously and their uptake by the myocardium reflects perfusion in different parts of the heart. Multiple images are obtained in different projections to evaluate separate parts of the heart. The major use of these techniques has been in the evaluation of coronary artery insufficiency. In a normal person the distribution of these agents during rest and exercise appears homogeneous, with no areas of defect. In patients with coronary artery insufficiency, the scans appear abnormal or normal in the resting studies, depending on the degree of insufficiency. However, when these agents are injected after exercise, the majority of patients with coronary artery insufficiency will demonstrate areas of decreased perfusion in the myocardium. This test is being used as a complementary examination to the exercise ECG in many cardiac units. Thallium scanning has also been applied to the early detection of myocardial infarction. Thallium images are obtained very soon after the administration of the radionuclide.

Another major group of radiopharmaceuticals which have been used for the early diagnosis of myocardial infarction are the bone-seeking agents (see bone section, page 297). Although ^{99m}Tc pyrophosphate has been the agent most commonly used in the past for this purpose, any of the ^{99m}Tc-tagged phosphates appear to be quite satisfactory. The area of infarction and the surrounding regions reveal uptake of these agents approximately 10 to 15 hours from the onset of symptoms. This uptake has been attributed to calcific deposits in these areas. The studies are performed 1½ to 2 hours after the intravenous injection of ^{99m}Tc-tagged phosphate.

With the introduction of portable scintillation cameras, it is possible to obtain these studies at the bedside with minimal discomfort to the patient.

Liver Scans

Liver scanning can be divided into two general categories: scanning for demonstration of anatomical changes and scanning for the evaluation of biliary patency. In order to outline the liver, particles which are phagocytized by the reticuloendothelial system of the liver are used. Of these agents, colloidal gold 198 and ^{99m}Tc sulfur colloid have been used most extensively. Scans are obtained about 10 minutes after intravenous injection of the particles. No preparation is needed for this study. When ^{99m}Tc sulfur colloid is used as a scanning agent, the spleen also appears on the scan. Normally the distribution of the activity is homogeneous throughout the organ. In patients with metastasis, areas of defect appear in the background of normal liver activity. However, defects in the liver are nonspecific and can be seen in any disease state such as abscesses or cysts, etc.

Evaluation of the Biliary Tract

For evaluation of the biliary tract, ^{131}I rose bengal is used; hence Lugol's solution must be given before the study. This agent is rapidly cleared by hepatic cells and excreted into the gastrointestinal tract. The study is performed 10 to 15 minutes after the agent is injected. Thirty minutes after injection there should be evidence of activity in the small bowel. In patients with biliary tract obstruction no activity is seen in the region of the small bowel. In a situation like this, studies are repeated in 4, 24, and sometimes 48 hours for a conclusive result. With the introduction of computerized tomography and ultrasonic techniques, this test may be used less frequently in the future. In recent years ^{99m}Tc-tagged agents have been introduced and tested in patients. Some of these radio-pharmaceuticals appear quite promising in the evaluation of the biliary tract.

The Spleen

In the past, red cells damaged by heat or chemicals and tagged with radioactive chromium or mercury were used for spleen scans. However, nowadays, other agents which are picked up by RES (reticuloendothelial system) are preferably utilized for this purpose, so that both the liver and the spleen are visualized in the scans. The normal spleen has an ovoid or comma shape. Scanning is helpful in the evaluation of splenic size, shape, and position. This technique has also been used in the detection of intrasplenic space-occupying lesions such as malignancy, hematoma due to rupture, and infarction.

The Pancreas

Although rarely done today, pancreas scanning has been useful for the detection of carcinoma of the pancreas. The agent used for this study is selenomethionine (^{75}Se), which is incorporated by the pancreas. The normal pancreas appears in a variety of shapes with no defect in the scan. Areas of abnormality are devoid of activity. These defects are nonspecific, and half of them result from diseases other than carcinoma.

The Kidney

Two types of agents are used to evaluate the kidneys in nuclear medicine. The first group comprises radiopharmaceuticals that bind to the kidney for several hours and outline the renal parenchyma (parenchymal agents). Chloromeridine-tagged mercury-197 is the best example of this category of agents. However, recently ^{99m}Tc-tagged chemicals such as ^{99m}Tc iron-ascorbate DTPA (diethylenetriamine-pentacetic acid) and ^{99m}Tc dimercaptosuccinate have been added to this group. The second group includes functional agents, of which ^{131}I hippuran and ^{99m}Tc DTPA have been used widely in nuclear medicine. These radiopharmaceuticals are excreted by the parenchyma and outline the draining system. With chloromeridine mercury-197 and ^{99m}Tc-tagged parenchymal agents, scans are usually obtained 1 to 3 hours after injection. With ^{131}I hippuran and ^{99m}Tc DTPA the images are obtained immediately after intravenous injection of these agents. Prior to introduction of radiohippuran, Lugol's solution should be administered to the patient. Scans with mercury and ^{99m}Tc-tagged agents show uniform outline of the kidney. Areas of abnormality such as carcinoma and cysts, etc., appear without activity. Normal hippuran and DTPA studies show uniform, progressive, symmetrical accumulation of tracer in the kidney and later in the pelvis and ureters. When kidney function is impaired there is delay in the appearance of this agent in the kidney area, and some-

times delayed scans are obtained in 24 hours to complete these studies. Hippuran and DTPA studies are useful in the detection of obstruction of the ureter. Hippuran has been used for evaluation of renal hypertension; however, more investigative work in this area is needed.

Nervous System

Brain studies are based on the fact that intracranial lesions alter the blood brain barrier, so that the administered radiopharmaceutical will be able to localize in or around the lesion. This study is mainly useful in detection and localization of primary or secondary brain tumors as well as cerebral vascular disease. ^{99m}Tc pertechnetate or other ^{99m}Tc-tagged radiopharmaceuticals are the agents of choice today in many laboratories. If ^{99m}Tc pertechnetate is used, perchlorate solution should be given to the patient 20 to 30 minutes prior to administration of ^{99m}Tc to block choroid plexus uptake, which may interfere with interpretation of the scans. In some laboratories, after a rapid bolus IV injection of ^{99m}Tc, multiple serial pictures of cerebral perfusion are obtained. These can add to the information obtained from static scans, which are usually done 1 to 2 hours after introduction of the agent.

Normally there should be no activity in the brain substance. In patients with brain tumor or stroke, the area of the lesion appears radioactive when compared with normal brain. In patients with brain tumor, lesions are usually seen whenever the first scan is obtained. However, in patients with stroke, the scan done immediately after the incident is usually normal, and in 7 to 10 days most of these patients will show areas of irregular radionuclide uptake on their brain scans.

Skeletal System

The localization of bone-seeking agents such as calcium, strontium, fluorine, and recent ^{99m}Tc-tagged agents is noted in almost all osseous lesions including malignancy, osteomyelitis, and healing fractures. This has been attributed to reactive bone formation around bony lesions. Until recently, Strontium-85 and Fluorine-18 were the agents of choice for bone scanning. However, with the introduction of ^{99m}Tc-tagged phosphate agents, the former elements are becoming generally outmoded in many laboratories. When Fluorine-18 or ^{99m}Tc-tagged agents are used, patients are scanned 2 to 3 hours after injection and no preparation is necessary except to ask the patient to void before the scan, because these agents are cleared by the kidneys into the bladder. The normal bone scan demonstrates a uniform pattern of uptake in the spine, ribs, and other flat bones. Regions of active growth, such as ends of long bones, show increased activity. Areas of abnormality appear more active than normal background. In patients with malignancy, metastasis to the bone, if present, is clearly outlined on bone scans. Bone scans are the most sensitive means of detecting early lesions in the bones, especially when routine roentgenograms are negative.

NON-IMAGING IN-VIVO STUDIES

Measurement of Red Cell Mass

Measurement of red cell mass involves labeling of the patient's own red blood cells with 51 Cr sodium chromate. Ten to 15 milliters of the patient's blood are withdrawn and added to a solution of acid citrate dextrose (as an anticoagulant). The radioactive 51 Cr is added to this combination and the content of the vial is kept at room temperature for a period of 30 minutes. During this time, chromate penetrates the red cell membrane and binds to hemoglobin. This phenomenon only takes place when the valence of the chromium is +6. When ascorbic acid is added at the end of 30 minutes, the untagged chromium is converted to chromium with a +3 valence. A small fraction of this preparation is kept as a standard and the remainder is injected into the patient. After 10 to 15 minutes, a blood sample is withdrawn, and radioactivity in the sample and the standard is measured. From these counts the red cell mass is calculated from the following basic formula:

$$\text{Red Cell Mass} = \frac{\text{Total Radioactivity of Tagged RBCs Injected}}{\text{Radioactivity / ml. of RBCs After Mixing}}$$

Plasma Volume

For this purpose an already prepared solution of ^{131}I or ^{125}I is used. A sample of this solution is injected intravenously and a fraction is kept as a standard for later calculation. Fifteen minutes later a blood sample is withdrawn and the plasma volume is calculated according to the following formula:

$$\text{Plasma Volume} = \frac{\text{Radioactivity of Injected Tracer}}{\text{Radioactivity / ml. Plasma After Mixing}}$$

The plasma volume also can be measured, indirectly, after red cell mass is calculated from the 51 Cr-tagged red blood cells. With this approach, the patient's hematocrit is used to calculate the plasma volume.

Measurement of Total Blood Volume

The total blood volume can be measured by using both the tagged red cells and the radioiodinated albumin combined. However, for the sake of simplicity, the whole blood volume is commonly calculated indirectly by adding the red cell mass (using 51 Cr) and the plasma volume which has been estimated by taking the peripheral hematocrit into consideration.

Red Cell Survival and Sequestration

The measurement of the life span of red blood cells is important in some hematologic disorders when shortened survival of the cells is suspected. In this study a sample of the patient's own cells is tagged with 51 Cr sodium chromate in a manner similar to that described for red cell mass determination. The entire preparation is injected into the patient. Blood samples are drawn from the patient daily for a week, then three times a week for the second and third week, and, if needed, twice a week for the fourth and fifth week. From these samples the half-time survival of the red cells is calculated. The normal red cells survive approximately 120 days within circulation. Because of elution of 51 Cr from the red cells, the survival time value obtained with the 51 Cr technique is approximately half of this number (half-life of 28 to 30 days).

In patients with shortened red cell survival (hemolytic anemia), the half-time calculated by this technique is shorter than normal. The degree to which the spleen is responsible for the destruction of red blood cells is often important in the management of patients with hemolytic anemias. If evidence is found for excessive trapping of the red cells by the spleen, removal of this organ should be considered to reduce the red cell destruction. Such evidence can be obtained by external monitoring over the splenic and cardiac areas after the patient has received 51 Cr-tagged red blood cells. From the ratios of the values obtained in these areas, the presence of red cell sequestration can be determined.

Schilling Test

In patients who lack intrinsic factor in their gastric juice, which is essential for the absorption of vitamin B-12, radioactive 57 cobalt cyanocobalamin is important in diagnosis. A fasting patient is given a small oral dose of 57 cobalt-labeled vitamin B-12 and the collection of urine is immediately started. Two hours later, 1 mg. of nonradioactive B-12 is injected intramuscularly for the purpose of saturating the tissue-binding sites, thereby reducing the degree of removal by the liver or other organs of the radiolabeled B-12. The 24-hour urine content of the radioactivity is measured and the percentage of administered dose which was excreted in the urine is calculated. This measurement is only valid if the urine is collected accurately for this period. Normal individuals excrete between 7 to 40 percent of the injected activity. Patients with pernicious anemia will excrete 0 to 3 percent of the radioactivity in 24 hours. In some patients, the diagnosis of intrinsic factor deficiency can be further confirmed by adding this factor to the radioactive B-12 in the second stage of this examination. When the study is repeated with intrinsic factor, the absorption of vitamin B-12 approaches the normal range. However, in patients with an absorptive defect in the small intestine, the addition of intrinsic factor does not correct the percentage of activity in the urine.

TREATMENT WITH RADIONUCLIDES

Because of their versatility, radioactive agents can be administered by different routes for the treatment of various disorders. The major disorders which benefit from these agents include: (1) hyperthyroidism, (2) thyroid cancer, (3) polycythemia vera, and (4) malignant effusion of the pleural and the peritoneal cavities. The radioactive isotopes used generally emit beta rays, which are more destructive than gamma rays.

HYPERTHYROIDISM. [131]I (sodium iodide) is mainly used for the treatment of hyperthyroidism and thyroid cancer. In patients with hyperthyroidism, usually a relatively small dose of this radionuclide results in the cure of the majority of these patients. In some patients who are resistant to single dose treatment two or more administrations may be necessary to obtain a satisfactory result.

THYROID CANCER. Radioisotopic treatment of patients with thyroid cancer usually follows surgical removal of the cancer and part or most of the thyroid gland. In these patients the radionuclide is administered in two stages. The first stage involves the administration of enough radioactivity to irradiate the remaining functioning thyroid gland and render the patient hypothyroid. This is usually accomplished by a relatively large dose of [131]I. The second stage is accomplished by the administration of another large dose while the patient has become significantly hypothyroid. The second dose is used to destroy the cancer cells in the original site as well as in metastatic sites.

- The urine of patients with cancer who have been treated with a large dose of ^{131}I, contains a significant amount of radioactivity and should be handled carefully to prevent contamination.

POLYCYTHEMIA VERA. Patients with polycythemia vera may benefit from the intravenous administration of 32-P sodium phosphate. A small dose of the agent is administered and the desired effect (gradual decline of red cell production) is usually observed several weeks later. Since 32-P emits only beta rays, these patients are not a source of radiation to the others.

MALIGNANT EFFUSIONS. Intracavitary administration of radioactive agents is useful only for the treatment of malignant effusions in the pleural and peritoneal cavities. The advantage of 32-P over 198 Au is its lack of gamma ray emission, so that the radiation is confined only to the patient's body. 198 Au colloidal gold has both gamma and beta rays, which makes the patient a significant source of radiation until considerable decay of the radioactivity has taken place. Both of these agents are administered by

physicians in the nuclear medicine laboratory after a secure catheter or needle is in place.

- These patients should be watched very carefully for leakage of the liquid from the site of administration or other areas for several days. Any leakage should be reported immediately to the staff of the nuclear medicine laboratory and the radiation safety office of the institution.

RADIATION PROTECTION AND THE CARE OF PATIENTS WHO HAVE RECEIVED RADIOACTIVE MATERIALS

We have always been exposed to small but definite amounts of radiation (called background radiation) from the radioactivity in natural materials and our own bodies and from cosmic rays from outer space. In addition to background radiation, most of us are exposed to radiation from medical diagnostic x-ray examinations, nuclear weapon testing fallout, radium dial wristwatches, and so forth. Some of us are further exposed to radiation because of the nature of our work.

This section contains suggestions and rules for controlling radiation exposures and reducing hazards from the use of radioactive isotopes in the hospital environment. When radioactive materials are properly controlled, the risks from radiation exposure are very small. However, without control, these materials can be dangerous to patients, health care personnel, and the public.

Because radiation cannot be seen or felt, it is extremely important that common sense rules of radiation safety always be observed by personnel working near sources of radiation. The best way to ensure proper patient care and, at the same time, to keep radiation exposure of personnel at safe, low levels is to understand and carefully observe the rules outlined in this section. It is the responsibility of all personnel who may be exposed to radiation in every institution to follow such precautions.

LARGE AMOUNTS OF RADIOACTIVE MATERIALS
Precautions

**NOTIFY THE RADIOLOGY DEPARTMENT
RADIOISOTOPE SECTION IMMEDIATELY:**

In case of any doubt as to safe procedure.
In case of any emergency.
If any unexpected complications arise.
In case of death,
    Before postmortem care is given,
    Before an autopsy is performed,
    Before the body is released.
During Day: Call Radioisotope Section, Radiology
    Department
During Night: Call Radiologist on CALL.

GENERAL RULES FOR RADIATION PROTECTION
To Be Observed By All Personnel

EXTENT OF HAZARD

1. The degree of possible hazard associated with a patient who has received radioactive isotopes will depend on the amount and kind of radioactive material administered, where and how it was given, and how long a time has elapsed since its administration.

2. The amounts of radioisotopes contained in patients after treatment or diagnostic study is completed can be classified as follows:

	HALF-LIFE GREATER THAN 15 HOURS	HALF-LIFE LESS THAN 15 HOURS
Small Amount	Less than 0.2 mCi	Less than 10 mCi
Moderate Amount	0.2 to 5 mCi	More than 10 mCi
Large Amount	More than 5 mCi	

IDENTIFICATION OF PATIENTS WHO HAVE RECEIVED RADIOISOTOPES

1. Small Amounts
   a. Patients may contain small amounts of radioisotopes after diagnostic studies. For these patients, the Doctor's Progress Sheet in the patient's Hospital Chart is marked to indicate the amount and type of radioactive material administered.
   b. Patients who contain small amounts of radioactive material can be given normal hospital care and attention without any appreciable hazard to personnel.

2. Moderate and Large Amounts
   Patients containing radioactive materials in moderate to large amounts may present a radiation hazard unless certain simple precautions are followed. Patients may be treated with systemic radionuclides, that is, materials administered as solutions (such as iodine-131, colloidal gold-198, or phosphorus-32) or encapsulated radionuclides (such as radium-226, radon-222, cesium-137, iodine-125, californium-252, gold-198 seeds, or iridium-192). To make sure that these patients are identified, the Doctor's Order Sheet is marked to indicate the amount and type of radioactive material administered. In addition, in order to provide instructions for the safe care of these patients, the following steps are taken:
   a. An appropriate Precaution Sheet, listing special rules to be observed, is inserted into the Hospital Chart.
   b. For patients who contain *moderate or large amounts* of radionuclides, the Hospital Chart is marked with an appropriate label showing the standard radiation symbol. A label is placed on the chart cover and on the Precaution Sheet.
   c. All patients who contain *large amounts* of radioactive material will have a wrist band attached to them by the doctor who administers the radionuclide. The band will indicate the date and the nature and amount of radioactivity.
   d. A precaution tag will be attached to the bed of each patient containing a *large amount* of radioactive material.

   • WHEN YOU SEE THE RADIOACTIVE LABEL ON A CHART, ON A PATIENT, OR ON A PATIENT'S BED, IT IS YOUR RESPONSIBILITY TO LOOK FOR, READ, AND FOLLOW INSTRUCTIONS GIVEN ON THE PRECAUTION SHEET.

RADIOACTIVE EXCRETA

1. There will be some radioactivity in the excreta of all patients who have received radioactive materials except for those instances in which the radioactive material is encapsulated.

   • In all cases other than these exceptions, contamination should be avoided by wearing rubber gloves when handling the patient's excreta, vomitus, or body fluids. If linens become wet with patient excreta, notify the Nuclear Medicine Section, Radiology Department.

2. In some instances it will be necessary to save patients' excreta in containers provided by the Radiology Department. In these cases, special instructions will be issued. When feasible, the patient should be encouraged to collect his own urine.

DISCHARGE OF PATIENTS WHO HAVE RECEIVED RADIOACTIVE MATERIALS FROM THE HOSPITAL

No patient who has received a large amount of radioactive material may be discharged from the Hospital before the time and date indicated on the Precaution Sheet. Additional special arrangements must be made with the Radiotherapy Physics Section for patients being treated with iodine-125.

GENERAL RULES FOR RADIATION PROTECTION (CONTINUED)

DEATH OF PATIENTS CONTAINING RADIOACTIVE MATERIALS

1. If a patient containing more than 5 millicuries of systemic radioactive material dies in the hospital, the physician signing the death certificate should note from the wrist band and the Hospital Chart that the patient contains radioactivity and inform the pathologist of this fact. The Nuclear Medicine Section of the Radiology Department should also be notified.
2. If a patient containing any encapsulated radioactive material dies, the Radiation Therapy Physics Section must be notified.
3. If there is no autopsy, and the body contains more than 30 millicuries of systemic radioactivity, the physician signing the death certificate should notify the Nuclear Medicine Section, Radiology Department, so that the proper Statement to the funeral director can be prepared.
4. If there is an autopsy, and the body contains more than 5 millicuries of systemic radioactivity, it may be necessary for the pathologist to take special precautions while performing the autopsy.

SPECIAL MEDICAL PROCEDURES

Special medical procedures may be necessary with patients containing radioactive materials which may involve the removal of body fluids containing radioactivity. In such cases, advice on the radiation safety of the procedure should be obtained from the Nuclear Medicine Section, Radiology Department.

EMERGENCY SURGERY

If emergency surgery is required for a patient containing a *large amount* of systemic radioactivity, the Nuclear Medicine Section, Radiology Department should be notified.

ADMISSION OF PATIENTS WHO WILL BE TREATED WITH ENCAPSULATED RADIONUCLIDES

Because of the radiation hazard involved in admitting patients for treatment with certain radionuclides, the following procedures are advised:

1. The physician should notify the Admissions Office in advance when admitting patients.
2. The admission clerk must assign a patient scheduled to receive an encapsulated radionuclide application to a private room.
3. The admission clerk must assign a patient scheduled to receive a dose of iodine-131 greater than 8mCi to a private room.
4. For a patient scheduled to receive a californium-252 application, the admission clerk will attempt to assign the patient to a private room having as many outside walls as possible.
5. Physicians in charge will confirm BEFORE the radioactive application is made that the patient's accommodations are such that no radiation hazard will exist.

MONITORING OF VICINITY

The vicinity of patients treated with large amounts of radioactivity will be carefully monitored with a suitable radiation detecting instrument to insure that no member of the general population is likely to receive a dose in excess of 100 millirems. Reports of the survey will be attached to the patient's chart and a copy will be sent to the Radiation Survey Office. After the patient is discharged, a survey will be made by the Radiology Department to ensure that no radiation hazard remains.

VISITOR LIMITATIONS

Unless precautions to the contrary are posted, there are no limitations for visitors to patients containing radioactive materials.

RADIATION HAZARDS

When there is any doubt as to whether an unusual situation exists that may constitute a radiation hazard with systemic radionuclides, call the doctor responsible in the Nuclear Medicine Section, Radiology Department. Regarding patients being treated with encapsulated radionuclides, call the Radiation Therapy Physics Section.

RADIATION PRECAUTIONS: SPECIAL INSTRUCTIONS
For Nurses and Patient-Care Attendants

1. It is very important to provide the patient who contains radioactivity with proper nursing care and at the same time to limit radiation exposure to as low a level as is reasonable. To do this, read and observe all General Rules in this section and consult the PRECAUTION SHEET that is in the patient's Hospital Chart.

2. There is no appreciable hazard to hospital personnel from radiation in the vicinity of the patient except for patients who have received large amounts (see page 300) of radioactive materials. Do not stay in the immediate vicinity (within three feet) of patients who have received large amounts of radioactivity longer than is necessary to give proper care and attention. The hazard is very slight, however. A nurse could stand continuously at the bedside of a typical patient being treated with radium for 10 hours before her radiation exposure would exceed the Dose Limiting Recommendations of the National Committee on Radiation Protection for the average dose for occasionally exposed individuals for one year. It should be noted that the radiation exposure diminishes rapidly as the distance from the patient is increased. At a distance of 3 feet from the patient, it would require 40 hours to exceed the recommended annual limit. Any nurse who is exposed frequently to radiation would be considered to be a Radiation Worker and should be monitored continuously by the Radiation Safety Office.

   - Special instructions limiting the time a nurse may spend near a patient should be issued when necessary.

3. Body fluids and excreta of patients who have received radioactive nuclides (except encapsulated sources) should be assumed to be radioactive.

   - Avoid direct contact with patient's blood, urine, vomitus and other body fluids. Wear rubber gloves if such contact is anticipated.
   - If bed clothing or patient's clothing becomes wet from body fluids and hence contaminated with radioactivity, notify the Nuclear Medicine Section, Radiology Department, and save for radioactive monitoring by the Nuclear Medicine Section, Radiology Department.
   - If dressings covering the site of administration of gold-198 become stained, notify the Nuclear Medicine Section, Radiology Department.
   - Wash hands after bathing patient. Wear rubber gloves when giving patient other personal attention. Patients who have received large amounts of iodine-131 should not be bathed until 24 hours after the time of administration of the radioactivity.
   - Bedpans should be handled with rubber gloves and thoroughly flushed before returning to general use. For patients who have received large amounts of iodine-131 the bedpan should be flushed out thoroughly after every use and the same bedpan should be reserved for the same patient during his hospitalization.
   - If a spill of any type occurs, mop up immediately. Save all liquids and the mop used. Notify the Nuclear Medicine Section, Radiology Department, immediately so that measurements can be made to evaluate any possible hazard.

4. Needles, seeds, or capsules containing radioisotopes in patients who are being treated with encapsulated sources of radioactivity may sometimes become dislodged or displaced. If there is any indication that this has happened, notify the Radiotherapy Department, Physics Section, immediately. These sources can be handled safely with tongs or forceps but should never be picked up or touched directly.

5. If a patient who contains more than 5 millicuries of systemic radioactivity dies, notify the Department of Radiology, Nuclear Medicine Section. If a patient containing encapsulated radionuclides dies, notify the Radiotherapy Department, Physics Section. Observe all General and Special Rules in this section while preparing the patient for the morgue. Clearly mark the tags that are to be placed on the cadaver, the shroud, and the icebox door with "CAUTION—RADIOACTIVITY."

(Courtesy Hospital of the University of Pennsylvania)

BIBLIOGRAPHY
BOOKS

Baum, L.: Basic Nuclear Medicine, Appleton-Century-Crofts, New York, 1975.

Blahd, W. H.: Nuclear Medicine, 2nd ed. New York, McGraw-Hill, 1971.

Chesney, D. N., and Chesney, M. O.: Care of the Patient in Diagnostic Radiography. London, Blackwell Scientific Pubs., 1978.

Freeman, L. M., and Blaufox, M. D.: Physicians Desk Reference for Radiology and Nuclear Medicine. Oradell, N. J., Medical Economics, Inc., 1971.

Gottschalk, A., and Potcher, J. E.: Diagnostic Nuclear Medicine. Williams and Wilkins, Baltimore, 1976.

Hale, J.: Radiation Protection. Prepared for the personnel of the Hospital of the University of Pennsylvania.

Maynard, C. D.: Clinical Nuclear Medicine. Philadelphia, Lea and Febiger, 1969.

Mulherin, L. E.: Practical Points in Radiation Oncology. New York, Medical Examination Pub. Co., 1979.

National Council on Radiation Protection and Measurements: Precautions in the Management of Patients Who Have Received Therapeutic Amounts of Radionuclides. Washington, D. C., Oct. 1, 1970.

Noz, M. E., and Maguire, G. Q. Jr.: Radiation Protection in the Radiologic and Health Sciences. Phila., Lea and Febiger, 1979.

Wagner, H. N. (ed.): Principles of Nuclear Medicine. New York, H. P. Pub. Co., 1975.

ARTICLES

Abrams, H. L., and McNeil, B. J.: Medical implications of computed tomography ("cat scanning"). New Eng. J. Med., Part I, *298*:255-260, Feb. 2, 1978; Part II, *298*:310-316, Feb. 9, 1978.

Braunstein, P., and Whelan, C. A.: Newer diagnostic tests and techniques used in nuclear medicine. Postgrad. Med., *60*:84-90, Aug. 1976.

Breeding, M. A.: Patients receiving radioactive iodine and phosphorus. Nursing '77, 7:56, Aug. 1977.

Croll, M. N.: Radionuclides in common use. Am. Fam. Phys., *12*:164-167, Nov. 1975.

Eymontt, M. J., and Eymontt, D.: Preparing your patient for nuclear medicine. Nursing '77, 7:46-49, Dec. 1977.

Levinson, C.: Thallium-201 myocardial imaging. Heart & Lung, *6*:115-120, Jan.-Feb. 1977.

Mould, R. F.: Danger! Guard against radiation. Nurs. Mirror, *147*:15-18, Aug. 31, 1978.

Robbins, S. E., and Crawford, D.: Nursing and the Pion Irradiation Project. AJN, *76*:1445-1449, Sept. 1976.

Rose, J. C.: Nutritional problems in radio-therapy patients. AJN, *78*:1194-1196, July 1978.

Schreier, A. M., and Lavenia, J.: The nurse's role in nutritional management of radiotherapy patients. NCNA, *12*:173-182, Mar. 1977.

Stillman, M. J.: Experiences in clinical problem solving. "Rose S: A patient undergoing radiation therapy." RN, *41*:65-71, Feb. 1978.

Swartz, H. M., and Reichling, B. A.: Safety of x-ray examination or radioisotope scan. JAMA, *239*:2031-2032, May 12, 1978.

Trevis, S., and Maltz, D. L.: Radionuclide angiocardiography. Postgrad. Med., *56*:99-107, July, 1974.

Wagner, H. N., Jr., and North, W.: What is nuclear medicine all about? Disease-A-Month, Year Book, Chicago, Nov. 1976.

Zaret, B. L., and Cohen, L. S.: Cardiovascular nuclear medicine. 1. Evaluation of cardiac performance. Mod. Concepts of Cardiovasc. Disease, *46*:33-36, July 1977; 2. Evaluation of perfusion and viability, *46*:37-41, Aug. 1977.

Perioperative Management of the Surgical Patient

UNIT FIVE

17

PREOPERATIVE NURSING MANAGEMENT

Major surgery and the trauma it implies give rise to numerous pathophysiological disturbances that are related in many ways to stress. Stress, with its varied physical and psychic components, finds expression in numerous neuroendocrine changes that are triggered by a wide range of stimuli including anxiety, pain, tissue damage, blood loss, anoxia, and a myriad of effects related to general anesthesia, nutritional deprivation, immobilization, medication, and infection. In view of the many ramifications of stress, it goes without saying that the nursing care of patients in the preoperative and postoperative periods should be designed to reduce stress and its deleterious effects.

PSYCHOSOCIAL NURSING ASSESSMENT

Any kind of surgical procedure is always preceded by some type of emotional reaction in a patient, whether it is obvious or hidden, normal or abnormal. For example, preoperative anxiety is an anticipatory response to an experience that the patient may view as a threat to his customary role in life, his body integrity, or even life itself. The extent of the patient's reaction is based on many factors, including the discomforts and sacrifices he anticipates — whether physical, financial, psychological, or social — and the surgical outcome he imagines. Will the operation improve his present condition? Will he be disabled? Is this just a temporary measure in a chronic condition?

Preoperative Anxiety and Nursing Approach

From the psychological point of view, it is known that a mind that is not at peace influences directly the functioning of the body. Therefore, it is imperative to know what anxieties the patient is experiencing. By taking a careful nursing history, the nurse will elicit patient concerns that can have a direct bearing on the course of his surgical experience. Undoubtedly, a patient facing surgery is beset by fears; fears of the unknown, of death, of anesthesia, of cancer. Add to this, worries about the possible loss of a job, the need to support a family, or the possibility of permanent incapacity and one can get a sense of the enormous emotional strain created by the prospect of surgery. Emotional upsets are more apparent in illness. Consequently, the nurse who learns this early will be more tolerant and understanding.

Fear is expressed in different ways by different individuals. For example, fear may be expressed indirectly by the patient who asks a lot of questions, repeating them constantly even though answers were given previously. For another person, the reaction may be withdrawal — deliberately avoiding communication, perhaps by concentrating on a book. Still others may talk incessantly about trivialities. Often such behavior ends abruptly as the patient turns to the nurse and says, "I guess you can tell I'm a bit nervous about my operation." The need to keep the outlet of communication open is never greater than at this time. To belittle the patient's fears by saying, "Oh, there's nothing to be afraid of," immediately closes the door and causes the patient to lapse into his own less effective means of coping with his worries.

Such breakdowns in satisfactory interrelations leave the patient upset, bewildered, and even unable to follow simple directions. Often in the course of conversation, something which was mentioned by a nurse or a physician becomes exaggerated out of all proportion to its importance. For example, if an operation is postponed because of a filled schedule, and the patient is merely told that "something had come up," he may begin to worry that the reason for the delay is a deterioration in his condition.

Let us examine the causes of fear that a preoperative patient may experience.

Fear of anesthesia was justified years ago, when little was known about the control and the effect of anesthetic agents. But with refined methods, tested drugs, and skilled anesthesiologists, the hazards are minimized. The ease with which a patient accepts an anesthetic today is attributed to the adequate physical and mental preparation that he receives. The price of poor preparation is a difficult period of induction, followed by an unpleasant emergence from the anesthetic agent. The nurse in daily association with each patient can do much to dispel false conceptions and misinformation. In instances in which the anesthesiologist visits the patient the day before surgery, real confidence is established, and the patient accepts the anesthetic more gracefully.

Another fear of anesthesia stems from the patient's concern that he will reveal secrets or lose control of his behavior while succumbing to the anesthetic agent. This patient needs to be assured by the nurse that such behavior happens very seldom and that if it does, the patient's utterances are not disclosed.

Often the fear of the anesthetic is secondary to the *fear of pain or of death*. Will I feel the knife? What if the anesthesia wears off? The patient needs reassurance that the anesthesiologist will be in constant attendance to take care of these problems. Some surgeons will not operate on a patient who is convinced that he will die. This is a real fear, and it cannot be dismissed lightly. Good rapport between patient and nurse, together with tact on the nurse's part, may bring him to a realization that his fear is magnified. It will help him greatly if those responsible for his care build up his confidence.

The *fear of the unknown* is the worst of all. This fear stems partly from a belief on the patient's part that he is not being told "everything" about his diagnosis or illness. Therefore, the more understanding one has of the probabilities for the future, the better is the adjustment. The nurse can do much to allay the anxieties of the patient and induce a certain peace of mind. A patient frequently expresses fears and misgivings to the nurse but hides them from the surgeon. In such circumstances the nurse communicates these evidences of anxiety privately to the surgeon.

The *fear of destruction of body image* occurs more frequently than it did a few years ago because surgery in many instances has become more radical. Then too, there is greater emphasis today on youth, the body beautiful, and more revealing clothing, as is verified by magazine and television advertising. Consequently, any surgical encroachment on the body is viewed with distress by many patients.

Fear of separation from former activities, family, and friends may compound the concerns and anxieties of the preoperative patient.

In addition to the above fears, the average patient has many *worries* to deal with. He may have financial problems, family responsibilities, and employment obligations; in addition to these, he may fear a poor prognosis or the probability of a handicap in the future. These problems can be investigated by the nurse. If the difficulty is of such a nature that a medical social worker can give assistance, the aid of such a person is enlisted. If the worry stems from fear of what the prognosis is likely to be, the physician is informed.

When some of these fears have been expressed, brought to light, and examined in their proper perspective, it is possible and even essential to get the patient to reveal what the operation means to him. Have him express his thoughts about the importance and the meaning of this surgery for the immediate future as well as the more distant future. Most fears are manifestations of concern over losing control over one's person, either physically or socially. The patient may be concerned about losing some of his independence, his integrity, and his control over his effectiveness in coping with his environment. The nurse may be in a position to elicit these concerns from the patient. The importance of adequate lines of communication between surgeon and nurse as they work together to prepare the patient for surgery must be emphasized here.

Psychological preparation for subsequent stress includes permitting the patient some degree of worrying. This is more desirable than having little or no anticipatory fear. Moderately fear-arousing information allows the patient to increase his tolerance for stress by developing effective ways of coping with his problems. Absence of worry will deprive the patient of the motivation to prepare himself psychologically for a stressful experience, with the result that when a crisis develops, he will have a low tolerance for stress.

The significance of *spiritual therapy* must not be forgotten. Regardless of the religious affiliation of the patient, the nurse recognizes that faith in a Higher Power can be as therapeutic as medication. Every attempt must be made to help the patient obtain the fullest spiritual help that he requests. This may be accomplished by participating in prayer, by reading passages from the Scriptures, or by calling a clergyman. Faith has great sustaining power; thus, the beliefs of each individual patient should be respected and supported.

The interval of time preparatory to surgery in some

instances may become very extended. *Recreation and diversion* can be provided by such activities as reading, listening to the radio, watching television, engaging in handcrafts, games, and so forth. The nurse can arrange for individuals with similar interests to meet. Many times patients can help one another.

Perhaps the most valuable facility at the disposal of the nurse is the ability to *listen* to the patient. By engaging in conversation and using the principles of tactful interviewing, the nurse can acquire invaluable bits of information. An unhurried, understanding, and kind nurse invites confidence on the part of the patient.

Every patient should be treated as an individual who has fears and hopes quite distinct from the fears of hopes of the next person. Understanding and helping one patient may require a completely different approach from that used with another. Providing time to answer questions and offering psychological support will insure a smoother postoperative course for the surgical patient. He will sleep better, recall fewer fearful images, experience less postoperative urinary retention, and need less anesthetic and pain medication. He will recover more rapidly and be discharged from the hospital sooner.

DENIAL OF ANXIETY. The preceding discussion of preoperative anxiety emphasizes the most common problems of the patient facing an operation. The opposite reaction of denying anxiety can also provide obstacles to effective treatment, such as in the case of a person who notices abnormal signs or symptoms but puts off seeking treatment. Denial is a reaction noted in many persons when they are suddenly confronted with potentially shocking information. Usually this reaction does not last longer than a few days or a few weeks, but nevertheless such denial and delay may have serious consequences. This is an area where the nurse's responsibility extends outward in all contacts with members of the community. Any questionable abnormal finding relating to one's body should be checked as soon as possible by a knowledgeable person in the health field.

NURSING ASSESSMENT AND PHYSICAL PREPARATION OF THE SURGICAL PATIENT

Physical Assessment and Diagnostic Tests

Before treatment is initiated, the patient is given a physical examination, during which time vital signs are noted and a data base established for future comparisons. Many diagnostic tests may be performed, such as blood counts, roentgenographic studies, gastric analyses, tissue biopsies, and stool and urine studies. In all of these tests the nurse is in a position to help the patient understand the need for the diagnostic studies. There is also an opportunity during the physical examination or while bathing the patient to note significant physical findings

such as a rash or pressure sores that may be contributing to the patient's condition.

These preliminary contacts with the staff during the examination and the diagnostic tests provide the patient with an opportunity to ask questions and to get acquainted with those who will be caring for him. In their efforts to establish rapport with the patient, the physician and nurse must respect the patient's feelings and his sense of modesty.

Assessment of Fluid and Nutritional Status

The nutritional state of the patient is directly related to the success of surgery and the reparative process in the tissues. If the person is in optimum health, the body is in homeostasis, with adequate amounts of fluids, electrolytes, protein, vitamins, and calories. As the patient undergoes an operation, his body may remain in homeostasis, provided that therapy is instituted to replace any losses. However, if a malnourished or dehydrated patient requires surgery, additional time is needed to replace deficits in order to get him in the best possible condition. This is especially true with respect to protein deficiency, since protein is essential for tissue repair. Protein deficiency may result from anorexia concomitant with the aging process, chronic debilitating illness, cancer, or frequent vomiting. Or it may be caused by poor food habits and a diet in which meats and eggs are almost absent. Proteins may also be lost in severe burns and through draining abscesses or wounds.

Protein replacement is a slow process and may take several days or weeks. The replacement may be accomplished by means of (1) a diet high in protein (meat, milk, eggs and cheese), carbohydrates, and calories but low in fat, (2) supplementary liquid feedings such as milk enriched with skim milk powder, or (3) protein hydrolysates given orally or by infusion. Hypertonic parenteral therapy may be given through a polyethylene tubing placed percutaneously in a large bore vein such as the subclavian (using a cutdown). Such therapy requires special dressing care (page 730).

The nursing challenge is to encourage the patient to eat by serving him attractive and palatable meals made up of small, manageable servings. If the patient is on parenteral therapy or is given gastrostomy feedings or infusions, he needs diversion and encouragement when he becomes depressed. The method of giving fluids will depend on the type of replacement therapy. If a nasogastric tube is being used, liquids will be taken more readily if the patient is in a sitting position. If gastrostomy feedings are used, then the reclining position is better.

Vitamins are required for specific purposes. Thiamine (vitamin B_1) is necessary for oxidizing carbohydrates and maintaining normal gastrointestinal function. A deficiency in vitamin B_1 is noted in chronic gastrointestinal and liver diseases. Ascorbic acid (vitamin C) is required for wound healing and collagen formation. Vitamin K is necessary for blood clotting and prothrombin production. These vitamins may be given orally or parenterally.

Loss of body fluids results in electrolyte imbalances. The replacement of these fluids is discussed in Chapter 8. The nurse records all intake and output and keeps a daily record of the patient's weight. Periodic evaluations are made to note the patient's progress and readiness for surgery. Dental caries and poor mouth hygiene may contribute to general debilitation and should be corrected (Chapter 33).

Effect of the Aging Process

It is important for the nurse to remember that in the older person, reactions to injury are less pronounced and slower in appearing. The aged do not tolerate dehydration well. The possibility of long-established diabetes, anemia, obesity, hypoproteinemia, etc., must be considered. Certain drugs are dangerous because they are poorly tolerated. Scopolamine, morphine, and the barbiturates are likely to cause confusion and disorientation, even excitement and apprehension. Some drugs have a cumulative effect. Sleeping and eating habits and the use of alcohol and laxatives, as well as the nightly "sleeping" medicine, must not be dismissed as unimportant (see page 311).

Obesity

If the patient is overweight and if preoperative time permits, physicians will insist that a prescribed and systematic program of weight reduction be undertaken in order that the surgical risk may be lessened. Obesity increases the seriousness of complications to a great extent. During surgery, fatty tissues are not highly resistant to infection; the surgeon faces increased technical and mechanical problems, and therefore dehiscence and wound infections are more common. The obese patient is difficult to care for because of his weight; he breathes poorly when lying on his side and thus is subject to hypoventilation and postoperative pulmonary complications, distention, and phlebitis. In addition, cardiovascular, endocrine, hepatic, and biliary diseases are more common in obese patients. It has been estimated that for each 30 pounds of excess weight, about 25 additional miles of blood vessels are needed. The increased demands on the heart are obvious.

Cardiovascular Disease

Since the margin of safety is lessened when a patient exhibits signs of cardiovascular disease, this condition demands greater than usual diligence during all phases of management and care. Depending upon the severity of symptoms, surgery may be deferred until maximal benefits have been obtained from medical treatment. At times, surgical treatment can be modified to meet the likely tolerance of the patient. For example, in an obese patient with acute obstructive cholecystitis and possible diabetes and coronary artery disease, simple gallbladder drainage with removal of calculi may be done rather than a more extensive operation.

Of particular significance in the patient with cardiovascular disease is the necessity to avoid sudden changes of position, prolonged immobilization, hypotension or hypoxia, and overloading of the body with fluids or blood.

Diabetes

In uncontrolled diabetes, the chief life-threatening hazard is that of hypoglycemia, which may develop during anesthesia or postoperatively. It results from inadequate intake of carbohydrates or from insulin overdosage. Other hazards which threaten but occur less rapidly are acidosis and glucosuria. In general, the surgical risk of the patient with controlled diabetes is not greater than that of the nondiabetic patient. (See Chap. 39.)

Upper Respiratory and Pulmonary Disease

Since it is necessary to maintain adequate ventilation during all phases of surgical treatment, surgery is usually contraindicated when the patient has a respiratory infection. Respiratory difficulties increase the possibility of atelectasis, bronchopneumonia, and respiratory failure when anesthetics are superimposed. Patients with pulmonary problems are evaluated by testing pulmonary function and determining blood gas values to note the extent of respiratory insufficiency. Antibiotics may be given for infections. Elimination of smoking and administration of bronchodilators may be prescribed for treating bronchospasm.

Hepatic and Renal Disease

The *liver* is important in the biotransformation of anesthetic compounds. Therefore, any disease of the liver has an effect on anesthetic intake. Acute liver disease is associated with a high surgical death rate; hence, preoperative improvement in liver function is desired. Careful assessment is made utilizing various liver function tests. (See Chap. 38.)

The *kidney* is involved in the excretion of anesthetic drugs and their metabolites. Acid-base and water metabolism are also important considerations in anesthetic administration. Surgery is contraindicated when a patient has acute nephritis, acute renal insufficiency with oliguria or anuria, or other acute renal problems, unless the surgery is a lifesaving measure or is necessary to improve urinary function, as in a prostatectomy.

Alcoholism

The acutely intoxicated person is susceptible to injury. If surgery is required, local or regional block anesthesia is used for minor surgery; for more extensive injury, surgery is postponed if possible. Otherwise, the stomach must be intubated and aspirated before general anesthesia is administered, in order to prevent vomiting and aspiration.

The person with a history of chronic alcoholism often suffers from malnutrition and other systemic problems; therefore, the surgical risk is increased. In view of this, delirium tremens may be anticipated on the second or third day postoperatively; it is associated with a significant mortality rate.

Prior Drug Therapy

Attention should be given to the history of drug usage by the patient. Potent medications have an effect on physiological functions; interactions of such drugs with anesthetic agents have caused serious problems such as arterial hypotension and circulatory collapse or depression.

The potential effects of prior drug therapy are evaluated by the anesthesiologist, who considers the length of time the patient has used the drugs, his condition, and the nature of the proposed surgery. Drugs that cause particular concern are:

Adrenal steroids —It is not advisable to discontinue corticosteroids before surgery. If steroid therapy has been used for a chronic problem over a period of time, it is usually advisable to give a "burst" of high dose steroid immediately before and after surgery.

Diuretics —In particular, the thiazide drugs may cause excessive respiratory depression during anesthesia; this results from an electrolyte imbalance.

Phenothiazines —These drugs may increase the hypotensive action of anesthetics.

Antidepressants —In particular, monoamine oxidase (MAO) inhibitors increase the hypotensive effects of anesthetics.

Insulin —Interaction between anesthetics and insulin must be considered when a diabetic patient is undergoing surgery.

Antibiotics —"Mycin" drugs such as neomycin, kanamycin, and, less frequently, streptomycin, may present problems; when these drugs are combined with a curariform muscle relaxant, nerve transmission is interrupted and apnea due to respiratory paralysis may result. Dripps and his colleagues call attention to the possibility of respiratory insufficiency "occurring most often in patients with peritonitis when (antibiotics) irrigation is done at wound closure —respiratory difficulty may occur in the recovery room."* For the reasons cited, it is imperative that the patient's drug history be assessed by the nurse and anesthesiologist.

*Dripps, R. D., et al.: Introduction to Anesthesia, 5th ed. Philadelphia, W. B. Saunders, 1977, p. 32.

OPERATIVE PERMIT (INFORMED CONSENT)

Before the surgeon has the right to operate, it is necessary to obtain a voluntary and informed consent from the patient. Such written permission, witnessed by the physician, nurse, or other authorized person, protects the patient against unsanctioned surgery and protects the surgeon and the hospital against claims of an unauthorized operation. In the best interests of all parties concerned, sound medicolegal principles are followed.

Prior to signing the permit, the patient should be told in clear and simple terms, by means of diagrams or models if necessary, what the surgeon proposes. This explanation usually is offered by the surgeon, who should also inform the patient of possible complications, disfigurement, disability, and removal of body parts, as well as what to expect in the early and late postoperative periods. Permission should be repeated for each operation, for each procedure in which it is necessary to enter a body cavity (cystoscopy, paracentesis, etc.), and when general anesthesia is given, as for a closed reduction of a fracture.

The patient may sign his own permit for operation if he is of age and is mentally capable. If he is a minor or is unconscious or irresponsible, permission must be obtained from a responsible family member. If he is an emancipated minor (married or independently earning his own living) he may sign his own permit. In an emergency, it may be necessary for the surgeon to operate as a lifesaving measure without a permit. However, every effort should be made to contact the patient's family. In such a situation, consent by telephone, telegram, or letter is acceptable.

No patient should be forced to sign an operative permit. Refusing to have an operation is a person's privilege. However, such information must be relayed to the surgeon so that other arrangements can be made; for instance, additional explanations may be offered to the patient and his family or the operation may be rescheduled at a more suitable time.

- The informed consent is placed in a prominent place on the patient's chart and accompanies the patient to the operating room.

PREOPERATIVE NURSING INTERVENTION

The preparation and care of the patient before operation are guided by an understanding that he is a unique, multifaceted individual.

The twin objectives of preoperative care are:
- *to present the patient in the best possible physical and psychosocial condition for his operation;*
- *to initiate every effort which will eliminate or reduce postoperative discomforts and complications.*

The length of time that the patient spends in the hospital before surgery should be reduced to the barest minimum, not only for reasons of economy, but also to reduce the likelihood of hospital-acquired infections.

Surgeons and hospitals differ in the details of preparation for operation, but the general principles remain the same: to make the patient as clean as possible, externally and internally, and to cause the least possible amount of physical and mental exhaustion for the patient in the process.

The rationale for preoperative procedures is obvious. All sources of infection must be eliminated, hence the scrupulous cleanliness of the operative site. The intestines and the bladder must be empty to prevent their contents from being discharged involuntarily while the patient is under the influence of the anesthetic and to prevent them from being inadvertently incised, as sometimes occurs in an abdominal operation when these organs are distended. This is especially true of the bladder and explains why it is so important that it be emptied before a patient is sent to the operating room for a laparotomy.

Any preparation of the patient before operation is to be carried out in the most efficient and skillful way.

- Approach the patient with an air of decision and interest in his well-being; to do so will gain his confidence — lost confidence is not easily regained.
- Determine exactly what procedures are to be performed and proceed with them in a systematic manner.
- Explain what you are about to do so that the patient is prepared for each step.
- Always work quietly, thoroughly, and neatly; bustle, confusion, and noise will only disturb and unsettle the patient.

During this period of preparation, from the time of admission to the actual operation, one of the most important responsibilities of the nurse is to observe the patient very closely for any unfavorable signs. Any sneezing, sniffling, and coughing must be reported, since operating on a patient with such symptoms may lead to postoperative pulmonary complications.

Nutrition

When the operation is scheduled for the morning, the meal on the preceding evening may be an ordinary light diet. Water may, and should, be given freely up to 4 hours before operation. In dehydrated patients, and especially in older ones, fluids by mouth often are encouraged before operation. In addition, fluids may be administered by vein, especially in patients to whom fluids cannot be given by mouth. If the operation is scheduled to take place after noon and does not involve any part of the gastrointestinal tract, the patient may be given a soft diet for breakfast.

Enema

A warm cleansing enema may be given the evening before operation, and may be repeated if ineffectual. Unless the condition of the patient presents some contraindication, the toilet, and not the bedpan, should be used in evacuating the enema.

Preoperative Skin Preparation

The aim of preoperative skin care is to render the skin as free as possible of microorganisms without causing damage to its physical and physiological integrity.

When there is time, such as in surgery of a non-emergency nature, the patient may use a soap containing a detergent-germicide to cleanse the skin area for several days before surgery in order to reduce the number of skin organisms.

Prior to surgery, the patient should take a warm, relaxing bath or shower, using betadine soap. Although it is preferable that this be done on the day of surgery, the time schedule may require that the shower be taken the night before. The purpose for recommending that the cleansing shower be taken as close to surgery as possible is to reduce the risk of skin contamination of the surgical wound. A shampoo the day before operation is advisable unless the condition of the patient does not make it feasible.

It has been customary as part of routine preoperative care to shave the skin in the vicinity of the operative site. However, this practice is now under critical study. Research results seem to indicate that injury to the skin caused by the razor serves as a portal of entry for bacteria and that the injured tissue may act as a substrate for bacterial growth. In addition, it has been reported that the longer the interval between the shave and the operation, the higher the rate of postoperative wound infection. Therefore, many hospitals have instituted the policy of limiting the timing of the preoperative shave to no more than one hour before surgery. Research appears to indicate that, contrary to former belief, skin that is well cleansed but unshaven is less often implicated in wound infections than shaved skin. Nonetheless, most patients in most hospitals are given a skin shave prior to surgery at the request of the surgeon.

The patient is told about the shaving procedure, placed in a comfortable position, and not exposed unduly. Any adhesive or grease may be readily removed with a sponge moistened in benzene or ether, if the odor is not objectionable to the patient. All hair must be shaved from the area to be operated upon. A sharp razor should be used and a thorough shave given to a wide area, including the operative site and the surrounding region, to reduce sources of contamination. Preparation of specific operative sites is illustrated in the chart on pp. 314–315.

Scratches should be avoided, and any skin eruptions should be reported because they are potential sites of infection.

In most hospitals, a male nurse or nursing assistant takes care of male patients. Skin shaving may be done by a special "prep" team, by the nurse assigned to the patient, or by a member of the operating room team. Disposable "prep" trays guarantee individualized equipment.

Usually nothing further is required in the way of local preparation other than thorough shaving and cleansing of the part until the patient reaches the operating room.

DEPILATORY CREAM. Chemical compounds (creams to remove hair) are safe for preparing the skin of the surgical patient. As an economy measure, long hairs may be cut before the cream is applied in order to reduce the amount of cream used.

The depilatory cream usually comes in a collapsible tube and is expressed on the body surface. The cream is spread in a smooth layer of about 1.25 cm. (½ inch) in depth over the entire operative site. A wooden tongue blade or a gloved hand can be used to apply the cream. After the cream has been allowed to remain on the skin for 10 minutes, it is scraped off gently with the tongue blade or multiple moistened gauze sponges. When all cream and hair have been removed, the skin is then washed with soap and water and patted dry.

There are several advantages in using a depilatory cream for preoperative skin preparation. The end result is a clean, smooth, and intact skin. Scrapes, abrasions, cuts, and inadequate hair removal are eliminated. It is more comfortable for the patient, since he is less apprehensive and often finds this method relaxing. There is even the possibility of the patient's preparing himself in selected operative procedures. Depilatory creams are more effective and safer for use on uncooperative or agitated patients. This method is no more expensive than other methods. A disadvantage is that a few patients have had some transient skin reactions involving the rectal and scrotal areas.

PATIENT EDUCATION IN THE PREOPERATIVE PERIOD

General Principles

The value of preoperative instruction to the patient has long been recognized. However, each patient should be taught as an individual, in terms of his anxieties, needs, and hopes. The background information of one patient is usually very different from that of the next patient. Once these differences are recognized and particular needs are assessed, a program of instruction can be planned and then implemented at the proper time. If the patient is taught essential information several days before he needs

it, he may not remember what he was told. If he is instructed too close to the time of surgery, he may not be in prime learning condition because of the effect of the preanesthetic medication.

If instruction is offered at a time when the patient is most receptive and can participate in the learning process, the chances are that he will retain more of the information. In actuality, instruction is spaced over a period of time to allow the patient to assimilate information and to ask questions as they arise. Frequently, teaching sessions are combined with various preparation procedures to allow for an easy flow of information. In essence, the nurse must make a judgment about how much the patient wants and needs to know. In some instances, too much explanation can be worse than not enough.

Limiting teaching to a description of the various steps of a procedure is not as helpful as telling the patient what sensations he will experience. For example, telling the patient that preoperative medication will relax him before the operation is not as effective as informing him that the medication will make him feel light-headed and sleepy. Once he knows what to expect, he will anticipate these reactions, which in turn will cause him to attain a higher degree of relaxation than might otherwise be expected.

Effective preoperative patient instruction has many advantages: (1) recuperation is more rapid; (2) drugs are used less frequently and in lower concentration; (3) fewer complications occur; and (4) hospitalization is shortened.

Deep Breathing and Coughing

The nurse first demonstrates to the patient how to take a deep breath slowly (maximal sustained inspiration) and how to exhale slowly, explaining that the purpose is to promote lung ventilation and blood oxygenation following general anesthesia. The patient is placed in a sitting position to provide maximum lung expansion. After practicing deep breathing several times, he is instructed to breathe deeply, exhale through his mouth, take a short breath, and cough from deep in the lungs. (See figure in chart on page 316.) If there is to be a thoracic or abdominal incision, the nurse can demonstrate how the incision line can be splinted so that pressure is minimized and pain is controlled. For an abdominal or chest incision, the patient can put the palms of his hands together, interlacing his fingers snugly. Placing the hands across the incisional site acts as an effective splint when he coughs. Of course he needs to know that medications will be given to control pain.

When a deep breath is taken before coughing, the cough reflex is stimulated. The purpose of coughing is to mobilize secretions so that they can be removed; not to do so may cause hypostatic pneumonia and other lung complications.

PREOPERATIVE SKIN PREPARATION

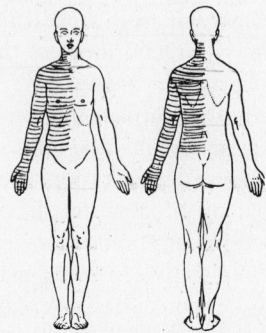

Shoulder prep. Shave fingertips to hairline, midline chest to midline spine on operative side and to iliac crest, including axilla.

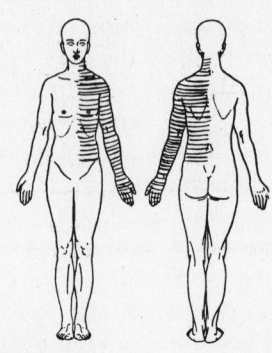

Upper arm prep. Shave fingertips to neckline (hairline), on operative side from midline chest to midline spine on operative side from axilla to iliac crest. Trim and clean fingernails. Use brush on hand and nails.

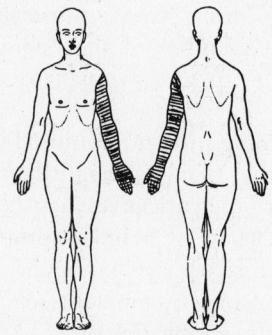

Hand prep. Shave fingertips to shoulder. Trim and clean fingernails. Use brush on hand and nails.

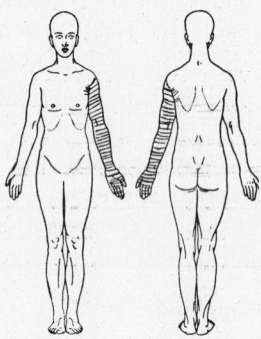

Forearm and elbow prep. Shave from fingernails to shoulder including axilla. Trim and clean fingernails. Use brush on hand and nails.

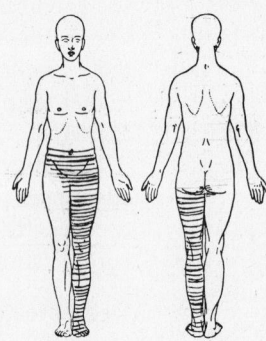

Saphenous vein ligation prep. Shave from umbilicus to toes of affected leg, or both legs. Include pubis and perineal area. Prep entire leg posteriorly.

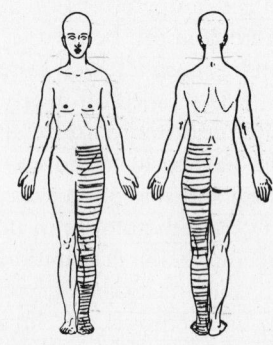

Thigh prep. Shave from toes to 3 inches above the umbilicus, midline front and back. Complete pubic shave. Clean and trim toenails. Use brush on foot and nails.

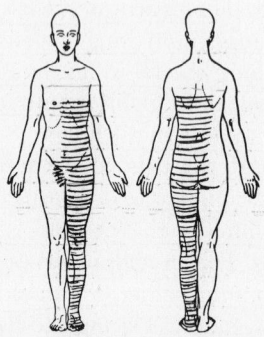

Hip prep. Shave toes to nipple line to at least 3 inches beyond midline back and front. Complete pubic shave. Clean and trim toenails. Use brush on foot and nails. Hip fractures—all preps done in the operating room.

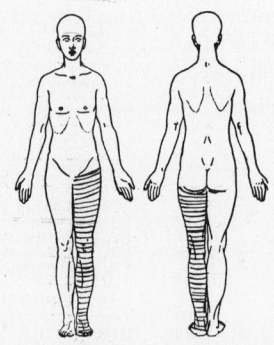

Knee and lower leg prep. Shave entire leg, toes to groin. Clean and trim toenails. Use brush on foot and nails.

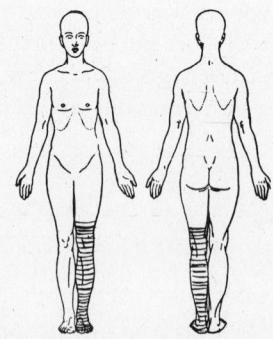

Ankle and foot prep. Shave entire leg, toes to 3 inches above the knee. Clean and trim toenails. Use brush on foot and nails.

(From Committee on Control of Surgical Infections of the Committee on Pre- and Postoperative Care, American College of Surgeons: Manual on Control of Infection in Surgical Patients, Philadelphia, J. B. Lippincott Co., 1977.)

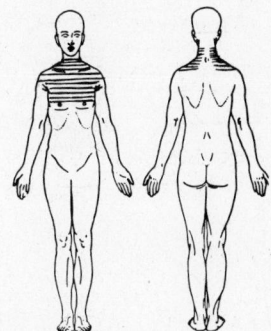

Thyroid prep. Shave from chin line to nipples, including axillary region. Extend to back of neck and upper shoulder as sketched.

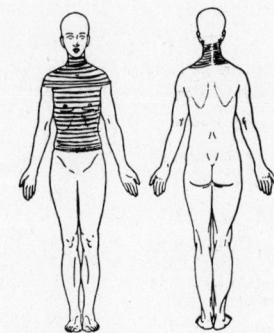

Parathyroid prep (as for sternal splitting). Shave from chin line to umbilicus, shoulder to shoulder in the front. Extend to back of neck and upper shoulder in back as shown. Prep laterally for chest tubes if so ordered.

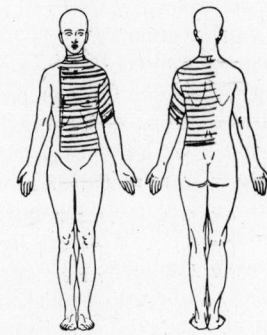

Thoracotomy prep. Shave from chin line to iliac crest, from nipple on unaffected side to at least 2 inches beyond the midline in back. Include axilla and entire arm to elbow.

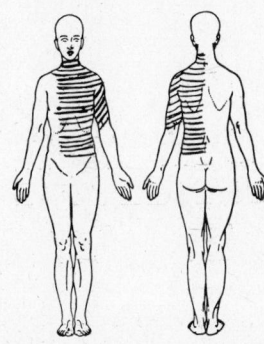

Mastectomy prep. Shave from upper neck to iliac crest, from nipple line on unaffected side to midline of back (affected side). Prep axilla and entire arm to elbow on affected side.

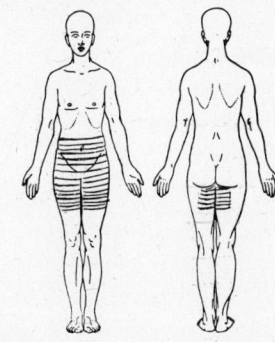

Lower abdominal prep (as for hernia, femoral vein ligation, femoral embolectomy). Shave from 2 inches above the umbilicus to mid-thigh, including the pubic area. Femoral ligation—shave to midline of thigh posteriorly. Hernia and embolectomy—shave to costal margin and down to knee as ordered.

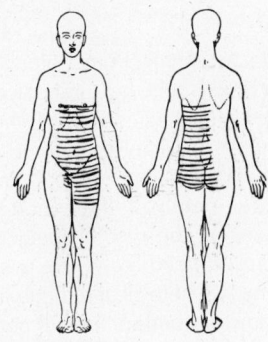

Flank prep (as for renal procedures, adrenalectomy, sympathectomy). Shave from nipple line to pubis and 3 inches beyond the midline in back. Shave pubic area. Shave upper thigh on the affected side.

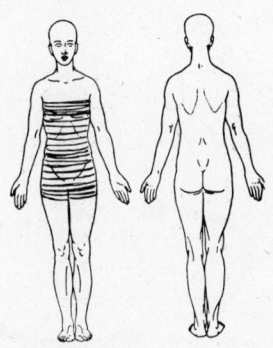

Abdominal prep. Shave from 3 inches above the nipple line to upper thighs, including pubis.

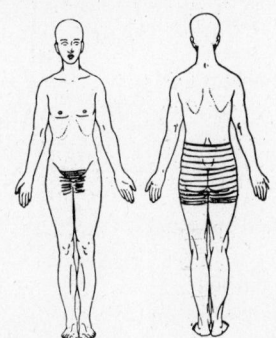

Perineal prep (as for hemorrhoidectomy, fistula-in-ano). Shave pubis, perineum, and perianal area. Shave from the waist in back to at least 3 inches below the groin.

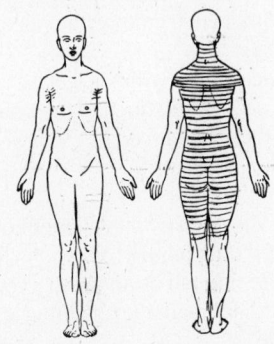

Spine prep. Shave entire back including shoulders and neck to hairline and down to knees and to both sides, including axillae.

315

A. DIAPHRAGMATIC BREATHING

Diaphragmatic breathing refers to a flattening of the dome of the diaphragm during inspiration with resulting enlargement of the upper abdomen as air rushes in. During expiration, the abdominal muscles contract.

1. Practice in the same position you would assume in bed following surgery: semi-Fowler, propped in bed with the back and shoulders well supported with pillows.
2. With the hands in a loose-fist position, allow the hands to rest lightly on the front of the lower ribs—fingernails against lower chest to feel the movement (A).
3. Breathe out gently and fully as the ribs sink down and inward toward midline.
4. Then take a deep breath through your nose and mouth, letting the abdomen rise as the lungs fill with air.
5. Hold this breath for a count of 5.
6. Exhale and let out *all* the air through the nose and mouth.
7. Repeat 15 times with a short rest after each group of five.
8. Practice this twice a day preoperatively.

B. COUGHING

1. Lean forward slighlty from a sitting position in bed, interlace the fingers together, and place the hands across the incisional site to act as a splint when coughing (B).
2. Breathe with the diaphragm as described in A.
3. With the mouth slightly open, breathe in fully.
4. "Hack" out sharply for three short breaths.
5. Then, keeping the mouth open, take in a quick deep breath and immediately give a strong cough once or twice. This will help clear secretions from the chest. It may cause some discomfort but will not harm incision.

C. LEG EXERCISES

1. Lie in a semi-Fowler position and perform the following simple exercises to improve circulation.
2. Bend the knee and raise the foot—hold it a few seconds, then extend the leg and lower it to the bed (C).
3. Do this about five times with one leg, then repeat with the other leg.
4. Then trace circles with the feet by bending them down, in toward each other, up, and then out (D).
5. Repeat these five times.

D. TURNING TO THE SIDE

1. Turn on your side with the uppermost leg flexed most and supported on a pillow.
2. Grasp the side rail as an aid to maneuver to the side.
3. Practice diaphragmatic breathing and coughing while on your side.

E. GETTING OUT OF BED

1. Turn on your side.
2. Push yourself up with one hand as you swing your legs out of bed.

F. USING THE URINAL (FOR MALE PATIENT)

When in bed for a period of time have the nurse explain the method for using the urinal in bed.

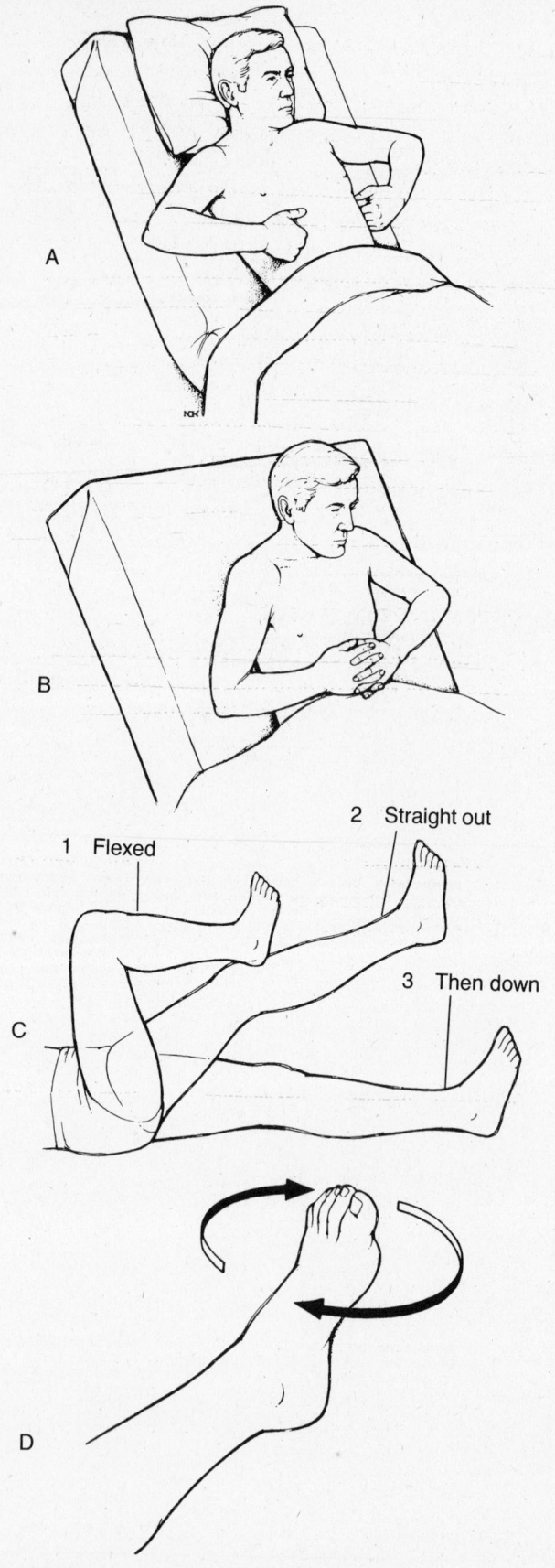

Turning and Active Body Movement

The patient is shown how to turn from side to side and how to assume Sims' lateral position. This position will be used postoperatively (even before he is conscious) and assumed every second hour to improve circulation, prevent venous stasis, and contribute to optimal respiratory exchange.

Exercises of the extremities include extension and flexion of the knee and hip joints (similar to bicycle riding while lying on the side). The foot is rotated as though tracing the largest possible circle with the great toe. (See chart, page 316.) The elbow and shoulder are also put through the range of motion. At first the patient will be assisted and reminded to do these exercises, but later he is encouraged to do them himself.

The nurse is reminded to use proper body mechanics and to instruct the patient to do the same. When he is placed in any position, the body is to be maintained in proper alignment. Turning and exercising promotes circulation and respiratory function. Muscle tone is maintained so that ambulation will be made easier.

Medications and Pain Control

The patient should be told that he will receive a preanesthetic medication to help him relax and perhaps feel sleepy. He is also warned that it may make him thirsty. Postoperatively, he can expect medications to keep him comfortable but not to prevent him from regaining activity and maintaining an adequate air exchange.

Visiting Information and Spiritual Resources

The patient feels more at ease when he knows at what point postoperatively he can expect his family or friends. It helps him to know that his family will be kept informed regarding the acute phases of his surgical experience. He appreciates information regarding the availability of a spiritual adviser of his preference.

Special Equipment

If the patient knows beforehand that he will be on assisted breathing and that drainage tubes will be in place along with any special equipment required, he is more likely to accept these accoutrements postoperatively without too much concern.

The patient is brought to the operating room about 20 minutes before the anesthesia is to be started. Previous to this the nurse clothes the patient in the regulation short gown, leaving it untied and open in the back. Occasionally, long leggings are added. In the case of a female

TABLE 17-1.   CATEGORIES OF CONTEMPLATED SURGERY BASED ON URGENCY

CLASSIFICATION	INDICATION FOR SURGERY	EXAMPLES
I. Emergency—Requires immediate attention	Without delay	Extensive burns Major bone fractures Fractured skull Gunshot wounds Stab wounds Bladder or intestinal obstruction Severe bleeding Serious eye injuries
II. Urgent—Requires prompt attention	Within 24-28 hrs.	Acute gallbladder infection Kidney or ureteral stones Bleeding hemorrhoids or uterine tumors Cancer
III. Required—Requires operation	Plan hospital admission within a few weeks or months	Eye cataracts Thyroid operations Tonsillectomy Gallbladder problems without acute inflammation Prostatic hypertrophy without bladder obstruction Spinal fusion Bone deformities
IV. Elective—Should be operated on	Failure to have surgery is not catastrophic	Repair of scars Simple hernia Vaginal repair Superficial cysts
V. Optional—The decision rests with the patient	Personal preference	Cosmetic surgery

patient, long hair is plaited in two braids, any hairpins are removed, and the head and the hair are entirely covered with a disposable paper cap. The mouth must be inspected and all dentures or plates, chewing gum, etc., removed. If these items were left in the mouth, they could easily fall to the back of the throat during induction of anesthesia and cause respiratory obstruction.

Jewelry should not be worn to the operating room; even wedding rings should be taken off. If a patient has any real objection to the removal of a ring, a narrow tape may be tied to the ring and then fastened securely around the patient's wrist. All articles of value, including dentures and prosthetic devices are labeled clearly with the patient's name and stored in a safe place according to local hospital policy.

All patients (except those with urologic problems) should void immediately before being sent to the operating room. The bladder must be empty, but catheterization should not be resorted to except in an emergency, or when it is desirable to have an indwelling catheter in place to ensure bladder collapse. In this instance, such a catheter would be connected to a closed drainage system. The urine voided is measured and the amount and the time of voiding are recorded on the preoperative check slip or the anesthesia chart.

For patients with vascular problems that could lead to deep vein thrombosis, elastic stockings may be applied and the legs elevated. However, controversy has developed over these practices, some studies supporting them and others indicating no beneficial effects.*

Preanesthetic Medication—Pharmacokinetics

The main purpose of preanesthetic medication is to reduce the patient's anxiety so that induction and maintenance of anesthesia will be smooth. As with other management modalities, medication is prescribed on an individual basis to meet the needs of the particular patient.

BARBITURATES. For sedation, *barbiturates* are commonly used, mainly pentobarbital (Nembutal) and secobarbital (Seconal Sodium). However, it is worthwhile to note that studies have shown that the reassuring visit of the anesthesiologist and operating room nurse prior to the operation has a more calming effect than the barbiturates. Nonetheless, the night before surgery, a hypnotic is usually given to allay insomnia which is brought about by new and different surroundings, apprehension over pending surgery, and disturbing hospital sounds.

OPIATES. Drugs such as morphine and meperidine (Demerol) may be prescribed before an operation to reduce the amount of general anesthetic required. These drugs also can be used to produce analgesia in patients who have pain before the operation. At the same time it is important to realize that analgesic doses may depress respiration and the cough reflex and present an increased risk of respiratory acidosis and aspiration pneumonitis. Full doses may cause hypotension, nausea, vomiting, constipation, and abdominal distention.

ANTICHOLINERGICS. Drugs of this type may be prescribed to reduce respiratory tract secretions and to prevent or treat severe reflex slowing of the heart during anesthesia. Atropine is the most popular of the medications prescribed, although it should be given only when required. Scopolamine is another common preanesthetic medication given for sedation and amnesia. This drug may cause irritability and restlessness, reactions which can be controlled by the intravenous injection of physostigmine (Antilirium).

Because the belladonna alkaloids (atropine and scopolamine) have varying effects on pulse rate, as well as other shortcomings, a quaternary ammonium compound, glycopyrrolate (Robinul), is an anticholinergic drug which is gaining in popularity because it is twice as potent as an antisialogogue (reducing secretions) and acts three times as long.

TIMING OF ADMINISTRATION OF DRUGS. Because preanesthetic medications should be given from 45 to 75 minutes before anesthesia is begun, it is most important that the nurse give this medication precisely at the prescribed time; otherwise, its effect will have worn off or—what happens more often—it will not have begun to act when anesthesia is started.

After the preanesthetic medication is given, the patient is kept in bed, because he will begin to feel light-headed and drowsy. (If the patient is unattended, the side rails are placed in position.) If he receives atropine or Robinul, he may be told it will make his mouth dry. During this time, the nurse observes the patient for any untoward reaction to the medications. His environment should be kept quiet to assist in relaxing him.

Very frequently operations are delayed or schedules changed, and it becomes impossible to request that a medication be given at a specific time. In these situations the preoperative medication is prescribed "on call from operating room." Although this is far from ideal and should be avoided whenever possible, the nurse can help by having the medication ready to give and by administering it as soon as the patient is called for. It usually takes 15 to 20 minutes to get a patient ready for the operating room. If the nurse gives the medication before attending to the other details of preparing the patient, he will have at least partial benefit from the preoperative medication and will have a smoother and more pleasant anesthetic and operative course.

---

*Rosengarten, D. S., et al.: The failure of compression stockings (Turbigrip) to prevent deep venous thrombosis after operation. Brit. J. Surg., 57:296–299, Apr. 1976.

Patient: Date:

Division:

	Remarks	Yes	No

PATIENT PREPARATION

1. Operative area prepared

2. Operative area inspected by head nurse or supervisor
    (not necessary if done by "Prep" team)

3. Oral hygiene given
    Dentures removed

    Dentures present

    Capped teeth present

    "Removable bridgework" removed

4. Hair prepared—covered if necessary

    Hairpins removed

5. Jewelry:
    Removed

    Ring tied or taped on

    Other (medal, etc.) present

6. Voided, catheterized, or indwelling catheter

    Amount

    Time

7. Medications
    Those given in past 8 hrs. recorded

    Preanesthetic medication given
        Time   A.M.   P.M.

8. Side rails applied after giving preanesthetic medication

9. Identification wristlet applied

10. Colored nail polish removed (from at least 2 fingers)

CHART PREPARATION

1. Operative permit (Informed Consent) signed and on chart

2. Morning T.P.R. recorded

3. Morning B.P. recorded

4. Laboratory blood studies on chart

5. Laboratory urine studies on chart

6. Doctor's Order Sheet on chart

Figure 17-1.   Preoperative check list which is attached to the patient's chart and is checked immediately before the patient is taken to the operating room.

Preoperative Record

A preoperative check list is completed and attached to the chart (Fig. 17-1). The completed chart accompanies the patient to the operating room. The informed consent also is attached as are all laboratory reports and nurses' records. Any unusual last minute observations that may have a bearing on the anesthesia or surgery are to be placed to the front of the chart in a prominent place.

Transportation to the Presurgical Suite

The patient is transferred to the holding area or pre-surgical suite in bed or on a previously prepared stretcher. The stretcher should be as comfortable as possible, with a sufficient number of blankets to ensure against chilling from drafty corridors. A small pillow at the head usually is acceptable. The top covers of the stretcher should be long enough to tuck in at both the patient's feet and shoulders. Preferably the nurse who has cared for the patient up to this time should accompany him to the operating room. An attendant always remains with the patient in the holding area until relieved by one of the anesthesiologists. The chart is given to the anesthesiologist or an operating room nurse; it never should be left with the patient.

It is important that someone be with the preoperative patient at all times. Even though he has had preoperative medication, appears to be dozing, and seems to be secure on the stretcher with a strap in place, he should not be left alone. It is desirable to have the patient brought directly to the induction room, where he is greeted by name and made to feel that he is in safe hands. The area must be quiet if the preoperative medication is to have maximal effect. The patient should not hear undesirable sounds or conversations which might be misinterpreted or exaggerated.

It is assumed that preoperative preparation has covered every contingency before the patient comes to the operating room. However, as the patient waits with his eyes closed, he is often reviewing some personal thoughts; a question or concern about a particular thing may occur to him and may assume an exaggerated importance. Someone should be available to answer or attempt to find the answer to his question.

Reassurance is given not only verbally but also by facial expression, manner, and a touch or warm grasp of the hand. It is important for the patient to have the security of seeing a familiar face — the nurse who helped to prepare him before he was sent to the operating floor, or the anesthesiologist who visited with him the day before and discussed anesthetic management.

Attention to physical needs will add greatly to comfort. The patient should be kept out of drafts and covered with a blanket if he is cold. If he is too warm, some of the covering can be removed, although unnecessary exposure should be avoided and the patient's modesty respected. Knee straps should be applied loosely to minimize circulatory impairment as well as nerve injury. If it is necessary to discuss something that the patient should not hear, this should be done well out of the patient's hearing range; even if he appears to be asleep, he may be acutely aware of all conversation.

ATTENDING TO THE PATIENT'S FAMILY

Most hospitals have a special waiting room where the family can wait while the patient is having surgery. This room may be equipped with comfortable chairs, television, telephones, and facilities for light refreshment. Volunteers may remain with the family, serve them coffee, boost their morale, and even keep them informed of the patient's progress. After surgery, the surgeon may meet the family here, join them for coffee, and report his findings.

The family never should judge the seriousness of an operation by the length of time the patient is in the operating room. He may be in surgery much longer than the actual operating time for several reasons:

1. It is customary to send for the patient some time in advance of the actual operating time.
2. Anesthesiologists often make additional preparations that may take from ½ to 1 hour.
3. Occasionally, the surgeon takes longer than he expected with the preceding case, hence delaying the time of beginning the next operation.
4. After surgery, the patient is taken to the recovery room to ensure satisfactory emergence from the anesthetic.

Those waiting to see the patient after the operation should be forewarned that the patient may be returned to his room with a variety of equipment in place, including blood transfusion lines, suction bottles, nasal tube, airway, oxygen tent, tracheostomy tube, monitoring equipment, etc. If the prognosis for the patient is more negative than positive, it is not within the prerogative of the nurse to relay this information to the family, even when the odds appear in the patient's favor.

BIBLIOGRAPHY

Perioperative Care

BOOKS

American College of Surgeons: Manual on Control of Infection in Surgical Patients. Philadelphia, J. B. Lippincott, 1976.

Artz, C. P., et al.: Brief Textbook of Surgery. Philadelphia, W. B. Saunders, 1976.

Artz, C. P., and Hardy, J. D.: Management of Surgical Complications. Philadelphia, W. B. Saunders, 1975.

Atkinson, L. J., and Kohn, M. L.: Berry and Kohn's Introduction to Operating Room Technique, 5th ed. New York, McGraw-Hill, 1978.

Dripps, R. D., Jr., et al.: Introduction to Anesthesia, 5th ed. Philadelphia, W. B. Saunders, 1977.

Fay, M. R.: Introduction to Recovery Room Nursing. Denver, Col., Assoc. of Operating Room Nurses, 1977.

Gruendemann, B. J., et al.: The Surgical Patient, 2nd ed. St. Louis, C. V. Mosby, 1977.

Hardy, J. D., ed.: Rhoads Textbook of Surgery, 5th ed. Philadelphia, J. B. Lippincott, 1977.

LeMaitre, G. D., and Finnegan, J. A.: The Patient in Surgery, 3rd ed. Philadelphia, W. B. Saunders, 1975.

Meltzer, L. E., ed., et al.: Concepts and Practices of Intensive Care for Nurse Specialists, 2nd ed. Bowie, Md., Charles Press Pub. 1976.

Peacock, E. E., Jr. and Van Winkle, W., Jr.: Wound Repair. Philadelphia, W. B. Saunders, 1976.

Rhodes, M. J., et al.: Alexander's Care of the Patient in Surgery, 6th ed. St. Louis, C. V. Mosby, 1978.

Thorek, P.: Surgical Diagnosis, 3rd ed. Philadelphia, J. B. Lippincott, 1977.

Walraven, G., et al.: Manual of Advanced Prehospital Care. Bowie, Md., Robert J. Brady Co., 1978.

Zschoche, D. S., ed.: Mosby's Comprehensive Review of Critical Care. St. Louis, C. V. Mosby, 1976.

Preoperative Care

ARTICLES

A better way to calm the patient who fears the worst. RN, *40*:47-54, Apr. 1977.

Burke, J. F.: Preventive antibiotics in surgery. Postgrad. Med., *58*:65-68, Sept. 1975.

Damsteegt, D.: Pastoral roles in presurgical visits. AJN, *75*:1336-1337, Aug. 1975.

Dzuirbejko, M. M., and Larkin, J. C.: Including the family in preoperative teaching. AJN, *78*:1892-1894, Nov. 1978.

Girard, N. J.: Home visits give continuity of care. AORN J., *24*:1057-1062, Dec. 1976.

Group teaching can supplement patient interviews. AORN J., *26*:223-226, Aug. 1977.

Gruendemann, B. J.: The impact of surgery on body image. Nurs. Clin. N. Am., *10*:536-543, Dec. 1975.

_____: Preoperative group sessions part of nursing process. AORN J., *26*:257-262, Aug. 1977.

Gurewich, V., et al.: Hemostatic effects of uniform, low-dose subcutaneous heparin in surgical patients. Arch. Intern. Med., *138*:41-44, Jan. 1978.

Hoopes, N. M., and McConnell, M.: An approach to preoperative visits. AORN J., *26*:1048-1052, Dec. 1977.

Irving, J.: When fear is healthy. Psych. Today, *1*:46-49, 60, 61, Apr. 1968.

Furst, J. B.: Emotional stress reactions to surgery: Review of some therapeutic implications. NY State J. Med., *78*:1083-1085, 1975.

Laird, M.: Techniques for teaching pre- and postoperative patients. AJN, *75*:1338-1340, Aug. 1975.

Marcinek, M. B.: Stress in the surgical patient. AJN, *77*:1809-1811, Nov. 1977.

Mehaffy, N. L.: Assessment and communication for continuity of care for the surgical patient. Nurs. Clin. N. Am., *10*:625-633, Dec. 1975.

Ridgeway, M.: Preop interviews assure quality care. AORN J., *24*:1083-1085, Dec. 1976.

Silva, M. C.: Preoperative teaching for spouses. AORN J., 1081-1086, May, 1978.

Skillings, I. L.: Emotional support for surgery patients. AORN J., *26*:263-265, Aug. 1977.

Strauss, R. J., and Wise, L.: Operative risks of obese patients: nursing care. AORN J., *25*:1053-1057, May 1977.

Winslow, E. H., and Fuhs, F. F.: Preoperative assessment for postoperative evaluation. AJN, *73*:1372-1374, Aug. 1973.

Wyatt, S., and Cullop, M. E.: Problems with patient visits by RR nurses. AORN J., *27*:1087-1091, May 1978.

Informed Consent

Gargaro, W. J., Jr.: Informed consent. Cancer Nurs., *1*:81-82, Feb. 1978.

_____: How much to tell the patient. Cancer Nurs. *1*:167-168, April, 1978.

Howard, R. B.: More on informed consent. Postgrad. Med., 65:25, Jan. 1979.

Kelly, L. Y.: The patient's right to know. Nurs. Outlook. *24*:26-32, Jan. 1976.

_____: Keeping up with your legal responsibilities. Nursing '76, *6*:81, 83, 85-7 passim, Mar. 1976.

Lafout, E. G.: The fiction of informed consent. JAMA, *235*:1579-1584, Apr. 12, 1976.

Mangold, W. J., Jr.: Informed consent and its implications in family practice. J. Fam. Pract., *2*:103-105, 1975.

Meisel, A.: Informed consent—the rebuttal. JAMA, *234*:615, Nov. 10, 1975.

Miller, R., and Willner, H. S.: The two-part consent form: A suggestion for promoting free and informed consent. New Eng. J. Med., *290*:964-966, April 25, 1974.

Preoperative Skin Preparation

MacClelland, D. C.: Are current skin preparations valid? AORN J., *21*:55-60, Jan. 1975.

Seropian, R., and Reynolds, B. M.: Wound infections after preoperative depilatory versus razor preparation. Am. J. Surg., *121*:251-254, Mar. 1971.

18

MANAGEMENT OF THE PATIENT UNDERGOING ANESTHESIA

THE ANESTHESIOLOGIST AND THE PATIENT

The surgical patient usually is interested in and concerned about the anesthesia that he is to receive. He has heard friends or relatives discuss the subject on the basis of personal experience or hearsay, and not infrequently has formed opinions as to the merits or demerits of various methods in use. Therefore, it is helpful for the anesthesiologist to visit the patient in his room before the operation and to point out that the purpose of the visit is to allay any fears that may exist in the patient's mind. Choice of anesthetic agent is discussed and the patient has an opportunity to disclose idiosyncrasies as well as types of medications he is currently taking that may affect the choice of an agent (see page 311).

During this essential visit, the anesthesiologist determines the condition of the patient's lungs and inquires about any preexisting pulmonary infections and the extent to which the patient smokes. The patient's general physical condition must also be ascertained because this may affect the management of anesthesia (Table 18-1).

The preoperative visit from the anesthesiologist builds up confidence and enables the patient to recognize a familiar face as he is being wheeled onto the operating floor. Uncertainty and anxiety are relieved to a certain degree, and a smoother course can be anticipated.

In the anesthetizing room the patient is transferred to the operating table and a last-minute check of his condition is made; blood pressure and pulse and respiratory rates in particular are noted. Induction of the anesthetic is usually done in the operating room.

An anesthesiologist is specifically trained in the art and the science of anesthesiology. After consulting with the surgeon, he usually selects the anesthesia and deals with any technical problems relating to the administration of the anesthetic agent and supervision of the patient's condition during the operation. Such "sharing" of responsibility obviously benefits the patient.

During the course of surgery, the anesthesiologist monitors the patient's blood pressure, pulse, and respirations as well as the electrocardiogram, tidal volume, blood gas levels, blood pH, alveolar gas concentrations, and body temperature. Monitoring by electroencephalograph may be required in some instances. Should the body's physiological mechanisms become incapable of maintaining these functions within safe limits, the anesthesiologist would then resort to the use of devices which ventilate the patient's lungs and circulate and aerate his blood.

TYPES OF ANESTHESIA

Anesthetics are divided into two classes according to whether they suspend sensation in (1) the whole body (general anesthesia) or in (2) parts of the body (local, regional, epidural, or spinal anesthesia).

General anesthesia can be obtained by inhalation or by intravenous or rectal techniques.

Liquid anesthetics produce anesthesia when their vapors are inhaled. Included in this group are ethyl ether, halothane, trichloroethylene, and enflurane. All are given with oxygen and usually with nitrous oxide as well.

Gas anesthetics are administered by inhalation, always in combination with oxygen. This group of anesthetics includes nitrous oxide and cyclopropane.

These substances, when inhaled, enter the blood through the pulmonary capillaries and, when in sufficient concentration, act on the cerebral centers in such a manner as to produce loss of consciousness and of sensation. When administration of the anesthetic is discontinued, the vapor or gas is eliminated by way of the lungs.

Physiologic and Physical Factors

General anesthetics produce anesthesia because they are delivered to the brain at high partial pressure. Relatively large amounts of anesthetic must be given during induction and the early maintenance phases because the anesthetic is recirculated and deposited in body tissues. As these depots become saturated, smaller amounts of the anesthetic agent are required to maintain anesthesia, since equilibrium or near equilibrium has been achieved between brain, blood, and other tissues. It is apparent that anything that diminishes peripheral blood flow, such as vasoconstriction or a condition of shock, may cause only small amounts of anesthetic to be required. Conversely, when peripheral blood flow is unusually high, as in the muscularly active or apprehensive patient, the brain receives a smaller quantity of anesthetic, with the result that induction is slower and larger than usual quantities of anesthetic are required.

Stages of Inhalation Anesthesia

Anesthesia generally is described as consisting of four stages, each of which presents a definite group of signs and symptoms (Table 18-2). Generally, these stages are seen best when ether is the anesthetic used. When narcotics and neuromuscular blockers (relaxants) are given, several of these stages are absent.

STAGE I: BEGINNING ANESTHESIA. As the patient breathes in the anesthetic mixture, a feeling of warmth steals over his body, dizziness is experienced, and a feeling of detachment develops. He experiences a ringing, roaring or buzzing in his ears and, though still conscious, is aware that he is unable to move his extremities easily. During this stage, noises are exaggerated; even low voices or minor sounds appear distressingly loud and unreal. For this reason, unnecessary noise or motion must be prevented when anesthesia is started.

STAGE II: EXCITEMENT. This stage—characterized variously by struggling, shouting, talking, singing, laughing, or even crying—frequently may be avoided by judicious suggestion before anesthesia is begun and by the smooth and rapid administration of the anesthetic. The pupils become dilated but contract if exposed to light; the pulse rate is rapid and respiration irregular.

Because of the uncontrolled movements of the patient during this stage, the anesthesiologist always should be attended by someone ready to help restrain the patient. A strap is in place across the thighs of each patient, and the hands are fixed to an intravenous armboard. Also, the patient lies on a conduction strap for the purpose of avoiding burns during use of diathermy, ECG leads, etc. The patient should not be touched except for purposes of restraint, and under no circumstances should there be palpation of the operative site.

TABLE 18-1. CLASSIFICATION OF PHYSICAL STATUS FOR ANESTHESIA PRIOR TO SURGERY

CLASSIFICATION	DESCRIPTION	EXAMPLE
I. Good	No organic disease, no systemic disturbance	Uncomplicated hernias, fractures
II. Fair	Mild to moderate systemic disturbance	Mild cardiac (I and II), mild diabetes
III. Poor	Severe systemic disturbance	Poorly controlled diabetes, pulmonary complications, moderate cardiac (III)
IV. Serious	Systemic disease threatening life	Severe renal disease, severe cardiac disease (IV), decompensation
V. Moribund	Little chance of survival but submitting to operation in desperation	Massive pulmonary embolus, ruptured abdominal aneurysm with profound shock
E. Emergency	Any of the above when surgery is done in an emergency situation	Hitherto uncomplicated hernia which is now strangulated and associated with nausea and vomiting; designation 1(E). If classification is III and, an emergency, the designation is 3(E).

From: American Society of Anesthesiology, Inc.: Codes for the Collection and Tabulation of Data Relating to Anesthesia, Inhalation Therapy and Therapeutic and Diagnostic Blocks.

TABLE 18-2. STAGES OF ANESTHESIA

STAGE	DEFINITION	PAIN	PUPIL SIZE; REACTION TO LIGHT	BLOOD PRESSURE	PULSE	LID REFLEX	RESPIRATION	REFLEXES PHARYNX-LARYNX	PRECAUTIONS
Stage I Induction Amnesia and Analgesia	From beginning of administration of anesthetic agent to loss of consciousness	Pain sensation is not absent but altered	Size is normal. Contracts in response to light.	Normal	Rapid	Attempt of lid to close when passively opened	Regular	Normal	
Stage II Delirium	From time of loss of consciousness to onset of a regular pattern of breathing	Response to stimuli uninhibited	Becomes dilated. Contracts when exposed to light.	Higher	Rapid; sometimes irregular	Lost	Irregular	Vomiting may occur Retching	Avoid stimulation because patient may respond violently Proper restraints Quiet O.R. Hypnotic suggestion
Stage III Plane I	Onset of regular breathing	Pain response diminishes	Eyes may oscillate; present with ether, cyclopropane, fluroxene; absent with halothane, enflurane.	Normal	Steady Slow	Abolished	Regular: Inspiration longer than expiration	Gradually abolished	
Plane II		Responds to rough tissue handling	Eyes cease to move; pupils progressively dilate with ether, cyclopropane, and fluroxene. Pupils more or less constricted with other agents.	Normal	Steady Slow		Regular; inspiration and expiration equal, or expiration more prolonged	Laryngospasm no longer develops	Muscle tone lessens—surgical handling of tissues tolerated
Plane III	Intercostal activity begins to decrease		Reaction to light is lost.	Normal or low	Steady Slower		Expiration longer than inspiration		Little muscle tone
Plane IV	Paralysis of intercostal muscles to cessation of spontaneous respiration			Low	Weak and thready	Reflexes absent		Reflexes absent	Imperative to lighten anesthesia; ventilate lungs with 100 percent oxygen
Stage IV	Cessation Premortem		Become widely dilated. Do not contract when exposed to light.				Cessation		

STAGE III: SURGICAL ANESTHESIA. Surgical anesthesia is reached by continued administration of the vapor or gas. The patient is unconscious, lying quietly on the table. The pupils are small but retain contractile power on exposure to light. Respiration is regular, pulse rate is about normal and of good volume, and the skin is pink or slightly flushed. By proper administration of the anesthetic this stage may be maintained for hours in one of several planes (1, 2, 3, 4), depending upon the depth of anesthesia needed.

STAGE IV: DANGER. This stage is reached when too much anesthesia has been given. Respiration becomes shallow, the pulse weak and thready; the pupils become widely dilated and no longer contract when exposed to light. Cyanosis develops and, unless prompt action is taken, death follows rapidly. If this stage should develop, the anesthetic is discontinued immediately and artificial respiration is given. Stimulants, although rarely used, may be administered for circulation if an overdosage of anesthetic has been given. Narcotic antagonists can be used if these agents are at fault.

During smooth administration of an anesthetic, there is, of course, no sharp division between the various stages. The patient passes gradually from one stage to another, and it is only by close observation of the signs exhibited by the patient that an anesthesiologist can control the situation. The condition of the pupils, the blood pressure, and the respiratory and cardiac rates are probably the most reliable guides to the patient's condition.

Other Physiologic Changes

The administration of an anesthetic is attended by other physiologic activities that have not been mentioned. Some anesthetics, especially ether, produce hypersecretion of mucus and saliva. This may be minimized by the preoperative administration of atropine. Vomiting or regurgitation occurs frequently, especially when the patient comes to the operating room with a full stomach. If gagging occurs, the patient's head is turned to the side, the head of the table is lowered, and a basin is provided to collect the vomitus. Suction apparatus should always be available.

During anesthesia, the patient's temperature may fall, and therefore every precaution must be taken against chilling. Warm cotton blankets should be available. Glucose metabolism is much reduced, and as a result, acidosis may develop.

In addition to the dangers of the anesthetic itself, the anesthesiologist must guard against asphyxia. This may be caused by foreign bodies in the mouth, spasm of the vocal cords, swallowing of the tongue, or aspiration of vomitus, saliva, or blood. These complications are avoided by the use of an endotracheal tube with an inflated cuff.

ADMINISTRATION OF THE ANESTHETIC

Open-Drop Method

Only on rare occasions is this method now used for administering volatile liquid anesthetics. Such an occasion would be the administration of halothane when very brief anesthesia is required, such as for myringotomy or an eye examination in children. The fluid is dropped slowly on eight layers of gauze which is placed over the patient's nose and mouth. While the patient inhales the vapor that evaporates from the gauze, oxygen is delivered under the mask to minimize hypoxia. Care must be taken to prevent any of the anesthetic from entering the eye. If this occurs, the eye should be irrigated immediately with saline solution.

Vapor or Gas Administration with Mask

Liquid anesthetics may also be given by mixing the vapors with oxygen or nitrous oxide-oxygen and then having the patient inhale the mixture. The vapor is conducted to the patient by a tube and a mask.

Gases (nitrous oxide, ethylene, cyclopropane, and oxygen) are contained in tanks under pressure and are allowed to escape at the proper rate or pressure through valves opening into a mixing chamber and then usually into a large rubber bag. The bag is connected by a flexible tube to a mask, which is put over the patient's face. A reservoir containing liquid anesthetic often is incorporated in the breathing circuit, so that, by turning a valve, a regulated amount of vapor may be given with the gas.

Endotracheal Anesthesia

The endotracheal technique for administering anesthetics consists of introducing a soft rubber or plastic tube into the trachea, either by exposing the larynx with a laryngoscope or by passing the tube "blindly." It may be inserted through either nose or mouth (Fig. 18-1).

The technique has many advantages, and the most important is the most obvious—a clear airway is maintained. Thus, there is minimal danger of respiratory obstruction, either from the tongue's falling back against the posterior pharyngeal wall (swallowing the tongue) or from spasm of the vocal cords. However, there is danger if the tube kinks, ends up in a bronchus, or becomes plugged with secretions, e.g., mucus, blood, or pus.

The endotracheal method has its greatest use in chest surgery, in which the thorax is open and the patient must depend on the anesthesiologist to assist him in breathing, or to take over breathing completely by rhythmic compression of the breathing bag. Many other types of operation have been made possible or safer by this technique, including neurosurgical, dental, plastic, and nose and throat procedures, in which the anesthesiologist does not have immediate access to the patient's face. It is also effective when there is danger of the airway's becoming

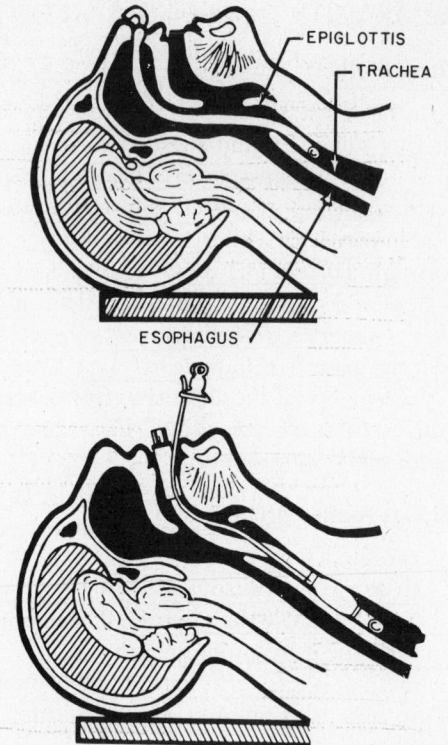

Figure 18-1. Endotracheal anesthesia. *(Top)* Magill tube in proper position, intranasal intubation being used. Note metal elbow at proximal end of tube. This adaptor is used to keep the tube from entering the nose beyond reach of extubation and also used to attach to anesthetic circuit. *(Bottom)* Oral intubation. Tube in position with cuff inflated.

compromised, which may occur in the obese patient or the patient with an anatomical abnormality. Endotracheal anesthesia is used today in the vast majority of longer operations regardless of the site, because most patients are paralyzed with muscle relaxants.

Another important advantage of tracheal intubation is that it provides a convenient method of aspirating secretions, blood, or other foreign material from the trachea and the bronchi. This is not only important in anesthesia, but it is invaluable in the nursing care of very ill patients in the recovery room or intensive care unit.

The advantages normally overshadow the disadvantages of this technique. Care must be taken in inserting the tube to prevent injury to the lips, tongue, and teeth. Other complications must be prevented during intubation, such as increased resistance to breathing, obstruction or dislodgment of the tube, and coughing. Additional complications may develop after removal of the tracheal tube: (1) laryngospasm, which may occur in the lightly anesthetized patient and can be treated by administration of 100 percent oxygen or use of succinylcholine intravenously; (2) tracheal collapse; (3) edema or infection of the larynx or the trachea; (4) hoarseness; and (5) sore throat.

GENERAL ANESTHESIA

INHALATION VOLATILE LIQUIDS

Diethyl Ether

Diethyl ether is a clear, volatile, flammable fluid. It may be given by any of the methods mentioned.

ADVANTAGES. Ether produces anesthesia with muscular relaxation suitable for surgical operations.

It is not highly toxic and has a wide margin of safety between the dosage required for anesthesia and the toxic dose. Signs of toxicity usually appear in sufficient time to allow for resuscitation of the patient and to avoid a fatal outcome.

No accurate statistics are available, but various authors give mortality figures ranging from 1 death in 16,000 to 1 in 30,000.

In emergencies, ether may be given by unskilled persons under the guidance of the surgeon.

DISADVANTAGES. Ether vapor, especially in high concentration, irritates the respiratory mucous membrane. Its administration may be followed by increased secretions in the respiratory tract and by nausea and vomiting in the postoperative period. In addition, some rise in blood glucose may be noted. The period of induction and of emergence is longer than for most of the other anesthetics (Table 18-3). Ether is seldom used these days because of the hazard of explosion and other unpleasant effects.

Halothane (Fluothane)

This anesthetic, introduced in 1956, is a potent nonflammable halogenated hydrocarbon which must be administered by way of precisely calibrated vaporizers.

ADVANTAGES. Halothane is useful because it is easy to administer, allows for rapid induction and emergence from anesthesia, is nonflammable, and has a low incidence of postoperative nausea and vomiting.

DISADVANTAGES. Halothane provides relatively poor muscular relaxation of the abdominal muscles, hence is frequently used with a neuromuscular blocking agent. When the patient emerges from anesthesia, he frequently shivers, a reaction thought to be of neurologic origin rather than the result of lowered body temperature as commonly found. Methylphenidate (Ritalin) is given to combat shivering. Because of some undesirable effects on the liver, halothane is not recommended for patients with a history of hepatic dysfunction or those who have had a previous bad hepatic reaction to the anesthetic.

Methoxyflurane (Penthrane)

Methoxyflurane is a halogenated ether that was synthesized in 1958 and put into practice in 1959.

TABLE 18-3. VOLATILE LIQUIDS AS AGENTS OF GENERAL ANESTHESIA

AGENT	ADMINISTRATION	ADVANTAGES	DISADVANTAGES	IMPLICATIONS
1. *Diethyl ether*	Open-drop; inhalation	Excellent relaxant Wide margin of safety Inexpensive Relatively nontoxic Used for all types of surgery	Slow induction: 10 minutes Long recovery; not eliminated for approximately 8 hours Irritating to skin, eyes May cause metabolic acidosis Causes nausea and vomiting Flammable	*Protect eyes by keeping them closed.* *Expect nausea and vomiting—turn head to side to prevent aspiration of vomitus.* *Practice safeguards in view of flammability.*
2. *Halothane* (Fluothane)	Inhalation; special vaporizer	Not explosive or flammable Induction rapid and smooth Useful in almost every type of surgery Low incidence of postoperative nausea and vomiting	Requires skillful administration to prevent overdosage Has caused liver damage in a few cases May produce hypotension (low blood pressure) Requires special vaporizer for administration	*In addition to observing pulse and respiration postoperatively, it is important that blood pressure be determined frequently.*
3. *Methoxyflurane* (Penthrane)	Inhalation; special vaporizer	Nonflammable Seldom causes postoperative nausea and vomiting Analgesic action continues several hours after surgery Excellent muscle relaxation	Requires skillful administration Renal damage may occur	*Prolonged postoperative depressant action calls for careful observation by recovery room personnel.*
4. *Enflurane* (Ethrane)	Inhalation	Rapid induction and recovery Potent analgesic Nonflammable and nonexplosive	Respiratory depression may develop rapidly along with EEG abnormalities	*Observe for possible respiratory depression.*

ADVANTAGES. Methoxyflurane is nonflammable and provides excellent muscular relaxation as well as anesthesia. Induction and emergence from anesthesia are slow when compared with other inhalation agents. For this reason, the anesthetic can be terminated up to a half hour before the operation ends.

DISADVANTAGES. There is evidence that renal damage has resulted from the use of methoxyflurane. In some cases, renal damage has persisted for many months. When very ill patients have been given methoxyflurane, recovery has been accompanied by shivering. Nausea and vomiting occur, but to a lesser degree than is seen following ether or cyclopropane.

Because of the renal toxicity noted above, methoxyflurane is rarely used.

Enflurane (Ethrane)

Enflurane is a fluorinated hydrocarbon.

ADVANTAGES. Similar to halothane in its advantages, enflurane is nonflammable and is a good muscle relaxant. Induction and recovery are rapid.

DISADVANTAGES. Respiratory depression may develop rapidly, along with EEG abnormalities. Analgesia could be better.

INHALATION GASEOUS ANESTHETICS

The main gases used as agents for general anesthesia are nitrous oxide and cyclopropane (Table 18-4). It might be well to note at this point that to avoid confusion in identifying containers holding the various gases used in a

TABLE 18-4.   GASES AS AGENTS OF GENERAL ANESTHESIA

AGENT	ADMINISTRATION	ADVANTAGES	DISADVANTAGES	IMPLICATIONS
1. *Nitrous oxide* (N_2O)	Inhalation (semi-closed method)	Induction and recovery rapid Nonflammable Useful with oxygen for short procedures Useful with other agents for all types of surgery	Poor relaxant Weak anesthetic May produce hypoxia	*Most useful in conjunction with other agents.*
2. *Cyclopropane* (C_3H_6)	Inhalation (closed method)	Good relaxant Useful in all types of surgery	Explosive Powerful depressant; therefore should be administered skillfully Frequently produces disturbances in heart rhythm May cause broncho-spasm	*Employ precautions against explosions.* *Because cyclopropane may be followed by hypotension, it is important to observe blood pressure postoperatively.*

hospital, the Division of Simplified Practices of the National Bureau of Standards, Washington, D.C. has recommended the following color markings for tanks containing these gases:

Oxygen . . . . green
Carbon dioxide . . . . gray
Nitrous oxide . . . . light blue
Cyclopropane . . . . orange
Helium . . . . brown
Ethylene . . . . red
Carbon dioxide & oxygen . . . gray and green
Helium & oxygen . . . . brown and green

Nitrous Oxide

This general anesthetic causes the least disturbance of bodily function if it is given with a concentration of oxygen not less than that of air (21 percent).

ADVANTAGES. The onset of and emergence from anesthesia are rapid and usually uneventful. Therefore, nitrous oxide is useful for short procedures on outpatients. It has a fairly pleasant smell, is nonexplosive, and can be used with the electrocautery.

DISADVANTAGES. Nitrous oxide is a weak anesthetic. Its lack of potency can be overcome by adequate preanesthetic medication or by supplementation with an anesthetic vapor, such as ether, or an intravenous barbiturate or narcotic. Without these, if nitrous oxide alone is used for induction, it may be necessary to reduce the oxygen to 10 percent or less. This is dangerous in any individual particularly those suffering from heart or lung disease or anemia.

Cyclopropane

Cyclopropane is much more potent than nitrous oxide or ethylene and can produce anesthesia in concentrations of 15 to 20 percent. The remainder of the anesthetic mixture will consist of oxygen; therefore, a more than adequate supply of oxygen should be available at all times.

ADVANTAGES. Cyclopropane is relatively nonirritating. It is a powerful depressant to breathing.

DISADVANTAGES. Frequently, marked disorders of heart rate and rhythm occur during cyclopropane anesthesia. These increase with respiratory depression and deepening of anesthesia.

EXPLOSIBILITY

Flammable agents are being used less and less and, in fact, have been abandoned in many hospitals. However, whenever these agents are used, the hazard of explosion is always present. Although such accidents are extremely rare, special precautions are required, as is indicated in the chart on page 329.

NEUROMUSCULAR BLOCKERS (MUSCLE RELAXANTS)

Neuromuscular blockers interfere with the passage of impulses from the motor nerve to the skeletal muscle. Muscle relaxants make it possible to give a lighter degree of anesthesia since a less potent anesthetic agent can be used at a reduced dosage. Purified curare was the first widely used muscle relaxant; tubocurarine was isolated as the active principle. Since then, succinylcholine has been introduced because it acts more rapidly than curare. The full effect of a dose occurs in 60 to 90 seconds after administration and persists for 1 to 2 minutes. Return to normal occurs in about 3 to 5 minutes. Serious depression of respiration may occur if the dose that is given is too great; thus careful observation of breathing is of great importance. Newer relaxants are pancuronium (Pavulon) and gallamine (Flaxedil).

PRECAUTIONS FOR FLAMMABLE ANESTHETICS

Equipment: Containers of flammable liquids, gas cylinders, and anesthesia machines should be stored in a well ventilated place away from heat sources.
Oil or grease should never be applied to equipment, since they may be ignited by oxidizing gases under pressure.

Atmosphere: Good ventilation is effective in reducing accumulation of explosive concentrations of anesthetic gases. Air conditioning does not offer complete protection.

Ignition Sources:

1. Lighted cigarettes or flames of any sort (striking a match) are prohibited, as are electrocautery procedures when flammable gases are being used.
2. The current National Electrical Code of NFPA and local fire codes and regulations must be followed, including:
   a. Explosion-proof motors, switches, housings, and outlets
   b. Grounded conduits
   c. Heavy duty cords with grounded wires
3. Any potential for static sparks must be reduced in areas where flammable anesthetics are used.
   a. Conductive flooring, equipment and footwear should be used.
   b. Conductive floors must be kept clean and free from dirt, wax, blood, grease. (These elements impair conductivity.)
   c. Flooring should be tested periodically for conductivity.
   d. Wool blankets and loose-hanging silk, nylon, and other synthetics are not to be used. (These fabrics may be worn provided that they are in contact with the skin and beneath outer cotton garments. Nylon stockings are permissible since they are in close contact with the skin.)
   e. Humidity should be kept at 50% or higher.
   f. Gas machines are not to be covered with dust protectors, since such covers may generate a spark when removed.
   g. Adhesive tape should not be placed on the wall or anywhere else, since tape may set off a spark when removed.
   h. Adhesive tape should not be unrolled or torn near the patient on the operating table.
   i. No one should touch the patient in the vicinity of the breathing mask since such action may set off a spark.

INTRAVENOUS BARBITURATE ANESTHESIA

General anesthesia also can be produced by the intravenous injection of various substances such as thiopental (Table 18-5). A short-acting barbiturate, thiopental sodium (Pentothal) is the most commonly used anesthetic for this purpose. This substance leads to unconsciousness within 30 seconds.

ADVANTAGES. The onset of anesthesia is pleasant; there is none of the buzzing, roaring, or dizziness known to follow administration of an inhalation anesthetic. For this reason induction of anesthesia with an intravenous agent is preferred by patients who have experienced various methods. The duration of action is brief, and the patient awakens with little nausea or vomiting. Thiopental often is given with other anesthetic agents in prolonged procedures.

Intravenous anesthesia has the advantage of being nonexplosive, of requiring little equipment, and of being easy to administer. The low incidence of postoperative nausea and vomiting makes the method useful in eye surgery, in which retching endangers vision in the operated eye. It is useful for short procedures, but is used less often for abdominal surgery. It is not indicated for chil-

TABLE 18-5.   INTRAVENOUS BARBITURATE AS AN AGENT OF GENERAL ANESTHESIA

AGENT	ADMINISTRATION	ADVANTAGES	DISADVANTAGES	IMPLICATIONS
Thiopental sodium (Pentothal)	Intravenous injection	Rapid induction Nonexplosive Requires little equipment Low incidence of postoperative nausea and vomiting	Powerful depressant of breathing Poor relaxant Sometimes produces coughing, sneezing, and laryngospasm Not useful for children because of small veins	*Requires intelligent and close observation because of potency and rapidity of drug action.*

dren, who have small veins and who are more susceptible to respiratory obstruction. The reasons in both instances are apparent.

DISADVANTAGES. Thiopental is a powerful depressant of breathing, and its chief danger lies in this characteristic. It should be administered by skilled anesthesiologists and nurse anesthetists and only when some method of giving oxygen is available immediately should trouble arise. Sneezing, coughing, and laryngospasm are sometimes noted.

SPINAL ANESTHESIA

It must never be forgotten that the patient under spinal, regional, or local anesthesia is awake and aware of his surroundings. Careless conversation, unnecessary noise, unpleasant odors—all are noticed by the patient on the operating table and reflect discredit on the operating room staff. Quiet must be insisted upon. The diagnosis must not be made aloud if the patient is not to be made aware of it at this time.

Anesthesia of the lower extremities, abdomen, and even of the chest may be induced by the introduction of anesthetic drugs into the subarachnoid space (Fig. 18-2). A spinal puncture is made, with sterile precautions, and the drug is injected in solution through the needle. As soon as the injection has been made, the patient is placed on his back. If a relatively high level of block is desired, the head and the shoulders are lowered, depending on the height of anesthesia desired. In a few minutes anesthesia and paralysis appear, first of the toes and the perineum and then gradually of the legs and the abdomen. The drugs generally used are procaine, tetracaine (Pontocaine), and lidocaine (Xylocaine) Table 18-6).

ADVANTAGES. Spinal anesthesia is easy to administer, is inexpensive, and requires a minimum of equipment. The anesthesia produced is rapid in onset, and there is excellent muscular relaxation. The patient may remain awake, if that is desirable. It is a relatively safe anesthesia in experienced hands. Mortality figures compare favorably with those of the safer general anesthetics.

DISADVANTAGES. Soon after the administration of the drug there may be a marked fall in blood pressure, caused by paralysis of the vasomotor nerves. This phenomenon is noted most often when the anesthesia ascends to the upper abdomen and chest. The preoperative administration of drugs such as ephedrine or phenylephrine (Neosynephrine) may prevent this marked decrease in blood pressure. Inhalation of oxygen, intravenous administration of saline or plasma, and the injection of stimulant drugs such as ephedrine or phenylephrine, are of value once blood pressure has fallen.

Nausea, vomiting, and pain may occur during surgery under spinal anesthesia. As a rule, these reactions result from traction on various structures, particularly those within the abdominal cavity. Such reactions may be avoided by the simultaneous intravenous administration of a weak solution of thiopental and inhalation of nitrous oxide.

When the anesthetic drug reaches the upper thoracic and cervical cord in high concentration, a temporary, partial, or complete respiratory paralysis may occur. This complication is treated by maintaining artificial respiration until the effects of the drug on the respiratory nerves have worn off.

Such postoperative complications as headache, paralysis, or meningitis may occur; the latter two now are extremely rare. Several factors are involved in the incidence of headache: the size of the spinal needle used, the leakage of fluid from the subarachnoid space through the puncture site, and the degree of the patient's hydration. Any measure that can increase cerebrospinal pressure is

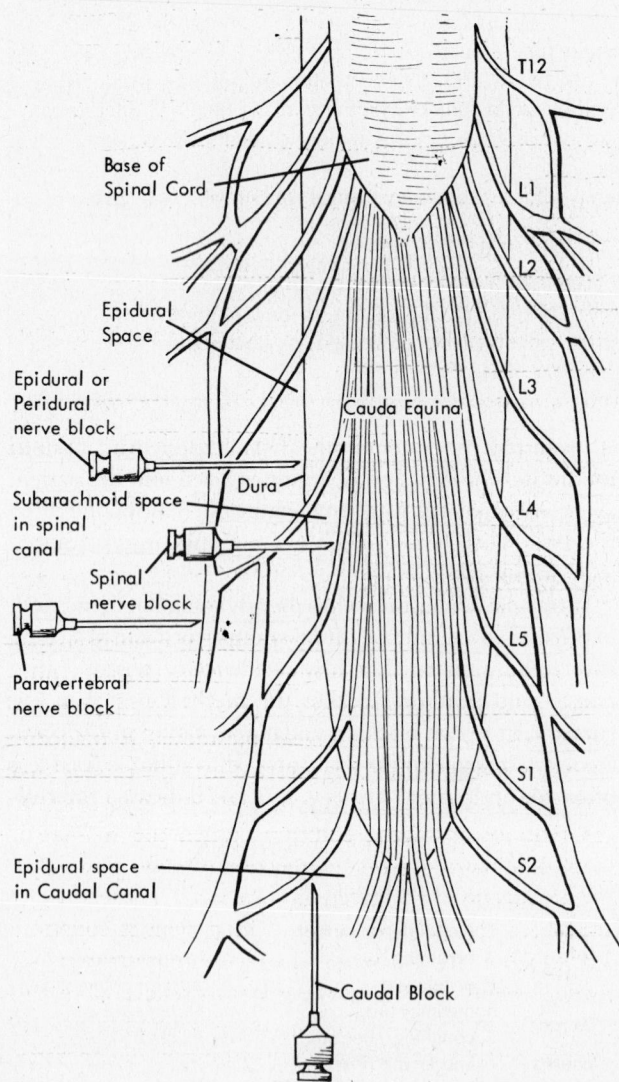

T12

Base of
Spinal Cord

L1

L2

Epidural
Space

L3

Cauda Equina

Epidural or
Peridural
nerve block

Subarachnoid space
in spinal
canal

Dura

L4

Spinal
nerve block

L5

Paravertebral
nerve block

S1

Epidural space
in Caudal Canal

S2

Caudal Block

Figure 18-2. Sites of injection for spinal, epidural, and paravertebral anesthesia, showing position of needle for the several types. Letters indicate vertebral level of injection. (Injections for paravertebral anesthesia may be made at any level.)

TABLE 18-6. SPINAL ANESTHESIA

AGENT	ADVANTAGES OF SPINAL ANESTHESIA (INCLUDES ALL AGENTS)	DISADVANTAGES OF SPINAL ANESTHESIA (INCLUDES ALL AGENTS)
Procaine (Novocaine)	Easily administered by a physician	Blood pressure may fall rapidly unless watched carefully and treated with such drugs as ephedrine, etc.
Tetracaine (Pontocaine)	Inexpensive	
Dibucaine (Nupercaine)	Minimum of equipment required	
Xylocaine (Lidocaine)	Rapid onset	If the spinal anesthesia ascends to the chest, there may be respiratory difficulties.
	Excellent muscular relaxation	Occasionally, postoperative complications occur, such as headache; rarely, meningitis or paralysis.

helpful in relieving headache. These include keeping the patient flat and quiet, providing body hydration, applying a tight abdominal binder, and injecting fluid into the epidural space.

Nursing Assessment After Spinal Anesthesia

In addition to taking the blood pressure, the nurse should observe these patients closely and record the time when motion and sensation return in the legs and the toes. When there is complete return of sensation in the toes (in response to pin-prick) the patient may be considered to have recovered from the effects of the spinal drug.

"Serial" or Continuous Spinal Anesthesia

The tip of a plastic catheter may be left in the subarachnoid space during operation, so that more anesthetic may be injected as needed. Greater control of dosage is afforded by this technique. However, there is greater potential for postanesthetic headache because of the large gauge needle used.

Epidural or Peridural Anesthesia

This anesthesia is obtained by the injection of a local anesthetic into the spinal canal in the space surrounding the dura mater (Fig. 18-2). Interest in this approach has increased because of a desire to find a method of anesthesia without undesirable neurologic sequelae, notably headache, that occasionally result from subarachnoid injection.

Advantages of epidural anesthesia appear to be the absence of neurologic complications and slightly less disturbance of blood pressure. One disadvantage lies in the greater technical problem of introducing the anesthetic into the epidural rather than the subarachnoid space. Another is that the level of anesthesia is less controllable.

REGIONAL ANESTHESIA

Regional anesthesia is a form of local anesthesia in which an anesthetic agent is injected into or around nerves so that the area supplied by these nerves is anesthetized. The effect depends on the type of nerve involved. Motor fibers are the largest and have the thickest myelin sheath. Sympathetic fibers are the smallest and have a minimal covering. Sensory fibers are intermediary. Thus a local anesthetic blocks motor nerves least readily and sympathetic nerves most readily. An anesthetic cannot be regarded as having "worn off" until all three systems (motor, sensory, and autonomic) are no longer affected by the anesthetic. There are many types of regional anesthesia, depending upon the various nerve groups that are injected.

Brachial Plexus Block

A brachial plexus block produces anesthesia of the arm.

Paravertebral Anesthesia

Paravertebral anesthesia produces anesthesia of the nerve supplying the chest, abdominal wall, and the extremities.

Transsacral (Caudal) Block

A transsacral block produces anesthesia of the perineum and, occasionally, the lower abdomen.

An addition to obstetric anesthesia has been an adaptation of the caudal block analogous to the change from a single-injection spinal to a serial spinal. This adaptation is called *continuous* or *serial caudal* anesthesia. A malleable needle or plastic catheter is inserted into the caudal canal and is allowed to remain in place, attached by a tube to a reservoir of anesthetic solution. When the woman in labor complains of pain, an injection is made, and subsequent injections are given as indicated. These may be continued for 20 to 30 hours. The patient is conscious during labor, and the fetus is spared the depression caused when general anesthetics are given to relieve labor discomfort. The mechanism of labor is changed somewhat by this method. The second stage is longer, and operative deliveries are more frequent. The method is not entirely without harm. Infections have occurred at the site of the injection. The level of anesthesia may become too high, and respiratory and circulatory difficulties may follow. A drop in blood pressure can endanger the fetus. Convulsions can occur as a result of absorption of the local anesthetic into the bloodstream, hence the nurse should report at once any marked restlessness, anxiety, tremor or twitching. Lumbar epidural anesthesia is now frequently used for the first and second stages of labor, supplanting the caudal technique.

LOCAL INFILTRATION ANESTHESIA

Infiltration anesthesia is the injection of a solution containing the local anesthetic into the tissues through which the incision is to pass. Often it is combined with a local regional block by injection of nerves immediately supplying that area. Local anesthesia is popular for several reasons:

(1) It is simple, economical, and nonexplosive. The amount of equipment is minimal. Postoperative care is lessened.
(2) Undesirable effects of general anesthesia are avoided.
(3) It is ideal for short and superficial operations.

In operations upon the abdominal viscera, complete anesthesia is not obtained by infiltration or local block of the anterior abdominal wall, because the viscera are supplied by nerves that have not been affected by the anesthetic. For this reason, a separate injection must be made into the region of the splanchnic nerves which supply the abdominal organs, except those of the pelvis. This injection may be made from the back (posterior-splanchnic anesthesia), or anteriorly, after the abdomen is opened.

Local anesthesia is often administered in combination with epinephrine. Epinephrine causes constriction of blood vessels, which prevents rapid absorption of the anesthetic drug and thus prolongs its local action; absorption into the bloodstream, which could cause convulsions, is also prevented.

Contraindications for Local Anesthesia

Local anesthesia is the anesthesia of choice in any operation in which it can be used. However, it is contraindicated for operations upon highly nervous, apprehensive patients. The emotional trauma experienced by these individuals during local anesthesia may be harmful. A patient who begs to be put to sleep rarely does well under local anesthesia.

For some kinds of operations, local anesthesia is impractical because of the number of injections and the amount of anesthetic required, for example, in a radical mastectomy.

Technique of Local Anesthesia

The technique for the introduction of local infiltration requires few materials. For the ordinary case the following are all that are needed:

1. Solution of local anesthetic in various concentrations (0.5–2.0 percent)
2. Sterile beaker or medicine glass
3. Sterile syringes and needles to fit
4. Sterile sponges and drape

The skin is prepared as for any operation, and a small-gauge needle is used to inject a little of the anesthetic into the skin layers. This produces blanching or a wheal. The anesthetic then is carried ahead of the needle in the skin until an area as long as the proposed incision is anesthetized. A larger, longer needle then is used to infiltrate deeper tissues with the anesthetic. The action of the drug is almost immediate, so that the operation may begin as soon as the injection is finished. Anesthesia lasts anywhere from ¾ hour to 3 hours depending upon the anesthetic and the use of epinephrine.

Lidocaine (Xylocaine)

Lidocaine has achieved wide usage because of rapid onset of action, freedom from local irritative effect, and longer duration of action as compared with procaine (Table 18-7). Lidocaine frequently is used intravenously to treat ventricular arrhythmias such as premature ventricular contractions and ventricular tachycardia. It may be given intravenously to depress the cough reflex; this permits patients to tolerate endotracheal tubes and oral airways at lighter planes of anesthesia.

Mepivacaine (Carbocaine)

Mepivacaine is most similar to lidocaine. It is found to act equally fast but to increase the duration of anesthesia by approximately 20 percent. Tissue irritation appears to be minimal.

Procaine (Novocaine)

Procaine is the least toxic of the local anesthetics. It is used in ½ and 1 percent solutions, and as much as 1 gm. may be injected without toxic effects over a period of an hour, if the injection rate is slow. It has supplanted cocaine for general use (see Table 18-7).

ADVANTAGES. Procaine may be sterilized by heat, is only slightly toxic, and produces anesthetic effects sufficiently potent for all ordinary requirements, but of relatively brief duration. In many places this drug is no longer used, having been supplanted by lidocaine (Xylocaine).

Tetracaine (Pontocaine) and Bupivacaine (Marcaine)

The chief use of *tetracaine* is for spinal anesthesia, the advantage being that it can give up to 2 hours of anesthesia.

Bupivacaine is more potent and has a longer action time than lidocaine or mepivacaine; however, the onset may be somewhat slower (see Table 18-7).

TABLE 18-7. LOCAL ANESTHETIC AGENTS

AGENT	ADMINISTRATION AND ACTION	ADVANTAGES	DISADVANTAGES	IMPLICATIONS
Lidocaine (Xylocaine) and *mepivacaine* (Carbocaine)	Topical or injection	Rapid Longer duration of action (compared with procaine) Free from local irritative effect	Occasional idiosyncrasy	*Useful topically for cystoscopy Injected for use in dental work and surgery*
Bupivacaine (Marcaine)	Parenteral	Duration is 2-3 times longer than lidocaine or mepivacaine	Use cautiously in persons with known drug allergies or sensitivities	*A period of analgesia persists after return of sensation; therefore need for strong analgesics is reduced*
Procaine (Novocaine)	Solution, ½, 1, or 2% subcut., IM, IV, or spinal	Low toxicity Inexpensive	Some idiosyncrasy Skin rash	*Usually given with epinephrine, causing vasoconstriction, thereby slowing absorption and prolonging nerve-deadening effect*

ARTIFICIAL HYPOTENSION DURING OPERATION

There are times during surgery when it is desirable to lower blood pressure in order to reduce bleeding at the operative site, since this allows for more rapid surgery with less blood loss. In such operations as brain surgery, radical neck dissection, and radical pelvic surgery, artificially induced hypotension has been used.

Deliberate hypotension is accomplished by inhalation or intravenous injection of drugs that affect the sympathetic nervous system and peripheral smooth muscle. Halothane is the inhalational anesthetic agent commonly used. This anesthetic is supplemented with other measures to lower blood pressure, such as a head-up position, positive pressure applied to the airway, and administration of a ganglionic blocking drug such as pentolinium (Ansolysen) or sodium nitroprusside.

MALIGNANT HYPERTHERMIA OCCURRING DURING GENERAL ANESTHESIA

Instances of severe hyperthermia during surgery have been reported in which the temperature has reached over 43.3° C. (110° F.). The mortality rate is approximately 60 to 70 percent. Reasons for the phenomenon are related to a biochemical disturbance in skeletal muscle involving calcium distribution. However, careful monitoring can anticipate and sometimes minimize the increase in temperature. When hyperthermia occurs, the anesthetic is discontinued and the operation is halted.

Measures to combat the temperature rise include use of a hypothermia blanket, infusion of iced saline solution, and administration of high concentrations of oxygen and sodium bicarbonate to combat metabolic acidosis. These methods require monitoring: electrocardiogram, temperature probe, placement of arterial and central venous lines, and bladder catheterization.

POSITION ON OPERATING TABLE

The position in which the patient is placed on the operating table depends upon the operation to be performed as well as the physical condition of the patient (Fig. 18-3). Factors to consider include:

1. The patient should be in as comfortable a position as possible, whether asleep or awake.
2. The operative area must be adequately exposed.
3. Circulation should not be obstructed by an awkward position or undue pressure on a part.
4. There should be no interference with the patient's respiration as a result of pressure of the arms on the chest or constriction of the neck or chest caused by a gown.
5. Nerves must be protected from undue pressure. Improper positioning of the arms, hands, legs, or feet may cause serious injury or paralysis. Shoulder braces must be well padded to prevent irreparable nerve injury, especially when the Trendelenburg position is necessary.
6. Concern for the patient as an individual must be practiced, particularly with the very thin, the elderly, or the obese patient.
7. Every patient needs *gentle* restraint before induction, in case of excitement.

DORSAL RECUMBENT POSITION. The usual position is flat on the back; one arm is at the side of the table, with the hand placed palm down; the other is carefully posi-

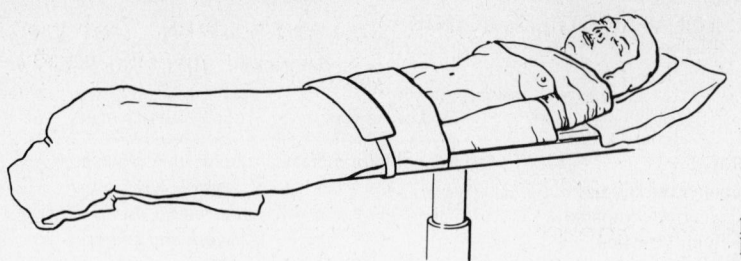

(Left) Patient in position on the operating table as prepared for a laparotomy. Note the strap above the knees.

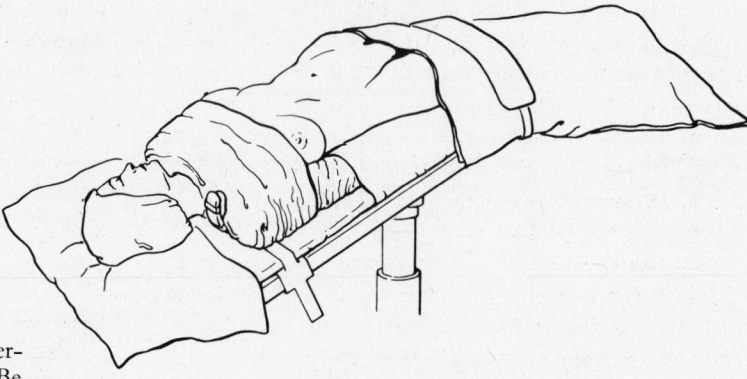

(Right) Patient in Trendelenburg position on operating table. Note padded shoulder braces in place. Be sure that brace does not press on brachial plexus.

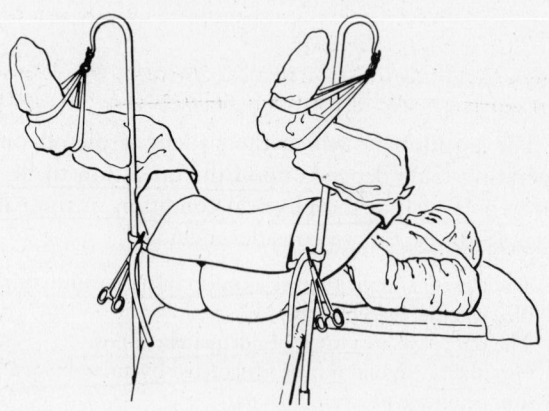

(Left) Patient in lithotomy position. Note that the hips extend over the edge of the table.

(Right) Patient on operating table for kidney operation, lying on his well side. Table is broken to spread apart space between the lower ribs and the pelvis. The upper leg is extended; the lower leg is flexed at the knee and the hip joints; a pillow is placed between the legs. Note the sandbag, which helps to support patient's chest.

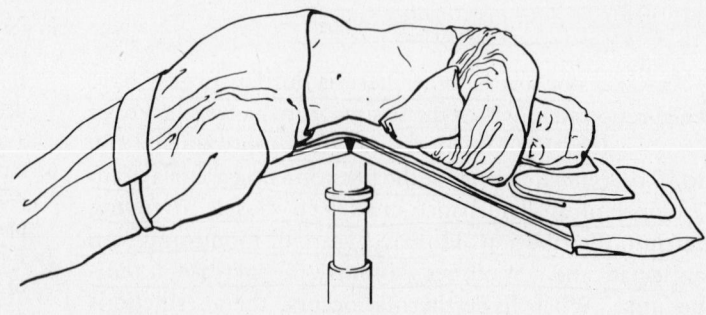

Figure 18-3.   Positions on the operating table.

334

tioned on an armboard for intravenous infusion (Fig. 18-3). This position is used for most abdominal operations, except for those upon the gallbladder and the pelvis and for the operations described below.

TRENDELENBURG POSITION. This position usually is employed for operations on the lower abdomen and the pelvis in order to obtain good exposure by displacing the intestines into the upper abdomen. In this position the head and body are lowered, so that the plane of the body meets the horizontal at an angle. The knees are flexed by "breaking" the table, and the patient is held in position by padded shoulder braces (Fig. 18-3).

LITHOTOMY POSITION. In this position the patient is lying on his back with the legs and thighs flexed at right angles. The position is maintained by placing the feet in stirrups. Nearly all perineal, rectal, and vaginal operations require this posture (Fig. 18-3).

FOR KIDNEY OPERATIONS. The patient is placed on his well side in Sims's position with an air pillow 12.5-15 cm. (5 or 6 inches) thick under the loin, or he is placed on a table with a kidney or back lift (Fig. 18-3).

FOR CHEST AND ABDOMINOTHORACIC OPERATIONS. The position varies with the operation to be performed. The surgeon and the anesthesiologist place the patient on the operating table in the proper position.

OPERATIONS ON THE NECK. Such operations, for example, those involving the thyroid, are performed with the patient on his back, the neck extended somewhat by a pillow beneath the shoulders and the head and chest elevated, in order to reduce venous pressure.

OPERATIONS ON THE SKULL AND THE BRAIN. Such procedures demand special positions and apparatus, usually adjusted by the surgeon.

BIBLIOGRAPHY

BOOKS

Anesthesia

Aldrete, J. A., et al., eds.: Low Flow and Closed System Anesthesia. New York, Grune and Stratton, 1979.

Collins, V. J.: Principles of Anesthesiology, 2nd ed. Philadelphia, Lea and Febiger, 1976.

Dripps, R. D., et al.: Introduction to Anesthesia, 5th ed. Philadelphia, W. B. Saunders, 1977.

Lichtiger, M., and Moya, F.: Introduction to the Practice of Anesthesia. Hagerstown, Md., Harper and Row, 1978.

ARTICLES

A plea for moderation in anesthesia standards. AORN J., 26:1025, Dec. 1977.

deJong, R.: Toxic effects of local anesthetics. JAMA, 239:1166-1168, Mar. 20, 1978.

OR Standards: Standards for cleaning and processing anesthesia equipment. AORN J., 25:1268-1270, June 1977.

Ozuna, J. M., and Foster, C.: Hypothermia and the surgical patient. AJN, 79:646-648, Apr. 1979.

Smith, B. J.: Safeguarding your patient after anesthesia. Nursing '78, 8:53-56, Oct. 1978.

White, M. J., and Wolf-Wilets, V. C.: Memory loss following halothane anesthesia. AORN J., 26:1053-1064, Dec. 1977.

19

INTRAOPERATIVE NURSING MANAGEMENT

The center of attention and activity in the operating room is the patient who is undergoing a surgical procedure for the repair, correction, or relief of a physical problem. Although the immediate concern is physiological and its focus is on anatomical body structures, the psychological impact of the patient's condition has a tremendous effect on his behavior and requires careful consideration in planning nursing care.

Throughout the surgical experience, the nurse functions as the patient's chief advocate. The "caring" and concern of nursing management extends from the time when the patient is prepared for and instructed about the forthcoming surgery, through the more immediate preoperative period, into the operative phase and the recovery from anesthesia, and on through convalescence. Throughout this continuum, priority is given to the patient, his safety, his understanding of the care he is receiving, and the biophysical and psychosocial needs he is experiencing. Because the operation is usually a unique experience in the patient's life, he needs the security of knowing that someone is protecting his best interests at this time, especially when he is unable to make decisions for himself.

PERIOPERATIVE NURSING

To describe the wide variety of nursing functions associated with the patient's surgical experience, a relatively new descriptive phrase has been established —*perioperative nursing*. The word "perioperative" is an encompassing term that incorporates the three phases of the surgical experience —namely, preoperative, intraoperative, and postoperative. Each of these phases begins and ends at a

336

particular time in the sequence of events that constitute the surgical experience, and each includes a wide range of behaviors and nursing activities that the nurse performs using the nursing process as reflected in the standards of practice. (See Fig. 19-1 and the Chart on page 337.)

The *preoperative phase* of the perioperative nursing role begins when the decision for surgical intervention is made and ends with the transference of the patient to the operating room table. The scope of nursing activities during this time can be as broad as establishing a baseline assessment of the patient, in the clinical setting or at home, and carrying out a preoperative interview. Or it may be as limited as doing a preoperative patient assessment in the holding area or surgical suite.

The nursing functions included in the *intraoperative phase* of the perioperative role begin when the patient is transferred to the operating room table and end when he is admitted to the recovery area. In this phase, the scope of nursing activity can be as broad as providing for the patient's safety throughout the surgical procedure or as limited as positioning the patient on the operating room table according to basic principles of body alignment.

The *postoperative phase* of the perioperative nursing role begins with the admission of the patient to the recovery area and ends with a follow-up evaluation in the clinical setting or at home. The scope of nursing activities during this period may be as broad as assessing the postoperative status of the patient in terms of the effects of the anesthetic agents and the impact of surgery on body image, etc., as well as evaluating the family's perception of the surgery. Or it can be as limited as communicating pertinent information about the patient's surgery to personnel in the recovery area.

The whole spectrum of perioperative nursing func-

THE PERIOPERATIVE ROLE: A CONTINUUM

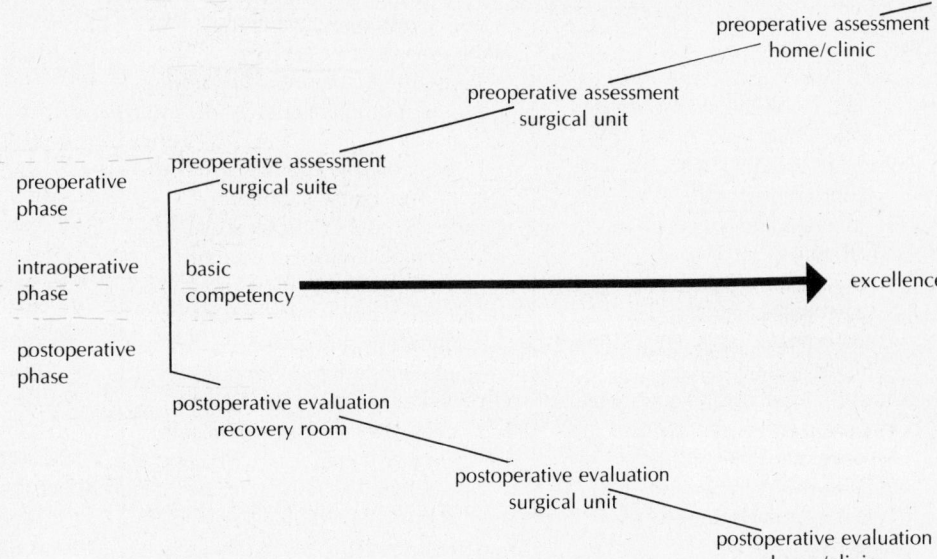

Figure 19-1. The perioperative role: A continuum. (From: Operating room nursing: Perioperative role, AORN Journal, *27*: May 1978)

tions, especially those related to meeting the life-sustaining needs of the surgical patient, has undergone extensive study and analysis by educators and practitioners associated with the AORN (Association of Operating Room Nurses). One result of this study was a resolution issued in 1973 listing the reasons for retaining registered nurses in the operating room. On the basis of knowledge, experience, and responsibility, these nurses are able to:

- Independently assess patient needs
- Make collaborative decisions relative to total intraoperative care
- Make decisions and take action in emergency situations
- Establish and maintain inter- and intradepartmental functioning for continuity of care
- Provide for and contribute to the patient's safety through control of his internal and external environment, biological testing, and product evaluation
- Assist the patient with the management of anxiety through the application of the principles of biological, physical, and social sciences
- Provide efficient patient care in the operating room through organizational skills, preoperative and postoperative visits, and sound principles of management
- Conduct and participate in research projects directed toward improvement of patient care through the application of scientific principles
- Control hospital costs through budget preparation and implementation
- Participate in architectural design of operating suites affecting efficiency and quality in patient care
- Participate in supervision and instruction of ancillary and allied health personnel in the operating room
- Evaluate and modify the quality of patient care within the operating room.*

*Necessity for the registered nurse in the operating room—Delegates approve statements. AORN J., *17*:188–189, Apr. 1973.

PRINCIPLES OF PERIOPERATIVE ASEPSIS

As was indicated earlier, in all phases of the surgical experience, the main priority for all personnel is patient safety—which includes protection of the patient from infection. Inherent in this goal is strict adherence to the practice of asepsis.

The successful practice of aseptic surgery requires the strict observance of rigorous standards for *preoperative* sterilization of surgical materials and of precautions against infection, both *during* the course of the operation, and *after* the operation, when the wound must be guarded until such time as it is healed.

To provide the best possible conditions for performing a surgical operation, the operating room is placed in a section of the hospital where it is free from such hazards as contaminating particles, dust, other pollutants, radiation, noise, etc. Strict building codes must be set and adhered to in the selection of materials for construction and in determining room size and air circulation patterns. Electrical hazards, conductivity checks, emergency exit clearances, and storage of equipment and anesthetic gases are checked periodically by the state and the Joint Commission for the Accreditation of Hospitals.

In surgical practice, asepsis is a tool designed to reduce to the barest minimum the contamination of surgical wounds. Although postoperative wound infection may be caused by natural skin flora or a previously existing infection, it is the responsibility of the personnel in the operating room to utilize aseptic principles to minimize this risk. These principles will be described and illustrated in detail in the pages which follow, in terms of the various protocols and practices to be carried out.

EXAMPLES OF NURSING ACTIVITIES IN THE PERIOPERATIVE ROLE

Preoperative Phase	Intraoperative Phase	Postoperative Phase

PREOPERATIVE ASSESSMENT
Home/clinic
  1. initiates initial preoperative assessment
  2. plans teaching methods appropriate to patient's needs
  3. involves family in interview
Surgical unit
  1. completes preoperative assessment
  2. coordinates patient teaching with other nursing staff
  3. explains phases in perioperative period and expectations
  4. develops a plan of care
Surgical suite
  1. assesses patient's level of consciousness
  2. reviews chart
  3. identifies patient
  4. verifies surgical site
PLANNING
  determines a plan of care
PSYCHOLOGICAL SUPPORT
  1. tells patient what is happening
  2. determines psychological status
  3. gives prior warning of noxious stimuli
  4. stands near/touches patient during procedures/induction
  5. communicates patient's emotional status to other appropriate members of the health care team
	MAINTENANCE OF SAFETY
	  1. assures that the sponge, needle, and instrument counts are correct
	  2. positions the patient
	    a. functional alignment
	    b. exposure of surgical site
	    c. maintenance of position throughout procedure
	  3. applies grounding device to patient
	  4. provides physical support
	PHYSIOLOGICAL MONITORING
	  1. calculates effects on patient of excessive fluid loss
	  2. distinguishes normal from abnormal cardiopulmonary data
	  3. reports changes in patient's pulse, respirations, temperature, and blood pressure
	PSYCHOLOGICAL MONITORING (PRIOR TO INDUCTION AND IF PATIENT CONSCIOUS)
	  1. provides emotional support to patient
	  2. continues to assess patient's emotional status
	  3. communicates patient's emotional status to other appropriate members of the health care team
	NURSING MANAGEMENT
	  1. provides physical safety for the patient
	  2. maintains aseptic, controlled environment
	  3. effectively manages human resources
		COMMUNICATION OF INTRAOPERATIVE INFORMATION
		  1. gives patient's name
		  2. states type of surgery performed
		  3. provides contributing intraoperative factors, i.e., drain, catheters
		  4. states physical limitations
		  5. states impairments resulting from surgery
		  6. reports patient's preoperative level of consciousness
		  7. communicates necessary equipment needs
		POSTOPERATIVE EVALUATION
		Recovery area
		  determines patient's immediate response to surgical intervention
		Surgical unit
		  1. evaluates effectiveness of nursing care in the OR
		  2. determines patient's level of satisfaction with care given during perioperative period
		  3. evaluates products used on patient in the OR
		  4. determines patient's psychological status
		  5. assists with discharge planning
		Home/clinic
		  1. seeks patient's perception of surgery in terms of the effects of anesthetic agents, impact on body image, distortion, immobilization
		  2. determines family's perception of surgery

(Source: Operating room nursing: Perioperative role. AORN Journal, *27*:May 1978)

Preoperative Protocol

Prior to the operation, all surgical material must be sterilized; this includes any instruments, needles, sutures, dressings, gloves, covers, etc. that may come in contact with the wound and exposed tissues. In addition, the surgeon, the surgical assistants, and the nurses must prepare themselves by scrubbing their hands and arms with soap and water ("scrubbing") and donning long-sleeved sterile gowns and gloves. Head and hair are covered with a cap, and a mask is worn over the nose and mouth to prevent bacteria from the upper respiratory tract from entering the wound. The patient's skin, over an area considerably larger than that requiring exposure during the course of the operation, also requires meticulous cleansing followed by the application of an antiseptic agent. The rest of the patient's body is covered with sterile drapes.

Intraoperative Protocol

During the operation, none of the personnel who have scrubbed touch anything that has not been sterilized. Nonscrubbed personnel refrain from touching or contaminating anything that is sterile.

Postoperative Protocol

After the operation, the wound is protected from possible infection by means of sterile dressings and by the use of antiseptics and sterile saline when the wound is cleansed and the dressings changed. Particular care is taken to protect the unhealed wound from coming in contact with anything that is not sterile. In wounds that become infected, it may be necessary to remove and destroy microorganisms that are already in the tissues by removing or "debriding" devitalized tissues. To prevent subsequent infection from without, rigid aseptic technique must be followed during the course of treatment.

When infection has already developed in tissues, antimicrobials specific for the offending organism are prescribed, and heat is applied and/or drainage established to assist the body in eliminating the offending organisms.

Environmental Controls

In addition to the above protocols, the implementation of aseptic principles requires meticulous housekeeping in the operating room. Floors and horizontal surfaces are cleaned frequently with detergent soap and water or detergent germicide, and sterilizing equipment is inspected regularly to assure optimum operation and performance. Although sterilization of linens is no longer done on the operating room floor (it may be done in central supply service, or prepackaged sterilized items may be used), instruments are cleaned and sterilized in a unit close to the operating room. The use of peel-apart individually wrapped sterile items has replaced the transfer forceps which was formerly used to transfer a sterile item from a stock container or table to the operating field, a procedure that carried a much greater danger of contamination.

Many operating rooms are equipped with laminar airflow systems which filter out a high percentage of dust and bacteria. Originally designed for spacecraft, these systems use high efficiency particulate air (HEPA) filters to remove more than 99 percent of airborne particles measuring 0.3 microns or more. Laminar flow also changes air more effectively—about 200 times an hour as compared with air conditioning, which exchanges air 12 times per hour.

Unfortunately, in spite of all these precautions, postoperative wound infections may occasionally occur during an operation, appearing days or weeks later in the form of an incisional infection or abscess.

- Constant surveillance and conscientiousness in carrying out aseptic practices must be stressed continually, since errors and misjudgment can occur as a result of human failure.

Basic Rules of Surgical Asepsis

General

- Sterile surfaces or articles may touch other sterile surfaces or articles and remain sterile; unsterile contact at any point renders a sterile area contaminated.
- If there is any doubt about the sterility of an article or area, it is considered unsterile.
- Whatever is sterile for one patient (an opened sterile tray or tables with sterile supplies) can be used for this patient only. Unused sterile supplies must be discarded or resterilized if they are to be used again.

Personnel

- Scrubbed personnel remain in the area of the operation; if a "scrubbed" person leaves the room, that person's "sterile" status is lost. To return to the operation, this person is required to go through the procedure of scrubbing, gowning, and gloving.

- Only a small part of a "scrubbed" person's body is considered sterile: from front waist to the shoulder area; forearms and gloves.
- Therefore the gloved hands must be kept in front and above the waistline.
- In some clinics, a special wraparound gown is worn which extends the sterile area.
- The "circulator" and any unscrubbed personnel remain on the periphery of the surgical operating area at a safe distance in order not to contaminate any sterile area.

Draping

- During draping of a table or patient, the sterile drape is held well above the surface to be covered and is placed from front to back.
- Only the top of the patient or table which is draped is considered sterile; drapes hanging over the edge are not regarded as sterile.
- Sterile drapes are to be kept in position by the use of clips or adherent material; drapes are not to be moved during the operation. A tear or puncture of the drape permitting access to an unsterile surface underneath renders the area unsterile.

Delivery of Sterile Supplies

- Packages are wrapped or sealed in such a way that they can be opened easily without risk of contaminating contents.
- Sterile supplies, including solutions, are delivered to a sterile field or handed to a "scrubbed" person in such a way that sterility of the object or fluid remains intact.
- Edges of wrappers covering sterile supplies or outer lips of bottles or flasks containing sterile solutions are not considered sterile.
- The unsterile arm of the "circulator" must not extend over a sterile area. Sterile articles are to be dropped at a reasonable distance from the edge of the sterile area.

Fluids

- Sterile fluids are poured from a point high enough to prevent accidental touching of the sterile receiving cup or basin, but not so high as to produce splashing (this may cause fluid to touch an unsterile surface and then flow back into the receptacle, causing contamination).

Principles Regarding Health and Operating Room Attire

Good health is essential for any person in the operating room. Colds, sore throats, and infected fingers are distinct sources of pathogenic organisms and must be reported. A series of wound infections in postoperative patients were traced in one instance to a mild throat infection in an operating room nurse. Therefore, the importance of reporting any seemingly slight ailment without delay can be readily understood.

1. **CLOTHING.** Street clothes are never worn in the operating room. Only approved clean operating room attire is permitted. Likewise, OR attire is not worn out of the operating room. Written policies describe the practice which all persons are required to follow. Dressing rooms are located near the operating suite and are reached from an outer corridor. Clothing is changed in the dress-

ing room before entering and upon leaving the operating room.

Close-fitting cotton dresses, pants suits, and jumpsuits are available in a variety of styles. When pants are worn, the ankles should have close-fitting cuffs (drawstring or knitted) to contain organisms shed from the perineum and leg. Shirts and waist drawstrings should be tucked inside the pants to prevent any accidental contact with sterile areas and again to contain skin sheddings. Fresh OR attire is put on each time the person enters the operating room; when this clothing is removed it is bagged and sent to the hospital laundry.

2. MASK. Masks are worn at all times in the operating room for the purpose of minimizing airborne contamination. Droplets containing microorganisms from the oropharynx and nasopharynx must be contained and filtered. Therefore the mask must not leak air. At the same time, it should not interfere with breathing or hinder speech or vision, and must be compact and comfortable. Forced expiration, such as that produced by talking, laughing, sneezing, and coughing, should be avoided, since it deposits additional organisms on the mask. Many effective disposable masks are available that have high filtration efficiency: 95+%. Tests prove their superiority over gauze masks.

Since the mask loses much of its effectiveness when it becomes moistened, it should be changed between operations and more often if necessary. The mask should be either on or off; it must not be allowed to hang around the neck. When the mask is removed, only the strings are handled in order to prevent contamination of the hands. Mask strings are tied snugly; top strings are tied at the back of the head and bottom strings are tied at the back of the neck.

3. HEADGEAR. Headgear should completely cover the hair (head and neckline), so that single strands of hair, bobbypins, clips, or particles of dandruff or dust do not fall on sterile fields. The styles of headgear available are disposable, lint-free, soft, and clothlike.

4. SHOES. Shoes should be comfortable and supportive; clogs, tennis shoes, sandals, and boots are not permitted because they are unsafe and difficult to clean. Shoes are covered with disposable or canvas shoe covers. Conductive covers establish an electrical ground for the wearer. The black strips provided with some conductive shoe covers should be placed inside the shoe in contact with the sole of the foot. Shoe covers are worn one time only and are removed upon leaving the restricted area. Conductometers are usually located at the entrance to the operating room area.

GUIDELINES: "SCRUBBING" FOR AN OPERATION

Action	Rationale
1. The nails are kept short and free of nail polish; special attention is given to the subungual space (beneath nail) with a sterile nail cleaner early in the scrub.	1. Scrubbing can cause nail polish to chip and peel; this would produce nicks in which microbes could breed.
2. A soft but firm-bristled brush or one of the numerous polyurethane disposable sponges which are impregnated with soap is used for scrubbing.	2. The brush or special sponge facilitates removal of dead skin, soil, and resident organisms.
3. There are many acceptable antiseptic detergents, such as the iodophors.	3. Broad-spectrum microbicidal solution is preferred where gram-negative nosocomial infections predominate.
4. Hands and arms must be well lathered and rinsed frequently. No chemical agent can be relied upon as a substitute for conscientious mechanical cleansing of the skin.	4. Microbes are removed by two actions: a. Physical mechanical separation b. Chemical antisepsis from action of antimicrobial solution
5. The duration of the scrub may be determined by setting a time limit for the conscientious scrubbing of one part after another in a prescribed manner, or by counting a certain number of strokes per part. A practical, reliable, and effective procedure should be followed. Because the moisture and warmth present under surgical gloves provide an ideal growing medium for bacteria, it is essential that a prescribed scrub be done between operations.	5. Individual conscientious attention to detail is important. Hospital policy is followed.
6. Following the scrub, hands and arms are rinsed thoroughly; soap and brush are left in sink or discarded in appropriate container. The elbow or the knee is used to turn the water off. Hands are held higher than the elbows and away from the body.	6. This allows water to run off at the elbow and prevents contaminated water from above the elbow from running down to the scrubbed hands.
7. When drying hands, care is taken to prevent the towel from touching the scrub dress or suit. One hand, then the arm, are dried with a towel, proceeding from fingertips to elbow; the other hand and arm are dried in similar fashion using a dry segment of the towel.	7. Proceeding from the fingertips to the elbow will prevent above-elbow sources of contamination from affecting scrubbed hands and lower arms.

After the hands and arms are scrubbed using an antiseptic detergent, a sterile gown and gloves are put on. These are worn to allow the wearer to participate in or observe the surgical operation while maintaining a state of asepsis in as practical a way as possible.

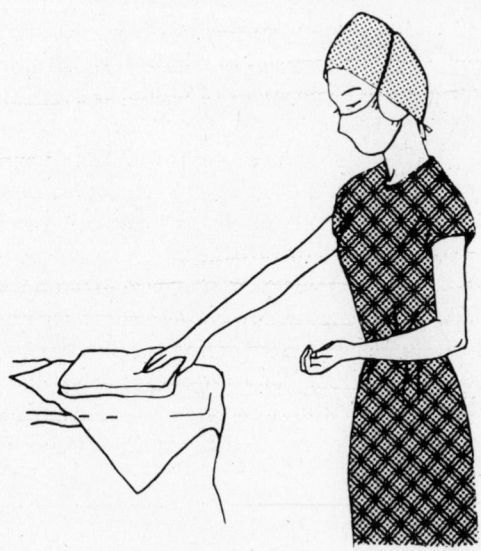

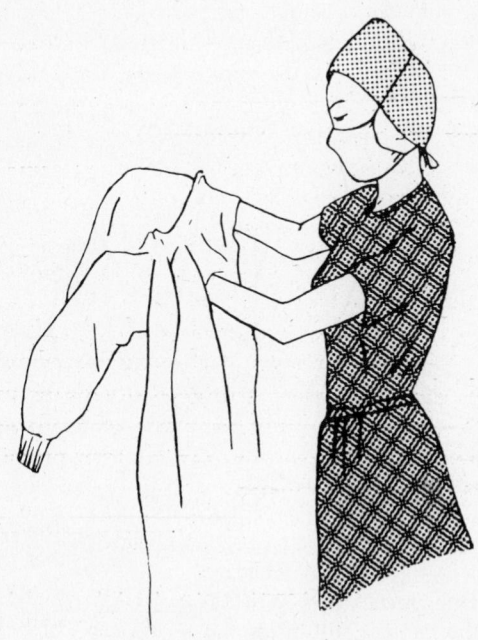

1. The sterile gown may be obtained from an open pack or it may be handed by someone already scrubbed.

2. Since gowns are folded inside out (to eliminate the need to touch the outside of the garment), the gown can be held by the neckband and allowed to unfold from the extended hands. As the gown unfolds, the armholes should face the wearer. The hands are held upward and slipped into the armholes—but only as far as the sleeve cuff.

3. The circulating nurse can assist by reaching inside the gown and pulling the sleeves over the hands. (Sleeves are pulled to the hands, not over them when the "closed glove technique" is to be used. See page 342.)

4. To secure the gown, the tapes at the back are tied. If the gown has tapes at the waist, the circulating nurse reaches for the ends of the tapes without touching the gown, draws the tapes back, and ties them. (Gowns may be fastened with Velcro, which eliminates the need for tapes.)

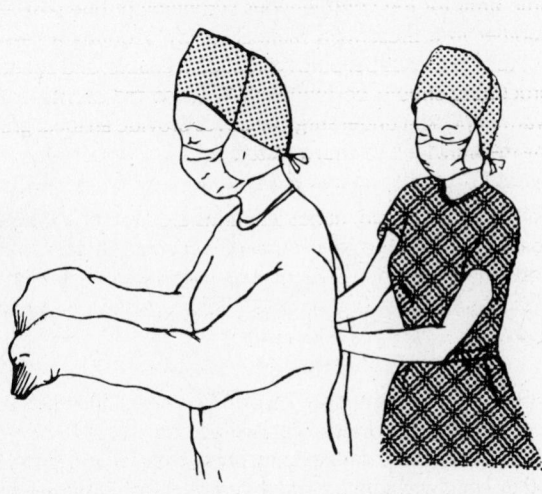

Note: A gown is sterile only as long as it is dry and not torn. If it is wet from perspiration or from any other cause, it must be considered contaminated.

When the gown is donned, the hands are slid into the sleeve only as far as the cuff seam, which is then grasped by the thumb and index finger through the fabric.

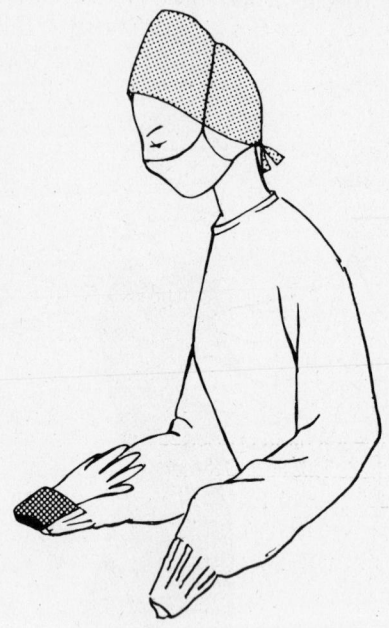

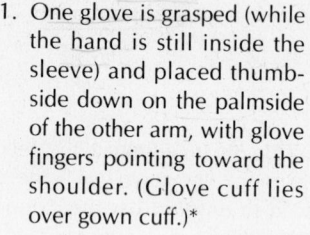

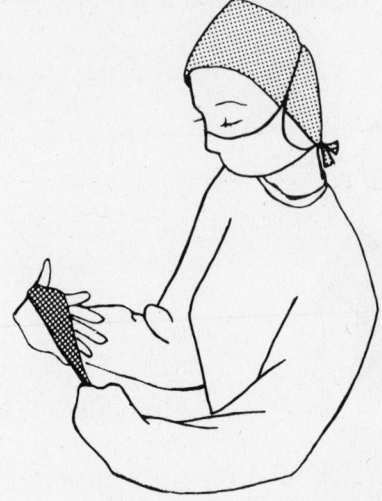

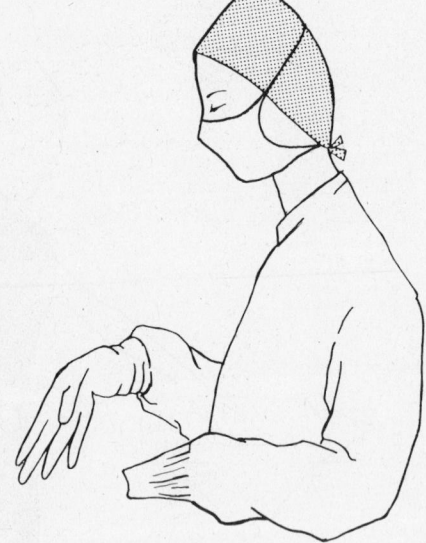

1. One glove is grasped (while the hand is still inside the sleeve) and placed thumb-side down on the palmside of the other arm, with glove fingers pointing toward the shoulder. (Glove cuff lies over gown cuff.)*

2. The wrist edge of the glove that is against the sleeve is grasped with the finger that holds the seam, and the uppermost glove wrist edge is grasped with the sleeve-covered fingers of the other hand.

3. The glove wrist is pulled over the gown cuff, care being taken not to fold the gown cuff back or to expose the fingers inside it.

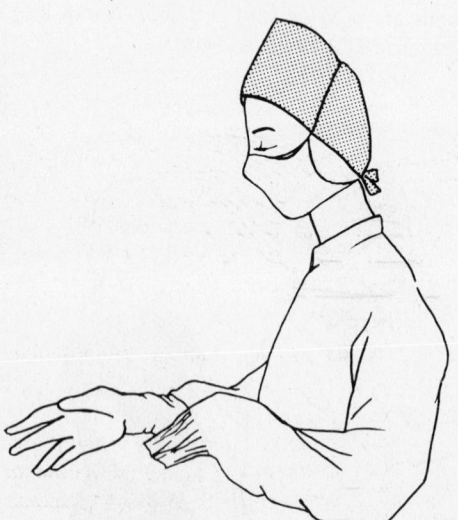

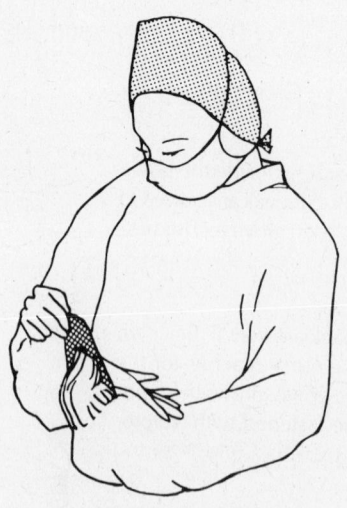

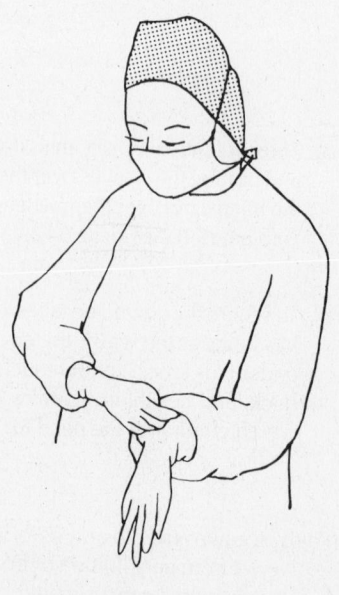

4. As cuff is drawn onto wrist, fingers are directed into cots in glove and the glove is adjusted to the hand.

5. The second glove is put on in the same manner, using the newly gloved hand to hold the glove.

*Shaded or crosshatched areas of the glove (representing the inside of glove) are considered unsterile.

PUTTING ON STERILE GLOVES: OPEN METHOD

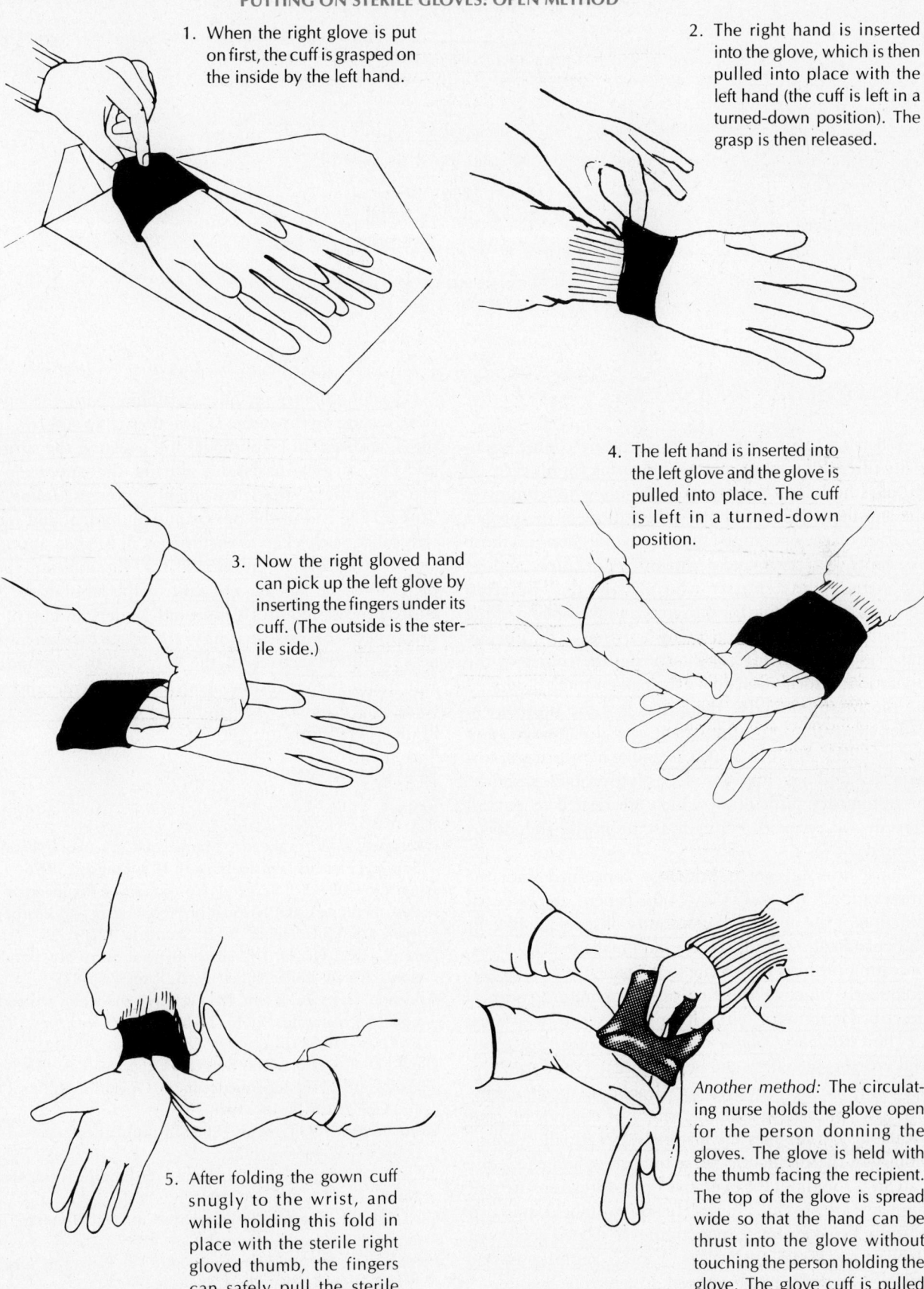

1. When the right glove is put on first, the cuff is grasped on the inside by the left hand.

2. The right hand is inserted into the glove, which is then pulled into place with the left hand (the cuff is left in a turned-down position). The grasp is then released.

3. Now the right gloved hand can pick up the left glove by inserting the fingers under its cuff. (The outside is the sterile side.)

4. The left hand is inserted into the left glove and the glove is pulled into place. The cuff is left in a turned-down position.

5. After folding the gown cuff snugly to the wrist, and while holding this fold in place with the sterile right gloved thumb, the fingers can safely pull the sterile glove cuff over the gown cuff.

Another method: The circulating nurse holds the glove open for the person donning the gloves. The glove is held with the thumb facing the recipient. The top of the glove is spread wide so that the hand can be thrust into the glove without touching the person holding the glove. The glove cuff is pulled up over the gown cuff.

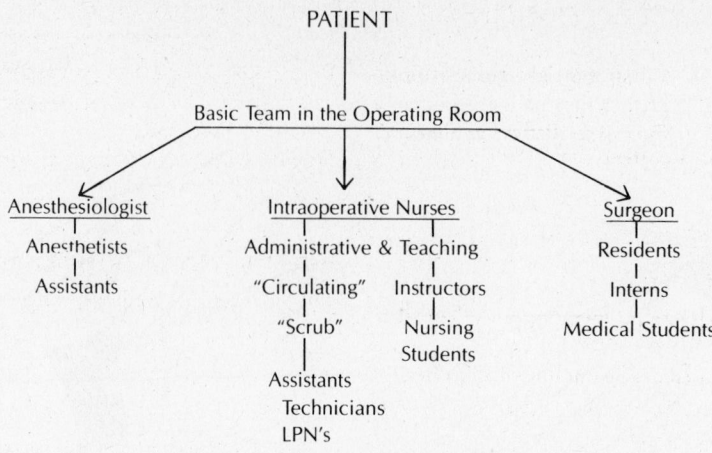

Figure 19-2. Basic operating room team.

INTRAOPERATIVE PATIENT CARE

When a patient arrives in the operating room, essentially three different groups are preparing for his care: (1) the anesthesiologist and those assistants who administer the anesthetic agent and place the patient in the proper position on the operating table, (2) the surgeon and those assistants who scrub and perform the operation, and (3) the intraoperative nurses who manage the operating room, are responsible for the safety and well-being of the patient, and coordinate the many activities of the operating personnel (see Fig. 19-2). During the course of the operation, information about the patient must be shared by the anesthesiologist, the nurse, and the surgeon, in order to assure optimum patient care. In addition, any pertinent developments such as undue hemorrhage, unexpected findings, fluid and electrolyte problems, shock, or respiratory difficulties, which are related to patient care in the recovery room must be noted and documented.

Since nursing care is primarily concerned with the observation, care, and safety of the patient, the essential function of the nurse is to constantly observe the patient and coordinate various services and management of the operating room as they relate to the patient's well-being. Frequently, nursing function in the operating room is described in terms of "circulating" and "scrub" activities.

The *"circulating" nurse* manages the operating room and protects the safety and health needs of the patient by assessing the environment for cleanliness, proper temperature, humidity, lighting, safety of equipment, and availability of supplies and materials. It is also the responsibility of the circulating nurse to observe and check the patient throughout the operative procedure to ensure that his needs are provided for and his rights upheld. It is also necessary to coordinate the activities of related personnel (laboratory, x-ray, medical, etc.) and to monitor aseptic practices in order to avoid breakdowns in technique.

"Scrub" activities include "scrubbing" for the operation, setting up the sterile tables, preparing sutures, ligatures, and special equipment, and assisting the surgeon and the surgical assistants during the operation by providing the required instruments, sponges, drains, etc. Toward the end of the operation, equipment and materials must be checked to ensure that all needles, sponges, and instruments are accounted for. In addition, specimens must be labeled and sent to the laboratory. The entire process requires a thorough understanding of the principles of asepsis, anatomy, and tissue care; an awareness of the objectives of the surgery; an aptitude for anticipating needs and working as a skilled member of a team; and the ability to handle any emergency situation in the operating room.

BIBLIOGRAPHY

BOOKS

Altemeier, W. A., et al., eds.: Manual on Control of Infection in Surgical Patients. Philadelphia, J. B. Lippincott, 1976.

American College of Surgeons Committee on Preoperative and Postoperative Care: Manual of Preoperative and Postoperative Care. Philadelphia, W. B. Saunders, 1977.

Artz, C., and Hardy, J.: Management of Surgical Complications, 3rd ed. Philadelphia, W. B. Saunders, 1975.

Atkinson, L. J., and Kohn, M. L.: Berry and Kohn's Introduction to Operating Room Technique, 5th ed. New York, McGraw-Hill, 1978.

Davis, D. L., et al.: The Surgical Experience: A Model for Professional Nursing Practice in the Operating Room. Denver, Col., AORN, Inc. 1978.

Gruendemann, B. J., et al.: The Surgical Patient, 2nd ed. St. Louis, C. V. Mosby, 1977.

———: Nursing Audit: Challenge to the Operating Room Nurse. Denver, Col., AORN, Inc. 1974.

Lach, J.: O.R. Nursing: Preoperative Care and Draping Technique. Chicago, The Kendall Co., 1974.

LeMaitre, G. D., and Finnegan, J. A.: The Patient in Surgery, 3rd ed. Philadelphia, W. B. Saunders, 1975.

Meshelany, C.: Infection Control Manual. Oradell, N. J., Med. Economics, 1977.

Metzger, R. S., and Robertson, P. A.: Intraoperative Learning. Denver, Col., AORN, Inc. 1977.

Rhodes, M. J., et al.: Alexander's Care of the Patient in Surgery, 6th ed. St. Louis, C. V. Mosby, 1978.

ARTICLES

General

AORN standards of nursing practice: Operating room. AORN J., *24*:798-808, Oct. 1976.

Brown, M. E.: Transfer of asepsis principles by students. AORN J., *27*:970-976, Apr. 1978.

Davis, L.: Bicentennial forecast: Operating room nursing. Surgical Team, *5*:34-37, Nov.-Dec. 1976.

Davis, J. E.: Why a mandate for the circulator? AORN J., *23*:1185-1193, June 1976.

Fay, M.: The challenge of operating room nursing. Nursing '77, *7*:98-100, Oct. 1977.

Gruendemann, B. J.: The impact of surgery on body image. Nurs. Clin. N. Am., *10*:635-643, Dec. 1975.

McConnell, E. A.: Nursing care in the surgical reception area. AORN J., *27*:1315-1320, June 1978.

Nolan, M. G., et al.: Perspectives in operating room nursing. Nurs. Clin. N. Am., *10*:673-679, Dec. 1975.

Regan, W. A.: When the surgeon isn't the captain. RN, *41*:23, Jan. 1978.

Sabo, B.: Hazards of macroshock in the operating room. AORN J., *24*:892-898, Nov. 1976.

Tenzer, I. E.: Nursing students learn operating room skills. AORN J., *26*:62-70, July, 1977.

Asepsis, Antisepsis, Infection

Brown, M. E.: Transfer of asepsis principles by students. AORN J., *27*:970-976, Apr. 1978.

Floor cleaning effect on wound infections. AORN J., *23*:1271-1272, June 1976.

Huth, M. E.: Principles of asepsis, AORN J., *24*:790-796, Oct. 1976.

MacClelland, D. C.: Are current skin preparations valid? AORN J., *21*:55-60, Jan. 1975.

Polk, H. C., Jr., et al.: Operating-room-acquired infection: Its epidemiology and prevention. *In* Nyhus, L. M., ed.: 1977 Surgery Annual. New York, Appleton-Century-Crofts, *9*:83-101, 1977.

Nursing Process

Fehlau, M. T.: Applying the nursing process to patient care in the operating room. Nurs. Clin. N. Am., *10*:617-623, Dec. 1975.

Jacob, J. L.: Documenting patient care in the operating room. AORN J., *26*:659-663, Oct. 1977.

Mehaffy, N. L.: Assessment and communication for continuity of care for the surgical patient. Nurs. Clin. N. Am., *10*: 625-633, Dec. 1974.

Phippin, M. L.: Intraoperative nursing assessment. AORN J., *28*:160-166, July 1978.

Skin Preparation, Gowning, and Gloving

AORN Standards for preoperative skin preparation of patients. AORN J., *23*:974-975, May 1976.

AORN Standards — OR wearing apparel, draping and gowning materials. AORN J., *21*:594-596, Mar. 1975.

Dineen, P.: An evaluation of the duration of the surgical scrub. Surg. Gyn. & Obstet., *129*:1181-1184, Dec. 1969.

Errera, D.: Panels discuss bacterial-hazard control, infection management in surgical patient. Hosp. Topics, *52*:43-49, Jan. 1974.

MacClelland, D. C.: Are current skin preparations valid? AORN J., *21*:55-60, Jan. 1975.

McBride, M. E., et al.: An evaluation of surgical scrub brushes. Surg. Gyn. & Obstet., *133*:934-936, Dec. 1973.

Nurses discuss problems in asepsis. AORN J., *26*:928-930, Nov. 1977.

Peterson, A. F., et al.: Comparative evaluation of surgical scrub preparations, Surg. Gyn. & Obstet., *146*:63-65, Jan. 1978.

Sterilization

Alertness advised in use of packaged materials in surgery. AORN J., *24*:1130-1134, Dec. 1976.

AORN Standards for cleaning and processing anesthesia equipment. AORN J., *25*:1268-1274, June 1977.

AORN Standards for in-hospital packaging material. AORN J., *23*:978-979, May 1976.

Experts appraise antiseptic agents (chlorhexidine preparations). Cont. Surg., *11*:29-31, Sept. 1977.

Litsky, B. Y., and Litsky, W.: Thermocouple-pyrometer data for evaluating in-hospital packaging material. AORN J., *23*:1175, June 1976.

MacClelland, D. C.: Sterilization by ionizing radiation. AORN J., *26*:675-684, Oct. 1977.

Polk, H. C., Jr., et al.: Operating room-acquired infection: Its epidemiology and prevention. *In* Surgery Annual. 1977, pp. 83-101.

Revised guidelines for EO sterilization. AORN J., *24*: 1086-1088, Dec. 1976.

Rodman, M. J.: Lasting scrub solution kills broad range of pathogens (Hibiclens). RN, *40*:29, July 1977.

Ryan, P.: In-hospital packaging rationale. AORN J., *23*: 980-988, May 1976.

20

POSTOPERATIVE NURSING MANAGEMENT

Nursing care in the postoperative period is directed toward the reestablishment of the patient's physiological equilibrium and the prevention of pain and complications. Careful assessment and immediate intervention will assist the patient in his return to normal function as quickly, safely, and comfortably as possible.

Considerable effort should be expended on *anticipation* and *prevention* of difficulties in the postoperative period. The nursing care of the patient after operation is second in importance only to the operation itself.

REMOVING THE PATIENT FROM THE OPERATING TABLE

The patient is moved from the operating table to the bed or the stretcher with the least possible delay and exposure. Exposing a perspiring patient can lead to pulmonary complications and postoperative shock. The site of the operation should be kept in mind every time a newly operated patient is moved. Many wounds are closed under considerable tension, and every effort should be made not to place any further strain on the sutures. Thus, in thyroid operations, the patient's head is not allowed to hyperextend; in breast amputations, the arm of the operated side is held close to the body; in nephrectomy, the patient is not allowed to lie on the affected side.

Serious arterial hypotension may occur when a patient is moved from one position to another, such as from a lithotomy position to a horizontal position, from a lateral to a supine position, or from a prone to a supine position.

Even moving the anesthetized patient to the stretcher can precipitate this problem. Thus, the patient must be moved slowly and carefully.

As soon as the patient is placed on the stretcher or bed, he is covered with lightweight blankets that have been arranged previously on the stretcher. The wet and soiled gown should be removed, a dry gown applied, and the bedding tucked in along the sides as well as at the bottom. On the stretcher the patient is held with straps above the knees and the elbows. The straps serve the double purpose of securing the blankets and of restraining the patient, should he pass through a stage of excitement as he recovers from the anesthetic. Side rails should be raised to the position affording protection.

RECOVERY ROOM

The recovery room is a unit usually located on the same floor as the operating rooms, or as near to them as possible. Patients who are still under anesthesia or are recovering from it are placed in this unit for easy access to (1) nurses who are especially prepared in caring for the immediate postoperative patient, (2) anesthesiologists and surgeons, and (3) special equipment, medications, and replacement fluids. In this setting, the newly operated patient is given the best care available by those best qualified to give it.

The room should be quiet, neat and clean, and free of unnecessary equipment. It should also have: (1) walls and ceiling painted in soft, pleasing colors, (2) indirect lighting, (3) soundproof ceiling, (4) equipment that controls or eliminates noise, e.g., synthetic emesis basins, rubber bumpers on beds and tables, and (5) isolated quarters (glass encased) for noisy patients. These seemingly luxurious features may be added at little extra cost, yet psychologically they are of real value to the patient.

Equipment includes every type of breathing aid: oxygen, laryngoscopes, tracheotomy sets, bronchial instruments, catheters, mechanical ventilators, and suction equipment; another necessity is equipment for meeting circulatory needs, such as blood pressure apparatus, parenteral equipment, universal donor blood, plasma expanders, intravenous trays and cutdown trays, cardiac arrest equipment, defibrillator, venous catheters, and tourniquets. Surgical dressing materials, narcotics, and emergency drugs should also be available, as well as catheterization sets and drainage equipment. In addition, monitoring devices may be at hand to provide an accurate and instant appraisal of the patient's condition.

The recovery bed should be one that affords easy access to the patient, is safe and easily movable, can readily be placed in shock position, and possesses features that facilitate care, such as available receptacles for intravenous poles, side guards, wheel brakes, and chart storage rack.

The temperature of the room should be about 20-22.2° C. (68-70° F.) and there should be an abundance of fresh air but no drafts.

A patient remains in this unit until he has fully recovered from the anesthetic agent, that is, has a stable blood pressure, good air passage, and a reasonable degree of consciousness.

IMMEDIATE POSTOPERATIVE NURSING CARE

Transfer of the postoperative patient from surgery to the recovery room is the responsibility of the anesthesiologist, with a member of the surgical team in attendance. Additional assistance may be provided by a nurse assigned to this particular patient. Transfer of the patient is done expeditiously with special attention paid in transit to comfort, safety, and general condition. Various tubes and receptacles are handled carefully for optimum function.

The recovery room nurse who receives the patient reviews the following with the physician: (1) the patient's general condition: age, airway, blood pressure, pulse, and respiration; (2) the operation performed; (3) the kind of anesthetic used; (4) any untoward problem(s) that occurred in the operating room that may have a bearing on postoperative care, e.g., extensive hemorrhage, shock, cardiac arrest; (5) any pathology encountered (if malignancy, whether the patient or his family have been informed); (6) any tubing, drains, catheters, infusions, or other supportive aids which may have been instituted in the operating room; (7) complications to anticipate; (8) special symptoms to watch for; (9) immediate postoperative directives (in writing); and (10) anything special the surgeon or anesthesiologist wishes to be notified about.

Postanesthesia Recovery Room Scoring Guide

Many hospitals use a scoring system to determine the patient's general condition and his readiness to be released from the Recovery Room. As the patient progresses through the recovery period, his physical signs are observed and evaluated by means of an objective scoring guide, which provides a set of criteria useful to the recovery room staff in assessing the patient's condition following surgery and anesthesia. This evaluation system, a modification of the Apgar score, makes possible a more objective evaluation of the patient's physical condition in the recovery area.

The patient's score is taken at stated intervals, such as every 15 or 30 minutes, and totaled on the official scorecard. (See chart, page 349.) A patient with a total score of less than 7 must remain in the recovery room until his condition improves or he is transferred to an intensive care area.

Respiratory Considerations

• *The chief immediate postoperative hazards are those of shock and hypoxemia due to respiratory difficulties.*

Shock can be avoided largely by the timely administration of intravenous fluids and blood and by appropriate drugs. The *respiratory difficulties* may be treated as they arise, or better, the patient can be treated so that they do not arise. These disturbances are confined almost entirely to those patients who are under prolonged or deep anesthesia. Patients given local anesthesia or nitrous oxide usually are "awake" a few minutes after leaving the operating room. However, those patients who have experienced prolonged anesthesia usually are completely unconscious, with all muscles relaxed. This relaxation extends to the muscles of the pharynx; therefore, when the patient lies on his back the lower jaw and the tongue fall backward, and the air passages close more or less completely (Fig. 20-1A). Signs of this difficulty include choking, noisy and irregular respirations, and, in a short time, a blue duskiness (cyanosis) of the skin.

• The treatment of hypopharyngeal obstruction involves tilting the head back and pushing forward on the angle of the lower jaw as if to push the lower teeth in front of the upper teeth (Fig. 20-1 B, C).

This maneuver pulls the tongue forward and opens the air passages. At times it may be necessary to grasp the tongue between layers of gauze and pull it forward for a time. This maneuver prevents respiratory obstruction and should be continued when necessary until the patient has regained reflex functions sufficiently to carry on normal respiration.

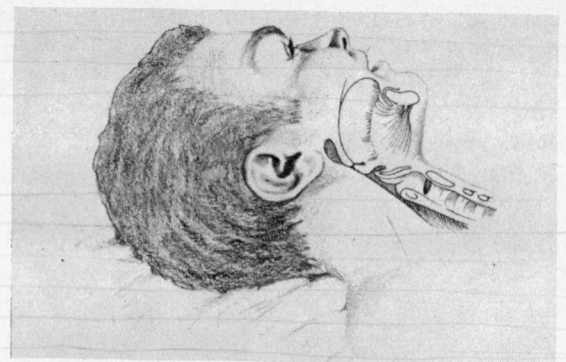

A. Hypopharyngeal obstruction always occurs when the neck is flexed and almost always when the head is in the midposition.

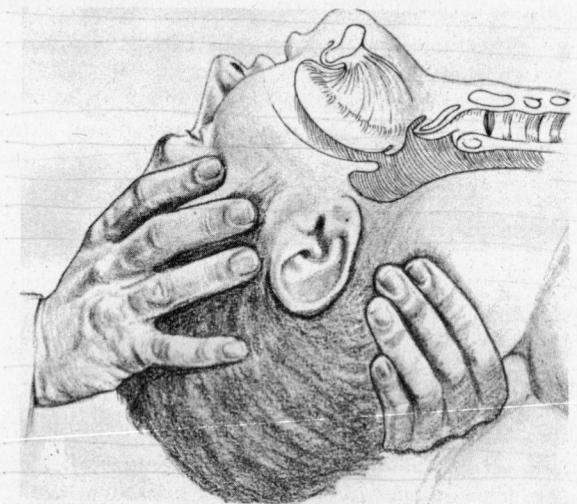

B. Tilting the head back to stretch the anterior neck structure will cause base of the tongue to be lifted off the posterior pharyngeal wall.

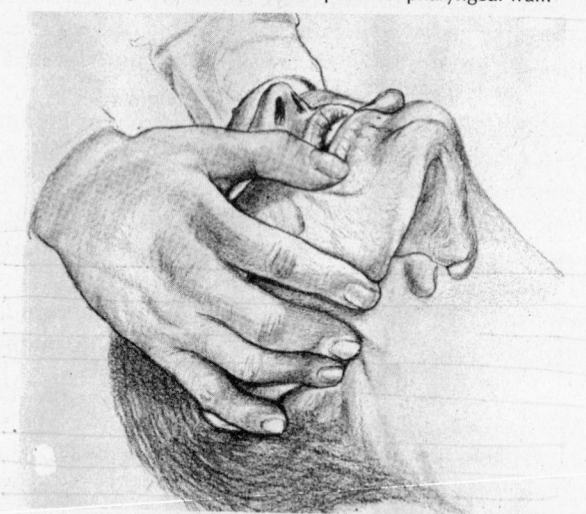

C. Opening the mouth is necessary to correct valve-like obstruction of the nasal passage during expiration, which occurs in about 30 percent of unconscious patients. Open the patient's mouth (separate lips and teeth) and move the lower jaw forward so that the lower teeth are in front of the upper teeth. To regain backward tilt of the neck, lift with both hands at the ascending rami of the mandible.

Figure 20-1. Reprinted with permission from Nursing Update, May 1972, copyright © Miller and Fink Publishing Corp., Darien, Conn. All rights reserved.

Often the anesthesiologist leaves a hard rubber or plastic "airway" in the mouth (Fig. 20-2) or a rubber nasal catheter in the nose. Either device can be used to maintain a patent airway. Such a device should not be removed until there are signs, such as gagging, that reflex action is returning.

Occasionally a patient may be brought to the recovery room with an endotracheal tube still in place and may require continued mechanical ventilation. The nurse will then assist in the preparation of the respirator and in the weaning and extubation procedures.

Not infrequently respiratory difficulty is produced by an excessive secretion of mucus. Turning the head to the side allows the collected fluid to escape from the side of the mouth. If the patient's teeth are clenched, his mouth may be opened by the method described in Figure 20-3A. If vomiting occurs, the head should be turned sharply to the side and the vomitus collected in the emesis basin. The face should be wiped with gauze or paper wipes.

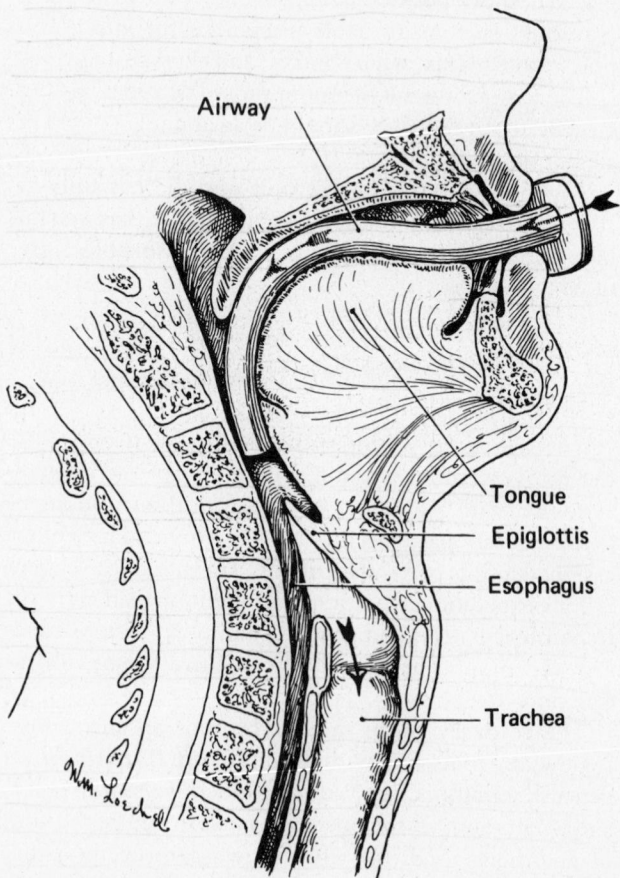

Airway

Tongue

Epiglottis

Esophagus

Trachea

Figure 20-2. Diagrammatic view showing a method by which an "airway" prevents respiratory difficulty after anesthesia. The airway passes over the base of the tongue and delivers air into the pharynx in the region of the epiglottis. Patients are often brought from the operating room with an airway in place. This should remain in place until the patient recovers sufficiently to breathe normally. Usually, as the patient regains consciousness, the airway causes irritation; then it should be removed.

POST-ANESTHESIA RECOVERY ROOM SCORING CARD

Patient: *Smith, Raymond*
Room: *B 1083*
Date: *3/7/ -*

Final Score: *10*
Physician: *Dr. J. Evans*
Nurse: *Mrs. Peggy Fay, R.N.*

Physical Signs → TIME ↓	ACTIVITY		RESPIRATION		CIRCULATION		CONSCIOUSNESS		COLOR		TOTAL SCORE
	Score	Comment	Score	Comment	Score	Comment	Score	Comment	Score	Comment	
Admission (A.M.) 11:15 P.M.	1	Spinal anesth.	1	chest & abdom. pain	1		1	Semi-conscious	1		5
½ Hour (A.M.) 11:45 P.M.	1		1		2		1		1	slight pallor	6
½ Hour A.M. P.M.											
Dismissal A.M. 12:15 (P.M.)	2		2		2		2	alert verbally responsive	2	color improved	10
FINAL SCORE A.M. P.M.	2		2		2		2		2		10

PHYSICAL SIGNS AND CRITERIA FOR THEIR ASSESSMENT

1. ACTIVITY
Muscle activity is assessed by observing the ability of the patient to move his extremities spontaneously or on command.
Score: 2—able to move all extremities
1—able to move 2 extremities
0—not able to control any extremity

2. RESPIRATION
Respiratory efficiency evaluated in a form that permits accurate and objective assessment without complicated physical tests.
Score: 2—able to breathe deeply and cough
1—limited respiratory effort (dyspnea or splinting)
0—no spontaneous respiratory effort

3. CIRCULATION
Use changes in arterial blood pressure from preanesthetic level.
Score: 2—systolic arterial pressure between plus or minus 20% of preanesthetic level (Riva-Rocci method)

1—systolic arterial pressure between plus or minus 20% to 50% of preanesthetic level
0—systolic arterial pressure between plus or minus 50% or more of the preanesthetic level

4. CONSCIOUSNESS
Determination of the patient's level of consciousness.
Score: 2—full alertness seen in patient's ability to answer questions and acknowledge his/her location
1—aroused when called by name
0—failure to elicit a response upon auditory stimulation
Physical stimulation should not be considered reliable since even a decerebrated patient might react to it.

5. COLOR
This is an objective sign that is easy to recognize.
Score: 2—normal skin color and appearance
1—any alteration in skin color: pale, dusky, blotchy, jaundiced, etc.
0—frank cyanosis

*(Adapted from Fay, M. R.: Introduction to Recovery Room Nursing, Denver, Assoc. of O.R. Nurses, 1977, pp. 11, 29)

Mucus or vomitus obstructing the pharynx or the trachea should be aspirated with a pharyngeal suction tip (Fig. 20-3B) or a nasal catheter introduced into the nasopharynx or the oropharynx. In most recovery rooms, wall suction or suction machines are available for this purpose. The catheter can be passed into the nasopharynx or the oropharynx at a safe distance of 15 to 20 cm. (6 to 8 inches) if secretions are obtained at this level.

• The only sure way of knowing whether a patient is breathing or not is to place the palm of the hand over the patient's nose and mouth in order to feel the exhaled breath. Movements of the thorax and the diaphragm do not necessarily mean that a patient is breathing.

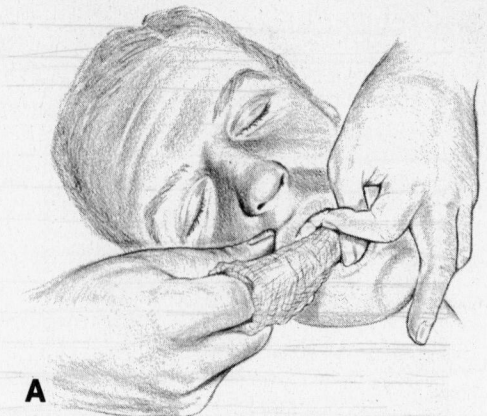
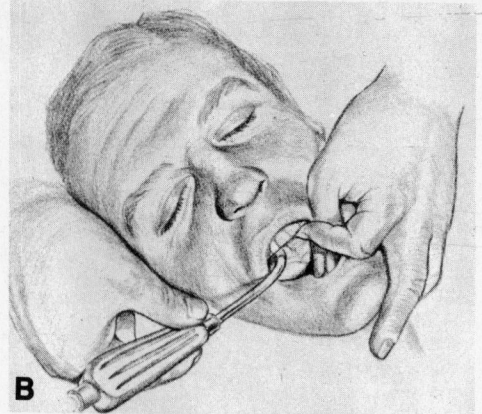

Figure 20-3.   *A.* To maintain a patent airway, it may be necessary to clear the upper airway manually or with suction. If the teeth are clenched, place your thumb against the lower teeth and your index finger against the upper teeth; open the mouth by crossing thumb and index finger for better leverage. If the teeth are tightly clenched, insert the tip of your index finger behind the last molar and pry open. Circumstances may permit only manual clearing, as illustrated. When possible, use mechanical suction *B.* or catheter. Suction equipment powerful enough to clear semi-solid materials from the pharynx should produce a negative pressure of at least 300 mm. Hg when occluded and a flow of at least 30 liters per minute when open. (Reprinted with permission from Nursing Update, May 1972. Copyright © Miller and Fink Publishing Corporation, Darien, Conn. All rights reserved)

Other Considerations

The function of the recovery room nurse cannot be limited to bedside procedures, safety measures, and the relief of pain; an understanding of the significance of psychological support is also important. If the nurse has never seen the patient before, a definite handicap is immediately presented. The nurse who knows the patient and accompanies him through the immediate preoperative and operative experiences is in a unique position to offer valuable support. In the absence of such continuous care by one nurse, pertinent nurses' notes on the chart help the recovery room nurse to recognize the particular needs of each individual patient.

OBJECTIVES OF POSTOPERATIVE NURSING CARE

The major goal of postoperative nursing care is to assist the patient to return to normal function as rapidly, safely, and comfortably as possible. The specific objectives related to this goal may be listed as follows:

1. To assist the patient in maintaining optimum respiratory function.
2. To assess the cardiovascular status of the patient and correct any deviations.
3. To promote the comfort and safety of the patient.
4. To promote the nourishment of the patient through proper nutrition, elimination, and maintenance of fluid and electrolyte balance.
5. To enhance wound healing and avoid or control infection.
6. To encourage activity through early exercises, ambulation, and rehabilitation.
7. To minister to the psychosocial well-being of the patient and his family.
8. To document all phases of the nursing process and report pertinent data.

1. ***To assist the patient in maintaining optimum respiratory function.***

Maintaining a patent airway is discussed in the section immediately preceding this.

POSITIONING.   Until the patient regains consciousness, the bed is kept flat. Unless contraindicated, the unconscious patient is positioned on his side with a pillow at his back and with his chin extended to minimize any danger of aspiration. His knees are flexed to reduce strain on abdominal sutures.

CLEARING THE AIRWAY.   If the patient vomits, he should be turned on his side and the nature and amount of the vomitus should be recorded. At the end of the vomiting episode the patient's lips and mouth should be wiped with paper tissues and gauze. To relieve thirst, his lips should be moistened.

If frequent aspiration of the nasopharynx and oropharynx is indicated, a clean aspirating catheter should be used and a basin of water kept nearby to flush and clean the catheter. Caution is necessary in suctioning the throat of a patient who has had a tonsillectomy, since the operative area may become irritated, causing bleeding and added discomfort.

PROMOTING LUNG EXPANSION.   To encourage lung expansion and exchange of gas, a variety of measures may be followed. For example, having the patient yawn or take sustained maximal inspirations (SMI) will create a negative intrathoracic pressure of minus 40 mm. Hg and will expand lung volume to total capacity. During this maneuver, right atrial and pulmonary artery pressures decrease while venous return and cardiac output (CO) increase.

Incentive Spirometry. Probably the most effective method of promoting lung expansion is incentive spirometry, which involves the use of special equipment to aid the patient in reliably producing the yawn maneuver and maximizing voluntary lung expansion (Fig. 20-4).

An example of this type of equipment is the Spirocare® Incentive Breathing Exerciser, an electric device which functions on a feedback system. When the patient is inhaling, the digital electronic circuitry approximates the patient's breathing performance. An automatic record is made of the number of patient maneuvers and the Exerciser is set for the preselected patient target. This number is illuminated on the panel, showing the patient very vividly what his breathing goal is. When he inhales, the lower registers are the first to light up; subsequent higher numbers are illuminated until the prescribed goal is reached. The combined features of the equipment offer the following advantages: (1) the patient is encouraged to actively participate in his own treatment, (2) it assures that the maneuver will be physiologically appropriate and repeated, and (3) it makes a record of the frequency of performance, which provides data for assessment by the nurse, physician, and respiratory therapist.

Intermittent Positive Pressure Breathing (IPPB). IPPB therapy has been used extensively as a means of promoting lung expansion. However, its effectiveness in reducing postoperative pulmonary complications continues to be scrutinized. Often when it is used, the patient is not instructed to hold his breath at the end of inspiration and he may not be encouraged to cough following the treatment. These oversights defeat the purpose of IPPB. In addition, when used improperly, IPPB may cause air swallowing, with resultant gastric dilatation and further ventilatory compromise. Similarly, the use of the *blow bottles* technique is being studied for its actual effectiveness in reducing postoperative pulmonary complications. When used correctly—that is, when the patient takes sustained deep breaths and then slowly blows the air out—a slight increase in functional residual capacity is achieved. Unfortunately, the patient usually blows out with greater attention to expiration than inspiration, which leads to rapid reduction in lung volume and results in closure of airways.

REBREATHING CARBON DIOXIDE. Another less frequently used method for stimulating deep respirations is to have the patient inhale carbon dioxide. This may be accomplished by means of a face mask attached to a gas tank or simply by instructing the patient to blow in and out of a paper bag. Most studies indicate that the tidal volume is not increased to total lung capacity and that

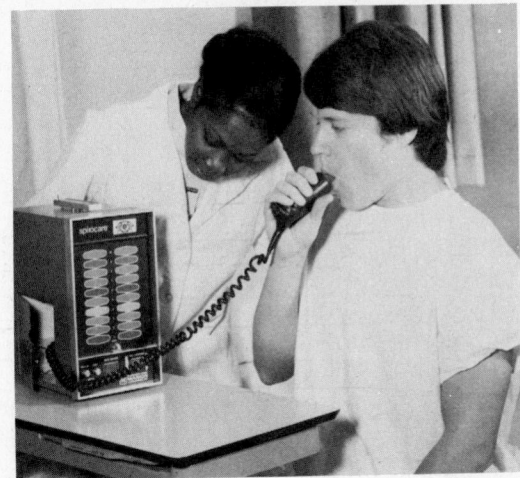

Figure 20-4. Incentive spirometry.

hypoxemia will be produced with dead space rebreathing. Because of this, the actual volume of carbon dioxide rebreathing is questionable and may even be hazardous in patients with cardiorespiratory diseases.

DOXAPRAM. Finally, in patients *unable* to cooperate in incentive breathing exercises, doxapram may be helpful; this is a selective respiratory stimulant given intravenously to stimulate carotid chemoreceptors, which then mediate increases in the rate and depth of ventilation. (See Respiratory Complications, page 372.)

2. *To assess the cardiovascular status of the patient and correct any deviations.*

The basic consideration in assessing cardiovascular function is monitoring of the patient for signs of shock and hemorrhage. The chief guides are the patient's appearance and determinations of pulse, respiration, blood pressure, temperature, central venous pressure, and blood gas. CVP and blood gas readings are monitored if required by the patient's condition. The pulse and respiration should be noted at frequent intervals for the first 2 hours, and every ½ hour for the next 2 hours. Thereafter, they may be taken less frequently if they remain stable. The blood pressure is taken as often as indicated.

• A temperature over 37.7° C. (100° F.) or under 36.1° C. (97° F.), respirations over 30 or under 16, and a systolic blood pressure under 90 are usually considered reportable at once.

However, the patient's preoperative or baseline blood pressure should be known in order to make effective postoperative comparisons.

• A blood pressure that shows a downward trend of 5-10 mm. Hg at each reading should also alert the nurse to a problem.

The general condition of the patient is assessed and recorded, including whether his color is good or cyanotic; his skin cold and clammy or warm and moist; or if there is excessive mucus in the throat and in the nostrils.

3. *To promote the comfort and safety of the patient.*

A patient coming out of anesthesia may display restless behavior. If it is at all possible, he should not be restrained, but he must be protected from injuring himself or interfering with IV therapy since an infusion is usually running. If the arm is splinted, the needle will not be dislodged. However, the patient can pull the needle out with his free hand.

Patients who have had hyoscine (scopolamine) or amobarbital (Amytal) before operation should be watched closely for several hours after they have recovered from the effects of the anesthesia. Not infrequently, these drugs cause a type of delirium. Patients have been known to get out of bed and do other injurious things while under their influence.

If the patient has been placed between blankets, they should be removed on complete recovery from the anesthesia—when the temperature, pulse, and respirations are within normal limits. Or the blankets may be removed when they are the cause of excessive perspiration. Recovery beds should be made in such a manner that the patient is left between sheets when blankets are withdrawn. Cool sheets usually are a gratifying change and often very soothing. However, care must be taken that the change is not too abrupt. Remember that patients who have been anesthetized are susceptible to chills and drafts. Remember also that the obese patient perspires profusely and so loses fluid and salt much more rapidly than the patient who is of normal weight.

Hampered by dressings, splints, or drainage apparatus, the patient very frequently is quite unable to shift his position. Lying constantly in the same position may lead to pressure sores or hypostatic pneumonia, to mention only two of the more serious resulting complications.

- The helpless patient must be turned from side to side at least every 2 hours, and his position must be changed as soon as he becomes uncomfortable.

Simple comfort measures include turning a pillow from side to side so that the patient can rest against a cool surface and providing proper support for the arms and hands, as well as for the feet, so that the patient can stretch his foot muscles and spread his toes.

It is comforting and soothing to the patient coming out of anesthesia to have cool cloths applied to his forehead. Moistening the patient's lips with a cool gauze sponge when water by mouth is *not* permitted may also be comforting. When convenient, a soothing back rub with lotion or alcohol is appreciated.

- The extremities may be stroked very lightly with alcohol. *They never should be rubbed vigorously.* To do so may dislodge a thrombus and result in embolism and death.

RESTLESSNESS AND DISCOMFORT. Restlessness is a postoperative symptom that should not be passed over lightly. The most common cause probably is general discomfort from the operation due to the patient's lying in one position on the operating table, the surgeon's handling of tissues, and the body's reaction to recovering from the anesthetic. These discomforts may be relieved by giving the prescribed postoperative sedation and changing the patient's position frequently. At the same time, the nurse will assess other possible contributing causes such as tight drainage-soaked bandages. Reinforcing or changing the dressing completely will make the patient more comfortable. Urinary output is noted and the patient is observed for urinary retention. Overdistention of the bladder is to be avoided. If possible, the patient should be helped to assume as normal a position as possible for voiding. Various techniques are tried to encourage voiding before resorting to catheterization.

Flatulence and hiccups are other causes of discomfort. Their recognition and treatment are discussed on page 356. Probably the most serious cause of restlessness is hemorrhage. This is discussed on page 370.

PAIN. Morphine or meperidine hydrochloride (Demerol) often are prescribed for pain and immediate postoperative restlessness. The time of administration frequently is left to the judgment of the nurse, but one should realize that pain in the first 24 hours after an operation requires relief by narcotics, and these drugs should not be denied when the patient is in pain. Complete pain relief in the operative region is seldom attainable; however, changing the patient's position, washing his face, and rubbing his back with a soothing lotion may be useful in assuaging general discomfort temporarily and rendering the hypodermic medication more effectual when it is given.

4. *To promote nourishment of the patient through proper nutrition, elimination, and maintenance of fluid and electrolyte balance.*

FLUID BALANCE. Any drainage apparatus such as nasogastric tube, cholecystostomy or choledochostomy tubes, catheters, enterostomy drains, and chest tubes, should be attached when drainage is to be collected. In case of underwater drainage tubes, such as those used after thoracotomy, clamps should be available to occlude the tube in order to prevent air from entering the chest if the drainage receptacle is accidentally disturbed or the apparatus disconnected.

If permissible, the patient should be offered water in small quantities when nausea ceases. If small amounts are retained by the patient, the quantity given at one time may be increased gradually. Water is best either hot or cold; otherwise, it is likely to cause nausea. There are times when a large glass of water will do a patient no harm, even when he is nauseated, but this never should be given unless prescribed. At times, patients ask for cracked ice, and usually it does no harm when given in small amounts. If orders are that the patient is to have nothing by mouth, cracked ice wrapped in a piece of gauze is refreshing and soothing to the lips.

DIET. Following surgery, the more rapidly the patient can accept his usual diet, the more quickly will his normal gastrointestinal function resume. The best method for the postoperative patient to take food is by mouth. This stimulates digestive juices and promotes gastric function and intestinal peristalsis. Exercise in bed or early ambulation also assists the digestive process and prevents such problems as distention "gas pains" and constipation. Chewing of food prevents parotitis (inflammation of the parotid glands), a formerly common postoperative problem which occurred in dehydrated patients who also practiced poor mouth hygiene.

The return to a normal dietary pattern should proceed at the pace set by the individual patient. Of course, the nature of surgery and the type of anesthesia directly affect the rate of return. Once the patient has completely recovered from the effects of anesthesia and is no longer nauseated, steps may be taken to restore his normal diet.

Liquids are usually the first substances desired and tolerated by the patient after operation. Water, fruit juices, and tea with lemon and sugar may be given in increasing amounts if vomiting does not occur. The fluids administered should be cool, not ice cold or tepid. Since fluids supply relatively few calories, and are tolerated well, gelatin, junket, custard and even buttered toast, milk, and creamed soups may be added gradually. As soon as the patient tolerates soft foods well, solid food may be given.

A well balanced diet should be provided and should include foods that have been selected and preferred by the patient. Usually it takes 2 to 3 days for appetite to return, so that attractive trays are a therapeutic consideration.

- When surgery has been done on the gastrointestinal tract, fluids and food are not given until peristalsis returns.

The nurse can determine when peristaltic bowel sounds return by listening to the abdomen with a stethoscope. This activity of bowel sounds is reported so that the proper diet modification can be prescribed.

Usually a nasogastric or gastrointestinal tube is in place for the first 24 to 48 hours following gastrointestinal surgery. Such decompression tubes remove flatus and secretions. Attention is given to the maintenance of proper fluid and electrolyte balance and an attempt is made with parenteral fluids and perhaps even hyperalimentation to achieve this nutritional level (see Chap. 35).

When nothing is given by mouth postoperatively, conscientious mouth hygiene is required (page 694).

URINATION. The length of time a patient may be permitted to go without voiding after operation varies considerably with the type of operation performed. Following gynecologic and abdominal operations, catheterization may be required at the end of 8 or 10 hours (sometimes sooner), whereas after other operations it may be put off for 16 to 18 hours.

- Generally speaking, every effort must be made to avoid the use of a catheter.

All known methods to aid the patient in voiding should be tried—letting water run, applying heat, etc. A patient should never be given a cold bedpan. When a patient complains of not being able to use the bedpan, it may be permissible to use a commode rather than resort to catheterization. Male patients sometimes are permitted to sit up or stand beside the bed, but safeguards should be taken to prevent any accidents due to the patient's falling or fainting.

- All urine, whether voided or catheterized, must be measured and the amount noted on the nurse's record.
- An input and output chart should be kept on all patients following urological or complex operative procedures and on all aged persons.

DEFECATION. Each defecation is recorded. If the bowels do not move spontaneously every other day, a cleansing enema usually is given. As a rule, cathartics are not given to postoperative patients, especially if the operation has been on the abdomen.

5. *To enhance wound healing and avoid or control infection.*

Dressings are inspected periodically to detect signs of undue hemorrhage or abnormal drainage. For incisions on the anterior part of the body, the posterior area is checked for signs of bleeding, since gravity assists in permitting seepage to accumulate in an area quite removed from the incision. Dressings should be reinforced, if necessary, and the time noted on the nurses' record.

Dressings and care of the incision are discussed further on pages 361–364.

6. *To encourage activity through early exercises, ambulation, and rehabilitation.*

POSITIONING. Following surgery, the patient may be placed in a variety of positions to promote comfort and ease pain.

Dorsal Position. The patient lies on his back without elevation of the head. In most cases this is the position in which the patient is placed immediately after operation. The head usually is turned to one side to facilitate easy evacuation of vomitus and to prevent its aspiration into the lungs. Bed covers should not restrict the movement of the toes and the feet of the patient.

This position may be employed to advantage many times when the necessity for drainage does not require the Fowler position. It is believed that when the patient is flat in bed, respiration often is more free and turning is easier, advantages that are important in the prevention of respiratory complications.

Sims' or Lateral Position. The patient lies on either side with the upper arm forward. The under leg is slightly flexed, while the upper leg is flexed at the thigh and the knee. The head is supported on a pillow, and a second pillow is placed longitudinally under the flexed knee. This position is used when it is desirable to have the patient change position frequently, to aid in the drainage of cavities, such as chest and abdomen, and to prevent postoperative pulmonary, respiratory, and circulatory complications.

Fowler Position. Of all the positions prescribed for a patient, perhaps the most common, as well as the most difficult to maintain, is the Fowler position. The difficulty in most instances lies in trying to make the patient fit the bed rather having the bed conform to the needs of the patient. The patient's trunk is raised to form an angle of from 60 to 70 degrees with the horizontal plane. This is a comfortable sitting position. Patients with abdominal drainage usually are put in Fowler position as soon as they have recovered consciousness, but great caution must be observed in raising the bed.

- It is not unusual for a patient to feel faint after the head of the bed is raised; for this reason a close watch must be kept on pulse rate and color. If the patient complains of any dizziness, the bed must be slowly lowered.

However, if the condition of the patient is good, the head of the bed may be raised within 1 to 2 hours.

The nurse must determine whether the patient is in correct position and comfortable. Often very short people are most uncomfortable in the ordinary hospital bed and must be supported by pillows. It is advisable to place a support against the feet to prevent the patient from slipping down in bed, to prevent foot drop, and to make the patient feel more secure.

It is the nurse's responsibility to see that the Fowler position is maintained at all times. No matter how correctly placed or how well supported by pillows the patient is, he will slip down in the course of time. Thus, it will be necessary to move the patient up in bed frequently and to readjust the pillows.

Jackknife, or Semi-Fowler Position. This position is one used to relieve tension following the repair of inguinal or abdominal hernia. It is achieved by raising the head of the patient about 25 to 30 cm. (10 to 12 inches) and flexing the knees.

AMBULATION. Most surgical patients are allowed and encouraged to be out of bed within 24 to 48 hours after operation.

- The advantage of early ambulation is that it reduces postoperative complications such as atelectasis, hypostatic pneumonia, gastrointestinal discomfort, and circulatory problems.

Atelectasis and hypostatic pneumonia are relatively infrequent when the patient is ambulatory, since ambulation increases respiratory exchange and aids in preventing stasis of bronchial secretions within the lung. Ambulation also reduces the possibility of postoperative distention because it helps to increase the tone of the gastrointestinal tract and the abdominal wall. Therefore, frequent enemas are unnecessary.

Thrombophlebitis or phlebothrombosis are less frequent because ambulation, by increasing the rate of circulation in the extremities, prevents stasis of venous blood. Clinical as well as experimental evidence shows that the rate of healing in abdominal wounds is more rapid when ambulation is started early, and the occurrence of postoperative evisceration in a series of cases actually was less frequent when patients were allowed to be out of bed soon after operation. Statistics also indicate that pain is decreased when early ambulation is allowed. Comparative records show that the pulse rate and the temperature return to normal sooner when the patient attempts to regain his normal preoperative activity as quickly as possible. Finally, there are the further advantages to the patient of a shorter stay in the hospital, with the consequent lower expense.

However, early ambulation should not be overdone. The condition of the patient must be the deciding factor and a progression of steps must be followed in getting the patient out of bed.

1. First of all, the patient must be placed almost upright in bed until all suggestion of dizziness has passed. This position can be obtained by raising the head of the bed.
2. Then, he may be placed completely upright and turned so that his legs hang over the edge of the bed.
3. After this preparation, the patient may be helped to stand beside his bed.

When the patient has become accustomed to the upright position, he may start to walk. The nurse should be at his side to give support, both physical and moral. Care must be taken not to tire the patient, and the extent of the first few periods of ambulation will vary with the type of operation and the physical condition and age of the patient.

BED EXERCISES. When early ambulation is not feasible because of circumstances already mentioned, *bed exercises* may achieve the same desirable results to some extent. General exercises should begin as soon after operation as possible — preferably within the first 24 hours — and they should be done under supervision to ensure their adequacy. These exercises are done to promote circulation and prevent the development of contractures and other deformities as well as to permit the patient the fullest return of his physiologic functions. Such exercises include:

1. Deep breathing exercises for complete lung expansion

2. Arm exercises through full range of motion, with specific attention to abduction and external rotation of the shoulder
3. Hand and finger exercises
4. Foot exercises to prevent foot drop and toe deformities and to aid in maintaining good circulation. A plastic ball under the covers may be a help in reminding the patient to exercise his leg muscles. Grasping the ball with the toes contracts calf muscles, stimulates circulation, and reduces venous stasis.
5. Exercises to prepare the patient for ambulation activities
6. Abdominal and gluteal contraction exercises

7. *To minister to the psychosocial well-being of the patient and his family.*

Almost all postoperative surgical patients need psychological support during the immediate postoperative period. When the patient's condition permits, a close member of his family may see him for a few moments. Thus, the family is reassured, and the patient feels more secure.

The questions posed by an awakening patient often indicate his deep feelings and thoughts. Perhaps he shows concern about the outcome of the operation or about his future — whatever his expression, the nurse should be in a position to answer his query reassuringly without going into a discussion of details. The immediate postoperative period is not the time for discussion of operative findings or prognosis. On the other hand, these questions ought not to be dismissed lightly, for they may offer clues that suggest the method to select in directing future treatment and rehabilitation.

8. *To document all phases of the nursing process and to record and report pertinent data.*

The determination of the significance of the signs and symptoms noted in assessing the patient is a matter of judgment. When viewed in isolation, one sign may be of little importance, but in the broader context it may be the missing link in a very important total evaluation.

There are a few general rules that may be of some assistance in guiding the nurse to make accurate value judgments. Of course, any severe symptom always is important.

- Any apparently slight symptom that tends to recur repeatedly or to increase in severity should be regarded as significant — for example, hiccups may or may not be of importance, depending on their duration.
- A symptom seemingly may be of no consequence in itself but when associated with other definite changes may foretell danger. For example, a repeated sigh means nothing, but, when accompanied by great restlessness, increasing pallor, rising pulse rate, etc., it becomes one of the clinical signs of dangerous hemorrhage.
- Any progressive and steady changes for the worse in the general condition of the patient, even with no outstanding symptoms evident, is of the gravest importance.
- The patient's complaints and statements never should be passed over without investigation.

Recording information accurately and concisely not only informs all medical and nursing personnel of the patient's condition, but also satisfies medicolegal requirements.

If a physician is to be notified for any reason, all necessary information should be at hand before the telephone is picked up, including the latest vital signs and monitor readings. It is also advisable to take the patient's chart, including nursing records, to the telephone in order to refer to them should questions arise.

POSTOPERATIVE DISCOMFORTS

Vomiting—Aspiration

In past years, vomiting was a common and expected postoperative occurrence, particularly following the use of ether as an anesthetic agent. However, with the advent of other anesthetic agents and antiemetic drugs, vomiting has become a less common postoperative phenomenon, although inadequate ventilation during anesthesia can increase the incidence of vomiting. Also the vomiting that occurs as the patient comes out of anesthesia is frequently an attempt to relieve the stomach of the mucus and saliva swallowed during the anesthetic period.

Other causes of postoperative vomiting include an accumulation of fluid in the stomach, inflation of the stomach, and the ingestion of food and fluid before peristalsis returns. Psychological factors also may play a role; if the patient expects to vomit postoperatively, he usually will. Thus, helpful preoperative instruction can reduce the probability of vomiting after surgery.

When vomiting is likely because of the nature of surgery, a nasogastric tube is passed beforehand and remains in place throughout the operative procedure and the immediate postoperative period. Otherwise, simple symptomatic therapy is usually all that is required. Many authorities believe that most antiemetic drugs (usually derivatives of phenothiazine) promote more undesirable effects, such as hypotension and respiratory depression. If a medication is required, short-acting barbiturates are often prescribed.

- The most important nursing intervention required when vomiting occurs is to prevent aspiration of vomitus, which can cause asphyxiation and death. (See pages 372-373.)

Such precautions are also necessary even before the patient begins to vomit. After the airway is removed, the patient is usually turned to the side-lying position to provide effective drainage from the throat and to help prevent the tongue from slipping backwards and irritating the pharynx or possibly obstructing the airway.

- Following the slightest indication of nausea, the patient is turned completely on his side to increase mouth drainage.

If the patient is in a prone position, such as is generally used for children following tonsillectomy, adequate mouth drainage is provided by the position itself. However, to facilitate breathing, a pillow may be placed under the abdomen to permit the chest to expand.

Vomiting requires no special treatment beyond washing out the mouth and withholding fluids for a few hours. The main danger, as was already indicated, is from aspiration of the vomitus.

Under emergency conditions, since a patient who is brought to the operating room may have food in the stomach, some anesthesiologists administer preoperative oral antacids to counteract the acid-aspiration syndrome. Otherwise, if acid from the vomitus is inhaled into the lungs, it causes an asthma-like attack, with severe bronchial spasms and wheezing. Patients can subsequently develop pneumonitis and pulmonary edema and become extremely hypoxic.

Abdominal Distention

Postoperative distention of the abdomen is another common occurrence. The trauma to the abdominal contents by manipulation during the operation produces a loss of normal peristalsis for 24 to 48 hours, depending on the type and the extent of the operation. Even though nothing is given by mouth, swallowed air and gastrointestinal secretions enter the stomach and the intestines, and if not propelled by peristaltic activity, they collect in the intestinal coils producing distention and causing the patient to complain of fullness or pain in the abdomen. Most often the gas collects in the colon; hence, a rectal tube may be expected to give relief (Fig. 20-5).

After major abdominal surgery, distention may be avoided by having the patient turn, exercise, and move frequently and by using a gastric or an intestinal tube, whereby the air that is swallowed (swallowed air provides most of the gas that produces distention) may be aspirated from the stomach and the upper intestine. Certain patients swallow air as a part of an anxiety reaction. If these characteristics can be recognized, the nasogastric tube may be used for a longer time than usual, until full peristaltic activity (passage of flatus) is resumed.

Thirst

Thirst is a troublesome symptom after many general anesthetics, and even after some cases of local anesthesia. It stems largely from the dryness of the mouth and the pharynx caused by the inhibition of mucous secretion after the usual preoperative medication of atropine. Many patients operated on under local anesthesia complain of thirst during the operation. In addition, there is a considerable loss of body fluids due to perspiration, increased mucous secretion in the lungs, and loss of blood, so that the factor of fluid imbalance also contributes to thirst. To combat the loss of fluids, solutions are given into the vein for the first few hours after operation. Even though an adequate amount of fluid is taken by this method, often it does not relieve the thirst.

Since a sticky, dry mouth demands moisture, fluids may be given to most patients as soon as the postoperative nausea and vomiting have passed. Sips of water or hot tea with lemon juice help to dissolve the mucus better than cold water. Ice chips seem to increase thirst and leave the mouth more parched. As soon as the patient can take water by mouth in sufficient quantities, parenteral administration is discontinued.

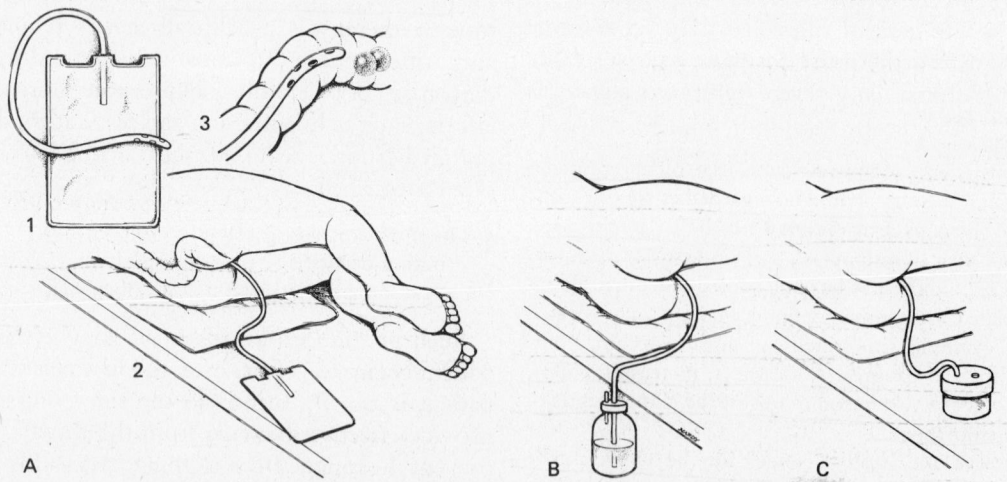

Figure 20-5. Rectal intubation. *A.* (1) rectal tube attached to plastic bag; (2) tube in place, patient lying on left side; (3) enlargement of lower colon showing gas bubbles which will be tapped by rectal tube. *B.* Tubing connected to a water bottle with vent. *C.* Tubing connected to a plastic receptacle.

Hiccup (Singultus)

Hiccup occurs occasionally after abdominal operations. Often it occurs in mild transitory attacks that cease spontaneously or with very simple treatment. When hiccups persist they may produce considerable distress and serious effects such as vomiting, acid-base and fluid imbalance, malnutrition, exhaustion, and possibly wound dehiscence.

Hiccup is produced by intermittent spasms of the diaphragm and is manifested by a coarse sound (an audible "hic"), a result of the vibration of the closed vocal cords as the air rushes suddenly into the lungs. The cause of the diaphragmatic spasm may be any irritation of the phrenic nerve from its center in the spinal cord to its terminal ramifications on the undersurface of the diaphragm. This irritation may be (1) direct—such as a stimulation of the nerve itself by a distended stomach, peritonitis or subdiaphragmatic abscess, abdominal distention, pleurisy, or tumors in the chest pressing on the nerves; (2) indirect—such as from toxemia or uremia that stimulates the center; or (3) reflexive in nature—such as irritation from a drainage tube, exposure to cold, drinking very hot or very cold fluids, or obstruction of the intestines.

TREATMENT. The multitude of remedies suggested for the relief of this condition is proof that no one treatment is effective in every case. The best remedy, of course, is removal of the cause, which in some cases is simple—for example, gastric lavage for gastric distention, shortening or removal of drainage tubes causing irritation. At other times the removal of the cause is almost impossible; then attention must be directed toward the treatment of the hiccup itself. Probably the most efficient of the older and simpler remedies is to hold the breath while taking large swallows of cold water.

After studying the problem, a group of anesthesiologists have recommended treatment ranging from the simplest to the most drastic until relief is obtained. Their suggestions, in order, are:

1. Finger pressure on the eyeballs, applied through closed lids for several minutes
2. Induced vomiting
3. Gastric lavage
4. Intravenous injection of atropine
5. Inhalation of carbon dioxide (by breathing in and out of a paper bag or by mechanical means)
6. A phrenic nerve block (should the above measures not work)
7. A phrenic nerve crush as a final resort

Phenothiazine drugs, especially thorazine, have been helpful on occasion. It has also been suggested that an interruption of the reflex arc that results in the intermittent spasm of the diaphragm may be accomplished by the introduction of a rubber catheter 7.5 to 11 cm. (3 to 4½ inches) long into the pharynx. The catheter may be introduced either through the nose or through the mouth to tickle the pharynx (Fig. 20-6).

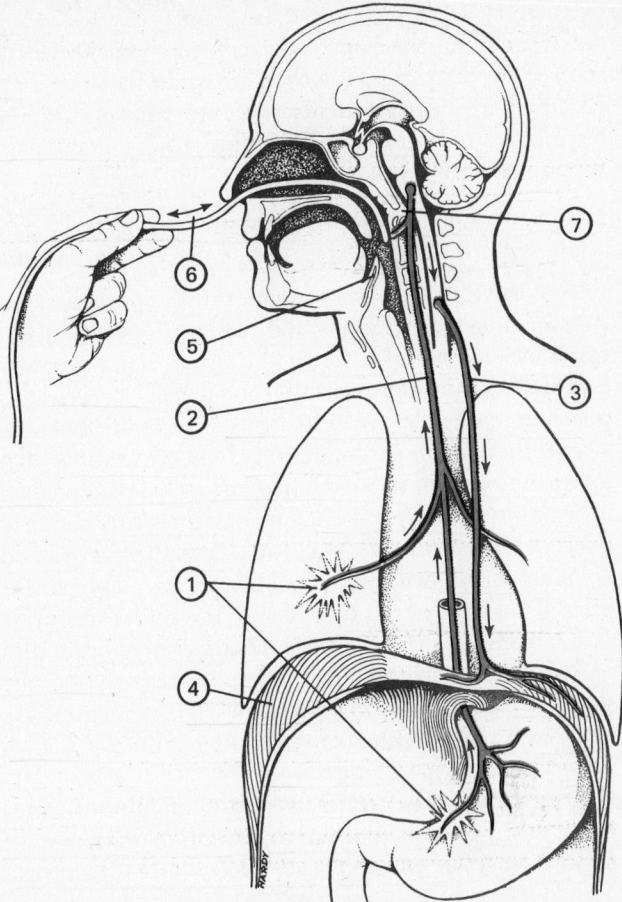

Figure 20-6. Controlling hiccups. Irritations in chest or abdomen (1) are transmitted by the vagus nerve (2). The reflex arc is completed by the transmission of the impulses to the diaphragm by the phrenic nerve (3). This causes contraction of the diaphragm (4) resulting in sudden intake of breath, which in turn is suddenly interrupted by rapid closure of the glottis (5). This is the hiccup.

Introduction of the No. 16F catheter into the nasopharynx about 7.5-10 cm. (3 to 4 inches) (6) stimulates the pharyngeal branches of the vagus nerve (7) and interrupts the reflex arc, stopping the hiccups.

Constipation

The causes of constipation after operation may be minor or serious. The irritation and the trauma to the bowel at the time of the operation may inhibit intestinal movement for several days, but usually peristaltic function returns after the third day, following the combined effect of early ambulation, perhaps a simple enema, and an increase in diet. Local inflammation, peritonitis, or abscess may cause constipation, in which case treatment of the causal condition is indicated.

• Constipation has been described as a constant symptom of complete intestinal obstruction.

It must be borne in mind also, that many people are constipated habitually, and often give a history of having taken some form of laxative drug every day for years. Attempts should be made to correct their bowel habits as soon as is practical. However, in some instances, especially with elderly patients, these attempts may not be feasible. Liquid petrolatum (paraffin oil) or enemas usually are effective in evacuating the lower bowel.

- Cathartic drugs should never be given except when prescribed by the physician.

FECAL IMPACTION. An avoidable cause of postoperative constipation is fecal impaction. This complication is a result of neglect and never should occur. Early ambulation and regard for proper fluids and diet can prevent this problem in the majority of patients. Those affected usually are individuals past middle age, weakened somewhat by operation, whose bowel movements have been small in amount for several days. Enemas appear to be fairly effective, but distention usually continues, accompanied by general and local abdominal discomfort. The patient often states that he feels that the bowel wants to move but that movement gives no relief. Diarrhea may occur and persist, due to irritation of the upper rectum and the sigmoid by dammed-up fecal material. The diagnosis is made easily by inserting the gloved finger into the rectum and palpating a hard fecal mass.

Treatment. The treatment of the condition is to remove the impaction. Enemas of 180 ml. (6 oz.) of liquid petrolatum (oil enema) often are effective in softening the mass and helping in its discharge. The harder masses may not be moved by this treatment. In these patients, the impaction may be broken up with the gloved finger, or by injecting from 30 to 60 ml. (1 to 2 oz.) of hydrogen peroxide into the rectum. The foaming action of the drug tends to break up the fecal masses, which then may be evacuated.

Diarrhea

After operation, diarrhea is rare. When it does occur, the patient may have five to ten liquid stools a day, each small in amount. This should be reported at once. Fecal impaction seems to be the most frequent cause of this complication in the aged.

Local irritation, such as a pelvic abscess, is the most frequent cause of diarrhea after operations in which peritonitis was found. Insertion of a gloved finger into the rectum will reveal a tender mass bulging into the rectum. Surgical drainage usually is required, although at times these abscesses rupture spontaneously and drain into the rectum.

CARE OF THE WOUND

A *wound* may be described as a disruption in the continuity of cells; it follows then, that *wound healing* is the restoration of that continuity.

When wounds occur, a variety of effects may result: (1) immediate loss of all or part of organ functioning, (2) sympathetic stress response, (3) hemorrhage and blood clotting, (4) bacterial contamination (when the bacterial count approaches $10^3/cm.^3$, the body's defense is usually effective; a septic wound usually contains bacteria within the range of 10^7 to $10^9/cm.^3$), and (5) death of cells. Careful asepsis is the most important factor in keeping these effects to a minimum and promoting the successful care of wounds.

Careful Asepsis

In the operating room an attempt is made to exclude bacteria from wounds by the practice of strict aseptic technique. When airborne organisms enter a wound they are usually destroyed by the body's natural powers of resistance. Traumatic wounds are potentially infected wounds. Therefore, the surgeon is concerned with the removal of as much of the infection as possible and with the protection of the wound from further invasion by bacteria.

Wound Classification

Wounds are classified as (1) incised, (2) contused, (3) lacerated, or (4) puncture wounds, according to the manner in which they were made.

Incised wounds are made by a clean cut with a sharp instrument, for example, those made by the surgeon in every operation.

Contused wounds are made by blunt force and are characterized by considerable injury of the soft parts, hemorrhage, and swelling.

Lacerated wounds are those with jagged, irregular edges, such as would be made by glass, barbed wire, etc.

Puncture wounds result in small openings in the skin, for example, those made by bullets or knife stabs.

Clean wounds (those made aseptically) usually are closed by sutures after all bleeding vessels have been ligated carefully. All other wounds are potentially infected and cannot be closed until every effort has been made to remove all devitalized tissue and infection. Therefore, a formal operation is performed for the purpose of cutting out the infected and devitalized tissue. This operation is called *debridement*. Often a small drain is inserted before the wound is sutured to prevent lymph and blood from collecting and retarding the healing process.

Physiology of Wound Healing

Many tissues of the body are repaired by varying degrees of regeneration. This is true of epidermis, tracheobronchial epithelium, alimentary tract epithelium, skeletal muscle, adipose tissue, liver, and bone. For those tissues and organs which do not undergo cell regeneration following injury, the repair process takes the form of scar formation.

There are many variables in the repair process which, if manipulated in a prescribed way, will enhance healing. These measures include keeping the wound clean, removing necrotic tissue and foreign matter, taking steps to reduce bacterial contamination (such as antibiotic therapy) and closing the wound as soon as possible. It is recommended that the fewest possible sutures, made of the finest suture material, be used to maintain the tissues of the wound in close approximation.

When a wound occurs, hemorrhage results and a clot develops to fill the defect. Fibrinogen produces a network of molecules to bring the wound edges in loose approximation. A scab is formed as fibrin and other proteins dry at the surface. This seal prevents fluid loss and bacterial invasion.

Meanwhile, nearby blood vessels leak serum protein which contains albumin, globulin, and antibodies. Due to heightened metabolism, signs of inflammation become apparent—heat, redness, swelling, and pain. Repair actively accelerates with a migration of white blood cells into the wound. Neutrophils break down and ingest cellular debris. These phagocytes are followed by monocytes which become macrophages in the wound and continue the process of digesting debris.

The healing process moves upward from the depths of the wound. Epidermal cells migrate from the edges of the wound, proliferating by mitosis and preparing for the fibroblasts to begin reconstruction. This process begins within 24 to 48 hours after injury. Concurrent with cell migration, fixed basal cells begin rapid mitosis and fill in spaces left by the migrating cells. Fibroblasts and epithelial buds grow upward as epithelial cells grow inward from the periphery to cover granulation tissue (reparative fibrous connective tissue). Granulation tissue includes blood vessels and lymphatics which proliferate from the less traumatized tissue at the base of the wound. When resurfacing of the wound is accomplished, additional mitosis takes place to thicken the new epithelial layer. Upon completion of this process, the scab or the surface sloughs off and the new epidermal cells begin to keratinize.

HEALING BY FIRST INTENTION (PRIMARY UNION). Wounds made aseptically, with a minimum of tissue destruction and properly coapted, as with sutures, heal with very little tissue reaction "by first intention" (Fig. 20-7A). When wounds heal by first intention, granulation tissue is not visible and scar formation is minimal.

HEALING BY SECOND INTENTION (GRANULATION). In wounds in which pus formation (suppuration) has occurred or in which the edges have not been approximated, the process of repair is less simple and is delayed longer. When an abscess is incised, it collapses partly, but the dead and the dying cells forming its walls are still being thrown out into the cavity. For this reason rubber tubes, rubber tissue, or gauze packing often is inserted into the abscess pocket to allow the pus to escape easily.

Gradually the necrotic material disintegrates and escapes, and the abscess cavity fills with a red, soft, sensitive tissue that bleeds very easily. It is composed of minute thin-walled capillaries, growing off from the parent vessels, each bud surrounded by cells that later form connective tissue. These buds, called granulations, enlarge until they fill the area left by the destroyed tissue (Fig. 20-7B). The cells surrounding the capillaries change their round shape; they become long and thin, intertwining with

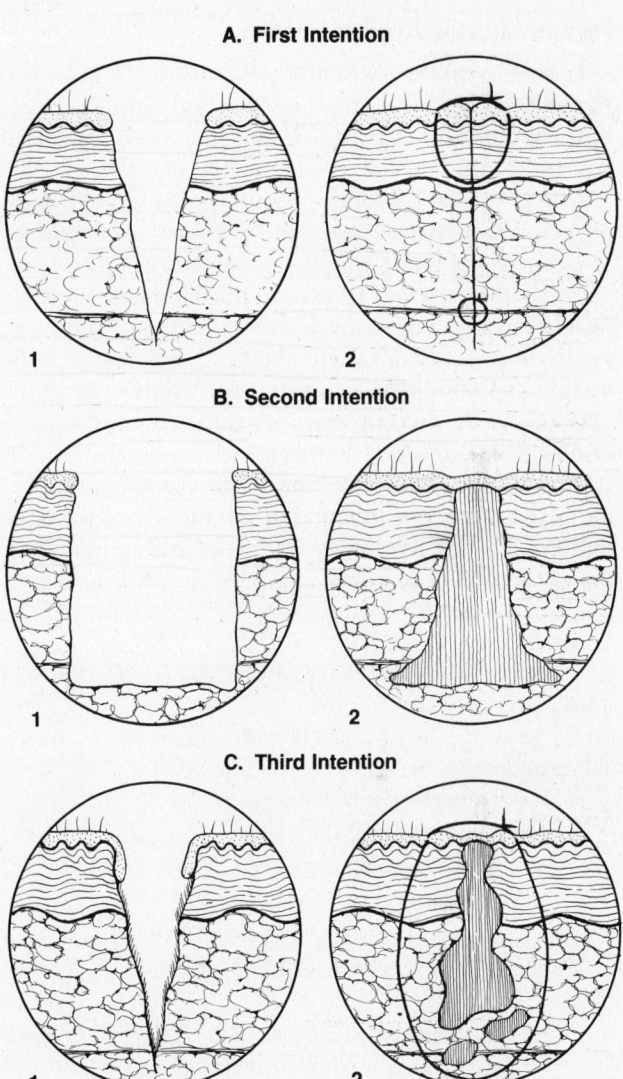

A. First Intention

1   2

B. Second Intention

1   2

C. Third Intention

1   2

Figure 20-7. Schematic representation of healing by first, second, and third intention. When a clean incision through epidermis, dermis, and subcutaneous tissue (A, 1) is closed immediately and heals without complication, a minimal quantity of scar tissue unites the edges firmly (A, 2). In open wounds with tissue loss (B, 1), wound contraction and epithelialization are the major factors in wound closure. The epithelial surface lacks a normal epidermal-dermal junction and can be unstable; the scar is large and wedge shaped (B, 2). When a wound remains open for a few days and is closed secondarily (C, 1), the initial scar is larger than in primarily healed wounds (C, 2). Within a few days, however, third intention wounds epithelialize and eventually may remodel to resemble primary wounds. (Hardy, J. D.: Rhoads Textbook of Surgery, 5th ed. Philadelphia, J. B. Lippincott, 1977, page 190)

each other to form a *scar* or *cicatrix*. Healing is complete when skin cells (epithelium) grow over these granulations. This method of repair is called *healing by granulation,* and it takes place whenever pus is formed or when loss of tissue has occurred for any reason.

HEALING BY THIRD INTENTION (SECONDARY SUTURE). If a deep wound either has not been sutured early or breaks down and then is resutured later, two apposing granulation surfaces are brought together. This results in a deeper and wider scar (Fig. 20-7C).

Factors Affecting Wound Healing

In healthy tissue a wound heals at its normal optimal rate. There is no way in which this rate can be accelerated, but certain aids can be introduced to assist the reparative process and prevent delay in healing. This includes providing an adequate nutritional level through proper diet. Protein elements and vitamin C are examples of essential needs. Resting the part or organ (depending upon its location and function) also favors healing, as does assuring adequate circulation of blood to and from the tissue in order to supply nutrients, leukocytes, antibodies, and other requirements and to remove the products of tissue metabolism. Circulatory impairment results in a poor blood supply which can interfere with wound healing. Blood flow may be accelerated by applying heat as prescribed, although this must be done with caution. Venous return may be promoted by elevating the part. Whole blood may be given in an effort to maintain the red blood cell count at a level as near normal as possible; the wounds of anemic patients are known to heal less readily.

Systemic disorders such as hemorrhagic shock and septicemia along with their sequelae of acidosis and hypoxia are depressants of cell function which directly affect wound healing. Renal failure and hepatic disease also inhibit tissue repair as do immunosuppressive therapy and cancer chemotherapy.

In the operating room, tissues that are handled with care will repair more rapidly than those handled roughly. Keeping the wound free from starch or talcum powder (from gloves) is also important, since foreign bodies will adversely affect the healing process.

Numerous factors can impair wound healing, such as age, edema, certain drugs which may mask the presence of infection (steroids) or cause hemorrhage (anticoagulants), and overactivity on the part of the patient which may prevent the wound edges from approximating and thus delay wound repair.

Local factors also may affect wound healing, such as poor dressing technique in which a saturated dressing is not changed frequently enough, or too small a dressing is applied, permitting bacterial contamination to take place. A dressing also may be too tight and hence may reduce the blood supply to the part.

Broad-spectrum or specific antibiotics can be effective if given immediately before surgery to patients with specific pathology or bacterial contamination. The use of

---

EFFECTIVE METHODS OF LOWERING INCIDENCE OF WOUND INFECTION

Method	Rationale
PREOPERATIVE	
Shorter preoperative hospitalization	Reduces exposure of patient to nosocomial infections.
Treatment of coexistent infections	Infections, such as respiratory, can initiate pulmonary complications.
Limited shaving of skin hairs	The fewer nicks and cuts in the skin, the less opportunity for infection.
Shorter time between shaving and operation	The longer the time between shaving and the operation, the greater the incidence of infection.
Thorough cleansing of operative site—Betadine shower the evening before and repeated preoperative cleansing with antiseptic detergents	Resident bacteria and skin contaminants are reduced to a minimum.
INTRAOPERATIVE	
Flawless aseptic technique	Any breaks in technique can initiate infection by introducing contaminants.
Powder or talcum washed off sterile gloves	Foreign particles in a wound, such as talcum or starch, will adversely affect the healing process.
Bleeding controlled with meticulous hemostasis	Bacterial infection is enhanced with ferric iron.
Drains eliminated in clean wounds	Drains are associated with higher wound infection rates.
Closure delayed in contaminated wounds	Permits healing from the base of wound to exterior—otherwise, pocket of infection may develop.

antibiotics in the wound area shortly after it is closed is not effective because of intravascular coagulation. If sepsis occurs, specific cultures are done to determine the antibiotic to which the bacteria are most sensitive.

Despite the many problems that can interfere with proper wound healing, the most important development in the management of surgical wounds has been the use of parenteral hyperalimentation (page 728) which makes it possible for even a malnourished patient to be operated upon with a greater margin of safety.

The Purposes of an Effective Dressing

A dressing is applied to a wound for one or more of the following reasons: (1) to provide proper environment for wound healing, (2) to absorb drainage, (3) to splint or immobilize the wound, (4) to protect the wound and new epithelial tissue from mechanical injury, (5) to prevent adherence of dressing to the wound due to ingrowth of new tissue, (6) to protect wound from bacterial contamination and soil from feces, vomitus, and urine, (7) to promote hemostasis, as in a pressure dressing, (8) to maintain proper moisture conditions at wound surface, and (9) to provide mental and physical comfort for the patient.

Whenever possible or feasible, some surgeons prefer to eliminate dressings, either shortly after surgery or within the immediate postoperative period. Examples of circumstances in which dressings are not necessary are facial lacerations, pedicle flap (see skin grafts, page 1072), or skin grafts on a smooth surface.

When the initial dressing on a clean, dry incision is removed, usually it is not replaced. Generally, initial dressings on clean, dry incisions are left in place until the sutures are removed, and if a dressing is replaced at all, its purpose is more esthetic than useful.

The apparent advantages of not using any dressings are these: (1) eliminates the conditions necessary for growth of organisms (warmth, moisture, and darkness), (2) allows for better observation and early detection of wound difficulties, (3) facilitates bathing, (4) tends to minimize the operative procedure, (5) avoids adhesive tape reaction, (6) appears to be more comfortable for the patient and facilitates his activity, and (7) is economical.

The suture line is gently cleansed and swabbed with half-strength hydrogen peroxide every 4 hours until drainage ceases. When sutures are removed (before 7th day), center sutures are removed first and replaced with steri-strips (Fig. 20-8) to keep the tender incision line reinforced. Incision line may be swabbed thereafter with tincture of benzoin for protection until complete healing has taken place.

Substitute materials, such as sprayed plastic dressings, can also be used, and they seem to provide satisfactory service for clean and dry incisions. This dressing usually lasts from 5 to 7 days. Depending upon the product, it

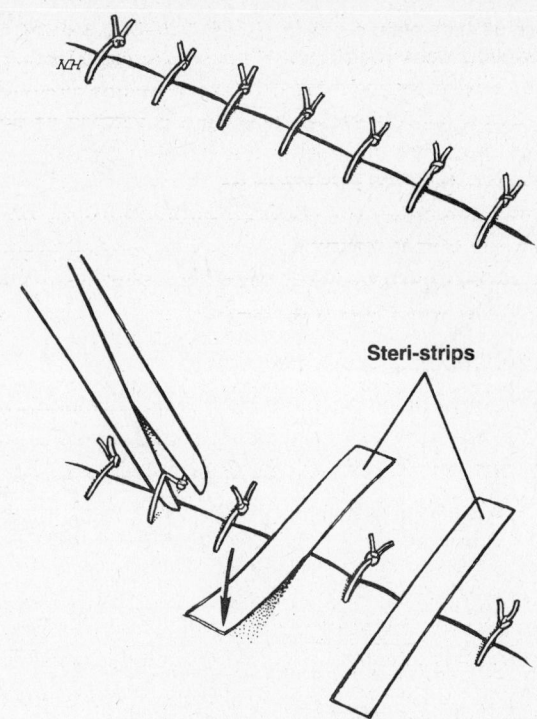

Figure 20-8. Steri-strips.

either peels off or can be wiped off with a dissolvent. On clean, dry wounds it seems superfluous to be concerned with the ability of the dressing to absorb secretions, since there are practically no secretions to be absorbed. Texture, comfort, and perhaps screening ability against microorganisms (although this latter is a doubtful prerequisite) are more important in such dressings.

Newer products such as polyethyl glycol (liquid) and hydron (powder) are being investigated as spray-type plastic wound coverings which are flexible and transparent, and which allow fluid to be transmitted through the dressing.

In spite of the advantages of not using a dressing, most surgeons prefer to apply a dressing at the time of operation and a second dressing between 4 and 6 days later, after the removal of sutures. Stitches (black silk, nylon, or fine wire) or metal skin clips used to approximate the skin edges are of little value after the sixth or seventh day and are therefore removed.

The dressings are purely protective from a functional point of view, and they give the patient a sense of security which is not present if wounds are treated without dressings.

Surgical Dressing Technique

Because of the dangers of contamination and spread of infection, the most desirable and safe technique is to use a sterile dressing pack for each patient. A surgical dressing cart may be used as a stock table to hold the individually

**Loosen all ends of tape.
Gently pull toward wound**

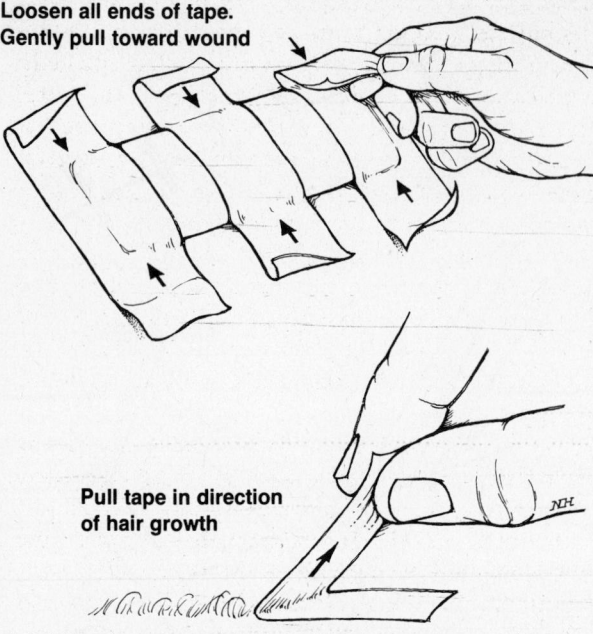

**Pull tape in direction
of hair growth**

Figure 20-9.   Removing adhesive tape.

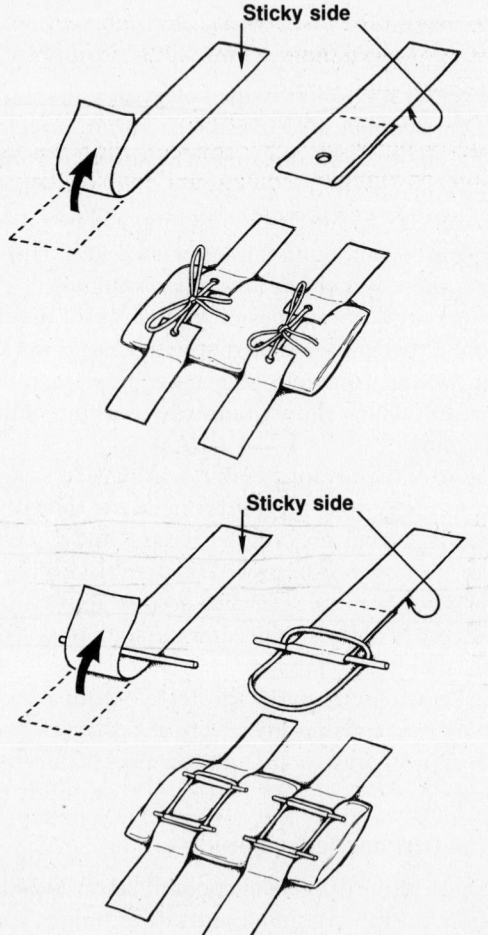

Sticky side

Sticky side

Figure 20-10.   Montgomery straps.

wrapped sterile supplies, including individual flasks of antiseptic solution.

NURSING RESPONSIBILITY.   The nurse should be available to assist the physician in the changing of dressings for several reasons:

(1) The "team" working together assures the patient of expert care.
(2) The nurse, as a colleague, is better informed concerning the patient and therefore can provide more knowledgeable care.
(3) The nurse can anticipate and obtain additional sterile materials as needed and can ensure the proper disposal of contaminated articles.
(4) Although all initial postoperative dressings are done by the surgeon, subsequent applications may be done by the nurse.
(5) The condition of surgical dressings should be noted on the patient's chart as carefully as any medication or treatment, and pertinent observations should be documented by the nurse.

PREPARATION OF THE PATIENT.   The patient should be told that his dressing is to be changed and that it is a simple procedure associated with little discomfort. The dressing change should be scheduled for a suitable time. *Dressings should not be done at mealtime.* If the patient is in an open unit, the curtains are drawn to ensure privacy and to accommodate the patient's sense of modesty. In this regard, the patient should not be exposed unduly. When the dressing has a foul odor or the patient is unusually squeamish, it is better to wheel the bed to the treatment room, away from other patients. At no time should the incision be referred to as a "scar," since for some patients the term has ugly or undesirable connotations.

REMOVAL OF ADHESIVE.   The adhesive is removed by pulling it parallel with the skin surface and not at right angles (Fig. 20-9). Nonirritating solvents available in aerosol containers aid in removing adhesive tapes painlessly and quickly.

The old dressing and the pledgets used in cleaning the wound are removed by means of a forceps and are then deposited in a waterproof bag for easy disposal by burning. Such dressings are never touched by ungloved hands because of the danger of transmitting pathogenic organisms. After instruments are used in the changing of dressings, they are placed in a receptacle such as an emesis basin, not on surfaces where contamination of clean areas is possible. If instruments are disposable, they are discarded in the proper receptacle.

A SIMPLE DRESSING.   For the routine dressing, an individual sterile pack usually contains scissors, forceps, hemostat, and grooved director as well as cotton balls, dressings, and perhaps a solution container. When the tray has been properly opened the person changing the dressing grasps a cotton ball with a forceps and holds it over the emesis basin as the assistant pours a small quantity of the desired antiseptic. After the wound and surrounding skin are cleansed with an antiseptic, the stitches are removed, a new dressing is applied, and tape is used to keep it in place (see page 364).

Surgical tape is available for patients who are allergic to the rubber base in the usual adhesive tape. 3M brand Micropore surgical tape is porous in structure and thus permits ventilation and prevents maceration. Tension sutures are allowed to remain in place for a longer period of time in some instances.

- *If there is any doubt concerning the sterility of an instrument or a dressing, it should be considered unsterile. In no circumstances should the nurse touch soiled dressings with ungloved hands.*

THE DRESSING OF DRAINING WOUNDS. It may be necessary to dress draining wounds within 24 hours of the operation. Nothing causes a patient more unnecessary discomfort than a dressing saturated with drainage fluids. It dries on the edges and becomes stiff and scratchy, and the odor frequently is very offensive if not actually nauseating. The nurse may relieve such a situation by changing the outer layers of the dressing at frequent intervals between dressings.

When it is necessary to dress the wound daily, adhesive strips fastened with either tapes or laces (Montgomery straps, Fig. 20-10) are more convenient than simple adhesive strips. These should not be applied so tightly that the dressings beneath are unable to retain drainage.

When the edges of the wound gape and the gauze is adhering to the tissues, the patient may be spared considerable pain if the dressings are moistened with peroxide

of hydrogen. For this purpose a syringe and a basin containing the solution must be provided along with a waste pan to prevent the solution from soiling the bed.

When *drainage tubes* are being shortened, the nurse should have a sterile safety pin (or Klip) ready to insert in the new tube end. If the tubes are removed, the surgeon frequently inserts a piece of rubber tissue or packing to prevent the drainage tract from closing too quickly.

The drainage from an infected wound frequently proves to be irritating to the surrounding skin. Often this situation may be avoided by the use of a protective ointment or dressing. Petrolatum gauze, nitrofurazone (Furacin roll), and zinc oxide ointments are effective preparations.

When the discharge from the wound contains any digestive enzymes, as in pancreatic or intestinal fistulae and ileostomy or cecostomy wounds, more active measures to protect the skin must be taken. In some cases, the enzyme-containing secretion may be aspirated by constant portable suction (see below). In others, the skin surrounding the wound may be protected by such adhering ointments as zinc oxide ointment or by a creamy paste mixture of aluminum hydroxide gel and kaolin (Protogel) or of magnesium and aluminum hydroxides (Maalox), which both soothe the skin and neutralize the enzymes in the secretions. These must be applied to an absolutely dry skin surface.

When a drainage tube is attached to drainage tubing and a bag or bottle, it is necessary to check the tubing frequently for kinking, coiling, and looping that could restrict the flow of drainage.

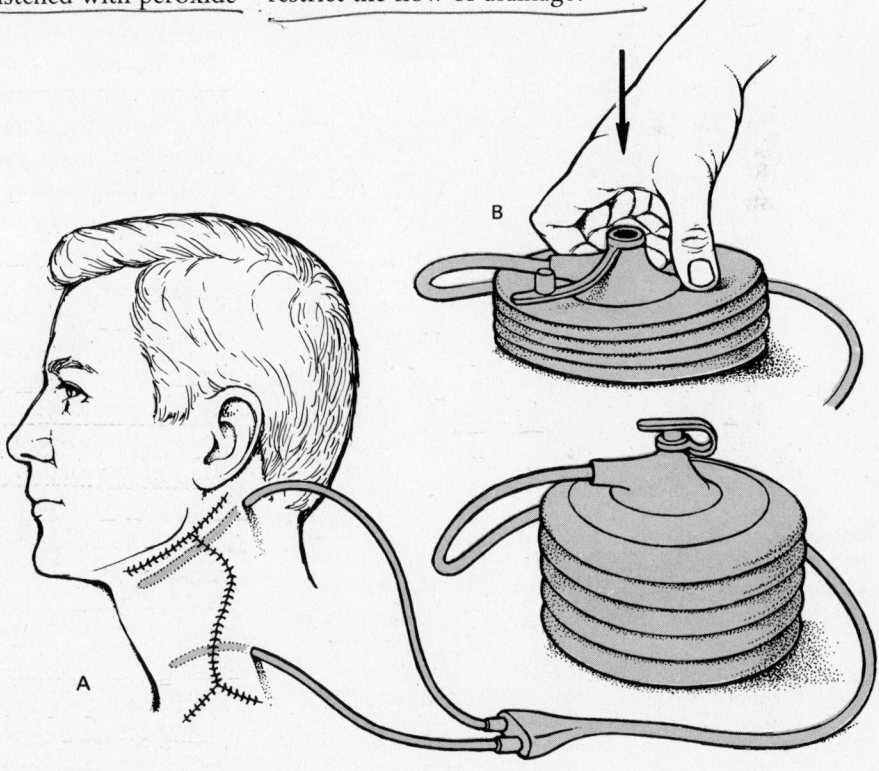

Figure 20-11. Portable wound suction. *A.* Two perforated catheters are draining the incisional area following a radical neck dissection. By means of a Y-tube, drainage is drawn into a portable wound suction receptacle. When full, open top plug of receptacle and empty.

B. To reestablish negative pressure, compress receptacle as indicated and replace plug; suction drainage will resume.

PORTABLE WOUND SUCTION. The principle involved in portable wound suction is the use of gentle, constant suction to effect drainage of serosanguineous fluid and to collapse the skin flaps against the underlying tissue. The apparatus is equipped with small multiple, perforated, inert polyethylene tubes. Such tubes are inserted in the drainage areas in the operating room, and the wound is completely closed (Fig. 20-11). An electric suction machine may be connected to the device or operated as an independent unit, depending upon the nature of the suction required and whether drip irrigation is to be used.

Portable suction has several advantages over conventional wound suctioning. It is silent, saves space, and is disposable. It is light in weight and permits the patient to ambulate.

THE COMPLETION OF A DRESSING. Dressings are held in place by adhesive which comes in many types and widths. If the patient is sensitive to the adhesive material, hypoallergenic tape should be used.

The correct way to apply tape is to place the tape at the center of the dressing and then press the tape down on both sides, applying tension evenly away from the midline (Fig. 20-12). Unfortunately, the wrong method of

applying tape is more common—fixing one end of the tape to the skin and then pulling it tight over the dressing, often wrinkling and pulling the skin in the process. The resulting continuous and forceful traction produces a shearing effect, causing the epidermal layer to slip sideways and become prematurely separated from the deeper dermal layers.

A commercial silicone aerosol is available that can be sprayed over the adhesive used to hold dressings in place; the silicone waterproofs the dressing so that the patient can bathe or swim, and isolates the area from contamination. The spray is odorless, colorless, nonstaining, noninflammatory, heat stable, and also nonallergenic.

Elastic adhesive bandage (Elastoplast, Microfoam-3M) is preferable for holding dressings in place over mobile areas such as the neck or the extremities—or where pressure is required. When the dressing is completed, the soiled dressings are wrapped in a waterproof bag and deposited in the large covered utility can to await its removal to the incinerator.

POSTOPERATIVE COMPLICATIONS

The danger inherent in surgery involves not only the risk of the operative procedure, but also the very definite hazard of postoperative complications that may prolong convalescence or even adversely affect the surgical outcome. The nurse plays an important part in the prevention of these complications and in their early treatment should they arise. The signs and symptoms of the more common postoperative complications are discussed below. In each instance the most effective method of prevention and the usual treatment are emphasized.

It should be borne in mind constantly that attention must be paid to the patient as an individual as well as to his particular surgical condition.

SHOCK

One of the most serious postoperative complications is shock, which may be described as failure to provide adequate cellular oxygenation accompanied by failure to remove the waste products of metabolism. Shock can occur in association with many kinds of major illness—hemorrhage, trauma, burns, infection, and heart disease—and results from a failure of three aspects of circulation—the heart pump, peripheral resistance, and blood volume. Thus, while there are many kinds of shock, the basic definition centers on an inadequate blood flow to vital organs or the inability of the tissues of these organs to utilize oxygen and other nutrients.

Shock may be classified as hypovolemic, cardiogenic, neurogenic, or septic. The changes involved in each type are summarized in Figure 20-13 and Table 20-1.

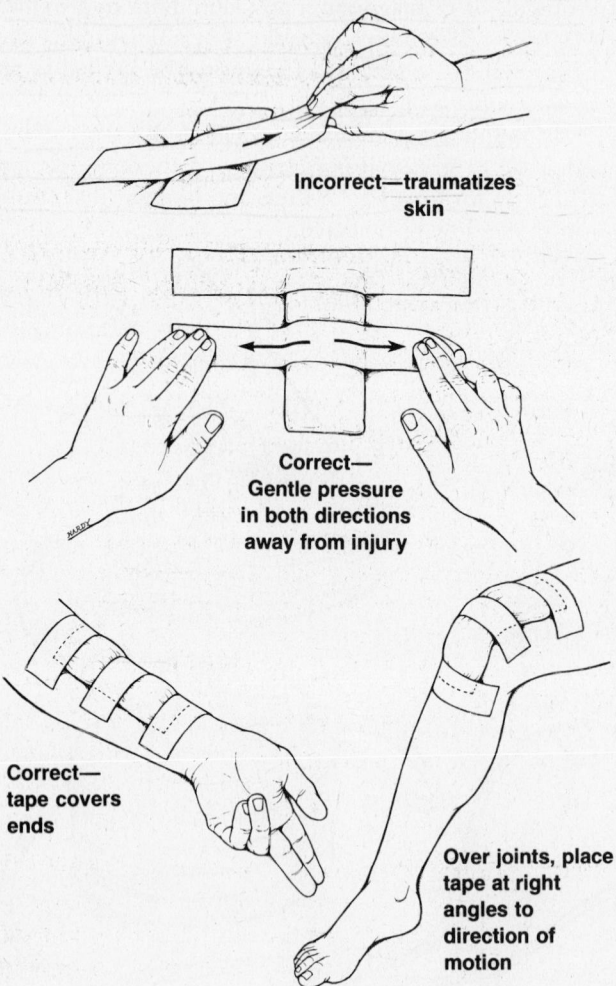

Incorrect—traumatizes skin

Correct—
Gentle pressure in both directions away from injury

Correct—
tape covers ends

Over joints, place tape at right angles to direction of motion

Figure 20-12. Application of adhesive tape.

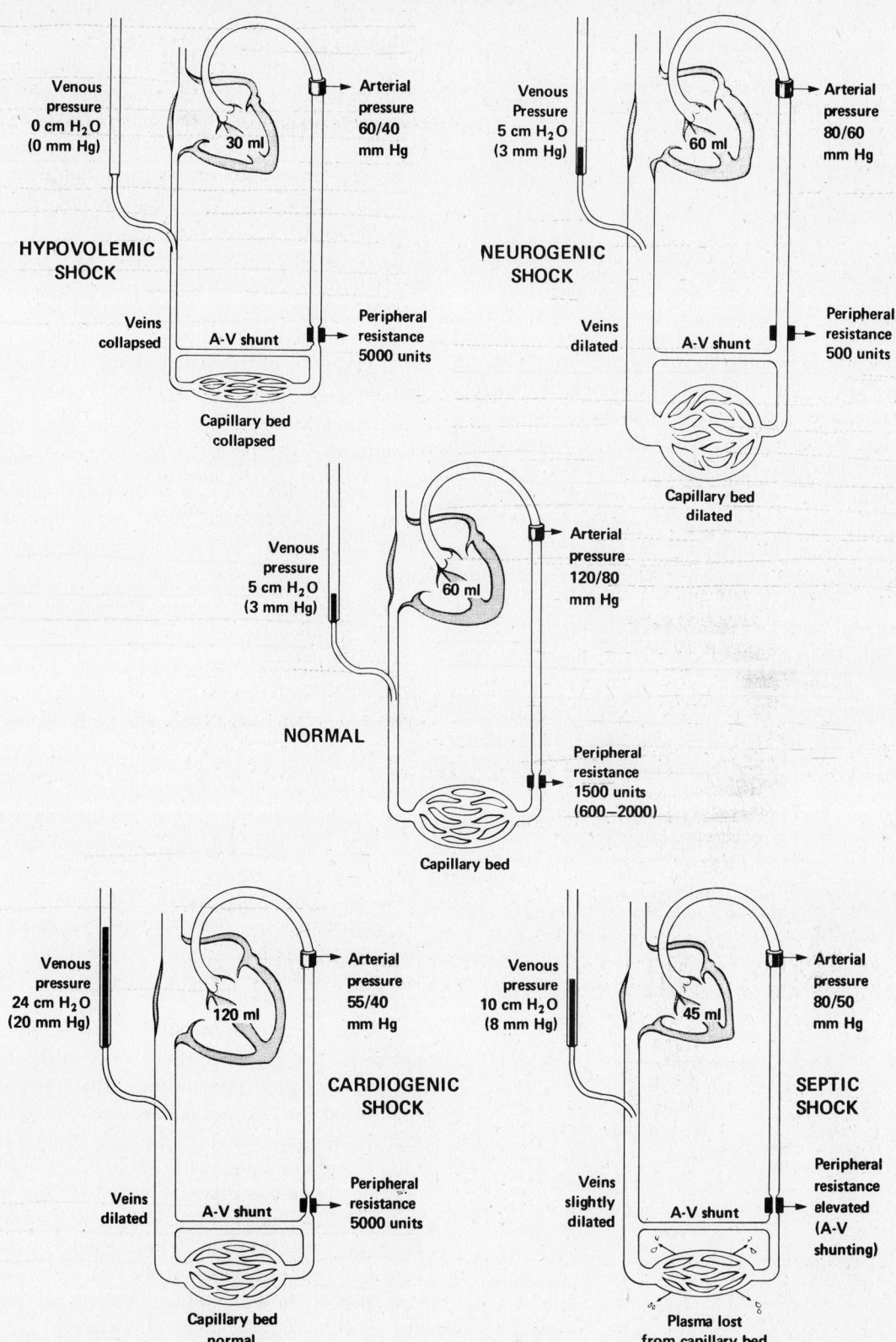

Figure 20-13. Hemodynamic changes in shock. (From Dunphy and Way: Current Surgical Diagnosis and Treatment. Los Altos, California, Lange Medical Publishers, 1973)

TABLE 20-1. MAJOR CHANGES IN THE PRINCIPAL TYPES OF SHOCK

TYPE	CARDIAC FUNCTION	ARTERIOLAR RESISTANCE	VENOUS RESERVOIR
Hypovolemic	↑	↑	↓↓
Cardiogenic	↓↓	↑	↑
Neurogenic	↑	↓↓	↑
Septic	↓	↓	↓

(From Dunphy and Way: Current Surgical Diagnosis and Treatment. California, Lange Medical Publishers, 1973.)

↑ increase   ↓ decrease   ↓↓ very low

HYPOVOLEMIC SHOCK. Hypovolemic shock is caused by decreased fluid volume due to loss of blood, plasma, or water. Fluid volume is frequently decreased after surgery for a number of reasons. At times more blood is lost at operation than is realized. In addition, the handling of body tissues may cause local trauma and loss of blood and plasma from the circulation, thereby creating a decrease in the circulating blood volume. Hypovolemic shock is characterized by a fall in venous pressure, a rise in peripheral resistance, and tachycardia. (For additional symptoms see Table 20-2.)

CARDIOGENIC SHOCK. This type of shock results from cardiac failure or an interference with heart function (poor heart-pump function causing diminished cardiac output), as in myocardial infarction, arrhythmias, tamponade, pulmonary embolism, advanced (late) hypovolemia, or epidural and general anesthesia. The signs are

TABLE 20-2. CLASSIFICATION AND SYMPTOMS OF HYPOVOLEMIC SHOCK

	MILD	MODERATE	SEVERE
Percent of blood volume loss	Up to 20%	20 to 40%	40% or more
Decreased perfusion	Skin, fat, skeletal muscle, bone	Liver, intestine, kidneys	Brain, heart
Pulse	Rapid	Rapid—weaker, thready	Very rapid—irregular
Respirations	Deep and rapid	Shallow and rapid	Even more shallow and rapid
Blood pressure	120/80	60-90 mm. Hg systolic	Under 60 mm. Hg systolic
Skin	Cool, pale	Cold, pale, moist	Cold, clammy cyanotic lips and nails
Urinary output	Above 50 ml./hr.	10-25 ml./hr.	10 ml. or less/hr. → anuria
Level of consciousness	Anxious but oriented and alert	Restless, mentally "fuzzy," vertigo	Lethargic → comatose

increased pressure in the venous bed and an increase in peripheral resistance.

NEUROGENIC SHOCK. Neurogenic shock occurs as a result of a failure of arterial resistance (such as may be caused by spinal anesthesia, quadriplegia). It is characterized by a fall in blood pressure due to pooling of blood in dilated capacitance vessels (those with the ability to change volume capacity). Heart activity increases and thus maintains a normal output (stroke volume); this helps in filling the dilated vascular system as it attempts to preserve perfusion pressure.

SEPTIC SHOCK. Septic shock results most frequently from gram-negative septicemia (infection, peritonitis, etc.). Hypovolemia develops along with depressed cardiac function.

Symptoms

Even though shock can result from widely different causes (trauma, systemic infection, or cardiac dysfunction), clinical manifestations are generally similar.

- The classical signs of shock are: pallor, cool, moist skin, rapid breathing, ischemia of the eyelids, lips, gums, and tongue, a weak thready pulse, small pulse pressure, and usually a low blood pressure.

Medical and Nursing Assessment of the Patient in Shock

Before treatment can be instituted promptly and intelligently it is necessary to monitor and evaluate the patient. Such an assessment includes the following:

1. **SKIN.** A cold, pale, moist skin indicates vasoconstriction with increased arteriolar resistance and is suggestive of hypovolemic shock. Warm, red skin indicates a decrease in arteriolar resistance and may be seen in septic and neurogenic shock.

2. **RESPIRATIONS.** Hyperventilation is an early sign of septic shock.

3. **PULSE AND BLOOD PRESSURE.** Alone, these signs may not be reliable guides to the severity of shock, but their progressive pattern is significant. That is, if each 5- to 15-minute interval shows a fall in pulse and blood pressure, then such signs are indicative of shock. A pulse of 80 per minute and a blood pressure of 120/80 are normal. When systolic pressure is between 90 and 60 mm. Hg (in the normotensive individual), shock is well advanced. (For the hypertensive person, 30 mm. Hg below the base-line systolic pressure is a sign of shock.)

4. **URINARY OUTPUT.** Since the output of urine is one of the most valuable indices of adequacy of vital organ perfusion, an indwelling catheter is recommended for any patient susceptible to shock. A drop in renal artery pressure and flow produces renal artery vasoconstriction and results in decreased glomerular filtration and decreased urine output. Normal urine flow is 50 ml. per

PATHOPHYSIOLOGY OF SHOCK

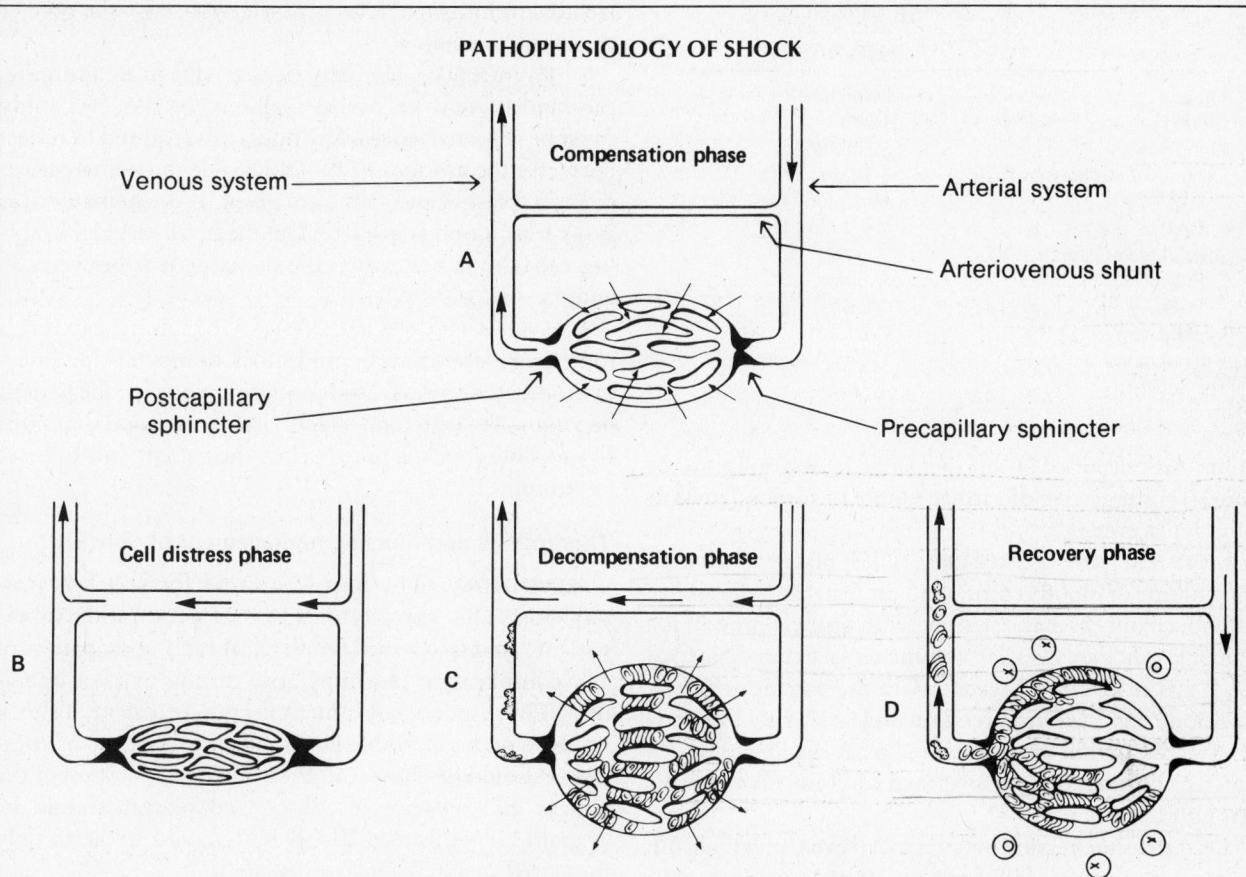

Figure 20-14. Microcirculatory changes in shock. *A.* Compensation phase; *B.* cell distress phase; *C.* decompensation phase; *D.* recovery phase. (From Dunphy and Way: Current Diagnosis and Treatment. Los Altos, California, Lange Medical Publishers, 1973)

When the body sustains an insult such as hemorrhage, extensive burns, or heart failure, a compensatory reaction occurs. The adrenal cortex releases catecholamines to constrict arterioles and venules in the major organs of the body (kidneys, liver, intestines, etc.) so that more blood is diverted to the brain and heart.

PATHOPHYSIOLOGICAL CONSEQUENCES OF SHOCK

The greatest impact of all types of shock is exerted on the microcirculation (arterioles, capillaries, venules—microvasculature), which reacts to shock in a series of steps. The first phase involves a response to the hypovolemia, as is seen in the contraction of the precapillary arteriole sphincters (Fig. 20-14A). This causes capillary pressure to fall, with the result that fluid moves into the vascular spaces and increases the blood volume. By such compensatory action, blood volume returns to normal and the precapillary sphincters relax. However, if shock is more prolonged, recovery is prevented and the next phase, cell distress, is entered (Fig. 20-14B). In this phase, arteriovenous shunts open and divert arterial flow

directly back into the venous system. Meanwhile the cells in the bypassed segment of microcirculation rely on anaerobic metabolism for energy. Glucose and oxygen are reduced markedly for the cells, and waste products such as lactate increase. Histamine is released and the postcapillary sphincter closes. Capillary flow is slowed considerably and the bed constricts with very few capillaries remaining open. In the decompensation phase (Fig. 20-14C), just before the death of the cell, acidosis (decreasing serum pH) causes the precapillary sphincter to open. Fluid and protein are lost in the interstitial space and the capillary expands with agglutinated red blood cells (sludge). White cells and platelets gather in the venules where acidosis is most profound. Arteriovenous circulation continues to supply essential oxygen to the vital areas of heart and brain. In the recovery phase (Fig. 20-14D), if the blood volume is restored during the decompensation phase before the effects on microcirculation are still reversible, badly damaged cells can be repaired. Cell aggregates can be filtered out by the lungs and into the systemic circulation. However, if there is an overabundance of dead cells, secondary morbidity results.

TABLE 20-3. NORMAL VALUES

MEASUREMENTS	NORMAL VALUE
Pulse	80/minute
Blood pressure (arterial)	120/80
Urine flow	50 ml./hr.
Central venous pressure	5-12 cm. (H_2O)
PAP	10-15 mm. Hg
PWP	8 mm. Hg
Arterial blood gases	
PO_2	100 mm.
PCO_2	40 mm. Hg
pH	7.4
Arterial blood lactate	12 mg./100 ml.
Hematocrit	35-45%

hour. An output of 30 ml. per hour or less (oliguria or anuria) is suggestive of cardiac failure or inadequate volume replacement.

5. CENTRAL VENOUS PRESSURE. CVP places a value on the volume of blood returning to the heart and the ability of both chambers in the right heart to propel blood. It is a valuable guide to vascular volume replacement. Normal CVP is 5 to 12 cm. of water. With the patient in supine position, any venous pressure under 12 cm. water is considered within the normal range. A reading above 12 cm. is considered fluid overload. A low CVP means strong pump action.

Left atrium pressure readings are even more useful. Some intensive care units are equipped to measure pulmonary artery pressure (PAP) and pulmonary wedge pressure (PWP), which is left atrial pressure. These are more accurate in indicating the heart's pumping ability. Normal PAP measures 5 to 15 mm. Hg; normal PWP, 8 mm. Hg.

6. ARTERIAL BLOOD GASES. The partial pressures of oxygen (PO_2) and carbon dioxide (PCO_2) are useful indices in providing therapy. An arterial oxygen tension below 60 mm. Hg indicates a marginal respiratory reserve (see Table 20-3 for normal values). A PCO_2 over 45 mm. Hg indicates serious hypoventilation. In shock, PCO_2 is usually within normal limits.

7. SERUM LACTATE. In 1964 Peretz showed the close correlation (in a person in shock) between arterial blood lactate levels and survival. Later a correlation was shown between lactate elevation and oxygen debt; the higher the

TABLE 20-4. EQUIPMENT NEEDED TO TREAT SHOCK

For blood studies:	Sphygmomanometer—
Prothrombin time	stethoscope
Type and cross match	Indwelling catheter; urinometer
Hemoglobin	Suction equipment
Hematocrit	Nasal oxygen equipment
pH	CVP tray
BUN	Defibrillator
Serum electrolytes	
Lactic acid levels	

lactate level (normal level is 12 mg./100 ml.), the greater the oxygen need.

8. HEMATOCRIT. Hematocrit is useful in determining the kind of fluid to use in replacement. (Such a study must be repeated since a few hours are required to reflect correctly the amount of blood loss.) If the hematocrit is over 55, plasma and saline are given. If the hematocrit is 20 or less, blood is needed. The maximal oxygen-carrying capacity is best when the hematocrit is between 35 and 45.

9. LEVELS OF CONSCIOUSNESS. Consciousness levels may range from alert in mild shock to mental cloudiness in moderate shock. As the condition worsens, the patient becomes lethargic and reacts only to noxious stimuli. Irreversible shock is noted when the patient fails to react to stimuli.

Therapeutic and Nursing Management of Shock

PREVENTION. The best treatment for shock is prophylaxis. This consists of adequate preparation of the patient, mental as well as physical, and anticipation of any complication that may arise during or after operation. Thus, special equipment for the treatment of shock must be on hand (Table 20-4). The proper type of anesthesia should be chosen after careful consideration of the patient and his disease. Blood and plasma should be available if indicated. Blood loss should be accurately measured or intelligently estimated.

- If the amount of blood loss exceeds 500 ml., replacement is usually indicated.

Obviously, the individual patient and the particular circumstances must be considered in determining replacement therapy. An older, malnourished person is more likely to require this therapy than a patient whose health is generally good.

Operative trauma should be kept at a minimum as the first step in avoiding shock. After operation, factors that may promote shock are to be prevented. Pain is controlled by making the patient as comfortable as possible and by using narcotics judiciously. Exposure should be avoided, and lightweight, unheated covers should be used to prevent vasodilation. In the recovery room the patient can be watched and cared for by nurses trained especially in the recovery of patients from anesthesia. In addition, a quiet room helps to reduce mental trauma. Any moving of the patient is done gently. He is placed in the dorsal recumbent position to facilitate circulation. Monitoring of vital signs is continued until the patient's recovery indicates that shock is unlikely.

TREATMENT. (See *Emergency Treatment of Shock,* Chap. 61.) The patient is kept warm, but overheating is avoided to prevent cutaneous vessels from dilating and depriving vital organs of blood. An infusion of 5 percent dextrose in water is started. The patient is placed flat in bed with his legs elevated as in Figure 20-15. (Avoid the Trendelenburg position.) The patient's respiratory and circulatory status is monitored constantly: respiration, pulse, blood pressure, skin, urinary output, level of consciousness, CVP (PAP, PWP, and CO [cardiac output] if available).

The basic approach to the treatment of shock is to determine its cause and correct it if possible.

1. ***The first objective of treatment is to ensure the adequacy of the airway.*** When the patient is ventilating adequately, blood gas determinations are made to determine adequacy of pulmonary function, and the patient is given oxygen by nasal catheter or endotracheal tube.

2. ***The second objective is to restore blood volume.*** Of the total blood volume, under normal conditions, 20 percent is in the capillaries, 10 percent in the arterial system, and the balance in the veins and heart. In shock, there is dilatation of the capillary beds, so that a considerable volume of blood can be accommodated.

Two kinds of fluids are used: crystalloids and colloids. Crystalloids are electrolyte solutions that diffuse into interstitial spaces. An example is lactated Ringer's Injection, a buffering solution, in which lactate is metabolized and excess hydrogen ions are neutralized.

Three parts crystalloids are lost to extravascular space for every one part that remains in the vascular system. This means that for every 2,000 ml. given, 500 ml. increase the vascular volume. For hemorrhagic shock, crystalloids are given initially to lower blood viscosity and aid in microcirculation. After blood typing and cross matching are done, blood is given to bring oxygen to the tissues.

Colloids are blood, plasma, serum albumin, and plasma substitutes such as dextran: these remain in the intravascular compartment. Blood of the same type as the patient's should be administered in preference to the generally used O-Rh-negative blood. Burn shock requires large amounts of colloid replacement.

Dextran is the most commonly used plasma substitute. Clinical dextran (molecular weight of 70,000) stays in the vascular system for 24 hours but interferes with blood typing and coagulation. Low molecular weight dextran (40,000) remains in the vascular system for about 8 hours but interferes less with blood typing and coagulation.

Cardiogenic shock has been recognized as being due to fluid overload. However, blood replacement may be necessary for proper resuscitation. It is essential that metabolic acidosis be corrected; therefore, blood pH must be monitored. (Acidosis has an adverse effect on myocardial contractility.) Alkalosis interferes with the ability of the red blood cells to give up oxygen to the cells, hence this is even more serious — since shock can be aggravated.

Digitalis and dopamine are the drugs of choice, but CVP must be carefully monitored.

3. ***The third objective is to administer vasodilators.*** This is done after vascular volume has been returned to normal and the CVP is normal. Vasopressors are not used for the patient in shock (except in cardiogenic shock) because they tend to intensify vasoconstriction in the microcirculatory beds.

Vasodilators are given to reduce peripheral resistance which in turn decreases the work of the heart and increases cardiac output and tissue perfusion. The drug usually used is isoproterenol (Isuprel), which stimulates myocardial contractility and lowers peripheral resistance. Some clinics advocate the use of steroids, others use combinations of pharmocotherapeutic agents such as phentolamine (Regitine) and *l*-norepinephrine (Levophed).

Nursing management requires constant monitoring of the blood pressure when vasodilators are used. The patient is kept flat during their administration. If the systolic blood pressure falls below 70, the drug is stopped and fluids are increased.

4. ***The fourth objective is to provide psychological support and minimize the patient's energy expenditure.*** Promote rest for the patient and assess his reactions to treatment. Offer support and reassurance to relieve apprehension. Administer sedatives cautiously as prescribed for pain, so that circulation is not further depressed. Keep the patient warm, because hypothermia

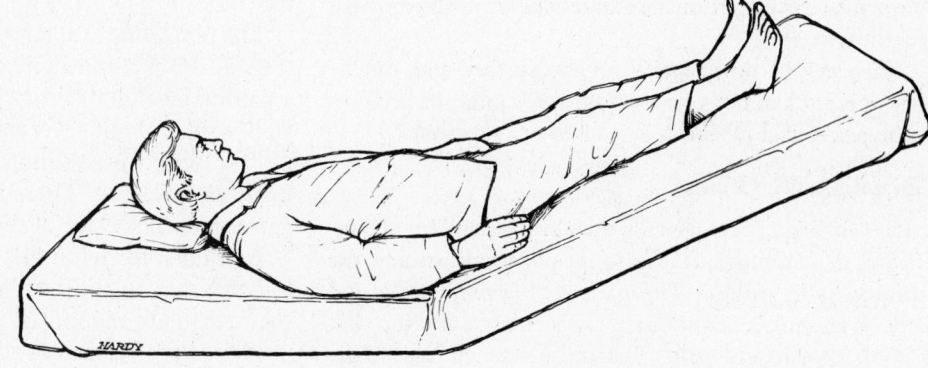

Figure 20-15. Proper positioning of the patient who shows signs of shock. The lower extremities are elevated to an angle of approximately 20 degrees; knees are straight, trunk horizontal, and head slightly elevated.

increases hemoglobin saturation but decreases tissue oxygenation. However, proper balance must be maintained, because hypothermia also affects peripheral circulation. Turn the patient every 2 hours and encourage deep breathing to promote optimum cardiopulmonary function. Exercises and gentle massage help to prevent pressure sores.

5. *The fifth objective is to prevent complications.* Observe all parameters and monitor the patient closely in the 24-hour period following shock, since complications may develop. Peripheral and pulmonary edema due to fluid overload is the most common complication that results from administering fluids faster than the body can accommodate them. (See page 584, pulmonary edema.)

Shock lung (a condition of respiratory failure associated with shock) is another complication which may occur if the following symptoms are noted: dyspnea, hyperventilation, tachypnea, rising blood pressure, and anxiety. This is in part related to the rapid infusion of crystalloid solutions during resuscitation from shock.

Oxygen toxicity may occur from oxygen therapy that is given in too high concentration. Convulsions may result following the initial warning signs of muscular twitchings of the face (around lips, eyes, forehead).

HEMORRHAGE

Classification

Hemorrhage is classified as (1) *primary,* when it occurs at the time of the operation; (2) *intermediary,* when it occurs within the first few hours after an operation, because of the return of blood pressure to its normal level and the consequent washing out of the insecure clots from untied vessels; and (3) *secondary,* when it occurs some time after the operation, as a result of the slipping of a ligature because of infection, insecure tying, or erosion of a vessel by a drainage tube.

A further classification frequently is made according to the kind of vessel that is bleeding. *Capillary* hemorrhage is characterized by a slow general ooze; *venous* hemorrhage bubbles out quickly and is dark in color; *arterial* hemorrhage is bright in color and appears in spurts with each heartbeat.

When the hemorrhage is on the surface and can be seen, it is spoken of as *evident;* when it cannot be seen, as in the peritoneal cavity, it is spoken of as *concealed.*

Clinical Manifestations

Hemorrhage presents a more or less well-defined syndrome, depending on the amount of blood lost and the rapidity of its escape. The patient is apprehensive and restless, and moves continually; he is thirsty; and the skin is cold, moist, and pale. The pulse rate increases, the temperature falls, respirations are rapid and deep, often of the gasping type spoken of as "air hunger." As the hemorrhage progresses, cardiac output decreases, arterial and venous blood pressure and the hemoglobin of the blood fall rapidly, the lips and the conjunctivae become pallid, spots appear before the eyes, a ringing is heard in the ears, and the patient grows weaker but remains conscious until near death.

Management

Often the signs of hemorrhage after an operation are masked by the effects of the anesthetic or shock; therefore, the treatment of the patient is in a general way almost identical to that described for shock, viz., (1) place the patient in shock position (Fig. 20-15) and (2) administer morphine to keep the patient quiet. The wound always should be inspected to find the site of the bleeding if possible. A sterile gauze pad and a snug bandage are indicated, as well as elevation of the part, arm, or leg.

- Giving a transfusion of blood and determining the cause of hemorrhage are the most logical therapeutic measures.
- In giving fluids by vein in cases of hemorrhage, remember that too large a quantity of fluid or too rapid administration may raise the blood pressure enough to start the bleeding again, unless the hemorrhage has been well controlled.

FEMORAL PHLEBITIS OR THROMBOSIS

Pathophysiology

Femoral phlebitis or thrombosis occurs most frequently after operations upon the lower abdomen or in the course of septic diseases such as peritonitis and ruptured ulcer. A mild to severe inflammation of the vein occurs in association with a clotting of blood. The complication may result from a number of causes, including injury to the vein by tight straps or leg-holders at the time of operation, pressure from a blanket-roll under the knees, concentration of blood by loss of fluid or dehydration, or, more commonly, the slowing of the blood flow in the extremity due to a lowered metabolism and depression of the circulation after operation. It is probable that several of these factors may act together to produce thrombosis. The left leg is affected more frequently.

The first symptom may be a pain or a cramp in the calf (Fig. 20-16). Pressure here gives pain, and a day or so later a painful swelling of the entire leg occurs, often associated with a slight fever and sometimes with chills and perspiration. The swelling is due to a soft edema that pits easily on pressure. There is marked tenderness over the anteromedial surface of the thigh.

A milder form of the same disease is termed *phlebothrombosis,* to indicate intravascular clotting without marked inflammation of the vein. The clotting occurs usually in the veins of the calf, often with few symptoms except slight soreness of the calf. The danger from this type of thrombosis is that the clot may be dislodged and produce an embolus. It is believed that most pulmonary emboli arise from this source. (See Figure 20-16.)

Medical and Nursing Management

The treatment of thrombophlebitis or phlebothrombosis may be considered as (1) preventive and (2) active.

PREVENTION. Efforts directed toward preventing the formation of a thrombus include such measures as adequate administration of fluids after operation to prevent blood concentration, leg exercises, elastic stockings (see below), and early ambulation to prevent stagnation of the blood in the veins of the lower extremity. Some clinics use low-dose heparin prophylactically to prevent deep vein thrombosis and major pulmonary embolism following general surgical operations. This method has not yet been generally accepted.

Leg exercises can be taught before surgery. If the patient recognizes their significance in preventing circulatory complications, he will often initiate his own exercises. To avoid thrombus formation, leg straps should not be fastened in the recovery room, particularly with stretchers that are equipped with side rails. Not only are the straps restrictive, but they can constrict and impair circulation.

Another important nursing measure is to avoid the use of blanket-rolls, pillow-rolls, or any form of elevation which can constrict vessels under the knees. Even the practice of "dangling" (having the patient sit on the edge of the bed with his legs hanging over the side) can be dangerous and is not recommended because pressure under the knees can impede circulation.

ACTIVE TREATMENT. Some surgeons believe that ligation of the femoral veins is an important therapeutic method. The rationale behind this method of therapy is to prevent pulmonary embolism by eliminating the cause (thrombi that could become detached from femoral veins and circulate in the blood).

Anticoagulant therapy has taken a prominent place in the prophylaxis and the treatment of phlebitis and phlebothrombosis. Heparin, given intravenously by the drip method or subcutaneously in an oily menstruum, reduces the coagulability of the blood rapidly and is used most often when an immediate effect is desired. Repeated checks of the coagulation time of the blood are necessary to control its administration. Dicumarol or drugs with a similar action are used for the same purpose. It is given by mouth and does not become effective for about 24 hours. Daily dosage is controlled by daily estimations of the prothrombin time of the blood (see also page 657).

Wrapping the legs from toes to groin with elastic stockings has been practiced both as a prophylactic and as an active treatment of phlebitis and thrombosis. These stockings prevent swelling and stagnation of venous blood in the legs and do much to relieve pain in the phlebitic extremity. However, to be effective, elastic stockings must be used in combination with leg elevation and leg exercises. Early ambulation is helpful, but the nurse also needs to be aware of the problem which can result when a patient with a protuberant abdomen walks a few steps and then sits with legs dependent; namely, the pressure of the abdomen can obstruct venous flow. Several recent research studies have questioned the value of elastic stockings, suggesting an actual danger when they are not applied correctly. Some clinics now do not advocate the use of elastic stockings for any surgical patient.

PULMONARY EMBOLISM

An *embolus* is a foreign body in the bloodstream, formed by a blood clot that becomes dislodged from its original site and is carried along in the blood.

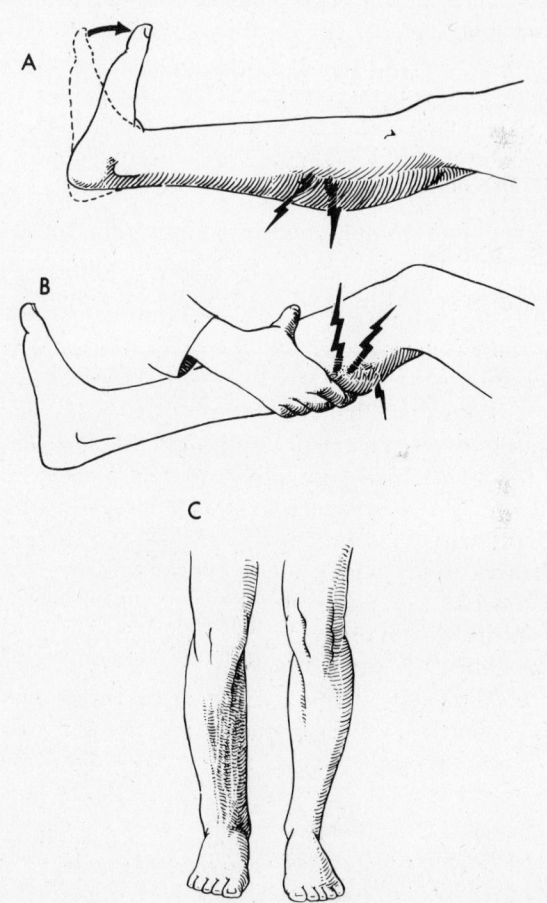

Figure 20-16. Nursing assessment of signs and symptoms of phlebothrombosis. Signs of phlebothrombosis of the calf muscle veins: *A*, Homans' sign, pain in the calf on dorsiflexion of the foot with the leg in extension; *B*, tenderness of the calf muscles on gentle compression; *C*, slight swelling about the ankle and prominence of the veins. (Gius, J. A.: Fundamentals of General Surgery, Chicago, Year Book Medical Pub., 1966)

When the clot is carried to the heart, it is forced by the blood into the pulmonary artery, where it plugs the main artery or one of its branches. The symptoms produced may be among the most sudden and startling in surgical practice. A patient passing an apparently normal convalescence suddenly cries out with sharp, stabbing pains in the chest and becomes breathless, cyanotic, and anxious. The pupils dilate, cold perspiration appears, the pulse becomes rapid and irregular, then imperceptible, and death usually results. If death does not occur within 30 minutes, there is a chance of recovery.

Fortunately, pulmonary embolism is usually a less dramatic event than that described above and may be heralded by no more than mild dyspnea, arrhythmia, or seemingly innocent chest pain. Keen alertness on the part of the nurse is necessary to detect these subtle emboli in order that treatment may be initiated and further embolization avoided.

- Thus, one of the many reasons for getting the patient out of bed as soon after surgery as possible is to avoid a pulmonary embolism.

(See pages 491–493 for therapeutic and nursing management.)

RESPIRATORY COMPLICATIONS

Respiratory complications are among the most frequent and serious problems with which the surgical team has to deal.

RISK FACTORS AFFECTING POSTOPERATIVE PULMONARY COMPLICATIONS

Type of surgery	greater incidence following all forms of abdominal surgery when compared with peripheral surgery
Location of incision	the closer the incision to the diaphragm, the higher the incidence of pulmonary complications
Preoperative respiratory problems	
Age	greater risk over age 40 than under age 40
Sepsis	
Obesity	weight greater than 110 percent of ideal body weight
Prolonged bed rest	
Duration of operation	over 3 hours
Aspiration	
Dehydration	
Malnutrition	
Hypotension and shock	

Experience has shown that such complications may be avoided in large measure by careful preoperative observation and teaching and by taking every precaution during and after the operation. It is well known that those patients who have some respiratory disease before operation are more apt to develop serious complications after operation. Therefore, only emergency operations are performed when acute disease of the respiratory tract exists. The nurse may aid by reporting any symptom, such as cough, sneezing, inflamed conjunctivae and nasal discharge, to the surgeon before the operation.

During and immediately after the operation, every effort should be made to prevent chilling. Aspiration of the nasopharynx in the recovery room removes secretions that would otherwise cause respiratory problems in the postoperative period. Occasionally, when secretions form that cannot be coughed up by the patient, aspiration may be carried out through a bronchoscope, and, in very debilitated patients in whom retained secretions are a complicating factor, a tracheostomy may be performed so that aspiration of the trachea is done directly through the tube as necessary.

Following upper abdominal surgery, total lung capacity (TLC) is reduced, for the following reasons:

1. Deep breathing may be quite painful.
2. Abdominal excursions with respiration normally are twice those of the chest cage. After surgery, they are greatly inhibited.
3. Spontaneous deep breaths are abolished (normally taken every 5 to 10 minutes).
4. Sigh mechanism is also abolished.

Complications are described briefly here and in more detail in Chapters 24 and 25.

ATELECTASIS. When the mucus plug closes one of the bronchi entirely, there is a collapse of the pulmonary tissue beyond, and a massive *atelectasis* is said to result (Fig. 20–17). (See also page 412.) The principal factors predisposing to postoperative atelectasis are diagramed in Figure 20–17.

BRONCHITIS. This pulmonary complication may appear at any time after operation, usually within the first 5 to 6 days. The symptoms vary according to the disease. A simple bronchitis is characterized by a cough that produces considerable mucopus, but without marked temperature or pulse elevation.

BRONCHOPNEUMONIA. Bronchopneumonia is perhaps the second most frequent pulmonary complication. Besides a productive cough, there may be considerable temperature elevation, with an increase in the pulse and the respiratory rates.

LOBAR PNEUMONIA. Lobar pneumonia is a less frequent complication after operation. Usually it begins with a chill, followed by high temperature, pulse, and respiration. There may be little or no cough, but the

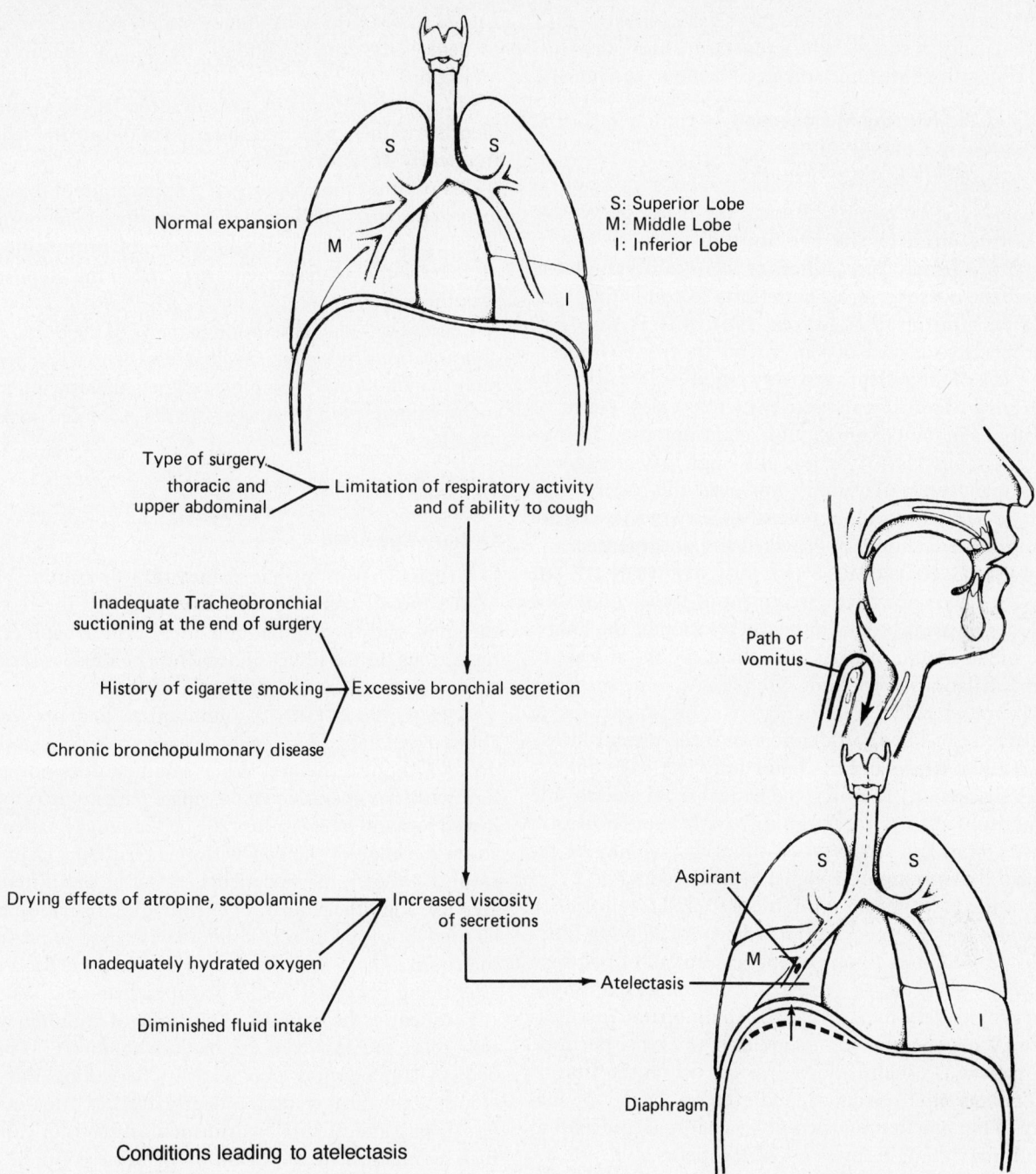

S: Superior Lobe
M: Middle Lobe
I: Inferior Lobe

Normal expansion

Type of surgery,
thoracic and
upper abdominal → Limitation of respiratory activity
and of ability to cough

Inadequate Tracheobronchial
suctioning at the end of surgery

History of cigarette smoking → Excessive bronchial secretion

Chronic bronchopulmonary disease

Drying effects of atropine, scopolamine → Increased viscosity
of secretions

Inadequately hydrated oxygen

Diminished fluid intake → Atelectasis

Conditions leading to atelectasis

Path of
vomitus

Aspirant

Diaphragm

Figure 20-17.   Atelectasis.

respiratory embarrassment, the flushed cheeks, and the evident illness of the patient make a combination of clinical signs that is distinctive. The disease runs its usual course with the added complication of the operative wound.

HYPOSTATIC PULMONARY CONGESTION.   Hypostatic pulmonary congestion is a condition that may develop in old or very weak patients. Its cause is a weakened heart and vascular system that permit a stagnation of secretions at the bases of both lungs. It occurs most frequently, per-

haps, in elderly patients who are not mobilized effectively. The symptoms frequently are not marked for a time—perhaps a slight elevation of temperature, pulse, and respiratory rate, and also a slight cough. However, physical examination reveals dullness and rales at the base of the lungs. If the condition goes untreated, the outcome may be fatal.

PLEURISY.   Pleurisy is not an uncommon occurrence after operation. Its chief symptom is an acute, knifelike pain in the chest on the affected side that is particularly excruciating when the patient takes a deep breath. Also, there usually is some slight temperature and pulse rise, and respirations are rapid and more shallow than normal.

Medical and Nursing Management of Pulmonary Complications

Awareness of the many possible respiratory complications enables the nurse to initiate the many preventive measures cited in the previous discussion (pages 313, 316). Timely recognition of signs and symptoms allows the nurse to direct her efforts to combating specific respiratory difficulties. Not only is the first postoperative day one of concern, but the first postoperative week of the patient's recovery requires close observation and careful management. The early signs of elevations in temperature, pulse, and respiration are significant. Chest pain, dyspnea, and cough may or may not accompany these elevations; however, the patient may seem to be restless and apprehensive. Such indications are important and should be reported and documented.

MEASURES TO PROMOTE THE FULL AERATION OF THE LUNG. The prophylactic treatment of these conditions includes measures to promote full aeration of the lungs. The nurse should instruct the patient to take at least 10 deep inhalations every hour. Frequently, some surgeons recommend IPPB treatments or some apparatus (a spirometer or blowbottle) into which the patient blows in an effort to expand the lungs fully (see page 351 for fuller discussion). Turning the patient from side to side sometimes results in coughing, with expulsion of a mucus plug, and recovery. At times mucus may be removed by aspiration through a bronchoscope.

The increased metabolism, more complete pulmonary aeration, and the general improvement of all body functions incidental to getting the patient up out of bed have led many surgeons to regard ambulation as one of the best prophylactic measures against pulmonary complications. When the wound or condition otherwise permits, the patient is usually allowed to get up on the first or second day after operation, and even on the day of surgery. This practice is especially valuable in preventing pulmonary complications in older patients.

INDICATIONS FOR SPECIFIC MEASURES. A most effective method of treating *bronchitis* is the inhalation of cool mist or steam, which may be administered by electric vaporizers. The apparatus must be kept filled with water and precautions must be taken to prevent the patient from being burned.

In *lobar* and *bronchopneumonia,* the patient is encouraged to take fluids; expectorant and antibiotic drugs also are given. Distention is watched for and prevented, if possible, so as to avoid added respiratory or cardiac embarrassment.

For *pleurisy,* analgesics, hot or cold applications, or, if necessary, a procaine intercostal block may be administered to provide symptomatic relief. A search is made to detect any possible underlying disease (pneumonia, infarction).

Pleurisy with effusion may result secondary to a primary pleurisy. In these patients aspiration of the pleural space is frequently necessary.

Many times the pulmonary complication of *hypostatic pulmonary congestion* becomes more serious than the original surgical condition, in which case the prime objective of therapeutic management is to treat the hypostatic pneumonia.

Because of reduced aeration in many of the pulmonary complications, which means that less oxygen reaches the blood, many clinics employ oxygen therapy in treatment. Principles and management are presented on pages 415–416.

URINARY PROBLEMS

Urinary Retention

Urinary retention may follow any operation, but it occurs most frequently after operations on the rectum, the anus, and the vagina, and after herniorrhaphies and operations on the lower abdomen. The cause is thought to be a spasm of the bladder sphincter.

NURSING MANAGEMENT. Quite often, patients are unable to void in bed but, when allowed to sit or stand up, do so without difficulty. When standing does not interfere with the operative result, male patients may be allowed to stand by the side of the bed or female patients to sit on the edge of the bed with their feet on a chair or a stool. However, many patients cannot be permitted this activity, and other means of encouraging urination must be tried. Some people cannot void with another person in the room. These patients should be left alone for a time after being provided with a warm bedpan or urinal.

Frequently the sound or the sight of running water may relax the spasm of the bladder sphincter. Using a bedpan containing warm water or irrigating the perineum with warm water frequently initiates urination for female patients. A small warm enema often is of value in such a situation. If the retention of urine continues for some hours, the patient complains of considerable pain in the lower abdomen, and the bladder frequently can be palpated and seen in outline distending the lower anterior abdominal wall.

When all conservative measures have failed, catheterization must be resorted to. If the patient has voided just before operation, this procedure may be delayed in most cases for 12 to 18 hours. There are two reasons for wishing to avoid catheterization: (1) there is the possibility of infecting the bladder and producing a cystitis, and (2) experience has shown that once a patient has been catheterized, frequently subsequent catheterizations are needed.

Many patients may exhibit a palpable bladder, with lower abdominal discomfort, and still void small amounts of urine at frequent intervals. The alert nurse does not mistake this for normal functioning of the bladder. This voiding of 30 to 60 ml. (1 to 2 oz.) of urine at intervals of 15 to 30 minutes is, rather, a sign of an overdistended bladder, the very distention being sufficient to allow the escape of small amounts of urine at intervals. The condition usually is spoken of as the "overflow of retention." A catheter usually relieves the patient by draining from 600 to 900 ml. (20 to 30 oz.) of urine from the bladder. "Incontinence of retention" may be evidenced by a constant dribble of urine, yet the bladder remains overdistended. Because distention injures the bladder, catheterization is indicated. There often is a definite psychic element in urinary retention.

At times, following extensive surgery, the surgeon may anticipate voiding difficulties and insert an indwelling catheter before the patient emerges from anesthesia. Usually the surgeon desires to be notified if an amount less than 30 ml. of urine per hour is collected in the calibrated receptacle.

Urinary Incontinence

Incontinence of urine is a frequent complication in the aged, either after operation or after shocking injuries. It is probably due to weakness with loss of tone of the bladder sphincter. This symptom frequently disappears as the patient gains in strength and normal muscular tone is regained.

TREATMENT. (See page 202 for bladder training, which is helpful for patients with urinary incontinence.)

Urinary Infection

(See discussion in Chapter 43.)

GASTROINTESTINAL COMPLICATIONS

Nutritional Considerations

Surgery of the gastrointestinal tract frequently disrupts the normal physiological processes of digestion and absorption. Complications arising from this disruption may take several forms depending on the location and extent of surgery. For example, oral surgery may present problems of chewing and swallowing, requiring that diet be modified to accommodate the difficulty. Other surgical procedures, such as gastrectomy, small bowel resection, ileostomy, colostomy, etc., have a more drastic effect on the gastrointestinal system and require more extensive dietary considerations, as indicated in Table 20-5.

Intestinal Obstruction

Intestinal obstruction is a complication that may follow abdominal operations. It occurs most often after operations on the lower abdomen and the pelvis, and

TABLE 20-5. DIETARY SUPPORT OF COMMON COMPLICATIONS IN SURGICAL TREATMENT*

PROCEDURE	COMPLICATIONS	DIETARY SUPPORT
Radical oropharyngeal surgery	Difficulty in mastication and swallowing	*Diet:* Liquid consistency—tube feedings *Fluid by mouth:* Fruit juices as tolerated Coffee, tea, gelatin, ice cream
Gastrectomy	*Small pouch:* "Dumping syndrome" Epigastric fullness, distention; pallor, sweating, tachycardia, hypotension, diarrhea	Low carbohydrate Moderate fat High protein Small frequent feedings Periodic injections of B_{12}
Small bowel resection	Poor absorption Weight loss (absorptive capacity improves with time)	*Immediate support after surgery:* Long-term parenteral nutrition *Later:* oral intake of high protein, high-calorie, low-fat diet Medium chain triglycerides
Ileostomy Colostomy	Initial loss of water and electrolytes	Daily replacement of electrolytes, full liquid diet, high in protein
Bypass surgery	For relief of pain and obstruction Malabsorption syndrome Maldigestion, diarrhea	Feedings by natural route High protein, high vitamin C Adequate vitamins and minerals

*Valassi, K.: Nutritional management of cancer patients in a variety of therapeutic regimens. Arch. Phys. Med. & Rehab., *58*:Sept. 1977.

especially after operations in which drainage has been necessary. The symptoms usually appear between the third and the fifth days but may occur at any time, even years after the operation. The cause is some obstruction of the intestinal current—frequently a loop of intestine that has become kinked from inflammatory adhesions or is involved with peritonitis or generalized irritation of the peritoneal surface.

Usually there is no temperature or pulse elevation. At first the pains are localized, a point which should be noted by the nurse, because the localization of the early pains represents in a general way the loop of intestine that is just above the obstruction.

Usually, the patient continues to have abdominal pains, with shorter and shorter intervals between. When a stethoscope is placed on the abdomen, sounds may be heard that give evidence of extremely active intestinal movements, especially during an attack of pain. The intestinal contents, being unable to move forward, distend the intestinal coils, are carried backward to the stomach, and are vomited. Thus, vomiting and increasing distention gradually become more prominent symptoms. Hiccup often precedes the vomiting in many patients. The bowels do not move, and enemas return nearly clear, showing that a very small amount of the intestinal contents has reached the large bowel. Unless the obstruction is relieved the patient continues to vomit, distention becomes more pronounced, the pulse becomes rapid, and the end is a toxic death.

TREATMENT. Sometimes the distention of the intestine above the obstruction can be prevented by the use of constant-suction drainage with the Miller-Abbott, Harris or Cantor tubes or simple nasogastric tube, in which case the inflammatory reaction of the bowel at the site of the obstruction may subside and the obstruction is relieved. However, at times it is necessary to relieve the obstructed intestine by operation. In addition, intravenous infusions of prescribed solutions usually are given. (See the section on intestinal obstruction for a more complete discussion of the treatment and postoperative care, pages 788-791.)

WOUND COMPLICATIONS

Hematoma (Hemorrhage)

The nurse should know the location of the patient's incision so that the dressings may be inspected for hemorrhage at intervals during the first 24 hours after operation. Any undue amount of bleeding should be reported. At times concealed bleeding occurs in the wound, beneath the skin. This hemorrhage usually stops spontaneously but results in clot formation within the wound. If the clot is small, it will be absorbed and need not be treated. When the clot is large, the wound usually bulges somewhat, and healing will be delayed unless it is removed. After several stitches are removed, the clot is evacuated, after which the wound is packed lightly with gauze. Healing occurs usually by granulation, or a secondary closure may be performed.

Infection (Wound Sepsis)

Staphylococcus aureus accounts for many postoperative wound infections. Other infections may result from *Escherichia coli, Proteus vulgaris, Aerobacter aerogenes,* and *Pseudomonas aeruginosa,* and, occasionally, from other organisms. The most important area of prevention lies in meticulous wound management and surgical technique. In addition, housekeeping cleanliness and environmental disinfection are important. When the inflammatory process occurs, it usually begins to show symptoms in 36 to 48 hours. The patient's pulse rate and temperature increase, and the wound usually becomes somewhat tender, swollen, and warm. At times, when the infection is deep, there may be no local signs. When a diagnosis of wound infection is made, the surgeon usually removes one stitch or more and, under aseptic precautions, separates the wound edges with a pair of blunt scissors or a hemostat. Once the infection is opened, a drain of rubber or gauze is inserted. In addition, many surgeons require some form of warm antiseptic solution with which to flush the wound. The surgeon may take a culture of the infected wound and prescribe specific antibiotics. It may be necessary to continue hot wet dressings if so prescribed. (See Risk Factor Chart.)

Disruption, Evisceration, or Dehiscence

This complication is especially serious in the case of abdominal wounds. It results from sutures giving way and from infection, and, more frequently, after marked distention or cough. It may also occur because of increasing age and the presence of pulmonary or cardiovascular disease in abdominal surgical patients.

The earliest sign is usually a gush of serosanguineous peritoneal fluid from the wound. The rupture of the wound may occur suddenly, coils of intestine escaping onto the abdominal wall. Such a catastrophe causes considerable pain and often is associated with vomiting. Frequently the patient says that something gave way. When the wound edges part slowly, the intestines may protrude gradually or not at all, and the presenting symptom may be the sudden drainage of a large amount of peritoneal fluid into the dressings.

- When disruption of a wound occurs, the surgeon is notified at once. The protruding coils of intestine should be covered with sterile dressings.

An abdominal (scultetus) binder, properly applied, is an excellent prophylactic measure against an accident of this kind, and often it is used along with the primary dressing, especially for operations on individuals with weak or pendulous abdominal walls. It is often used also as a firm binder when rupture of a wound has occurred. Vitamin deficiency or lowered serum protein or chloride may require correction.

Keloid

Not infrequently in an otherwise normal wound the scar develops a tendency to excessive growth. Sometimes the entire scar is affected; at other times the condition is segmented. This keloid tendency is unexplainable, unpredictable, and unavoidable in some individuals.

Much investigation has been done along the lines of prevention and cure. Careful closure of the wound, complete hemostasis, pressure support without undue tension on the suture lines—all are reputed to combat this distressing wound complication.

RISK FACTORS CONTRIBUTING TO WOUND SEPSIS	
Local	**General**
Wound contamination	Debilitation
Foreign body	Dehydration
Faulty suturing technique	Malnutrition
Devitalized tissue	Anemia
Hematoma	Advanced age
"Dead" space	Extreme obesity
	Shock
	Length of preoperative hospitalization
	Length of operation
	Associated diseases, i.e., diabetes mellitus

POSTOPERATIVE PSYCHOSIS

Postoperative psychosis (mental aberrations) may be physiologic or psychologic in origin. Cerebral anoxia, thromboembolism, and fluid-electrolyte imbalances are recognized physical factors in postoperative central nervous system impairment. Emotional factors such as fear, pain, and disorientation can contribute to postoperative depression and anxiety.

The individuals most susceptible to psychologic disturbances are older patients and those in the lower socioeconomic levels. Disfiguring surgery or operations for cancer also predispose to intense emotional problems. Dressings that obscure vision or confinement in a body cast can result in behavioral changes because of the reduced sensory input.

The highest incidence of psychotic sequelae appears to occur in those individuals who have had open-heart surgery. Several factors seem significantly related to neurologic damage: age (the older, the more likely), length of extracorporeal circulation (the longer, the greater the likelihood), mean arterial pressure of less than 50 mm. Hg during perfusion, and the possibility of air emboli. Even sensory-overload of the ICU unit is believed to contribute to postcardiotomy delirium.

Nursing Intervention—Preoperative and Postoperative

The patient should be thoroughly informed before the operation about what to expect after surgery. Frequent contact provides reassurance to the patient and allows the nurse to gain significant information about the patient's psychological status as she assesses his responses and thoughts. The judicious use of narcotics can also reduce confusion and disorientation.

Orienting the patient to time, day, and place can help him to accept unfamiliar surroundings. Studies have indicated that thorough preoperative briefing of the patient and his family can usually counteract many of the potential postoperative psychological stresses. In addition, a positive attitude conveyed by all personnel who come in contact with the patient will foster positive feelings in the patient.

For overt psychosis, the patient may require major tranquilizers. Since postoperative psychosis does occur, it is helpful when discussing this with patients to indicate that it is transient. If a patient has illusions or hallucinations, it is often reassuring to him to know that these aberrations are occasionally experienced and do not reflect on his sanity.

RESTRAINT. In the postoperative care of these patients, it is wise for the nurse to explain the necessity for the patient's remaining in bed until the surgeon permits him to get up. Often patients prefer to get out of bed to void or to get a drink of water rather than bother the nurse. This may lead to serious complications that a few words of explanation can prevent. However, some patients, especially older patients and those who are disoriented, may find it impossible to grasp this. For such patients, the simplest form of restraint is the use of a bed with side rails or side protection. This permits the patient to move about in bed but prevents him from getting out of bed easily and injuring himself.

The room should be lighted to reduce the incidence of visual hallucinations. It is desirable to have a family member stay with the patient as much as possible, since the presence of another person has a reassuring and quieting effect.

To protect both patient and nurse, it often becomes necessary to apply some form of restraint in cases of delirium. In the milder forms, a restraining sheet may be used—an ordinary sheet folded lengthwise to a width of approximately 30 to 37.5 cm. (12 to 15 inches), applied firmly over the thighs and held in place by wrapping each end round the bed frame.

The psychological effect of being restrained can be severe; therefore, any form of restraint should be applied *only as a last resort.* All other means of making the patient quiet should be tried first. If possible, he should be isolated from other patients. Any potentially harmful article in his vicinity should be removed.

When restraints are used, the patient should be in a comfortable and natural position, and care should be taken that the part is not so constricted as to interfere with the circulation. Restraint to the chest should be avoided, if possible. The appearance of cyanosis in hand or foot indicates that the appliance is too tight. The appliances should be padded carefully and placed so as to prevent chafing or pressure sores. The skin underneath them should be inspected frequently, bathed carefully, and massaged at least every 2 or 3 hours. Even though restraints are applied, the patient never should be left unwatched. Any patient requiring restraint should have constant and careful nursing attention.

Delirium

Postoperative delirium occurs occasionally in several groups of patients. The most common types of delirium are: toxic, traumatic, and alcoholic (delirium tremens).

TOXIC. Toxic delirium occurs in conjunction with the signs and the symptoms of a general toxemia. This patient is very ill, usually with a high temperature and pulse rate. The face is flushed, and the eyes are bright and roving. The patient moves incessantly, often attempting to get out of bed and disarranging the bedclothes continually. A marked degree of mental confusion is present. These states are seen most often in patients with general peritonitis or other septic conditions.

In such patients, elimination is promoted by encouraging the intake of fluids, and the causative condition is treated by antimicrobial therapy. At times, however, the outcome is fatal.

TRAUMATIC. Traumatic delirium is a mental state resulting from sudden trauma of any sort, especially in highly nervous people. The malady may take the form of wild maniacal excitement, simple confusion with hallucinations and delusions, or melancholic depression. Sedative drugs—chloral hydrate, paraldehyde, and morphine—are used in treatment. Usually the state begins and ends suddenly.

DELIRIUM TREMENS. Individuals who have used alcohol habitually over a long period of time are poor surgical risks. Not only is their resistance lower than normal, but the effects of alcohol have most likely damaged practically every organ. In addition, these patients take anesthesia poorly.

After operation the patient may do well for a few days, but the prolonged abstinence from alcohol causes him to become restless, nervous, and irritated easily by little things. His facial expression may change entirely. He sleeps poorly and often is disturbed by unreal dreams. When approached by the doctor or the nurse he appears to awake suddenly, asks "Who are you?" and, when he is told where he is, will appear to be fairly normal for a short time. These symptoms should be watched for in patients who have been alcoholics, because active treatment at this stage may avoid the more violent delirium.

Active delirium tremens may come on suddenly or gradually. After a period of restless, nervous, semi-delirium, the patient finally loses entire control of his mental functions and "horrors reign supreme." His mind is a chaos of everchanging ideas. He talks incessantly and tries to get out of bed to get away from the hallucinations of fear and persecution that torment him continually. If attempts are made to restrain him, he may fight maniacally and often will injure himself and others. In this stage the patient is obviously sick. He is sleepless, perspires freely and displays a marked tremor in his extremities. Finally, after many hours of torture, the patient becomes stuporous.

Treatment and Nursing Management. When possible, the treatment of these patients should begin 2 or 3 days before operation with a most thorough elimination from the kidneys, the bowels, and the skin. These measures should be continued after operation, especially if any of the early signs of the condition develop. Sedative drugs and/or tranquilizers should be given to keep the patient quiet. The chief cause of the symptoms in chronic alcoholics has been shown to be a depletion of the carbohydrate stores of the body and an inadequate ingestion of vitamins. Therefore, glucose is given intravenously, and vitamins are administered in concentrated form by mouth and by injection.

BIBLIOGRAPHY

ARTICLES

Postoperative Care

Croushore, T. M.: Postoperative assessment: The key to avoiding the most common nursing mistakes. Nursing '79, 9:47-51, Apr. 1979.

DelGuercio, L. R. M., and Cohn, J. D.: Monitoring: Methods and significance. Surg. Clin. N. Am. 56:977-994, Aug. 1976.

Fay, M. R.: Nursing process in the recovery room. AORN J., 24:1069-1075, Dec. 1976.

Felton, C. L.: Hypoxemia and oral temperatures. AJN, 78:56-57, Jan. 1978.

Garrett, J. J.: Oliguria in postoperative patients. Nurs. Clin. N. Am. 10:59-67, Mar. 1975.

Johnson, M.: Outcome criteria to evaluate postoperative respiratory status. AJN, 75:1474-1475, Sept. 1975.

Johnson, J. E., et al.: Sensory information, instruction in a coping strategy, and recovery from surgery. Research in Nurs. & Health, 1:4-17, Apr. 1978.

Hudson, S.: Teach breath control to ease your patients' postoperative pain. RN, 40:37-38, Jan. 1977.

Karetzky, M. S., and Khan, A. U.: Review of current concepts in aspiration pneumonia. Heart & Lung, 6:321-326, Mar.-Apr. 1977.

McConnell, E. A.: After surgery. Nursing '77, 7:32-39, Mar. 1977.

———: Nursing audit for recovery room. AORN J., 26:525-530, Sept. 1977.

Marcott, M.: Postoperative extubation. RN, 40:43-47, Sept. 1977.

Metheny, N. A.: Water and electrolyte balance in the postoperative patient. Nurs. Clin. N. Am., 10:49-57, Mar. 1975.

Mitchell, M.: Immediate recovery room care. Nurs. Care, 9:30-31, June 1976.

King, J.: Nursing grand rounds. Nursing '77, 7:29-33, Apr. 1977.

Sandham, G., and Reid, B.: Some Q's and A's about suctioning. Nursing '77, 7:60-65, Oct. 1977.

Sladden, A.: Maintenance of a patent airway. Hosp. Med., 13:56-67, Aug. 1977.

Smith, B. J.: Safeguarding your patient after anesthesia. Nursing '78, 8:53-56, Oct. 1978.

Taggart, B.: Body image. J. Pract. Nurs., 27:25-28, Aug. 1977.

Postoperative Complications

Archibald, L. H., et al.: Complications of general surgery. *In* Meltzer, et al.: Concepts and Practices in Intensive Care for Nurse Specialists, 2nd ed. Bowie, Md., Charles Press, 1976, pp. 405-436.

Campbell, G. G.: Respiratory failure in surgical patients. Curr. Prob. in Surg., *13*:1-67, Feb. 1976.

Cullen, D. J.: Recovery room complications, AORN J., *26*:746-762, Oct. 1977.

Durkin, D. M.: Pulmonary fat embolism: A complication of fracture. Heart & Lung, *5*:477-481, May-June 1976.

Marengo-Rowe, A. J., and Leveson, J. E.: Evaluation of the bleeding patient. Postgrad. Med., *62*:171-177, July 1977.

Schmidt, G. B.: Prophylaxis of pulmonary complications following abdominal surgery, including atelectasis, ARDS, and pulmonary embolism. *In* Nyhus, L. M., ed. Surgery Annual: 1977. New York, Appleton-Century-Crofts, 1977.

Wounds, Infections

Altemeier, W. A.: Operative procedure, wound classification, and risk of infection. Contemp. Surg., *10*:46-49, Mar. 1977.

Aspinall, M. J.: Scoring against nosocomial infections. AJN, *78*:1704-1707, Oct. 1978.

Bryant, W. M.: Wound healing. Clin. Symp., *29*:2-36, Nov. 3, 1977.

Choice of antimicrobial drugs. Med. Letter, *30*:1-8, Jan. 13, 1978.

Crow, S.: Control of surgical nosocomial infections. AORN J., *28*:148-158, July 1978.

Current concepts in healing wounds (symposium): Contemp. Surg., *13*:73-98, Oct. 1978.

Green, J. W., and Wenzel, R. P.: Postoperative wound infection. Ann. Surg., *185*:264-268, Mar. 1977.

Jenny, J.: What you should be doing about infection control. Nursing '76, *6*:78-79, Nov. 1976.

LaForce, F. M.: The hospital infection control committee: A personal view. Hosp. Pract., *12*:135-148, Mar. 1977.

Manson, H.: Exorcising excoriation from fistulae and other draining wounds. Nursing '76, *6*:57-60, Mar. 1976.

Meakins, J. L.: Pathophysiologic determinants and prediction of sepsis. Surg. Clin. N. Am., *56*:847-857, Aug. 1976.

Pachter, H. L., and Riles, T. S.: Low-dose heparin: Bleeding and wound complications in the surgical patient—a prospective randomized study. Ann. Surg., *186*:669-674, Dec. 1977.

Postoperative wound sepsis rate can be cut by simple measures. JAMA, *239*:9-10, Jan. 2, 1978.

Ryan, G. B.: Inflammation and localization of infections. Surg. Clin. N. Am., *56*:831-846, Aug. 1976.

Schilling, J. A.: Wound healing. Surg. Clin. N. Am., *56*:850-874, Aug. 1976.

Symposium on surgical infections. Surg. Clin. N. Am., *55*: Dec. 1975.

Tobey, L. E., and Covington, T. R.: Antimicrobial drug interactions. AJN, *75*:1470-1473, Sept. 1975.

Veterans Ad Hoc Interdisciplinary Adv. Comm. on Antimicrobial Drug Usage: 1. Prophylaxis in Surgery, JAMA, *237*:1003-1008, Mar. 7, 1977.

Wayne State University Symposium on Sepsis: Heart & Lung, *5*:May-June, 1976.

Problems Affecting Oxygen-Carbon Dioxide Exchange and Respiration

UNIT SIX

21

MANAGEMENT OF PATIENTS WITH CONDITIONS OF THE UPPER RESPIRATORY AIRWAY

PROBLEMS OF THE NOSE

EPISTAXIS (NOSEBLEED)

Pathophysiology. A hemorrhage from the nose, referred to as epistaxis, is caused by the rupture of tiny, distended vessels in the mucous membrane of any area of the nose. Rarely does epistaxis originate in the densely vascular tissue over the turbinates. Most commonly, the site is the anterior septum, where three major blood vessels enter the nasal cavity: (1) the anterior ethmoidal artery on the forward part of the roof, (2) the sphenopalatine artery in the posterosuperior region, and (3) the internal maxillary branches (the plexus of veins located at the back of lateral wall under inferior turbinate).

Epistaxis may result from injury or disease, although the usual cause of small nosebleeds is "picking" of the nose. Other local causes are deviated septum, perforated septum, cancer, and trauma. Epistaxis may also occur as a symptom of acute rheumatic fever, acute sinusitis, arterial hypertension, and hemorrhagic diseases.

Emergency Therapy. In providing emergency care, remember that cessation of bleeding is aided by having the patient sit upright and by promoting vasoconstriction in the nasal mucous membrane. The patient should breathe through his mouth, refrain from talking, and compress the soft outer portion of the nose against the midline septum for 5 or 10 minutes continuously. Saturating a piece of cotton with a local vasoconstricting drug such as Neo-Synephrine and then inserting the cotton into the nostril may be helpful.

Instruct the patient not to blow his nose during or after a nosebleed. Provide tissues and an emesis basin into which he can expectorate any blood that collects in the nasopharynx. Should these measures fail, the problem should be reported to the physician, who may control the epistaxis by applying aqueous epinephrine 1:1000 to a cotton pledget, inserting it in the nostril near the bleeding source, and applying pressure. The physician may then cauterize the site (if the bleeding point is visible) using an electric cautery (after injection of a local anesthetic) or a chemical agent such as a silver nitrate stick, a chromic acid bead, or trichloroacetic acid.

Subsequent Therapy. For subsequent therapy, the objectives are to ease pain, identify the bleeding site, and control bleeding.

TO EASE PAIN. It may be necessary to administer morphine (very judiciously), if pain is troublesome. Another method may be to apply cotton pledgets saturated with a solution of cocaine and epinephrine in order to shrink nasal mucosa and provide comfort.

ANATOMY OF THE UPPER RESPIRATORY TRACT

NOSE

The nose has two passages, called *nares,* separated in the middle by the septum. These passages open externally through the anterior nostrils and posteriorly into the nasopharynx. Between these two openings the air passages expand into broad chambers, on the lateral walls of which are three turbinate bones and into which open the paranasal sinuses, cavities within the hollow bones that surround the nasal passages.

PARANASAL SINUSES

The paranasal sinuses include the frontal sinuses, located in the lower forehead between and above the eyes; the ethmoidal group of sinuses, both anterior and posterior, extending along the roof of the nostrils; the sphenoid sinuses, opening at the rear; and, located on either side of the nose, the maxillary sinuses (Fig. 21-1). The same type of ciliated epithelium that lines the nasal passages also lines these paranasal sinuses.

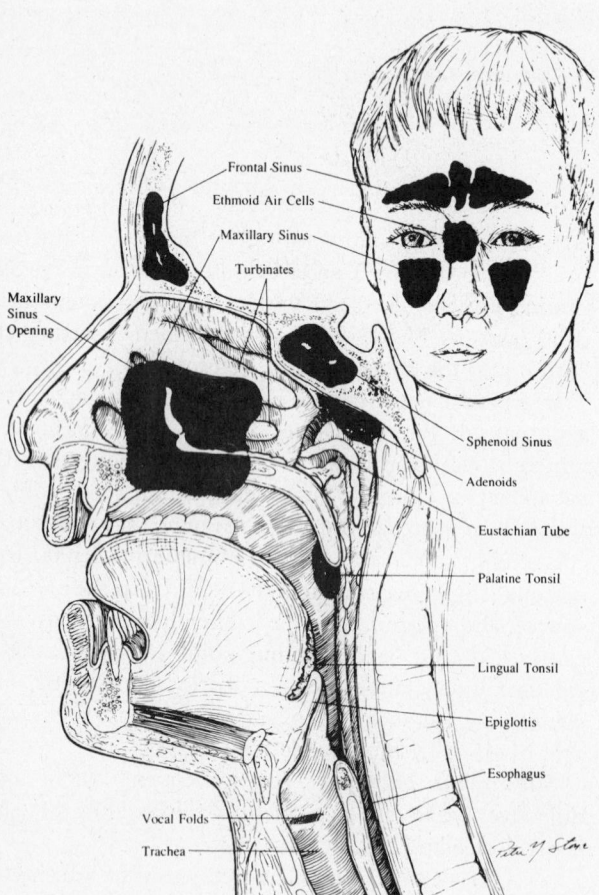

Figure 21-1. Anatomical features of the upper respiratory tract. (From Patient Education Chart material courtesy of and available from *Medical Times*, 80 Shore Road, Port Washington, N.Y. 11050)

A prominent function of the sinuses is to help give resonance and timber to speech. One notes how "nasal" the voice is when an individual has a head cold and sinusitis.

TURBINATE BONES (CONCHAE)

The turbinate bones, or conchae (the name suggested by their shell-like appearance), are adapted by shape and position to increase the mucous membrane surface of the nasal passages and to obstruct slightly the current of air flowing through them (Fig. 21-1). The sense organs of smell are located in the olfactory membrane, which covers the roof of the nose and the superior turbinate bones.

The current of air entering the anterior nostrils is deflected upward to the roof of the nose and follows a circuitous route before it reaches the nasopharynx. On its way, it comes into contact with a large surface of moist, warm mucous membrane that catches practically all of the dust and germs in the inhaled air. This air is moistened and warmed to body temperature and brought into contact with sensitive nerves. Some of these nerves detect odors and others provoke sneezing to expel irritating dust.

PHARYNX

The pharynx, or throat, is limited below by the larynx and the upper end of the esophagus. Its upper extension is the nasopharynx, into which open the posterior nostrils and the eustachian tubes from the middle ears. The nose and the nasopharynx are lined with the same type of ciliated epithelium as that which lines the trachea and bronchial tree; but the pharynx, which serves as both a respiratory and an alimentary passage, is lined with squamous (flat-celled) epithelium.

TONSILS AND ADENOIDS

The tonsils are two almond-shaped bodies, one on each side at the back of the throat. The adenoid, or pharyngeal tonsil, is located in the roof of the nasopharynx. The tonsils and the adenoids constitute only two of a ring of similar masses of lymphoid tissue that completely encircles the throat. These organs are important links in the chain of lymph nodes guarding the body from invasion by organisms entering the nose and the throat.

LARYNX

The larynx is a cartilaginous epithelium-lined structure forming the upper extremity of the trachea. The vocal cords, controlled by muscular attachments, are mounted in its lumen. Over it, preventing the entry of ingested food or liquid, is attached a valve flap called the *epiglottis.* The whole function of the larynx is to permit vocalization. It is the "voice box."

TO IDENTIFY THE BLEEDING SITE. Identifying the bleeding site may prove difficult; perhaps only the bleeding area can be determined. A light source such as a concave head mirror whose rays are parallel to the line of vision may be used to view deep, narrow spaces of the nasal cavity. If bleeding is occurring from the posterior regions, drug-moistened cotton pledgets may be inserted into the nostril to reduce the blood flow and improve the view. Suction can remove excess blood and clots from the field of inspection. The search may shift from the anteroinferior quadrant to the anterosuperior, then to the posterosuperior, and finally to the posteroinferior area. The field can be kept clear by using suction and by shifting the cotton tampons. However, only about 60 percent of the total nasal cavity can actually be seen.

TO CONTROL BLEEDING. When the origin of the bleeding cannot be found, the nose is sprayed with a topical anesthetic and a decongestant and then packed with gauze impregnated with petrolatum. A postnasal packing may be inserted with a balloon-inflated catheter or by the methods shown in Fig. 21-2. Pressure may be increased by moistening the gauze. The packing can be kept in place for 48 hours or up to 5-6 days if necessary.

RHINITIS

Pathophysiology. Rhinitis is an inflammatory lesion involving the mucous membrane of the nose. It is sometimes a manifestation of allergy (page 1107), in which instance the condition is referred to as "allergic rhinitis," but usually it is due to an infection. The most common variety of infection causing viral rhinitis is "coryza" (the common cold). Rhinitis also is encountered with regularity in the early stages of measles and other specific viral infections. Bacterial rhinitis is usually caused by a gram-positive bacterium and is characterized by a purulent nasal discharge. The infection is often secondary to a viral upper respiratory infection. If untreated, rhinitis

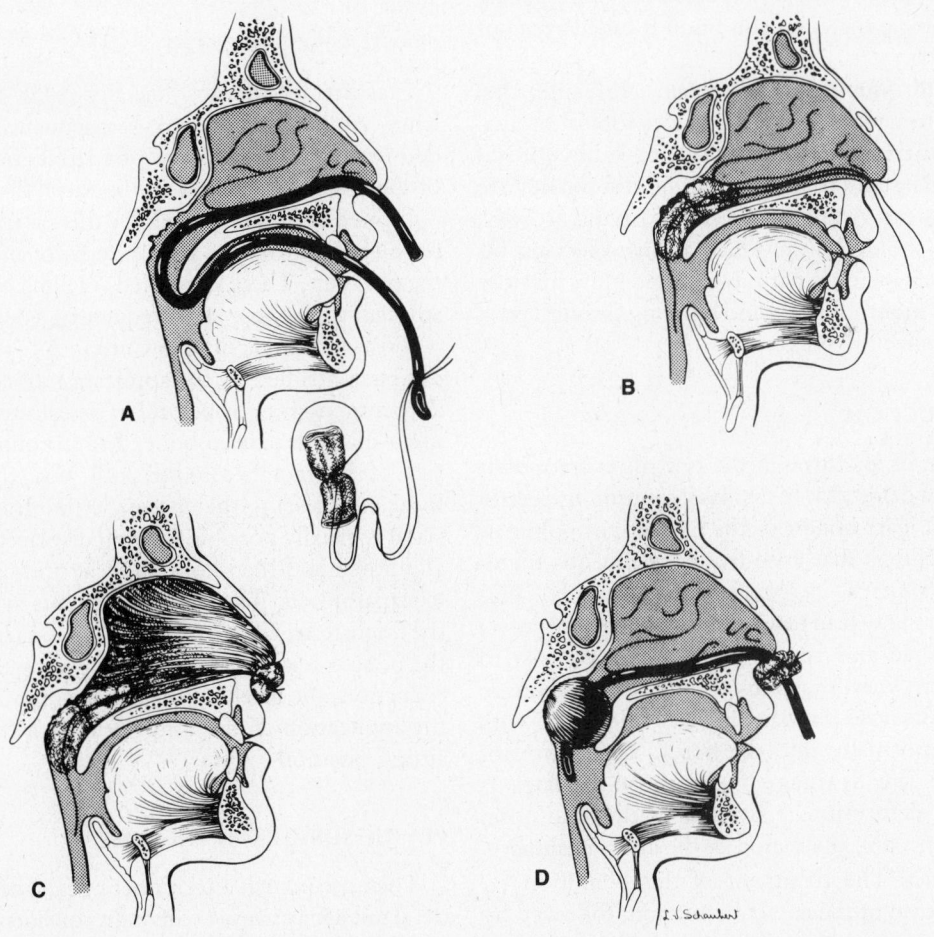

Figure 21-2. Packing to control bleeding from the posterior nose. *A.* Catheter inserted and pack attached. *B.* Pack drawn into position as catheter is removed. *C.* Strip tied over a bolster to hold pack in place with anterior pack installed "accordion pleating" style. *D.* Alternative method using balloon catheter instead of gauze pack. (Reproduced, with permission, from Dunphy, J. E., Way, L. W. [editors]: Current Surgical Diagnosis & Treatment, 3rd ed. Copyright 1977 by Lange Medical Publications, Los Altos, Calif.)

can lead to sinusitis, otitis media, bronchitis, and pneumonia.

In acute rhinitis, the nasal mucous membrane becomes congested, swollen, and edematous for a short period of time and then quickly returns to normal. After repeated attacks, however, particularly in cases which originate as a result of chronic sinusitis, this swelling becomes obstinate, and the patient has a "chronic catarrh." Persons with this problem say that they are "subject to colds." The fact is that, excluding the recurring attacks of allergic rhinitis, their attacks are acute exacerbations of the same "cold."

If continued, chronic rhinitis leads to the deposition of abnormally large amounts of connective tissue in the nasal mucous membrane, which greatly thickens it and, in addition to hypertrophy, causes the formation of spurs and polyps on the nasal septum. Wasting or atrophy of the mucous membrane, the cartilage, and the bones lining the nasal passages eventually may occur, with the result that these passages become large empty caverns, in which an abundant exudate builds up on the walls, giving off a disagreeable odor. This condition is called *ozena* or atrophic rhinitis.

Therapy and Nursing Intervention. In acute viral rhinitis, symptomatic treatment includes topical or systemic vasocontricting medications to relieve nasal obstruction, analgesics for headache, and rest to alleviate general discomfort. Adults are advised to avoid crowds.

The patient should be cautioned against blowing his nose too frequently or too hard. He should blow his nose by opening his mouth slightly and blowing through both nostrils to equalize the pressure.

NASAL OBSTRUCTION

The passage of air through the nostrils is frequently obstructed by a deflection of the nasal septum, hypertrophy of the turbinate bones, or the pressure of polyps — grape-like swellings that arise from the mucous membrane of the sinuses, especially the ethmoids. This obstruction also may lead to a condition of chronic infection of the nose and result in frequent attacks of nasopharyngitis. Very frequently the infection extends to the sinuses of the nose (mucous-lined cavities filled with air that drain normally into the nose). When sinusitis develops and the drainage from these cavities is obstructed by deformity or swelling within the nose, pain is experienced in the region of the affected sinus.

Management. The treatment of this condition requires the removal of the nasal obstruction, followed by measures to overcome whatever chronic infection exists. In many patients the underlying nasal allergy is the lesion requiring treatment. At times it is necessary to drain the nasal sinuses by a radical operation. The operations performed depend on the type of nasal obstruction found. Usually they are performed with local anesthesia.

If a deflection of the septum is the cause of the obstruction, the surgeon makes an incision into the mucous membrane and, after raising it from the bone, removes the deflected bone and cartilage with bone forceps. The mucosa then is allowed to fall back in place and is held there by tight packing. Generally the packing used is soaked in liquid petrolatum to facilitate its removal in 24 to 36 hours. This operation is called a *submucous resection* or septoplasty.

Nasal polyps are removed by clipping them at their base with a wire snare. Hypertrophied turbinates may be treated by astringent applications to shrink them close to the side of the nose.

After these procedures, the head of the bed is elevated to promote drainage and to help in alleviating the patient's discomfort due to edema. Frequent oral hygiene care should be given because the patient breathes through his mouth.

FRACTURES OF THE NOSE

Fractures of the nose usually result from direct violence. As a rule, no serious consequences result, but the deformity that may follow often gives rise to obstruction of the nasal air passages and to facial disfigurement.

Immediately after the injury there is usually considerable bleeding from the nose externally and internally into the pharynx. There is marked swelling of the soft tissues adjacent to the nose and, frequently, a definite deformity.

Treatment and Nursing Care. As a rule, the bleeding can be controlled by the application of cold compresses. A roentgenogram is helpful in determining the displacement of the fractured bones and in ruling out an extension of the fracture into the skull. With the application of local anesthesia to the nose or with intravenous anesthesia, it is usually possible to bring displaced fragments into alignment and then hold them by intranasal packing or external splints. The important points in the reduction of the fracture are to reform the nasal passages and to realign the bones so as to prevent a disfiguring deformity. After reduction, the swelling that occurs may be decreased by the application of ice compresses with the patient in the sitting position.

PLASTIC SURGERY OF THE NOSE

The nose is such a prominent organ of the face that its deformity may cause the patient considerable embarrassment. The deformity may result from congenital causes, from disease, or from injury.

Deformities resulting from congenital causes often may be corrected by simple operations (rhinoplasty) in which the nose is straightened or lengthened by either removing offending bone or supplying new tissue (usually costal cartilage). The incisions are so placed as to be inconspicuous. In deformities resulting from injury or disease, various types of plastic surgery may be employed. Skin, tube, or sliding grafts may be used to cover the defects left by scars, malignancy, or injuries. In some instances, especially in older people with malignancy, artificial appliances may be modeled and held in place with the rims of glasses. (See Reconstructive Surgery, page 1070.)

Nursing Management. Before surgery, a photograph of the patient's face and nose may be taken to serve as a permanent record and to be used as an aid in determining goals of treatment.

After operation, the patient usually is placed flat on his back with the head slightly elevated. Ice compresses are used frequently to reduce bleeding, swelling, and pain. A splint may be taped to the nose and in some instances, pressure dressings may be placed over the eyes.

• Hemorrhage is the chief postoperative complication.

It must be remembered that the spitting up or the vomiting of blood that has run back into the pharynx is as much a symptom of nasal hemorrhage as is the flow at the nares. Frequent swallowing, followed by belching, often is indicative of bleeding that results in an accumulation of blood in the stomach.

In patients for whom local anesthesia has been used, the blood sometimes trickles down the throat, but the patient is not sufficiently aware of it to show a swallow reflex.

• If the bleeding is excessive or continuous, or if any of the constitutional signs of hemorrhage appear, the surgeon should be called and the following items made available: fresh packing, a light, a head mirror, a nasal speculum, and packing forceps.

Patients may have a liquid diet on the day of operation and whatever they prefer after that. Sedatives often are necessary on the day and the night of operation, but after that there is little need for them. The patient should be warned that he will be tempted to blow his nose because of a full feeling caused by the packing. He should be cautioned against blowing his nose until the surgeon grants permission. Packing is removed usually after 24 hours.

Convalescence and Patient Education. Swelling and discoloration may be noticed for a few days but will subside by the end of the first week. Usually, normal activities may be resumed after 2 weeks. During that time, heavy weights should not be lifted.

The patient should be urged to have follow-up visits with the surgeon and to avoid any pressure on the nose for a few weeks, such as may be caused by eyeglasses. If the patient wears contact lenses, he should consult the surgeon as to when he may resume wearing them.*

SPECIFIC INFECTIONS OF THE UPPER RESPIRATORY TRACT

COMMON COLD

The phrase "common cold" is a general term which patients use in different ways, usually when referring to symptoms of upper respiratory infection.

Manifestations and Pathophysiology. These symptoms are nasal discharge and obstruction, sore throat, sneezing, malaise, fever, chills, and often headache and muscle aching. As the cold progresses, cough usually appears. Most specifically, the term *cold* refers to afebrile, infectious acute coryza. More broadly the word refers to acute upper respiratory infection, whereas terms such as *rhinitis, pharyngitis, laryngitis, chest cold,* etc., distinguish the sites of the major symptoms.

The symptoms last 5 days to 2 weeks. If there is significant fever or more severe constitutional problems with the respiratory symptoms, we are no longer dealing with a common cold but with one of the other acute upper respiratory infections. Many different viruses (over 100) are known to produce the symptoms of the common cold and about 10 percent of colds seem to be associated simultaneously with more than one virus. Also allergic conditions affecting the nose can mimic the symptoms of a cold.

Community Health and Social Significance. Colds are highly contagious, since patients shed virus for about two days before the symptoms appear and during the first part of their symptomatic phase. Colds prevail among 15 percent of the work population at any time during the winter and account for almost half of all work absences and one quarter of the total time lost from work.

Three waves of colds appear yearly in the United States—in the fall just after the opening of school, in midwinter, and in spring. Immunity after recovery is variable, depending on many factors including natural host resistance and the specific virus that caused the cold in the first place. The major complication of a cold is the secondary bacterial infection that can affect the ears, nose, sinuses, bronchi, or lungs.

Management. Management of the common cold consists of adequate fluid intake, rest, prevention of chilling, aqueous nasal decongestants, vitamin C, bron-

---

*An excellent pamphlet for patient education is "Facts About Plastic Surgery of the Nose," American Academy of Facial Plastic and Reconstruction Surgery, Inc.

chodilators and expectorants as needed. Warm salt water gargles soothe the sore throat, and acetylsalicylic acid relieves the general constitutional symptoms. Antibiotics are not indicated in the uncomplicated common cold.

Using disposable tissues and disposing of them hygienically, covering the mouth when coughing, and avoiding crowds are about all that can be offered in the way of prevention.

STREPTOCOCCAL SORE THROAT

Ranking high among the most uncomfortable, debilitating, and dangerous of the upper respiratory tract infections are those produced by the Group A streptococcus. This type of infection is characterized by the abrupt onset of sore throat, chilly sensations or frank chills, temperature elevations above 38.3° C. (101° F.), headache, loss of appetite, and general malaise. The pharynx is diffusely reddened; the tonsils and the tonsillar nodes beneath the angles of the mandible are enlarged, and the uvula is edematous. A patchy or confluent exudate covers the tonsils and the pharynx. The face is flushed, and individuals who are not immune to the exotoxin of the Group A streptococcus (i.e., who are "Dick positive") are likely to develop the typical rash of scarlet fever. The blood leukocyte count generally exceeds 12,000.

Nursing Management and Chemotherapy. The nursing care of patients with acute pharyngitis, including the type due to the hemolytic streptococcus, is discussed in detail on pages 389-390.

- Early chemotherapy in patients with hemolytic streptococcal infection is of the utmost importance from the standpoint of preventing its most serious complications—acute rheumatic fever and acute glomerulonephritis.

Penicillin is the drug of choice, given for 10 days. Antibiotics that may serve as adequate substitutes for penicillin in the event of sensitivity include erythromycin, tetracycline, chlortetracycline, and oxytetracycline.

HERPES SIMPLEX INFECTION

The herpes simplex virus most commonly produces the familiar *herpes labialis* (cold sore, fever blister, or canker), but in children who are reacting to this virus for the first time, the infection may take the form of an acute herpetic gingivostomatitis. Small vesicles, single or clustered, may erupt on the lips, the tongue, the cheeks, and the pharynx. These soon rupture, forming sore, shallow ulcers that are covered with a gray membrane.

Herpes infections appear often in association with other febrile infections, such as streptococcus pneumonia, meningococcic meningitis, and malaria. The virus remains latent in cells of lips or nose and is activated by febrile illnesses. The herpes virus does not yield in the slightest to any of the chemotherapeutic agents that have become available to date. Analgesics and codeine are helpful in relieving pain and discomfort. Applications of drying lotions or liquids may help to dry the lesions.

SINUSITIS

The sinuses are involved in a high proportion of upper respiratory tract infections. If their openings into the nasal passages are clear, the infections within them recover promptly; but if their drainage is obstructed by a deflected septum or by hypertrophied turbinates, spurs, or polyps, sinusitis may persist as a smoldering secondary infection or it may flare up into an acute suppurative process.

Acute Sinusitis

Pathophysiology and Manifestations. Acute sinusitis may be localized in one sinus or may involve several. If all are involved, the condition is called *pansinusitis.* The most prominent symptom of acute sinusitis is pain. Since the location of the pain is diagnostically important, it should be noted by the nurse. In *frontal sinusitis,* the patient complains of frontal headache; in *ethmoidal sinusitis,* the pain is usually in or about the eyes; in *maxillary sinusitis,* pain may be referred to the brow but usually is lateral to the nose and sometimes is accompanied by aching of the upper teeth of the corresponding side; in *sphenoidal sinusitis,* occipital headache may result. Aside from being located in a specific area, pain also may be referred, for example, to the forehead. Nasal congestion and discharge are usually, but not necessarily, present. The patient feels generally miserable, quite apart from pain. Fever, however, if present at all, is usually mild. This may be the case even in the presence of an acute suppurative infection, or "empyema," of a sinus.

- The most dangerous variety of sinusitis is empyema of a frontal sinus, because it may rupture posteriorly, producing a brain abscess.

A careful history and diagnostic assessment should be done to rule out other local or systemic disorders such as tumor, fistula, allergy, and viral infections.

Management. The treatment of acute sinusitis is bed rest and the establishment of free drainage of the sinuses involved. This usually can be accomplished by nasal instillations or sprays of phenylephrine hydrochloride (Neo-Synephrine, 0.25 percent) or by oral decongestants such as pseudoephedrine or a similar vasoconstrictor drug. Depending on the type of infecting organism and the extent of the infection, the patient may be instructed to apply local therapy of this sort at intervals of 1 to 4 hours until drainage is established. The use of penicillin usually speeds recovery and definitely diminishes the chance of complications that can follow the extension of a bacterial sinusitis. If allergy is suspected as the basis of the inflammatory process, one of the antihistaminic agents (e.g., tripelennamine [Pyribenzamine]) in oral doses may be beneficial, at least symptomatically, in very early stages.

Chronic Sinusitis

Pathophysiology and Manifestations. Chronic sinusitis usually manifests itself by persistent nasal obstruction due to discharge and edema of the nasal mucous membrane. The patient experiences cough, because of the constant dripping of the discharge backward into the nasopharynx, and headaches, which are apt to be most pronounced on awakening in the morning. Fatigue is also common, as are dullness and nasal stuffiness.

Management. Treatment of chronic sinusitis includes measures to facilitate drainage, antibacterial therapy, and antiallergic measures. Increased humidity, steam inhalations, increased fluid intake, and local heat applications will assist in promoting drainage. Local use of vasoconstricting drugs in the form of sprays or nose drops may be tried.

- However, overuse or prolonged use of vasoconstrictive nasal drugs may aggravate rhinitis and sinusitis by causing rebound congestion, which leads to further overuse.

Oily nose drops are to be avoided. Sterile Ringer's solution used with a nasal douche can be obtained in any drugstore and is a soothing method of cleansing the nose. Structural deformities that obstruct the ostia of the sinus may require surgical attention: polyps may require excision or cauterization, a deflected septum may have to be removed or a narrowed ostium widened.

For drainage of the maxillary sinus, the incision is made along the upper gum line above the canine teeth (Caldwell-Luc operation). To drain the frontal sinus an incision is made through the inner third of the eyebrow.

Some victims of severe chronic sinusitis obtain relief only by moving to a dry climate.

PREVENTION OF UPPER RESPIRATORY INFECTIONS

The prevention of most upper respiratory tract infections is difficult, since their causes are legion. The responsible pathogen usually cannot be identified and vaccines are unavailable except in rare instances. Allergies, pathology of the septum and the turbinate, emotional problems, and various systemic illnesses may be predisposing factors in isolated cases.

The following hygienic measures tend to support the body's defenses and reduce susceptibility to respiratory infections:

- Practice good health measures — nutritious diet, appropriate exercise, adequate rest and sleep.

- Avoid excesses in alcohol and smoking.
- Correct air dryness by proper home humidification, especially during cold weather.
- Avoid air contaminants (dust, chemicals) when possible.
- Avoid unnecessary chilling of the skin, especially the feet; chilling lowers resistance.
- Obtain influenza vaccination if and when directed by the physician.

PROBLEMS OF THE PHARYNX AND THE TONSILS

ACUTE PHARYNGITIS

Acute pharyngitis, caused by several viruses and bacteria, is a febrile inflammation of the throat. The pharyngeal membrane becomes fiery red; the lymphoid follicles of the throat and the tonsils become swollen and flecked with exudate; and the cervical lymph nodes may become tender and enlarged. Uncomplicated viral infections usually subside promptly, within 3 to 10 days after the onset. But pharyngitis caused by certain of the more virulent bacteria, such as beta hemolytic streptococcus, or hemolytic *Staphylococcus aureus,* is a more severe illness during the acute stage and far more important because of the incidence of dangerous complications. These complications include sinusitis, otitis media, mastoiditis, cervical adenitis, rheumatic fever, nephritis, and, in the rare case of infection by the diphtheria bacillus, paralysis. A throat culture is the chief means of determining the causative organism (Fig. 21-3). When this is obtained, proper therapy can be prescribed. Note that if one member of a family has a proved streptococcal infection, all other family members, whether symptomatic or not, should also have throat cultures done. Those with positive cultures are treated with penicillin.

Nursing Management. The patient should be kept in bed during the febrile stage of illness. When he is ambulatory he needs periods of rest. Medical asepsis must be observed to prevent the spread of infection. The skin should be examined once or twice daily for possible rash, because acute pharyngitis may precede some other communicable disease.

Aside from throat cultures, it may be necessary to secure nasal swabbings and blood cultures for further laboratory investigation to determine the nature of the causative organism.

Warm saline gargles or irrigations are employed, depending on the severity of the lesion and the degree of pain. Recognizing that the benefits of this treatment depend on the degree of heat that is applied, the nurse should ensure that the temperature of the solution is sufficiently high to be effective, i.e., approaching the limits of tolerance, which vary with each patient, usually between 40.6–43.3° C. (105°–110° F.). A throat irrigation,

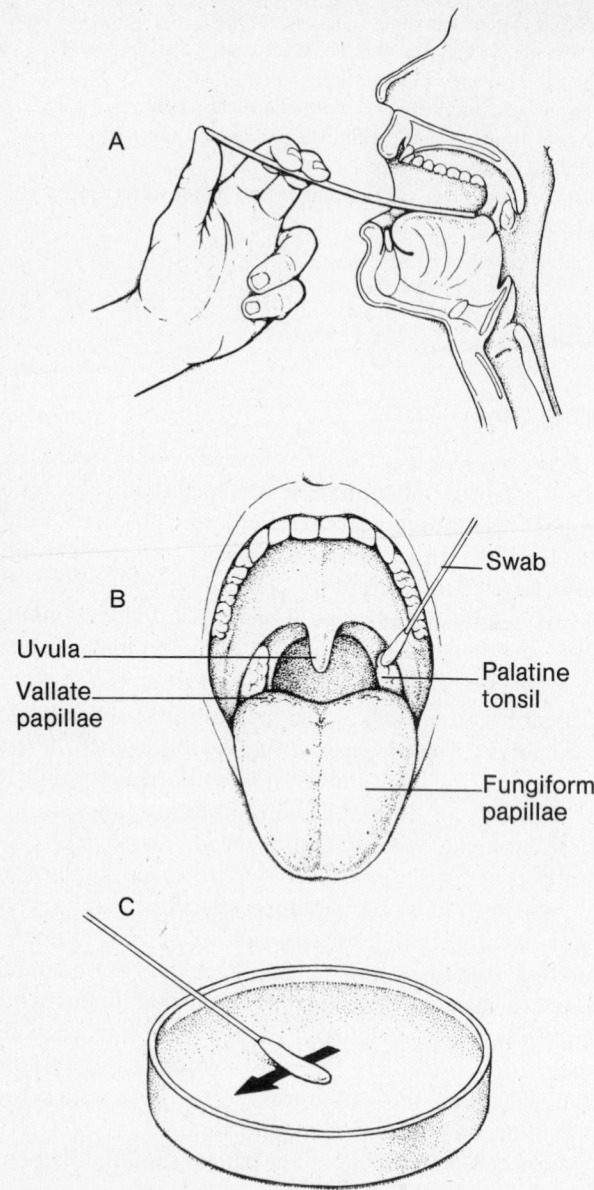

Figure 21-3. Taking a throat culture. When obtaining a throat culture from a patient who "gags," it is helpful to have him close his eyes. Since anticipation is lessened, the culture can be obtained with only a slight gag.

A. Grasp the tongue blade so that the thumb pushes the end upward (as a fulcrum) while the fingers push the middle section downward.

B. Vigorously rub a cotton or dacron swab over each tonsillar area and the posterior pharynx.

C. Streak the swab on a blood agar plate and place in an incubator for 24 hours. A gross reading of the plate can then be made.

properly performed, is an effective means of reducing spasm in the pharyngeal muscles and relieving soreness of the throat. However, unless the purpose of the procedure, and its technique, are understood clearly by the patient, the results may be less than satisfactory. If throat irrigation is a new experience for the patient, the nurse

should explain the procedure and its purpose before commencing.

Symptomatic relief in patients with severe sore throat also may be afforded by applying an ice collar and administering analgesic drugs, e.g., acetylsalicylic acid or acetaminophen given at 3- to 6-hour intervals and, if required, codeine sulfate, 3 or 4 times daily. Antitussive medication, in the form of codeine or hydrocodone bitartrate (Hycodan), may be required to control a persistent and painful cough that often accompanies acute pharyngitis. One of the barbiturates, e.g., pentobarbital (Nembutal) may be prescribed for the patient as a soporific at bedtime.

If a bacterial etiology is suspected or demonstrated, treatment may include the administration of antimicrobial agents.

A liquid or a soft diet is provided during the acute stage of the disease, depending on the patient's appetite and the degree of discomfort caused by swallowing.

The patient should be encouraged to drink to the limit of tolerance, the minimum intake during the febrile stage exceeding, if possible, 2,500 ml. each day. Often, the patient can achieve this goal more easily if the rationale of therapy is explained adequately to him. His personal tastes should be considered and indulged when possible.

Mouth care may add greatly to the patient's comfort and may aid in preventing the development of fissures of the lips and pyoderma about the mouth when bacterial infection is present.

Convalescence and Patient Education. Resumption of activity should be permitted gradually. Unusually conservative management is indicated in patients with hemolytic streptococcus infection in view of the possible development of complications such as nephritis and rheumatic fever, which may have their onset 2 or 3 weeks after the pharyngitis has subsided. Local extension of an apparently quiescent pharyngitis may develop in the form of sinusitis, otitis media, mastoiditis, or cervical adenitis. Daily assessment of morning and evening temperatures should be continued until convalescence is complete, and the patient or his family should be familiarized with symptoms that deserve investigation because they could lead to possible complications.

CHRONIC PHARYNGITIS

Incidence, Pathophysiology, and Manifestations. This disease is common in adults who work in dusty surroundings, use the voice to excess, and suffer from chronic cough. Its incidence also is high among habitual users of alcohol and tobacco.

Three types of chronic pharyngitis are recognized: (1) hypertrophic, characterized by general thickening and congestion of the pharyngeal mucous membrane; (2) atrophic, probably a late stage of type one (the membrane is thin, whitish, glistening, and, at times, wrinkled); and (3) chronic granular ("clergyman's sore throat"), with numerous swollen lymph follicles on the pharyngeal wall.

Patients with chronic pharyngitis complain of a constant sense of irritation or fullness in the throat, of mucus which collects in the throat and can be expelled by coughing, and of difficulty in swallowing.

Management and Patient Education. The treatment of chronic pharyngitis consists of avoiding alcohol and tobacco, resting the voice, and correcting any upper respiratory, pulmonary, or cardiac condition that might be responsible for a chronic cough.

Nasal congestion may be relieved by nasal instillations or sprays containing ephedrine sulfate, phenylephrine hydrochloride (Neo-Synephrine) or tuaminoheptane sulfate (Tuamine) in saline, and, in the early stages, if there is a history of allergy, one of the antihistaminic drugs such as tripelennamine (Pyribenzamine) every 4 to 6 hours by mouth. The attendant malaise is controlled effectively by aspirin or acetaminophen. Contact with others should be avoided, at least until the fever has subsided completely, in order to prevent the infection from spreading.

DISEASES OF THE TONSILS AND THE ADENOIDS
Tonsils

The tonsils are a pair of lymphatic tissue structures, one of which is situated on each side of the oropharynx; they frequently serve as the seat of acute infection (Fig. 21-4).

Chronic tonsillitis occurs less commonly and may be mistaken for other disorders, such as allergy, asthma, and sinusitis. A thorough physical examination is given and a careful history is taken to rule out related or systemic conditions. A culture of the organisms at the tonsillar site is done to determine the presence of bacterial infection. Medical therapy with appropriate antibiotics is initiated.

Tonsillectomy is usually not done unless medical treatment is unsuccessful and there is severe hypertrophy or peritonsillar abscess which occludes the pharynx, making swallowing difficult and endangering the airway. Enlargement of the tonsils is per se rarely an indication for their removal; most children have normally large tonsils, which decrease in size as the child grows older.

Despite the continuing debate over the effectiveness of many tonsillectomies, the operation is still the most common nondiagnostic surgical procedure done in the United States.

Adenoids

The adenoids consist of an abnormally large lymphoid tissue mass near the center of the posterior wall of the nasopharynx. Unusually enlarged adenoids may cause

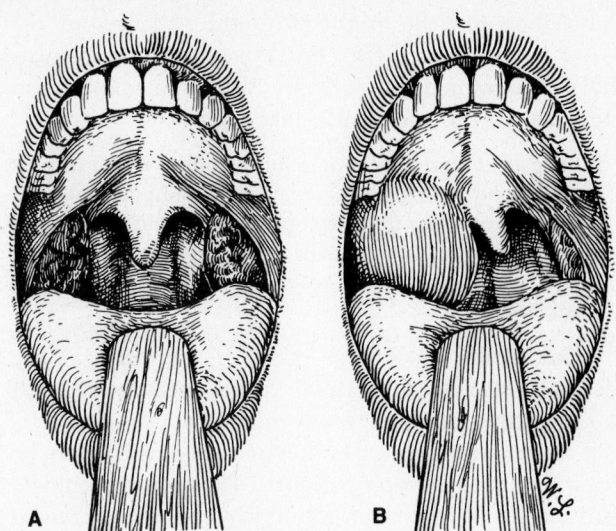

Figure 21-4. Views of oral pharynx. *A.* Showing enlargement of the tonsils. *B.* Showing peritonsillar abscess on the right side.

nasal obstruction. As a chronic problem, adenoid hypertrophy may cause mouth-breathing, earache, draining ears, frequent head colds, bronchitis, fetid breath, voice impairment, snoring, and noisy respiration. Infection of the adenoids frequently accompanies acute tonsillitis.

Extension of the infection to the middle ears by way of the eustachian tubes may result in acute otitis media, the potential complications of which include spontaneous rupture of the eardrums and further extension into the mastoid cells, causing acute mastoiditis. Or the infection may reside in the middle ear as a chronic, low-grade smoldering process that eventually may lead to permanent deafness. Consequently, if adenoiditis is not controlled by antibiotics, and there are recurrent episodes of suppurative otitis media which is causing a hearing loss, it is important for the patient to have a comprehensive audiometric examination (page 1150). If there is conductive hearing loss, an adenoidectomy may diminish the frequency of otitis media.

Management Following Tonsillectomy and Adenoidectomy

Continuous nursing care is required in the immediate postoperative and recovery period because of the significant risk of hemorrhage. For the patient undergoing general anesthesia, atropine is usually given to decrease the amount of mucous secretion. After the operation, the most comfortable position is prone with the head turned to the side to allow for drainage from the mouth and pharynx. The airway is not removed until the patient demonstrates that his swallowing reflex has returned. An ice collar should be applied to the neck and a basin and tissues provided for the expectoration of blood and mucus.

Bleeding may be bright red if the patient spits the blood out at once. Often, however, the blood is swallowed and immediately becomes brown in color due to the action of the acid gastric juice.

• If the patient vomits large amounts of altered blood or spits bright blood at frequent intervals, or if the pulse rate and temperature rise and the patient is restless, the surgeon should be notified immediately and the following items made available: a light, a head mirror, gauze, curved hemostats, and a waste basin.

Occasionally it may be necessary to suture or ligate the bleeding vessel. In such cases the patient must be taken to the operating room and given anesthesia.

If there is no bleeding, water and cracked ice may be given the patient as soon as desired. The patient should be instructed to refrain from too much talking and coughing, because this can produce throat pain. Alkaline mouthwashes may be useful in coping with the thick mucus that may be present after a tonsillectomy.

A liquid or semiliquid diet is given for several days, excluding orange or lemon juice and other acids. Ice cream, ice sherbet, gelatin desserts, custards, and junkets are very acceptable foods, especially for children.

Codeine is usually prescribed for pain; however, acetylsalicylic acid is contraindicated because it tends to increase bleeding.

Patient Education. The patient may be discharged from the hospital on the day after the operation, but he should convalesce at home for several days. This means getting plenty of rest, eating soft food, drinking fluids, and resuming activity gradually. Any bleeding should be reported to the physician; delayed hemorrhage may occur up to a week after operation.

PERITONSILLAR ABSCESS (QUINSY)

Pathophysiology and Manifestations. Peritonsillar abscess, or quinsy, is an abscess that develops above the tonsil in the tissues of the anterior pillar and soft palate (Fig. 21-4B, page 391). As a rule, it is secondary to a tonsillar infection. The usual symptoms of an infection are present, together with such local symptoms as difficulty in swallowing (dysphagia), thickening of the voice, drooling, and local pain. An examination shows marked swelling of the soft palate, often to the extent of half-occluding the orifice from the mouth into the pharynx.

Management. A considerable measure of relief may be obtained by throat irrigations or the frequent use of mouthwashes or gargles, using saline or alkaline solutions at a temperature of 40.6° to 43.3° C. (105° to 110° F.). This treatment hastens the pointing of the process.

The abscess should be evacuated as soon as possible. The mucous membrane over the swelling first is sprayed with topical anesthetic and then injected with local anes-

thesia; after a small incision has been made, the points of a blunt hemostat are forced into the abscess pocket and opened as they are withdrawn. This operation is performed best with the patient in the sitting position, since this will make it easier for him to expectorate the pus and blood that accumulate in the pharynx. Almost immediate relief is experienced. After-treatment includes warm gargles at intervals of 1 or 2 hours for 24 to 36 hours.

Some laryngologists advocate bilateral tonsillectomy for acute peritonsillar abscess; they claim that this is necessary to prevent recurrences and eliminate unsuspected asymptomatic pockets of infection.

Antibiotics, usually penicillin, are extremely effective in the control of the infection in peritonsillar abscess. Given early in the course of the disease, the abscess may be aborted, and incision can be avoided. If antibiotics are not given until later, the abscess must be drained, but improvement in the inflammatory reaction is rapid.

PROBLEMS OF THE LARYNX

The larynx, or voice box, serves as a passageway for air between the pharynx and the trachea. Because of its unique structure, the larynx also acts as a guard at the entrance of the trachea (windpipe), controlling air flow and preventing anything other than air from entering the lower passages. When a foreign body touches the sensitive laryngeal mucosa, the cough reflex is triggered. Exhalation of air through the larynx enables it to become an organ of speech, sounds being created as a result of vocal cord vibrations. Speech patterns are produced with the aid of the pharynx, palate, teeth, tongue, and lips. The larynx may be viewed directly with a laryngoscope or indirectly with a laryngeal mirror (Fig. 21-5).

LARYNGITIS

Pathophysiology and Management. Inflammation of the larynx often occurs as a result of voice abuse or as a part of an upper respiratory infection. It may also be caused by an isolated infection involving only the vocal cords.

Acute laryngitis is manifested by hoarseness or complete loss of the voice (aphonia) and by severe cough. The treatment is bed rest, steam or aerosol therapy, and abstinence from talking and smoking. If the laryngitis is part of a more extensive respiratory infection due to a bacterial organism, or if it is severe, appropriate antibacterial chemotherapy should be instituted.

Chronic laryngitis, marked by persistent hoarseness, may follow repeated attacks of acute laryngitis. It is sometimes a complication of chronic sinusitis and chronic bronchitis. The condition also may be induced by the frequent inhalation of irritating gases, the exces-

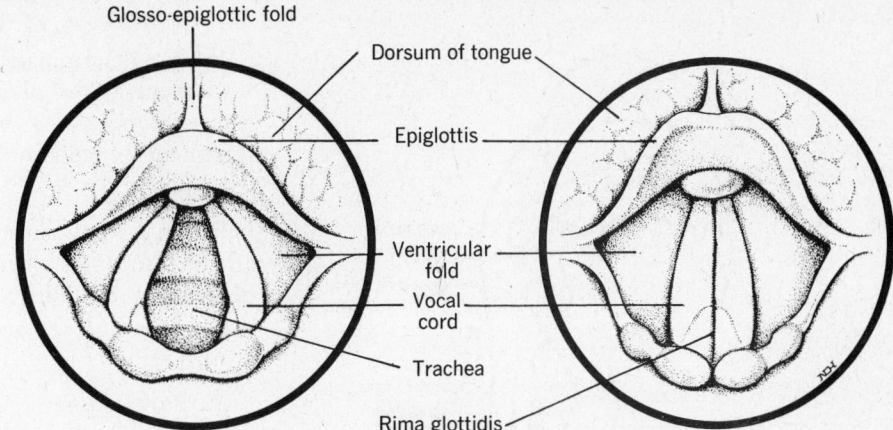

Glosso-epiglottic fold

Dorsum of tongue

Epiglottis

Ventricular fold

Vocal cord

Trachea

Rima glottidis

Figure 21-5. Interior of the larynx, as seen with laryngoscope: *left,* rima glottidis wide open; *right,* rima closed. (From Chaffee and Greisheimer: Basic Physiology and Anatomy, 3rd ed. Philadelphia, J. B. Lippincott, 1974)

sive use of tobacco or alcohol, or the habitual overuse of the voice, as in the case of public speakers. Laryngoscopic examination of the patient with chronic laryngitis is always indicated in order to eliminate the possibility of tuberculosis or tumor of the larynx. The treatment of the condition is rest of the voice, elimination of any primary respiratory tract infection that may be present, and restriction of smoking.

LARYNGEAL OBSTRUCTION

Edema of the larynx (or glottis) is a serious, often fatal, condition. The larynx is a stiff box that will not stretch, and the space within it between the vocal cords, through which the air must pass, is narrow. Swelling of the laryngeal mucous membrane, therefore, may close this orifice tightly, leading to suffocation. Edema of the glottis occurs rarely in patients with acute laryngitis, occasionally in patients with urticaria, and more frequently in severe inflammations of the throat — for example, erysipelas and scarlet fever. It is an occasional cause of death in severe anaphylaxis (angioneurotic edema).

When caused by an allergic reaction, treatment includes applying an ice pack to the neck and administering epinephrine, 1:1000 subcutaneously, or adrenal corticosteroid.

Foreign bodies frequently are aspirated into the pharynx, the larynx, or the trachea, and cause a two-fold problem. First, they obstruct the air passages and cause difficulty in breathing that may lead to asphyxia; later they may be drawn farther down, entering the bronchi or one of their branches and causing symptoms of irritation, such as a croupy cough, bloody or mucous expectoration, and paroxysms of dyspnea. The physical signs and roentgenograms confirm the diagnosis.

In emergencies, when the signs of asphyxia are evident, immediate treatment is necessary. Frequently, if the foreign body has lodged in the pharynx, it may be dislodged by the finger. If the obstruction is in the larynx or the trachea, an immediate tracheotomy is necessary. Or the "Heimlich maneuver" may be used (see Fig. 61-2).

- To perform the Heimlich maneuver, stand behind the person who is choking and place both arms around his waist, with one hand grasping the other wrist. Then quickly and forcefully apply pressure against the victim's diaphragm, pressing slightly upward, just below the ribs. The pressure will compress the lungs and expel the aspirated object.

CANCER OF THE LARYNX

If detected early, cancer of the larynx is readily curable. It occurs about 10 times more frequently in males than in females and most commonly in men from 50 to 65 years of age. It represents about 3 to 5 percent of all cancers.

In the United States, approximately 9,000 new cases are discovered each year, and 3,000 persons with cancer of the larynx will die annually.

Predisposing Factors and Symptoms

Factors which contribute to laryngeal cancer are irritants such as cigarette smoke, alcohol, vocal straining, chronic laryngitis, and noxious fumes, and family predisposition. A malignant growth may occur on the vocal cords (intrinsic) or on another part of the larynx (extrinsic). Hoarseness is noted early in the patient with intrinsic cancer since accurate approximation of the cords during phonation is interrupted by the presence of the tumor. Affected voice sounds are not early signs of extrinsic cancer; however, the patient may complain of pain and burning of the throat when drinking hot liquids and citrus juices. Later a lump may be felt in the neck. Later, too, dysphagia (swallowing difficulty), dyspnea, hoarseness, and foul breath may be noticed. Enlarged cervical nodes, weight loss, general debility, and the discomfort of pain radiating to the ear may all be suggestive of metastasis.

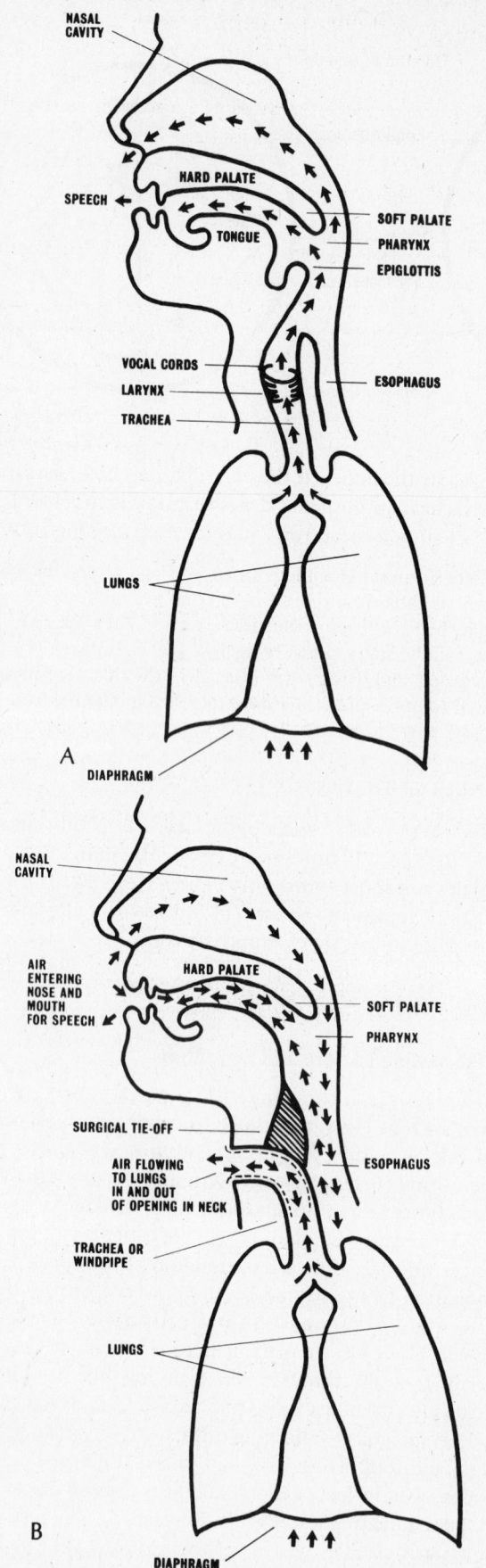

Figure 21-6. Diagram showing direction of air flow before (A) and after (B) a total laryngectomy. (American Cancer Society)

Management

Precise determination of the exact location and involvement of the malignancy is done by indirect and direct laryngoscopy, biopsy, and x-ray before specific treatment by radiation or surgery is prescribed.

1. Radiation. Good results have been produced by radiation therapy in patients in whom only one cord was affected and was normally mobile (i.e., moved with phonation). In addition, these patients retain a practically normal voice. A few may develop chondritis or stenosis; a small number may later require laryngectomy.

2. Partial Laryngectomy (Laryngofissure, Thyrotomy). This is recommended in the early stages, especially in intrinsic cancer of the larynx (limited to the vocal cords), and has a cure rate of more than 80 percent. In this operation, the thyroid cartilage of the larynx is split in the midline of the neck and the portion of the vocal cord that is involved with tumor growth is removed. Sometimes a tracheostomy tube (see page 451) is left in the trachea when the wound is closed; it is usually removed after a few days.

3. Total Laryngectomy. For extrinsic cancer of the larynx (extension beyond the vocal cords), the entire larynx is removed; this includes the thyroid cartilage, the vocal cords, and the epiglottis. Many surgeons recommend that a neck dissection be performed on the same side as the lesion even though no lymph nodes are palpable. The rationale for this approach is that as many as 35 percent of patients have had metastases to the cervical lymph nodes. Obviously, the problem is more complex when a lesion involves midline structures or both cords. With or without neck dissection, a laryngectomy requires a permanent tracheal stoma (Fig. 21-6). The opening of the larynx is closed by sutures.

4. Total Laryngectomy with Laryngoplasty. In this delicate three-stage procedure (Assai operation), a dermal tube is fashioned from the upper end of the trachea into the hypopharynx. By closing the permanent tracheostomy opening with his finger, the patient can exhale air up through the dermal tube and into the pharyngeal cavity. The sound produced is transformed into speech which is almost normal and far superior to esophageal speech.

5. Supraglottic (Horizontal) Laryngectomy. This recently developed procedure is used in the management of certain extrinsic tumors. After adequate resection, sufficient normal larynx is left so that the cords remain intact and their function is maintained. During surgery a radical neck dissection is also done on the involved side. Postoperatively, the patient may experience some difficulty in swallowing for the first two weeks. The chief advantage of this operation, of course, is that it preserves the voice. The major problem is that there may be local recurrence; therefore, patients have to be selected carefully.

Nursing Assessment and Preparation for Surgery

To plan appropriate nursing care, it is important to consult with the surgeon regarding the nature of the surgery recommended for a particular patient. Some patients experience loss of speech, whereas others do not. Thus the nursing care plan is based upon the surgical plan of therapy.

Since surgery of the larynx is done most commonly for a tumor that may be malignant, the nurse is faced with a patient who is worried for many reasons: Will the surgeon be able to remove all of the tumor? Is it cancer? Will I die? Will I choke? Will I ever speak again? Therefore, the psychological preparation of the patient is as important as the physical. If the patient is going to have a complete laryngectomy, he should know that he will lose his natural voice completely and that, with training, there are ways in which he can carry on a fairly normal conversation. (He also will not be able to sing, laugh, or whistle.) Until he receives this training, the patient needs to know that the nurse can be reached by the call light and that he can communicate in the immediate postoperative phase by writing.

The physician describes the nature of the surgery and tells the patient that he will lose his ability to vocalize speech. He should be reassured that much can be done for him through a rehabilitation program, and he should be referred to a speech pathologist before surgery.

Thorough mouth hygiene prior to surgery is imperative. Usually antibiotics are prescribed to reduce further the possibility of infection. In men, preoperative shaving includes the beard and the hair on the neck and the chest down to the nipple line.

Postoperative Nursing Management

If a laryngofissure has been performed, a tracheostomy tube will be in place for 2 or 3 days (page 451). The physician may insert a nasogastric tube, and feedings are given under the same precautions that prevail in gastrostomy feedings (see page 727). Intravenous therapy may be given concurrently. Oral feedings often are started on the first day after operation if acceptable to the patient. Speaking is deferred until the physician permits whispering (2 to 3 days). This is followed by gradual resumption of the use of the voice.

If the patient has had a total laryngectomy, a laryngectomy tube will most likely be in place. (In some clinics a laryngectomy tube is not used, in others it is used temporarily, and in many it is used permanently.) The laryngectomy tube (which is shorter than a tracheostomy tube but has a larger diameter) is the only airway the patient has. The care of this tube is the same as for a tracheostomy tube (see page 453).

Respiratory effectiveness is promoted by positioning the patient in the semi-Fowler to Fowler position following recovery from anesthesia. The patient is observed for restlessness, labored breathing, apprehension, and increased pulse rate, since these suggest respiratory or circulatory problems. Medications that depress respirations are to be avoided. Like other surgical patients, the laryngectomy patient needs to be turned and reminded to cough and take deep breaths. Early ambulation, also, will help in preventing atelectasis and pneumonia.

Wound drains that may be in place assist in removal of fluid and air from the dead space. Portable suction may also be used. Drainage is observed, measured, and recorded; when drainage amounts to less than 50 to 60 ml./day, drains usually are removed.

The stoma is kept clean by daily cleansing with saline solution or diluted hydrogen peroxide; antibiotic ointment may then be applied around the stoma and suture line.

Vitamins may be given as supplemental feedings, and infusions often are necessary to keep up fluid, electrolyte, and nutritional balance. Since a "magic slate" is often used for communication, it is well to remember which hand the patient uses for writing so that the opposite arm will be used for intravenous feedings. When notes are the means of communication, they should be destroyed to assure the patient's privacy. If the patient is not able to write, flash cards can be used. The phone to the patient's room may be disconnected since he is unable to talk.

Nutrition is maintained by means of a tube passed through a cervical pharyngostomy or by nasogastric catheter. Usually a nasogastric catheter is passed by the physician after operation, and liquid feedings are given. Thereafter, the nurse is permitted to remove and pass this tube because there is no possibility of its getting into the trachea, the trachea now being sutured permanently to the skin as a tracheostomy. After a few days the patient can be taught to pass his own feeding tube. Good mouth hygiene must be followed rigidly. After about 7 days, when the incision has healed, the surgeon may allow the patient to begin oral feedings. Then he begins to develop his ability to belch. About an hour after he has eaten, the nurse can remind him to belch. Later this conscious action is transformed into simple explosions of air from the esophagus for speech purposes. At this point the speech pathologist works wih him in an attempt to make his speech intelligible and as close to normal as is possible.

- Through the postoperative period, be alert for the possible serious complication of rupture of the carotid artery, particularly if wound infection is present. Should this occur, apply direct pressure over the artery, summon assistance, and provide psychological support to the patient until the vessel can be ligated.

The laryngectomy tube may be removed when the stoma is well healed, usually within three to six weeks after the operation.

Laryngectomy Patient Education

Speech Rehabilitation. The patient should be reassured that much can be done for him through a rehabilitation program. Ideally, the speech pathologist sees the patient before the operation, in order to counsel him and to enlarge upon what the physician has told him. The speech pathologist reassures the patient that with speech therapy the sound source can be replaced with either laryngeal or esophageal speech or by using one of the different types of artificial larynxes.

The partially laryngectomized patient has little difficulty, because in a matter of a few days his voice will improve. However, the completely laryngectomized patient often is depressed and needs encouragement. The rehabilitative management of this patient requires a team that includes the surgeon, the nurse, the patient's family, persons who have had laryngectomies (Fig. 21-7), and the speech pathologist.

There are two methods of learning to speak after a laryngectomy. The first method relies on laryngeal or esophageal speech. The patient takes air into his mouth, and then by compression of the lips or by strong articulation of "plosive" speech sounds such as "p," "t," or "k," he can air-charge, or inflate, his esophagus. By lip compression or the plosive sound method the air is sent posteriorly towards the esophagus. As air gets into the upper part of the esophagus, the increased pressure at that point will be released and will produce a vibration or tone. This tone is made at the narrowing between the pharynx and esophagus. The resultant voice sounds low pitched because the neoglottis from which the sounds are now emitted is indeed different from the normal vocal cords. In a few months time the new speech becomes automatic and the individual does not have to think about getting an adequate air charge before talking.

Another method of vocalization after a laryngectomy is by means of an artificial larynx. Most laryngectomees are able to learn the esophageal method of voice produc-

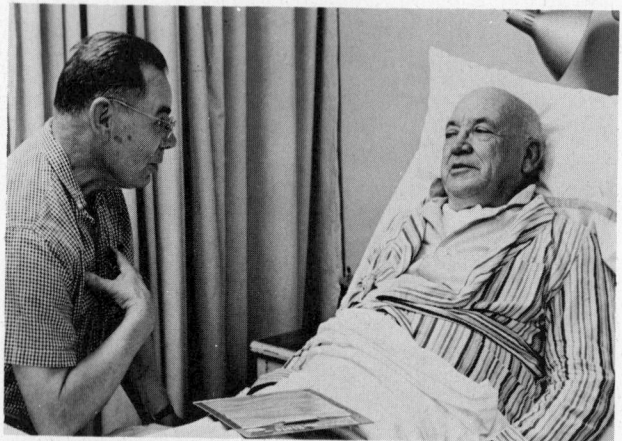

Figure 21-7. A special kind of caller. During recovery, a former laryngectomee may visit the "new" laryngectomee. This caller will use esophageal speech and answer questions written by the patient. Such contact with a former patient has been very effective in encouraging the new patient when he needs it most. (Courtesy, International Association of Laryngectomees)

tion. However, if the patient is unable to attain esophageal speech due to various reasons (advanced emphysema, asthma, stenosis of the esophagus, hearing loss, etc.), an artificial larynx can be used. A variety of artificial larynxes are available. One type consists of a vibrator powered by batteries, which is placed against the side of the neck. When it is turned on, the air inside the mouth is vibrated and the patient articulates in a somewhat normal fashion.

Another device, also battery-powered, utilizes a plastic tube that is inserted into the side and well to the back of the mouth, providing a continuous sound source in the mouth. The individual merely articulates this sound, shaping it in a normal manner to form audible speech.

The International Association of Laryngectomees is a voluntary organization that sponsors "Lost Chord" or "New Voice" clubs to encourage and give opportunities for laryngectomized persons to learn to speak again.

Tracheostomy and Stomal Care. The nurse conveys optimism to the patient, assuring him that he will be able to carry on most of his preoperative activities. The patient needs specific information about what to expect from his tracheostomy (see page 451). He will frequently cough up rather large amounts of mucus through this opening. Because the air passes directly into the trachea without being warmed and moistened by the respiratory mucosa, the tracheobronchial tree compensates by secreting excessive amounts of mucus. Therefore, the patient will have frequent coughing episodes, and he may be somewhat troubled by the brassy sounding, mucus-producing cough. However, he should be assured that these problems diminish in time as the tracheobronchial mucosa adapts to the patient's altered physiology.

When the patient coughs, the orifice should be wiped clean and cleared of mucus. In addition, the skin around the stoma should be washed twice daily. If crusting occurs, the skin around the stoma can be lubricated with an ointment (prescribed by the physician) and the crusts removed with sterile tweezers. It is necessary that a bib be worn in front of the tracheostomy to keep the mucus from soiling the clothing. The bib may be a simple gauze dressing taped over the neck or one made of other porous fabric.

One of the most important factors in decreasing cough and mucus production as well as crusting around the stoma is to provide adequate humidification of the environment. Mechanical humidifiers and cool mist or steam vaporizers are excellent sources of humidification and are absolutely essential for the patient's comfort. Some system of humidification should be set up in the home *before the patient is discharged from the hospital.* An air-conditioned atmosphere may be distressing to the newly laryngectomized patient, since the air may be too cool or too dry and thus too irritating.

Changes in Taste and Smell. The patient can expect to have a diminished sense of taste and smell for a period after the operation. Because he is breathing directly into the trachea, air is not passing through the nose to the olfactory end organs. Because taste and smell are so closely connected, his taste sensations are altered. However, in time the individual usually accommodates to this problem and his olfactory sensation adapts to meet his needs.

Hygienic and Recreational Measures. Special precautions need to be taken in a shower to prevent water from entering the stoma. Wearing a loose-fitting plastic bib or simply holding one's hand over the opening is effective. However, swimming is not recommended, because the laryngectomee can drown without getting his face wet. Barbers and beauticians need to be cautioned so that hair sprays, loose hair, and powder do not get near the stoma, since they could cause blockage, irritation, and possibly infection.

Recreation and exercise are important. Golf, bowling, bridge, spectator activities, and walking can be enjoyed safely. Moderation in order to prevent fatigue is important because, when tired, the laryngectomee has more difficulty speaking with his new voice. At such times, he can easily become discouraged and depressed.

Follow-up and Emergency Care. It is important for the laryngectomee to visit his physician regularly for physical examinations and for advice concerning any problems relating to his convalescent program. He should also carry proper identification, such as a card, to alert a first-aider to the special requirements of resuscitation should this need arise. On the back of the card can be included the name of a responsible person to notify in the event of emergency.

BIBLIOGRAPHY

BOOKS

Archer, W. H.: Oral and Maxillofacial Surgery, 5th ed. Philadelphia, W. B. Saunders, 1975.

Ballenger, J. J.: Diseases of the Nose, Throat, and Ear. Philadelphia, Lea and Febiger, 1977.

Boone, D. R.: The Voice and Voice Therapy, 2nd ed. Englewood Cliffs, N.J., Prentice-Hall, 1977.

Bull, T. R.: Color Atlas of E.N.T. Diagnosis. Chicago, Year Book Med. Pub. 1974.

Bull, T. R., and Cook, J. L.: Speech Therapy and ENT Surgery. Philadelphia, J. B. Lippincott, 1976.

Dingman, R. O., and Natvig, P.: Surgery of Facial Fractures. Philadelphia, W. B. Saunders, 1978.

DeWeese, D. D., and Saunders, W. H.: Textbook of Otolaryngology. St. Louis, C. V. Mosby, 1977.

English, G. M.: Otolaryngology. Hagerstown, Md., Harper and Row, 1976.

International Association of Laryngectomees: Helping Words for the Laryngectomee. New York, International Assoc. of Laryngectomees, 1964.

Jaffe, B. F.: Diseases and Surgery of the Nose. Clinical Symposia, vol. 26. Summit, N.J., Ciba Pharmaceutical Co. 1974, pages 2-32.

Lynch, M. A., ed.: Burket's Oral Medicine, 7th ed. Philadelphia, J. B. Lippincott, 1977.

ARTICLES

Nose and Throat

Carpenter, J. L., and Artenstein, M. S.: Use of diagnostic microbiologic facilities in the diagnosis of head and neck infections. Otolaryngol. Clin. N. Am., *9*:611-629, Oct. 1976.

Dobie, R. A.: Rehabilitation of swallowing disorders. Am. Fam. Phys., *17*:84-95, May 1978.

Komaroff, A. L.: A management strategy for sore throat. JAMA, *239*:1429-1432, Apr. 3, 1978.

Kutnick, S. L., and Kerth, J. D.: Acute sinusitis and otitis: Their complications and surgical treatment. Otolaryngol. Clin. N. Am., *9*:689-701, Oct. 1976.

McCurdy, J. A.: The tonsillectomy-adenoidectomy dilemma. Am. Fam. Phys., *16*:137-141, Sept. 1977.

Paradise, J. L., et al.: History of recurrent sore throat as an indication for tonsillectomy. New Eng. J. Med., *298*:409-413, Feb. 23, 1978.

Paradise, J. L., and Bluestone, C. D.: Toward rational indications for tonsil and adenoid surgery. Hosp. Pract., *11*:79-87, Feb. 1976.

Removal of inhaled objects often delayed. (Editorial): JAMA, *238*:296-297, July 25, 1977.

Ruben, R. J.: Otolaryngologic problems of the old. Hosp. Pract., *12*:73-87, Aug. 1977.

Shank, J. C.: Streptococcal infection and the chronic carrier state. Am. Fam. Phys., *15*:87-92, Jan. 1977.

Sheffield, R. W., et al.: Complications of sinusitis. Postgrad. Med., *63*:93-101, Mar. 1978.

Tonsillectomy—trials and tribulations. Report on the National Institutes of Health Consensus Conference on Indications for Tonsillectomy and Adenoidectomy. JAMA, *240*:1961-1962, Oct. 27, 1978.

Wang, R. M.: Streptococcal sore throat. AJN, 77:1796-1798, Nov. 1977.

Larynx

Brown, M. H., and Kiss, M. E.: Nursing patient-care outcome audit criteria: Laryngectomy with radical neck dissection. Cancer Nurs., *1*:331-334, Aug. 1978.

DeSanto, L. W., et al.: Cancers of the larynx: Glottic cancer. Surg. Clin. N. Am., *57*:611-620, June 1977.

_____: Cancers of the larynx: Supraglottic cancer. Surg. Clin. N. Am., *57*:505-514, June 1977.

Harvey, T. G.: A symposium on laryngectomy: The team approach, diagnosis and surgical management. Nurs. Mirror, *141*:48-50, Dec. 4, 1975.

Marlowe, F. I.: Laryngeal rehabilitation: A historical perspective. ENT J., *57*:366-371, Sept. 1978.

Nicholson, E. M.: Personal notes of a laryngectomee. AJN, *75*:2157-2158, Dec. 1975.

Owlett, A.: A symposium on laryngectomy: The team approach, speech rehabilitation. Nurs. Mirror, *141*:53-54, Dec. 4, 1975.

Stillman, M. J.: Joseph K.: A laryngectomee. RN, *40*:65-72, Nov. 1977.

Vaughan, C. W., et al.: Laryngeal carcinoma: Transoral treatment utilizing the CO_2 laser. Am. J. Surg., *136*:490-493, Oct. 1978.

Weaver, A. W., and Fleming, S. M.: Partial laryngectomy: Analysis of associated swallowing disorders. Am. J. Surg., *136*:486-489, Oct. 1978.

AGENCIES

American Academy of Ophthalmology and Otolaryngology, 15 Second St., S.W., Rochester, Minn. 55901.

International Association of Laryngectomees, % American Cancer Society, 777 Third Avenue, New York, N.Y. 10017.

22

ASSESSMENT OF RESPIRATORY FUNCTION

PHYSIOLOGIC OVERVIEW

The cells of the body derive their necessary energy from the oxidation of carbohydrates, fats, and proteins. For this process, as for any type of combustion, oxygen is required. Certain vital tissues such as those of the brain and the heart, cannot survive for long without a continuing supply of oxygen. As a result of oxidation in the body tissues, carbon dioxide is produced and must be removed from the cells to prevent buildup of acid waste products.

Oxygen is supplied to cells and carbon dioxide is removed from cells via circulating blood. No cell is far removed from a capillary, the thin walls of which present little resistance to the passage of dissolved gases. The concentration of oxygen in the tissues, where it is being consumed by cellular metabolism, is lower than it is in the blood within the capillaries. As a result, oxygen diffuses from the capillary blood, through the capillary wall into the interstitial fluid, and then through the membrane of the tissue cell into the cell sap where it can be used by the mitochondria for cellular respiration. The movement of carbon dioxide proceeds in the opposite direction, from cell to blood. This movement also occurs by diffusion, since carbon dioxide concentration inside the cell is greater, due to metabolism, than it is in the blood passing through the tissue capillary. An average resting adult utilizes approximately 250 ml. O_2/min. and produces approximately 200 ml. CO_2/min. With strenuous exercise, these values may increase up to tenfold. As a result of the exchange of O_2 and CO_2 in tissue capillaries, arterial blood loses about 25 percent of its oxygen, whereas carbon dioxide content is increased about 15 percent.

After these capillary exchanges, blood enters the veins (where it is called venous blood) and travels to the lung capillaries. The oxygen concentration in blood within lung capillaries is lower than it is in the lung gas spaces. As a result, oxygen diffuses from the gas spaces into the blood. Carbon dioxide, since its concentration in the blood is higher than it is in the gas spaces of the lung, diffuses from the blood into the lung gas. Movement of fresh air in and out of the airways (called ventilation) intermittently replenishes the oxygen in and removes the carbon dioxide from the gas within airspaces of the lung. This overall process by which exchanges take place between atmospheric air and the cells of the body is called respiration.

Anatomy of the Lung

The lungs are elastic structures enclosed in the thorax, an airtight chamber with distensible walls. Ventilation involves movements of the walls of the thorax and of its floor, the diaphragm. The effect of these movements is to alternately increase and decrease the capacity of the chest. When the capacity of the chest is increased, air enters through the trachea, because of the lowered pressure within, and inflates the lungs. When the chest wall and diaphragm return to their previous positions, the elastic lungs recoil and force the air out via the bronchi and trachea.

The outer surfaces of the lungs are enclosed by a smooth, slippery membrane, the *pleura,* which also extends to cover the interior wall of the thorax and the superior surface of the diaphragm. The pleura is termed *parietal pleura* where it lines the thorax, and *visceral pleura* where it covers the lungs. Between the two pleural surfaces is a small amount of fluid that lubricates the surfaces and allows them to slide freely during ventilation.

The *mediastinum* is the wall that divides the thoracic cavity into two halves. It is composed of two layers of pleura between which lie all of the thoracic structures except the lungs.

Each lung is divided into subsections called lobes. The left lung consists of upper and lower lobes, whereas the right lung has upper, middle, and lower lobes. Each lobe is further subdivided into 2 to 5 segments. Lobes of the lungs are separated by fissures which are extensions of the pleura. A schematic diagram of the airways and the lobes of the lungs is shown in Figure 22-1.

The airways through which gases enter and leave the alveoli are called *bronchioles.* The bronchioles join to form larger and larger bronchi and eventually form one main bronchus for each lung. The two primary bronchi then unite to form the trachea, which is continuous with the oropharynx and the mouth. The walls of the airways contain smooth muscle which can, upon contraction or relaxation, cause a change in the caliber of the airway. These smooth muscles are innervated by both the parasympathetic and sympathetic nervous systems. The airways also contain bronchial glands which secrete mucus into the lumen. The bronchi and bronchioles are lined with cells whose luminal surfaces are covered with short "hairs" called *cilia.* These cilia maintain a constant whipping motion which serves to propel mucus and substances from the inside of the lungs towards the mouth.

The human lung is made up of a large number (300 million) of tiny air sacs which are called *alveoli.* They are scarcely visible to the naked eye (approximately ¼ mm. in diameter). Their elastic walls are lined by a single layer of epithelial cells and contain a network of pulmonary capillaries. Certain cells in the walls of the alveoli secrete a lipid-containing material onto the surface of each alveolus. This thin layer of lipid rich material is called the *alveolar surfactant.* So numerous are these alveoli that if their surfaces were united to form one sheet, it would cover an area of over 90 square yards.

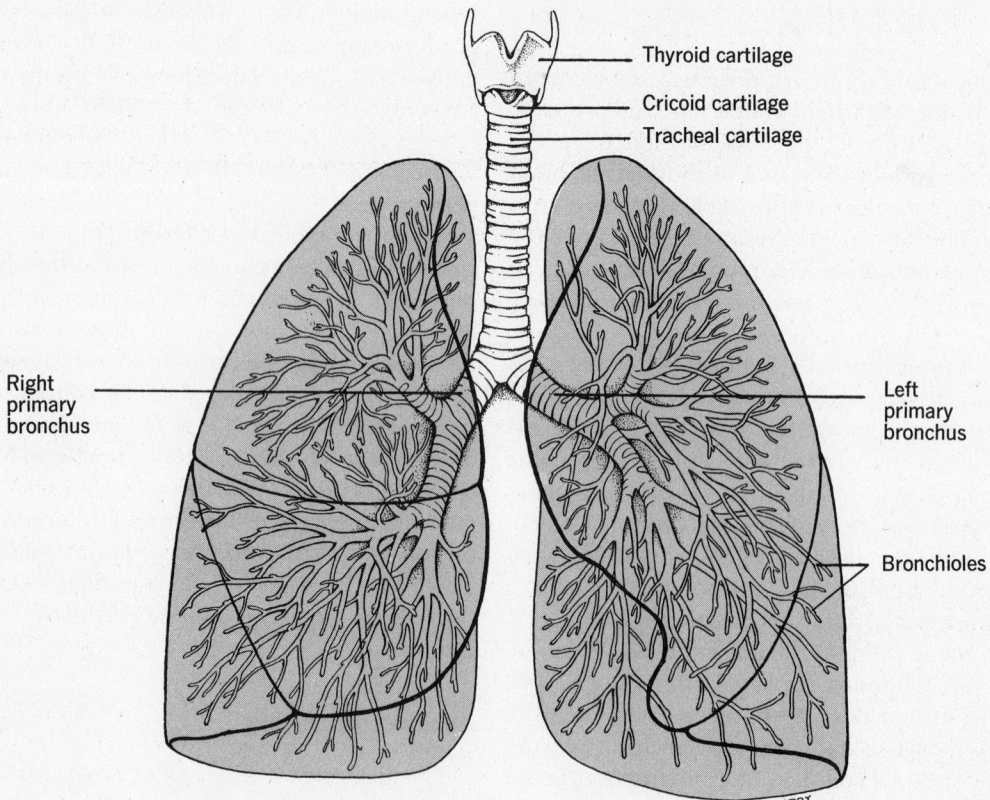

Figure 22-1.   Larynx, trachea, and bronchial tree (anterior view). (From Chaffee, E. E., and Greisheimer, E. M.: Basic Physiology and Anatomy, 3rd ed. J. B. Lippincott, 1974)

Mechanics of Ventilation

During inspiration, air flows from the environment into the trachea, bronchi, bronchioles, and alveoli. During expiration, alveolar gas travels the same route in reverse.

The physical factors that govern airflow into and out of the lungs are collectively referred to as the mechanics of ventilation. Air flows from a region of higher pressure to a region of lower pressure. During inspiration, contraction of the diaphragm and other muscles of respiration enlarges the thoracic cavity and thereby lowers the pressure inside the thorax to a level below that of atmospheric pressure. Therefore, air is drawn through the trachea and bronchi into the alveoli.

During normal expiration, the muscles of respiration relax and the thoracic cavity decreases in size. The alveolar pressure now exceeds atmospheric pressure, and air flows from the lungs into the atmosphere.

The rate of inspiratory or expiratory airflow is equal to the pressure gradient between the atmosphere and the alveoli divided by the airflow resistance of the airways:

$$\text{Flow} = \Delta \text{Pressure/Resistance}$$

Resistance is determined chiefly by the radius of the airway through which the air is flowing. Any process that changes bronchial diameter will therefore affect airway resistance and alter the rate of airflow for a given pressure gradient during respiration. Common factors that may alter bronchial diameter include contraction of bronchial smooth muscle as in asthma, thickening of bronchial mucosa as in chronic bronchitis, or obstruction of the airway due to mucus, tumor, or a foreign body. Loss of lung elasticity such as is seen in emphysema may also alter bronchial diameter since the lung connective tissue encircles the airways and helps to keep them open during both inspiration and expiration. With increased resistance, greater than normal respiratory effort is required by the patient to achieve normal levels of ventilation.

The pressure gradient between the thoracic cavity and the atmosphere causes airflow in and out of the lungs and also stretches the lung tissue itself. The pressure required to stretch the lung is determined by the properties of its elastic tissue. A measure of how easily lungs can be stretched is called *lung compliance*. It equals change in volume of the lung divided by change in pressure (after correction for the portion of the pressure that is required to cause air flow). A compliant lung (high compliance) distends easily when a pressure is applied, whereas a noncompliant lung (low compliance) requires a greater than normal pressure to distend it. The major factors that determine lung compliance are connective tissue (collagen and elastin) and the surface tension in the alveoli. The surface tension at the surface of the alveoli is normally maintained at a low level by the presence of the alveolar lining material (lung surfactant). Increased connective tissue or increased alveolar surface tension results in low compliance. In respiratory distress syndrome of the newborn (hyaline membrane disease), there is a surfactant deficiency and lungs are stiff (low compliance). In pulmonary fibrosis, connective tissue proliferates and compliance is decreased. Lungs with low compliance require a greater than normal energy expenditure to achieve normal levels of ventilation.

Pulmonary Circulation

Almost the entire cardiac output ordinarily passes through capillaries of the lung and is capable of exchanging gases with the alveoli. Pulmonary artery pressure is normally about 25 mm. Hg systolic compared with 120 mm. Hg in the systemic arteries. Since flow in the pulmonary and systemic circuits is almost the same, the resistance to blood flow in the pulmonary vasculature is roughly one fifth of that in the systemic circulation. In an upright individual, blood flow to the top of the lungs (apex) is somewhat less than that to the base of the lungs, because of the effects of gravity.

A small percentage of the cardiac output even in normal people bypasses alveoli, does not participate in gas exchange, and returns to the left heart where it mixes with oxygenated blood. This fraction of the cardiac output that bypasses ventilated alveoli is referred to as a right-to-left shunt.

The pulmonary capillary bed has an important metabolic role, which includes the regulation of the concentration of many vasoactive compounds present in the blood. The lung removes and inactivates serotonin and norepinephrine (potent vasoconstrictors) from the circulating blood. The pulmonary endothelium is selective since compounds with similar structure, such as histamine and epinephrine, are not removed from the blood. The lung converts angiotensin I (an inactive compound) to angiotensin II by the action of converting enzyme located on the pulmonary capillary endothelium. Bradykinin may be inactivated by the same enzyme. These metabolic functions of the capillary endothelium are not unique to the lung and may occur in other capillary beds. However, because of the vast pulmonary capillary endothelial surface area and because all of the cardiac output goes to the lungs, the lung becomes most important for these metabolic processes.

The lung has mechanisms that help to match blood flow to ventilation. With decreased ventilation to a region of the lung, the oxygen concentration in those alveoli decreases. The resulting hypoxia causes local blood vessels to constrict, which diminishes the blood flow to the region. In this way, blood flow and ventilation become better matched. With decreased perfusion to a region of the lung, the carbon dioxide concentration in the alveoli decreases. The hypocapnea causes local bronchi to constrict, which diminishes ventilation to the region and helps to match regional ventilation to blood flow.

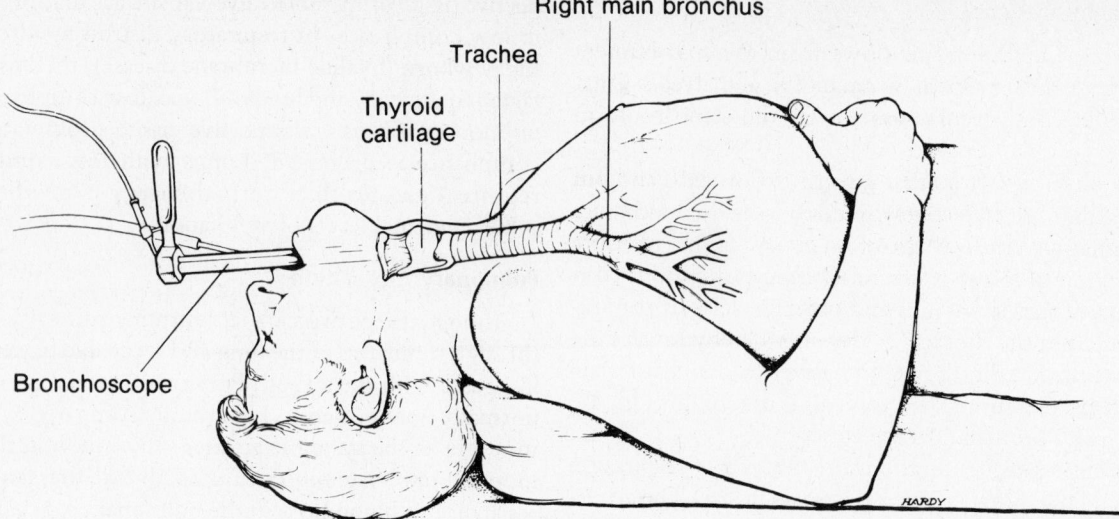

Figure 22-2. Introduction of the rigid bronchoscope.

DIAGNOSTIC ASSESSMENT OF RESPIRATORY FUNCTION

Aside from the general physical examination of the chest, which was discussed in Chapter 5, a wide range of diagnostic studies, described in the following pages, may be conducted in patients with thoracic conditions.

Radiographic Examinations of the Chest

Normal pulmonary tissue is radiolucent; therefore, densities produced by tumors, foreign bodies, etc., can be detected by means of radiographic examination. A chest x-ray may reveal extensive pathology in the lungs in the absence of symptoms. Radiographs are taken after full inspiration (deep breath) since the lungs are best demonstrated when they are well aerated. Also, the diaphragm is at its lowest level and the largest expanse of lung is visible.

Tomography (Planigraphy). Tomography provides films of sections of the lungs at different planes within the thorax. It is valuable in demonstrating the presence of solid lesions, calcification, or cavitation within a lesion.

Computerized Tomography. Computerized tomography is an imaging method in which the lungs are scanned in successive layers by a narrow beam x-ray. A computer printout is obtained of the absorption values of the tissues in the plane that is being scanned. It may be used to define pulmonary nodules, small tumors adjacent to pleural surfaces that are not visible on routine chest x-rays, and to demonstrate mediastinal abnormalities and hilar adenopathy. (See Chapter 16.)

Fluoroscopy. Fluoroscopy is helpful in evaluating a lesion that has been previously identified by x-ray. It is also useful in the study of pulmonary dynamics (the motion of pulmonary structures; diaphragmatic motion) and in detecting regional variations in ventilation.

Bronchogram. A bronchogram provides an outline of the bronchial tree after a radiopaque medium that coats the bronchial mucosa has been instilled directly into the trachea, bronchi, and the entire bronchial tree. This is a diagnostic test for any disease that alters the caliber or patency of the bronchial tree or causes displacement there. It reveals anomalies of the bronchial tree and is important in the diagnosis of bronchiectasis, since involved segments cannot always be outlined by other methods.

The procedure must be carried out while the patient is in a fasting state to reduce the possibility of aspiration of gastric contents. Preoperative medication may include atropine to decrease secretions and vagally mediated reflex bradycardia, codeine to suppress the cough reflex, and diazepam (Valium) for sedation.

A topical anesthetic is sprayed into the nose, mouth, and posterior pharynx to prevent gagging and coughing when the tube is passed. The contrast medium may be instilled by dripping it over the glottis, by slowly injecting it through a tube in the trachea, or by injecting it through a needle inserted percutaneously into the trachea below the glottis.

NURSING SUPPORT. After such a roentgenogram, food and fluids are withheld until the patient demonstrates he has a cough reflex. Once the cough reflex has returned, the patient should be encouraged to cough and clear the bronchial tree. Postural drainage may be required. A slight temperature elevation is common following this procedure.

Angiographic Studies of the Pulmonary Vessels

Pulmonary angiography is the rapid injection of a radiopaque medium into the vasculature of the chest. It can be performed by venous injection into one or both arms (simultaneously) through a needle or catheter, by introducing a catheter into the main pulmonary artery or its branches, or by introducing a catheter into the great veins or heart proximal to the pulmonary artery.

These procedures include pulmonary angiography, angiocardiography, aortography, bronchial arteriography, superior vena cava angiography, and azygography. Pulmonary angiography is most commonly used to investigate thromboembolic disease of the lungs and congenital abnormalities of the pulmonary vascular tree and to detect abnormal vasculature arising from tumors.

Bronchoscopy

Bronchoscopy is the direct inspection and observation of the larynx, trachea, and bronchi through either a flexible or a rigid bronchoscope.

The *diagnostic purposes* of bronchoscopy are (1) to examine tissues or collected secretions (2) to determine the location and extent of a pathological process, and (3) to determine whether a tumor can be resected surgically.

Therapeutically, bronchoscopy is used (1) to remove foreign bodies from the tracheobronchial tree, (2) to remove secretions obstructing the tracheobronchial tree such as occur in cystic fibrosis, intractable asthma, and pulmonary suppurative disease (saline and mucolytic agents may be administered through the bronchoscope to aid in the removal of these secretions), (3) to provide postoperative treatment in atelectasis, and (4) to fulgurate and excise lesions.

The *rigid bronchoscope* (Fig. 22-2) is a hollow metallic tube used mainly for the removal of foreign bodies or for patients having some encroachment on the tracheal lumen.

The *fiberoptic bronchoscope* is a thin, flexible bronchoscope that can be directed into the segmental bronchi (Fig. 22-3). Because of its smaller size, flexibility, and excellent optical system, it allows increased visualization of the peripheral airways. Fiberoptic bronchoscopy is better tolerated by patients than rigid bronchoscopy, allows biopsy of previously inaccessible tumors, is safer in the very ill, and can be performed at the bedside or through endotracheal or tracheostomy tubes for patients on ventilators or in whom it is desirable to ensure airway patency.

Nursing Support. An informed consent is obtained before the procedure. Food and fluids are withheld for 6 hours before the test. The patient is told what to expect, in order to reduce fear and correct misapprehensions. Preoperative medication (usually atropine and a sedative or narcotic) are given to reduce secretions and relieve anxiety.

• *Caution:* Sedation given to patients with respiratory insufficiency may precipitate respiratory arrest.

Contact lenses, dentures, and other prostheses are removed. The examination is usually done under local anesthesia, but general anesthesia may be given, especially when the rigid bronchoscope is used.

If local anesthesia is used, the pharynx is sprayed with a topical anesthetic (lidocaine [Xylocaine]), and the solution is dropped on the epiglottis and vocal cords and into

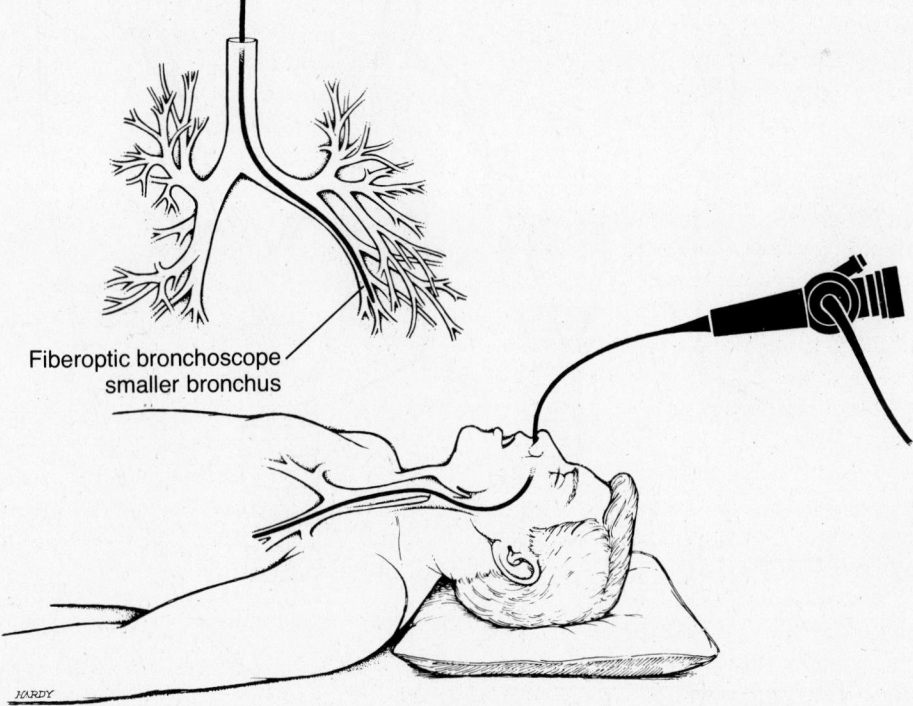

Fiberoptic bronchoscope
smaller bronchus

HARDY

Figure 22-3. Fiberoptic bronchoscopy.

the trachea. Diazepam (Valium) may be administered intravenously for additional sedation and for amnesia.

Following the procedure, the patient is given nothing by mouth until the cough reflex returns. Once the patient demonstrates that he can cough, cracked ice may be given, and eventually fluids. Difficulty in breathing, particularly in children, is looked for and reported promptly. The patient should also be observed for evidence of cyanosis, hypotension, tachycardia, arrhythmias, and hemoptysis.

Esophagoscopy

Esophagoscopy is the viewing of the interior of the esophagus through a lighted tube. It is used in removing foreign bodies, in inspecting lesions of the esophagus such as ulcers, diverticuli, and tumors, and often in making a positive diagnosis by removing small bits of tissue for microscopic examination (biopsy). The care before and after the procedure is the same as for bronchoscopy.

Sputum Studies

Sputum may be obtained for study to identify pathogenic organisms and to determine whether malignant cells are present. It may also be used to assess for hypersensitivity states (in which there is an increase of eosinophils). Periodic sputum examinations may be called for in patients receiving antibiotics, steroids, and immunosuppressive drugs for prolonged periods, since these agents give rise to opportunistic infections. In general, sputum cultures are used in diagnosis, for drug sensitivity testing, and as a guide in treatment. Sputum can be obtained by expectoration, which can be induced by the use of aerosols with saline, propylene glycol, or some other agent. Other methods of collecting sputum specimens include: endotracheal aspiration (page 423), bronchoscopic removal (page 403), bronchial brushing (page 406), gastric aspiration (usually for tuberculosis organisms (page 722), or transtracheal aspiration (page 405).

Generally, a morning specimen is preferable. The patient is instructed to clear his nose and throat and rinse his mouth in order to decrease contamination of the sputum. He then takes a few deep breaths, coughs (rather than spits), using his diaphragm, and expectorates into a sterile container.

The specimen should be sent to the laboratory immediately; allowing it to stand for several hours in a warm room will result in the overgrowth of contaminant organisms and may make culture more difficult (especially for *Mycobacterium tuberculosis*).

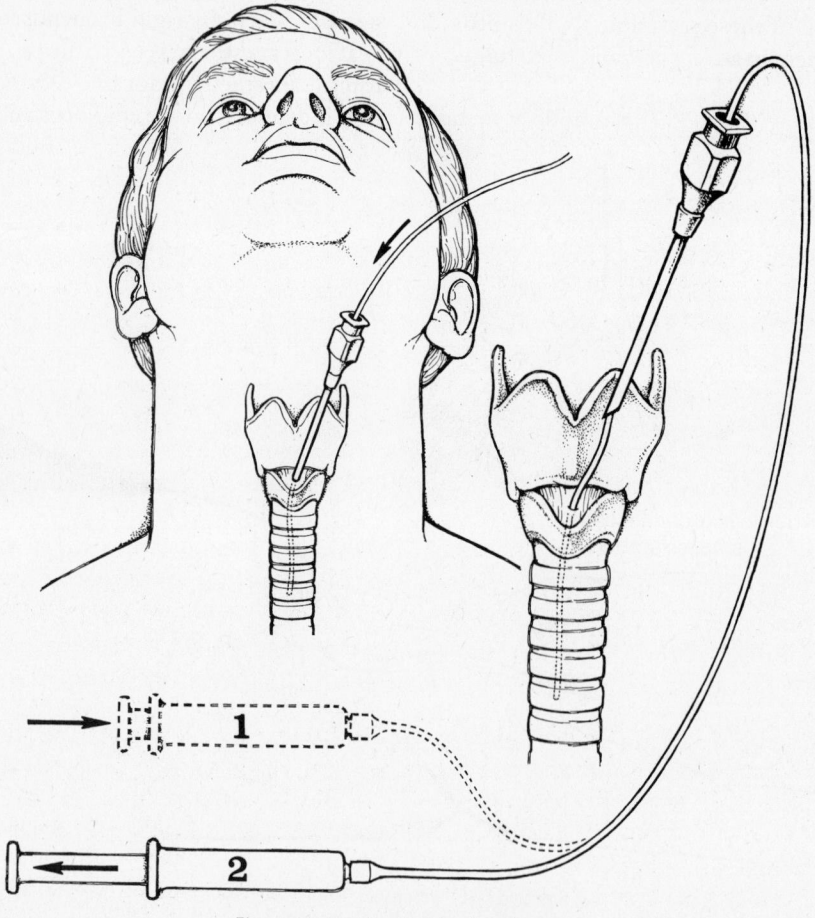

Figure 22-4. Transtracheal aspiration.

Often a qualitive study is done to determine whether the secretions are saliva, mucus, or pus. Usually they separate into layers that are seen readily when a conical glass container is used. A yellow-green color of the material expectorated usually implies infection, i.e., bronchitis or pneumonia.

For quantitative studies, the patient is given a special container in which to expectorate. This is weighed at the end of 24 hours, and the amount and the character of the contents are described and recorded. Such a specimen is disposed of by wrapping it in paper and sending it to the incinerator. To prevent odors, all sputum containers should be covered. Malodorous discarded mouth wipes should be removed and good room ventilation assured. Of course, frequent oral hygiene is a nursing priority for these patients.

Transtracheal aspiration of sputum is accomplished by transtracheal puncture through the cricothyroid membrane and by the introduction of a fine catheter through the needle into the trachea (Fig. 22-4). The needle is withdrawn, leaving the catheter in place. Sterile saline (3 to 5 ml.) is injected into the catheter to induce coughing. Then material is aspirated back through the catheter into a syringe. The contents of the syringe are expressed into a sterile culture tube. The catheter is withdrawn and pressure is applied over the puncture site.

This technique may also be used to promote coughing and sputum production in thoracotomy patients. In this instance, the catheter may be left in place for periodic instillation of saline to induce coughing.

Transtracheal aspiration bypasses the oropharynx and thus avoids specimen contamination by mouth flora. It is of special value to the immunocompromised patient with pneumonia who does not produce sputum.

Examination of Pleural Fluid (Thoracentesis)

A thin layer of pleural fluid normally remains in the pleural space. A sample of this fluid can be obtained by thoracentesis or by tube thoracotomy. *Thoracentesis* is the aspiration of pleural fluid for diagnostic or therapeutic purposes (Fig. 22-5). Frequently a needle biopsy of the pleura is taken at the same time. Guidelines for assisting the patient undergoing a thoracentesis are presented on pages 407–408. Studies on pleural fluid include gram stain culture and sensitivity, acid–fast staining and culture, differential cell count, cytology, specific gravity, total protein, and lactic dehydrogenase (LDH).

Pleural Biopsy

Pleural biopsy is accomplished via (1) needle biopsy of the pleura or (2) pleuroscopy, which is a visual exploration of the pleural space through a fiberoptic bronchoscope inserted into the pleural space. Pleural biopsy is done when there is pleural exudate of undetermined etiology and when there is need for pathological tissue staining or tissue culture for tuberculosis and fungi.

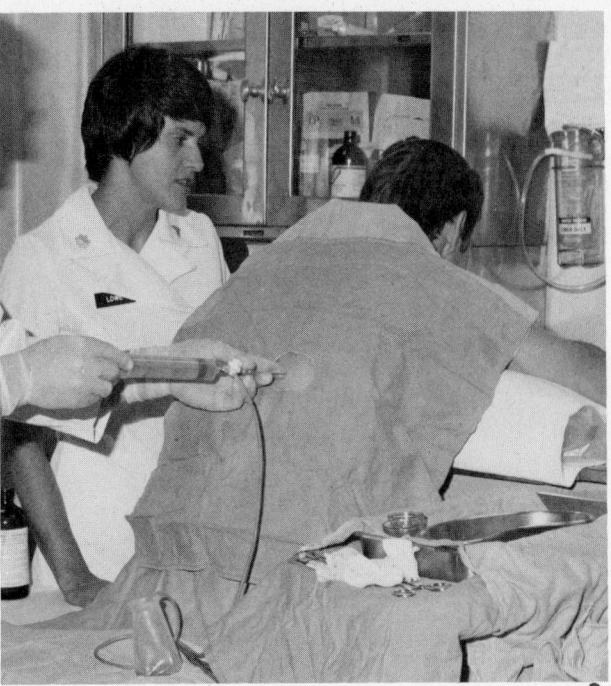

Figure 22-5. The patient is having a diagnostic thoracentesis performed. (Courtesy, Walter Reed Army Medical Center, Washington, D.C.)

Pulmonary Function Tests

Pulmonary function tests are done to detect abnormalities in respiratory function and to determine the extent of the abnormality. Such tests may measure lung volume and capacity, flow measurements, compliance and resistance, diffusion characteristics, oxygen consumption, respiratory quotient, ventilation, and perfusion. The newer tests include more sophisticated measurements. Pulmonary function tests are useful in following the course of a patient with established respiratory disease and assessing response to therapy. They are useful as screening tests in potentially hazardous industries such as coal mining and those which involve exposure to asbestos.

Most pulmonary function tests require some type of spirometer which has a volume-collecting device attached to a recorder that demonstrates volume and time simultaneously. There is a wide variety of tests ranging from the simple to the complex. A number of function tests are carried out since no single measurement can be done to evaluate pulmonary function. Usually, test results are interpreted on the basis of degree of deviation from normal, taking into consideration the patient's height, weight, age, and sex. Normal values have been established on nomograms, which are available in manufacturer's handbooks or with pulmonary function equipment.

Since there is a wide range of normal values, pulmonary function tests may not detect early localized

TABLE 22-1. VENTILATORY FUNCTION TESTS

DESCRIPTION	TERM USED	SYMBOL	REMARKS
The maximum volume of air exhaled from the point of maximum inspiration	Vital capacity	VC	Slow vital capacity may be normal or reduced in COPD* patients.
Vital capacity performed with a maximally forced expiratory effort	Forced vital capacity	FVC	Forced vital capacity is often reduced in COPD due to air trapping.
Volume of air exhaled in the specified time during the performance of forced vital capacity	Forced expiratory volume (qualified by subscript indicating the time interval in seconds)	FEV_t, usually FEV_1	A valuable clue to the severity of the expiratory airway obstruction.
FEV_T expressed as a percentage of the forced vital capacity	Ratio of timed forced expiratory volume to forced vital capacity	$FEV_t/FVC\%$, usually $FEV_1/FVC\%$	Another way of expressing the presence or absence of airway obstruction.
Mean forced expiratory flow between 200 and 1,200 ml. of the FVC	Forced expiratory flow	$FEF_{200-1200}$	Formerly called maximum expiratory flow rate (MEFR). An indicator of large airway obstruction.
Mean forced expiratory flow during the middle half of the FVC	Forced mid-expiratory flow	$FEF_{25-75\%}$	Formerly called maximum mid-expiratory flow rate. Slowed in small airway obstruction.
Mean forced expiratory flow during the terminal portion of the FVC	Forced end-expiratory flow	$FEF_{75-85\%}$	Slowed in obstruction of smallest airways.
Volume of air expired in a specified period during repetitive maximal effort	Maximal voluntary ventilation	MVV	Formerly called maximum breathing capacity. An important factor in exercise tolerance.

(From American Lung Association: Chronic Obstructive Pulmonary Disease, 5th ed., 1977.

*Chronic obstructive pulmonary disease.

changes. The patient with respiratory symptoms (dyspnea, wheezing, cough, sputum production) should undergo a complete diagnostic evaluation, even though the results of pulmonary function tests are "normal."

Table 22-1 lists and describes the most frequently used pulmonary function tests.

Arterial Blood Gas Studies

Measurements of blood pH and of arterial oxygen and carbon dioxide tensions are made when managing patients with respiratory problems. Arterial blood gas studies aid in assessing the degree to which the lungs are able to provide adequate oxygen and remove carbon dioxide, and the degree to which the kidneys are able to reabsorb or excrete bicarbonate ions to maintain normal body pH. Serial blood gas analysis is also a sensitive indicator of whether or not the lung has been damaged following chest trauma. (See page 442 for a discussion of arterial blood gas measurement and the technique of arterial puncture).

Radioisotope Diagnostic Procedures (Lung Scan)

A *perfusion lung scan* is done by injecting a radioactive isotope (technetium) into a peripheral vein and then taking a scan of the chest and body to detect radiation. The isotope particles pass through the right heart and are distributed into the lungs in amounts proportional to the regional blood flow, making it possible to trace and measure the blood perfusion through the lung. This procedure is used clinically to measure the integrity of the pulmonary vessels relative to blood flow and to evaluate blood flow abnormalities as seen in pulmonary emboli. (See Chapter 16.)

A *ventilation scan* is done after the perfusion scan. The patient takes a deep breath of a mixture of oxygen and radioactive gas (^{133}Xe) which diffuses throughout the lungs. A scan is done to detect ventilation abnormalities, especially in patients who have regional differences in ventilation, e.g., emphysema.

Lung Biopsy Procedures

When the chest x-ray is inconclusive or reveals pulmonary density (indicating an infiltrate; lesion), it is desirable to examine lung tissue to establish the nature of the lesion. In the past, diagnostic thoracotomy was done to obtain pulmonary tissue. This procedure, though reliable, involved considerable risk and was expensive and uncomfortable. There are now two nonoperative lung biopsy techniques which are being used because they yield accurate information with low morbidity: (1) transcatheter bronchial brushing or (2) percutaneous (through the skin) needle biopsy.

In *transcatheter bronchial brushing* a fiberoptic bronchoscope is introduced into the bronchus under fluoroscopic monitoring. A small brush is attached to the end of a flexible wire which is inserted through the fiberscope.

GUIDELINES FOR ASSISTING THE PATIENT HAVING A THORACENTESIS

A thoracentesis (aspiration of fluid or air from the pleural space) is done on patients with various clinical problems. It may be a diagnostic or therapeutic procedure for:

(1) removal of fluid and air from the pleural cavity
(2) diagnostic aspiration of pleural fluid
(3) pleural biopsy
(4) instillation of medication into pleural space

The responsibilities of the nurse in relation to the patient having a thoracentesis and the rationale of her participation are summarized below.

Nursing Activities	Amplification/Rationale
1. Ascertain in advance whether chest roentgenograms have been ordered and completed and consent form has been signed.	1. Posteroanterior and lateral chest x-rays are used to localize fluid and air in the pleural cavity and to aid in determining the puncture site.
2. Determine whether the patient is allergic to the local anesthetic agent to be used. Give sedation if prescribed.	
3. Inform the patient about the procedure and indicate how he can be helpful. Explain: a. The nature of the procedure b. The importance of remaining immobile c. Pressure sensations to be experienced d. That no discomfort is anticipated after the procedure	3. An explanation helps to orient the patient to the procedure, assists him to mobilize his resources, and gives him an opportunity to ask questions and verbalize anxiety.
4. Make the patient comfortable with adequate supports. If possible, place him upright and in one of the following positions: a. Sitting on the edge of the bed with the feet supported and his arms and head on a padded over-the-bed table. b. Straddling a chair with his arms and head resting on the back of the chair. c. Lying on his unaffected side if he is unable to assume a sitting position.	4. The upright position facilitates the removal of fluid that usually localizes at the base of the chest. A position of comfort helps the patient to relax.
5. Support and reassure the patient during the procedure. a. Prepare the patient for cold sensation of skin germicide solution and of pressure sensation from infiltration of local anesthetic agent. b. Encourage the patient to refrain from coughing.	5. Sudden and unexpected movement by the patient can cause trauma to the visceral pleura with resultant trauma to the lung.
6. Expose the entire chest. The site for aspiration is determined from chest x-rays and by percussion. If fluid is in the pleural cavity, the thoracentesis site is determined by chest x-ray and physical findings, with attention to site of maximal dullness on percussion.	6. If air is in the pleural cavity, the thoracentesis site is usually in the 2nd or 3rd intercostal space in the midclavicular line. Air rises in the thorax because the density of the air is much less than the density of liquid.
7. The procedure is done under aseptic conditions. After the skin is cleansed, a local anesthetic is injected slowly with a small caliber needle into the intercostal space by the physician.	7. An intradermal wheal is raised slowly; rapid injection causes pain. The parietal pleura is very sensitive and should be well infiltrated with anesthetic before the thoracentesis needle is passed through it. To minimize intercostal artery laceration, the needle is inserted into the intercostal space just above the lower rib.
8. The physician advances the thoracentesis needle with the stylet in place. When the pleural space is reached, the stylet is removed and suction may be applied with the syringe. a. A 50-ml. syringe with a 3-way adapter (stopcock) is attached to the needle (one end of the adapter is attached to the needle and the other to the tubing leading to a receptacle that receives the fluid being aspirated). b. If a considerable quantity of fluid is removed, the needle is held in place on the chest wall with a small hemostat.	a. When a large quantity of fluid is withdrawn, a 3-way adapter serves to keep air from entering the pleural cavity. b. The hemostat steadies the needle on the chest wall. Sudden pleuritic chest pain or shoulder pain may indicate that the visceral or diaphragmatic pleurae are being irritated by the needle point.

(Continued)

GUIDELINES FOR ASSISTING THE PATIENT HAVING A THORACENTESIS (Continued)

Nursing Activities	Amplification/Rationale
9. After the needle is withdrawn, pressure is applied over the puncture site and a small sterile dressing is fixed in place.	
10. The patient is placed on bed rest. A chest x-ray is usually obtained following thoracentesis.	10. Chest x-ray verifies that there is no pneumothorax. Sometimes a minimal leak may be determined best on expiratory x-ray.
11. Record the total amount of fluid withdrawn and the nature of the fluid, its color, and its viscosity. If requested, prepare samples of fluid for laboratory evaluation. A small amount of heparin may be needed for several of the specimen containers in order to prevent coagulation. A specimen container with formalin may be needed if a pleural biopsy is to be obtained.	11. The fluid may be clear, serous, bloody, purulent, etc.
12. Evaluate the patient at intervals for faintness, vertigo, tightness in chest, uncontrollable cough, blood-tinged frothy mucus, and a rapid pulse.	12. Pneumothorax, tension pneumothorax, subcutaneous emphysema, or pyogenic infection may result from a thoracentesis. Pulmonary edema or cardiac distress can be produced by a sudden shift in mediastinal contents when large amounts of fluid are aspirated.

The area under suspicion is brushed back and forth so as to catch pieces of tissue on the bristles of the brush. The catheter may be irrigated with saline to secure material for additional studies.

This procedure is useful for cytologic evaluations of lung lesions and for the identification of pathogenic organisms (*Nocardia, Aspergillus, Pneumocystis carinii,* and other pathogens). It is especially useful in the immunologically compromised patient.

Nursing support for this procedure includes reinforcing the patient's understanding and seeing that the consent form has been signed. Following the procedure, the patient may have a mild sore throat and transient hemoptysis. Fluids and food are withheld for several hours following the procedure. Possible complications include anesthetic reactions, laryngospasm, hemoptysis, and rarely, pneumothorax.

Another method of bronchial brushing involves the introduction of the catheter through the transcricothyroid membrane by needle puncture. Following this procedure the patient is instructed to hold his thumb over the puncture site while coughing to prevent air from leaking into the surrounding tissues.

Percutaneous needle biopsy may be accomplished with a cutting needle or by aspiration with a spinal-type needle that provides a tissue specimen for histologic study. It is indicated when a lung lesion is suspected and routine sputum samples and bronchoscopic washings are negative.

Meperidine may be given as premedication. The skin over the biopsy site is cleansed and anesthetized, and a small incision is made. The biopsy needle is inserted through the skin into the pleura while the patient holds his breath in midexpiration. Under fluoroscopic monitoring, the needle is guided into the periphery of the lesion and the mass is biopsied. Possible complications include pneumothorax, pulmonary hemorrhage, and empyema.

Lymph Node Biopsy

The scalene lymph nodes are enmeshed in the deep cervical pad of fat overlying the scalenus anterior muscle. They drain the lungs and mediastinum and may show histologic changes due to intrathoracic disease. When these nodes are palpable on physical examination, a biopsy may be in order. A biopsy of these nodes may be done to detect lymph node spread of pulmonary disease and to establish a diagnosis or prognosis in such diseases as Hodgkin's disease, sarcoidosis, fungal disease, tuberculosis, and carcinoma.

Mediastinoscopy is the endoscopic examination of the mediastinum for exploration and biopsy of mediastinal nodes. Biopsy is usually done through a suprasternal incision. Mediastinoscopy is carried out to detect mediastinal involvement of pulmonary malignancy and to obtain tissue for diagnostic studies of other conditions; e.g., sarcoidosis.

ASSESSMENT OF RESPIRATORY SYMPTOMS

The major symptoms of respiratory disease are cough, sputum production, chest pain, hemoptysis, wheezing, and dyspnea. The constitutional symptoms of bronchopulmonary disease are anorexia, fever, weight loss, fatigue, malaise, weakness, and sweating. These clinical manifestations are related to the duration and severity of the disease. When data on patients with these symptoms is collected, analyzed, and interpreted, it is important to determine body location, quality, quantity, chronology, and factors aggravating or alleviating the problem.

Cough

Cough results from irritation of the mucous membranes anywhere in the respiratory tract. The stimulus producing a cough may arise from an infectious process or from an airborne irritant such as smoke, smog, dust, or a gas. "The cough reflex is the watchdog of the lungs" and is the patient's chief protection against the accumulation of secretions in the bronchi and bronchioles.

On the other hand, the presence of cough may indicate serious pulmonary disease. Of equal importance is the type of cough. A dry, irritative cough is characteristic of upper respiratory infection of viral etiology. Laryngotracheitis causes an irritative, high-pitched cough. Tracheal lesions produce a brassy cough. An acute dry cough often occurs in the early stages of virus infections that involve both upper and lower respiratory tracts. A severe or *changing* cough may indicate bronchogenic carcinoma. Pleuritic chest pain accompanying coughing may indicate pleural or chest wall (musculoskeletal) involvement.

Nursing Assessment. Evaluate the character of the cough. Is it dry? hacking? brassy? wheezing? loose? severe? Note the time of coughing. Coughing at night may herald the onset of left-sided heart failure or bronchial asthma. A cough in the morning with sputum production is indicative of bronchitis. A cough that worsens when the patient is supine may indicate a postnasal drip (sinusitis). Coughing after food intake may indicate aspirated material in the tracheobronchial tree. A cough of recent onset is usually from an acute infectious process.

Sputum Production

A patient who coughs long enough will almost invariably produce sputum. Violent coughing results in bronchial spasm, obstruction, and further irritation of the bronchi. A severe, repeated, or uncontrolled cough that is nonproductive is potentially harmful. Sputum production is the reaction of the lungs to any constantly recurring irritant. It may also be associated with a nasal discharge. If there is a profuse amount of purulent sputum (thick yellow or green), the patient probably has a bacterial infection. Rusty sputum indicates the presence of bacterial pneumonia, if the patient has not received antibiotics. A thin, mucoid sputum frequently results from viral bronchitis. A gradual increase of sputum over a period of time may reveal the presence of chronic bronchitis or bronchiectasis. Pink-tinged mucoid sputum is suggestive of a lung tumor, whereas profuse frothy pink material, often welling up into the throat, may indicate pulmonary edema. Malodorous sputum

and bad breath point to the presence of lung abscess or an infection caused by fusospirochetal or other anaerobic organisms.

Nursing Management. If the sputum is too thick to raise it is necessary to decrease its viscosity by increasing its water content through adequate hydration (drinking water) and inhalation of aerosolized solutions. These may be delivered via any type of nebulizer. Methods of assisting the patient to cough productively are discussed on pages 422 and 431.

Smoking is definitely contraindicated since it paralyzes ciliary action, increases bronchial secretions, causes inflammation and hyperplasia of the mucous membranes, and reduces production of surfactant. Thus bronchial drainage is impaired. If smoking is stopped, sputum volume will decrease and resistance to bronchial infections will improve.

The patient's appetite may be depressed because of the odor of the sputum and the taste it leaves in the mouth. Adequate mouth hygiene, proper environment, and wise selection of food will stimulate appetite. After the patient's mouth is carefully cleansed and rinsed, sputum cups and emesis basins should be removed before the next meal arrives. Serving citrus juices at the beginning of the meal will make the mouth feel better and will help to make the patient more receptive to the rest of the meal.

Dyspnea

Dyspnea (shortness of breath) is a symptom common to many pulmonary and heart conditions, particularly when there is increased lung rigidity and airway resistance. The right ventricle of the heart will ultimately be affected by lung disease since it must pump blood through the lungs. Sudden dyspnea in a healthy person may indicate pneumothorax (air in the pleural cavity). Sudden shortness of breath in an ill or postoperative patient may denote pulmonary embolism. Orthopnea (inability to breathe except in an upright position) is characteristic of cardiogenic pulmonary congestion. Shortness of breath with an expiratory wheeze is seen in chronic obstructive pulmonary disease (asthma, bronchitis, emphysema). A wheezing respiration may result from a narrowing of the airway or localized obstruction of a major bronchus by a tumor or foreign body. The presence of both inspiratory and expiratory wheezing usually signifies asthma, if the patient is not in congestive heart failure. Shortness of breath is quite commonly related to tension and anxiety. In general, the acute diseases of the lungs produce a more severe grade of dyspnea than do the chronic diseases.

Nursing Assessment. Determine the circumstances which produce the patient's dyspnea. How much exertion triggers shortness of breath? Is there an associated cough? Is dyspnea related to other symptoms? What was the mode of onset: sudden or gradual? At what time of day or night is it obvious? Is it worse when the patient is flat in bed? Does it occur at rest? with exercise? walking (how far?) climbing stairs? running?

The treatment of dyspnea depends on the success with which its cause can be alleviated. Relief of the symptom is sometimes achieved by placing the patient at rest with his head elevated and, in severe cases, by administering oxygen.

Chest Pain

Chest pain associated with pulmonary conditions may be sharp, stabbing, and intermittent, or dull, aching, and persistent. The pain usually is felt on the side where the pathology is located, but it may be referred elsewhere, for example, to the neck, the back, or the abdomen. Chest pain is experienced by many patients with pneumonia, pulmonary embolism with lung infarction, and pleurisy and is a late symptom of bronchogenic carcinoma. In carcinoma the pain may be dull and persistent because of invasion into the chest wall, mediastinum, or spine.

Lung disease does not always produce thoracic pain since the lungs and the visceral pleural covering lack sensory nerves and are insensitive to pain stimuli. But the parietal pleura has a rich supply of sensory nerves which are stimulated by inflammation and stretching of the membrane. Pleuritic pain due to irritation of the parietal pleura is sharp and seems to "catch" on inspiration; patients say it is "like the stabbing of a knife." They are more comfortable when they lie on the affected side, a posture that tends to "splint" the chest wall, restrict the expansions and contractions of the lung, and reduce the friction between the injured or diseased pleurae on that side. Pain associated with cough may be lessened by manual splinting of the rib cage as is illustrated in Figure 23-6.

Nursing Assessment. Assess the quality, intensity, and radiation of pain. Look for factors that precipitate it. Determine whether there is a relationship between pain and the patient's posture. Also evaluate the inspiratory and expiratory phase of respiration and its effect on pain. (See guidelines, page 519.)

Analgesic medications are effective in relieving chest pain, but care must be taken not to depress the respiratory center or a productive cough. For relief of extreme pain a regional anesthetic block may be done by injecting procaine along the intercostal nerves that supply the painful area.

Hemoptysis

Hemoptysis (expectoration of blood from the respiratory tract) is a symptom of pulmonary or cardiac disorders. It varies from blood-stained sputum to a large sudden hemorrhage and always merits investigation.

The most common pulmonary causes are (1) pulmonary infection (tuberculosis), (2) bronchiectasis and lung abscess, (3) neoplasms, and (4) vascular lesions. Frank bloody sputum may indicate pulmonary infarction. The onset of hemoptysis is usually sudden and may be intermittent or continuous. Three investigations are usually done to determine the cause: blood examination, chest x-ray, and bronchoscopy. A careful history and physical examination are necessary to establish a diagnosis of the underlying disease, irrespective of whether the bleeding produced a fleck of blood in the sputum or a massive hemorrhage. The amount of blood produced is not necessarily in positive correlation with the seriousness of the cause.

Nursing Assessment. Determine first where the blood is coming from. Has it come from the gums, nasopharynx, lungs, or stomach? The nurse may be the only witness to the episode. The following points should be borne in mind in making and recording observations. In patients whose bloody sputum originates from the nose or the nasopharynx, expectoration is usually preceded by considerable sniffing, and blood may appear in the nares. Blood from the lung is usually bright red, frothy, and mixed with sputum. Initial symptoms include a tickling sensation in the throat, a salty taste, a burning or bubbling sensation in the chest, and perhaps chest pain, in which case the patient tends to splint the bleeding side. The term *hemoptysis* is reserved for the coughing of blood arising from a pulmonary hemorrhage. This blood has an alkaline pH (greater than 7.0).

In contrast, if the hemorrhage is in the stomach, the blood is vomited (*hematemesis*) rather than coughed up. Blood that has been in contact with gastric juice is sometimes so dark that it is referred to as "coffee-ground" material. This blood has an acid pH (less than 7.0).

Management. A patient who has experienced a hemoptysis, whatever its cause, should be placed immediately at complete bed rest; his respiratory movements should be reduced. He should be placed on his affected side (if known) to protect the contralateral lung from aspiration of blood. The patient is instructed to remain quiet and is given the prescribed sedative, tranquilizer, or analgesic as directed. If there is a sudden increase in bleeding, endotracheal intubation is carried out quickly to control the airway. Equipment for performing an emergency laryngoscopy and bronchoscopy should be in readiness for the removal of blood clots and identification of the bleeding site. If the patient shows the initial signs of asphyxia, a balloon embolectomy catheter may be placed in the bronchus and the balloon inflated to occlude the bleeding site. Surgical intervention may eventually become necessary.

The nurse must realize that hemoptysis is one of the most frightening of all the symptoms that patients experience. Fright promotes hyperventilation, which is the opposite of what is desired, namely, a minimum of thoracic movement. Therefore a calm, reassuring approach is definitely part of the therapy.

Collection of Fluid and Air in the Pleural Cavity

Hydrothorax is a collection of watery fluid in the pleural cavity (pleural effusion) which may occur in such medical conditions as cardiac or renal failure, hepatic or pancreatic disease, lung and pleural tumors, etc. The presence of fluid may cause respiratory difficulties and require aspiration (thoracentesis). (See page 478 for the management of pleural effusion.)

Pneumothorax (air in the pleural cavity) may occur spontaneously from rupture of a lung alveolus (see below); it may occur after thoracentesis, pleural biopsy, or percutaneous needle biopsy. It may be secondary to infection or result from high positive end-expiratory pressure of a ventilator. Or it may arise from trauma, the air

entering the pleural cavity through a resulting wound or from the injured lung.

Hemothorax (blood in the pleural cavity) also accompanies chest trauma. Aspiration of the air and blood permits reexpansion of the lung and a return to a more physiologic state. (Pneumothorax and hemothorax due to chest injuries are discussed on page 499.)

Spontaneous pneumothorax is the spontaneous appearance of air in the pleural cavity as a result of rupture of the visceral pleura or of emphysematous blebs or bullae. It may occur in healthy adolescents and young adults without pulmonary disease as well as in older persons with chronic pulmonary disease. The patient complains of sudden chest pain and mild to severe dyspnea.

Treatment depends on the etiology of the pneumothorax and on its size and duration. If the pneumothorax is small and the patient is relatively

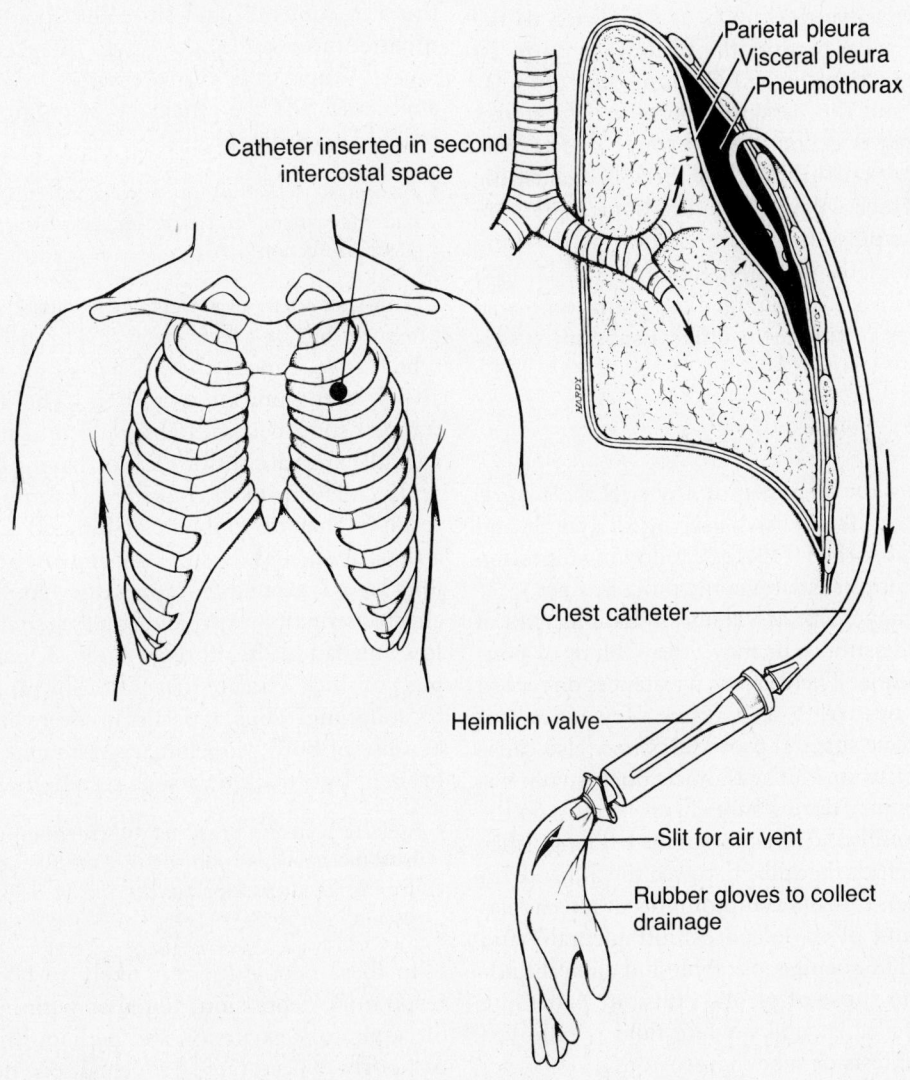

Figure 22-6. Ambulatory treatment of spontaneous pneumothorax.

asymptomatic, no intervention is required. However, a larger area will require that the air be removed via thoracentesis. If a significant air leak occurs, it may be necessary to insert into the pleural cavity a chest catheter that is attached to some type of drainage system. Occasionally, a thoracotomy and pleural abrasion are indicated in selected cases of spontaneous pneumothorax, especially for a recurrent condition. Recurrence is a problem with spontaneous pneumothorax and may affect either side of the chest.

In some instances of spontaneous pneumothorax, it may be possible to treat the patient on an outpatient basis by means of an intercostal drainage tube and a flutter valve. A 16 French catheter is inserted into the 2nd intercostal space anteriorly for men and in the 5th intercostal space laterally for women (for cosmetic reasons). The chest catheter is attached to underwater drainage temporarily and the patient is observed for a few hours. A chest x-ray is obtained. If the lung shows adequate reexpansion, the underwater drainage is discontinued and a disposable flutter valve (Heimlich) is connected to the chest tube. The valve permits the pleural cavity to be drained without suction (Fig. 22-6). Immediate ambulation is possible and the patient is permitted to return home. The patient is encouraged to cough and to perform the Valsalva maneuver (exhale forcibly against the closed glottis), which will increase intrathoracic pressure and aid in the expulsion of air. As soon as the lung expansion is complete, the chest tube is removed (3-4 days) and the patient is encouraged to return to normal activity. This type of treatment offers a substantial savings in cost.

Chylothorax

Chylothorax is the presence of chyle in the pleural cavity. (Chyle, a milky fluid consisting of lymph and emulsified fat, is absorbed from food following digestion and enters the venous system via the thoracic duct.)

Chylothorax may occur as a result of malignancies of the lung and mediastinum or may follow blunt or penetrating chest trauma. There are even instances on record of chylothorax occurring as a result of yawning or stretching. Thoracic surgical procedures may also cause chylous pleural effusions. (The thoracic duct is vulnerable to traumatic injury during surgical procedures on the heart and great vessels and resection of the left lung, since it crosses to the left of the spine between the 5th and 7th thoracic vertebrae). Usually symptoms occur after a relatively large amount of chyle collects intrapleurally and causes dyspnea. The roentgenographic and clinical findings are similar to those of pleural effusion. A definite diagnosis is made when milky white fluid is removed either by thoracentesis or tube thoracostomy.

The objectives of therapy are to reduce chyle formation and reexpand the lung. Reduction of lymph flow is achieved by reducing the patient's activities and maintaining him on intravenous hyperalimentation to decrease the volume of chyle. Pulmonary reexpansion is achieved by repeated thoracenteses or closed tube thoracostomy.

Atelectasis

Atelectasis refers to the collapse of an alveolus or of multiple alveolar units (Fig. 22-7); it may result from pressure on the lung tissue which restricts normal lung expansion on inspiration. Such pressure may be produced by a variety of causes: fluid accumulation within the thorax (pleural effusion), air in the pleural space (pneumothorax), an extremely large heart, a pericardium distended with fluid (pericardial effusion), tumor growth within the thorax, or an elevated diaphragm that is displaced upward as the result of abdominal pressure. Under such circumstances there is crowding of the intrathoracic contents, and since the spongy lung tissue is most compressible, the lung collapses without resistance. Where it is compressed it becomes airless, or atelectatic, and the efficiency of pulmonary function is reduced accordingly.

- Atelectasis caused by pressure is encountered most often in patients with pleural effusion due to cardiac failure, or in pleural infection.

Another form of atelectasis is caused, not by external pressure, but by obstruction of a bronchus, the effect of which is to impede the passage of air to and from the alveoli communicating with it. The alveolar air thus trapped soon becomes absorbed into the bloodstream, and, all external communication having been blocked, its replacement from the outside air is impossible. The net result is that the portion of lung so isolated becomes airless: it shrinks in size, causing the remainder of the lung to overexpand (compensatory emphysema). Bronchial obstruction capable of causing atelectasis may follow inhalation of a foreign body. It may result from a plug of thick exudate that is not, or cannot be, expelled by coughing. Thus, it occurs in severe bronchial asthma, because of both bronchiolar spasm and plugging of the bronchi by a thick tenacious secretion.

- Atelectasis due to bronchial obstruction by secretions is the usual mechanism producing the "massive collapse" occasionally observed postoperatively and in debilitated bedridden patients.

In these people there is likely to be long continued respiratory depression, together with inadequate depth of respiratory excursion and perhaps unusually profuse or poorly expectorated bronchial secretions. Tumors of the bronchi often make their presence known first by an atelectasis resulting from their obstructive growth.

Clinical Manifestations. If collapse occurs suddenly, and if sufficient lung tissue is involved, the following may be anticipated: marked dyspnea, cyanosis, prostration, and pleural pain which usually is referred to the lower chest. Fever commonly occurs. Tachycardia and dyspnea are unusually prominent. The patient characteristically sits bolt upright in bed, appears anxious and cyanotic, and has difficulty in breathing. The chest wall on the affected side moves little, if at all, whereas on the opposite side the excursion appears excessive. Lungs that have collapsed because of the obstruction of a bronchus should be reexpanded as rapidly as possible to avoid the common complications of pneumonia or lung abscess.

Management. If atelectasis has resulted from a pleural effusion or pressure pneumothorax, the fluid or air may be removed by needle aspiration. If bronchial obstruction is the cause, it must be removed in order to permit air to enter the lung again. Methods to accomplish this include aspirating secretions, encouraging the patient to cough, and using an aerosol ultrasonic nebulizer, followed by postural drainage and chest percussion. The patient should be turned frequently in an effort to stimulate coughing. If possible, he should be assisted out of bed and walked. If these methods fail to remove the obstruction, a bronchoscopy is done. If bronchoscopy is not successful, it may be necessary to use an endotracheal tube and mechanical ventilation for a few days (page 450).

The incidence of postoperative pulmonary atelectasis has been reduced significantly as a result of the more conservative and judicious use of preoperative and postoperative sedation and by early ambulation of postoperative patients, along with the use of incentive spirometry. (See page 372 for a discussion of postoperative atelectasis.)

All stuporous, debilitated, and heavily sedated patients should be turned frequently in bed, a procedure that affords increased respiratory excursion on the uppermost side. Judicious use of nasopharyngeal and nasotracheal suction is also very helpful in stimulating patients to cough and in removing tenacious secretions (see page 423).

PREVENTION OF RESPIRATORY DISEASE

Cigarette smoking, exposure to environmental air pollution (dust, fumes, and gases), and respiratory tract infections play a role in the development of respiratory disease.

Cigarette smoking is the most important risk factor for diseases of the lung, especially lung cancer, emphysema, and chronic bronchitis. According to the "Surgeon General's Report on Smoking and Health" (1979), the lighted cigarette generates about 4,000 compounds which can be separated into gas and particulate phases. Carbon mon-

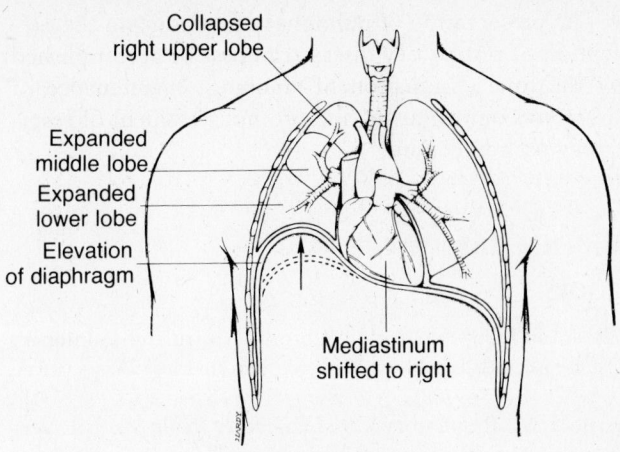

Collapsed right upper lobe

Expanded middle lobe

Expanded lower lobe

Elevation of diaphragm

Mediastinum shifted to right

Figure 22-7. Atelectasis.

oxide (the gas phase), nicotine, and tar (the particulate phase) are the most likely contributors to the health hazards of smoking. It is generally accepted that most cases of bronchogenic carcinoma are attributable to inhalation of carcinogenic pollutants (smoke, environmental toxins) by a susceptible host. The inhalation of cigarette smoke impairs alveolar macrophage function and reduces ciliary action. This results in a reduction in the tracheobronchial mucociliary clearance—the mechanism that normally removes particles from the respiratory tract. Inhalation of cigarette smoke also produces an increase in airway resistance.

There appear to be negative health effects from "passive smoking"—the inhalation by the nonsmoker of fumes from nearby cigarettes, pipes, and cigars. Passive smoking may be hazardous to persons with respiratory disease. In addition, an estimated 2 million Americans are sensitive to tobacco smoke and suffer smoke-caused asthma attacks. Research also indicates that respiratory illness is twice as common in young children whose parents smoke at home as it is in children with nonsmoking parents.

Air pollution presents its own hazard to health. The air may be polluted by hundreds of substances, but in the United States the five "criteria pollutants" that are generally monitored are carbon monoxide (CO), sulfur dioxide (SO_2), total suspended particulate (TSP), ozone, or photochemical oxidants (O_3), and nitrogen dioxide (NO_2). The major pollution problems are from air pollutants emitted from motor vehicles and heat or power generators. When the air is significantly polluted it is known to increase morbidity and mortality due to aggravation of chronic pulmonary disease.

Exposure to environmental toxic factors (industrial and agricultural chemicals) may lead to significant respiratory impairment. The risk of developing occupational respiratory disease is increased by smoking. The pneumoconioses are almost entirely preventable by the maintenance of a safe working environment.

The preservation of pulmonary function and the prevention of respiratory disease can best be accomplished by the total elimination of smoking, maintenance of clean environmental air, and prompt treatment of respiratory tract infection.

BIBLIOGRAPHY

BOOKS

American Lung Association: Chronic Obstructive Pulmonary Disease, 5th ed. New York, American Lung Association, 1977.

Arnold, V.: Respiratory Care Laboratory Skills Manual. Ventura, Calif., Respiratory West Co., 1977.

Burton, G. G., Gee, G. N., and Hodgkin, J. E.: Respiratory Care. A Guide to Clinical Practice. Philadelphia, J. B. Lippincott, 1977.

Effler, D. B. (ed.): Blades' Surgical Diseases of the Chest. St. Louis, C. V. Mosby, 1978.

Fraser, R. G., and Pare, J. A. P.: Diagnosis of Diseases of the Chest, 2nd ed., Philadelphia, W. B. Saunders, 1977.

Guenter, C. A., and Welch, M. H.: Pulmonary Medicine. Philadelphia, J. B. Lippincott, 1977.

Lane, D. J.: Respiratory Disease. London, William Heinemann Medical Books, Ltd., 1976.

Lillington, G. A., and Jamplis, R. W.: A Diagnostic Approach to Chest Diseases. Baltimore, Williams and Wilkins, 1977.

MacDonnell, K. F., and Segal, M. S.: Current Respiratory Care. Boston, Little, Brown, 1977.

O'Connor, A. B., ed.: Nursing in Respiratory Diseases, 2nd ed. New York, American Journal of Nursing Co., 1977.

Report of the Surgeon General: Smoking and Health: A Report of the Surgeon General. Washington, D.C., U.S. Public Health Service, 1979.

Ruppel, G.: Manual of Pulmonary Function Testing. St. Louis, C. V. Mosby, 1975.

von Hippel, A.: A Manual of Thoracic Surgery. Springfield, Charles C Thomas, 1978.

ARTICLES

Assessment of Respiratory Function

Boysen, P. G., et. al.: Prospective evaluation for pneumonectomy using the [99m]Technetium quantitative perfusion lung scan. Chest, 72:422-425, Oct. 1977.

Foley, M., Tomashefski, J., and Underwood, E., Jr.: Pulmonary function screening tests in industry. AJN, 77:1480-1484, Sept. 1977.

Katz, S.: What is the air quality index? Am. Fam. Phys., 18:121-122, Oct. 1978.

Krausz, M., and Manny, J.: A safe method of thoracentesis. J. Thorac. Cardiovasc. Surg., 72:323-325, Aug. 1976.

Light, R. W.: Pleural effusions. Med. Clin. N. Am., 61:1339-1352, Nov. 1977.

Shank, J. C., and Latshaw, R. F.: Pleural effusion. Am. Fam. Phys., 17:143-149, Mar. 1978.

Zavala, D. C.: Diagnostic fiberoptic bronchoscopy: Techniques and results of biopsy in 600 patients. Chest, 68:12-19, July 1975.

AGENCIES

Governmental

National Heart, Lung and Blood Institute, National Institutes of Health, Bethesda, Md. 20205

Voluntary

American Association for Respiratory Therapy, 7411 Hines Place, Suite 101, Dallas, Tex. 75235

American Lung Association, 1740 Broadway, New York, N.Y. 10019

American Thoracic Society, 1740 Broadway, New York, N.Y. 10019

23

MANAGEMENT OF PATIENTS WITH IMPAIRED RESPIRATORY FUNCTION

SPECIAL MANAGEMENT IN RESPIRATORY CONDITIONS

A wide variety of treatment modalities can be used in caring for patients with different types of respiratory conditions. The most common modalities include oxygen therapy, intermittent positive pressure breathing (IPPB), and physical therapy such as postural drainage, percussion and vibration, breathing exercises, and physical conditioning.

OXYGEN THERAPY

Oxygen therapy is the administration of oxygen at a concentration or pressure greater than that found in the environmental atmosphere. It is particularly useful in the treatment of hypoxemic states which result in inadequate transport of oxygen by the blood. The goal in oxygen therapy is to treat the hypoxemia while decreasing the work of breathing and the stress on the myocardium. Oxygen transport to the tissues depends upon many factors: cardiac output, arterial oxygen content, and metabolic requirements. All of these must be considered when oxygen therapy is contemplated. (Respiratory physiology and oxygen transport are discussed in Chapter 22.)

Patient Assessment. A change in the patient's respiration is often evidence of the need for oxygen therapy.

Other clinical signs of hypoxia include changes in mental status, dyspnea, increase in blood pressure, changes in heart rate, arrhythmias, cyanosis (late), and cool extremities. However, the signs and symptoms of oxygen need may depend upon how suddenly this need develops. With rapidly developing hypoxia there are changes in the central nervous system since the higher centers are more sensitive to oxygen deprivation. The clinical picture may resemble that of drunkenness, the patient exhibiting similar signs of incoordination and impaired judgment. Longstanding hypoxia (as seen in chronic obstructive pulmonary disease and chronic congestive heart failure) may produce fatigue, drowsiness, apathy, inattentiveness, and delayed reaction time. The need for oxygen is assessed by arterial blood gas analysis (page 442) as well as by clinical evaluation.

Precautions. Excessive oxygen may produce toxic effects on the lungs and central nervous system and/or result in depression of ventilation in certain conditions, namely chronic obstructive pulmonary disease (pages 481–488). In these patients the stimulus for respiration is a decrease in blood oxygen rather than an elevation in carbon dioxide levels. Thus, sudden administration of a high concentration of oxygen will remove the respiratory drive that has been created largely by the patient's chronic low oxygen tension. This can cause a progressive increase in arterial PCO_2, ultimately leading to death from carbon dioxide narcosis. (See page 445 and page

415

474.) Therefore, oxygen should be administered with care and its effects on each patient should be carefully assessed.

As a general rule, with pulmonary patients, oxygen therapy should only be given to raise the arterial PO_2 to 60 torr. At this level the blood is 80 to 90 percent saturated, and higher PO_2 values will not add further significant amounts of oxygen to the red cells or plasma. Instead of helping, increased amounts of oxygen may possibly suppress ventilation.

With the use of oxygen, by any method, the patient should be assessed frequently for signs of oxygen need: mental aberration, disturbed consciousness, abnormal color, perspiration, changes in blood pressure, and increasing heart and respiratory rates.

Other precautions to be taken with oxygen involve the careful handling of oxygen equipment. Since oxygen supports combustion, there is always danger of fire when oxygen is used. Thus, "No Smoking" signs must be posted when oxygen is in use. It is also important to realize that the oxygen therapy equipment is a potential source of bacterial cross infection. Thus, the breathing circuits should be changed and sterilized daily.

Methods of Administration

Oxygen is dispensed from a cylinder or from a piped-in system. A reduction gauge is necessary to reduce the pressure to a working level and a flow meter regulates the control of oxygen in liters per minute. Oxygen is moistened by passing it through a humidification system to prevent the mucous membranes of the respiratory tree from becoming dry.

Oxygen may be administered by a variety of means: nasal cannula (or prongs), oropharyngeal catheter, various types of face masks, and tent. It may also be applied directly to the endotracheal or tracheal tube via a T-piece or hyperinflation bag. The method selected depends on the concentration of oxygen required. The appropriate form of oxygen therapy is best determined after obtaining arterial blood gases which will indicate the patient's oxygenation status and acid-base balance.

The *nasal cannula* is used when the patient requires a low-to-medium concentration of oxygen for which precise accuracy is not essential. This method is relatively simple to use and allows the patient to move about in bed, talk, cough, and eat without interruption of oxygen flow. Flow rates in excess of 6 liters per minute may lead to air swallowing and may cause irritation to the nasal and pharyngeal mucosa.

The *oropharyngeal catheter* is employed for short-term use to administer moderate to moderately high concentrations of oxygen. To insert the catheter, measure the distance from the external nares to the tip of the ear lobe. Lubricate the catheter with a water soluble lubricant and pass it through the nose into the oropharynx. Look into the oropharynx (using a tongue depressor and flashlight) to check on the position of the catheter. Pull the catheter back slightly until the tip is not visible. It should not extend beyond the uvula in order to prevent gastric distention. Be sure the patient is not coughing, gagging, or swallowing air during this procedure. Secure the catheter to the bridge of the nose or face with hypoallergenic tape. Change the catheter every 8 to 12 hours and place it in alternate nostrils to prevent catheter encrustation and ulceration of the nasal mucosa. This method of oxygen administration can lead to discomfort and irritation of the nasal mucosa. When nasal oxygen is administered (either by cannula or oropharyngeal catheter), the percentage of oxygen reaching the lungs varies with the depth and rate of respiration.

A *face mask* is used when high concentrations of oxygen are required in the acute phase of certain diseases. A rebreathing bag permits the patient to inhale a high concentration of oxygen from a reservoir bag. Perforations on both sides of the mask serve as exhalation ports. The mask must fit snugly to ensure an airtight seal between the face and the mask. The mask is placed on the patient's face and the liter flow adjusted (per order) so that the rebreathing bag will not collapse during the inspiratory cycle. With a well-fitting rebreathing bag that is adjusted correctly, inspired oxygen concentrations of 30 to 60 percent can be achieved.

The disadvantages of a face mask are the mechanical restrictions it imposes on eating, drinking, and talking. There is also a certain amount of discomfort associated with the use of a mask for any length of time.

The *venturi mask* is a face mask designed to administer precisely controlled oxygen concentrations. It is so constructed that there is a constant flow of room air mixed with a fixed concentration of oxygen. It is used primarily for patients with chronic obstructive pulmonary disease. The venturi mask, which employs the principle of air entrainment, provides a high air flow with controlled oxygen enrichment, allowing a fixed low oxygen concentration with a flow-rate surplus according to the patient's needs. Excess gas leaves the mask through the perforated cuff, carrying with it the expired carbon dioxide. It allows inhalation of a constant oxygen concentration regardless of the depth or rate of respiration.

The patient's skin should be checked for irritation, and the mask should fit snugly enough to prevent oxygen flow into the eyes. The mask must be removed in order that the patient may eat, drink, take medications, etc., and it becomes uncomfortable after prolonged use.

The *aerosol mask* provides oxygen in concentrations of 35 percent or greater with high humidity by administering aerosol mist that is either heated or unheated.

Oxygen tents are rarely used for adults, since oxygen concentration within the tent is variable. Difficulties in caring for the patient within the tent and the danger of fire are additional disadvantages.

HAZARDS OF INTERMITTENT POSITIVE PRESSURE BREATHING THERAPY

I. Adverse Effects of Positive Pressure
    A. Pulmonary effects
        1. Hyperinflation with air trapping may result in:
            a. dyspnea and discomfort in chest
            b. growth of bullae
            c. pneumothorax
        2. Pulmonary edema, if very high pressures are used
    B. Circulatory effects
        1. Decreased venous return may result in:
            a. hypotension
            b. increased intracranial pressure
        2. Physical (and pharmacologic) disturbance of heart may cause:
            a. arrhythmias
            b. coronary insufficiency
        3. Changes in fluid balance
            a. diuresis
            b. fluid retention, as from increased antidiuretic hormone secretion
            c. secondary electrolyte imbalance
    C. Gastrointestinal effects
        1. Gastric insufflation
        2. Abdominal distention, with possibility of adverse effects on abdominal incisions
        3. Nausea, vomiting, pulmonary aspiration
    D. Effects on blood gases
        1. Hypoventilation with deterioration in blood gases
        2. Hyperventilation may result in:
            a. hyperoxia with depression of hypoxic respiratory drive

           b. hypocapnia with depression of respiratory drive
           c. respiratory alkalemia, causing paresthesias, lightheadedness, liability to seizures, etc.

II. Adverse Effects of Aerosols
    A. Bronchodilators
        1. Systemic side effects, such as tachycardia, arrhythmias, nervousness
        2. Tachyphylaxis (with over-frequent use)
    B. Mucokinetics
        1. Toxic effects, such as nausea, bronchial irritation
        2. Loosening of secretions with distal retention, causing hypoxemia
        3. Sodium chloride retention may result in hypernatremia
    C. Danger of delivering unhumidified gas which dries mucosa
    D. Danger of delivering hot, dry gas if heated humidifier becomes empty, causing dehydration, irritation, and crusting of mucosa
    E. Danger of delivering infected aerosol, resulting in nosocomial pneumonia

III. General Adverse Effects
    A. Patient may become claustrophobic, or distressed by IPPB
    B. Patient may not relax, and may fight machine, resulting in dyspnea, increased work of breathing, and deterioration in pulmonary function
    C. Patient may become "addicted" to machine, resulting in overuse and dependency

(From: Ziment, I.: Intermittent positive pressure breathing. *In* Burton, G. G., Gee, G. N., and Hodgkin, J. E.: Respiratory Care. Philadelphia, J. B. Lippincott, 1977, page 571.)

INTERMITTENT POSITIVE PRESSURE BREATHING

Intermittent Positive Pressure Breathing (IPPB) is the breathing of air or oxygen (or a combination of both) under pressure. During inhalation, the air or oxygen is delivered by a pressure-cycled respirator, after which the patient exhales into the atmosphere. IPPB is prescribed as a mode of delivering aerosols to the lungs and/or assisting ventilation in order to decrease the work of breathing.

Since there are numerous IPPB devices on the market, the individual who administers the treatment should understand the mechanical functioning of the machine as well as the objective of therapy for the individual patient. Usually the respiratory therapist administers the IPPB treatment, but the nurse should become familiar with the use of these machines and know the effects of therapy on the patient. The role of the nurse is to (1) calm the anxious dyspneic patient and (2) reinforce the teaching concerning the use of the machine. The patient must be encouraged to relax and synchronize his breathing with the machine's cycling. IPPB treatments require careful surveillance and must never be regarded as routine or boring, since there are specific hazards associated with the use of these units, which are summarized in the chart above.

There is currently a great deal of controversy surrounding the use of IPPB. A search of recent literature does not reveal with certainty that IPPB is more effective in delivering aerosols than the hand-held nebulizers. Data is also inconclusive about whether or not IPPB decreases the work of breathing for prolonged periods. Some patients appear to respond symptomatically and feel that IPPB helps in loosening sputum and inducing expectoration.

An added concern is the possibility that IPPB machines can be a potent source of infection, since microorganisms may collect in the nebulizer devices. These residual organisms multiply in a warm, moist medium, become aerosolized during treatment, and are inhaled into the lung. Thus, pulmonary infection and superinfection may result. To avoid such outcomes, meticuluous cleaning and sterilization routines must be followed.

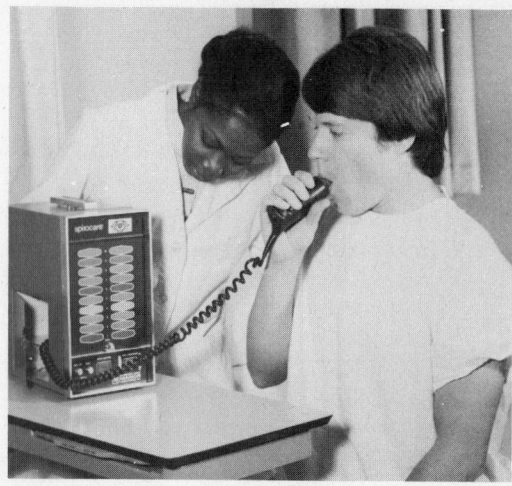

Figure 23-1. The incentive spirometer stimulates the patient to achieve maximum inspiration. The advantages of this type of therapy are that no compressed gases are necessary, most models are relatively inexpensive, and the patient can work independently, since the control mechanism is built in.

Incentive Spirometer

The incentive spirometer is a piece of equipment that maximizes voluntary lung inflation (Fig. 23-1). It is used in the prevention and treatment of atelectasis, especially in the postoperative patient. The patient is placed in a sitting or semi-Fowler's position, since the diaphragmatic excursion is greater with this posture. However, this treatment may be done with the patient in any position. The tidal volume of the spirometer is set according to the manufacturer's instruction (often 500 ml. to start). The purpose of the device is to measure a gradually increasing tidal volume as the patient takes deeper and deeper breaths. The patient takes a deep breath from the mouthpiece, pauses at peak inflation, then relaxes and exhales. To avoid fatigue he should take several normal breaths before attempting another with the incentive spirometer. The tidal volume is periodically increased as tolerated. The patient is encouraged to cough after a deep breath since deep lung inflation may loosen secretions so that they can be expectorated. A counter on the incentive spirometer indicates the number of breaths the patient has taken. Ten breaths per hour while the patient is awake is a frequent goal.

CHEST PHYSICAL THERAPY

Postural Drainage

Because the patient is usually in an upright position, secretions are likely to accumulate in the lower part of the lung. When postural drainage is used, the patient is positioned sequentially in different postures (Fig. 23-2), so that the force of gravity helps to drain secretions from the smaller bronchial airways to the main bronchi and trachea. The secretions are then removed by coughing. Inhalation of the prescribed bronchodilators before postural drainage assists in draining the bronchial tree.

Postural drainage exercises can be directed at any of the segments (bilateral) of the lung. Usually the lower and middle lobe bronchi empty more effectively when the head is down; the upper lobe bronchi empty more effectively when the head is up. Frequently the patient is placed in five positions, one for drainage of each lobe: head down, prone, right and left lateral, and sitting upright.

Nursing Implications. The nurse should be aware of the patient's diagnosis as well as the lung lobes or segments involved, the cardiac status, and any structural deformities of the chest wall and spine. To determine the area(s) needing treatment and the effectiveness of treatment, the chest should be auscultated before and after the procedure.

Postural drainage is usually done four times daily, before meals and at bedtime. If prescribed, bronchodilator aerosol medications may be inhaled before postural drainage to reduce bronchospasm, decrease thickness of mucus and sputum, and combat edema of the bronchial walls. The patient should be made as comfortable as possible in each position and an emesis basin or sputum cup and paper tissues should be available. The patient is instructed to remain for 5 to 10 minutes in each position and to breathe slowly through his nose and blow out through his mouth while assuming the postures. If he cannot tolerate the position, he should be helped to assume a modified posture.

When the patient changes positions, he should be instructed to cough as follows:

1. Assume a sitting position and bend slightly forward.
2. Keep the knees and hips flexed to promote relaxation and lessen the strain on the abdominal muscles while coughing.
3. Inhale slowly through the nose and exhale through pursed lips several times.
4. Cough twice during each exhalation while contracting (pulling in) the abdomen sharply with each cough.

It may be necessary to use chest percussion and vibration to loosen bronchial secretions and mucus plugs that adhere to the bronchioles and bronchi and to propel sputum in the direction of gravity drainage.

Following the procedure, the amount, color, viscosity, and character of the ejected sputum is noted; the patient's color and pulse are evaluated the first few times the exercises are performed. It may be necessary to administer oxygen during postural drainage.

If the sputum is foul-smelling, this procedure should be carried out in a room away from other patients, and deodorizers should be used. After postural drainage, the patient may find it refreshing to brush his teeth and use a mouthwash before resting in bed.

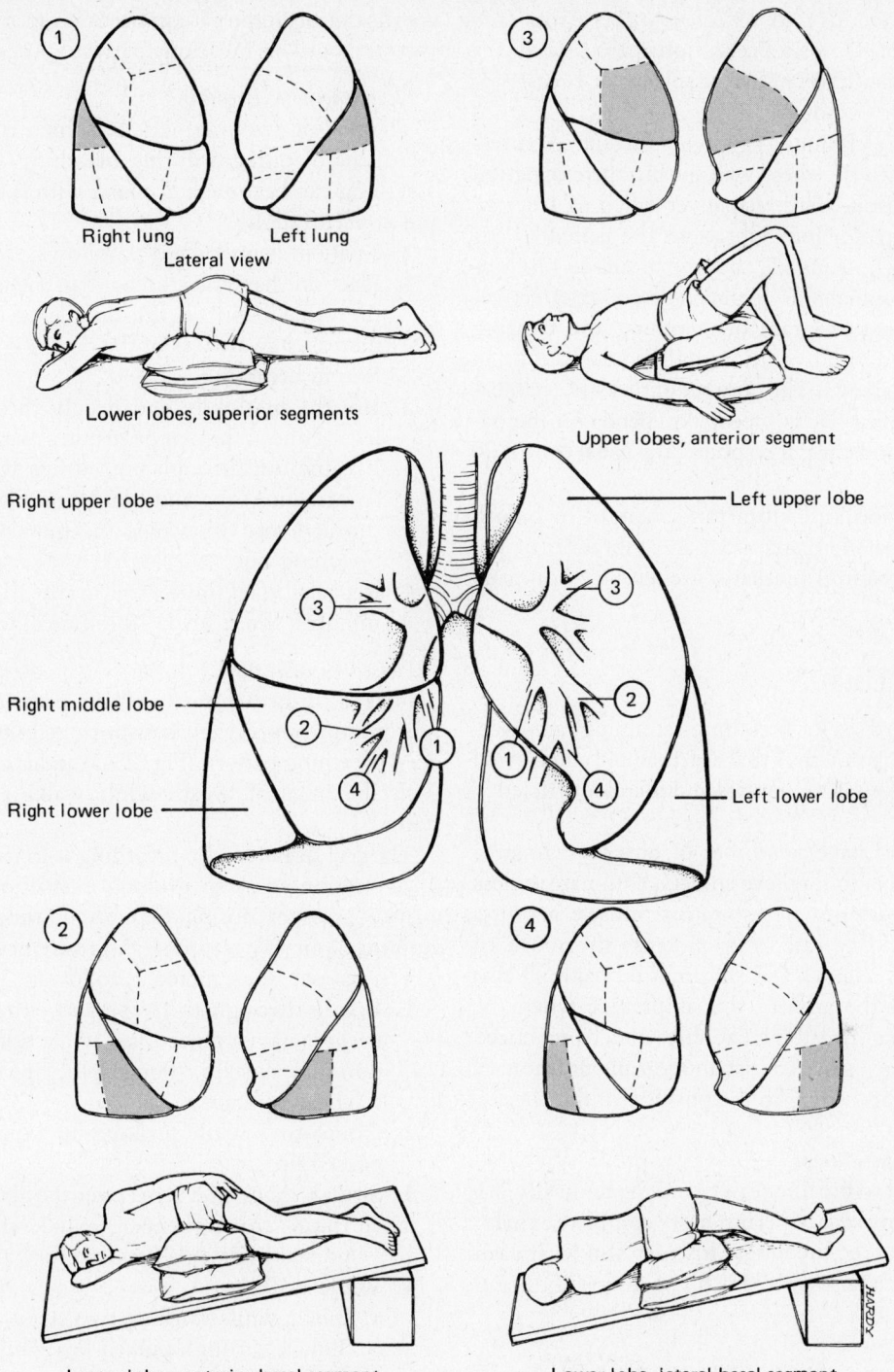

Right lung   Left lung
Lateral view
Lower lobes, superior segments

Upper lobes, anterior segment

Right upper lobe — Left upper lobe

Right middle lobe

Right lower lobe — Left lower lobe

Lower lobes, anterior basal segment   Lower lobe, lateral basal segment

Figure 23-2. Postural drainage.

Percussion and Vibration

To aid in the loosening and removal of thicker secretions the chest may be tapped (percussion) and vibrated by the therapist or nurse. Percussion and vibration help to dislodge mucus adhering to the bronchioles and bronchi.

Percussion is carried out by cupping the hands and lightly striking the chest wall in a rhythmical fashion. The wrists are alternately flexed and extended so that the chest is cupped or clapped in a painless manner. A linen towel may be placed over the segment of the chest that is being cupped. The patient uses diaphragmatic breathing during this procedure to promote relaxation (see Breathing Exercises). As a precaution, percussion over the sternum, spine, liver, kidneys, spleen, or breasts (in female) should be avoided.

Vibration is the technique of applying manual compression and tremor to the chest wall during the exhalation phase of respiration. This maneuver helps to free the mucus. After three or four vibrations the patient is encouraged to cough, using his abdominal muscles. (Contracting the abdominal muscles increases cough effectiveness.) A scheduled program of coughing and clearing sputum, together with hydration, will reduce sputum in the majority of patients. The number of times the percussion and vibration cycle is repeated depends on the patient's tolerance and clinical response; the usual time is 20 to 30 minutes.

After percussion and vibration, changes in breath sounds are evaluated. (Percussion and vibration of the patient on a mechanical ventilator are discussed on page 463.)

BREATHING EXERCISES

Breathing exercises (or breathing retraining) are exercises and breathing practices that are designed and carried out to correct respiratory deficits and increase efficiency in breathing.

These exercises have a number of purposes: to promote muscle relaxation, relieve anxiety, eliminate useless uncoordinated patterns of respiratory muscle activity, slow the respiratory rate, and decrease the work of breathing. Slow, relaxed, and rhythmical breathing also helps to control the anxiety that is present when the patient is dyspneic. Breathing exercises may be practiced in several positions, since air distribution and pulmonary circulation vary according to the position of the chest.

Instructions to the Patient

Tell the patient to breathe slowly and rhythmically in a relaxed manner in order to permit more complete exhalation and emptying of the lungs. Instruct him to always inhale through the nose since this filters, humidifies, and warms the air. If the patient becomes short of breath have him stop until his breathing pattern comes under control.

Diaphragmatic Breathing

The *goal* of diaphragmatic breathing is to increase the use of the diaphragm during breathing. Diaphragmatic breathing can become automatic with sufficient practice and concentration.

The patient is instructed as follows:

1. Place one hand on stomach (just below the ribs) and the other hand on the middle of the chest. This increases awareness of the diaphragm and its function in breathing.
2. Breathe in slowly and deeply through the nose, letting the abdomen protrude as far as it will.
3. Breathe out through pursed lips while tightening (contracting) the abdominal muscles. Press firmly inward and upward on the abdomen while breathing out.
4. Repeat for 1 minute; follow by a rest period of 2 minutes. Work up to 10 minutes, four times daily.

Pursed Lip Breathing

Pursed lip breathing (positive pressure breathing), which improves oxygen transport, helps to induce a slow deep breathing pattern (Fig. 23-3) and is useful in coping with shortness of breath while walking and climbing stairs.

The *goal* of pursed lip breathing is to train the muscles of expiration so as to prolong exhalation and increase airway pressure during expiration, thus lessening the amount of airway trapping and resistance.

The patient is instructed as follows:

1. Inhale through the nose and exhale slowly and evenly against pursed lips while tightening the abdominal muscles. (Pursing the lips increases intratracheal pressure.)
2. Count to 7 while prolonging expiration through pursed lips.
3. Sit in a chair; fold arms over the abdomen.
   Inhale through nose; exhale slowly through pursed lips while bending forward; count to 7.
4. While walking
   a. Inhale while walking two steps.
   b. Exhale through pursed lips while walking four or five steps.

Many patients will require additional oxygen using a low flow technique while doing breathing exercises.

NURSING THE PATIENT UNDERGOING CHEST SURGERY

PREOPERATIVE ASSESSMENT

Fortunately the lungs have a large functional reserve. Newer techniques of anesthesia, respiratory therapy, skillful surgery and intensive postoperative care have

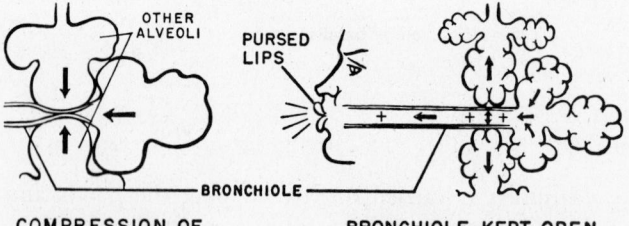

OTHER ALVEOLI

PURSED LIPS

BRONCHIOLE

COMPRESSION OF BRONCHIOLE ON FORCED EXPIRATION

BRONCHIOLE KEPT OPEN BY POSITIVE PRESSURE DURING EXPIRATION

Figure 23-3. Effect of pursed lip breathing. (Courtesy, American Lung Association.)

made possible more extensive thoracic surgery. The details of preoperative management may be of greater importance than those in other surgical procedures, since chest operations are of greater magnitude and may present a narrower margin of safety.

The patient is evaluated during the preoperative period for preexisting ventilatory impairment, particularly obstructive pulmonary disease. (Chronic obstructive pulmonary disease is the most common complicating disease in persons undergoing thoracic surgery.)

A battery of preoperative tests is done to determine the preoperative status of the patient and assess his physical assets and liabilities. The initial investigation starts with the history and physical examination—the foundation of preoperative evaluation. The general appearance of the patient, his behavior, and his mental alertness will indicate whether a significant surgical risk is involved. The decision to perform any pulmonary resection is based on the patient's cardiovascular status and pulmonary reserve. Pulmonary function studies (especially lung volume and vital capacity) are done to determine whether the contemplated resection will leave sufficient functioning lung tissue. Such tests are especially important in determining whether the patient who is a candidate for pneumonectomy can tolerate whole lung removal.

Preoperative studies are done to provide a baseline for comparison during the postoperative period and to reveal any unsuspected abnormalities. These studies include chest x-rays, ECG (for arteriosclerotic heart disease; conduction defects), BUN and serum creatinine (renal function), glucose tolerance or blood sugar (diabetes), assessment of blood electrolytes, serum protein studies, and blood volume determinations. Arterial blood gases are assessed to provide a more complete picture of the functional capacity of the lung.

Nursing Assessment

Chest auscultation should give an estimate of the intensity of breath sounds in the different regions of the lungs. (See Chapter 5.) When the chest is auscultated it is important to note whether breath sounds are normal, indicating a free flow of air in and out of the lungs. (In the emphysematous patient, the breath sounds may be markedly decreased or even absent upon auscultation). Rales, rhonchi, wheezes and hyperresonance are noted, along with decreased diaphragmatic motion. Unilateral diminished breath sounds and rhonchi can be the result of occlusion of the bronchi by mucus plugs. Evidence of retained secretions may be evaluated during auscultation by asking the patient to cough and noting any signs of rhonchi or wheezing.

The nursing assessment may also include the following:
- What signs and symptoms are present—cough, expectoration (amount), hemoptysis, chest pain, dyspnea?
- What is the smoking history? How long has the patient been smoking? How much is he currently smoking?
- What is the patient's cardiopulmonary tolerance while resting, eating, bathing, walking?
- What is his breathing pattern? How much exertion is required to produce dyspnea?
- What is the physiologic age of the patient—e.g., general appearance, mental alertness, behavior, degree of nutrition?
- What other medical conditions exist; allergies, etc.?
- What are his personal preferences and dislikes?

Improvement of Ventilation

An important preoperative objective is to improve alveolar ventilation and to reduce the presence of respiratory secretions as much as possible. To achieve this goal, the therapeutic regimen includes *cessation of smoking,* which is a bronchial irritant, fluid intake and humidification to loosen secretions, bronchodilators for relief of bronchospasm, and postural drainage and chest percussion following administration of bronchodilators for clearance of secretions. The volume of sputum is measured daily in patients who expectorate large volumes of secretions. Such measurements are carried out to determine if the amount is decreasing. Antimicrobials are given for infection. Intermittent positive pressure breathing may be employed for the delivery of aerosol drugs, to improve clearance of secretions, and to improve ventilation. The use of the incentive spirometer to maximize voluntary lung inflation, as a means of preventing atelectasis (page 412), and of the ultrasonic nebulizer for humidification and mobilization of secretions is taught and performed both in side-lying and sitting positions.

Preoperative Patient Teaching

The patient is informed of what to expect in the postoperative period; i.e., the possible presence of chest tube(s) and drainage bottles, the usual postoperative administration of oxygen to facilitate breathing, and the possible use of a ventilator. The importance of frequent turning to promote drainage of lung secretions is explained.

Since a coughing schedule will be necessary in the postoperative period to bring up secretions, the patient should be instructed in the technique of coughing and warned that the coughing routine may prove to be uncomfortable.

Huffing Technique*
1. Show the patient how to take a deep diaphragmatic breath and exhale forcefully against his hand. Explain that he should exhale forcefully in a quick, distinct pant, or "huff."

*Cimprich, B., Eagdos, D., and Langan, R.: A preoperative teaching program for the thoracotomy patient. *Cancer Nursing,* 1:35–39, Feb. 1978.

2. Have the patient practice doing small "huffs" and progress to one strong "huff" as he exhales.
3. This type of forceful exhalation stimulates pulmonary expansion and assists in alveolar inflation.

Coughing Technique

1. Sit the patient upright with knees flexed and body bending slightly forward.
2. Splint the incision with your (nurse's) hands; later the patient should support his own chest incision with his hands or a pillow while coughing.
3. Tell the patient to take three short breaths followed by a deep inspiration (inhaling slowly and evenly through the nose.)
4. Then instruct him to contract (pull in) the abdominal muscles and cough twice forcefully, with his mouth open and tongue out.

Psychological Support

Usually, several days are allotted to the preoperative phase, which provides time for the nurse to talk with the patient. By listening, the nurse may be able to discover how the patient really feels about his illness and the proposed treatment. He may reveal significant reactions: the fear of hemorrhage because of bloody sputum, the discomfort of a chronic cough and chest pain, the social stigma attached to foul-smelling sputum, the fear of death because of dyspnea and tumor—all contribute to his psychological status.

The nurse may help the patient to overcome many of his fears and to mobilize his intellectual functions in order to cope with the stress of surgery. This is done by correcting any false impressions, by offering reassurance about the capability of the surgical team, by reporting special problems to the appropriate services, and by dealing honestly with questions about possible pain and discomfort. The management and control of pain should begin before surgery by informing the patient that he, himself, can overcome many postoperative problems by following certain routines related to deep breathing, coughing, turning, and moving.

OPERATIVE PROCEDURES (Fig. 23-4)

Lobectomy. When the pathology is limited to one area of a lung, a lobectomy (removal of a lobe of a lung) is done. This operation, which is more common than pneumonectomy, may be carried out for bronchogenic carcinoma, giant emphysematous blebs or bullae, benign tumors, metastatic malignant tumors, bronchiectasis, and fungus infections.

A thoracotomy incision is used, its exact location depending on the lobe to be resected. When the pleura is entered, the involved lung collapses and the lobar vessels and the bronchus are ligated and divided. After the lobe is removed, the remaining lobes of the lung are reexpanded. Frequently, two chest catheters are inserted for drainage (Fig. 23-5). The upper tube is for the removal of air; the lower one is for drainage of fluid. Frequently only one well-placed catheter is needed. The chest tube is connected to a chest drainage apparatus for several days.

Pneumonectomy. The removal of an entire lung (pneumonectomy) is done chiefly for cancer when the lesion cannot be removed by a lesser procedure. It also may be performed for lung abscesses, bronchiectasis, or extensive unilateral tuberculosis. The removal of the right lung is more dangerous than the removal of the left since the right lung has a larger vascular bed and its removal imposes a greater physiologic burden.

A posterolateral or anterolateral thoracotomy incision is made, sometimes with resection of a rib. The pulmonary artery and the pulmonary veins are ligated and severed.

The main bronchus is divided and the lung removed.

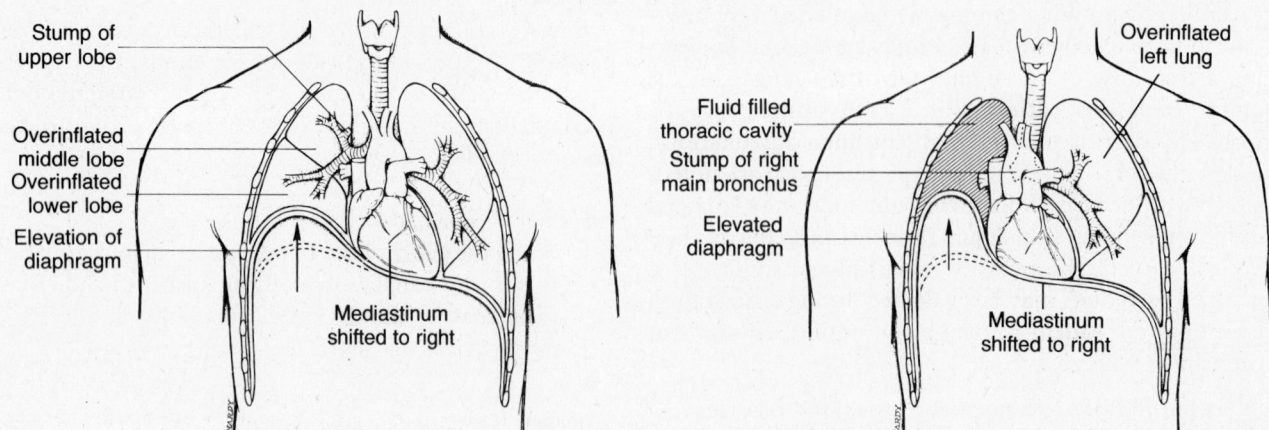

Figure 23-4. Operative procedures. (*Left*) Lobectomy. (*Right*) Pneumonectomy. The thorax fills up, over a period of time, with serosanguineous fluid.

The bronchial stump is stapled and usually no drains are used because the accumulation of fluid in the empty hemithorax is the desired end result.

Segmentectomy (Segmental Resection). Some lesions are confined to a segment of lung. Bronchopulmonary segments are subdivisions of the lung that function as individual units. They are held together by delicate connective tissue; disease processes may be limited to a single segment. Care is used to preserve as much healthy and functional lung tissue as possible, especially in patients who already have a limited cardiorespiratory reserve. Single segments can be removed from any lobe, but the right middle lobe, since it has only two small segments, invariably is removed entirely. On the left side, corresponding to a middle lobe, is a "lingular" segment of the upper lobe. This can be removed as a single segment or by *lingulectomy*. This segment is frequently involved in bronchiectasis.

Wedge Resection. A wedge resection of a small, well-circumscribed lesion may be done without regard for the location of the intersegmental planes. The pleural cavity usually is drained because of the possibility of an air or blood leak. This procedure is done for random lung biopsy and for the excision of small peripheral nodules.

POSTOPERATIVE PROGRAM FOLLOWING THORACIC SURGERY

Regardless of the surgical procedure, certain objectives and problems are common to all patients undergoing thoracic surgery.

After the operation, the major nursing objective is to restore normal cardiopulmonary function as quickly as possible. This is accomplished by (1) maintaining a patent airway, (2) providing for maximum expansion of the remaining lung tissue, (3) recognizing early signs and symptoms of untoward complications, and (4) providing supportive and rehabilitative measures.

Maintenance of a Patent Airway

Every means possible must be utilized to maintain a patent airway. First, secretions must be suctioned from the tracheobronchial tree before the endotracheal tube is removed. In fact all secretions should be aspirated by suctioning until the patient can cough up secretions effectively. Endotracheal secretions are present in excessive amounts in post-thoracotomy patients due to trauma to the tracheobronchial tree during operation, diminished lung ventilation, and diminished cough reflex. Excessive secretions will produce airway obstruction causing air in the alveoli distal to the obstruction to become absorbed and the lung to collapse. Atelectasis, pneumonia, and respiratory failure may follow.

Technique for endotracheal suctioning
(Sterile technique is to be used. This procedure should be learned under expert clinical supervision.)

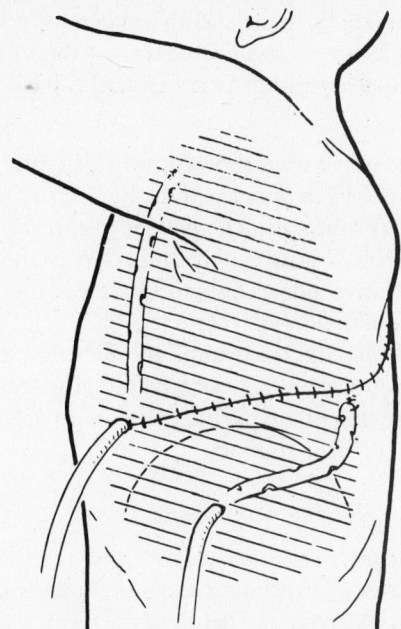

Figure 23-5. Postoperative drainage of the chest. The upper drainage tube is used for the escape of air from leaks in the resected lung. The tip is anchored in the parietal pleura near the apex and brought out through the anterior end of the incision. The lower tube is usually for serosanguineous drainage. (From Johnson, Julian, and Kirby, C. K.: Surgery of the Chest. Chicago, Year Book Publishers, 1970)

1. Place the patient in a sitting or semi-Fowler's position. Attach the sterile catheter to a "Y" or "T" tube that has been connected to a suction device.
2. Oxygenate the patient several minutes before each suctioning procedure.
3. Give the patient a gauze square, and instruct him to pull his tongue outward; this tilts the epiglottis forward. If the patient cannot comply, have another person do this.
4. Pass a lubricated (with water-soluble gel) catheter through the nostril to the pharynx. Check the position of the tip of the catheter; it should be in the lower pharynx.
5. Instruct the patient to take a deep breath. This opens the epiglottis and helps the catheter to move in the direction of the negative pressure generated by inspiration.
6. Advance the catheter into the trachea only during inspiration.
7. Apply suction intermittently by closing the open end of the "Y" or "T" catheter with the finger and slowly rotating the catheter between the thumb and forefinger.
8. Avoid prolonging suction more than 5 to 10 seconds, since cardiac arrest may ensue in patients with borderline oxygenation.
9. While the catheter is being withdrawn, apply gentle suction to clear the tracheal walls of secretions.

10. Ventilate the patient with oxygen for several minutes before a second passage of the catheter (if a second aspiration is necessary.) Check the pulse rate.

Most postoperative thoracotomy patients are given humidified oxygen because of the hypoxemia secondary to abnormal shunting. The patient's ventilation mechanism is impaired primarily because of pain and splinting of the operative side. This can lead to as much as a 30 percent reduction in vital capacity. Thus ventilator assistance may be necessary until the patient can support adequate ventilation. The arterial blood gases as well as clinical assessment are parameters used to determine the need for ventilator support.

Continuing Nursing Assessment

The blood pressure, pulse, and respiration are monitored every 15 minutes and more frequently as indicated. The character and depth of the respiration and the patient's color serve as important criteria in evaluating whether the lungs are being adequately expanded. Arrhythmias can occur at any time but frequently are seen between the second and sixth postoperative day. The heart rate and rhythm are monitored by auscultation and electrocardiography, since arrhythmias are apt to develop after thoracic surgery. Frequent monitoring of blood gases, serum electrolytes, hemoglobin, and hematocrit is also continued.

Coughing Technique

The patient must be encouraged to cough effectively, since ineffective coughing will result in exhaustion and retention of secretions, which can lead to atelectasis and pneumonia. Since it is difficult to cough in a supine position, the patient should be helped to a sitting position on the edge of the bed, with his feet resting on a chair.

Coughing should be carried out at least every hour (as described on page 422) during the first 24 hours and when necessary thereafter. If audible rales are present it may be necessary to use chest percussion with the cough routine until the lungs are clear. To lessen incisional pain during coughing, the nurse should support the incision firmly over the operated side and against the opposite chest (Fig. 23-6).

After helping the patient to cough, the nurse should listen to both lungs, both anteriorly and posteriorly, with a stethoscope to determine whether there are any changes in breath sounds, since diminished sounds may indicate collapsed or hypoventilated alveoli. Aerosol therapy may be used to reduce the viscosity of the secretions and to prevent excessive drying of secretions.

Control of Pain

Pain following a thoracotomy may be severe depending on the type of incision and the patient's reaction to and ability to cope with pain. Pain can lead to postoperative complications if it reduces the patient's ability to breathe deeply and cough, and if it further limits chest excursions so that effective ventilation is decreased. Immediately after the surgical procedure and before the incision is closed, the surgeon may do a nerve block with a long-acting local anesthetic which can reduce postoperative pain and improve pulmonary function. Small and rather frequent doses of narcotic will permit the patient to breathe more deeply and cough more effectively. However, it is important to avoid depressing the respiratory system with too much narcotic, since the patient should not be so somnolent that he does not cough.

Other pain relief measures include supporting the chest tube so that it will not pull against the chest wall when the patient moves, changing the patient's position, and intermittently elevating the patient's head.

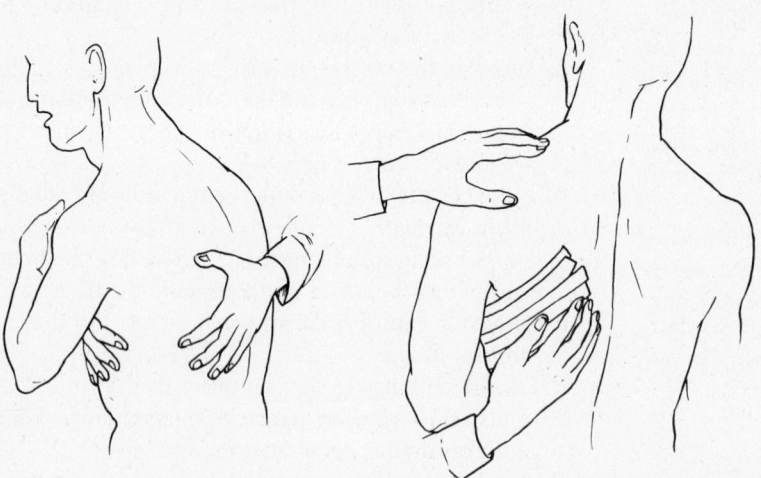

Figure 23-6. Techniques for support of incision while patient with thoracic surgery coughs. (*Left*) The nurse's hands should support the chest incision anteriorly and posteriorly. The patient is instructed to take several deep breaths, inhale, and then cough forcibly. (*Right*) With one hand, exert downward pressure on the shoulder of the affected side while firmly supporting beneath the wound with the other hand. The patient is instructed to take several deep breaths, inhale, and then cough forcibly. (From Barrett, R. J., and Tuttle, W. M.: Preoperative and postoperative care of the thoracotomy patient. Surg. Clin. N. Am., 39:1609.)

• A word of warning: do not confuse the restlessness of hypoxia with restlessness due to pain. Dyspnea, restlessness, increasing respiratory rate, increasing blood pressure, and tachycardia are warning signs of impending respiratory insufficiency (page 445).

Positioning the Patient

The patient with limited pulmonary reserve may not be able to tolerate being turned on the unoperated side, since this position may limit ventilation on that side. The patient's position is varied from horizontal to semi-erect, in order to allow residual air to rise to the upper portion of the pleural space and be removed via the upper chest catheter. Since remaining in one position tends to promote the retention of secretions in the dependent portion of the lungs, the patient may be placed upright to cough. However, the surgeon should be consulted concerning individual patient positioning.

Turning Procedure
1. Instruct the patient to bend his knees and use his feet to push.
2. Have the patient shift his hips and shoulders to the opposite side of the bed while pushing with his feet.
3. Bring the patient's arm over his chest, pointing it in the direction towards which he is being turned, and have him grasp the side rail with his hand.
4. Turn patient in "log roll" fashion to prevent twisting at the waist and possible pulling of the incision, which could be painful.

Fluids and Nutrition

During the operation or immediately after, the patient usually receives a blood transfusion, followed by an intravenous infusion to "keep the vein open" until the blood volume can be reassessed. The rate of administration is slow (10 ml./hour), especially when there is evidence of limited cardiopulmonary reserve and when the pulmonary vascular bed has been greatly reduced, as in pneumonectomy.

• *Caution: Pulmonary edema due to overinfusion is a real danger.* The early symptoms of such a complication are cyanosis, dyspnea, rales, and bubbling sounds in the chest, as well as frothy sputum. This constitutes an emergency and is to be reported immediately.

Chest Drainage

The normal breathing mechanism operates on the principle of negative pressure (the pressure in the chest cavity is lower than the pressure of the outside air, causing air to rush into the lungs). Whenever the chest is opened, from any cause, there is a loss of negative pressure which can result in the collapse of the lung. The collection of air, fluid, or other substances in the chest can compromise cardiopulmonary function and even cause collapse of the lung, because these substances take up space. Three types of pathologic substances collect in the pleural space: solids (fibrin or clotted blood), liquids (serous fluids, blood, pus, chyle), and gas (air from the lung, tracheobronchial tree, or esophagus).

Surgical incision of the chest wall almost always causes some degree of pneumothorax. Air and fluid collect in the intrapleural space, restricting lung expansion and reducing air exchange. It is necessary to restore pleural negative pressure and prevent this from happening. Therefore, during or immediately after thoracic surgery, chest catheters are positioned strategically in the pleural space (Fig. 23-6), sutured to the skin, and connected to some type of drainage apparatus in order to remove the residual air and drainage fluid from the pleural or mediastinal space. This assists in the reexpansion of remaining lung tissue.

A chest drainage system must be capable of removing whatever collects in the pleural space so that a normal pleural space and normal cardiopulmonary function may be restored and maintained. There are many types of commercial chest drainage systems in use, most of which use the water-seal principle (see below). The chest catheter is attached to a bottle, using a one-way valve principle. Water acts as a seal and permits air and fluid to drain from the chest, but air cannot reenter the submerged tip of the tube. The care of the patient with water-seal chest drainage is discussed in the guidelines on pages 427-428.

Principles of Chest Drainage

Chest drainage can be categorized into three types of mechanical systems (Fig. 23-7):

The single-bottle water-seal system
The end of the drainage tube from the patient's chest is covered by a layer of water which permits drainage and prevents lung collapse by sealing out the atmosphere. Functionally, drainage depends on gravity, on the mechanics of respiration, and, if desired, on suction by the addition of *controlled* vacuum.

The tube from the patient extends approximately 2.5 cm. (1 inch) below the level of the water in the container. There is a vent for the escape of any air that might be leaking from the lung. The water level fluctuates as the patient breathes; it goes up when the patient inhales and down when the patient exhales. At the end of the drainage tube, bubbling may or may not be visible. Bubbling can mean either persistent leakage of air from the lung or other tissues or a leak in the system.

The two-bottle system
The two-bottle system consists of the same water-seal chamber plus a fluid collection bottle. Drainage is similar to that of a single unit, except that when pleural fluid

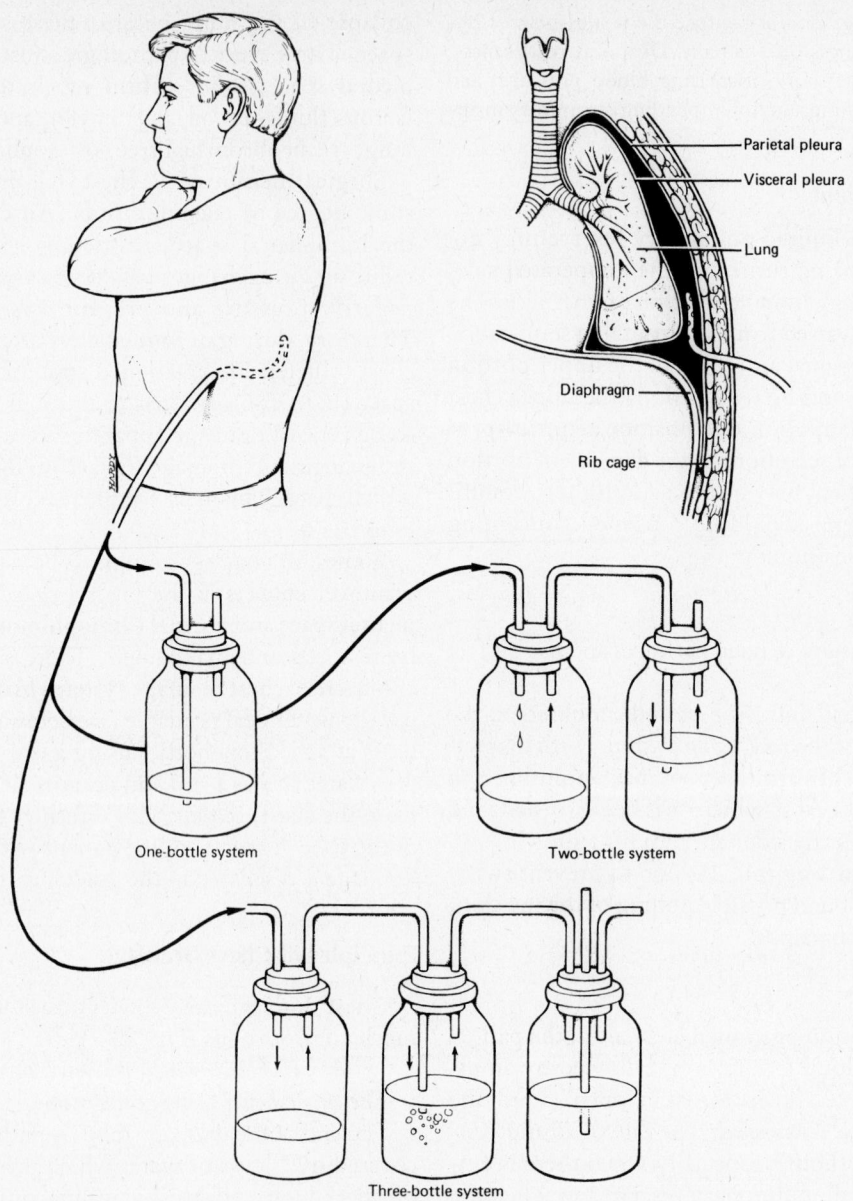

Parietal pleura

Visceral pleura

Lung

Diaphragm

Rib cage

One-bottle system

Two-bottle system

Three-bottle system

Figure 23-7.   One, two, and three bottle chest drainage systems.

drains, the underwater seal system is not affected by the volume of drainage.

Effective drainage depends on gravity or on the amount of suction added to the system. When vacuum (suction) is added to the system from a vacuum source such as wall suction, the connection is made at the vent stem of the underwater seal bottle. The amount of suction applied to the system is regulated by the wall gauge.

The three-bottle system

This system is similar in all respects to the two-bottle system, except for the addition of a third bottle to control the amount of suction applied. The amount of suction is determined by the depth to which the tip of the venting

glass tube is submerged. (For example, submersion to 10 cm. below the surface of the water will equal 10 cm. of water suction applied to the patient.)

In the three-bottle system (as in the other two), drainage depends on gravity or the amount of suction applied. The amount of suction in this system is controlled by the manometer bottle. The mechanical suction motor or wall suction creates and maintains a negative pressure throughout the entire closed drainage system.

The manometer bottle regulates the amount of vacuum in the system. This bottle contains three tubes: (1) A short tube above the water level comes from the water-seal bottle. (2) Another short tube leads to the vacuum or suction motor or wall suction. (3) The third tube is a long tube (standpipe) which extends below the water level in the bottle and which is open to the atmosphere outside the bottle. This is the tube that regulates the amount of vacuum in the system. This is regulated by the depth to which this tube is submerged — the usual depth is 20 cm. (7.6 inches).

When the vacuum in the system becomes greater than the depth to which the tube is submerged, outside air is sucked into the system. This results in constant bubbling in the manometer (or pressure-regulator) bottle, which indicates that the system is functioning properly.

- *Note:* When the motor is off or the wall vacuum is turned off, the drainage system should be open to the atmosphere so that intrapleural air can escape from the system. This can be done by detaching the tubing from the suction port to provide a vent.

GUIDELINES TO THE NURSE'S ROLE IN THE MANAGEMENT OF THE PATIENT WITH WATER-SEAL CHEST DRAINAGE

An intrapleural drainage tube is used after most intrathoracic procedures. One or more chest catheters are held in the pleural space by suture to the chest wall and are attached to a drainage system. The purposes are:

1. To remove solids, liquids, and gas from the pleural space or thoracic cavity and the mediastinal space.
2. To bring about reexpansion of the lung and restore normal cardiorespiratory function after surgery, trauma, or medical conditions.

PROCEDURE

Nursing Action	Rationale/Amplification
1. Attach the drainage tube from the pleural space to the tubing that leads to a long tube with end submerged in sterile normal saline.	1. Water-seal drainage provides for the escape of air and fluid into a drainage bottle. The water acts as a seal and keeps the air from being drawn back into the pleural space.
2. Tape the places where the tubing is connected, if needed. Some connectors hold without taping. a. The tube should be approximately 2.5 cm. (1 inch) below the water level. b. The short tube is left open to the atmosphere.	2. Taping the connecting points of the tubing will make certain that the tubing remains airtight to reestablish negative (intrapleural) pressure. a. If the tube is submerged too deep below the water level, a higher intrapleural pressure is required to expel air. b. Venting the short glass tube lets air escape from the bottle.
3. Mark the original fluid level with tape on the outside of the drainage bottle. Mark hourly/daily increments (date and time) at the drainage level.	3. This marking will show the amount of fluid loss and how fast fluid is collecting in the drainage bottle. It serves as a basis for blood replacement, if the fluid is blood. Grossly bloody drainage will appear in the bottle in the immediate postoperative period and if excessive may require reoperation. Drainage usually declines progressively in the first 24 hours.
4. Fasten the tubing to the drawsheet with rubber bands and safety pins so that flow by gravity will occur. The tubing should not loop or interfere with the movements of the patient.	4. Kinking, looping, or pressure on the drainage tubing can produce back pressure, and may thus possibly force drainage back into the pleural space or impede drainage from the pleural space.
5. Encourage the patient to assume a position of comfort. Encourage good body alignment. When the patient is in the lateral position, place a rolled towel under the tubing to protect it from the weight of the patient's body. Encourage the patient to change position frequently.	5. The patient's position should be changed frequently to promote drainage and the body should be kept in good alignment to prevent postural deformities and contractures. Proper positioning helps breathing and promotes better air exchange. Pain medication may be needed to enhance comfort and deep breathing.
6. Put the arm and shoulder of the affected side through range-of-motion exercises several times daily. Some pain medication may be necessary.	6. Exercise helps to avoid ankylosis of the shoulder and assists in lessening postoperative pain and discomfort.
7. "Milk" the tubing in the direction of the drainage bottle hourly.	7. "Milking" the tubing prevents it from becoming plugged with clots and fibrin. Constant attention to maintaining the patency of the tube will facilitate prompt expansion of the lung and minimize complications.

(Continued)

GUIDELINES TO THE NURSE'S ROLE IN THE MANAGEMENT
OF THE PATIENT WITH WATER-SEAL CHEST DRAINAGE (CONTINUED)

Nursing Action	Rationale/Amplification
8. Make sure there is fluctuation ("tidaling") of the fluid level in the long glass tube.	8. Fluctuation of the water level in the tube shows that there is effective communication between the pleural cavity and the drainage bottle, provides a valuable way of checking the drainage system, and is a gauge of intrapleural pressure.
9. Fluctuations of fluid in the tubing will stop when: a. the lung has reexpanded b. the tubing is obstructed by blood clots or fibrin c. a dependent loop develops d. suction motor or wall suction is not working properly	
10. Watch for leaks of air in the drainage system as indicated by constant bubbling in the water-seal bottle. a. Clamp the tubing (*momentarily*) close to the chest to look for air leak only if so directed by the physician. b. Report excessive bubbling in the water-seal chamber immediately. c. "Milking" of chest tubes in patients with air leaks should only be done if requested by the surgeon.	10. Leaking and trapping of air in the pleural space can result in tension pneumothorax. If the leak is in the patient and the tube is clamped for more than a few seconds, air may back up in the pleural cavity and extend the patient's pneumothorax.
11. Observe and report immediately signs of rapid, shallow breathing, cyanosis, pressure in the chest, subcutaneous emphysema, or symptoms of hemorrhage.	11. Many clinical conditions may cause these signs and symptoms, including tension pneumothorax, mediastinal shift, hemorrhage, severe incisional pain, pulmonary embolus, and cardiac tamponade. Surgical intervention may be necessary.
12. Encourage the patient to breathe deeply and cough at frequent intervals. If there are signs of incisional pain, adequate pain medication is indicated.	12. Deep breathing and coughing help to raise the intrapleural pressure, which allows emptying of the accumulation in the pleural space and removes secretions from the tracheobronchial tree, so that the lung expands and atelectasis is prevented.
13. Stabilize the drainage bottle on the floor or in a special holder. *Caution visitors and personnel against handling equipment or displacing the drainage bottle.*	13. If any part of the apparatus is damaged, the closed system of drainage will be destroyed and the patient will be endangered by atmospheric pressure in the pleural space and resultant collapse of the lung. The drainage system must be kept airtight to reestablish negative intrapleural pressure.
14. If the patient has to be transported to another area, place the drainage bottle below the chest level (as close to the floor as possible), if he is lying on a stretcher. Hemostats (clamps) should be attached to the patient's gown while he is transported.	14. The drainage apparatus must be kept at a level lower than the patient's chest to prevent backflow of fluid into the pleural space.
15. When assisting the surgeon in removing the tube: a. Instruct the patient to perform the Valsalva maneuver (forcible exhalation against a closed glottis, holding one's breath). b. The chest tube is clamped and quickly removed. c. Simultaneously a small bandage is applied and made airtight with vaseline gauze covered by 4" x 4" gauze and thoroughly covered and sealed with adhesive tape.	15. The chest tube is removed as directed when the lung is reexpanded (usually 24 hours to several days). During removal of the tube the chief priorities are prevention of entrance of air into the pleural cavity as the tube is withdrawn and prevention of infection.

Postoperative Considerations

Patient Education. Usually, patients who have had pulmonary resections are able to return to sedentary occupations about 2 to 3 weeks after discharge and to heavy labor in about 6 to 8 weeks after discharge. Some individuals, usually those with preexisting lung disease, who have had extensive resection, may experience a significant reduction in exercise capacity. This is usually permanent, and their tolerance at 8 to 12 weeks posthospitalization is at approximately the level at which it will remain. Social and occupational counseling may be necessary.

The following regimen may be stressed as part of patient teaching:
1. Practice deep breathing exercises for the first few weeks at home.

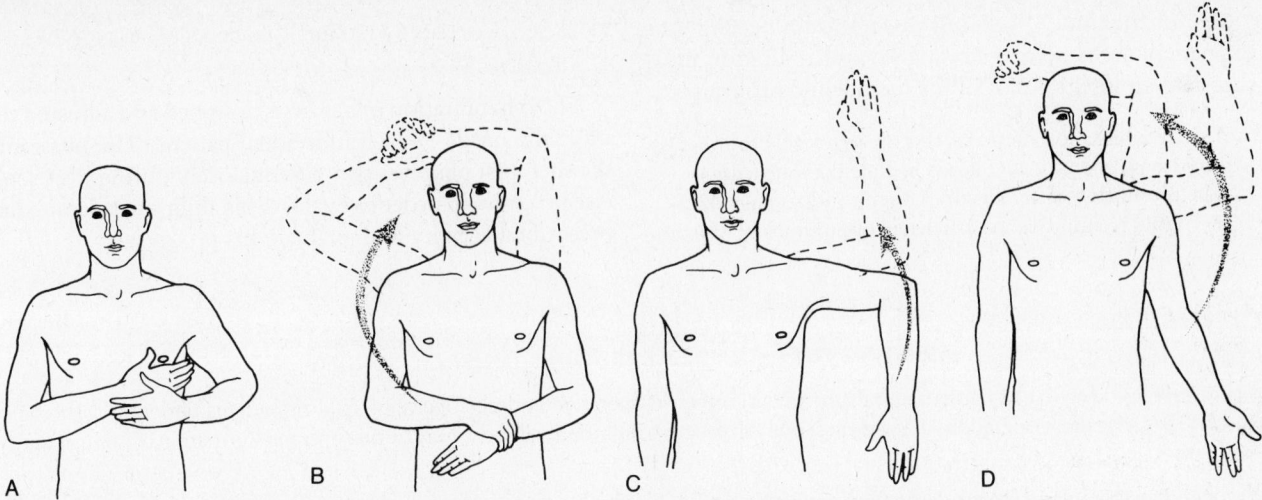

Figure 23-8.   Arm and shoulder exercises are done following thoracic surgery to restore movement, prevent painful stiffening of the shoulder, and improve muscle power. *A, B*. Hold hand of the affected side with the other hand, palms facing in. Raise the arms forward, upward, and then overhead, while taking a deep breath. Exhale while lowering the arms. Repeat five times. *C*. Raise arm sideward, upward, and downward in a waving motion. *D*. Place arm at side. Raise arm sideward, upward, and over the head. Both exercises can also be done while lying in bed. (Adapted from Cameron, M.: What patients need most before and after thoracotomy. Nursing '78, *8*:28-36, May 1978)

2. Practice good body alignment by standing up straight with shoulders held back (preferably in front of a full-length mirror).
3. Practice exercises that were done while in the hospital.
4. Practice good oral hygiene by brushing teeth well and visiting the dentist frequently.
5. Remain away from crowds during upper respiratory epidemics.
6. Seek medical attention at the onset of an upper respiratory infection.
7. Avoid areas where the air is filled with dust, smoke, and irritating chemicals.
8. Avoid anything that may cause spasms of coughing.
9. Avoid smoking after chest surgery.
10. Maintain good nutrition.
11. Obtain adequate rest. A good plan should include an early afternoon nap for the first few weeks following discharge from the hospital.
12. Report for follow-up care by the surgeon or clinic as necessary.

Complications of Thoracic Surgery.   Complications following thoracic surgery include hemorrhage, respiratory insufficiency, respiratory failure (see pages 445-449), bronchopulmonary fistula, pneumonitis, atelectasis, and cardiac arrhythmias. Gastric distention and renal failure are other complications which may occur.

Ambulation.   If shock has not occurred and the patient does not have heart disease or a limited cardiovascular reserve, he may get out of bed on the evening of the day after surgery, upon the physician's request. Since the chest tube is well secured, this activity need not be restricted. Postural and breathing exercises are started as prescribed in order to produce better lung ventilation, restore motion and muscle tonus in the shoulder girdle and trunk, and maintain normal posture. (See Fig. 23-8 and Table 23-1.) Chest x-rays are taken frequently to ensure full expansion of the patient's lungs and to rule out any unwanted collections of air or fluid.

TABLE 23-1.   SKELETAL EXERCISES DESIGNED TO RESTORE FUNCTION FOLLOWING THORACIC SURGERY

MUSCLE AFFECTED BY THORACOTOMY	FUNCTION	ACTIVITIES TO RESTORE FUNCTION
Trapezius	Promotes arm extension, abduction, and reach extension.	Extend the arm up and back, out to the side and back, down at the side and back.
Rhomboideus major	Adducts and slightly elevates scapula.	Place hands in small of back. Push elbows as far back as possible.
Latissimus dorsi	Depresses the shoulder.	Sit erect in an armchair; place the hands on the arms of the chair directly opposite either side of the body. Press down on hands, consciously pulling the abdomen in and stretching up from the waist. Inhale while raising the body until the elbows are extended completely. Hold this position a moment, and begin exhaling while lowering the body slowly to the original position.
Serratus anterior	Rotates scapula and fixes it against the rib cage.	Reach over head and "push" in an upward and outward motion.

Rehabilitation. Rehabilitation should begin when the patient seeks help; consequently, rehabilitation measures are an integral part of his therapeutic program.

Basic rehabilitation measures that are applicable to most patients with pulmonary conditions include the following:
1. The promotion of an effective cough routine (page 422)
2. Activities to improve the efficiency of pulmonary function

3. Skeletal exercises for retraining injured muscles and preventing deformities.

The rehabilitation program is designed and adjusted to meet the needs of each individual patient. The nurse or the therapist observes the patient closely during his exercise program in order to evaluate his ability to tolerate the prescribed activity and evaluate his progress.

ASSISTING THE PATIENT UNDERGOING THORACIC SURGERY

The Challenge: Meticulous attention must be given to the preoperative and postoperative care of patients undergoing thoracic surgery, because these operations are wide in scope, obstructive pulmonary disease may be present, and the margin of safety is apt to be narrow.

Preoperative Objective: To ensure optimal patient condition for surgery.

A. Determine the preoperative status of the patient, his physical assets and his liabilities.
  1. Assist the patient undergoing diagnostic studies.
    a. History and physical examination
    b. Chest roentgenogram
    c. Pulmonary function studies (page 405)—to ascertain if patient will have adequately functioning lung tissue after the operation
    d. Special diagnostic studies as required
    e. Baseline studies to ascertain any unsuspected abnormalities and to serve as a baseline reference during the postoperative period when indicated.
      (1) ECG—to disclose presence of arteriosclerotic heart disease or conduction defect
      (2) Blood urea nitrogen—to obtain a "rough" measurement of renal function
      (3) Blood sugar or glucose tolerance—to detect unrecognized diabetes
      (4) Blood electrolytes, serum protein studies, and blood volume determinations as indicated
      (5) Arterial blood gas studies
  2. Nursing assessment of the patient.
    a. What signs and symptoms are present—cough, expectoration, hemoptysis, chest pain?
    b. What is his smoking history—how long and how much?
    c. What is the patient's cardiopulmonary tolerance while bathing, eating, walking, etc.?
    d. What is the "physiologic age" of the patient—general appearance, mental alertness, behavior, degree of nutrition?
    e. What is his breathing pattern?
    f. How much exertion is required to produce dyspnea?
    g. What are his personal preferences and dislikes?

B. Improve alveolar ventilation.
  1. Encourage the patient to stop smoking, since this increases bronchial irritation.
  2. Employ all measures to minimize pulmonary secretions.
    a. Measure sputum daily in patients with large volume of secretions to determine whether volume of secretions is decreasing.
    b. Instruct the patient to cough against a closed glottis to increase intrapulmonary pressure.
    c. Humidify the air to loosen secretions.
    d. Administer bronchodilators for bronchospasm.
    e. Give antibiotics for infection.
    f. Give expectorants, enzymes, and mucolytic agents as directed.
    g. Employ IPPB therapy to improve pulmonary ventilation (page 417).
    h. Carry out postural drainage on patients with bronchiectasis, chronic bronchitis, or other conditions with increased mucus production.
    i. Teach diaphragmatic breathing during preoperative period (see page 420).
    j. Set up a schedule of breathing exercises that encourage the use of abdominal muscles (page 420).

C. Evaluate cardiovascular and pulmonary status so that complications may be anticipated and prevented.
  1. Study the results of diagnostic tests to learn of existing deviations from normal.
  2. Observe the patient and his reactions to various activities of daily living.
  3. Give cardiac drugs to patients in congestive heart failure.
  4. Correct anemia, dehydration, and hypoproteinemia—intravenous infusions, tube feedings, blood transfusions as indicated.

D. Prepare the patient for the surgical experience by reassurance, explanation, and skillful preoperative nursing care.
  1. Orient the patient to events in the postoperative period.
    a. Cough and breathing routine
    b. Presence of chest tube and drainage bottles
    c. Oxygen therapy
    d. Measures used to control discomfort
    e. Leg exercises and range of motion exercises for affected shoulder.
  2. Encourage expression of psychological and safety needs.
  3. See that consent form has been signed.

ASSISTING THE PATIENT UNDERGOING THORACIC SURGERY (CONTINUED)

Postoperative Objectives: To restore normal cardiopulmonary function as quickly as possible.

A. Maintain an open airway.

B. Maintain constant nursing surveillance of the patient.
1. Take blood pressure, pulse, respirations every 15 minutes or more frequently, as indicated; extend time interval according to the patient's clinical status.
2. Evaluate character of respirations and patient's color.
3. Evaluate character of drainage from the chest drainage bottles.
4. Elevate the head of the bed to a 30-to-40-degree angle when the patient is oriented and his blood pressure is stabilized.

C. Aspirate all secretions with suctioning until patient is able to raise secretions effectively. (Endotracheal secretions are present in excessive amounts in post-thoracotomy patients due to trauma to the tracheobronchial tree during operation, diminished lung ventilation, and cough reflex.)
1. Carry out tracheal aspiration on "wet" semicomatose patients to prevent atelectasis.
2. Indications for tracheal aspirations are determined by chest auscultation. (See page 423 for technique of tracheal aspiration.)
3. Look for changes in the color and consistency of aspirates or sputum. Colorless fluid sputum is not unusual; opacification or coloring of sputum may indicate dehydration or infection.

D. Monitor the patient's ECG, since cardiac arrhythmias are more frequently seen after thoracic surgery (especially atrial fibrillation and atrial flutter). A patient with total pneumonectomy is especially prone to cardiac irregularity.

E. Give oxygen in the immediate postoperative period to assure maximum oxygenation—respirations are still depressed and residual secretions in the peripheral respiratory passages may partially block gas exchange. Monitoring by means of arterial blood gas analysis is usually done.

F. Give aerosol therapy to reduce viscosity of secretions.

G. Administer IPPB treatments as directed, in order to help expand the lung.

H. Listen to both sides of the chest with a stethoscope to determine if there are any changes in breath sounds.
1. Are breath sounds normal, indicating free flow of air in and out of lungs?
2. Are breath sounds distant? wheezing? rales present?

I. Encourage and promote an effective cough routine.
1. Sit patient on side of bed with feet supported on a chair if his condition permits.
2. Support the chest firmly over the operated side and against opposite chest to lessen incisional pain (Fig. 23-7).
3. Instruct the patient to cough against a closed glottis (pull in the abdominal muscles) to increase intrapulmonary pressure.
4. Assist the patient to cough at least every 1 to 2 hours during the first 24 hours and when necessary thereafter.

J. Maintain surveillance and careful management of the chest drainage system.*
1. Monitor the chest drainage system which is used to eliminate any residual air or fluid following thoracotomy.
2. Check amount and character of drainage immediately after the operation and at necessary intervals thereafter—drainage should progressively decrease after first 12 hours.
3. Persistence of bloody drainage indicates bleeding. Prepare for blood replacement and possible reoperation to achieve hemostasis.
4. See page 427 for summary of the nurse's role in the management of the patient with water-seal drainage.

K. Provide intelligent pain relief, since pain limits chest excursions and thereby decreases ventilation.
1. Severity of pain varies with type of incision and the patient's reaction to and ability to cope with pain.
2. Narcotics and analgesics may assist patient to cough more effectively.
3. Narcotics and analgesics may make some patients too somnolent to cough.
4. Watch for signs of respiratory depression.
5. Assist patient having an intercostal nerve block for pain control.

L. Record hourly urinary output; the patient should excrete at least 30 ml. of urine hourly after surgery.

M. Administer blood and parenteral fluids at a slower rate after thoracic surgery—pulmonary edema due to transfusion overload is an ever present threat; following pneumonectomy the pulmonary vascular system has been greatly reduced.

N. Maintain care in positioning the postoperative thoracotomy patient.
1. Position patient flat in bed at intervals unless this produces dyspnea.
2. Position patient in a semi-Fowler's position to permit residual air to rise to upper portion of pleural space and be removed via the upper chest catheter.
3. Patients with limited respiratory reserve may not be able to turn on unoperated side, since this may limit ventilation of the operated side.

O. Anticipate and forestall complications.
1. Hemorrhage
2. Respiratory acidosis
3. Pneumonitis; atelectasis
4. Cardiac arrhythmias
5. Renal failure
6. Pulmonary edema

(Continued)

---

*A patient with a pneumonectomy usually does not have water-seal chest drainage, since it is desirable that the pleural space fill with an effusion which eventually obliterates this space. Some surgeons do use a "modified" water-seal system.

ASSISTING THE PATIENT UNDERGOING THORACIC SURGERY (CONTINUED)

7. Gastric distention (Utilize nasogastric tube during the first 24 hours as directed.)

P. Restore normal range of motion and function of shoulder and trunk.
   1. Teach breathing exercises to mobilize thorax (page 420).
   2. Encourage skeletal exercises to promote abduction and mobilization of shoulder.
   3. Ambulate as soon as pulmonary and circulatory systems are compensated.

4. Encourage progressive activities according to development of fatigue.

Q. Patient Teaching Aspects
   1. There will be some intercostal pain for a period of time which can be relieved by local heat and oral analgesia.
   2. Weakness and fatigability are common during the first three weeks following a thoracotomy.
   3. Range of motion exercises for the arm and shoulder on the affected side should be carried out several times daily to prevent "frozen shoulder."

*A patient with a pneumonectomy usually does not have water-seal chest drainage, since it is desirable that the pleural space fill with an effusion which eventually obliterates this space. Some surgeons do use a "modified" water-seal system.

BIBLIOGRAPHY

BOOKS

Arnold, V.: Respiratory Care Laboratory Skills Manual. Ventura, Calif., Respiratory West Co., 1977.

Brashear, R. E., and Rhodes, M.: Chronic Obstructive Lung Disease. St. Louis, C. V. Mosby, 1978.

Burton, G. G., Gee, G. N., and Hodgkin, J. E.: Respiratory Care. A Guide to Clinical Practice. Philadelphia, J. B. Lippincott, 1977.

Collis, J. L., Clarke, D. B., and Smith, R. B.: d'Abreu's Practice of Cardiothoracic Surgery. Baltimore, Williams and Wilkins, 1976.

Effler, D. B., ed.: Blades' Surgical Diseases of the Chest. St. Louis, C. V. Mosby, 1978.

Fraser, R. G., and Pare, J. A. P.: Diagnosis of Diseases of the Chest, 2nd ed. Philadelphia, W. B. Saunders, 1977.

Guenter, C. A., and Welch, M. H.: Pulmonary Medicine. Philadelphia, J. B. Lippincott, 1977.

Hunsinger, D. L., et al.: Respiratory Technology: A Procedure Manual, 2nd ed. Reston, Reston Publishing Co., Inc., 1976.

Kirsh, M. M., and Sloan, H.: Blunt Chest Trauma. Boston, Little, Brown, 1977.

Lane, D. J.: Respiratory Disease. London, William Heinemann Medical Books, Ltd., 1976.

Lawrence, W., and Terz, J. J.: Cancer Management. New York, Grune and Stratton, 1977.

MacDonnell, K. F., and Segal, M. S.: Current Respiratory Care. Boston, Little, Brown, 1977.

Melamed, M., et al.: The Adult Postoperative Chest. Springfield, Charles C Thomas, 1977.

O'Connor, A. B., ed.: Nursing in Respiratory Diseases, 2nd ed. New York, American Journal of Nursing Co., 1977.

Report of the Surgeon General: Smoking and Health: A Report of the Surgeon General. Washington, D.C., U.S. Public Health Service, 1979.

Sabiston, D. C., and Spencer, F. C.: Gibbon's Surgery of the Chest. Philadelphia, W. B. Saunders, 1976.

Salmon, S. S., and Jones, S. E.: Adjuvant Therapy of Cancer. New York, North-Holland Pub. Co., 1977.

Shibel, E. M., and Moser, K. M.: Respiratory Emergencies. St. Louis, C. V. Mosby, 1977.

Straus, M. J., ed.: Lung Cancer. Clinical Diagnosis and Treatment. New York, Grune and Stratton, 1977.

von Hippel, A.: A Manual of Thoracic Surgery. Springfield, Charles C Thomas, 1978.

ARTICLES

Therapeutics

Boysen, P. G., et. al.: Prospective evaluation for pneumonectomy using the ^{99m}Technetium quantitative perfusion lung scan. Chest, 72:422-425, Oct. 1977.

Light, R. W.: Pleural effusions. Med. Clin. N. Am., 61:1339-1352, Nov. 1977.

Rau, J., and Rau, M.: To breathe or be breathed: Understanding IPPB. AJN, 77:613-617, Apr. 1977.

Shank, J. C., and Latshaw, R. F.: Pleural effusion. Am. Fam. Phys., 17:143-149, Mar. 1978.

Waterson, M.: Teaching your patients postural drainage. Nursing '78, 8:51-53, Mar. 1978.

Zavala, D. C.: Diagnostic fiberoptic bronchoscopy: Techniques and results of biopsy in 600 patients. Chest, 68:12-19, July 1975.

Surgical Procedures

Benfield, J. R., et al.: An interdisciplinary perspective of lung cancer. Curr. Probl. Cancer, 1:3-53, Apr. 1977.

Cameron, M. I.: What patients need most before and after thoracotomy. Nursing '78, 8:28-36, May, 1978.

Cimprich, B., Gaydos, D., and Langan, R.: A preoperative teaching program for the thoracotomy patient. Cancer Nurs., 1:35-39, Feb. 1978.

Fontana, R. S.: Early diagnosis of lung cancer. Am. Rev. Resp. Dis., 116:399-402, Sept. 1977.

Garrett, G.: Left upper lobectomy for carcinoma. Nurs. Times, 72:29-32, 23 Sept. 1976.

Gross, N. J., and DeMeester, T. R.: Lung cancer: An immunologic viewpoint and the prospects for immunotherapy. Surg. Clin. N. Am., 56:219-231, Feb. 1976.

Harmon, H., Fergus, S., and Cole, F. H.: Pneumonectomy: Review of 351 cases. Ann. Surg. 183:719-722, June 1976.

Holmes, E. C.: Immunology and lung cancer. Ann. Thorac. Surg., *21*:250-258, Mar. 1976,

Kaplan, J. A., Miller, E. D., and Gallagher, E. G.: Postoperative analgesia for thoracotomy patients. Anesth. Analg., *54*:773-777, Nov.-Dec. 1975.

Kirsh, M. M., et al.: Carcinoma of the lung: Results of treatment over ten years. Ann. Thorac. Surg., *21*:371-377, May 1976.

————: Major pulmonary resection for bronchogenic carcinoma in the elderly. Ann. Thorac. Surg., *122*:369-373, Oct. 1976.

McKneally, M. F., et al.: Regional immunotherapy with intrapleural BCG for lung cancer. Thorac. Cardiovasc. Surg., *72*:333-338, Sept. 1976.

Mercier, C., et al.: Outpatient management of intercostal tube drainage in spontaneous pneumothorax. Ann. Thorac. Surg., *22*:163-165, Aug. 1976.

Mittman, C., and Bruderman, I.: Lung cancer: To operate or not. Am. Rev. Respir. Dis., *116*:477-496, Sept. 1977.

Ross, W. M.: How to deal with bronchogenic carcinoma in the elderly. Geriat., *31*:107-110, June 1976.

Wilson, R. F., Gibson, D. B., and Antonenko, D.: Shock and acute respiratory failure after chest trauma. J. Trauma, *17*:697-705, Sept. 1977.

AGENCIES

Governmental

National Heart, Lung and Blood Institute, National Institutes of Health, Bethesda, Md. 20205

Voluntary

American Association for Respiratory Therapy, 7411 Hines Place, Suite 101, Dallas, Tex. 75235

American Lung Association, 1740 Broadway, New York, N.Y. 10019

American Thoracic Society, 1740 Broadway, New York, N.Y. 10019

RESPIRATORY INTENSIVE CARE NURSING

A large percentage of patients requiring intensive care need airway assistance and ventilation. The purpose of this chapter is to expand the nurse's understanding of these acute problems in order to provide optimum care to these critically ill persons. Detailed descriptions of techniques of respiratory care are included as well as the underlying factors that predispose patients to these problems.

First, however, it is necessary to gain an understanding of the basic terminology and concepts encountered in respiratory care.

TERMINOLOGY AND PHYSIOLOGIC CONCEPTS APPLIED TO RESPIRATORY THERAPY

Mechanics of Ventilation

Ventilation in its simplest definition is the movement of air in and out of the lungs by means of inspiration and expiration.

Inspiration. Air flows from the atmosphere to the lungs in response to pressure gradients. As air is breathed in, the diaphragm and external intercostal muscles contract, causing the intrapleural pressure to become more negative. This negative pressure expands the alveoli, which in turn causes atmospheric air to flow into the lungs. When equilibrium between the airway pressure and intrapleural pressure is achieved, the flow of air stops.

Expiration. Normally, expiration is passive. When the inspiratory muscles relax, the contraction of the lungs squeezes air out of them. When the pressure gradient between the alveolar and intrapleural pressure is gone, the flow of air stops.

434

Tidal Volume and Dead Space

Tidal volume is that volume of air which is inspired during normal respiration. It is usually equal to 7 to 8 milliliters per kilogram of body weight. Part of the tidal volume enters the alveoli and the rest stays in the conducting airways. Dead space is the term applied to the volume of air in the conducting airways (nose, mouth, pharynx, larynx, trachea, and the bronchus down to the terminal bronchioles). The portion of the tidal volume that occupies the dead space cannot take part in oxygen uptake or carbon dioxide elimination.

If the blood supply to some alveoli stops for some reason or other, the gas occupying those alveoli cannot participate in gas exchange. These alveoli, then, function as dead space. To distinguish between the two types of dead space, the first is called *anatomical dead space* and the second *physiological dead space*. In a normal adult the anatomical dead space is approximately 150 ml. and the physiological dead space is insignificant.

Minute Ventilation

The volume of air expired by the nose and mouth each minute is referred to as *minute ventilation*. Minute ventilation is subdivided into alveolar ventilation and dead space ventilation, the normal distribution being two thirds to the alveoli and one third to dead space.

Ventilation Pattern

The normal pattern of ventilation includes approximately 6 to 10 deep breaths or sighs per hour, each considerably larger than tidal volume. If no breaths are larger than tidal volume, alveolar collapse occurs, because not all alveoli are opened with each breath. Alveolar collapse (atelectasis) produces unventilated areas with continued blood flow. Periodic deep breaths serve to keep all alveoli open. This is the reason for encouraging postoperative patients to take deep breaths and for using incentive spirometry to increase tidal volume.

Vital Capacity

Vital capacity is the *maximum* volume of gas that can be expelled from the lungs by a forceful expiratory effort following a *maximum* inspiration. To measure the vital capacity, the patient is asked to inhale maximally and exhale *fully* through a gas meter (respirometer). The normal vital capacity is about 70 ml./kg. of body weight.

Vital capacity is decreased in most lung diseases, abdominal distention, obesity, muscle weakness, and chest trauma and following upper abdominal or thoracic surgery. If the vital capacity is less than 10 ml./kg. body weight, respiratory assistance is usually required.

Inspiratory Force

Deep breaths may be decreased or eliminated by central nervous system depression, disease, or drugs; when this occurs, vital capacity is not a useful measurement because a conscious cooperative effort is required for the test. In the unconscious or uncooperative patient the measurement of inspiratory force is substituted for vital capacity. *Inspiratory force* is the maximum negative pressure that the patient can exert against an occluded airway. The minimal safe value is −25 cm. H₂O. Lower values indicate insufficient muscle strength for deep breaths or effective coughing.

Functional Residual Capacity (FRC)

Functional residual capacity is the volume of gas left in the lungs at the end of a normal expiration. It is usually approximately 2.5 liters. The actual volume depends on age, height, weight, sex, and body build. Functional residual capacity is less in the supine than in the erect position and decreases even more in the head down position. In acute respiratory failure it is markedly diminished. Emphysematous patients on the other hand have increased FRC.

Closing Capacity

Small airways (0.5 to 0.9 mm. in diameter) are easily collapsible. They are kept open by the pull of fibrous tissues attached to their outer surfaces and this mechanism works only if the volume of the lung is above a certain value. If the lung volume is less than this, the airways close (collapse).

The volume of the lung at which a significant number of small airways close is known as the *closing capacity*. In a healthy young adult it is about 2 liters, and since the lung volume at the end of a normal expiration (FRC) is about 2.5 liters, the small airways always remain open. With advancing age, the closing capacity gradually increases and may exceed the functional residual capacity. When this happens, significant numbers of small airways close at the end of a normal expiration, and some alveoli may be poorly ventilated. In respiratory distress syndrome, extensive small airway closure occurs, leading to hypoxia.

Compliance

Compliance of the lung is the change in lung volume per unit change in pressure. It is a measure of the stiffness of the lung. The lower the compliance, the smaller the change in lung volume per unit change in pressure due to increased stiffness of the lung.

The pressure change is the difference in pressure between the alveoli and the pleura at the beginning and end of inspiration. Pleural pressure is not routinely measured in clinical practice and consequently compliance of the lung itself cannot be calculated. However, the combined compliance of the lung and the chest wall is easy to calculate. Acute changes in the compliance of the chest wall are uncommon and when they occur the reason is generally obvious (e.g., tight chest bandage). Changes in the compliance of the lung and chest wall, therefore, usually reflect changes in the compliance of the lung.

Compliance of the lung and chest wall is easily measured when the patient is mechanically ventilated. The tidal volume is divided by the maximum pressure required to ventilate the patient. Example: If the tidal volume is 0.45 liters and the maximum pressure is 15 cm. of water, the compliance is $0.45 \div 15 = 0.03$ liters per cm. of H₂O. Low compliance is a characteristic finding in pneumothorax, hemothorax, pleural effusion, and most acute illnesses of the lung. Compliance is useful in assessing the progress of the disease in respiratory distress syndrome.

Diffusion

Diffusion is the physical process by which gases move across the alveolar membrane. Gases move from a region of high pressure (tension) to a region of low pressure. Oxygen tension is about 104 mm. Hg in the alveoli and 40 mm. Hg in venous blood. Oxygen, therefore, moves from the alveoli into the blood. Carbon dioxide tension is about 40 mm. Hg in the alveoli and 45 mm. Hg in venous blood. Carbon dioxide, therefore, moves from the venous blood into the alveoli.

Perfusion

Perfusion is the filling of the pulmonary capillaries with venous blood which has returned to the heart from the general circulation. The blood is pumped into the lungs by the right ventricle through the pulmonary artery. The pulmonary artery divides into the right and left branches to supply the two lungs. These two branches divide further to supply all parts of each lung.

The systolic and diastolic blood pressures in the pulmonary artery are about 22 mm. Hg and 8 mm. Hg respectively. Compared with 120 and 80 mm. Hg in the aorta, the pulmonary artery pressure is low. Consequently, in an erect position, the pulmonary artery pressure is not enough to supply blood to the apex of the lung against the force of gravity. Thus, when a person is in an erect position, the lung may be divided into three sections: an upper part with poor blood supply, a lower part with maximum blood supply, and the section in between the two with an intermediate supply of blood. When an individual turns to one side, more blood passes to the dependent lung.

Perfusion is also influenced by alveolar pressure. The pulmonary capillaries are sandwiched between adjacent alveoli. If the alveolar pressure is sufficiently high, the capillaries will be squeezed. Depending on the pressure, some capillaries will be completely collapsed, whereas others will be narrowed.

Pulmonary artery pressure, gravity, and alveolar pressure determine the patterns of perfusion. In lung disease these factors vary and the perfusion of the lung may become very abnormal.

Shunting

Normally about 2 percent of the blood pumped by the right ventricle does not perfuse the alveolar capillaries. This blood, which cannot participate in gas exchange with alveolar gas, is called *shunted blood*. It drains into the left heart through the bronchial, pleural, and thebesian veins. In some pathological states of the heart and great vessels (ventricular septal defect, patent ductus arteriosus) and lung diseases (pulmonary edema, atelectasis) the amount of blood shunted exceeds the normal 2 percent.

The shunted blood, which contains the same amount of oxygen as venous blood, mixes with the blood returning from the alveoli to produce arterial blood. The oxygen content of the arterial blood depends on both the oxygen content and the volume of each fraction. Severe hypoxia results when the amount of blood shunted exceeds 20 percent. The hypoxia is not significantly improved by breathing even 100 percent oxygen because the oxygen does not come in contact with the shunted blood.

Distribution of Ventilation and Perfusion

Ventilation is the flow of gas in and out of the lung, and perfusion is the filling of the alveolar capillaries with blood. We have seen how the pulmonary artery pressure, gravity, and alveolar pressure lead to uneven perfusions of the lung. Now we will discuss some of the factors leading to uneven ventilation of the lung and mismatching of ventilation and perfusion.

The main factors controlling the distribution of ventilation are:
1. Patency of the airways
2. Local changes in compliance within the lung
3. Gravity

Any factor which reduces the airway caliber (mucosal edema, inflammation, secretion, bronchospasm) will raise the resistance to airflow and decrease the ventilation of the corresponding alveoli. Similarly, any area in which the local compliance has decreased (i.e., that portion of the lung has become more stiff) will receive less ventilation than the surrounding more expandable portions of the lung.

The effect of gravity on ventilation is complex. Because of the consistency of the lung, its weight is distributed within the chest cavity in such a manner that the intrapleural pressure is less negative at the bottom (-2.5 cm. of H_2O) than at the top of the lung (-10 cm. of H_2O) in the erect position. The pressure within the airways is, however, the same in all parts of the lung. Consequently, the alveoli at the apex are larger than the alveoli at the base of the lung. When one applies these facts to the pressure-volume relationship of the lung, it becomes clear why, in the early phase of inspiration, more of the tidal volume is distributed to the basal region of the lung. The basal region of the erect lung, therefore, receives more blood and air than the apex.

For optimum gas exchange the perfusion of each alveolus must be matched by optimum ventilation. In addition to the pressure-volume relationship of the lung, there are other mechanisms such as changes in caliber of airways or capillaries which ensure that ventilation and perfusion are properly matched in the normal lung.

Mismatching of ventilation and perfusion leads to hypoxia. It appears to be the main cause of hypoxia following thoracic or abdominal surgery and most types of respiratory failure. Its effects are similar to those of shunts, except that breathing 100 percent oxygen eliminates hypoxia due to mismatched ventilation and perfusion.

Partial Pressure

Partial pressure is the pressure exerted by each type of gas in a mixture of gases. The partial pressure of a gas is proportional to the concentration of that gas in the mixture. The total pressure exerted by the gaseous mixture is equal to the sum of the partial pressures.

The air we breathe is a gaseous mixture consisting mainly of nitrogen (78.62%) and oxygen (20.84%), with traces of carbon dioxide (.04%), water vapor (.05%), helium, argon, etc. The atmospheric pressure at sea level is about 760 mm. of Hg (mm. of Hg = torr). From this data we may calculate the partial pressure of nitrogen and oxygen. Partial pressure of nitrogen is 79 percent of 760 (.79 × 760) = 600 torr, and that of oxygen is 21 percent of 760 (.21 × 760) = 160 torr.

The following is a reference list of expressions related to partial pressure:

P = pressure

PO_2 —partial pressure of oxygen

PCO_2 —partial pressure of carbon dioxide

P_AO_2 —partial pressure of alveolar oxygen

P_ACO_2 —partial pressure of alveolar carbon dioxide

P_aO_2 —partial pressure of arterial oxygen

P_aCO_2 —partial pressure of arterial carbon dioxide

P_vO_2 —partial pressure of venous oxygen

P_vCO_2 —partial pressure of venous carbon dioxide

P_{50} —oxygen tension at 50% hemoglobin concentration

torr —mm. Hg

Once the air enters the trachea it becomes fully saturated with water vapor, which displaces some of the gases in order that the air pressure within the lung may remain equal with the air pressure outside (760 torr). Water vapor exerts a pressure of 47 torr when it fully saturates a mixture of gases at the body temperature of 37° C. (98.6° F.). Nitrogen and oxygen are therefore now responsible for the remaining 713 torr (760 − 47) pressure. Once this mixture enters the alveoli, it is further diluted by carbon dioxide. In the alveoli, the water vapor continues to exert a pressure of 47 torr. The remaining 713 torr pressure is now exerted as follows: nitrogen, 569 torr (74.9%); oxygen, 104 torr (13.6%); and carbon dioxide, 40 torr (5.3%).

When a gas is exposed to a liquid, the gas will dissolve in the liquid until an equilibrium is reached. The dissolved gas also exerts a partial pressure. At equilibrium, the partial pressure of the gas in the liquid is the same as the partial pressure of the gas in the gaseous mixture. Oxygenation of venous blood in the lung illustrates this point. In the lung, venous blood and alveolar oxygen are separated by a very thin alveolar membrane. Oxygen diffuses across this membrane to dissolve in the blood until the partial pressure of oxygen in the blood is the same as that in the alveoli (104 torr). However, since carbon dioxide is manufactured in the cells, venous blood contains carbon dioxide at a higher partial pressure than that in the alveolar gas. In the lung, carbon dioxide diffuses out of venous blood into the alveolar gas. At equilibrium, the partial pressure of carbon dioxide in the blood and in alveolar gas is the same (40 torr).

The entire sequence of changes in partial pressure readings (in torr) may be summarized as follows:

	ATMOSPHERIC AIR	TRACHEAL AIR	ALVEOLAR AIR
PH_2O	3.7	47.0	47.0
PN_2	597.0	563.4	569.0
PO_2	159.0	149.3	104.0
PCO_2	0.3	0.3	40.0
Total	760.0	760.0	760.0

Bicarbonate. A third component of blood, important in the assessment of respiratory function, is bicarbonate (HCO_3), which acts mainly as a buffer in maintaining acid-base balance as reflected in the blood pH (the concentration of hydrogen ions in the blood). Normal blood pH has a limited range of 7.38 to 7.44. An excess of hydrogen ions results in a pH below 7.38 (acidosis); a deficit of hydrogen ions results in a pH above 7.44 (alkalosis). The role of bicarbonate in regulating hydrogen ion concentration can be expressed chemically as:

$$\underset{\text{(carbon dioxide)}}{CO_2} + H_2O \rightleftharpoons \underset{\text{(carbonic acid)}}{H_2CO_3}$$

$$\rightleftharpoons \underset{\substack{\text{(hydrogen} \\ \text{ions)}}}{H^+} + \underset{\substack{\text{(bicarbonate} \\ \text{ion)}}}{HCO_3^-}$$

The relationship of bicarbonate to carbon dioxide can also be ascertained from this formula, and it is this relationship that has a direct bearing on the assessment of respiratory function. In normal blood concentrations, the ratio of bicarbonate to carbonic acid (dissolved carbon dioxide) is 20 to 1. If there is an excess of carbon dioxide due to poor respiratory function (respiratory acidosis) then the balance between the bicarbonate and carbonic acid is upset, at which point the kidneys, in an attempt to reestablish the correct ratio, will excrete less or no bicarbonate. A more complete explanation of the role of bicarbonate in carbon dioxide transport is found on page 439.

Oxygen Transport

Oxygen and carbon dioxide are carried simultaneously by virtue of their abilities to dissolve in blood or to combine with some of the elements of blood. Oxygen is carried in the blood in two forms: (1) as physically dissolved oxygen in the plasma; (2) in combination with the hemoglobin of the red blood cells. Each 100 ml. of arterial blood carries 0.3 ml. of O_2 physically dissolved in the plasma and 19 ml. of O_2 in combination with hemoglobin. Note that the volume of O_2 carried by hemoglobin is considerably greater than that carried in physical solution.

The volume of oxygen physically dissolved in the plasma varies directly with the P_aO_2. The higher the P_aO_2, the greater the oxygen dissolved. For example, it is found that at a P_aO_2 of 10 mm. Hg, 0.03 ml. of oxygen is dissolved in 100 ml. of plasma. At 20 mm. Hg, twice this amount is dissolved in plasma and at 100 mm. Hg, ten times this amount. Therefore, the amount of dissolved oxygen is directly proportional to the partial pressure, and this is true no matter how high the oxygen pressure rises. For example, in a hyperbaric chamber in which a subject is breathing oxygen at 3 atmospheres, the P_aO_2 would be 2,000 mm. Hg. The dissolved oxygen would be 6 ml. of oxygen per 100 ml. of blood.

The volume of oxygen that combines with hemoglobin also depends on P_aO_2, but only up to a P_aO_2 of about 150 mm. Hg. Above this P_aO_2, hemoglobin is 100 percent saturated, by which we mean that hemoglobin will not combine with any additional oxygen. When hemoglobin is 100 percent saturated, 1 gram of hemoglobin will combine with 1.34 ml. of oxygen. Therefore, in a person with 14 gm. percent of hemoglobin, each 100 ml. of blood will contain about 19 ml. of oxygen associated with hemoglobin. If the P_aO_2 is less than 150 torr, the percentage of hemoglobin saturated with oxygen is lower. For example, at a P_aO_2 of 100 torr (normal value) saturation is 97 percent, and at a P_aO_2 of 40 torr, the saturation is 70 percent.

The oxygen dissociation curve of hemoglobin (Fig. 24-1) shows the relationship between the partial pressure of oxygen and the percentage saturation of the hemoglobin more clearly.

The unusual shape of the oxygen dissociation curve is a distinct advantage to the patient for several reasons:
1. If the arterial PO_2 decreases from 100 to 80 mm. Hg as a result of lung disease or heart disease, the hemoglobin of the arterial blood will still be almost maximally saturated (94 percent), and the tissues will not suffer from anoxia.
2. When the arterial blood passes into tissue capillaries and is exposed to the tissue tension of oxygen (about 40 mm. Hg), hemoglobin gives up large quantities of oxygen for utilization by the tissues.

Oxygen Dissociation Curve

The oxygen dissociation curve indicates the methods used by the body to release oxygen to the tissues so that the oxygen obtained from the lungs is stored and then released to the tissues in amounts sufficient for their needs. The oxygen dissociation curve in Figure 24-1 is marked to show three levels of sufficiency: (1) normal levels — P_aO_2 above 70; (2) relatively safe levels — P_aO_2 45 to 70; and (3) dangerous levels — P_aO_2 below 40.

Figure 24-2 shows that at a normal pH of 7.40, the steep part of the curve is between a P_aO_2 of 40 torr (75 percent hemoglobin saturation) and 20 torr (33 percent hemoglobin saturation). P_{50} refers to the oxygen tension (27 torr) at 50 percent hemoglobin saturation. When we talk about changes in P_aO_2 and saturation, we talk about changes in P_{50}.

The oxygen hemoglobin dissociation curve will shift to either the right or the left depending upon the presence of the following: CO_2; hydrogen ion concentration (acidity); temperature; 2-3 diphosphoglycerate and steroids.

A rise in these factors will shift the curve to the right, so that more oxygen is then released to the tissues at the same P_aO_2. A reduction in these factors will cause the curve to shift to the left, making the bond between oxygen and hemoglobin stronger, so that less oxygen is given up to the tissues at the same P_aO_2. In the diagram,

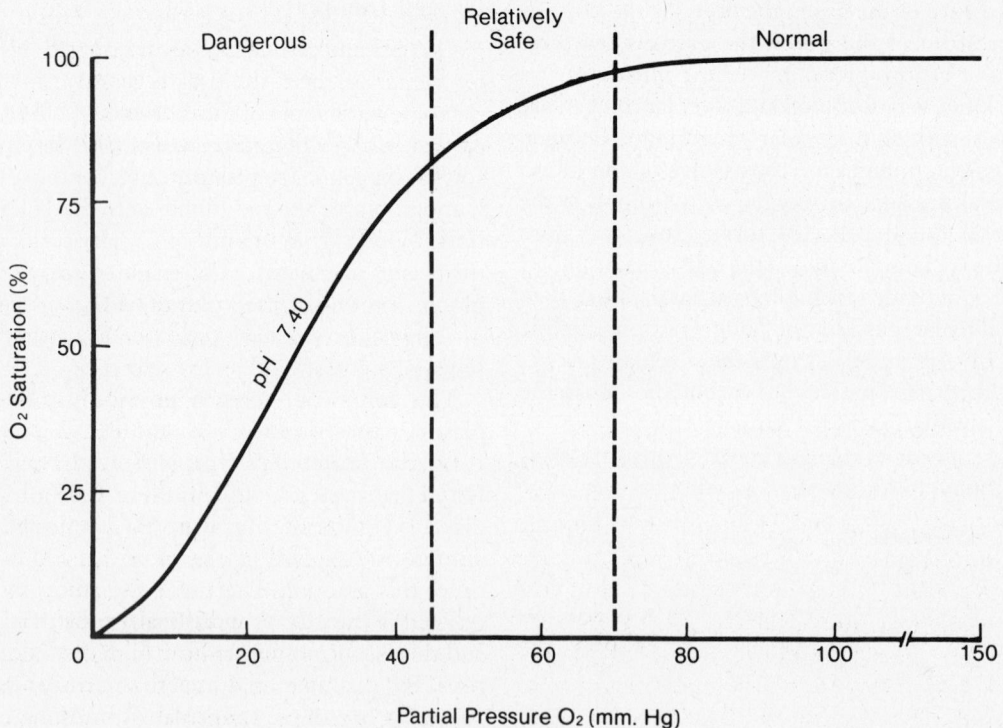

Figure 24-1. Oxygen-hemoglobin dissociation curve showing levels of pH that are normal, relatively safe, and dangerous.

ARTERIAL OXYGENATION

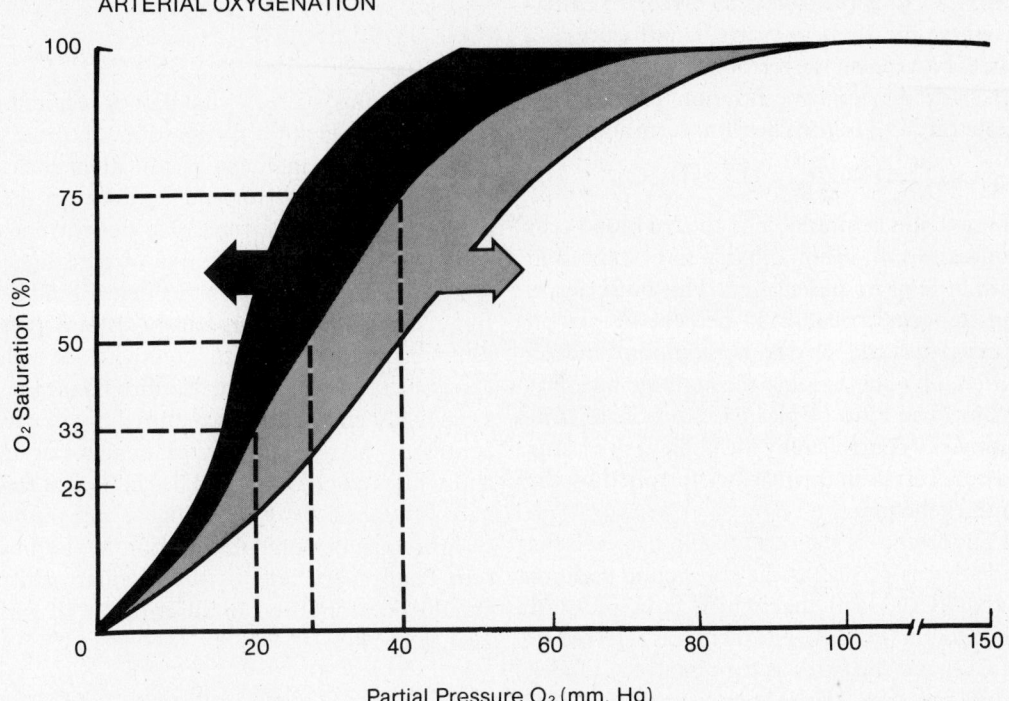

Figure 24-2. Oxygen-hemoglobin affinity: A normal pH shows the steep arc of the curve between a PO_2 of 40 mm. Hg (75 per cent saturation) and 20 mm. Hg (33 per cent hemoglobin saturation). The diagram shows that at 75 per cent hemoglobin saturation the PO_2 is 57 mm. Hg; when it shifts to the left, the PO_2 in the diagram is 25 mm. Hg. P_{50} is normally 27 mm. Hg. A shift to the right gives a higher P_{50} and a shift to the left gives a lower P_{50}. (Adapted from Shapiro, B.: Clinical Application of Blood Gases. Chicago, Year Book Medical Publishers.)

the normal (middle) curve shows that 75 percent saturation occurs at a P_aO_2 of 40 torr. If the curve shifts to the right, the same saturation (75 percent) occurs at the higher P_aO_2 of 57 torr. If the curve shifts to the left, 75 percent saturation occurs at a P_aO_2 of 25 torr.

Clinical Significance. With a normal hemoglobin of 15 gm./100 ml. and a P_aO_2 level of 40 torr (oxygen saturation 75 percent), there is adequate oxygen available for the tissues, but there is no reserve. With a catastrophe (e.g., bronchospasm, aspiration, hypotension, or cardiac arrhythmias), which reduces the intake of oxygen from the lungs, tissue hypoxia would result. The normal value of P_aO_2 is 60 to 80 torr (90 percent saturation). With this level of oxygenation, there is a 15 percent margin of excess oxygen available to the tissues.

An important consideration in the transport of oxygen is the cardiac output, which determines the amount of oxygen delivered to the body. Oxygen flux is the term given to the amount of oxygen delivered to the body per minute. For example in a person with a hemoglobin concentration of 14 gm. percent and hemoglobin saturation of 97 percent, each 100 ml. of arterial blood will contain $(14 \times 1.34 \times .97) = 18.2$ ml. of oxygen combined with hemoglobin. Each liter (1,000 ml.) of blood will contain 182 ml. of oxygen. If the cardiac output is 5 liters per minute, the oxygen flux is 910 ml. per minute

(182×5). If the cardiac output falls to 2.5 liters per minute, oxygen flux falls to 450 ml. This is why cardiac output measurements are so important. Not all of the oxygen delivered to the body is used up. In fact, only 250 ml. of oxygen is used up per minute. The rest of the oxygen returns to the right heart, and the PO_2 of venous blood drops to about 40 mm. Hg.

Carbon Dioxide Transport

Simultaneously with the diffusion of oxygen from the blood into the tissues, carbon dioxide diffuses in the opposite direction, e.g., from tissue cells to blood, and is transported to the lung for excretion. The amount of carbon dioxide in transit is one of the major determinants of the acid-base balance of the body. Normally only 6 percent of the venous CO_2 is removed and enough remains in the arterial side to exert a pressure of 40 torr. (Torr is gas tension in mm. Hg). Most of the carbon dioxide (95 percent) enters the red blood cells, and the small portion (5 percent) that remains dissolved in the plasma (PCO_2) is the critical factor that will determine carbon dioxide movement in or out of the blood. The dissolved carbon dioxide takes the form of carbonic acid (H_2CO_3), which is a volatile acid, i.e., it undergoes a chemical reaction that changes it from a liquid to a gas (as CO_2), which explains why the blood concentration of carbonic acid (H_2CO_3) is controlled by alveolar ventilation. This is where bicarbonate exerts its influence as a stabilizing force. Note again the relationships of carbonic acid (H_2CO_3), hydrogen ion concentration ($pH^\pm$ or pH), and bicarbonate (HCO_3) in the chemical formula

$$CO_2 + H_2O \rightleftharpoons H_2CO_3 \rightleftharpoons H^+ + HCO_3^-$$

The bicarbonate and hemoglobin in the red blood cells allow great quantities of carbon dioxide to be carried in the blood with little or no pH change. This buffering is essential, and it occurs because 30 percent of carbon dioxide is carried directly on the hemoglobin and 65 percent is buffered by hemoglobin through the bicarbonate mechanism. The ratio of plasma bicarbonate concentration (primarily controlled by the kidney) to plasma carbonic acid concentration (primarily controlled by the lungs) determines the pH.

Of critical importance is the relationship between the carbon dioxide that is carried as the compound sodium bicarbonate ($NaHCO_3$) and that which is in physical solution in the plasma (PCO_2). The former is referred to as the bound CO_2 and the latter as the dissolved. Under normal conditions the ratio of the bound to the dissolved CO_2 is remarkably constant at 20:1. Such a ratio is essential to maintain normal acid-base balance of the blood. (The plasma bicarbonate ion concentration is primarily controlled by the renal system, but to a lesser extent is affected by the respiratory system.)

The whole process of oxygen and carbon dioxide transport together with formation of bicarbonate (HCO_3) is summarized as follows:

Tissue Level:
1. CO_2 enters the red blood cells, combines with H_2O to form carbonic acid (H_2CO_3).
2. At the same time, hemoglobin releases O_2 to the tissues and becomes reduced hemoglobin (HHb).
3. H_2CO_3 dissociates into H^+ and bicarbonate (HCO_3^-).
4. Reduced hemoglobin (HHb) and HCO_3^- are carried in the venous system to the lungs.

Lung Level:
1. Reduced hemoglobin takes up O_2 and gives off H^+.
2. HCO_3^- combines with $H^{+'}$ to give H_2CO_3.
3. H_2CO_3 dissociates into H_2O + CO_2 (expired air).

In summarizing respiratory gas transport, it is important to emphasize that the many processes described do not take place in intermittent stages but occur rapidly, simultaneously, and continuously.

MONITORING IN RESPIRATORY INTENSIVE CARE

Monitoring is a very vital part of respiratory intensive care nursing. Prompt recognition, accurate assessment, and proper management of any adverse changes in the critically ill patient depend entirely on the quality of monitoring. For good reasons, the current trend is towards greater sophistication in monitoring.

There are certain vital signs that should be monitored frequently if not continuously. Blood pressure, heart rate, respiratory rate, and temperature belong to this category. Frequent electrocardiograms are also necessary. Daily chest x-ray is required on all patients on the ventilator. Serum electrolytes, hematocrit, hemoglobin, and white cell count should be checked at frequent intervals. The total daily fluid intake and output and daily weight must be noted to monitor the fluid balance. Certain respiratory and cardiovascular parameters also should be monitored in all critically ill patients (Table 24-1, page 445).

CHEST AUSCULTATION

Care of the critically ill patient requires frequent inspection and auscultation of the chest. The important factor to consider is whether breath sounds are present or absent. Presence of normal breath sounds is proof that air is entering the lungs. Absence of breath sounds in areas where they should be heard suggests that although perfusion is present the alveoli are not getting air. Serial auscultation of the chest will allow the nurse to confirm the presence of air exchange, to know when tracheobronchial aspiration is required, and to prevent ventilatory catastrophes. Changes in the aforementioned factors indicate that treatment needs to be modified.

Breath Sounds and Their Significance

Normal Breath Sounds. There are three categories of normal breath sounds: (1) vesicular, (2) bronchial or tracheal, and (3) bronchovesicular.

Vesicular breath sounds are heard over most of the lung fields and appear breezy and swishy in character. Inspiration is high-pitched and predominates over expiration. Expiration is low-pitched and both shorter and fainter than inspiration.

Bronchial or tracheal breathing is heard normally over the trachea and main bronchi. Inspiration is louder than expiration and high-pitched. Expiration is of increased duration, so much so that it actually is longer than inspiration. Its pitch is higher and of greater intensity. It has a harsh, tubular quality.

Bronchovesicular breath sounds represent an intermediate stage. They are heard normally in the second interspace anteriorly, in the interscapular area posteriorly, and often at the medial right apex. Inspiration is unchanged from that of vesicular breathing, but expiration is as loud, equal in length, and similar in pitch.

Abnormal Breath Sounds. Rales are abnormal additional or adventitious sounds and are always pathologic. They may be subdivided into (1) rhonchi—continuous coarse sounds; and (2) moist rales—interrupted crackling sounds. These abnormal sounds indicate the presence of fluid somewhere in the respiratory tract. The fluid or exudate may result from infection, inflammation, aspiration, edema, or retained secretions.

- The presence of rhonchi implies disease of the larger bronchi. Moist, medium, and fine rales imply bronchiolar and alveolar disease. Rhonchi are usually heard earlier in inspiration than are rales, since sound is produced when the column of inspired air meets the exudate at its anatomic location.

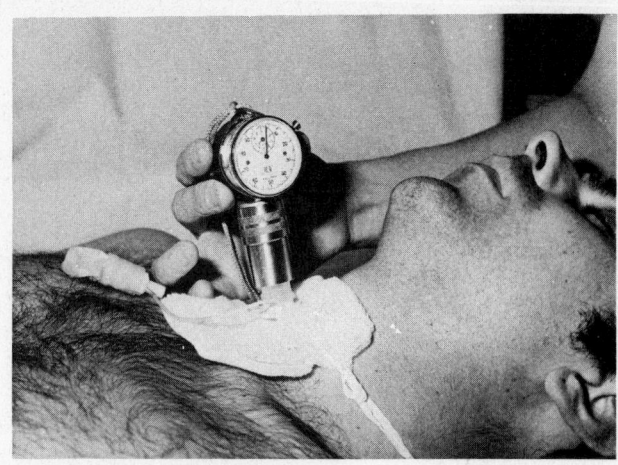

Figure 24-3. The Wright respirometer connected to a tracheostomy tube with the cuff inflated. The small dial measures the tidal volume and vital capacity. The large dial measures the minute volume.

PULMONARY FUNCTION MONITORING

Tidal Volume

The volume of each breath is referred to as the *tidal volume*. The instrument commonly used to measure volumes at the bedside is known as the Wright respirometer (Fig. 24-3).

If the patient is breathing via an endotracheal tube or tracheostomy the respirometer is directly attached to it and the exhaled volume is read off the dial. In others, the respirometer is attached to a face mask, which is placed to cover the nose and mouth so that it is airtight, and the exhaled volume is measured as before.

The tidal volume may vary from breath to breath. To make the measurement reliable the volumes of several breaths must be measured and the range of tidal volumes together with the average tidal volume must be noted. The normal tidal volume is 7 to 8 ml. per kg. body weight. When the tidal volume falls below 5 ml. per kg. body weight, mechanical ventilation is usually required.

Respiratory Rate

Respiratory rate is important, for together with tidal volume it determines minute ventilation (see below) and is useful in the diagnosis of the etiology of respiratory failure. The normal adult who is resting comfortably breathes at 18 to 20 breaths per minute. Except for occasional sighs the breathing is reasonably regular. Raised intracranial pressure, brain injury, and drug overdose are conditions associated with slow breathing. It is typical of narcotic overdose. Rapid breathing is commonly seen in pneumonia, pulmonary edema, metabolic acidosis, septicemia, and rib fracture.

When the rate of breathing falls outside the range of 14 to 25, mechanical ventilation may be necessary. Some patients who are breathing spontaneously may develop respiratory arrest. It is most likely to occur in patients with brain injury or following neurosurgery. Therefore, these patients require continuous monitoring of their respiration. There are instruments now available which will carry out this function.

Minute Ventilation

Minute ventilation is the volume of air breathed per minute. It is equal to the product of the tidal volume and the respiratory rate. Minute ventilation consists of the dead space ventilation ("wasted" ventilation) and alveolar ventilation. Alveolar ventilation is responsible for carbon dioxide elimination and oxygenation of the blood.

The body tends to keep the arterial PCO_2 at 40 torr (mm. Hg). It does this by maintaining the alveolar ventilation, and therefore the CO_2 elimination, reasonably constant. This implies that if the dead space increases, the minute ventilation must increase to compensate for the wasted ventilation of the dead space. If the patient cannot increase minute ventilation, carbon dioxide accumulates in the body and the PCO_2 will increase.

When the minute ventilation exceeds 10 liters per minute, mechanical ventilation is usually required. When a patient is mechanically ventilated the tidal volume and respiratory rate are chosen to provide a minute ventilation that maintains the arterial PCO_2 at 40 torr. Occasionally a higher or lower PCO_2 is desirable.

Vital Capacity

Vital capacity, like tidal volume, is measured with a Wright respirometer. The patient is asked to inspire maximally and exhale fully through the respirometer. The normal value depends on age, sex, body build, and weight. In an adult, if the vital capacity is less than 10 ml. per kg. of body weight, mechanical ventilation is usually required.

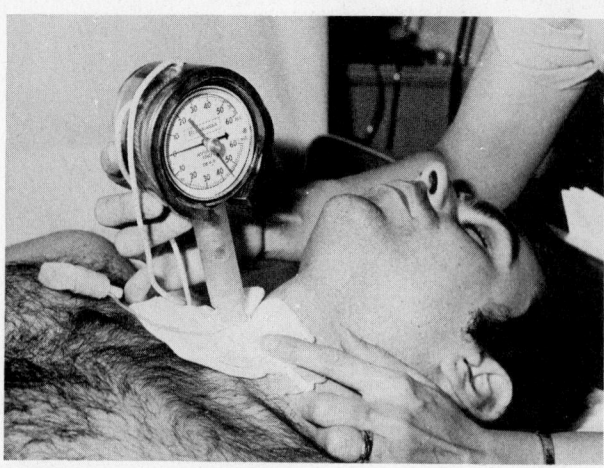

Figure 24-4. Measurement of inspiratory force. The inspiratory force manometer is connected to the tracheostomy tube. The tracheostomy cuff should be inflated. Plug the hole in the connector between the tracheostomy and manometer so that the airway is obstructed on inspiration. Negative inspiratory force is reflected at −45 cm. H₂O pressure. Allow the patient to breathe between measurements by unplugging the hole.

Inspiratory Force

Inspiratory force quantitates the effort a patient is making during inspiration. It does not require patient cooperation and hence is useful in the unconscious patient. The equipment needed for this measurement includes (1) a manometer that measures negative pressure and (2) adapters for connection to an anesthetic mask or a cuffed endotracheal tube. The manometer is attached and the airway is completely occluded (Fig. 24-4). This is continued for 10 to 20 seconds while the inspiratory efforts of the patient are registered on the manometer. The normal inspiratory pressure is −100 cm. of H₂O. If the negative pressure registered after 15 seconds of occluding the airway is less than −25 cm. of H₂O, mechanical ventilation is usually required for that patient.

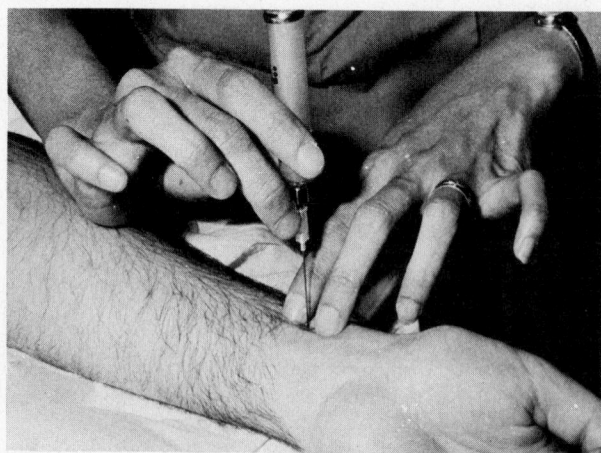

Figure 24-5. Technique of arterial puncture for blood gas analysis.

Compliance

Compliance is a measure of how stiff the lung is. Compliance of the lung and chest wall is easily obtained in patients on ventilation. The tidal volume delivered to the patient is divided by the maximum pressure required to deliver that volume. If the patient is on PEEP (see page 449), this pressure must be subtracted from the maximum pressure developed during ventilation. The greater the stiffness, the greater the pressure required to ventilate the lungs and the lower the compliance. As the condition of the lung improves, the compliance increases and the pressure required to ventilate the lung decreases.

Arterial Blood Gases

Arterial oxygen and carbon dioxide tensions (P_aO_2, P_aCO_2) and pH must be measured at frequent intervals when managing patients with respiratory problems. The P_aO_2 indicates the degree of oxygenation of the blood and the P_aCO_2 indicates adequacy of alveolar ventilation. Whenever changes are made in the inspired oxygen concentration, tidal volume, or respiratory rate, arterial blood gases should be measured after allowing 20 to 30 minutes for alveolar and blood gases to equilibrate.

About 3 ml. of arterial blood is required for gas analysis. Arterial puncture is performed on areas where good pulses are palpable (e.g., radial, brachial, or femoral artery).

Procedure:

- With the left hand, feel along the course of the artery and palpate for pulsation with the middle and index fingers. With the right hand, hold a No. 20 gauge needle and heparinized glass syringe (0.05 ml. of 1 percent sodium heparin for every ml. of blood) at a 90-degree angle to the surface. Anchor the wrist to the surface to allow finer control of the needle.
- With the right hand insert the needle between the closely approximated middle and index fingers of the left hand, aiming at the pulsating artery (Fig. 24-5). It is easier to obtain a sample with a glass syringe, because once the artery is punctured, arterial pressure will push up the plunger of a glass syringe; as a result, air is less likely to enter the sample. After the blood is obtained, apply pressure on the punctured area for 5 minutes to avoid a hematoma.
- Cap the syringe, and place the arterial blood sample in an iced container while awaiting analysis. The lower temperature reduces the metabolism and minimizes the alteration of the true values of oxygen, carbon dioxide, and pH.

Precautions:

1. Use aseptic technique.
2. Avoid frequent puncture in the same place because of the danger of local aneurysmal dilatation.
3. Do not insert the needle deeper than 0.5 cm. (unless necessary), since in most cases this artery is located close to the surface.
4. Know the anatomy in order to avoid trauma to adjacent nerves.
5. Palpate for the presence of the ulnar artery before puncturing the radial artery.

If repeated arterial blood gas determinations are planned, an arterial catheter may be left in the radial artery. However, this may compromise the blood flow through the artery. Before the catheter is inserted, an Allen test is done to check the adequacy of blood flow through the ulnar artery, so that the perfusion of the hand is not compromised even if the radial artery is blocked. The Allen test is done by causing the hand to blanch and then occluding the radial artery and watching the blood flow to the hand by way of the ulnar artery. This ensures collateral circulation even if thrombosis of the radial artery should occur. It is performed in the following manner:

- If the patient is conscious, ask him to clench his fist while the nurse obliterates the radial and ulnar pulses simultaneously at the wrist. Then ask the patient to unclench his fist and observe the blanching of the palm. Release pressure on the ulnar artery while compressing the radial artery and watch for the return of skin color. If flow through the ulnar artery is good, flushing of the palm will be seen instantaneously.
- If the patient is unconscious, elevate his hand above the heart and squeeze or compress the hand until blanching occurs. Now obliterate the radial and ulnar pulses simultaneously at the wrist. Lower the hand while compressing the radial and ulnar arteries. Then release the pressure on the ulnar artery and watch for the return of skin color as above.

Inspired Oxygen Concentration

The air we breathe contains 21 percent of oxygen by volume. In other words, the fraction of oxygen in inspired air is 0.21 (Fraction = %/100). The fraction of inspired oxygen (F_IO_2) may be increased by adding oxygen to the inspired air (see oxygen therapy for respiratory failure). If the F_IO_2 is not adequate, hypoxia and death will result. Too high an F_IO_2, on the other hand, will lead to needless oxygen toxicity. To ensure that the F_IO_2 is just right, an oxygen analyzer must be used from time to time to measure the concentration of oxygen in the inspired gas.

Alveolar-Arterial Oxygen Tension Difference

The difference in oxygen tension between the alveolar gas (P_AO_2) and arterial blood (P_aO_2) is a measure of the efficiency of the lung as an oxygenator. A sample of arterial blood is easily obtainable to measure the P_aO_2. Unfortunately, a representative sample of alveolar gas cannot be obtained to measure the P_AO_2. However, if the values of the F_IO_2 and P_aCO_2 (CO_2 tension in arterial blood) are known, an acceptable value of P_AO_2 may be calculated from the following formula:

$$P_AO_2 = (713 \times F_IO_2) - P_aCO_2 \times 1.25)$$

Example: If a man breathing room air ($F_IO_2 = .21$) has an arterial blood carbon dioxide tension ($P_A\text{-}CO_2$) of 40 torr (mm. Hg) then his P_AO_2 is 99.73 torr.

$$P_{(A-a)}O_2 = P_AO_2 - P_aO_2$$

The normal lung is an efficient oxygenator and the normal range $P_{(A-a)}O_2$ is 5 to 15 torr. Shunts and mismatched ventilation/perfusion renders the lung an inefficient oxygenator. This will become evident by widening of the $P_{(A-a)}O_2$.

Pulmonary Capillary Wedge Pressure (PCW Pressure)

Pulmonary capillary wedge pressure is obtained by using a specially designed cardiac catheter known as the Swan-Ganz catheter. In its simplest design it is a double lumen catheter (Fig. 24-6). The larger of the two lumens is open at both ends and is used for measuring pressures and obtaining pulmonary arterial blood samples. The lumen must be flushed continuously or intermittently with heparinized solution. The other lumen is used to inflate a balloon situated at the tip of the catheter with about 1 ml. of air. When the balloon is inflated it has a diameter of 11 to 13 mm. and it surrounds and hides the tip of the catheter.

The catheter is inserted via a large peripheral vein under continuous monitoring of the ECG and the venous pressure through the catheter lumen. When the catheter tip enters the thorax the venous pressure tracing will show fluctuation with respiration. The balloon is now inflated and the catheter advanced. Blood flow carries the balloon as if it were an embolus and guides the catheter through the right atrium and tricuspid valve into the right ventricle and thence into the pulmonary artery. During insertion the position of the balloon and catheter tip at any moment is reflected in the pressure tracing (Fig. 24-6). The balloon will finally end up (like an embolus) in one of the branches of the pulmonary artery, where it obstructs the flow of blood through that artery; it is now said to be wedged. The pressure recorded is called the pulmonary capillary wedge (PCW) pressure.

The balloon serves three purposes: (1) it guides the catheter; (2) it covers the tip of the catheter and prevents it from irritating the myocardium, which greatly reduces the incidence of arrhythmias; and (3) it is used to obtain the wedge pressure.

- If the catheter is left wedged for too long, pulmonary infarct may result. Therefore, keep the balloon deflated when the wedge pressure is not measured. After the catheter has been in the patient for some time, it softens and may be carried forward to wedge in a smaller artery even when the balloon is not inflated. In order to detect this early, monitor the pulmonary arterial tracing continuously. If the tracing disappears, flush the catheter with heparinized solution. If this does not help, withdraw the catheter a few centimeters until the pulmonary arterial tracing reappears.

The pulmonary capillary wedge (PCW) pressure is important for two reasons. First, it is one of the factors

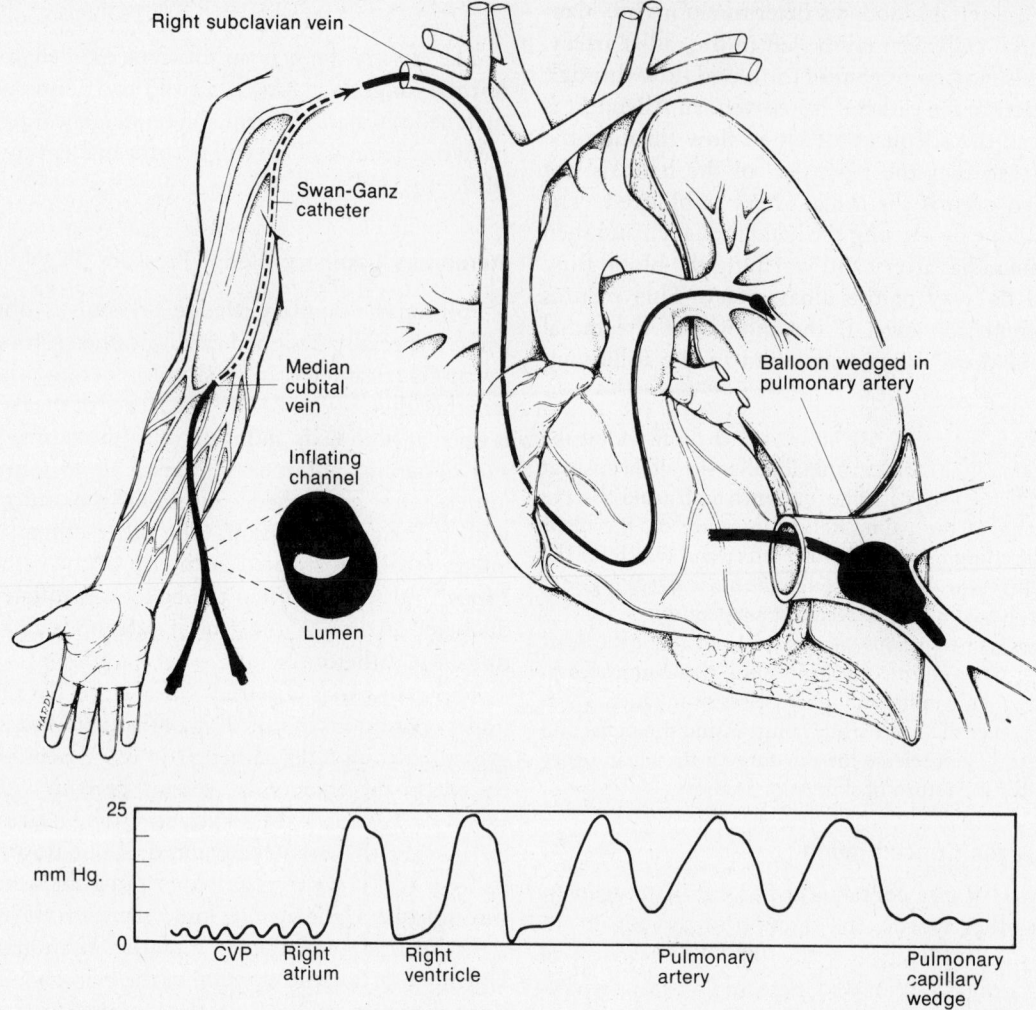

Figure 24-6.   Insertion of a Swan-Ganz catheter. The position of the catheter is reflected by the pressure tracings. Capillary wedge pressure is obtained by inflating the balloon.

controlling fluid shift in the lung. The normal PCW pressure is about 6 to 12 mm. Hg. If the PCW pressure exceeds 18 mm. Hg, pulmonary congestion usually follows because of the movement of fluid out of the capillaries. When the PCW pressure is in excess of 25 or 30 mm. Hg, pulmonary edema may occur.

The second reason for the importance of the PCW pressure is that it reflects the left atrial pressure and therefore indirectly reflects the left ventricular function. When the PCW pressure is combined with measurements of cardiac output, important conclusions regarding the cardiovascular status may be drawn. If the cardiac output is low and the PCW pressure is high (more than 20 mm. Hg), left ventricular failure is indicated (if mitral valve is normal). PCW pressure is also useful in the diagnosis of cardiac tamponade, pulmonary embolism, and acute mitral regurgitation.

Cardiac Output

Cardiac output is the volume of blood delivered to the tissues by the heart every minute. Introduction of the triple (three) lumen Swan-Ganz catheter with a thermistor (electronic heat-sensing device) has made cardiac output measurements relatively simple. The third lumen of this type of catheter opens some distance from the tip and is used for measuring central venous pressure (CVP) or administering fluids. The thermistor is situated 4 cm. from the tip of the catheter and measures the temperature of the blood that flows by.

When 5 or 10 ml. of a cold solution are injected through the CVP line of the catheter, the solution mixes with some blood, which is consequently cooled. This cooled blood is ejected into the pulmonary artery, where the temperature drop is detected by the thermistor. The electrical signals arising from the thermistor can be used to trace the curve of this temperature drop on a graph paper (thermodilution curve) and can also be processed by an integrator circuit to yield the cardiac output in digital form.

The cardiac output determines the amount of nutrients delivered to the tissues. We are primarily concerned with oxygen delivered to the tissues. The amount of oxygen present in the cardiac output is known as *oxygen flux*. Oxygen flux depends on the hemoglobin concentration (mg.%) and oxygen saturation of hemoglobin (which is determined by the P_aO_2 and P_{50}) and cardiac output.

Cardiac output depends on the cardiac function, tone of the blood vessels, and blood volume. Low blood volume may result from blood loss in accidents, major surgery, hemorrhage from peptic ulcer, esophageal varices, or diverticulitis. Fluid loss seen in intestinal obstruction, peritonitis, severe diarrhea, diabetes, chronic renal failure, dialysis, or injudicious use of diuretics may also lead to low blood volume. Whatever the cause of low blood volume, it leads to low cardiac output.

Poor cardiac function is most frequently due to ischemic heart disease, hypertension, or valvular defects. Hypoxia itself may lead to poor cardiac function and may set up a vicious cycle. When cardiac function is so poor that the cardiac output is inadequate for the needs of the body, cardiac failure is present.

Low cardiac output is often the cause of the patient's being critically ill and is a persistent problem in his management. The use of mechanical ventilators and PEEP (page 449) may also lead to low cardiac output. Since the output of the right and the left ventricles must be equal, pulmonary perfusion is equal to the cardiac output. When the cardiac output falls, pulmonary perfusion also falls and may lead to hypoxia because of ventilation abnormalities. For these reasons, frequent measurement of cardiac output is very important for the proper management of these patients.

For a summary of the parameters involved in the monitoring of respiratory care, see Table 24-1.

CAUSES OF RESPIRATORY FAILURE

Respiratory failure exists whenever the exchange of oxygen for carbon dioxide in the lungs cannot keep up with the rate of oxygen consumption and carbon dioxide production in the cells of the body. This results in a fall in arterial oxygen tension (hypoxemia) and a rise in arterial carbon dioxide tensions (hypercapnia).

One must distinguish between acute respiratory failure and acute exacerbation of chronic respiratory failure. Acute respiratory failure is the respiratory failure appearing in the individual whose lung was structurally

TABLE 24-1. PARAMETERS FOR MONITORING RESPIRATORY CARE

Basic Monitoring	*Fluid Balance*
Blood pressure	Fluid intake
Heart rate	Fluid output
Respiratory rate	Weight
Temperature	
Electrocardiogram	*Blood Tests*
	Electrolytes
Respiratory Parameters	Hemoglobin and hematocrit
Chest auscultation	White cell count
Tidal volume	
Vital capacity	*Urinalysis*
Respiratory force	
Compliance	*Cardiovascular Parameters*
Inspired oxygen concentration	Pulmonary capillary wedge
Alveolar to arterial oxygen	pressure
tension difference	Cardiac output
Chest X-ray	

and functionally normal before the onset of the present illness. Chronic respiratory failure is the respiratory failure seen in individuals with chronic lung diseases such as chronic bronchitis, emphysema, and black lung disease (coal miner's disease). These patients develop a tolerance to the gradually worsening hypoxia and hypercapnia. Following acute respiratory failure, the lung usually returns to its original state. In chronic respiratory failure the structural damage is irreversible. The principles of management of these two conditions are different; this discussion will be confined to acute respiratory failure.

Causes of acute respiratory failure are numerous and may be subdivided into various categories. One major group includes those diseases in which respiratory failure results from inadequate ventilation; the lung itself remains structurally normal in the early stages. One of the most important causes of inadequate ventilation is upper airway obstruction. Its etiology, diagnosis, and management are discussed on page 449.

Central nervous system depression will also result in inadequate ventilation. The respiratory center, which controls every breath, lies in the lower part of the brain stem (pons and medulla). Drug overdose, head injury, cerebrovascular accidents, brain tumors, encephalitis, meningitis, hypoxia, and hypercapnia are all capable of depressing the respiratory center. In these patients, respiration becomes slow and shallow. Respiratory arrest may occur in severe cases.

The impulses arising in the respiratory center travel in nerves that extend from the brain stem down the spinal cord to receptors in the muscles of respiration. Any disease of the nerves, spinal cord, muscles, or neuromuscular junction involved in respiration would seriously affect ventilation. Polyneuritis, myasthenia gravis, damage to the cervical segment of the spinal cord, and poliomyelitis are examples of such diseases.

Respiratory failure due to inadequate ventilation should be looked for in the immediate postoperative period, especially following major thoracic or upper abdominal surgery. The reasons for respiratory failure during this period are numerous. The effects of anesthetic drugs (morphine, pentothal, droperidol) are long-lasting. They depress respiration by their own effects or by enhancing the effects of narcotics used for pain control. Pain in the thoracic and abdominal area interferes with deep breathing and coughing. Muscle relaxants (drugs which paralyze muscles) are frequently used during anesthesia. Some patients may have difficulty in breaking down or excreting these drugs, so that their effects last longer than usual, making patients weak in the postoperative period. Ventilation/perfusion abnormality also accounts for respiratory failure following major abdominal and thoracic operations.

Pleural effusion, hemothorax, and pneumothorax are a group of conditions that interfere with ventilation by preventing expansion of the lung. They are usually produced by an underlying lung disease or pleural disease.

Trauma resulting from motor vehicle accidents is a very common cause of acute respiratory failure. In this type of accident head injury, unconsciousness, and bleeding from nose and mouth lead to upper airway obstruction and respiratory depression. Hemothorax, pneumothorax, and rib fractures may occur and may be responsible for inadequate ventilation. Flail chest may also occur and may lead to respiratory failure.

There are many acute diseases of the lung that may lead to acute respiratory failure. Of these diseases, pneumonia is perhaps the commonest. It is usually caused by viral or bacterial activity. Chemical pneumonitis is pneumonia produced by the inhalation of irritant fumes or the aspiration of acidic gastric material. Bronchial asthma, atelectasis, pulmonary embolism, and pulmonary edema are some other conditions that cause acute respiratory failure.

ADULT RESPIRATORY DISTRESS SYNDROME (RDS)

Most patients in acute respiratory failure get better with the proper management of airway ventilation and oxygenation. However, a small group of patients do not respond to this treatment. They become severely hypoxic (P_aO_2 to 50 mm. Hg) in spite of adequate ventilation with 100 percent oxygen. These symptoms are caused by widespread injury to the alveolar capillary bed. Adult respiratory distress is the name given to this clinical picture.

Clinical Manifestations

The clinical features of the syndrome include initial severe illness with no pulmonary component, followed by a latent period in which pulmonary abnormalities are minimal. There is a subsequent period of progressive respiratory disease with dyspnea and hypoxia. The x-ray will show bilateral involvement of the lungs leading to pulmonary edema.

Adult respiratory distress syndrome frequently results from pneumonia or shock. The pneumonia is usually caused by a virus but may be caused by microorganisms such as bacteria, rickettsia, or leptospira. Chemical pneumonitis, which follows inhalation of noxious fumes or aspiration of acidic gastric material, accounts for some patients' having pneumonia. Shock is usually due to blood loss but may be caused by septicemia.

Motor vehicle accident or gunshot injuries account for the incidence of shock due to blood loss. However, blood loss occurring during childbirth, ruptured aortic aneurysm, ruptured esophageal varices, peptic ulceration, and major surgery may also lead to shock. Adult RDS may also follow massive fat embolism, acute pancreatitis, massive blood transfusions, and extracorporeal circulation for open-heart surgery.

Pathophysiology

In spite of the different causes the clinical picture, pathophysiology, and pathology are similar. RDS appears 6 to 48 hours after the onset of the illness. The patient develops respiratory distess; the rate of breathing increases (tachypnea) and may reach 40 breaths per minute. Each breath is shallow and labored (dyspnea) and may be associated with grunting. Retraction of the intercostal and suprasternal areas is seen during inspiration. Widening of the alae nasi and contractions of the accessory muscles of respiration are other signs of respiratory distress.

Cyanosis appears and fails to respond to oxygen therapy. Evidence of cerebral hypoxia such as anxiety, confusion, irritability, lack of cooperation, drowsiness, and mental obtundation may appear. Hypoxia of the heart will result in tachycardia, arrhythmias, and hypotension.

Auscultatory findings are minimal in the early stages, but later bronchial breathing may be heard. In the early stages chest x-ray may show patchy alveolar infiltrates in both lungs which later become more diffuse.

As was mentioned before, the arterial oxygen tension (P_aO_2) is low (usually around 50 torr) even when the patient is breathing 100 percent oxygen. In other words, the alveolar to arterial oxygen gradient, $P_{(A-a)}O_2$, is widened. Severe hypoxia is the result of extensive shunting in the lungs. The functional residual capacity (FRC) is markedly diminished. When the FRC falls below the closing capacity, small airways close and the air in the corresponding alveoli is absorbed leading to their atelectasis. Oxygen cannot reach the alveolar capillaries, and the blood passing through these capillaries constitutes shunted blood.

Pulmonary edema (fluid in the alveoli) and interstitial

TABLE 24-2. INDICATIONS FOR RESPIRATORY SUPPORT*

		ACCEPTABLE RANGE	CHEST PHYSICAL THERAPY OXYGEN CLOSE MONITORING	ENDOTRACHEAL INTUBATION TRACHEOSTOMY VENTILATION
Muscle Power	1. Respiratory rate per minute	12-25	25-35	>35
	2. Vital capacity ml./kg. (ideal body weight)	70-30	30-15	<15
	3. Inspiratory force in negative cm. H$_2$O	100-50	50-25	<20
Oxygenation	Alveolar to arterial O$_2$ tension gradient in mm. Hg**	50-200	200-350	>450
	pO$_2$ mm. Hg	100-75 air	200-75 (on mask O$_2$)	<70
Ventilation	pCO$_2$ mm. Hg	35-45	45-60	>60†

*(Adapted from Pontoppidan, H.: Treatment of respiratory failure in nonthoracic trauma. J. Trauma, *8*:940, 1968.)
**After 15 minutes of 100% O$_2$.
†Except in chronic hypercapnea.

Recognition of Respiratory Complications: Table 24-2 shows objective practical guidelines used in the bedside evaluation of the patient's respiratory status. (*The trend of change in values is of utmost importance.*) The first column refers to the values of normal acceptable range. The second column lists borderline values where chest physical therapy, oxygen, and close monitoring are essential. The third column lists values which indicate the necessity of intubation, tracheostomy, or ventilation.

edema (fluid in the lung substance) are also seen and contribute to hypoxia. As a result of all of these changes the lung becomes more stiff (low compliance).

Adult respiratory distress syndrome used to be associated with high mortality. The use of positive end expiratory pressure (PEEP) has increased the survival rate.

MANAGEMENT OF RESPIRATORY FAILURE

The principles of management of acute respiratory failure are the following:

1. Treat the cause.
2. Maintain a good airway.
3. Provide adequate ventilation.
4. Provide optimum oxygen.
5. Carry out chest physiotherapy.

Treatment of the cause may involve evacuating the pleural cavity, giving antibiotic treatment for infection, reversing effects of drugs or accelerating their excretion, decreasing raised intracranial pressures, etc. Diseases such as bronchial asthma and pulmonary edema require specific therapy. In some illnesses, such as polyneuritis and poliomyelitis, one has to wait for the illness to resolve.

To maintain a good airway it may be necessary to intubate the patient or to do a tracheostomy. Once the airway is clear, adequacy of ventilation must be assessed by measuring the respiratory rate, tidal volume, vital capacity, inspiratory force, and arterial carbon dioxide tensions (P$_a$CO$_2$). Depending on the results the patient is allowed to breathe spontaneously or is helped by a ven-

tilator (see Table 24-2) and by being monitored in the intensive care unit.

The arterial oxygen tension (P$_a$O$_2$) will show the degree of oxygenation.

Administration of Oxygen

The concentration of oxygen in air is 21 percent. Another way of expressing the same fact is to say that the fraction of inspired oxygen (F$_I$O$_2$) is 0.21. The F$_I$O$_2$ may be increased by the addition of oxygen to inspired air. The oxygen must always be humidified to prevent drying of the upper airway or secretions in the airway. Nasal prongs, nasal catheters, or face masks are commonly used to administer oxygen to the spontaneously breathing patient.

With nasal prongs or catheters the F$_I$O$_2$ varies between 0.24 to 0.44 (24% to 44%).

The actual F$_I$O$_2$ depends on:

1. Flow rate of oxygen
2. Degree of mouth breathing
3. Patency of nasal passages
4. Depth of insertion of nasal catheter

Table 24-3 shows the approximate F$_I$O$_2$ obtained with various flow rates of oxygen delivered with nasal prongs or catheters. When blood is taken to measure arterial blood gases, always note the flow rate of oxygen or, better still, measure the F$_I$O$_2$ with an oxygen analyzer. It may be necessary to pass a small cannula into the pharynx to obtain a sample of well mixed inspired gas.

When a higher concentration or a very precise concentration of oxygen needs to be delivered, face masks

TABLE 24-3. GUIDELINES FOR ESTIMATING F_IO_2 IN ADULTS WITH LOW-FLOW OXYGEN DEVICE

A. NASAL CANNULA OR CATHETER 100% O_2		B. OXYGEN MASK 100% O_2		C. MASK WITH RESERVOIR BAG 100% O_2	
FLOW RATE IN LITERS	F_IO_2	FLOW RATE IN LITERS	F_IO_2	FLOW RATE IN LITERS	F_IO_2
1 L	24%	5-6 L	40%	6 L	60%
2 L	28%	6-7 L	50%	7 L	70%
3 L	32%	7-8 L	60%	8 L	80%
4 L	36%			9 L	90%
5 L	40%			10 L	99+%
6 L	44%				

Note: Normal respiratory pattern is assumed.

With these basic guidelines for the concentration of oxygen administration we are capable of increasing or decreasing the inspired oxygen concentrations within reasonable predictable limits in correlation with the arterial blood gas results.

are preferable. The various types of face masks available include aerosol face masks, venturi face masks, and face masks with reservoir bags which may or may not allow rebreathing. The aerosol face masks are light and acceptable to most patients. They provide oxygen concentration of 60 percent to 80 percent with flow rates of 8 to 10 liters per minute of 100 percent oxygen. The flow rates must be equal to or greater than the minute ventilation of the patient. Table 24-3 (B) shows the relationship of flow rates to the F_IO_2.

Some masks are fitted with a reservoir bag which fills with oxygen and functions as a reservoir of oxygen. These masks may be provided with valves which keep the exhaled gas from entering the reservoir and thus prevent rebreathing of the exhaled gas. The inspired oxygen concentration is usually above 60 percent with these masks (Table 24-3 [C]).

The aerosol masks and masks with reservoir bags must fit tightly over the face in order to function properly.

Ventimasks are based on the Venturi principle. These masks are so constructed that as the oxygen flows at a set rate through an orifice it traps and mixes a precise amount of the surrounding air to give the desired oxygen concentration. Masks are available which provide 24, 26, 35 and 40 percent oxygen. Ventimasks need not fit tightly over the face.

If the patient has an endotracheal tube or a tracheostomy, a T-bar (Briggs adapter) is used for the administration of oxygen (Fig. 24-7). Since the upper airway is bypassed in these patients the inspired air must be humidified.

The percentage of oxygen inspired by the patient depends on (1) the diluter valve setting of the nebulizer, (2) the output of the nebulizer, (3) the reservoir tube on the expiratory limb, and (4) the inspiratory effort of the patient.

The diluter valve setting puts an upper limit on the inspired oxygen concentration. This concentration may be reduced by air pulled in via the expiratory limb during the inspiratory effort of the patient. By increasing the nebulizer outflow and by using a reservoir tube on the expiratory limb, air dilution may be reduced or completely eliminated.

Humidification

The air we breathe contains water in the form of vapor. This is referred to as humidity. The amount of water vapor present in the air at any time varies with the weather conditions and greatly influences our comfort. A given volume of air at a given temperature cannot contain more than a certain amount of water vapor, and when it contains the maximum amount of water vapor it is said to be 100 percent saturated.

If the temperature of this sample of air is raised, more water vapor will have to be added to it to saturate it to 100 percent. Whatever the temperature and percentage saturation of the air we breathe, it is rendered 100 percent saturated at body temperature when it passes through the nose and reaches the lower part of the trachea.

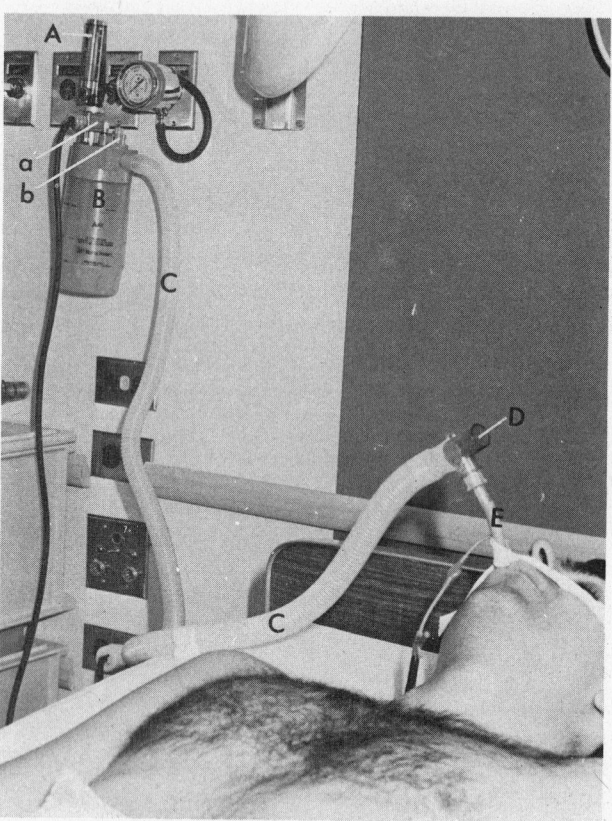

Figure 24-7. The T-bar. Lettered items are as follows: (A) oxygen flow meter; (B) Nebulizer—(a) heater, (b) diluter valve; (C) disposable hose; (D) T-bar; (reservoir tube, 50-200 ml. can be attached at (D); (E) endotracheal tube.

The oxygen that is commercially available is totally devoid of water vapor (100 percent dry) and humidifiers are required to provide the water vapor that will make oxygen breathing comfortable and prevent drying up of the respiratory tract and the secretions therein. If the patient is using his own airway, a simple humidifier may be used that will add some water vapor to the oxygen and allow the patient's airway to saturate it to 100 percent. A simple humidifier is formed by bubbling oxygen through water. Its efficiency is increased by various methods that make the bubbles very small. Many disposable simple humidifiers are available which produce 80 to 100 percent saturated oxygen at room temperature (100 percent saturated oxygen at room temperature becomes 37 percent saturated at body temperature unless more water vapor is added).

A patient breathing via an endotracheal tube or a fresh tracheostomy must be provided with 100 percent saturated air at body temperature. This may be achieved by heating the water in the humidifier to a temperature above that of the body and letting the humidified oxygen cool to body temperature as it passes through the delivery tube. Many mechanical ventilators use this technique.

Alternatively, a nebulizer may be used to provide humidity. A nebulizer produces small particles of water, some of which evaporate to produce water vapor. Suspension of small particles in gas is referred to as an *aerosol*. There are several types of nebulizers. The Puritan nebulizer is capable of delivering aerosol for a long period. It also traps air which dilutes the oxygen. By adjusting a valve on the nebulizer, it is possible to set the nebulizer to deliver 40, 60, 70, or 100 percent oxygen. Because of air entrapment, when the nebulizer is set at 40 percent and 10 liters of 100 percent O_2 per minute are run through, 40 liters per minute of 40 percent oxygen with water particles are delivered by the nebulizer.

Positive End Expiratory Pressure (PEEP)

Positive end expiratory pressure (PEEP) means the airway pressure remains higher than atmospheric pressure at the end of expiration. Normally, during spontaneous breathing or during mechanical ventilation, at the end of expiration the airway pressure equals the atmospheric pressure (zero end expiratory pressure). The airway pressure is measured in centimeters of water (cm. H_2O). The usual range of PEEP used is 5 to 15 cm. H_2O. However, higher PEEP values (20 to 35 cm. H_2O) are also used.

PEEP may be applied to a patient on a mechanical ventilator. Such a patient would have positive airway pressure during inspiration and expiration and at the end of expiration. The term "continuous positive pressure ventilation" (CPPV) is sometimes used to describe this situation. When PEEP is applied to a patient who is breathing spontaneously (via his or her own airway, an endotracheal tube, or a tracheostomy) it is called CPAP (continuous positive airway pressure).

However, PEEP can be regulated so that a spontaneously breathing patient on PEEP will have zero airway pressure during the inspiratory phase. We cannot strictly apply the term CPAP to this method. The term sPEEP (spontaneous PEEP) has been used by some to describe the situation.

When PEEP is applied, the FRC is increased, so that small airway closure is prevented. PEEP also splints the airways. With PEEP, shunting is decreased and compliance is improved. The end result is improved oxygenation, as is demonstrated by the decrease in the alveolar to arterial oxygen tension gradient $P_{(A-a)}O_2$. With improved oxygenation the F_IO_2 may be reduced to less toxic levels.

PEEP may produce some undesirable results. A fall in cardiac output may be seen when more than 5 cm. of H_2O PEEP are used.

- The amount of oxygen carried to the tissues per minute (oxygen flux) depends as much on the cardiac output as on the degrees of oxygenation. Care must be taken not to compromise oxygen flux by decreasing the cardiac output.

Other complications reported with PEEP include pneumothorax, pneumomediastinum, and interstitial emphysema.

UPPER AIRWAY OBSTRUCTION

The trachea, larynx, pharynx, nose, and mouth constitute the upper airway. It is vital that this pathway remain patent at all times. The swallowing reflex, the cough reflex, and the tone of the muscles of the pharynx and the larynx ensure that patency is maintained.

However, airway obstruction sometimes does occur. Food particles, vomitus, blood clots, or any other particle that enters the trachea or larynx can obstruct the airway.

Epiglottitis, laryngeal edema, laryngeal carcinoma, and peritonsillar abscess are conditions in which the airway is obstructed by masses arising from the walls of the airway. Thick secretions may also cause airway obstruction. Sometimes obstruction may be produced by collapse of the walls of the airway. Such is the case with retrosternal goiter, enlarged mediastinal lymph nodes, hematomas around the upper airway and thoracic aneurysm, all of which push upon the wall of the upper airway, leading to its collapse. Upper airway obstruction is very commonly seen in mentally obtunded (unconscious, comatose) patients. These patients lose their protective reflexes as well as the tone of the pharyngeal muscles, with the result that the tongue falls back and obstructs the airway.

Nursing Assessment for Upper Airway Obstruction

Observe the patient for the following signs of upper airway obstruction.

1. Inspiration will cause indrawing of parts of the upper chest, sternum, and intercostal spaces.
2. Exhalation will be characterized by a jerky protrusion and prolonged, somewhat sustained contraction of the abdominal muscles, followed by a brief relaxation before another contraction.
3. Seesaw movement of the chest and abdomen may ensue (combination of 1 and 2 above). (As the inspiratory muscles contract, an inward thoracic depression results while relaxed abdominal muscles are jerkily pushed up. Exhalation is produced by a labored and prolonged abdominal muscle contraction, causing a jerky upward push of the thorax.)
4. Tracheal tug, or indrawing of the suprasternal notch may occur.

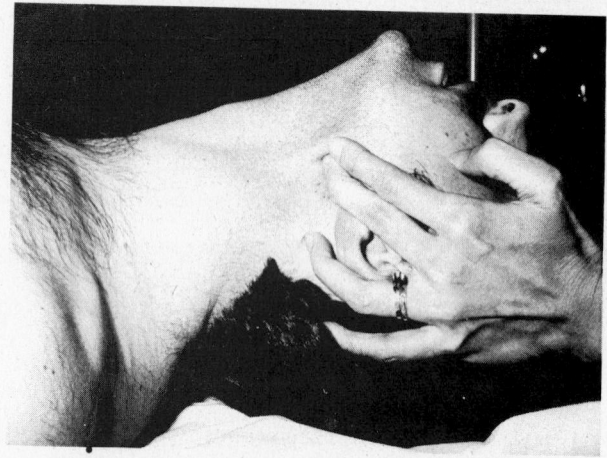

Figure 24-8. To clear upper airway of obstruction, extend the head and push mandible forward.

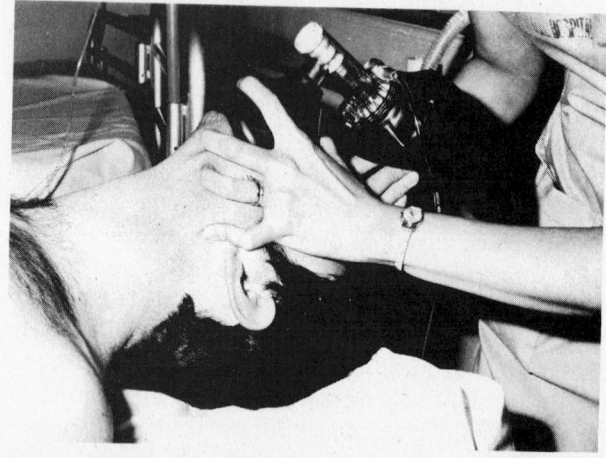

Figure 24-9. Bag and mask ventilation. The head is extended and the mask is sealed to the face by pressing the left thumb on the bridge of the nose and the index finger on the chin. The remaining three fingers pull the chin and mandible upward to maintain the head in extension. The right hand then squeezes the bag.

Management of Upper Airway Obstruction

As soon as upper airway obstruction is diagnosed, measures must be taken to correct it.

- The mouth is opened to see if the tongue has fallen back or if there are secretions, blood clots, or any particles obstructing the airway. Secretions must be suctioned and any particulate matter in the pharynx must be removed immediately with forceps or by suctioning.
- Extension of the head is the simplest way of relieving upper airway obstruction caused by the tongue's falling back. The head must be extended at the atlanto-occipital joint. This will increase the distance between the chin and the cervical spine, which puts the muscles that support the tongue under tension and pulls the tongue forward.
- If simple extension of the head is not adequate to clear the airway, the mandible should be forced forward. This maneuver is designed to put further tension on the musculature that supports the tongue. It is best executed by standing behind the patient and placing the tips of the index finger and middle finger on each side along the ascending ramus of the mandible. The mandible is lifted upwards by exerting pressure on the ascending ramus of the mandible and at the same time tilting the head backward (Fig. 24-8). The fingers and the palm of each hand are applied on each side of the face in order to maintain the extension of the head.
- If this maneuver is not adequate and partial airway obstruction still exists, then an oral airway may have to be inserted and/or endotracheal intubation done. Unconsciousness and loss of protective airway reflexes require endotracheal intubation to maintain a patent airway and prevent aspiration. Temporary relief is obtained by pulling the tongue out with thick gauze.
- If assisted ventilation is required, a resuscitator bag and mask are used initially prior to intubation and mechanical ventilation. The mask is sealed onto the patient's face by pressing the mask with the left thumb on the bridge of the nose while the index finger presses around the lips. At the same time the rest of the fingers of the left hand pull on the chin and the angle of the mandible to maintain the head in extension (Fig. 24-9). The right hand inflates the lungs by periodically squeezing the bag.

Endotracheal Intubation

Endotracheal intubation refers to the passing of a tube through the mouth or nose into the trachea. It is done to provide an airway when the patient is having respiratory difficulty that cannot be treated by simpler methods. It is the method of choice in emergency care. Endotracheal intubation can be used as a means of assisting respiration for patients who cannot maintain an adequate airway on their own (comatose patients; those with upper airway obstruction), and it provides an excellent means for suctioning secretions from the pulmonary tree.

An endotracheal tube usually is passed by means of a laryngoscope. A cuff around the tube is inflated to prevent leakage around the outer part of the tube and to minimize the possibility of subsequent aspiration. (Suctioning of the tracheobronchial secretions is done through the tube.) Warm humidified oxygen can be introduced through the tube, or the tube may be connected to ventilatory equipment. Endotracheal intubation may be used for up to 72 hours. Then a tracheostomy should be considered.

As in any other treatment modality there are disadvantages associated with endotracheal or tracheostomy tubes. For one thing, the tube causes discomfort. But, more important, the cough reflex is depressed because closure of the glottis is hindered, and this prevents the generation of the high intrathoracic airway pressure necessary to produce an expulsive cough. Secretions tend to become thick and viscid because the warming and humidifying effect of the upper respiratory tract has been bypassed. The swallowing reflexes, composed of the glottic, pharyngeal, and laryngeal reflexes, also are depressed because of prolonged disuse and the mechanical trauma due to the presence of the endotracheal or tracheostomy tube. Ulceration and stricture of the larynx or trachea may develop. Finally, the patient is not able to talk. For nursing management of the patient on endotracheal intubation see the outline below.

Tracheostomy

A tracheotomy is an operation in which an opening is made into the trachea. When an indwelling tube is inserted into the trachea, the term "tracheostomy" is used. A tracheostomy may be either temporary or permanent.

A tracheostomy is done to bypass an upper airway obstruction, to remove tracheobronchial secretions, to permit the use of mechanical ventilation, to prevent aspiration of oral or gastric secretions in the unconscious or paralyzed patient (by closing off the trachea from the esophagus), and to replace an endotracheal tube. There are many disease processes and emergency conditions that make a tracheostomy necessary.

The procedure is usually done in the operating room or in an intensive care unit where the patient's ventilation can be well controlled. An opening is made in the 2nd and 3rd tracheal rings. After the trachea is exposed, a cuffed tracheostomy tube of an appropriate size is inserted (Fig. 24-10). The cuff is an inflatable attachment to a tracheostomy or endotracheal tube which is designed to provide the snug fit required for mechanical ventilation.

The tracheostomy tube is held in place by tapes fastened around the patient's neck. Usually a square of sterile gauze is placed between the tube and the skin before the tape is tied (Fig. 24-10 B).

Immediate Postoperative Care. The patient requires continuing nursing monitoring and assessment. The newly made opening must be kept patent by proper suctioning of secretions. (See page 452). After the vital signs are stable, the patient may be placed in a semi-Fowler's position to facilitate respiration, promote drainage, minimize edema, and prevent strain on the suture lines. Analgesic and sedative drugs are given with caution since it is undesirable to depress the cough reflex.

NURSING MANAGEMENT OF THE PATIENT UNDERGOING ENDOTRACHEAL INTUBATION

1. Check symmetry of chest expansion.
   a. Auscultate breath sounds of anterior and posterior chest bilaterally.
   b. Do this immediately and then every 30 minutes to 1 hour.
2. Ensure a high humidity.
   a. A visible mist should be seen from the T-bar or inspiratory limb of the respirator.
   b. The oxygen concentration is prescribed by physician depending upon arterial blood gas analysis (page 442).
3. Secure the tube to the face with tape and mark the proximal end for position maintenance.
   a. Cut proximal end of tube if it is longer than 7.5 cm. (3 inches) to prevent kinking.
   b. An oral airway or mouth bite should be in place to stabilize the tube and prevent the patient from biting on the tube.
4. If the cuff is not of the low pressure type, deflate the cuff every 2 hours.
   a. Thoroughly suction the endotracheal tube and then the oropharynx prior to deflation.
   b. Use sterile suction technique and airway care to prevent iatrogenic contamination and infection.

5. "Sigh" or hyperinflate the patient every hour to open up atelectatic alveoli.
   a. A self-inflating bag is used if the patient is on T-bar or pressure controlled ventilator.
   b. Volume respirators have a built-in sighing mechanism.
6. Give oral hygiene and suction the oropharynx whenever necessary.
7. To extubate the patient (remove the tube):
   a. Have self-inflating bag and mask ready in case ventilatory assistance is required immediately after extubation.
   b. Suction the tracheobronchial tree and oropharynx before deflating the cuff.
   c. Give oxygen for a few breaths, and then remove the tube.

Care of Patient Following Removal of the Endotracheal Tube

1. Give heated humidity and oxygen via face mask.
2. Monitor respiratory rate and quality of chest excursions. Note stridor, color change, change in mental alertness or personality.
3. Give coughing and deep breathing exercises for the next few days.

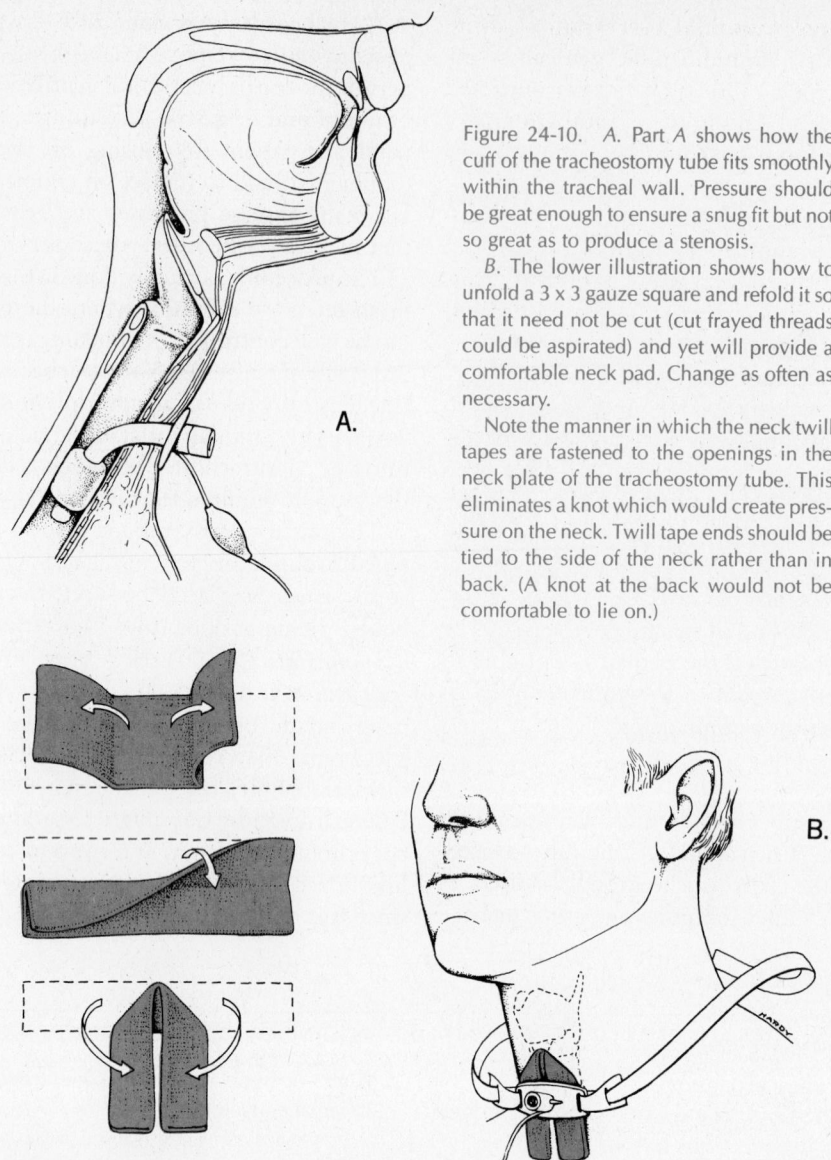

Figure 24-10. *A.* Part *A* shows how the cuff of the tracheostomy tube fits smoothly within the tracheal wall. Pressure should be great enough to ensure a snug fit but not so great as to produce a stenosis.

B. The lower illustration shows how to unfold a 3 x 3 gauze square and refold it so that it need not be cut (cut frayed threads could be aspirated) and yet will provide a comfortable neck pad. Change as often as necessary.

Note the manner in which the neck twill tapes are fastened to the openings in the neck plate of the tracheostomy tube. This eliminates a knot which would create pressure on the neck. Twill tape ends should be tied to the side of the neck rather than in back. (A knot at the back would not be comfortable to lie on.)

Another objective of nursing care is to alleviate the apprehension of the patient. He needs reassurance for he may have a real fear that he will asphyxiate while he is asleep. Since the patient cannot speak, paper and pencil or magic slate should be kept near him so that he has a means of communication. A tap bell or other signaling device should be within his reach.

Removal of Secretions; Tracheostomy Suction

When a tracheostomy is present, it is necessary to suction the patient's secretions, since his own cough mechanism is not as effective. Tracheostomy suctioning is performed every 1 to 2 hours or whenever secretions are present. Unnecessary suctioning can initiate bronchospasm and cause mechanical trauma to the tracheal mucosa.

All equipment that comes into direct contact with the patient's airway must be sterile, in order to prevent overwhelming pulmonary and systemic infections. The following equipment is used: (a) suction catheters, (b) gloves, (c) 5 to 10 ml. syringe, (d) normal saline poured in a cup for irrigation, (e) the patient's own self-inflating bag (hand resuscitator) with supplemental oxygen (the bag should be changed daily to reduce infection), and (f) suction machine.

- Explain the procedure to the patient before beginning and reassure him during suctioning, since he most likely is apprehensive about choking and about his inability to communicate.
- Begin by washing hands thoroughly. Then open sterile package containing catheter and gloves. Connect the catheter end (not tip) to suction tubing before putting on the gloves. It is all right to touch one end of the catheter with a bare hand, since the catheter end will not enter the patient's airway. Put the

glove on the hand that will guide the suction catheter. With the gloved hand, pull the catheter from the package, being careful not to contaminate it. Wet the catheter tip with sterile saline to lubricate it.

- One nurse should suction the patient while a second nurse ventilates and oxygenates him with a self-inflating bag. Before deflating the cuff, suction around the pharynx to remove regurgitated stomach contents or other secretions. Discard the catheter.

- Take patient off the mechanical ventilator or T-bar. The free end of the connection respirator should be anchored to the machine without contamination. Then deflate the cuff.

- Inflate the patient's lungs with the self-inflating bag containing supplemental oxygen to prevent hypoxia and sudden cardiovascular collapse during suctioning. Insert a second sterile catheter deep into the airway. Then apply suction while gently rotating the catheter out of the bronchial tree. (Suction superficial secretions first.) The aspiration should not exceed 10 to 15 seconds, since the patient can become hypoxic with subsequent arrhythmias and cardiac arrest. Give the patient a breath with the machine or the self-inflating bag with supplemental oxygen after each suction; always inflate the tracheostomy cuff before giving this breath.

- Instill about 2 to 3 ml. of sterile normal saline into the trachea as illustrated in Figure 24-12, page 464.

- It is important not to tire the patient. When suction is completed, return the patient to the ventilator. Reinflate the cuff until the air leak disappears. Listen to the breath sounds bilaterally with a stethoscope. Respiration should be quiet and essentially effortless at the end of inspiration. Check exhaled tidal volume and thoracic expansion.

(The care of the patient with a tracheostomy is summarized below and on page 454.)

THE CARE OF THE PATIENT WITH A TRACHEOSTOMY

Tracheostomy Care	Rationale
A. Tracheostomy cuff 1. Cuffed tube (air injected into cuff) is required during prolonged mechanical ventilation.	1. The purpose of a cuffed tube is to prevent air from leaking during positive pressure ventilation and to prevent tracheal aspiration of gastric contents. A good seal is indicated by the disappearance of any air leakage from the tracheostomy or disappearance of the harsh gurgling sound of air coming from the throat.

2. Types of cuff:
   a. Low pressure cuff (preferred)
 	
   b. High pressure cuff
	2. a. Low pressure cuffs exert minimal pressure on the tracheal mucosa and thus reduce the danger of tracheal ulceration and stricture. Periodic deflation is not necessary.
	   b. Recommend periodic deflation of high pressure cuff to allow return of circulation in the tracheal wall.

3. Indications for cuff deflation	3. a. Allowed during spontaneous ventilation if there is no danger of aspiration.
	   b. Periodic deflation for 2 to 3 minutes every 1 to 2 hours if possible during controlled ventilation provided satisfactory air exchange and chest expansion are still present. Deflation is controlled by adjusting the volume and air flow on the ventilator.
	   If the patient has stiff lungs, in spite of respiratory adjustment, air exchange will not be satisfactory with deflated cuff because high airway pressures are needed. Therefore, in these patients, the cuff should be kept inflated.

B. Dressing and skin care
 	
  1. Wash hands.
  2. Explain procedure to patient.
 	
  3. Remove twill tapes (if soiled) by untying.
  4. Hold tube in place and replace tape immediately.
	B. The tracheostomy dressing is changed PRN to keep the skin clean and dry. Do not allow moist or soiled dressings to remain on the skin.
	
	  2. A patient with a tracheostomy is apprehensive and requires continuing assurance and support.
	
	  4. Tracheostomy tube can be dislodged by movement or forceful cough. It is difficult to reinsert the tracheostomy tube in a fresh tracheostomy. Airway catastrophe may occur if the tracheostomy tube is dislodged.

(Continued)

THE CARE OF THE PATIENT WITH A TRACHEOSTOMY (CONTINUED)

Tracheostomy Care (Continued)   **Rationale (Continued)**

5. Clean tracheostomy area with water and peroxide solution.
6. Place clean twill tapes in position to secure tracheostomy tube. Make a horizontal slit 2.5 cm. (1 inch) from end of tape. Insert this end of the tie through the side opening of the outer cannula. The opposite end of the tie can be threaded through the slit end, drawn securely, and fastened at the side of the neck.
7. Remove soiled dressing and discard.
8. Put on sterile gloves.
9. Cleanse wound with sterile applicators or textile cleaners moistened with dilute hydrogen peroxide.
10. Cleanse entire flange of tracheostomy tube with sterile textile cleaner or sterile applicator moistened with dilute hydrogen peroxide. Do not allow solution to enter tracheostomy.
11. Use neosporin or betadine ointment on the edge of the tracheostomy wound.
12. Use sterile tracheostomy dressing from the wrappers and fit securely under the twill tapes and flange of tracheostomy tube so that the incision is covered (Fig. 24-11B).

10. Fluid entering the tracheostomy will irritate the respiratory tract.

12. Dressings which will shred are not used around a tracheostomy because of the danger that pieces of material, lint, or thread may get into the tube, and eventually the trachea, causing obstruction or abscess formation. Special dressings that do not have a tendency to shred are used.

C. Changing of tracheostomy tube
1. Varies from 3 to 5 days.

2. Only a skilled physician should change a fresh tracheostomy.
3. A nurse can change the tracheostomy tube if a patent stomal tract has developed.
4. Have resuscitation equipment ready.

5. Procedure:
  a. Suction tracheostomy and oropharynx.
  b. Cut off twill ties.
  c. Remove tracheostomy tube.
  d. Insert new tracheostomy tube with obturator following the curvature of the tube until it is set in place.
  e. Remove stylet, inflate cuff, tie twill ties.
  f. Apply tracheostomy dressing.

1. Depends upon amount of crust and thickened secretions adhering to the tracheostomy tube.
2. Because airway problems can develop. Original stomal tract may be hard to find.

4. In case airway problems develop in the process of changing.

THE PATIENT REQUIRING MECHANICAL VENTILATION

Assessment of the Patient Requiring Mechanical Ventilation. A mechanical ventilator is a positive pressure breathing device which can maintain respiration automatically for prolonged periods. It is indicated when the patient is unable to maintain safe levels of arterial carbon dioxide and/or oxygen by spontaneous breathing.

An outline for evaluating clinical and pulmonary function for patients on mechanical ventilation is located on page 456. It will enable the nurse to intelligently care for the patient and allow early recognition of his problems and progress.

Managing the Patient on Mechanical Ventilation. Numerous factors influence the management of the patient on a mechanical ventilator. Table 24-4 and the tabular material found on pages 455-463 present a summary view of factors that must be considered when nursing care is provided.

Adjustment of the Ventilator. The ventilator is adjusted so that the patient is comfortable and "in phase" with the machine (Fig. 24-11). Minimal alteration of the normal cardiovascular and pulmonary dynamics is

ASSESSMENT OF PATIENTS REQUIRING MECHANICAL VENTILATION

General Assessment

1. Assess the level of responsiveness. Restlessness may indicate early hypoxia, whereas drowsiness may signify increasing PCO_2 due to hypoventilation. Determine whether the drowsiness is due to hypoventilation or to lack of sleep, which is a problem inherent in many intensive care units as a result of frequent interruptions to monitor vital signs, do blood work, and administer medications. A check of arterial blood gases will reveal the presence or absence of increasing PCO_2.

2. Determine the degree of respiratory distress. Observe to see the degree of muscle power the patient exerts while breathing.

3. Monitor the patient's temperature. The onset, degree, and pattern of rise in temperature will show the patient's progress and response to therapy. A high temperature causes an increase in oxygen consumption. Very low temperatures may cause some degree of cardiorespiratory depression or arrhythmia.

Assessment of Respiratory Function

1. Check respiratory rate.
2. Note color.
3. Auscultate the chest. (Note air entry and presence or absence of added sounds.)
4. Note bedside pulmonary functions:
   a. Tidal volume
   b. Vital capacity
   c. Minute volume
   d. Inspiratory force
5. Note color, quantity, and consistency of sputum.
6. Note quality of cough effort in its ability to bring up secretions.
7. Provide humidity to the inspired gases. Low humidity will cause drying and inspissation of pulmonary secretions.

8. Know the changes in airway pressure on the machine. Decreased airway pressure may be due to presence of a leak with subsequent low tidal volume. Increased airway pressure may be due to:
   a. Secretions
   b. Airway obstruction
   c. Pulmonary edema
   d. Bronchospasm
   e. Pneumothorax
   f. Flail chest
9. Check chest x-ray evaluation.
10. Check laboratory evaluation.
    a. Culture and sensitivity of tracheobronchial secretions every 3 days
    b. WBC and differential
11. Arterial blood gas assessment: PO_2, PCO_2, pH, base excess or deficit, Hgb or hematocrit.

Assessment of Cardiovascular and Renal Function

1. Systemic BP
2. Heart rate
3. CVP
4. ECG
5. Fluid and electrolyte balance
6. Hypo- and hyperkalemia
7. Presence of ostomies
8. Urine output/hour and specific gravity
9. Serum creatinine and BUN
10. Total protein

Assessment of Neurological Status (pages 83-88)
   a. Motor and sensory function
   b. Pupillary size and light reflex

sought. Arterial blood gases should be satisfactory and auscultation of the chest should indicate good bilateral gas exchange.

The following guidelines are recommended for the initial adjustment of the ventilator for a patient:

1. Set the machine to deliver tidal volume required (10 to 15 ml./kg.).
2. Adjust the machine to deliver 100 percent inspired oxygen or whatever is necessary to maintain normal P_aO_2 (70 to 100 torr).
3. Record peak inspiratory pressure.
4. Adjust inspiratory-expiratory ratio. Within the above criteria, make a setting that will provide satisfactory blood gases, with adequate tidal volume and inspiratory-expiratory ratio at the minimum airway pressure.
5. If the patient is not controlled, adjust sensitivity so that the patient can trigger the machine with a minimum effort. Adjust the rate to provide normal PCO_2 (38 to 42 torr).
6. Record minute volume and measure PCO_2, pH and PO_2 after 20 minutes of continuous ventilation at 100 percent inspired O_2 concentration. Estimate inspired O_2 concentration required to maintain PO_2 between 70 to 100 mm. Hg.

7. After results of arterial blood gases on 100 percent inspired oxygen are obtained, adjust F_IO_2 accordingly and recheck PO_2. Maintenance F_IO_2 can then be assessed.
8. Added mechanical dead space may be required to maintain normal arterial PCO_2 when large tidal volumes are used.
9. Use 100 percent F_IO_2 setting to follow progress of pulmonary status. True physiologic shunt can be estimated from the arterial blood gases and an F_IO_2 of 100 percent.

● Rule out the possibility of an impending catastrophe whenever a patient becomes out of phase with the ventilator. The "out of phase" patient usually has hypoxemia, air leak, obstruction, and inadequate flow rate, minute volume, or inspiratory-expiratory ratios.

If, after life-threatening situations have been corrected, the patient is still out of phase with the ventilator or is breathing too fast, then sedatives and muscle relaxants are given to provide optimum ventilation.

Factors Causing the Patient to "Fight the Ventilator." The patient is in synchrony with the respirator when thoracic air expansion coincides with the inspiratory phase of the machine and exhalation occurs passively. The patient "fights" the ventilator when he is out of phase with the machine. This is manifested when (1) the patient attempts to breathe in during the ventilator's mechanical expiratory phase; (2) the respirator is triggered faster than 18 times/minute; and/or (3) there is jerky and increased abdominal muscle effort.

The following factors contribute to this problem: increased secretions, low F_IO_2, hypercarbia, inadequate minute volume, and pulmonary edema. These must be corrected (see Table 24-5) before the ordered sedation or muscle relaxant is given to the patient. Otherwise, the basic problem is masked and the patient will continue to deteriorate.

Life-threatening problems, of course, require immediate correction (see Table 24-6). Thus the nurse must be constantly on the watch for these difficulties and must be prepared to act.

Weaning the Patient from the Mechanical Ventilator

Weaning takes place in four stages. The patient is gradually weaned from the (1) ventilator, (2) cuff, (3) tube, and (4) oxygen.

Weaning from Ventilator. Weaning from mechanical ventilation should be done at the earliest possible time consistent with patient safety. It is essential that the decision be made from a physiologic rather than from a mechanical viewpoint. A total understanding of the patient's clinical status is required in making this decision.

Weaning is started when the patient is recovering from the acute stage of his medical and surgical problems and when the etiology of respiratory failure is sufficiently reversed.

The objective measurements of the patient's ventilatory capacities should include the following:
1. An ability to generate a minimum vital capacity of 15 ml./kg. body weight, or a vital capacity twice as large as the predicted normal resting tidal volume. The minimum required volume is usually in the range of 1000 ml. in a normal adult.
2. An inspiratory force of at least −20 cm. water pressure. Occasionally tidal volume can be used as an added criterion. If tidal volume is used, it must be measured during the patient's quiet respiration. Do not ask the patient to take a deep breath because the volume thus obtained will be difficult to interpret since it is between his actual tidal volume and vital capacity.
3. A minimum ratio of 2 between the vital capacity and tidal volume is necessary before weaning is attempted.

When the physician decides that the patient has adequate ventilatory capacity, weaning can be initiated. Baseline measurements are noted: (a) vital capacity, (b) inspiratory force, (c) respiratory rate, (d) resting tidal

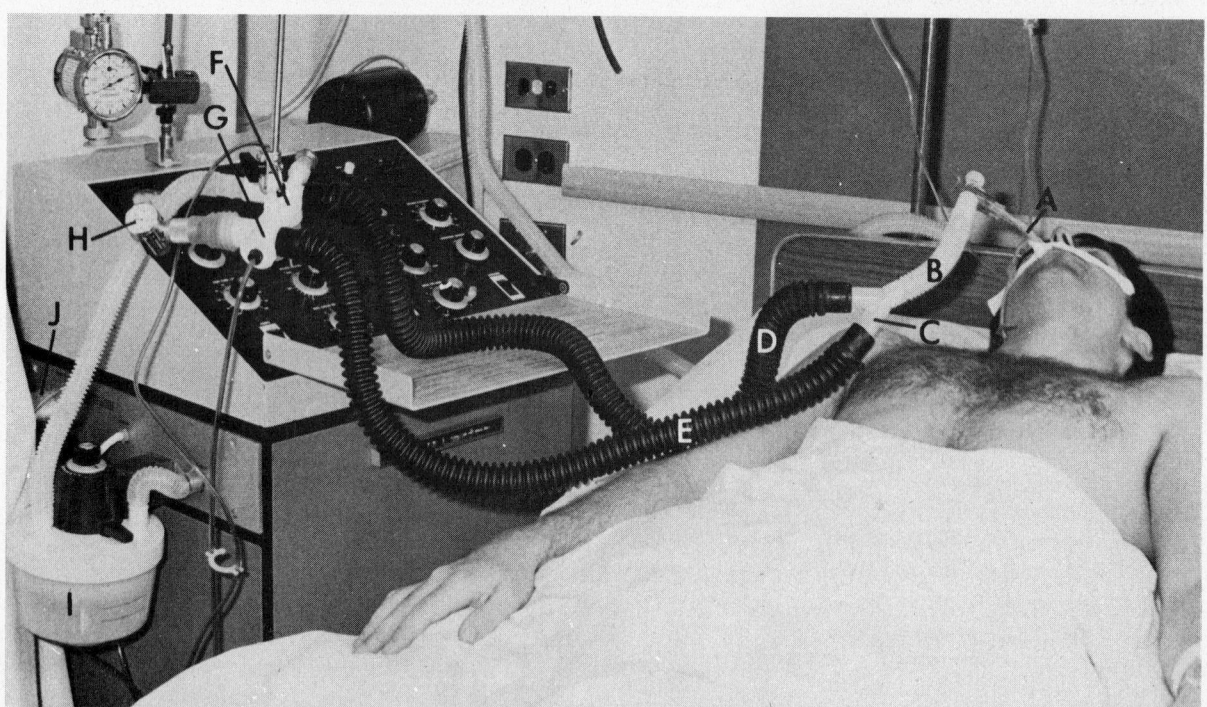

Figure 24-11.   Patient on MAI mechanical ventilator: Lettered items are as follows: (A) endotracheal tube; (B) mechanical dead space; (C) Y piece; (D) inspiratory hose; (E) expiratory hose; (F) inspiratory valve; (G) expiratory valve; (H) Wright respirometer; (I) cascade humidifier; (J) knob for PEEP (positive end expiratory pressure).

TABLE 24-4. MANAGING THE PATIENT ON A VENTILATOR

Type of ventilator	1. Volume-controlled ventilator (MAI; Ohio 560, Emerson). Will deliver set tidal volume with varying pressures. 2. Pressure-controlled ventilator. Preset pressure is achieved at varying tidal volumes.		2. The sigh is given by machine or manual hand-bag ventilation. 3. Sigh volume is 3 times tidal volume every 5-10 minutes.
Fraction of inspired oxygen (F_1O_2)	Interpretation of PO_2 will depend upon the concentration of inspired O_2. Normal values: 1. F_1O_2—room air 21% O_2 PO_2—100 mm. Hg or 105 minus half of patient's age 2. F_1O_2 = 100% PO_2 = 500 mm. Hg	*Mechanical dead space*	Refers to the volume of tubing from endotracheal or tracheostomy tube connector to the Y piece. *Purpose:* 1. To rebreathe exhaled CO_2. 2. Serves as a pliable connector from tracheostomy tube to Y piece; thus prevents discomfort when patient moves.
Tidal volume (V_T) *Respiratory rate* *Sensitivity setting*	10-15 ml./kg. body weight 10-12/minute 1. Increased sensitivity indicates that very low negative pressure is required to trigger machine. 2. Do not allow patient to generate more than -2 cm. H_2O to trigger the ventilator.		*Caution:* The volume of mechanical dead space should not be larger than one third of the set tidal volume, especially at 21% of F_1O_2, because hypoxic oxygen concentrations may result due to exhaled CO_2 dilution. Should not be used to correct metabolic alkalosis.
Type of ventilation	1. Controlled. The machine ventilates the patient according to set tidal volumes and respiratory rate. These patients usually require medication with morphine, curare, or pancuronium. 2. Assist Control. The patient triggers the machine.	*Flow rate*	*Slow* 1. Opens up more alveoli because of a more even air flow distribution within the respiratory tract. 2. If flow rate is too slow it will prolong inspiration and may hinder venous return. *High* 1. Shortens inspiratory time. 2. Preferential flow of gases to alveoli with least resistance and may not open atelectatic alveoli at all.
Inspiration to exhalation ratio	1. Should be 1:3, 1:2 or 1:1 (1 second of inspiration to 3 seconds of exhalation, etc.) 2. Inspiration should never be longer than exhalation, because venous return to the right side of the heart occurs on exhalation. Prolonged inspiration prevents venous return and may cause hypotension. 3. Patients with obstructive lung disease need longer exhalation time to keep the bronchi open and allow exit of more air.	*Expiratory retard*	1. Used only when prescribed by physician. 2. Keeps the terminal bronchioles patent, preventing early closure on exhalation; thus, more air can be exhaled.
Minute volume (V_E)	Tidal volume × respiratory rate/minute. Normal = 6-8 L./minute.	*Humidity and temperature*	1. Heated humidity is provided for all intubated and tracheotomized patients to avoid thick and viscid secretions. 2. Daily clinical evaluation of the viscosity of the patient's secretions provides a guideline for the effectiveness of humidification and nebulization.
Airway pressure	Normal = 15-20 cm./H_2O Low airway pressure is seen with air leak. High airway pressure is seen in: 1. Increased secretions 2. Airway obstruction 3. Bronchospasms 4. Pulmonary edema 5. Pneumothorax 6. Flail chest 7. Patient out of phase with respirator	*Positive end expiratory pressure*	1. A positive pressure of 5, 10, or 15 cm. H_2O is maintained at the end of exhalation instead of a normal 0 cm. H_2O pressure. 2. Increases functional residual capacity.
Sigh	1. The lungs are hyperinflated periodically to open collapsed alveoli.	*Synchronization of patient with ventilator*	1. Inspiratory and expiratory time of the patient and respirator should be synchronized. 2. Asynchrony (out of phase) with ventilator will result in altered cardiopulmonary hemodynamics and cause arrhythmias, hypotension, and increased airway pressure.

volume, (e) minute ventilation ($f \times V_T$), (f) arterial blood gases, (g) F_IO_2.

The patient is then attached to a T-bar, on spontaneous ventilation, with warmed and humidified oxygen. The F_IO_2 or fraction of inspired oxygen concentration given will depend upon the patient's previous satisfactory arterial PO_2. Do not wean the patient from oxygen therapy while weaning from mechanical assistance of ventilation. It is unreasonable to expect a patient to assume the work of breathing and, at the same time, to meet the increased cardiovascular demands of decreased inspired oxygen concentrations. During the weaning process the patient must be maintained on the same oxygen therapy, whether he is on the ventilator or off.

F_IO_2 can be increased or decreased by either adjusting the flow rate of oxygen, adjusting the diluter valve setting, or adding or reducing a reservoir tube. While the patient is on the T-bar, close monitoring should be done. Psychological support and assurance are necessary.

It is of the utmost importance to follow the trend of the values obtained for the following rather than rely on isolated measurements: (1) vital capacity, (2) inspiratory force, (3) respiratory rate, (4) resting tidal volume, (5) minute volume, (6) blood gases, (7) F_IO_2.

The second set of blood gases should be drawn 20 minutes after the patient has been on spontaneous ventilation at a constant F_IO_2. (It takes 15 to 20 minutes for alveolar arterial equilibration to take place.)

While the patient is on the T-bar he should be observed for signs of hypoxemia or increasing fatigue as manifested by the following: (1) bradycardia, PVCs (premature ventricular contractions), or any sign of increasing cardiac irritability, (2) restlessness, (3) a respiratory rate greater than 35 per minute, and (4) labored respiration. Fatigue or exhaustion is, initially, manifested by an increased respiratory rate associated with a gradual reduction in tidal volume. Later there is a slowing of the respiratory rate.

Serial blood gas analysis and periodic measurements of: (1) inspiratory force, (2) vital capacity, (3) tidal volume, (4) respiratory rate, and (5) minute volume should be continued until they stabilize at satisfactory levels. The frequency of these measurements depends upon the patient's clinical progress.

TABLE 24-5. FACTORS THAT MAKE THE PATIENT FIGHT THE VENTILATOR

PROBLEM	NURSING ACTION
1. Increased secretions Volume ventilator—airway pressure is increased but tidal volume is maintained. Pressure ventilator—secretions will make the patient cough or generate increased intrapulmonary pressure, which will oppose the preset pressure on the ventilator; thus the inspiratory volume is reduced. The reduced tidal volume will promote progressive atelectasis and shunting.	1. Suction as often as necessary. 2. Hourly, hand ventilate with self-inflating bag for 5-10 minutes. 3. Chest physical therapy. 4. Frequent change of position. 5. Adequate humidification and nebulization. 6. For pressure ventilator—adjust flow rate and preset pressure to maintain an adequate chest expansion and satisfactory air entry heard on auscultation. 7. If suctioning of trachea does not improve phasing with ventilator call the physician.
2. Low F_IO_2—may manifest initially with tachycardia, hyperventilation, or arrhythmias.	1. Measure inspired oxygen concentration and arterial blood gases. 2. Call respiratory therapist to check accuracy of delivered F_IO_2. 3. Call physician for differential diagnosis and management.
3. Hypercarbia—may be manifested initially by hyperventilation, tachycardia, arrhythmias, increased blood pressure, and increasing drowsiness.	1. Measure arterial blood gases. 2. Call respiratory therapist to check mechanical dead space, accuracy of valves, and ventilator performance. 3. Call physician for differential diagnosis and management.
4. Inadequate minute volume $V_E = V_T \times RR$	1. Measure exhaled tidal volume and respiratory rate if minute volume is lower than 6 L./minute. Increase delivered tidal volumes to 10-15 ml./kg. at a rate of 10-12/minute. 2. Call respiratory therapist for accuracy of ventilator performance. 3. Call physician for differential diagnosis and management.

5. Pulmonary edema—may be manifested as follows:
a. High airway pressure
b. Poor compliance
c. Tracheal secretion
  (1) Foamy or pink frothy secretions
  (2) Abundant watery, and bright red fluid
d. Engorged neck veins
e. Dusky, cyanotic color
f. Chest, full of wet rales
g. Tachycardia, hypotension
h. Marked restlessness
	1. 100% F_IO_2.
	2. Hand ventilate with self-inflating bag. Use volume controlled respirator and PEEP (positive end expiratory pressure).
	3. Suction trachea.
	4. Elevate head of bed (sitting up position).
	5. Call physician. Give specific drug therapy as directed. (See page 584.)

The appearance of signs of exhaustion and hypoxemia correlated with a deterioration of the above measurements suggest the need of immediate ventilatory support. The patient should be placed back on the ventilator each time signs of fatigue or deterioration develop.

Patients who have had short-term ventilatory assistance usually can be extubated within 2 or 3 hours of weaning and allowed spontaneous ventilation via a mask with humidified oxygen. Patients who have had prolonged ventilatory assistance usually require more gradual weaning, which may take several days. They are weaned primarily during the day and placed back on the ventilator at night to sleep.

During the times that the patient is on spontaneous ventilation, the diluter valve, flow rate, and reservoir tube can be adjusted according to the results of the blood gases. IPPB should be given every hour during the day while the patient is on spontaneous ventilation with a T-bar and also after the endotracheal tube has been removed.

Some patients are difficult to wean from mechanical ventilation. A device incorporated into the respirator called "IMV—Intermittent Mandatory Ventilation," will allow the patient to breathe spontaneously as desired, but also delivers a mandatory hyperinflation at regular intervals. IMV is indicated if the patient satisfies all the criteria for weaning but cannot sustain adequate spontaneous ventilation for long periods of time. Upon initiation of IMV the machine is set at a slower rate but larger tidal volume than the patient's spontaneous respiratory activity. It then can be adjusted to maintain satisfactory arterial blood gases.

Following initiation of IMV, serial determinations of the following are made and recorded: (1) respiratory rate, (2) minute volume (V_E), (3) tidal volume (V_T), (4) F_IO_2, and (5) arterial blood gases.

If there is no deterioration in these parameters, and as the patient's tidal volume improves, the rate of the ventilator is progressively decreased and the patient is allowed to rely more on spontaneous respiration until weaning is complete.

Successful weaning from the ventilator should be vigorously followed by intensive pulmonary care. Continue (1) oxygen therapy, (2) arterial blood gas evaluation, (3) IPPB, (4) chest physical therapy, and (5) adequate hydration and humidification. Remember that these patients still have minimum pulmonary function and need vigorous supportive therapy before they return to normal.

Weaning from the Cuff. While the patient is on the ventilator, the cuff is kept inflated to avoid aspiration and prevent an air leak and thus to allow adequate chest expansion. Patients with tracheostomies should exercise the larynx by phonation (although no sound or voice comes out) in order to maintain active pharyngeal and laryngeal reflexes. This helps to reduce the chances of aspiration.

Weaning from the Tube. The tracheostomy or endotracheal tube can be removed if the following criteria are present: (1) spontaneous ventilation is adequate; (2) the pharyngeal and laryngeal gag reflexes are active; (3) the patient is maintaining an adequate airway and can swallow, move his jaw, or clench his teeth; and (4) voluntary cough is effective in bringing up secretions. If these are ineffective, the tracheostomy tube is needed so that tracheobronchial secretions can be suctioned. In these patients a fenestrated tracheostomy tube is used in order to minimize resistance to air flow. The presence of an endotracheal or tracheostomy tube prevents closure of the epiglottis, making the cough less forceful.

Before the patient is weaned from the tracheostomy tube, he is given a trial of mouth or nose breathing. This can be accomplished by: (1) changing to a smaller size tube to reduce resistance to air flow while at the same time plugging off the tracheostomy (deflate the cuff) or (2) removing the tracheostomy tube completely.

Weaning from Oxygen. This is the last step. The patient has been weaned from the ventilator, cuff, and tube. His respiratory function has been checked, and oxygen has been given according to the result of the blood gas determinations. The F_IO_2 is then gradually reduced until the PO_2 is in the 70 to 100 mg./Hg range while the patient is breathing room air. If the PO_2 is less than 70 on room air, supplementary oxygen is recommended.

CHEST PHYSICAL THERAPY IN INTENSIVE CARE

The various types of chest physiotherapy include relaxation, breathing exercises, mobilizing and postural exercises, and postural drainage with cupping and chest wall vibrations. These measures may be used to treat both medical and surgical conditions.

The patient is encouraged to breathe deeply and cough effectively. To do so he is taught to relax and avoid splinting while the abdominal and chest wounds are stabilized. The breathing technique should be one of sustained maximum inspiration with slow inspiratory flow, maximum inspiratory volume, and a peak inspiratory hold. The patient should be encouraged to practice for several minutes every hour while awake, for the first 3 to 4 days following surgery.

In both medical and surgical patients, when there is evidence of retained secretions, atelectasis, or pneumonia, postural drainage should be initiated. The patient is positioned so that the drainage of secretions from the affected area is assisted by gravity. As is shown on page 419, there is a drainage position described for each lung segment. The appropriate position is assumed by the patient, and a combination of sustained maximum inspirations, chest-wall vibrations upon expiration, and/or cupping over the affected area are performed. The treatment plan is modified according to the tolerance of the patient and the presence of any medical contra-indications.

Alternate Method of Care for Intubated Patients (Bag-Inflation)

The bag-inflation technique requires two persons, one to inflate the patient's lung, and the other to apply chest wall vibrations during exhalation.

The procedure is carried out as follows:
- The patient is placed in the side-lying position, and the nurse inflates the patient's lungs with the manual resuscitation bag. The maximum inflation volume should be held at a plateau for a second or so to allow time for poorly ventilated alveoli to fill.
- At the end of the inflation plateau, just as the bag pressure is released, the physical therapist should start to vibrate the chest wall to augment the peak expiratory flow rate and help mobilize secretions. This vibratory compression (produced by molding the hands to the chest wall and tensing the arm and shoulder muscles) is continued to the end of expiration. This helps to dislodge the secretions from the bronchial walls, from which they are expelled by coughing or sterile aspiration.
- Approximately 4 to 6 inflation-expiration cycles are per-

formed, and then the patient is suctioned. However, if secretions are heard at any time, the trachea is suctioned before inflation is started again.
- Each time, after completing this procedure, the therapist listens with a stethoscope while the nurse inflates the lungs. Air entry should be good. The procedure is continued as long as rattling secretions are present and as tolerated by the patient.
- When one side of the chest is clear, the patient is turned and the procedure is repeated on the other side. (The complete procedure is presented in Figure 24-12).

This technique should only be carried out by persons skilled in the technique of "bagging," since inability to coordinate the manual ventilation with the patient's own respiratory efforts can result in increased airway pressures, bronchospasm, excessive coughing, and an increased level of agitation in the patient. If the technique results in any of the above, or if the patient is being ventilated with PEEP, or if his condition is unstable, it is advisable to simply "sigh" the patient 5 or 6 times on the mechanical ventilator, following saline instillations and in combination with chest wall vibrations and/or cupping.

- Caution should be exercised in patients who cannot tolerate vigorous coughing spells, such as those in frank congestive heart failure, those who have recently suffered a myocardial infarction, and those with increased tendency to bronchospasm. Chest physical therapy is also contraindicated in the presence of hypotension, unstable vital signs, medical and surgical catastrophes, and dialysis.

TABLE 24-6. LIFE-THREATENING PROBLEMS WHILE ON MECHANICAL VENTILATION

Call the physician the moment any life-threatening situation arises following this sequence of priorities:

Priority I. Evaluate the patient's current status and compare it to an earlier observation:
1. level of responsiveness
2. degree of distress
3. color
4. degree of neck vein distention
5. chest expansion
6. abdominal movements.

Priority II. Correlate airway pressures on the machine, central venous pressure, pulse rate, and bilateral breath sounds (heard via auscultation).

Priority III. Disconnect patient from the machine and ventilate him with self-inflating bag at high F_IO_2's.
Note: 1. Compliance and chest expansion in relation to amount of inflating pressure
2. Expiratory time
3. Bilateral breath sounds

Priority IV. 1. Pass a catheter through the endotracheal tube and feel for areas of resistance or obstruction.
2. Suction around the pharynx first, then deflate the cuff and note if there is improvement in air exchange with the cuff deflated. (This is true if obstruction is due to the cuff.)

Priority V. If patient is ventilating well on the self-inflating bag, check the machine while another person ventilates the patient by hand.

PROBLEM	RECOGNITION OF THE PROBLEM	NURSING INTERVENTION

Airway Leak
1. Patient-connected Problem
  a. Inadequate cuff inflation
  b. Inadequate coaptation, or fit, of tracheostomy tube (loose tie around the neck)
  c. Changes in the patient's position can
	Clinical manifestations depend on amount of leak.
	Early Signs
	  1. Absent or inadequate chest expansion
	  2. Absent or decreased breath sounds
	  3. Marked apprehension, if patient is conscious
		1. Disconnect patient from ventilator.
		2. Inflate patient's chest with self-inflating bag at high F_IO_2's.
		3. Search for source of leak from the patient and from the machine. Once corrected, adequate chest expansion is seen.
		  a. Exhaled volume as measured with

TABLE 24-6. (CONTINUED)

PROBLEM	RECOGNITION OF THE PROBLEM	NURSING INTERVENTION

create a leak around tracheostomy.
2. Ventilator-connected Problem
  a. Disconnected or loose-fitting ventilator hose and tubes
  b. Malfunction of inspiratory and expiratory valves
  c. Improperly sealed humidifier
	4. a. Pressure-controlled ventilator—inspiration is prolonged or continuous
	   b. Volume-controlled ventilator—normal cycle
	5. Zero or markedly reduced airway pressure
	6. Sounding of safety alarm in some machines
	7. Measured exhaled volume is reduced
	
	Late Signs
	  1. Arrhythmia 3. Cyanosis
	  2. Hypotension 4. Death
		Wright respirometer should tally with dialed tidal volume on machine.
		  b. Dialed tidal volume is reduced by 3 ml. for every cm. H_2O peak airway pressure due to gas compression in the system.

Airway Obstruction	Manifestations will vary according to:
	  1. Pressure-controlled ventilator
	  2. Volume-controlled ventilator
	  3. Presence or absence of muscle power
	  4. Complete or partial airway obstruction
		1. Disconnect patient from ventilator. Confirm and correct obstruction.
		2. Use self-inflating bag; note compliance.
		3. Partial obstruction will require greater pressure to expand chest.
		4. Complete obstruction makes it impossible to inflate chest or bag.
		5. In partial obstruction, exhalation characterized by delayed and reduced bag expansion.
		6. Pass catheter down endotracheal or tracheostomy tube, feeling for points of resistance or obstruction.

1. Complete airway obstruction in a patient who is on a ventilator and has no muscle power.	1. Pressure-controlled ventilator:
	The preset airway pressure is easily reached without any visible chest expansion or any inspiratory or expiratory air exchange on auscultation. Inspiratory time is very short.
	2. Volume-controlled ventilator:
	Acute high increase in airway pressure occurs without chest expansion or audible air exchange.
	There is no visible muscle effort in chest or abdomen.
		7. Note improvement in airway pressure and chest expansion while doing the following maneuvers to relieve obstruction:
		  a. Suction inside tube and around pharynx. Deflate cuff.
		  b. Straighten tube to relieve kinked areas in the pharynx, mouth, or connectors.
		  c. Tilt back head, if patient's head is flexed.

2. Complete airway obstruction in a patient who is on a ventilator and has muscle power.	1. Same as 1 and 2 when patient has no muscle power.
	2. Seesaw movement of chest and abdomen. (During inspiration, the chest is depressed. With expiration there is jerky protrusion and prolonged sustained contraction of the abdominal muscles followed by a brief relaxation before another protrusion and contraction.)
	3. Use of accessory muscles of respiration
	4. Extreme anxiety and respiratory distress
	5. Initial increase in BP and PR; later, decrease in BP and pulse rate
	6. Patient is out of phase with machine.
		d. Adjust tracheostomy tube to fit snugly. (Loose fit will cause air leak and possible obstruction of the lumen against wall.) If patient ventilates well on the self-inflating bag, obstruction may be on the machine.
		  e. Drain condensed water in the loop of ventilator tubing.
		  f. Check valves
		  g. Determine whether the connections are wrong or out of adjustment.

Hemothorax
Blood accumulates in pleural cavity causing collapse of the lung and hypovolemia or shock.
	1. Auscultation of chest reveals absent breath sounds at bases and midlung fields (on affected side).
	2. Increased airway pressure
	3. Signs of bleeding and hypovolemia, (e.g., an increase in pulse rate and a decrease in BP)
	4. Chest x-ray will show density on affected side.
		1. If patient is out of phase with ventilator:
		  a. Disconnect from ventilator.
		  b. Ventilate by hand with self-inflating bag at high inspired oxygen concentrations.
		  c. Call physician.
		2. If patient is synchronous with ventilator, call physician.
		3. In the meantime, differentiate from other life-threatening situations while on ventilator (see pages 460-463).
		4. Assist with the following:
		  a. Chest tube drainage. The needle trochar is inserted at 5th and 6th intercostal space in the midaxillary line.
		  b. Restore blood volume with blood and fluids.
		  c. Prepare for possible thoracic surgical exploration to ligate bleeder(s).

(Continued)

TABLE 24-6. (CONTINUED)

PROBLEM	RECOGNITION OF THE PROBLEM	NURSING INTERVENTION

Tension Pneumothorax
Pathophysiology:
1. Any direct or indirect communication of a bronchus, bronchiole, or alveolus with the pleural cavity produces a closed pneumothorax.
2. When the visceral pleura acts as a valve, air is permitted to enter the pleural cavity on inspiration but not permitted to escape on exhalation.
3. Successive increments of air build up the intrapleural tension.
4. The progressive buildup of intrapleural tension collapses the lung on the affected side.
5. The mediastinum shifts to the opposite side. This will *kink* or collapse the great veins and thus will seriously interfere with cardiac filling.
6. Death rapidly follows unless tension pneumothorax is promptly relieved.
	1. Acute onset of respiratory distress while on ventilator
	2. Chest
	  a. Unilateral tension pneumothorax
	  Inspection: unequal chest expansion
	  Auscultation:
	    (1) Unequal breath sounds
	    (2) Absent or distant breath sounds on affected side
	    (3) Inspiration—short, crepitant rales
	    (4) Exhalation—absent breath sounds or brief, muffled, crepitant rales
	  b. Bilateral pneumothorax
	  Same chest findings as above but on both sides.
	3. Rapid progressive increase in airway pressure
	  Volume ventilator: increase in airway pressure is shown on manometer.
	  Pressure ventilator: reaches the maximum pressure limit with little alveolar expansion. Short inspiratory time.
	4. Distended neck veins
	5. Increased CVP
	6. Hypotension
	7. Diagnostic thoracentesis at the 2nd and 3rd intercostal spaces will push out bevel of syringe due to increased intrathoracic pressure.
	8. Chest x-ray: shows pneumothorax and possible displacement of trachea away from the affected side
	9. Subcutaneous emphysema
		1. Disconnect patient from ventilator.
		2. Ventilate patient by hand with self-inflating bag.
		3. Call physician.
		
		4. Assist physician with insertion of chest tubes with underwater seal drainage.

Flail Chest (from trauma)	These signs and symptoms will be manifested if the patient is on spontaneous ventilation or on an inadequate pressure-controlled ventilator.
	1. Progressive increase in respiratory distress; increased respiratory rate and reduced tidal volumes
	2. Increase use of all accessory muscles of respiration
	3. a. Inspiration—as chest expands, flail section sinks in, impairing ability to produce negative intrapleural pressure which is necessary to draw air into the lungs.
	  b. Expiration—flail segment bulges outward, thus impairing ability to exhale.
	  In severe flail chest, air may shift uselessly from side to side.
	4. Accumulation of secretions due to decreased intrapleural negative pressure, and impaired ability to cough them up.
	5. Rhoncal breath sounds and varying degrees of rales noted on chest auscultation.
	6. Neck veins engorged
	7. Increased CVP
		1. Ventilate by hand with self-inflating bag.
		2. Suction secretions.
		3. Call physician.
		4. Attach patient to volume-controlled ventilator.

TABLE 24-6. (CONTINUED)

PROBLEM	RECOGNITION OF THE PROBLEM	NURSING INTERVENTION
	8. Cardiac output, BP, and pulse rate initially increased followed by falling BP and pulse rate when the patient can no longer compensate. 9. Progressive reduction in arterial PO_2 10. Progressive signs of hypoxemia—restlessness followed by drowsiness leading to coma and death.	
Cardiac Tamponade: (Accumulation of excessive fluid in the pericardial space) 1. Increased intrapericardial pressure causes compression of the vena cava and atria and thereby impedes venous return to the heart. 2. Cardiac compression lowers cardiac output. This leads to a fall in BP and a reduction in coronary filling. 3. These are factors which predispose to myocardial hypoxia and failure.	1. Progressively rising venous pressure (CVP). Neck veins distended (pathognomonic) 2. Heart sound distant 3. Quiet fatigue 4. Decreased arterial and pulse pressure 5. Signs of respiratory insufficiency, but mechanical ventilation will aggravate hypotension.	1. Call physician. 2. Assist with pericardiocentesis (page 597).

SUMMARY: NURSING MANAGEMENT OF THE PATIENT ON MECHANICAL VENTILATOR

1. A nurse should be in constant attendance while the patient is on a mechanical ventilator.
2. Take vital signs every 5-30 minutes: BP, pulse and respirations, CVP, temperature.
3. Auscultate chest frequently (every 15 minutes). Note any change in breath sounds.
4. Aspirate tracheobronchial tree as necessary. Suction around pharynx before cuff deflation. Use sterile technique in airway care and suction. Note added breath sounds and the quality of air exchange before and after tracheobronchial aspiration. Record color and quantity of sputum aspirated.
5. Periodically deflate endotracheal or tracheostomy cuff with high pressure cuffs. Reinflate cuff with identical volume. At the same time check for air leaks. Stop inflation when significant air leak is gone.
6. Flush arterial line with heparinized saline every hour or maintain a slow continuous microdrip.
7. Total fluid balance every 8 hours.
8. Record urine specific gravity with hourly urinary output.
9. Give mouth care every 4-8 hours to all debilitated and paralyzed patients.
10. In all paralyzed and comatose patients, perform eye care every 12 hours. Use lubricating ointment and tape the eyelids closed.
11. Change respiratory therapy equipment every day.
12. Note end inspiratory pressure and tidal volume hourly.
13. Empty condensed water from ventilatory tubing p.r.n.
14. Check pressure of humidifier every 2 hours. Be sure a visible mist is produced if nebulizer is used.
15. Record humidifier volume and refill every 8 hours. If refilling is necessary, empty residual water and replace with sterile distilled water. The emptying helps prevent accumulation of pseudomonas which thrive in warm, moist places.
16. Check temperature of inspired air as often as necessary. Temperature of inspired air should be as close to body temperature as possible in order to provide more humidity. An increase in body temperature will develop if the air is higher than body temperature.
17. Check oxygen lines and flow meters hourly to be sure that they are properly connected and functioning as prescribed.
18. Change patient's position in bed hourly while he is awake, or hourly around the clock if comatose.
19. Coordinate chest physiotherapy with position change, airway suctioning, and IPPB treatments. The frequency of this is to be determined by the clinical status of the patient.
20. Put all joints of comatose or paralyzed patients through a passive full range of motion several times daily (see page 183). Attention should be directed to the care of the skin of the dependent parts.
21. Assess neurological signs every hour when indicated (page 83).
22. Note amount and quality of drainage in nasogastric tubes and any ostomies.
23. Send all stools to the lab for guaiac test. This is done to evaluate early bleeding due to stress ulcers.
24. Weigh the patient daily.
25. Help the patient to ambulate as soon as possible.
26. Give diet as tolerated. This will depend upon severity of illness.
27. Plan nursing care so that patient has periods of uninterrupted sleep.
28. Notify the physician immediately if a change occurs in the level of responsiveness; also keep him informed of the occurrence of tachycardia, bradycardia, hypotension, confusion, agitation, tarry stools, arrhythmia, high or low CVP, or labored ventilation.

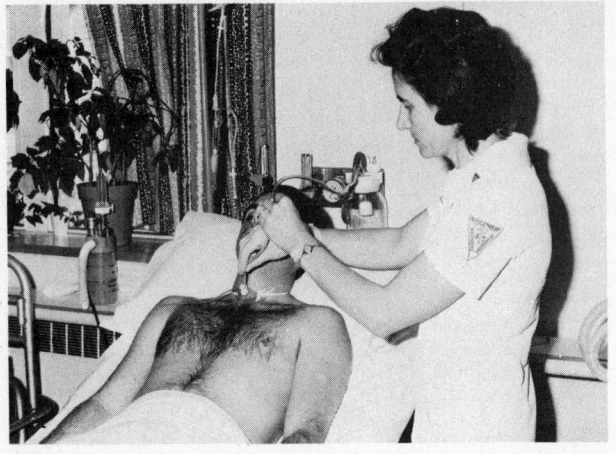

1. Prior to the bag-squeezing procedure, the trachea and then the oropharynx are suctioned.

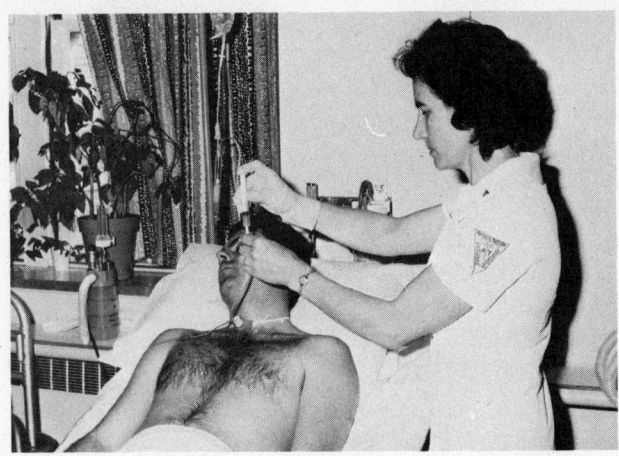

2. About 2-3 ml. of saline are instilled into the trachea.

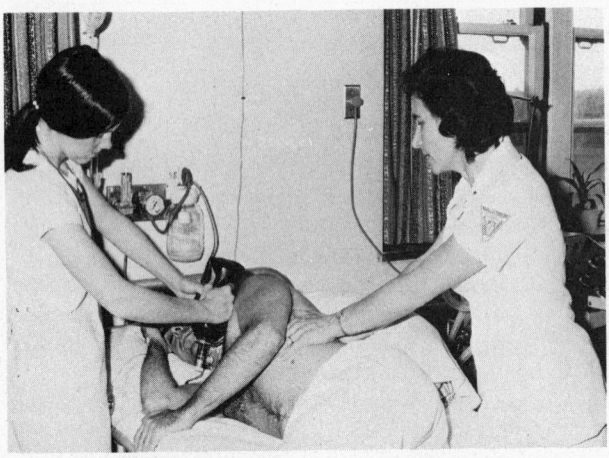

3. The patient is positioned on the right side for mobilization of secretions from left lung. Photo shows sigh volume being delivered.

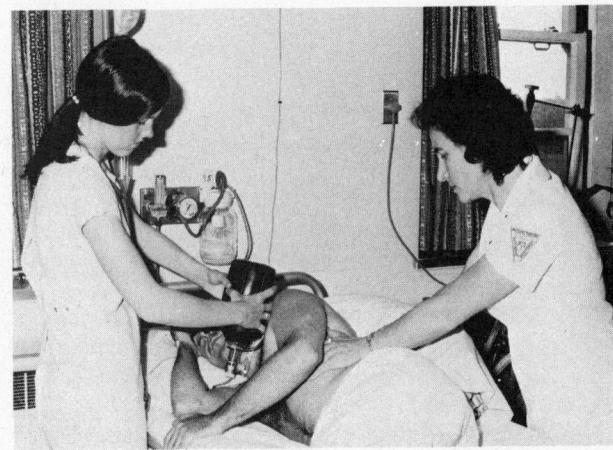

4. The pressure on the bag is released, allowing for exhalation and mobilization of secretions as vibration of the chest wall is carried out.

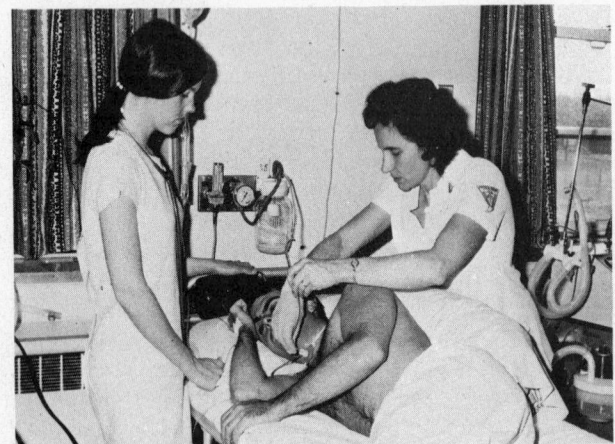

5. The patient is suctioned for mobilization of secretions.

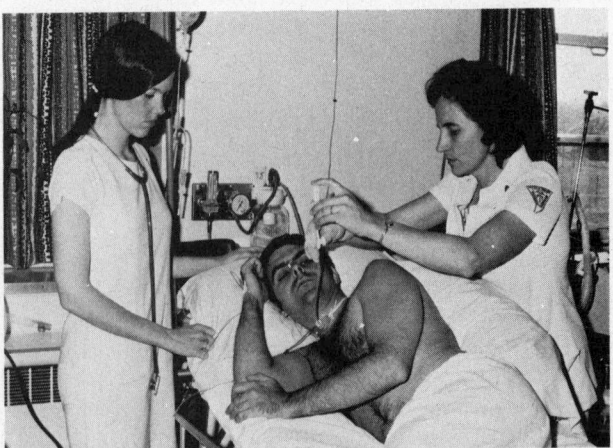

6. Saline is instilled before the patient turns to the left side.

Figure 24-12. Technique for chest physical therapy in the critically ill patient.

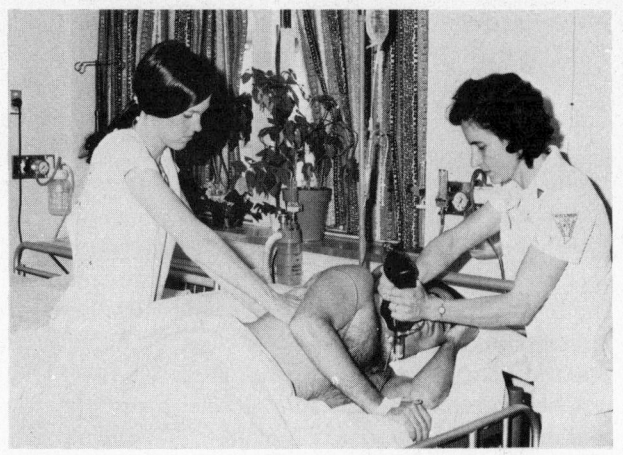

7. While patient lies on left side, sigh volume is delivered via resuscitation bag.

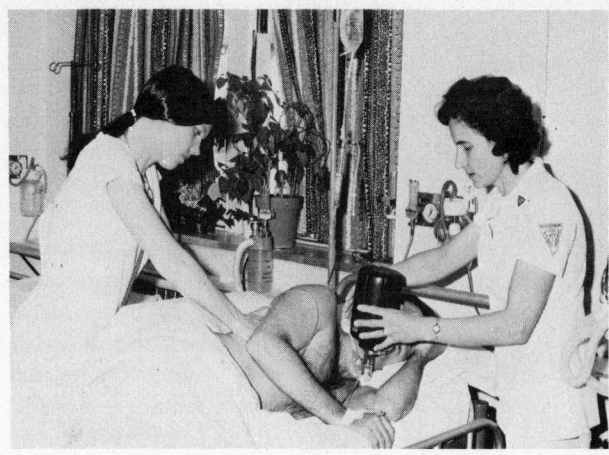

8. Pressure on the bag is released, allowing for exhalation, while vibration of chest wall is carried out to mobilize secretions from the right lung.

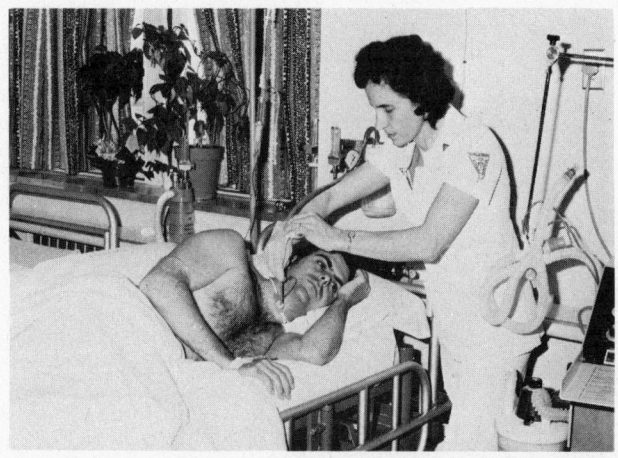

9. Mobilized secretions are suctioned from the trachea and then the oropharynx.

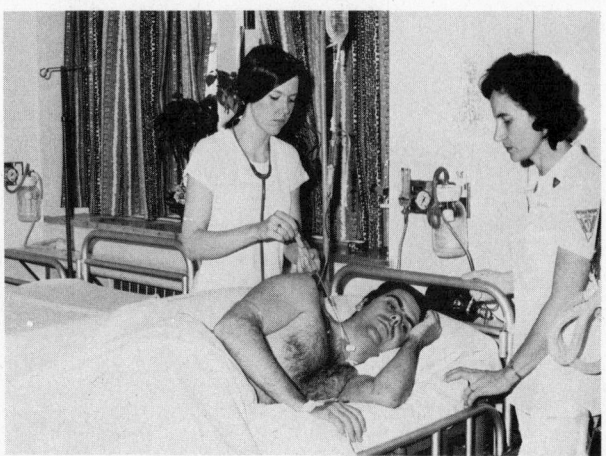

10. Pressure is released from the tracheostomy tube cuff.

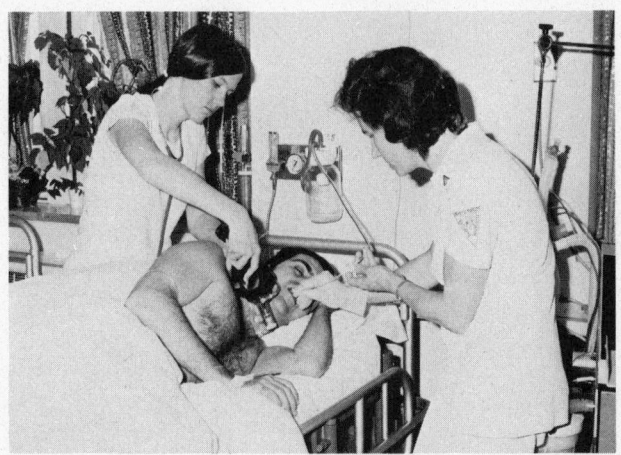

11. Sigh volume is delivered via bag with cuff deflated, while secretions released from around the cuff are suctioned from mouth.

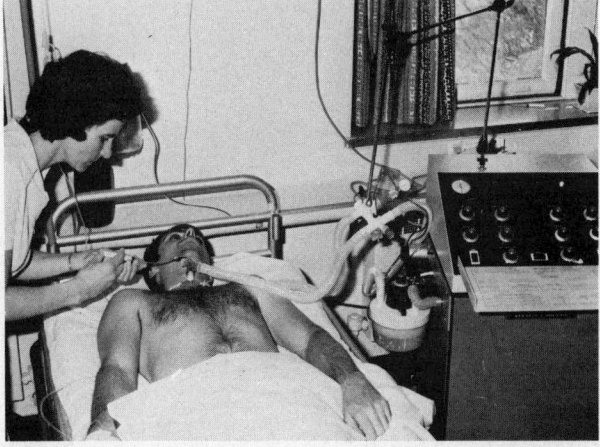

12. Patient is placed back on ventilator. Cuff is inflated with minimum pressure until air leak disappears and satisfactory chest expansion is achieved.

THE CLINICAL PROBLEM OF ASPIRATION

Aspiration is the inhalation of stomach contents; it is a serious complication and may cause death. It can occur when there is loss of protective airway reflexes, such as is seen in patients who are unconscious from drugs, alcohol, stroke, or cardiac arrest, or in instances when a nonfunctioning nasogastric tube allows the gastric contents to drain around the tube and cause silent aspiration.

Massive inhalation of gastric contents, if untreated, will, in a period of several hours, result in the clinical syndrome of tachycardia, dyspnea, cyanosis, hypertension, and finally death. The primary factors responsible for morbidity and mortality after aspiration of gastric contents are the volume of aspirated gastric contents and their character. A full stomach contains solid particles of food. If these are aspirated, the problem then becomes one of mechanical blockage of the airways and secondary infection. A fasting stomach contains gastric juice which, if aspirated, may prove destructive to the alveoli and capillaries. The presence of fecal contamination (more likely seen in intestinal obstruction) will increase the likelihood of mortality because the endotoxins produced by intestinal organisms may be absorbed systemically, or the thick proteinaceous material found in the intestinal contents may obstruct the airway, leading to atelectasis and secondary bacterial invasion.

Chemical pneumonitis may develop from aspiration and may result in destruction of alveolar-capillary endothelial cells, with a consequent outpouring of protein-

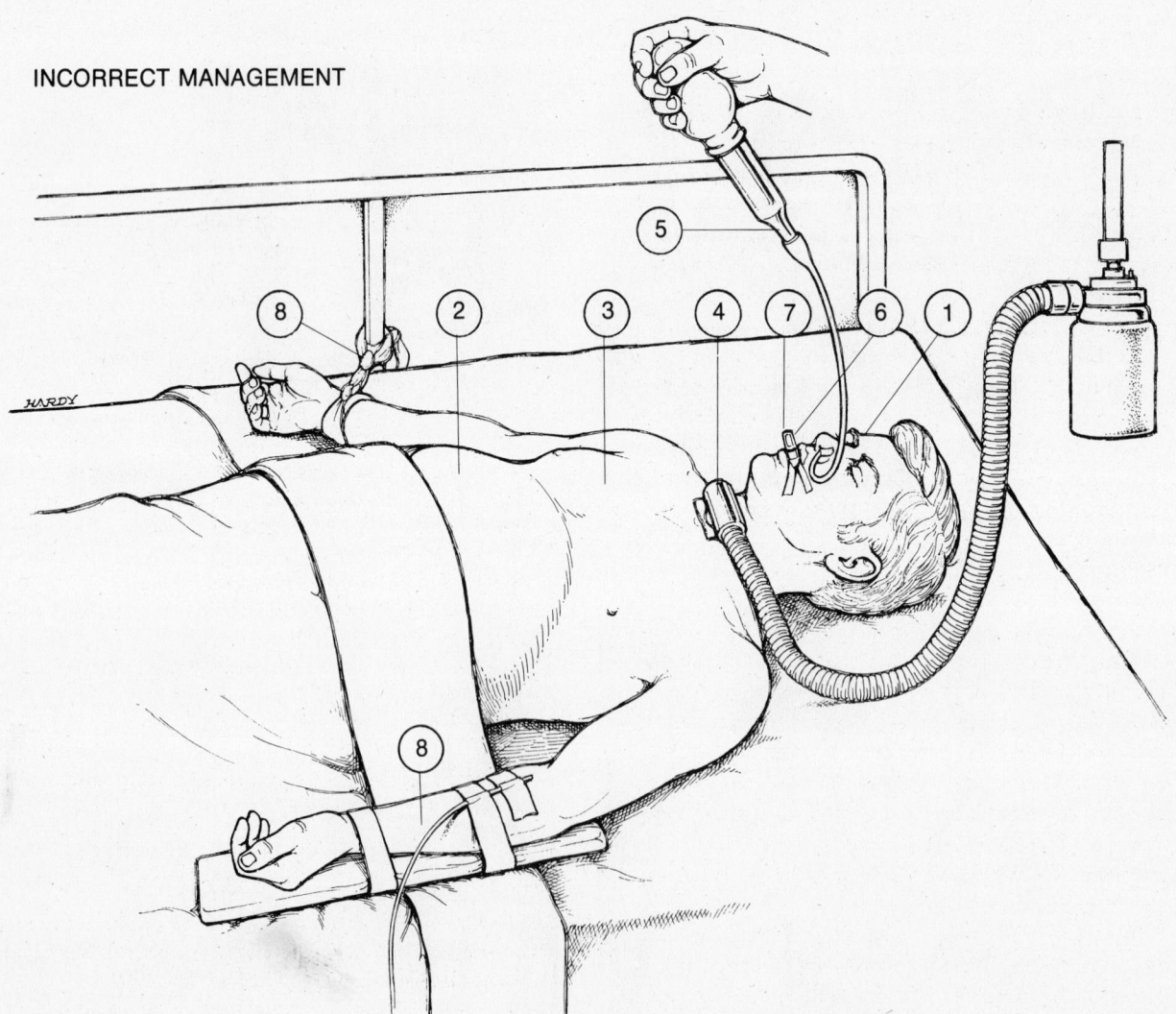

INCORRECT MANAGEMENT

Figure 24-13.   Factors that promote aspiration. (1) The patient is obtunded. (2) He has a distended abdomen. (3) He is in a supine position. (4) The tracheostomy tube has been inserted for a prolonged time. (5) The volume of the required calorie intake is being pumped or forced through the nasogastric tube. (6) Improper suctioning of oral and pharyngeal secretions causing marked stimulation of the gag reflex will promote vomiting and aspiration. (7) As a finale, an oral airway was inserted and taped to the patient to facilitate suction of oral secretions. (8) The patient's right hand is restrained while the left is immobilized because of the presence of an IV.

rich fluids into the interstitial and intra-alveolar spaces. This results in loss of surfactant, which in turn causes early closure of the airway. Finally the impaired exchange of oxygen and carbon dioxide causes respiratory failure.

Preventive Measures

When Reflexes Are Lacking. Aspiration is likely to occur if the patient cannot adequately coordinate his protective glottic, laryngeal, and cough reflexes. This hazard is increased if the patient has a distended abdomen, is in a supine position, and has his upper extremities immobilized by intravenous infusions or hand restraints. A normal person, when vomiting, can take care of his airway by sitting up or turning on his side and coordinating his breathing, coughing, gag, and glottic reflexes. If these reflexes are active, do not insert an oral airway. If an airway is in place, pull it out the moment the patient gags on it so as not to stimulate the pharyngeal gag reflex and promote vomiting and aspiration. Catheter suction of oral secretions should be executed with minimal pharyngeal stimulation yet at the same time should be effective.

During Tube Feeding. The patient who is receiving tube feedings should be positioned upright during the feeding and for 30 minutes thereafter to allow the stomach to partially empty. Small volumes given under low pressure will help to prevent aspiration.

With Delayed Emptying Time of Stomach. A full stomach may cause aspiration because of increased intra- or extragastric pressure. The following clinical situations cause delayed emptying time of the stomach and may contribute to aspiration: intestinal obstruction, increased gastric secretions during anxiety, stress, or pain, or abdominal distention because of ileus, ascites, peritonitis, drugs, severe illness, or vaginal delivery.

During Labor and Delivery. The patient during labor and delivery is a candidate for regurgitation and aspiration due to (1) loss of the protective reflexes of the upper airway because of general anesthesia, excessive narcotics, and sedatives; (2) the lithotomy position; (3) delayed emptying time of the stomach, because of labor contractions and the enlarged uterus. Increased intra-abdominal pressure while straining during delivery or manual pressure on the uterus to help expel the baby along with stimulation of the gag reflex also contribute to the problem.

Following Prolonged Endotracheal Intubation. Prolonged endotracheal intubation or tracheostomy can depress the laryngeal and glottic reflexes because of disuse. Patients with prolonged tracheostomies should be made to phonate and exercise their laryngeal muscles. The pharynx should be suctioned before deflating the cuff to prevent aspiration of regurgitated material. Bear in mind that improperly administered IPPB treatments

---

| **REMEMBER!!!** |
| 1. Massive aspiration is fatal. |
| 2. Small localized aspiration from regurgitation can cause pneumonia and respiratory distress. |
| 3. Silent regurgitation often takes place unobserved and may be more common than we think. |

by mask can distend the stomach and promote aspiration.

Figure 24–13 shows the different factors that promote aspiration. As you see, the stage is set for aspiration to take place. Awareness of the problem and better communication among physicians, nurses, and paramedical personnel will prevent this catastrophe from occurring. The best treatment for this iatrogenic disaster is prevention.

BIBLIOGRAPHY

BOOKS

Burton, G. G., Gee, G. N., and Hodgkin, J. B.: Respiratory Care. Philadelphia, J. B. Lippincott, 1977.

Gaskell, D. V., and Webber, B. A.: The Brompton Hospital Guide to Chest Physiotherapy. Philadelphia, J. B. Lippincott, 1975.

MacDonnell, K. F., and Segal, M.: Current Respiratory Care. Boston, Little, Brown, 1977.

McPherson, S. P.: Respiratory Therapy Equipment. St. Louis, C. V. Mosby, 1977.

Rau, J. L., Jr.: Respiratory Therapy Pharmacology. Chicago, Year Book Medical Publishing Co., 1978.

Rogers, R. M., ed.: Respiratory Intensive Care. Springfield, Charles C Thomas, 1977.

Shapiro, B. A., Harrison, R. A., and Walton, J. R.: Clinical Application of Respiratory Care. Chicago, Year Book Medical Publishing Co., 1977.

Shibel, E. M., and Moser, K. M.: Respiratory Emergencies. St. Louis, C. V. Mosby, 1977.

Wade, J. F.: Respiratory Nursing Care. St. Louis, C. V. Mosby, 1977.

Ziment, I.: Respiratory Pharmacology Therapeutics. Philadelphia, W. B. Saunders, 1978.

ARTICLES

Ashbaugh, D. G., et al.: Continuous positive pressure breathing (CPPB) in adult respiratory distress syndrome. J. Thor. Cardiovasc. Surg., 57:31–41, Jan. 1969.

Bakow, E. D.: Sustained maximal inspiration—a rationale for its use. Resp. Care, 22:379–382, Apr. 1977.

Drummond, G. B., and Milne, A. C.: Oxygen therapy after thoracotomy. Brit. J. Anaesth, 49:1093–1100, Nov. 1977.

———, and Wright, D. J.: Oxygen therapy after abdominal surgery. Brit. J. Anaesth., 49:789–796, Aug. 1977.

Gillick, J. S.: Spontaneous positive end-expiratory pressure (sPEEP). Anes. Analg., *56*:627-632, Sept.-Oct. 1977.

Hathaway, R.: The Swan-Ganz catheter: A review. Nurs. Clin. N. Am., *13*:339-407, Sept. 1978.

Levy, M. M., and Stubbs, J. A.: Nursing implications in the care of patients treated with assisted mechanical ventilation modified with positive-end expiratory pressure. Heart Lung, 7:299-305, Mar./Apr. 1978.

Loh, L., Sykes, M. K., and Chakrabarti, M. K.: The assessment of ventilator performance. Brit. J. Anaesth., *50*:63-71, Jan. 1978.

Rigg, J. R. A., and Jones, N. L.: Clinical assessment of respiratory function. Brit. J. Anaesth., *50*:3-12, Jan. 1978.

Sahn, S. A., Lakshminarayan, S., and Petty, T. L.: Weaning from mechanical ventilation. JAMA, *235*:2208-2212, May 17, 1976.

Swan, H. J. C., and Ganz, W.: Use of balloon flotation catheters in critically ill patients. Surg. Clin. N. Am., *55*:501-520, June 1975.

Sweetwood, H.: Acute respiratory insufficiency: How to recognize this emergency . . . how to treat it. Nursing '77, 7:24-31, Dec. 1977.

Weisel, R. D., Berger, R. L., and Hechtman, H. B.: Measurement of cardiac output by thermodilution. N. Eng. J. Med., *292*:682-684, Mar. 27, 1975.

Woods, S. L.: Monitoring pulmonary artery pressures. AJN, 76:1765-1771, Nov. 1976.

25

MANAGEMENT OF PATIENTS WITH CONDITIONS OF THE CHEST AND LOWER RESPIRATORY TRACT

PULMONARY INFECTIONS

ACUTE TRACHEOBRONCHITIS

Acute tracheobronchitis, an acute inflammation of the mucous membranes of the trachea and the bronchial tree, often follows infections of the upper respiratory tract. A patient with a viral infection has a lessened resistance and can readily develop a secondary bacterial infection. Thus the adequate treatment of upper respiratory infections is one of the major factors in the prevention of acute bronchitis. Aside from infection, inhalation of physical and chemical irritants, gases, or other air contaminants can also cause acute bronchial irritations.

Clinical Manifestations. The patient's symptoms result from the mucopurulent sputum that is secreted by the hyperemic edematous mucosa of the bronchi. The patient has a dry, irritating cough and expectorates a scanty amount of mucoid sputum at first. He complains of sternal soreness from coughing, and has fever, headache, and general malaise. As the infection progresses, the sputum is more profuse and purulent and the cough becomes looser. Acute tracheobronchitis can be a serious disease in very young children. The child is acutely ill and may have noisy strident respirations with intercostal retraction. Strict nursing vigilance and prompt action are required if these symptoms of respiratory obstruction appear.

Management. The treatment is largely symptomatic. Therefore, the nurse's observations are important in determining the therapeutic plan. The patient is placed on bed rest. Moist heat to the chest will relieve the soreness and pain, and hot drinks may prove soothing. Cool vapor therapy or steam inhalations are beneficial in relieving the laryngeal and tracheal irritation. Increasing the vapor pressure (moisture content) in the air will reduce irritation.

Cough depressants should not be given or should be given only with caution, when the cough becomes productive. Antihistamines especially may be excessively drying, making secretions more difficult to expectorate. An expectorant such as potassium iodide may be given and the fluid intake increased to "thin" the viscous and tenacious secretions. Usually recovery ensues within 7 to 10 days. Broad-spectrum antibiotics may be ordered if the patient does not improve promptly.

A primary nursing function is to caution the patient

469

against overexertion and chilling, which can induce a relapse or extension of the infection. Aged individuals are prone to develop bronchopneumonia as a complication. They are not always able to cough effectively and therefore tend to retain the mucopurulent exudate. These patients should be turned and should assume the sitting position at frequent intervals. Adequate opportunity for convalescence should be provided after the acute infection subsides, in order to avoid its recurrence.

PNEUMONIA

Pneumonia is an inflammatory process of the lung substance that is commonly caused by infectious agents. It is classified according to its causative agent, if known: for example, it may be a *bacterial, viral, fungal,* or *lipid pneumonia*. There is also a *chemical* pneumonia, such as that seen after ingestion of kerosene or inhalation of irritating gases. Radiation pneumonitis may follow radiation therapy for breast or lung cancer and usually occurs 6 weeks or more after completion of radiotherapy.

If a substantial portion of one or more lobes is involved, the disease is referred to as *lobar pneumonia. Bronchopneumonia* implies that the pneumonic process is distributed in patchy fashion, having originated in one or more localized areas within the bronchi and extended to the adjacent surrounding lung parenchyma. Of these two types, bronchopneumonia is more common than lobar pneumonia.

In recent years, with the use of immunosuppressive drugs, antileukemic drugs, or corticosteroids over long periods of time, an increase in the incidence of pneumonia due to more unusual organisms such as fungi, cytomegalovirus, or *Pneumocystis carinii* has occurred.

Pneumonia is spread by droplets or by contact with patients or carriers, since the pathogens producing pneumonia may be carried in the nasopharynx of a healthy person. The pathogens may invade tissues when the host's natural resistance is lowered. Colds and upper respiratory tract infections lead to more serious illnesses by allowing bacterial invasion of the lower respiratory tract. More often, pneumonia arises from endogenous flora of the patient whose resistance has been altered.

Pneumonia accounts for 10 percent of hospital admissions and along with influenza, is the fifth leading cause of death in the United States (the fourth in persons over 65). See Table 25-1 for a summary of the pneumonias.

Prevention and Persons at Risk

The nurse should be acquainted with the factors and circumstances that commonly predispose the person to pneumonia in order to identify the high-risk individual and engage in anticipatory and preventive nursing.

- Any condition producing mucus or bronchial obstruction and interfering with normal drainage of the lung (cancer,

chronic obstructive pulmonary disease) renders the individual susceptible to pneumonia.
- Any patient who is permitted to lie passively in bed for prolonged periods, relatively immobile and breathing shallowly, is highly vulnerable to the risk of bronchopneumonia.
- Any person who has a depressed cough reflex (due to drugs or weakness) or has aspirated foreign material into the lungs during a period of unconsciousness (head injury, anesthesia) or has an abnormal swallowing mechanism is very likely to develop bronchopneumonia.
- Persons who are intoxicated frequently are particularly susceptible to this infection, since alcohol suppresses the body's reflexes, white cell mobilization, and tracheobronchial ciliary motion.
- Any person scheduled to receive a sedative should be observed for respiratory rate and depth before the drug is given; if respiratory depression is apparent, the drug should not be administered. Respiratory depression predisposes to the pooling of bronchial secretions and subsequent development of pneumonia.
- An important preventive measure is the frequent suctioning of secretions in patients who are unconscious or have poor cough and gag reflexes; this reduces the likelihood that secretions will be aspirated or accumulate in the lungs and induce bronchopneumonia.

Postoperative pneumonia should be anticipated in the elderly and forestalled by frequent mobilization, coughing, and breathing exercises. In very ill persons, the oropharynx is likely to be colonized by gram-negative bacteria.

Infectious Disease Precautions

The infective organisms can become disseminated by means of airborne droplets or through contact with articles contaminated by the patient's respiratory secretions.

- Thorough handwashing should therefore be carried out after each contact with the patient or his surroundings. The patient should be instructed to use tissues when coughing. Used paper tissues and disposable sputum cups should be securely wrapped in paper and burned. Proper room ventilation to the outside will decrease the number of airborne droplets in the room.

Bacterial Pneumonia (*Streptococcus pneumoniae*)

Streptococcus pneumoniae pneumonia is the most common bacterial pneumonia and is most prevalent during the winter and spring months when upper respiratory infections are most frequent. It may occur as a lobar or bronchopneumonic form in patients of any age. A history of recent respiratory illness can often be elicited.

Streptococcus pneumoniae, the infecting agent that causes almost 90 percent of the cases of bacterial pneumonia, is a gram-positive, capsulated, nonmotile coccus that resides naturally in the upper respiratory tract. *S. pneumoniae* is commonly referred to as the pneumococcus.

Pathophysiology. The altered physiology occurring with the pneumonic process is a ventilation problem.

The pneumococci gain access to the alveoli where an inflammatory reaction occurs which produces an exudate that pours into the air spaces. White blood cells, mostly neutrophils, also migrate into the alveoli, so that the lung segment assumes a more solid structure as the air-containing spaces become filled. Areas of the lung are not adequately ventilated because of secretions, mucosal edema, and bronchospasm. These conditions cause partial occlusion of the bronchi and/or alveoli, producing a drop in the alveolar oxygen tension. Venous blood coming into the lungs passes through the underventilated area and goes out of the lung to the left side of the heart without being oxygenated. In essence, the blood is shunted from the right to the left side of the heart. This mixing of oxygenated and unoxygenated blood eventually results in arterial hypoxemia.

Clinical Manifestations. The onset of acute pneumococcal pneumonia is precipitous. The patient has a sudden onset of shaking chill, rapidly rising fever (38.5-40.5° C. [101-105° F.]), and stabbing chest pain that is aggravated by respiration and coughing. He appears severely ill with marked tachypnea (25-45/minute) accompanied by respiratory grunting and flaring nares. He often lies on his affected side in an attempt to splint his chest. The pulse is rapid and bounding. The cheeks are flushed, the eyes bright, and the lips and nail beds cyanotic. The patient prefers to be propped up in bed because of his cough, which is short, painful, and incessant. He sweats profusely and is often cyanotic. The sputum is purulent and sometimes blood-tinged or rusty.

Other signs occur in patients who suffer from a condition such as cancer or those who are undergoing treatment with immunosuppressants which lower their resistance to infection and to organisms heretofore not considered serious pathogens. Such patients present with fever, rales, and physical signs of lobar consolidation (tactile and vocal fremitus, bronchial breathing, and percussion dullness).

In older patients or those with chronic obstructive pulmonary disease, the symptoms may develop insidiously. Purulent sputum may be the only signal of pneumonia in these patients. It is difficult to detect subtle changes in their conditions as they already have seriously compromised pulmonary function. Assess these patients for unusual behavior, alterations in mental status, stupor, and congestive heart failure. A restless, excited delirium may be exhibited especially in alcoholic patients.

Diagnostic Assessment. Diagnosis is made by history (particularly of recent respiratory infection), physical examination, and chest x-rays, and is confirmed by examination of a gram-stained specimen of sputum.

• In order to get a good sample of sputum, have the patient rinse his mouth with water to minimize contamination by normal oral flora. Instruct him to breathe deeply several times and then to cough deeply and expectorate the raised sputum into a sterile continer.

Sputum may also be obtained by transtracheal aspiration (page 405) in patients who cannot raise sputum or those who are obtunded, have abnormal host defense mechanisms, or have developed pneumonia after antimicrobial therapy or while hospitalized.

Bacteriologic diagnosis may also be based on a blood culture, since bloodstream invasion occurs frequently with bacterial pneumonia.

Management. The treatment of pneumonia depends upon laboratory identification of the agent causing the infection. Penicillin G is usually the antibiotic of choice. If the patient is seriously ill the drug may be given intravenously. Erythromycin or a cephalosporin (cephalothin or clindamycin) may be alternative drugs for persons who are sensitive to penicillin.

Supportive Nursing Management. The patient is placed on bed rest until infection shows signs of clearing. He is observed carefully and continually until his clinical condition improves. Lethal complications may develop during the first few days of antibiotic treatment. The patient is watched for continuing or recurring fever. Inadequate lung drainage or poor blood supply to the involved lung may reduce the amount of antibiotic agent reaching the invading organism. Resistant or recurring fever may be due to drug allergy (assess for skin rash), drug resistance or slow response of the susceptible organism, super-infection, infected pleural effusion, or pneumonia due to unusual organisms (such as *Pneumocystis carinii* or fungi).

• Failure of the pneumonia to resolve raises the suspicion of underlying carcinoma of the bronchus.

ELIMINATION AND CONTROL OF SECRETIONS. Retained secretions interfere with gas exchange. A high level of fluid intake (within level of cardiac reserve) is encouraged, since adequate hydration thins and loosens pulmonary secretions and also replaces fluid losses due to fever, diaphoresis, dehydration, and dyspnea. The air is humidified in order to loosen secretions and improve ventilation. A high humidity face mask (using either compressed air or oxygen) delivers warm humidified air to the tracheobronchial tree and liquefies secretions.

The patient is encouraged to cough in the following manner:
1. Inhale slowly through the nose.
2. Exhale and cough forcefully while contracting (holding in) the abdomen. (This tightens the glottis and raises intra-pulmonary pressure.)

Chest physiotherapy (percusssion and postural drainage) is also important in loosening and mobilizing secretions. The chest is vibrated and clapped and the patient is then placed in the proper position to drain the involved lung. Postural drainage uses the principle of gravity that

TABLE 25-1.   COMMONLY ENCOUNTERED PNEUMONIAS

TYPE (BACTERIAL)	ORGANISM RESPONSIBLE	MANIFESTATIONS
Streptococcal pneumonia	*Streptococcus pneumoniae*[1]	May be history of previous respiratory infection Sudden onset, with shaking and chills Rapidly rising fever Cough, with expectoration of rusty or green (purulent) sputum Pleuritic pain aggravated by cough Chest dull to percussion; rales, bronchial breath sounds
Staphylococcal pneumonia	*Staphylococcus aureus*	Often prior history of viral infection Insidious development of cough, with expectoration of yellow, blood-streaked mucus Onset may be sudden if patient is outside hospital Fever Pleuritic chest pain Pulse varies; may be slow in proportion to temperature
Klebsiella pneumonia	*Klebsiella pneumoniae* (Friedländer's bacillus—encapsulated gram-negative aerobic bacillus)	Onset sudden with high fever, chills, pleuritic pain, hemoptysis Dyspnea, cyanosis Copious pink, gelatinous or loose, thin sputum expectorated Profound prostration and toxicity
Pseudomonas pneumonia	*Pseudomonas aeruginosa*	Hectic fever, cough, hypoxia, apprehension, confusion, cyanosis

[1]Formerly classified in the genus *Diplococcus* (pneumococcus)

permits secretions to flow from the smaller bronchi to the larger bronchi to be expectorated or suctioned. If the patient is too weak to cough effectively, the mucus may have to be removed by nasotracheal suctioning or by bronchoscopic aspiration.

OXYGENATION.   The patient who is hypoxic should be given oxygen. Arterial blood gas analysis is done to determine oxygen need and evaluate oxygen effectiveness. A high concentration of oxygen is to be avoided in persons with chronic obstructive pulmonary disease since it may worsen alveolar ventilation by removing the patient's only remaining ventilatory drive and lead to respiratory decompensation. Respiratory support mea-

sures such as endotracheal intubation, high inspiratory oxygen concentrations, and positive end-expiratory pressure may be required for some patients. These treatment modalities are discussed in chapter 24.

PAIN RELIEF.   Pleuritic pain may be relieved by codeine or intercostal nerve block. Evaluate the patient's sensorium before administering sedatives or tranquilizers, in order to assess for signs and symptoms of pneumococcal meningitis. Restlessness, confusion, and aggression may well be due to cerebral hypoxemia, in which case sedatives are inappropriate.

Avoid suppressing the cough reflex. However, serious hypoxia may follow paroxysms of coughing especially in

CLINICAL FEATURES	TREATMENT	COMPLICATIONS
Herpes simplex lesions often present on face or lips Usually involves one or more lobes	Penicillin G Alternate drug therapy in penicillin-allergic patient (erythromycin, clindamycin, cephalothin)	Shock Pleural effusion Superinfections Pericarditis Otitis media Empyema
Frequently seen in hospital setting (ventilator therapy; postoperative) May follow influenza especially in pregnant women or leukemic patients Staphylococcal pneumonia is a necrotizing infection Treatment must be vigorous and prolonged due to disease's tendency to destroy the lungs Organism may develop rapid drug resistance Prolonged convalescence usual	Nafcillin, methicillin, clindamycin, vancomycin	Effusion/pneumothorax Lung abscess Empyema Meningitis
Tends to attack chronically ill, debilitated, alcoholic, and elderly men or those with chronic obstructive pulmonary disease Tissue necrosis occurs rapidly in lungs with cavity formation in some patients May be rapidly fulminating, progressing to fatal outcome High mortality rate	Gentamicin, cephalothin, cefazolin, kanamycin	Lung abscesses, either single or multiple Persistent cough with expectoration remains for prolonged period Empyema Pericarditis
Usually acquired in the hospital Susceptible persons: those with preexisting lung disease, cancer (particularly leukemia); those with homograft transplants, burns; debilitated persons; patients receiving prolonged courses of antibiotics and treatment such as tracheostomy, suctioning Respiratory equipment may be contaminated with these organisms	Gentamicin, carbenicillin	Multiple lung abscess formation High fatality rate

(Continued)

persons with preexisting heart conditions. Nonproductive paroxysms of coughing may be controlled with codeine. This may, however, be contraindicated in patients with chronic obstructive pulmonary disease (COPD) in whom opiates or other central nervous system depressants cause further hypoventilation.

Abdominal distention may be distressing since the patient may swallow air during intervals of severe dyspnea. It impairs respiratory movement by elevation of the diaphragm. A nasogastric tube may be passed for acute gastric dilation.

DIET. Initially, the dyspneic patient is anorexic and prefers a liquid diet. With improvement, a normal diet is offered. Persons with congestive heart failure may be on a low sodium diet. (See also Guidelines for Caring for a Patient with Bacterial Pneumonia, pages 476–477.)

Assessment for Complications. Patients should respond to treatment within 24 hours after antibiotic therapy is initiated. Complications of pneumonia include sustained *hypotension and shock* (especially in gram-negative bacterial disease in the elderly). This complication is encountered chiefly in patients who have received no specific treatment, have been treated too little or too late, have received chemotherapy to which the infecting organism is resistant, or are suffering another debilitating disease which complicates the pneumonia.

TABLE 25-1. (CONTINUED)

TYPE (NONBACTERIAL)	ORGANISM RESPONSIBLE	MANIFESTATIONS
Mycoplasma pneumonia	*Mycoplasma pneumoniae*	Gradual onset, severe headache, irritating hacking cough producing scanty, mucoid sputum Anorexia; malaise Low grade fever
Viral pneumonia	Influenza viruses Parainfluenza viruses Respiratory syncytial viruses Adenovirus Varicella, rubella, rubeola, herpes simplex, cytomegalovirus, Epstein-Barr virus	Cough Constitutional symptoms may be pronounced (severe headache, anorexia, fever, and myalgia)
Pneumocystis carinii pneumonia	*Pneumocystis carinii*	Insidious onset Increasing dyspnea and nonproductive cough Tachypnea; progresses rapidly to intercostal retraction, nasal flaring, and cyanosis Lowering of arterial oxygen tension Chest x-ray will reveal diffuse, bilateral interstitial pneumonia
Fungal pneumonia	*Aspergillus fumigatus*	Hectic fever, productive cough, chest pain, hemoptysis Chest x-ray reveals broad range of abnormalities from infiltration to consolidation, cavitation, and empyema

To combat peripheral collapse and maintain arterial blood pressure, a vasoconstrictor agent is given intravenously in the form of a constant infusion and at a rate that is readjusted constantly in accordance with the pressure response. Corticosteroid drugs may be administered parenterally to combat shock and toxicity in patients with pneumonia who are extremely ill and in apparent danger of succumbing to the infection.

Atelectasis (from obstruction of bronchus by accumulated secretions) may occur at any stage of acute pneumonia. Pleural effusion (page 478) also is fairly common and may signal the beginning of empyema. A diagnostic thoracentesis is usually necessary to evaluate an effusion. A chest tube may be required to control pleural infection by establishing proper drainage of the empyema.

Delirium is another possible complication and is considered a medical emergency when it occurs. It may be caused by hypoxia, meningitis, or the delirium tremens of alcoholism. The patient with delirium is given oxygen, adequate hydration, and mild sedation and is observed constantly. Congestive heart failure and arrhythmias are also complications of pneumonia.

Vaccine for Pneumococcal Disease. Polyvalent polysaccharide vaccine against diseases caused by *Streptococcus pneumoniae* has recently been licensed in the United States. The vaccine contains 14 particular types of pneumococci which cause at least 80 percent of all bacteremic pneumococcal disease in this country. It appears to induce satisfactory antibody response in persons over 2 years of age.*

Patient Education. After the fever subsides, the patient may gradually increase his activities. Fatigue and weakness may be prolonged after pneumonia. Breathing exercises to clear the lungs and promote full lung expansion are encouraged (page 420). The patient is instructed to return to the clinic or physician's office for follow-up chest x-rays.

Explain to the patient that it is wise to stop smoking since cigarette smoking destroys tracheobronchial cilial action, which is the first line of defense of the lungs. It also irritates the mucous cells of the bronchi and inhibits the function of alveolar macrophage (scavenger) cells. Review with the patient the principles of good nutrition and rest, since one episode of pneumonia may make him susceptible to recurring respiratory infections. He should be encouraged to obtain influenza vaccine at the pre-

*Recommendation of the Public Health Service Advisory Committee on Immunization Practices. Pneumococcal polysaccharide vaccine. Morbidity and Weekly Report, Vol. 27, Jan. 27, 1978.

CLINICAL FEATURES	TREATMENT	COMPLICATIONS

Occurs most commonly in children and young adults
Cold agglutinin antibody titer elevated
	Tetracycline or erythromycin	Rare:
		    pleural effusion
		    meningoencephalitis
		    myelitis
		    Guillain-Barré syndrome

In majority of patients influenza begins as an acute coryza; others have bronchitis, pleurisy, etc., while still others develop gastrointestinal symptoms Risk of developing influenza related to crowding and close contact of groups of individuals	Treat symptomatically Does not respond to treatment with presently available antimicrobials Prophylactic vaccination recommended for high risk persons (over 65; chronic cardiac or pulmonary disease, diabetes and other metabolic disorders)	May develop a superimposed bacterial infection Bronchopneumonia Pericarditis; endocarditis
Usually seen in host whose resistance is compromised and who has received steroids in recent past Organism invades lungs of patients who have suppressed immune system (from cancer, leukemia) or following immunosuppressive therapy for cancer, organ transplant, or collagen disease Frequently associated with concurrent infection by viruses, (cytomegalovirus) bacteria, and fungi Diagnosis made by lung biopsy	Pentamide isethionate	Patients are critically ill Death may be due to asphyxia
Neutropenic individual most susceptible May develop *Aspergillus* as a superinfection	Amphotericin B Granulocyte transfusions may be beneficial	High fatality rate Invades blood vessels and destroys lung tissue by direct invasion and vascular infarction

scribed times, because influenza increases susceptibility to secondary bacterial pneumonia, especially staphylococcus, *Haemophilus influenzae,* and *Streptococcus pneumoniae.*

Mycoplasma Pneumonia (Primary Atypical Pneumonia)

Mycoplasma pneumoniae is one of the chief causes of primary atypical pneumonia. Mycoplasmas are small organisms surrounded by a triple-layered membrane without a cell wall. The organisms grow on a special culture medium but differ from viruses. Mycoplasma pneumonia occurs most frequently in older children and young adults.

It is probably spread by infected respiratory droplets, through person-to-person contact. Often these patients develop positive cold agglutinin titers in their serum but specific complement fixation antibody titers of acute and convalescent titers are diagnostic.

The inflammatory infiltrate is primarily interstitial rather than alveolar. It spreads throughout the entire respiratory tract, including the bronchioles. Generally it has the characteristics of a bronchopneumonia.

Clinical Manifestations. Usually the patient has had an upper respiratory infection, and the onset of his pneumonic symptoms is gradual. The predominant symptoms are a harassing and nonproductive cough, a feeling of tightness in the chest, and generalized aching and prostration, along with tracheal pain when coughing. After a few days, mucoid or mucopurulent sputum is expectorated. The patient complains of headache that is aggravated by the cough.

Nursing Management. The objective of nursing care is to promote the patient's rest and comfort. Warm moist inhalations are helpful in relieving bronchial irritation. Mycoplasma pneumonia responds to erythromycin and tetracycline. Other "atypical" pneumonias are viral in origin and do not respond to antibiotics. The nursing care and treatment (with the exception of antibacterial therapy) is the same as that given to the patient who has a bacterial pneumonia (pages 471–477).

PLEURISY

Pleurisy (pleuritis) is inflammation of the visceral and parietal pleurae. When these inflamed membranes rub together during respiration (particularly inspiration) the result is severe, sharp, "knifelike" pain. The pain may become minimal or absent when the breath is held, or it may be localized or radiate to the shoulder or abdomen. Later, as pleural fluid develops, the pain lessens. In the early dry period, the pleural friction rub can be heard with the stethoscope, only to disappear later as fluid appears to separate the roughened pleural surfaces.

Pleurisy may develop with pneumonia or upper respiratory infection, tuberculosis, collagen disease, after trauma to the chest or pulmonary infarction or embolism, in primary and metastatic cancer, in the viral disease known as epidemic pleurodynia, and after thoracotomy.

Careful x-ray and sputum examinations and thoracentesis with pleural fluid examination and possibly pleural biopsy are indicated in order to discover the underlying condition.

Management. The objective of treatment is to discover the underlying condition causing the pleurisy. As the underlying disease is treated (pneumonia, infarction) the pleuritic inflammation usually resolves. At the same time it is necesary to watch for signs of pleural effusion: shortness of breath, pain, and decreased local excursion of the chest wall.

Since this patient has real pain on inspiration, the nurse can offer suggestions to enhance comfort, such as turning frequently on the affected side in order to splint the chest wall; this will lessen the stretch of the pleura. The nurse

---

GUIDELINES FOR CARING FOR THE PATIENT WITH BACTERIAL PNEUMONIA
Objectives, Principles, and Rationale of Care

I. To assist with collection of laboratory data for the identification of the causative organism:
   A. Bacteriological study of sputum
      1. Instruct patient to cough productively so that specimens will consist of bronchial secretions.

      Specific antimicrobial therapy depends upon the nature and sensitivity of organisms isolated from the culture and the sensitivity tests of the sputum specimen.

      2. If patient is too ill to raise sputum, aspirate trachea with catheter or use transtracheal aspiration.

      Tracheal aspiration can produce a paroxysm of coughing that produces sputum.

      3. Collect sputum in sterile containers.
   B. Hemogram and urinalysis
   C. Bacteriological study of blood
   D. Posteroanterior and lateral chest x-rays

II. To provide specific therapy to eradicate the organism:
   A. Give prescribed antibiotic at correct time intervals.
      1. Penicillin is usually drug of choice.
      2. Clindamycin, cephalothin, erythromycin can be given if patient is allergic to penicillin.

      Pneumococci are highly susceptible to the action of penicillin. Parenteral antimicrobial therapy is given to severely ill patients; the dosage and route of administration depend upon severity of pneumonia and the appearance of complications.

   B. Observe patient for nausea, vomiting, diarrhea, anal pruritus, skin rash, and soft tissue reactions.

III. To evaluate the patient's response to therapy:
   A. Take T.P.R. and B.P. at regular 4-hour intervals and more frequently if indicated.

      Lethal complications may develop during the early period of antimicrobial treatment.

      1. Watch for continuing or recurring fever from drug allergy, drug resistance or slow response to therapy, inadequate/inappropriate antimicrobial therapy, superinfection, failure of pneumonia to resolve.

      The temperature curve provides an index of the patient's response to therapy and his progress.
      Hypotension occurring early in the course of the illness may indicate hypoxia or bacteremia.
      Salicylates should be given with caution since they produce a drop in temperature and thus interfere with evaluation of the temperature curve.

   B. Evaluate for evidences of peripheral vascular collapse.

      If hypotension is present, there is a decrease in coronary and brain oxygenation, which may produce serious effects.

      1. Combat shock immediately and vigorously with pressor amines, IV fluids, and blood.
      2. Give penicillin IV if shock is present.
   C. Assess patient for evidence of delirium.

      Delirium is considered a grave prognostic sign and may be due to hypoxia, hypercapnia, meningitis, or the delirium tremens of alcoholism.

   D. Auscultate chest for rales, signs of consolidation or pleural effusion.

IV. To provide supportive care and relieve the patient's discomfort:
   A. Assist the patient to cough productively.
      1. Splint the patient's chest while he is coughing.

      Depression of the cough reflex may produce retention of pulmonary secretions and lead to atelectasis.

(Continued)

2. Give codeine as prescribed.
3. Humidify air to loosen secretions and improve ventilation. Encourage high level of fluid intake.
4. Employ postural drainage and percussion to mobilize secretions.

B. Use measures to reduce pleuritic pain.
   1. Use hot and cold applications as prescribed.
   2. Assist with intercostal nerve block with procaine.
   3. Use analgesics with caution to prevent depression of cough reflex and CNS respiratory drive.

C. Maintain fluid and electrolyte balance.
   1. Offer 2,000-3,000 ml. of fluids daily.
   2. Administer IV fluids and electrolytes if patient is seriously ill or vomiting.

D. Give oxygen as indicated for dyspnea, circulatory disturbance, or delirium.
   1. Monitor arterial blood gases to determine oxygen need and evaluate oxygen effectiveness.

Elderly patients have a diminished cough reflex and may require vigorous measures (suctioning, bronchoscopy) for removal of secretions.

Pain and cough result from pleuritic invasion by pneumococci. The discomfort of pleuritic pain can interfere with the mechanics of ventilation. Pleuritic pain causes shallow breathing; the aeration of the pulmonary alveoli is diminished and this contributes to the development of ventilation-perfusion imbalance and hypoxemia.
Fluid loss is high because of fever, dehydration, dyspnea, and diaphoresis.

Restlessness, confusion, and aggressiveness may be due to cerebral hypoxia.
A patient suffering from pneumonia who has preexisting chronic obstructive pulmonary disease (bronchitis, emphysema) is apt to develop CO_2 narcosis when receiving oxygen (see pages 415-416). A mechanical ventilator may be required for patients with coexisting chronic ventilatory insufficiency.

V. To be alert for complications:
   A. Pleural effusion; atelectasis
   B. Sustained hypotension and shock
   C. Delayed resolution
   D. Superinfection
      1. Pericarditis
      2. Bacteremia
      3. Meningitis
   E. Toxic delirium (a medical emergency)
   F. Congestive heart failure; arrhythmias
   G. Acute respiratory failure

Approximately 15 to 20 percent of patients with pneumonia develop complications. Patients should respond to treatment within 24 to 48 hours.

VI. To educate the patient concerning prevention of pulmonary disease.
   A. Fatigue and weakness may be prolonged after pneumonia.
   B. Try to stop smoking.

Cigarette smoking destroys tracheobronchial cilial action which is the first line of defense of the lungs; smoking also irritates mucous cells of bronchi and inhibits function of alveolar scavenger cells (macrophages).

   C. Keep up natural resistance (adequate rest, good nutrition).
   D. Obtain influenza vaccine at prescribed times.

One episode of pneumonia appears to make the individual susceptible to recurring respiratory infections.
Influenza increases susceptibility to secondary bacterial pneumonia.

   E. Avoid overfatigue, chilling, and excessive alcohol intake, which lower resistance to pneumonia.
   F. Report any signs and symptoms of a respiratory infection to the physician.

Colds and upper respiratory tract infections may lead to bacterial invasion of lower respiratory tract.

   G. Urge patients to have follow-up examinations after recovery and dismissal from the hospital.
   H. Avoid obliteration of cough reflex and aspiration of secretions.

Pneumonia frequently coexists with other pulmonary pathology, namely, cancer of the lung.

can also teach the patient to use his hands to splint the rib cage while coughing.

Prescribed analgesics and applications of heat or cold will provide symptomatic relief. Indomethacin, an anti-inflammatory drug, may give pain relief while allowing the patient to cough effectively. If the pain is severe, a procaine intercostal block may be required. Since pain upon breathing produces anxiety, the patient will require support and understanding.

PLEURAL EFFUSION

Pleural effusion, a collection of fluid in the pleural space, is rarely a primary disease process but is usually secondary to other diseases. Normally the pleural space may contain a small amount of fluid acting as a lubricant that allows the visceral and parietal surfaces to move without friction.

In certain intrathoracic and systemic diseases, large quantities of fluid may accumulate in the pleural space. The effusion can be a relatively clear fluid which may be a transudate or an exudate, or it can be blood, pus, or chyle. A *transudate* (filtrates of plasma that move across intact capillary walls) occurs when factors influencing formation and reabsorption of pleural fluid are altered. A transudate indicates that a condition like ascites or a systemic disease like congestive heart failure or renal failure underlies the fluid accumulation. An *exudate* (extravasation of fluid into tissues/cavity) usually results from inflammation and may indicate that the pleural effusion has accumulated as a result of local inflammatory processes within the pleural space or in either adjacent tissues or the subdiaphragmatic area (subdiaphragmatic abscess, liver abscess). Pleural effusion may be a complication of tuberculosis, pneumonia, congestive heart failure, pulmonary viral infections, and neoplastic tumors. In fact 50 percent of patients with cancer of the lung develop pleural effusion. In approximately one in four patients, pleural effusion is secondary to carcinoma.

Clinical Manifestations. The accumulation of fluid manifests itself by shortness of breath and an increasing pulse rate. There is dullness or flatness to percussion over the areas of fluid with minimal or absent breath sounds. Sometimes the patient has a slight dry cough. Confirmation of the presence of fluid is obtained by chest x-ray, ultrasound, physical examination, and thoracentesis. Tests made of pleural fluid include bacterial cultures, gram stain, acid-fast bacillus stain (for tuberculosis), red cell count, white cell count, chemistry studies (glucose, amylase, lactic dehydrogenase, protein), and pH.

Management. The objectives of treatment are to discover the underlying cause, to prevent fluid collection from recurring, and to relieve discomfort and dyspnea. Specific treatment is directed to the underlying cause, e.g., congestive heart failure, cirrhosis, etc.

Thoracentesis is done to remove fluid, to collect a specimen for analysis, and to relieve dyspnea. However, if the underlying cause is a malignancy, the effusion may recur within a few days or weeks. Repeated thoracenteses result in pain, depletion of protein and electrolytes, and sometimes pneumothorax. In this event the patient may be treated with chest tube drainage connected to an underwater seal drainage system or suction to evacuate the pleural space and reexpand the lung. Sometimes radioactive isotopes or cytotoxic or other chemically irritating drugs are instilled in the pleural space to prevent further accumulation of fluid. After drug instillation, the chest tube is clamped and the patient is assisted to assume various positions to assure uniform drug distribution and to maximize drug contact with the pleural surfaces. The tube is unclamped as prescribed and chest drainage is usually continued several days longer. Other modalities of treatment for malignant pleural effusions include radiation of the chest wall, surgical pleurectomy, and diuretic therapy.

If the pleural fluid is an exudate, more extensive diagnostic procedures are done in order to determine the cause. Therapy for pleural disease is then instituted.

LUNG ABSCESS

Pathogenesis. A *lung abscess* is a localized, pus-containing necrotic lesion in the lung characterized by cavity formation. It may occur from aspiration of vomitus or infected material (nasotracheal secretions; blood) from the upper respiratory tract. After aspiration, pneumonitis develops, and the area of pneumonia cavitates because the microorganisms have necrotizing potential; hence a lung abscess may develop very rapidly. A lung abscess may also occur secondarily to bronchial obstruction due to a tumor. Stasis of secretions occurs with infection or necrosis within the tumor mass. Or, it may be a sequela of necrotizing pneumonias, tuberculosis, pulmonary embolism, or chest trauma.

In the initial stages the cavity in the lung may or may not communicate with a bronchus; eventually, however, it becomes surrounded, or "encapsulated," by a wall of fibrous tissue, except at one or two points where the necrotic process extends until it reaches the lumen of some bronchus or the pleural space and thus establishes a communication with the respiratory tract, the pleural cavity, or both. In the first instance, its purulent contents are evacuated continuously in the form of sputum, whereas if a pleural exit is accessible, empyema results; if both types of communication are furnished, the problem becomes one of *bronchopleural fistula*.

Clinical Manifestations. The majority of patients have a cough which produces a small amount of sputum, a low grade fever, and malaise. In time the sputum may become voluminous, purulent, and malodorous. This occurs frequently when bronchial communication is established and the abscess begins to drain. The patient may complain of a pleuritic type of chest pain. Sometimes the onset is acute, with chills, high fever, cough, and malaise. Physical examination reveals an area of consolidation and pleural thickening, dullness to percussion, and suppressed breath sounds. Clubbing of the fingers may occur.

Confirmation of the diagnosis is made by chest roentgenography, sputum culture, and direct visualization with fiberoptic bronchoscopy, which is necessary to rule out the possibility of tumor or a foreign body in the lung.

Preventive Measures. The following principles will reduce the risk of suppurative lung disease:

1. Patients who must have teeth extracted while their gums and teeth are infected may be given appropriate antibiotic therapy before any dental manipulations.
2. The patient should be instructed to maintain good dental and oral hygiene, since anaerobic bacteria play a role in the pathogenesis of lung abscess.
3. Appropriate antimicrobial therapy should be given to patients with pneumonia.
4. Bronchoscopy is called for if inhalation of foreign material is suspected.
5. A patient with impaired cough reflexes and loss of glottis closure or one who has swallowing difficulties is apt to aspirate foreign material and hence to develop lung abscess.
6. Other persons at risk include alcoholics, patients with seizure disorders, stroke, drug addiction, or esophageal disease, as well as patients being fed by nasogastric tube or those who have received general anesthesia.

Management. The objectives of treatment are to establish adequate drainage of the abscess and to eradicate infection. Drainage of lung abscesses is usually established through the tracheobronchial tree. Most lung abscesses resolve through frequent bronchoscopy (to maintain bronchial communication with the abscess), postural drainage, and appropriate antibiotic therapy.

Usually sputum specimens are obtained by transtracheal aspiration since an expectorated sputum specimen will be contaminated by the indigenous flora of the mouth and gingivae. Usually several species of bacteria are present in a lung abscess. Antimicrobial therapy is given according to sputum culture and sensitivity. Penicillin G is the treatment of choice for anaerobic pulmonary abscesses. High intravenous doses are generally required, because the antibiotic must penetrate necrotic tissue and abscess fluid. Alternative drugs (clindamycin, chloramphenicol) are used for penicillin-sensitive patients.

After the patient shows signs of improvement as demonstrated by normal temperature, abatement of leukocytosis, and improvement in the chest x-ray (resolution of surrounding infiltrate, diminution in size of cavity,

and absence of fluid), the antibiotic is administered orally rather than intravenously. If treatment is stopped too soon, a relapse may occur. The duration of antibiotic therapy may be from 6 to 12 weeks.

Surgical intervention is indicated only when medical therapy has been proved inadequate by failure of the cavity to resolve or by a continuing septic condition. Pulmonary resection (lobectomy) is the procedure usually performed when there is a thick-walled abscess with purulent drainage. If the patient's condition is critical, tube thoracostomy is used.

Patient Education. After surgery there is usually a somewhat prolonged period of drainage before the wound closes entirely. It may be necessary to teach a family member to change the simple dressings frequently enough to prevent excoriation of the skin and an offensive odor. If possible, the patient should be placed under the supervision of a community health nurse or some helping agency that will assist the family in meeting any problems that may arise. The patient is encouraged to have patience, since it takes time for chest x-rays to indicate that the condition has cleared. The patient should receive nutritional counseling for attaining and maintaining an optimal state of nutrition.

EMPYEMA

Empyema is a collection of infected pleural exudate between the visceral and parietal pleurae (the pleural cavity). At first the pleural fluid is thin, with a low leukocyte count, but frequently it progresses to a fibropurulent stage and finally to a stage where it encloses the lung within a thick exudative membrane.

In most instances empyema is associated with an underlying pulmonary infection. Organisms may invade the pleural space by direct extension or as the result of the rupture of a lung abscess. Empyema may also follow thoracic surgery or penetrating wounds of the chest. The character of the exudate varies according to the infecting organism.

Symptoms. The patient has fever, pleural pain, dyspnea, anorexia, and weight loss. Chest auscultation reveals the absence of breath sounds and there is flatness to chest percussion as well as decreased fremitus (vocal vibration felt by palpation). If the patient has received antibiotic therapy the clinical manifestations may be altered. The diagnosis is established by white blood count and differential counts, chest x-ray, and the examination of the pleural exudate by needle aspiration.

Management. The objectives of treatment are to remove the infected material and to approximate (bring closer together) the pleural surfaces. This is accomplished by adequate drainage and by appropriate antibiotics selected on the basis of the causative organism. Large doses of the drug are usually given.

Drainage of the pleural fluid or pus depends on the stage of the disease and is accomplished by

1. needle aspiration (thoracentesis) if the fluid is not too thick,
2. closed-chest drainage using a large diameter intercostal tube attached to underwater drainage (page 425), or
3. open drainage via rib resection to remove the thickened pleura, pus, and debris and to resect the underlying diseased pulmonary tissue.

If the inflammation has been long-standing, an exudate can form over the lung and interfere with its normal expansion. This will have to be removed surgically (decortication). (See page 423 for the nursing management following thoracotomy.) The drainage tube is left in place until the pus-filled space is obliterated completely; otherwise it will recur. The complete obliteration of the pleural space is checked by x-ray. This process may take a prolonged period of time. Breathing exercises, particularly those emphasizing exhalation against resistance, help to restore normal respiratory function.

BRONCHIECTASIS

Bronchiectasis is an abnormal and persistent dilatation of the bronchi resulting from inflammatory damage to their walls. Bronchial dilatation may be caused by a variety of causes, including pulmonary infections and obstruction of the bronchus, aspiration of foreign bodies, vomitus, or material from the upper respiratory tract, and pressure from tumors, dilated blood vessels, and enlarged lymph nodes. A person may be predisposed to bronchiectasis as a result of respiratory infection in early childhood, measles, influenza, tuberculosis, and IgA deficiency. Following surgery, bronchiectasis may develop when the patient's cough is ineffective, with the result that mucus obstructs the bronchus and leads to atelectasis.

Pathophysiology. The infection damages the bronchial wall, causing loss of its supporting structure and producing thick sputum that may ultimately obstruct the bronchi. The walls become permanently distended by severe coughing. The infection extends to the peribronchial tissues, so that in the case of saccular bronchiectasis, each dilated tube virtually amounts to a lung abscess, the exudate of which drains freely through the bronchus. The lower lobes are most frequently involved.

The retention of secretions and obstruction ultimately lead to collapse of the distally situated lung (atelectasis). Inflammatory scarring or fibrosis replaces functioning lung tissue. In time the patient develops respiratory insufficiency with decreased vital capacity, decreased ventilation, and an increased ratio of residual volume to total lung capacity. There is impaired mixing of inspired gas (ventilation-perfusion imbalance) and hypoxemia.

Clinical Manifestations. Characteristic symptoms of bronchiectasis include chronic cough and the production of purulent sputum in copious amounts. A high percentage of patients with this disease experience hemoptysis. Clubbing of the fingers is also very common. The patient is likely to be subject to repeated episodes of pulmonary infection.

Many persons with bronchiectasis pass unrecognized, since their symptoms are mistaken for those of simple chronic bronchitis. A definite clue is offered by the prolonged history of productive cough, with a sputum consistently negative for tubercle bacilli. The diagnosis is established on the basis of bronchography (page 402) and bronchoscopy (page 403). These give proof of the presence or absence of bronchial dilatation.

Preventive Measures. All respiratory infections should be promptly treated. Bronchial secretions can be removed (by expectorants, postural drainage, therapeutic bronchoscopy) in order to avoid bronchiectasis. If a child has a prolonged cough and fever the family should be urged to seek medical treatment. All unconscious persons should be turned (prone position to lateral) to drain all bronchial segments. The educational programs concerning immunization should be continued to prevent pertussis and measles (which may lead to bronchiectasis) so that these severe viral infections will not occur.

Management. The objectives of treatment are to prevent and control infection and to promote bronchial drainage to rid the affected portion of the lung(s) of excessive secretions. Infection is controlled with antibiotics. Patients may be put on a year-round regimen of antibiotics, alternating types of drugs at intervals. Some clinicians use antibiotics throughout the winter or when acute upper respiratory infections occur.

Postural drainage of the bronchial tubes underlies all treatment considerations because draining the bronchiectatic areas by gravity reduces the amount of secretions and the degree of infection. (Sometimes mucopurulent sputum must be removed by bronchoscopy.) The affected chest area may be percussed or "cupped" to assist in raising secretions.

The patient is started out with short periods of postural drainage and the time is increased steadily. Bronchodilators may be given to persons who also have obstructive airway disease. Patients with bronchiectasis almost always have associated bronchitis. Beta-sympathomimetics may be used for bronchodilation and to increase the mucociliary transport of secretions.

To make sputum expectoration easier, the water content of the sputum is increased by aerosolized nebulizer treatments and by an increase in oral fluid intake. A face tent is ideal for providing extra humidification for aerosols. The patient should not smoke since this impairs bronchial drainage by paralyzing ciliary action, increasing bronchial secretions, and causing inflammation of the mucous membranes resulting in hyperplasia of the mucous glands. Patients with bronchiectasis should be immunized against influenza.

Surgical intervention may be indicated for the patient who continues to expectorate fairly large amounts of sputum and experience repeated bouts of pneumonia and hemoptysis in spite of a good medical regimen, provided the disease involves only one or two areas of the lung and can be removed in toto without producing respiratory insufficiency. The goal of surgical treatment is to conserve normal pulmonary tissue and avoid infectious complications.

All diseased tissue is removed provided that the postoperative lung function will be adequate. It may be necessary to remove a segment of a lobe (segmental resection), a lobe (lobectomy), or an entire lung (pneumonectomy). *Segmental resection* is the removal of an anatomical subdivision of a pulmonary lobe. The chief advantage is that only diseased tissue is removed, with greater conservation of healthy lung tissue. Bronchography aids in the delineation of the segment. The operation is preceded by a period of preparation, which is exceedingly important. The objective is to obtain a dry (as dry as possible) tracheobronchial tree in order to prevent complications (atelectasis, pneumonia, bronchopleural fistula, and empyema). This is accomplished by means of postural drainage or, if the abscess is suitably situated, by direct suction through a bronchoscope. A course of antibacterial therapy may be started.

Following the operation, the care is the same as for any chest surgical patient, as is discussed on pages 423 to 432.

Patient Education. The patient is taught postural drainage exercises. He is encouraged to have regular dental care and to avoid all pulmonary irritants (cigarette smoke, noxious fumes). Other aspects of health teaching are included under emphysema on page 489.

CHRONIC OBSTRUCTIVE PULMONARY DISEASE

Chronic obstructive pulmonary disease (COPD) is a broad classification which includes a group of conditions associated with chronic obstruction of airflow entering or leaving the lungs. Airway obstruction is diffuse airway narrowing, causing increased resistance to airflow. Included are chronic bronchitis, emphysema, and asthma. Basically the person with COPD has (1) excessive secretion of mucus within the airways not due to specific causes (bronchitis), (2) an increase in the size of the air spaces distal to the terminal bronchioles with loss of alveolar walls and elastic recoil of the lungs (emphysema), and (3) narrowing of the bronchial airways that varies in severity (asthma). As a result there is a subsequent derangement of airway dynamics—e.g., obstruc-

tion to airflow. There is often an overlap of these conditions. Whereas bronchitis and emphysema are discussed in the following pages, asthma is dealt with in Chapter 50, since the triggering device in asthma is allergic in orgin.

Studies support the theory that COPD is a disease of genetic and environmental interaction; cigarette smoking and air pollution may contribute to its development. This is a disease spectrum that may span 20 to 35 years. It appears to begin fairly early in life and is a slowly progressive disorder that is present many years before the onset of clinical symptoms and impairment of pulmonary function.

CHRONIC BRONCHITIS

Manifestations and Pathophysiology. Chronic bronchitis is characterized by excessive mucus secretion, cough, and dyspnea associated with recurring infections of the lower respiratory tract and often with reduced ability to ventilate the lungs. The patient's major problem is the protracted and abundant production of inflammatory exudate that fills and obstructs the bronchioles and is responsible for a persistent, productive cough and shortness of breath. This constant irritation leads to hypertrophy of mucus-secreting glands, goblet cell hyperplasia, and increased mucus production leading to bronchial plugging and bronchial narrowing. Alveoli adjacent to the bronchioles may become damaged and fibrosed. Further bronchial narrowing follows as a result of these fibrotic changes in the airways. In time, irreversible lung changes may occur, with resultant emphysema or bronchiectasis.

A wide range of viral, bacterial, and mycoplasmal infections can produce acute episodes of bronchitis. Bronchitis is encountered in persons who smoke heavily or are exposed to air pollutants in their work. Hereditary factors also play a part in its development. Exacerbations of chronic bronchitis are most apt to occur during the winter months. The inhalation of cold air produces bronchospasm in sensitive persons. Progressive bronchitis will almost invariably result in chronic obstructive pulmonary disease.

Preventive Measures. Because of the disabling nature of chronic bronchitis, every effort should be directed toward its prevention. An important feature is the avoidance of respiratory irritants, particularly tobacco smoke. Persons who are prone to respiratory infections should be immunized against common viral agents with influenza vaccines and with vaccine for *Streptococcus pneumoniae*. All persons with acute upper respiratory infections should receive proper treatment including antibiotics based on cultures and sensitivity studies at the first sign of purulent sputum.

Management. The main objectives of treatment are to maintain the patency of the peripheral bronchial tree and to facilitate removal of bronchial exudates. Changes in the sputum pattern (nature, color, amount, thickness) and in the cough pattern are important signs to note. Recurrent bacterial infections are treated with antibiotic therapy that is directed by sensitivity studies.

To facilitate the removal of bronchial exudates, bronchodilators are administered to relieve bronchospasm and reduce airway obstruction; thus gas distribution and alveolar ventilation are improved. IPPB treatments facilitate removal of secretions and deliver aerosolized bronchodilators to the obstructed airways more effectively (page 417). Postural drainage and chest percussion following treatments are usually helpful. Water (given orally or parenterally if bronchospasm is severe) is an important part of therapy, since proper hydration helps the patient to bring up secretions. Steroid therapy may be used when the patient fails to respond to more conservative measures. In some instances in which there is an underlying bronchiectasis, postural drainage is most important. The patient must stop smoking, since smoke inhalation causes bronchoconstriction, paralysis of ciliary activity, and inactivation of surfactant. Smokers are also more susceptible to bronchial infection. Basically the medical treatment, nursing management, and patient education are similar to that for the patient with pulmonary emphysema (page 484).

PULMONARY EMPHYSEMA

Pulmonary emphysema is a complex and destructive lung disease characterized by destruction of the alveoli, enlargement of airspaces, and loss of airway support by the lung parenchyma. It appears to be the end stage of a process which has slowly progressed for many years. In fact, by the time the patient develops symptoms, pulmonary function is often irreversibly impaired. It is a leading cause of disability under Social Security and is the most common respiratory cause of death in the United States.

Cigarette smoking is the major cause of chronic obstructive pulmonary disease (emphysema). However, in a small percentage of patients there is a familial predisposition to emphysema associated with a plasma protein abnormality, a deficiency of alpha$_1$-antitrypsin. The genetically susceptible individual is sensitive to environmental influences (smoking, air pollution, infectious agents, allergens) and, in time, develops chronic obstructive symptoms, namely emphysema. It is imperative that the carriers of this genetic defect be identified to permit genetic counseling and that the environmental factors be modified to delay or prevent overt symptoms of disease.

Pathophysiology and Manifestations

In emphysema the major site of obstruction is the airways where mucus plugging and inflammatory narrowing occur. In later stages the obstruction is caused by loss of the supporting tissues of the airway (elasticity of the lung) with resultant bronchial collapse during expiration. There is dilatation of all of the finer air passages as well as dilatation and coalescence (fusing together) of the alveoli with loss of inherent elasticity and increased dead space. The alveolus is the site in the lung where venous blood and environmental air complete the process of gas exchange. In order for gas exchange to be effective, the alveoli must be adequtely ventilated with air. Interference with alveolar ventilation may occur if there is bronchial obstruction or uneven expansion of the lungs with poor air distribution.

The person with emphysema has a chronic obstruction (marked increase in airway resistance) to the inflow and outflow of air from the lungs. The lungs are in a state of chronic hyperexpansion. In order to get air into and out of the lungs, negative pressure is required during inspiration and an adequate level of positive pressure must be attained and maintained during expiration. The rest position is one of inflation. Instead of being an involuntary act, expiration becomes a muscular act. The patient becomes increasingly short of breath, the chest becomes rigid, and the ribs are fixed at their joints. This accounts for the "barrel chest" of many of these patients (Fig. 25-1A) although in some instances the barrel chest may be due to dorsal kyphosis. Some patients bend forward to breathe, using the accessory muscles of respiration. There is retraction of the supraclavicular fossae on inspiration (Fig. 25-1B). In advanced disease there is also contraction of the abdominal muscles on inspiration. There is a progressive reduction of the vital capacity. Full deflation becomes increasingly difficult and finally impossible. The total vital capacity may be normal, but the 1-second vital capacity is low. The patient moves air more slowly and inefficiently and has to work hard to do it.

The alveolar integrity begins to break down. As the walls of the alveoli are destroyed (a process accelerated by recurrent infections), the internal surface of the lungs, i.e., the area available for the exchange of oxygen and carbon dioxide between the atmosphere and the blood, continually decreases. In late stages of the disease there is interference with carbon-dioxide diffusion, and the increased carbon-dioxide tension causes a mild to severe *pulmonary acidosis*. There is also impairment of oxygen diffusion with inadequate oxygen saturation of the arterial blood. The increased CO_2 level within the poorly ventilated alveoli is increased to such a degree that the partial pressure of O_2 and CO_2 in the alveoli is the opposite of normal; hence, little if any diffusion takes place in the affected areas of the lung (i.e., O_2 does not enter the blood and CO_2 does not leave it).

As the alveolar walls continue to rupture, the pulmonary capillary bed is reduced. The pulmonary blood flow is speeded and the right ventricle is forced to maintain a higher blood pressure in the pulmonary artery. Thus right-sided heart failure (cor pulmonale) is one of the complications of emphysema. The presence of leg edema (dependent edema), distended neck veins, or pain in the region of the liver suggests the development of cardiac failure.

Secretions are increased and retained, since the person is unable to make a forceful cough to expel them. Chronic and acute infections thus take hold in the emphysematous lungs, adding to the air transfer problem.

Classification.   There are two main pathologic types of emphysema, which are classified on the basis of the kind of changes taking place in the lung: (1) panlobular (panocinar) and (2) centrilobular (centriacinar).

In the *panlobular (panocinar) type,* there is destruction of the respiratory bronchiole, alveolar duct, and alveoli. All air spaces within the lobule are more or less enlarged. This patient typically has a hyperinflated chest and marked dyspnea on exertion. Sometimes he is referred to as a "pink puffer." This patient remains "pink," or well-oxygenated, until the disease becomes terminal.

In the *centrilobular (centriacinar) form,* the pathological changes take place mainly in the center of the secondary lobule while the peripheral portions of the acinus are preserved. Frequently there is a derangement of ventilation/perfusion ratios producing chronic hypoxia, hypercapnia, and polycythemia. This leads to cyanosis, peripheral edema, and respiratory failure. The patient may be called a "blue bloater." In addition to the management outlined on page 484, the blue bloater usually receives diuretic therapy for edema. Both types of emphysema may occur in the same patient.

Clinical Manifestations.   Dyspnea is the presenting symptom in emphysema and has an insidious onset. The patient usually has a history of cigarette smoking and a long history of chronic cough, wheezing, and increasing shortness of breath, especially with respiratory infection. In time even the slightest exertion, such as bending over to tie his shoelaces, produces dyspnea and fatigue (exertional dyspnea). The emphysematous lung is not contracted on expiration and the bronchioles are not effectively emptied of their secretions.

The patient readily develops inflammatory reactions and infections due to the pooling of these secretions. After these infections, the patient experiences a prolonged wheezing expiration. Anorexia and weakness are common complaints.

Assessment

The patient's symptoms and the clinical findings on physical examination provide the initial clues to the individual's problem. Other aids in diagnosis include roent-

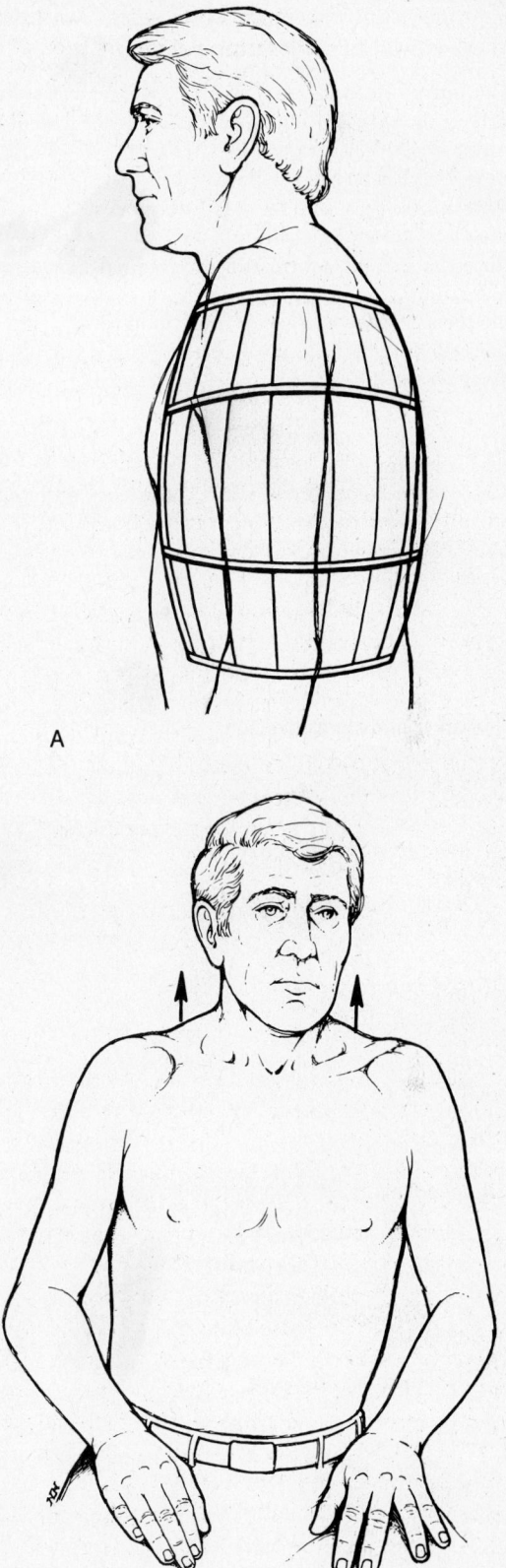

A

B

Figure 25-1.   Comparison of typical findings in the patient with pulmonary emphysema. *A.* The common "barrel chest" condition of the patient with emphysema showing characteristic increase of anteroposterior diameter. *B.* Another posture of the patient with emphysema showing elevation of shoulder girdle and retraction of the supraclavicular fossae on inspiration.

genography, pulmonary function tests, and blood gas studies, as well as the electrocardiogram.

The nurse's observations, nursing history, and subsequent recording should yield an understanding of the patient and his disease.

- How long has he had respiratory difficulty?
- What are the pulse and the respiratory rates?
- Are the respirations even?
- Does the patient contract his abdominal muscles during inspiration?
- Are the accessory muscles of respiration used?
- Does exertion increase the dyspnea?
- What are the limits to his exercise tolerance?
- Is cyanosis evident?
- Are the patient's neck veins engorged?
- Is he coughing?
- What are the color, amount, and consistency of the sputum?
- What is the status of the patient's sensorium?
- Is there increasing stupor? apprehension?

- At what times during the day does he complain most of fatigue and shortness of breath?
- Have his habits of eating or sleeping been affected?
- What does he know about the disease and his condition?

Management

The major objectives of treatment are to improve the quality of life, to slow the progression of the disease process, and to treat the obstructed airways so as to relieve hypoxia. The therapeutic approach includes (1) treatment measures designed to improve ventilation and decrease the work of breathing, (2) prevention and prompt treatment of infection, (3) use of physical therapy techniques to conserve and increase pulmonary ventilation, (4) maintenance of proper environmental conditions to facilitate breathing, (5) supportive and psychological care, and (6) an ongoing program of patient education (Fig. 25-2).

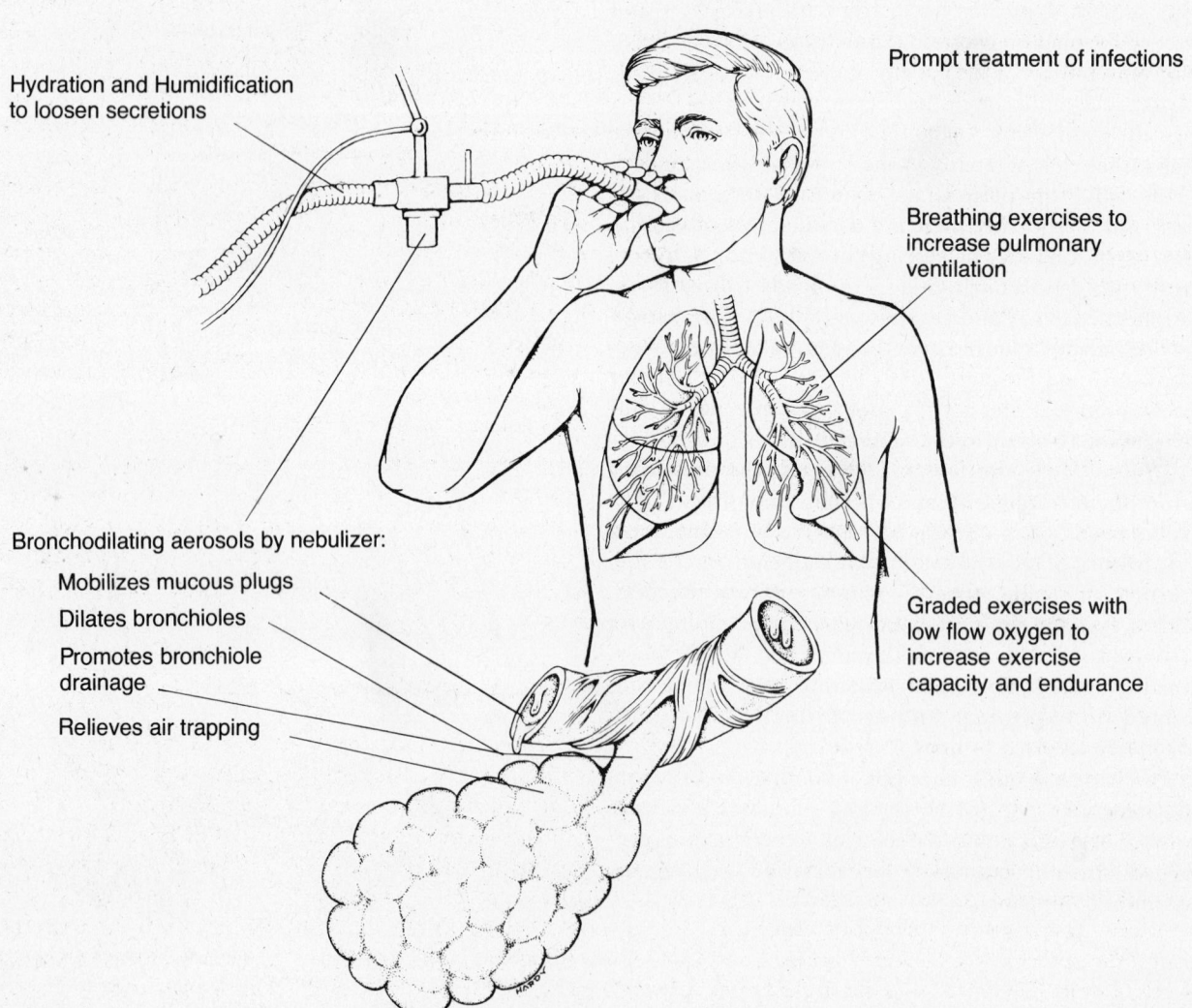

Figure 25-2. Supporting the patient with emphysema.

Measures to Improve Ventilation and Decrease Work of Breathing

Removal of Bronchial Secretions. A major goal in the treatment of emphysema is to diminish the quantity and tenacity of sputum in order to improve pulmonary ventilation and gas exchange. All pulmonary irritants must be eliminated, particularly cigarette smoking, which is the most persistent source of pulmonary irritation. A high fluid intake (2½ to 3 liters or 10 to 12 glasses) daily is encouraged to liquefy secretions. An added reason for encouraging fluid intake is the tendency for the patient to breathe through the mouth, which accelerates water loss.

Inhaling nebulized water is also helpful since it humidifies the bronchial tree, adding water to the sputum and decreasing its viscosity, so that evacuation of sputum is facilitated.

Bronchodilators. Bronchospasm, present in many forms of pulmonary disease, causes reduction of the caliber of the small bronchi, resulting in stasis of secretions and infection. (Bronchospasm is detected by auscultation with a stethoscope.)

Bronchodilators are administered to dilate the airways, because they combat both bronchial mucosal edema and muscular spasm and thus help in reducing airway obstruction and clearing secretions. Bronchodilator drugs may be administered orally, subcutaneously, intravenously, rectally, or via nebulization (conversion into a spray). Nebulized drugs may be delivered by pressurized aerosols, hand-bulb nebulizers, pump-driven nebulizers, or IPPB. Table 25-2 lists the commonly used nebulized drugs. These bronchodilators may produce unwanted side effects, which include tachycardia, cardiac arrhythmias, and central nervous system excitation. The methylxanthines may also produce gastrointestinal disturbances such as nausea and vomiting. Since side effects are common, the drug dosage is carefully adjusted for each patient, in accordance with his tolerance and clinical response. Nursing assessment is an important guide. The relief of bronchospasm is confirmed by measuring improvement in expiratory flow rates and by assessing whether the patient has a reduction in dyspnea.

Aerosolization (process of dispensing in a fine mist) of saline bronchodilators and mucolytics is frequently used to aid in bronchodilatation. The particle size in the aerosol mist must be small enough to allow the medication to be deposited deep within the tracheobronchial tree.

Nebulized aerosols relieve bronchospasm, decrease mucosal edema and liquefy bronchial secretions. This facilitates the process of bronchial clearance, helps to control the inflammatory process, and improves ventilatory function. Hand-bulb nebulizers and metered-dose aerosol devices give the patient quick relief. Electrically powered nebulizers, air-powered nebulizers, and positive pressure breathing devices (IPPB) may be useful if the patient has more marked ventilatory impairment. Oxygen is forced into the lungs and accumulated carbon dioxide is flushed out of the residual air spaces. The improvement of the oxygen saturation of the arterial blood and the reduction of its carbon-dioxide content assists in relieving the patient's hypoxia and gives considerable relief from constant respiratory fatigue. IPPB treatments driven with oxygen must be given with extreme caution in patients who have chronically elevated CO_2 tensions and are breathing on hypoxic stimuli. It is possible to use IPPB driven with compressed air in such circumstances. However the role of IPPB in the treatment of patients with emphysema is not clear. IPPB may transiently decrease the work of breathing and improve ventilation. There usually is short-term improvement. With long-term use there may be lack of improvement and even detrimental effects. (See page 417 for hazards of IPPB therapy.)

The ultrasonic nebulizer creates a fog; water is bombarded with high-frequency sound waves that produce pure droplets far smaller than those produced by ordinary nebulizers. Various agents may be nebulized, including bronchodilators, antifoaming agents, mucolytics, steroids, water, or saline or propylene glycol solutions. Nebulized inhalant treatments (IPPB, etc.) should be given before meals to improve lung ventilation and thus reduce the fatigue that accompanies eating. Following inhalation of bronchodilator aerosols, the patient is advised to inhale moisture to help liquefy secretions. Then expulsive coughing and/or postural drainage will aid him in expectorating secretions. Help the patient to do this in such a manner that it will not be exhausting to him.

Bronchoscopic removal of secretions may be necessary for the patient who is unable to cough and raise sputum. For the patient who develops acute respiratory failure (page 445) endotracheal intubation or tracheostomy is indicated to permit more effective suctioning of secretions, to prevent mucous plugging, and to provide ventilatory assistance.

Prevention and Treatment of Infection

Bronchial infections must be controlled to diminish inflammatory edema and to permit recovery of normal ciliary action. Minor respiratory infections which are of no consequence to the person with normal lungs can produce fatal disturbances of pulmonary function in the person with emphysema. The cough associated with bronchial infection introduces a vicious cycle with further trauma and damage to the lungs, further progression of symptoms, increased bronchospasm, and further increase in susceptibility to bronchial infection. Therefore respiratory infections are a constant threat.

TABLE 25-2. COMMONLY USED NEBULIZED DRUGS

	PHARMACOLOGIC EFFECTS	INDICATIONS	UNDESIRED EFFECTS	NURSING IMPLICATIONS
Bronchodilators and Decongestants				
Racemic epinephrine	Sympathomimetic acting on alpha (vasoconstrictor), beta$_1$ (cardiac stimulation) and beta$_2$ (bronchial smooth muscle relaxation) receptors	Bronchospasm in asthma or bronchitis, laryngeal or tracheal edema	Tachycardia, arrhythmias, elevation of blood pressure, headache, nausea, vomiting, tachyphylaxis, paradoxical increase in bronchospasm	Use extreme caution in patients who are elderly, or who have heart or thyroid disease; discontinue treatment and observe pulse and blood pressure closely if major undesired effects occur.
Isoproterenol	Sympathomimetic acting on beta$_1$ and beta$_2$ receptors	Bronchospasm	Tachycardia, arrhythmias, headache, nausea, excitement, tremors	Use caution in patients who are elderly or who have heart or thyroid disease; discontinue and observe pulse if arrhythmias or other major undesired effects occur.
Isoetharine	Sympathomimetic, claimed to act more selectively on beta$_2$ than on beta$_1$ receptors	Bronchospasm	Tachycardia, headache, excitement	Although safer than the preceding drugs, caution should still be used in patients with heart disease.
Phenylephrine	Sympathomimetic acting on alpha receptors to cause vasoconstriction	Used only as a topical decongestant, usually in combination with another adrenergic drug	Mostly those of other drugs used in combination	Depends on other drugs used in combination.
Terbutaline	Sympathomimetic with selective beta$_2$ activity	Bronchospasm	Rare	Not yet clinically available but probably safer than other less selective agents.
Proteolytics				
Acetylcysteine	Derivative of naturally occurring protein; breaks disulfide bonds in mucoproteins and thus lowers viscosity of mucus; liquefaction starts 1 minute following nebulization and reaches maximum in 5 minutes; action is immediate in direct instillation	Abnormally thick or inspissated secretions in airways	Nausea, bronchospasm	Should be used with caution in patients with asthma or other bronchospastic disorders and should probably be administered with a bronchodilator; should be used with caution in patients who cannot cough up secretions and should be followed by vigorous suctioning to prevent "drowning" patient in liquefied secretions.
Dornavac	Purified enzyme which breaks DNA bonds and is therefore only effective in liquefaction of extremely purulent secretions that are rich in DNA	Thick, purulent secretions, as in lung abscess, bronchiectasis, and cystic fibrosis	Bronchospasm (rare)	Allergic reaction to beef protein is rare, but patient should be observed closely for increased dyspnea or wheezing during treatment.
Antifoaming Agent				
Ethyl alcohol	Reduces surface tension and therefore collapses foam that may obstruct airways	Pulmonary edema due to left ventricular failure	None	None

(Continued)

TABLE 25-2. (CONTINUED)

	PHARMACOLOGIC EFFECTS	INDICATIONS	UNDESIRED EFFECTS	NURSING IMPLICATIONS
Corticosteroids				
Beclomethasone	Synthetic corticosteroid with potent anti-inflammatory activity; effective when administered by inhalation	Patients with steroid-dependent asthma	Oral moniliasis	Should *not* be used in patients with status asthmaticus or other acute episodes of asthma.
Miscellaneous				
Cromolyn sodium	Inhibits release of histamine from mast cells in the respiratory tract when inhaled as a dry powder; prevents acute attacks *only,* and must be used for 2-4 weeks to demonstrate effectiveness	Asthma	Cough, bronchospasm	Should *not* be used in patients with status asthmaticus or other acute episodes of asthma; may have to be given in combination with bronchodilator if administration brings about bronchospasm.

Some physicians keep the patient on a program of continuous or intermittent prophylactic broad-spectrum antibiotic, whereas others administer antibiotics at the first sign of an infection. The latter approach is more acceptable, because the continued use of antibiotics can cause more organisms to develop antibiotic resistance.

In emphysema, infection does not manifest itself in the same way as it does elsewhere in the body. The patient should be instructed to report to the physician immediately if the sputum becomes discolored, since purulent expectoration or a change in the character or color of the sputum is evidence of infection. He should be taught that any worsening of his symptoms (increased tightness of the chest, increase in dyspnea, and fatigue) is also suggestive of infection and must be reported. Steroids may be given to the patient who does not improve with bronchodilators, antibiotics, etc. Viral infections are hazardous to these patients because they are so often followed by infections due to *Streptococcus pneumoniae, Hemophilus influenzae,* etc. Persons who are prone to respiratory infections should be immunized against influenza and *Streptococcus pneumoniae.* During highly polluted or heavily pollinated days (in the spring) these persons should avoid outdoor exposure since it may increase bronchospasm. Outdoor periods of high temperatures associated with high humidities should likewise be avoided.

Physical Therapy

Physical therapy techniques include breathing exercises and general physical conditioning exercises intended to conserve and increase pulmonary ventilation.

Breathing Exercises and Retraining. Most persons with chronic obstructive pulmonary disease breathe shallowly from the upper chest, in a rapid and inefficient manner. This type of upper chest breathing can be changed to the lower costal and diaphragmatic type with breathing exercises and practice. Training in diaphragmatic breathing reduces the respiratory rate, increases tidal volume and alveolar ventilation, and causes a reduction of functional residual capacity.

Pursed-lip breathing helps the patient to control the rate and depth of respiration and to relax, which enables him to gain control of his dyspnea and feelings of panic.

A patient with emphysema has definite periods of the day when his exercise tolerance is decreased. This is especially true on arising in the morning, because bronchial secretions and edema collect in the lungs during the night while he is lying on his back. He often will be unable to shave or to wash. Activities requiring the arms to be supported above the level of the thorax may produce distress. These activities may be tolerated better after the patient has been up and moving around for an hour or more. Because of these limitations, the patient has the right to participate in planning his nursing care with the nurse and in determining the best time for bathing and shaving. A hot beverage on arising will assist him to expectorate and will shorten the period of disability noted on arising.

Another period of increased disability occurs immediately after meals, particularly the evening meal. Fatigue from the day's activities coupled with abdominal distention limits his exercise tolerance. The patient's chief complaint at this time is fatigue. This is another way of saying, "I am dyspneic": dyspnea is the underlying cause of his fatigue.

Exercises and Physical Conditioning. There is a close relationship between physical fitness and respiratory fitness. Graded exercises and physical conditioning programs employing treadmills, stationary bicycles, measured level walks, etc., have been shown to improve symptoms and to increase work capacity and exercise tolerance. It is useful for the patient to have a physical activity that he can do on a regular sustained basis. A lightweight portable oxygen system is available for the ambulatory patient who requires oxygen therapy during physical activity to improve hypoxia. This type of rehabilitation improves the quality of life.

Psychosocial Support

Any factor that interferes with normal breathing quite naturally induces anxiety, depression, and changes in behavior. Many persons find the slightest exertion exhausting. Constant shortness of breath and fatigue may render the patient irritable and apprehensive to the point of sheer panic. His enforced inactivity (and reversal of family roles due to loss of employment), the frustration of having to work to breathe, and the realization that he faces a prolonged, unrelenting disease may cause the patient to react with anger, depression, and demanding behavior. Sexual ability may be compromised, which also diminishes self-esteem.

It is important for the nurse and other health care personnel to adopt a cautiously hopeful and encouraging attitude and keep the patient active up to his level of symptom tolerance. Emphasis should be on controlling his symptoms and increasing self-esteem and sense of mastery and of well-being. Supportive medical and nursing care and ongoing patient teaching help to relieve somewhat an almost overwhelming burden.

Patient Teaching

To help the patient live better, it is essential that he be educated about his disease process. One of the major teaching factors is helping the patient to accept realistic long-range goals. If he is severely disabled, the objective of treatment is to preserve his present pulmonary function and relieve his symptoms as much as possible. If his disease is mild, the objective is to increase his exercise tolerance and prevent further loss of pulmonary function. The patient has to be told what to expect. He and those caring for him need patience to achieve these goals. A summary of patient education in emphysema is found on page 489.

The patient should be instructed to avoid excessive heat and cold. Heat increases the body temperature, hence raises the oxygen requirements of the body; cold tends to promote bronchospasm. High altitudes aggravate the hypoxia. Bronchospasm may also be initiated by such air pollutants as fumes, smoke, dust, and even talcum and lint.

Protection of the lung is basic for the preservation of lung function. Patients with emphysema should be informed unequivocally that, for them, smoking is contraindicated. Cigarette smoking profoundly affects the ciliary cleansing mechanism of the respiratory tract, the function of which is to keep the breathing passages free of inhaled irritants, bacteria, and other foreign matter. This is one of the major defense mechanisms of the body. When this cleansing mechanism is damaged by smoking, airflow is obstructed and air becomes trapped behind the obstructed airway. The air sacs greatly distend and the lung capacity is diminished. Cigarette smoking also irritates the goblet cells and mucous glands, causing an increased accumulation of mucus. The mucus accumulation produces more irritation, infection, and damage to the lung capacity. Frequently the patient is unaware of what is happening until he notices that extra physical effort produces respiratory distress. At this point the damage may be irreversible. Therefore, patients with emphysema should definitely refrain from smoking.

Patients with emphysema should restrict themselves to a life of moderate activity, ideally in a climate with minimal shifts in temperature and humidity. Stress situations that might trigger a coughing episode or emotional disturbance should be avoided.

PULMONARY HEART DISEASE (COR PULMONALE)

Cor pulmonale is a condition in which the right ventricle enlarges (with or without failure) as a result of diseases that affect the structure or function of the lung or its vasculature. Any disease that affects the lungs and has associated hypoxemia may result in cor pulmonale. The most frequent cause is chronic obstructive pulmonary disease (emphysema, chronic bronchitis) in which changes in the airways and retained secretions reduce alveolar ventilation. Other causes are conditions that restrict or compromise ventilatory function leading to hypoxia or acidosis (deformities of the thoracic cage; massive obesity) or conditions that reduce the pulmonary vascular bed (primary idiopathic pulmonary artery hypertension; pulmonary embolus). Certain disorders of the nervous system, respiratory muscles, chest wall, and pulmonary arterial tree may be responsible for cor pulmonale. Left-sided heart failure or valvular diseases like mitral stenosis may, in advanced disease, transmit pressures backward producing similar pulmonary artery hypertension.

Pathophysiology. Pulmonary disease can produce a chain of events that will in time produce hypertrophy and failure of the right ventricle. Any condition that deprives the lungs of oxygen can cause hypoxemia (decreased arterial oxygen saturation) and hypercapnea (increased carbon dioxide in the blood) resulting in ventilatory insufficiency. There may be associated reduction of the pulmonary vascular bed, as in emphysema or pulmonary emboli. The result is increased resistance in the pulmo-

Teaching the emphysematous patient is one of the most important aspects of his care. The patient becomes an active participant in planning his care when he understands the objectives of his therapy and has guidelines set forth to achieve them.

Objective: To improve the quality of life.

I. To delay the progression of the disease process.

  A. Avoid exposure to respiratory irritants (fumes, dust, smoke, cold, etc.)

    1. Stop smoking and avoid smoke-filled rooms.

    2. Stay indoors in a clear environment with windows closed during periods of heavy air pollution.

    3. Stay out of extremely cold weather or keep a scarf over nose and mouth to warm inspired air; this avoids provoking airway irritation.

    4. Try to avoid abrupt changes in environmental temperature.

    5. Stay out of excessively dry air.

    6. Have a home humidifier system and possibly an electronic air filter.

  B. Prevent and eliminate bronchial infections.

    1. Report any evidence of respiratory infection to the physician promptly.

    2. Take prescribed antimicrobial at first sign of infection.

      a. Have a home supply available.

      b. Have periodic sputum cultures when receiving long-term antimicrobial therapy.

  C. Reduce bronchial secretions.

    1. Maintain an adequate fluid intake (10 to 12 glasses daily); mark down the amount of liquid consumed daily.

    2. Take bronchodilators only as directed.

    3. Follow postural drainage exercises as prescribed.

      a. Stay in each position 5 to 10 minutes.

      b. Use controlled cough after each position.

    4. Avoid drugs (cough suppressants, antihistamines, anticholinergics) which suppress cough and dry secretions.

  D. Avoid activities that produce excessive dyspnea.

    1. Live within the limitations that emphysema imposes.

    2. Learn to relax and work at a slower pace. Obtain vocational counseling to secure a sedentary job (if patient has a demanding manual job).

    3. Adjust activities according to individual fatigue patterns.

    4. Use pursed-lip breathing in a slow and relaxed manner during periods of breathlessness and physical exertion.

    5. Avoid emotional stress or cope as positively as possible with stresses that trigger attacks of dyspnea.

  E. Maintain general health at the highest attainable level.

    1. Follow good habits of nutrition.

      a. Have rest periods before, during, and after meals if eating produces dyspnea.

      b. Avoid excessively hot or cold fluids and foods that may provoke irritating cough.

      c. Avoid gas-producing foods, because they hamper abdominal breathing.

      d. Take small, frequent feedings to help lessen pulmonary fatigue.

      e. Take liquid supplements or "breakfast bars" if weight loss and fatigue during eating occur.

    2. Avoid overfatigue, which is a factor in producing respiratory distress.

    3. Use good oral hygiene frequently to prevent respiratory infections.

    4. Avoid contact with persons having respiratory infections.

    5. Obtain immunization with influenza vaccine at prescribed times, if advised by physician.

  F. Understand the importance of preserving existing function.

    1. Become familiar with the nature of the disease and the reasons for the therapeutic regimen.

    2. Accept the fact that therapy and medical supervision must be continued for a lifetime.

    3. Secure vocational rehabilitation services if a job change is indicated.

II. To increase pulmonary ventilation.

  A. Use nebulization treatment consistently and faithfully.

    1. Do the procedure immediately upon arising in the morning and before meals when indicated.

    2. Learn how to assemble and disassemble equipment.

    3. Use the exact amount of medication prescribed by the physician.

    4. Inhale and exhale as evenly as possible during the treatment.

    5. Try to cough *productively* after the treatment.

      a. Breathe slowly and deeply, using diaphragmatic breathing.

      b. Hold breath several seconds.

      c. Cough—2 short, forceful coughs with the mouth open: the first cough loosens mucus and the second cough moves it.

      d. Pause and inhale by sniffing quietly; inhaling vigorously may initiate unproductive coughing, which is energy consuming.

      e. Rest.

    6. Practice oral hygiene after each treatment.

    7. Clean respiratory therapy equipment daily.

  B. Do breathing exercises to strengthen muscles of expiration.

    1. Learn the importance of slow and relaxed breathing.

    2. Practice diaphragmatic breathing (see page 420).

    3. Practice pursed-lip breathing (see page 420).

    4. Do resistive exercises (candle- and bottle-blowing).

    5. Consciously use pursed-lip breathing during episodes of dyspnea.

    6. Maintain muscle tone of the body by regular exercise.

nary circuit, with a subsequent rise in pulmonary blood pressure. Right ventricular hypertrophy may then result and may be followed by right ventricular failure. In short, cor pulmonale results from pulmonary hypertension that causes the right side of the heart to enlarge because of the increased work required to pump blood against high resistance through the pulmonary vascular system.

Clinical Manifestations. Usually the symptoms of cor pulmonale are those of underlying lung disease. Chronic obstructive pulmonary disease produces shortness of breath and cough. As the right ventricle fails, the patient develops edema of the feet and legs, distended neck veins, an enlarged palpable liver, pleural effusion, ascites, and heart murmur. Headache, confusion, and somnolence may be manifested as a result of carbon dioxide narcosis.

Therapeutic Approach. The objectives of treatment are to improve the patient's ventilation and to treat both the underlying lung disease and the manifestations of heart disease. In chronic obstructive pulmonary disease the airways have to be opened to improve gas exchange. With improved oxygen transport, the reactive pulmo-

nary hypertension that leads to cor pulmonale is relieved. In short, the lung must be treated first. Additional measures include bronchial hygiene and the administration of bronchodilators, chest physical therapy, and assessment of arterial blood gases to determine the adequacy of alveolar ventilation and to monitor low-flow oxygen for patients with chronic hypoxia. If the patient is in respiratory failure, endotracheal intubation and mechanical ventilation may be necessary. If the patient is in heart failure, the improvement of hypoxemia and hypercapnia will be necessary to improve cardiac action and output. In addition he is placed on bed rest, and sodium restriction and diuretic therapy are employed to reduce peripheral edema and the circulatory load on the right heart. Digitalis therapy is also prescribed depending on the patient's condition and the results of blood gas analysis, serum electrolyte determinations, and ECG assessment. Digitalis is given with caution, since digitalis toxicity (see page 579) is a serious problem in the management of respiratory failure due to hypoxia, acidosis, and electrolyte abnormalities. The use of low-flow oxygen up to periods of 18 hours a day has been beneficial in ameliorating and preventing long-term consequences of cor pulmonale; i.e., heart failure, polycythemia, edema, and internal pulmonary artery changes due to elevated pressures. The patient's prognosis depends on whether or not the hypertensive process is reversible. (The management of the patient with respiratory failure is discussed on page 447.)

Patient Education. There is an interrelationship between infection, air pollution, and cardiopulmonary disease. The patient should be counseled to stop smoking and to avoid exposure to air pollutants, e.g., smoke, fumes. Respiratory infections should be treated promptly.

PULMONARY EMBOLISM

Pulmonary embolism refers to the obstruction of one or more pulmonary arteries by a thrombus (or thrombi) which originates somewhere in the venous system or in the right side of the heart, becomes dislodged, and is carried to the lung. An infarction of lung tissue due to interruption of the lung's blood supply may result. Pulmonary embolism is a common disorder and is often associated with advanced age and postoperative states. It may occur in an apparently healthy person.

The majority of thrombi originate in the deep veins of the legs. Other sources include the pelvic veins and the right atrium of the heart. Stasis, or slowing of blood flow, due to damage to the blood vessel wall (particularly the endothelial lining) and changes in the blood coagulation mechanism, are factors favoring venous thrombogenesis.

PULMONARY EMBOLISM: PERSONS AT RISK

The following events and conditions predispose to thrombophlebitis and pulmonary embolism.

Venous stasis (slowing of blood flow in veins)
　Prolonged immobilization
　Prolonged periods of sitting/traveling
　Varicose veins
Hypercoagulability (due to release of tissue thromboplastin following injury/surgery)
　Injury
　Tumor
　Increased platelet count (polycythemia; splenectomy)
Venous Endothelial Disease
　Thrombophlebitis
　Vascular Disease
　Foreign bodies (IV/central venous catheters)
Certain Disease States (combination of stasis, coagulation alterations, and venous injury)
　Heart disease (especially congestive heart failure)
　Trauma (especially fracture of hip, pelvis, spine, lower extremities)
　Postoperative state/postpartum period
　Diabetes
　Chronic obstructive pulmonary disease
　Previous pulmonary embolism
Other Predisposing Conditions
　Advanced age
　Obesity
　Pregnancy
　Oral contraceptives
　History of preceding thrombophlebitis
　Constrictive clothing

Pathophysiology

Following a massive embolic obstruction of the pulmonary arteries, there is an increase in alveolar dead space since the area, though continuing to be ventilated, receives little or no blood flow. In addition, a number of vasoactive and bronchoconstrictive substances are released from the clot. These substances compound the ventilation-perfusion imbalance, causing venous admixture and shunting.

The hemodynamic consequences are increased pulmonary vascular resistance due to reduction in the size of the pulmonary vascular bed, a consequent increase in pulmonary arterial pressure, and, in turn, an increase in right ventricular work to maintain pulmonary blood flow. When the work requirements of the right ventricle exceeds its capacity, right ventricular failure occurs. When this happens there is a decrease in cardiac output followed by a drop in systemic blood pressure and the development of shock.

Clinical Manifestations

The symptoms of pulmonary embolism depend upon the size of the thrombus and the area of the pulmonary artery occluded. A massive embolism occluding the bifurcation of the pulmonary artery can produce pronounced dyspnea, sudden substernal pain, rapid and weak pulse, shock, syncope, and sudden death.

If one or more branches of the right or left pulmonary arteries are obstructed, the patient experiences dyspnea, mild substernal pain, anxiety, weakness, and tachycardia. Usually these symptoms are the result of pulmonary infarction. There may also be fever, cough, and hemoptysis. The patient's respiratory rate is accelerated out of proportion to the degree of fever and tachycardia. If the terminal pulmonary arteries are occluded, a pleuritic type of pain develops, together with cough and hemoptysis. Multiple small emboli can lodge in the terminal pulmonary arterioles producing multiple small infarctions. The clinical picture may simulate that of bronchopneumonia or heart failure. In some instances, however, the disease presents in an atypical fashion with few signs and symptoms.

Diagnostic Assessment

A diagnosis of pulmonary infarction may be suspected in patients who have combined symptoms of pleurisy, cough, hemoptysis, tachycardia, pallor, and perhaps signs of shock, especially if phlebitis is present in the legs or if these symptoms occur during the postoperative period.

The chest x-ray may show the presence of a consolidation and elevation of the diaphragm on the affected side, but most of the radiographic changes are subtle or nonspecific. Bronchoconstriction may lead to a focal decrease in breath sounds and wheezing, whereas loss of surfactant may be associated with fine rales in the affected lung area. Radioisotope lung scanning and pulmonary angiography usually confirm the presence of emboli. A phlebogram may be done to detect "silent" thrombi in the legs. An electrocardiogram may also reflect changes due to the embolism. However, it is necessary to compare the results with a previous ECG in order to determine whether there is any correlation between the changes and the suspected embolism.

Preventive Measures

The ideal method of treatment is prevention. Effort is directed towards preventing venous stasis in patients on bed rest by ambulation or by active and passive leg exercises. When the legs are moved in a "pumping" exercise, the leg muscles assist in increasing venous flow. Patients with conditions predisposing to slowing of venous return (varicosities, polycythemia, fractures, congestive heart failure) may wear elastic stockings to increase blood flow to the deep leg veins. The patient should not be permitted to "dangle" his legs and feet in a dependent position while sitting on the edge of the bed. His feet should be on the floor or on a chair. A liberal fluid intake is encouraged since dehydration predisposes to embolism. Intravenous catheters (for parenteral therapy or CVP measurement) should not be left in veins for prolonged periods.

The American Heart Association recommends that patients who are over 40 and hemostatically competent, and who are undergoing major elective abdominothoracic surgery, be given low doses of heparin to diminish postoperative deep thrombus and pulmonary embolism. The heparin is given subcutaneously 2 hours before surgery and continued every 12 hours until the patient is discharged. Low-dose heparin is thought to enhance the activity of antithrombin III, a major plasma inhibitor of clotting factor X_a. (This regimen is not recommended for patients who are experiencing an active thrombotic process or those undergoing major orthopedic surgery, open prostatectomy, or operations on the eye or brain.)

Assessment for Thrombus

The nurse should examine each susceptible patient for a positive Homan's sign which may or may not indicate impending thrombosis of the leg veins (see pages 370-371).

1. Position the patient on his back.
2. Lift the leg and dorsiflex the foot.
3. Note if there is pain in the calf during this maneuver (positive Homan's sign); it may indicate deep venous thrombosis.
4. Conduct another clinical assessment by tapping on the anterior tibial crest to see if this elicits pain.

5. Apply a blood pressure cuff around the patient's calf and inflate it. Pain on inflation of the cuff (80 to 100 mm. Hg) is significant as is tenderness along the course of a vein, pain in the calf or foot area, and/or edema in the ankle or calf area. It is best to compare both extremities.

6. Look for swelling and palpable veins. Clinical evidence of phlebitis in one leg does not necessarily indicate that this is the site of the embolus; the other leg, even though normal on examination, may be the site.

Emergency Treatment

Pulmonary embolism is a true medical emergency.

The immediate objective of treatment and care is to stabilize the cardiorespiratory system. The majority of patients who succumb from massive pulmonary embolism do so in the first 2 hours following the embolic event.

- Nasal oxygen is administered immediately to relieve respiratory distress and cyanosis.
- An infusion is started to open an intravenous route for drugs/fluids that will be needed.
- A central venous catheter is inserted into a vein and threaded into the superior vena cava or right atrium while another catheter (radial, brachial, femoral) is placed in an artery to monitor the blood pressure and blood gases.
- If the patient has suffered massive embolism and is hypotensive, an indwelling urethral catheter is inserted to monitor urinary volume.
- The blood pressure is maintained by a slow infusion (IV) of isoproterenol (has a dilating effect on pulmonary vessels and bronchi) or dopamine.
- The ECG is monitored continuously for arrhythmias and ST-segment changes caused by right bundle branch block, which is frequently observed in massive pulmonary embolism.
- Sodium bicarbonate may be administered to correct metabolic acidosis. Digitalis glycosides, intravenous diuretics, and antiarrhythmic agents are given when appropriate.
- Blood is drawn for serum electrolytes, BUN, CBC, and hematocrit.
- If clinical assessment and arterial blood gases indicate the need, the patient is placed on a volume-controlled ventilator.
- Small doses of intravenous morphine are given to relieve the patient's anxiety, to alleviate chest discomfort, to help him accept the discomfort of the endotracheal tube, and to ease his adaptation to the mechanical ventilator.

Antiembolism Drugs. Another important aspect of treatment is the prevention of further embolization. Remember that a thrombus is not static but is continuously changing and will continue forming both at the site of origin and in the lungs where it has lodged. Anticoagulants are given to prevent recurrence and extension of the thromboembolism. Heparin (effect is observed within 15 minutes after injection) is usually given intravenously, either by bolus injection or continuous intravenous infusion. The dose(s) are given to maintain the Lee-White clotting times at approximately 2 to 2½ times that of normal or the activated partial thromboplastin time at 1½ to 2½ times the control value. As soon as the patient is stabilized he is placed on an oral anticoagulant such as warfarin sodium (Coumadin). This dosage is controlled by prothrombin activity and is continued for several weeks. Bear in mind that many drugs, including some sleeping pills, barbiturates, aspirin, phenylbutazone, d-thyroxine, quinidine, and antibiotics used to reduce the number of bacteria in the colon, increase the body's susceptibility to anticoagulants. (See page 638 for discussion of anticoagulant therapy.)

Thrombolysins (capable of breaking up a thrombus) may be used. Urokinase and streptokinase are enzymatic activators that are being tried to dissolve clots. Recently there have been encouraging attempts to prevent further embolization with dextran and salicylates (which reduces platelet aggregation).

Surgical Intervention

If the patient has persistent hypotension, shock, and respiratory distress, and if angiograms reveal an embolus occupying a large part of the major pulmonary arteries, embolectomy may be indicated. This requires cardiovascular surgery using the cardiopulmonary bypass technique (page 553). Another surgical approach utilized when pulmonary emboli recur despite adequate anticoagulation is an interruption of the inferior vena cava. This method prevents dislodged thrombi from being swept into the lungs. This can be done by total ligation or the use of teflon clips applied to the vena cava to divide the caval lumen into small channels without occluding caval blood flow. The use of transvenous devices which occlude or filter the blood through the inferior vena cava is a fairly safe procedure for the prevention of recurrent pulmonary embolism. One such technique is the insertion of a prosthetic umbrella device through a cervical incision in the internal jugular vein (Fig. 25-3). The device is advanced through the superior vena cava and the right atrium into the inferior vena cava where it is brought into an open position. The perforated umbrella permits the passage of blood, but prevents the passage of large thrombi.

Following the surgical procedure, the patient's central venous pressure and urinary output are monitored. An adequate blood pressure must be maintained to ensure perfusion of the vital organs. The legs are kept elevated for 7 to 10 days during the initial development of collateral return.

A newer technique has recently been developed in which a vacuum cupped catheter is introduced transvenously into the affected pulmonary artery. Suction is applied to the end of the embolus and the embolus is aspirated into the cup. The surgeon maintains suction to hold the embolus within the cup, and the entire catheter is withdrawn through the right heart and out the femoral venotomy. An inferior caval filter is often inserted at the same time to protect against a recurrence.

Patient Education

The following patient instructions are intended to help prevent recurrences:

- When taking anticoagulants, look for bruising and try to protect yourself from bumping into objects, etc. that can cause bruising.
- Use a toothbrush with a soft bristle.
- Do not take aspirin or antihistamine drugs while receiving heparin. Always check with the physician before taking any medication.
- Avoid sitting with your legs crossed or sitting for prolonged periods.
- When traveling, change your position regularly, walk occasionally, and do active exercises of the legs and ankles while sitting. Drink plenty of liquids while traveling to avoid hemoconcentration due to fluid loss.
- Report dark, tarry stools to the physician/clinic immediately.

OCCUPATIONAL LUNG DISEASES

Diseases of the lungs can occur in a variety of occupations as a result of exposure to organic or inorganic (mineral) dusts and noxious gases (fumes and aerosols). The effect of inhaling these materials depends upon the composition of the inhaled substance, its antigenic (precipitating an immune response) or irritating properties, the dose inhaled, the length of time inhaled, and the host's response (individual's susceptibility to the irritant). There are a growing number of occupational lung diseases due to new and untested industrial substances (presumed to be harmless). The problem may be compounded by smoking, which appears to have a synergistic effect on occupational lung disease and may increase the risk of lung cancers in people exposed to asbestos.

The Pneumoconioses

Pneumoconiosis refers to a non-neoplastic alteration of the lung resulting from exposure to inorganic dust, e.g., "dusty lung." The most common pneumoconioses are silicosis, asbestosis, and coalworker's pneumoconiosis.

Silicosis is a chronic pulmonary disease caused by inhalation of silica dust (silicon dioxide particles). Since the earth's crust is composed of silica and silicates, exposure is encountered in almost any form of mining, i.e., gold, coal, tin, and copper mining, and quarrying. Stonecutting, the manufacture of abrasives and pottery, and foundry work are other occupations presenting exposure hazards. When the silica particles, which have fibrogenic properties, are inhaled, nodular lesions are produced throughout the lungs. With the passage of time and exposure, the nodules enlarge and coalesce. Dense masses form in the upper portion of the lungs, resulting

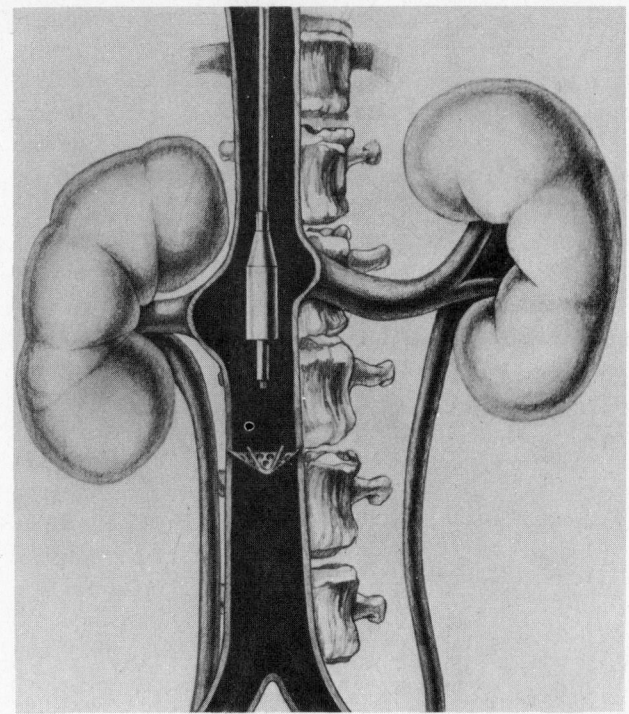

Figure 25-3. Interruption of the inferior vena cava to prevent pulmonary embolism. An umbrella-shaped filter is compressed within an applicator catheter and inserted through an incision in the right internal jugular vein. It is advanced under fluoroscopic control to a position below the renal veins. The filter fixes itself to the wall of the inferior vena cava upon ejection from the applicator, and the applicator is then withdrawn. (Mobin-Uddin Vena Cava Umbrella Filter, Courtesy Edwards Laboratories Division of American Hospital Supply Corp.)

in loss of pulmonary parenchymal volume. Restrictive lung disease (inability of the lungs to expand fully) and obstructive lung disease from secondary emphysema result. Cavity formation is likely to be the result of superimposed tuberculosis. Ten to 20 years of exposure are usually required before the disease develops and shortness of breath is manifested. Fibrotic destruction of pulmonary tissue can lead to emphysema, pulmonary hypertension, and cor pulmonale. There is no specific therapy for silicosis; thus it is essential to avoid inhaling silica dust. With cavitary lesions or advanced fibrosis, many physicians treat the patient for tuberculosis even when cultures are negative.

Asbestosis is a disease characterized by diffuse pulmonary fibrosis due to the inhalation of asbestos dust. The use of asbestos is almost indispensable in modern industry and exposure occurs in numerous occupations including asbestos mining and manufacturing, demolition work, roofing, etc. Materials such as shingles, cement, vinyl asbestos tile, fireproof paint and clothing, brake linings, filters, etc., all contain asbestos. The risk appears to lie in the manufacture, cutting, and demolition of asbestos-containing materials.

The asbestos fibers are inhaled and enter the alveoli, which, in time, are eventually obliterated by fibrous tissue that surrounds the asbestos particles. There is fibrous pleural thickening and pleural plaque formation. The altered physiologic pattern is that of restrictive lung disease with decrease in lung volume, diminished gas transfer, and hypoxemia. The patient has progressive dyspnea, mild to moderate chest pain, anorexia, and weight loss. Cor pulmonale and respiratory failure occur as the disease progresses. It has been found that a high incidence of bronchogenic cancer and an increase of cancer of the stomach, colon, and rectum are associated with significant exposure to asbestos. The treatment is symptomatic and avoidance in general is essential.

Coal worker's pneumoconiosis (CWP, "black lung") is a variety of respiratory disease found in coal workers in which there is an accumulation of coal dust in the lungs causing a tissue reaction to its presence. Coal miners are exposed to dusts that are mixtures of coal, kaolin, mica, and silica. The first physiologic reaction to the deposition of coal dust in the alveoli and respiratory bronchioles is an increase of macrophages which engulf (by phagocytosis) the particles and transport them to the terminal bronchioles where they are removed by mucociliary clearance. In time, the clearance mechanisms are unable to handle the excessive dust load, and the macrophages aggregate in the respiratory bronchioles and alveoli. Fibroblasts appear and a network of reticulin is laid down surrounding the dust-laden macrophages. The respiratory bronchioles and the alveoli become clogged with coal dust, dying macrophages, and fibroblasts, which leads to the formation of the coal macule, the primary lesion of CWP. (Macules appear as blackish dots on the lungs.) As the macules enlarge, there is a dilation of the weakening bronchiole with subsequent development of a focal emphysema.

The patient with complicated coal worker's pneumoconiosis has massive lesions of dense fibrotic tissue containing black material. These masses eventually destroy blood vessels and the bronchi of the affected lobe. The patient develops dyspnea, cough, and sputum production with expectoration of varying amounts of black fluid (melanoptosis). Eventually cor pulmonale and respiratory failure result. The treatment is symptomatic.

Other Inhalation Disorders

Organic Dust Exposure. The inhalation of organic dusts results in hypersensitivity reactions at the alveolar level. The best known example is *farmer's lung,* which occurs with exposure to moldy hay containing thermophilic actinomycetes (*Microsporum faeni; Thermoactinomyces vulgaris*). This induces an allergic inflammatory reaction with granuloma involving the interstitial tissues of the lung. Within a few hours of heavy exposure, the patient develops chills, fever, malaise, myalgia, arthralgia, chest tightness, dry cough, and dyspnea.

Treatment is directed towards removing the patient from further exposure. Corticosteroids may be administered to decrease systemic toxicity and promote resolution of the pulmonary disease. The patient is treated symptomatically, with oxygen, bronchodilator therapy, and physiologic monitoring as required.

Inhalation of Irritant Gases. The inhalation of gases, aerosols, or fumes is a hazard inherent in many occupations. The nature of the gas and the duration and intensity of exposure are important factors determining the type of problems that may develop. In an industrial setting, chlorine, ammonia, sulfur dioxide, ozone, nitrogen dioxide, phosgene, and smoke may produce a chemical pneumonitis.

These irritant gases produce tracheobronchitis or bronchitis with a variety of pulmonary manifestations: cough, dyspnea, chest pain. Inhalation of nitrogen or sulfur dioxide is especially dangerous since these gases may initiate physiologic changes leading to pulmonary edema. Heavy exposure causing wheezing and prolonged symptoms will require hospitalization and early treatment with steroids to prevent bronchiolitis obliterans.

TUMORS OF THE CHEST

A chest tumor may be *primary,* arising within the lung or the mediastinum, or it may represent a metastasis from a primary tumor site elsewhere. Metastatic tumors of the lungs occur frequently, since the bloodstream transports free cancer cells from primary cancers elsewhere in the body. Such tumors grow in and between the alveoli and the bronchi, which they push apart in their growth. This process may occur over a long period of time causing few or no symptoms.

Primary tumors of the lung may be benign or malignant. Most arise from the bronchial epithelium. Bronchial adenomas are slow growing, usually benign tumors, but they are very vascular, and therefore produce symptoms of bleeding and bronchial obstruction. Bronchogenic carcinoma is a malignant tumor arising from the bronchus. Such a tumor is epidermoid, usually located in the larger bronchi, or is an adenocarcinoma, arising further out in the lung. There are also several intermediate or undifferentiated types of lung cancer, identifiable by cell type.

CANCER OF THE LUNG (BRONCHOGENIC CARCINOMA)

Lung cancer is the number one cancer killer among men in the United States and has shown an alarming increase among women. In fact, in one year lung cancer deaths in women increased 7.6 percent. The incidence has more than doubled in both men and women. The survival rate is low and has only slightly increased since the 1940s.

Persons at Risk. Bronchogenic cancer is 10 times

more common in cigarette smokers than in nonsmokers, the prevalence being related to the length of time and the intensity of smoking. Epidermoid carcinoma, involving the larger bronchi, is thought to be almost entirely associated with heavy (1 pack/day) cigarette smoking. Few cases of this type of cancer have been reported in nonsmokers.

Adenocarcinoma of the peripheral bronchi is not associated with any known cause and occurs equally in smokers and nonsmokers. Another risk factor is occupational exposure to asbestos, radioactive dusts, coal gas, etc. Some health experts think that inhalation of asbestos may become a major health problem since research evidence suggests it causes death from respiratory illness and lung cancer.

Clinical Manifestations. The disease begins insidiously (over several decades) and often is asymptomatic until late in its course. The signs and symptoms depend on the location and size of the tumor, the degree of obstruction, and the existence of metastases to regional or distant sites.

The earliest symptom of lung cancer is cough, which is present in about 90 percent of the patients. It is frequently ignored as a "cigarette cough." Starting as a hacking, nonproductive cough, it later progresses to a point where it produces a thick purulent sputum as secondary infection occurs.

• Thus, a cough that changes in character should arouse suspicion of lung cancer.

A wheeze in the chest (occurs when a bronchus becomes partially obstructed by the tumor) is noted in about 20 percent of patients, and spitting of blood or blood streaks in the sputum is common. In a few patients, recurring fever due to a persisting infection in an area of pneumonitis distal from the tumor is the early symptom. In fact, cancer of the lung should be suspected in persons with repeated unresolved upper respiratory infections. Pain is a late manifestation and is often found to be related to bone metastasis. Headaches, diplopia, and other central nervous system manifestations may be grave indications of metastasis. General symptoms of weight loss, fatigue, and anorexia appear late.

Diagnostic Assessment. If the patient with pulmonary symptoms is a heavy smoker, cancer of the lung can be suspected. Chest x-rays are done to search for pulmonary density, solitary peripheral nodule (coin lesion), atelectasis, and infection. Cytologic examination of fresh sputum obtained by cough or saline washings from a suspected bronchus may be done. Bronchoscopy with a flexible fiberoptic instrument allows a detailed study of the bronchial segments and identification of the source of malignant cells. Lung scans are part of the diagnostic workup. A bone scan or bone marrow study is done for detection of bone metastasis, and liver scanning is used to verify metastatic spread to the liver. Detection of central

nervous system metastases is accomplished by brain scanning, computerized tomography, and other neurological diagnostic procedures. Mediastinoscopy may be used to evaluate tumor spread to hilar lymph nodes of the right lung, and mediastinotomy gives access to the hilar lymphatics of the left lung.

Before surgery, the patient is evaluated to determine whether the tumor is resectable and whether he can tolerate the physiologic impairment resulting from such surgery. Pulmonary function tests are done so that calculations of the total lung capcity and residual air volume can be made. The patient's ability to move air (vital capacity, FEV_1) is important since the ability to generate an effective cough is imperative in the postoperative period.

Classification and Staging. The four major cell types of lung cancer (which differ significantly) are epidermoid (squamous cell) carcinoma, small cell (oat cell) carcinoma, adenocarcinoma, and large cell (anaplastic) carcinoma (Table 25-3), shows the World Health Organiza-

---

TABLE 25-3. HISTOPATHOLOGICAL TYPES
OF LUNG TUMORS

I. EPIDERMOID CARCINOMAS
II. SMALL CELL ANAPLASTIC CARCINOMAS
  1. Fusiform cell type
  2. Polygonal cell type
  3. Lymphocyte-like ("oat-cell") type
  4. Others
III. ADENOCARCINOMAS
  1. Bronchogenic
    a. acinar $\Big\}$ with or without mucin formation
    b. papillary
  2. Bronchiolo-alveolar
IV. LARGE CELL CARCINOMAS
  1. Solid tumors with mucin-like content
  2. Solid tumors without mucin-like content
  3. Giant cell carcinomas
  4. "Clear" cell carcinomas
V. COMBINED EPIDERMOID AND ADENOCARCINOMAS
VI. CARCINOID TUMORS
VII. BRONCHIAL GLAND TUMORS
  1. Cylindromas
  2. Mucoepidermoid tumors
  3. Others
VIII. PAPILLARY TUMORS OF THE SURFACE EPITHELIUM
  1. Epidermoid
  2. Epidermoid with goblet cells
  3. Others
IX. "MIXED" TUMORS AND CARCINOSARCOMAS
  1. "Mixed" tumors
  2. Carcinosarcomas of embryonal type ("blastomas")
  3. Other carcinosarcomas
X. SARCOMAS
XI. UNCLASSIFIED
XII. MESOTHELIOMAS
  1. Localized
  2. Diffuse
XIII. MELANOMAS

From Kreyberg, L., Liebow, A. A. and Vehlinger, E. A. Histological Typing of Lung Tumors. Geneva, World Health Org., 1967.

tion classification of lung tumors by histological type. Many tumors contain more than one cell type. The different cell types display different biological behavior and have prognostic significance. Therefore, different approaches to treatment may be indicated by the cell type.

The stage of the tumor refers to the anatomical extent of the tumor and indicates the presence or absence of spread to the regional lymph nodes and the presence or absence of metastases. Staging is accomplished by tissue diagnosis, lymph node biopsy, and mediastinoscopy. Staging is important in determining whether or not tumor resection should be attempted. Prognosis appears most favorable for epidermoid and adenocarcinoma, whereas undifferentiated small cell (oat cell) tumors appear to have a poor prognosis.

Management

The treatment varies with the cell type and stage of disease. In general, treatment may involve surgery and/or radiotherapy, chemotherapy and immunotherapy.

Surgery. Surgical resection is the preferred method of treatment if the tumor is resectable. The usual operation for small, apparently curable tumor of the lung is lobectomy (removal of a lobe of the lung). An entire lung may be removed (pneumonectomy) in combination with other surgical procedures such as resection of involved mediastinal lymph nodes. Before surgery, the cardiopulmonary reserve of the patient must be determined. (See page 420 for the preoperative and postoperative management of the patient undergoing chest surgery.)

Radiation. Radiation therapy is useful in controlling radio-responsive neoplasms that cannot be resected. The oat cell and epidermoid tumors are usually radiation sensitive. Respite may be obtained from cough, chest pain, dyspnea, hemoptysis, and bone and liver pain. Relief of symptoms may last from a few weeks to many months and is important in improving the quality of the remaining period of life.

TABLE 25-4. DRUGS WITH ACTIVITY* AGAINST BRONCHOGENIC CANCERS OF ALL CELL TYPES

ALKYLATING AGENTS	ANTIBIOTICS	NATURAL PRODUCTS	MISCELLANEOUS
Ifosphamide	Mitomycin C	Vincristine	Nitrosoureas
Mechlorethamine	Adriamycin	Vinblastine	Methotrexate
Cyclophosphamide	Bleomycin	Podophyllotoxins	Procarbazine
Busulfan	Daunomycin		Hexamethylmelamine
Phenylalanine mustard			Fluorouracil

*Activity = measurable regression of > 50% tumor size.

(From Benfield, J. R., et al.: An interdisciplinary perspective of lung cancer. *In* Hickey, R. C., et al., eds.: Current Problems in Cancer. Copyright © 1977 Year Book Medical Publishers, Inc., Chicago. Used by permission.)

Attention should be paid to the patient's nutrition, to signs of anemia, control of infection, and psychological outlook. (See pages 292-294 for management of the patient receiving radiation therapy.)

Chemotherapy. At the present time chemotherapy is used for patients with widespread lung cancer who are not candidates for surgical resection or high-dose radiation. Combinations of two or more drugs may be more beneficial than single dose regimens. A large number of drugs are reported to have some activity against lung cancer (see Table 25-4). These agents are toxic and have a narrow margin of safety. Chemotherapy may give palliation, especially from pain, but does not cure and rarely prolongs life. It is valuable in reducing pressure symptoms of lung cancer and in treating brain, spinal cord, and pericardial metastasis. (See pages 264-273 for chemotherapy for the patient with cancer.)

Immunotherapy. It has been observed that immunologic responsiveness is suppressed in persons with lung cancer and that this affects their prognosis. Immunotherapy may be tried in an attempt to reverse this immunosuppression. The objective of immunotherapy is to restore or augment the normal mechanisms of host defense against the tumor. A living vaccine (bacille Calmette-Guerin [BCG]) may be introduced into the pleural space (via chest tube or thoracentesis) or by cutaneous immunization to scarification sites in the hope that a local bacterial infection may cause regional activation of the immune system and destroy tumor cells that may have escaped surgical resection. Approximately 14 days following BCG injection, a course of isoniazid is administered to prevent overgrowth of BCG organisms. Immunotherapy is monitored by skin tests and lymphocyte culture studies. Although this modality of treatment is fairly recent, there are indications that immunotherapy can prolong survival for patients with lung cancer.

TUMORS OF THE MEDIASTINUM

Most mediastinal tumors are adjacent to vital structures and have an unpredictable manner of growth. They include neurogenic tumors, thymic tumors, and mesodermal and endocrine tumors. Thymic tumors have the highest percentage of malignancy.

Cysts of the mediastinum usually are small when benign. Dermoid cysts occasionally develop, and these may ulcerate into the air passages.

Manifestations. Nearly all the symptoms of mediastinal tumors are due to the pressure of the mass against important intrathoracic organs. Among these pressure symptoms are chest pain; bulging of the chest wall; orthopnea (an early sign due to pressure against the trachea, a main bronchus, the recurrent laryngeal nerve, or the lung); cardiac palpitation, anginal attacks, and various other circulatory disturbances; cyanosis; superior vena caval syndromes, i.e., swelling of the face, the neck, and the upper extremities and the marked distention of the veins of the neck and the chest wall (evidence of the closure of large veins of the mediastinum by extravascular compression or intravascular invasion); and dysphagia due to pressure against the esophagus.

Diagnosis. Roentgenograms are of great value in the diagnosis of mediastinal tumors and cysts. Lateral and oblique films and tomography are used to localize the tumor.

The biopsy of an enlarged lymph node removed from above the clavicle or one removed during mediastinoscopy may reveal the diagnosis. Blood studies are of value in excluding leukemia, and sputum examinations aid in ruling out tuberculosis.

Management. Most mediastinal tumors are benign and operable. The location of the tumor in the mediastinum will dictate the type of incision. Most incisions are median sternotomies. The care is the same as for any patient who is undergoing thoracic surgery (pages 420-432). If the tumor is malignant and infiltrating, radiotherapy and chemotherapy are the therapeutic modalities used when complete surgical removal is not feasible.

AN ASPIRATED FOREIGN BODY IN THE LUNG

Foreign bodies are frequently aspirated into the lung, especially by children. When this occurs, the object usually lodges in the right main bronchus, because of its more vertical position. However, a foreign body can enter any segment of the lung depending on the size and character of the object, the position of the person when the aspiration occurs, and whether or not the object could be dislodged by coughing.

The complete closure of the larynx, trachea, or bronchus by a foreign body may result in sudden death. However, the usual result is that the lobes communicating with the occluded bronchus collapse as the air contained in them becomes absorbed into the bloodstream. Sometimes, the foreign object acts as a check valve, allowing air to pass by during inspiration (the bronchial diameter enlarges) but obstructing the exhalation of air during expiration (the bronchial diameter decreases). An inspiratory and expiratory x-ray is helpful in this circumstance, since the lung or the segment beyond the obstruction will not decrease fully during expiration.

A small solid object such as a pin, a tack, or a tooth in a bronchus causes trouble, not from the obstruction of a bronchus, but from infection. For a short time following the aspiration there may be symptoms of choking, gagging, and coughing. But these symptoms, often mild, abate and for a time become forgotten. For weeks the only suggestion of trouble may be a persistent cough.

Such substances as peanuts, grains of corn, etc., on the other hand, produce a severe bronchitis with high irregular fever and all the symptoms and signs of severe pneumonitis. Whether the foreign body is composed of organic or inorganic material, signs of obstructive emphysema, atelectasis, or lung abscess eventually appear.

Management. The patient is x-rayed to check the presence and position of the foreign body (foreign bodies often shift in position). The prognosis is serious unless the foreign body is removed early, for rarely is it coughed up spontaneously. Therefore, bronchoscopy is indicated when this diagnosis is suspected.

Prevention. Prevention is extremely important and consists of teaching children not to put small toys, coins, buttons, pencil caps, and such articles in their mouths. Open safety pins should never be put on a pillow near a baby, nor should a child be permitted to play with a button box. Parents require considerable education in such details of child training, and no small part of their responsibility in this regard is the example that they set for their offspring.

CHEST TRAUMA

Injuries to the chest may cause minor or serious disturbances of cardiorespiratory function, depending on which part of the complex mechanism is involved. Thus, a fall against the side of a bathtub may fracture one or two ribs with painful but rather slight disturbance of respiratory function, whereas an automobile accident in which the driver of the car is thrown against the steering wheel may crush the chest causing cardiac and lung injuries that may be rapidly fatal. In the United States approximately 25 percent of traffic accident fatalities are due to chest trauma alone and in an additional 50 percent chest trauma is a major factor leading to death. There is frequent association of other injuries, most commonly major fractures, cerebrocranial injuries, and abdominal trauma. In high speed accidents there is an abrupt application of a shearing force to the intrathoracic structures as the person rapidly decelerates (a fast-stop situation). This compresses all of the structures within the rib cage, especially the lungs. Other causes of trauma to the chest are falls, crushing injuries, blows to the chest, and knife and gunshot wounds.

The most serious consequences of chest trauma are acute respiratory failure from damage to the chest wall, airways, diaphragm and lungs and shock due to large vessel and extrathoracic injuries. Frequently, acute respiratory failure and shock are encountered in combination. This situation is particularly lethal.

Chest injuries may be caused by *blunt trauma,* which does not penetrate but injures by force, and by *penetrating injuries.* Both types of injuries can cause serious respiratory and hemodynamic dysfunction.

Immediate Management. In the treatment of injuries to the chest, efforts are made to correct disturbances of cardiorespiratory function caused by the trauma. The first requirement is to evaluate the patency of the airway by assessing for signs of obstruction, sternal retraction, stridor, wheezing, and cyanosis. To restore and maintain cardiopulmonary function, an adequate airway is created, ventilation is ensured, and hypovolemia and low cardiac output are corrected. These treatment efforts along with control of hemorrhage are usually carried out simultaneously by the emergency department team. The patient is completely undressed to avoid missing additional injuries. Pain is treated cautiously to avoid depression of the cough reflex. Nerve block may be used effectively. Many injuries involving the chest may have associated head and abdominal injuries that require urgent attention.

Principles of care are essentially those pertaining to postoperative thoracic care, discussed on pages 423-432.

RIB FRACTURES

Rib fractures are the most common chest injury and should be taken seriously, since they may result in underlying lung contusion (page 500). Such injuries are of special concern in middle-aged and elderly persons who may already have seriously reduced vital capacity. The fifth to the ninth ribs are the ribs most commonly broken. If the rib fragments are driven inward, there may be lacerations of the pleura, pneumothorax, hemothorax, or hemopneumothorax.

If the patient is conscious, he will experience severe pain over the area of fracture that is aggravated by coughing, deep breathing, and motion. To reduce the pain the patient will try to limit his respiratory excursion and coughing by breathing in a shallow manner. This results in diminished ventilation, collapse of unaerated alveoli, and subsequent atelectasis. Because the patient is reluctant to cough, secretions accumulate, which also can lead to atelectasis. Respiratory insufficiency and failure can be the outcome of such a cycle. Following blunt chest trauma serial analysis of arterial blood gases is a sensitive indicator to determine whether or not the lung has been injured.

Management. If there are no complications (pneumothorax; hemothorax), the objective is to relieve the pain so that the patient can breathe effectively. Relief of pain can be achieved by repeatedly blocking the intercostal nerves that transmit painful sensations from the affected area. Nerve block also abolishes muscle splinting that limits respiratory excursion. Injections of the intercostal nerve(s) may be done at the angle of the rib. In some instances the intercostal block will include two intercostal nerves above and two below the ribs that are injured. Narcotic drugs must be used in small doses and with caution because of their tendency to suppress the cough and depress respiration. Usually the pain abates in five to seven days and discomfort can be controlled with non-narcotic analgesia. Most rib fractures heal in three to six weeks.

FLAIL CHEST

Flail chest is the loss of stability of the chest wall with subsequent respiratory impairment (Fig. 25-4). It is usually the result of multiple rib fractures. When this happens one portion of the chest wall no longer has a bony connection with the rest of the rib cage.

Pathophysiology. During inspiration, as the chest expands, the detached part of the chest (flail segment) will show a paradoxical movement in that it is pulled inward during inspiration. This impairs the ability to produce the negative intrapleural pressure required to draw in air. The mediastinum shifts to the normal side. On expiration, since the intrathoracic pressure will exceed atmospheric pressure, the flail segment will bulge outward, impairing the patient's ability to exhale. At the same time, the mediastinum shifts to the injured side. This paradoxical action (air moves between the lungs) results in increased dead space ventilation, retained airway secretions, increasing lung resistance and compliance and reduction in alveolar ventilation. The patient fatigues rapidly because of decreased efficiency of ventilation and increased muscle effort. There is a vicious cycle of decreased ventilation and increased fatigue and oxygen need.

The diagnosis is made by inspection of the *entire* chest, observing for paradoxical motion, and by palpation of the thorax.

Management. If only a small segment of the chest is involved, the objectives are to clear the airway (coughing, deep breaths, gentle suctioning) in order to aid in the expansion of the lung and to relieve pain.

When a severe flail is encountered, a tracheostomy is performed. (Tracheostomy decreases airway resistance and reduces respiratory dead space.) Positive pressure ventilation using a volume type mechanical ventilator is used to internally splint the chest wall and to correct abnormalities in gas exchange. This "floats out" the flail segment. Optimum expansion helps to overcome increased turbulence and resistance to airflow and to expand the alveoli when compliance is reduced by injury. This therapy expands the lungs, ventilates the patient, and corrects anoxia and acidosis, since respiratory insufficiency leads to acidosis.

A more recent treatment of flail chest has been the combination of intermittent mandatory ventilation (IMV)—a technique that allows the patient to breathe spontaneously from a constant gas flow between cycles on the ventilator—and positive end expiratory pressure

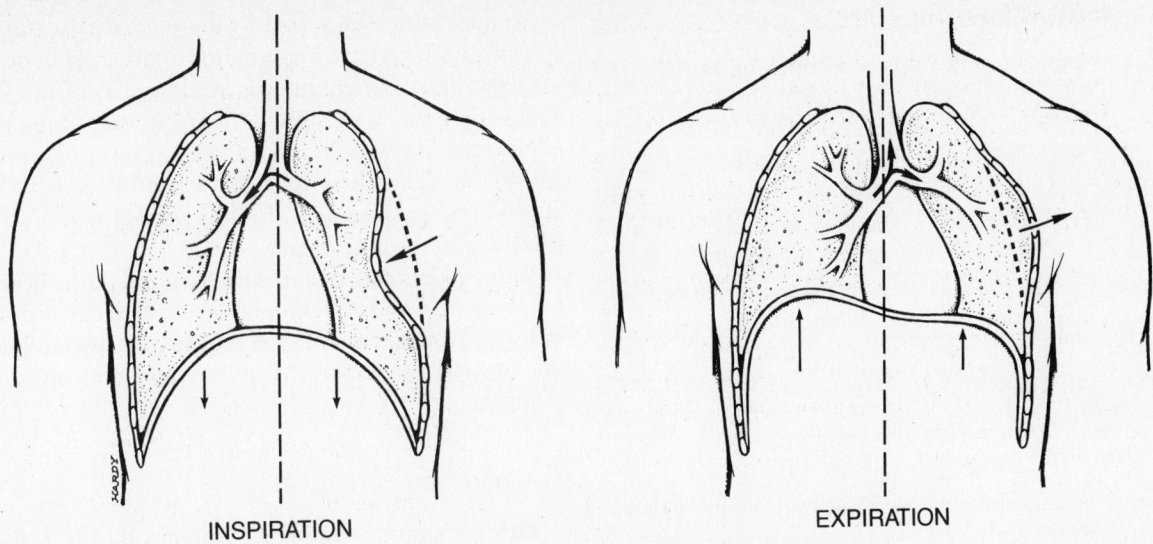

INSPIRATION   EXPIRATION

Figure 25-4.   Flail chest and pathophysiologic effects.

(PEEP), which maintains the pressure above at-mospheric levels throughout the entire ventilatory cycle. The use of IMV and PEEP appears to reduce the duration of ventilator support.

If pneumothorax, hemothorax, or hemopneu-mothorax accompanies flail chest, a chest tube is inserted before mechanical ventilation is started. Serial blood gas determinations are essential in determining the adequacy of therapy. With any thoracic injury there may be under-lying pulmonary contusion. Since a contused lung is swollen, engorged, and edematous, fluid restriction and diuretics may be prescribed to keep the lung dry. (Pulmo-nary contusion is discussed on page 500.)

HEMOTHORAX AND PNEUMOTHORAX

Severe chest injuries usually are accompanied by the collection of blood in the chest cavity (hemothorax) as the result of torn intercostal vessels, lacerations of the lungs, or the escape of air from the injured lung into the pleural cavity (pneumothorax). Often, both blood and air are found in the chest cavity (hemopneumothorax). The lung on that side of the chest is compressed, which interferes with its normal function.

The seriousness of the problem depends upon the amount and rate of thoracic bleeding. Needle aspiration (thoracentesis) or chest tube drainage of the blood or air allows decompression of the pleural cavity so that the lung is able to reexpand and again perform its function in respiration.

Chest Tube Drainage: A large diameter intercostal tube (catheter) is usually inserted in the 2nd intercostal space or in the 5th space in the axilla. This usually brings about prompt and effective decompression of the pleural cavity (drainage of blood/air).

TENSION PNEUMOTHORAX

In some patients, air may be drawn into the pleural space from the lacerated lung or through a small hole in the chest wall. In either case, the air that enters the chest cavity with each inspiration is trapped there: it cannot be expelled through the air passage or small hole in the chest wall.

A tension (pressure) thus is built up within the pleural space, which produces a collapse of the lung and may even push the heart and the great vessels toward the unaffected side of the chest. This not only interferes with respiration, but also disrupts circulatory function, be-cause with increased intrathoracic pressure, venous re-turn to the heart is compromised causing decreased cardiac output and impairment of peripheral circulation. The clinical picture is one of air hunger, agitation, hypo-tension, and cyanosis.

- *Relief of this "tension pneumothorax" must be looked on as an emergency measure.*

Immediate thoracentesis is done to relieve the positive pressure or "tension" within the chest. If the lung ex-pands and there is no continuing leakage from the lung, further drainage may be unnecessary. If the lung is still leaking, as evidenced by the reaccumulation of an inex-haustible volume of air during the thoracentesis, then constant egress of this air must be provided by a large-bore chest tube with underwater seal drainage.

In an emergency situation a tension pneumothorax can be quickly converted to a simple pneumothorax by inser-tion of a large-bore needle into the pleural space, which relieves the pressure and vents the intrathoracic air to the outside. Then a chest tube can be inserted and connected to suction in order to remove the remaining air and fluid and reexpand the lung.

SUCKING WOUNDS OF THE CHEST

Open pneumothorax implies an opening in the chest wall large enough to allow air to pass freely in and out of the thoracic cavity with each attempted respiration. Since the rush of air through the hole in the chest wall produces a sucking sound, such injuries are termed "sucking wounds" of the chest. In such patients not only is the lung collapsed, but the structures of the mediastinum (heart and great vessels) are pushed toward the uninjured side with each inspiration and in the opposite direction with expiration. This is termed *mediastinal flutter,* and it produces serious circulatory embarrassment.

To stop the flow of air through the opening in the chest wall is a lifesaving measure.

In such an emergency, anything may be used that is large enough to fill the hole—a towel, a handkerchief, or the heel of the hand. If the patient is conscious, tell him to inhale and strain against a closed glottis. This action assists in the reexpansion of the lung and the ejection of the air from the thorax. In the hospital, the opening is plugged by sealing it with gauze impregnated with petrolatum jelly. A pressure dressing is applied by circumferential strapping. Usually a chest tube is inserted to permit egress of air and fluid.

PENETRATING WOUNDS OF THE CHEST

Stab wounds are a common cause of penetrating wounds of the chest, most of which are caused by knives and switch blades. The appearance of the external wound may be very deceptive, since pneumothorax, hemothorax, and cardiac tamponade along with severe and continuing hemorrhage can occur from any small wound, even one caused by an icepick.

The objective of immediate management is to restore and maintain cardiopulmonary function. After an adequate airway is ensured and ventilation is corrected, the patient is examined for shock and intrathoracic and intra-abdominal injuries. The patient is undressed completely so that additional injuries will not be missed, for approximately 10 to 15 percent of stab wounds of the chest have associated intra-abdominal injuries.

After the status of the peripheral pulses is assessed, an intravenous line is secured. Blood is withdrawn for chemistries, typing, and crossmatching. Simultaneously a central venous pressure line is established. An indwelling catheter is inserted to monitor urinary volume and to collect a urine sample for laboratory study.

Shock is treated simultaneously with colloid solutions, crystalloids, blood, or vasopressors as indicated by the condition of the patient. Chest x-rays are taken and other diagnostic procedures are carried out (esophagogram, flat plate of the abdomen, arteriogram) as dictated by the needs of the patient.

A chest tube is inserted in the pleural space in most patients with penetrating wounds of the chest in order to achieve rapid and continuing reexpansion of the lungs. Frequently this will cause a complete evacuation of hemothorax and will decrease the incidence of clotted hemothorax. The chest tube allows early recognition of continuing intrathoracic bleeding, which will make surgical exploration necessary.

If the patient has a penetrating wound of the heart and great vessels and the esophagus and tracheobronchial tree, surgical intervention is required. Associated intra-abdominal wounds also necessitate abdominal exploration.

PULMONARY CONTUSION

Pulmonary contusion is damage to the lung parenchyma that results in leakage of blood and fluid. It may occur any time when there is rapid compression and decompression of the chest wall—e.g., a steering wheel injury or the blast effect from gunshot wounds.

Pathophysiology. The primary pathologic defect is the abnormal accumulation of fluid in the interstitial and intra-alveolar spaces. It is thought that injury to the lung parenchyma and its capillary network results in a serum protein and plasma leak. The extravascular serum protein exerts an osmotic pressure that enhances loss of fluid from the capillaries. Blood, edema, and cellular debris (from cellular response to injury) enter the lung and accumulate in the bronchioles and alveolar surface where they interfere with the efficiency of gas exchange. There is an increase in pulmonary vascular resistance and pulmonary artery pressure. The patient experiences systemic hypoxia and carbon dioxide retention. Occasionally a contused lung occurs on the other side of the point of body impact. This is called a contrecoup contusion.

Management. Pulmonary contusion may be mild, moderate, or severe. The efficiency of gas exchange is determined by arterial blood gas measurements. The chest x-rays will reveal pulmonary infiltration. The patient experiences tachypnea, tachycardia, rales on auscultation, pleuritic chest pain, and copious secretions that are sometimes bloody or blood-tinged.

In mild cases of pulmonary contusion, ultrasonic mist nebulization is used to keep the secretions fluid. Postural drainage, physiotherapy, and sterile endotracheal suctioning are used to remove the secretions. Pain is managed by intercostal nerve blocks or by narcotics. Usually antimicrobial therapy is given, for a damaged lung is susceptible to infection. Oxygen by mask or canula is usually given for 24 to 36 hours. Fluids are restricted because the injury is thought to be due to an abnormal collection of fluid in the interstices of the lung.

If moderate lung contusion is encountered, in addition to the above symptoms, the patient will have a large

26

ASSESSMENT OF CARDIOVASCULAR FUNCTION

PHYSIOLOGIC OVERVIEW

The heart is a hollow muscular organ located in the center of the thorax where it occupies the space between the lungs and rests upon the diaphragm. It weighs approximately 300 grams (10.6 ounces). The function of the heart is to pump blood to the tissues, supplying them with oxygen and other nutrients and at the same time removing carbon dioxide and other waste products of metabolism. Actually, there are two pumps within this organ, located on the right and left sides of the heart. The output of the right heart is distributed entirely to the lungs via the pulmonary artery, whereas the output of the left heart is distributed to the remainder of the body via the aorta. These two pumps eject blood simultaneously at approximately the same rate of output.

The pumping action of the heart is accomplished by the rhythmical contraction and relaxation of its muscular wall. During contraction of the muscle, the chambers inside the heart become smaller, as the blood is ejected. During relaxation of the muscles of the heart wall, the heart chambers fill with blood in preparation for the subsequent ejection. A normal adult heart beats approximately 60 to 80 times per minute, ejects approximately 70 ml. from each side per beat, and has a total output of approximately 5 liters/minute. Therefore, in a normal human life time of 70 years, the heart beats approximately 2½ billion times and pumps 180 million liters of blood. Failure of this pump for just several minutes is catastrophic.

Anatomy and Physiology of the Heart

The space in the middle of the chest between the two lungs is called the *mediastinum*. The bulk of the mediastinal space is occupied by the heart, which is encased in a thin fibrous sac called the *pericardium*. The pericardium is not essential for the proper functioning of the heart, but serves as an envelope to protect its surface. The space between the surface of the heart and the pericardial lining is filled with a very small amount of fluid, which lubricates the surface and tends to reduce friction during cardiac muscle contraction.

The right and left sides of the heart are each composed of two chambers, an *atrium* (pl. atria) and a *ventricle*. The common wall between the right and left chambers is called the *septum*. The ventricles are the chambers that eject blood into the arteries. The function of the atria is to receive incoming blood from the veins and to act as temporary storage reservoirs for subsequent emptying into the ventricles. The relationship of the four chambers of the heart is shown in Fig. 26-1.

The atria and ventricles are easily distinguished by the greater thickness of the muscle that forms the ventricular wall. The left ventricular wall is approximately 1 cm. (½ inch) thick, which is about 2½ times as thick as the wall of the right ventricle. The greater thickness of the left ventricular wall corresponds to the greater pressure against which it has to pump. The left ventricle extends further from the midline in the chest and is responsible for the impulse (apex beat) that is usually apparent on the left side of the thorax.

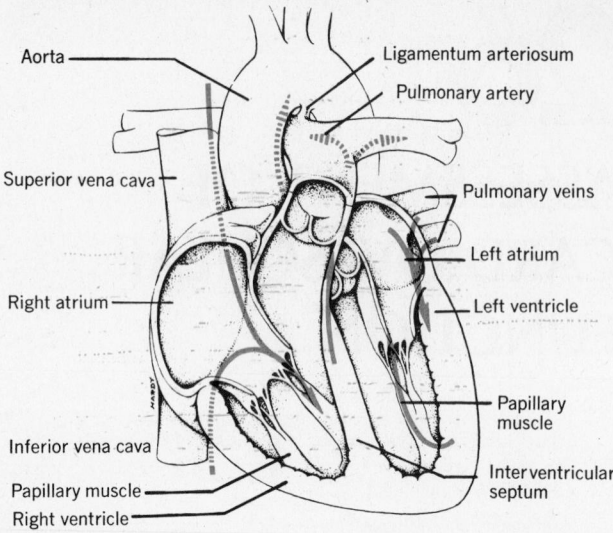

Aorta

Ligamentum arteriosum

Pulmonary artery

Superior vena cava

Pulmonary veins

Left atrium

Right atrium

Left ventricle

Papillary muscle

Inferior vena cava

Papillary muscle

Interventricular septum

Right ventricle

Figure 26-1.   Interior of the heart. Arrows indicate the direction of blood flow. (From Chaffee, E. E., and Greisheimer, E. M.: Basic Physiology and Anatomy. Philadelphia, J. B. Lippincott, 1974)

THE HEART VALVES.   The atrial and ventricular chambers are separated from each other by thin leaflets of fibrous tissue which function as valves, permitting blood to flow in only one direction, from the atria into the ventricles, as shown in Figure 26-1. On the right side of the heart, the valve between the atrium and the ventricle is called the *tricuspid valve*, so named because it is composed of three leaflets (cusps). On the left side of the heart, the valve between the atrium and the ventricle is called the *mitral* or *bicuspid valve* and is composed of only two cusps. The mitral and tricuspid valves are together identified as the *atrioventricular valves*. There are also valves, called the

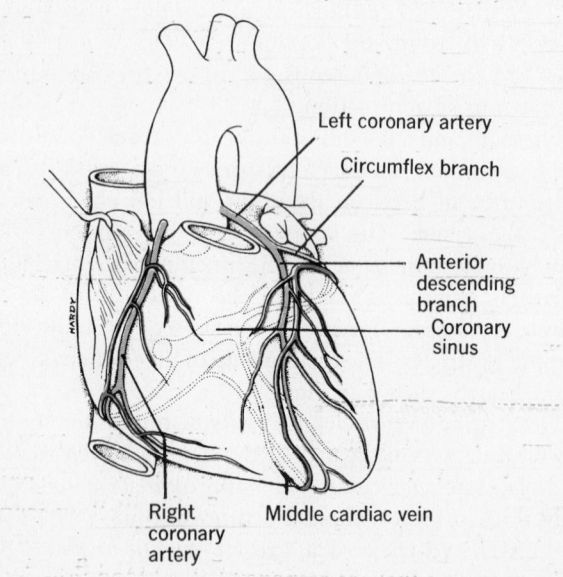

Left coronary artery

Circumflex branch

Anterior descending branch

Coronary sinus

Right coronary artery

Middle cardiac vein

Figure 26-2.   Diagram of the coronary arteries arising from the aorta and encircling the heart. The coronary sinus and some of the coronary veins also are shown. (From Chaffee, E. E., and Greisheimer, E. M.: Basic Physiology and Anatomy. Philadelphia, J. B. Lippincott, 1974)

semilunar valves, situated between each ventricle and its corresponding artery. The valve between the right ventricle and the pulmonary artery is called the *pulmonic valve;* the valve between the left ventricle and the aorta is called the *aortic valve*. The semilunar valves also allow only unidirectional flow of blood, that is, from the ventricle into the artery. Both of the semilunar valves are normally composed of three cusps. There are no valves between the large veins and the atria.

When the ventricles contract, blood tends to push the atrioventricular valve leaflets the wrong way back into the atrial cavity. Normally, the leaflets are maintained in their proper position by the papillary muscles, specialized bundles of muscle tissue that tether the free edge of the cusps to the ventricular wall. Malfunctioning of the papillary muscles results in failure of the valve to maintain its proper closed position during ventricular contraction and, therefore, the unidirectional flow of blood is not maintained. The semilunar valves, on the other hand, are constructed so that tethers are not required.

THE CORONARY CIRCULATION.   The heart muscle (myocardium) is metabolically active in that its requirements for oxygen and nutrients are large and continuous. These required substances are supplied to the heart muscle by blood flowing in the coronary arteries (Fig. 26-2). As a manifestation of its large metabolic requirements, the heart uses approximately one half of the oxygen delivered through the coronary arteries in contrast to other organs which (on the average) use only one quarter of the oxygen delivered to them. The coronary arteries arise from the aorta near its origin at the left ventricle. The wall of the left side of the heart is supplied in large part through the left coronary artery which divides into several large branches that run down and across the left side of the myocardium. The right heart wall is supplied similarly from a separate right coronary artery. Blockage of any of these arteries or their branches will deprive the muscle supplied by the vessel of its necessary oxygen and nutrients and result in severe damage to or the death of those muscle fibers.

CARDIAC MUSCLE.   The specialized muscle tissue composing the wall of the heart is called *cardiac muscle*. Microscopically, cardiac muscle resembles striated (skeletal) muscle, which is under conscious control. However, heart muscle is not under conscious control and in that sense resembles smooth (involuntary) muscle. The cardiac muscle fibers are arranged in an interconnected manner (called a syncytium) so that they can contract and relax in coordination. The sequential pattern of contraction and relaxation of individual muscle fibers insures the rhythmic behavior of the heart muscle as a whole and enables it to function as a pump. The heart muscle itself is called the *myocardium*. The segment of cells on the inner surface of this muscle, which is in contact with the blood, is called the *endocardium,* and the portion of cells on the outer surface of the heart is called the *epicardium*.

ELECTROMECHANICAL COUPLING. In the normal cardiac muscle cell, an electrical voltage exists between the inside and the outside of the cell across its membrane. When the magnitude of this voltage is reduced (depolarization), contraction of the muscle cell results. The membrane voltage of a cardiac muscle cell is normally reduced when the voltage of a neighboring cell is reduced (although it can also be reduced by external electrical stimulation). Sufficient depolarization of a single cardiac muscle will therefore result in depolarization and contraction of the entire myocardium.

The reduction in membrane voltage of a cardiac muscle cell changes the permeability of the membrane and allows an uptake of calcium into the cell. This increase in intracellular calcium concentration leads to shortening of the muscle fibers and development of tension (contraction). After a short time period, the membrane voltage returns to its original value, the calcium that had accumulated in its interior is removed, and the cell relaxes. This interaction between changes in membrane voltage and muscle contraction is called *electromechanical coupling*.

Normal electromechanical coupling and contraction of the heart are dependent on the composition of the fluid (extracellular fluid) surrounding the heart muscle cells. The composition of this fluid is in turn influenced by the composition of the blood. A change in blood calcium concentration may therefore alter contraction of the heart muscle fibers. A change in blood potassium concentration is also important since potassium affects the normal electrical voltage of the cell.

Conduction System of the Heart

Cardiac muscle cells have an inherent rhythmicity, which is illustrated by the fact that a segment of myocardium removed from the rest of the heart will continue to contract rhythmically if maintained under the proper conditions. Membrane voltage changes accompany these rhythmic contractions. The membrane voltage change that ordinarily initiates the heartbeat arises from those cells of the myocardium that have the fastest intrinsic rate of contraction. These specialized cells, located at the junction of the superior vena cava and the right atrium, are known as the *sinoatrial (SA)* node and function as the pacemaker for the entire myocardium (Fig. 26–3). The sinoatrial node initiates approximately 70 to 80 impulses per minute in a resting normal heart but can change its rate in response to needs of the body. The electrical signal initiated by the SA node is conducted along the myocardial cells of the atrium to the atrioventricular (AV) junction. The *AV junction* (located in the right atrial wall near the tricuspid valve) is another group of specialized muscle cells similar to the SA node but with an intrinsic rate of

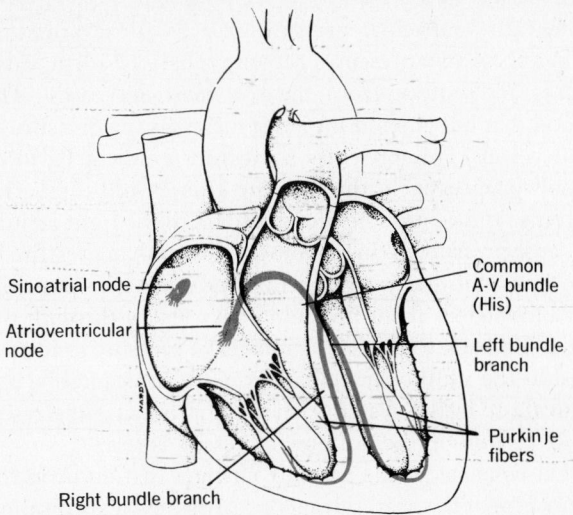

Figure 26-3. Conducting system. Diagram shows relationships of the sinoatrial node, the atrioventricular node, the common atrioventricular bundle and its branches. (From Chaffee, E. E., and Greisheimer, E. M.: Basic Physiology and Anatomy. Philadelphia, J. B. Lippincott, 1974)

about 50 to 60 impulses per minute. The AV junction coordinates the incoming electrical impulses from the atria and relays an electrical impulse to the ventricles. This electrical impulse is conducted away from the AV junction through a bundle of specialized muscle fibers (called the atrioventricular bundle or the bundle of His) that travel in the septum separating the left and right ventricles. The His bundle divides into right and left bundle branches near the apex of the heart. The fibers in the right and left bundle branches are called Purkinje fibers. The right bundle fans out into the right ventricular muscle. The left bundle divides again into the left anterior and left posterior bundle branches, which fan out into the left ventricular muscle. Further spread of depolarization through the rest of the myocardium takes place by conduction through the muscle fibers themselves.

If the SA node malfunctions, the AV node generally takes over the pacemaker function of the heart. Should both the SA and AV nodes fail in their pacemaker function, the myocardium will continue to beat at a rate of about 40 beats per minute, which is the intrinsic rate of electrical depolarization of the ventricular myocardial cells.

Cardiac Hemodynamics

What determines the direction of blood flow from the heart through the circulation and then back to the heart? The important principle is that fluid will flow from a region of higher pressure to a region of lower pressure. The pressures that are responsible for blood flow in the normal circulation are generated by contraction of the ventricular muscle. During contraction, blood is forced from the ventricle into the aorta during the period of time when left ventricular pressure exceeds aortic pressure. When these two pressures become equal, the aortic valve closes and output from the left ventricle ceases. The blood that has entered the aorta increases the pressure in that vessel. This provides a pressure gradient to force blood progressively through the arteries and capillaries and into the veins. The blood returns to the right atrium because pressure in this chamber is lower than pressure in the veins. Similarly, a gradient of pressure is responsible for blood flow from the pulmonary artery through the lung and back to the left atrium. The pressure gradients within the pulmonary circulation are considerably less than those in the systemic circulation because the resistance to flow in the pulmonary vessels is less.

Let us consider the pressure changes that occur in the chambers of the heart during the cardiac cycle, beginning with the period when the ventricles are relaxed. This period is called *diastole*. During diastole, the atrioventricular valves are open, and blood returning from the veins flows into the atrium and then into the ventricle. Towards the end of this diastolic period, the atrial muscle contracts in response to a signal initiated by the sinoatrial node. This contraction raises the pressure inside the atrium and forces an increment of blood into the ventricle. At this point, the ventricles themselves begin to contract in response to propagation of the electrical impulse that began in the SA node some milliseconds previously. The period of contraction of the ventricles is called *systole*. During systole, the pressure inside the ventricle rapidly rises, forcing the atrioventricular valves to close. The consequence of this action is that no further filling of the ventricle from the atrium can occur and blood ejected from the ventricle cannot flow back to the atrium. The rapid rise of pressure inside the ventricles forces the pulmonic and aortic valves to open, and blood is ejected into the pulmonary artery and aorta. The exit of blood is at first rapid, and then, as the pressures in each ventricle and its corresponding artery approach equalization, the flow of blood gradually decreases. At the cessation of systole, the ventricular muscle relaxes and the pressure within the chamber rapidly decreases. This decrease in pressure creates a tendency for blood to come back from the artery into the ventricle, which forces the semilunar valves to close. Simultaneously, as the pressure within the ventricle drops to below atrial pressure, the atrioventricular valves open, the ventricles begin to fill, and the entire sequence is repeated. It is important to note that the mechanical events related to filling and ejection by the heart are closely coupled to the corresponding electrical events that cause cardiac contraction and relaxation.

The events just described lead to the repetitive rise and fall of pressures inside the ventricles. The maximum pressure reached is called *systolic pressure* and the minimum pressure is defined as *diastolic pressure*.

Cardiac Output

Cardiac output is the amount of blood pumped by either of the ventricles during a given period of time. The cardiac output of a typical adult is normally about 5 liters/minute but varies greatly depending on the metabolic needs of the body. Cardiac output equals the stroke volume times the heart rate. *Stroke volume* is the amount of blood ejected per heartbeat. Cardiac output can be affected, therefore, by changes either in stroke volume or heart rate. The resting heart rate of an average adult is approximately 72 beats/minute and the average stroke volume is about 70 ml./beat.

CONTROL OF HEART RATE. Since the function of the heart is to supply blood to all tissues of the body, its output must vary as the metabolic needs of the tissues themselves change. For example, during exercise, the total cardiac output may increase fourfold to 20 liters/minute. This increase is normally accomplished by approximately doubling both the heart rate and the stroke volume. Changes in heart rate are accomplished by reflex controls mediated by the autonomic nervous system, including its sympathetic and parasympathetic divisions. The parasympathetic nerves which travel to the heart through the vagus nerve can slow the cardiac rate, whereas sympathetic nerves increase it. These nerves exert their effect on heart rate through their action on the sinoatrial node to either decrease or increase its rate of intrinsic depolarization. The balance between these two reflex control systems normally determines the heart rate. The heart rate is also stimulated by an increased level of circulating catecholamines (secreted by the adrenal gland) as well as by the presence of excess thyroid hormone which produces a catecholamine-like effect.

CONTROL OF STROKE VOLUME. Stroke volume is primarily determined by three factors: (1) intrinsic contractility of the cardiac muscle, (2) the degree of stretch of the cardiac muscle prior to its contraction, and (3) the pressure against which the heart muscle has to eject blood during contraction.

Intrinsic contractility is a term used to denote the force that can be generated by the contracting myocardium under any given condition. It is increased by circulating catecholamines, sympathetic neuronal activity, and certain drugs (such as digitalis). It is depressed by hypoxia and acidosis. Increased contractility results in increased stroke volume.

The precontraction length of the ventricular muscle fibers is determined by the volume of blood within the ventricle at the beginning of systole (or end of diastole). This volume, the ventricular end-diastolic volume, is called *preload*. The larger the preload, the greater will be the stroke volume. The relationship between increased stroke volume and increased ventricular end-diastolic volume for a given intrinsic contractility is called Starling's Law of the Heart. This effect is due to a greater initial length which leads to a greater degree of shortening of cardiac muscle. This results from increased interaction between thick and thin filaments of the sarcomeres (similar to that discussed more fully in the chapter on skeletal muscle physiology).

The pressure against which the left ventricle ejects blood is the pressure in the aorta; right ventricular ejection works against the pressure in the pulmonary artery. The greater these pressures, the greater will be the tension in the ventricular wall during contraction. This tension is called *afterload*. Increased afterload leads to decreased stroke volume.

The heart can achieve a greatly increased stroke volume, as during exercise, by increasing preload (through increased venous return), by increasing contractility (through sympathetic nervous discharge), and by decreasing afterload (through peripheral vasodilatation with decreased aortic pressure).

The fraction of the end-diastolic volume that is ejected with each stroke is called the *ejection fraction*. With each stroke, 0.56 to 0.78 of the end-diastolic volume is ejected by the normal heart. The ejection fraction can be used as an index of myocardial contractility; it is decreased if contractility is depressed.

Generation of Heart Sounds

The normal heart sounds are produced in the heart primarily by closure of the heart valves. Abnormal sounds may be produced in diseased hearts due to turbulent flow through abnormal valve openings (*murmurs*), friction between the heart and its surrounding tissue (*rubs*), and abnormal vibrations of the heart wall (*gallops*). The first heart sound, S_1, coincides with closure of the atrioventricular valves and is a normal heart sound. The major component of this sound is the vibration of the leaflets of the atrioventricular valves as they close, although vibration of the myocardial wall may also contribute. The second heart sound, S_2, occurs upon closure of the semilunar valves. Although the aortic and pulmonary valves close almost simultaneously, the pulmonic valve usually lags slightly behind the aortic valve. Therefore, two components of the second sound can frequently be heard separately. The brief lag ordinarily increases slightly during inspiration and decreases during expiration. The time between the first and second heart sounds corresponds roughly to the duration of systole. This is normally shorter than the time between S_2 and S_1, which corresponds roughly to the duration of diastole. A composite drawing showing the relationships among electrical events, ventricular pressures and volumes, and heart sounds is given in Figure 5-21.

S_1 and S_2 are normal heart sounds. Two other heart sounds are frequently heard during examination of the heart and denote some abnormality of the heart function.

These sounds, S_3 and S_4, occur during the diastolic period. The third heart sound, S_3, is due to rapid filling of the ventricles in abnormal hearts with flabby and/or dilated walls. Because of the flabbiness, the ventricular walls vibrate excessively when blood enters at the beginning of diastole. The fourth heart sound, S_4, is also due to vibration of ventricular walls. S_4 occurs at the time of atrial contraction in hearts that are stiffer than normal and is caused by a rush of blood into a partially filled ventricle. When S_3 and/or S_4 are heard together with the first and second heart sounds, an effect may be produced that sounds like a gallop. The S_3 gallop is usually found in patients with congestive heart failure, and the S_4 gallop is often heard in patients with high blood pressure.

Another class of abnormal heart sounds are the heart murmurs. These are caused by the turbulence in the flow of blood across either the semilunar or atrioventricular valves. In diseased valves that fail to open adequately (stenosis), a murmur is produced by the forward flow of blood across the valve. With diseased valves that fail to close normally (insufficiency or regurgitation), murmurs are also heard due to the backward flow of blood through the valve. Occasionally, murmurs are heard in normal hearts and are called *outflow* or *ejection murmurs*.

In abnormal conditions when the pericardium or the myocardium has been damaged, the heart may rub against its pericardial sac. This may generate a sound that has a harsh quality and is termed a rub.

THE CARDIAC PATIENT AND THE NURSE

Over 10 million people in this country are affected by chronic heart disease. Cardiovascular disease ranks first among the leading causes of death in the United States, Canada, and Western Europe. However, cardiovascular deaths in the United States have declined 14 percent during the past five years and the downward trend appears to be accelerating. This dramatic development may be due in part to a change in the American life style (exercise, diet) in response to research and public education and/or to advances in diagnosis, medical treatment, and surgical techniques in repairing congenital and acquired cardiovascular abnormalities.

Safe and effective nursing care in cardiac conditions requires a thorough appreciation of the pathologic and physiologic processes involved. And, if the nurse is to contribute materially toward the recovery of the patient, the rationale of prescribed treatment must be understood.

The symptoms of heart disease vary from patient to patient. However, most cardiovascular symptoms are likely to be included in this brief list: fatigue, chest pain, dyspnea, orthopnea, cough, palpitation, edema, and cyanosis.

Symptomatic relief is a major objective of nursing, but objectives change as the patient's problems and needs change. With the passage of time therapeutic priorities must be revised in accordance with these needs.

Facets of nursing care to be considered, apart from observation, identification, interpretation, and relief of symptoms, include teaching methods aimed at preventing symptomatic recurrences and the instruction of patients regarding health measures designed to retard the progression of heart disease. One important nursing goal is to equip the patient with knowledge and motivation to participate effectively in his own plan of care.

The nursing care of the patient with heart disease is never routine because there are too many variables in heart disease. In making modifications in the nursing management of these patients, the nurse must ask, "Which is easier for *this* patient?" Will it be less stressful for the patient to feed himself or to be fed? Will the patient become more upset by being shaved, by not being shaved, or by receiving help?"

In giving the cardiac patient the nursing support he requires, the nurse demonstrates interest in him as a person and gives him the feeling of being understood. This is most important in helping the patient to cope with his anxiety. The relief of anxiety is a major factor in caring for any patient with a cardiac condition.

ASSESSING RISK FACTORS IN CARDIOVASCULAR DISEASE

The nurse has a great responsibility for health assessment and health maintenance. Preventive cardiac nursing is found in all facets of caring for people—both in and out of the hospital. In working with patients and their families the nurse is likely to encounter many individuals with cardiovascular symptoms who have not sought but obviously need diagnostic, therapeutic, or preventive services. To identify patients at risk, the nurse is particularly alert for symptoms of edema and shortness of breath. Upon hearing a person blame his exertional dyspnea on a "cold," "too many cigarettes," or "old age," the nurse, knowing that dyspnea never is normal, should attempt to convince the person to seek immediate medical attention.

HYPERTENSION. Over 24 million persons in this country have hypertension or hypertensive heart disease. Hypertension is a major risk factor in coronary artery disease and can cause stroke, congestive heart failure, and kidney failure. One in every six adults has some elevation of blood pressure which is often untreated, since hypertension produces no characteristic symptoms. Risk factors associated with the hypertension-prone individual include a family history of toxemia of pregnancy, obesity, elevated blood sugar, and elevated pulse rate. For a more detailed discussion of hypertension, see pages 628–635.

ATHEROSCLEROSIS. Study has shown that the serum cholesterol level is the best single screening test for the detection of hyperlipidemia (elevated blood lipids), which leads to the development of coronary heart disease. A preventive approach to atherosclerotic heart disease should be started at *birth* with a lifelong plan to limit calories, saturated fat, cholesterol, and excess carbohydrates.

CORONARY HEART DISEASE. Even with improvement in therapy there is a high mortality rate for patients with coronary heart disease. Risk factors to identify individuals who are coronary-prone include an elevated serum cholesterol, increasing levels of blood pressure, cigarette smoking, electrocardiographic abnormalities, obesity, genetic factors (diabetes, hypertension), and stress. The nurse can help identify these susceptible individuals and can encourage them to seek medical assistance for preventive measures and to change their life styles in order to cope with stress in a more positive manner.

OBESITY. Obesity often is associated with an elevated blood pressure, increased cardiac load, impaired glucose tolerance, and altered blood lipid metabolism. Thus the individual who is overweight becomes susceptible to heart disease.

CIGARETTE SMOKING. Convincing evidence points to an association between cigarette smoking and deaths from the complications of coronary heart disease. Any cigarette smoker with symptoms of angina pectoris or a history of myocardial infarction should be informed of this relationship in no uncertain terms and strongly urged to discontinue the use of tobacco. It has been demonstrated that men who quit smoking before the development of overt coronary disease will have a lower incidence of disease than do the men who continue to smoke. Better still, nurses should endorse community health efforts to stop children and young persons from *starting* to smoke.

LACK OF EXERCISE. There is also a definite relationship between habitual lack of exercise and cardiac morbidity and mortality. Sedentary work and living habits are common in this country and may well be a serious challenge to preventive medicine in the future. Physical exercise is beneficial because it increases cardiac output and coronary blood flow. It behooves the nurse to participate in a daily program of exercise and to encourage this activity in others. Exercise also helps overweight persons to expend energy and thus aids in a weight reduction program.

RHEUMATIC FEVER. The nurse should instruct parents regarding the potential dangers associated with pharyngitis (sore throat) and tonsillitis. Streptococcal infection can result in rheumatic fever with rheumatic heart disease in which heart valves become scarred and deformed. This is considered a *preventable* heart disease.

Were every patient with streptococcal pharyngitis to receive prompt and adequate treatment with penicillin, rheumatic fever would virtually cease to exist. *Thus it is advisable to take throat cultures on all patients with acute pharyngitis* (page 390). In addition, the nurse plays an important role in the instruction of patients who have had rheumatic fever by pointing out the purpose and the importance of continuing antibiotic prophylaxis for an indefinite period of time.

CONGENITAL HEART DISEASE. Detection of congenital heart disease begins before the baby is born. Young women of childbearing age can be taught that some drugs are teratogenic (tending to produce physical defects in the fetus). No pregnant woman should take any medication without the physician's advice. Some patients require genetic counseling especially if there is familial clustering of congenital heart disease. Siblings of a child with congenital heart disease are at risk for a similar type of lesion. It is thought that congenital malformations of the heart result from developmental abnormalities and/or possible genetic predisposition.

Upon encountering a person who is in the first trimester of pregnancy and has been exposed to German measles (rubella), the nurse should advise an immediate visit to the physician's office or clinic for prophylactic injections of gamma globulin. Evidence indicates that if rubella is contracted in the early stages of pregnancy the offspring is more likely to be afflicted with congenital defects than would otherwise be the case. There are active vaccines now available for both rubella (German measles) and rubeola (measles). The widespread use of these vaccines should make the prevention of measles possible in the future.

Early diagnosis is the key to the successful treatment of congenital heart disease. Correction is most likely to be accomplished by early surgery, i.e., surgery carried out before the patient develops pulmonary hypertension. With the school nurse and the community health nurse continually on the lookout for children who become cyanotic or unduly breathless on exertion, this diagnostic possibility is not likely to be overlooked. Moreover by being familiar with normal growth and development, the nurse should be quick to perceive the possibility of congenital heart disease in a child who appears not to be developing normally.

SYPHILIS. The nurse who participates in the treatment of patients with early syphilis must educate these individuals concerning the potential long-range effects of this infection and how they can be avoided if the disease is eradicated completely by adequate therapy. Stress to the patient the desirability of complete cooperation with his physician throughout the follow-up period and until such time as he may receive his final discharge from the clinic. With careful attention, syphilitic aortitis and aortic aneurysms can be prevented.

CARDIAC DECOMPENSATION (Congestive Heart Failure). Patients who repeatedly return to their physician or hospital in a recurrent state of cardiac decompensation need continuing reevaluation and repeated preventive teaching. A detailed description of the previous day's meals should be requested on the occasion of each visit in order to determine to what extent the patient has been adhering to his low-sodium diet. Although meticulous about his diet, does he relieve his dyspepsia with antacid powders that contain sodium? Is he keeping track of his weight to detect water retention and to control edema? These and many other considerations require repeated discussion. Repetition is essential to the process of learning and therefore is an important principle in preventive teaching.

MENOPAUSE. Following menopause there is an increasing incidence of coronary heart disease in women. A young woman who has had a hysterectomy with bilateral oophorectomy should be provided with estrogen replacement. Such therapy may have to be considered in the normally menopausal woman who has other risk factors.

ASSESSMENT OF CARDIAC FUNCTION

There are numerous diagnostic studies that help to determine accurately the nature and the exact location of cardiovascular defects. To begin with, a complete history of the patient is taken, from birth to the present. Then a physical examination is carried out including an electrocardiogram which is basic to the initial clinical workup and subsequent evaluation of the patient. Fluoroscopy (often with barium swallow) and x-ray study of the chest are carried out to determine heart size and chamber enlargement. Other tests are conducted as the patient's symptoms and condition warrant.

Chest X-ray and Fluoroscopy

A *chest x-ray* is usually ordered to determine the size, contour, and position of the heart. It reveals cardiac and pericardial calcifications and demonstrates physiological alterations in the pulmonary circulation.

Fluoroscopy provides visual observation of the heart on a luminescent x-ray screen. It shows heart and vascular pulsations and is useful in the assessment of unusual cardiac contours. Fluoroscopy is a useful tool in the placement and positioning of intravenous pacemaking electrodes and for guiding the catheter in cardiac catheterization, etc.

Electrocardiography

The *electrocardiogram* is a visual representation of the electrical activity of the heart as reflected by changes in electrical potential at the skin surface. The ECG is recorded as a tracing on a strip of paper or appears on the screen of an oscilloscope. In order to facilitate the interpretation of the ECG, data about the patient's age, sex, blood pressure, height, weight, symptoms, and medications (especially digitalis and antiarrhythmic drugs) should be noted on the ECG requisition. Electrocardiography is particularly useful in the evaluation of conditions that interfere with normal heart functions, such as disturbances of rate or rhythm, disorders of conduction, enlargement of heart chambers, presence of a myocardial infarction, and electrolyte imbalances. This procedure is discussed in detail in Chapter 27.

AMBULATORY MONITORING. Ambulatory cardiac monitoring is being done with increasing frequency to obtain evidence of arrhythmias that are transient in nature, to assess patients who suffer from transient dizziness and weakness, or to evaluate antiarrhythmic drugs. Ambulatory monitoring is also used after a myocardial infarction to assess for ventricular irregularities or to evaluate pacemaker function.

The patient wears a miniaturized tape recording device with a single or double lead system that is attached to the belt or worn on a shoulder device. Various systems are available which record the patient's ECG continuously for up to 24 hours while he is going about his daily activities. It is useful also in determining the effects of stress.

COMPUTER ANALYSIS OF ECG. Computer analysis of electrocardiograms is now available in some centers. It provides computer assistance for interpretation of electrocardiograms that helps to strengthen diagnostic competence and permits the analysis of large numbers of ECGs. It is especially useful in providing ECG analysis in outlying areas where such services have been lacking. The computer requires the same informational input that human interpreters need: age, body build, diagnosis, drugs used, etc. Computer analysis is not meant to replace interpretation by a physician.

Exercise Stress Testing

Exercise testing is a noninvasive means of assessing certain aspects of cardiac function. The purposes are to search for ischemic changes in the ECG and to screen for ischemic heart disease, to evaluate patients with chest pain, to assess the results of therapy, and to aid in developing individual physical fitness programs.

Exercise testing may be done by having the patient walk on a treadmill, pedal a stationary bicycle, or climb a set of stairs. The patient is exercised by increasing the walking speed and incline of the treadmill or by increasing the load against which the bicycle is pedaled. ECG electrodes are applied to the patient and tracings are made before, during, and after exercise testing. Blood pressure, skin temperature, physical appearance, and the occurrence or worsening of chest pain are monitored during and following the test.

The patient is instructed to avoid smoking, eating, and drinking for four hours prior to the test. Following the test the patient should be instructed to rest for a period of time and to avoid stimulants, eating, or extreme temperature changes (i.e., hot or cold showers, going out into the cold).

Vectorcardiography

The vectorcardiogram presents a three-dimensional view of the electrical forces of the heart: horizontal or transverse, frontal, and left sagittal or lateral planes. This diagnostic modality amplifies understanding of the ECG and gives more accurate diagnostic information in certain areas of cardiac diagnosis.

Echocardiography (Ultrasonic Examination of the Heart)

Ultrasound is acoustic energy propagated at frequencies of more than 1 million cycles per second. In echocardiography, high frequency sound waves are sent into the heart through the chest wall and are recorded as they return. The ultrasound is generated by a hand-held transducer (a device that converts one form of energy to another form of energy) applied to the front of the chest. An ECG is recorded simultaneously to time events within the cardiac cycle. Motions of the echoes are traced on an oscilloscope and recorded on film. This is the same sonar principle by which submarines detect ships. It is a safe, noninvasive method that gives information similar in many respects to the data obtained with angiocardiography. Echocardiography is especially useful in the diagnosis and differentiation of heart murmurs. An echogram can detect whether the heart is dilated, the walls or septum are thickened, or pericardial effusion is present. It has also been used to study the motion of prosthetic heart valves.

Phonocardiography

Phonocardiography is the graphic recording of heart sounds and pulse waves and their relation to time. It helps to identify, accurately time, and differentiate various sounds and murmurs. It provides a permanent record for future comparison.

Angiocardiography

Angiocardiography is a technique of injecting dye into the vascular system at appropriate sites to outline the heart and blood vessels. It is accompanied by *cineangiograms* (rapidly changing films or movies on an intensified fluoroscopic screen) which record the passage of the contrast media through the vascular tree. This procedure is useful for providing information regarding structural abnormalities such as occlusions, defects, or fistulae or abnormal heart-valve function. Angiography is especially useful in identifying obstructive coronary lesions.

SELECTIVE ANGIOCARDIOGRAPHY. Selective angiocardiography is the injection of a contrast medium through a catheter directly into one of the heart chambers, coronary arteries, or great vessels. The angiocardiogram is recorded by means of a rapid film changer or motion picture camera.

AORTOGRAPHY. An aortogram is a form of angiography that outlines the lumen of the aorta and the major arteries arising from it. In *thoracic aortography* a contrast medium is used to study the aortic arch and its major branches by means of rapid serial roentgenography. The translumbar or retrograde brachial or femoral approach may be used.

CORONARY ARTERIOGRAPHY. In coronary arteriography a radiopaque catheter is introduced into the right brachial artery (via open arteriotomy) or femoral artery (via cutaneous puncture), and is passed into the ascending aorta and manipulated into the appropriate coronary artery under fluoroscopic control. Coronary arteriography is used as an evaluation tool before coronary artery surgery. It is also used to study suspected congenital anomalies of the coronary arteries.

NURSING IMPLICATIONS IN ANGIOCARDIOGRAPHY. When dye is used, the patient is kept in a fasting state prior to x-ray study in order to minimize the danger of pulmonary aspiration should emesis occur. The vital signs are recorded every 15 minutes or more often, as the patient's condition indicates, until they are stable. The puncture or cutdown site is checked for bleeding, and the distal extremity is checked for normal color and intact pulses. The patient may complain of mild headache and/or discomfort in the groin or other site, depending on the route by which the dye was administered.

Heart Catheterization

Heart catheterization is a diagnostic procedure in which a catheter(s) is introduced into the heart and blood vessels in order to (1) measure oxygen concentration (tension), saturation, and pressure in the various heart chambers; (2) detect shunts; (3) provide blood samples for analysis; and (4) determine cardiac output and pulmonary blood flow. Cardiac catheterization is done also to evaluate the patient with chest pain (unstable angina) and to assess heart status before heart surgery. Angiography is usually combined with heart catheterization for coronary artery visualization. During the procedure the patient is monitored electrocardiographically by means of an oscilloscope. Appropriate resuscitative equipment should be readily available when heart catheterization is done.

RIGHT-HEART CATHETERIZATION. Right-heart catheterization involves passing a radiopaque catheter from an antecubital or femoral vein into the right atrium, right ventricle, and pulmonary vasculature. This is carried out under direct visualization with a fluoroscope. Pressures within the right atrium are measured and recorded, and blood samples are removed for measurment of the hematocrit and oxygen saturation. The catheter is then passed through the tricuspid valve, and similar tests are performed on the blood within the right ventricle. Finally, the catheter is introduced into the pulmonary artery, i.e., through the pulmonic valve, and as far as possible beyond that point, where "capillary" samples are obtained and "capillary" pressures (also known as wedge pressure) are recorded. Then the catheter is withdrawn.

Right-heart catheterization is considered a relatively safe procedure. Complications, when they do occur, include cardiac arrhythmias, venous spasm, infection of the cutdown site, cardiac perforation, and, rarely, cardiac arrest.

LEFT-HEART CATHETERIZATION. Left-heart catheterization is usually done by retrograde catheterization of the left ventricle or by transseptal catheterization of the left atrium. In the retrograde technique, the catheter is inserted under direct vision into the right brachial artery (arteriotomy) and advanced under fluoroscopic control down into the ascending aorta and into the left ventricle; or the catheter may be introduced percutaneously by puncture of the femoral artery.

In the transseptal approach the catheter is passed from the right femoral vein (percutaneously or by saphenous vein cutdown) into the right atrium. A long needle is passed up through the catheter and is used to puncture the septum separating the right and left atria. The needle is withdrawn and the catheter is advanced under fluoroscopic control into the left ventricle. In both of these techniques the patient is monitored by electrocardiogram.

Left-heart catheterization gives hemodynamic data; e.g., it permits flow and pressure measurements of the left heart. It is most often performed to evaluate the function of the left ventricular muscle and the mitral and aortic valves or the patency of the coronary arteries. It is used to evaluate patients before and after cardiac surgery. Usually the right side of the heart is catheterized before the left side is done. Complications include arrhythmias, myocardial infarction, perforation of the heart or great vessels, and systemic embolization.

Following the catheterization, the catheter is slowly withdrawn, the artery is repaired, and the cutdown site is closed and dressed.

NURSING MANAGEMENT IN CARDIAC CATHETERIZATION. Prior to cardiac catheterization the patient always undergoes a complete history, physical examination, electrocardiogram, chest x-ray, and blood tests to assure that he is in the best cardiac condition for the test. Heart failure, an arrhythmia, or electrolyte imbalance increase the risk of the procedure. Determine whether the patient has any allergies (especially to iodine).

- Withhold food and fluids for 6 hours before the procedure to ensure a basal metabolic rate and to prevent vomiting and aspiration.

- Prepare the patient for the boredom of the procedure and warn him that he will be lying on a hard table for a prolonged period. (Right and left catheterization with angiography can rarely be completed in less than 2 hours.)
- Prepare the patient for certain sensations he may experience during the catheterization. Knowing what to expect can help the patient to cope with the experience.

  An occasional thudding sensation (palpitation) may be felt in the chest because of extra systoles that almost always occur, particularly when the catheter tip touches the myocardium.

  When dye is injected into the right heart (during angiography) there may be a strong desire to cough.

  The injection of contrast medium into either side of the heart may produce a feeling of heat, particularly in the head, which leaves in a minute or less.
- In the postcatheterization period, watch the puncture (or cutdown) sites for hematoma formation, check the peripheral pulses, and report any complaint of pain, numbness, or tingling in the extremities.
- Watch for arrhythmias by listening to the apical rate and evaluating the pulse following the procedure.
- Check the peripheral pulses in the affected extremity (dorsalis pedis, posterior tibial pulse in the lower extremity; radial pulse in the upper extremity).
- Evaluate extremity temperature and color and complaints of pain, numbness, or tingling sensations to determine signs of arterial insufficiency.
- If protocol requires, see that patient remains in bed with little movement of the involved extremity until the following morning.
- Report any complaint of chest pain immediately.

Circulation Time

Circulation time measures the velocity of blood flow and helps to diagnose right- and left-heart failure. Two methods are used:

Arm-to-tongue: A rapid intravenous injection of dehydrocholic acid (Decholin) is made in a peripheral vein. The interval between the moment the injection starts and the end point (when the patient complains of a bitter taste) is measured with a stopwatch. The normal arm-to-tongue time is approximately 8 to 16 seconds.

Arm-to-lung: Either paraldehyde or ether is injected intravenously. The time from the moment the injection begins to the end point (when the patient smells or tastes the ether or when the odor of the drug is detected on his breath) is measured with a stopwatch. The normal arm-to-lung time is approximately 4 to 8 seconds.

A prolonged arm-to-lung time points to right-sided congestive failure. If the arm-to-lung time is normal and the arm-to-tongue time is prolonged, isolated left-sided failure can be suspected. Usually cardiac failure is a combination of left and right failure, and only the arm-to-tongue time is determined. At present this test is seldom used and appears to have limited value.

Central Venous Pressure

Central venous pressure (CVP) is the pressure within the right atrium or in the great veins within the thorax. It represents the filling pressure of the right ventricle and indicates the ability of the right side of the heart to manage a fluid load. It serves as a guide to fluid replacement in seriously ill patients and is a measurement of effective circulating blood volume. CVP may also be used for total parenteral nutrition (hyperalimentation), long-term chemotherapy, and fluid therapy. It also serves as a guide (in conjunction with other parameters) in the early recognition of congestive (left-sided) heart failure, because commonly right-sided heart failure is the result of left-sided heart failure.

A catheter is threaded through an arm or neck vein into the superior vena cava just above or within the right atrium. Vascular pressure is measured by the height of a column of water.

CVP is a dynamic or changing measurement. The change in CVP correlated with the patient's clinical status is a more useful indication of adequacy of venous blood volume and alterations of cardiovascular function than is a single measurement of CVP. A lowered CVP indicates that the patient is hypovolemic, and this is verified when a rapid intravenous infusion causes the patient to improve. A rising CVP may be due to either hypervolemia or poor cardiac contractility.

Laboratory Studies

BLOOD STUDIES. *Blood electrolyte studies,* particularly of potassium, sodium, and calcium, are frequently carried out on cardiac patients. The evaluation of serum potassium is especially important in patients treated with digitalis and/or diuretics.

The *C-reactive protein* (CRP) is a sensitive indicator of inflammation of infectious or noninfectious origin.

The *antistreptolysin titer* is a blood measurement of antibodies against streptococcus. This test shows whether a patient has had a recent streptococcal infection. (Streptococcal infection is an antecedent of acute rheumatic fever.)

The *sedimentation rate* reveals the speed of sedimentation of red blood cells and is elevated when an inflammatory process is present.

The *blood culture* is performed to detect the presence of bacteria in circulating blood. Its major usefulness in cardiology is in the diagnosis of infective (bacterial) endocarditis.

ENZYME AND ISOENZYME TESTS. *Enzymes* are complex protein substances that have a specific action in promoting chemical changes. The heart muscle is rich in enzymes that promote different biochemical reactions. When myocardial tissue is damaged, certain cardiac enzymes are released into the bloodstream and result in elevated peripheral blood enzyme levels. The enzymes creatine phosphokinase (CPK), serum aspartate aminotransferase (AST)—previously known as serum glutamic oxaloacetic transaminase (SGOT)—and lactic dehydrogenase (LDH) are found in increased serum levels at different times during the course of an acute myocardial infarction. However, these enzymes are also present in a variety of tissues and may also be elevated as a result of damage to skeletal muscles, liver, brain, kidneys, and other organs. Hence, false positive results may occur with these tests.

Isoenzymes promote the same biochemical reactions but exist in slightly different forms that are chemically or physically distinct from each other. Isoenzymes can be identified by electrophoresis to reveal the specific tissue that is damaged. Improved techniques have led to the identification and quantification of the isoenzymes of CPK and LDH. The isoenzyme CPK-MB is present in significant amounts only in the myocardium. It is the most sensitive indicator currently available for the diagnosis of myocardial infarction. It usually becomes elevated 4 to 6 hours after the onset of myocardial infarction, and peak activity is observed within 12 to 24 hours.

LDH has five different isoenzymes designated LDH_1 to LDH_5. Heart muscle is particularly rich in LDH_1 and it is this isoenzyme blood level which is elevated earliest in the presence of heart damage, as with infarction.

In summary, the determination of CPK-MB and LDH isoenzymes is more specific in the evaluation of the presence or absence or myocardial infarction than are the determinations of total enzymes.

Cardiovascular Nuclear Medicine: Radionuclide Angiography

A radionuclide (usually technetium ^{99m} (tagged to serum albumin) is injected into a peripheral or central vein and is recorded sequentially either by a video storage system or directly with a rapid-sequence photocamera as it passes through the cardiac chambers. This is useful in determining the presence, direction, and magnitude of intracardiac shunts. Since cardiovascular nuclear medicine focuses on function, nuclear medicine techniques can yield information on ventricular motion and can study regional myocardial blood flow (myocardial perfusion imaging).

A radionuclide may be injected during exercise testing in a patient with angina pectoris. Obstruction of the coronary arteries can be detected by lack of uptake of the tracer in areas of the heart supplied by these arteries. Radioactive tracers may also be used to delineate the acutely infarcted myocardium. (See Chapter 16.)

NURSING ASSESSMENT OF THE CARDIAC PATIENT

When a patient is hospitalized for a cardiac condition, it often is a life-threatening situation. The nurse's observations are important for the patient's diagnostic and therapeutic regimen. No symptom is unimportant. Although there are some exceptions, the symptoms of heart disease usually correlate with the degree of heart disease present. The symptoms most commonly seen in heart disease are precordial pain, dyspnea, palpitation, weakness or fatigue, light-headedness, syncope, epigastric discomfort, and cough. The following is an outline of salient observations that have first priority in patient assessment. This knowledge helps the nurse to determine the patient's primary problems and gives direction in establishing objectives and in planning and evaluating nursing care.

Skin color and temperature; change in skin color
Pallor, flushing, cyanosis

• Look in mouth, since there is less color variation in mucous membranes; examine nail beds and palms.

Petechiae, jaundice
Sweating, cold, clammy, warm, or dry skin

Heart rate
see also auscultation of the chest, page 64

• Take apical and radial pulse rates.
  a. Rates less than 60 beats/min. (bradycardia) are most commonly due to sinus bradycardia, nodal rhythm, and heart block.
  b. Rates more than 100 beats/min. (tachycardia) most commonly are due to sinus tachycardia or atrial arrhythmias.
• Examine the radial, brachial, carotid, femoral, popliteal, posterior tibial, and dorsalis pedis pulses.
• Feel the pulses bilaterally. Peripheral pulses should be equal. Assess for differences in timing and intensity.
• Note amplitude (fullness) which depends on pulse pressure (difference between systolic and diastolic pressures); this gives an estimate of stroke volume.
  a. Small volume pulse may be from low stroke volume and peripheral vasoconstriction (myocardial infarction, shock, constrictive pericarditis, vasoconstrictive drugs).
  b. Large volume pulse produced by large stroke volume (aortic regurgitation, pregnancy, thyrotoxicosis), bradycardia, patent ductus arteriosus.
• Examine venous pulse; arterial and venous pulsations are visible in the neck.
  a. Examine internal jugular veins since pressure waves in internal jugular veins follow those of right atrium.
  b. See page 70 for bedside technique of measuring venous pressure.

Heart rhythm

• Notify physician and secure a full 12-lead electrocardiogram and a rhythm strip during episodes of palpitation to help establish diagnosis.

Respirations

- Rate and depth
- Character
- Presence of Cheyne-Stokes respirations
- Position assumed by patient
- Factors precipitating or relieving dyspnea

Blood pressure

- Take on both arms; subsequently blood pressure is taken on right arm.
- Take on both legs at initial evaluation.
  a. Place patient on abdomen.
  b. Apply a wide cuff to mid-thigh.
  c. Place stethoscope in popliteal fossa.
- Measure blood pressure with patient supine and standing.
- Document site of blood pressure measurement and position of patient. (See also page 68 for further discussion of technique of blood pressure measurement.)

Presence of pain

(for detailed discussion see Guidelines on Nursing Assessment of the Patient with Chest Pain, page 519, and Figure 26-4, page 520)

Location	Intensity
Radiation	Circumstances precipitating
Quality	and relieving pain
Duration	

Cough

- Cough of early congestive failure is usually nonproductive.
- Nocturnal cough may be related to pulmonary edema.

Hemoptysis

(coughing up of blood)

- Small quantities of dark, clotted blood may indicate severe mitral stenosis but are more common with pulmonary embolism and pulmonary infarction.
- Pink, frothy sputum indicates acute pulmonary edema.
- Mixture of blood and pus indicates pulmonary suppuration.
- Frank hemoptysis is usually due to lung pathology.

Edema

(abnormal accumulation of serous fluid in the connective tissues)

- Results from heart failure most commonly.
- In heart conditions the location of edema is influenced by gravity; fluid collects in lower parts of the body (dependent edema).
  a. Evaluate for edema of ankles and feet in the ambulatory patient.
  b. Evaluate for edema of sacral area and posterior thighs in patient confined to bed.
- Avoid undue pressure on edematous area since edematous patients are prone to develop pressure sores.

Fatigue

- Fatigue associated with heart disease is produced by low cardiac output.

- Undue fatigue related to effort usually indicates advanced heart disease.

Syncope or fainting

- May be caused by anoxemia or reduced cardiac output with resulting inadequate circulation to the brain's vital centers.
- Also seen in arrhythmias, atrioventricular block, carotid sinus sensitivity, and cerebrovascular obstructive disease.

Distention of neck veins

- May be produced by pressure on liver, congestive heart failure, pericardial compression due to effusion or constrictive pericarditis.

Abdominal pain or discomfort

- Epigastric (upper abdominal) pain may be due to myocardial infarction, distention of liver capsule from congestive heart failure.
- Severe abdominal pain may be from dissecting abdominal aorta, rupture of aortic aneurysm, systemic embolism from infective endocarditis.
- Intermittent abdominal pain (related to food intake) may indicate circulatory insufficiency of mesenteric arteries.

Other manifestations of heart disease

- Digital clubbing (clubbing of fingers) is due to cyanotic congenital heart disease, bacterial endocarditis, certain forms of lung pathology.
- Jaundice is seen in congestive heart failure associated with severe liver congestion.

Note frequency and severity of symptoms, precipitating causes, and emotional reaction of the patient.

SUMMARY POINTS IN CARDIAC ASSESSMENT

Skin color and temperature
Heart rate
Heart rhythm
Respirations
Blood pressure
Presence of pain
Cough
Hemoptysis
Edema
Fatigue
Syncope or fainting
Distention of neck veins
Abdominal pain or discomfort
Other manifestations of heart disease

GUIDELINES: NURSING ASSESSMENT OF THE PATIENT WITH CHEST PAIN

Objective: To differentiate the serious conditions which carry the risk of sudden death from those of less serious causes.

Underlying Considerations:

1. There is little correlation between the severity of chest pain and the gravity of its cause.
2. There is poor correlation between the location of the chest pain and its source.
3. The patient may have more than one clinical problem occurring simultaneously.

	LOCATION AND RADIATION	CHARACTER AND DURATION	PRECIPITATING EVENTS	METHOD OF RELIEF
Angina pectoris	Substernal or retrosternal pain spreading across chest. May radiate to *inside* of either arm or to both arms, neck, or jaws.	*Pressure; squeezing, heavy discomfort.* Usually subsides within 1-10 minutes.	Related to exertion, emotion, eating, cold.	Cessation of all effort at once Sublingual nitrates
Myocardial infarction	Substernal or over precordium. May spread widely throughout chest; painful disability of shoulders and hands may be present.	Crushing, vise-like, gripping *More severe and prolonged than angina.*	Occurs spontaneously. Unrelated to emotion, exercise. Associated with dizziness, perspiration, and nausea.	Morphine Analgesics
Pericardial chest pain	Substernal or to left of sternum. May be felt in epigastrium. May be referred to neck, arms, back. *Listen for presence of friction rub (page 595)*	Sharp intermittent pain. Made worse by swallowing, coughing, *rotation of trunk.*	Often severe and sudden in onset. Pain increases with inspiration and motion of trunk.	Possible relief with bending forward
Pain of pulmonary origin	Arises from inferior portion of the pleura. May be referred to costal margins or upper abdomen. Patient may be able to localize the pain.	Stabbing, knife-like. Accentuated by respiratory movements.	Frequently associated with cough. Patient has anxious expression.	Codeine Intercostal nerve block
Esophageal pain (hiatus hernia, reflux esophagitis)	Substernal. May be projected around chest to shoulder.	Burning; *a sense of fullness or a knot.* May simulate the pain of angina.	Brought on by food intake or lying down, especially after a large meal. May occur without provocation.	Relief with antacids or sitting up
Chest wall pain	Costochondral or sternocostal junctions.	Aching or soreness; of variable duration. Muscles tender on palpation. Generally long-lasting.	Provoked by movement of chest wall.	Relief with heat, muscle relaxants, and correct posture and work habits
Anxiety	Over left chest; variable. Does not radiate. Assess for hyperventilation, sighing respirations, palpitation. Patient may complain of numbness and tingling of hands and mouth.	Sharp, stabbing, or vague chest discomfort. Less than 1 minute to several hours or days.	Related to fatigue or emotion (sometimes neither).	Lying down Sedation

Other considerations

A. Arthritis and bursitis — Local pain with tenderness. Accentuated by movement.

B. Biliary disease — Referred to scapulae and shoulders; associated with indigestion and a sense of fullness.

C. Cervical disc — May cause pain in chest, midscapular and postscapular areas.

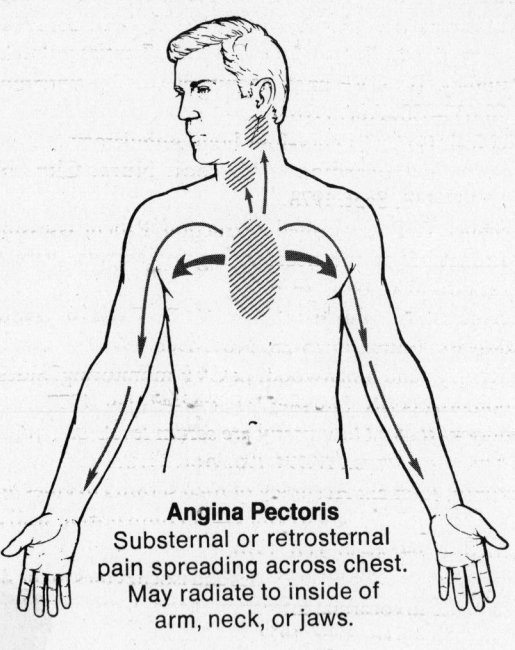

Angina Pectoris
Substernal or retrosternal
pain spreading across chest.
May radiate to inside of
arm, neck, or jaws.

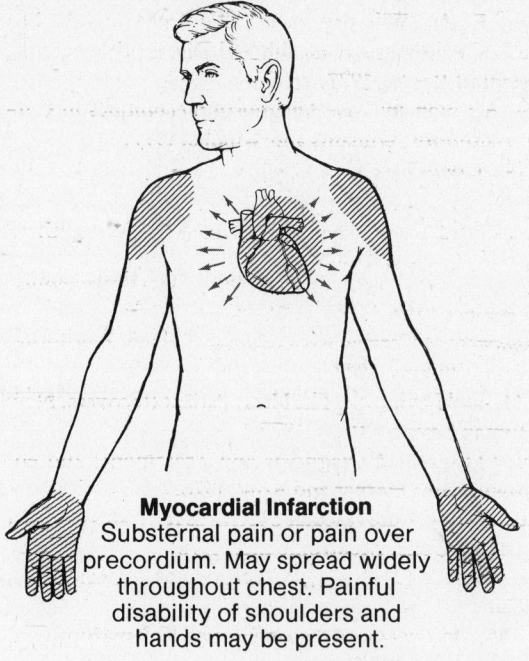

Myocardial Infarction
Substernal pain or pain over
precordium. May spread widely
throughout chest. Painful
disability of shoulders and
hands may be present.

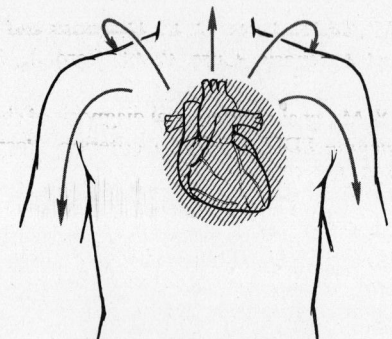

Pericardial Chest Pain
Substernal pain or pain to the left of sternum. May
be felt in epigastrium and may be referred
to neck, arms, and back.

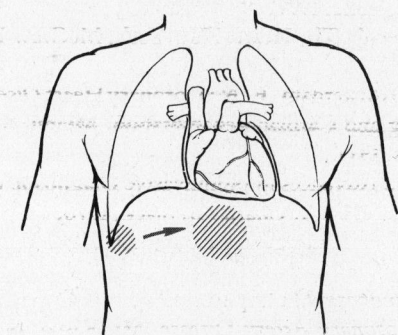

Pain of Pulmonary Origin
Pain arises from inferior portion of pleura.
May be referred to costal margins or upper abdomen.
Patient may be able to localize the pain.

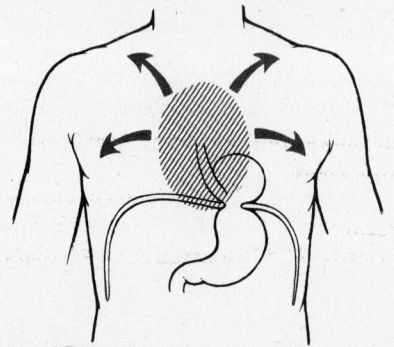

Esophageal Pain (*Hiatus Hernia, Reflux Esophagitis*)
Substernal pain. May be projected around chest
to shoulders.

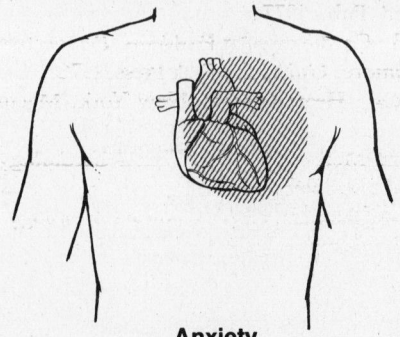

Anxiety
Pain over left chest. May be variable. Does not
radiate. Assess for hyperventilation, sighing
respiration, palpitations. Patient may complain
of numbness and tingling of hands and mouth.

Figure 26-4. Assessment of chest pain.

BIBLIOGRAPHY

BOOKS

Amsterdam, E. A., Wilmore, J. H., and DeMaria, A. N.: Exercise in Cardiovascular Health and Disease. New York, Yorke Medical Books, 1977.

Benchimol, A.: Non-Invasive Diagnostic Techniques in Cardiology. Baltimore, Williams and Wilkins, 1977.

Brest, A. N.: Congestive Heart Failure. New York, Medcom Press, 1975.

Caird, F. I., Dall, J. L. C., and Kennedy, R. D.: Cardiology in Old Age. New York, Plenum Press, 1976.

Chung, E. K.: Non-Invasive Cardiac Diagnosis. Philadelphia, Lea and Febiger, 1976.

———: Principles of Cardiac Arrhythmias, 2nd ed. Baltimore, Williams and Wilkins, 1977.

Croog, S. H., and Levine, S.: The Heart Patient Recovers. New York, Human Sciences Press, 1977.

Fowler, N. O.: Cardiac Diagnosis and Treatment, 2nd ed. Hagerstown, Md., Harper and Row, 1976.

Gill, C., et al.: The Cardiovascular System as It Relates to Heart Pacing. Minneapolis, Medtronic Inc., 1975.

Gazes, P. C.: Clinical Cardiology. Chicago, Year Book Medical Pub., 1975.

Gotto, A. M., Jr., et al.: Atherosclerosis. Kalamazoo, The Upjohn Company, 1977.

Hammer, J., ed.: Recent Advances in Cardiology. New York, Churchill Livingstone, 1977.

Hurst, J. W., ed., et al.: The Heart. New York, McGraw-Hill, 1978.

James, W. E., and Amsterdam, E. A.: Coronary Heart Disease, Exercise Testing and Cardiac Rehabilitation. Miami, Symposia Specialists, 1977.

Kingsley, B., et al.: Advances in Noninvasive Diagnostic Cardiology. Thorofare, N. J., Charles B. Slack, 1976.

Mason, D. T.: Cardiac Emergencies. Baltimore, Williams and Wilkins, 1978.

Morse, D., and Goldberg, H.: Important Topics in Congenital, Valvular and Coronary Artery Disease. Mt. Kisco, N. Y., Futura Pub. Co., 1975.

O'Connor, A. B., ed.: Advances in Cardiovascular Nursing. New York, American Journal of Nursing Co., 1975.

Ravin, A., et al.: Auscultation of the Heart, 3rd ed. Chicago, Year Book Med. Pub., 1977.

Russek, H. I., ed.: Cardiovascular Problems: Perspectives and Progress. Baltimore, University Park Press, 1976.

Silber, E. N., et al.: Heart Disease. New York, Macmillan, 1975.

Sokolow, M., and McIlroy, M. B.: Clinical Cardiology. Los Altos, Lange Medical Pub., 1977.

Willerson, J. T., and Sanders, C. A.: Clinical Cardiology. New York, Grune and Stratton, 1977.

ARTICLES

Ariet, M., and Crevasse, L. E.: Status report on computerized ECG analysis. JAMA, 239:1201-1202, Mar. 20, 1978.

Hamer, J., ed.: Recent Adv. Cardiol., 7:entire volume, 1977.

Haughey, B.: CVP lines: Monitoring and maintaining. AJN, 78:635-638, Apr. 1978.

McNeal, G. J.: Twenty-four hour ambulatory monitoring. A new electrocardiographic tool. Nurs. Clin. N. Am., 13:437-448, Sept. 1978.

Mechner, F.: Programmed Instruction. Patient assessment: Examination of the heart and great vessels. Part 1. AJN, 76:1807-1830, Nov. 1976.

Merrill, S. A., and Froelicher, V. F.: Exercise testing. Cardiovasc. Nurs., 13:23-28, Nov.-Dec. 1977.

Murray, J., and Smallwood, J.: CVP monitoring: Sidestepping potential perils. Nursing '77, 7:42-47, Jan. 1977.

Pennock, R. S.: How useful are serum levels of cardiac drugs? Am. Fam. Phys., 17:194-196, Apr. 1978.

Raffetto, J., et al.: Accuracy of total serum enzymes and myocardial specific isoenzymes—A comparative study. Nebr. Med. J., 64:36-38, Feb. 1978.

Rappaport, E.: Serum enzymes and isoenzymes in the diagnosis of acute myocardial infarction. Mod. Concepts Cardiovasc. Dis., 46:43-46, Sept. 1977.

Roe, C. R.: Diagnosis of myocardial infarction by serum isoenzyme analysis. Ann. Clin. Lab. Sci., 7:201-209, May-June 1977.

Shah, P. M., and Roberts, D. L.: Diagnosis and treatment of aortic valve stenosis. Curr. Probl. Cardiol., 2:3-49, Sept. 1977.

Van Diji, Y. M., et al.: Differential diagnosis of chest pain. Use of isoenzyme LDH$_1$ level as a criterion. Postgrad. Med., 65:189-192, Jan. 1979.

AGENCIES

Governmental

National Heart, Lung and Blood Institute, National Institutes of Health, Bethesda, Md. 20205

Voluntary

American College of Cardiology, 9650 Rockville Pike, Bethesda, Md. 20012

American Heart Association, 7320 Greenville Ave., Dallas, Tex. 75231

Mended Hearts, 721 Huntington Ave., Roxbury, Mass. 02115

27

ELECTRO-CARDIOGRAMS AND HEART ARRHYTHMIAS

ESSENTIALS OF BASIC ELECTROCARDIOGRAPHY

Thousands of lives are being saved today because of the ability of the modern nurse to interpret electrocardiograms and initiate emergency treatment. Since the nurse is frequently the only person at the patient's bedside when a life-threatening ECG abnormality occurs, she is now expected to have some basic knowledge of electrocardiography.

An electrocardiogram is nothing more than a recording of the heart's electrical impulse (Fig. 27-1). The heart is stimulated to contract and thus pump blood to the body organs because of an electrical pulsation which begins at the top of the heart and travels downward. In order to record this impulse, an electrode need not be placed directly on the heart but can be placed on the extremities where the heart's activity can be sensed.

Conduction System of the Heart

The normal electrical impulse of the heart, which inscribes the ECG and causes the heart to contract, begins in the SA node (other terms used are *sinoatrial node, sinus node,* or *normal physiological pacemaker*) which occupies the superior aspect of the right atrium. After beginning in the SA node the impulse travels across the atria so that they contact and pump blood into the ventricles. The impulse then hits the AV node (atrioventricular node) which lies between the atria and ventricles. The impulse is somewhat delayed in the AV node and then travels down the ventricles causing them to contract and thus pump blood to the body organs.

Both the SA and AV nodes are connected to two main nerve systems which control the rate at which the heart beats (Fig. 27-2). The sympathetic nerves cause the heart rate to increase, whereas the parasympathetic system slows the heart rate. (The vagus nerve constitutes the parasympathetic system in the heart.)

Clinical Uses of the ECG

An electrocardiogram can be helpful in the diagnosis of the following conditions:

1. Myocardial infarction and arteriosclerotic heart disease
2. Cardiac arrhythmias
3. Cardiac enlargement
4. Electrolyte abnormalities (especially potassium and calcium)
5. Pericarditis (inflammation of the pericardial sac which surrounds the heart)
6. Pericardial effusion (fluid in the pericardial sac which can restrict the heart's pumping ability)

This chapter will emphasize myocardial infarction and the subsequent arrhythmias since they are life-threatening and fall into an area where the nurse may be forced to act immediately and without consultation.

522

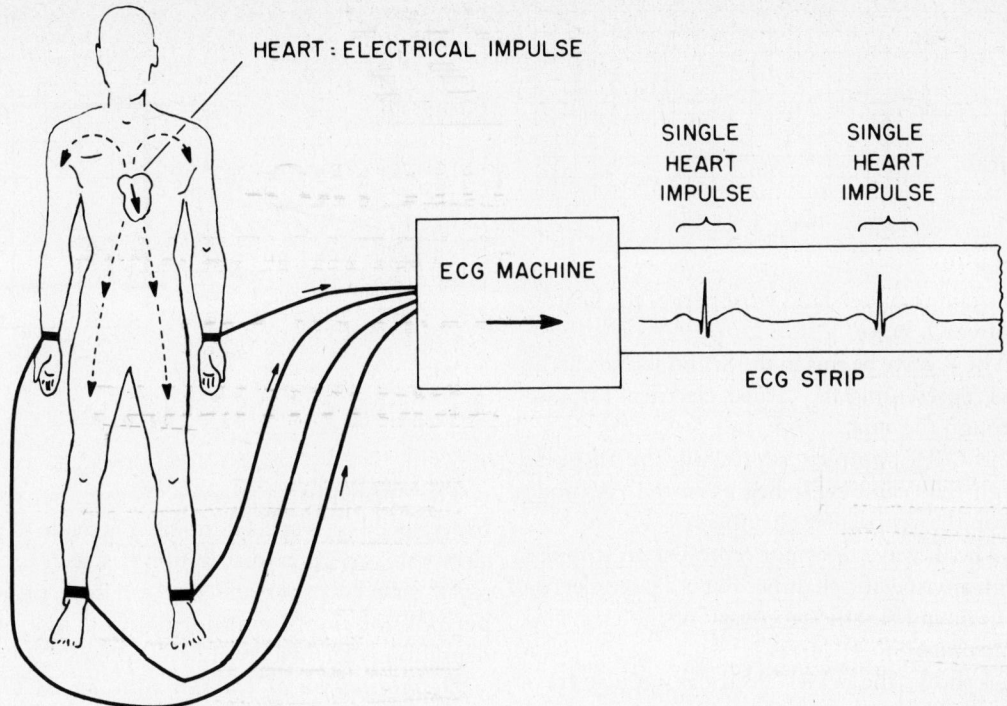

Figure 27-1. Transmission of heart's impulse to ECG paper. The ECG wires on the extremities sense the electrical impulse as it travels from the top of the heart to the bottom. The impulse is sent through the ECG machine where a picture of the heart's activity is recorded.

A Normal ECG

Figure 27-3 represents a normal ECG. It can be seen that each heartbeat is manifested as three major deflections which have been labeled as the P wave, the QRS complex, and the T wave. The QRS complex is in turn composed of three parts: the Q wave is the first downward deflection, the R wave is the first upward deflection, and the S wave is the first downward deflection after the R wave.

ECG Waves Related to Heart Anatomy. It is ex-

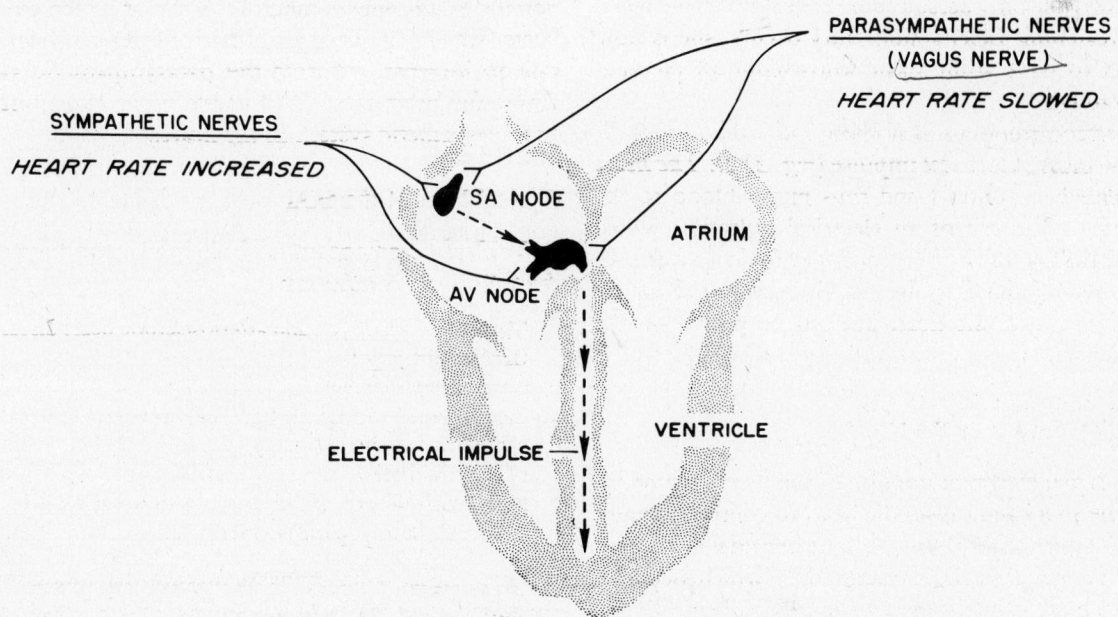

Figure 27-2. Conduction system of the heart. Pictured is the pathway of the normal electrical impulse which inscribes the ECG and causes the heart to contract and pump blood. Also shown are the nerves which regulate the heart rate.

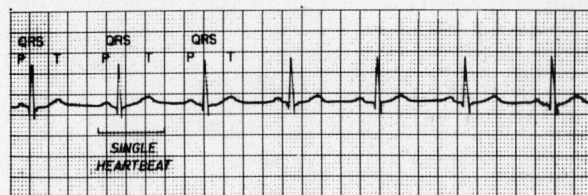

Figure 27-3.   A normal ECG.

tremely important to understand what part of the heart is represented by each wave.

P wave — The P wave begins in the SA node and can be thought of as representing the cardiac electrical impulse traveling through the *atria.*

QRS — The QRS complex represents the impulse going through the *ventricles.* It begins in the AV node which lies atop the ventricular chambers.

T wave — The T wave does not represent an impulse going through any specific chamber but is a pure electrical phenomenon and signifies recovery of the electrical forces (*repolarization*).

Figure 27-4 shows the heart's electrical impulse traversing the areas of the heart to give the various deflections of a normal single heartbeat.

ECG Paper.   Before discussing the various abnormalities that may occur with each wave, it is necessary to define the various squares on the ECG paper (Fig. 27-5). The *vertical* lines measure the *magnitude* of the heart's electrical impulse and the *horizontal* lines represent the *time* it takes for an impulse to travel over cardiac tissue.

In the vertical axis each small block is 1 mm., and 1 darker large block is 5 mm. In the horizontal direction 1 small block is 0.04 second, whereas a darker large block is 0.20 second.

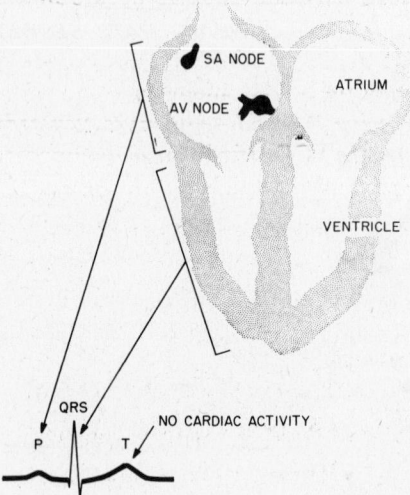

Figure 27-4.   ECG waves related to heart anatomy. The electrical impulse is shown traveling through the chambers of the heart and thus inscribing the normal ECG of 1 heart beat. The P wave represents atrial activity and the QRS complex is derived from ventricular stimulation.

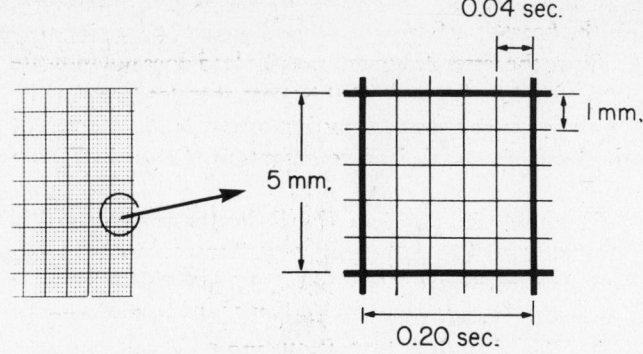

Figure 27-5.   Meaning of blocks on ECG paper. All one really needs to remember is that 1 small block is 1 mm. tall and .04 second wide.

The normal paper speed is 25 mm. per second. If the paper speed on a special monitor is made to go at a very slow rate, more cardiac activity is seen on a relatively small strip of paper and one can scan prolonged time periods for impulse abnormality. This form of condensation is termed "trend recording."

Determination of Cardiac Rate on ECG Paper.   A quick rough determination of the cardiac rate can be obtained by dividing the number of heavily lined large blocks (Fig. 27-6) between each pair of QRS complexes into 300. Thus, if there are 2 *large* blocks between each pair of QRS complexes, the rate would be 150 beats per minute (300 divided by 2 = 150). If there are 3 large blocks between each pair of QRS complexes, the rate would be 100 beats per minute (300 divided by 3 = 100). If there are 2½ blocks between each pair of QRS complexes, the rate would be 120 beats per minute. The figure 300 is used because 300 large blocks represent one minute on the ECG paper. Therefore, by dividing the number of large blocks between each pair of QRS complexes into 300, one arrives at the number of complexes that occur in one minute.

ECG Leads

Standard ECG machines have a dial which turns to one of 12 *leads* (I, II, III, AVR, AVL, AVF, V1, V2, V3, V4, V5, V6). Each lead "sees" and records the heart's electri-

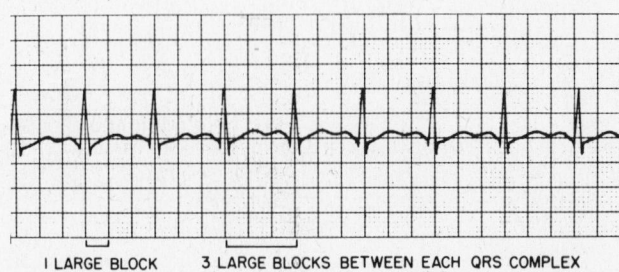

I LARGE BLOCK   3 LARGE BLOCKS BETWEEN EACH QRS COMPLEX

Figure 27-6.   Determination of rate. There are 3 large blocks between each pair of QRS complexes. By dividing 300 by 3, the rate is 100 beats per minute.

cal impulse from a different anatomical position relative to the heart's surface.

Since the letter designation of the lead does not indicate very clearly what part of the heart each lead represents one must memorize the position of each lead. The part of the heart that each lead represents is shown in Figure 27-7.

Knowing the position of each lead is very helpful in localizing cardiac pathology. For example, leads II, III, and AVF in Figure 27-7 record the inferior portion of the heart. Therefore, if a myocardial infarct shows up on the ECG strip only in leads II, III, and AVF, we know that the patient' infarction is limited to the inferior wall of the heart.

Localization of pathology is also helpful in the diagnosis of many types of congenital heart disease. If a patient has pulmonic stenosis (the blood in the right side of the heart is impeded by the small pulmonic valve located between the right ventricle and the pulmonic artery), the right-sided leads, V1 and AVR, will show larger complexes because the cardiac tissue in the right heart enlarges in order to force blood past the small valve opening.

Lead II is one of the most useful leads in detecting arrhythmias, since the P wave, the key to the diagnosis of arrhythmias, is relatively clearly shown.

Significance of Each ECG Wave and Interval

P Wave (Fig. 27-8A). Since the P wave represents the atrial contraction, enlargement of the P wave deflection indicates enlargement of the atrium, such as might occur in mitral stenosis. (The atrium enlarges in mitral stenosis because the mitral opening between the atrium and ventricle is small, causing the blood to back up, which in turn forces the atrial wall to expand.) The P wave is usually considered enlarged if it is over 3 mm. (3 small blocks) tall and/or 0.12 second (3 small blocks) wide.

PR Interval (Fig. 27-8B). The PR interval starts at the beginning of the P wave and extends to the onset of the Q wave. The PR interval is principally important in that it increases in length in arteriosclerotic heart disease

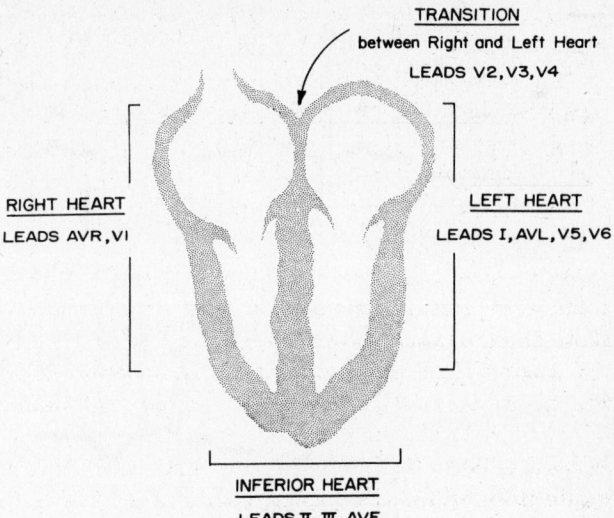

Figure 27-7. ECG leads related to heart anatomy.

and in other diseases of the heart such as rheumatic fever. This interval is prolonged because the heart tissue covered by the PR interval (namely atrium and AV node area) is scarred or inflamed, and the impulse is forced to travel at a slower rate.

At normal rates the PR interval should not be over 0.20 second (5 small blocks).

The QRS Complex (Fig. 27-8C). As was previously mentioned, the QRS consists of three deflections. The Q wave is the first downward stroke. When it becomes large in some leads it is indicative of an old myocardial infarction. The R wave is the first upward deflection of the QRS; it increases in amplitude when the ventricle enlarges, such as occurs in most types of heart diseases. (Overwork of a specific part of the heart causes enlargement.) An R wave may become small when the heart is compressed by fluid, such as occurs in a pericardial effusion.

ST Segment (Fig. 27-8D). The ST segment begins at the end of the S wave and terminates at the beginning of the T wave. The ST segment is elevated above the baseline on the ECG strip in an acute myocardial infarction or pericarditis and becomes depressed when the

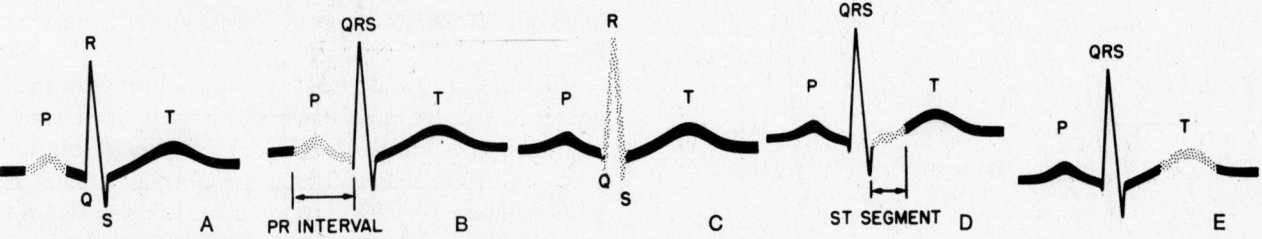

Figure 27-8. Parts of a heartbeat. (*A*) The *P wave*; (*B*) the *PR interval* (extends from the beginning of the P wave to the onset of the Q wave); (*C*) the *QRS complex* (even when the complex does not have a discrete Q or S wave, it is still referred to as the QRS complex to denote a ventricular impulse and to provide simplicity and uniformity); (*D*) the *ST segment* (begins at the termination of the S wave and ends at the beginning of the T wave); (*E*) the *T wave*.

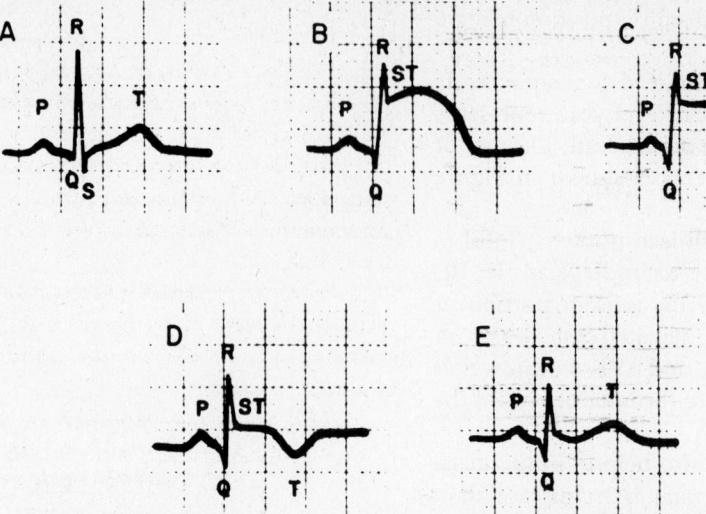

Figure 27-9. ECG interpretation of myocardial infarction. *A.* Normal tracing. *B.* Hours after infarction, the S-T segment becomes elevated. *C.* Hours to days later, the T wave inverts and the Q wave may become larger. *D.* Days to weeks later, the S-T segment returns to near-normal. *E.* Lastly, the T wave becomes upright again, but the Q wave may remain permanently large.

heart muscle is getting a decreased supply of oxygen or when a patient is taking digitalis. The ST segment becomes long in hypocalcemia. (Hypocalcemia occurs most commonly in chronic renal disease because the scarred kidneys cannot excrete phosphate. Since phosphate and calcium maintain a reciprocal balance in the body fluids, the elevated phosphate causes a depression in the calcium level.) The ST segment becomes shorter in hypercalcemia which is most commonly seen in metastatic carcinoma because the tumor erodes the bones and spills calcium into the serum.

T Wave (Fig. 27-8E). The T wave represents no cardiac activity but reflects the *electrical* recovery of the ventricular contraction. (An electrical impulse is the flow of electrons and the T wave is inscribed on the ECG when these electrons migrate back to their resting position after traversing the heart muscle to make it contract.) The T wave is flat when the heart is not receiving enough oxygen (arteriosclerotic heart disease) and may be inverted in a myocardial infarction.

The T wave should not be over 10 mm. high (10 small blocks) in the precordial leads (those that are placed on the chest) and should not be over 5 mm. in the remaining leads. The T wave may be made tall by an elevated serum potassium.

ECG INTERPRETATION OF MYOCARDIAL INFARCTION

One of the most important points to remember about interpreting an ECG in a myocardial infarction is that the ECGs of some of these patients show *no changes* on the initial tracing. Therefore, if a person has symptoms compatible with a heart attack and has a normal ECG, he nevertheless should be admitted to the hospital for observation and further electrocardiograms.

Usually the first finding in an infarct is elevation of the ST segment. This is followed by T wave inversion, which in turn is followed by a large Q wave. As the infarct heals, the Q wave may remain as the only stigma of an old coronary occlusion. This sequence is shown in Figure 27-9.

Since a large Q wave is many times indicative of an old infarction (except in AVR where a large Q wave is normal), the question is often asked: How large can a Q wave be before it is considered abnormal? (A normal ECG will have small Q waves in many of the leads.) A Q wave can be considered abnormal if it is over 0.04 second wide (1 small block is 0.04 second) or if it is greater in depth than one third the height of the QRS complex (Fig. 27-10).

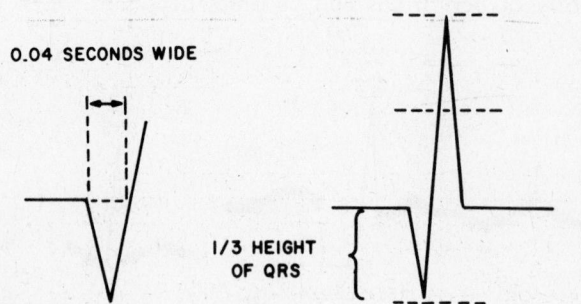

Figure 27-10. Abnormal Q wave. A Q wave is considered abnormal when it is over .04 second (1 small block on the ECG paper) or over one-third the height of the QRS complex. This usually indicates an old myocardial infarction.

Normal Pathway   Sinus Tachycardia Pathway

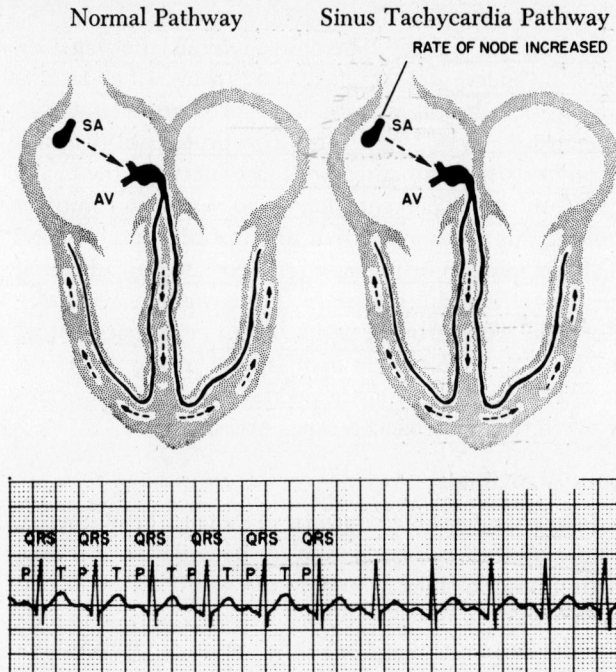

Figure 27-11.   Sinus tachycardia: (*top*) pathway; (*bottom*) ECG.

ECG INTERPRETATION OF CARDIAC ARRHYTHMIAS

Familiarity with the various arrhythmias and their treatment is an essential component of acute nursing care. A patient may die in seconds if certain arrhythmias are not immediately terminated. Also, many patients will present with episodic syncope or seizures, which can be secondary to arrhythmias (which cause decreased circulation to the brain). If the patient appears well but presents with a history of syncope or seizures, he may be placed on a portable ECG machine such as a Holter monitor. This machine allows one to record the patient's ECG over a 10 to 24 hour period to determine if the patient is manifesting any arrhythmia activity which may have caused his previous symptoms.

The arrhythmias can best be understood and remembered by knowing the focus in the heart from which the rhythm originates.

- A good general rule is that the lower the ectopic focus resides in the heart, the more lethal the arrhythmia becomes.

The following arrhythmias will be discussed: (1) sinus tachycardia, (2) sinus bradycardia, (3) sinus arrhythmia, (4) premature atrial contractions (PACs), (5) paroxysmal atrial tachycardia (PAT), (6) atrial flutter, (7) atrial fibrillation, (8) AV blocks (first, second, and third degree), (9) premature ventricular contractions (PVCs), (10) ventricular tachycardia, and (11) ventricular fibrillation.

Sinus Tachycardia

Sinus tachycardia can be defined as a cardiac rate of over 100 beats per minute. All the complexes are normal, but their rate is excessive. The impulse begins normally in the SA node but comes at a faster rate secondary to increased sympathetic nerve stimuli. Some of the most common causes of sinus tachycardia are exercise, anxiety, fever, and shock.

Mechanism of Sinus Tachycardia.   The pathway of sinus tachycardia is the same as that of a normal sinus rhythm (Fig. 27-11), but the number of impulses per minute is greater.

ECG of Sinus Tachycardia.   In sinus tachycardia the P wave, the QRS complex, and the T wave are all normal. The only abnormality is a rate of over 100 (Fig. 27-11).

Treatment of Sinus Tachycardia.   Since sinus tachycardia is usually a compensatory rhythm, treatment is directed at the primary causes, which usually are not cardiac.

Sinus Bradycardia

Sinus bradycardia is defined as a heart rate below 60 when all the complexes are normal. Sinus bradycardia is seen *normally* in well trained athletes or secondary to certain drugs such as digitalis or morphine. This arrhythmia is also seen in myocardial infarction, in which instance it could be detrimental to the patient who already is in a compromised cardiac state. Because of the slow rate and low cardiac output, sinus bradycardia may

Normal Pathway   Sinus Bradycardia Pathway

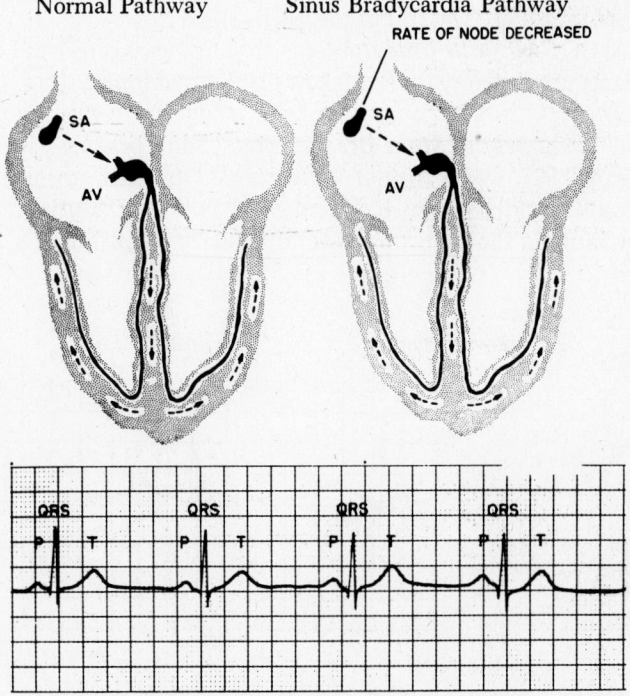

Figure 27-12.   Sinus bradycardia: (*top*) pathway; (*bottom*) ECG.

Normal Pathway   Sinus Arrhythmia Pathway

RATE OF NODE IRREGULAR

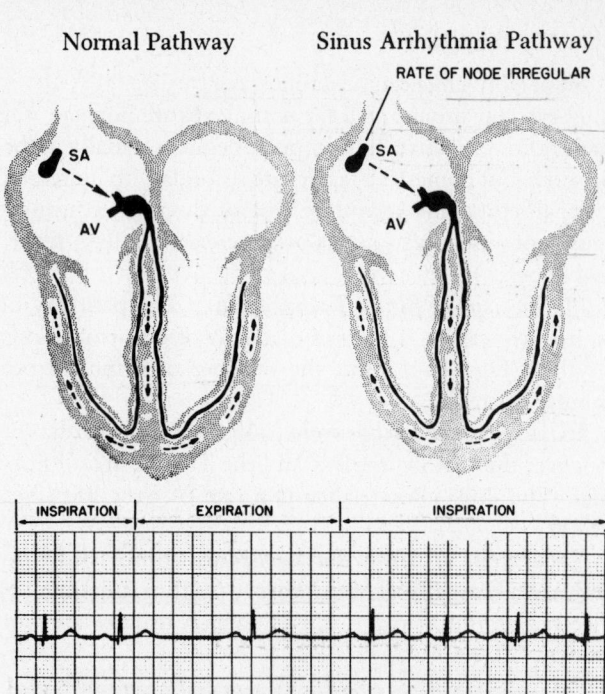

INSPIRATION   EXPIRATION   INSPIRATION

Figure 27-13.   Sinus arrhythmia: *(top)* pathway; *(bottom)* ECG.

cause fainting (Stokes–Adams syndrome) or congestive heart failure. (The term congestive failure is used when the heart cannot pump all the fluid presented to it, resulting in stasis or "congestion" of the blood in the lungs and other body tissues.)

Mechanism of Sinus Bradycardia.   The pathway of sinus bradycardia is identical to that of normal sinus rhythm (Fig. 27-12), but the rate is slower.

ECG of Sinus Bradycardia.   In sinus bradycardia the only abnormality is a rate below 60 beats per minute (Fig. 27-12).

Treatment of Sinus Bradycardia.   Sinus bradycardia rarely has to be treated. However, if this arrhythmia causes symptoms such as congestive failure or fainting, treatment should be initiated immediately. The quickest

way of increasing the heart rate is to give 0.5–1.0 mg. of atropine by IV push. (Atropine inhibits the vagal or "slowing" nerve and therefore makes the heart go faster.) If the patient becomes resistant to atropine, the rate can be increased by adding 1 mg. of isoproterenol (Isuprel) (stimulates the sympathetic or "fast" nerve of the heart) to 250 ml. of 5 percent glucose in water and initially running this solution at about 10 drops per minute. Then the heart rate can be increased or decreased by adjusting the rate of fluid administration. The advantage of starting treatment with atropine is that it can be prepared more quickly and is less toxic than Isuprel to the heart. An electrical pacemaker may be necessary in refractory cases or when the fluid load becomes excessive.

Sinus Arrhythmia

Sinus arrhythmia is characterized by a heart rhythm that is normal in every way except for irregularity. It is normally found in children and young adults.

On inspiration the heart rate increases, and on expiration the heart rate decreases. Inspiration tends to inhibit the vagus nerve (the vagus nerve slows the heart) and causes an acceleration of the cardiac rate.

Mechanism of Sinus Arrhythmia.   The pathway of sinus arrhythmia is the same as that of normal sinus rhythm (Fig. 27-13); the only differential point is the regularity of the impulses.

ECG of Sinus Arrhythmia.   In sinus arrhythmia all the complexes are normal but the rate is irregular — varying with respiration. The rate increases with inspiration and decreases on expiration (Fig. 27-13). Since sinus arrhythmia is usually normal, no treatment is necessary.

Sick Sinus Syndrome

The sick sinus syndrome refers to an SA node which is diseased and which conducts at a slow rate or fails to conduct completely for various periods of time (Fig. 27-14). When this occurs, the patient may become dizzy or even faint because of poor cerebral perfusion. The most common cause of the sick sinus syndrome is ar-

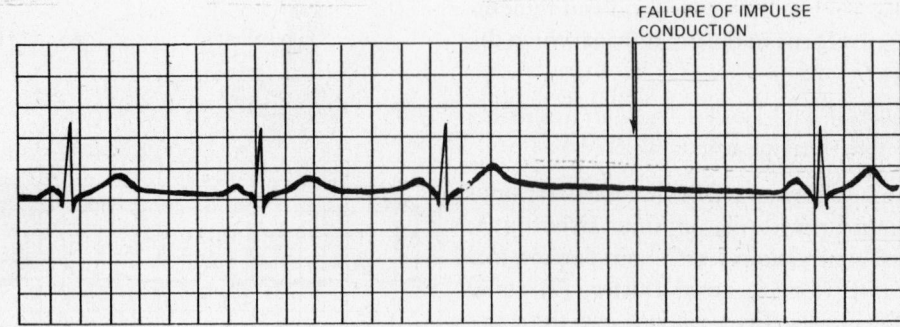

FAILURE OF IMPULSE CONDUCTION

Figure 27-14.   An example of the sick sinus syndrome, in which the sinus node fails to propagate an impulse, so that the P wave and QRS segment are absent.

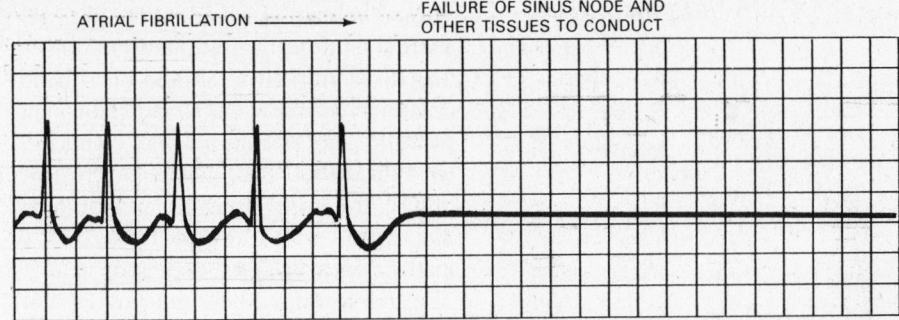

Figure 27-15. In the ECG shown above atrial fibrillation has stopped abruptly and the diseased sinus node has failed—leaving the patient without a heartbeat. This ECG illustrates the importance of having a pacemaker in these patients. Drugs used to treat the atrial fibrillation further suppress the SA node, and there must be a backup system (pacemaker) to establish impulse formation.

teriosclerosis, which leads to ischemia or scarring of the node.

The sick sinus syndrome may be associated with a tachycardia which may stop abruptly (either by cardioversion or spontaneously), and, since the sinus node is diseased, the heart may not begin to beat on its own (Fig. 27-15). It is thought that the tachycardia precipitates the sinus arrest by constantly firing impulses into the sinus node (atrial fibrillation with ectopic impulses originating in the atrium fires impulses *both* down into the ventricles and back into the SA node), which becomes depressed because of the constant activation.

The sick sinus syndrome with tachycardia is very difficult to treat, because many drugs used to treat the tachycardia (propranolol or digitalis) will tend to further suppress the already compromised SA node, which leads to more asystole. The treatment for a diseased sinus node associated with tachycardia is the implantation of a pacemaker. With the pacemaker in place, one can treat the tachycardia with depressant drugs and, when the tachycardia abates, the pacemaker can activate the heart if the SA node fails.

Premature Atrial Contractions (PACs)

Premature atrial contractions are beats that occur early in the cycle. They constitute a very common rhythm disturbance and are seen in both normal and abnormal hearts. PACs rarely cause symptoms and are felt to be of little consequence except when they occur frequently, at which time they may tend to deteriorate into other more serious arrhythmias.

Mechanism of PAC. PACs begin in the atrium, but *outside* the sinus node where normal impulses originate. Thus the source of the beat is ectopic (Fig. 27-16).

ECG of PAC. Since the atrial pathway is abnormal, the P wave is distorted, but since ventricular activation is undisturbed, the QRS complex is normal in configuration (Fig. 27-16).

Treatment of PAC. Most of the time, PACs do not need to be treated; however, when the patient requires therapy many clinicians give quinidine, which is a good suppressant of atrial ectopic beats.

Paroxysmal Atrial Tachycardia (PAT)

PAT is a common arrhythmia seen in young adults and many times, as with PACs, is found in normal hearts. The patient with PAT will usually complain of a pounding or fluttering in the chest associated with shortness of breath and faintness. These symptoms are caused by the rapid heart rate, which range from 140 to 250 per minute with an average of about 180.

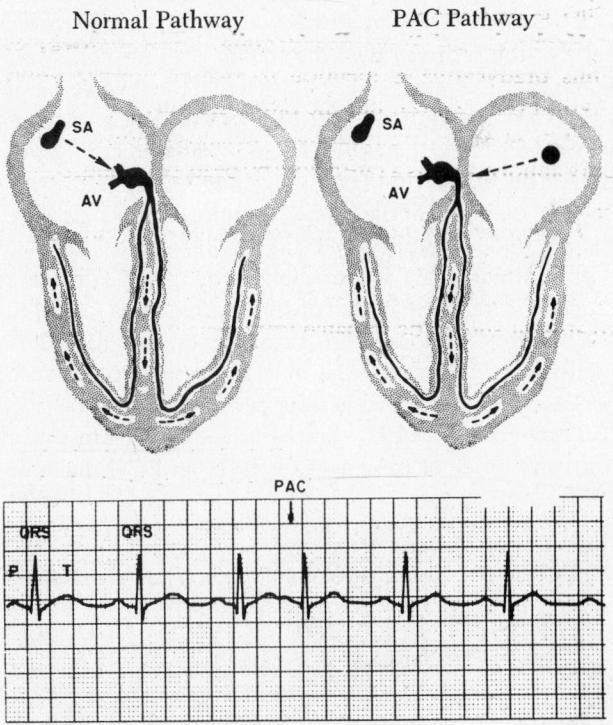

Normal Pathway   PAC Pathway

Figure 27-16. Premature atrial contraction (PAC): (*top*) pathway; (*bottom*) ECG.

Normal Pathway   PAT Pathway

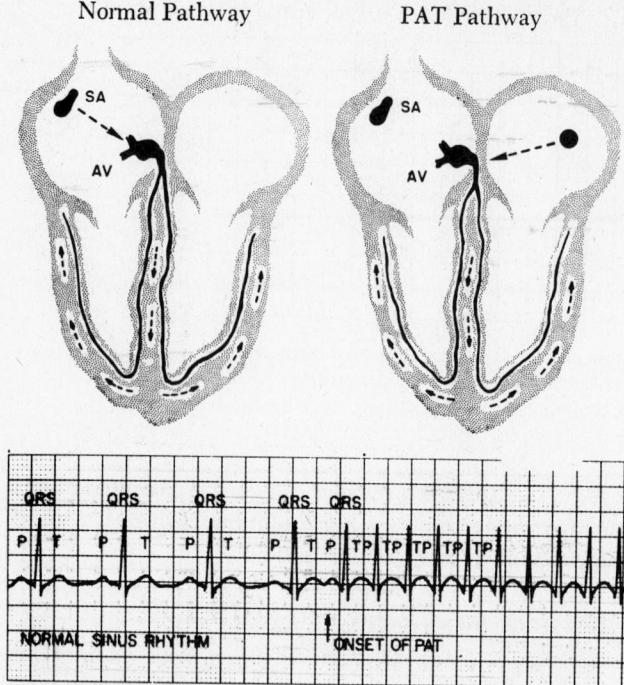

Figure 27-17.   Paroxysmal atrial tachycardia (PAT): (*top*) pathway; (*bottom*) ECG.

Mechanism of PAT.   PAT begins in an ectopic focus of the atrium outside the sinus node (Fig. 27-17). Its pathway over the heart is similar to that of a PAC and may be thought of as a rapid succession of PACs.

ECG of PAT.   The P wave (atrial wave) is distorted because the pathway over the atrium is abnormal. Most of the time the rate is so fast in PAT that the P wave is not seen, since it is buried in the previous complex. If the P waves were seen they would be abnormal in configuration. The QRS complex (ventricular wave) is normal because the route of the cardiac impulse after penetrating the AV node is undisturbed (Fig. 27-17).

In summary, PAT is characterized on the ECG by (1) a rate that is higher than that of sinus tachycardia (over 140 per minute), (2) normal QRS complexes, and (3) abnormally shaped P waves that in many cases are not seen because they are buried in the preceding T waves.

Treatment of PAT.   Since cardiac arrest can occur with any mode of treatment for PAT, an ECG machine

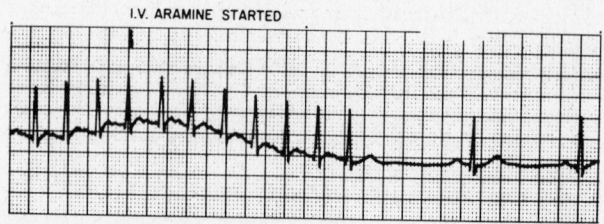

Figure 27-18.   Termination of PAT. The ECG illustrates PAT being terminated with a slow I.V. infusion of Aramine.

should remain attached to the patient, an IV should be started, and appropriate resuscitation equipment, including the defibrillator, should be at hand. If the patient is relatively asymptomatic and stable, simple sedation and waiting 5 to 10 minutes may result in spontaneous conversion of PAT. One may begin treatment by stimulating the right carotid sinus (an area of dense nerve supply in the carotid artery) for several seconds or by gagging the patient with a tongue depressor in an effort to terminate the arrhythmia. These maneuvers work by stimulating the vagus nerve, which puts a "brake" on the heart.

If the above two procedures are not effective, and if the blood pressure is low (most patients with PAT have systolic pressures of 90 to 100 mm. Hg.), one can start a slow drip of IV phenylephrine (Neo-Synephrine) or metaraminol (Aramine). Gradually increase the rate of the infusion until the PAT terminates (Fig. 27-18), at which time the IV should be stopped. This is usually a matter of seconds. Do not raise the systolic blood pressure above 180. These drugs work by increasing the blood pressure, which in turn stimulates the vagus nerve to inhibit the ectopic focus in the atrium. If the patient is already hypertensive (rare), hypertensive agents should not be used.

Some authorities have gotten away from using vasopressor agents such as Aramine in PAT because of the occasional report of a cerebral vascular accident, but these have usually occurred as a result of using the hypertensive drugs in bolus form. Instead of Aramine, these physicians prefer a fast-acting digitalis preparation which works in part by its stimulating effect on the vagal nerve.

In the unusual case in which the above are ineffective or contraindicated, 1 to 3 mg. of propranolol (Inderal), a sympathetic nerve blocker, can be given IV at a rate no greater than 1 mg. per minute. In the extreme case in which the patient is in congestive heart failure, DC synchronized electrical shock (cardioversion) should be instituted instead of giving Inderal. The initial shock can be 50 to 100 watt-seconds (joules). The electrical shock stops the heart and allows it to begin again normally at the SA node.

Atrial Flutter

As the name implies, *atrial flutter* is a rapid, regular "fluttering" of the atrium. The P waves take on a "sawtooth" appearance because they are coming from a focus other than the sinus node and also because they are coming at a very rapid rate.

Mechanism of Atrial Flutter.   As in PAC or PAT, the impulse comes from *one* ectopic focus in the atrium (Fig. 27-19), but the *atrial* rate (not pulse or ventricular rate) is between 250 and 350 per minute in contrast to the average atrial rate of about 180 per minute for PAT.

An easy but oversimplified arbitrary rule to help distinguish the atrial arrhythmias from each other is as follows:

1. The *atrial* rate in sinus tachycardia goes up to 140/minute.
2. The *atrial* rate in PAT is between 140-250/minute.
3. The *atrial* rate in atrial flutter is between 250-350/minute.

ECG of Atrial Flutter.

Atrial flutter occurs usually in a pathological heart (usually arteriosclerotic or rheumatic), as contrasted to PAT, which many times is associated with a normal heart. Since the abnormality is above the AV node, the QRS complex (ventricular wave) is normal in configuration (Fig. 27-19).

Since the P waves are coming so rapidly, the AV node cannot accept and conduct each one and, therefore, there is usually some degree of "blockage" at the AV node. For example, if the atrial rate is 300, the ventricular rate (which will be the same as the pulse rate) might be 150 since the AV node is not able to conduct every atrial impulse because of the excessive rapidity. In this instance the "block" is said to be 2:1, since there are 2 atrial impulses per 1 ventricular response. The 2:1 ratio is the most common block in atrial flutter. Since the P waves in PAT do not occur as fast as in atrial flutter, most cases of PAT exhibit no block and all the impulses are transmitted by the AV node to the ventricles.

Treatment of Atrial Flutter.

The classic initial treatment of atrial flutter has always been digitalis, which partially blocks the AV node; this allows fewer P waves to pass through the ventricles and thus slows the pulse rate. It is important to slow down a fast pulse rate (ventricular rate) because the heart is not given enough time to fill itself with blood when it is contracting rapidly. If the heart is not filling properly, the blood backs up in the body tissues, leading to congestive failure.

Atrial flutter responds very well to cardioversion at a relatively low wattage (50-100 watts per second), and this is the treatment of choice if the patient is tolerating the arrhythmia poorly.

- *It should be noted that when a patient is taking digitalis, cardioversion can be dangerous, since a lethal arrhythmia may be precipitated.*

Atrial Fibrillation

Atrial fibrillation is disorganized and uncoordinated twitching of atrial musculature. It is usually seen in patients with arteriosclerotic or rheumatic heart disease.

Mechanism of Atrial Fibrillation.

Arteriosclerosis leads to scarring of the atrium and thus to disruption of the normal course of the P wave (atrial wave). In this condition, the QRS (ventricular wave) is of normal configuration since the conduction tissue beyond the AV node has not yet been critically involved with the arteriosclerotic process (Fig. 27-20).

ECG of Atrial Fibrillation.

In atrial fibrillation, as the name implies, normal P waves have been replaced by irregular rapid waves each of which is different in configuration from the other. The P waves (often called fibrillatory waves) assume different shapes because they are

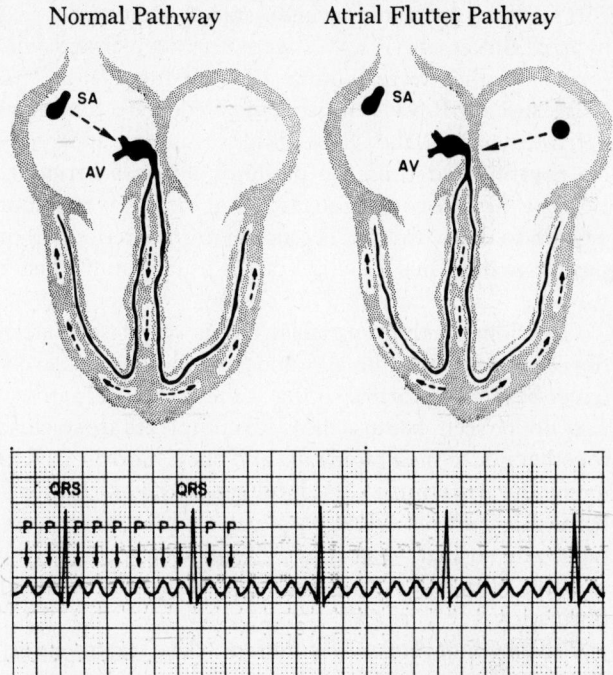

Figure 27-19.   Atrial flutter: (*top*) pathway; (*bottom*) ECG. The arrows indicate the P waves that are coming from the fast ectopic focus in the atrium. Notice that not every P wave stimulates a QRS complex (ventricular wave). Since the abnormality present in the heart is above the AV node, the QRS complexes that appear are normal in configuration.

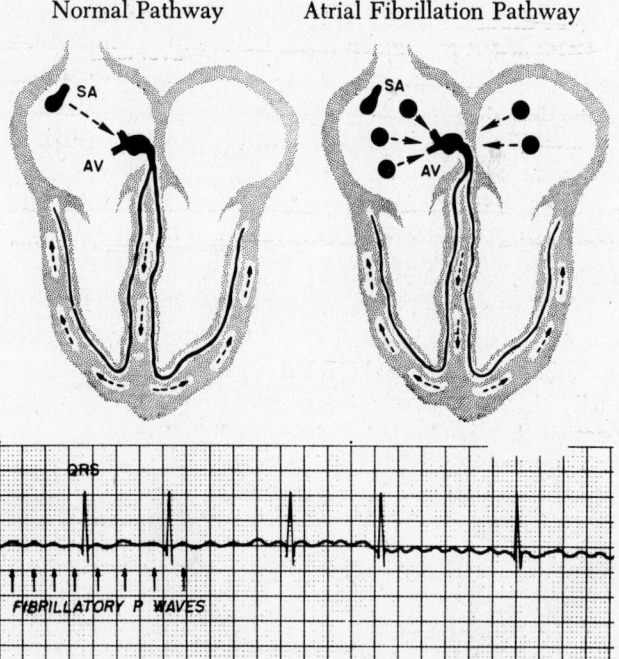

Figure 27-20.   Atrial fibrillation: (*top*) pathway; (*bottom*) ECG. Note the small, irregular fibrillating P waves (*arrow*). As with atrial flutter, only an occasional P wave travels through the AV node to form a QRS complex, but since these complexes come at irregular intervals in atrial fibrillation, the ventricular rate is irregular. Each P wave is different in shape because it is coming from a different focus in the atrium.

coming from different foci in the atrium. Remember that in atrial flutter, the P waves were very regular and uniform since they were coming from one focus.

Because the P waves in atrial fibrillation are coming at variable intervals, the QRS complexes assume an irregular rhythm and thus the patient's pulse is *irregular*. Because they are coming so fast, all of the P waves do not pass on to the ventricles, because of normal refraction of the AV node. Thus the atrial rate is usually much faster than the ventricular rate (Fig. 27-20).

Occasionally, the ventricular rate is very fast in atrial fibrillation because the AV node is blocking relatively fewer beats than normal. If this is the case, atrial activity may not be seen, because the QRS complexes are so close together due to their rapid rate, and one is hard pressed to define the arrhythmia. A helpful general rule to remember is that if *normal* QRS complexes are present at a very rapid rate so that atrial activity cannot be seen and the rhythm is *irregular*, the probable diagnosis is atrial fibrillation.

Treatment of Atrial Fibrillation. The treatment depends on the patient's clinical condition, cardiac rate, and drug status. Many patients with atrial fibrillation are in congestive failure, have a rapid cardiac rate, and either have not been given digitalis or have had too little. (Excessive digitalis can also occasionally cause atrial fibrillation.)

For the average patient who is not critical and not on digitalis, the following treatment is common: 0.5 mg. of IV digoxin is given over a 5-minute period under ECG control. After 2 hours, an additional 0.25-0.5 mg. is administered, depending on the ECG and the patient's condition (total IV dose before oral maintenance therapy is 0.75-1.5 mg.).

If atrial fibrillation is an immediate life-threatening emergency (rare), cardioversion may be instituted, starting with 100 watt-seconds. As with atrial flutter, cardioversion becomes somewhat of a risk when the patient is taking digitalis. In contrast to atrial flutter, atrial fibrillation is more difficult to correct to normal sinus rhythm with electric countershock.

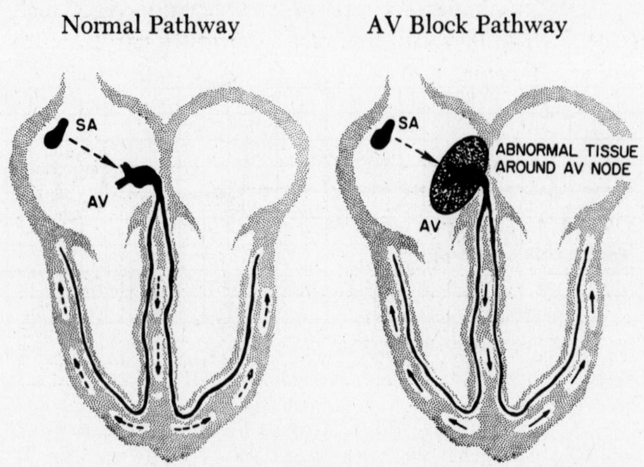

AV Block

Atrioventricular (AV) block means that the AV node is diseased and has difficulty conducting the atrial waves (P waves) into the ventricles. The most common causes are arteriosclerosis and its congener myocardial infarction. AV blocks are divided into 1st, 2nd, and 3rd degree blocks.

Mechanisms of AV Blocks. Abnormal tissue around and in the AV node causes physiological blockage of the atrial impulse into the ventricles (Fig. 27-21). In a 1st degree block the impulses are merely slowed, but all enter the ventricles. In 2nd degree block only a portion of the atrial impulses penetrate to the ventricles, and in 3rd degree block no atrial impulse enters the ventricles, so that the atria and ventricles are beating independently.

1st Degree AV Block. In 1st degree block the PR interval is prolonged. (The PR interval represents the impulse going through the atrium and the area of the AV node.) Since the atrial and AV nodal tissue are diseased, the electrical impulse takes a longer time to traverse its pathway and this is reflected by an increased length in the PR interval on ECG (Fig. 27-22). In contrast to 2nd and 3rd degree block, all P waves penetrate the ventricles to form QRS complexes. At normal rates, the PR interval should not be over 0.20 second (5 small blocks on the ECG paper when each block equals 0.04 second).

2nd Degree AV Block. A 2nd degree block means that some P waves do not pass through the ventricles, but others do. Figure 27-23 shows a 2:1, 2nd degree block, meaning that every second P wave does not penetrate the ventricles. A 2nd degree block can also be 3:1, 4:1, or any such combination. The essential point (which distinguishes 2nd degree block from 3rd degree block) is that some P waves conduct QRS complexes and others do not.

3rd Degree AV Block. A 3rd degree block (also called a complete AV block) means that *no* P waves penetrate the AV node to the ventricles; therefore, the P waves and QRS are beating *independently*. P waves are

Normal Pathway   AV Block Pathway

Figure 27-21.   Mechanism of AV blocks.

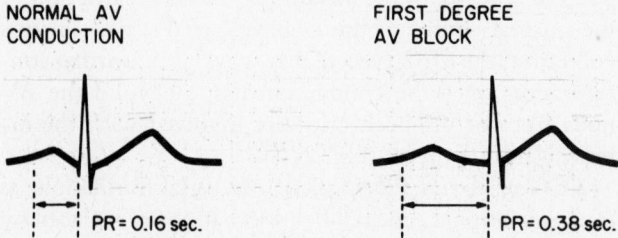

NORMAL AV CONDUCTION   FIRST DEGREE AV BLOCK

PR = 0.16 sec.   PR = 0.38 sec.

Figure 27-22.   1st degree AV block. Since the tissue around the AV node is abnormal, the impulse takes longer to traverse this area which leads to a prolonged PR interval.

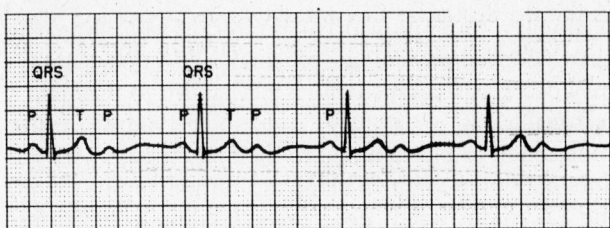

Figure 27-23.   2nd degree AV block. Some P waves pass through to the ventricles but others do not.

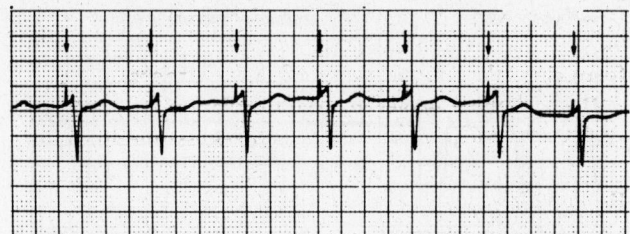

Figure 27-25.   Normal pacemaker function. In this ECG each QRS complex is preceded by a small vertical line (*arrows*) which represents the electrical stimulus of the artificial pacemaker.

seen before the QRS complexes, but the PR interval varies and there is no constant relationship of the P waves to the QRS complexes (Fig. 27-24). The pulse rate is usually slow since the AV node and ventricles are beating at their own inherent rhythm, which is between 30 to 60 beats per minute.

Treatment of AV Blocks.   No treatment is needed for a 1st degree heart block. When certain types of 2nd degree heart block occur in a myocardial infarction, many cardiologists insert a pacemaker which is activated when the cardiac rate falls to unacceptable levels. If it is desired to increase the rate in a 2nd degree block while awaiting the pacemaker, atropine, 0.5-1.0 mg., may be given IV. If the rate cannot be maintained with atropine, 1.0 mg. of isoproterenol (Isuprel) added to 250 ml. of 5 percent glucose in water may be infused by the "piggy-back" technique to stimulate the heart to function at an acceptable rate.

A 3rd degree heart block in a myocardial infarction is frequently treated with a pacemaker, but the drugs mentioned above should be used to increase the rate while awaiting insertion of the pacemaker wires.

The ECG of a patient with a normally functioning artificial pacemaker shows a *vertical line* just at the beginning of the QRS complex (Fig. 27-25).

Pacemaker difficulties are not uncommon, and it is important to identify these on the ECG. One of the most common causes of nonpacing is failure of the pacemaker wire to remain in contact with the heart wall, which may occur when the patient performs a sudden movement. This is readily identified on the ECG when the small vertical pacemaker stimulus is *not* followed by a QRS complex, as in the ECG in Figure 27-26.

Lack of contact between pacing catheter and heart wall is not the only thing that can go wrong with artificial pacing. Other common causes of pacemaker failure are breakage of the wires to the heart (or disconnection from the pacemaker) or battery failure of the pacer. This situation is easily recognized by the absence of vertical pacer lines on the ECG strip as shown in Figure 27-27.

Premature Ventricular Contractions (PVCs)

Premature ventricular contractions represent one of the most easily recognized rhythm disturbances seen on an ECG. They occur in all forms of heart disease and are seen in the majority of patients with myocardial infarcts. PVCs are seen frequently in normal hearts and can be secondary to smoking or intake of coffee or alcohol. PVCs are not usually symptomatic but, when frequent, may cause palpitations.

Mechanism of PVCs.   As the name indicates, premature ventricular contractions come early in the cycle and originate in the ventricle *below* the AV node (Fig. 27-28). It will be remembered that a normal ventricular complex (the QRS) begins *in* the AV node.

ECG of PVCs.   Since a PVC does not begin normally and therefore does not follow the true conduction path in the ventricle, it has a wide and bizarre QRS configuration (Fig. 27-28).

Treatment of PVCs.   If a patient has an infarct, premature ventricular contractions are usually vigorously treated since *they can precipitate ventricular fibrillation by hitting a T wave.*

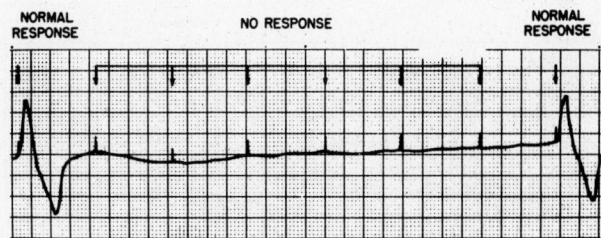

Figure 27-26.   Poor pacemaker contact. Notice that the first and last pacemaker stimuli are followed by ventricular complexes and that the other pacemaker deflections failed to produce a cardiac impulse because of the lack of pacemaker contact with the heart wall.

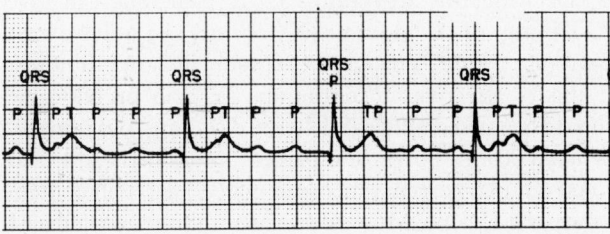

Figure 27-24.   3rd degree AV block. The P waves and QRS complexes are beating independently of each other.

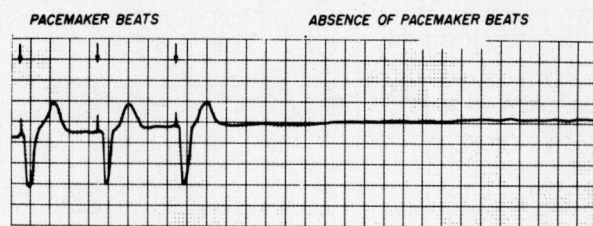

PACEMAKER BEATS   ABSENCE OF PACEMAKER BEATS

Figure 27-27. Malfunctioning pacemaker. Notice the eventual absence of pacemaker stimuli which in this case resulted in cardiac standstill. This patient had a faulty pacemaker.

PVCs are especially dangerous when they do the following:

1. Occur more frequently than once in ten beats.
2. Occur in groups of two or three.
3. Land near the T wave.
4. Take on multiple configurations, since this indicates that the PVCs are coming from different foci, which in turn means that the ventricle is more irritable.

"Vigorous treatment" consists of administering lidocaine (Xylocaine) as outlined in the next section, under ventricular tachycardia.

It should be noted that PVCs are usually seen with a cardiac rate of over 60 per minute and that Xylocaine (a cardiac muscle suppressant) is the drug of choice because the PVCs are most likely coming from an irritable focus such as an infarct. If, on the other hand, the rate is *slow*

Normal Pathway   PVC Pathway

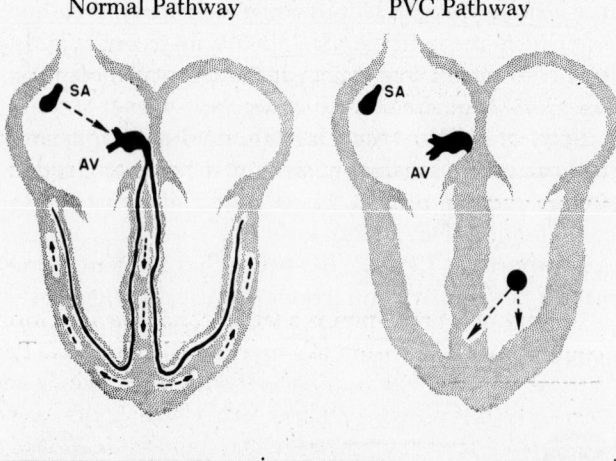

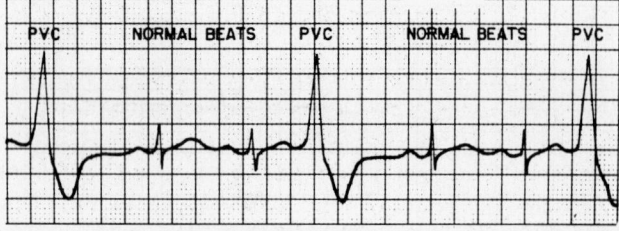

PVC | NORMAL BEATS | PVC | NORMAL BEATS | PVC

Figure 27-28. Premature ventricular contractions (PVC): (top) pathway; (bottom) ECG. PVCs come early in the cycle and are wider than the normal beat.

secondary to a myocardial infarction involving the heart's normal physiologic pacemaker (SA node), PVCs may occur as a compensatory mechanism to maintain a reasonable rate so as to provide some type of cardiac contraction to pump blood to the body tissues. A PVC does not pump as much blood as a normal impulse from the SA node, but it does provide some circulation. Therefore, in *sinus bradycardia,* since the PVCs are pumping needed blood and since they usually do not land on a T wave (which could trigger ventricular fibrillation) Xylocaine would be contraindicated since it would decrease circulation by extinguishing the PVCs. Therefore, if the rate is slow, resulting in compensatory PVCs, the treatment of choice would be *atropine* to increase the sinus node rate, which in turn would terminate the inefficient ectopic beats by replacing them with normal impulses. Thus, when PVCs are compensatory and caused by a slow firing SA node, the treatment is to speed the rate with 0.5-1.0 mg. of IV atropine and not to give Xylocaine, which would only further depress cardiac activity.

Ventricular Tachycardia

Ventricular tachycardia is one of the dreaded complications of a myocardial infarct and can be considered as multiple (3 or more) consecutive premature ventricular contractions occurring from an ectopic focus below the AV node in the ventricles which causes the complexes to be wide and bizarre in configuration. Ventricular tachycardia is very dangerous because it leads to a reduced cardiac output (the ventricles are not being stimulated normally from the AV node but from a focus further down in the ventricular wall, which leads to an incomplete and inefficient contraction of the heart muscle) and is a precursor of ventricular fibrillation in which there is no cardiac output.

Mechanism and ECG of Ventricular Tachycardia. Since this arrhythmia begins below the AV node, the atria are beating independently and in 20 percent of cases in which the ventricular rate is not too fast and the ventricular complexes are not too wide, P waves can be seen which are independent of the QRS complexes. (Fig. 27-29). Notice that the rate is fast and that the QRS is wide. A width of .12 second (three small blocks) or more is considered abnormal for a QRS complex.

Treatment of Ventricular Tachycardia. If the patient is tolerating this arrhythmia fairly well, one can give 75-100 mg. of IV lidocaine (Xylocaine) as a bolus over a 2-minute period. This can be repeated in 2 or 3 minutes. If this is effective, a continuous IV drip of lidocaine should be started with the delivery of 1-3 mg. per minute. When a 50-ml. bottle of 2 percent lidocaine is added to 1,000 ml. of 5 percent glucose in water, 1 ml. will contain 1 mg. of lidocaine. Most IV sets are calibrated to deliver 1 ml. in 10 drops of fluid. If this concentration results in too much fluid for the patient, the amount of Xylocaine

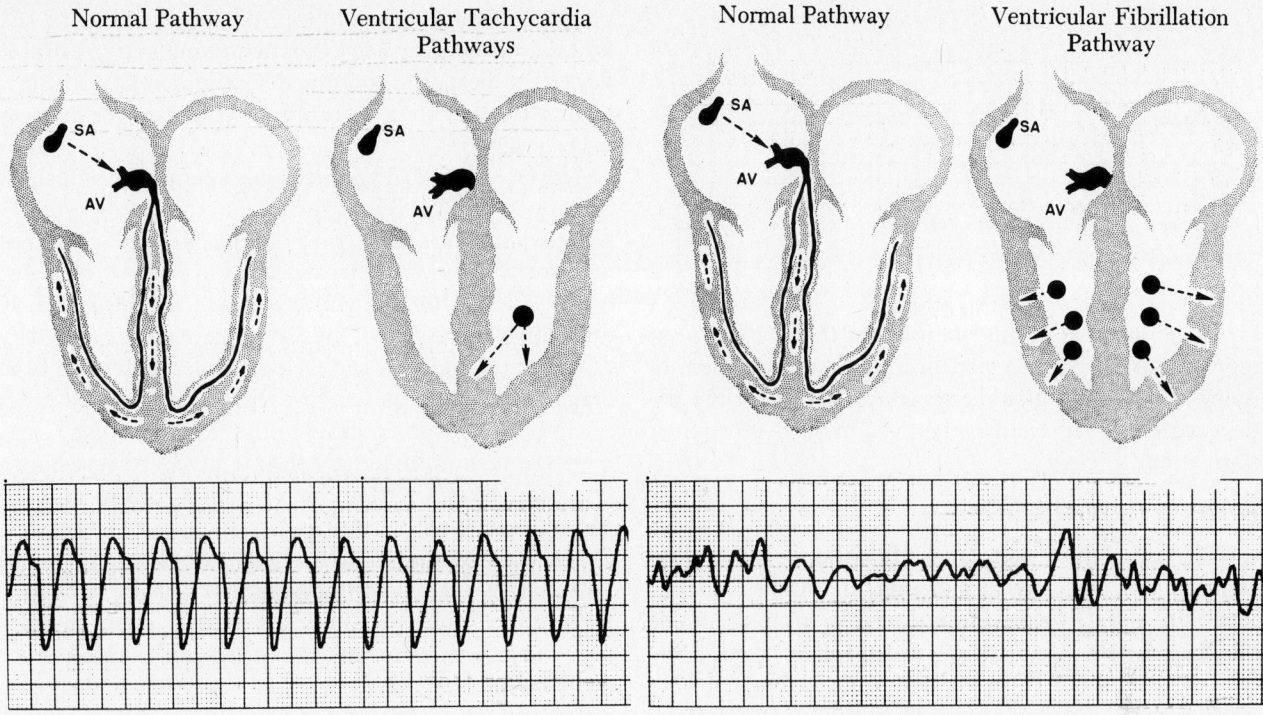

| Normal Pathway | Ventricular Tachycardia Pathways | Normal Pathway | Ventricular Fibrillation Pathway |

Figure 27-29.   Ventricular tachycardia: (*top*) pathway; (*bottom*) ECG.

Figure 27-30.   Ventricular fibrillation: (*top*) pathway; (*bottom*) ECG. The complexes are completely distorted and irregular.

should be increased in the IV solution. Because the heart muscle is weakened, the cardiac patient should not receive excessive fluid since this may precipitate congestive failure.

If the patient is tolerating ventricular tachycardia poorly when first seen, or if lidocaine fails to convert this arrhythmia, *cardioversion* should be performed.

Cardioversion is begun by first reassuring the patient, if he is lucid enough to understand the situation, and is carried out as follows:

- Allow the patient to receive oxygen before and after the procedure but not during it, since an electrical spark from the paddles may ignite the oxygen and cause severe facial burns.
- Make sure the paddles are clean, because surface debris will interfere with the flow of electricity into the heart.
- Apply electrode paste to all of the paddle surface, but make sure there is no excess around the edges of the paddles. (If there is excess paste around the paddle edge, the discharge may run across the skin, causing a burn.) The paste (which acts as an electrical conductor) should be rubbed into the skin very thoroughly, since this allows more electricity to penetrate the body surface. Firm contact between the paddles and skin also helps the electricity to penetrate better into the myocardium.
- There are several different paddle placements, but the quickest one involves placing one paddle just to the right of the sternum at the 2nd interspace and the other paddle just under the left nipple.
- Set machine's synchronization mechanism so that the electrical shock discharges on the R wave. If the electrical impulse

from the machine hits the T wave, the ventricular tachycardia may be converted to ventricular fibrillation.

- On many machines, the R wave must be upright before there is synchronization; hence one may have to switch to a lead in which the R waves are not inverted.

Usually, an initial shock at 200 watt-seconds (joules) will accomplish conversion. If 200 watt-seconds is unsuccessful, one should then change to 400 watt-seconds. Valium or a short-acting barbiturate should be given if the patient is conscious, since this helps to produce amnesia for the procedure.

Ventricular Fibrillation

Ventricular fibrillation is a lethal condition seen most commonly in the setting of a myocardial infarction. The patient will die within minutes if the arrhythmia is not terminated. It is extremely important for the nurse to be cognizant of this rhythm, since she is usually the first one to see the patient and should institute therapy immediately.

Mechanism of Ventricular Fibrillation.   In ventricular fibrillation, the heart is being stimulated simultaneously from *numerous ectopic foci throughout the ventricles*. Therefore, there is no effective contraction of the cardiac musculature and thus no pulse (Fig. 27-30).

ECG of Ventricular Fibrillation.   As shown in Figure 27-30, ventricular fibrillation is recognized by its *totally irregular appearance*. It is extremely important to be

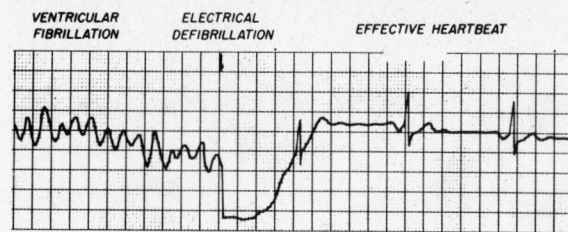

VENTRICULAR FIBRILLATION   ELECTRICAL DEFIBRILLATION   EFFECTIVE HEARTBEAT

Figure 27-31.   Electrical defibrillation.

sure that the chaotic undulations on the ECG do not represent artifacts, since patient motion or movement of monitor wires can give the same appearance. If the patient is alert or has a pulse, the rhythm *is not* ventricular fibrillation.

Electrical Defibrillation

The treatment of ventricular fibrillation is *electrical defibrillation* at 400 watts per second, the highest energy capability of the machines now available. In children, one may begin with 200 watts per second. If successful, the defibrillation shock stops the erratic uncoordinated electrical activity of the ventricle. After a moment the heart resumes its normal innate rhythm from the SA node (Fig. 27-31).

Electrical defibrillation differs from cardioversion in that no timing is necessary with the defibrillation shock since there are no T waves in ventricular fibrillation.

The principles of paddle placement (Fig. 27-32) are the same as those discussed under ventricular tachycardia (page 534).

"DIGITALIS EFFECT" AND TOXICITY

When a patient presents with an abnormal cardiac rhythm, one should remember that almost *every* arrhythmia can be produced by excessive digitalis. An-

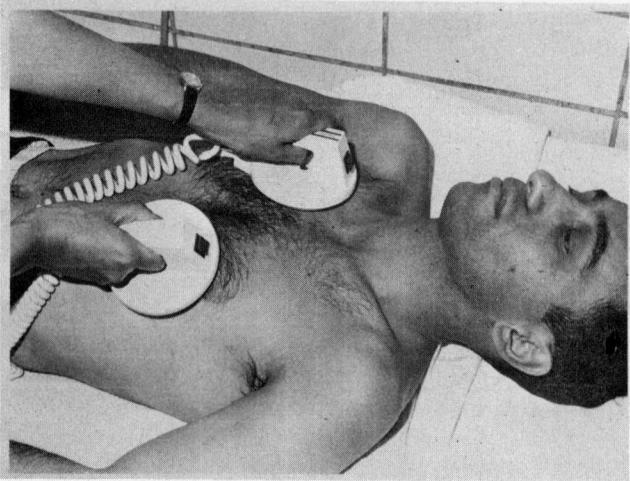

Figure 27-32.   Paddle placement in ventricular defibrillation.

orexia is a common symptom of digitalis toxicity and is often followed by nausea and vomiting in two or three days if the digitalis is continued. Green or yellow vision is a fairly distinct (but uncommon) complaint of digitalis overdosage.

The ECGs of many patients taking digitalis will show a depression of the ST segments, but this does *not* represent toxicity. This is known as "digitalis effect" and is not necessarily related to the therapeutic level of digitalis. Normal levels of digitalis often will produce a fairly distinctive depression of the ST segment characterized by "scooping," which is said to look as if a finger had been dragged through the end of the QRS complex (Fig. 27-33A). This is in contrast to the "horizontal" ST segment depression frequently seen in myocardial ischemia (Fig. 27-33B, C). Often the ST depressions of digitalis and ischemia will be similar.

The most common arrhythmia associated with digitalis toxicity is *ectopic ventricular* beats. Even more characteristic of digitalis toxicity are ectopic beats that are *multifocal*, which means that they are coming from different locations in the ventricles and thus will take on different configurations in the ECG (Fig. 27-34).

Probably the next most common arrhythmia in digitalis toxicity is a complete AV block. This is frequently seen in a patient who is being treated for atrial fibrillation. Digitalis is being used to decrease the ventricular rate so that the heart can have time to fill with blood and thus increase the output. In this situation, digitalis toxicity is identified by *"regularization"* of the previous irregular *ventricular* rate of atrial fibrillation (Fig. 27-35). (The ventricular rate of atrial fibrillation is normally irregular, and since the AV node area is blocked, no atrial waves penetrate to the ventricles and the AV node must initiate the impulses, which are regular.)

- Therefore, when one sees a regular ventricular rate in a patient with atrial fibrillation, the first thought should be digitalis toxicity.

Potassium and digitalis have a reciprocal relationship which is reflected in their effect on the heart; thus, if the serum potassium is low, digitalis will have a greater chance of causing toxicity.

Treatment

If the patient is hemodynamically stable with his digitalis induced arrhythmia, it is probably best to simply withhold the digitalis and await body excretion of the drug. If the patient's potassium is low, replacement would be indicated.

If a patient is doing poorly with his arrhythmia, initial treatment with *potassium* or *Dilantin* would be appropriate. (Potassium, which prolongs impulse conduction, would be contraindicated if the serum potassium were above a high normal level or if a significant degree of AV

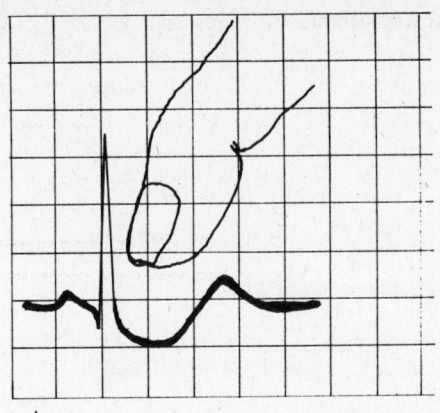
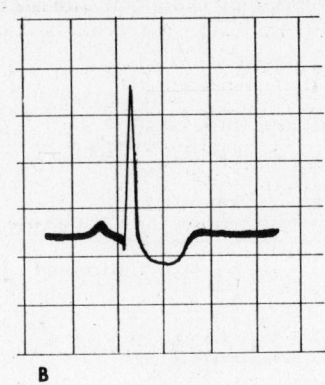
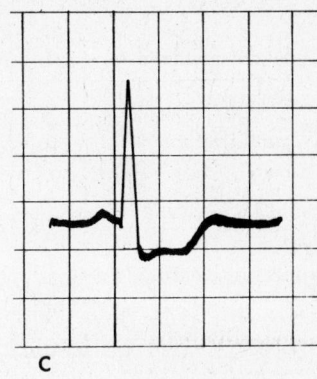

Figure 27-33.   A. The ST segment depression of digitalis often appears as if someone had dragged his finger through the end of the QRS complex into the T wave.

B. Digitalis effect: Notice the rounded scooped appearance of the ST segment.

C. Ischemic effect: In contrast to digitalis effect, the ST segment depression is horizontal.

block were present.) The average dose of potassium chloride would be about 40mEq. in one liter of saline over four to six hours. If potassium is not effective, 125–250 mg. of Dilantin IV over three to five minutes under ECG control is sometimes helpful. Dilantin decreases myocardial excitability and increases the rate of impulse formation through the AV node, both effects being opposite to

that of digitalis. If potassium and Dilantin are not effective, lidocaine, propranolol (Inderal), and pacing can also be used in digitalis toxicity.

• Cardioversion is contraindicated in digitalis toxicity because of the danger of converting relatively benign arrhythmias to more lethal ones. If all modalities fail and the situation seems terminal, cardioversion or defibrillation should be attempted.

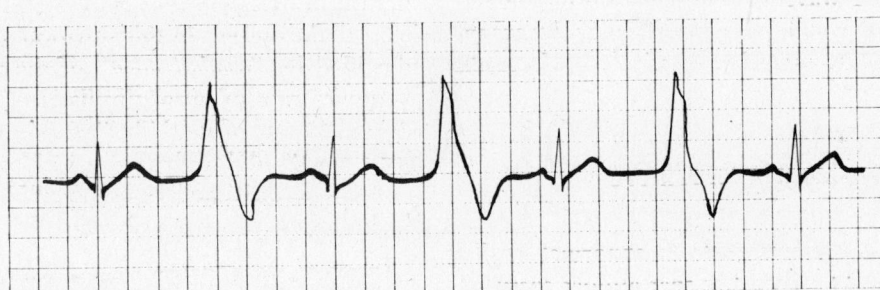

Figure 27-34.   The ectopic ventricular contractions shown above are secondary to digitalis toxicity.

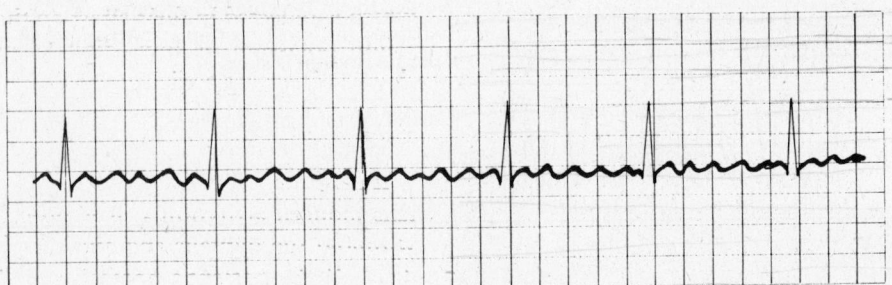

Figure 27-35.   Atrial fibrillation with a regular ventricular response which is often secondary to digitalis toxicity.

Summary: Emergency Diagnosis and Treatment of Arrhythmias

Type of Arrhythmia	Appearance of ECG	Treatment	Pathway
Normal rhythm		None.	
Sinus tachycardia		Treat cause.	
Sinus bradycardia		Atropine, Isuprel, or pacemaker when condition is pathological.	
Sinus arrhythmia		None.	
PAC's		Usually none. Quinidine may be used.	
PAT		Carotid sinus pressure or metaraminol (Aramine).	
Atrial flutter		Digitalis if rate is above 100. Cardioversion is very effective.°	
Atrial fibrillation		Digitalis if rate is above 100, and if fibrillation is not caused by too much digitalis. Cardioversion may be effective.°	
AV Blocks 2nd degree		Atropine, Isuprel, or pacemaker.	
3rd degree		Atropine, Isuprel, or pacemaker.	
PVC's		No treatment if benign. Lidocaine (Xylocaine) in most patients. Atropine if basic rhythm is slow.	
Ventricular tachycardia		Cardioversion° or lidocaine.	
Ventricular fibrillation	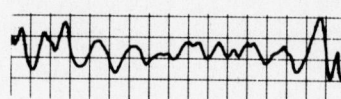	Electrical defibrillation.	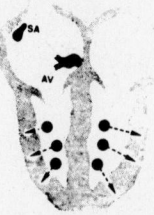

° Cardioversion can be dangerous when the patient is taking digitalis.

538

BIBLIOGRAPHY

BOOKS

Andreoli, K., et al.: Comprehensive Cardiac Care, 4th ed. C. V. Mosby, St. Louis, 1979.

Chung, E.: Electrocardiography. Hagerstown, Md., Harper and Row, 1974.

———: Principles of Cardiac Arrhythmias, 2nd ed. Baltimore, Williams and Wilkins, 1977.

Delman, A. J. and Stein, E.: Dynamic Cardiac Auscultation and Phonocardiography. Philadelphia, W. B. Saunders, 1979.

Dubin, D.: Rapid Interpretation of EKGs, 3rd ed. Tampa, Fl., Cover Publishing Co., 1974.

Friedman, H.: Diagnostic Electrocardiography and Vectorcardiography, 2nd ed. New York, McGraw-Hill, 1977.

Goldman, M.: Principles of Clinical Electrocardiography, 9th ed. Los Altos, Lange Medical Pub., 1976.

Hurst, W.: The Heart. New York, McGraw-Hill, 1978.

Marriott, H.: Practical Electrocardiography, 6th ed. Baltimore, Williams and Wilkins, 1977.

Meltzer, L., Pinneo, R., and Kitchell, J.: Intensive Coronary Care, 3rd ed. Bowie, Md., Charles Press Publishers, 1977.

Phibbs, B.: The Cardiac Arrhythmias, 3rd ed. St. Louis, C. V. Mosby, 1978.

Schamroth, L.: An Introduction to Electrocardiography, 5th ed. Oxford, Blackwell Scientific Pub., 1976.

Stein, E.: The Electrocardiogram. Philadelphia, W. B. Saunders, 1976.

ARTICLES

Basta, L.: The ambulatory patient with ectopic beats and episodic tachyarrhythmias. Am. Fam. Phys., *15*:94-98, Feb. 1977.

Chung, E.: Artificial cardiac pacing. Postgrad. Med., *59*:83-90, June 1976.

Dolgin, M.: The peculiarities of cardiac arrhythmias. Consultant, *16*:167-175, May 1976.

Driefus, L.: Chronic atrial arrhythmias. Heart & Lung, *3*:26-31, July-Aug. 1977.

Galen, R.: Myocardial infarction: A clinician's guide to the isoenzymes. Resident & Staff Phys., *23*:67-72, May 1977.

Glasser, S., and Martinez-Lopez, J.: Atrial flutter. Postgrad. Med., *62*:61-67, Aug. 1977.

Grace, W.: Protocol for the management of arrhythmias in acute myocardial infarction. Crit. Care Med., *2*:235-242, Sept.-Oct. 1974.

Kastor, J.: Atrioventricular-block. New Eng. J. Med., *292*:572-574, Mar. 13, 1975.

Kleiger, R.: Arrhythmias, Part 1. Heart & Lung, *6*:60-88, Jan.-Feb. 1977.

———: Arrhythmias, Part 2. Heart and Lung, *6*:249-262, Mar.-Apr. 1977.

Krikler, D.: A fresh look at cardiac arrhythmias. Lancet, vol. 1: (7862). May 4, 1974, p. 851; May 11, 1974, p. 913; May 18, 1974, p. 974; May 25, 1974, p. 1074.

McNeal, G. P.: Tracing arrhythmias. AJN, *79*:98-100, Jan. 1979.

Narula, O.: Sick sinus syndrome. Primary Cardiol., *4*:27-31, Jan. 1975.

Tai, A., et al.: Step-by-step protocols for arrhythmias. Patient Care, *11*:100-123, Feb. 25, 1977, pages 100-123.

Uhley, H.: Clinical application of electrocardiographic trend recording. Heart & Lung, *5*:267-72, Mar.-Apr. 1976.

Winslow, E. F., and Powell, A. H.: Sick sinus syndrome. AJN, *76*:1262-1265, Aug. 1976.

28

MANAGEMENT OF THE PATIENT IN THE CARDIAC CARE UNIT

THE CARDIAC CARE UNIT

The cardiac care unit, or coronary care unit (CCU) is an area in a hospital that is equipped with special electronic devices used in monitoring patients with actual or potential heart problems. It is staffed by nurses with clinical expertise in cardiovascular nursing. Since the advent of the CCU in the early 1960s, mortality of cardiac patients has dramatically decreased. Some authorities suggest that this decreased mortality ranges from 10 to 24 percent in myocardial infarction (MI) patients. The main objective of the unit is to prevent, detect, and treat cardiac arrhythmias, which were originally the leading cause of death of the patient with MI. Additional objectives are to prevent, detect, and treat complications that occur because of the myocardial infarction. (More information regarding this disease is presented in Chapter 30.)

In order to meet these objectives, the CCU is generally a confined area with limited access from other parts of the hospital. It affords a quiet, temperature-controlled environment, often with private rooms. Resuscitative equipment and electrocardiographic monitoring devices with automatic alarm systems are provided. The usual equipment includes individual oscilloscopes at each patient's bed and a base oscilloscope with multiple channels at the nurses' station which displays the individual patient's electrocardiogram.

The most important aspect of the CCU, however, is not the equipment but the special nurses who care for the patients in this unusual environment. They must be well prepared to manage, diagnose, and intervene without immediate consultation with physicians, if an emergency occurs. The nurse must be knowledgeable in basic anatomy, physiology, and pathophysiology of the cardiovascular system and must be familiar with the methods and goals of medical therapy and appropriate nursing support. Additional facets of the knowledge base include the ability to make assessments and diagnoses and to plan and evaluate care. The nurse who functions in the CCU is sensitive to the special psychological needs of the patients, the families, and the staff members. The benefits of the care in this specialized unit are directly proportional to the knowledge, skills, and commitment of the nursing staff.

CARE OF THE PATIENT WITH MYOCARDIAL INFARCTION

The patient is usually admitted to the CCU for an actual or potential myocardial infarction (MI). The condition, which is also known as a coronary occlusion or "heart attack," occurs when the coronary arteries which supply blood to the myocardium have such a severely compromised flow that they are unable to maintain the survival of the myocardial muscle. Two coronary arteries originate at the base of the aorta as it leaves the left ventricle. The right coronary artery supplies blood to the right atrium and ventricle and, in the majority of people, to the posterior surface of the left ventricle. The left coronary artery has two main branches. These supply the left atrium and remaining left ventricle and the septum. Coronary artery disease (CAD) occurs when there is partial or total obstruction of these vessels. Atherosclerosis, the leading cause of CAD, is characterized by a narrowing of the lumen of the artery due to complex

540

deposits known as "atherosclerotic plaques." Obstruction of the vessel occurs and the portion of the myocardium that it supplies becomes ischemic and finally necrotic. When this tissue death occurs, the normal conduction of electrical activity of the heart may be inhibited and lethal arrhythmias may occur. (See Chapter 27 for interpretation of the electrocardiogram and heart arrhythmias.)

Arrhythmias are probably the leading cause of death following an MI, and CCUs have been established primarily to monitor the electrical activity of the heart so that irregularities of rhythm can be identified and immediate—often lifesaving—measures instituted. At present, care in the CCU is focused on the prevention, early recognition, and treatment of arrhythmias and the identification and treatment of secondary complications. Arrhythmias are discussed in Chapter 27.

Nursing Assessment

One of the most important aspects of care of the patient on admission to the CCU is the nursing assessment. This serves to establish a baseline of information regarding the present status of the patient so that any deviations may be immediately noted. The nursing assessment is orderly and inclusive and has as its objective the identification of the priority of needs of the cardiac patient.

Systematic assessment of the patient includes a careful history, particularly as it relates to the description of symptoms compatible with possible myocardial infarction: chest pain, dyspnea, palpitations, faintness (syncope), and/or sweating (diaphoresis). Each symptom must be evaluated with regard to time, duration, and precipitating and relieving factors.

In addition, there are several areas in the physical examination that relate directly to the needs of the patient in CCU. These include:

1. Radial arterial pulse. Rate, rhythm, and volume are assessed. Many cardiovascular disorders will be reflected here; for example, a rapid, regular but weak pulse indicates low volume and reduced cardiac output; a slow, regular, and strong pulse may indicate heart block; and an irregular pulse indicates cardiac arrhythmia.

2. Jugular venous pressure. The assessment of the pressure in this vessel gives a convenient reflection of the pressure in the right side of the heart. Elevation of venous pressure may indicate the failing ability of the heart to pump and empty its contents. The examination is done with the patient at rest with the head and chest supported at a 45-degree angle. With normal venous pressures, distention of the veins is seen slightly above the clavicle. More extensive venous distention should be noted. (Fig. 28-1).

3. Heart location. The size of the heart may be assessed by identifying its location by means of palpation. The apex beat, often referred to as the point of maximum

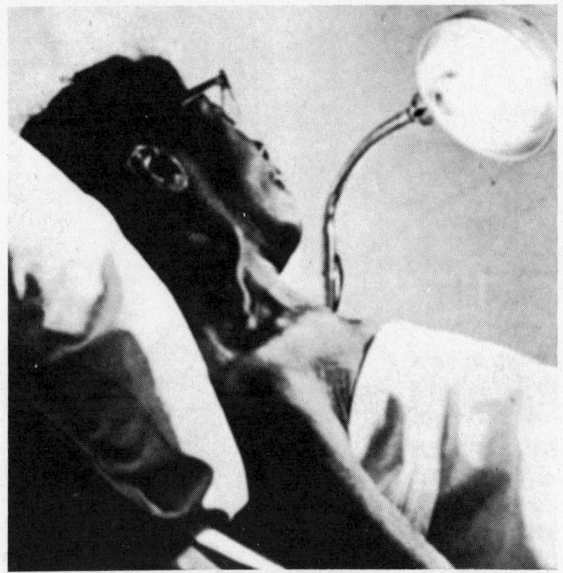

Figure 28-1. This photo illustrates distended neck veins with the patient in a semireclined position, indicating that the heart is incapable of receiving and pumping adequately all the incoming venous blood. (Reproduced with permission of the American Heart Association)

impulse (PMI), is normally found at the 5th intercostal space in the midclavicular line (Fig. 28-2). A movement to the left and down may indicate left ventricular enlargement.

4. Heart sounds. Auscultation is the method used in identifying the normal heart sounds. A stethoscope of good quality and proper fit is essential for the interpretation of heart sounds. The chest piece must have a bell to identify low-pitched sound and should possess a diaphragm for the auscultation of high-pitched sounds. It is important to apply the bell of the stethoscope lightly to the skin and firmly to the diaphragm in order to hear the sounds correctly. The first heart sound (S_1), heard best over the base and indicating the beginning of systole,

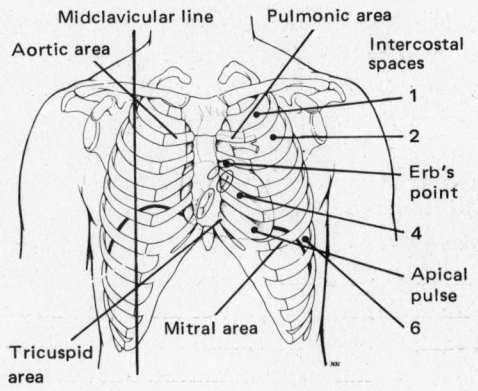

Figure 28-2. The apex beat, often referred to as the point of maximum impulse (PMI), is normally found at the 5th intercostal space in the midclavicular line.

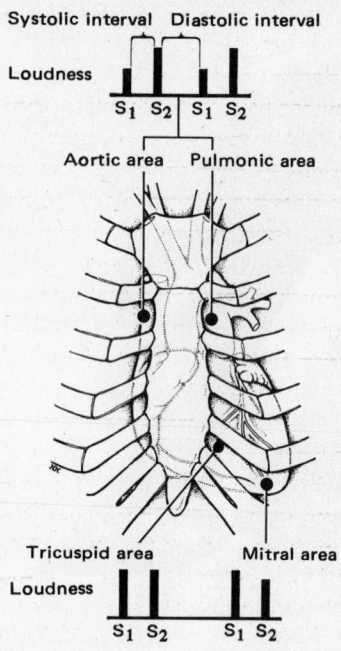

Systolic interval Diastolic interval

Loudness

S₁ S₂ S₁ S₂

Aortic area Pulmonic area

Tricuspid area Mitral area

Loudness

S₁ S₂ S₁ S₂

Figure 28-3. Identification of first and second heart sounds.

and S_2 together sound like the syllables *LUB DUB*. The S_1 *(LUB)* is louder at the apex, the S_2 *(DUB)* louder at the base. The S_3 sound follows closely after S_2 and has a cadence similar to the spoken word *Ken-tuck-y* (S_1-S_2-S_3). The S_4 sound precedes the S_1 and has the cadence of the spoken word *Ten-nes-see* (S_4-S_1-S_2). Other sounds, i.e., murmurs, created by blood flowing around an obstruction or flowing backward through an incompetent valve, are noted. All nurses who care for patients in the CCU must become skillful in the identification of heart sounds and murmurs.

5. Edema. The patient should be evaluated for signs of edema caused by the decreasing ability of the heart to work effectively as a pump. This may be noted in the extremities, particularly at the pretibial area (Fig. 28-4). An enlarged liver is also a sign of failing circulatory status and is palpated in the right upper quadrant (Fig. 28-4).

Early assessment of the patient not only serves to establish priorities of needs and provide baseline data for further nursing plans, but also initiates a relationship between the patient and the nurse that can promote confidence in the nursing staff of the CCU.

Nursing Management

The nursing intervention is designed to support the therapeutic goals of the patient. These are generally to:

- Maintain the present condition of the patient so that healing of the damaged myocardium may occur
- Prevent complications: arrhythmias, congestive heart failure, cardiogenic shock, and others, and

should be identified first. The second sound (S_2), heard best at the base of the heart and indicating the beginning of diastole, is identified next (see Fig. 28-3). Abnormal sounds are noted. These include the third heart sound (S_3), known as *ventricular gallop*, and the fourth heart sound (S_4), known as an *atrial or presystolic gallop*. The S_1

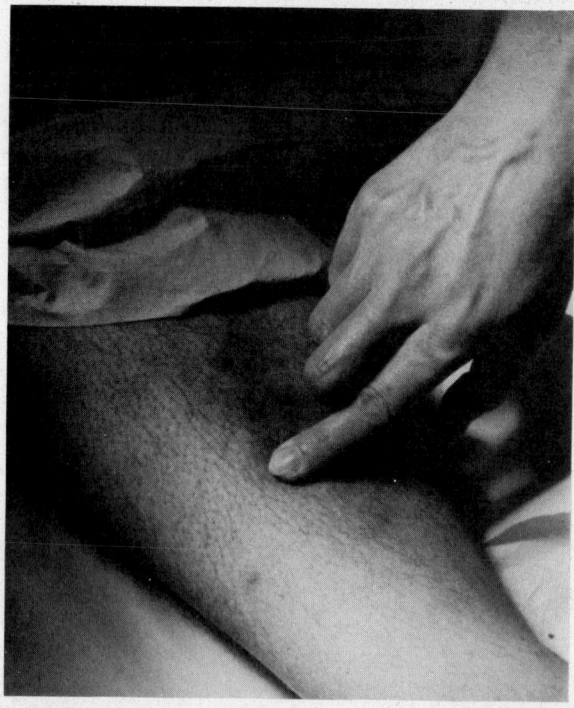

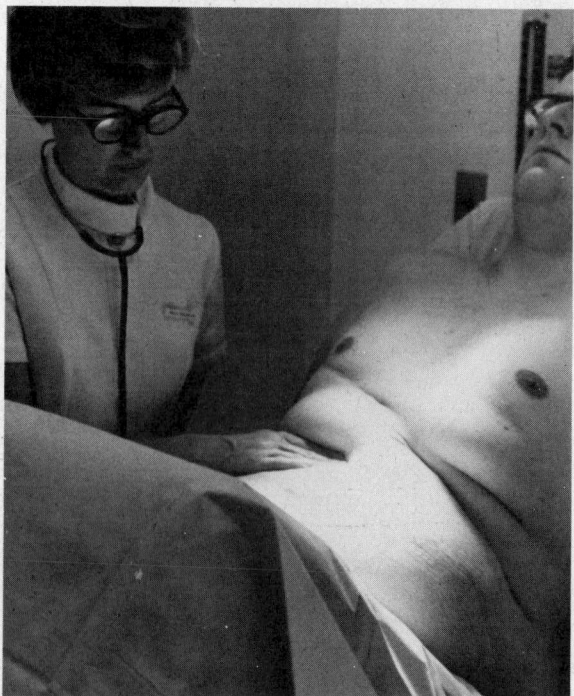

Figure 28-4. A nurse clinician tests for pretibial edema (*left*) and palpates for an enlarged liver in the right upper quadrant (*right*).

- Facilitate the return to normal functioning as soon as possible through the rehabilitative process.

With these broad objectives in mind, the nursing process during the early phase of the illness includes monitoring of the cardiovascular function, maintenance of adequate fluid and oxygen intake, and support of patient rest. When considering a plan of care for these patients, it is important to determine the priority of a given need as well as its long-term importance.

Continuous Monitoring. The priority of early and continuous monitoring of the patient cannot be overemphasized. The current practice is to begin monitoring even before the patient is admitted to the hospital. Thus, community paramedical teams are often taught this skill. The patient is generally reassured by this procedure and feels less anxious, since it has been shown that the patient usually views the equipment as important to maintaining his life. The nurse may allay much needless anxiety in some patients by explaining as fully as possible the nature of the equipment. The nurse is the one who assumes the primary and continuing responsibility for recognizing any malfunctioning of the equipment. (See Chapter 27 for more information.)

Maintaining Fluid and Oxygen Intake. The second priority of care is the maintenance of adequate fluid and oxygen intake. An intravenous line is started immediately in order to provide a readily available route for the administration of fluids and/or medications which may become vital in an emergency. In a line that is only to be "kept open" as a potential route, fluid is administered at a very slow rate, and heparin or another similar drug is added to prevent clotting. The nurse ensures that this line is maintained in a viable condition at all times.

The patient is generally started on oxygen on admission to the CCU. (Portable oxygen may already have been instituted prior to admission.) Oxygen therapy is essential for several reasons. The primary rationale is to provide more oxygen to the myocardium in order to prevent further damage to the muscle, prevent arrhythmias, and reduce pain. In addition, increased perfusion of oxygen will be provided to other organs and the peripheral body structures.

Oxygen is given by nasal cannula or face mask. The rate is regulated by body needs, which are usually determined by the measurement of the amount of oxygen in the blood—arterial blood gas evaluation. In the absence of laboratory results, the rate is 8 to 10 liters per minute by mask and 3 to 5 liters per minute by cannula. (See Chapter 24).

Promoting Rest. The promotion of patient rest is the third important nursing goal in the initial period following myocardial infarction. Rest has both a physical and an emotional component. The physical benefits of rest result from a decrease in stress which helps to lower blood pressure and heart rate and prevent further damage to the myocardium. (Emotional rest is discussed on page 575.) An important aspect of rest is the administration of an analgesic for pain and sedatives to promote relaxation. Both should be given as prescribed and as needed. It is also important to keep the unit as quiet and as nonstressful as is possible in such a technological environment. For elimination, the patient is generally allowed to use a bedside commode, since this method has been shown to be much more acceptable and no more stressful than the use of a bedpan. Laxatives and stool softeners are generally given to prevent excessive straining during bowel movements.

The patient is usually transported to the CCU on a stretcher and lifted from it. The most comfortable position in bed includes some elevation of the head in order to facilitate breathing. There is a difference of opinion about the level of activity that should be allowed during the first few days following an MI. (See rehabilitation after MI on pages 576-577.) All activities are modified to meet individual needs.

Dietary Support. Another consideration related to the early care of the patient is diet. The type of diet provided is one that will impose the least possible work effort and muscular strain on the heart. In the acute stage of myocardial infarction, depending on the extent of the damage, the diet for the first 24 hours may consist of clear liquids providing approximately 500 to 1,000 calories chiefly in the form of clear soups, fruit juices, ginger ale, or weak tea.

Although the patient is encouraged to maintain fluid intake, there remains some controversy about whether iced beverages cause arrhythmias. Most studies indicate that they do not; however, the nonuse of iced beverages in the early hours of the first day may be part of the CCU policy. If sodium restriction is necessary, the total amount of sodium in the diet should be checked. If the patient's condition progresses satisfactorily, after 48 hours the calorie level may be increased to 1,500 calories. This intake should be planned with caution in order to avoid any metabolic overload which might increase the oxygen uptake of the heart.

A full liquid diet will include skim milk and blenderized soups and will slowly progress to a soft diet that allows appropriate choices from meats, vegetables, and fruits with low connective tissue and fiber content for ease of digestion. Such foods might be cooked vegetables that are low in roughage, cooked cereals, puddings, and gelatin desserts.

In both the acute and subacute stage, fats should be kept to approximately 25 to 30 percent of total calorie intake and should consist predominantly of polyunsaturated fat, with cholesterol levels that do not exceed 300 mg. per day. When the patient is discharged from the hospital, the dietitian should include the patient's family in the dietary counseling. The nurse may often need to reinforce and supplement the patient's knowledge when questions are raised by the patient concerning his prescribed diet.

MAJOR COMPLICATIONS OF MYOCARDIAL INFARCTION

Complications of myocardial infarction include congestive heart failure, shock, pulmonary embolism, and heart block. It should be noted that these complications, all of which reflect the underlying pathophysiology of the damaged myocardium, are linked in a circular pattern of interrelationships. These interrelationships are demonstrated in Figure 28-5.

Congestive Heart Failure

Congestive heart failure (CHF) is the syndrome of physiological reactions that occurs when the heart ceases to function effectively as a pump to maintain adequate circulation of the blood. In the CCU the major cause of CHF is massive damage to the myocardium following a myocardial infarction. Many authorities believe that after an MI all patients have a certain amount of congestive heart failure, the degree being determined by the size of the infarction. (See page 577 for a discussion of congestive heart failure.)

Measurements of circulatory function during a myocardial infarction have been shown to be valuable therapeutically and are commonly utilized in patients with complicated myocardial infarctions. The two most common measurements made are those of pressure and cardiac output. The pressure of blood in the right atrium is assessed by the measurement of central venous pressure (CVP), and in the left atrium by estimation of pulmonary capillary ("wedge") pressure. Cardiac output may also be determined through the use of catheters and equipment designed for safe bedside use. Both measurements can be made with the Swan-Ganz catheter (see page 443), which is threaded through the right side of the heart into the pulmonary artery. The Swan-Ganz catheter can measure the left ventricular end-diastolic pressure (LVEDP) and is the most accurate indicator for the presence of heart failure.

Management. The treatment of congestive heart failure (CHF) is directed at three main objectives:

1. To provide rest for the heart,
2. To reduce the amount of circulating blood volume,
3. To increase cardiac output by strengthening muscle contraction or decreasing peripheral resistance.

To accomplish these objectives, the patient is placed on bed rest and the head of the bed is elevated. Diuretic therapy is given (to increase urinary output) and digitalis is sometimes administered to increase the force of myocardial contractions.

- Patients with MI appear to be sensitive to digitalis and must be monitored for rhythm disturbances when this drug is used.

Oxygen is also usually indicated.

Nitroprusside is a vasodilator which is used in several clinical situations; in the CCU it is used most often for left ventricular failure. In a compromised ventricle, nitroprusside improves hemodynamic action by reducing the impedance to left ventricular ejection, which increases cardiac output. Some authorities believe that the reduced need for myocardial oxygen may reduce the size of the infarction, and this hypothesis is the subject of extensive clinical investigations.

The nursing responsibility when the patient is receiving nitroprusside is directed toward strict monitoring of the circulatory status. Ideally, this is done by observing the internal cardiac pressure readings with a Swan-Ganz catheter. When this method is not available, the standard methods for measuring systemic blood pressure should be used frequently, along with careful assessment of the clinical signs of poor tissue perfusion, such as change in mental status and diminished urinary output.

- Since nitroprusside is a potent vasodilator, hypotension, with inadequate oxygenation of the tissues, is always a potential problem; the nurse must be aware of this complication.

Since the use of nitroprusside is becoming more common in the treatment of congestive failure as a complication of myocardial infarction, the nurse must be familiar with the values and problems associated with the use of this drug and should follow the findings of the clinical results of the testing.

Cardiogenic Shock

Cardiogenic shock (power failure), the end stage of left ventricular dysfunction, occurs when the left ventricle is extensively damaged by myocardial infarction. The heart muscle loses its contractile power and the result is a

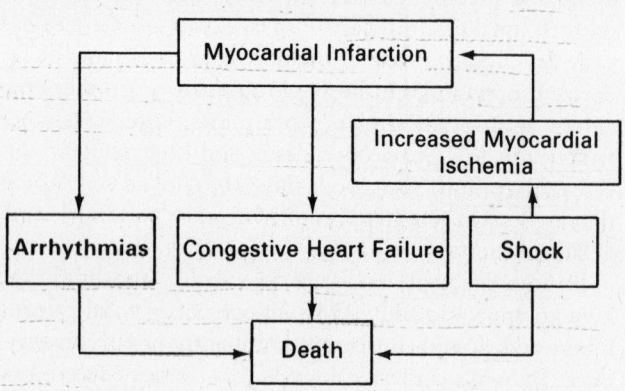

Figure 28-5. Model of interrelationship of complications of myocardial infarction.

marked reduction in cardiac output with decreased perfusion to vital organs (heart, brain, and kidneys). The degree of pump dysfunction is related to the extent of damage to the heart muscle.

Pathophysiology. The symptoms and signs of cardiogenic shock reflect the circular nature of the pathophysiology of the condition. The damage to the myocardium results in a decrease of the cardiac output, which in turn reduces the arterial blood pressure in the vital organs. Flow to the coronary arteries is reduced, and this results in a decrease in the oxygen supply to the myocardium, which in turn increases ischemia and further reduces the heart's ability to pump. Thus, a "vicious cycle" is set in motion.

- The classic signs of cardiogenic shock are low blood pressure, rapid and weak pulse, signs of cerebral anoxia manifested by confusion and agitation, and decreased urinary output.

Arrhythmias are common and result from a decrease of oxygen to the myocardium. As in congestive heart failure, the use of the Swan-Ganz catheter to measure left ventricular pressure is important in assessing the severity of the problem and evaluating management. Continuing elevation of left ventricular end-diastolic pressure (LVEDP) accompanied by a fall in arterial blood pressure indicates the failure of the heart to function as an effective pump.

Management. There are many approaches to the treatment of cardiogenic shock. Any major arrhythmia is corrected, since these may have caused or contributed to the shock. If low intravascular volume is suspected, or found, through pressure readings (i.e., hypovolemia), the patient is treated by infusion of volume expanders. If hypoxia is present, oxygen is given, often under positive pressure when regular flow is insufficient to meet tissue demands.

Drug therapy is selected and guided by cardiac output and mean arterial blood pressure. With respect to specific medications, there continues to be controversy about the best approach. One group of drugs used are the catecholamines, which raise the blood pressure and increase the cardiac output. This, however, tends to increase the workload of the heart, and many studies are currently being done to test vasodilator drugs that impede the resistance to the circulation and thereby reduce the workload of the heart. The latter approach is gaining widespread support.

Other therapeutic modalities employed in treating cardiogenic shock involve the use of circulatory assist devices. The most frequently used mechanical support system is the Intra-aortic balloon pump (IABP) (Fig. 28-6). The IABP uses internal counterpulsation to augment the pumping action of the heart by the regular inflation and deflation of a balloon located in the descending thoracic aorta. The device is connected to a control

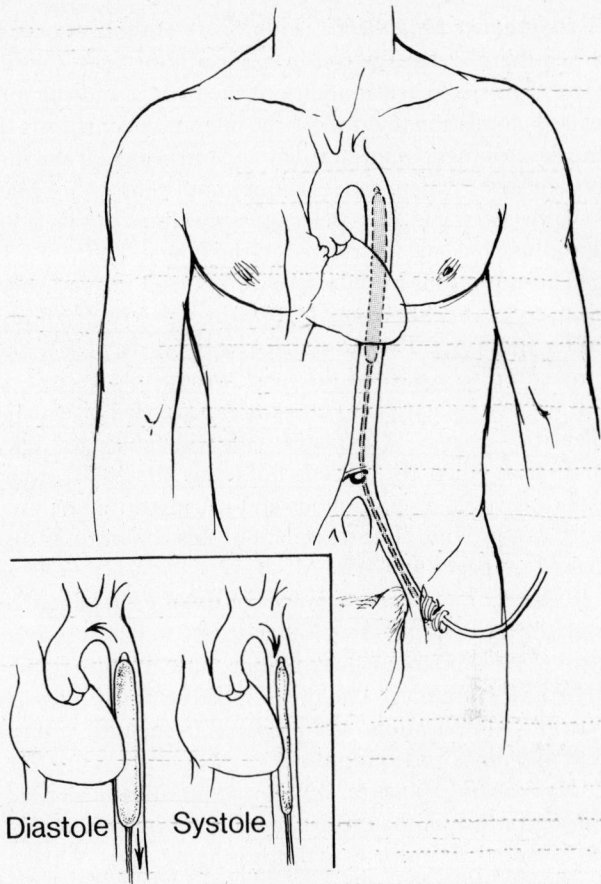

Diastole **Systole**

Figure 28-6. The intra-aortic balloon pump augments diastole which results in increased perfusion of the coronary arteries and myocardium and a decrease in the left ventricular workload.

box that directs its activities by synchronization with the electrocardiogram. Hemodynamic monitoring is also essential to determine the patient's circulatory status during the use of the IABP. The balloon inflates during ventricular diastole and deflates during systole at a rate equal to the heart rate. The IABP augments diastole, which results in increased perfusion of the coronary arteries and myocardium and a decrease in the left ventricular workload. Studies have indicated that prompt use of this method of treatment reduces the mortality rate of patients with cardiogenic shock.

Nursing Implications. Cardiogenic shock, with an untreated mortality of over 90 percent, is described as the most lethal complication of acute myocardial infarction in the hospitalized patient. The patient with this complication requires constant nursing care and observation. Careful assessment and recording of intake and urinary output are essential. The patient must be closely monitored for arrhythmias, which must be corrected immediately.

Other Complications

Pulmonary Embolism. Pulmonary embolism occurs when there is damage to the endocardium from the infarct. The decreased mobility of the patient and the impaired circulation that follow the infarction contribute to the development of intracardiac and intravascular thrombosis. As the patient moves about more, a thrombus may become detached (the detached thrombus is called an embolus) and may be carried to the lungs.

The symptoms of pulmonary embolism include chest pain, cyanosis, shortness of breath, rapid respirations, and hemoptysis. The pulmonary embolus may block the circulation to a part of the lung, producing an area of pulmonary infarction. The pain experienced is usually pleuritic—that is, it increases with respiration and may disappear when the patient holds his breath. Cardiac pain, however, is continuous and usually does not vary with respirations. The treatment of this condition is discussed on pages 490–493.

Systemic embolism may occur from the left ventricle, and the resulting vascular occlusion may present as stroke, renal infarct; it may compromise the blood supply to an extremity. The nurse must be aware of such possible complications and prepared to identify and report any signs and symptoms.

Myocardial Rupture. When an infarction extends through much of the cardiac muscle, the heart may rupture leading to immediate death in most cases. Cardiac rupture, although fairly rare, can occur during the first week following a myocardial infarction.

Death is caused by cardiac tamponade (the heart is bleeding into its pericardial sac); thus, pericardiocentesis (aspiration of the pericardial cavity) and repair of the myocardium can be life-saving measures. The clinician detects this condition by noticing a sudden increase in the distention of the neck veins, a decrease in heart sounds, and a reduction of blood pressure. Pericardiocentesis is performed by placing a long No. 18 needle (spinal needle) just to the left of the xyphoid and directing it under the rib cage to the left shoulder (pages 597–598).

Heart Block. Heart block may follow acute myocardial infarction as a result of damage to the conduction system which may interfere with the normal impulse from the atria to the ventricles. This damage may occur above or below the atrioventricular node, the latter being the more serious. When second or third degree heart blocks are present, the heart rate is slowed and cardiac output is decreased. This may precipitate congestive heart failure, cardiogenic shock and death.

The usual treatment of choice is artificial pacemaking (pages 588–591). Although there continues to be controversy regarding the usefulness of artificial pacing in reducing mortality due to heart block, this treatment is used more and more. The nurse who functions in the CCU must be prepared to care for patients with pacemakers and must be alert to the most common complication, ventricular arrhythmias resulting in cardiac arrest; emergency equipment must be available.

EMERGENCY INTERVENTION IN CARDIAC ARREST

A complication of myocardial infarction that requires immediate action is cardiac arrest. This is a sudden cessation of effective heart action with lack of circulation. In the CCU this is most commonly caused by failure of the electrical conduction system due to the damaged myocardium. (This should be differentiated from cardiogenic shock, page 544, which occurs when the heart has lost its muscular ability to pump.) Most often, cardiac arrest in the CCU is preceded by premature ventricular contractions (PVC) that result in ventricular fibrillation (VF). Ventricular fibrillation is a continuous ineffective

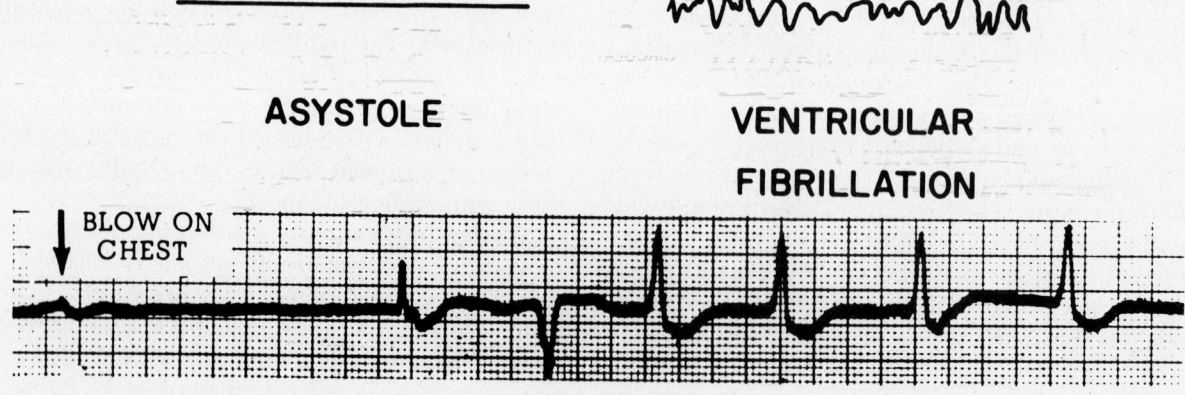

Figure 28-7.   The two principal types of cardiac arrest are indicated. In both cases the heart is not pumping blood into the body tissues. Occasionally a person can have a fairly normal ECG even though the heart is not contracting effectively; this also is termed a cardiac arrest. The electrical impulse in this case is traversing the heart, but the myocardium fails to contract satisfactorily. This is termed electromechanical dissociation.

The ECG shows a patient's heart (asystole) that was started with a sharp blow to the anterior chest wall.

movement of the heart muscle sometimes described as a "quiver."

Diagnosis must be made immediately so that conversion to effective heart action may be accomplished before irreversible cerebral damage is caused by anoxia. The main symptom is immediate loss of consciousness. Other symptoms include absence of carotid or femoral pulses, absence of audible heart signs, absence of breath sounds, convulsions, dilation of pupils, and grey, ashen color. In the CCU, the electrocardiographic monitor will show a waving line in ventricular fibrillation or a flat line in ventricular standstill (see Fig. 28-7).

In a witnessed cardiac arrest, a precordial thump should be attempted. This sharp, quick single blow to the midportion of the sternum will generate a small electrical stimulus which may restore normal beat (Fig. 28-8). If

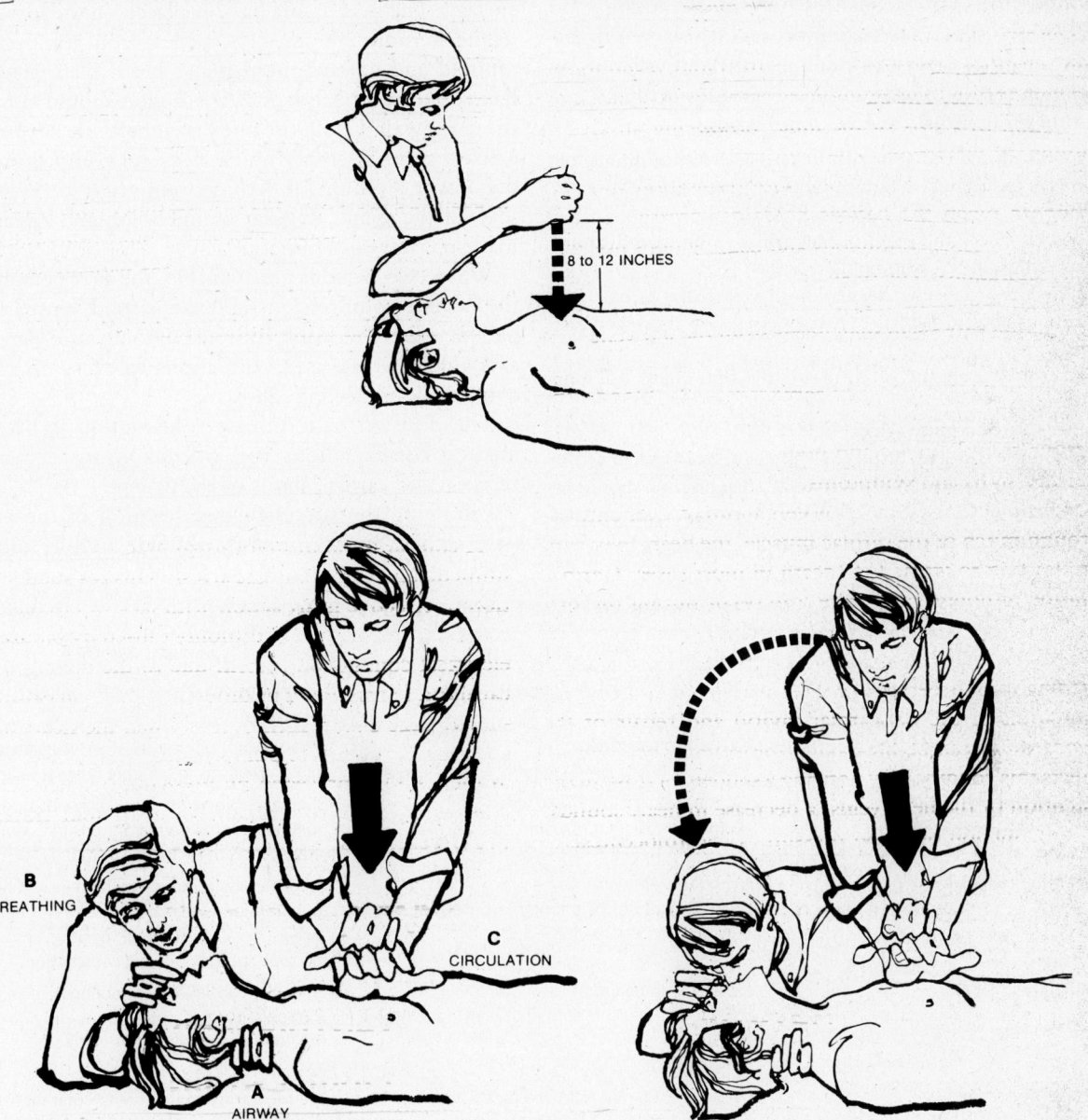

Figure 28-8.   Emergency intervention in cardiac arrest. (*Top*) Precordial thump.
(*Left*) Two-rescuer cardiopulmonary resuscitation:
    5 chest compressions
      Rate of 60/minute
      No pause for ventilation
    1 lung inflation
      After each 5 compressions
      Interposed between compressions
(*Right*) One-rescuer cardiopulmonary resuscitation:
    15 chest compressions (rate of 80/minute)

(Reprinted from the Supplement to Journal of the American Medical Association, Feb. 18, 1974. © The American Medical Association. Reprinted with permission from the American Heart Association)

this is not effective, direct electrical defibrillation should be done. If the equipment is not available, or until it is, supportive cardiopulmonary resuscitation (CPR) should be started. (Electrical defibrillation is discussed on page 536.)

Cardiopulmonary Resuscitation

Basic cardiopulmonary resuscitation (CPR) consists of the following ABC sequence: Airway, Breathing, and Circulation. The resuscitation process consists of maintaining an open airway, providing artificial ventilation by means of rescue breathing, and providing artificial circulation by external cardiac compression.

The recommended approach to cardiac arrest in monitored patients is as follows:
1. Give a single precordial thump (Fig. 28-8).
2. Quickly check the monitor for cardiac rhythm, and simultaneously check carotid pulse.
3. If there is ventricular fibrillation or ventricular tachycardia without a pulse, deliver countershock as soon as possible (see page 536).
4. If the pulse is absent, tilt the head, give four quick, full lung inflations.
5. Check carotid pulse again.
6. If the pulse is absent, begin one-rescuer or two-rescuer CPR.

Note: It must be emphasized strongly that no time should be lost by waiting to assess the results of the precordial thump or by delivering repeated precordial thumps.

The first step in CPR is to open an airway. Remove any material from the airway, tilt the head back, and pull the jaw forward. Insert an oropharyngeal airway if available. Ventilate the patient 12 breaths per minute using direct mouth-to-mouth breathing or by using the bag and mask technique.

The next step after ventilation is external cardiac compression. This must be done with the patient on a firm surface. The heel of one hand is placed on the lower half of the sternum 3.8 cm. (1½ inches) from the tip of the xiphoid and toward the patient's head. Place the other hand on top of the first one. The fingers should not touch the chest wall. Using the body weight while keeping the elbows straight, apply quick, forceful compressions to the lower sternum, 3.8 to 5.0 cm. (1½ to 2 inches) toward the spine. Regular compression and release are made 60 times per minute.

When two persons are available, the first person does the cardiac compressions and the second ventilates the patient after five compressions. If only one person is available, the rate is 2 ventilations to every 15 cardiac compressions (see Fig. 28-8).

The decision to terminate resuscitation is based on medical considerations and will take into account the cerebral and cardiac status of the patient.

Following the successful resuscitation of the patient with cardiac arrest, the nurse should carefully monitor

TABLE 28-1.   ESSENTIAL EMERGENCY DRUGS FOR RESUSCITATION

DRUG	ROUTE AND DOSAGE	EFFECTS AND USES
atropine sulfate	I.V. bolus, 0.5 mg., may repeat	Decreases vagal tone in pronounced bradycardia.
calcium chloride	I.V. bolus, intracardiac 1 Gm. (10 ml. of a 10% solution), may repeat	Positive inotrope for asystole; increases force of contractions in a feebly beating heart.
dopamine HCl (Intropin)	I.V. infusion at 5 mcg./kg./min. up to 20 to 50 mcg./kg./min.	Increases blood pressure and perfusion; maintains renal perfusion; positive inotropic effect; increases cardiac output.
epinephrine HCl (Adrenalin)	I.V. bolus, intracardiac 0.5 to 1 mg. (5 to 10 ml. of a 1:10,000 solution), may repeat	Asystole, ventricular fibrillation (with bicarbonate); increases amplitude of fibrillatory waves, positive inotrope, positive chronotrope, peripheral vasoconstriction.
isoproterenol (Isuprel)	I.V. bolus, intracardiac 0.2 mg. I.V. infusion titrated to heart rate, blood pressure 2 mg./500 ml. D_5W	Asystole, cardiovascular collapse; positive inotrope, positive chronotrope, increases cardiac output and blood pressure.
lidocaine (Xylocaine)	I.V. bolus: 100 mg. followed by I.V. infusion 1 to 2 Gm. in 500-ml. D_5W at 2 to 3 mg./min.	Ventricular irritability, ventricular tachycardia, PVCs, raises fibrillation threshold.
metaraminol (Aramine)	I.M.: 2 to 10 mg.; I.V.: 15 to 100 mg. in 500-ml. D_5W/NSS	Vasopressor increases peripheral resistance, improves cardiac contractility and cardiac, cerebral, and renal blood flow.
norepinephrine levarterenol (Levophed)	I.V. infusion titrated to blood pressure, 2 to 4 ampuls in 500-ml. D_5W	Vasopressor, increases peripheral pressure and perfusion.
sodium bicarbonate 50 mEq. (8.4%, 50-ml. solution)	I.V. bolus, 1 mEq./kg. initially, repeat in 10 minutes if necessary. Further doses based on blood-gas analysis. If tests unavailable, use ½ initial dose evey 10 minutes.	Reverse metabolic acidosis; facilitates defibrillation (with epinephrine).

the patient's condition, since he is at great risk for another cardiac arrest. Continuation of ECG monitoring is essential and any abnormalities of rhythm must be corrected. Electrolyte and acid-base balances must be established and maintained. Hemodynamic monitoring should be initiated if it was not previously instituted. Selected drugs are used during and after resuscitation (see Table 28-1), and these should be immediately available in the cardiac care unit.

The nurse who works in the CCU must be aware that patients who witness a cardiac arrest are very distressed by the experience and often exhibit anger or lack of identification with the victim. Both are useful defense mechanisms. Following such an event, there may be an increase in patient requests for sedation, and these should be met, if compatible with the individual patient's total condition.

PSYCHOLOGICAL PROBLEMS IN THE CARDIAC CARE UNIT

During the Acute Phase

Of great concern to the nurse in the CCU are the psychological problems of the patient with a myocardial infarction. Problems that are apt to occur early in the hospitalization can be recognized and in some instances prevented. In this regard, the nurse helps the patient and his family to cope with such difficulties. It has been suggested that the typical patient reacts to an MI with a pattern of four basic responses — anxiety, denial, depression, and chronic behavioral traits (Fig. 28-9).

Anxiety. Anxiety occurs early in the CCU and, in fact, is probably pronounced at the time of admission.

Such fears are caused by the prospect of death or by the symptoms which may herald death, such as breathlessness, severe chest pains and complications of the MI (arrhythmias, cardioversion, or pacemaker insertion). The patient is "scared" and fears death, pain, and the strange environment. Although the patient may appear tense, restless, and watchful, he may or may not voice his feelings and uneasiness. The nurse should explain all interventions to the patient and provide reassurance by accenting positive factors in the situation. Medications for pain relief and sedation are given as frequently as needed.

Denial. The second predictable psychological reaction is denial, which usually appears on the second or third day of hospitalization and may be either conscious or unconscious. The patient may begin to deny that he ever had a heart attack, or he may say that the diagnosis is incorrect. There is controversy regarding the usefulness of this defense mechanism. Nurses caring for these patients are aware that denial is a common reaction that accounts for the calm nature of the patient even when his condition is serious. It is not considered helpful to the patient to insist that he is being foolish in his denial. Nonetheless, the nurse should be honest in explaining the patient's condition to him in order to establish the reality of the situation.

Depression. Depression is the expected response on the third or fourth post MI day and occurs soon after denial, when the reality of the illness has set in. At this time, the patient has often passed the critical stage and is beginning to evaluate the changes in life style which the illness could cause. Changes in self-concept and self-perception, concerns about earning or living or fulfilling former role requirements, and doubts about the ability to

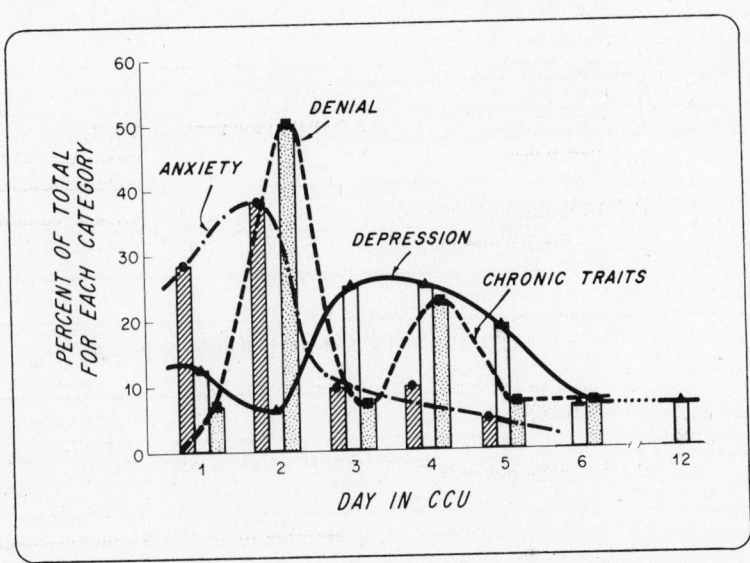

Figure 28-9. Hypothetical schedule of onset of emotional and behavioral reactions of a coronary care unit (CCU) patient. (© Reprinted with permission, American Heart Association)

resume the usual activities of living may trouble the patient. It is interesting to note that women experience depression in a less acute manner than male patients. The best approach of the nurse during this period is to listen carefully to the problems expressed by the patient and to answer questions and concerns as honestly as possible.

Chronic Behavioral Traits. Following depression, the patient often exhibits chronic traits which may be manifested in behavior problems. One of the more se-rious problems is the patient who wants to discharge himself from the hospital against the advice of his physician. This may be attributed to the fact that the patient believes he is not seriously ill. He may still be in a denial state and may complain about being in the CCU. Often, *"significant others"* (wife, clergy, children) may be able to convince the patient that remaining in the unit is in his best interest. Other behavior problems often relate to overt sexual comments or actions directed to the nursing

---

TEACHING GUIDE FOR MYOCARDIAL INFARCTION PATIENTS IN THE CORONARY CARE UNIT

	TAUGHT BY NURSE	UNDERSTANDING DEMONSTRATED BY PATIENT*
	(Check when done)	
1. TRANSFER:	—	—
a. Emphasize that transfer is a sign of progress.		
b. Discuss the average length of stay in this coronary care unit (CCU) and in this hospital after myocardial infarction (MI).		
c. Explain criteria for transfer and when transfers usually occur.		
d. Discuss whether or not monitoring will be continued.		
e. Describe what occurs during the transfer process.		
2. UNIT TO WHICH PATIENT WILL BE TRANSFERRED:	—	—
a. Inform the patient of the location of the new unit.		
b. Describe the type of room (private, semi-private, or ward), location of bathrooms, and TV and telephone use.		
c. Discuss liberalization of visiting privileges.		
3. PHYSICIANS:	—	—
a. Identify which physicians will see patient after transfer.		
b. Explain how to contact physician after transfer.		
4. NURSES:	—	—
a. Identify the nurses and describe their specialized training in the care of the MI patient after transfer.		
b. Explain the change in nurse-patient ratio from CCU to new unit.		
c. List what symptoms and/or feelings to report to the nurse.		
5. REST, ACTIVITY, AND REHABILITATION:	—	—
a. Advise that some patients feel anxious or depressed after transfer and that these feelings are normal.		
b. Explain the importance of continuing rest.		
c. Explain the level of self-care activity patient can expect at transfer and for remainder of hospitalization.		
d. Discuss the educational program available to patients and to families in the unit to which transfer will occur.		

*by repeating information back to the nurse

(Chart courtesy of Jean Toth, RN, MSN, CCRN)

staff by male patients. These expressions may reflect anxiety related to threats to the male role and should be managed with understanding.

Relationship to Transfer

The patient must be prepared for transfer from the specialized care of the coronary care unit to a nursing unit where he will be more independent. The patient to nurse ratio in the nonacute setting is much higher, and the patient may feel more vulnerable. Symptoms of stress may occur, including insomnia, arrhythmias, and possible extension of the infarction. Increased urine catecholamines, suggesting increased stress, have been found in transfer patients. Efforts are currently being made by the nursing staff of the CCU to prepare the patient for transfer. The chart on page 550 is a teaching guide designed to orient coronary care patients to changes both in the environment and in the care that they will receive in the progressive care unit. The care of the patient after transfer from the CCU is discussed on pages 575-577.

Related Stress Problems of Nursing Staff

Nurses working in the CCU frequently report high levels of stress. Although many reasons for this reaction have been identified, the chief cause probably is the continual care of critically ill patients who need constant supervision. Other sources of stress that are cited are overwhelming workloads, too much responsibility, poor communication with physicians and staff in other units, limited work area, and inadequate continuing education programs. This high stress level found in the CCU often causes a high "turnover" rate among the nursing staff, which can prove costly to the institution because of the expense involved in preparing a nurse to function in the unit. One of the best methods of dealing with stress in the CCU is recognition of the potential sources of stress through open group discussions in unit conferences, inservice education, and other similar activities. Consideration of the emotional needs of the nursing staff is essential for maintaining a therapeutic environment that will ensure good care of the patient with a myocardial infarction.

BIBLIOGRAPHY

BOOKS

Andreoli, K. G., et al.: Comprehensive Cardiac Care, 4th ed. St. Louis, C. V. Mosby, 1979.

Bolooki, H.: Clinical Application of Intra-Aortic Balloon Pump. Mount Kisco, N.Y., Futura Publishing Co., 1977.

Cromwell, R. L., et al.: Acute Myocardial Infarction, Reaction and Recovery. St. Louis, C. V. Mosby, 1977.

Foster, W. T.: Principles of Acute Coronary Care. New York, Appleton-Century-Crofts, 1976.

Gentry, W. D., and Williams, R. B.: Psychological Aspects of Myocardial Infarction and Coronary Care. St. Louis, C. V. Mosby, 1975.

Hamilton, A. J.: Selected Subjects for Critical Care Nurses. Missoula, Mont., Mountain Press Publishing Co., 1975.

Hamilton, W. P., and Lavin, M. A.: Decision Making in the Coronary Care Unit. St. Louis, C. V. Mosby, 1976.

Hurst, J. W.: The Heart. New York, McGraw-Hill, 1978.

Malasanos, L., et al.: Health Assessment. St. Louis, C. V. Mosby, 1977.

Mason, D. T.: Cardiac Emergencies. Baltimore, Williams and Wilkins, 1978.

Pantridge, J. F., et al.: The Acute Coronary Attack. New York, Grune and Stratton, 1975.

Stephenson, H. E.: Cardiac Arrest and Resuscitation. St. Louis, C. V. Mosby, 1974.

Turner, G. O.: The Cardiovascular Care Unit, A Guide for Planning and Operation. New York, John Wiley and Sons, 1978.

ARTICLES

Cassem, N. H., and Hackett, T. P.: Psychological rehabilitation of myocardial infarction patients in the acute phase. Heart & Lung, 2:382-388, May-June 1973.

Eckhardt, E.: Intra-aortic balloon counterpulsation in cardiogenic shock. Heart & Lung, 6:93-98, Jan.-Feb. 1977.

Manzi, C.: Cardiac emergency. How to use drugs and CPR to save lives. Nursing '78, 8:30-39, Mar. 1978.

Preston, T. A.: The use of pacemaking for the treatment of acute arrhythmias. Heart & Lung, 6:249-255, Mar.-Apr. 1977.

Rogove, H. J., et al.: Cardiopulmonary resuscitation (CPR) in the hospital. Cardiovasc. Nurs., 13:6-12, Mar.-Apr. 1977.

Tanner, G.: Heart failure in the patient. AJN, 77:230-234, Feb. 1977.

Toth, J. E.: Effect of structured preparation for transfer on patient anxiety after leaving coronary care unit. Unpublished manuscript, Catholic University of America, Washington, D.C. 1978.

Walinsky, P.: Acute hemodynamic monitoring. Heart & Lung, 6:838-844, Sept.-Oct. 1977.

Winslow, E. H.: A symposium on teaching and rehabilitating the cardiac patient. Nurs. Clin. N. Am., 11:211-383, June 1976.

Ziesche, S., and Franciosa, J.: Clinical application of sodium nitroprusside. Heart & Lung, 6:99-103, Jan.-Feb. 1977.

29

MANAGEMENT OF THE CARDIOVASCULAR SURGERY PATIENT

STRIDES IN CARDIOVASCULAR SURGERY

Each historical event of any consequence depends upon a chain of events which precedes it; thus each era of cardiovascular surgery stands upon the successes and failures of a previous era. The triumphs of interpleural thoracic surgery in the 1930s, which led to safe anesthesia and the use of adequate blood transfusion, were followed by the surgical procedures for the treatment of ductus arteriosus and coarctation of the aorta. Most of the common inborn heart defects and many of the more rare forms as well, can be treated by corrective or palliative operations today.

In the 1940s there were successes with closed mitral valve repairs. Out of this era came recognition of a need for grafts of artificial materials and the design of mechanical valve prostheses. The development and use of cardiac catheterization led to precise information about hemodynamic states within the heart. Improved radiologic techniques led to visualization of the size and shape of cardiac cavities and vascular channels. During this decade aortic valves also were successfully repaired. Hypothermia was used to increase the operating time upon the open heart. This was an important stage prior to the development and successful employment of the heart-lung machine in the early 1950s.

Throughout the decade of the fifties, numerous groups of surgeons and engineers worked diligently to perfect the heart-lung machine. Bubble oxygenators, vertical screens, and rotating discs have been used. The membrane oxygenator now being used allows for more prolonged use of the heart-lung machine. While these devices were being perfected, simplified, and redesigned to meet current needs, the catheterization of coronary arteries and injection with small amounts of contrast medium was being developed to detect the localization of obstructive or constrictive lesions. The perfection of this cineangiocardiographic technique led to the events of the 1960s which remain outstanding today.

It was during the late 1960s that a number of surgeons performed the saphenous vein-coronary artery bypass procedure in an attempt to enhance the quality and quantity of life for persons crippled by the effects of ischemia and angina. In order to restore adequate or improved blood flow to ischemic hearts, it is estimated that over 100,000 aortocoronary bypass grafts were performed in the United States by 1974. During the same time sequence, the first cardiac transplantation was performed.

A review of cardiovascular surgery in the 1970s shows that aortocoronary bypass grafting has escalated to the extent that in less than a decade it has involved more than 400,000 patients. Serious questions have been raised which leave the medical profession in the throes of weighing the benefits and the risks of this surgery and of determining who the recipient should be and whether the surgery should be performed in selected centers. Because of a renewed national emphasis on cost controls for health care and the relatively high expense of cardiovascular surgery, the efficacy of bypass surgery continues to be debated, and specific criteria have been recommended. Heart transplantation serves a small population. Moral and ethical questions are being addressed more aggressively, in terms of human experimentation. Problems associated with immunologic response are being resolved slowly, but the supply versus the demand of donor hearts leaves scientists in the late 1970s experimenting with alternatives.

With the perfection and simplification of assistive devices such as the intra-aortic balloon, patients' hearts have been "rested" to provide healing time by diminishing workload. The search for a mechanical heart is ongoing. A partial artificial heart, the left ventricular assist device (LVAD), is being tried as a compromise designed to relieve the ailing heart on a short-term basis (see Fig. 29-1). This device consists of a plastic pump that contains valves from the heart of a pig and is electrically powered by a bedside console. It allows the ailing heart to rest and regain its strength and shows potential for use in the initial critical period following open-heart surgery.

The Report of the Inter-Society Commission for Heart Disease Resources (1975) indicates the scope of cardiac surgery. See Table 29-1 which has been adapted from this report.

Intra-aortic balloon counterpulsation (IABC) has proved most effective when employed as a protective adjunct during stressful diagnostic and therapeutic procedures in instances in which myocardial tissue is temporarily but reversibly injured.

Although IABC alone has not improved the prognosis of cardiogenic shock following myocardial infarction, it has been beneficial when used during surgical procedures to increase survival when the patient has suffered an acute MI. It is used as an assistive device prior to, during, and following surgery.

The number of cardiac transplants performed has increased since 1968. The criteria for transplantation restrict selection to those patients who are incapacitated and who face the prospect of imminent death. Cardiac transplants are absolutely contraindicated in patients with intercurrent infection or a pulmonary vascular resistance greater than 10 units; patients with diabetes dependent on insulin are usually not considered for surgery.

The cause of death in patients with transplanted hearts can be rejection, acute or chronic pulmonary hypertension or rheumatic fever, infection, cerebral vascular accident (CVA), and coronary artery disease of the transplanted heart.

Some patients return to work. One five-year survivor works eight hours a day.

1 year survival rate	43 percent
2 year survival rate	39 percent

Among patients operated on in 1973-1974, the survival rate was 50 percent in the first year.

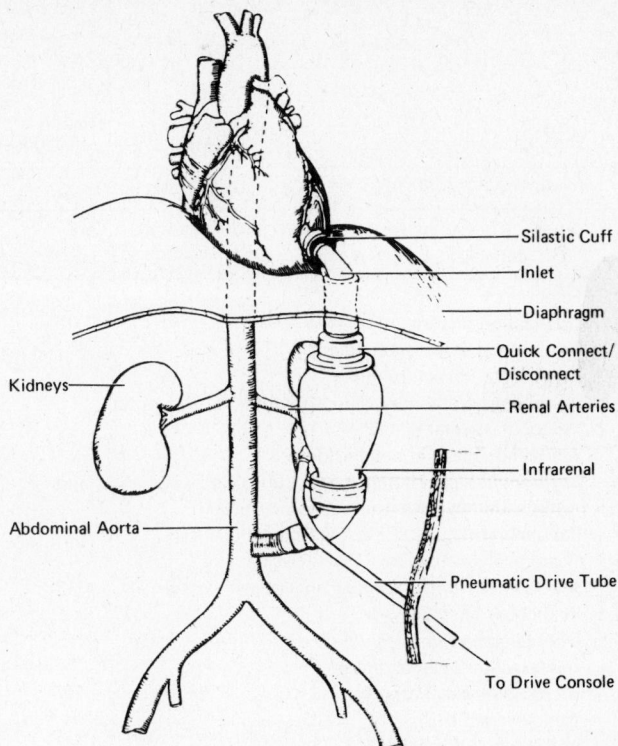

Figure 29-1. Left ventricular assist device.

CARDIOVASCULAR PROCEDURES

Cardiovascular surgery has been performed to increase the life spans and activity levels of many individuals who would otherwise have died or been very restricted in life style. The treatment of coronary artery disease has made marked advances since the development of selective coronary angiography to document anatomical defects of the coronary arteries. This diagnostic technique has proved to be a safe and reliable method for pinpointing lesions of the coronary arteries, valve defects, and left ventricular function.

Cardiopulmonary Bypass

Many of the cardiac surgical procedures are performed while the patient is placed on partial or complete cardiopulmonary bypass (extracorporeal circulation — meaning "outside the body"). In this procedure, the patient is placed on a machine which consists of a mechanical pump that simulates the pumping action of the left ventricle and an oxygenator that simulates the function of the lungs. The blood is removed from the systemic circulation via cannulas inserted into the inferior and superior venae cavae. By means of the force of gravity or with the aid of a pump, the blood enters the venous reservoir and is then filtered, passed through the oxygenator and heat exchanger, and returned to the patient via a cannula in the ascending aorta or the femoral artery.

TABLE 29-1.   SCOPE OF CARDIAC SURGERY

A.   CONGENITAL DISEASE OF THE HEART AND GREAT VESSELS

1. CONDITIONS FOR WHICH SURGICAL PROCEDURES ARE ESTABLISHED	2. CONGENITAL DISORDERS FOR WHICH PROCEDURES ARE BEING DEVELOPED
Patent ductus arteriosus	Single ventricle
Coarctation of aorta	Atresia of aortic isthmus
Atrial septal defect (secundum)	Underdeveloped right ventricle
Atrial septal defect (primum)	Taussig-Bing complex
Anomalous pulmonary venous return (total and partial)	Ebstein's anomaly
Ventricular septal defect	
Atrioventricularis communis defect	
Aortic stenosis (including valvar, subvalvar, supravalvar, and idiopathic hypertrophic subaortic stenosis)	
Pulmonary stenosis (including infundibular and supravalvar stenosis)	
Tetrology of Fallot (including anatomical variants)	
Pulmonary atresia	
Double outlet right ventricle	
Transposition of great arteries	
Tricuspid atresia	
Truncus arteriosus	
Aortal septal defect	
Mitral stenosis	
Mitral insufficiency	
Congenital origin of left coronary artery from pulmonary artery	
Coronary arteriovenous fistula	
Wolff-Parkinson-White syndrome	

B.   ACQUIRED DISEASE OF THE HEART AND GREAT VESSELS

1. CONDITIONS FOR WHICH SURGICAL PROCEDURES ARE ESTABLISHED	2. PROCEDURES WITH UNCERTAIN FUTURE
Constrictive pericarditis	Allotransplantation of the heart
Heart block	Prosthetic replacement of the heart
Mitral stenosis	
Mitral regurgitation	
Aortic stenosis	
Aortic regurgitation	
Ventricular aneurysm	
Ventricular septal defect	
Coronary bypass grafts for arterial reconstruction	
Myocardial trauma (cardiac rupture)	
Traumatic rupture of aorta	
Fusiform and saccular thoracic aneurysms	
Dissecting aortic aneurysm	
Tricuspid stenosis	
Tricuspid insufficiency	
Aneurysm of sinus of Valsalva (with or without fistula)	
Massive pulmonary embolism (acute and chronic)	
Resection of dyskinetic areas of myocardium (for cardiac failure or focus of arrhythmia)	

Report of the Inter-Society Commission for Heart Disease Resources:
   Optimal resources for cardiac surgery, guidelines for program planning and evaluation.
   Circulation, 52:A23-A37, Nov. 1975.

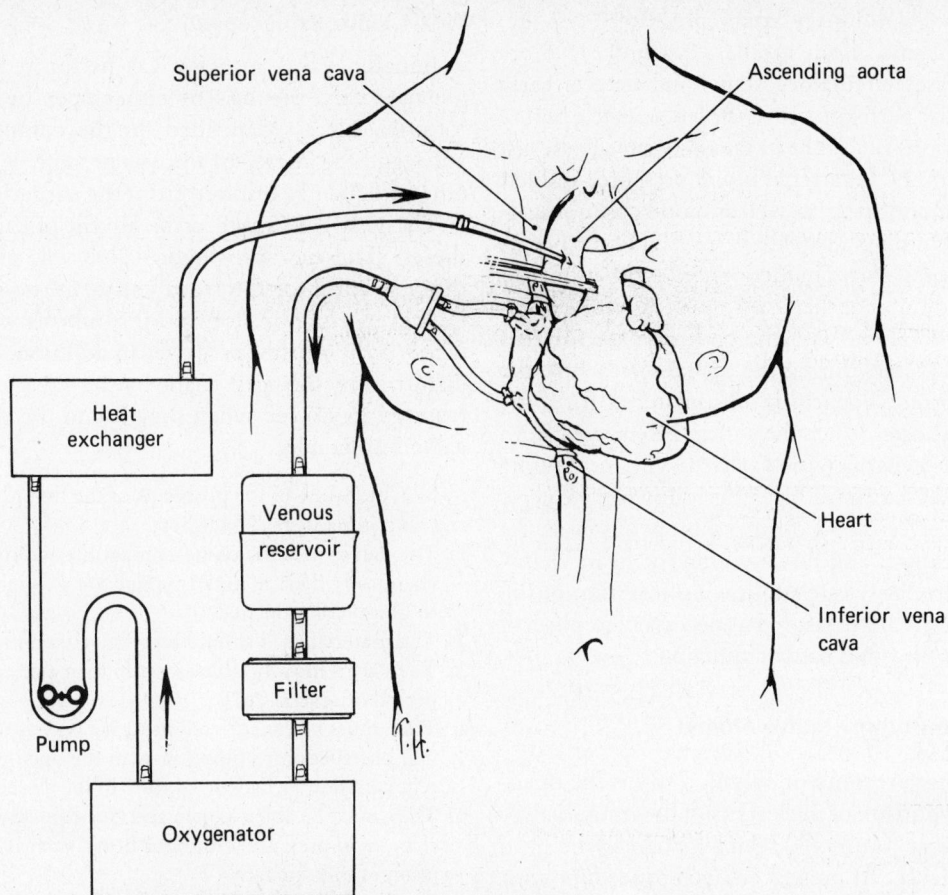

Figure 29-2.   Schematic drawing of the heart-lung bypass.

The oxygenated blood is used by the tissues of the body and then returned to the pump or heart-lung machine where the process is once again repeated (Fig. 29-2).

At present there are four types of oxygenators used in cardiopulmonary bypass: (1) the screen oxygenator, (2) the disc oxygenator, (3) the bubble oxygenator, and (4) the membrane oxygenator.

The screen oxygenator provides gas exchange by filming the blood in thin layers over stainless steel screens enclosed in a plastic case. The blood is pumped to the top of the oxygenator whence it then flows down the sides of the screen by gravity and is oxygenated by the gas to which it is exposed.

The disc oxygenator uses rotating discs instead of screens. The discs continually rotate through blood collected in the bottom of the cylinder. As the blood flows over the discs it picks up oxygen which enters a side port of the cylinder.

The bubble oxygenator bubbles oxygen through a long column of blood in a chamber. The blood is foamy when it reaches the top of the chamber and is defoamed when it passes over steel wool or a polypropylene mesh with a silicone antifoam compound on its surface.

The membrane oxygenator uses a semipermeable membrane which separates blood from gas containing oxygen, eliminating direct blood gas interface which occurs in the other oxygenators. Oxygen diffuses across the membrane into the blood in a manner similar to the physiologic process which takes place between the alveoli and capillaries in the lungs. This type of oxygenator is widely used today in all medical centers, since it provides effective gas exchange and allows prolonged cardiopulmonary bypass without many of the complications that can be encountered, such as damage to blood cells.

In treating acquired heart disease, most of the procedures are performed through a midline sternotomy incision. Prior to induction of anesthesia, an indwelling catheter is placed in the patient's bladder to accurately assess urinary output. A rectal probe and an esophageal probe are inserted (after induction) to record temperature. The patient's ECG is continuously monitored and displayed. The arterial blood pressure is measured by means of an arterial catheter and the venous pressure via a CVP catheter (page 516). A Swan-Ganz catheter (flow-directed balloon-tipped catheter) may also be in place to measure pulmonary artery pressures (systolic, diastolic, mean, and mean capillary wedge). It more accurately assesses circulatory status and detects early changes in cardiac performance of the left ventricle before overt complications such as heart failure occur. These last three parameters: ECG, arterial blood pressure, and left atrial pressure monitoring, as well as blood gas monitoring, aid in determining adequate peripheral tissue perfusion during bypass. After induction and intubation, the patient is placed on a mechanical ventilator by the anesthesiologist, who along with the perfusionist monitors all of these parameters during the operation. Before the cannula is inserted, heparin is administered for anticoagulation purposes. When the patient is removed from the bypass, the heparin is neutralized with protamine sulfate to prevent excessive bleeding following surgery. The patient receives blood during the operation as the need arises. Pressures and flows within the heart chambers and the coronary vessels following insertion of the vein or artery graft are measured as necessary to observe adequate blood flow and cardiac function.

Mitral Commissurotomy (Valvulotomy)

Mitral commissurotomy or valvulotomy is the opening of the fused portion of the leaflets of the mitral valve. The fusion is most commonly seen in patients who have had rheumatic fever. At present an open procedure with cardiopulmonary bypass is more widely performed since it provides the surgeon with a better view of the valve.

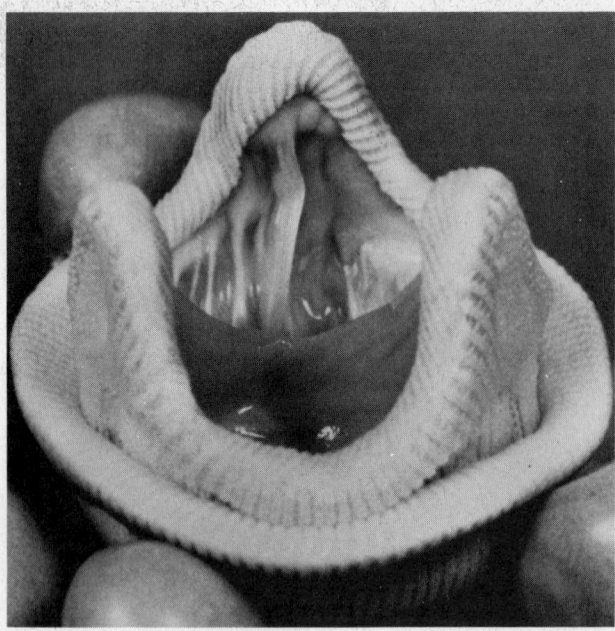

Figure 29-3. Porcine heart valve.

Heart Valve Replacement

Initially, valve surgery was performed primarily to alleviate valve stenosis by either open or closed valvulotomy. Success depended on the competency of the valve and the degree of fibrosis present. Valve incompetency frequently resulted from the surgery.

The year 1954 marked the advent of caged ball prostheses. The first prosthetic valve was inserted in the thoracic aorta for the treatment of aortic regurgitation. However, embolization and thrombosis were disadvantages of the prosthetic valve. In addition, patients were disturbed by the noise made by the valve and some even resorted to suicide when they found the clicking of the valve intolerable.

To avoid some of the problems of the first prosthetic valves, certain criteria were established:
1. The valves must be tissue-compatible and must be made of chemically inert materials which are reasonably atraumatic to blood components.
2. The material used should be relatively nonthrombogenic.
3. The valves must be able to retain their size and shape over a period of several years.
4. They must be constructed in such a way as to present minimal obstruction to blood flow in the open position and no regurgitation or backward flow in the closed position.
5. They must be able to open and close quickly in response to changes of pressure within the heart, such as take place with changes in heart rate.
6. They must be secured in an area that is accessible and must remain secure for a period of several years.
7. They should function quietly so as not to disturb the patient or require any appreciable modification of the patient's life style.

More recently, valves have been devised from biological tissue. Xenografts (grafts from a species other than man) have been made using porcine or bovine heart valves (Fig. 29-3). These valves have been shown to be effective in patients with clotting problems.

MITRAL VALVE REPLACEMENT. Mitral valve replacement is recommended for patients with mitral valve disease when they begin to develop persistent symptoms during normal or less than normal activity. When patients find that they are requiring more and more frequent rest periods in order to accomplish their usual tasks and must alter their way of life to cope with daily activities, surgical intervention may be advised, but only after a prolonged trial of maximal medical therapy with drugs such as digitalis and diuretics.

AORTIC VALVE REPLACEMENT. Patients with aortic stenosis or insufficiency due to any cause usually lead an asymptomatic life followed by an abrupt onset of symptoms which tend to be incapacitating.

In aortic stenosis the clinical manifestations are angina, syncope, and congestive heart failure. The average life expectancy after the development of the major symptoms of aortic stenosis is about 3 or 4 years. Left ventricular failure is a late and ominous symptom. There is a 5 to 20 percent incidence of sudden death in patients with aortic stenosis.

Patients with aortic insufficiency are less prone to die suddenly. They have a long period before becoming symptomatic. Left ventricular failure is more common than in aortic stenosis and usually progresses slowly. Life expectancy is about 6 years following onset of failure as opposed to 4 years following onset of angina.

Aortic valve replacement is recommended as an elective procedure when a patient with aortic stenosis or regurgitation develops significant symptoms of angina, syncope, or congestive failure. It is felt, however, that better long-term results with prosthetic valve replacement can be achieved if surgery is performed earlier in the disease, before severe irreversible left ventricular dysfunction occurs.

Repair of Traumatic Lesions of the Heart

Traumatic lesions of the heart are becoming more common as accidents due to high speed transportation increase and crime rates rise. A wide variety of injuries are possible, such as laceration of a coronary artery or rupture of the chordae tendineae, papillary muscles, or valve cusps (blunt, nonpenetrating injuries). Survival from penetrating injuries such as gunshot or stab wounds depends largely on the location of the injury, the size of the wound, and the availability of emergency medical and surgical management of cardiac tamponade and/or shock.

Pericardiectomy

Pericardiectomy is performed to remove tight adhesions which constrict the outflow of blood from the cardiac chambers. As the constriction becomes tighter there may also be a reduction in venous return. Constrictive pericarditis can develop following an inflammation of the pericardium. Removal of the pericardial sac is done very gently and slowly. The left ventricle is freed first, so that the increased flow to the right side of the heart is prevented from overloading the lungs and causing pulmonary edema. This method also allows the left ventricle to accommodate to the increased load that it will receive as the constriction is removed.

Removal of Cardiac Tumors

Cardiac tumors, especially primary tumors, are rare. The most common benign tumor is the myxoma, which is an intercavitary tumor that is formed on a stalk, or pedicle. It is often difficult to diagnose myxomas because of their similarity to thrombi. However, successful removal of these tumors has been achieved. The most

common malignant primary tumor of the heart is sarcoma. Secondary malignant tumors of the heart are usually due to metastasis from a primary lesion elsewhere in the body.

Embolectomy

Embolectomy can be performed to remove pulmonary emboli that may originate when a blood clot breaks away from the wall of a vessel, as in thrombophlebitis. The clot travels to the lung via the venous circulation and lodges in the pulmonary artery or one of its branches. When it obstructs blood flow to the lungs, a life-threatening situation exists. If the patient develops refractory shock, removal of the clot or clots may be attempted by placing the patient on cardiopulmonary bypass. An incision is made in the pulmonary artery and the clot is extracted. Following the closing of the artery, the vena cava is ligated to prevent further clots from entering the pulmonary circulation.

Ascending Aorta Repair

Diseases of the ascending aorta, primarily aneurysms, are surgically repaired by cross clamping the area above the aneurysm, removing the diseased or affected portion, and replacing it with a teflon or dacron graft.

Coronary Artery Revascularization

Coronary artery revascularization is indicated in coronary artery disease when there is evidence that severe arteriosclerotic disease is causing incapacitating angina which is refractory to medical therapy. A series of surgical procedures has been established. One of the first was the Vineburg procedure, an indirect method of implanting the internal mammary artery into the ischemic myocardium. As with any collateral circulation, a period of time had to be allowed for the development of increased blood flow to the area of the diseased coronary arteries following the operation. Although the Vineburg procedure has largely been replaced by direct methods, it served as a beginning for the development of other significant procedures. A modification was subsequently made in the Vineburg procedure using multiple myocardial tunnels for implantation of four or five branches of the left internal mammary arteries.

The saphenous vein coronary artery bypass graft procedure (CABG), a direct method, provides a means of prompt myocardial perfusion. Suturing a segment of reversed saphenous vein and anastomosing it to the side of the involved coronary artery, below the site of the occlusion where there is good distal run-off, provides for immediate coronary revascularization. Since more than one coronary artery may be involved, the procedure may

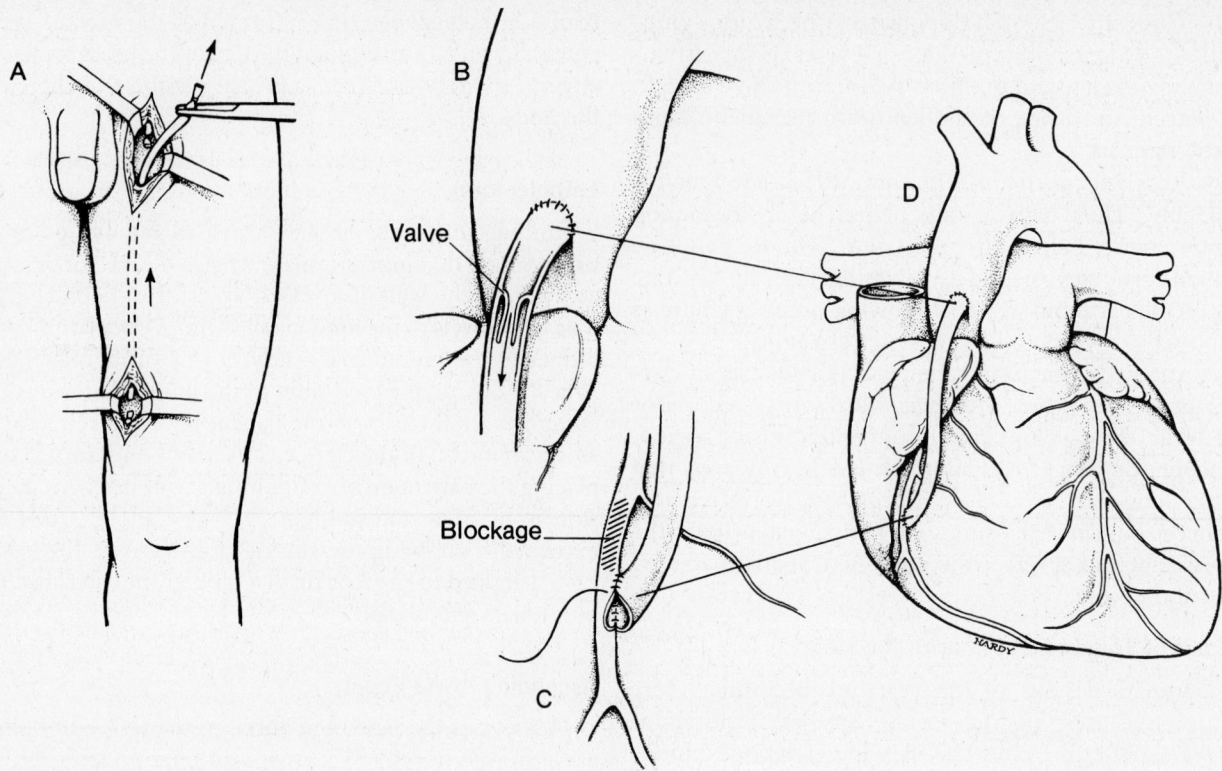

Figure 29-4. Saphenous vein revascularization procedure. (A) Saphenous vein is removed from the patient's leg. The vein is reversed so that valves will not interfere with blood flow. (B) The distal end of vein is sutured to the ascending aorta. (C) At a point distal to the blockage, the vein is sutured to the coronary artery by end-to-end anastomosis. (D) The completed bypass reestablishes the flow distal to the blockage.

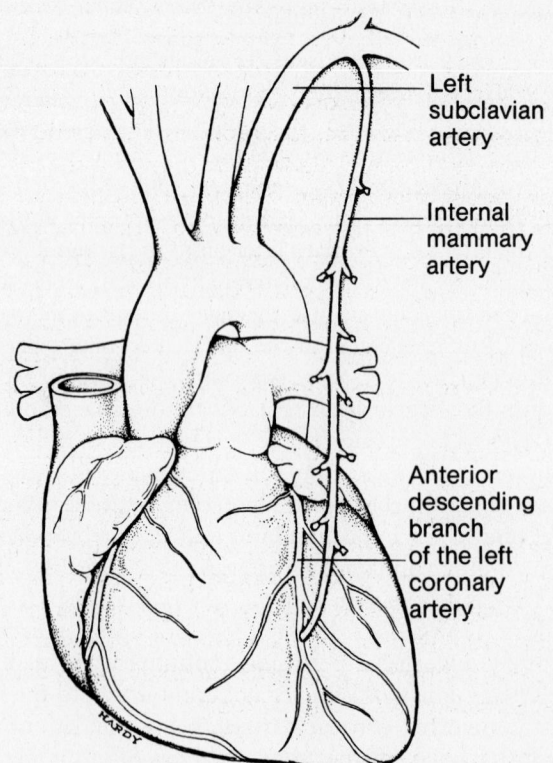

Figure 29-5. Mammary artery revascularization procedure, showing mammary artery anastomosis to the anterior descending branch of the left coronary artery.

involve placement of two, three, or more grafts (see Fig. 29-4).

Another direct procedure uses the internal mammary artery in bypass grafting rather than or in addition to the saphenous vein (Fig. 29-5). This method promises to have a patency rate superior to that of the vein grafts. However, it is a more time-consuming procedure and it is difficult to bring the mammary artery to portions of the right coronary artery that need revascularization. The most suitable procedure for the individual patient is determined by the location of the lesions as shown by precise angiography.

Selection of the patient for coronary artery revascularization should be based on the extent of the disability caused by the angina. The history of the patient as well as the social picture must be weighed and presented to the individual, if compliance in the medical, surgical, and postoperative regimes is to be effective. All of the clinical data, and particularly the cineangiography, are reviewed by the team to determine need and to select the procedure for the individual. In centers where there is an active team of surgeons, nurses, and technicians who work well together, the mortality rate is low and the complications are kept to a minimum. Although much progress has been made since the advent of coronary artery surgery, future research may be directed toward minimizing

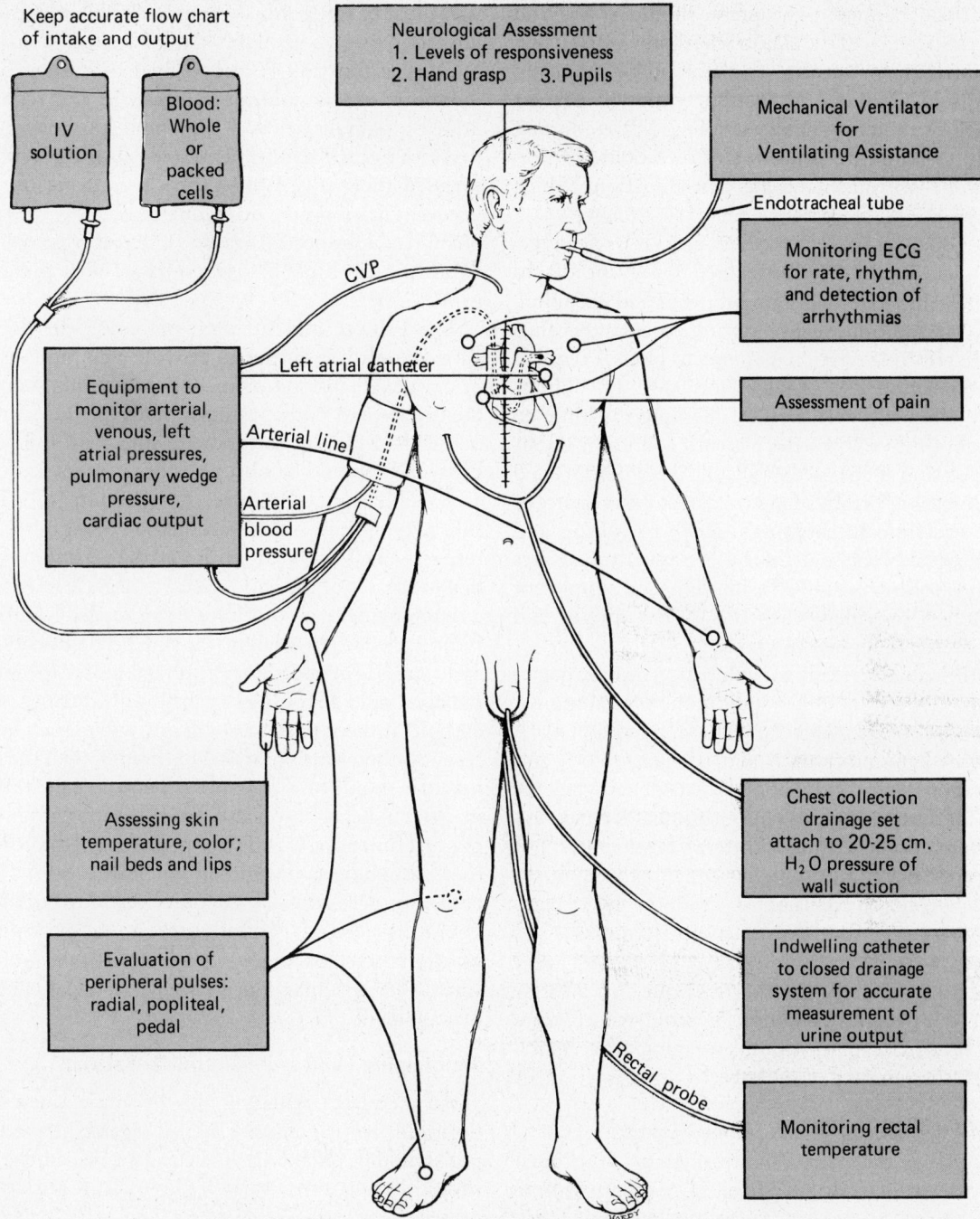

Keep accurate flow chart of intake and output

IV solution

Blood: Whole or packed cells

Neurological Assessment
1. Levels of responsiveness
2. Hand grasp   3. Pupils

Mechanical Ventilator for Ventilating Assistance

Endotracheal tube

CVP

Monitoring ECG for rate, rhythm, and detection of arrhythmias

Equipment to monitor arterial, venous, left atrial pressures, pulmonary wedge pressure, cardiac output

Left atrial catheter

Arterial line

Arterial blood pressure

Assessment of pain

Assessing skin temperature, color; nail beds and lips

Chest collection drainage set attach to 20-25 cm. H$_2$O pressure of wall suction

Evaluation of peripheral pulses: radial, popliteal, pedal

Indwelling catheter to closed drainage system for accurate measurement of urine output

Rectal probe

Monitoring rectal temperature

Figure 29-6.   Postoperative care of the cardiovascular surgery patient.

- relieving pain,
- maintaining adequate cerebral circulation, and
- observing for possible complications.

Providing for Adequate Tissue Oxygenation

All body tissues require an adequate supply of oxygen and nutrients for survival. To achieve this end after surgery, endotracheal intubation with ventilator assistance may be left intact from 8 to 48 hours in the postoperative period, depending upon the results of blood gas measurements. Recent studies have shown that patients who are stable following surgery may be extubated as early as 6 hours following surgery, which reduces their anxiety regarding their ability to communicate with the staff. A patient should normally awaken within an hour or two after cardiac surgery. If he does not, the following possibilities should be considered: (1) prolonged drug or anesthetic effect, (2) embolic damage, (3) hypoxia, (4) previous brain damage. The nurse should assess and maintain the patency of the endotracheal tube by (1) using the sigh mechanism on the ventilator or by manually using the self-inflating bag (Ambu) with 100 percent oxygen prior to and following suctioning, (2) suctioning frequently to minimize collection of secretions, (3) observing and reporting blood gas determinations which are compared with the baseline data.

Since an open airway enhances O_2 and CO_2 exchange, the endotracheal tube must be secured to prevent it from slipping into the right mainstem bronchus and occluding the airway. In addition, suctioning at frequent intervals is essential to remove secretions and mucus plugs. Frequent change of position also provides for optimum pulmonary ventilation and perfusion by allowing the lungs to expand more fully. When the patient's condition stabilizes, his position is changed every one to two hours and the nurse listens to breath sounds to detect the presence of wheezes and fluid in the lungs. Deep breathing and coughing are also encouraged to open the alveolar sacs and provide for increased perfusion. Physical support of the incision is provided when the patient coughs and breathes deeply at regular intervals.

When the patient is ready for extubation he may gag or "fight" the respirator. Other indications for calling for extubation are an adequate tidal volume, toleration of O_2 with warmed humidification and adequate blood gas determinations. Early extubation is considered when the patient's condition is stable. This means that the patient's pressures are not fluctuating and are within 20 percent of his preoperative volumes — and hence are high enough to maintain peripheral perfusion as indicated by urinary output, provided that there are no dangerous arrhythmias. With these parameters as guidelines, early extubation has been performed without any adverse effects on the patient's condition or prognosis. During this time the nurse assists with the weaning process and, eventually, the removal of the tube.

Assessing Cardiac Output

In evaluating the patient's cardiac status, the nurse primarily determines the effectiveness of cardiac output through clinical observations and routine measurements. Serial readings of blood pressure, heart rate, central venous pressure, arterial pressure, and left atrial or pulmonary artery pressure from modules are observed and recorded. The Swan-Ganz catheter (page 443) when inserted in the pulmonary artery indicates left ventricular filling pressure by measuring pulmonary artery pressure (PAP) and pulmonary artery wedge pressure (PWP). At the end of the diastolic phase and before the next systolic contraction occurs, the pulmonary vascular bed, the left atrium, and the left ventricle act for a moment as a single chamber. The changes in the left side of the heart, therefore, are reflected in the mean pulmonary artery and pulmonary artery wedge pressures. Sterility of catheter

sites must be scrupulously maintained in order to prevent infection.

Cardiac function is also related to kidney function; therefore, urinary output is measured and recorded. If urine output falls below 30 ml./hour, this may indicate a decrease in cardiac output. Urine specific gravity is also assessed (normally 1.010-1.025) as is urine osmolality. Underhydration may be manifested by low urinary output and a high specific gravity, whereas overhydration is exhibited by high urinary output with low specific gravity.

The growth and function of body cells depend on adequate cardiac output to provide a continuous supply of oxygenated blood to meet the changing demands of the organs and body systems. Since the buccal mucosa, nail beds, lips, and earlobes are sites with rich capillary beds, they should be observed for cyanosis or duskiness as possible signs of reduced heart action. Moist or dry skin may indicate either vasodilation or vasoconstriction respectively. Venous distention of the neck veins or of the dorsal surface of the hand raised to heart level may signal a changing demand or diminishing capacity of the heart. If cardiac output has fallen, the skin becomes cool, moist, and cyanotic or mottled. Peripheral pulses (pedal, tibial, radial) should be routinely palpated as a further check for emboli. If these pulses are absent, which may be due to recent catheterization of that extremity, then the carotid, brachial, popliteal, or femoral pulse is palpated. Irregularities in heart action also serve as important indicators of heart function. When poor perfusion of the heart exists there may be irregularities in the heart action. The most common arrhythmias encountered during the postoperative period are bradycardias, tachycardias, and ectopic beats. Continuous observation of the monitor for various arrhythmias is an essential part of patient care and management.

Maintaining Fluid and Electrolyte Balance

An adequate circulating blood volume is necessary for optimum cellular activity. In this regard, intake and output should be quickly reviewed and replacement therapy should be instituted early if flow sheets are utilized to determine positive or negative fluid balance. An adult's total body weight is composed of between 50 and 70 percent fluid. Anything that alters fluid volume or composition can have a marked effect on homeostasis. All intravenous fluids, including flush solutions provided through arterial and venous catheters, as well as through a nasogastric tube, if present, must be considered as intake. The hydration status of the individual may be monitored by means of a number of parameters: pulmonary wedge and left atrial pressure and CVP readings, weight, electrolyte levels, hematocrit readings, distention of neck veins, tissue edema, liver size, and breath sounds (i.e., fine rales, wheezing).

Chest drainage tubes provide a route for evacuation of

blood and air from the pleural cavity. Drainage is usually bloody and copious initially but gradually decreases. Chest drainage tubes should be secured tightly at connection sites and at the skin; the collection device is positioned below chest level in a safe manner (page 427). The tubes are "milked," or "stripped," at regular intervals to maintain patency. Drainage of blood and fluid to prevent pooling is facilitated by turning the patient from side to side or, alternately, from side to flat in bed to a semi-Fowler's position. An accurate account of chest tube drainage is essential in the immediate postoperative period. Bloody drainage should not exceed 200 ml./hour for the first four to six hours. Sudden cessation of drainage, on the other hand, may be due to kinked or blocked chest tubes.

Electrolytes are found in both extracellular and intracellular body fluids. A specific concentration is necessary in both compartments in order to sustain life. The nurse should be alert to changes in serum electrolytes, report changes promptly, and institute treatment as prescribed. Especially important are dangerously high or low levels of potassium, sodium, or calcium.

Hypokalemia (low potassium) may be caused by: inadequate intake, diuretics, vomiting, diarrhea, excessive nasogastric drainage, and stress due to surgery—increased aldosterone secretion produces decreased potassium-ion (K^+) and increased sodium-ion (Na^+) retention. The patient must be observed carefully when serum potassium rises or falls outside the normal level ($K^+ = 3.5\text{-}5.0$ mEq./L.). Some cardiac surgeons feel that it is important to maintain the K^+ level at 4.5 mEq. or higher in order to avoid arrhythmias in the postoperative period. The following effects of low K^+ may be noted: digitalis toxicity, arrhythmias, metabolic alkalosis, a weakened myocardium, and cardiac arrest. One possible specific ECG change is the presence of a U wave that is more than 1 mm. high (Fig. 29-7). (A U wave is a positive deflection following the T wave). Additional signs are A-V block, flat or inverted T waves, and low voltage. Intravenous potassium replacement should be administered at a rate usually not to exceed 15 to 20 mEq./hour (40-120 mEq. is diluted in 1,000 ml. of IV solution; or a more concentrated solution may be given through a central rather than peripheral catheter, when closely monitored).

Hyperkalemia (high potassium) may be caused by: increased intake, red cell breakdown caused by the pump, acidosis, renal insufficiency, tissue necrosis, and adrenal cortical insufficiency. The patient who exhibits symptoms of high K^+ may exhibit mental confusion, restlessness, nausea, weakness, and paresthesia of the extremities. ECG changes specific for hyperkalemia are: tall peaked T waves, increased amplitude, a widening of the QRS complex, and a prolonged Q-T interval (Fig. 29-8). The nurse should be prepared to administer an ion-exchange resin, sodium polystyrene sulfonate (Kayexal-

ate), which binds the potassium, or to give IV sodium bicarbonate or IV insulin and glucose to drive the potassium back into the cells from the extracellular fluid.

Both *hypernatremia* (high sodium) and *hyponatremia* (low sodium) may be seen following cardiac surgery; however, the latter is more commonly observed. Hyponatremia may result from a reduction of total body sodium or an increase in water intake which causes a dilution of body sodium. The patient must be observed for sodium values outside the normal limits (i.e., $Na^+ = 135\text{-}145$ mEq./L.). Replacement of sodium is instituted as directed if there is a true loss from the body. Diuretics are given as directed when reduction in sodium is due to increased water intake. Symptoms of hyponatremia for which the patient is observed are weakness, fatigue, confusion, convulsions, and coma.

Hypocalcemia (low calcium) is caused by (1) alkalosis, which reduces the amount of Ca^{++} in the extracellular fluid, and (2) multiple blood transfusions. When large amounts of citrated blood are given, the level of ionized Ca^{++} is reduced as some of the citrate binds calcium. The calcium level should be checked to see that it is within normal limits ($Ca^{++} = 9.0\text{-}11.5$ mg./100 ml.). Symptoms exhibited with reduced calcium levels may be: (1) numbness and tingling in the fingertips and toes, ears, and nose, (2) carpal pedal spasm, and (3) muscle cramps and tetany. Replacement therapy is indicated immediately.

Hypercalcemia (high calcium) can cause arrhythmias that imitate those caused by digitalis toxicity. Calcium is known to potentiate, or enhance, the action of digitalis. Therefore, the nurse must be alert to signs of digitalis toxicity (page 579) and must institute treatment for hypercalcemia immediately, since this condition may lead to asystole and death.

Relieving Pain

Deep pain may not be reflected in the immediate area of injury but in a broader, more diffuse area. Patients who have had cardiac surgery experience pain caused by the

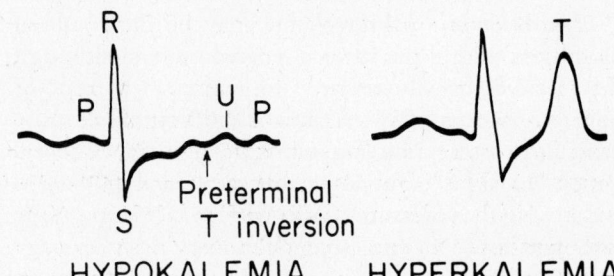

Figure 29-7. (Left) Effect of hypokalemia on ECG. Note elevated U wave. (From Sharp, L., and Rabin, B.: Nursing in the Coronary Care Unit. Philadelphia, J. B. Lippincott.)

Figure 29-8. (Right) Effect of hyperkalemia on ECG. (From Sharp, L., and Rabin, B.: Nursing in the Coronary Care Unit. Philadelphia, J. B. Lippincott.)

severance of intercostal nerves along the incision route and irritation of the pleura by the chest catheters. It is essential to observe and listen to the patient for verbal and nonverbal clues of pain. The nurse should accurately record the nature, type, location, and duration of the pain. (Incisional pain must be differentiated from anginal pain.) The patient is medicated as often as prescribed to reduce the amount of pain and to help him perform deep breathing and coughing exercises more successfully. If pain inhibits his performance of these activities, his progress will be jeopardized.

Pain produces tension which may stimulate the central nervous system to release adrenalin and thus constrict the arterioles. Certain narcotics have a depressant effect on respirations. Morphine sulfate alleviates anxiety and pain and induces sleep, which reduces the metabolic rate and the need for oxygen. Following the administration of narcotics, any observations indicating relief of apprehension and pain are documented in the patient's record.

Maintaining Adequate Cerebral Circulation

The brain is dependent upon a continuous supply of oxygenated blood. It does not have the capacity to store oxygen and must rely on adequate continuous perfusion by the heart. Thus it is important to observe the patient for any symptoms of hypoxia: restlessness, headache, confusion, dyspnea, hypotension, and cyanosis. An assessment of the patient's neurological status is made hourly in terms of level of consciousness, response to verbal commands and painful stimuli, pupillary size and reaction to light, movement of extremities, hand grasp ability, presence of pedal and popliteal pulses, and temperature and color of extremities. Any indication of a changing status is documented and reported immediately to the surgeon, since it may signal the beginning of a complication in the postoperative period.

POSSIBLE COMPLICATIONS FOLLOWING CARDIOVASCULAR SURGERY

Hypovolemia. Hypovolemia may be the result of blood loss during the surgical procedure, and although the blood is usually replaced to within 10 percent of normal, the loss of extracellular fluid volume is more difficult to assess. Nursing management includes observation for signs of hypovolemia: arterial hypotension and low venous pressure (CVP) with an increasing pulse rate, and low left atrial and pulmonary artery wedge pressures. The nurse should be prepared to administer blood to maintain adequate blood balance and additional solutions to replace any deficits in electrolytes and protein.

Persistent Bleeding. Hemorrhage may be the result of tissue fragility, trauma to tissues, or some unexplained clotting defect. Therefore, accurate measurement of blood loss is important. Appropriate treatment may include the administration of protamine sulfate, vitamin K, and blood products (fresh frozen plasma, platelets, or specific blood factors). One may be expected to transfuse until the venous pressure is 12 to 15 cm. H_2O or the left atrial pressure is 10 to 14 mm. Hg. All the while, preparations are made for the potential return of the patient to surgery should this be deemed necessary.

Cardiac Tamponade. Cardiac tamponade results from bleeding into the pericardial sac or accumulation of fluids in the sac which compresses the heart and prevents adequate filling of the ventricles. Nursing management includes observation for signs of tamponade, which is reflected by arterial hypotension accompanied by a rising left atrial pressure; muffled heart sounds; weak, thready pulse; neck vein distention; and falling urinary output. A reduction in the amount of drainage in the chest-collection device may cause one to suspect that the fluid is accumulating elsewhere. A chest x-ray is done to assess fluid accumulation at the mediastinum. Once the nurse is assured that the chest tubes are patent by "milking" or "stripping" them, and has checked to see that they are free from kinking or obstruction, preparation should be made for pericardiocentesis (page 597).

Cardiac Failure. The failing heart's diminished pumping action results in an elevated hydrostatic pressure created by the backing up of blood in the vessels (page 577); fluid is then forced out into the extracellular space. Nursing management includes observation for signs of cardiac failure: (1) a falling mean arterial pressure, (2) a rising venous pressure, and (3) an increasing tachycardia. The patient may exhibit symptoms of restlessness and agitation, peripheral cyanosis, venous distention, labored respirations, tissue edema, and ascites. Diuretic therapy and rapid digitalization may be necessary to avoid acute failure.

Myocardial Infarction. A myocardial infarction may occur during the postoperative period. However, symptoms may be masked by the usual postoperative discomfort. The patient may be suspected of having sustained an infarction if the mean arterial pressure falls in the presence of normal circulating volume and a normal venous pressure. Nitroglycerin may be used to counteract vasospasm. Serial ECGs may be obtained to determine how serious the injury is. A careful assessment of the pain is made in order to differentiate it from the usual incisional pain, and the patient is medicated cautiously. Shock, if present, should be treated as directed. It may be necessary to reduce the rate at which the patient increases his activity in order to allow the heart adequate time for healing. Other drugs used in the treatment of MI, besides nitroglycerin, are phentolamine (Regitine), trimethaphan camsylate (Arfonad), and nitroprusside, when indicated.

Renal Failure. A low cardiac output prior to and following open heart surgery can cause impairment of renal function. In addition, trauma to blood cells during cardiopulmonary bypass can cause hemolysis of red blood cells. This leads to a buildup of toxic substances due to the kidney's inability to excrete waste products. Use of vasopressor agents to increase blood pressure can also lead to reduction of the blood flow to the kidneys. Nursing management includes accurate measurement of urine output. An output of less than 20 ml./hour can indicate hypovolemia. Specific gravity tests should be carried out to determine the kidneys' ability to concentrate urine in the renal tubules. Rapid-acting diuretics and/or inotropic drugs (digitalis, isoproterenol) may be used to increase cardiac output and renal blood flow. The nurse should be aware of the BUN and serum creatinine levels as well as urine and serum electrolytes. It may be necessary to restrict fluids and limit the use of drugs that are normally excreted by the kidneys. The patient may be prepared for peritoneal dialysis or hemodialysis if indicated (pages 916–917).

Hypotension. Hypotension may be caused by inadequate cardiac contractility and volume and by mechanical ventilation, when the patient "fights" the respirator or when positive end expiratory pressure (PEEP) is used, causing a reduction in cardiac output. The circulating blood volume can decrease after the patient has been removed from cardiopulmonary bypass. Normally, as the blood is rewarmed, vasodilation takes place and fluid replacement is instituted to supply an adequate blood volume.

Nursing management includes the monitoring of vital signs: left atrial pressure (LAP), CVP, and pulmonary artery mean and wedge pressures, as well as arterial pressure. It is essential to check tube drainage, since hypotension may be seen when there is excessive drainage from the chest tubes. The nurse may have to give blood as directed in order to maintain left atrial pressure at a level that will provide a blood circulating volume adequate for good tissue perfusion. Symptoms of pulmonary edema may be observed if the left atrial pressure is greatly increased. Knowing what the patient's left atrial pressure should be and assisting in the treatment of low output syndrome are the nurse's responsibilities. An attempt is made to maintain the patient's blood pressure at a desirable level by closely titrating the rate and amount of vasopressor being administered.

Embolization. The usual embolic sites are the lungs, coronary arteries, mesentery, extremities, kidneys, spleen, and brain. Embolization may result from injury to the intima of the blood vessels, dislodgment of a clot from a damaged valve, venous stasis aggravated by certain arrhythmias, loosening of mural thrombi, and coagulation problems. Air emboli may occur as an effect of cardiopulmonary bypass. Nursing management implies initiating preventive measures early: (1) applying antiembolic stockings, (2) discouraging leg crossing, (3) avoiding use of the knee gatch on the bed, (4) omitting pillows in the popliteal space, and (5) instituting passive exercises followed by active exercises to promote circulation and prevent loss of muscle tone.

Symptoms of embolization, which vary according to site, should be watched for: (1) midabdominal or midback pain; (2) pain, cessation of pulses, blanching, numbness, or coldness of an extremity; (3) chest pain and respiratory distress with pulmonary embolus or myocardial infarction; and (4) one-sided weakness and pupillary changes such as occur in cerebral vascular accident.

Postperfusion Syndrome. Postperfusion or postpericardotomy syndrome occurs in approximately 10 to 40 percent of patients who undergo cardiac surgery. Its precise etiology is unknown. A common factor appears to be trauma with residual blood in the pericardial sac following surgery. It is characterized by fever, pericardial pain, pleural pain, dyspnea, pleural effusion and pericardial friction, and arthralgia. There may be a combination of these signs and symptoms. Leukocytosis is present along with elevation of the sedimentation rate. These symptoms frequently appear after the patient is discharged from the hospital.

The syndrome must be differentiated from other postoperative complications (incisional pain, myocardial infarction, pulmonary embolus, bacterial endocarditis, pneumonia, or atelectasis). The treatment is dependent on the severity of the symptoms. Salicylates and bed rest usually lead to a dramatic improvement in symptoms. Other symptoms are treated as they occur.

Psychosis. Psychosis may result from anxiety, sleep deprivation, increased sensory input, and disorientation to night and day when the patient loses track of time. An important finding is that patients who do not or cannot express anxiety before surgery are more prone to develop psychosis in the postoperative period. Psychosis may appear after a brief lucid interval. Characteristic signs of psychosis include: (1) transient perceptual distortions, (2) visual and auditory hallucinations, and (3) disorientation and paranoid delusions. The nurse should be watchful for signs of denial and should provide an opportunity for emotional expression during the preoperative period. Careful explanations of all procedures and of the need for the patient's cooperation help to keep him oriented throughout his postoperative course. Continuity of care, if at all possible, is desirable; a familiar face and a nursing staff with a consistent approach will prove to be assets in the delivery of nursing care. The use of a well designed and individualized nursing care plan will provide guidelines to assist the nursing team in the coordination of their efforts for the emotional well-being of the patient.

As you are about to leave the hospital, you will have some questions and concerns which you may need to discuss with your physician and nurse. The following guidelines may be helpful as a beginning. Please read carefully.

	General information	Specific instructions
1. Diet: _No added salt_	Maintain ideal weight with a well balanced diet as prescribed.	Avoid salty foods such as bacon, peanuts, and pretzels. Do not add salt in cooking or at the table.
2. Activity A. Walking, Exercise	All activity should be gradually increased within limits. Walk outside if not too cold or windy.	A) Continue to increase your walking time each day. Rate at which you walk is important to exercise your heart.
B. Stairs		B) Climb stairs 1–2x/day the first week
C. Recreation	Don't sit with legs down for too long a period. Get up and walk around to maintain blood flow.	C) Avoid large crowds, movies, and restaurants at first.
D. Marital Relations		D) May be resumed when you feel up to it
E. Hobbies	Don't spend too long on your feet.	E) Needlepoint and knitting at first.
F. Driving	May ride in a car up to an hour at a time, then get out and walk around	F) Avoid driving until you have returned for your checkup. Your physician will instruct you as to when you may resume driving.
3. Medications*	Dosage	
A. _Digoxin_ (for heart action)	0.25 mg.	1 pill daily at same time 9 am.
B. _Isordil_ (vasodilator)	5 mg. (2.5–10 mg. q. 4–6 hr.) normal range	Take 1 tablet (5 mgm.) 4x each day 6 a.m.–12 p.m.–6 p.m.–12 a.m.
C. _____ (for angina pain)		
D. _Lasix_ (for diuretic action)	40 mg. (20–80 mg. q.i.d. or b.d.) normal range	q.i.d. 9 a.m.
** E. _KCl Elixir_ (potassium replacement)	20 mEq. (20–80 mg.)	Take 3x/day after each meal. (9am.–1pm.–6pm.)
*** F. _Coumadin_ (anticoagulant)	7.5 mg. (2.5–7.5 mg. q.i.d.)	Take at the same time each day. 6p.m.
**** G. _Keflex_ (antibiotic)	250 mg.	q.i.d.
H. _____ (for relief of pain)		
I. _Dalmane_ (sedative or tranquilizer)	15 mg.	Take 1 capsule at bedtime if you have difficulty in sleeping.
J. _Minipress_ (antihypertensive)	$\ddot{\text{i}}$ mg. $\dot{\text{i}} - \ddot{\text{iii}}$ mg. (for pulmonary hypertension)	b.d. 9am.–6pm. for blood pressure.
K. _Iron caps_ (other)		Take 1 capsule 2x/day (9 a.m.–6 p.m.)
4. Return to Work	You and your physician will determine when you are physically able to return to employment.	6 wks. to 2 mos. if you feel able.

* Written guidelines will be given to you regarding the action of the drugs you will be taking and the side effects they may produce.

** This can be eliminated if long-term diuretics are supplemented with Aldactone or Dyrenium.

*** You will need a weekly prothrombin time test for the first 2 months, and then when your physician feels it is necessary.

**** Usually not needed unless a stitch abscess or urinary tract infection cause continuing problems.

POSTSURGICAL CONVALESCENCE AND PATIENT INSTRUCTION

Long-range plans should be discussed with the patient during the convalescent period. It is much easier to talk about the future while the patient is still recuperating than to try to fit it all in on the last day of hospitalization. Frequently the patient is too excited on the day of discharge to learn about modifications of life style that may be necessary.

As soon as the patient is up and moving around, plans for discharge should begin. The patient whose activity was greatly restricted prior to surgery because of his cardiac condition often needs much more encouragement and emotional support at this stage. He is more fearful of performing those activities which previously caused exacerbation of his symptoms.

The nurse must often be firm but kind in assisting the patient to relinquish dependence upon the health team and develop more self-reliance. If this approach is not instituted during the period of hospitalization, the patient may continue to use the illness as a crutch. It is often difficult for family members not to give in to the patient's desires, especially when they know that he has undergone major surgery.

One necessary adjunct to the patient's care is a set of guidelines, preferably written ones, which can be followed at home (see page 566).

BIBLIOGRAPHY

BOOKS

Borman, J. B.: Recent Trends in Cardiovascular and Thoracic Surgery. New York, Grune and Stratton, 1975.

Chow, R.: Cardiosurgical Nursing Care. New York, Springer Pub. Co., 1976.

Hudak, C. M., Lohr, T., and Gallo, B.: Critical Care Nursing, 2nd ed. Philadelphia, J. B. Lippincott, 1977.

Little, D. E., and Carnevali, D. L.: Nursing Care Planning. 2nd ed. Philadelphia, J. B. Lippincott, 1976.

Mason, D. T.: Advances in Heart Disease, Clinical Cardiology Monographs, Vol. 1. Philadelphia, J. B. Lippincott, 1977.

Moos, R. H., ed.: Coping with Physical Illness. New York, Plenum Medical Book Co., 1977.

Sanford, J. P., et al., eds.: The Science and Practice of Clinical Medicine, Vol. 3: Clinical Cardiology. Willerson, J. T., and Sanders, C. A., eds. New York, Grune and Stratton, 1977.

Turner, G. O.: The Cardiovascular Care Unit, A Guide For Planning and Operation. New York, John Wiley and Sons, 1978.

ARTICLES

Ashburn, W. L., et al.: Left ventricular ejection fraction—A review of several radionuclide angiographic approaches using the scintillation camera. Progress in Cardiovasc. Dis., 20:267-284, Jan.-Feb. 1978.

Adams, N. R., et al.: Reducing the perils of intracardiac monitoring. Nursing '76, 6:66-74, Apr. 1976.

Blackburn, G., et al.: Nutritional support in cardiac cachexia. J. Thorac. & Cardiovasc. Surg., 73:489-496, Apr. 1977.

Boisvert, C.: Convalescence following coronary surgery, a group experience. Can. Nurse, 72:26-27, Nov. 1976.

Bolooki, H., et al.: Clinical and hemodynamic criteria for use of the intra-aortic balloon pump in patients requiring cardiac surgery. J. Thorac. & Cardiovasc. Surg., 72:756-758, Nov. 1976.

Chun, P. K. C., and Nelson, W. P.: Common cardiac prosthetic valves. JAMA, 238:401-403, Aug. 1977.

DeBakey, M. E., and Lawrie, G. M.: Aortocoronary-artery bypass, assessment after 13 years. JAMA, 239:837-839, Feb. 27, 1978.

Hart, L., and Frantz, R.: Characteristics of postoperative patient-education programs for open-heart surgery patients in the United States. Heart & Lung, 6:137-142, Jan.-Feb. 1977.

Kinney, M. R.: Effects of preoperative teaching upon patients with differing modes of response to threatening stimuli. Internat'l. J. Nurs. Studies, 14:49-59, Jan. 1977.

Klineberg, P., et al.: Early extubation after coronary artery surgery. Crit. Care Med. 5:272-274, Nov.-Dec. 1977.

Lamb, J.: Intra-arterial monitoring. Nursing '77, 7:65-71, November, 1977. Vol. 7 No. 11

Lasater, K. L., and Grisanti, D. J.: Postcardiotomy psychosis: Indications and interventions. Heart Lung 4:724-729, Sept.-Oct. 1975.

Levinson, C.: Thallium-201 myocardial imaging. Heart & Lung, 6:115-120, Jan.-Feb. 1977.

Long, M. L., et al.: Cardiopulmonary bypass. AJN, 74:861-867, May 1974.

McIntosh, H. D., and Garcia, J. A.: The first decade of aortocoronary bypass grafting, 1967-1977. Circulation, 57:405-431, Mar. 1978.

Matloff, J. M., and Chaux, A.: What is the current status of prosthetic cardiac valve replacement. Controversies in Cardiol., 8:241-268, 1977.

Miller, Sr. P., and Shada, E.: Preoperative information and recovery of open-heart surgery patients. Heart Lung, 7:486-493, May-June 1978.

Rakoczy, M.: The thoughts and feelings of patients in the waiting period prior to cardiac surgery, a descriptive study. Heart Lung, 6:280-287, Mar.-Apr. 1977.

Roberts, W. C.: Prosthetic heart valves, which ones and why. Hosp. Pract., 13:63-69, Jan. 1978.

Strong, A. B.: Caring for cardiac catheterization patients. Nursing '77. 60-64, November 1977. Vol. 7, No. 11.

Verderber, A.: Cardiopulmonary bypass: Postoperative complications. AJN, 74:868-869, May 1974.

Winslow, E. H., and MacVaugh, H.: Coronary artery surgery, operative technique and patient education. Nurs. Clin. N. Am., 11:371-383, June 1976.

Woods, S.: Monitoring pulmonary artery pressures. AJN, 76:1765-1771, Nov. 1976.

AGENCIES

Governmental

National Heart, Lung and Blood Institute, National Institutes of Health, Bethesda, Md. 20205

Voluntary

American College of Cardiology, 9650 Rockville Pike, Bethesda, Md. 20012

American Heart Association, 7320 Greenville Ave., Dallas, Tex. 75231

Mended Hearts, 721 Huntington Ave., Roxbury, Mass. 02115

30

MANAGEMENT OF PATIENTS WITH CARDIAC DISORDERS

CORONARY ARTERY DISEASE

CORONARY ATHEROSCLEROSIS

The most common heart disorder in the United States is coronary atherosclerosis, a form of arteriosclerosis. This pathological condition of the coronary arteries is characterized by an abnormal accumulation of lipid substances and fibrous tissue in the vessel wall which leads to changes in arterial structure and function and reduction of blood flow to the myocardium. Causes of atherosclerotic heart disease probably involve alterations in lipid metabolism, blood coagulation, and the biophysical and biochemical properties of the arterial walls. Hyperlipidemia is a contributing factor in the development of atherosclerosis.

Hyperlipidemia. The association of elevated blood cholesterol with coronary artery disease has served to focus clinical attention on a mixed group of biochemical substances called lipids that have a common property of being more soluble in fat or organic solvents than in water. In the blood, the principal lipids are cholesterol, triglycerides (free fatty acids esterified to glycerol), and phospholipids (lipid esters of phosphoric acid). To render them sufficiently water soluble for transport in the blood, the lipids are attached (complexed) to a variety of proteins, the resulting complex being called a lipoprotein.

The lipoproteins can be separated into families either by protein electrophoresis, which causes these electrically charged molecules to migrate in an electrical field, or by high speed centrifugation, which separates the lipoproteins according to density. Each method employs a different set of names; however, in this discussion the terms that electrophoresis apply to are used, because this assay is available in many clinical laboratories. Table 30-1 summarizes the four families of lipoproteins according to the chief lipid carried, the appearance of the plasma, and the major clinical features often associated with an increase in the particular lipoprotein level in the blood.

For clinical purposes, hyperlipidemia may be suspected if the *fasting* blood cholesterol and/or triglyceride levels are elevated. Inspection of plasma chilled to 4° C. (39.2 F.) overnight may indicate elevated lipoprotein. Precise analysis sometimes requires ultracentrifugation. In nonfasting states, blood triglycerides are normally elevated above fasting levels. These triglycerides are contained in chylomicrons, particles of newly absorbed (dietary) fat which appear one to four hours after a meal.

Hyperlipidemia may be primary or secondary. Primary hyperlipidemia is generally a hereditary disorder. The secondary type occurs as a manifestation of numerous other diseases including hypothyroidism, nephrotic syndrome, diabetes mellitus, and alcoholism. Therapy consists in treating the basic disorder.

The primary hyperlipidemias have been classified by

TABLE 30-1. CHARACTERISTICS OF LIPOPROTEIN FAMILIES

| | | ELEVATED LEVELS | |
LIPOPROTEIN	PRINCIPAL LIPID	PLASMA APPEARANCE	CLINICAL FEATURES
Chylomicrons	Dietary fat	Creamy supernatant layer	Xanthomata Enlarged liver Pancreatitis
Beta	Cholesterol	Clear	Premature atherosclerosis Xanthomata
Prebeta	Triglyceride	Turbid	Glucose intolerance Hyperuricemia Premature atherosclerosis
Alpha	Phospholipids	Clear	Normal lifespan

TABLE 30-2. CHARACTERISTICS OF PRIMARY HYPERLIPIDEMIAS*

THIN	CHOLESTEROL	TRIGLYCERIDE	CHYLOMICRON	†DOMINANT LIPOPROTEIN FAMILY
I (rare)	++	++++	+++	Chylomicron
II (common)	++++	+	0	Beta
III (uncommon)	++	++	+	"Floating" beta
IV (common)	+	+++	0	Prebeta
V (uncommon)	++	++++	++	Chylomicron Prebeta

*The plus signs and zero signs signify amount.
†The column entitled Dominant Lipoprotein Family represents quantitatively the most important member of a mixture of proteins determined by electrophoresis. "Floating" beta represents a broad beta band that often does not clearly separate from the prebeta region.

Frederickson and co-workers* into five types, summarized in Table 30-2. Of the two common types of primary hyperlipidemia, one is hypercholesterolemic and the other is hypertriglyceridemic. Since the disorders are often familial, relatives should be surveyed. Typing of hyperlipidemias is useful because treatment, largely dietary, varies with the type. For instance, Type IV is treated primarily with a low carbohydrate diet. Type I is treated with a very low fat diet, and Type II with a low cholesterol, high carbohydrate diet which is low in fat from animal sources. Details concerning these diets are available in dietary textbooks. (See also page 570.)

Adjunctive drug therapy is also used when dietary treatment is inadequate. Nicotinic acid, clofibrate, cholestyramine, and/or d-thyroxine may be administered, each differing in pharmacologic action. These agents are shown to be biochemically effective in that elevated lipoprotein concentration tends to return toward normal

*Fredrickson, D. S., et al.: Fat transport in lipoproteins—an integrated approach to mechanisms and disorders. New Eng. J. Med., *276*:34–44, Jan. 5, 1967; 94–103, Jan. 12, 1967; 148–156, Jan. 19, 1967; 215–225, Jan. 26, 1967; 273–281, Feb. 2, 1967.

and manifestations of the abnormalities such as xanthomas (yellow papules in the skin due to lipid deposits) may disappear. Drug treatment also varies with the type of hyperlipidemia.

The question of the usefulness of diet and drugs in reversing coronary artery disease is still under investigation. The search for persons who have primary hyperlipidemias assumes importance, because dietary changes effected early in life may well yield a harvest of health. Such measures may constitute a major step toward the positive goal of prevention, as opposed to amelioration, of coronary artery disease.

Pathophysiology. Atherosclerosis begins when waxy cholesterol plaques which look like pearly gray mounds of tissue become deposited on the inner lining of the arteries. These deposits interfere with the absorption of nutrients by the endothelial cells that compose the vessel lining and obstruct blood flow by protruding into the lumen of the vessel. The vascular endothelium in involved areas becomes necrotic, then scarred, further compromising the lumen and impeding the flow of blood. At sites such as these, where the lumen is narrowed and the wall rough, there is a great tendency for clots to form, which explains the fact that intravascular coagulation, followed by thromboembolic disease, is among the most important complications of atherosclerosis (and of all the diseases that man is heir to!).

Our knowledge of the process by which plaques grow is limited. Among suspected mechanisms are thrombus formation on the surface of the plaque followed by fibrous organization of the thrombus, hemorrhage into a plaque, and continuing lipid accumulation. If the fibrous cap of the plaque ruptures, the lipid debris is swept into the bloodstream and obstruction of the arteries and capillaries distal to the ruptured plaque results.

Another form of arteriosclerosis is characterized by thickening and calcification of the arterial media, converting the vessel into a relatively inflexible tube with a very narrow lumen. Hypertension, it seems, plays a role in promoting atherosclerosis and is responsible for most of its major dangers and complications (see page 628).

CLINICAL MANIFESTATIONS. Coronary atherosclerosis produces symptoms and complications through narrowing of the arterial lumen and obstruction of blood flow to the myocardium. This impediment to blood flow progresses, to the extreme detriment of the muscle cells that depend for their survival on the native components of blood and on various other constituents that it transports. The major manifestation of ischemia of the myocardium is chest pain. Recurrent chest pain due to ischemia without irreversible damage to myocardial cells is termed *angina pectoris*. More severe ischemia with cell damage is termed *myocardial infarction*. Irreversibly damaged myocardium undergoes degeneration and is replaced by scar tissue. If the damage to the myocardium is extensive, the heart eventually may fail, that is, it may be unable to support the body's needs for blood by providing an adequate cardiac output.

Dietary Considerations as a Preventive Aspect of Coronary Heart Disease

Dietary fat is becoming a significant risk factor in coronary heart disease and a possible risk factor in cancer. Therefore, the control of fat is an important factor in preventive nutrition.

Dietary fat is regulated by changing either the total amount or the type of fat in the diet or by changing both. Assisting the patient to modify dietary fat intake through effective counseling requires an understanding of the differences between saturated and polyunsaturated fatty acids, cholesterol, medium chain triglycerides, and different other fractions as well as their functions in the human body.

The five types of lipid profiles are indicated in Table 30-2. Proponents of this method view the classification by types as a potentially important key to the prevention and control of coronary heart disease. No single diet or

TABLE 30-3.   COMPOSITION OF LIPIDS PRESENT IN PLASMA

α = *Lipoproteins–high density lipoproteins (HDL)*	
Protein	35-60%*
Phospholipid	34-44%
Cholesterol	20-28%
Triglyceride	17%
β = *Lipoproteins–low density lipoproteins (LDL)*	
Protein	20-25%
Phospholipid	25%
Cholesterol	46%*
Triglyceride	14%
Very low density lipoproteins (VLDL)	
Protein	10%
Phospholipid	20%
Cholesterol	5%
Triglyceride	65%*
Chylomicrons (Nonmigrating)	
Protein	2%
Phospholipid	6-9%
Cholesterol	2%
Triglyceride	85-95%*

*The highest component in each type of lipid.

drug will be effective in all conditions in lowering the particular elevated lipid abnormality, but in most people with such an abnormality the level can be brought within the upper average range.

The compositions of the various types of lipids are indicated in Table 30-3. The α-lipoproteins (HDL) are highest in protein, and the β-lipoproteins (LDL) are highest in cholesterol. The very low density lipoproteins (VLDL) and chylomicrons are higher in triglycerides.

For patients in whom diet alone cannot normalize the specific lipid, there are several medications that have a synergistic effect when taken with the prescribed diet. These are usually grouped into two types: those that decrease lipoprotein synthesis, such as nicotinic acid and clofibrate, and those that increase lipoprotein catabolism, such as cholestyramine, sitosterol, and D-thyroxine.

Risk Factors and Prevention of Atherosclerotic Heart Disease

Epidemiological studies and observations reveal that there are risk factors for atherosclerosis that tend to make an individual more prone to develop coronary heart disease, angina pectoris, and myocardial infarction. These risk factors include:

Elevated serum cholesterol
Elevated blood pressure
Cigarette smoking
Elevated serum or plasma triglycerides
Elevated blood sugar (diabetes mellitus)

Obesity ✓
Physical inactivity ✓
Positive family history
Stress: Type A behavior
Age
Sex M>F

The more risk factors a person has, the greater is the likelihood of his having angina pectoris and/or myocardial infarction. Persons at risk should have periodic medical examinations, change their life styles, and alter their dietary habits.

Behavior Patterns of Coronary Prone Individuals. It is believed that stress and certain behaviors contribute to the pathogenesis of coronary (atherosclerotic) heart disease. Psychobiological and epidemiological studies have investigated behaviors that characterize the coronary prone person. Individuals who manifest these behaviors (competitive striving for achievement, exaggerated sense of time urgency, aggressiveness and hostility) are classified as Type A coronary-prone individuals.* It appears that in addition to reducing other risk factors (smoking, dietary fats) some effort should be made to correct the life style and alter the behavior and long-term habit structure of this individual.

ANGINA PECTORIS

Angina pectoris is a clinical syndrome characterized by paroxysms of pain or a feeling of pressure in the anterior chest. The cause is considered to be insufficient coronary blood flow and/or inadequate oxygen supply to the myocardial muscle. (Myocardial oxygen utilization is directly related to coronary blood flow.)

Angina is usually caused by atherosclerotic heart disease and almost invariably is associated with a significant obstruction of a major coronary artery. (The characteristics of the various types of angina are listed in the chart on this page.)

Any number of factors can produce anginal pain. Physical exertion can precipitate an attack by increasing myocardial oxygen demands. Exposure to cold or even the drinking of iced beverages can cause vasoconstriction and an elevated blood pressure with increased oxygen demand. Eating a heavy meal increases the blood flow to the mesenteric area and places a heavier demand on the heart. Stress and any emotion-provoking situation causing the release of adrenalin and increased blood pressure may accelerate the heart rate, and a bout of anginal pain can result. If blood flow from the left ventricle is obstructed, as in aortic stenosis, the oxygen needs of the myocardium are drastically increased.

*Glass, D.: Behavior Patterns, Stress and Coronary Disease. Hillsdale, New Jersey. Lawrence Erlbaum Associates, 1977.

Clinical Manifestations

Ischemia of the heart muscle produces *pain* varying in severity from upper substernal pressure to agonizing pain that is accompanied by severe apprehension and a feeling of impending death. The pain is usually felt deep in the chest behind the upper or middle third of the sternum (retrosternal). Although the pain frequently is localized, it may radiate to the neck, jaw, shoulders, and inner aspects of the upper extremities. The patient often experiences a tightness, a choking or strangling sensation that has a viselike, insistent quality. A feeling of weakness or numbness in the arms, wrists, and hands may accompany the pain. Along with the physical pain, the patient also has a sense of impending death, an apprehension which is so characteristic of angina that if it occurs alone, as it sometimes does, it is sufficient for diagnosis.

The diagnosis is made by an evaluation of the clinical manifestations and the nitroglycerin test, i.e., determining if relief is obtained by the use of nitroglycerin. The patient's response to exertion or stress may also be tested by means of electrocardiographic monitoring while he exercises on a bicycle or treadmill.

TYPES OF ANGINA

UNSTABLE ANGINA (preinfarction angina; crescendo angina)

Progressive increase in frequency, intensity, and duration of anginal attacks

Increasing danger of myocardial infarction within 3 to 18 months

NOCTURNAL ANGINA

Pain occurring at night usually during sleep; may be relieved by sitting upright

Commonly due to left ventricular failure

ANGINA DECUBITUS

Angina while lying down

INTRACTABLE OR REFRACTORY ANGINA

Severe incapacitating angina

PRINZMETAL'S VARIANT ANGINA

Spontaneous type of anginal pain accompanied by ST segment elevation in ECG

Thought to be due to coronary artery spasm

Associated with high risk of infarction

Nursing Assessment

If the patient is in the hospital, the nurse should observe and record all facets of his activity with particular regard for the activities that have been found to precede and precipitate attacks of anginal pain.

When do attacks tend to occur?
  Following a meal?
  After engaging in certain activities?

After physical activities in general?

After visits from members of the family or others?

Where is the pain located?

How does the patient describe the pain?

Was the onset of pain gradual or sudden?

How long did it last — seconds? minutes? hours?

Was the pain steady and unwavering in quality?

Is the discomfort accompanied by other symptoms such as sweating, light-headedness, nausea, palpitation, shortness of breath?

How many minutes after taking nitroglycerin did the pain last?

What was the mode of abatement?

The answers to these questions, ascertained from observation, can form a basis for designing a logical program of prevention.

If a patient senses that an attack is imminent, he should cease all movement, in order to reduce to a minimum the oxygen requirements of the ischemic myocardium. This is done with the hope that oxygen needs can be met by the limited supply available at the moment and the impending attack can thus be averted.

Management

The objectives of treatment are to decrease the oxygen demands of the myocardium and to increase the oxygen supply.

DECREASING OXYGEN DEMANDS OF THE MYOCARDIUM. The patient must understand the symptom complex and the need to avoid activities known to cause anginal pain. He needs to become aware of the factors producing this pain: sudden exertion, walking against the wind, exposure to cold, emotional excitement, etc., and he must learn to change, modify, or adapt to these stresses.

There are patients whose attacks occur predominantly in the morning. This idiosyncrasy obviously calls for a change in the schedule of daily activities. As a first step, the patient should plan to rise earlier each morning so that he may complete his shaving, washing, and dressing in a more leisurely fashion. Ideally, he should maintain this unhurried pace throughout the entire day — performing his scheduled tasks and meeting whatever commitments he has without haste or a sense of pressure. Any patient with angina pectoris should be instructed to initiate all movements with deliberation, avoid exposure to cold, avoid tobacco, eat regularly but lightly, and maintain a proper weight. Other measures to decrease the oxygen demands of the myocardium include lowering the patient's blood pressure, correcting aortic stenosis, and treating hyperthyroidism.

Pharmacologic Therapy: Nitroglycerin. The nitrates are still the mainstay of treatment for angina pectoris. Glyceryl trinitrate (Nitroglycerin) is given to reduce myocardial oxygen consumption, which decreases ischemia and relieves anginal pain. Nitroglycerin

has an effect on the peripheral circulation. By increasing the capacity of the venous bed, it causes venous pooling of blood throughout the body. As a result, less blood is returned to the heart and there is a reduction in filling pressure and stroke output in the left ventricle. Nitrates also relax the systemic arteriolar bed and thus cause a fall in blood pressure. These effects decrease myocardial oxygen requirements, bringing about a more favorable balance between supply and demand.

Nitroglycerin taken sublingually (under the tongue) or in the buccal pouch alleviates the pain of ischemia within 3 minutes.

- The patient should be instructed to keep the tongue still and to avoid swallowing saliva until the nitroglycerin tablet is dissolved. If the pain is severe, the tablet can be crushed between the teeth to hasten sublingual absorption.
- As a precaution, the patient should carry the medication at all times in a securely capped dark glass bottle, not in a metal or plastic pillbox. The drug should be kept in its original container. If it is transferred to another bottle, evidence indicates that it will lose a large amount of its potency.

Nitroglycerin is volatile and is inactivated by heat, moisture, air, light, and time. If the nitroglycerin is fresh, the patient will feel a burning sensation under the tongue and often a feeling of fullness or throbbing in the head.

Instead of following a fixed dosage, the patient regulates drug usage, taking the smallest dose that relieves pain. He is instructed to take the drug in anticipation of any activity that may produce pain. Since nitroglycerin will increase the patient's tolerance for exercise and stress when taken prophylactically (e.g., before exercise, stair climbing, sexual intercourse), it is best that it be taken *before* the pain develops.

- The patient should note how long it takes for the nitroglycerin to relieve the discomfort. If the pain lasts more than 20 or 30 minutes after the nitroglycerin has been taken, an impending myocardial infarction may be suspected.

Side effects of nitroglycerin include flushing, throbbing headache, hypotension, and tachycardia. The use of long-acting nitrate preparations is controversial. Isosorbide dinitrate appears to be effective for up to 2 hours if taken sublingually but has an uncertain effect if taken orally.

TOPICAL NITROGLYCERIN OINTMENT. Nitroglycerin is also available in a lanolin-petrolatum base which, when applied to the skin, appears to protect against anginal pain and promote its relief. It is especially useful when patients experience nocturnal angina or are involved in periods of extended activity (e.g., golfing) since it has a prolonged effect of at least 3 hours.

The amount of ointment applied is measured with a calibrated strip of paper that comes with the product. The measured dose is smoothed onto the skin in a thin uniform layer. Most patients prefer to apply it on the chest site where anginal pain originates. The dose is usually increased until headache or an excessive effect on blood pressure or heart rate occurs and then is reduced to the largest dose which does not produce these side effects.

Beta-Adrenoreceptor Blockade. If the patient continues to have chest pain despite treatment with nitroglycerin and modification of life style, the beta-adrenergic blocking agent propranolol hydrochloride (Inderal) is given. This drug appears to reduce myocardial oxygen consumption by blocking the sympathetic impulses to the heart. The result is a reduction in heart rate, blood pressure, and myocardial contractility that establishes a more favorable balance between myocardial oxygen needs and the amount of oxygen available. This helps to control chest pain and allows the patient to work or exercise. Propranolol may be given with sublingual isosorbide dinitrate for anti-anginal and anti-ischemia prophylaxis. Propranolol is cleared by the liver at varying rates, depending on the individual patient. It is usually given at 6-hour intervals. Side effects include musculoskeletal weakness, hypotension, bradycardia, and mental depression.

When propranolol is started, blood pressure and heart rate should be taken (while the patient is in an upright position) 2 hours after the medication has been administered. If the blood pressure drops significantly, a vasopressor may be needed. If severe bradycardia occurs, atropine is the drug of choice. It is also important to remember that propranolol can precipitate congestive heart failure and asthma.

- Caution the patient not to stop taking propranolol abruptly, since there is evidence that angina may worsen and myocardial infarction develop if this drug is abruptly discontinued.

INCREASING OXYGEN SUPPLY TO THE MYOCARDIUM. Several measures are necessary in order to increase the oxygen supply to the myocardium. For one thing, if anemia is present, it must be corrected. It is also important that the patient stop smoking, since smoking produces tachycardia and raises the blood pressure, thus increasing the work of the heart. Obese individuals must lose weight to reduce cardiac work.

Physical conditioning should be encouraged since it increases exercise capacity and produces a lower heart rate and blood pressure in response to a given exercise. (See page 576 for rehabilitation of the heart patient.)

Surgical Treatment

Angina pectoris may persist for many years in a stable form with brief attacks. However, it is a serious disease. In the unstable stage the episodes of chest pain become more frequent and intense, occurring without apparent provocation. When symptoms cannot be controlled despite an adequate trial of drug therapy, some form of surgical revascularization is considered that can correct the basic problem by bringing a new blood supply to the ischemic myocardium (see pages 557–559).

Patient Education

The education of the patient with angina is designed to acquaint him with the basic nature of his illness and to furnish him with the facts he needs if he is to reorganize his living habits in a way that is effective; i.e., that will reduce the frequency and severity of anginal attacks, delay the progress of the underlying disease, if possible, and help protect him from other complications. The factors outlined below are important in the education of the patient with angina pectoris.

PATIENT EDUCATION IN ANGINA

Goal: To improve the quality of life and promote health

I. To prevent an episode of anginal pain:
   A. Use moderation in all activities of life.
      1. Participate in a normal daily program of activities which do not produce chest discomfort, shortness of breath, and undue fatigue.
      2. Exercise before work, after work, or before meals.
      3. Avoid exercises requiring sudden bursts of activity. Avoid all isometric exercise.
      4. Avoid activities that require heavy effort.
      5. Alternate activity with periods of rest. Some fatigue is normal and temporary.
   B. Shun situations that are emotionally stressful.
   C. Avoid overeating.
      1. Eat smaller portions.
      2. Avoid excessive caffeine intake (coffee, cola drinks) that can increase the heart rate and produce angina.
      3. Refrain from engaging in physical exercise for 2 hours after meals.
      4. Do not use "diet pills," nasal decongestants, or any over-the-counter medications that can increase the heart rate.
   D. Stop smoking since smoking increases the heart rate, blood pressure, and blood carbon monoxide levels.
   E. Try to avoid cold weather if possible.
      1. Wear a scarf over nose/mouth during very cold weather to warm the air.
      2. Walk more slowly in cold weather.
      3. Dress warmly in winter.
   F. Follow general principles of good hygienic living.

II. To cope with an attack of anginal pain:
   A. Carry nitroglycerin at all times.
      1. Keep nitroglycerin in a tightly capped dark-colored glass bottle.
      2. Discard the cotton filler/packing.   *(Continued)*

PATIENT EDUCATION IN ANGINA (CONTINUED)

  3. Avoid opening the bottle unnecessarily.
  4. Try to avoid carrying your supply right next to your body.
  5. Discard tablets after 5 months.
  6. If tablets are fresh, they should cause a burning sensation when placed under the tongue.

B. Place nitroglycerin under the tongue at first sign of chest discomfort.
  1. Do not swallow saliva until the tablet has dissolved.
  2. Stop and rest until all pain subsides.
  3. The upright position potentiates the effect of nitroglycerin.
  4. Usually another nitroglycerin tablet may be taken in 3 to 5 minutes if pain relief is not obtained. If pain persists, call the physician. If the anginal discomfort is unrelieved by the usual number of nitroglycerin tablets, or if it recurs after a short interval, go to the nearest emergency facility.

C. Take nitroglycerin prophylactically to avoid pain known to occur with certain activities (stair climbing, sexual intercourse).

D. Be alert for the side effects of nitroglycerin: headache, flushing, and dizziness.

MYOCARDIAL INFARCTION

Myocardial infarction refers to the process by which myocardial tissue is destroyed in regions of the heart that are deprived of an adequate blood supply because of a reduced coronary blood flow. The cause of the reduced blood flow is either a critical narrowing of a coronary artery due to atherosclerosis or, less commonly, a complete occlusion of an artery due to embolus or thrombus. Decreased coronary blood flow may also result from shock and hemorrhage. In this situation, there is a profound imbalance between myocardial oxygen supply and demand.

"Coronary occlusion," "heart attack," and "myocardial infarction" are all used synonymously, but the latter is the preferred term. In the United States, well over a million of these attacks occur annually.

The pathophysiology of atherosclerotic heart disease is discussed on page 569. The risk factors are found on page 570.

Clinical Manifestations

The patient with myocardial infarction is usually male, is over 40, and has atherosclerosis of the coronary vessels, often with arterial hypertension. However, attacks also occur in women and in younger men in their early thirties or even twenties.

In a typical patient, the pain starts suddenly, usually over the lower sternal region and the upper abdomen, and is continuous; but it may increase steadily in severity until it becomes almost unbearable. It is a heavy, viselike pain, which may radiate to the shoulders and down the arms, usually the left arm. Unlike the pain of true angina, it begins spontaneously (not following effort, emotional upset, etc.), persists for hours or days, and is relieved neither by rest nor by nitroglycerin. The pulse may become very rapid, irregular, and feeble, even imperceptible, and the heart may dilate. Gallop rhythm (accentuated third heart sound making the three heart sounds similar to those of a galloping horse) often develops.

The person with a severe occlusion may be in shock; he appears ashen and breaks out in a clammy sweat. Vomiting is common. In a few hours body temperature rises, blood pressure falls to an unusually low point, the leukocyte count rises to 15,000 or 20,000 cu. mm. Changes may be seen in the electrocardiogram within 2 to 12 hours (but may take as long as 72 to 96 hours). These changes reveal not only the presence but also the location of the infarct. Serum enzymes and isoenzymes are elevated and can be correlated with the patient's clinical course (see page 516). Even if the ECG is normal, elevation of serum enzymes reveals that caution is indicated in the handling of this person.

A significant percentage of patients with acute myocardial infarction diagnosed on the basis of subsequent ECGs deny having experienced any pain or discomfort whatever. These are the so-called silent myocardial infarction patients, who are admitted to the hospital for observation solely on the basis of their histories.

Prognosis

Studies show that the extent of the myocardial damage and the severity of coronary artery obstruction are important predictors of survival. Approximately 70 percent of patients dying from coronary atherosclerotic heart disease never reach a hospital. The highest mortality occurs during the first hour after onset of symptoms. A large percentage of all *sudden* deaths occur in patients with coronary atherosclerotic heart disease (CAHD). Other patients live a few days and succumb as the result of cardiogenic shock, arrhythmias, congestive heart failure, and other complications.

Of those persons who live long enough to get to a hospital, a much higher percentage survive, especially if an intensive coronary care unit is available. A small infarct may heal, with scar formation, leaving the patient fairly well, but a second occlusion often occurs later, or the patient develops heart failure. In fact a recurrent infarction within 5 months after recovery from an acute myocardial infarction carries a significant fatality rate. Of those who recover, the majority can return to normal duties.

Immediate Emergency Care

To reduce the awesome mortality rate of coronary arteriosclerotic heart disease, every effort must be made to identify and treat the individual who is in danger of sudden death from myocardial infarction, namely, the patient who has had a previous myocardial infarction, angina pectoris, or other conditions known to be risk factors (see page 570). Over half the persons reaching cardiac care units have significant prodromal, or warning, symptoms. The major complaints of these patients were *changing anginal patterns* and *unusual fatigue*. All persons, especially those at risk, must learn to recognize the early manifestations of life-threatening illness. Persons with symptoms must be advised to proceed immediately to a health care facility, especially if new symptoms develop or if old symptoms change in quality or duration.

An important achievement is the development of mobile heart units equipped with monitoring and resuscitative equipment.

The emphasis in these units is being shifted from resuscitation to prevention of electrical arrest, since a large percentage of the persons seen within the first hour of the attack have some form of bradycardia, which for the most part can be relieved by atropine. (See page 527.) Hypotension may accompany early bradycardia, which may lead to the extension of the initial area of infarction and to an increase of shock and pump failure. It may be that bradycardia is an important precursor of ventricular fibrillation.

Sinus arrest, transient heart block, and ventricular irritability are also encountered during the first few hours of acute coronary symptoms. Ideally all patients with myocardial infarctions should be admitted to a cardiac care unit (see page 540). It is believed that this action would prevent many of the deaths that occur from arrhythmias following myocardial infarctions.

The manner in which the medical team handles the patient when he enters the hospital may influence the outcome of his illness. It is important that the patient's emotional needs be met, as well as his physiologic needs, since myocardial infarction gives rise to extreme anxiety. Although time and deliberate speed are important, the patient should be greeted and oriented. Frenzied activity evokes more anxiety and fear, which has the effect of mobilizing the patient's catecholamines (i.e., norepinephrine and epinephrine), the action of which increases the heart rate and the force of myocardial contraction and thus accelerates metabolic processes. This results in an inadequate supply of blood to the myocardium. Serious complications (arrhythmias, congestive heart failure) can be provoked.

Management Objectives

The most critical period for the patient with a myocardial infarction is the first 48 hours following the attack. The area of infarction can increase in size for several hours or days after the onset of the attack. Cardiogenic shock, and ventricular fibrillation are common causes of sudden death during this time period.

The objectives of management are designed to

- detect and treat arrhythmias
- alleviate shock
- relieve pain
- rest the myocardium
- prevent complications
- achieve physiologic and functional rehabilitation
- halt the progress of arteriosclerosis, the lesion that is basically responsible for the myocardial infarct

Since the patient usually receives this initial care in the cardiac care unit, a detailed discussion will be found on pages 540–551 of Chapter 28, Management of The Patient in the Cardiac Care Unit.

Management Following Discharge from the Cardiac Care Unit

Psychosocial Considerations. Nursing care in the cardiac care unit involves constant surveillance, monitoring, and attention to patient needs. When the patient is transferred from this atmosphere of total dependence to a regular unit, he no longer receives this type of continual care. As a result, he may feel anxious and/or angry. This anxiety may be manifested by chest pain, headache, dizziness, restlessness, insomnia, etc. By understanding the patient's feelings and behavior, the nurse can counteract his stress and better plan his care. The patient's negative behavior may derive partly from his incomplete internalization of the education that he received while in the CCU.

- Find out what the patient knows about his condition and correct any misconceptions. Help him to identify his stresses, and encourage him to ventilate and discharge his strong pent-up emotions. Above all, be encouraging and optimistic.

The goal is to assist the patient to develop healthy attitudes toward the illness and to prepare him to manage the self-care that will be required when he returns home.

Physical Considerations. On return from the CCU, physical and emotional rest are still important therapeutic considerations. The patient is usually permitted to ambulate and go to the bathroom. Physical activities are increased gradually, but the patient is instructed to avoid sudden effort, including the Valsalva maneuver (straining). Usually, a cholesterol-modified diet is prescribed and caffeine-containing beverages are forbidden.

The patient's progress is followed with the aid of repeated electrocardiograms and determinations of serum enzymes. Cardiac function is estimated on the basis of symptoms and physical signs. Gradually, self-confidence should be built up and a workable approach to work, recreation, and hobbies, should be established that will allow a return to a normal or near-normal life style.

The patient's prognosis may be jeopardized by the advent, during the initial 2 weeks, of any one of several complications, including arrhythmias, thromboembolism, congestive failure, and myocardial rupture. To be on the alert for any such development is an important nursing responsibility.

Rehabilitation

The goals of rehabilitation for the patient with myocardial infarction are to extend and improve the quality of life. The immediate objectives are to return the patient as rapidly as possible to a normal or near-normal life style. This includes training the patient for physical activity, educating him and his family, and initiating psychosocial and vocational counseling when necessary.

Actually, cardiac rehabilitation begins as soon as the acute episode occurs. During this stage the nurse can assist the patient toward the realization of his goal of independence even when he is on strict bed rest. This is achieved by directing his thinking toward the time when he will be active again. The goal here is not to change the patient's life style but to make necessary modifications. It is best to avoid remonstrating about what the patient should not do. Instead, he should be encouraged to develop short-term and long-range goals based upon his needs. It is important to explain the nature of the disease, answer questions honestly, and reassure the patient that most persons return to a useful economic life and resume their usual activities. These are positive approaches in preventing the patient from becoming a cardiac cripple.

There is a divergence of opinion concerning the amount of activity the patient may participate in following a myocardial infarction. Although dangerous complications occur early, the scar formation over the infarcted area is seen at the beginning of the third week. The necrotic debris is resolved by the fourth week, while the development of the scar continues. Thus, there is an area of ischemia in some patients for varying lengths of time which affects the individual's exercise prescription.

PHYSICAL CONDITIONING. Physical conditioning or exercise training is done to improve cardiac efficiency and enhance the patient's ability to perform work at reduced heart and blood pressure rates. This will reduce the oxygen requirements of the heart and enable the patient to perform more physical activity before developing symptoms of myocardial ischemia; e.g., chest pain, ECG changes. Physical conditioning may be divided into the acute phase, convalescent phase (up to eight weeks), and maintenance phase (lifelong).

As soon as the patient is *stable* and the physician permits, the arms are put through range of motion exercises. Active motion of the muscles of the shoulder girdle helps to prevent anterior chest wall pain which may be interpreted as being cardiac in origin. The patient may be able to sit in a chair for 20 to 30 minutes several times a day beginning a few days after admission. As soon as he is able (depending on his signs and symptoms, clinical condition, ECG, serum enzymes) he is encouraged to participate in self-care activities. Early mobilization under supervision is usually permitted after an uncomplicated myocardial infarction. Mobilization begins with walking and progresses to stair climbing. Prolonged immobilization has a deconditioning effect and also contributes to anxiety and depression.

- Evaluate the patient closely and carefully during physical activity for chest pain, dyspnea, weakness, fatigue, and an increase in heart rate of more than 20 beats from baseline or greater than 120 beats per minute.
- Watch also for a fall in systolic blood pressure, the development of an arrhythmia or conduction disturbance, or an increase in ST segment displacement or T wave abnormality on the monitor. If these occur, the activity is stopped immediately, and the patient's clinical status is reevaluated.

Isometric exercises are contraindicated because they may impose stress on the left ventricle by raising the blood pressure while at the same time decreasing coronary perfusion. The performance of the Valsalva maneuver (straining) is to be avoided.

A treadmill test with ECG monitoring is done to help in developing guidelines for the design of an appropriate exercise program for the patient. Submaximal testing is done before the patient leaves the hospital and maximal testing before he returns to work. The patient who demonstrates low functional capacity with ischemic ST segment depression and premature ventricular beats will need a different activity program than the patient who has good functional capacity with no significant ECG abnormalities. The level of the patient's physical activity before infarction is also considered.

In general, the activity (walking) is increased in distance and speed. The cardiovascular benefits of exercise depend on whether or not the patient can exercise long enough to reach and maintain the prescribed pulse rate for a period of 15 minutes. (The patient is taught to monitor his pulse during physical activity.)

Several months after myocardial infarction the maintenance phase begins. As a result of physical training the patient may participate in activities that promote endurance—jogging, running, swimming, cycling. These appear to be useful for heart and lung conditioning. In general, the best type of exercise consists of rhythmic and repetitive movements (calisthenics, walking, running) that require maximal or submaximal effort. Short bursts of intensive effort are to be avoided since they produce a marked rise in blood pressure.

SEXUAL ACTIVITY. Many patients fear that sexual activity will be harmful to their heart condition and will precipitate chest pain.

If the patient can walk vigorously around the block or climb a flight of stairs without symptoms (rapid heart rate, chest pain, etc.) sexual activity may usually be resumed. Some modifications may be necessary—i.e. intercourse after a night's sleep and followed by a rest

---

PATIENT EDUCATION IN MYOCARDIAL INFARCTION

A patient with heart disease should learn to regulate his activity according to his individual response. The goal is always to improve the quality of life and promote health.

I. To modify activities during convalescence so that complete recovery is realized.
  A. Myocardial healing starts early but is not complete for varying periods; usually 6 to 8 weeks.
  B. A myocardial infarction usually requires some modification of the life style; adaptation to a heart attack is an ongoing process.
    1. Avoid any activity that produces chest pain, dyspnea, or undue fatigue.
    2. Avoid extremes of heat and cold and walking against the wind.
    3. Take off weight as directed.
    4. Stop smoking.
    5. Alternate activity with rest periods. Some fatigue is normal and expected during convalescence.
    6. Avoid overprotection. Emphasize areas of competency.
    7. Eat 3 or 4 meals daily, each containing the same amount of food.
      a. Avoid large meals and hurrying while eating.
      b. Restrict caffeine-containing beverges, since caffeine can affect heart rate, rhythm, and blood pressure.
      c. Stay within prescribed diet, modifying calories, fat, and sodium as prescribed.
    8. Make every effort to comply with medical regimen, especially in taking medications.
    9. Pursue a pleasurable hobby that affords release of tension.

PATIENT EDUCATION IN MYOCARDIAL INFARCTION (CONTINUED)

II. To undertake an *orderly* program of increasing activity and exercise for long-term rehabilitation.
  A. Engage in a regimen of physical conditioning with a gradual increase in activity levels.
    1. Walk daily, increasing distance and time as prescribed.
    2. Monitor your pulse during physical activity until you reach the maximal level of activity.
    3. Avoid activities that tense the muscles; isometric exercise, weight lifting, any activity that requires sudden bursts of energy.
    4. Avoid physical exercise immediately after a meal.
    5. Exercise before work, after work, or before retiring.
    6. Shorten work hours when first returning to work.
    7. Sexual relations may be resumed upon advice of physician, usually after exercise tolerance is evaluated. (See page 576.)
  B. Plan and participate in a *daily* program of exercise that develops into a program of regular exercise for a lifetime.
  C. Notify your physician when the following symptoms occur:
    1. Chest pressure or pain not relieved in 15 minutes by nitroglycerin. (Report to nearest emergency facility.)
    2. Shortness of breath
    3. Fainting
    4. Slow or rapid heart beat
    5. Swelling of feet and ankles

---

period; use of more passive positions to decrease cardiac work load. Sexual relations should be avoided after drinking alcohol or ingesting a large meal, if the situation produces anxiety or if abnormal symptoms develop and persist.

Patient Education

Certain general principles for living are usually prescribed at this stage, the character of which must vary widely from patient to patient, owing to marked differences in practical considerations and individual personalities. Questions that will arise may concern such matters as requirements for rest, criteria for controlling activities, and recommendations as to diet and the use of tobacco.

Obesity increases the work of the heart and should be brought under control, speedily and permanently. Arterial hypertension also imposes a myocardial burden and must be treated. Anemia, of course, should be corrected. With respect to smoking, it may be pointed out that most sudden deaths that occur in individuals with a past history of a myocardial infarction are due to cardiac arrhythmias, notably ventricular fibrillation, and that many of the individuals so afflicted are habitually heavy smokers. Smoking increases peripheral and coronary vasoconstriction and may produce a tachycardia. Logically, any individual who has sustained a myocardial infarction is well advised to eliminate the use of tobacco. (See also the summary of patient education in myocardial infarction below.)

CARDIAC FAILURE

In heart failure, the heart is unable to pump sufficient blood to meet the needs of the tissues for oxygen and nutrients. The cardiac output is frequently lower than normal, although heart failure can occur when there is high cardiac output in conditions when the metabolic requirements of the tissues are abnormally high. There are two predominant patterns of heart failure. The first has low cardiac output as its primary feature. If the low cardiac output develops acutely and is accompanied by low systemic arterial blood pressure, it is termed *cardiogenic shock*. The second pattern, *congestive heart failure*, is characterized by manifestations that are related primarily to retention of fluid in the lungs and/or peripheral tissues.

The underlying mechanism of heart failure involves the impaired contractile properties of the heart, which lead to a lower than normal stroke volume for any given conditions of preload and afterload. Dilatation of the ventricle usually results from inability of the heart to eject its usual volume of blood; i.e., ejection fraction is decreased. Because of ventricular dilatation, the preload is increased, which has the effect of augmenting the stroke volume (see Starling's Law of the Heart, page 510). Dilatation, therefore, tends to compensate for the decreased contractility of the heart. An increase in heart rate usually occurs in heart failure and also helps to restore cardiac output towards normal levels.

Etiology and Pathogenesis of Heart Failure

Heart failure most commonly occurs with disorders of cardiac muscle that result in decreased contractile properties of the heart. Frequent underlying conditions that lead to disordered muscle function include coronary atherosclerosis, arterial hypertension, and inflammatory or degenerative muscle disease. Coronary atherosclerosis leads to myocardial dysfunction by interfering with the normal blood supply to cardiac muscle. Hypoxia, acidosis (due to accumulation of lactic acid), and nutrient deprivation of heart muscle result. Myocardial infarction (death of myocardial cells) frequently precedes the development of overt heart failure. Systemic or pulmonary hypertension (increased afterload) increases the work requirement of the heart and this in turn leads to hypertrophy of myocardial muscle fibers. This effect (i.e., myocardial hypertrophy) can be considered a compensatory mechanism since it increases the contractility of the heart. However, for reasons that are not clear, the hypertrophied cardiac muscle does not function normally, and heart failure may eventually result. Heart failure associated with inflammatory and degenerative diseases of the myocardium is due to direct damage to myocardial fibers with a resultant decrease in contractility.

Heart failure may occur as a result of heart disease that only secondarily affects the myocardium. The mechanisms involved include impediment to flow of blood through the heart (e.g., stenosis of a semilunar valve), inability of the heart to fill with blood (e.g., pericardial tamponade, constrictive pericarditis, or stenosis of A-V valves), or abnormal emptying of the heart (e.g., insufficiency of A-V valves). Sudden increases in afterload due to elevated systemic blood pressure ("malignant" hypertension) may result in heart failure in the absence of myocardial hypertrophy.

A number of systemic factors can contribute to the development and severity of heart failure. Increased metabolic rate (e.g., fever, thyrotoxicosis), hypoxia, or anemia require an increased cardiac output to satisfy systemic oxygen demand. Hypoxia or anemia also may decrease the supply of oxygen to the myocardium. Acidosis (respiratory or metabolic) and electrolyte abnormalities may decrease myocardial contractility. Cardiac arrhythmias, which may be present independently or secondary to heart failure itself, decrease the efficiency of overall myocardial function.

Pathophysiology and Clinical Manifestations

The low output state in heart failure results in widespread manifestations due to diminished tissue and end-organ perfusion. Some commonly encountered effects related to low perfusion are dizziness, confusion, fatigue, exercise or heat intolerance, cool extremities, and oliguria. Renal perfusion pressure falls, which results in the release of renin from the kidney, which in turn leads to aldosterone secretion, sodium and fluid retention, and increased intravascular volume. The group of manifestations related to low cardiac output are sometimes referred to as "forward heart failure."

The dominant feature in congestive heart failure is increased intravascular volume. In this syndrome, congestion of tissues results from increased atrial and venous pressures due to decreased ventricular ejection fraction in the failing heart. Increased pulmonary venous pressure can lead to transudation of fluid from pulmonary capillaries (pulmonary edema), manifested by cough and shortness of breath. Increased systemic venous pressure can result in generalized peripheral edema and weight gain. This syndrome is sometimes referred to as "backward heart failure." Forward and backward heart failure usually coexist in most patients with heart failure.

The right and left ventricles can fail separately. Since the outputs of the ventricles are coupled, failure of either ventricle may lead to decreased tissue perfusion. The congestive manifestations, however, may differ according to whether right or left ventricular failure exists. Pulmonary congestion predominates when the left ventricle fails, whereas congestion of viscera and peripheral tissues predominates when the right ventricle fails.

Management

The basic objectives in the treatment of patients with congestive heart failure are:

1. To promote rest to reduce the work load on the heart.
2. To administer pharmacologic agents to increase the force and efficiency of myocardial contraction, which will improve the heart's effectiveness as a pump.
3. To eliminate the excessive accumulation of body water by means of diuretic therapy, diet, and rest.

Rest to Reduce Cardiac Work

If the cardiac load is to be decreased, it is essential that the patient have both physical and emotional rest. Rest reduces the work of the heart, increases heart reserve, and reduces the blood pressure. Periods of recumbency also promote diuresis by improving renal perfusion. Rest also decreases the work of the respiratory muscles and oxygen utilization. The heart rate is slowed, which prolongs the diastolic period of recovery and thus improves the efficiency of heart contraction. The patient will be impressed when he hears that each day of complete rest spares the heart approximately 25,000 contractions.

POSITIONING. The head of the bed may be elevated on 20- to 30-cm. (8-10 inch) blocks or the patient may be placed in a comfortable armchair. In this position the venous return to the heart and the lungs is reduced, pulmonary congestion is alleviated, and impingement of the liver on the diaphragm is minimized. The lower arms should be supported with pillows to eliminate the fatigue caused by the constant pull of their weight on the shoulder muscles. The orthopneic patient may sit on the side of his bed with his feet supported on a chair, his head and arms resting on an over-the-bed table, and his lumbosacral spine supported by a pillow. If pulmonary congestion is present, positioning the patient in an armchair is advantageous since this position favors the shift of fluid away from the lungs. Edema, which usually occurs in dependent parts of the body, shifts from the extremities to the sacral areas when the patient is confined to bed.

A bedside commode is advocated to avoid straining during bowel movements which can precipitate a pulmonary embolism.

- Remember that there are dangers inherent in bed rest: pressure sores (especially in edematous patients), phlebothrombosis, and pulmonary embolism. Changes of position, deep breathing, elastic stockings and leg exercises all help to improve muscle tone, aid in venous return to the heart, and increase the sense of well-being.

RELIEVING NIGHTTIME ANXIETY. Patients in congestive heart failure are very apt to be restless and anxious at night. Raising the head of the bed and keeping a night light on are helpful. The presence of a member of the family provides necessary reassurance to some persons. The patient should be observed for possible respiratory irregularities, such as Cheyne-Stokes respirations, a phenomenon that may occur in cardiac failure. If such a respiratory disturbance is present it may be worthwhile to test the effect of oxygen inhalations administered (as prescribed) each night just before the hour of sleep. Oxygen may be given during the acute stage to diminish the work of breathing and increase the comfort of the patient. Small doses of morphine may be ordered for extreme dyspnea and chloral hydrate may be given as needed for sleep.

- It should be recalled that the patient with hepatic congestion is unable to detoxify drugs with normal rapidity and should be medicated with caution. As a result of cerebral hypoxia, with superimposed nitrogen retention, the patient may react unfavorably to soporific drugs, becoming confused and increasingly anxious in response to medication. Such a patient should not be restrained; restraints are likely to be resisted, and resistance inevitably increases the cardiac load.

If the patient insists on getting out of bed at night, he should be seated comfortably in an armchair. As his cerebral and systemic circulations improve, the quality of his sleep will improve.

AVOIDING STRESS. Rest is not possible without relaxation. Emotional stress produces vasoconstriction, elevates the arterial pressure, and speeds the heart. Promoting the physical comfort and avoiding situations that tend to promote anxiety and agitation may help the patient to relax. The period of rest is continued for a few days to a few weeks until the congestive heart failure is controlled.

Pharmacologic Therapy: Digitalis

Cardiac glycosides (digitalis) and diuretics form the basis of the pharmacologic treatment of congestive heart failure.

Digitalis increases the force of myocardial contraction and slows the heart rate. Several effects are produced: an increase in cardiac output; decreases in heart size, venous pressure, and blood volume; and diuresis, which relieves edema. The effect of a given dose of digitalis depends on the state of the myocardium, electrolyte and fluid balance, and renal and hepatic function.

A loading dose of digitalis may be given to induce the full therapeutic effect of the drug. This is usually done in the treatment of more severe forms of congestive heart failure. Otherwise the patient is started without a loading dose. A maintenance dose is given and continued daily. In either case, the patient is observed closely and given a daily dose just adequate to replace the amount of drug that is destroyed or excreted, in order to maintain the digitalis effect without toxicity. The optimal dosage is the amount that relieves the patient's signs and symptoms of congestive failure or slows the ventricular response to atrial arrhythmias *without causing toxicity*. The patient is closely observed for relief of his signs and symptoms; lessening dyspnea and orthopnea, decrease in rales, and relief of peripheral edema.

DIGITALIS TOXICITY. Anorexia, nausea, and vomiting are early effects of digitalis toxicity. There may be alterations in the heart rhythm, especially bradycardia, premature ventricular contractions, and bigeminy (double beat).

- The apical heart rate is taken before digitalis is administered. If there is slowing of the heart rate and/or rhythm, the drug is withheld and the physician is notified.

TABLE 30-4. DIGITALIS AND CARDIAC GLYCOSIDE PREPARATIONS

I. ACTIONS OF DIGITALIS

1. Increases force and velocity of myocardial contractions
   a. Increases cardiac output by enhancing force of contraction of ventricle
   b. Slows heart rate
   c. Decreases heart size
   d. Decreases venous pressure
   e. Promotes diuresis
   f. Slows the ventricular rate in the setting of supraventricular arrhythmias

II. CLINICAL USES

   a. Congestive heart failure
   b. Atrial fibrillation; atrial flutter
   c. Supraventricular tachyarrhythmias
   d. Before cardiac surgery

III. PREPARATIONS

The choice of drug depends on the speed of onset desired, duration of action required, and individual patient response. The recommended dosage varies considerably.

Oral

Digitalis
Digitoxin
Digoxin
Lanatoside C
Acetyldigitoxin (Acylanid)
Gitalin (Gitaligin)

Parenteral

Ouabain
Deslanoside (Cedilanid-D)
Digitoxin
Digoxin (Lanoxin)

IV. NURSING CONSIDERATIONS AND ACTIONS

SPECIAL PRECAUTION: *The incidence of digitalis toxicity is high. Toxic effects do not always appear in a predictable manner.*

1. Watch for toxic effects; *arrhythmias* (most important toxic effect), *anorexia*, nausea, vomiting, bradycardia, headache, malaise.
2. Assess clinical response of patient by relief of symptoms (dyspnea, orthopnea, rales, hepatomegaly, peripheral edema).
3. Elderly patients may tolerate digitalis therapy poorly; assess for bradycardia, impaired renal function.
4. Monitor serum potassium levels in patients receiving digitalis, especially those receiving both digitalis and diuretics. There is a predisposition to arrhythmias if the state of potassium balance is not evaluated and corrected.
5. Assess for symptoms of electrolyte depletion in patients taking digitalis: lassitude, apathy, mental confusion, anorexia, decreasing urinary output, azotemia.
6. The following factors may increase sensitivity to digitalis: myocardial infarction, potassium depletion, kidney or hepatic disease, diuretic therapy, diarrhea, loss of appetite, advancing age, hypoxia and hypercapnia in pulmonary disease, acidosis, alkalosis.

Table 30–4 summarizes the major cardiac glycosides, along with their actions and the nursing surveillance required when these drugs are administered. (For a more detailed discussion of digitalis toxicity, see page 536.)

Diuretic Therapy

Diuretics are given to promote the excretion of sodium and water through the kidneys. These drugs may not be necessary if the patient responds to restricted activity, digitalis, and a low sodium diet.

- When diuretics are given they should be administered early in the morning so that the resultant diuresis will not interfere with the patient's nighttime rest.
- An input and output record is kept, since the patient may lose a large volume of fluid after a single dose of a given diuretic.
- As a basis for evaluating the effectiveness of therapy, patients receiving diuretic drugs are weighed daily at the same time. In addition, skin turgor is examined for evidences of edema or dehydration. The pulse rate is also monitored.

The dosage schedule is determined by the patient's daily weight, physical findings, and his symptoms. Table 30–5 summarizes the diuretics in common use.

DIURETIC SIDE EFFECTS. Prolonged diuretic therapy may produce *hyponatremia* (deficiency of sodium in the blood), which results in apprehension, weakness, fatigue, malaise, muscle cramps and twitching, and rapid thready pulse.

Profuse and repeated diuresis can also lead to *hypokalemia* (potassium depletion). Signs are weak pulse, faint heart sounds, hypotension, muscle flabbiness, diminished tendon reflexes, and generalized weakness. This poses new problems for the cardiac patient, because among the complications of hypokalemia are marked weakening of cardiac contractions and the precipitation of digitalis toxicity in individuals receiving digitalis, both of which increase the likelihood of dangerous arrhythmias.

- Periodic assessment of the electrolytes will alert to hypokalemia and hyponatremia.
- To lessen the risk of hypokalemia and its attendant complications, patients receiving diuretic drugs may be given a potassium supplement (potassium chloride). Bananas, orange juice, dried prunes, raisins, apricots, dates, figs, peaches, and spinach are good dietary sources of potassium.

Other problems associated with diuretic administration are hyperuricemia, volume depletion, hyperglycemia, and diabetes mellitus.

The elderly male patient requires ongoing nursing surveillance inasmuch as the incidence of urethral obstruction due to prostatic hypertrophy is high in this age group. Signs of bladder distention should be sought regularly by palpation over the bladder.

Dietary Support in Congestive Heart Failure

The rationale of dietary support is to provide the type of diet that will cause the heart the least possible work effort and muscular strain, to maintain the good nutritional status of the patient, and to provide a diet suited to the patient's likes and dislikes or cultural food habits. (The diet in the acute phase of myocardial infarction is discussed on page 543.)

TABLE 30-5. COMMONLY USED DIURETICS

Definition: Diuretics are agents which increase the rate of urine flow.

Action: Dependent upon functionally active kidneys; most diuretics decrease the reabsorption of electrolytes (principally sodium) by the kidneys, promoting water loss as a secondary action.
In the treatment of hypertension the naturetic (sodium excretion) effect is probably the action of importance.
In edema states, the salt and water actions are both important.

Special Precaution: Some diuretics may produce electrolyte depletion including potassium loss, which causes weakness and induces cardiac arrhythmias. Vigorous diuresis can produce hypovolemia.

Dosage Determination: (1) Patient's daily weight; (2) clinical signs and symptoms; (3) physical examination; (4) state of renal function

DIURETIC	ACTION	NURSING IMPLICATIONS
Thiazides and Related Drugs Chlorothiazide (Diuril) Hydrochlorothiazide (HydroDIURIL, Esidrix, Oretic) Methyclothiazide (Enduron) Polythiazide (Renese) Chlorthalidone (Hygroton) Quinethazone (Hydromox)	Increases renal excretion of sodium (nateresis), potassium, chloride, bicarbonate (alkaline urine) with accompanying "osmotic" water loss. Used principally in states of edema and hypertension. Most widely used for prolonged administration.	Monitor for electrolyte depletion. Watch for signs and symptoms of electrolyte imbalance: hyponatremia, hypokalemia, hypochloremic alkalosis. Adverse reactions may occur, manifested by gastrointestinal, central nervous system, hematologic, and cardiovascular signs and symptoms. Supplementary potassium is usually given with these diuretics.
Potassium-Sparing Diuretics Spironolactone (Aldactone)	Inhibits action of aldosterone in distal tubule and reduces reabsorption of sodium and chloride. Gives gradual diuretic effect. Used in treatment of cirrhosis and edema when other diuretics are toxic or ineffective.	Monitor for electrolyte depletion. Usually used in combination with thiazide diuretic. Watch for side effects—skin rash, gynecomastia.
Triamterene (Dyrenium)	Inhibits reabsorption of sodium ions in exchange for potassium and hydrogen ions in distal tubule.	Usually used as an adjunct to thiazide therapy. May cause elevation in blood uric acid. Watch for nausea, vomiting, diarrhea, weakness, headache, and skin rash.
Potent Diuretics Furosemide (Lasix) Ethacrynic Acid (Edecrin)	Usually reserved for patients who do not respond to classical thiazide diuretics. Blocks the reabsorption of sodium and water in proximal renal tubule and interferes with reabsorption of sodium in ascending limb of loop of Henle and in the most proximal portion of the distal tubule. Associated with sodium, potassium, chloride, and hydrogen ion loss (acid urine). Have an almost immediate action (within 5 minutes) when given IV.	Monitor for electrolyte depletion: may produce *profound diuresis* with hyponatremia, hypokalemia, hypochloremic alkalosis, and circulatory collapse. Potent and rapid-acting. Especially useful in acute pulmonary edema. Watch for nausea, vomiting, diarrhea, skin rash, pruritus, blurring of vision, postural hypotension, vertigo, hearing loss. Furosemide is chemically related to sulfonamides; consider cross allergies. Administer early in the day to avoid nocturia and consequent loss of sleep.

If sodium restriction is indicated for the prevention, control, or elimination of edema, such as in hypertension or congestive heart failure, *sodium* should be specified in describing the regimen (rather than "low salt" or "salt free"), and the quantity should be indicated in milligrams. Very often mistakes are made in hospital units because of inconsistencies in the translation of salt to sodium. It is important to realize that salt is not 100 percent sodium. There are only 393 mg., or approximately 400 mg., of sodium in one gram (1,000 mg.) of salt.

In some hospital manuals the level of sodium restriction may be prescribed in units of mEq. The following method may be useful in converting mg. of sodium to mEq. and vice versa:

To convert mg. to mEq. of sodium:

$$1,000 \div 23 = 43.5$$
mg. sodium $\div$ atomic weight $=$ mEq. sodium

To convert mEq. to mg. of sodium:

$$43.5 \times 23 = 1,000$$
mEq. sodium $\times$ atomic weight $=$ mg. sodium

Therefore, a diet containing

20 mEq. Na = 460 mg. Na
40 mEq. Na = 920 mg. Na
90 mEq. Na = 2,070 mg. Na

When food composition tables are consulted to determine the sodium content of menu items, the sodium content can be calculated in milligrams (mg.) and then converted to milliEquivalents (mEq.).

Although the major source of sodium in the average American diet is salt, many types of natural foods contain varying amounts of sodium. Therefore, even if no salt is added in cooking and if salty foods are avoided, the daily diet may still contain approximately 1,000 to 2,000 mg. of sodium.

Other sources of sodium can be found in some processed foods. Added food substances such as sodium alginate, which improves texture; sodium benzoate, which acts as a preservative; or di-sodium phosphate, which improves cooking quality in certain foods — all increase the sodium intake when included in the daily diet. Therefore, patients on low sodium diets should be advised not to buy processed foods and to check labels carefully for such words as "salt" or "sodium." For diets that call for less than 1,000 mg. of sodium, low sodium milk and bread and salt-free butter should be considered.

Patients on sodium restricted diets should also be cautioned against buying nonprescription medications such as alkalizers, cough syrups, laxatives, sedatives, or salt substitutes, because these products contain sodium or excessive amounts of potassium. Any over-the-counter medication of this type should not be purchased without first consulting the physician.

When diets are very restrictive of both fat and sodium, the patient may find the food unpalatable and may refuse to eat. A variety of flavorings and herb seasonings may be used to improve the taste of the food and encourage the patient to accept the diet. Every effort should be made to take into account the patient's likes and dislikes.

Patient Education

After the patient's congestive failure is under control he is encouraged to gradually resume the activities he was accustomed to prior to his illness, particularly his job. The patient's earlier life style should be retained if possible. However, some modifications in his habits, work, and interpersonal relationships usually have to be made. Any activity that produces symptoms must be curtailed or other adaptations made. The patient should be helped to identify his emotional stresses and to explore ways in which these may be ventilated and discharged.

All too frequently patients keep returning to the clinic and hospital for recurring episodes of congestive heart failure. Not only does this create psychological, sociological, and financial problems, but the physiological burden on the patient can be serious. Previously normal organs of the body may ultimately be damaged. Repeated attacks can lead to pulmonary fibrosis, liver cirrhosis, enlargement of the spleen and kidneys, and even brain damage due to insufficient oxygen during acute episodes. *To ensure that the patient will persevere in his therapy requires patient education, involvement, and cooperation.* Many of the recurrences of congestive heart failure appear to be preventable. These include failure to follow the drug therapy *properly,* dietary indiscretions, inadequate medical follow-up, excessive physical activity, and failure to recognize recurring symptoms. A summary of what the patient should know about his condition is given on page 583.

It must be emphasized that cough medicines, alkalizers, pain remedies, etc., contain fairly large amounts of sodium. The patient must be warned against using these products and advised to rinse his mouth with clear water when using toothpaste and mouthwashes. In some areas the drinking water has a high sodium content. To find out what this content is, the patient should contact his local health department. As an added precaution for older patients whose eyesight is dimming and whose fingers are less nimble as a result of arthritis, the printing on the drug bottle should be large and easily readable and the bottle should be equipped with an easy-open stopper.

Congestive heart failure can be controlled. The patient must never become lax in following his therapeutic program. Careful follow-up of patients with heart lesions, maintenance of correct weight, sodium restriction, prevention of infection, avoidance of noxious agents such as

---

PATIENT EDUCATION IN CONGESTIVE HEART FAILURE

A patient with heart disease should learn to regulate his activity according to his individual response. The goal is always to prevent progression of disease and the development of congestive heart failure.

I. To live within the limits of the cardiac reserve:
  A. Obtain adequate rest.
    1. Have a regular daily rest period.
    2. Shorten working hours if possible.
    3. Avoid emotional upsets.
  B. Accept the fact that taking digitalis and restricting sodium intake will be a permanent way of life.
    1. Take digitalis daily, exactly as prescribed.
      a. Do not substitute another brand of digitalis for the one that you are taking.
      b. Check your own pulse rate.
      c. Have a check-off system so that you are sure the medicine(s) have been taken.
    2. Take diuretic as prescribed.
      a. Weigh at the same time daily to detect any tendency toward fluid accumulation.
      b. Report weight gain of more than 0.9 to 1.4 kg. (2 to 3 pounds) in a few days.
      c. Know the signs and symptoms of potassium depletion; if taking oral potassium, keep a check-off system along with diuretic medication.
  C. Restrict sodium as directed.
    1. Consult the written diet plan and the list of permitted and restricted foods that have been provided for you.

PATIENT EDUCATION IN CONGESTIVE HEART FAILURE (CONTINUED)

    2. Look at all labels to ascertain sodium content (antacids, laxatives, cough remedies, etc.)
    3. Avoid using the saltshaker.
    4. Avoid excesses in eating and drinking.
  D. Review activity program.
    The patient is instructed as follows:
      a. Increase walking and other activities gradually, provided that they do not cause fatigue and dyspnea.
      b. In general, continue at whatever activity level you can maintain without the appearance of symptoms.
      c. Avoid extremes of heat and cold which increase the work of the heart. Air conditioning may be essential in a hot, humid environment.
      d. Keep regular appointment with physician or clinic.

II. To be alert for symptoms that may indicate recurring congestive heart failure.
    1. Recall the symptoms you experienced when you first became ill; reappearance of previous symptoms may indicate a recurrence.
    2. Report immediately to the physician or clinic any of the following:
      a. Gain in weight.
      b. Loss of appetite.
      c. Shortness of breath upon activity.
      d. Swelling of ankles, feet or abdomen.
      e. Persistent cough.
      f. Frequent urination at night.

---

coffee and tobacco, avoidance of unregulated or excessive exercise—all aid in preventing the onset of congestive heart failure. In patients with valvular heart disease, surgical correction of the defect at the appropriate time may spare the heart and prevent failure.

The Patient with Severe or Chronic Congestive Heart Failure

Severe or chronic heart failure that does not yield to conventional measures will require additional treatment such as the use of vasodilators to increase cardiac output by dilating peripheral blood vessels and reducing *impedance* (resistance) to left ventricular outflow.

Sodium nitroprusside has a vasodilator effect in both the arterial and venous vascular beds by relaxing vascular smooth muscle. This results in venous pooling and a reduction in peripheral vascular resistance. It decreases left ventricular filling pressure and increases cardiac output. This aids renal blood flow and thus causes diuresis. Sodium nitroprusside, given by intravenous infusion, is potent and rapid-acting. The flow rate is monitored by an infusion pump or microdrip regulator and is titrated according to the patient's blood pressure response. If available, the patient's pulmonary artery pressures and cardiac output are monitored (see page 443).

• If hypotension occurs, the infusion is stopped, the patient's legs are elevated, and intravenous fluids are given for rapid volume expansion.

Long-acting nitrates (Isorbide dinitrate) act primarily on the veins and help to lower left ventricular end diastolic pressure and relieve pulmonary congestion. Nitroglycerin ointment appears to have a similar beneficial action. These drugs are discussed on pages 572-573.

Other drugs include phentolamine, which acts chiefly on arterioles to raise cardiac output; orally administered hydralazine, which produces systemic arteriolar dilatation, and prazosin (Minipress), which causes systemic vasodilatation of both the arteriolar and venous systems. These drugs are being used as impedance reduction therapy and to raise cardiac output in ambulatory patients with chronic heart failure.

ACUTE PULMONARY EDEMA

Pathophysiology

Pulmonary edema is the abnormal accumulation of fluid in the lungs, either in the interstitial spaces or in the alveoli.

Pulmonary edema represents the ultimate stage of pulmonary congestion, in which fluid has leaked through the capillary walls and is permeating the airways, giving rise to dyspnea of dramatic severity. Pulmonary congestion, it will be recalled, occurs when the pulmonary vascular bed has received more blood from the right ventricle than the left can accommodate and remove. The slightest imbalance between inflow on the right side and outflow on the left side of the heart may have drastic consequences: for example, if with each heartbeat the right ventricle pumps out just one more drop of blood than the left, within the space of only 3 hours the pulmonary blood volume will have expanded 500 ml.!

Noncardiac pulmonary edema has a wide variety of causes: toxic inhalants, drug overdose, neurogenic pulmonary edema. Clinical management is directed towards reducing pulmonary blood flow and pulmonary arterial pressure.

The most common cause of pulmonary edema is cardiac disease—atherosclerotic, hypertensive, valvular, myopathic. Most patients with pulmonary edema have chronic heart disease of a type that imposes a strain on the left ventricle, such as arterial hypertension or aortic valve disease. The development of pulmonary edema signifies that cardiac function has become grossly inadequate. There is an elevated left ventricular end diastolic pressure and a rise in pulmonary venous pressure. This produces an increase in hydrostatic pressure, which results in transudation of fluid. Impaired lymphatic drainage contributes to the accumulation of fluid in the lung tissues.

The pulmonary capillaries, engorged with an excess of blood that the left ventricle has been incapable of discharging, no longer are able to retain their contents. Fluid, first serous and later bloody, escapes into the adjacent alveoli through the communicating bronchioles and bronchi. It then mixes with air and, churned by respiratory agitation, is expelled from the mouth and nostrils, producing the ominous "death rattle." Because of the fluid buildup, the lungs become stiff and cannot expand, and air cannot enter. The result is severe hypoxia.

However, death from pulmonary edema is by no means inevitable. If appropriate measures are taken, and taken promptly, many attacks can be aborted and many patients can survive this complication to benefit from measures directed against its return. Fortunately, pulmonary edema usually does not develop precipitously but is preceded by the premonitory symptoms of pulmonary congestion. Moreover, even after it has become well established, it usually does not progress to a fatal termination with lightning rapidity; its course may occupy a period of many minutes, even hours, during which time treatment may prove to be effective.

Clinical Manifestations

The typical attack of pulmonary edema occurs at night after the patient has been lying down for a few hours. Recumbency increases the venous return to the heart and favors the resorption of edema fluid from the legs. The circulating blood becomes diluted, and its volume expands. The venous pressure mounts and the right atrium fills with increasing rapidity. There is a corresponding increase in the right ventricular output, which eventually surpasses the output from the left ventricle. The pulmonary vessels become engorged with blood and proceed to leak. Meanwhile the patient has become increasingly restless, oppressed with anxiety, and unable to sleep.

There is a sudden onset of breathlessness and a fearful sense of suffocation. The patient's hands become cold and moist; the nail beds become cyanotic and the complexion turns gray. In addition, the pulse is small and rapid and the neck veins distended. There is incessant coughing, which produces increasing quantities of mucoid sputum. As the pulmonary edema progresses, the patient's anxiety develops into near panic and he becomes confused, then stuporous. He breathes noisily and moistly, nearly suffocated by the blood-tinged frothy fluid that now is pouring into his bronchi and trachea. He literally is drowning in his own secretions. The situation is precarious and demands immediate action.

Management

The objectives of therapy are to improve ventilation and oxygenation, reduce pulmonary congestion, and increase myocardial contractility. A combination of the following measures helps to implement these objectives.

POSITIONING. Proper positioning can help reduce venous return to the heart.

- Place the patient upright, with his legs and feet down. This has the immediate effect of decreasing venous return, lowering the output of the right ventricle, and decongesting the lungs.
- Then place the patient in an upright position in bed to allow blood to pool in the dependent portions of the body (Fig. 30-1). As long as blood accumulates in the periphery, correspondingly less blood returns to the heart. The upright position also improves lung volume and vital capacity.

OXYGENATION. Oxygen is administered in high concentration by face mask to relieve hypoxia and dyspnea. It must be given with high enough pressure to overcome the pressure barrier from the edema fluid and to provide oxygenation of the blood. If signs of hypoxemia persist, oxygen is delivered by intermittent or continuous positive pressure. If respiratory failure occurs despite optimal management, endotracheal intubation and mechanical ventilation are required. The use of positive end expiratory pressure (PEEP) is effective in reducing venous return, lowering pulmonary capillary pressure, and improving oxygenation (see page 449). Oxygenation is monitored by measurement of arterial blood gases.

MORPHINE. Morphine is given intravenously in small doses to reduce anxiety and dyspnea and to decrease peripheral resistance so that blood can be redistributed from the pulmonary circulation to the periphery. This action decreases pressure in the pulmonary capillaries and decreases transudation of fluid.

- Morphine is not given if pulmonary edema is caused by cerebral vascular accident or if chronic pulmonary disease or cardiogenic shock is present.
- Watch for excessive respiratory depression and have a morphine antagonist (naloxone hydrochloride [Narcan]) available.

DIURETICS. Either furosemide or ethacrynic acid is given intravenously to produce a rapid diuretic effect. In addition, furosemide causes vasodilatation and peripheral venous pooling with a subsequent reduction in venous return that occurs even before the diuretic effect. Thus dyspnea is rapidly relieved and pulmonary congestion is decreased. Since a large volume of urine will accumulate within minutes after administration of a potent diuretic, an indwelling catheter must be inserted.

- Watch for falling blood pressure, increasing heart rate, and decreasing urinary output; these indicate that the total circulation is not tolerating diuresis.
- Patients with prostatic hypertrophy must be watched for signs of urinary retention.

AMINOPHYLLINE. When the patient is wheezing and bronchospasm appears to play a significant role, aminophylline may be given to relax bronchospasm.

- Give aminophylline *slowly* by vein, since arrhythmias, syncope, and sudden death may follow too rapid administration.

ROTATING TOURNIQUETS. The application of rotating tourniquets (or automatic inflating cuffs) on the extremities decreases venous return and right ventricular output, which aids in decongesting the lungs. The immediate effect is equivalent to removing about 1,000 ml. of circulating blood. Rotating tourniquets are an adjunct to pharmacologic therapy.

- Tell the patient the purpose of the treatment and that the skin of the extremities may become discolored.
- Take an initial blood pressure reading to serve as a baseline for future comparisons.
- Mark the peripheral pulses, if time permits.
- If tourniquets are used (instead of cuffs) they are positioned over a small towel as high as possible on three extremities. The arterial pulse should not be occluded. One extremity should be free of a tourniquet during each time interval. (A

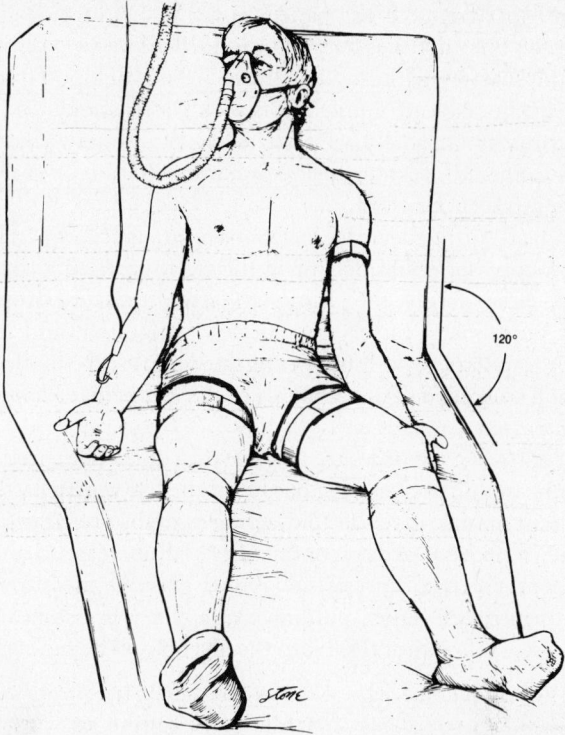

Figure 30-1. The patient with pulmonary edema is placed upright to reduce venous return to the heart. The administration of oxygen improves arterial hypoxemia and cardiac function. The application of rotating tourniquets brings about a rapid decrease in venous return and may result in dramatic clinical improvement. (Courtesy, Am. Fam. Phys.)

tourniquet is not placed on an extremity in which an IV line is inserted.)
- Release one tourniquet every 15 minutes; then apply a tourniquet to the previously free extremity. The venous outflow in any one extremity may be occluded for 45 minutes and unoccluded for 15 minutes. However, tourniquets may have to be rotated at 5-minute intervals on elderly patients or those with poor circulation in order to prevent gangrene and other complications.
- Rotate the tourniquets in a consistent clockwise pattern.
- Monitor the blood pressure every few minutes, since the use of tourniquets may precipitate hypotension in some patients.
- When the patient's symptoms have been relieved, discontinue the use of the tourniquets by removing them one at a time at 15-minute intervals. Simultaneous removal of all tourniquets could precipitate a recurrence of pulmonary edema.
- Examine each extremity after the tourniquet is removed for color, warmth, and the presence of a palpable pulse.

When an automatic rotating tourniquet machine is used, the cuffs are inflated and deflated automatically in sequence. The nurse follows the protocol of the machine's manufacturer in applying the cuffs, adjusting the pressure, checking for leaks in the system, etc. Clinical assessment of the patient is the same as for manual rotating tourniquets (see above).

PHLEBOTOMY. If the patient is refractory to management it is sometimes helpful to reduce the venous return to the heart by withdrawing 250 to 500 ml. of blood from a peripheral vein (a phlebotomy or venesection). Phlebotomy is especially valuable when pulmonary edema has followed overtransfusion or administration of excessive intravenous fluid.

The resulting decrease in venous return is accompanied by a corresponding decline in the right ventricular output. Accordingly, the pulmonary artery pressure drops, the pulmonary vessels become less congested, and the lung capillaries, no longer congested, reabsorb the fluid that has escaped. The edema clears; the immediate danger has passed.

DIGITALIS. In order to improve the contractile force of the heart and increase the output of the left ventricle, the patient may be given a rapid-acting digitalis preparation. The improved cardiac contractility will increase cardiac output, enhance diuresis, and reduce diastolic pressure in the ventricles. Thus, pulmonary capillary pressure and the transudation of fluid into the alveoli will be reduced.

- Digitalis must be given with extreme caution to patients with acute myocardial infarction, since these patients are sensitive to digitalis and may develop toxic arrhythmias.
- The serum potassium level is measured at intervals because diuresis may have produced hypokalemia. If this occurs, a potassium supplement is given to prevent digitalis toxicity.
- If the patient has been on digitalis, the drug is usually withheld until the possibility of digitalis intoxication is ruled out.

VASODILATOR THERAPY. In instances in which the patient has not responded to treatment, vasodilator drugs have been used to reduce impedance (resistance) to left ventricular ejection of blood. The drug action allows more complete ventricular emptying and increases venous capacity, so that left ventricular filling pressure is reduced and a dramatic decrease in pulmonary congestion may be achieved rapidly. Sodium nitroprusside may be given intravenously by means of carefully monitored infusions. The dosage is titrated to keep the arterial systolic pressure at the prescribed level, and the patient is monitored by measuring pulmonary artery pressures (Swan–Ganz, page 443) and cardiac output.

PSYCHOLOGICAL SUPPORT. Extreme fear and anxiety are cardinal features of pulmonary edema. These emotions, which are self-perpetuating, make the condition more severe. Reassuring the patient and providing skillful anticipatory nursing are integral parts of the therapy.

Prevention

Like most medical and surgical complications, pulmonary edema is easier to prevent than to treat. Thus, if recognized in its *early* stages, when the presenting symptoms and signs are solely those of pulmonary congestion, the situation may be corrected by relatively simple measures. These include: (1) placing the patient in an upright position; (2) eliminating overexertion and emotional stress to reduce the left ventricular load, and (3) administering morphine to reduce anxiety and dyspnea.

The long-range approach to the prevention of pulmonary edema must be directed at its precursor, namely, pulmonary congestion. See measures to prevent congestive heart failure (page 582) and the various facets of patient teaching (page 583).

In addition to these measures it may be wise for the patient to sleep with the head of his bed elevated on 25-cm. (10-inch) blocks. It is especially important to take extreme precautions when giving infusions and transfusions to cardiac patients and elderly persons.

- Intravenous fluids are given at a slower rate, with the patient positioned upright in bed and kept under close nursing surveillance, in order to prevent circulatory overloading, which could precipitate acute pulmonary edema.

Surgical treatment may be necessary to eliminate or to minimize valvular defects that limit the flow of blood into or out of the left ventricle, since such defects impair the cardiac output and predispose the patient to the development of pulmonary congestion and edema.

ARRHYTHMIAS*

An *arrhythmia* is a clinical disorder of the heartbeat that may include a disturbance of rate, rhythm (sequence), or both. Arrhythmias are derangements of heart function and not of heart structure.

Pathophysiology

The rate and the rhythm of the heartbeat depend on the speed and the regularity with which the electrical impulses are generated by the pacemaker (normally the SA node) and on the functional integrity of the conduction system that distributes these impulses through the myocardium. The activity of the SA node, as was previously pointed out, is subject to the influence of the autonomic nervous system. It responds to chemical changes in the blood and is highly susceptible to the action of some drugs (digitalis, quinidine, atropine). Its normal activity may be altered and its conduction pathways interrupted as a result of disturbances of other organ systems (central nervous system disturbances and endocrine and renal disorders). Its function as a pacemaker can be usurped by the AV node or by some other "hyperirritable" focus elsewhere in the conduction system. When the SA node or AV node fails to produce an electrical impulse, pacemakers with slower rates may control cardiac activity. Other causes of arrhythmias are digitalis intoxication, infection, disturbances of electrolyte balance, anemia,

*Specific arrhythmias are discussed on pages 527–538.

and cardiac surgery. Of course, arrhythmias may be due to organic heart disease: atherosclerotic, congenital, hypertensive, or inflammatory. Pacemaker malfunction may produce serious arrhythmias.

Types of Arrhythmias

The classification of arrhythmias is based on the disturbed physiology. There may be a disturbance of impulse formation in which the heartbeat is activated for one or more beats by a pacemaker other than the SA node. There may be disturbances in conduction in which there is a delay in the transmission of impulses, failure of some impulses to be conducted, or a blockage of impulse at the affected site. Or, there may be a combination of abnormally rapid impulse formation and decreased ability to conduct the impulses.

Clinical Manifestations

The signs and symptoms depend on the ventricular rate, the condition of the heart, and the patient's psychological reaction. Clinical manifestations of rapid arrhythmias include *anxiety* and *palpitation*, in which the patient is aware of a rapid, forceful, or irregular heartbeat. The patient may complain of nervousness and uneasiness and of pounding, jumping, or "stopping" sensations in his chest. There may be dizziness, fainting, throbbing in the head and neck, shortness of breath, and precordial discomfort and pain. Symptoms and signs of bradycardia (slow heart action) are shortness of breath, fatigue on exertion, dizziness, and fainting which may lead to convulsive seizures.

Clinical Effects of Arrhythmias

Some arrhythmias are relatively harmless, whereas others are harbingers of cardiac arrest. In general, arrhythmias impair the pumping action of the heart and reduce cardiac output, which has the effect of lowering the blood pressure and decreasing blood perfusion of the brain, heart, kidneys, gastrointestinal tract, muscles, and skin. Cardiac arrhythmias can also produce transient cerebral ischemia attacks which result in a complete cerebral vascular accident (stroke), or they can precipitate congestive heart failure or angina pectoris in certain patients. Bradyarrhythmias (rate below 60) may predispose to electrical instability of the heart. Obviously, a marked degree of disability may accompany an arrhythmia.

Nursing Assessment

- Evaluate the patient's general appearance.
   Is there pallor, cyanosis, or sweating? (These signs may result from arteriolar constriction.)
- How does the patient describe his symptoms?
- Observe the carotid pulsation.
   Is it rapid and vigorous or irregular with varying amplitude?
- Listen to the heart with a stethoscope, noting rate, the pres-

ence of irregularity, and an increase in the intensity of the first heart sound (see page 71).

- Take the blood pressure and pulse. The carotid pulse should be counted if the radial pulse cannot be counted. Bear in mind that abnormal beats may not be detectable at the wrist since a very weak pulse wave often fails to reach the periphery; in this event, the apical and radial rates will not correspond. Both pulses must be counted independently and simultaneously by two observers for at least one minute in order to determine the pulse deficit. The greater the deficit, the less efficient the ventricular contractions are assumed to be, and the less favorable the clinical evaluation of cardiac function.
- Evaluate the patient for mental confusion, which indicates cerebral ischemia.
- Note the presence of chest pain.
   The presence of chest pains with an arrhythmia is usually due to myocardial ischemia.
- Note any signs and symptoms of congestive heart failure which may indicate that the arrhythmia is causing serious effects.

If possible, an electrocardiogram should be taken during an episode of arrhythmia. Arrhythmias are likely to be transient and elusive; hence an ECG recording is most informative during the course of an arrhythmic episode.

Patients with arrhythmias are prone to be anxious. Anxiety tends to beget more symptoms that promote increasing anxiety, which further aggravates symptoms until fear and anxiety can outweigh all other factors. It is important that this vicious cycle be broken. By displaying a supportive attitude, offering calm explanations, and conveying optimism, the nurse can help to alleviate this acute problem.

The common disturbances of rhythm, their ECG interpretations, and their treatment are discussed on pages 527–538.

Instant Telemetry

Transient heart arrhythmias can be difficult to detect because it is not always possible to take an electrocardiogram at the moment when they are occurring. By means of a battery-operated telemetry system, the ECG signals can be obtained without the use of electrode paste or limb leads. The patient can transmit his own ECG with an instant telemetry system. He presses the sensor across the lower part of his sternum, turns on the unit, and places the telephone transmitter over the speaker. His ECG is transmitted by telephone to a receiver located in a cardiac care unit (CCU) or a medical facility. The nurse in the CCU records the rhythm strip that has been transmitted and consults the physician. This telemetry method permits early recognition of arrhythmias.

The patient may wear a portable electrocardiographic monitor so that his cardiac rhythm may be recorded on magnetic tape as he goes about his daily routine. He keeps a diary of the times (and concomitant activities) when he feels his symptoms. This technique is described on page 514.

PACEMAKER THERAPY

A *pacemaker* is an electronic device that provides repetitive electrical stimuli to the heart muscle for the control of heart rate. It initiates and maintains the heart rate when the natural pacemakers of the heart are unable to do so. Pacemakers are generally used when a patient has an arrhythmia or the forerunner of an arrhythmia that causes failure of cardiac output (such as can be seen in bradycardias, particularly complete heart block, tachyarrhythmias, and arrhythmias following myocardial infarction). Temporary pacing is also done to control the heart rate during open heart surgery or thoracotomy.

Pacemaker Design

Pacemakers consist of two component parts: (1) the electronic pulse generator which contains the circuitry and batteries that generate the electrical signal, and (2) the pacemaker electrodes (also called leads or wires) which transmit the pacemaker impulses to the heart. The stimuli from the pacemaker travel through a flexible catheter electrode that is threaded through a vein into the right ventricle or introduced by direct penetration of the chest wall. The pulse generator is usually implanted in a subcutaneous pocket in the pectoral or axillary region.

Pacemaker generators are insulated to protect against body moisture and warmth. The pulse generator (or pacemaker) contains its own supply of power that is provided by battery cells. The main power sources in current use are mercury-zinc batteries (lasting 3 to 4 years), lithium cell units (lasting up to 10 years), and a nuclear-powered pacemaker (^{238}plutonium source) lasting 20 years to a lifetime. There are also pacemakers that can be recharged externally. Since pacemakers rely on batteries, battery exhaustion (with the exception of nuclear power and rechargeable batteries) is inevitable. Therefore, the generator that contains the batteries must be replaced periodically.

Types of Pacemakers

The most commonly used pacemaker is the *demand* (synchronous; noncompetitive) pacemaker which is set for a specific rate and stimulates the heart when normal ventricular depolarization does not occur or if the heart rate drops below the specified rate. It functions only when the natural heart rate goes below a certain level. The *fixed* rate pacemaker (asynchronous; competitive) stimulates the ventricle at a preset constant rate that is independent of the patient's rhythm. It is used infrequently, usually in patients with complete and unvarying heart block.

TEMPORARY PACEMAKER SYSTEMS. Temporary pacing is usually an emergency procedure and permits the observation of the effects of pacing on heart function so that the optimum pacing rate for the patient can be selected before a permanent pacemaker is implanted. It is used in patients who have suffered myocardial infarction with conduction block, in patients with cardiac arrest with bradycardia and asystole, or in selected postoperative cardiac surgery patients. Temporary pacing may be done for hours, days, or weeks and is continued until the patient improves or a permanent pacemaker is implanted.

Temporary pacing may be carried out either by an endocardial (transvenous) approach or by the transthoracic approach to the myocardium. The transvenous electrode is passed under fluoroscopic guidance through any peripheral vein (antecubital, brachial, jugular, subclavian, femoral) and the catheter tip is positioned in the apex of the right ventricle. The most common complications occurring during pacemaker insertion are ventricular arrhythmia and, much less frequently, cardiac perforation. A defibrillator should be immediately available.

Nursing Management. The pacemaker generator and control unit can be attached around the patient's waist or to his right arm, with plenty of slack available so that the motion of the arm will not dislodge the catheter. No metal parts of the output terminal or pacemaker wires should be exposed. All such bare metal should be scrupulously covered with nonconductive tape in order to prevent accidental ventricular fibrillation from stray currents which might reach the heart if exposed metal parts were to come in contact with a metal conductor such as a bedrail. Aberrant current sources (from malfunctioning equipment) can travel over the surface of a damp skin and can also cause ventricular fibrillation. *The patient must be placed in an electrically safe environment.* The nurse attending the patient should have special training in protecting patients from electrical hazards. All monitoring and other electrical equipment should be grounded with three-pronged plugs inserted into a proper outlet.

It is important that the nurse be familiar with the complications of the procedure (page 589) and with the operating instructions for the pacemaker equipment being used. The vein through which the pacing wire has been inserted is monitored for evidence of phlebitis. In addition, it may be necessary to change the amplitude of the stimulation impulse and adjust the rate of stimulation as an emergency intervention. Special training in these techniques is necessary.

PERMANENT PACING. For permanent pacing, the endocardial lead is passed transvenously into the right ventricle and the pulse generator is implanted within the body underneath the skin below the right or left pectoral region or below the clavicle (Fig. 30-2). This is termed an endocardial or transvenous implant. This procedure is usually done under local anesthesia. Another method of permanent pacing is the implantation of the pulse generator in the abdominal wall. The electrode is passed trans-

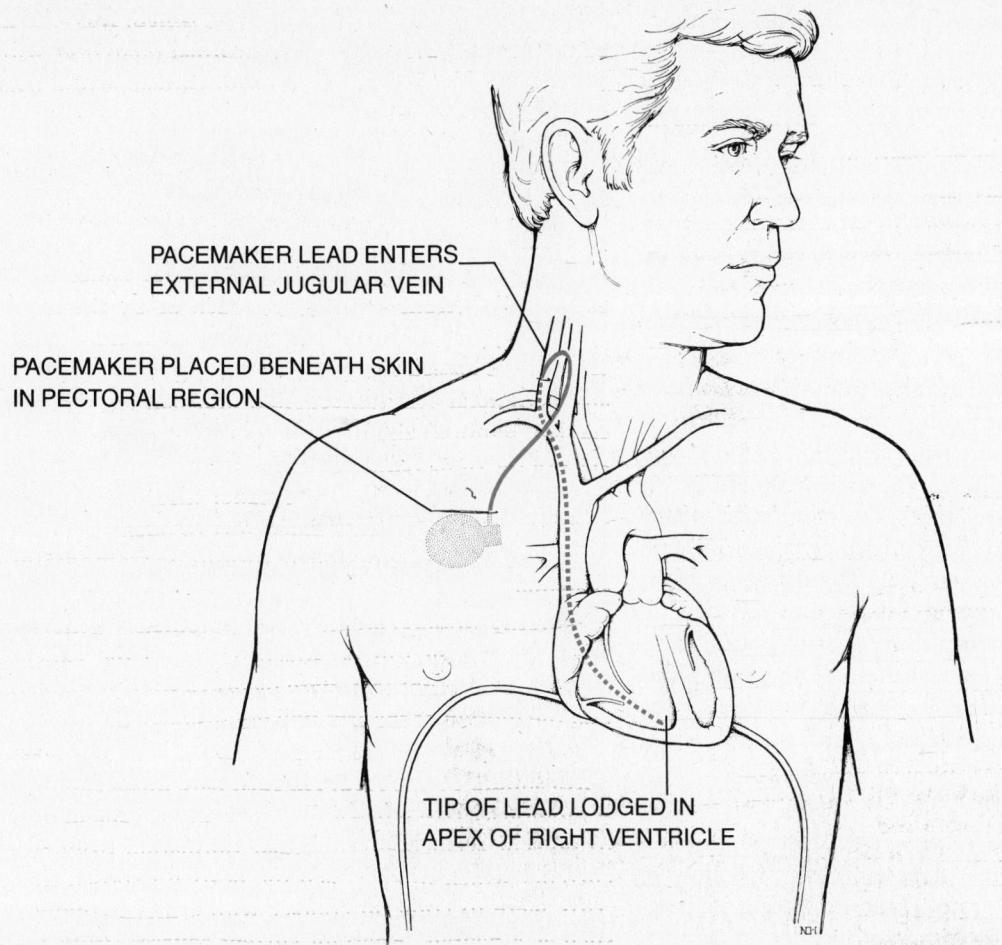

PACEMAKER LEAD ENTERS EXTERNAL JUGULAR VEIN

PACEMAKER PLACED BENEATH SKIN IN PECTORAL REGION

TIP OF LEAD LODGED IN APEX OF RIGHT VENTRICLE

Figure 30-2. Pacemaker therapy.

thoracically to the myocardium where it is sutured in place. For this method, termed an epicardial or myocardial implant, a thoracotomy is required to provide access to the heart. This procedure is frequently part of an open heart operation. Another electrode is screwed into the myocardium through a small incision in the subxiphoid area with minimal injury to heart muscle. This requires no sutures.

Nursing Management. Following the procedure the patient is monitored by electrocardiogram. After implantation the pacemaker rate tends to vary by 2 to 3 pulses and then stabilizes. An intravenous line is kept open to provide a readily accessible vein for drug administration in the event of an arrhythmia and for fluids to combat dehydration. Data about the model, date and time of insertion, location of the pulse generator, stimulation threshhold, and pacer rate should be noted on the patient's record and on a card at the head of the bed.

The incision site under the pressure dressing where the pulse generator is implanted is watched for evidences of bleeding, hematoma formation, and infection.

All electrical equipment used in the vicinity of the patient is grounded with 3-pronged plugs inserted into a proper outlet. Improperly grounded equipment can generate leakage currents capable of producing ventricular fibrillation. A biomedical engineer, electrician, or other qualified person should make certain that the patient is in an electrically safe environment.

After permanent pacemaker implantation, the patient initially will be aware of the pulse generator under his skin and will want to touch it frequently. Reassurance should be given that this is no cause for concern. Patients usually feel ambivalent about their pacemakers: they understand their benefits, but feelings of dependence, anxiety over altered life style, and awareness of changing body image may be troubling. To counter the uneasy feelings it is best to take a positive approach in talking with the patient. The patient will require support and should be informed that the pacemaker will improve his cardiac output and thus give him more energy. (See page 590 for patient education.)

Complications

Complications associated with implanted pacemakers relate to (1) their presence within the body and (2) improper functioning.

The following complications may arise from the presence of the pacemaker:

1. Local infection (sepsis or hematoma formation) may occur at the site of venous cutdown or subcutaneous pacemaker placement.
2. Arrhythmias—ventricular ectopic activity may follow irritation of the ventricular wall by the electrode. (Pacemakers can produce baffling arrhythmias.)
3. Perforation of the myocardium or right ventricle by the catheter may occur.
4. High ventricular threshold—may cause abrupt loss of pacing.

Pacemaker malfunction can arise from failure in one or more components of the pacing system. The majority of pulse generator failures are from depletion of the power supply—i.e., battery failure. The patient should be informed that the battery cells are sealed in the pulse generator. When it is time for a battery change, a new incision is made over the old incision. The old pulse generator is removed and the new unit is connected to the existing leads and reimplanted in the already existing pocket. This is usually done under local anesthesia. Other complications include fracture (breakage) or dislocation of the electrodes and electronic failure.

Pacemaker Surveillance

Pacemaker clinics have been established to monitor patients and to test pulse generators for warnings of impending pacemaker system failure. Testing of pacemaker pulse amplitude and duration and analysis of pulse contour require amplification equipment. With special equipment lead fracture and insulation disruption can be detected. A 12-lead ECG is done during each patient visit to the clinic.

Another method of follow-up is evaluation by transtelephone monitoring of the transmission of the generator's pulse rate. By means of special equipment the sound tone of the patient's pacemaker is transmitted over the telephone to a receiving system at a pacemaker clinic. The sounds are converted into an electronic signal and permanently recorded on an ECG strip. The pacemaker rate and other data concerning pacemaker function are obtained and evaluated by a cardiologist or a cardiovascular surgeon. This simplifies the diagnosis for a failing generator, provides reassurance, and improves the management of the person who is physically remote from pacemaker testing facilities.

Pacemaker Developments

EXTERNAL AND LONG-RANGE RECHARGING. There is now available an electronic pacemaker whose battery can be recharged externally. Like other pacemakers, the new device is implanted under the skin in the chest wall or in the abdomen. Its lead wires (one enclosed inside the other) are threaded through a vein so that one end is in the heart and the other attached to a battery. To recharge the

---

PATIENT EDUCATION— THE PATIENT WITH A PACEMAKER

1. Report to your physician/pacemaker clinic periodically as prescribed, so that the rate of the pacemaker and its function can be checked. This is especially important during the first month after implantation.
   a. Usually weekly monitoring is necessary during the first month after implantation.
   b. Check your pulse daily. Report *immediately* any sudden slowing or increasing of the pulse rate. This may indicate pacemaker malfunction.
   c. Weekly monitoring is resumed when battery depletion is anticipated. The time for reimplantation depends on the type in use.
2. Wear loose-fitting clothing around the area of the pacemaker.
   a. There will be a slight bulge over the pacemaker implant.
   b. If the area becomes reddened or painful, notify your physician.
3. Study the manufacturer's instructions and become familiar with your pacemaker.
4. Physical activity does not usually have to be curtailed, with the exception of heavy contact sports.
5. Carry an identification card/bracelet indicating your physician's name, type and model number of pacemaker, manufacturer's name, pacemaker rate, and hospital where pacemaker was inserted.
6. Although at this time electrical interference is not a major problem, it is usually advisable to avoid being close to microwave ovens, arc welders and large electrical generators, and electric cautery and diathermy equipment.
7. A weapons detector at airports will detect the presence of a pacemaker. Show your identification card and request scanning by a hand scanner.
8. Hospitalization is necessary periodically for battery changes/pacemaker unit replacement.

---

battery the patient dons a lightweight canvas shoulder harness and attaches the charger unit to it over the location of his implanted battery. The charger is linked to a small console which is plugged into an ordinary electric socket. When the unit is turned on, an electromagnetic field is generated which rejuvenates the power cell in the battery through the skin. Recharging the battery takes only about 90 minutes at home each week.

NUCLEAR-POWERED PACEMAKERS. Nuclear-powered pacemakers are now being implanted in patients in selected centers in this country. The nuclear heart pacer is designed to operate for at least 15 to 20 years. The design of the pacemaker's nuclear power source is based on the principle of thermoelectricity—the direct conversion of heat to electrical energy. When certain metals are joined together, they form a thermocouple which, when heated at one end, will generate an electrical current. The pacemaker's thermocouple is composed of a copper and nickel alloy and a nickel and chromium alloy drawn into wire strands and woven into a glass tape. The heat developed by the decay of the radioisotope nuclear fuel (plutonium 238) is used to heat the wires at one end. The electrical current, as in conventional pacemakers, is fed into a pulse generator which supplies the pacing pulses to the heart via conventional wire electrodes. The radiation exposure to the patient from the nuclear fuel is considered to be within acceptable levels.

ATRIOVENTRICULAR PACING. Pacemaker technology has fostered the growth of safe and effective pacemaker therapy for many complex cardiologic problems that include not only ventricular pacemakers but atrial pacemakers as well. Both of these types of pacemakers can in specific instances function in the same patient (i.e., atrioventricular sequential pacing).

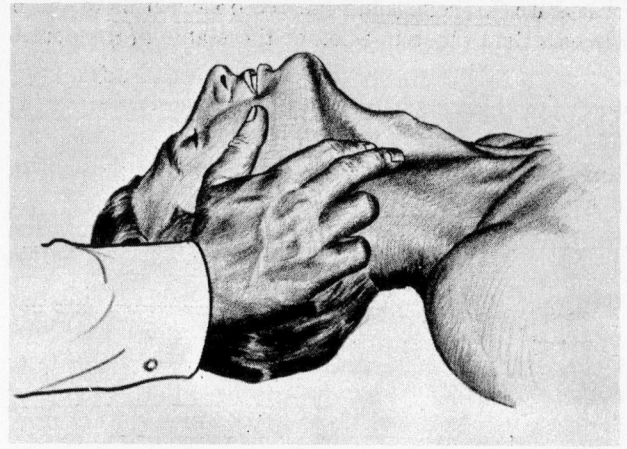

Figure 30-3. Method of carotid palpation. (From Cardiopulmonary Conference Proceedings, National Research Council, National Academy of Sciences, Washington.)

CARDIAC ARREST

Cardiac arrest is defined as the sudden, unexpected cessation of the heartbeat and effective circulation. All heart action may stop, or asynchronized muscular twitchings (ventricular fibrillation) may occur.

Factors that play a major role in the etiology of arrest include the following: cardiac arrhythmia precipitated by many causes (especially ischemic heart disease), extensive myocardial infarction with insufficient pump function to support life ("pump failure"), or shock of any cause (including sepsis, anaphylaxis, massive pulmonary embolism). Cardiac arrest may result from drowning, electric shock, carbon monoxide poisoning, other types of poisoning, and any condition in which there is anoxia, such as might occur in acute airway obstruction and during the administration of anesthesia.

There is an immediate loss of consciousness and an absence of pulses and audible heart sounds. Dilation of the pupils of the eyes begins within 45 seconds. Convulsions may or may not be present.

- There is an interval of approximately four minutes between the cessation of circulation and the appearance of irreversible brain damage. This varies with the age of the patient. During this period, the diagnosis of arrest must be made and the circulation must be restored.
- *The most reliable sign of arrest is the absence of a carotid pulsation* (Fig. 30-3). Valuable time should not be wasted taking the blood pressure or listening for the heartbeat.

Details of the resuscitation procedure may be found on pages 546-549.

ENDOCARDIAL DISEASE

Pathophysiology

The endocardium is the endothelial layer of tissue that lines the heart's cavities and covers the flaps of its valves. Of the diseases that affect it, the majority represent vari-

ous types and stages of inflammation, i.e., *endocarditis* or its aftermath. They include: (1) rheumatic endocarditis, one of the many complications of acute rheumatic fever; (2) infective endocarditis, produced by direct bacterial invasion of the endocardium, particularly that portion covering the valve leaflets; and (3) chronic valvular heart disease, based on structural deformities of the heart valves, whether of congenital origin or acquired as a result of either rheumatic or bacterial endocarditis in the past.

When an area of endocardium becomes inflamed, a fibrin clot, called a vegetation, may form. In time this clot becomes converted into a mass of scar tissue. The scarred endocardium becomes thickened, stiffened, contracted, and deformed. A fringe of vegetations ranging along the free margins of the valve flaps, marking the site of earlier erosions, represents the basic lesion of endocarditis and is the forerunner of chronic valvular heart disease.

Rheumatic Endocarditis

PATHOPHYSIOLOGY. Rheumatic fever is a sequel to a Group A streptococcal infection. It is considered a preventable disease. The most prominent symptom of rheumatic fever is polyarthritis, but the most serious damage occurs in the heart, where every structural component is likely to be the site of an inflammatory reaction. The heart damage and the joint lesions are not infectious in origin, in the sense that these tissues are not invaded and directly damaged by destructive organisms; rather, they represent a sensitivity phenomenon occurring in response to the *hemolytic streptococcus*. Blood leukocytes accumulate in the affected tissues and form nodules, which eventually are replaced by scars. The myocardium is certain to be involved in this inflammatory process; i.e., *rheumatic myocarditis* develops, which temporarily weakens the contractile power of the heart. The pericardium likewise is affected; i.e., *rheumatic pericarditis* also occurs during the acute illness. These myocardial and pericardial complications usually are without serious sequelae; on the other hand, the effects of *rheumatic endocarditis* are permanent and often crippling.

CLINICAL MANIFESTATIONS. Rheumatic endocarditis anatomically manifests itself first by tiny translucent vegetations, which resemble beads about the size of the head of a pin, arranged in a row along the free margins of the valve flaps. These tiny beads look harmless enough and may disappear without injuring the valve flaps, but more often they have serious effects. They are the starting point of a process that gradually thickens the flaps, rendering them just a little shorter, just a little thicker than normal, just a little shriveled along their edges—not much, but enough to prevent them from closing the orifice of the valve perfectly. The result is leakage, a condition called valvular regurgitation. The most common type of valvular regurgitation is mitral regurgitation.

In other patients the inflamed margins of the valve flaps become adherent, resulting in a narrowed, or "stenotic," valvular orifice. A small percentage of patients with rheumatic fever become critically ill with intractable heart failure, serious arrhythmias, and rheumatic pneumonia. These patients should be treated in an intensive care unit.

Most patients recover with gratifying speed and their recovery ostensibly is complete. However, although free of symptoms, the patient is left with certain permanent residuals that often gradually lead to progressive valvular deformities. The extent of cardiac damage, or even its existence, may not have been apparent on clinical examinations during the acute phase of the disease. Eventually, however, the heart murmurs that are characteristic of valvular stenosis, regurgitation, or both, become audible on auscultation and, in some patients, even detectable as "thrills" on palpation. The myocardium usually can compensate for these valvular defects very well for a time, despite its increased burden. As long as it can do so, the patient remains in apparent good health. However, sooner or later it fails to compensate—and decompensation, when it occurs, is signaled by the manifestations of congestive heart failure, as described on pages 577-578.

MANAGEMENT. The objectives of management are to observe for and control congestive heart failure and pericarditis (which may be life-threatening) and to give symptomatic relief to other manifestations.

The patient with rheumatic endocarditis should be confined to bed as long as he is febrile and has signs of active carditis. He should remain quiet thereafter until the erythrocyte sedimentation rate (a fair though nonspecific index of rheumatic activity) returns to normal. Salicylates are prescribed in large doses to suppress rheumatic

activity by controlling toxic manifestations, lessening constitutional symptoms, and improving the well-being of the patient. Corticosteroid therapy is given to the very ill person with carditis. However, treatment has no effect on valvular deformities that may occur.

The patient with rheumatic endocarditis, whose valve function is faulty but whose disease is quiescent, does not require therapy as long as the heart pumps effectively. Nevertheless, the danger exists of recurrent attacks of acute rheumatic fever, of bacterial endocarditis, or embolism from vegetations or mural thrombi in the heart, and of eventual cardiac failure. (The relation between valvular disease and congestive heart failure is discussed on page 598; the treatment of heart failure, on page 578.)

PREVENTION. The prevention of rheumatic fever is accomplished by (1) the prevention of streptococcal infections, especially in susceptible individuals and (2) early and adequate treatment of streptococcal infections in all individuals.

Persons who present a well-documented history of rheumatic fever (or chorea) or who show evidence of rheumatic heart disease should be given continuous prophylaxis with penicillin (or other suitable antibiotic) indefinitely. The patient must recognize and should accept the fact that he is a "rheumatic fever patient," and as such can lead a normal life only if he is willing to submit to certain limitations and inconveniences. In relation to this facet of patient education, the nurse is in a position to play a very important role.

A first line approach in preventing initial attacks of rheumatic fever is to recognize individuals with streptococcal infections, treat them adequately, and control epidemics in the community. Every nurse should be familiar with the symptoms and signs of streptococcal pharyngitis (see chart). *A throat culture is the only method by which diagnosis can be determined.*

PREVENTION OF RHEUMATIC HEART DISEASE

Rheumatic fever is a preventable disease. By eradication of rheumatic fever, the great cardiac crippler—*rheumatic heart disease*—would be virtually eliminated. Through the use of penicillin therapy in patients with streptococcal infections, almost all primary attacks of rheumatic fever could be prevented. The symptoms and signs of streptococcal pharyngitis are:

Fever (38.9° to 40° C., or 101° to 104° F.)
Chilliness
Sore throat (sudden in onset)
Diffuse redness of throat with exudate on oropharynx (may not appear until after the first day)
Enlarged and tender lymph nodes
Abdominal pain (more common in children)
Acute sinusitis and acute otitis media (may be due to streptococcus)

Infective Endocarditis

Infective endocarditis (bacterial endocarditis) is an infection of the valves and endothelial surface of the heart caused by direct invasion of bacteria or other organisms leading to deformity of the valve leaflets. It may be acute, subacute, or chronic. Acute endocarditis usually occurs on normal valves. Causative microorganisms include bacteria (streptococci, enterococci, pneumococci, staphylococci), fungi, and rickettsiae. The subacute form is usually caused by *Streptococcus viridans.*

ETIOLOGY. Infective subacute endocarditis usually develops in patients who have a history of valvular heart disease (particularly rheumatic heart disease with mitral or aortic involvement). Another predisposing factor is cardiac surgery, particularly when prosthetic materials are used.

Hospital-acquired endocarditis occurs most often in patients with debilitating disease, those with indwelling catheters, and those on prolonged intravenous or antibiotic therapy. Patients on immunosuppressive drugs or steroids may develop fungal endocarditis. Therefore, infective endocarditis often accompanies medical and surgical therapy and is more common in older persons probably due to decreased immunologic responses to infection, metabolic alterations arising from changes in the aging body, and increased instrumentation, especially in genitourinary disease. There is a high incidence of staphylococcal endocarditis among heroin addicts, the disease occurring for the most part on normal valves.

CLINICAL MANIFESTATIONS. The onset of infective endocarditis usually is insidious. The signs and symptoms develop from destruction of heart valves, from embolization of fragments of vegetations, and from toxicity of the infection.

The general manifestations include vague complaints of malaise, anorexia, weight loss, cough, and back and joint pain which may be mistaken for influenza. Fever is intermittent and may be absent in patients who are receiving antibiotics or corticosteroids or in those who are elderly or have congestive heart failure or uremia. Skin and nail manifestations are observed in some patients. Splinter hemorrhages (linear and hemorrhagic streaks) may be noted under the fingernails and toenails and petechiae may appear in the conjunctiva and mucous membranes. Hemorrhages with pale centers (Roth's spots) may be seen in the fundi of the eyes from emboli in the nerve fiber layer of the eye. Osler's nodes (painful, raised, tender, red lesions on the pads of fingers and toes) may occur and are thought to be secondary to acute vasculitis from an immunologic reaction. Janeway's lesions are hemorrhagic macular areas found on the palms or soles and are now thought to be a hypersensitivity reaction or deposit of immune complex.

The cardiac manifestations include heart murmurs, which may be absent initially. Changing murmurs may be encountered in the acute form and indicate valvular damage due to vegetations or to perforation of the valve or of the chordae tendinae. Heart enlargement or evidences of congestive heart failure are also seen.

The central nervous system manifestations include headache, transient cerebral ischemia, focal neurologic lesions, and strokes which may be caused by emboli involving the cerebral arteries.

Embolization may be a presenting symptom occurring at any time and involving other organ systems. The embolic phenomena may be manifested in the lung (recurrent pneumonia; pulmonary abscesses), kidney (hematuria; renal failure); spleen (left upper quadrant pain), heart (myocardial infarction), brain (stroke), or in the peripheral vessels.

MANAGEMENT. The objective of treatment is total eradication of the invading organism by adequate doses of an appropriate antimicrobial. The causative organism can be isolated through serial blood cultures. It is treated with a bactericidal (capable of destroying bacteria) agent or other appropriate drug based on proven sensitivity to the causative agent. The antibiotic is usually given parenterally in a continuous intravenous infusion for a period of 4 to 6 weeks. Thus it is important to note on the nursing care plan the date on which the intravenous needle or cannula was inserted. Bactericidal serum levels of the selected antibiotic are monitored by titering it against the causative organism. If the serum does not demonstrate bactericidal activity, increased dosages of the antibiotic are given or a different antibiotic is tried. There are numerous antimicrobial regimens currently in use, but penicillin is usually the drug of choice.

Blood cultures are taken periodically to monitor the course of therapy. Treatment with amphotericin B and surgery with valve replacement is usually required for the patient with fungal endocarditis.

EVALUATION OF THERAPY. The patient's temperature is monitored at regular intervals, since the course of fever is one determinant of the effectiveness of treatment. However, febrile reactions may also occur as a result of drug therapy. After adequate antimicrobial therapy is initiated, bacteria usually disappear. The patient should demonstrate an improved sense of well-being, better appetite, and decreased lethargy. During this time, the patient requires a great deal of psychosocial support, especially since he feels well but finds himself confined to the hospital with restrictive IV therapy.

COMPLICATIONS. Even though the patient may respond to the antimicrobial therapy, endocarditis can be very destructive to the heart and other organs. Congestive heart failure and cerebral vascular catastrophes may occur before, during, or after therapy. Valve stenosis or regurgitation, myocardial erosion, and mycotic aneurysms are some potential heart complications. A myriad of other organ complications can result from septic or nonseptic emboli, immunologic responses, or hemodynamic deterioration.

SURGERY. The advent of surgical valve replacement has favorably changed the prognosis of patients with severely damaged heart valves. Usually valve excision and replacement are required for (1) patients who develop congestive heart failure as a result of aortic or mitral valve involvement in spite of adequate medical treatment; (2) patients who have more than one serious systemic embolic episode; (3) persons with uncontrolled infection, recurrent infection, or fungal endocarditis. A large number of patients who have prosthetic valve endocarditis (infected prostheses) will require valve replacement.

PREVENTION. Infective endocarditis occurs most often in persons with structural abnormalities of the heart and great vessels, especially valvular heart disease. Any procedure that is associated with transient bacteremia may cause bacteria to lodge on damaged or abnormal valves. *Persons at risk are patients with structural abnormalities of the heart and great vessels, those with prosthetic heart valves, or patients with most types of congenital heart disease, rheumatic or other acquired valvular heart disease, and idiopathic hypertrophic or subaortic stenosis.*

Antibiotic prophylaxis (usually penicillin, penicillin plus streptomycin, or penicillin plus gentamicin) is recommended for persons at risk, for the following procedures and circumstances:*

1. Dental procedures causing gingival bleeding.
2. Surgery or instrumentation of the respiratory tract (tonsillectomy/adenoidectomy, bronchoscopy) or procedures involving disruption of respiratory mucosa; surgery or instrumentation of the genitourinary tract (especially urethral procedures including catheterization) or prostatic manipulation; or surgery or instrumentation of the gastrointestinal tract and gallbladder.
3. Cardiac surgery in which extracorporeal circulation is utilized, especially replacement of prosthetic valves. These recommendations apply to the recovery period as well.
4. Surgical procedures on infected or contaminated tissues.
5. Obstetrical infections (postpartum infection; septic abortion).

MYOCARDITIS

Acute *myocarditis* is an inflammatory process involving the myocardium. The heart is a muscle, hence its efficiency depends on the health of the individual muscle fibers. When the muscle fibers are healthy, the heart can function well in spite of severe valvular injuries; when the muscle fibers are poor, life is in jeopardy.

*From Statement Prepared by the Committee on Prevention of Rheumatic Fever and Bacterial Endocarditis of the American Heart Association: Circulation, 56:139A–143A, July 1977.

PATHOPHYSIOLOGY. Myocarditis usually results from an infectious process, particularly of viral, bacterial, mycotic, parasitic, protozoal, or spirochetal origin, or it may be produced by hypersensitivity states such as rheumatic fever. Therefore, myocarditis may be seen in patients with acute systemic infections, those receiving immunosuppressive therapy, or those with infective endocarditis.

Myocarditis can cause heart dilatation, mural thrombi, infiltration of circulating blood cells around the coronary vessels and between the muscle fibers, and degeneration of the muscle fibers themselves.

CLINICAL MANIFESTATIONS. The symptoms of acute myocarditis depend on the type of infection, the degree of myocardial damage, and the capacity of the myocardium to recover. Symptoms may be mild or absent. The patient may complain of fatigue and dyspnea, palpitations, and occasional precordial discomfort. Clinical examination may reveal cardiac enlargement, faint heart sounds, gallop rhythm, and a systolic murmur. A pericardial friction rub may be heard if the patient has associated pericarditis. Pulsus alternans (a pulse in which there is a regular alternation of weak and strong beats) may be present. Fever and tachycardia are frequently seen and evidences of congestive heart failure usually develop.

MANAGEMENT. The patient is given specific treatment for the underlying cause, if it is known, e.g., penicillin for hemolytic streptococci. He is placed on bed rest to decrease cardiac work, i.e., to reduce the heart rate, stroke volume, blood pressure, and heart contractility. Bed rest also helps to decrease residual myocardial damage and the complications of myocarditis. The treatment is essentially the same as that used for congestive heart failure (page 578). The pulse, heart sounds, and temperature are evaluated to determine whether the disease is subsiding and to assess for the occurrence of congestive heart failure. The apical rate should be taken since patients with myocarditis are apt to develop arrhythmias. If an arrhythmia occurs, the patient should be placed in a unit with continuous cardiac monitoring so that personnel and equipment are readily available if a life-threatening arrhythmia occurs.

When there is evidence of congestive heart failure, digitalis is given to slow the heart rate and augment myocardial contractility.

- Patients with myocarditis are sensitive to digitalis. There must be continuing nursing surveillance to assess the patient for digitalis toxicity (arrhythmia, anorexia, nausea, vomiting, bradycardia, headache, malaise).

Elastic stockings and passive and active exercises should be used since embolization from venous thrombosis and mural thrombi can occur.

PATIENT EDUCATION. The prevention of infectious diseases by means of appropriate immunizations and early treatment appears to be important in decreasing the incidence of myocarditis. Following a bout of myocarditis, there is usually some residual heart enlargement. Physical activity is increased slowly, and the patient is instructed to report any symptoms that occur with increasing activity such as a rapidly beating heart, etc. Competitive sports and alcohol must be avoided.

CARDIOMYOPATHIES

Myopathy refers to any disease of muscle. The cardiomyopathies are a group of diseases which affect the structure and function of the myocardium. The term *primary cardiomyopathies* is used if the condition is of unknown etiology. The term *secondary cardiomyopathies* implies that the myocardial involvement results from a known disease which is usually also manifested outside the heart. Arteriosclerotic disease of the coronary arteries, viral infections, alcoholism, neuromuscular disease, connective tissue disease, degenerative changes in the myocardium, metabolic disturbances, malnutrition, vasculitis, pregnancy, toxic agents, drugs, and other causes may all produce heart muscle disease. The manner in which they affect the heart muscle is not known. Explorations based on cellular and enzyme functions, infectious agents, and immunological causes are being sought.

CLINICAL MANIFESTATIONS. Most patients with myocardial disease have signs and symptoms of heart failure: dyspnea on effort, nocturnal dyspnea, cough, expectoration, and weakness. Physical findings reveal manifestations of systemic venous congestion: jugular vein engorgement, pitting edema, hepatic engorgement, tachycardia. Gallop rhythm is one of the identifying marks of myocardial disease. (Gallop rhythm is a tripling or quadrupling of heart sounds resembling the galloping of a horse.) It may be heard best with the bell of the stethoscope when the patient is in the left lateral position. The gallop impulses may be palpable as well as audible. The ECG may be normal in patients with heart muscle disease.

MANAGEMENT. Rest (physical and emotional) is an important aspect of management. Rest decreases the heart rate, stroke volume, arterial blood pressure, and heart size. Sodium restriction, digitalis, diuretics, and vasodilators are other treatment modalities. (See pages 577–583 on the patient with congestive heart failure.)

PERICARDITIS

Pericarditis refers to an inflammation of the pericardium, the membranous sac enveloping the heart. It may be a primary illness or may develop in the course of a variety of medical and surgical diseases.

The following are some of the causes underlying or associated with pericarditis.
1. Idiopathic or nonspecific causes
2. Infection
   Bacterial (streptococcus, staphylococcus, meningococcus, gonococcus, etc.)
   Viral (coxsackie, influenza, other)
   Mycotic (fungal), rickettsial, parasitic, etc.
3. Disorders of connective tissue — systemic lupus erythematosus, rheumatic fever, rheumatoid arthritis, polyarteritis
4. Hypersensitivity states — immune reactions, drug reactions, serum sickness
5. Diseases of adjacent structures — myocardial infarction, dissecting aneurysm, pleural and pulmonary disease (pneumonia)
6. Neoplastic disease (secondary to metastasis from lung cancer, breast cancer), leukemia; following radiation; primary (mesothelioma)
7. Trauma — chest injury; cardiac surgery; during cardiac catheterization, pacemaker implantation
8. Pericarditis associated with renal disorders (uremia).

CLINICAL MANIFESTATIONS. The characteristic symptom of the patient is *pain* and the characteristic sign is a *friction rub*. Pain is almost always present in acute pericarditis and is most common over the precordium. The pain may be felt beneath the clavicle and in the neck and left scapular region. Pericardial pain is aggravated by breathing, turning in bed, and twisting the body; it is relieved by sitting up. In fact, the patient prefers to adopt a forward-leaning or a sitting posture. Dyspnea may occur as the result of restriction of the heart contraction which leads to a decreased cardiac output. The patient may appear extremely ill. Pericarditis per se often gives rise to no signs other than fever and the production of a friction rub.

EXAMINATION FOR FRICTION RUB. A pericardial friction rub occurs when the pericardial surfaces lose their lubricating fluid because of inflammation. The rub is audible on auscultation and is synchronous with the heartbeat. A pericardial friction rub is diagnostic of pericarditis and should be searched for diligently.

• Place the diaphragm of the stethoscope tightly against the thorax and listen at the left sternal edge in the 4th intercostal space (Fig. 30-4). This is where the pericardium comes into contact with the left chest wall. A pericardial friction rub has a scratching or leathery sound which is heard "close to the ear." The rub is louder at the end of expiration and may be heard best while the patient is sitting.

NURSING ASSESSMENT. While observing the patient, try to discover whether or not the pain is influenced by respiratory movements, with or without the actual passage of air; by flexion, extension, or rotation of the spine, including the neck; by movements of the shoulders and arms; by coughing; or by swallowing. Recognizing these relationships may be very helpful in establishing a diagnosis.

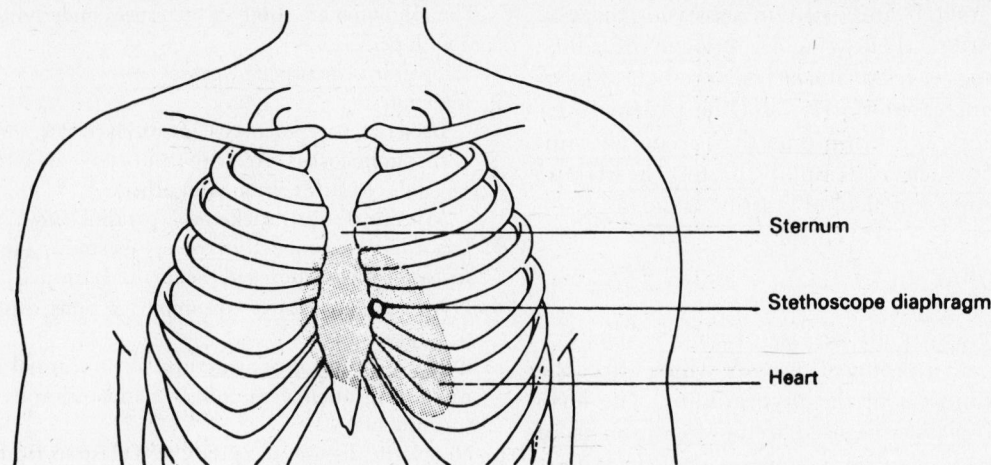

Figure 30-4. Auscultation for pericardial friction rub.

MANAGEMENT. The objectives of management are to determine the cause, to administer therapy for the specific cause (when known), and to be on the alert for cardiac tamponade (compression of the heart from fluid in the pericardial sac). The patient is placed on bed rest when cardiac output is impaired, until the fever, chest pain, and friction rub have disappeared.

Meperidine or morphine may be given for pain relief during the acute phase. Salicylates relieve pain and hasten reabsorption of fluid in the patient with rheumatic pericarditis. Corticosteroids are sometimes given to control

symptoms, hasten resolution of the inflammatory process in the pericardium, and prevent recurring pericardial effusion.

- Be alert to the possibility of cardiac tamponade. Use nursing assessment skills to anticipate and identify the triad of symptoms—falling arterial pressure, rising venous pressure, and a quiet heart sound.

Patients with infections of the pericardium are treated with the antimicrobial agent of choice based on identification and sensitivity tests. The pericarditis of rheumatic fever may respond to penicillin. Isoniazid, ethambutol, rifampin, and streptomycin in various combinations are used in the treatment of tuberculosis that produces pericarditis. Amphotericin B is used in fungal pericarditis and adrenal steroids are used in disseminated lupus erythematosus.

As the patient's condition improves, activity may be increased gradually. However, if pain, fever, or friction rub reappear, bed rest must be resumed.

Pericardial Effusion

Pericardial effusion refers to the escape of fluid into the pericardial sac. This may accompany pericarditis and advanced congestive heart failure.

CLINICAL MANIFESTATIONS. The characteristic sign of pericardial effusion is an extension of flatness (not dullness) to percussion across the anterior aspect of the chest wall. The patient may complain of a feeling of fullness within the chest or have substernal or an ill-defined pain.

Normally the pericardial sac contains less than 50 ml. of fluid. Pericardial fluid may accumulate slowly without noticeable symptoms. However, a *rapidly* developing effusion can stretch the pericardium to its maximum size and can cause decreased cardiac output and venous return to the heart. The result is *cardiac tamponade* (compression of the heart). (Cardiac tamponade is also discussed under

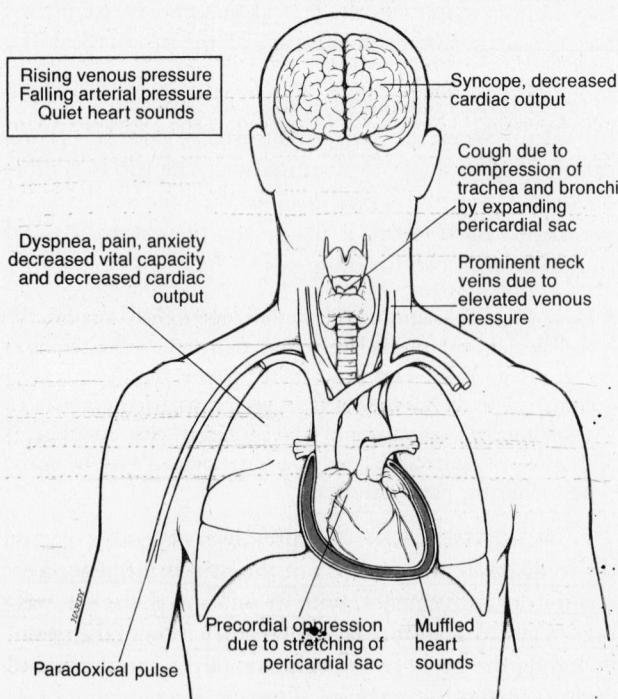

Rising venous pressure
Falling arterial pressure
Quiet heart sounds

Syncope, decreased cardiac output

Cough due to compression of trachea and bronchi by expanding pericardial sac

Dyspnea, pain, anxiety decreased vital capacity and decreased cardiac output

Prominent neck veins due to elevated venous pressure

Paradoxical pulse

Precordial oppression due to stretching of pericardial sac

Muffled heart sounds

Figure 30-5. Assessment for cardiac tamponade due to pericardial effusion. Pathophysiologic consequences of cardiac tamponade.

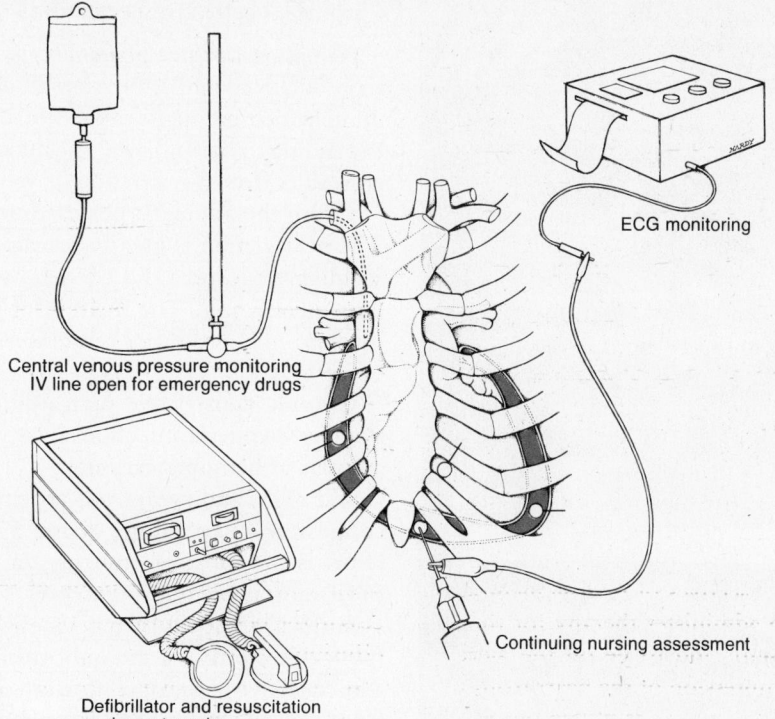

Central venous pressure monitoring
IV line open for emergency drugs

ECG monitoring

Defibrillator and resuscitation
equipment ready

Continuing nursing assessment

Figure 30-6.   Nursing support of the patient undergoing pericardiocentesis. (Small circles indicate sites for pericardial aspiration.)

Chest Injuries on page 501.) Signs include a feeling of precordial oppression, due to the stretching of the pericardial sac, and shortness of breath; the blood pressure drops and fluctuates. Blood pressure is lowest on inspiration (*pulsus paradoxus*), at which point the pulse may not be perceptible. The venous pressure tends to rise (20 cm. or more), or is evidenced by the engorged neck veins and enlarging liver. The heart sounds become feeble in intensity (quiet heart), and there are signs of cardiac enlargement and compression of the left lung posteriorly. (See Fig. 30-5 for assessment of cardiac tamponade due to pericardial effusion.)

• The important considerations are falling blood pressure, rising venous pressure (look at the neck veins), and quiet heart sounds. *This is a life-threatening situation, demanding close and constant observation.*

Pericardial Aspiration (Pericardiocentesis)

If the cardiac function becomes seriously impaired, a pericardial aspiration (puncture of the pericardial sac) is performed to remove fluid from the pericardial sac. The major purpose is to relieve cardiac tamponade which restricts normal heart action.

During the procedure the patient is monitored by ECG and central venous pressure measurements are made. A defibrillator is turned on, and other emergency resuscitative equipment should be readily available.

The head of the bed is elevated to a 45 to 60 degree angle so that the needle can be inserted into the pericardial sac more easily. A stable large bore needle is inserted and a slow intravenous drip of saline or glucose is started in order to provide immediate access to an intravenous route should it be necessary to administer emergency drugs or blood.

The pericardial aspiration needle is attached to a 50 ml. syringe by a three-way stopcock. The V lead (precordial lead wire) of the ECG is attached to the hub of the aspirating needle with alligator clips, because the monitoring of ECG oscillation is useful in determining whether or not the needle has contacted the myocardium. This is evidenced by an elevation of the ST segment or stimulation of premature ventricular contractions.

There are several possible sites for pericardial aspiration (Fig. 30-6). The needle may be inserted in the angle between the left costal margin and the xiphoid, near the cardiac apex, to the left of the 5th or 6th interspace at the sternal margin, or on the right side of the 4th intercostal space. The needle is advanced slowly until fluid is obtained.

A fall in central venous pressure associated with a rise in blood pressure indicates that relief of cardiac tamponade has occurred. The patient almost always feels immediate improvement. If there is a substantial amount of pericardial fluid, a small catheter may be left in place to drain recurrent bleeding or effusion.

During the procedure it is important to watch for the presence of bloody fluid. Pericardial blood does not clot

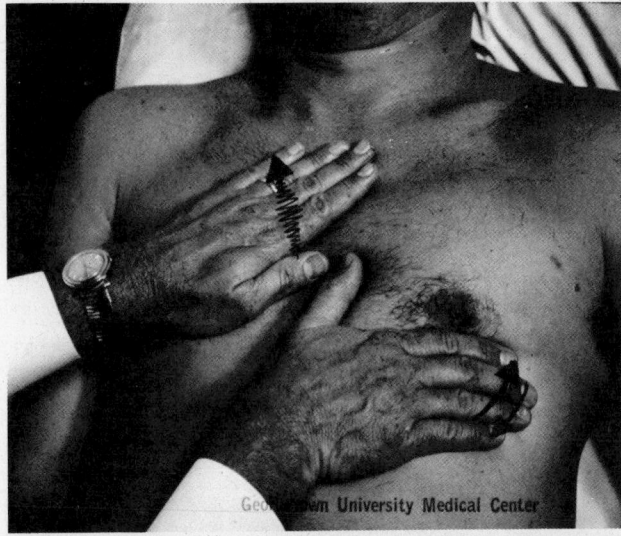

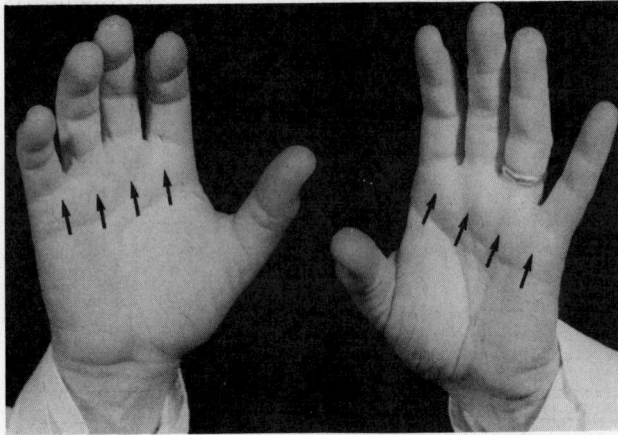

Figure 30-7.   Assessing for palpable thrill of aortic stenosis. The thrill is felt at the base of the heart, and its direction is toward the right shoulder and right side of the neck. The vibrations are best detected with the palmar surfaces of the hands. (From Shah, P. M., and Roberts, D. L.: Diagnosis and treatment of aortic valve stenosis. In Harvey, W. P., et al., eds.: Current Problems in Cardiology. Copyright © 1977 by Year Book)

readily, whereas blood obtained from inadvertent puncture of one of the heart chambers does clot. If blood accumulates rapidly, immediate thoracotomy and cardiorraphy (suturing of heart muscle) are indicated.

Pericardial fluid is sent to the laboratory for examination for tumor cells, bacterial culture, chemical and serological analysis, and differential cell count. A hematocrit is done if the fluid is bloody.

• Following pericardiocentesis, the patient will require careful monitoring of the blood pressure, venous pressure, and heart sounds to evaluate for the possible recurrence of cardiac tamponade (Fig. 30-7). A repeated aspiration is then necessary. If possible, the patient should be in an intensive care unit. Sometimes cardiac tamponade is treated by open pericardial drainage.

Chronic Constrictive Pericarditis

Chronic constrictive pericarditis is a condition in which there is chronic inflammatory thickening of the pericardium which compresses the heart and prevents it from expanding to normal size. The major hemodynamic deficit results from a restriction of ventricular filling.

Often the adherent pericardium becomes calcified. The heart action is greatly restricted by this tough, unyielding enclosure, and edema, ascites, and hepatic enlargement result. The fixation of the heart to the pericardium may produce a retraction of the chest wall with every beat.

Chronic constrictive pericarditis is caused by longstanding pyogenic infections, postviral infections, tuberculosis, or hemopericardium.

The signs and symptoms are predominantly those of congestive heart failure (page 578), but dyspnea on effort is the most prominent symptom. Chronic atrial fibrillation is commonly present.

Surgical removal of the tough encasing pericardium (pericardiectomy) is the only treatment of any benefit. The objective of the operation is to release both ventricles from the constrictive and restrictive inflammation. (See pages 560-564 for the care of the patient after cardiac surgery.)

ACQUIRED VALVULAR DISEASES OF THE HEART

The function of normal heart valves is to maintain the forward flow of blood from the atria to the ventricles and from the ventricles to the great vessels. Valvular damage may interfere with valvular function by stenosis (narrowing) of the valve or by impaired closure that allows backward leakage of blood (valvular insufficiency, regurgitation, or incompetence).

Acquired valvular heart disease often is a result of previous rheumatic carditis which has damaged one or more of the heart valves. The mitral valve is involved most frequently, followed by the aortic, tricuspid, and pulmonic valves. If the heart muscle remains strong, the circulatory apparatus can adjust itself efficiently even though a valve is injured badly. The details of such adjustment, called *compensatory changes,* include modifications in the rate and character of the heartbeat, changes in the blood, hypertrophy of the myocardium, redistribution of the blood in the body, etc. All of these changes lessen the unfavorable results of the valve defect.

Mitral Stenosis

Mitral stenosis is the progressive thickening and contracture of the mitral valve cusps, which causes narrowing of the orifice and progressive obstruction to blood flow. It is by far the most common of the late cardiac

valve (the normal direction), and back through the leaking tricuspid valve into the right atrium. The flow of venous blood from the systemic circulation is impeded, causing signs of general cyanosis and overfilling of all the veins of the body.

A pulse wave similar to that sent by the left ventricle throughout the arterial tree may be transmitted into the larger veins. Therefore, the liver, now swollen to perhaps two or three times its normal size, pulsates. The walls of the stomach, intestines, kidneys, and other abdominal organs, since they are turgid with venous blood, cannot function well and produce symptoms of chronic passive congestion. The skin of the legs and the dependent portions of the body becomes edematous. Fluid collects in the abdominal cavity (ascites) and in the pleural cavities (hydrothorax). If the heart responds to medical or surgical therapy, circulation improves, the congestion of the various organs is relieved, and all symptoms may abate.

MANAGEMENT. The treatment consists of surgical treatment of associated mitral valve disease, tricuspid valvuloplasty, or tricuspid valve replacement.

BIBLIOGRAPHY

BOOKS

Amsterdam, E. A., Wilmore, J. H., and DeMaria, A. N.: Exercise in Cardiovascular Health and Disease. New York, Yorke Medical Books, 1977.

Brest, A. N.: Congestive Heart Failure. New York, Medcom Press, 1975.

Caird, F. I., Dall, J. L. C., and Kennedy, R. D.: Cardiology in Old Age. New York, Plenum Press, 1976.

Chung, E. K.: Principles of Cardiac Arrhythmias, 2nd ed. Baltimore, Williams and Wilkins, 1977.

Cromwell, R. L., et al.: Acute Myocardial Infarction. Reaction and Recovery. St. Louis, C. V. Mosby, 1977.

Croog, S. H., and Levine, S.: The Heart Patient Recovers. New York, Human Sciences Press, 1977.

Fowler, N. O.: Cardiac Diagnosis and Treatment, 2nd ed. Hagerstown, Md., Harper and Row, 1976.

Gill, C., et al.: The Cardiovascular System as It Relates to Heart Pacing. Minneapolis, Medtronic Inc., 1975.

Gazes, P. C.: Clinical Cardiology. Chicago, Year Book Medical Pub., 1975.

Glass, D. C.: Behavior Patterns, Stress and Coronary Disease. Hillsdale, New Jersey, Lawrence Erlbaum Associates, Pub., 1977. (Distributed by John Wiley and Sons in New York.)

Gotto, A. M., Jr., et al.: Atherosclerosis. Kalamazoo, The Upjohn Company, 1977.

Hammer, J., ed.: Recent Advances in Cardiology. New York, Churchill Livingstone, 1977.

Hurst, J. W., ed., et al.: The Heart. New York, McGraw-Hill, 1978.

James, W. E., and Amsterdam, E. A.: Coronary Heart Disease, Exercise Testing and Cardiac Rehabilitation. Miami, Symposia Specialists, 1977.

Julian, D. G., ed.: Angina Pectoris. New York, Churchill Livingstone, 1977.

Kaplan, E. L., and Taranta, A. V.: Infective Endocarditis — An American Heart Association Symposium. Dallas, Tex., American Heart Association, 1977.

Kaye, D.: Infective Endocarditis. Baltimore, University Park Press, 1976.

Kingsley, B., et al.: Advances in Noninvasive Diagnostic Cardiology. Thorofare, N.J., Charles B. Slack, 1976.

Mason, D. T.: Cardiac Emergencies. Baltimore, Williams and Wilkins, 1978.

Morse, D., and Goldberg, H.: Important Topics in Congenital, Valvular and Coronary Artery Disease. Mt. Kisco, N.Y., Futura Pub. Co., 1975.

O'Connor, A. B., ed.: Advances in Cardiovascular Nursing. New York, American Journal of Nursing Co., 1975.

Pantridge, J. F., et al.: The Acute Coronary Attack. New York, Grune and Stratton, 1975.

Rahimtoola, S. H.: Infective Endocarditis. New York, Grune and Stratton, 1978.

Russek, H. I., ed.: Cardiovascular Problems: Perspectives and Progress. Baltimore, University Park Press, 1976.

Silber, E. N., et al.: Heart Disease. New York, Macmillan, 1975.

Sokolow, M., and McIlroy, M. B.: Clinical Cardiology. Los Altos, Lange Medical Pub., 1977.

Willerson, J. T., and Sanders, C. A.: Clinical Cardiology. New York, Grune and Stratton, 1977.

ARTICLES

Assessment/Diagnosis

Ariet, M., and Crevasse, L. E.: Status report on computerized ECG analysis. JAMA, 239:1201-1202, Mar. 20, 1978.

Hamer, J., ed.: Recent Advances in Cardiology, 7:entire volume, 1977.

Haughey, B.: CVP lines: Monitoring and maintaining. AJN, 78:635-638, Apr. 1978.

McNeal, G. J.: Twenty-four hour ambulatory monitoring. A new electrocardiographic tool. Nurs. Clin. N. Am., 13:437-448, Sept. 1978.

Mechner, F.: Programmed Instruction. Patient assessment: Examination of the heart and great vessels. Part 1. AJN, 76:1807-1830, Nov. 1976.

Merrill, S. A., and Froelicher, V. F.: Exercise testing. Cardio-Vac. Nurs., 13:23-28, Nov.-Dec. 1977.

Murray, J., and Smallwood, J.: CVP monitoring: Sidestepping potential perils. Nursing '77, 7:42-47, Jan. 1977.

Pennock, R. S.: How useful are serum levels of cardiac drugs? Am. Fam. Phys., 17:194-196, Apr. 1978.

Raffetto, J., et al.: Accuracy of total serum enzymes and myocardial specific isoenzymes — a comparative study. Nebr. Med. J., 64:36-38, Feb. 1978.

Rappaport, E.: Serum enzymes and isoenzymes in the diagnosis of acute myocardial infarction. Mod. Concepts Cardiovasc. Dis., 46:43-46, Sept. 1977.

Roe, C. R.: Diagnosis of myocardial infarction by serum isoenzyme analysis. Ann. Clin. Lab. Sci., 7:201-209, May-June, 1977.

Shah, P. M., and Roberts, D. L.: Diagnosis and treatment of aortic valve stenosis. Curr. Probl. Cardiol., *2*:3-49, Sept. 1977.

Van Diji, Y. M., et al.: Differential diagnosis of chest pain. Use of isoenzyme LDH₁ level as a criterion. Postgrad. Med., *65*:189-192, Jan. 1979.

Winslow, E. H.: Visual inspection of the patient with cardiopulmonary disease. Heart Lung, *4*:421-429, May-June 1975.

Atherosclerotic Heart Disease—Angina Pectoris/Myocardial Infarction

Abrams, J.: Current status of nitroglycerin ointment in angina pectoris. A new look at an old drug. Angiology, *28*:217-222, Mar. 1977.

Ahlquist, R. P.: Present state of alpha and beta adrenergic drugs. III, Beta blocking agents. Am. Heart J., *93*:117-120, Jan. 1977.

Aronow, W. S.: Treatment of angina pectoris. Pharmacologic approaches. Postgrad. Med., *60*:100-106, Nov. 1976.

Ball, K. P., and Turner, R.: Realism in the prevention of coronary heart disease. Prev. Med., *4*:390-397, Dec. 1975.

Cohen, B. D., Wallston, B. S., and Wallston, K. A.: Sex counseling in cardiac rehabilitation. Arch. Phys. Med. Rehabil., *57*:473-474, Oct. 1976.

Cook, C. I.: Self-concept of the myocardial infarction patient. Can. Nurse, *72*:37-38, Oct. 1976.

DeBusk, R.: How to individualize rehabilitation after myocardial infarction. Geriatrics, *32*:77-79, Aug. 1977.

Gillum, R. F., et al.: The pre-hospital phase of acute myocardial infarction and sudden death. Prev. Med., *5*:408-413, Sept. 1976.

Gottlieb, R. S., Duca, P. R., and Brest, A. N.: Pathophysiology and medical management of angina pectoris. Am. Fam. Phys., *16*:82-89, Oct. 1977.

Helfant, R. H.: Nitroglycerin: New concepts about an old drug. Am. J. Med., *60*:905-909, 31 May 1976.

Houser, D.: What to do first when a patient complains of chest pain. Nursing '76, *6*:54-56, Nov. 1976.

Johnston, B. L.: Eight steps in patient cardiac rehabilitation: The team effort—methodology and preliminary results. Heart Lung, *5*:97-111, Jan.-Feb. 1976.

Kotler, M. N., Segal, B. L., and Likoff, W.: Medical management of angina pectoris. Postgrad. Med., *61*:113-117, Mar. 1977.

Leon, A. S., and Blackburn, H.: Exercise rehabilitation of the coronary heart disease patient. Geriatrics, *32*:66-76, Dec. 1977.

Lethbridge, B., Somboon, O., and Shea, H. L.: The transfer process. Can. Nurse, *72*:39-40, Oct. 1976.

Luria, M. H., et al.: Acute MI: Prognosis after recovery. Ann. Intern. Med., *85*:561-565, Nov. 1976.

Madias, J. E., and Gorlin, R.: The myth of acute "mild" myocardial infarction. Ann. Intern. Med., *86*:347-352, Mar. 1977.

Merrill, S. A.: A nursing contribution to cardiac rehabilitation programs. Milit. Med., *142*:129-138, Feb. 1977.

Miller, A. J.: Rehabilitation and length of hospitalization after acute MI. Am. Heart J., *92*:547-548, Nov. 1976.

Miner, J. A., and Conti, R.: Topical nitroglycerin for ischemic heart disease. JAMA, *239*:2166-2167, May 19, 1978.

Murphy, M. L., et al.: Treatment of chronic stable angina. New Eng. J. Med., *297*:621-627, Sept. 22, 1977.

O'Rourke, R. A., and Schnitzle, R. N.: Angina pectoris: An overview. Angiology, *28*:135-141, Mar. 1977.

Parks, L.: Chest pain—a summary. Can. Nurse, *72*:35-36, Nov. 1976.

Puksta, N. S.: All about sex—after a coronary. AJN, *77*: 602-605, Apr. 1977.

Segal, B. L., Kotler, M. N., and Likoff, W.: Coronary risk factors and anginal pain patterns. Postgrad. Med., *61*:102-107, Mar. 1977.

Short, D.: The management of the patient with angina. Am. Heart J., *94*:135-139, Aug. 1977.

Vaisrub, S.: Variants of variance (editorial). JAMA, *237*:1127, Mar. 14, 1977.

Walton, C., and Hammond, B.: Angina: Teaching your patient how to prevent recurrent attacks. Nursing '78, *8*:32-38, Feb. 1978.

Wenger, N. K.: Critical evaluation of cardiac rehabilitation (editorial). Chest, *71*:317-318, Mar. 1977.

Weinberg, S. L.: Intermediate coronary care. Chest, *73*:154-157, Feb. 1978.

Woske, M., and Kratzer, J.: C. T. Cardiac Teaching: Preparing the patient for a different life. Nursing '77, *7*:25-26, May 1977.

Congestive Heart Failure/Pulmonary Edema

Biddle, T. L.: Hemodynamic concepts in treating acute pulmonary edema. South. Med. J., *70*:1342-1344, Nov. 1977.

Bussman, W., and Kaltenbach, M.: Sublingual nitroglycerin for left ventricular failure and pulmonary edema. Compr. Ther., *3*:29-36, Aug. 1977.

Cunningham, J. H., Richardson, R. H., and Smith, J. D.: Interstitial pulmonary edema. Heart Lung, *6*:617-623, July-Aug. 1977.

Diamond, N. J., Schofferman, J., and Elliott, J. W.: Arterial blood gases in acute pulmonary edema. JACEP, *5*:497-500, July 1976.

Drugs used in the care of the cardiac patient. Nurs. Clin. N. Am., *13*:473-497, Sept. 1978.

Frantz, A., and Galdys, M.: Keeping up with automatic rotating tourniquets. Nursing '78, *8*:31-35, Apr. 1978.

Haughey, E. J., and Sica, F. M.: Diuretics: How safe can you make them? Nursing '77, *7*:34-39, Feb. 1977.

Isacson, L. M., and Schulz, K.: Treating pulmonary edema. Nursing '78, *8*:42-45, Feb. 1978.

Jackson, F.: Pulmonary oedema. Practitioner, *219*:656-663, Nov. 1977.

Kemp, G., and Kemp, D.: Diuretics. AJN., *78*:1006-1010, June 1978.

Manzi, C. C.: Edema: How to tell if it's a danger signal. Nursing '77, *7*:66-70, April, 1977.

Mehta, J.: Vasodilators in the treatment of heart failure. JAMA, *238*:2534-2536, Dec. 5, 1977.

Miller, R. T., et al.: Afterload reduction in congestive heart failure. Adv. In Cardiol., *22*:199-204, 1978.

Weil, M. H., and Henning, R. J.: Acute circulatory failure (shock) associated with cardiogenic pulmonary edema. Crit. Care Med., *5*:215-219, Sept.-Oct. 1977.

Wolf, P. S.: Cardiac asthma — its origin, recognition and management. Ann. Allergy, *37*:250-254, Oct. 1976.

Ziesche, S., and Franciosa, J. A.: Clinical application of sodium nitroprusside. Heart Lung, *6*:99-103, Jan.-Feb. 1977.

Endocarditis/Pericarditis

Applefeld, M. M., and Woodward, T. E.: Infective endocarditis: A clinical overview. Curr. Prob. Cardiol., *2*:7-37, Apr. 1977.

Dunn, M., and Rinkenberger, R. L.: Clinical aspects of acute pericarditis. Cardiovasc. Clin., *7*:131-157, 1976.

Hancock, E. W.: Management of pericardial disease. Mod. Concepts Cardiovasc. Dis., *48*:1-6, Jan. 1979.

Kaplan, E. L.: Statement by AHA on prevention of bacterial endocarditis. Circulation, *56*:139A-143A, July 1977.

Pelletier, L. I., Jr., and Petersdorf, R. G.: Infective endocarditis: A review of 125 cases from University of Washington Hospitals 1963-1972. Medicine, *56*:287-313, July 1977.

Pacing

Czerwinski, B.: Trans-telephonic surveillance for pacemaker patients. AJN., *77*:829-830, May 1977.

Furman, S.: Cardiac pacing and pacemakers. VIII, The pacemaker follow-up clinic. Am. Heart J., *94*:795-804, Dec. 1977.

Furman, S., and Fisher, J. D.: Cardiac pacing and pacemakers. V., Technical aspects of implantation and equipment. Am. Heart J., *94*:250-259, Aug. 1977.

Mantini, E. L., et al.: A recommended protocol for pacemaker followup: Analysis of 1705 implanted pacemakers. Ann. Thorac. Surg., *24*:62-67, July 1977.

Manwaring, M.: What patients need to know about pacemakers. AJN, *77*:825-830, May 1977.

Parsonnet, V.: Permanent pacing of the heart. 1952-1976. Am. J. Cardiol., *39*:250-256, Feb. 1977.

Proctor, D., Fletcher, R. D., and Del Negro, A. A.: Temporary cardiac pacing. Nurs. Clin. N. Am., *13*:409-422, Sept. 1978.

Rossel, C. L., and Alyn, I. B.: Living with a permanent cardiac pacemaker. Heart Lung, *6*:273-279, Mar.-Apr. 1977.

Sweetwood, H.: Patients with pacemakers. Nursing '77, *7*:44-51, Mar. 1977.

What patients want to know about their pacemakers. Can. Nurse, *72*:27-29, Oct. 1976.

AGENCIES

Governmental

National Heart, Lung, and Blood Institute, Bethesda, Md. 20205

Voluntary

American Heart Association, National Center, 7320 Greenville Ave., Dallas, Tex. 75231

31

ASSESSMENT AND MANAGEMENT OF PATIENTS WITH VASCULAR DISORDERS AND PROBLEMS OF PERIPHERAL CIRCULATION

PHYSIOLOGIC OVERVIEW

The function of the vascular system is to provide a channel for the transport of blood from the heart to all the tissues of the body and then back to the heart. The vessels that transport the blood from the heart to the tissues are the *arteries*. The vessels that transport the blood from the tissues back to the heart are the *veins*. The vessels within the tissues that connect the arterial and venous systems are the *capillaries*.

The vascular system actually consists of two circulations that are connected in series. The *systemic circulation* carries blood from the left heart through the tissues and back to the right heart; as it makes its circuit, the blood supplies nutrients to and removes waste products from the organ systems of the body. The *pulmonary circulation*, also called the lesser circulation because of its shorter length, carries blood from the right heart through the lungs and back to the left heart.

The artery that receives the blood from the left ventricle is the largest artery in the body, the *aorta*. The large systemic veins that collect the blood and return it to the right atrium are the *vena cavae*, consisting of an inferior division that collects blood from the lower half of the body and a superior division that collects blood from the upper parts of the body. A schematic diagram of the circulation is shown in Figure 31-1.

The function of the lymphatic circulation is to provide a channel for the transport of lymph from tissues back into the vascular system. The lymph, composed of tissue

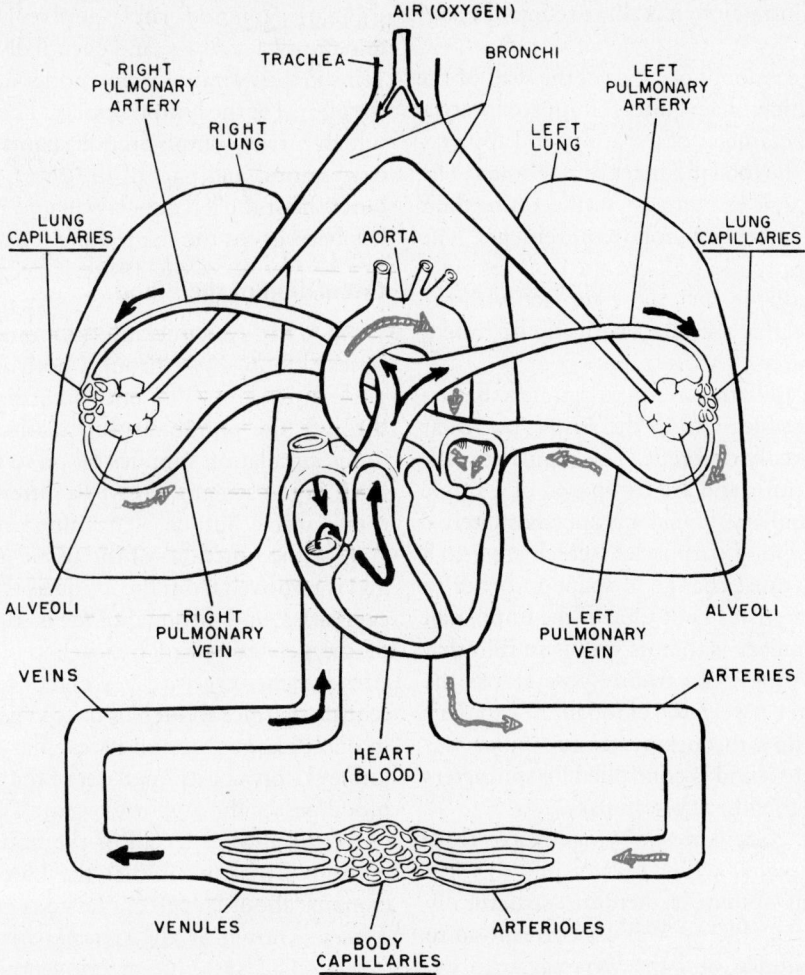

Figure 31-1.   Schematic drawing of systemic circulation. (Start at bottom of diagram.) Loaded with carbon dioxide, blood from the body capillaries goes through venules and veins into the right chamber of the heart (black arrows). It is pumped into the two lungs. Having dropped carbon dioxide and picked up oxygen, it goes back to the left chamber of the heart (red arrows). From there it is pumped through the aorta into the body circulation (arteries and arterioles) until it reaches the body capillaries, where it gives up oxygen and picks up carbon dioxide. (National Tuberculosis and Respiratory Disease Association)

fluids and certain waste products, is collected in lymphatic capillaries. It is then carried in lymphatic vessels through lymph nodes and ultimately returned to systemic veins.

Anatomy of the Vascular System

ARTERIES AND ARTERIOLES.   The systemic arteries are thick-walled structures that carry blood from the heart to the tissues. The aorta, which has a diameter of approximately 25 mm. (1 inch), gives rise to numerous branches, which in turn divide into smaller vessels that approach 4 mm. (0.16 inch) in diameter by the time they reach the tissues. Within the tissues, the vessels divide further, diminishing to approximately 30 microns in diameter; these vessels are called *arterioles*.

The walls of the arteries and arterioles are divided into three layers: an inner layer called the *intima*, which is in contact with the blood, a middle layer called the *media*, and an outer layer called the *adventitia*. The intima provides a smooth surface for contact with the flowing blood. It is composed of a single layer of flat endothelial cells. The adventitia is a layer of connective tissue that anchors the vessel to its surrounding structures. The media makes up the major portion of the vessel wall. In the aorta and other large arteries of the body, this layer is composed chiefly of elastic and connective tissue fibers that give the vessel considerable strength. There is much less elastic tissue in the smaller arteries and arterioles, and the media in these vessels is composed primarily of smooth muscle. This muscle is not under voluntary control but is subject to autonomic nervous system and hormonal influences. Since the smooth muscle can maintain a wide range of contraction, it is able to control vessel diameter.

Because of the large amount of muscle, the wall of the arteries is relatively thick; it accounts for approximately 25 percent of the total diameter of the artery and approximately 67 percent of the total diameter of arterioles. The muscle and adventitia of the arterial wall require their own blood supplies to meet metabolic requirements. The blood vessels that supply the wall are the *vasa vasorum*. The intima is thin and is in such close contact with the blood within the vessel that it can receive its nourishment directly from that source.

CAPILLARIES. The capillaries are small channels that are extensions of the arterioles within the tissue, but their wall structure is markedly different. The capillary walls lack muscle and adventitia and are composed of a single layer of cells. Since capillary diameter is approximately 6 to 8 microns, the red blood corpuscles (which are 7 to 8 microns in diameter) must change in shape in order to squeeze through the capillary bed. One of the important characteristics of a capillary is that its wall is so thin that nutrients, gases, and fluids can readily pass across the wall in either direction between the blood in the capillary and the tissue. Blood flow through systemic capillaries is known to be intermittent and is controlled by sphincters located at the arteriolar end of the capillary.

VEINS AND VENULES. Capillaries join together to form larger vessels called *venules,* which in turn join to form the veins. The venous system is therefore structurally analogous to the arterial system. Venules correspond to arterioles, veins to arteries, and the vena cavae to the aorta. Analogous types of vessels in the arterial and venous systems have approximately the same diameters.

However, the walls of the veins, in contrast to those of the arteries, are thinner and considerably less muscular. As an example, the wall of the average vein amounts to only 10 percent of the vein diameter, whereas the artery wall is 25 percent of its diameter. However, the wall of a vein, like that of an artery, is composed of three layers, as was described above, in the discussion of arteries.

The other major difference between the venous and arterial systems is the presence of valves in the veins. These valves are fibrous leaflets in the lumen of the vein that permit blood flow in one direction only. To perform this function, the valves remain open when blood is flowing from the tissues back towards the heart but close if blood attempts to flow in the opposite direction. In this respect they operate in a manner similar to what has been described previously for the semilunar valves of the heart.

LYMPHATIC VESSELS. The lymphatic circulation begins in the tissues and is a one-way system that carries lymph from tissues back to the venous circulation. Within the tissues, the lymphatic channels are composed of thin-walled capillaries similar to the blood capillaries. These capillaries join to form larger lymph vessels, which contain one-way valves, and eventually empty into the large veins in the thorax. Lymph nodes occur at intervals along the course of the lymph vessels. The largest lymph vessel, which carries lymph predominantly from the abdomen, extremities, and part of the chest, and empties into the junction of the left subclavian and internal jugular veins, has been given the name *thoracic duct*.

Circulation of the Blood

Since the systemic and pulmonary circulations are in series, blood flow through both must be equal over a period of time. The entire cardiac output must pass through the pulmonary circulation; however, the systemic circulation supplies blood to many organ systems. Each organ system receives a different percentage of the total cardiac output, determined roughly by the needs and/or the functions of the tissue (see Table 31-1). Oxygen is removed from the blood as it passes through tissue capillaries, and carbon dioxide is added to it. The amount of oxygen extracted by each tissue is different (*tissue arteriovenous oxygen difference*). For example, heart muscle tends to extract about half the oxygen from arterial blood in one passage through its capillary bed, whereas in the kidneys only about 7 percent of the oxygen is removed as blood passes through the organ. The average amount of oxygen removed by all of the body tissues is about 25 percent. This means that the blood in the vena cavae contains about 25 percent less oxygen than aortic blood. This is known as the *systemic arteriovenous oxygen difference.* The systemic arteriovenous oxygen difference increases when the amount of oxygen delivered to the tissues is decreased relative to their metabolic needs. More detailed information about the blood flow and oxygen extraction as blood passes through capillary beds in various tissues is summarized in Table 31-1.

MICROCIRCULATION. As was noted above, the extremely thin walls of capillaries are ideally suited for the exchange of material between the blood and tissue. The surface area for contact between capillary blood and tissue is very large. These factors combine to allow an efficient exchange in which oxygen and nutrients are absorbed from capillary blood by tissues for metabolic needs and carbon dioxide and other waste products of metabolism are released from tissue back into the capillary blood.

Within the tissue, plasma in the capillary is continually filtered and reabsorbed across the capillary wall. This filtered fluid, which has the same composition as plasma without its proteins, forms the interstitial fluid. Interstitial fluid is fluid within a tissue that surrounds the cells of the tissue. The pressure at the arterial end of the capillary is relatively high, compared with that at the venous end. This high pressure at the arterial end of the capillary tends to drive fluid out of the capillary blood and into the tissue

TABLE 31-1. TYPICAL VALUES FOR BLOOD FLOW AND OXYGEN CONSUMPTION
FOR VARIOUS ORGANS IN THE HUMAN

ORGAN	ORGAN WEIGHT (KG.)	BLOOD FLOW DURING REST				OXYGEN USAGE DURING REST			
		Organ Blood Flow (ml./min.)	Blood Flow Unit Wt. (ml./min./ 100 gm.)	% Total Card. Output	A-V O$_2$ Difference, ml./100 ml. Blood	Organ O$_2$ Usage (ml./min.)	O$_2$ Usage Unit Wt. (ml./min./ 100 gm.)	% Total O$_2$ Usage	
Brain	1.4	750	55	14	6.0	45	3.00	18	
Heart	0.3	250	80	5	10.0	25	8.00	10	
Liver	1.5	1,300	85	23	6.0	75	2.00	30	
G.I. tract	2.5	1,000	40						
Kidneys	0.3	1,200	400	22	1.3	15	5.00	6	
Muscle	35.0	1,000	3	18	5.0	50	0.15	20	
Skin	2.0	200	10	4	2.5	5	0.20	2	
Remainder (skeleton, bone marrow, fat, connective tissue, etc.)	27.0	800	3	14	5.0	35	0.15	14	
TOTAL	70 kg.	5,500 ml./min.		100		250		100	

(Folkow, B., and Neil, E.: Circulation. New York, Oxford University Press, Inc., 1971, page 12.)

(filtration). The plasma proteins in the capillary blood exert an osmotic force (osmotic pressure) that tends to pull fluid back into the capillary from the tissue space, but this osmotic force cannot overcome the high hydrostatic pressure at the arterial end of the capillary. At the venous end of the capillary, however, the osmotic force predominates over the low hydrostatic pressure in the capillary at that end and there is a net reabsorption of fluid from the tissue space back into the capillary. Virtually all of the fluid that is filtered at the arterial end of the capillary bed is reabsorbed at the venous end, except for a very small amount. This excess filtered fluid enters the lymphatic circulation. These processes of filtration, reabsorption, and lymph formation aid in the maintenance of tissue fluid volume and in the removal of tissue waste and debris.

Under certain abnormal conditions, the filtration of fluid may greatly exceed the amounts reabsorbed and carried away by lymph flow. This can result from leakage through damaged capillary walls, obstruction of lymphatic drainage, elevation of venous pressure, or decrease in plasma protein osmotic force. The accumulation of fluid that results from these processes is known as *edema.*

LYMPH CIRCULATION. As was mentioned above, lymph is formed when filtration exceeds reabsorption in a capillary bed. The lymph consists mainly of filtered fluid from the blood plus cellular debris, white blood cells, proteins, and fats. The lymph is carried by the lymphatic channels back into the venous system through a series of lymph nodes. The function of the lymph nodes is to filter particles and break them down so that they can be carried by the lymph back to the blood, where they can be further metabolized and excreted as necessary.

Hemodynamics

What are the physiologic factors that determine the rate of blood flow and the distribution of blood flow to the various organs? As was noted previously in the section on the heart (page 509) the rate of blood flow is equal to the pressure propelling the blood (ΔP) divided by the resistance to blood flow (R):

$$(1) \qquad \text{Flow} = \Delta P/R$$

The driving pressure is provided by contraction of the heart muscle. The factors that determine the resistance to blood flow during streamlined (nonturbulent) flow conditions can be summarized by the Poiseuille equation:

$$(2) \qquad R = \frac{8\eta L}{\pi r^4}$$

where r = radius of the vessel
L = length of the vessel
η = viscosity of the blood

Inspection of this equation shows that the resistance depends on the viscosity of the blood and the length of the vessel, but by far the most important factor is the vessel radius, since in the equation it is raised to the 4th power. Resistance to flow to any particular organ will therefore depend on the radius of the vessel supplying that organ. The total resistance to blood flow in the arterial system as a whole varies with the radii of all the blood vessels in the arterial circuit.

From equation (1), we can explain the events that occur

when resistance to flow in the arterial circulation is increased. In order to maintain total blood flow (cardiac output), the driving pressure has to increase. This is accomplished by increased force of contraction of the heart. Prolonged elevation of arterial resistance leads to cardiac muscle hypertrophy because of the necessity for chronically elevated force of contraction.

The Poiseuille equation applies when blood flows in a streamlined fashion without turbulence (laminar flow). Although most blood flow in the body is laminar and therefore can be described by the Poiseuille relationship, turbulent flow does occur in some portions of the vascular tree. This is seen at bifurcations where one artery divides into two, or where the intima of the blood vessel wall has been damaged and creates a localized obstruction to blood flow.

An important feature of arteries is that by contraction of the smooth muscle in their walls, their diameters can be altered, thereby altering the resistance to flow through them. It is by this mechanism that blood flow can be directed toward or away from an organ. The location in the arterial tree where the greatest changes in vessel diameter can take place is in the arterioles. Therefore, these vessels are best able to regulate local blood flow. As a consequence, blood pressure shows the greatest drop as it passes through this segment, and capillary pressure can be maintained relatively constant at a low level.

VASCULAR STORAGE OF BLOOD. Since the arteries are relatively thick-walled, muscular, elastic vessels, the volume of blood which they contain cannot be greatly increased. On the other hand, the veins, with their narrower walls, are much more compliant and distensible. The venous system, therefore, can serve as a temporary reservoir for blood and can return the blood to the heart quickly when necessary.

Blood Pressure

The energy required for pumping blood throughout the circulation comes from the heart muscle itself. Since the heart pumps blood by alternating contractions and relaxations, it creates fluctuations of pressure throughout the arterial system. During ventricular systole the pressure in the arterial system reaches a maximum, termed systolic blood pressure. During ventricular diastole, blood from the arterial system runs off into the capillary bed, and pressure within the arteries decreases. The minimum arterial pressure is called diastolic blood pressure.

The systolic and diastolic blood pressures can be measured in humans by applying pressure over an artery and stopping its blood flow. As the applied pressure is gradually reduced, one can hear sounds over the artery as flow starts to return. With further reduction in applied pressure, the sounds totally disappear when flow in the artery returns to normal. The pressure at which the sound begins to appear is the *systolic pressure,* and that at which the sounds disappear is *diastolic pressure.* These pressure measurements can be made on the arm or the leg with a device called a *sphygmomanometer.*

The pressure in the systemic veins is relatively close to atmospheric pressure, and pulsations of flow and pressure do not occur in these vessels. Valves are present in the veins so that blood can move in one direction only. The factors that influence propulsion of blood through the veins back toward the heart are the small pressure gradients transmitted through the capillaries, gravity, and compression of the veins by contraction of skeletal muscle during physical activity.

Control of the Circulation

A number of mechanisms influence resistance to flow in the circulatory system. These control mechanisms manifest themselves primarily by altering the tension in the smooth muscle of the arterial wall, which changes the radius of the vessel.

Minute-by-minute control of the resistance of the vascular tree is influenced by neural, hormonal, and local factors. Stimulation of the sympathetic nervous system dilates vessels in some circulatory beds and constricts vessels in others. The vessels that dilate are those necessary for "fight or flight"; for example, vessels to skeletal muscle dilate. Stimulation of the parasympathetic nervous system generally dilates vessels.

A number of hormonal substances affect resistance to blood flow in the vascular system. One of these is the hormone epinephrine, or adrenalin, a potent vasodilator in many vascular beds consistent with its role as a mediator of the "fight or flight" reaction. Angiotensin is another important hormonal regulator of resistance to blood flow, causing vasoconstriction. Blood levels of angiotensin in turn depend on release of the hormone renin by the kidney when blood pressure to the kidney falls.

Accumulation of tissue metabolites in general causes vasodilation of systemic vessels. For example, accumulation of lactic acid when oxygen supply to a tissue is inadequate leads to dilatation of local vessels so that oxygen supply is increased. Other local factors causing vasodilatation are products of inflammation, increased carbon dioxide, and chemical substances such as histamine and bradykinin. Vasoconstriction results from trauma to tissue, perhaps mediated by the release of substances such as serotonin.

Pathophysiology of the Vascular System

Edema. Edema refers to the abnormal accumulation of fluid within a tissue. It is formed whenever fluid is filtered from the vascular space faster than it is reabsorbed into capillaries or carried away by lymphatics. It is seen most commonly when pressure within the venous system is elevated, as with failure of the heart or damage to the valves of the veins. Because of gravity, venous pressure in the upright position is greatest in the lower extremities, and edema usually appears there first. This effect can be minimized by assuming the supine position and further decreased by elevating the legs above the level of the heart. Elevated venous pressure can also occur when a major vein is compressed from outside, such as by a tumor mass. Another cause of edema is the increased filtration of fluid that occurs when permeability of the capillaries is increased, leading to leakage of fluid into the tissues. This can be seen with localized inflammation or the administration of certain toxins and drugs. Localized edema due to a mosquito bite or a bee sting is a common example of this increased permeability phenomenon. A third general mechanism leading to edema is obstruction to the outflow of lymph, so that the excess fluid filtered from the capillaries cannot be carried away sufficiently rapidly. A tumor mass is a common cause of obstruction of the lymphatic channels. The final mechanism for edema formation is decreased osmotic pressure of the blood, such as is seen in patients with low plasma albumin due to liver or kidney disease.

Obstruction of Flow in the Vascular System. When an arterial channel is obstructed, blood flow is reduced or obliterated and the organ the vessel was serving is deprived of its normal blood supply. Obstruction to flow in the vascular system is usually due to one of two different processes. An *embolus* is a blood clot or other particle not normally present in the bloodstream that lodges in a branching artery or arteriole. The other type of obstruction is caused by the slow growth of an organizing clot, called a *thrombus,* on the interior wall of an artery. When either type of obstruction occurs, acute derangement of organ function or death of tissue may result secondary to deprivation of oxygen and nutrient supply. With chronic obstruction, blood supply may be restored either by revascularization through the original channel or by development of collateral channels to supply the organ by rerouting blood supply around the site of obstruction.

ASSESSMENT OF CIRCULATORY INSUFFICIENCY

Pain. Local and temporary deficiency of blood supply to the tissues due to constriction of vessels is called *ischemia.* When a person is reaching to perform work overhead, such as painting or hammering nails into the ceiling, a crampy pain ensues within a short time (30 seconds), and the arm must be lowered in order to obtain relief. The pain experienced is the result of ischemia in the arm muscles. The same type of crampy pain develops in the legs of patients with arterial insufficiency. This pain, called *intermittent claudication,* develops after a specific distance has been walked. If the claudication distance is 1 block, then every time the person walks 1

block, he must stop and rest for a few minutes after which he can again walk 1 block. If the arterial occlusion is in the superficial femoral artery, the patient will have calf claudication. If the blockage is in the pelvic (iliac) area, symptoms will be in the thigh. Should the arterial occlusion problem be in the abdominal aorta, the patient will have hip and buttock claudication.

The cause of ischemic pain is unknown; however, it is relieved by supplying oxygenated blood. Some suggest that pain is caused by the accumulation of large amounts of lactic acid in the tissues; others believe that histamine or other chemicals stimulate pain nerve endings.

As arterial insufficiency increases, rest pain may ensue and, since it is commonly present at night, can keep the patient from sleeping. This pain is not to be confused with night cramps. This latter condition may occur in either the normal or diseased leg and is frequently brought on by stretching the leg or the foot. It commonly awakens a person from sleep. Therapy consists of the use of diphenhydramine (Benadryl), quinine (or quinidine), or diazepam (Valium).

Skin Color and Temperature. Other signs of a deficient blood supply include coldness, numbness, pallor, loss of hair, and trophic skin changes. Even in a warm environment, the extremity affected may feel cool to the patient and to the touch. The usual healthy flesh color is blanched in appearance as superficial vessels are constricted.

With severe circulatory impairment, the foot will develop an intense reddish-blue, angry discoloration (*rubor*) on prolonged dependency due to overdilated capillaries. A bluish discoloration (*cyanosis*) occurs when there is a concentration of deoxygenated hemoglobin. Of course, skin pigment and skin thickness affect the degree of apparent discoloration.

Elevating an extremity in which there is impaired arterial circulation produces *cadaveric pallor;* lowering it to a dependent position thereafter is accompanied by delayed return of normal color and finally *dependent rubor.* Pulsations in the affected area are weak or absent and application of the oscillometer shows impaired arterial oscillations (pulsations).

Pulse Pressure. The state of pulsations in the peripheral arteries is an important means of assessing for vascular diseases (Fig. 31-2).

A method of recording the quality of pulsations felt is as follows:

> 0 — absence of pulsations
> 1 — marked impairment of pulsations
> 2 — moderate impairment of pulsations
> 3 — slight impairment of pulsations
> 4 — normal pulsations

The Doppler ultrasound enables one to detect peripheral flow in the pedal arteries even if no pulse is

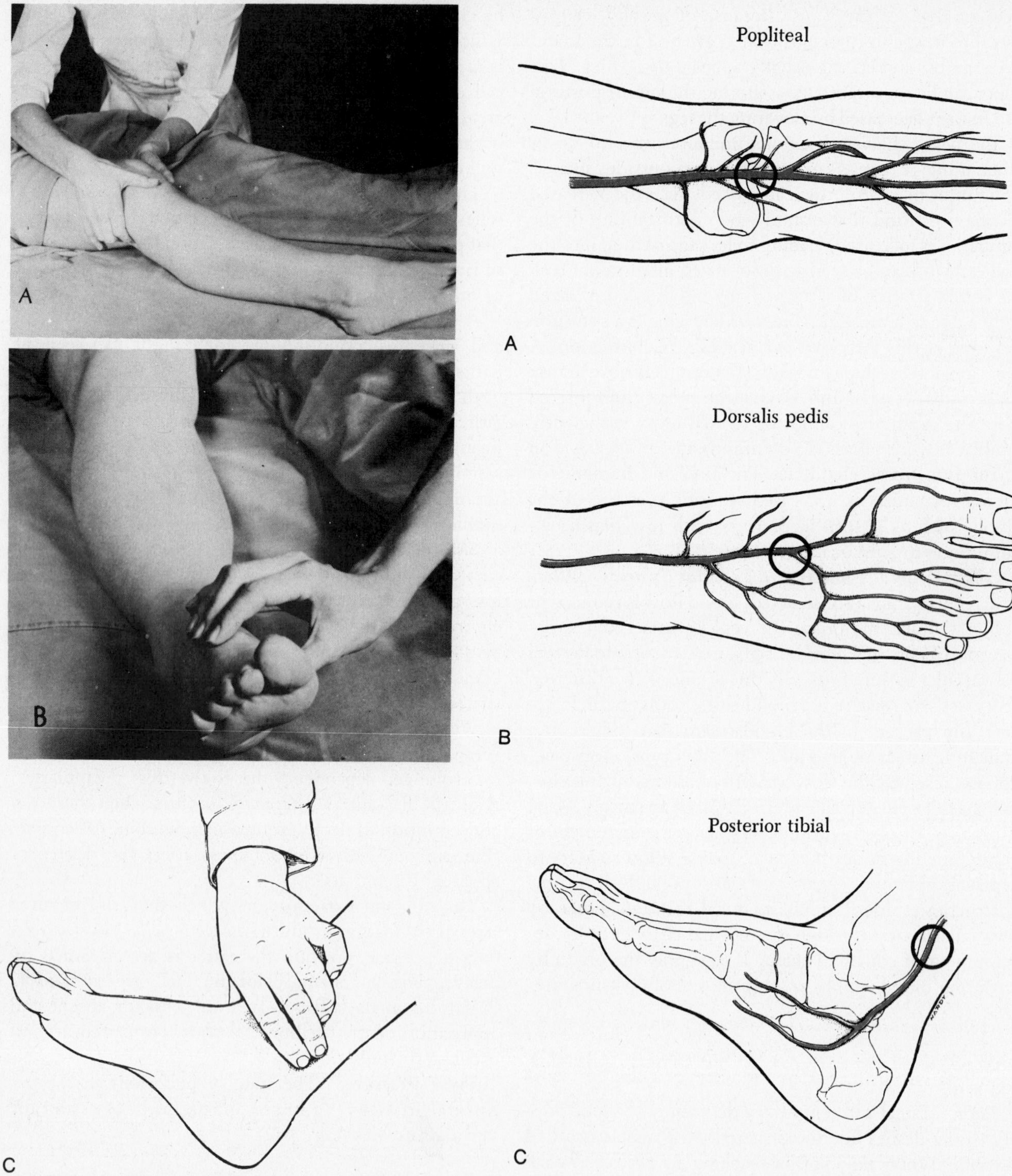

Popliteal

A

Dorsalis pedis

B

Posterior tibial

C

Figure 31-2. (A) Popliteal pulse. (B) Pedal pulse. (C) Posterior tibial pulse. (Photos from Ajemian, S.: Bypass grafting for femoral artery occlusion. American Journal of Nursing; 67:565.)

palpable. Ankle blood pressure can also be obtained with the Doppler. If ankle blood pressure is less than 50 percent of arm pressure, there is severe ischemia.

Other Signs. Arterial insufficiency may affect any area of the body, but the areas most commonly affected are the lower extremities. Mesenteric arterial insufficiency leads to abdominal pain, especially after meals and may result in mesenteric thrombosis. Narrowing of the carotid, basilar, vertebral, or cerebral arteries leads to cerebral symptoms such as dizziness, blurred vision,

TABLE 31-2. CLINICAL MANIFESTATIONS OF PERIPHERAL VASCULAR DISEASE

ARTERIAL INSUFFICIENCY *Embolism*	VENOUS INSUFFICIENCY *Thrombosis*
ACUTE	
1. Severe, steady pain	1. Steady pain, moderate to severe
2. Cold, pallid extremity	2. Skin warm; may be mottled, pale, or cyanotic
3. Diminution or loss of sensory and motor function	3. No significant neurologic deficit
4. Absent pulsation beyond embolus	4. Pulses present or diminished
5. Veins collapsed	5. Veins full (legs slightly dependent)
6. No swelling (unless ischemia is far advanced)	6. Usually moderate to severe swelling with tenderness over veins and muscles
CHRONIC	
1. Intermittent claudication progressing to pain at rest with severe ischemia	1. Aching, heavy sensation, muscle cramps
2. Extremity cool, distal pulsations diminished	2. Prominent superficial veins; usually warm feet
3. Delayed healing of minor traumatic lesions	3. Pigmentation and edema, lower leg
4. Atrophy of skin with loss of hair	4. Scaling, thickening, and scarring of skin
5. Pallor—when elevated Rubor—when dependent	5. Ulceration around ankle
6. Ulceration, superficial gangrene	

(Harvey, A. M., ed. The Principles and Practice of Medicine, 19th ed. New York, Appleton-Century-Crofts, 1976)

TABLE 31-3. ASSESSMENT OF ACUTE ARTERIAL OCCLUSION VS. DEEP VEIN THROMBOSIS

	ACUTE ARTERIAL OCCLUSION	DEEP VEIN THROMBOSIS
Onset	Sudden	Gradual
Color	Pale Later: mottled cyanotic	Slightly cyanotic Rubescent
Skin temperature	Cold	Warm
Leg size—diameter	May be reduced from normal	Enlarged
Superficial veins	Collapsed	Appear enlarged and prominent
Arterial pulsation	Pulse deficit in evidence	Normal and palpable (except in marked edema)
Effect of elevating leg	Condition worsens	Condition improves

blackouts (transient ischemic attacks) and finally to strokes (see Chapter 55 page 1222).

Arterial vs. Venous Insufficiency. There are various points of comparison to note between arterial and venous insufficiency in both acute and chronic conditions. A comparison of the clinical manifestations and the assessment evaluation are listed in Tables 31-2 and 31-3.

Peripheral Arteriography. A more definitive assessment of peripheral vascular disorders may be achieved with peripheral arteriography.

Arteriograms are done not solely to "map out" the arteries but also to obtain information for determining the best treatment plan, for instance, to investigate the feasibility of arterial reconstruction. According to the procedure, contrast medium can be injected into specific arteries to demonstrate stenosis, obstruction, thrombi, or aneurysms. The brachial and femoral arteries are commonly used for the extremities. To offset a burning sensation where the dye is injected, normal saline is usually injected, with the needle tip directed upstream. After the artery is entered, the syringe is switched (stopcock prevents air from entering) to one containing the contrast medium. When dye is injected directly into the vessel, the site should be observed for signs of local irritation which may occur if some of the medium has escaped into surrounding tissues. Usually, a warm feeling is experienced by the patient as dye is injected. A second sign to watch for is a reaction to the injected solution. Solutions containing iodine may cause a severe allergic reaction in some patients, resulting in dyspnea, nausea and vomiting, sweating, rapid heart rate, and numbness of the extremities. The reaction may appear at the time of the injection or may be delayed for a time and appear after the patient has left the x-ray department and has returned to his room. Any such reaction should be reported at once. These reactions are usually treated with epinephrine (Adrenalin), antihistaminic drugs, and steroids, and occasionally with oxygen inhalations.

MEASURES TO INCREASE BLOOD SUPPLY TO TISSUES

Arterial blood supply to a part can be enhanced when the part is placed at a lower level than the heart. For the lower extremities, this can be accomplished by elevating the head of the bed or allowing the patient to assume a sitting position with his feet resting on the floor. To promote circulation, particular exercises, including walking, may be recommended. The objective is to promote blood flow by muscular exercise and to encourage the formation of a secondary circulation (a collateral circulation) to substitute for those primary vessels that are occluded.

Buerger-Allen Exercises. The patient lies flat in bed with his legs elevated above the level of his heart for 2 minutes. Then, sitting on the edge of the bed with legs dependent, he exercises his feet for 3 minutes. He then lies flat for 5 minutes. This exercise may be repeated about 5 times and performed 3 times a day. Some physicians prefer not to time the exercises, but to have the patient or nurse observe the extremity for blanching when it is elevated, for redness when it is shifted to the dependent position, and lastly, for its appearance when it is placed at rest in the supine position.

Although these exercises are helpful, patients seldom have the patience to follow them. Therefore, the most practical method for developing collateral circulation is walking to the point of tolerance.

Other Measures. In the past, such therapy as contrast baths, hydrotherapy, and the use of so-called vasodilating drugs were used to increase blood supply, but today these measures have been largely discontinued since their efficacy is unproven and their use may actually result in harm or further compromise the arterial circulation.

Prevention of Vasoconstriction

Measures to prevent vasoconstriction include restricting the use of tobacco, avoiding exposure to cold, and eliminating practices such as crossing the legs or wearing tight garters or clothing.

Vasodilatation may be accomplished by interrupting sympathetic impulses. Nerve blocks (such as epidural block) or even cutting of the nerves (sympathectomy) has been used to improve circulation in superficial vessels. Surgical measures include lumbar sympathectomy (to relieve vasoconstriction in the lower extremities) and replacement of occluded arteries by grafts of plastic material or autogenous veins. If an arterial occlusion is the result of an embolus or thrombus and can be operated

upon quickly, the clot may be removed surgically and the artery preserved. Surgical removal (called *embolectomy* or *thrombectomy*) can be performed quickly under local anesthesia with the use of a Fogarty catheter. There is also a technique of surgically "reaming out" a narrowed vessel lumen to enhance blood flow (*endarterectomy*), but it has limited clinical application.

MANAGEMENT OF THE PATIENT WITH A PERIPHERAL VASCULAR PROBLEM

Psychosocial Considerations

Much of the progress made by patients with peripheral vascular conditions depends on nursing care. Because the problems of these individuals may appear minor when compared with those of other patients, they are often neglected; yet these persons may have long histories of circulatory difficulties and as a result may be depressed and greatly in need of help.

Treatment may be a long, slow process; setbacks are frequent, and this in itself can become discouraging. Usually this patient is past 50 and perhaps has other physical problems. Because peripheral vascular diseases are chronic or soon become chronic, the patient may have concerns about employment, financial insecurity, or the risk of being a burden to his family. Whatever the worry, all possible sources of concern for this person should be explored and relieved, if possible, inasmuch as emotional worries aggravate vascular disturbances.

The patient's stay in the hospital may be shortened if the physician is convinced that someone is able to take care of him at home. Many restrictions must be observed and precautions must be taken, as described in the following paragraphs. To ensure that the patient will be cared for adequately at home, instruction should be provided for him and for the person sharing responsibility for his care. His special problems and needs may be relayed to the visiting nurse.

Patient Teaching

Effect of Temperature. Changes in atmospheric temperature have a greater effect on a patient with a vascular disease than on the healthy person. Warmth is desirable in order to provide or maintain optimal circulation to the extremities and promote comfort. This should be achieved by warm clothing, such as long underwear, or a warm bath rather than by hot water bottles or electric pads applied to the ischemic area, because such measures may cause damage before the individual is aware of it. This is why it is desirable to instruct the patient to check the temperature of the bath with the elbow before he steps into the tub. Excessive heat increases metabolism, which in turn requires more oxygenated blood, a need which may not be met because of an occlusion. Too much heat injures the poorly oxygenated tissues, and even slight physical trauma may set the stage for the development of gangrene.

Exposure to chilling must be avoided, because this can cause vasoconstriction and result in further reduction of the circulation to an ischemic extremity. Therefore, in cold weather adequate clothing should be worn.

Cleanliness and Prevention of Infection. Sound hygienic habits will help to prevent many problems. However, as one ages, skin and vascular changes require changes in care. Vigorous rubbing of the skin after a bath must be replaced by gentle rubbing or patting. Since dryness occurs more frequently, superfatted soaps with a mild detergent action are preferred over other soaps. After a warm bath, softening lotions or creams are effective when applied gently to the skin. Scratching must also be avoided when itching occurs; calamine lotion may be effective in relieving pruritus.

Care of the Feet. An important facet of patient education concerns proper foot care. It must be realized that the chief objective is to protect the patient from foot trauma. The feet should be washed daily with neutral soap and warm water. They must be dried thoroughly, but not roughly. Lanolin or petrolatum can be used to prevent the skin from drying and cracking. Lamb's wool placed between the toes helps to prevent irritation and allows air to circulate.

Woolen socks can be worn in winter and white cotton socks in warm weather. A clean pair should be available every day. Bed socks may be worn, but hot-water bottles or electric heating pads should not be used. The patient must be instructed not to use strong antiseptics, such as tincture of iodine and Lysol. Corns and calluses require expert care. The trimming of toenails is done best after a footbath, when the nails are soft; they should be trimmed straight across. The patient also should be instructed not to cross his knees when sitting and to avoid long periods of immobility, such as may occur on plane or auto trips. Circular garters and constricting girdles or belts are to be avoided. Any signs of blister, ingrowing toenail, infection, etc., must be reported. The older person with impaired vision may need to have someone examine his feet periodically for signs of trauma.

Walking in bare feet or stocking feet is discouraged because of the possibility of injury from a bump or splinter. Shoes should provide support and should be comfortable and nonconstricting; new shoes should be broken in gradually and alternated with another pair. Leather soles are preferred to rubber soles, which can interfere with proper ventilation. Wet or damp shoes should be allowed to dry slowly on shoe trees to help retain their shape.

Prolonged standing should be avoided. Changing positions frequently and alternating between walking and sitting will prevent stasis. Moderate exercise is desirable. Good posture is recommended for sitting, standing, or lying. When sitting, the body should be upright with proper support to the back and thigh. Compression at the popliteal space constricts posterior vessels supplying the lower leg and causes stasis.

Because of the individual nature of vascular problems, it is necessary for the nurse and patient to obtain specific instruction regarding the position of the legs. Usually the legs of a patient with arterial insufficiency are best placed in the straight plane, although occasionally a slight downward placement may encourage further blood flow by gravity. The legs should never be elevated, since this further diminishes arterial flow to the periphery. A general rule cannot be followed, but instructions need to be individualized to meet each patient's requirements.

At night, bed clothing can be loosened around the feet to prevent constriction. A footboard will assist in maintaining proper position of the feet. A firm mattress ensures even distribution of body weight.

Maintaining Proper Nutrition. A diet high in protein is desirable to prevent tissue breakdown. Vitamins, particularly B and C, also are needed. Obesity should be avoided, inasmuch as excess weight increases congestion and affects proper functioning of the heart, which in turn affects circulation. A finding of elevated blood lipids (checked in the fasting state) indicates the need for a special diet. If the elevation is in the beta lipoprotein (cholesterol), then a low fat diet is recommended. If the elevation is in the prebeta fraction (triglyceride), then a low carbohydrate diet is prescribed. A balanced and varied diet that maintains a desirable weight for the patient and provides less fat, more protein, and a good selection of fruits and vegetables is recommended. The patient with diabetes mellitus requires special dietary care.

Dressings and Wound Care. If it is necessary to treat an extremity with moist dressings and there are no open wounds, surgically clean gauze and solution should be used. However, if there is an ulcer or an open infection, strict asepsis must be followed. In this case, sterile gloves should be used rather than forceps to change or apply dressings. The extremity must be supported adequately when bandage dressings are removed or applied. Often the surgeon débrides necrotic tissue and irrigates the wound. Petrolatum gauze or plain dressings moistened with saline solution at room temperature may be applied. If only some parts of an extremity are to receive moistened dressings, the best way to prevent areas from becoming wet is to apply petrolatum. A plastic wrapping can secure the dressings in place, but it should not be held in place with a constricting bandage.

Smoking. As a rule, tobacco in any form is denied patients with peripheral vascular problems. Vessel spasm definitely is related to smoking. A major nursing problem is to help the physician convince many avid smokers of the need to stop this habit.

THE PATIENT WITH PERIPHERAL VASCULAR PROBLEMS
Objectives and Principles of Medical and Nursing Management

SYMPTOMS

Intermittent claudication

Tingling and numbness of toes

SIGNS

Trophic changes

Differences in skin temperature and color

Absence of pulses

THE PROBLEM

1. Peripheral arterial insufficiency of the extremities represents only one part of the disease, which also affects other parts of the body such as the brain, heart, and internal organs.

2. A patient's arteriosclerosis is usually advanced before his symptoms become apparent.

3. The end result of uncontrolled circulatory impairment is gangrene.

MANAGEMENT AND THERAPEUTIC GOALS

A. To remove all vasoconstricting factors:
1. Encourage the patient to abstain completely from tobacco.
2. Avoid experiences that are emotionally upsetting to the patient.
3. For venous disease—instruct the patient to avoid wearing circular garters and constricting girdles or belts.

4. Keep the patient as comfortable as possible with the prescribed analgesic drugs.

B. To increase peripheral blood flow to the extremities:
1. Encourage the patient to take warm baths.
2. Teach the patient that heat applied to the feet by means other than warm clothing is contraindicated.
3. Increase collateral circulation:
   a. Engage in passive and active exercises as indicated.
   b. Progressively increase walking time.
4. If the patient has rest pain, he should sleep with the head of the bed elevated on blocks so that the entire bed is on a decline.

C. To decrease the metabolic demands of the body; it is necessary for the patient to:
1. Prevent injury and infection.
2. Learn hygienic care of his feet.
3. Remain on bed rest if ulceration or gangrene is present.
4. Avoid exposure to cold.
5. Reduce physical activity to allowed limits.

D. To prepare for surgical procedures that will increase circulation (when indicated):
1. Sympathectomy.
2. Bypass graft procedures.
3. Thromboendarterectomy.

DISEASES OF THE ARTERIES

ARTERIOSCLEROSIS AND ATHEROSCLEROSIS

Arteriosclerosis is the most common disease of the arteries; it literally means "hardening of the arteries" but more accurately refers to a group of processes in which there is a loss of elasticity in and thickening of the arterial walls. Three main forms of arteriosclerosis are distinguishable: (1) *atherosclerosis* (the most common), which is characterized by atheroma (patchy lipoidal degeneration of the intima); (2) Mönckeberg's medial sclerosis — calcification of the media of muscular arteries; and (3) *arteriosclerosis* —diffuse arteriolar sclerosis, which is characterized by fibromuscular or endothelial thickening of the walls of small arteries and arterioles.

All three forms of arteriosclerosis may occur in the same patient in different vessels. As was described above, the three kinds differ morphologically; however, since the most common form of arteriosclerosis is atherosclerosis (AS), the terms are often used interchangeably.

Pathophysiology and Etiology

The most common direct results of arteriosclerosis in smaller arteries include: narrowing, closure by thrombosis, and rupture. Its indirect results are malnutrition and the subsequent fibrosis of the organs that the sclerotic arteries supply with blood. All actively functioning tissue cells require an abundant supply of food and oxygen and are sensitive to any reduction in their supply. If such reductions are severe and permanent, these cells undergo ischemic necrosis and are replaced by fibrous tissue, which requires much less food. Thus arise the degenerative areas in the brain, the heart's weak myocardium, and the small, contracted kidneys.

Arteriosclerosis affects the entire arterial tree in varying degrees, some organs developing more fibrosis than others. Since the myocardium and the kidneys provide the most significant manifestations of this malady, the majority of arteriosclerotic conditions are grouped under the heading cardiovascular-renal diseases.

Atherosclerosis may appear in one of two forms, with the following characteristics: (1) diffuse weakening and destruction of the media (middle layer) causing dilatation and elongation of any of the major arteries (when exaggerated, these sites lead to aneurysms) and (2) diffuse degeneration involving the intima (inner wall) without weakening the media. The effect may be apparent only in microscopic examination but may be grossly visible in small segments of the arteries. Such atheromas or plaques may continue to increase until the vessel is completely occluded. These occlusions appear to occur more commonly at arterial bifurcations, because of constant trauma from the pulsating bloodstream.

The manner in which plaques form is not clearly understood. It is thought that they begin as yellow fatty streaks, possibly in childhood, and they appear to in-

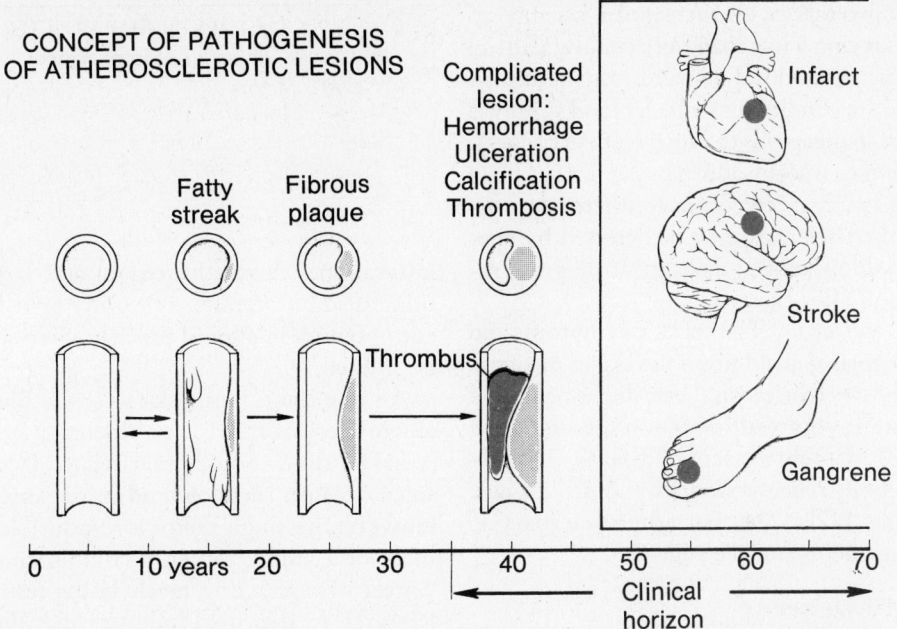

Figure 31-3. Schematic concept of the progression of coronary atherosclerosis. Fatty streaks constitute one of the earliest lesions of atherosclerosis. Many fatty streaks regress, whereas others progress to fibrous plaques and eventually to atheromata. These may then become complicated by hemorrhage, ulceration, calcification, or thrombosis and may produce myocardial infarction. (Adapted from Hurst, J. W., and Logue, R. B.: The Heart. McGraw-Hill.)

crease in number and size during the aging process. Fatty streaks can be produced in animals by feeding a diet high in cholesterol; this raises blood lipid levels, causing a condition called *hyperlipidemia* (see page 568). It is thought that this predisposes to the formation of plaques (Fig. 31-3).

As the disease progresses, there is a narrowing of the arterial lumen, which stimulates the development of collateral circulation. When the original artery approaches total occlusion, the reduced blood flow eventually leads to thrombosis. The end result is a completely occluded segment bypassed by collateral circulation (Fig. 31-4).

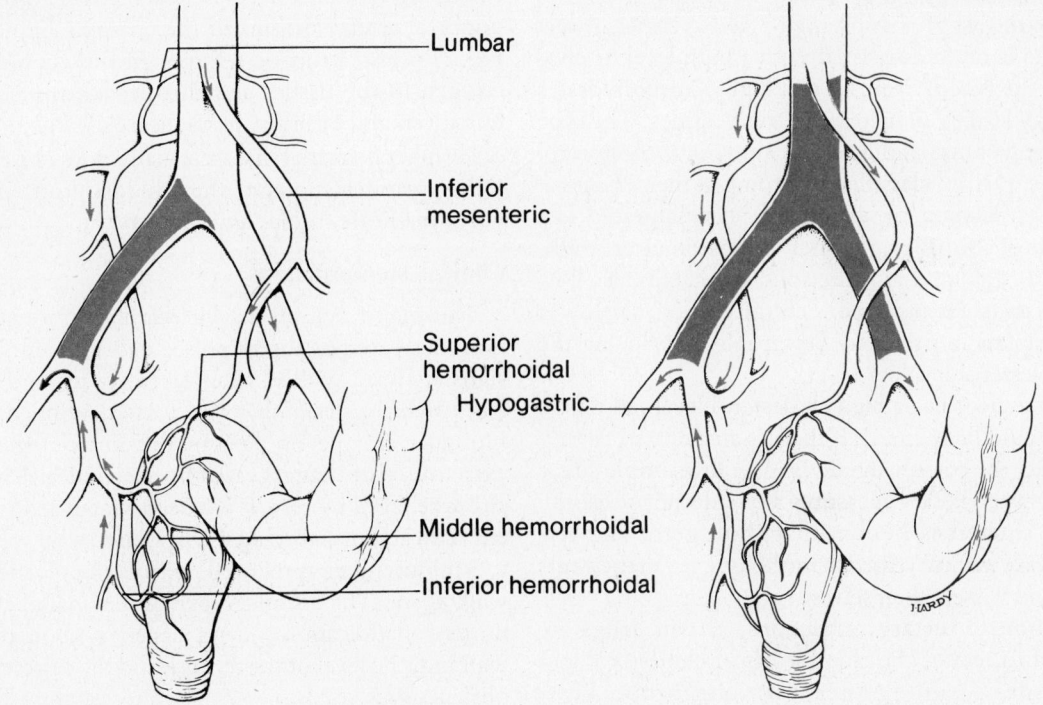

Figure 31-4. Development of collateral channels in response to occlusion of the right common iliac artery and the terminal aortic bifurcation.

Obviously the collaterals, with increased resistance to blood flow, are carrying a less than normal flow and are unresponsive to increased distal demands; this results in increasing ischemia (a condition in which blood supply is inadequate but not so meager as to cause death of tissues).

Presymptom Stage.   Many adults beyond 50 years of age have moderately advanced coronary atherosclerosis. Early coronary atherosclerosis may be detected by special tests such as angiography and electrocardiogram recordings during and after exercises.

Clinical Manifestations.   The specific symptoms and signs of atherosclerosis depend upon the organ or tissue affected. Coronary atherosclerosis (heart disease), angina pectoris, and acute myocardial infarction are discussed on pages 568-577. Cerebrovascular disease, including transient cerebral ischemic attacks and stroke, are discussed on pages 1222-1224. For atherosclerosis of the aorta including aneurysm, see page 623.

Prevention and Management

Many factors, both major and minor, contribute to the development of atherosclerosis. A moderate degree of atherosclerosis is considered to be an inevitable consequence of aging. Sex hormones also influence the development of atherosclerosis, since men are more prone to develop this condition than women of childbearing age, although in the later decades of life there is a narrowing of the differences between the sexes. Certain disease states such as hypertension and diabetes seem to predispose to atherosclerosis. People with diabetes mellitus have more extensive lesions, and at an earlier age, than nondiabetics. Smoking, too, seems to play a role in the development of atherosclerosis.

High on the list of possible major factors is diet. A diet high in fats is often associated with a high level of cholesterol in the bloodstream. A diet high in carbohydrates (sugar) may lead to an increase in triglycerides. The type of fat in the diet may influence the amount of cholesterol in the body. Fats are classified according to their chemical structure as *saturated* or *unsaturated*. The saturated fats include fats of animal origin, such as those in meat, milk, butter, and eggs, and also the solid vegetable oils. Unsaturated fats, such as corn oil, cottonseed oil, safflower oil, and the fats in fish, may be capable of reducing the blood cholesterol level.

When a patient has a high cholesterol level, all fats in the diet should be reduced. If there is an elevated fasting triglyceride, the patient should be on a low simple sugar diet. However, dietary measures alone do not solve the problem, since it is known that cholesterol and triglycerides are manufactured in the body, even in the walls of the blood vessels themselves.

In addition to dietary restrictions, certain drugs are being used to reduce the blood levels of cholesterol and triglycerides. Among these are clofibrate, cho-

RISK FACTORS IN ATHEROSCLEROSIS (in order of importance)	
1. Genetic factors	4. Increased serum lipids
2. Diabetes mellitus, gout	5. Obesity
3. Hypertension	6. Cigarette smoking
	7. Physical inactivity

lestyramine, dextrothyroxine, and large doses of nicotinic acid. Clofibrate is the only lipid-lowering drug in common use in clinical practice. Side effects continue to be studied.

Among the minor risk factors in the development of atherosclerosis are obesity, sedentary living, and psychosocial tensions. Some other related factors are intake of sugar, coffee, alcohol, and hard water, and hypoxia. However, no single factor is responsible for the development of a lesion; rather, a combination and possibly a variety of interacting mechanisms result in the disease. Research in this field indicates that the atherosclerotic process can be modified or reduced by avoiding or modifying one or more risk factors, for instance, lowering elevated blood pressure or altering the diet.

PERIPHERAL ARTERIAL OCCLUSIVE DISEASE

This disease, which predominantly affects the lower extremities, is usually found in individuals over 50 years of age. The age of onset and severity are influenced by heredity, smoking, dietary habits, and concomitant hypertension or diabetes. Obstructive lesions are usually confined to segments of the arterial system in the area extending from the aorta below the renal arteries to the popliteal artery (origins of the terminal branches). (See Fig. 31-5.) Obstruction reduces the flow of nutrients and oxygen to the tissues and thus leads to ischemia, malnutrition, and eventual tissue necrosis.

Peripheral arterial disease usually does not exist alone. Other manifestations of the atherosclerotic process involve the heart, brain, and kidneys.

Clinical Manifestations

The major symptoms include intermittent claudication, decreased or absent pulse, and rest pain. The major signs are bruit, pallor, cyanosis, atrophy, and necrosis.

Intermittent claudication, as was mentioned earlier, is muscular fatigue or pain in the muscle of the lower extremity that is aggravated by exertion such as walking and is relieved by rest. It is a deep-seated ache that worsens with activity, forcing the person to stop walking; in 3 to 5 minutes pain is relieved, permitting the individual to walk again. The distance a person can walk before intermittent claudication occurs depends upon the rate of walking, the level of the terrain, and the degree of arterial obstruction.

The cause of pain is not known; however it may be related to the accumulation of lactic acid during anaerobic metabolism. Another possible cause is the stimulation of nerve endings by bradykinin and histamine which are formed in tissues during muscle cell damage.

Impotence, the inability to attain or maintain a penile erection, may result from occlusion of the hypogastric artery or terminal aorta. However, impotence is frequently related to psychogenic causes.

Rest pain is felt as a continuous boring pain; numbness or paresthesias experienced in the lower foot indicate advanced ischemia. Pain is aggravated when the foot is elevated to the horizontal position, as when the patient goes to sleep. It disturbs sleep and is not relieved until the leg is placed in the dependent position.

Bruit is the sound produced by the blood as it flows through an irregular and stenotic arterial lumen. It can be heard (during systole) by lightly placing a stethoscope directly over the artery and indicates turbulence caused by dilatation (aneurysm) or stenosis at the site or in the adjacent area. The higher the pitch of bruit, the greater the stenotic involvement.

Pallor of the foot (or hand in the upper extremity) on elevation indicates arterial obstruction. In advanced degrees of obstruction, pallor will appear more quickly on elevation. Color returns when the extremity is returned to the dependent position. In the healthy person, exercise increases the pulse rate, but peripheral color changes and bruit are not elicited. However, in the ischemic extremity, exercise dilates the muscular bed, and a decreased or absent pedal pulse and marked lowering in ankle blood pressure result.

Cyanosis is another sign of atherosclerosis. When a person with advanced atherosclerosis places his leg in a dependent position, the skin of the foot becomes ruddy and cyanotic. This occurs because the flow of blood through the arterial system is delayed. As a result, the hemoglobin becomes deoxygenated so that by the time blood reaches the capillaries, it appears similar to the hemoglobin of venous blood.

Abnormal changes in the skin and nails (trophic changes) result from ischemia and tissue malnutrition. Skin appears smooth, shiny, hairless, and taut; a minor injury easily becomes infected because of insufficient blood supply. Because of the precarious nature of impaired tissue perfusion, a minor infection can develop into an ulcer, and later, gangrene.

Atrophy of the muscle of the foot results from progressive ischemia. Joint mobility is reduced.

Necrosis, the death of tissues, occurs first at the most distal joint and usually is instigated by trauma or pressure such as that from a shoe. Necrosis halts at the point where tissue is adequately nourished by blood.

Diagnostic Assessment. The presence, anatomical location, and physiologic extent of arterial occlusive dis-

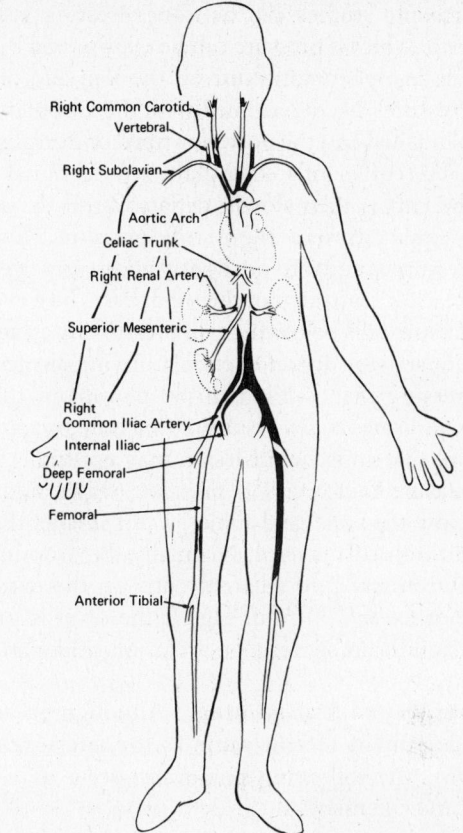

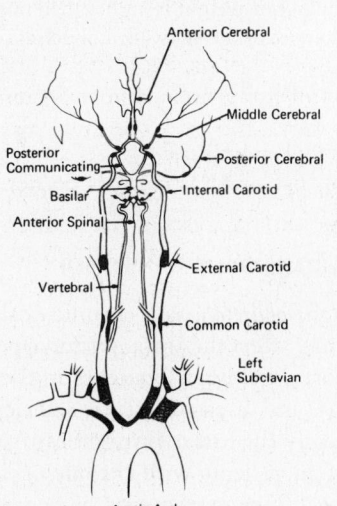

Figure 31-5. Common sites of artherosclerotic obstruction in major arterial systems of the body. (Figure above redrawn from Crawford, E. S., and DeBakey, M. E.: Surgical treatment of occlusive cerebrovascular disease. Mod. Treat., 2:36, Jan. 1965. Figure below from Beeson, P. B., and McDermott, W.: Textbook of Medicine. Philadelphia, W. B. Saunders, p. 1547.)

ease are determined by a careful clinical history and physical examination. Arteriography is used to confirm the diagnosis if surgery is contemplated. To determine the qualitative and quantitative extent of the problem, Doppler ultrasonic studies can be done. Resting arm and ankle systolic blood pressure can be determined by placing a standard pneumatic cuff on the arm and on each ankle. Pressures are determined with the Doppler probe over the brachial and the posterior tibial or dorsalis pedis arteries. The cuff is inflated until the arterial signal disappears; the cuff is then slowly deflated until the arterial velocity signal returns at the systolic pressure. Normally ankle pressure is equal to or slightly above arm pressure. In the presence of arterial occlusive disease, however, the ankle pressure falls below the arm pressure by an amount proportional to the degree of circulatory impairment. An ankle pressure that is less than 50 percent of the arm pressure indicates a severe degree of ischemia and the possibility that an ischemic lesion may not heal.

To measure four levels of pressure (thigh, above the knee, below the knee, and ankle), a cuff smaller than the standard thigh cuff is used. Normally the drop in pressure between any two adjacent cuffs on the extremity should not exceed 30 mm. Hg. If the drop is greater, there is significant stenosis or occlusion of the artery at the site.

Prevention and Management. Although prevention and management are the same as for arteriosclerosis (page 616), the following points can serve as a summary of management:

1. Cessation of smoking
2. Weight reduction if weight is higher than normal
3. An active exercise program (walk as much as can be tolerated each day)
4. Correction of lipoprotein abnormalities and diabetes mellitus
5. Meticulous foot and leg care
6. Realization that oral vasodilators do not appear to be beneficial

ARTERIOSCLEROSIS OBLITERANS (ASO)

Arteriosclerosis obliterans is a chronic occlusive arterial disease that may affect the aorta, terminal portions of the abdominal aorta, its major branches in the extremities, and the large and medium-sized arteries of the extremities, usually the lower extremities. Approximately 90 percent of all patients with chronic occlusive arterial disease of the lower extremities have arteriosclerosis obliterans.

Since etiologic factors are the same as for atherosclerosis, the reader is referred to page 614. Most patients with arteriosclerosis obliterans are between the ages of 50 and 70. Diabetes mellitus appears to increase the prevalence and severity of the disease, as does cigarette smoking.

Pathophysiology. The main physiologic disturbance in arteriosclerosis obliterans is obstruction of blood flow through large arteries, which leads to ischemia of the tissues supplied by these vessels.

Clinical Manifestations

Symptoms, which appear gradually in a series of episodes alternating with periods of partial regression, result from ischemia of tissues nourished by the affected arteries. Usually this effect is confined to the lower extremities. The earliest symptom is intermittent claudication (page 616), usually unilateral at first but later affecting both legs, one often more severely than the other. The distress most commonly affects the calf but may also occur in the foot, thigh, hip, and even the lower part of the back. The site of occlusion is almost always proximal to the pain zone. For example, intermittent claudication of the hip indicates occlusive disease of the lower aorta or the common iliac artery, whereas intermittent claudication of the thigh suggests occlusion of the iliac or common femoral artery. Superficial femoral occlusion produces claudication of the calf muscle.

A more advanced symptom is rest pain (pretrophic), which occurs most commonly at night. Because it becomes severe and persistent, it may awaken the individual and force him to sit up and rub his foot for hours in an attempt to get relief. Pain may also occur with ulceration and gangrene.

Other pain symptoms may be related to ischemic neuropathy and are manifested as steady or paroxysmal. The sensation may be numbness, coldness, or burning and may be so severe that it is difficult to relieve. Extreme sensitivity to cold may develop, so that the foot becomes excessively cold even on minimal exposure to a cold environment. Caution must be taken to avoid burns, which may occur when hot water baths are used to treat coldness of the feet. Stiffness and muscular weakness are other symptoms that may be noted.

Assessment

In the assessment of the patient, probably the most important finding is the impairment of arterial pulsations noted by palpation (page 609). These may be observed in one or both extremities. Pulsations of the posterior tibial, dorsalis pedis, popliteal, or femoral arteries are usually always palpable in a person at rest in a warm environment, *except* when occlusive arterial disease is present. However, it should be noted that 7 percent of people in the normal healthy population lack a dorsalis pedis pulse, and 3 percent lack a posterior tibial pulse. Occasionally, absence of pulsations may be noted in one or both ulnar or radial arteries. Sometimes subclavian occlusion leads to impairment or absence of all arterial pulsations in the upper extremity.

Bruits (systolic) may be heard over pulsating arteries, and color changes are apparent depending upon the degree of occlusion. Postural color changes are detectable if the disease is moderately extensive.

For example, if the feet are elevated for 1 minute and

are then suddenly placed in a dependent position, the following evaluation is made:

Failure of color to return in:	Degree of arterial insufficiency:
15 seconds	Moderate
30 seconds	Marked
60 seconds	Extreme

Ulceration or gangrene usually appears first in the terminal segment of the digits. The nail or nail bed is often the primary site following infection or loosening and sloughing of the nail. Pressure of a shoe in ordinary walking may initiate the process following ischemia. Gangrene may involve the distal part of the toe and progress to the entire toe, several toes, the lower foot, and even the leg, up to the knee. Ischemic ulcers are usually localized and hence do not cause systemic toxicity. They are quite painful.

Diagnostic Evaluation. Blood studies are done to see if there is coexisting diabetes mellitus. An electrocardiogram is suggested because coronary heart disease is frequently associated with arteriosclerosis obliterans. It is also helpful in evaluating operative risks if surgery is likely. Blood flow measurements may be done by means of plethysmography, Doppler techniques, or an electromagnetic flowmeter.

Angiography will show the arterial supply to the lower extremities from the level of the renal arteries to the feet. DeWolf suggests that angiography will provide the following information: (1) the exact location of the occlusion, (2) the length of the occlusion, (3) the condition of the vessels above and below the occlusion, (4) the location of other occlusions, (5) the extent of the collateral circulation, (6) reliable guidelines for short-term prognosis and an estimate of long-term prognosis, (7) a means of evaluating patients for surgical correction of arterial insufficiency, and (8) an estimate of the best level for amputation.

Management

The management of the patient must be individualized since no two patients are affected in the same way. Because this is a chronic progressive disease, medical and nursing measures are directed toward "caring" for the patient, since "curing" is not likely. Adequate nutrition is emphasized, exercise to stimulate collateral circulation is recommended, and diversional activities are suggested. All along the way, encouragement and understanding must be given. Although a damaged artery cannot be repaired, the destructive processes often can be reduced by early treatment and the organ dysfunctions already created may be relieved in part. The patient should avoid strenuous or fatiguing efforts, should rest each day, should retire early, take long vacations, and treat all minor illnesses as serious.

When the toes and feet are involved, preventive measures, such as practicing good foot hygiene and wearing proper shoes, should be taken.

The objectives of treatment are: (1) to arrest the progress of the disease, (2) to improve the flow of blood to the involved part, (3) to relieve pain and promote comfort, (4) to treat ulcers and gangrene, (5) to prevent injury and infection, and (6) to instruct the patient in the care of his specific condition and general related health measures.

To arrest the progress of the disease, dietary control may be required if the patient has a concomitant hyperlipoproteinemia. Furthermore, the type of hyperlipidemia must be determined before pharmacotherapy can be prescribed specifically.

Because of the importance of dietary compliance, a detailed dietary history should be taken. Consultation with a nutritionist may help in following through with dietary instruction. Aside from making adjustments in his diet, the patient should be discouraged from tobacco smoking. If diabetes mellitus is present, of course this should be treated to avoid cardiovascular complications. Anticoagulant therapy may be prescribed in acute processes but is not used in chronic arterial occlusion.

To improve blood circulation, the patient should be warned to avoid tobacco smoking, vasoconstricting drugs, and exposure to cold. Additional warmth may be provided to the extremity by keeping room temperature at 26.6° C. (80° F.). Heating cradles are sometimes used for the patient who is in bed, but since the risk of burning the skin by touching the cradle is great, they are best avoided.

The head of the bed may be elevated about 15 cm. (6 in.) with the patient in a low reclining position. This position will allow gravity to assist in improving arterial blood flow. When the patient is out of bed in a sitting position, pressure on the popliteal vessels in back of the knees should be avoided. Changing positions is important to prevent blood stasis, which can occur because of decreased venous pumping and the initiation of edema. In turn, pedal edema reduces and may even occlude arteriole blood flow. It is important for the nurse to understand the individual patient's peripheral vascular history, because proper positioning depends upon the unique hemodynamic pattern of the individual patient.

Exercises are prescribed specifically to meet the individual patient's needs. Buerger-Allen exercises may be recommended, although medical authorities are not in agreement about their benefit. Walking, even to the point of claudication, may be part of the daily exercise program. The objective is to improve collateral circulation.

Controversy continues over the benefits of vasodilating medications. Analgesics may be used when necessary for rest pain and tranquilizers may help in relieving anxiety. (See also Management, page 612 for the prevention of infection and patient teaching.)

Surgical Management and Anticipatory Nursing

In arteriosclerosis obliterans, the areas most often affected are the aorta at its bifurcation, the iliac arteries, and the superficial femoral arteries. Other sites commonly involved are the popliteal artery, the coronary artery, and the cerebral vessels. The segment showing severe degeneration of the artery is often found adjacent to other segments showing only minor pathology.

These facts have made it possible to treat arteriosclerosis surgically by one of several methods:

1. The circulation may be restored by the use of vascular grafts. In some cases of segmental occlusion, it may be possible to cut out the degenerated segment of artery and suture a graft in place end-to-end to replace the excised diseased segment. More often, grafts are implanted to "bypass" the obstructed diseased segment of vessel. The bypass graft has the advantage of reducing the amount of surgical trauma because it is not necessary to remove the obstructed segment of artery. The grafts commonly employed for leg bypass are autogenous vein grafts, usually the saphenous vein or reinforced umbilical vein, or prosthetic grafts of knitted Dacron or Teflon yarns or Goretex. Vein grafts are preferred, when possible, because long-term patency is better. For aorta-iliac bypass, the preferred grafting material is Dacron.

2. Patch grafts are used to increase the lumen diameter of small narrowed areas of the arteries. The artery is clamped above and below the short narrowed area and is then incised in the long axis of the vessel. A patch of woven Teflon material is sewed to the edges of the incision, thus increasing the diameter of the artery with a minimum of trauma. At times a piece of vein may be used for the patch graft instead of the Teflon material.

3. The obstruction in the vessel may be removed by making an incision into the artery after clamping above and below the plug in the vessel. By the use of special instruments, it is possible to shell out the atheromatous plug, which involves the intima and part of the media. The opening in the vessel is closed with fine silk sutures. The roughened lining of the reformed vessel becomes smooth after a very short time, and circulation is restored through the previously obstructed vessel. This procedure (endarterectomy) is not commonly used today as a primary, isolated procedure, because of the frequent recurrence of atherosclerosis at the same spot.

Preoperative Management. When the patient is prepared for surgery, several common problems need to be assessed on an individual basis. Since dehydration often occurs following extensive preliminary tests for renal function and arteriography, adequate fluids must be provided before and during the operation. Potassium should be assessed to see if there is a need for replacement; sodium may need to be restricted to control hypertension. The patient's history is assessed for relevant information such as cigarette smoking and medications taken (aspirin contributes to altered platelet activity).

Operative and Postoperative Management. The type of surgery done is determined by the treatment required for a particular occluded vessel. Plastic prosthesis, endarterectomy, and bypass operations are tailored to the need. Occasionally a lumbar sympathectomy is done for patients with marked distal ischemia before specific vascular surgery is performed.

At the time of surgery, heparin solution is sometimes used to prevent clotting locally. The nurse is alert for color and temperature changes in the legs after arterial surgery and looks for and records pulses in the feet and legs (Fig. 31-2).

- The disappearance of a pulse may indicate a thrombosis or obstruction of the artery or graft by a clot, and the surgeon should be notified at once.
- Another complication is paralysis of the lower extremities after operations upon the thoracic aorta. Prolonged occlusion of this vessel may produce ischemia of the spinal cord. This complication should be reported at once.

A prime objective of postoperative care is to insure adequate circulating blood volume through the arterial repairs. Oliguria is treated early by fluid replacement, constant monitoring of central venous pressure, and early use of mannitol, furosemide, or ethacrynic acid.

Exercises, particularly isometric muscle contractions, are encouraged shortly after surgery.

- Discourage the patient from maintaining a dependent leg position or crossing his legs for long periods, because the pressure on vascular structures may precipitate thrombosis. Edema of the leg can be minimized by elevating the legs above heart level when the patient is in bed. Well-supporting elastic stockings are helpful in combating stasis, particularly if the patient also has varicosities. Mini-dose heparin may be used if there is a history of previous venous problems.

SYMPATHETIC BLOCK OR SYMPATHECTOMY

Lumbar Sympathetic Block. A test used to evaluate the peripheral circulation of the legs is the *lumbar sympathetic block.* In this test, a local anesthetic is injected into the epidural space, so that the sympathetic ganglia that send fibers to the legs are blocked by the anesthetic; or, the solution may be injected as a spinal anesthetic, to block the sympathetic nerves that go to the legs. Since the sympathetic nerves control the tension in the muscles of the blood vessels, a block of these nerves should produce vasodilation and increased temperature in the legs if the vessels are normal. Arteriosclerotic vessels are incapable of vasodilation; hence there is either no increase in temperature in the legs or only a slight one. This test is often used to determine whether or not sympathectomy would be of benefit to the patient with impaired circulation of the legs.

Sympathectomy. Because the ischemia produced by the arteriosclerosis of the larger vessels is often associated with a spasm of the smaller, less-involved peripheral vessels, attempts have been made to increase the peripheral circulation by dividing the sympathetic nerve supply to these vessels. This procedure, *sympathectomy*, releases the constriction of the arterioles and permits an increased peripheral blood supply.

Sympathectomy (severing of sympathetic nerve fibers) has been performed for several decades, but unanimous agreement is still lacking regarding indications for its use and its specific mode of action. Sympathectomy is more likely to dilate skin arterioles than muscle arterioles and is therefore more useful if there is a skin lesion.

Lumbar sympathectomy increases blood flow to the lower extremities as a result of decreased peripheral resistance due to dilatation of the vascular tree distal to the popliteal artery. It is a useful adjunct in increasing blood supply to reconstructed segments after grafting or endarterectomy. Sympathectomy can be performed as an emergency treatment following severe vasospasm due to arterial embolism in a major vessel supplying an extremity, or due to freezing of an extremity.

When it is possible or desirable, procaine is first injected into the ganglia to determine whether the benefits of a sympathectomy can be expected.

Thoracic and Cervicothoracic Sympathectomy. This operation is less frequently performed than lumbar sympathectomy, probably because lasting improvement is not often achieved. Primarily, it is done for vascular insufficiency in the arm. The approach may be anterior or posterior. Depending upon the individual problems, ribs may or may not be removed. The type of incision and nature of the operation determine the postoperative nursing measures to be initiated. The principles of chest surgical care are followed in the posterior approach, in which case ribs are usually removed. In the anterior cervical approach, local anesthesia may be used. Postoperative position changes from lying to sitting must be done gradually to allow for circulatory adjustment. Failure to do this may cause the patient undue dizziness.

Lumbar Sympathectomy. The incision is an oblique one, similar to an extended McBurney incision (done for appendicitis) on either or both sides of the lower abdomen. Usually the peritoneum is not entered, but a retroperitoneal muscle-splitting approach provides adequate exposure under spinal anesthesia. The desired segments of ganglia are excised. Postoperatively, the nurse observes for the appearance of neuritis, which may result from manipulation during surgery. It may occur during hospitalization, or it may be a delayed type, occurring about the tenth postoperative day. The signs of such a complication are pain in the hip, anterior thigh, and medial leg area. The patient needs reassurance that the condition will remit spontaneously. He should be told to refrain from tiring activities, to develop hobby interests, and to avoid daytime naps if they interfere with night sleeping.

The patient may note a slight temperature increase in his feet and legs and perhaps a feeling of fullness. An elastic stocking may offer relief. Abdominal distention due to lessened peristalsis can be relieved in the initial postoperative period with neostigmine and a flatus rectal tube for flatus. On the operated side, the patient will notice that his foot does not perspire.

THROMBOANGIITIS OBLITERANS (TAO) (BUERGER'S DISEASE)

Thromboangiitis obliterans occurs less frequently today than it did 20 to 30 years ago, and is in fact rare today. Many patients formerly diagnosed as having Buerger's disease probably had another type of arteritis or premature atherosclerosis.

Buerger's disease is characterized by recurring inflammation in the arteries and veins of the lower and upper extremities, and results in thrombus formation and occlusion of the vessels. It is differentiated from other vessel diseases by its microscopic appearance. In contrast to arteriosclerosis obliterans, Buerger's disease has no lipid aggregates in the intimal coat, has more changes in the adventitia, and results in a thrombosis that contains many more cells. The disease begins in the small arteries and later progresses to the larger vessels. Although this condition is different from atherosclerosis, in older patients, atherosclerosis of the larger vessels may occur following involvement of the smaller vessels.

Etiology and Clinical Manifestations

The cause of the condition is unknown. It occurs most often in men between the ages of 20 and 35, and it has been reported in all races in many areas of the world. There is considerable evidence that heavy smoking is a factor, if not in the etiology at least in the progress of the disease. Most of the time the lower extremities are affected, but almost half of the time all four extremities may be involved.

As a rule, the patient appears for treatment when the disease has affected so many of the vessels of the extremity as to reduce the peripheral arterial circulation. At this point, the collateral circulation, which has been called upon more and more to take over the work of the damaged vessels, is being overtaxed.

Pain is the outstanding symptom. The patient complains of cramps in the legs after exercise (intermittent claudication), which are relieved by inactivity; often there is considerable burning pain that is aggravated by emotional disturbances, smoking, or chilling. Frequently, the patient notices painful red lumps under the skin; these heal and move to nearby areas in a migrating fashion as the phlebitis shifts.

As the disease progresses, definite cyanosis of the part appears when it is dependent, and ulceration with gangrene occurs, especially about the nails and the toes.

Management

The main objectives of patient care are to improve circulation to the extremities, prevent the spread of the disease, and protect the extremities from trauma and infection, to which they are dangerously susceptible. All attempts to help this patient end in failure if he continues to smoke; hence it is necessary to convince him of this most important facet of treatment. Unfortunately very few patients with this condition are able to give up smoking. Convincing the patient to do so represents a unique challenge.

Rest, adequate hydration, and scrupulous attention to cleanliness are essential. Daily washing of the feet with bland soap and warm water is desirable. After the feet are washed, they are dried, patted with a soft, nontraumatizing towel, and powdered. Clean socks or stockings are worn each day or changed as often as necessary. The patient should massage the extremities with a bland lubricating oil each day. Circumstances predisposing to trauma and infection must be strictly avoided. Shoes and stockings must be fitted accurately, and the feet must be protected adequately from both cold and incautious exposure to heat provided by mechanical warming devices or hot water.

Caustic antiseptics, such as iodine or phenol and its derivatives, never are applied to the feet if the peripheral circulation is inadequate, for tissue necrosis develops easily under these conditions. The patient must refrain from performing feats of minor surgery on corns and calluses. Caution must be exercised in the cutting of the toenails, which should be trimmed squarely. Circular garters and knee stockings should be avoided. Medical attention is indicated at the first sign of color changes in the feet; the development of a blister; an abrasion or infection; or changes in sensation, such as tingling, burning, numbness, or pain.

Vasodilators are rarely prescribed, because these drugs only cause dilatation of healthy vessels; therefore, vasodilators may even divert blood away from the partially occluded vessels, which makes the situation worse.

For patients with peripheral vascular disease with intermittent claudication, exercises are prescribed to promote the development of collateral circulation in the affected limbs. These exercises involve alternate raising and lowering of the legs in timed cycles, the rate and the duration of the exercises being regulated specifically for each individual patient on the basis of changes in skin color and subjective sensations of discomfort. It must be remembered, however, that one of the best exercises for developing collateral circulation is simply walking to the point of discomfort several times a day.

It is also important to remember that in no case of acute local circulatory insufficiency, whether due to an embolus or to intrinsic arterial disease, should heat be applied to the affected extremity. Heat merely increases tissue metabolism and raises the requirement for oxygenated blood, a demand which cannot be fulfilled.

It has been found worthwhile, in many types of peripheral obliterative arterial disease involving the legs, to perform a temporary sympathetic block by injecting the lumbar sympathetic ganglia and cord with procaine (see also page 620). This may be a helpful therapeutic procedure in acute occlusive processes, but is hardly worthwhile in the chronic situation, in which it is more often done as a test of vascular response. If results are definitely favorable, a lumbar sympathectomy may be performed for a more permanent effect.

Prognosis. If gangrene of a toe develops as a result of arterial occlusive disease in the leg, it is unlikely that toe amputation or even a transmetatarsal amputation will succeed. Usually a below-knee amputation, or occasionally an above-knee amputation, is necessary. The indications for amputation are worsening gangrene, especially if moist, severe rest pain, or sepsis secondary to gangrene. If any of these are present in a situation where bypass surgery is not feasible, then amputation becomes necessary.

AORTIC DISEASES

The aorta is the main trunk of the arterial system and is referred to in part as the ascending aorta (5 cm. [2 inches] contained in the pericardium), the aortic arch (extending upward, backward, and downward), and the descending aorta. The entire aorta is designated as thoracic above the diaphragm and abdominal below the diaphragm.

Aortitis

Aortitis is arteritis of the aorta, particularly of the aortic arch. Two types are known to occur: Takayasu's disease and syphilitic aortitis. Takayasu's disease, or occlusive thromboaortopathy, is uncommon; syphilitic aortitis is almost never seen today.

TAKAYASU'S DISEASE. Takayasu's disease is a chronic inflammatory disease of the aortic arch and its branches seen primarily in young or middle-aged females. It results in ischemic symptoms affecting the upper extremity, brain, and eyes. In the early stages, it may respond to corticosteroids.

SYPHILITIC AORTITIS. Syphilitic aortitis, unlike the arteriosclerotic type, usually begins before the age of 50. It starts at the root of the aorta and spreads in the form of a few discrete patches scattered over an otherwise normal intima. Its symptoms often are unusually severe, yet in some patients they are entirely absent. Although syphilitic aortitis was a fairly common entity three or four decades ago, it is rare today.

Manifestations. The most common symptoms of syphilitic aortitis are sensations of substernal oppression or weight, viselike feelings of constriction of the chest, or attacks of pain that are often agonizing. There are characteristic sudden attacks of dyspnea (often called *asthma*), which start abruptly, are agonizing, last from 5 to 15 minutes, and are accompanied by rapid pulse rate, high blood pressue, deep cyanosis, and profuse sweating.

Syphilitic aortitis leads to aortic insufficiency with the same symptoms and findings as those described under aortic insufficiency (page 600).

AORTIC ANEURYSMS

Classification of Aneurysms

Arteries are elastic tubes filled with blood flowing under high pressure. Should the wall of a vessel gradually become weak and yet not burst, the wall becomes distended at the weakened point. Such local distention is described as an *aneurysm* (Fig. 31-6). Very small aneurysms due to local infection are designated as *mycotic aneurysms*. An aneurysm which is somewhat larger but still limited in extent, projecting from one side of the vessel only, is called a *saccular aneurysm*. If the whole artery becomes dilated, a *fusiform aneurysm* develops. A wall of scar tissue at once begins to form around the developing aneurysmal sac, but never quite rapidly enough; there arises a slowly growing, pulsating tumor filled with blood communicating with the lumen of the vessel.

Possible causes for local weakness of the arterial wall that may result in aneurysm include trauma caused by a knife or missile, a local infection (either pyogenic or syphilitic), and arteriosclerosis. Some spots may have been congenitally weak.

Aneurysm of the Thoracic Aorta

Atherosclerosis, the most common cause of aneurysm of the thoracic aorta, affects about 85 percent of all patients with this disorder; approximately 5 percent of aneurysms are syphilitic in origin, 5 percent traumatic, and fewer congenital. Aneurysms at this location occur most frequently in men between the ages of 50 and 70.

Clinical Manifestations. Symptoms are variable and depend upon how rapidly the aneurysm dilates and how it affects surrounding intrathoracic organs. Many persons die as a result of asymptomatic aneurysm; however, *pain* usually is the most prominent pressure symptom. Such pain may be constant and boring in character, due to the erosion of a vertebra or rib by the pressure of the pulsating sac, or intermittent and neuralgic, due to pressure against nerves. Other conspicuous symptoms are *dyspnea,* the result of the pressure of the sac against the

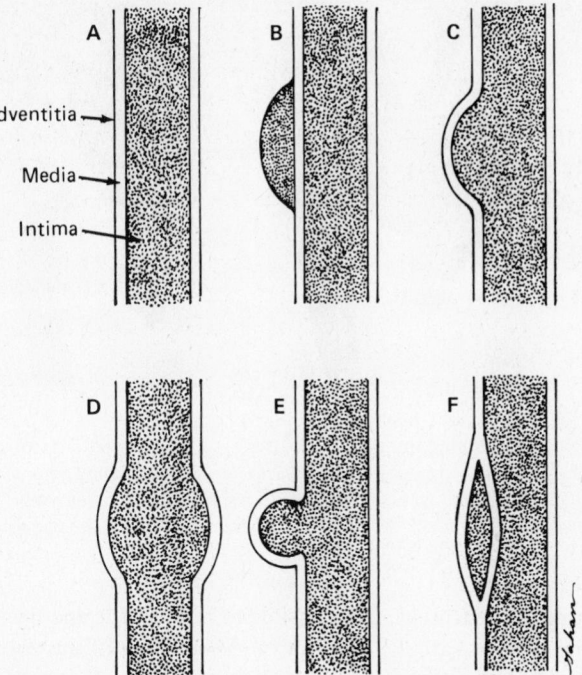

Figure 31-6. Characteristics of arterial aneurysm.
A. Normal artery
B. False aneurysm—actually a pulsating hematoma. The clot and connective tissue are outside the arterial wall.
C. True aneurysm. One, two, or all three layers may be involved.
D. Fusiform aneurysm—symmetrical spindle-shaped expansion of entire circumference of involved vessel.
E. Saccular aneurysm—a bulbous protrusion of one side of the arterial wall.
F. Dissecting aneurysm—this usually is a hematoma which splits the layers of the arterial wall.

trachea, a main bronchus, or the lung itself; *cough,* frequently paroxysmal and with a brassy quality ("goose cough"); *hoarseness,* weakness of the voice, or complete aphonia (evidences of pressure against the left recurrent laryngeal nerve); and *dysphagia,* due to impingement on the esophagus. In patients with syphilitic aneurysm, angina and paroxysmal dyspnea may also occur.

Signs of dilated superficial veins on the chest, the neck, or the arms, edematous areas on the chest wall, and often cyanosis are evidence that large veins in the chest are being compressed. The pupils of the eyes may be unequal because of pressure against the cervical sympathetic chain.

Tracheal tug is caused by adhesions between the sac and the trachea. The pulses at the two wrists differ markedly if the aneurysm impedes the blood flow into the left subclavian artery. Diagnostic evaluation of a descending aortic aeurysm is principally by roentgenoscopy.

Management. The poor prognosis for untreated patients (one third die from rupture; approximately half die of cardiovascular disease and arteriosclerosis) justifies

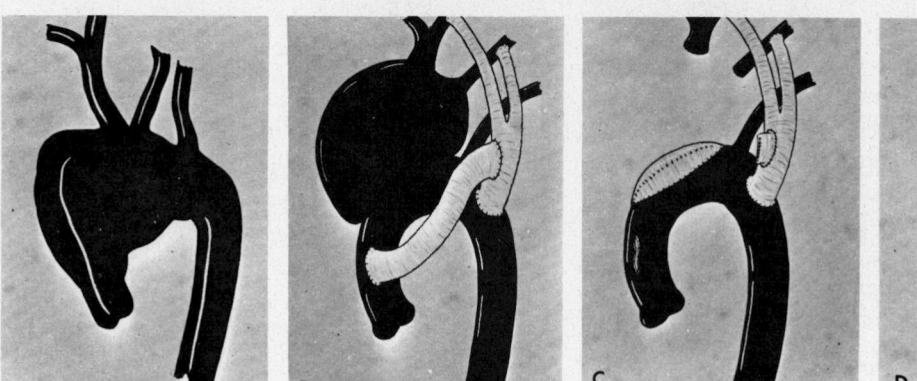

Figure 31-7. (A) Location and extent of aortic aneurysm. (B) Method of treatment utilizing temporary bypass graft to maintain normal aortic circulation during excision of aneurysm. (C) Completed procedure with patch graft angioplasty to repair excised segment of aortic arch and conversion of temporary bypass graft to innominate and left common carotid arteries into the permanent graft. (D) Temporary bypass grafts used to maintain normal aortic circulation during excision and graft replacement of aneurysm have been completely removed and aortic graft has been inserted. (From DeBakey, M. E.: Changing concepts in vascular surgery. Figs. 12B, 12E, 13C and 13D, J. Cardiov. Surg., 1:3-44.)

surgical treatment. It is possible to remove the aneurysm and restore vascular continuity. Aneurysms of the aortic arch are the most complicated and difficult to treat (Fig. 31-7).

(For nursing management, see page 559.)

Abdominal Aortic Aneurysm

The most common cause of abdominal aortic aneurysm is atherosclerosis; syphilis is present in less than one percent of patients. Four times more men than women are affected and the condition is most prevalent after age 60. Most of these aneurysms occur below the renal arteries. Untreated, the eventual outcome may be rupture and death.

Pathophysiology. The factor common to all aneurysms is a damaged media in the vessel. This may be caused by congenital weakness, trauma, or disease process. Once an aneurysm develops, the tendency is toward an increase in size.

Clinical Manifestations and Diagnosis. About two fifths of these patients display symptoms; the remainder are asymptomatic. At times the patient complains that he can feel his "heart beating" in his abdomen when he lies down. The most common symptom is *abdominal pain,* which may be persistent or intermittent and is often localized in the middle or lower abdomen to the left of the midline. The next most common symptom is *low back pain.* This is a serious symptom which usually signifies rapid expansion or impending rupture of the aneurysm. Symptoms vary according to where pressure is exerted on nearby organs. Less frequently, the patient complains of feeling an abdominal mass or abdominal throbbing. More than half of these patients exhibit hypertension. An interesting finding is the comparison of blood pressure readings of the thigh and arm. Ordinarily the systolic blood pressure of the thigh exceeds that of the arm by 15

mm. Hg or more. In about three quarters of patients with abdominal aortic aneurysm, the systolic pressure in the thigh is abnormally low in comparison with that in the arm.

A most important diagnostic indication of this aneurysm is the presence of a palpable mass with a definitely expansile pulsation. During physical examination of a patient, particularly of a male over 60 years of age, such a mass may present itself, even though there are no other symptoms to indicate its presence. Confirmation by a lateral abdominal x-ray may be helpful if the aneurysm is calcified. Abdominal aortogram by transfemoral or translumbar technique may confirm the presence of an aneurysm. However, ultrasonography is more accurate and less expensive in defining the size of an aneurysm in both transverse and longitudinal cross sections and is the best test for confirming the presence and checking the size of abdominal aortic aneurysms.

Management. The likelihood of rupture is significant in patients with an expanding or enlarging aneurysm. Long-term results are most satisfactory if surgery is carried out. Surgery is the treatment of choice for abdominal aneurysms greater than 5 cm. (2 inches) in diameter or those that are enlarging. This involves resection of the aneurysm and insertion of a bypass (synthetic) graft (Fig. 31-8). Although it is a major operation, elective aneurysm resection carries only about a one to two percent mortality risk.

Preoperative Management. Nursing assessment involves not only considering the possibility that the aneurysm might rupture, but also recognizing that the patient is an elderly person who most likely has atherosclerosis and may possibly have cardiovascular, cerebral, and pulmonary impairment. Before surgery, the patient is carefully monitored to determine the functional capacity of these systems as well as the renal and gastrointestinal systems. Signs of a rupturing abdominal aortic aneurysm include a constant intense back pain, falling blood pressure, decreasing red cell count and increasing white count, plus a soft abdomen. Another possible symptom is the formation of a hematoma—following a retroperitoneal rupture of an aneurysm, hematomas have been noticed in the scrotum, perineum, or penis. Signs of heart failure or loud bruit may suggest a rupture into the vena cava.

A variety of preoperative tests are done to determine baseline functioning: ECG, pulmonary function tests, blood gas determination, complete blood count, renal and liver function studies, state of hydration, baseline weight, and arteriogram or ultrasound studies.

Usually an enema is avoided in order to reduce the possibility of injury to the aneurysm. Antibiotics and a low residue diet are given for 2 to 3 days before the operation., The patient is prepared as for other abdominal surgery.

Postoperative Management. Care requires that the patient be carefully monitored to determine respiratory, cardiovascular, hemodynamic, and neurologic status. Renal assessment is facilitated by accurate recording of intake and output. Unless a complication arises or recovery is compromised by other preexisting conditions, convalescence is smooth.

Health Teaching. The patient may need instruction regarding the prescribed exercise schedule, which is determined in part by his cardiovascular condition. Dietary restriction or modification will also depend upon his cardiac and vascular health and the presence of hypertension. Sitting for long periods of time should be avoided; periods of sitting should be alternated with periods of light exercise. If the patient is a cigarette smoker, he will obviously be advised to abandon this habit. He should also be instructed to report any untoward signs to his physician immediately and encouraged to have follow-up examinations.

Ruptured Abdominal Aneurysm

Pain accompanied by signs of blood loss and shock is the predominant symptom of a ruptured aneurysm. Symptoms vary with intensity and hence will range from a rise in pulse rate and drop in blood pressure to shock and collapse. Surgical mortality for ruptured aneurysm is about 50 to 75 percent.

Rupture usually occurs in the retroperitoneal space where the surrounding structures, acting as a tamponade, can exercise control over the hemorrhaging artery for many hours. On the other hand, if the rupture occurs into the free peritoneal cavity, the patient may rapidly become exsanguinated and bleed to death. Rupture into the retroperitoneal duodenum will be evidenced by the passage of melena and the patient's going into shock. If leakage is slow retroperitoneally and the pa-

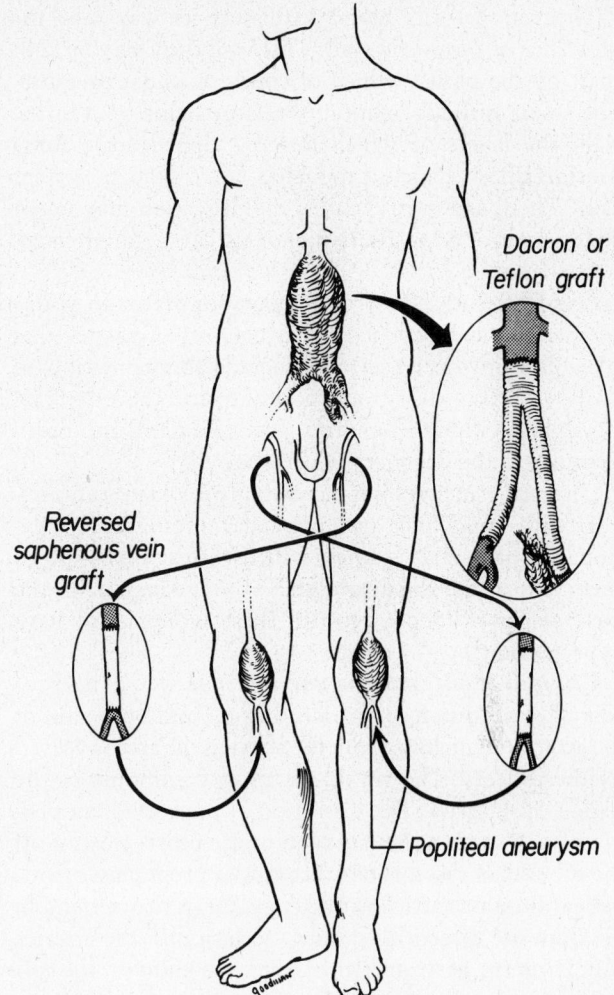

Figure 31-8. Surgical treatment of a patient who had a large abdominal aneurysm involving the iliac arteries plus bilateral symptomatic popliteal aneurysms. These were resected and the abdominal aneurysm was replaced with a Teflon graft. The popliteal aneurysms were replaced by saphenous vein grafts, which appear to function much better at the flexion crease than the synthetic graft. (Hardy, J. D., et al.: Aneurysms of the popliteal artery. By permission of Surgery, Gynecology, & Obstetrics, Mar. 1975, *140*:402)

tient's condition is fairly stable, surgical resection is usually effective. Through ongoing nursing assessment, the initial hemorrhage may be recognized at an early stage and the patient's life saved by alerting the physician immediately, so that surgical intervention can be carried out without delay.

Dissecting Aneurysm of the Aorta

Pathophysiology. On rare occasions, an aorta diseased by arteriosclerosis develops a tear in its intima due to a type of medial degeneration. This entity, which is often associated with hypertension, is three times more common in men than in women and occurs in the age group between 40 and 70. About 15 percent of dissections occur in persons under age 40.

The tear permits blood to dissect its way into the substance of the aortic wall. This wall then may be split apart by the blood, which of course is under pressure. The result is the formation of a large hematoma in the wall, the layers of which may be ripped apart for a considerable distance, producing severe and persistent pain. The location is variable; the dissection may occur on the anterior or posterior part of the chest or high in the epigastrium.

Less frequently, dissecting aneurysm occurs in younger persons with cystic medial necrosis. Changes that take place in the vessel wall include fragmentation of elastic lamellae, overproduction of mucin, and decreasing ability within the media to produce an inflammatory response to the degenerative process.

Dissecting aneurysm is increasingly noted in combination with congenital cardiovascular anomalies. Occasionally, pregnant women will manifest this type of aneurysm in the third trimester of pregnancy or in the early stages of labor. Most of these women also have hypertension.

Clinical Manifestations and Assessment. The process of dissection leads to shearing off and occlusion of the arteries branching from the aorta in the area involved by the process. The rip occurs most commonly in the region of the arch. The dissection of the aorta may progress backward in the direction of the heart, closing off the mouths of the coronary arteries or producing hemopericardium or aortic insufficiency. Or, it may extend in the opposite direction, causing occlusion of the arteries supplying the gastrointestinal tract, the kidneys, the spinal cord, and even the legs. Blood pressure may be unobtainable or may differ markedly from one arm to the other. Other symptoms are also variable depending upon where and how extensive the dissection is.

Diagnosis of a dissecting aneurysm is based on signs and symptoms closely resembling those of coronary occlusion (page 574) and on additional signs arising from multiple occlusions of the aortic branches. Pain, the predominant symptom, is usually severe and sudden in onset. It is described as "tearing" or "ripping" and is not relieved by the usual narcotic dosage. The location of pain is determined by the site of the ensuing dissection. In this type of aneurysm, as well as in cases of the syphilitic variety, a definitive diagnosis is made by aortography.

Management. The best results in treating the patient with a dissecting aneurysm are obtained by means of surgery; however, because the surgical mortality rate is high, recent approaches are aimed at reducing those factors which further the dissection once it has begun. Cardiac contraction and mean arterial pressures are such factors. Therefore, the following are recommended: reserpine, to decrease myocardial contraction; trimethaphan (Arfonad), to reduce cardiac output; propranolol (Inderal), to decrease myocardial contractility; plus alpha-Methyldopa (Aldomet) and thiazides (Diuril, HydroDiuril) to decrease blood pressure.

For long-term management, the patient (or a member of his family) must be instructed to take his blood pressure daily. Frequent follow-up visits are advised to determine the presence or absence of pain, the status of the peripheral pulses, and the presence of murmurs in the aortic area and to compare present x-rays with previous thoracic films. If saccular aneurysms develop, surgery is required.

Some authorities rely on the pharmacotherapeutic approach alone; others precede surgical intervention by a 2- to 3-week regime of drug therapy. Surgical treatment is determined by the type of aortic dissection in question; some surgeons advocate immediate surgery for ascending dissecting aneurysm and pharmacotherapy for descending aortic dissection. Surgery consists of excising the section of the aorta involved in the aneurysm and replacing the segment of vessel with a synthetic graft.

Other Aneurysms

Aneurysms may also arise in peripheral vessels, most often as a result of arteriosclerosis. These may involve such vessels as the renal artery, the subclavian artery, or (most frequently) the popliteal artery, in the area of the knee. Such aneurysms may be bilateral.

The aneurysm produces a pulsating mass and a disturbance of peripheral circulation distal to it. Pain and swelling develop because of pressure upon adjacent nerves and veins. Surgical repair of such aneurysms is now carried out with replacement grafts.

ARTERIAL EMBOLISM

Pathophysiology. Arterial emboli arise from thrombi that develop in the chambers of the heart as a result of atrial fibrillation or myocardial infarction secondary to occlusion of the coronary artery. These thrombi may become detached, and a detached thrombus is carried from the left side of the heart by way of the aorta into the arterial system, where it can plug an artery that is too small to allow it to pass. Emboli may also develop in advanced arteriosclerosis of the aorta due to roughening and even ulceration of the atheromatous plaques that form. Thrombi may form in these patients and break off, becoming emboli that can lodge in the arterial system, most often where vessels divide.

Clinical Manifestations. The symptoms of acute arterial embolism are acute pain and loss of function. The pain is severe and the loss of function is both motor and sensory. The patient shows a sudden paralysis and anesthesia of the part, which also appears pale and cold. These symptoms are due not only to the block of the artery by the embolus, but also to an associated vasomotor reflex that affects the arterial tree distal to the embolus.

Management. To relieve the vasoconstriction, the

sympathetic ganglia may be blocked with procaine. In addition, heparin is often given intravenously to reduce the tendency for a clot to form and extend within the vessel. In embolism of small arteries, these measures may be sufficient to prevent death of tissue, but in embolism of larger arteries, such as the aorta or the iliac arteries, surgery is usually undertaken as an emergency procedure (Fig. 31-9). The artery is exposed and the vessel is clamped or taped above and below the site of clot lodgement. An incision is made into the vessel and the clot is removed. This procedure (embolectomy) can be performed readily with the use of a Fogarty catheter. By this method, embolic material, whether proximal to the abdominal aorta or as far away as ankle level, can easily be extracted through an arteriotomy in the common femoral artery. The opening in the vessel is closed with a fine silk suture. As closure is made, a small amount of heparin solution is injected into the lumen of the vessel to minimize the tendency to thrombosis as the vessel is being closed.

During the postoperative period, every effort is made to encourage movement of the leg in order to stimulate circulation and prevent stasis. Since each patient problem is specific, the nurse collaborates with the surgeon with regard to appropriate patient activity. Anticoagulants (heparin) are given carefully, not only to prevent thrombosis of the operated artery, but also to diminish the development of thrombi at the original source of the embolus. The nurse frequently assesses the surgical wound for evidence of hemorrhage, which can occur when anticoagulants are given. Atrial fibrillation or coronary thrombosis are potential cardiac complications to watch for when monitoring the cardiovascular status of the patient.

ARTERIAL THROMBOSIS

Arterial thrombosis is another type of acute arterial occlusion that may develop in association with coronary occlusion. In the phase of depressed blood pressure, there is reduced peripheral circulation, which is manifested chiefly by arterial thrombosis in the degenerated vessels of the legs. The symptoms of arterial thrombosis are somewhat similar to those of acute arterial occlusion due to embolus, but treatment is made more difficult because the arterial occlusion has occurred in a degenerated vessel, requiring more extensive surgery (endarterectomy or graft), which can only be performed if the patient's arterial blood pressure can be restored.

VASOSPASTIC DISORDERS

Raynaud's Phenomenon

Raynaud's phenomenon is a form of intermittent arteriolar vasoconstriction that results in coldness, pain, pallor, and, occasionally, ulceration of the fingertips.

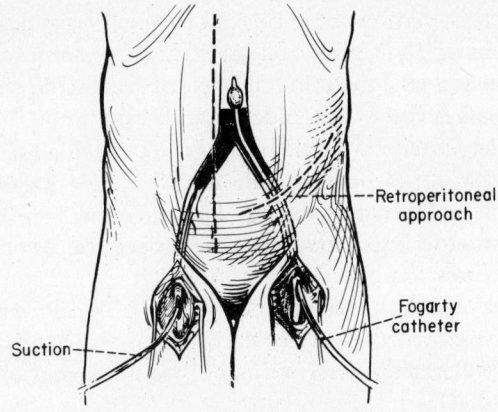

Figure 31-9. Aortic bifurcation embolectomy may be approached directly through the abdomen or in a retrograde fashion via the femoral arteries by suction or Fogarty catheter. (From Rhoads, et al.: Surgery. Philadelphia, J. B. Lippincott.)

Episodes may be triggered by emotional factors or by unusual sensitivity to cold. It is most common in females between the ages of 16 and 40 years and is seen much more frequently in cold climates and during the winter months. If the degree of vasoconstriction is moderate, there may still be some arterial flow. However, blood flow is relatively stagnant, producing a cyanotic (blue) color in the fingers. If the spasm is severe, the fingers become a dead-white color. After rewarming, the fingers develop a reactive hyperemia and appear red. Thus the characteristic color change of Raynaud's phenomenon is described as blue, white, and red. The involvement tends to be asymmetric — that is, some fingers may be involved while others appear normal. The thumbs are less often involved.

The condition was originally described by Maurice Raynaud over 100 years ago as bilateral, symmetrical gangrene and was called Raynaud's disease. Since this is not what we see today, the preferred term is Raynaud's phenomenon. Primary Raynaud's phenomenon does not indicate an underlying vascular disorder, whereas secondary Raynaud's phenomenon is a condition in which vasospasm is related to an underlying condition such as collagen vascular disease (scleroderma, SLE), thoracic outlet syndrome, Buerger's disease, or emboli, or to certain occupational activities such as typing or operating a jackhammer.

Raynaud's phenomenon occurs primarily in the hands and rarely in the feet. In patients who develop gangrene of the fingertips, there is probably an underlying problem such as a collagen vascular disease. (The Raynaud's phenomenon may precede the collagen vascular problem by as much as 10 years.) It is unusual for a patient to lose more than digits from gangrene with this problem.

The prognosis for the primary type of Raynaud's phenomenon varies: some patients slowly improve, some grow slowly worse, and others show no change. The etiology is unknown, but the vasoconstriction appears to be mediated through the release of catecholamines at the neuroarteriolar junction. The prognosis for the secondary type is that of the underlying disease.

Management. Avoidance of the particular stimuli that provoke vasoconstriction is the prime objective in controlling Raynaud's disease. *First,* an effort is made to avoid situations that may upset the patient. Since concern over serious complications such as gangrene and amputation may upset the patient, he needs to be reassured that loss of a large extremity never occurs in Raynaud's disease. A therapeutic environment is as important to this individual as insulin may be to the person who has diabetes.

Second, exposure to cold must be minimized. In areas where the fall and winter months are cold, the patient should remain indoors, which means no hiking or participation in winter sports. For those occasions when it is necessary to go outdoors, warm clothing must be worn. Attractive fleece-lined boots, gloves, and hooded jackets are effective as well as fashionable. Leotards and slacks can also be worn to keep the legs warm. Heated automobiles and heated shopping centers also help in reducing exposure to cold. The homemaker, who must avoid placing her hands in cold water, should always use tepid or warm water. Oven mitts may be worn to remove frozen packages and articles from the refrigerator. Cold beverages can be handled in insulated glasses or tumblers partially covered with knitted "pants."

A *third* aid in controlling this disease is the systemic administration of peripheral vasodilators (not always effective).

Fourth, since ulceration can easily develop following trauma to the digits, it is necessary for the patient to handle knives, needles, and other sharp objects carefully.

Pharmacotherapy includes administration of reserpine or other rauwolfia derivatives, methyldopa, griseofulvin, tolazoline (Priscoline) and phenoxybenzamine (Dibenzyline). Each of these medications has been reported to provide varying benefits.*

In severe cases, however, interruption of the sympathetic nerves by removal of the sympathetic ganglia or division of their branches is the only method affording much improvement. For the upper extremity, the ganglia are located in the upper part of the thorax and lower neck.

HYPERTENSIVE VASCULAR DISEASE (HYPERTENSION)

Incidence and Significance

Hypertensive vascular disease is defined as persistent levels of blood pressure in which the systolic pressure is above 150 mm. Hg and the diastolic pressure is above 90

*Fairbairn, J. F., et al.: Peripheral Vascular Diseases, 5th ed. Philadelphia, W. B. Saunders, 1979

mm. Hg. Hypertension is a major cause of heart failure, stroke, and kidney failure. It is called the "silent killer," because the individual is often symptom-free; it has been estimated by the National Heart, Lung and Blood Institute that 50 percent of persons with hypertension do not know they have it. Once a patient is identified as having hypertension, his blood pressure must be checked frequently, since it is a lifetime condition.

About 20 percent of the adult population develop hypertension; more than 90 percent of these have *essential* (primary) hypertension, which has no identifiable cause. The remainder develop elevations in blood pressure from some specific etiology, such as renovascular narrowing or parenchyma-renal disease. The rarer forms include aldosterone-producing adrenal tumor and pheochromocytoma.

Elevated blood pressure is associated with many disease states, such as thyrotoxicosis or preeclampsia, and it is corrected when the basic disease is corrected. Because of the frequency of hypertension, a national program for screening potential hypertensive individuals was launched in 1972 by a special committee under the Department of Health, Education and Welfare (see flow diagram, page 629).

Essential hypertension usually begins as a labile (intermittent) process in the late 30s to early 50s and gradually becomes "fixed." On occasion it appears abruptly and severely and takes an accelerated or "malignant" course that causes rapid deterioration of the patient.

Overstimulation with coffee, tobacco, and stimulatory drugs, as well as emotional disturbances and obesity, play a role, but the disease is strongly familial. It affects more women than men, but men, especially blacks, are less able to tolerate the disease.

Prolonged elevation of blood pressure eventually damages blood vessels throughout the body, most notably in the eyes, heart, kidneys, and brain, so that failing vision, coronary occlusion, congestive heart failure, renal failure, and strokes are the usual consequences of prolonged, uncontrolled hypertension.

Increased peripheral resistance controlled at the arteriolar level is the basic cause for the elevated blood pressure, but the causes of increased resistance are poorly understood. Drug therapy is aimed at reducing peripheral resistance, so as to lower the blood pressure and lessen the stresses on the vascular system.

Pathophysiology of Essential Hypertension

High blood pressure is a hereditary disease in which increased vasoconstrictor activity of the blood vessel results in an increase in blood pressure. The vasomotor center is situated in the medulla of the brain. Emanating from this vasomotor center are the sympathetic nervous system tracks, which go down the spinal cord and emerge from the spinal column to meet the sympathetic ganglia in the thorax and abdomen. Stimulation of the vasomotor center sets in motion impulses that travel down through the sympathetic nervous system to the sympathetic ganglia. At this point, the preganglionic neurons release acetylcholine, which stimulates the postganglionic nerve fibers in the blood vessel, where the release of catecholamines results in constriction of the vessel. Numerous influences may affect the response of the blood vessel to these vasoconstrictor stimuli.

In the hypertensive patient, many factors moderate the vasomotor and vasoconstrictor responses. Anxiety, fear, and undesirable noises represent a threat to the patient and may be registered as such on the cerebral cortex. Once recorded, these stimuli are quickly transferred through the internuncial neurons to the vasomotor center, which responds by dispatching vasoconstrictor impulses.

Occurring concurrently with sympathetic nervous system stimulation of the blood vessels is stimulation of the adrenal medulla, which secretes vasoconstrictors. These substances also mediate the release of corticotropin-releasing factor (CRF), which stimulates the pituitary gland in the brain to release adrenocorticotropic hormone (ACTH), which in turn stimulates the adrenal cortex to release hydrocortisone and other steroids which may enhance the response of the vasoconstrictor impulse. Vasoconstrictor impulses also result in ischemia of the kidney, causing the release of renin. Renin is converted to angiotensin, which in turn stimulates secretion of aldosterone by the adrenal cortex. This hormone promotes sodium and water retention by the kidney tubules. When the levels of aldosterone become quite high, the condition is referred to as a secondary hyperaldosteronism.

Sodium and water retention in the kidney increases the electrolyte concentration in the blood vessel wall to a level which enhances vasoconstrictor response of the blood vessel (arteriole) to sympathomimetic impulses. Thus, the vicious cycle of hypertensive vascular disease is established and may eventually lead to malignant hypertension, a very rapidly progressing disease which has a high mortality rate if not treated. When atherosclerotic disease of the large blood vessel occurs in addition to the hypertension, the prognosis is further affected, because these two diseases have an additive effect on morbidity and mortality.

Clinical Manifestations

The symptoms may be nonexistent or may be severe, with morning headaches, fatigability, nervousness, and irritability; if the heart is involved, dyspnea, edema, or the anginal syndrome and palpitations may occur. Nocturia and other signs of renal damage occur as the kidney becomes involved. There may be transient ischemic attacks such as giddiness and blackouts, indicating central nervous system involvement. On physical examination, no abnormalities other than high blood pressure may be found, but there may be changes in the retinae with hemorrhages, exudates, narrowed arterioles, and, in severe cases, papilledema. Cardiac enlargement and arrhythmias may be found, along with signs of congestive heart failure. In the older patient, evidences of arteriosclerosis may be seen, because prolonged hypertension seems to increase the rate at which the arteriosclerotic processes develop.

Diagnosis

A thorough physical examination including a moderate neurological testing examination is desirable. Eye grounds are checked and laboratory studies are done to determine target organ damage, such as sclerosis of the arterioles in the retina. Left ventricular hypertrophy (LVH) can be seen in the electrocardiogram; protein in the urine can be detected by urinalysis. Inability to concentrate the urine and an increase in the blood urea nitrogen may also be present. Special studies such as renograms, intravenous pyelograms, renal arteriograms,

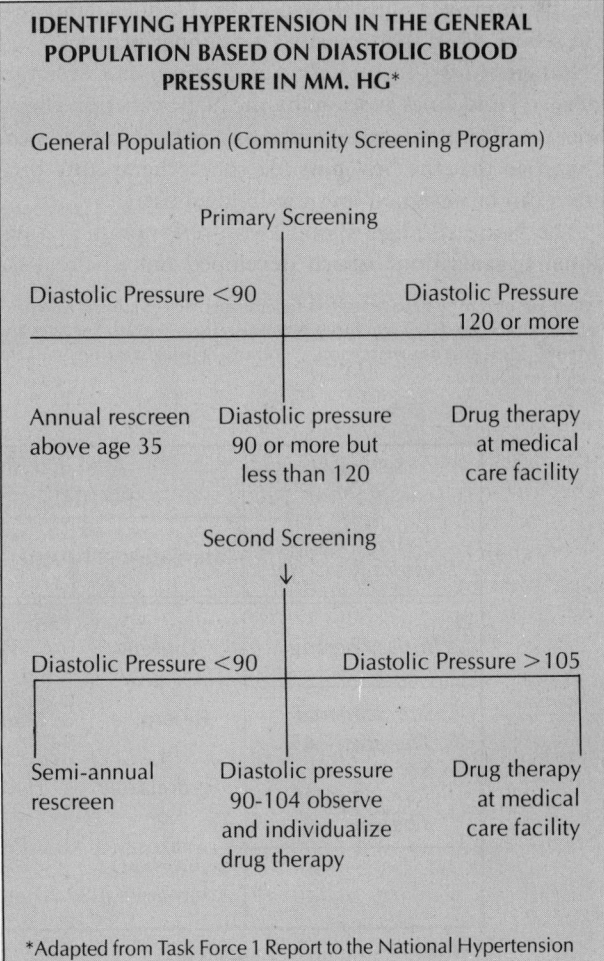

IDENTIFYING HYPERTENSION IN THE GENERAL POPULATION BASED ON DIASTOLIC BLOOD PRESSURE IN MM. HG*

General Population (Community Screening Program)

Primary Screening

Diastolic Pressure <90   Diastolic Pressure 120 or more

Annual rescreen above age 35   Diastolic pressure 90 or more but less than 120   Drug therapy at medical care facility

Second Screening

Diastolic Pressure <90   Diastolic Pressure >105

Semi-annual rescreen   Diastolic pressure 90-104 observe and individualize drug therapy   Drug therapy at medical care facility

*Adapted from Task Force 1 Report to the National Hypertension Information and Education Advisory Committee.

split renal function studies, and the determination of renin levels are done to identify patients with renovascular occlusion. If a stenosis of a renal artery is found, correction by surgery is possible. VMA (vanillylmandelic acid), catecholamine determination, and a Regitine test detect the rare pheochromocytoma tumors that secrete norepinephrine and epinephrine and can be treated surgically (page 870). Elevated aldosterone levels and decreased renin levels are highly suggestive of primary aldosteronism, an uncommon condition, but one which can be treated surgically. Of additional diagnostic significance is whether the patient is on oral contraceptives or is addicted to licorice, because either factor can cause an elevated pressure. Diabetes or hypercholesterolemia, even with moderate blood pressure elevations, greatly increases the risk of coronary disease.

Management

The objective of treatment is to lower the blood pressure to normal levels with the hope of alleviating symptoms and preventing the development or arresting the progress of vascular damage. In accelerated or malignant hypertension, which has a relatively short natural history and a limited life span, drug therapy has produced a greatly improved outlook, especially if kidney damage is not severe when the treatment gets under way.

Patient Classification, Initial Testing, and Management. Guidelines as set up by the National High Blood Pressure Program are followed and patient care is promoted so that the best possible chemotherapeutic program can be designed on an individual basis.

The National High Blood Pressure Program is a national organization* which developed out of the 1972

*Made up of representatives of five federal agencies: National Institutes of Health (NIH), Food and Drug Administration, Health Services and Mental Health Administration, Veterans Administration, and the Dept. of Defense.

conference of private and government groups directly concerned with hypertension. This group developed specific guidelines for primary and secondary hypertension screenings (see flow diagram page 629) and for the subsequent clinical evaluation and therapy of those found by the screenings to be hypertensive.

The guidelines may be summarized as follows:
1. Anyone found by primary screening to have a systolic blood pressure of 160 mm. Hg or higher or a diastolic pressure of 95 mm. Hg or higher is referred for a second examination.
2. Anyone with a diastolic pressure of 120 mm. Hg or higher is referred immediately for medical care.
3. On secondary screening, emphasis is placed on diastolic pressure, which is checked during the course of three relatively close visits.
    a. An overall average diastolic pressure of 105 mm. Hg or higher is referred for treatment.
    b. An average diastolic pressure of 95-105 mm. Hg is referred for further evaluation; this may mean immediate treatment or additional testing.
4. Six basic tests are recommended before treatment is indicated:
    a. Resting electrocardiogram
    b. Urinalysis for protein, hemoglobin, and glucose (dipsticks)
    c. Blood urea nitrogen or creatinine
    d. Serum potassium
    e. Microscopic urinalysis (red cells)
5. Less urgent but helpful tests include:
    a. Chest x-ray
    b. Creatinine clearance
    c. Serum uric acid
    d. Blood sugar (fasting or with standardized glucose load)
    e. Serum cholesterol
6. Recommended treatment is "stepped care" (Fig. 31-10). (For a detailed outline of chemotherapy for hypertension see Table 31-4.)

Severity	Mild and Moderately Severe (90-104) (105-120)			Severe (more than 120)
Diastolic Blood Pressure (mm. Hg)	* Alternative # 1	Alternative # 2	Alternative # 3	Alternative # 4
Initial Therapy	Diuretic +	Diuretic +	Diuretic +	Diuretic plus Guanethidine +
Supplemental Therapy — A	Reserpine +	Methyldopa +	Propranolol +	Methyldopa or
Supplemental Therapy — B	Hydralazine or Prazosin	Hydralazine or Prazosin	Hydralazine or Prazosin	Hydralazine +
	Alternative # 3	Alternative # 3	———	Propranolol

* When Tranquilizer Indicated

Figure 31-10. Regimens for the management of uncomplicated hypertension. In these regimens, alternative #4 usually requires the supervision of a specialist in the field because of the potency of the drugs being used. (From Hypertension Committee of AMA.)

TABLE 31-4. CHEMOTHERAPY FOR HYPERTENSION
(Antihypertensive Drugs)

Definition: Pharmacotherapy to lower blood pressure
Purpose: To maintain blood pressure within normal ranges, i.e., less than 90 mm. Hg (diastolic) by the simplest and safest means possible with the fewest side effects for each individual patient.

MEDICATION	MAJOR ACTION	ADVANTAGES	CONTRAINDICATIONS	EFFECTS AND NURSING CONSIDERATIONS
I. *Oral Diuretics* A. Thiazides and Related Drugs, i.e., Chlorthalidone (Hygroton) Quinethazone (Hydromox) Chlorothiazide (Diuril) Hydrochloro- thiazide (Esidrix; HydroDiuril)	At beginning of therapy: Decrease of blood volume, renal blood flow, and cardiac output Depletion of extra- cellular fluid Negative sodium balance (from natriuresis), mild hypokalemia Directly affects vascular smooth muscle	Effective orally Effective during long-term administration Mild side effects Enhance other anti- hypertensive drugs Counter sodium re- tention effect of other antihyperten- sive drugs	Gout Known sensitivity to sulfonamide- derived drugs Severely impaired kidney function	Dry mouth, thirst, weakness, drowsiness, lethargy, muscle aches, muscular fatigue, tachycardia, GI disturbance Orthostatic hypotension may be potenti- ated by alcohol, barbiturates, or narcotics Because thiazides cause sodium loss, patient is instructed to watch for pos- tural hypotension in the summer. (Eating salted pretzels in hot weather may avert this) Administer supplementary potassium
B. Loop Diuretics Furosemide (Lasix) Ethacrynic Acid (Edecrin)	Volume depletion Blocks reabsorption of sodium and water in kidney Antagonizes action of aldosterone	Action is rapid Potent-blocks To be used only when thiazides fail	Same as for thiazides	Volume depletion is rapid—profound diuresis Electrolyte depletion—replacement is required Thirst, nausea, vomiting, skin rash, postural hypotension Sweet taste noted; oral and gastric burning
C. Potassium- sparing Diuretics Spironolactone (Aldactone) Triamterene (Dyrenium)	Competitive inhibi- tor of aldosterone Acts on distal tubule independently of aldosterone	Spironolactone effective in treating hypertension ac- companying pri- mary aldosteronism Both spironolactone and triamterene re- tain potassium	Renal disease Azotemia Severe hepatic disease	Drowsiness, lethargy, headache—de- crease the dosage Diarrhea and other GI symptoms—give drug after meals Skin eruptions, urticaria Mental confusion, ataxia—perhaps dos- age needs to be reduced Gynecomastia (not for triamterene)
II. *Reserpine* (alkaloid of Rauwolfia serpentina)	Impairs intracellular storage of norepinephrine	Slows pulse, which counteracts tachy- cardia of hydralazine	History of depression Psychosis Obesity Chronic sinusitis Peptic ulcer	May cause severe depression; report manifestations since this may require that drug be omitted Nasal stuffiness which may require nasal vasoconstrictor Increases appetite—therefore suggest stricter diet Recurrence of peptic ulcer
III. *Methyldopa* (Aldomet)	Dopa—decarboxy- lase inhibitor	Effective in patients not controlled with thiazide-reserpine (with or without hydralazine) Useful in patients with renal failure Does not decrease cardiac output or renal blood flow Does not induce oliguria	Liver disease	Drowsiness, dizziness Dry mouth; nasal stuffiness (troublesome at first but then tends to disappear) Hemolytic anemia (a hypersensitization reaction)—positive Coombs' test—may not indicate drug discontinuance
IV. *Hydralazine hydrochloride* (Apresoline)	Decreases periph- eral resistance but concurrently ele- vates cardiac output Acts directly on smooth muscle of blood vessels	Used as a third drug of choice when patient does not respond to thiazide-reserpine, thiazide-methyl- dopa, thiazide- guanethidine	Angina or coronary artery disease Congestive heart failure Hypersensitivity	Headache, tachycardia, flushing and dys- pnea may occur—can be prevented by pretreating with reserpine Peripheral edema may require diuretics May produce lupus erythematosus-like syndrome

(Continued)

631

TABLE 31-4. CHEMOTHERAPY FOR HYPERTENSION (CONTINUED)
(Antihypertensive Drugs)

MEDICATION	MAJOR ACTION	ADVANTAGE	CONTRAINDICATIONS	EFFECTS AND NURSING CONSIDERATIONS
V. *Recently Approved Drugs*				
Propranolol (Inderal)	Blocks the sympathetic nervous system (beta adrenergic receptors), especially the sympathetics to the heart, producing a slower heart rate and lowered blood pressure	Reduces pulse rate in patients with tachycardia and blood pressure elevation and is useful as an adjunctive drug with those which act at the neuroeffector site of the blood vessel	Bronchial asthma Allergic rhinitis Right ventricular failure due to pulmonary hypertension Congestive heart failure	Mental depression manifested by insomnia, lassitude, weakness, and fatigue Lightheadedness and occasional nausea, vomiting, and epigastric distress Blood dyscrasias such as agranulocytosis and thrombocytopenic purpura do occur but are uncommon
Prazosin (Minipress)	Peripheral vasodilator acting directly on the blood vessel; similar to hydralazine	Acts directly on the blood vessel and is an effective agent in those patients with adverse reactions to hydralazine	Angina pectoris and coronary artery disease. Induces tachycardia if not preceded by administration of propranolol and a diuretic	Occasional vomiting and diarrhea, urinary frequency, and cardiovascular collapse especially if given in addition to hydralazine without lowering the dose of the latter. Patients occasionally experience drowsiness, lack of energy, and weakness
Clonidine Hydrochloride (Catapres)	Exact mode of action not understood, but acts through the central nervous system, apparently through centrally mediated alpha adrenergic stimulation in the brain, producing blood pressure reduction	Little or no orthostatic effect. Moderately potent and sometimes is effective when other drugs fail to lower blood pressure	Severe coronary artery disease, pregnancy, children	Most common side effects are dry mouth, drowsiness, sedation, and occasional headaches and fatigue. Anorexia, malaise, and vomiting with mild disturbance of liver function have been reported. Skin rash, dreams and nightmares, insomnia, and anxiety have been reported but are not common
VI. *Guanethidine* (Ismelin)	Prevents release of sympathetic transmitter, norepinephrine. It is a depressant of adrenergic activity Depletes tissue stores Causes venous pooling Decreases pulse rate, cardiac output, and renal blood flow	Potency	Pheochromocytoma, because it greatly enhances pressor effect of catecholamines	Severe orthostatic hypotension accentuated by alcohol, exercise, hot weather Warn against suddenly standing or standing for a long time Diarrhea and nausea, nocturia Failure of ejaculation; counsel about possible sexual dysfunction Fatigue and giddiness; blackout

Physical and Psychotherapeutic Measures. In all instances there are certain general health measures to be followed: overweight is corrected; overuse of stimulants and tobacco is curbed; serum cholesterol levels are lowered; dietary salt intake is reduced; other disease states such as anemia, thyrotoxicosis, and renal infection are corrected. Patients are also urged and educated to adopt a more tranquil outlook on life and its problems and to alter their habits so as to lead a well-balanced life with proper proportions of work, play, and rest. This is not easy, because many of these patients are tense, hard-driving individuals for whom relaxation is difficult.

Nursing Assessment

The guidelines just discussed will be helpful to the nurse in assessing the patient and directing him to the next step in seeking treatment for an elevated blood pressure. When medications have been prescribed, the nurse can be alert to unpleasant drug reactions such as lethargy or depression (see Table 31-4). All side effects should be reported so that the medication regime can be altered for optimum effect. Patience will be needed by the patient during early attempts at determining the best drug combinations for controlling blood pressure.

When a patient with possible high blood pressure is assessed, the following may serve as an effective guide in detecting problems:

1. Have the patient rest for 5-10 minutes, then take the blood pressure in both arms and a leg, in the supine position.
2. The following inconsistencies may be found:

a. High blood pressure in arms
Low blood pressure in arms

Suspect coarctation of aorta

b. Difference in pressure in the two arms

Suspect atherosclerotic plaque or a congenital narrowing of subclavian artery on one side.

c. From supine to upright position

Normal: A slight decrease in systolic and a slight increase in diastolic.

d. From supine to upright

If postural hypotension occurs on standing, suspect secondary hypertension, pheochromocytoma, or renal artery occlusive disease.

e. Be *consistent* in technique; for example, in determining diastolic reading always use the same index, such as the last audible sound or the first muffled sound.

Patient Education

Generally, patients taking medications as part of an antihypertensive program experience some degree of sedation, which may be too great for comfort. Many of these symptoms disappear as the patient adjusts to the medications or as the dosage is adjusted.

Sometimes, the patient is taught to measure blood pressure at home (Fig. 31-11). Some authorities believe that this involves the patient in his own care and emphasizes the fact that failing to take the medication can lead to a rise in blood pressure. It is difficult to convince many patients that the blood pressure is normally variable and does not stay fixed at one number. Patients must be encouraged to stick to their treatment programs. This is an important point for the nurse to emphasize. Should the patient discontinue the medications, the blood pressure will "escape," which means that it may become worse, is more difficult to control, and may even precipitate a coronary occlusion or myocardial infarction. Hence, the minimum drug therapy that must be continued under any circumstances is the daily administration of diuretics.

Salt restriction may be a problem for many patients, since processed foods frequently have salt added as a preservative and taste enhancer.

The patient is advised as follows:
- to avoid all processed foods except fruits and juices (check labels listing food ingredients)
- not to add salt to food during cooking and at the table
- to avoid milk and milk products, because of the naturally high sodium content of cow's milk and because most cheeses have added sodium chloride.

Salt substitutes with less sodium (Morton LITE-SALT) or no sodium (Co-salt) are available and recommended. For patients with renal damage, it is advisable to use caution in substituting potassium for sodium, particularly if potassium sparing diuretics are being taken (hyperkalemia is possible).

If a patient is overweight, it is prudent to reduce calories, which in effect also reduces the salt intake.

Neither coffee nor alcohol in moderation (up to 2 ounces a day) appears to affect blood pressure. Smoking cigarettes may raise the blood pressure. However, giving up smoking after many years will not appreciably affect blood pressure.

Patients with hypertension are cautioned not to perform isometric exercise, since sustained muscular contraction may precipitate angina, congestive failure, and cerebral hemorrhage.

Sexual intercourse may also cause significant elevations in blood pressure and pulse rate. The position assumed does not appear to have a significant effect on pulse or blood pressure.

Hypertensive Emergencies

Acute elevation of blood pressure associated with encephalopathy, eclampsia, malignant hypertension, and severe paroxysmal hypertension associated with pheochromocytoma demands prompt reduction of the blood pressure in order to prevent disabling or fatal cardiovascular catastrophies. Even moderate hypertension may be an emergency condition in the event of left ventricular failure with hypertensive heart disease and intracerebral or subarachnoid hemorrhage.

Diazoxide (Hyperstat) is a nondiuretic thiazide derivative considered by many to be the most effective and the safest medication for emergency reduction of blood pressure. It acts by relaxing smooth muscle in the arterioles, which causes an increase in cardiac output and a decrease in total peripheral resistance. There is a precipitous drop in blood pressure followed by a small increase before it levels.

- Diazoxide is given rapidly by the intravenous route in a peripheral vein. It is used on the hospitalized recumbent patient, who should be closely monitored since there is a risk of hypotension.
- After the medication is given, the patient should remain recumbent for one half hour; blood pressure is monitored every minute for 5 minutes, then every 5 minutes until it begins to rise, and then hourly.
- When the patient gets up, his blood pressure must be measured in the standing position and checked for stability before surveillance is lessened. If hypotension occurs, sympathomimetic drugs (norepinephrine) will restore blood pressure levels.

There are side effects associated with diazoxide, but patients on limited numbers of doses given for hypertensive crisis often do not experience them. One side effect is hyperglycemia, which can be controlled with insulin or some other hypoglycemic drug. The other is sodium and water retention which can be combated with furosemide or ethacrynic acid given before or concurrently with diazoxide.

Other drugs with various effects are used to treat hypertensive crisis; frequent monitoring of the patient is required.

Intramuscular reserpine (Serpasil) provides a satisfactory fall in blood pressure in about 85 percent of patients, but there is some delay in onset. Hydralazine (Apresoline) is a faster-acting drug which can be given intravenously or intramuscularly. It can cause postural

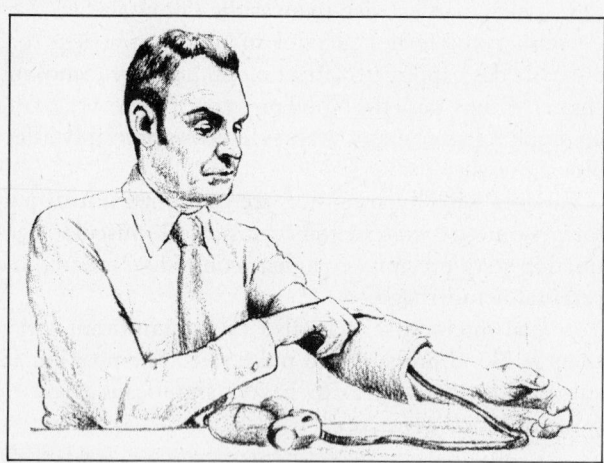

Keep your arm at the level of the heart and fit the cuff closely—but not too tightly—around your upper arm. You won't have to adjust the cuff again; simply slip it on and off at each reading.

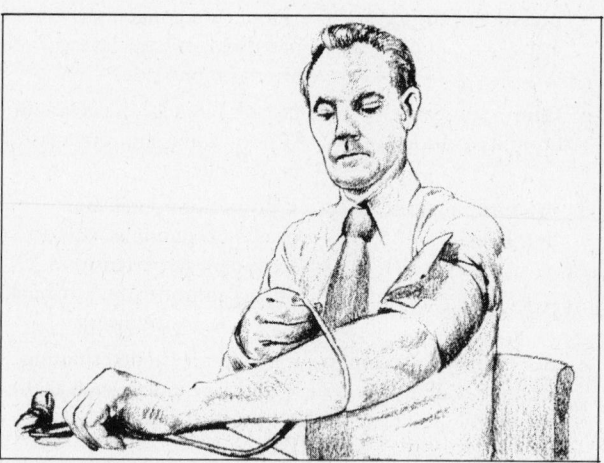

If you are not using a cuff design with the stethoscope sewn into it, you can slip two flat elastic bands up to the elbow and fasten the stethoscope diaphragm under them.

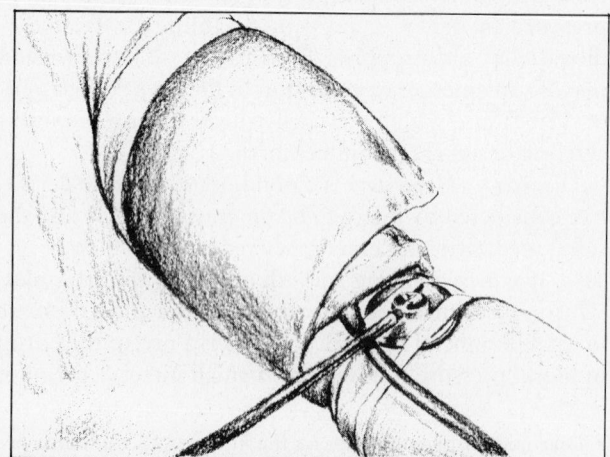

Place the diaphragm as shown, on the front surface of the upper arm directly above the elbow crease. Close the screw valve on the bulb, and squeeze the bulb to inflate the cuff. Listen through the stethoscope; when the cuff squeezes the artery so that the blood flow momentarily stops, you no longer hear the heartbeat. Pump the pressure up 20-30 mm.Hg above the last pulse heard.

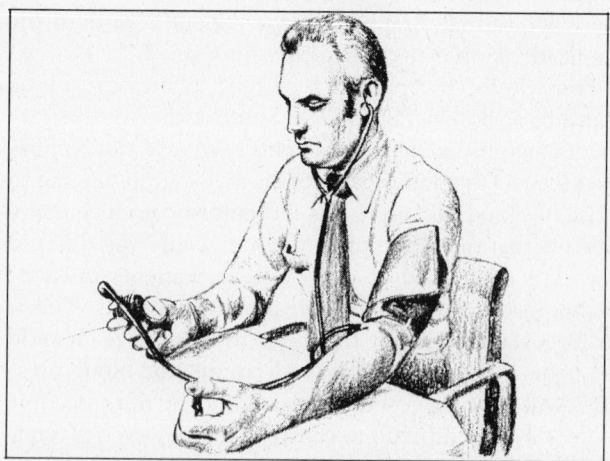

Open the valve slowly to release the cuff pressure, and listen for the first sound of the heart pumping blood through the arteries. At this moment the meter shows the systolic blood pressure. As you reduce the pressure, the pumping sound fades. At the point where you no longer hear it, the meter shows the diastolic pressure—the usual pressure on the arteries. Record your pressures immediately.

Figure 31-11. How to measure your own blood pressure at home. Since you must hold the arm you test completely still to avoid driving up the blood pressure, and you need one hand to pump up the cuff and then deflate it, and one to hold the stethoscope bell in place, you may feel that you really need an extra hand. It is possible, however, to take your own blood pressure without that extra hand. A, B, C, D. (Reproduced with permission of Patient Care magazine. Copyright © 1977, Patient Care Publications, Inc., Darien, CT. All Rights Reserved.)

hypotension and initiate angina; therefore, it is contraindicated for patients with coronary heart disease. Trimethaphan (Arfonad), given intravenously, acts quickly but its effect is short-lived and repeated doses are needed. Methyldopa (Aldomet) has a slower action, requiring 4 to 6 hours to lower blood pressure, but its effect lasts from 10 to 16 hours after intravenous injection.

VEIN DISORDERS

PHLEBITIS, VENOUS THROMBOSIS, THROMBOPHLEBITIS, AND DEEP VEIN THROMBOSIS (DVT)

Although the above terms do not necessarily represent an identical pathology, for clinical purposes they are used interchangeably when discussing the same process.

Etiology

Thrombosis (clot) and inflammation of the walls of veins (thrombophlebitis) can result from direct injuries to a vein (such as a perforating wound or a bruise), from an infection of the tissues surrounding the vessel, from continuous pressure against the vein by a tumor or aneurysm, and as a common complication of varicose veins. The condition is apt to arise in circumstances that promote stasis in the leg veins. Thus, it is not an uncommon complication of late pregnancy and should be anticipated in all patients who must be in bed for a prolonged period.

- For each bedfast patient, whether postoperative, postpartum, or ill with any condition that significantly reduces muscular movement, provision must be made for adequate venous drainage from the lower extremities, either by active or passive leg exercises or by postural changes.

Phlebitis may occur after unusual activity (or even without apparent cause) in a person used to a sedentary life. It is probable that stagnation of venous blood resulting from infrequent movement of the muscles may be a causal factor. It is for this reason that people are urged to move about intermittently when required to sit for long periods of time, as when riding in a car or plane or when watching television. The simple act of walking contracts muscles that press upon veins to empty them and thus promotes venous circulation and prevents venous stasis.

Pathophysiology

Venous thrombosis is a condition in which a clot forms in a vein, either secondary to phlebitis or due to partial obstruction of the vein. It is usually not possible to determine whether thrombus formation in the vein is the cause or result of inflammation of the vein wall (*thrombophlebitis*). The danger in this situation is that the clot, or a portion of it, may become detached and be swept into the pulmonary circulation, producing embolism. The thrombus is more likely to embolize if there is no inflam-

mation. The more inflammatory the process is (usually with more pain), the more adherent the clot will be to the wall of the vein and, therefore, the less likely to produce pulmonary emboli. This is the reason why deep vein thrombosis occurring secondary to bed rest (stasis) is more likely to result in pulmonary emboli (less inflammation and less adherence of the thrombus to the vein wall). Other complications of venous thrombosis are described in Figure 31-12.

Phlebitis and thrombosis occur most often in the veins of the leg, but also occur in veins of the femoral pelvis and, less often, in other areas of the body. The symptoms may be minimal, consisting of stiffness and soreness in the calf, progressing to swelling (edema), which may become quite marked in some patients. Pain in the upper posterior calf on dorsiflexion of the foot with the knee extended or slightly flexed is referred to as *Homans' sign*. At times, it is confused with sore musculature that results from wearing flat-heeled slippers during the postoperative period and may also be seen in instances of a torn calf muscle or hematoma. Hence, this sign is not pathognomonic of thrombophlebitis, which in fact is present in less than 50 pecent of such patients.

When the veins under the skin are involved (superficial thrombophlebitis) the area is red, hot, and tender. This type of thrombophlebitis may be treated at home with compresses, leg elevation, and anti-inflammatory drugs.

With deep thrombophlebitis, there is usually a slight elevation of temperature and pulse rate; in fact, this finding may be the first to draw attention to the possibility of

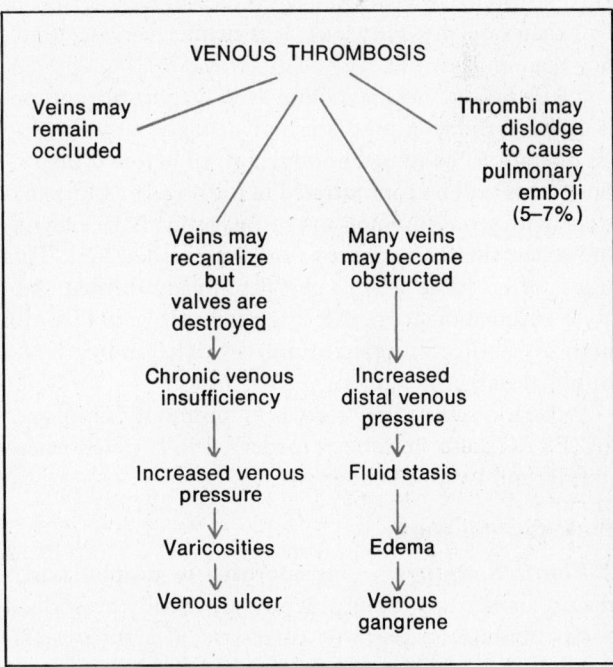

Figure 31-12. The seriousness of venous thrombosis is readily noted.

HIGH RISK FOR THROMBOPHLEBITIS

Bed rest—myocardial infarction, congestive heart failure, sepsis, traction

General surgery—in patients over 40 years old

Leg trauma—especially fractures, casts

Previous venous insufficiency

Obesity

Oral contraceptives

Malignancy

phlebitis in a postoperative patient. In addition, the nurse should look for early signs of edema, such as filling out of the concavity behind the medial malleolus.

Diagnostic Evaluation

Phlebography (venography) is the injection of a contrast solution into the venous system through a dorsal foot vein. The surgeon searches for four cardinal signs of phlebothrombosis: (1) constant filling defects, (2) termination of a dye column, (3) nonfilling of portions of, or of the entire venous system, and (4) diversion of dye to superficial channels. Unfortunately this is an invasive diagnostic method and may cause painful side effects.

Another method is to measure alterations in velocity of blood flow in leg veins by an *ultrasonic Doppler flowmeter.* This method is relatively inexpensive, very accurate, simple, rapid, and noninvasive but it requires skill on the part of the user (see pages 617–618).

Electrical impedance plethysmography is a diagnostic procedure in which the changes in electrical impedance in a current applied to a patient's legs is measured as he inhales or exhales deeply. However, it is neither very accurate, nor readily available.

^{125}I *fibrinogen,* a recent noninvasive diagnostic method, is useful in the asymptomatic high-risk patient following an operation. Labeled fibrinogen given before a thrombus forms will be concentrated in the area of clot formation. With serial scanning and comparison of one leg with the other, the formation of clots may be detected. This test is of no value when a clot has already formed. The chief disadvantages are that it is not sensitive to thrombi high in the ileofemoral region, is costly, and carries a minimal risk of hepatitis.

Other "noninvasive" tests not commonly employed are PVR (pulse volume recorder), PRG (phleborheogram), and isotope venogram.

Preventive Measures

Elastic Stockings. One approach to prophylaxis is the use of elastic stockings, which are usually prescribed for patients on a regimen of restricted activity, particularly those who are confined to bed. These stockings, by exerting a sustained, evenly distributed pressure over the entire surface of the calves, reduce the caliber of the superficial veins of the lower extremities, with the result that deeper venous blood flow is speeded and any tendency toward stagnation or pooling of blood in that area is reduced or abolished. It is important to note that any type of stocking, including the elastic type, can be converted into a tourniquet if applied incorrectly, i.e., rolled tightly at the top. In such instances, the stockings will produce stasis instead of reducing it. Elastic stockings are removed for a brief interval at least twice daily. While they are off, the skin should be inspected for signs of irritation and the calves examined for possible tenderness. Any skin changes or signs of tenderness should be reported.

Recent research studies have questioned the value of using elastic stockings and have indicated that the stockings may be ineffective or provide only modest benefit in some patients. There is some indication that on occasion stockings may even be dangerous. Because of differing opinions, the use of stockings will be determined by the patient's physician.

When elastic adhesive bandages (Elastoplast) are used, it is recommended that 10 cm. (4-inch) gauze bandage be applied loosely before the elastic adhesive bandage is put on. This will make it easier to remove the bandage with a blunt bandage scissors since skin and hair will not be pulled off.

An elastic bandage with good elasticity and with clips attached is useful and safer, particularly for elderly persons.

Body Position and Exercise. When the patient is on bed rest, the feet and lower legs should be elevated periodically above heart level. The superficial and tibial veins empty rapidly in this position and remain collapsed. A position with the head lower than the body is not recommended since respiratory difficulties may ensue.

Active and passive leg exercises, particularly those involving calf muscles, are done during the postoperative period to increase venous flow. Early ambulation is most effective in preventing venous stasis. Deep-breathing exercises are beneficial, since they produce increased negative pressure in the thorax which assists in emptying the large veins.

Intermittent Venous Compression. Although not commonly used, intermittent venous compression may help to prevent deep vein thrombosis. When this treatment plan is instituted, inflatable surgical plastic boots are placed on the patient's legs. The boots consist of a soft plastic inner boot and an inelastic outer boot which are attached at the top and heel. The leg appears to float, since pressure is exerted uniformly in all directions. Cyclic inflation and deflation of the boot provides intermittent repetitive compression of the feet and legs. Such comprssion can be used in the operating room and during the postoperative period until the patient is ambulatory. The boots can be removed and reapplied daily by the nurse to permit skin care. Although intermittent venous compression boots can be worn with comfort for long periods of time, their use is contraindicated in patients with acute thrombophlebitis and suspected deep vein thrombosis.

Nursing Assessment

Careful nursing assessment is invaluable in detecting early signs of venous disorders of the lower extremity. Particularly susceptible are patients with a history of varicose veins, hypercoagulation, cardiovascular disease, or recent major surgery or injury. Obese and elderly people and women taking oral contraceptives are also in the high risk group.

- Question the patient about the presence of leg pain, any functional impairment, or edema.
- Inspect the legs from the groin to the feet, noting asymmetry and measuring and recording calf circumference. (One early indication of edema is engorgement of the concavity behind the medial malleolus.)
- Note any increase in temperature in the affected leg. (To determine temperature differences more effectively, cool hands in cold water, dry, and place them simultaneously on both of the patient's ankles and then on the calves.)
- To identify areas of tenderness and any thromboses (as evidenced by cordlike venous segments), palpate the leg carefully using three or four fingers, advancing the hands back and forth from the ankle to the knee and then to the groin.

Management

The objectives of treatment are to prevent fatal pulmonary embolism and to prevent chronic venous insufficiency and its sequelae.

For acute thrombophlebitis, heparin is administered by intermittent intravenous infusion (every 4 hours) or by continuous infusion that is regulated to keep the partial thromboplastin time (PTT) between 50 and 80 seconds. (See also the discussion under anticoagulant therapy.)

After the desired response to heparin therapy has been achieved, the patient is placed on warfarin therapy. This continues for approximately 12 to 14 weeks.

If the use of heparin is contraindicated, dextran is an effective agent. The use of thrombolytic enzymes (urokinase or streptokinase) is accompanied by a higher incidence of bleeding and febrile reactions. Therefore, history of surgery, trauma, or childbirth within the previous 10 days would be a contraindication to their use. Fibrinolytic therapy is ineffective when clots have been present for at least four days. When thrombolytic agents are used, they are usually administered intravenously by infusion pump.

For a summary view of the clinical manifestations, diagnostic evaluation, and management of phlebitis, see Table 31-5.

Surgical Management

Although anticoagulants and prophylaxis (ambulation and elastic stockings) are the first line of defense against phlebitis and venous embolism, there are times when surgery is required in the management of these patients.

The surgical approach is necessary when (1) the patient cannot be given anticoagulants; (2) the danger of pulmonary embolism is extreme; (3) the venous drainage is so severely compromised that permanent limb damage will probably result; and (4) rarely, to remove life-threatening pulmonary emboli already present.

TABLE 31-5. PHLEBITIS

	SUPERFICIAL	DEEP

Clinical Manifestations	Local swelling; bumpy and knotty
	Red, tender, local induration
		"Heaviness" on standing
		Cramping leg pain
		Swelling:
		  Calf vein thrombus—none
		  Femoral vein thrombus—mild to moderate
		  Ileofemoral vein thrombus—severe
		Positive Homans' sign

Assessment	Venography—to rule out deep vein thrombosis	Blood flow studies to show inflow, filling and emptying Venography—to determine presence of phlebitis, recanalization, extent of occlusion
Management	Bed rest Warm moist compresses Legs elevated Then, elastic support after acute stage Heparin, intermittent or continuous Acetaminophen for pain Antibiotics if necessary If deep veins are patent, superficial phlebitic veins may be removed	Bed rest Warm moist compresses Foot of bed elevated to 15 cm. (6 in.) Surgery, possibly, to prevent embolic development

In those patients (groups 1 and 2 above) in whom pulmonary emboli must be prevented, venous interruption is performed. Most commonly, the inferior vena cava is ligated or plicated (narrowed from one large channel to three or four small channels), usually by a Teflon clip. Another method involves the insertion of an "umbrella" filter mounted on a catheter and passed into proper position under fluoroscopic control via the internal jugular vein (see page 492).

These procedures prevent large clots from traveling to the lung and causing blockage of the pulmonary artery. However one must keep in mind that large collateral venous pathways often develop within one year or so. Thus the benefit of vena caval ligation is not permanent.

In patients with severely compromised venous drainage (group 3), venous thrombectomy may be performed, although it is being used less frequently today.

Finally, for those patients who already have *life-threatening* pulmonary emboli (group 4), a pulmonary embolectomy may be required. Cardiopulmonary bypass is necessary, since the main pulmonary artery must be opened to remove emboli from both the right and left pulmonary arteries. This procedure is only rarely performed.

ANTICOAGULANT THERAPY FOR THROMBOEMBOLISM

Anticoagulant therapy is the administration of a medication to delay the clotting time of blood, to prevent the formation of a thrombus in postoperative patients, and to forestall the extension of a thrombus once it has formed. Anticoagulants cannot dissolve a thrombus that has already formed.

Measures for the *prevention* or reduction of blood clotting within the vascular system are indicated in patients with thrombophlebitis, patients suspected of recurrent embolus formation, those with persistent leg edema secondary to heart failure, and the elderly person with a hip fracture who is likely to be immobilized for a considerable time. The usual treatment consists of the single or combined administration of heparin or coumarin derivatives which reduce the normal activity of the clotting mechanism (see Table 31-6). The precise dose required to treat a thromboembolic problem without causing bleeding is difficult to determine.

Administration

Heparin is administered until clinical symptoms have disappeared (usually about 10 days). Generally, the patient with phlebitis is required to remain on bed rest, with the foot of the bed slightly elevated to promote venous drainage.

Continuous pump infusion is the preferred method for administering heparin (providing there are appropriate facilities and adequate personnel for monitoring). This method is preferred mainly because of the low incidence of hemorrhagic complications. Dosage is calculated on the basis of weight and any possible bleeding tendencies indicated by a pretreatment clotting profile. If renal insufficiency exists, lower doses are required. To prevent accidents or malfunction, the pump is placed out of reach of the patient. The nurse periodically checks for kinks or leaks in the tubing and inspects the entire system frequently to ensure that the exact dose is being administered. A calibrated burette chamber is usually located between the pump and the reservoir container (containing a 24-hour dose) to provide a means of monitoring the infusion rate. Periodic coagulation tests are obtained, including hematocrit and partial thromboplastin time (PTT). The nursing assessment also includes observing the patient for bleeding gums and ecchymotic areas and any signs of pain or ileus. In some instances, continuous infusion pumps are battery-powered to permit ambulation.

Intermittent intravenous injection is another means of administering heparin, in this instance as a dilute aqueous solution given every 4 hours. Administration may be facilitated by the use of a "heparin lock"—a small butterfly-type scalp vein needle with injection site at end of tubing (rubber diaphragm) usually inserted into the dorsum of the hand for intermittent therapy.

Subcutaneous injection of heparin may be administered at 8- or 12-hour intervals when given prophylactically or for long-term therapy. However, this method is not preferred for the management of acute problems.

Minidose heparin is the administration of small doses of heparin which can block the generation of large amounts of thrombin by inactivating coagulation Factors II, IX, X, XI, and XII. This method is used to reduce the incidence of postoperative thromboembolism. However, it is reportedly not as effective in hip surgery cases. No dietary restrictions are required with this form of therapy. Minidose heparin is injected into the lower abdomen or thigh. If minor ecchymosis or allergic reactions occur, it may be necessary to change to oral anticoagulants.

Oral anticoagulants, when used, require close laboratory monitoring.

Heparin therapy is usually given for a minimum of 7 to 10 days. Following hospitalization for venous thromboembolism, oral anticoagulant therapy may be continued for 3 or 4 months.

Anticoagulant therapy is contraindicated in conditions which increase the risk of hemorrhage. (See chart, page 639.)

Precautions and Nursing Assessment. *The principal complication of anticoagulant therapy is the occurrence of spontaneous bleeding anywhere in the body.* The earliest evidence of such a predisposition is obtained on routine examination of the urine; evidence of bleeding from the kidneys

TABLE 31-6. COMPARISON OF HEPARIN AND COUMARIN DERIVATIVES

	HEPARIN SODIUM	COUMARIN DERIVATIVES
Physiologic Action	Interferes with clotting reaction at many points but primarily acts as an antagonist to thrombin.	Blocks the formation of prothrombin from vitamin K, a conversion normally taking place in the liver.
Therapeutic Action		
Advantages	Used for short-term therapy primarily (may also be used for long-term therapy). Action is prompt and predictable. It can be used outside the body as well as inside: it may be used in certain dialysis procedures and in place of sodium citrate in donor blood.	Used for long-term therapy. Is given orally and provides efficient absorption from gastrointestinal tract. Uniform strength of medication because of synthetic production. Less expensive than heparin sodium. Control factor better than with heparin sodium. Sodium warfarin more completely absorbed than bishydroxycoumarin.
Disadvantages	Must be given parenterally, intravenously, or into the fat subcutaneously. A few patients have developed allergic reactions, and transient hair loss or osteoporosis has been reported (after several months of therapy).	Prolonged lag period (2-3 days) before the appearance of its effect. Unpredictable duration of anticoagulant action (at times persisting up to 3 weeks).
Administration	Test clotting and prothrombin time first. Clotting times are obtained every 4-6 hours, at which time repeat doses of heparin are given. The object is to get the clotting time 2 to 3 times the normal control (first clotting time). *Subcutaneous route*—least recommended because of erratic absorption, possible puncture of vessels, and discomfort. The average therapeutic dose is 20,000-30,000 units daily either by *continuous infusion* with an infusion pump or in divided doses by *intermittent IV injection* every 4-6 hours. *Prolonged Therapy:* May be given deep subcutaneously (into the fat) in lower abdomen. Use a fine, short, sharp needle (No. 25-27 gauge, 1.27-1.60 cm. [0.5-0.62 inches]). Grasp roll of fat gently, and in dartlike fashion insert needle at right angle to the skin surface. Following injection, do not rub site but firmly press site with an alcohol sponge. Each time use a new location on lower abdomen. *Note:* Intramuscular administration of heparin is avoided because of likelihood of local hematomas and tissue irritation.	Test prothrombin clotting time first. (See below.) Warfarin: Administer initial dose of 15-25 mg. Give a second dose, somewhat smaller, on following day (10 mg.). Adjust subsequent doses on basis of daily prothrombin determinations. Average dose usually 5 mg./day. Therapeutic level of hypoprothrombinemia may be reached in 3-4 days.
Antidote	Discontinue heparin. Protamine sulfate (acts as a base to neutralize acidic heparin). Blood transfusion when hemorrhage is present.	Administer vitamin K preparations: For mild bleeding control: Phytonadione tablets (oral use) (Mephyton) (vitamin K₁) For moderate to severe bleeding control: Phytonadione solution (Aqua-MEPHYTON) IV or IM.

Prothrombin Time is measured in seconds or percent of normal.
  Normal: 12.5 seconds or 100%
  Desired therapeutic range: 25-30 seconds when the control is 12 seconds (approximately 1½-2½ times the control in seconds). When the prothrombin time is measured in percent of normal, the desired therapeutic range is felt to be 20-30 percent.

(microscopic hematuria) is one of the first signs of danger. The nurse is alert for evidence of bruises, nosebleeds, and bleeding gums as early signs of a tendency to bleed. The effects of heparin can be abolished very promptly by the intravenous injection of protamine sulfate, the dosage of which should be approximately the same as that of the heparin given in the previous dose. The elimination of coumarin derivatives is more difficult, but effective mea-

<table>
<tr><td colspan="2">

**CONTRAINDICATIONS TO
ANTICOAGULANT THERAPY**
Risk Factors

Lack of patient cooperation

Bleeding from the following tracts:
    Gastrointestinal
    Genitourinary
    Respiratory

Hemorrhagic blood dyscrasias

Aneurysms

Severe trauma

Alcoholism

Compulsive drug use

Recent or impending surgery of:
    Eye
    Spinal cord
    Brain

Severe hepatic or renal disease

Recent cerebrovascular hemorrhage

Infections

Open ulcerative wounds

Occupations that involve a significant hazard of injury

</td></tr>
</table>

sures include administering phytonadione and possibly fresh whole blood or plasma.

Interaction between oral anticoagulants and other medications needs to be observed; for example: salicylates decrease prothrombin activity; vitamins in multivitamin combinations contain vitamin K, which will increase prothrombin activity; antibiotics can alter intestinal flora, which may interfere with the synthesis of vitamin K; mineral oil interferes with the absorption of fat-soluble vitamins, which may cause a vitamin K deficiency; mineral oil may also interfere with the absorption of anticoagulants; alcohol ingested in excessive amounts can decrease prothrombin activity; barbiturates increase the metabolism of coumarin drugs; and phenylbutazone (Butazolidin) augments the action of coumarin compounds. In addition, different individuals react differently to the various drugs.

Patient Education about Oral Anticoagulants

The patient should be informed about the medication he is taking, its purpose, and the need to take the correct amount at the specific times prescribed. He should also be aware that blood tests are scheduled periodically to determine how the blood is clotting and whether a change in medication dosage is required.

Specific teaching directives should include the following points:
- Take the anticoagulant tablet at the same time each day, usually between 8:00 and 9:00 A.M.
- Wear or carry identification indicating what anticoagulant is being taken.

- Since other medications affect the way the anticoagulant normally acts, do not take any of the following medications without the physician's consent: vitamins, cold medicines, antibiotics, aspirin, mineral oil, and phenylbutazone (Butazolidin).
- Remember that alcohol may alter the body's response to an anticoagulant.
- Avoid food fads, crash diets, or marked changes in eating habits.
- Do not take Coumadin unless so directed by the physician.
- Do not stop taking Coumadin (when prescribed) unless so directed by the physician or nurse.
- When seeking treatment from another physician, a dentist, or a podiatrist, indicate that an anticoagulant is being taken.
- Contact personal physician prior to dental extraction or elective surgery.
- If any of the following signs appear, report them immediately to the physician.
    faintness, dizziness, or increased weakness
    severe headaches or stomach pain
    red or brown urine
    any bleeding, such as cuts that do not stop bleeding
    bruises that increase in size, nosebleeds, or unusual
      bleeding from any part of the body
    red or black bowel movements
    skin rash
    pregnancy
- Be extra careful to avoid injury that can cause bleeding.
- Women should notify their physicians if they suspect that they are pregnant.

CHRONIC VENOUS INSUFFICIENCY

Pathophysiology and Clinical Manifestations

Recovery from an attack of phlebitis is not always a complete cure. When the main channel for the return of blood from the leg to the heart is blocked by the thrombus, smaller vessels dilate, especially the long superficial saphenous vein, to take up the burden of the increased venous flow. The deep vein blockage may be permanent or the clot may become recanalized so that blood can flow through or around the clot. However, with this process, the valves of the veins become perforated and incompetent and no longer can prevent backflow in the vessels. This results in chronic venous stasis, with swelling and edema, and a further difficulty — varicose superficial veins. The lower leg becomes pigmented, dry, and scaly and an ulceration frequently develops on the inner side of the leg, just above the ankle. This type of ulcer is really a stasis ulcer, but since a large part of the stasis is due to the phlebitis, such ulcers are called *postphlebitic ulcers*. They differ from the common "varicose ulcer" only in the fact that the venous stasis results from disease of the deep veins and not wholly from the dilated varicose superficial veins (see page 614).

Postphlebitic syndrome results in chronic venous stasis with associated changes, mainly on the medial lower leg: discoloration, swelling, ulceration, pain, venous congestion, and recurrent thromboses. The treatment of this type of venous stasis is much more difficult than treatment for stasis resulting from varicosities of only the superficial veins. In some patients there may be no visible or palpable superficial venous enlargement.

These changes take many years to develop. It may take 15 years to progress from edema through stasis pigmentation, stasis dermatitis, and finally stasis ulceration. Much of this process can be prevented by proper elastic support and periodic leg elevation. Much depends on which veins are affected and the extent of the problem. Gravity imposes overwhelming stress on the postphlebitic system. With increased pressure and stagnant blood in the dependent channels, edema results. Fibrosis follows each bout of edema. In addition, cutaneous reaction to chronic venous hypertension becomes critical. Itching, skin cracking, microscopic superficial infections, and reactions to medicaments used in treating the skin problem result. There is increasing pigmentation and the skin begins to atrophy and becomes susceptible to injury.

Management and Patient Teaching

Various measures have been suggested in the attempt to remove the venous stasis. These include ligation of the superficial femoral veins and the saphenous veins (long and short), if these are varicosed. Most often a more conservative method of therapy is applied, consisting largely of methods to prevent venous stasis by providing external pressure and gravity drainage of venous blood.

In order to impress upon the patient with phlebitis the necessity for thwarting venous stasis and edema of the legs, the following rules are suggested:

1. Prevent edema by wearing elastic stockings from the mid-foot to just below the knee. These work best when fitted to the individual. Details of care are described on page 646.
2. Mere standing or sitting produces increased venous stasis; therefore, some slight exercise should be attempted, such as walking, moving the toes in the shoes, etc. During the year following the attack of phlebitis, the legs should be elevated to a horizontal position on a chair (with full length support) at least 5 minutes out of every 2 hours.
3. At least 2 or 3 times a day the patient should lie down in order to elevate the legs above the head. He should lie on his back and elevate the leg on the back of the sofa or even against the wall, so that the venous blood is drained by gravity from the part.
4. At night, the foot of the bed should be elevated 15-20 cm. (6-8 inches) to promote venous drainage by gravity.
5. Patients with irritation of the skin of the leg should apply bland, oily lotions to prevent scaling and dryness.
6. Constricting bandages, panty girdles, and the indiscriminate use of tourniquets must be avoided.
7. Finally, the patient shoud be careful to avoid all trauma, bruising, scratching, or other forms of injury to the skin of the leg and the foot.

When these suggestions are carried out repeatedly, it is possible to avoid many of the complications that otherwise appear in the postphlebitic leg.

HEALTH TEACHING: CARE OF THE FEET AND LEGS FOR THE PERSON WITH A PERIPHERAL VASCULAR PROBLEM

CLEANLINESS
1. Wash feet at least once daily.
2. Use warm water and bland soap.
3. Dry feet thoroughly, especially between the toes. Blot and pat with a towel but do not rub.

WARMTH
1. Wear cotton hose, since they are comfortable and absorb moisture.
2. Prevent feet from getting cold; this reduces blood supply
3. Avoid applying heat to the feet or legs unless approved by a physician or nurse.
4. Avoid swimming in cold water.
5. Avoid sunburn.

SAFETY
1. Protect feet by performing exercises on level ground.
2. Avoid walking in crowds.
3. Use care in cutting toenails.
   a. First soak feet for 10 minutes in warm water to soften nails.
   b. Cut nails straight across; avoid cutting nails close to flesh.

COMFORT MEASURES
1. Wear shoes that provide adequate toe room, have a good arch, and feel comfortable.
2. Apply powder if feet tend to become moist.
3. Apply a thin coating of lanolin if feet are dry and scaly.

PREVENTING CONSTRICTION OF BLOOD VESSELS
1. Avoid circular garters that cut off blood supply to legs and feet.
2. Do not cross legs at knees.
3. Place a pillow at foot end of bed under covers to prevent top bedding from exerting pressure on toes.
4. Apply lamb's wool between toes if they rub each other.

EXERCISE
Walking stimulates circulation and promotes tissue repair.

MEDICAL ATTENTION
1. Report redness. blistering, swelling, or pain.
2. Report athlete's foot, peeling and itching between toes.
3. Do not use any medication on feet or legs unless prescribed by the physician.

SMOKING
Avoid tobacco in any form, since it aggravates peripheral vascular conditions.

LEG ULCERS

A leg ulcer is an excavation of the skin surface that is produced by the sloughing of inflammatory necrotic tissue. The most frequent cause is vascular insufficiency, either venous or arteriolar. It is estimated that of all leg

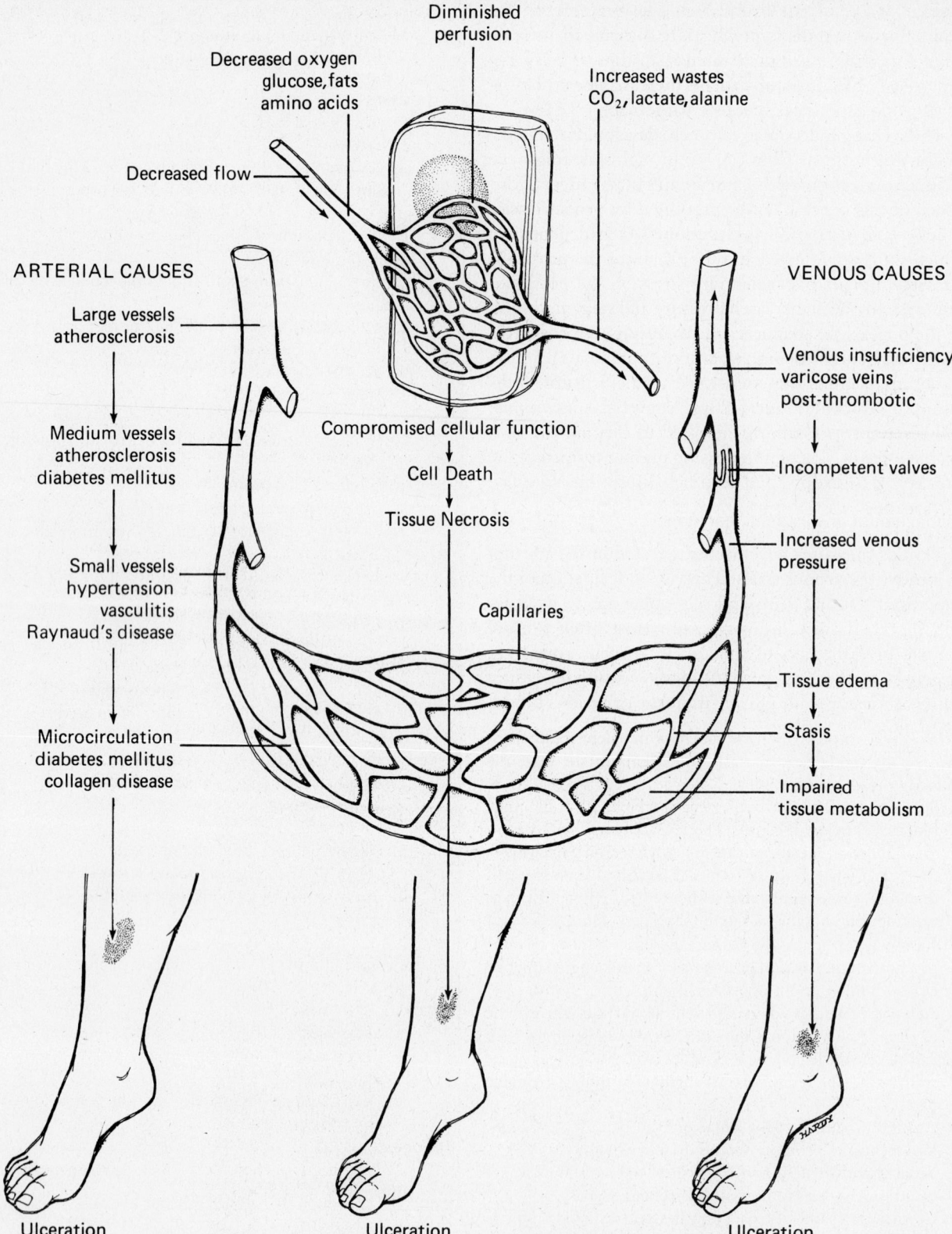

Diminished
perfusion

Decreased oxygen
glucose, fats
amino acids

Increased wastes
CO_2, lactate, alanine

Decreased flow

ARTERIAL CAUSES

Large vessels
atherosclerosis

Medium vessels
atherosclerosis
diabetes mellitus

Small vessels
hypertension
vasculitis
Raynaud's disease

Microcirculation
diabetes mellitus
collagen disease

Compromised cellular function

Cell Death

Tissue Necrosis

Capillaries

VENOUS CAUSES

Venous insufficiency
varicose veins
post-thrombotic

Incompetent valves

Increased venous
pressure

Tissue edema

Stasis

Impaired
tissue metabolism

Ulceration

Ulceration

Ulceration

Figure 31-13. Pathophysiology of leg ulcers. On the left are indicated some of the conditions that cause diminished blood flow to peripheral tissue. Oxygen and energy sources are further aggravated by capillary changes brought about by diabetes mellitus and collagen disease. Cellular function is compromised when insufficient oxygen and energy substrates are supplied. Tissue necrosis takes place and results in ulceration. A somewhat similar situation occurs when there is venous insufficiency brought about by a different hemodynamic pattern. Increased venous pressure reduces capillary flow. Edema and stasis result, impairing cellular metabolism and again leading to ulceration.

ulcers, postphlebitic and varicose ulcers account for about 70 percent; the remaining 30 percent, such as those caused by burns, sickle-cell anemia, and neurogenic disorders, are of nonvenous origin. Venous ulcers usually occur above the medial ankle (malleolus), whereas arterial ulcers occur farther from the ankle and sometimes higher.

The nursing challenge in caring for these persons is great, whether the older person is in the hospital or at home. The physical problem is often a long-term one that causes a substantial drain on the patient's physical, emotional, and economic resources.

Pathophysiology. Inadequate exchange of oxygen and nutrient substrates in the tissue is the metabolic abnormality underlying the development of leg ulcers. When the cellular metabolism cannot maintain energy balance, cell death results (necrosis). Alterations in blood vessels at the arterial, capillary, and venous level may affect cellular processes and lead to the formation of ulcers (Fig. 31-13).

Assessment. Because there are many causes of ulcers, it is important that a proper causative diagnosis be made so that appropriate therapy may be prescribed. The medical and nursing history of the person is important in determining venous or arterial insufficiency. Symptoms of aching, fatigue, heaviness, and especially swelling of the leg should be evaluated, and aortic, iliac, femoral, popliteal, and pedal pulses should be carefully checked. Note dependent redness. Look for chronic pitting or nonpitting edema. More conclusive diagnostic aids are Doppler ultrasound studies, arteriography, and venography. Laboratory tests can assist in determining whether infection is the primary cause of the ulcer; cultures may be required.

Management

Objectives of therapy can be successfully managed by simple therapy of the ulcer itself:

1. To control infection: Since all ulcers are infected, it is necessary to establish dependent drainage. Systemic antimicrobial therapy is used based on appropriate culture and sensitivity determinations. Topical antibiotics have not been as effective as desired.
2. To promote healing by keeping the wound clean: Cleansing requires very gentle handling; a mild soap, lukewarm water, and cotton balls are used. Flushing out of necrotic material can be done with hydrogen peroxide. Debriding can be performed using instruments to cut away devitalized tissue. It can also be done by applying isotonic saline dressings of fine mesh gauze to the ulcer bed. When dry, the dressing is removed along with the debris adhering to the gauze.

Enzymatic debridement may be preferred by some physicians and enzyme ointments may be used to treat the ulcer. The ointment is placed over the lesion but not over normal surrounding skin. The lesion and ointment are then covered with a saline-soaked sponge that has been thoroughly wrung out. A gauze dressing and a loose bandage are then applied. For the first 3 or 4 days, applications are made every fourth hour, then every eighth hour. When pink granulating tissue develops, saline wet dressings are used.

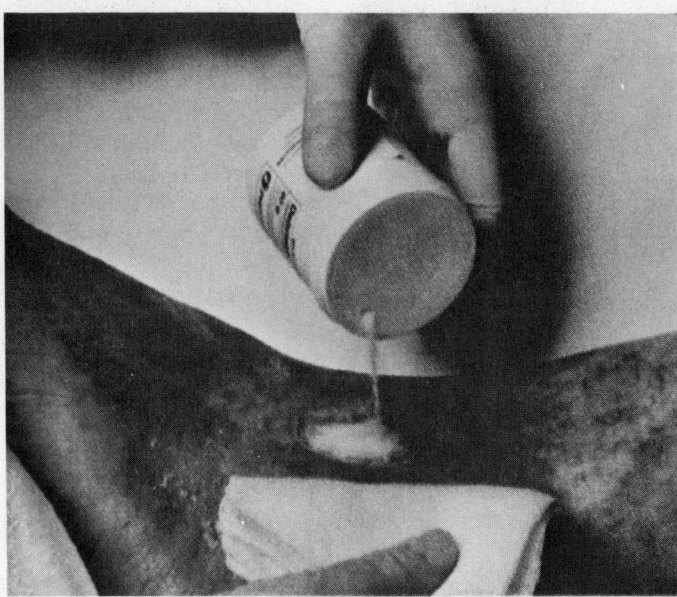

Figure 31-14. Method of applying dextranomer (Debrisan). A layer of dextranomer is poured into the lesion or ulcer after the wound has been cleansed with water and saline or another solution. The layer should be approximately 3mm. (1/8 inch) deep. (Courtesy, Pharmacia Laboratories, Div. of Pharmacia, Inc., 800 Centennial Ave., Piscataway, N.J. 08854)

A newer method of treating ulcers involves the use of dextranomer (Debrisan) beads, small highly porous spherical beads (0.1 to 0.3 mm. in diameter) that possess the ability to absorb wound secretions. Bacteria and products of tissue necrosis and protein degradation are actively suctioned into the bead layer, which changes color according to the infecting organism. When the beads are completely saturated they take on a greyish-yellow color, at which point their cleansing action stops. When the beads become saturated, they should be removed and a fresh layer should be applied (Fig. 31-14).

3. To provide rest: If there is arterial insufficiency, blood flow may be improved by elevating the head of the bed on 7.5- to 15-cm. (3- to 6-inch) blocks. Note whether such elevation increases dependent edema, since this must be avoided. Supplemental diuretics may be required.

4. To correct nutritional disturbances: Nutritional deficiencies must be determined and an adequate diet maintained. Such a diet should include vitamins (particularly vitamin C), protein, and minerals (iron).

5. To revascularize tissue by arterial reconstruction: Aortoiliac, aortofemoral, or femoropopliteal revascularization often are effective in correcting arterial insufficiency.

After 2 or 3 days of complete bed rest, an occlusive dressing may be applied. This can be an elastoplast bandage (Fig. 31-15), Unna boot, or a plaster of paris cast. Usually it requires 2 to 3 weeks for an average-sized ulcer (3 to 4 cm. in diameter) to heal. Once the cast or boot is removed, an elastic stocking is worn on the healed leg. Patient instruction is required for successful therapy.

VARICOSE VEINS

The Problem and Its Incidence

Varicose veins (varicosities) are abnormally dilated veins. Most commonly this condition occurs in the lower extremities or the lower trunk; however, it can occur elsewhere in the body, e.g., esophageal varices (page 819).

It is estimated that varicose veins affect one out of five individuals in the world. Occupation may be a factor in that the incidence of this problem is higher among sales-

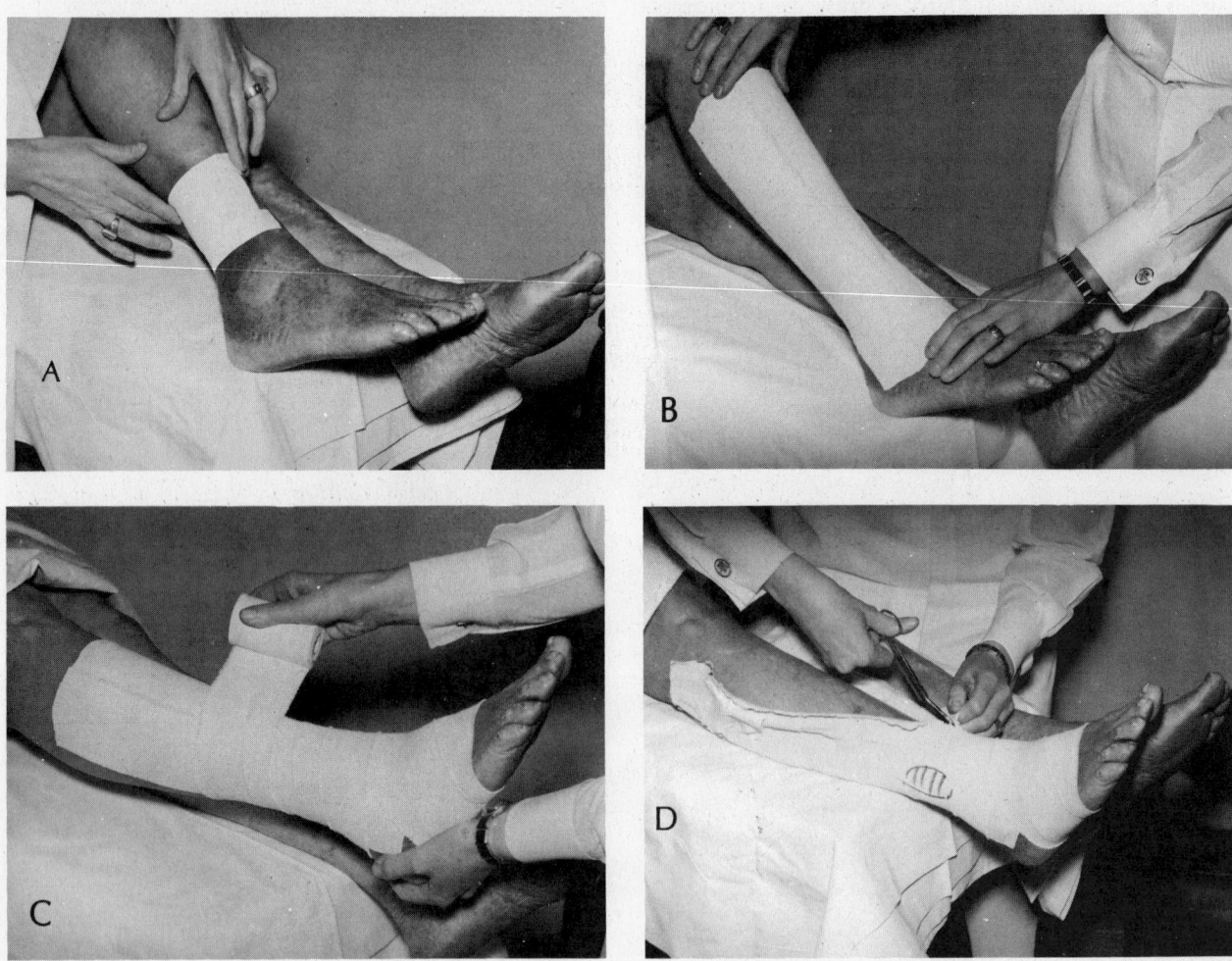

Figure 31-15. Elastoplast bandage: (A) After ointment has been applied, ulcer is covered with a Telfa or other nonadherent bandage and secured with nonallergic tape if plain adhesive irritates the patient's skin. (B) Strips of Elastoplast give support and protection. (C) Starting with a turn around foot, bandage is spiraled upward with firm, even pressure and fastened securely below knee. (D) After several days, bandages must be removed with special care; even slight trauma could cause injury. (From Wilson, S.: Chronic leg ulcers. American Journal of Nursing, 67:98.)

people, barbers, beauticians, elevator operators, nurses, and dentists than among individuals who sit most of the day. However, sedentary workers need to walk at periodic intervals to prevent stasis in the lower leg.

Pathophysiology and Manifestations

The blood flow in the veins is directed back toward the heart; its flow in the reverse direction is prevented by a series of cup-shaped valves (Fig. 31-16). A deficiency of these valves may be produced by disease, as in phlebitis, or by long-standing distention due to back pressure on the veins, as in pregnancy, obesity, or prolonged standing. A hereditary weakness of the vein wall may also contribute to the difficulty, and it is not uncommon to see this condition occur in families.

The veins most commonly affected in the lower extremities lie in the subcutaneous fatty tissues, especially the long saphenous vein. The dilatation of this vein produces a venous stasis with secondary edema, replacement fibrosis in the subcutaneous fatty tissue, pigmentation of the skin, and, because of these changes, lowered resistance to infection and to trauma.

The manifestations most often seen are disfigurement due to the large size of the vein, easy fatigue of the part, a heavy feeling, cramps in the legs at night, and pain during the menstrual period. The darkened, tortuous, swollen veins are more prominent when the patient stands, and a common reason for their treatment in women is cosmetic concern.

If varicose veins are untreated, the aforementioned changes in the lower leg may appear. Repeated attacks of inflammation are not uncommon and ulceration may develop.

Assessment

A common diagnostic test for varicose veins is the *Brodie-Trendelenburg test.* This is a test to demonstrate competence of the valves of the superficial veins and of the branches that communicate with the deep veins of the leg. With the patient lying down, the leg is elevated to empty the veins. A tourniquet is then applied around the upper thigh and the patient is asked to stand. If the valves of the communicating veins are incompetent, blood flows into the superficial vein from the deep veins; if the tourniquet is then released and blood flows rapidly from above into the superficial vein, the inference is that the valves of the superficial vein are also incompetent. This test is used to determine the type of treatment to be recommended for the varicose veins.

The *Perthes' test* is another diagnostic procedure that easily indicates whether the deeper venous system and communicating veins are competent. A tourniquet is applied just below the knee and the patient is requested to walk. If the varicose veins disappear, the deep system and communicating vessels are competent. If the vessels do

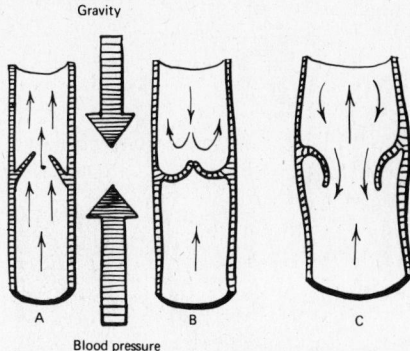

Figure 31-16. (*A, B*) *Competent* valves showing blood flow patterns when the valve is open (*A*) and closed (*B*) allowing blood to flow against gravity. (*C*) With faulty, or *incompetent*, valves, the blood is unable to move toward the heart.

not empty and become even more distended on walking, incompetency or obstruction is established.

A test done less often is phlebography, or venography, in which the veins are injected with a radiopaque substance to show evidence of occluded veins or old venous disease. Thermography and Doppler flow studies are other tests done by some physicians.

Preventive Suggestions and Health Teaching

Activities that cause venous stasis should be avoided; e.g., wearing tight garters or a constricting panty girdle that obstructs venous flow; crossing the legs at the thighs, particularly when the wearer is sitting; and sitting or standing for long periods of time. Frequent changes of position, elevating the legs when they are tired, and getting up to walk several minutes of every hour promote circulation. The patient should be encouraged to walk one or two miles a day if there are no contraindications. Walking up the stairs rather than using the elevator or escalator is helpful in promoting circulation. Swimming is also good exercise for the legs.

For primary varicose veins, it may be necessary to wear support hose or elastic stockings that are specifically prescribed by the physician. The overweight patient needs to be guided in a weight-reduction plan.

Surgical Treatment

In the treatment of secondary varicose veins, it is essential to remove the hydrostatic pressure of the column of blood in the veins. To accomplish this it is necessary to interrupt or remove the varicosities and the incompetent perforating veins. This can be done by one or a combination of three methods: (1) ligation, (2) stripping, or (3) sclerotherapy.

Ligation. Although a ligation is considered a minor surgical procedure, the patient receives a general anesthetic. The saphenous vein is ligated at its juncture with the femoral vein for two reasons: (1) to be certain that all tributaries are ligated to prevent their acting as initiating

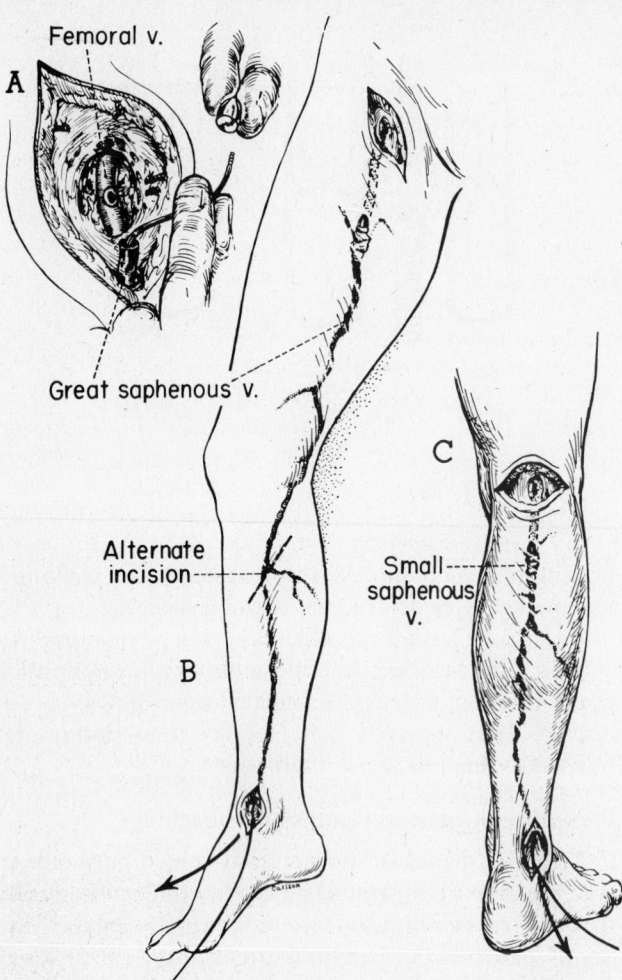

Figure 31-17. Ligation and stripping of the great and the small saphenous veins. (A) The tributaries of the saphenous vein have been ligated, and the saphenous vein has been ligated at the saphenofemoral junction. (B) Vein stripper has been inserted from the ankle superiorly to the groin. The vein is stripped from above downward. A number of alternate incisions may be needed to remove separate varicose masses. (C) The small saphenous vein is stripped from its junction with the popliteal vein to a point posterior to the lateral malleolus. (From Rhoads, et al.: Surgery. Philadelphia, J. B. Lippincott, 1970)

points for future varicosities and (2) to remove a cul-de-sac from which a thrombus could move into the femoral vein.

Stripping. The dilated saphenous vein with its incompetent valves may be removed by a procedure called *"stripping"* (Fig. 31-17). A metal or plastic stripper is inserted into the lower end of the vein in the groin and is threaded down the leg toward the knee and the ankle. If the vein is not too tortuous (twisted) it may be possible to thread the stripper through the entire vein down to the ankle. In other patients the stripper may be caught in vein pockets in the thigh or the leg. An incision is made at the lowermost point of the stripper, and the end of the stripper is pulled out of the vein. Tying the vein to the stripper and pulling downward causes the vein to be pulled out of

its location in the subcutaneous tissues. Pressure along the course of the vein is all that is necessary to control bleeding. After several incisions are made (usually longitudinal and not transverse, since the latter do not heal as well), tortuous veins may also have to be excised. The legs are dressed with gauze and elastic adhesive bandages.

Nursing Management. After the recovery period, the postanesthetic patient is encouraged to walk. Analgesics are permitted, and support and encouragement are offered by the nurse. Circulation is observed in order to detect the possibility of hemorrhage or a dressing that may be too constricting. Instruction is given to help the patient realize that varicosities may recur and that conservative measures practiced before the operation must be continued after he leaves the hospital.

Sclerotherapy. In *sclerotherapy* an irritating chemical is injected into the vein which irritates the vein wall and produces venous fibrosis, thereby obliterating the vein lumen. This treatment may be done by itself for small veins or in combination with ligation or stripping. When done alone, it is usually performed in the clinic or the physician's office. The drug currently favored is sodium tetradecyl sulfate (Sotradecol Sodium) 3 percent. About 0.5 ml. of the medication combined with an equal amount of air is drawn into a syringe and shaken until foamy. After this mixture is injected by means of a fine needle, pressure is applied. A final dressing is covered with a thin foam pad or gauze cotton roll to occlude the vein that has been injected, and an elastic or Velcro bandage is applied to encase the leg. An elastic stocking or flesh-colored elasticized tubular stockinette may then be applied.

The purpose of compression is to push the walls of the vein together so that fibrosis can fuse the opening completely. Physicians differ in the length of time recommended for compression, but usually it varies from 3 to 6 weeks. Walking 2 to 3 miles a day is recommended to encourage blood flow through the unoccluded veins.

If the patient experiences a burning sensation in the injected leg for 1 or 2 nights, a mild sedative and walking will relieve the problem. The bandage should be removed only by the physician. Because bathing may be a problem during this time, a plastic bag may be placed over the bandaged leg and secured above the bandage to allow the patient to shower.

The injection-compression method (sclerotherapy) appears to produce better results when the varicosities are in dilated collecting channels. The surgical stripping and excision methods are better for varicosities of the long and short saphenous channels.

Elastic Stockings

Elastic stockings are available in knee-length or groin-length sizes. The proper technique for putting on elastic stockings is as follows: prior to putting the stocking on, roll the stocking from top to toe. Insert both hands with palms together into the roll, spreading it wide enough to permit the toes of the leg to slip through the roll (Fig. 31-18). Using the thumbs as guides, gently pull the stocking over the heel, ankle, and calf, keeping the stocking smooth and straight. The short stocking should end about 5 cm. (2 inches) below the knee; the long stocking should end about 5 cm. (2 inches) below the groin. Check the stocking for twisting or tightness.

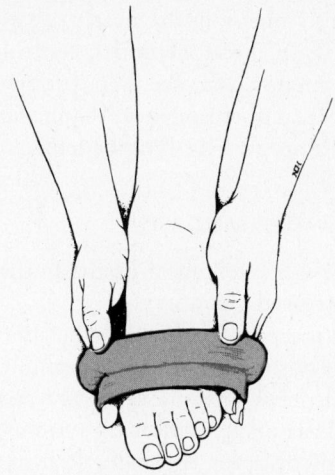

Figure 31-18. A support stocking can be rolled, spread apart, and unrolled as the hands hold it in place—moving from foot to ankle and up the calf.

THE LYMPHATIC SYSTEM

The lymphatic system consists of a set of vessels that spread throughout most of the body. These vessels start as lymph capillaries that drain tissue spaces. They unite to form the lymph vessels, which in turn pass through the lymph nodes and finally empty into the large thoracic duct that joins the jugular vein on the left side of the neck. *Lymph* is the fluid found in lymph vessels. *Tissue fluids* are found outside of vessels in the cellular interspaces. The lymphatic system of the abdominal cavity maintains a steady flow of digested fatty food (chyle) from the intestinal mucosa to the thoracic duct. In other parts of the body the lymphatic system's function is regional; the lymphatic vessels of the head, for example, empty into clusters of lymph nodes located in the neck, and those of the extremities into nodes in the axillae and the groin.

Assessment by Lymphangiography

Radiologic visualization of the lymphatic system is possible after the injection of contrast medium directly into lymphatic vessels in the hands and feet. This technique affords a means of detecting lymph node involvement by metastatic carcinoma, lymphoma, or infection in sites that are otherwise inaccessible to the examiner except by the direct surgical approach—for example, in the pelvis, the retroperitoneum, and deep in the axillae.

The first step in this procedure is the location of a lymphatic vessel in each foot (or hand) by injecting Evans blue dye intradermally between the first and the second digits. Approximately 15 to 20 minutes later, the skin proximal to the injection site is incised. A blue lymphatic segment is identified, isolated, cannulated with a 25- to 30-gauge needle and infused very slowly with a contrast medium containing iodine and oil (Ethiodol). Approximately 10 ml. of this material is injected into the foot (or 5 ml. into the hand) at a rate not exceeding 7 ml. per hour. Appropriate x-ray pictures are taken at the conclusion of the injection, 24 hours later, and periodically thereafter, as indicated. Injection of the feet delineates, for about an hour, the lymphatic channels in the legs and the thoracic duct and, for many weeks, the inguinal, abdominal, and supraclavicular lymph nodes. Similar delineation of lymphatic vessels in the upper extremity, and of the axillary and supraclavicular nodes, follows injection of the hand.

Apart from its diagnostic value in cases of unsuspected lymph-node disease, lymphangiography offers a means of evaluating the presence and the extent of metastases in patients who are known to have cancer. Moreover, since lymphomatous lymph nodes retain the contrast medium for 4 to 6 weeks after the injection, any change in their size that may occur in response to irradiation or chemotherapy can be measured and used as a criterion of therapeutic effect.

LYMPHANGITIS AND LYMPHADENITIS

Lymphangitis is an acute inflammation of the lymphatic channels. It arises most commonly from a focus of infection in an extremity. Usually it is caused by the streptococcus. The characteristic red streaks that extend up the arm or the leg from an infected wound outline the course of the lymphatics as they drain—toward nodes in the elbow or the axilla in the arm, or the knee or the groin in the leg. The presence of a lymphangitis indicates that the infection has not become localized but is extending at least to the lymph nodes. In some patients, the infection may progress and involve the bloodstream (septicemia).

The absorption of toxins produces high fever and often chills, in addition to the local symptoms of pain, tenderness, and swelling along the lymphatics involved. The lymph nodes located along the course of the lymphatic channels also become enlarged, red, and tender (acute lymphadenitis), and can become necrotic and form an abscess (suppurative lymphadenitis). The nodes involved most often are those in the groin, the axilla, or the cervical region.

Because these infections are nearly always caused by organisms that are brought under control rapidly by antibiotics, it is unusual to see them progress to abscess formation. Recurrent episodes of lymphangitis are often associated with progressive lymphedema.

LYMPHEDEMA—ELEPHANTIASIS

Lymphedema is a swelling of tissues in the extremities due to an increased quantity of lymph caused by an obstruction; it is especially marked when the extremity is in a dependent position. The most common type is congenital lymphedema (lymphedema praecox), which is due to hypoplasia of the lymphatic system of the lower extremity. This disorder is usually seen in females and appears first between the ages of 15 and 25.

The obstruction may be in both the lymph nodes and the lymphatic vessels, and at times it is seen in the arm, after a radical mastectomy for carcinoma, and in the leg in association with varicose veins or a chronic phlebitis. In the latter case the lymph block usually is due to a chronic lymphangitis. Lymph block due to a parasite (*Filaria*) is seen frequently in the tropics. When chronic swelling is present, there may be frequent bouts of acute infection characterized by high fever and chills. These lead to chronic fibrosis, thickening of the subcutaneous tissues, and hypertrophy of the skin. This condition, in which chronic swelling of the extremity recedes only slightly with elevation, is given the name *elephantiasis*.

Management

Obstruction of the lymphatic flow in an extremity means that the part involved may be traumatized easily. Conservative measures for treatment include prevention of infection (probably prophylactic antibiotic therapy), elevation of the involved extremity, weight reduction, and restriction of fluid and salt (with the use of diuretics if indicated). Local therapy includes using compression elastic bandages or stockings and pulsatile air pressure devices.

Often elephantiasis produces such marked disability that surgical relief is sought. Fortunately, only a small percent of patients with lymphedema require surgery. In fact, this type of surgery is rarely if ever performed today because prophylactic measures are used before the lymphedema becomes this severe. Indications include persistently increasing size of an extremity in spite of conscientious medical treatment, annoying functional impairment, recurrent bouts of infection, and psychological disturbances due to appearance and self-image.

In the operating room, thickened fibrosed subcutaneous fat and much of the excess skin are cut away, along with the fascia overlying the muscles (Kondolean procedure). Skin grafts are cut from the tissue removed and applied to the exposed muscles. Removing the sub-

cutaneous tissue in which the fluid collects allows the part to return to normal size and function.

Since this type of operation has not been consistently successful, newer approaches include transferring lymphatic channels from healthy areas. Another procedure is to bury an intact dermal flap into the deep tissues to provide a conduit for lymphatic drainage. A third approach is to transpose intact omentum into the lymphedematous extremity. (The lymph vessels of the omentum will then drain the extremity.)

In the postoperative care of these patients, if there are skin grafts in place, pressure dressings are applied until the grafts attach themselves to the underlying muscles. Transfusions may be necessary to prevent the shock that may result from the long operative procedure and rather profuse blood loss. The extremity is elevated for several weeks and then is lowered gradually. If the leg is involved, weight is borne only with support. Precautions to avoid injury must be observed carefully.

BIBLIOGRAPHY

BOOKS

Barker, W. F.: Peripheral Vascular Disease, 2nd ed. Philadelphia, W. B. Saunders, 1975.

Bergan, J. J., and Yao, J. S. T.: Venous Problems. Chicago, Year Book Med. Pub., 1978.

Fairbairn, J. F., et al.: Peripheral Vascular Diseases, 5th ed. Philadelphia, W. B. Saunders, 1979.

Hobbs, J. T., ed.: The Treatment of Venous Disorders. Philadelphia, J. B. Lippincott, 1977.

Perry, H. M., Jr., and Smith, W. M., eds.: Mild Hypertension: To Treat or Not to Treat. New York, Annals of the New York Academy of Sciences, Vol. 304, 1978.

Reid, W., and Pollack, J. G.: The Surgeons' Management of Gangrene. Kent, Eng., Pitman Medical, 1978.

Rushmer, R. F.: Cardiovascular Dynamics. 4th ed. Philadelphia, W. B. Saunders, 1976.

Rutherford, R. D.: Vascular Surgery. Philadelphia, W. B. Saunders, 1977.

U.S. Department of Health, Education, and Welfare, Pub. Health Service: Guidelines for Education of Nurses in High Blood Pressure Control. DHEW Pub. No. (NIH) 77-1241, 1977.

ARTICLES

General

Atchison, J. S., and Murray, J.: Post-vascular surgery. Nursing '78, 8:36-39, Dec. 1978.

Cudkowicz, L.: Current status of thrombolytic therapy. Heart & Lung, 7:97-100, Jan.-Feb. 1978.

Colon, V. F.: To help prevent circulatory problems on long trips. Med. Times, 105:52-54, Jan. 1977.

Deykin, D.: Antithrombotic therapy. Postgrad. Med., 65:135-146, Jan. 1979.

Eddy, M. E.: Teaching patients with peripheral vascular disease. Nurs. Clin. N. Am., *12*:151-159, Mar. 1977.

Hertzer, N. R.: Surgical management of intermittent claudication. Am. Fam. Phys., *16*:108-116, Sept. 1977.

Kanter, S. A.: Angiography management complications. AORN J., *26*:94-99, July 1977.

Miller, K. M.: Assessing peripheral perfusion. AJN, *78*:1673-1674, Oct. 1978.

Pierce, P. F.: Gains and losses of vascular surgery patients. Nurs. Clin. N. Am., *12*:119-127, Mar. 1977.

Precautions to be taken with fibrinolytic therapy. Rockville, Md., FDA Drug Bulletin, *8*:5, Jan.-Feb. 1978.

Ryzewski, J.: Factors in the rehabilitation of patients with peripheral vascular disease. Nurs. Clin. N. Am., *12*:161-168, Mar. 1977.

Smith, R. N.: Invasive pressure monitoring. AJN, *78*: 1514-1521, Sept. 1978.

Aneurysm

Cook, S., and Patrick, H.: A patient with abdominal aortic aneurysm. RN, *41*:71-76, Mar. 1978.

Kleiger, R., et al.: Management of dissecting aortic aneurysm. Arch. Int. Med., *138*:983-986, June 1978.

Lee, K. R., et al.: A practical approach to the diagnosis of abdominal aortic aneurysms. Surgery, *78*:195-201, Aug. 1975.

Long, D. G.: Managing the patient with abdominal aortic aneurysm. Nursing '78, *8*:21-27, Aug. 1978.

Nemir, P., Jr., and Vrachnos, T. C.: The surgical management of abdominal aneurysms. Hosp. Med., *12*:40-61, Jan. 1976.

Setki, G. K., et al.: Dissecting aortic aneurysms. Ann. Thorac. Surg., *18*:201-215, Aug. 1974.

The four faces of aneurysm. Emerg. Med., *8*:140-154, May 1976.

Anticoagulant and Thrombolytic Therapy

Caprini, J. A., and Zoellner, J. L.: Heparin therapy. Cardiovasc. Nurs., Part I: 13-16, May-June 1977; Part II: 17-20, July-Aug. 1977.

Coon, W. W.: Anticoagulant therapy for venous thromboembolism. Postgrad. Med., *63*:157-164, Apr. 1978.

Cudkowicz, L., and Sherry, S.: Current status of thrombolytic therapy. Heart & Lung, 7:97-100, Jan.-Feb. 1978.

Glazier, K. L., and Crowell, E. B.: Randomized prospective trial of continuous vs. intermittent heparin therapy. JAMA, *236*:1365-1367, Sept. 20, 1976.

Hoops, E. J., and Shinn, H.: Clotting and anticoagulants. Crit. Care Update, 4:20-26, Dec. 1977.

Lundin, D. V.: You can inject heparin subcutaneously. RN, *41*:51-54, Dec. 1978.

Moore, K., and Maschak, B. J.: The risks of anticoagulation. Nursing '77: 7:24-29, Sept. 1977.

New anticoagulant: streptokinase. Nurses' Drug Alert, 2:23-24, Mar. 1978.

Silverstein, A.: Neurological complications of anticoagulation therapy. Arch. Int. Med., *139*:217-219, Feb. 1979.

Simon, L., and Likes, K.: Hypothrombinemic response to ice cream. Drug Intelligence & Clin. Pharm., *12*:121-122, Feb. 1978.

Arterial Conditions

Barnes, R. W.: Evaluating peripheral arterial occlusive disease. Postgrad. Med., *59*:98-103, Feb. 1976.

de Wolfe, V. G.: Assessment of the circulation in occlusive arterial disease of the lower extremities. Mod. Concepts Cardiovasc. Dis., *45*:91-95, Apr. 1976.

Drugs for ischemic peripheral arterial disease. Med. Letter, *20*:11, Jan. 27, 1978.

Fagan-Dubin, L.: Atherosclerosis: A major cause of peripheral vascular disease. Nurs. Clin. N. Am., *12*:101-108, Mar. 1977.

Fenn, J. E.: Reconstructive arterial surgery. Nurs. Clin. N. Am., *12*:129-142, Mar. 1977.

Kessro, B.: Peripheral arterial insufficiency (Postoperative nursing care). Nurs. Clin. N. Am., *12*:143-149, Mar. 1977.

McIntyre, D. R.: A maneuver to reverse Raynaud's phenomenon of the fingers. JAMA, *240*:2760, Dec. 15, 1978.

Royster, T. S., et al.: Peripheral arterial disease. Postgrad. Med., *62*:153-159, Nov. 1977.

Sexton, D. L.: The patient with peripheral arterial occlusive disease. Nurs. Clin. N. Am., *12*:89-99, Mar. 1977.

Taggart, E.: The physical assessment of the patient with arterial disease. Nurs. Clin. N. Am., *12*:109-117, Mar. 1977.

Hypertension

Araoye, M. A., et al.: Furosemide compared with hydrochlorothiazide. JAMA, *240*:1863-1866, Oct. 20, 1978.

Bruckheim, A. H.: Practice patterns in the management of hypertension. Am. Fam. Phys., *17*:209-213, Mar. 1978.

Caldwell, J. R.: Practical approach to hypertension. 1. Diagnostic evaluation, *65*:66-77; 2. Treatment, *65*:81-92, Postgrad. Med., May 1979.

Devices for monitoring blood pressure at home. Med. Letter, *19*:55-56, July 1, 1977.

Dowdall, S. A.: Breathing techniques that help reduce hypertension. RN, *40*:73-76, Oct. 1977.

Finnerty, F. A., Jr.: Hypertension in the elderly. Postgrad. Med., *65*:119-125, May 1979.

Foster, S. B., et al.: Influence of side effects of antihypertensive medications on patient behavior. Cardiovasc. Nurs., *14*:9-14, May/June 1978.

Foster, S., and Kousch, D. C.: Promoting patient adherence. AJN, *78*:829-832, May 1978.

Frohlich, E. D.: Essential hypertension. Arch. Intern. Med., *137*:772-775, June 1977.

Geddes, L., and Whistler, S.: The error in indirect blood pressure measurements with the incorrect size of cuff. Am. Heart J., *96*:4-8, July 1978.

Gifford, R. W.: Managing hypertension. Postgrad. Med., *61*:153-163, Mar. 1977.

Grim, C. E., et al.: Diagnosis of secondary forms of hypertension. JAMA, *237*:1331-1336, Mar. 28, 1977.

Harvey, S.: Drugs in cardiovascular emergencies (hypertensive emergencies). Nurses' Drug Alert, 2:79-80, June 1978.

Hypertension compliance. Med. World News, *18*:20-29, May 30, 1977.

Hypertension Detection and Follow-up Program Cooperative Group: Patient participation in a hypertension control program. JAMA, *239*:1507-1514, Apr. 14, 1978.

Kohli, R. K., and Elwood, C. M.: Treating acute hypertensive crisis with sodium nitroprusside. Am. Fam. Phys., *15*:141-145, Jan. 1977.

Kosman, M. E.: Evaluation of a new antihypertensive agent (Prazosin). JAMA, *238*:157-159, July 11, 1977.

Metoprolol (Lopressor). Med. Letter, *20*:97-98. Nov. 3, 1978.

Moser, M.: Controlling your hypertension. Drug. Ther., *8*:85-95, Feb. 1978.

Onesti, G.: Antihypertensives and their modes of action. Drug Ther., *8*:35-48, Feb. 1978.

Pettinger, W. A.: Recent advances in the treatment of hypertension. Arch. Int. Med., *137*:679-681, May 1977.

Prazosin (Minipress) for hypertension. Med. Letter, *19*:1-2, Jan. 14, 1977.

Relaxation, biofeedback and exercise for the treatment of hypertension. Med. Letter, *20*:62-63, July 14, 1978.

Report of the Joint National Committee on Detection, Evaluation, and Treatment of High Blood Pressure. JAMA, *237*:255-261, Jan. 17, 1977.

Robertson, D., et al.: Effects of caffeine on plasma renin activity, catecholamines and blood pressure. New Eng. J. Med., *298*:181-183, Jan. 26, 1978.

Vidt, D. G.: Combination therapy in hypertension: A rational approach. Drug Ther., *8*:78-93, Aug. 1978.

Ward, G. W., et al.: Treating and counseling the hypertensive patient. AJN, *78*:824-828, May 1978.

Weiss, R. D., and Shah, S.: When "lymphoma" is not lymphoma. Postgrad. Med., *63*:101-109, May 1978.

Wollam, G. L., and Vidt, D. G.: The patient with resistant hypertension. Drug Ther., *8*:72-84, Feb. 1978.

Ziesche, S., and Franciosa, J. A.: Clinical application of sodium nitroprusside. Heart & Lung, *6*:99-103, Jan.-Feb. 1977.

Leg Ulcers

Conners, P.: Treating leg ulcers. Nursing '77, 7:66-67, May 1977.

O'Donnell, T. F., Jr.: Diagnosis and management of ulcerations of the lower extremity. Hosp. Med., *13*:53-74, Feb. 1977.

Pace, W. E.: Beads of a dextran polymer for the local treatment of cutaneous ulcers. J. Derm. Surg. & Oncol., *4*:678-682, Sept. 1978.

Romasz, R. S., et al.: Application of dextranomer beads (Debrisan) in the treatment of exudating skin leasions: Results of a cooperative study. Angiology (J. Vasc. Dis.), *29*:675-681, Sept. 1978.

Use of Elastic Stockings

Browse, N. L., et al.: The value of mechanical methods of preventing postoperative calf vein thrombosis. Brit. J. Surg., *61*:219-223, Mar. 1974.

Clagett, G. P., and Salzman, E. W.: Prevention of venous thromboembolism in surgical patients. New Eng. J. Med., *290*:93-96, Jan. 10, 1974.

Kerstein, M. D.: An update on the treatment of deep vein thrombosis and pulmonary embolism. Conn. Med., *42*:287-292, May 1978.

Lewis, C. E., Jr., et al.: Venous stasis on the operating table. Am. J. Surg., *124*:780-784, Dec. 1972.

Rosengarten, D. S., et al.: The failure of compression stockings (Turbigrip) to prevent deep venous thrombosis after operation. Brit. J. Surg., *57*:296-299, Apr. 1976.

Spiro, M., et al.: Effect of externally applied pressure on femoral vein blood flow. Brit. Med. J., *1*:719-723, Mar. 1970.

Varicose Veins

Britons use injections to treat varicose veins. JAMA, *237*:848-851, Feb. 28, 1977.

Hobbs, J. T.: Surgery and sclerotherapy in the treatment of varicose veins. Arch. Surg., *109*:793-796, Dec. 1974.

Tunick, A. M.: An internist looks at varicose veins. Contemp. Surg., *11*:11-15, Aug. 1977.

Venous Conditions

Coon, W. W.: Epidemiology of venous thrombo-embolism. Ann. J. Surg., *186*:149-164, July 1977.

Dardik, H., et al.: Current status—vascular graft materials. Contemp. Surg., *12*:9-20, Mar. 1978.

Fitzmaurice, J. B.: Venous thromboembolic disease: Current thoughts. Cardiovasc. Nurs., *14*:1-4, Jan.-Feb. 1978.

Geelhoed, G. W.: Prevention of thromboembolism. Am. Fam. Phys., *19*:147-153, Mar. 1979.

[125]I-fibrinogen for diagnosis of thromboembolism. Med. Letter, *20*:63-64, July 14, 1978.

Kerstein, M. D.: An update on the treatment of deep vein thrombosis and pulmonary embolism. Conn. Med., *42*:287-292, May 1978.

Lee, B. Y., et al.: Noninvasive prevention of deep vein thrombosis. Am. Fam. Phys., *14*:128-134, Nov. 1976.

Marder, V. J.: When to consider thrombolytic therapy. Pat. Care, *12*:190-205, July 15, 1978.

McConnell, E. A.: Fitting antiembolism stockings. Nursing '78, *8*:67-71, Sept. 1978.

Ream, I.: Counseling patients with leg pain. Nursing '77, 7:54-56, Oct. 1977.

Ryan, R.: Thrombophlebitis: assessment and prevention. AJN, *76*:1634-1636, Oct. 1976.

Tasapogas, M. J., and Jindal, P. K.: Fibrolytic therapy for deep vein thrombosis. Contemp. Surg., *10*:29-34, Mar. 1977.

32

ASSESSMENT AND MANAGEMENT OF PATIENTS WITH HEMATOLOGIC DISORDERS

PHYSIOLOGIC OVERVIEW

The hematologic system comprises the blood and the sites where blood is produced, including the bone marrow and lymph nodes. The blood is a specialized organ which differs from other organs in that it exists in a fluid state. The fluid consists of cellular components suspended in blood plasma. The blood cells are divided into erythrocytes (red blood cells, normally 5 million per mm.^{3} of blood) and leukocytes (white blood cells, normally 5,000–10,000 per mm.^{3} of blood). Thus, there are approximately 500–1,000 erythrocytes for each leukocyte. The cellular components of blood normally make up 40 to 45 percent of the blood volume. The fraction of the blood occupied by erythrocytes is called the *hematocrit*. Blood appears as a thick, opaque red fluid. Its color is imparted by the hemoglobin contained within the red blood cells.

The volume of blood in humans is approximately 7 to 10 percent of the normal body weight, which represents about 5 liters. The blood is recirculated through the vascular system and serves as a link between body organs, carrying oxygen absorbed from the lungs and nutrients absorbed from the gastrointestinal tract to the body cells for cellular metabolism.

It also carries waste products produced by cellular metabolism to the lungs, skin, liver, and kidneys for subsequent transformation and elimination from the body. The blood also carries hormones, antibodies, and other products of internal secretion to their sites of action or utilization.

In order to perform its functions, blood must remain in its normally fluid state. Because it is fluid, the danger always exists that trauma can lead to loss of blood from the vascular system. To prevent this, the blood has an intrinsic clotting mechanism that is activated when necessary to seal leaks in the blood vessels. When blood is withdrawn from the body, the clotting system is activated and the blood clots, unless an anticoagulant is present. The liquid portion that remains after the blood has clotted is termed blood *serum*.

Bone Marrow

The bone marrow occupies the interior of spongy bones and the central cavity of the long bones of the skeleton. The marrow accounts for 4 to 5 percent of the total body weight and therefore constitutes one of the larger organs of the body. The marrow can be either red or yellow. Red marrow is the site of active blood cell production and constitutes the major hematopoietic (blood producing) organ. Yellow marrow, on the other hand, is composed mainly of fat, and is not active in the production of blood elements. During childhood, the major portion of the marrow is red. As the individual ages, a large portion of the marrow in the long bones is converted into yellow marrow, but it retains the potential for reversion to hematopoietic tissue if necessary. Red marrow in the adult is confined chiefly to the ribs, vertebral column, and other flat bones.

The marrow is a highly vascularized organ which consists of connective tissue containing free cells. The most primitive of this population of free cells are the stem cells, which are precursors of three different cell lines. These cell lines comprise the erythroid series leading to the erythrocyte, the leukocytic series leading to the various types of leukocytes, and the megakaryocytic series which leads to the formation of platelets.

Erythrocytes

The normal red blood cell is a biconcave disk, its configuration resembling that of a soft ball compressed between two fingers. It has a diameter of about 8 microns but is a very flexible cell, so flexible that it is capable of passing easily through capillaries that may be as small as 4 microns in diameter. The volume of a red blood cell is about 90 cubic microns. The red blood cell membrane is so thin that gases such as oxygen and carbon dioxide can easily diffuse across it. Mature red blood cells consist primarily of hemoglobin, which makes up 95 percent of the cell mass. These cells have no nuclei and have many fewer metabolic enzymes than do most other cells. The presence of a large amount of hemoglobin enables the cell to perform its principal function, the transport of oxygen between lungs and tissues.

The oxygen-carrying pigment hemoglobin is a protein with a molecular weight of 64,000. The molecule is made up of 4 subunits, each containing a heme moiety attached to a globin chain. Iron is present in the heme portion of the molecule. An important property of the heme moiety is its ability to loosely and reversibly bind to oxygen. Hemoglobin can also combine with carbon monoxide, thereby blocking oxygen binding and preventing normal oxygen transport. When hemoglobin is combined with oxygen, it is called *oxyhemoglobin*. Oxyhemoglobin has a brighter red color than hemoglobin that does not contain oxygen (reduced hemoglobin), so that arterial blood is a brighter red than venous blood. Whole blood normally contains about 15 grams of hemoglobin per 100 milliliters of blood, or 30 micrograms hemoglobin per million erythrocytes.

Production of Erythrocytes (Erythropoiesis). Erythroblasts arise from the primitive stem cells in bone marrow. The erythroblast is a nucleated cell that in the process of maturing within the bone marrow accumu-

lates hemoglobin and gradually loses its nucleus. At this stage, the cell is known as a *reticulocyte*. Further maturation into an erythrocyte entails the loss of dark staining material and a slight shrinkage in size. The mature erythrocyte is then released into the circulation. Under conditions of rapid erythropoiesis, reticulocytes and other immature cells may be released prematurely into the circulation.

Differentiation of the primitive multipotential stem cell of the marrow into an erythroblast is stimulated by erythropoietin. The latter is a hormone produced by interaction of a plasma protein with a substance secreted into the blood by the kidney. Under conditions of prolonged hypoxia, as in the case of individuals dwelling at high altitudes or after severe hemorrhage, erythropoietin levels are increased and red blood cell production is stimulated.

For normal erythrocyte production, the bone marrow requires iron, vitamin B_{12}, folic acid, pyridoxine (vitamin B_6), and other factors. If any of these factors is deficient during erythropoiesis, decreased red blood cell production and anemia result.

Iron Stores and Metabolism. Total body iron content in the average adult is approximately 3 grams, most of which is present in hemoglobin or one of its breakdown products. Normally, about 0.5 to 1.0 mg. of iron is absorbed per day from the intestinal tract to replace losses of iron in the feces. Additional amounts of iron, up to 2 mg. per day, must be absorbed by the adult female to replace blood lost during menstruation. Iron deficiency in the adult (decreased total body iron content) generally indicates that blood has been lost from the body, for example, by hemorrhage or excessive menstruation.

The concentration of iron in blood is normally about 0.5 to 2.0 micrograms per milliliter. With iron deficiency, bone marrow iron stores are rapidly depleted, hemoglobin synthesis is depressed, and the red blood cells produced by the marrow are small and low in hemoglobin.

Vitamin B_{12} and Folic Acid Metabolism. Vitamin B_{12} and folic acid are required for DNA synthesis in many tissues, but deficiencies of either of these vitamins has the greatest effect on erythropoiesis. Vitamin B_{12} or folic acid deficiency is characterized by the production of abnormally large red blood cells (called megaloblasts). Because these cells are abnormal, many are sequestered in the bone marrow and their rate of release is decreased. This condition results in megaloblastic anemia.

Both vitamin B_{12} and folic acid are derived from the diet. Vitamin B_{12} combines with intrinsic factor produced in the stomach. The vitamin B_{12}-intrinsic factor complex is absorbed in the distal ileum. Folic acid is absorbed in the proximal small intestine. Deficiency of vitamin B_{12} most commonly occurs due to failure of the stomach to secrete intrinsic factor and is called pernicious anemia. Folic acid deficiency usually occurs as a result of inadequate folic acid in the diet.

Red Blood Cell Destruction. The average lifespan of a circulating red blood cell is 120 days. Aged red blood cells are removed from the blood by the reticuloendothelial system, particularly in the liver and the spleen. The reticuloendothelial cells produce a pigment called bilirubin from the hemoglobin that is released from the destroyed red blood cells. Bilirubin is a waste product that is excreted in the bile. The iron, freed from the hemoglobin during bilirubin formation, is carried in plasma bound to the protein called transferrin to the bone marrow, where it is reclaimed for production of new hemoglobin.

Function of Erythrocytes. The major function of the red blood cells is to transport oxygen from the lungs to the tissues. Erythrocytes are uniquely capable of performing this function because of their high concentration of hemoglobin. If hemoglobin were not present, the oxygen-carrying capacity of blood would be decreased by 99 percent and would not be sufficient to meet the metabolic needs of the body. An important property of hemoglobin is that it binds oxygen loosely and reversibly. As a result, oxygen readily binds to hemoglobin in the lungs and readily dissociates from hemoglobin in the tissues.

The transport of carbon dioxide by the blood is facilitated by the presence of the enzyme carbonic anhydrase. This enzyme catalyzes the conversion of carbon dioxide to bicarbonate ion and vice-versa:

$$CO_2 + H_2O \xrightarrow{\text{carbonic anhydrase}} HCO_3^- + H^+$$

As a result of this rapid conversion, the amount of CO_2 (or its equivalent bicarbonate ion) that can be carried by blood is greatly increased.

Leukocytes

Leukocytes are divided into two general categories, granulocytes and mononuclear cells. In normal blood, the total leukocyte count is 5,000 to 10,000 cells per cubic millimeter. Of these, approximately 60 percent are granulocytes and 40 percent are mononuclear cells. Leukocytes can be readily differentiated from erythrocytes by the presence of a nucleus, their larger size, and different staining properties.

Granulocytes. Granulocytes are defined by the presence of granules in their cytoplasm. The diameter of a granulocyte is generally two to three times that of an erythrocyte. Granulocytes are divided into three subgroups, which are characterized by their staining properties as seen on microscopic examination. Eosinophils have bright red granules in their cytoplasm, whereas the granules in basophils stain deep blue. The third, and by far the most numerous, cell in this series is the neutrophil, with granules that show a dull violet hue. The nucleus of the mature granulocyte generally has multiple lobes (usually 2 to 4) connected by thin filaments of nuclear material. Because of their nuclear characteristics, these cells are called polymorphonuclear leukocytes (abbreviated as PMN leukocyte). The immature granulocyte has a single-lobed ovoid nucleus and is called a band cell. Ordinarily, band forms account for only a small percentage of circulating granulocytes, although their percentage can increase greatly under conditions in which the rate of production of polymorphonuclear leukocytes is increased.

Granulocytes are produced in the bone marrow from precursor cells called myelocytes, which arise from the primitive stem cells. The bone marrow of normal adults contains approximately 20 to 30 granulocyte precursor cells for every circulating granulocyte. Normally the life span of granulocytes within the blood is only several hours. Consequently, the marrow of the normal adult must produce approximately 100 billion cells per day. The number of circulating granulocytes found in the healthy individual is maintained relatively constant, but in the presence of infection, large numbers of these cells are rapidly released into the circulation.

Mononuclear Leukocytes. Mononuclear leukocytes (lymphocytes and monocytes) are white blood cells with a single-lobed nucleus and a granule-free cytoplasm. In normal adult blood, lymphocytes account for approximately 30 percent and monocytes approximately 5 percent of the total leukocytes. Mature lymphocytes are small cells with scanty cytoplasm. They are produced primarily in the lymph nodes and in the lymphoid tissue of the intestine, spleen, and thymus gland from precursor cells which originated as marrow stem cells. Lymphocytes in the tissue give rise to plasma cells. Monocytes are the largest of the blood leukocytes. They are produced by the bone marrow and give rise to tissue histiocytes including Kupffer cells of the liver, peritoneal macrophages, alveolar macrophages, and other components of the reticuloendothelial system.

Function of the Leukocytes. The function of the leukocytes is to protect the body from invasion by bacteria and other foreign entities. The major function of neutrophilic polymorphonuclear leukocytes is to ingest foreign material (phagocytosis). When bacteria are ingested, the neutrophils can effectively kill them (bactericidal activity). Monocytes also are capable of phagocytosis but, compared with neutrophils, they phagocytize more slowly and are mobilized less rapidly. Consequently, neutrophils are the major leukocytes involved with acute infection, whereas monocytes predominate in chronic disease.

The function of lymphocytes is primarily to produce

substances that aid in the attack on foreign material. One group of lymphocytes (T lymphocytes) when confronted with foreign material release lymphokines, a group of substances that activate and attract phagocytic cells. B lymphocytes and plasma cells when activated produce antibodies that react with foreign material to make it more susceptible to phagocytosis. Eosinophils and basophils function as reservoirs of potent biological materials such as histamine, serotonin, and heparin. Release of these compounds alters the blood supply to tissues, such as occurs during inflammation, and helps to mobilize body defense mechanisms. The increase in the number of eosinophils in allergic states indicates that these cells are involved in the hypersensitivity reaction.

Platelets

Platelets are small particles, 2 to 4 microns in diameter, that are present in the circulating blood plasma. Their number varies normally between 150,000 and 500,000 per cubic millimeter of blood. They are formed from the fragmentation (the pinching off of bits of membrane and cytoplasm) of giant cells of the bone marrow called megakaryocytes. Megakaryocytes arise from the primitive marrow from stem cells.

Platelets are important in the formation of clots at the site of injury to blood vessels. Their granules contain adenosine diphosphate (ADP), calcium, serotonin, epinephrine, and other chemical substances. When tissues are injured, circulating platelets stick to the damaged blood vessel walls and release their granules. The serotonin and epinephrine cause vasoconstriction at the site of injury, and the ADP promotes release of the granules from other platelets. Additional substances released from platelets activate coagulation factors in the blood plasma.

Blood Coagulation

Blood coagulation is the process whereby the components of the liquid blood are transformed into a semisolid material called a blood clot. The blood clot is made up mainly of blood cells entrapped in a meshwork of fibrin. Fibrin is formed from proteins in the plasma as the result of a complex series of reactions.

At least 12 clotting factors are involved in the reaction cascade that forms fibrin. The clotting factors are listed in Table 32-1, and the extrinsic and intrinsic pathways for fibrin generation are shown diagramatically in Figure 32-1. When tissue is injured, the extrinsic pathway is activated by the release from the tissue of a substance called thromboplastin. As the result of a series of reactions, prothrombin is converted to thrombin, which in turn catalyzes the conversion of fibrinogen to fibrin. Calcium (Factor IV) is a necessary cofactor for many of these reactions. The intrinsic pathway is responsible for initiating the clotting of blood that comes into contact

with glass or other foreign surfaces, such as when blood is withdrawn from the body into a test tube. It is for this reason that anticoagulants must be used when drawing blood for chemical or other tests. The anticoagulants that are often used are either citrate, which binds the plasma calcium, or heparin, which prevents the conversion of prothrombin to thrombin. Citrate cannot be used as an anticoagulant in vivo because binding of plasma calcium would cause death. Heparin can be used clinically as an anticoagulant. Dicumarol is also used clinically for its anticoagulant action of interfering with the production of several of the plasma coagulating factors.

Clots that form in the body are eventually dissolved by the action of the fibrinolytic system, which consists of plasmin and other proteolytic enzymes. Through the action of this system, clots are dissolved as tissue is repaired, and the vascular system is returned to its normal baseline state.

Blood Plasma

After cellular elements are removed from blood, the remaining liquid portion is called *blood plasma*. It contains ions, proteins, and other substances. If plasma is allowed to clot, the remaining fluid is called *serum*. Serum has essentially the same composition as plasma except that its fibrinogen and several of the clotting factors have been removed.

Plasma Proteins. Plasma proteins consist largely of albumin and globulins. The globulins in turn consist of alpha, beta, and gamma fractions derived by a laboratory test called serum protein electrophoresis. Each of these groups is made up of distinct proteins. The gamma globulins, which consist largely of antibodies, are called immunoglobulins. These proteins are produced by the lymphocytes and plasma cells. Important proteins in the

TABLE 32-1.   CLOTTING FACTORS

FACTOR	ALTERNATIVE NAME
Factor I	Fibrinogen
Factor II	Prothrombin
Factor III	Thromboplastin (tissue), thrombokinase
Factor IV	Calcium
Factor V	Labile factor, proaccelerin, plasma Ac globulin
Factor VI	Serum Ac globulin, accelerin
Factor VII	Stable factor, proconvertin, SPCA (serum prothrombin conversion accelerator), cothromboplastin, autoprothrombin I
Factor VIII	Antihemophilic factor (AHF), antihemophilic globulin, thromboplastinogen, platelet cofactor I, plasma thromboplastic factor A
Factor IX	Plasma thromboplastin component (PTC), Christmas factor, platelet cofactor II, plasma thromboplastic factor B, autoprothrombin II
Factor X	Stuart-Prower factor
Factor XI	Plasma thromboplastin antecedent (PTA)
Factor XII	Hageman factor

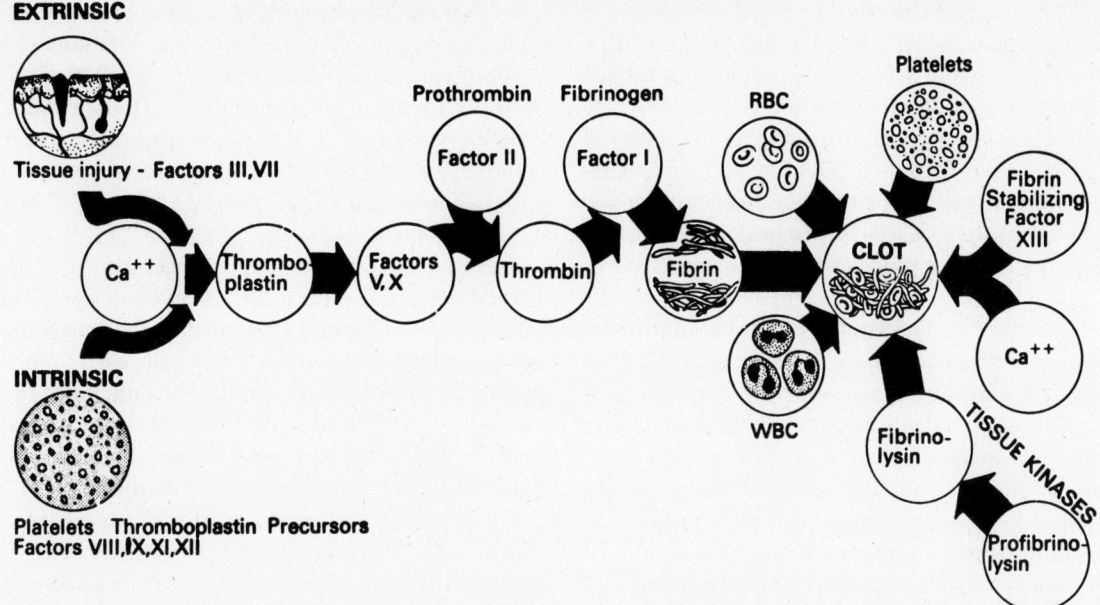

EXTRINSIC

Tissue injury - Factors III, VII

Prothrombin

Factor II

Fibrinogen

Factor I

RBC

Platelets

Ca⁺⁺

Thrombo-plastin

Factors V, X

Thrombin

Fibrin

CLOT

Fibrin Stabilizing Factor XIII

INTRINSIC

WBC

Fibrino-lysin

Ca⁺⁺

TISSUE KINASES

Platelets Thromboplastin Precursors
Factors VIII, IX, XI, XII

Profibrino-lysin

Figure 32-1. The blood-clotting mechanism. The schematic represents the factors essential to change blood into a solid gel. The entire chain reaction in which fibrinogen (a plasma protein) is converted to fibrin (the clot) takes place at the site of vessel damage. (Adapted from Feller, I., and Archambeault, C.: Nursing the Burn Patient. Ann Arbor, Michigan, The Institute for Burn Medicine, 1973)

alpha and beta fractions are the transport globulins and the clotting factors, which are made in the liver. The transport globulins carry various substances in bound form around the circulation. For example, thyroid-binding globulin carries thyroxin, and transferrin carries iron. The clotting factors, including fibrinogen, remain in an inactive form in the blood plasma until activated by the clotting cascade.

Albumin is particularly important for the maintenance of fluid volume within the vascular system. Capillary walls are impermeable to albumin, hence its presence in the plasma creates an osmotic force that keeps fluid within the vascular space. Albumin, which is produced in the liver, has the capacity to bind to a number of substances that are often present in plasma. In this way, it functions as a transport protein for metals, fatty acids, bilirubin, and drugs, among other substances.

Pathophysiology of the Hematologic System

Anemias. A frequent disorder of the hematologic system is a decrease in the number of circulating red blood cells. This condition, called anemia, can result from either underproduction of red blood cells by the bone marrow or increased destruction of circulating red blood cells. Underproduction of red blood cells can be due to a deficiency of cofactors for erythropoiesis including folic acid, vitamin B_{12} and iron. Red blood cell production may also be reduced if bone marrow is suppressed (by tumor or drugs) or is inadequately stimulated due to lack of erythropoietin such as occurs in

chronic renal disease. Increased destruction of red blood cells may occur because of an overactive reticuloendothelial system (e.g., hypersplenism) or because the bone marrow produces abnormal red blood cells (e.g., sickle cell anemia). Since the red blood cell and its contained hemoglobin are important for the delivery of oxygen to tissues, anemias may result in tissue hypoxia.

Bleeding Disorders. Bleeding disorders can be attributed to deficiency of either platelets or clotting factors in the circulating blood. Platelet function in the blood plasma can be reduced as the result of bone marrow insufficiency, increased splenic destruction, or abnormal circulating platelets. Deficiencies of clotting factors are usually due to underproduction of these factors by the liver. Hemophilia is a hereditary disorder that results from deficiency of clotting factors VIII and IX.

BLOOD STUDY PROCEDURES

Methods of Obtaining Blood

Venipuncture. Most routine hematologic studies are performed on venous blood, which is usually obtained from an antecubital vein, although occasionally, in very obese persons or those whose veins have been thrombosed by chemotherapy, it may be necessary to puncture one of the veins on the dorsum of the hand.

After a tourniquet has been tied around the upper arm, the arm and hand veins become prominent. The vein chosen for venipuncture should be straight, not tortuous, and should be well fixed in the subcutaneous tissue, so that it does not roll away. The skin below the vein is stretched with one hand while the opposite hand is used to push the needle through the skin and then slowly into the vein. Blood is immediately placed in a tube with the appropriate anticoagulant—EDTA (ethylenediamine-tetracetic acid) is usually used for blood cell counts and hemoglobin; citrate is used for coagulation studies; heparin may be used for glucose-6-phosphate dehydrogenase determination and hemoglobin electrophoresis.

Finger Puncture. The finger puncture method is used frequently for blood smears and counts. This method utilizes capillary blood, but for practical purposes the results are identical to those obtained with venous blood. Lances of various shapes are available. These make a puncture of 1-2 mm. Best results are obtained if the patient's hand is warm and if the pulp of the index or middle finger is punctured. The skin should be cleaned with alcohol first and then carefully wiped dry with a lint-free sponge. If any alcohol remains, it will alter red cell morphology. The drops of blood obtained by this method can be gently touched to glass slides or cover slips, for peripheral smears. Capillary blood can also be drawn into calibrated red cell and white cell pipettes and into microhematocrit tubes.

The most common hematologic tests are described in the chart on page 657.

Bone Marrow Aspiration

Bone marrow is usually aspirated from the sternum or iliac crest in adults. Most patients need no more preparation than a careful explanation of the procedure, but for some very anxious patients, meperidine (Demerol) or a minor tranquilizer may be useful. It is always important for physician and nurse to describe and explain the procedure as it is being performed. First, the skin area is cleansed as for any minor surgery. Then a small area is anesthetized with lidocaine (Xylocaine), through the

skin and subcutaneous tissue to the periosteum of the bone. The bone marrow needle is introduced with a stylet in place, and when the needle is felt to go through the outer cortex of bone and enter the marrow cavity, the stylet is removed, a syringe is attached, and a small volume (0.5 ml.) of blood and marrow is aspirated. The actual aspiration always causes brief pain, and the patient should be warned of this.

If a bone marrow biopsy is necessary, it is best performed after the aspiration and with a special needle. Several types of needles are available, the procedure varying according to the type of needle used. Since these needles are large, the skin should be punctured first with a surgical blade (No. 9 or 11) to make a 3- or 4-mm. incision. Only the iliac bone is used for this procedure (Fig. 32-2), since the sternum is too thin.

The procedures carry very little risk, except in patients with severe osteoporosis. Since patients with thrombocytopenia may bleed excessively, pressure should be applied to the site for 5 to 10 minutes after the needle has been removed. Most patients have no discomfort after a bone marrow aspiration, but the site of a biopsy may ache for a day or two.

ANEMIA

Anemia is a laboratory definition which implies a low red cell count and a below normal hemoglobin or hematocrit level. These levels are somewhat arbitrary since there is a range of normal values. Thus, a fall of 1 to 2 gm./100 ml. in a patient's hemoglobin level might still be within the normal range.

Pathophysiology

The appearance of anemia reflects either marrow failure or excessive red cell loss, or both. Marrow failure, i.e., reduced erythropoiesis, may occur as a result of a nutritional deficiency, toxic exposure, tumor invasion or, as in many instances, from causes unknown. Red cells may be lost through hemorrhage or hyperhemolysis (increased destruction). In the latter case the problem may be rooted in some red cell defect that is incompatible with normal red cell survival or explainable on the basis of some factor extrinsic to the red cell that promotes red cell destruction.

Red cell lysis occurs mainly within the phagocytic cells of the reticuloendothelial system, notably in the liver and spleen. As a by-product of this process, bilirubin, formed within the phagocyte, enters the bloodstream, and any increase in hemolysis is promptly reflected by an increase in plasma bilirubin. (This concentration normally is 1.0 mg./100 ml. or less; levels above 1.5 mg./100 ml. produce visible jaundice of the sclerae.)

If, as happens in certain specific hemolytic disorders, red cells are destroyed within the circulating blood-

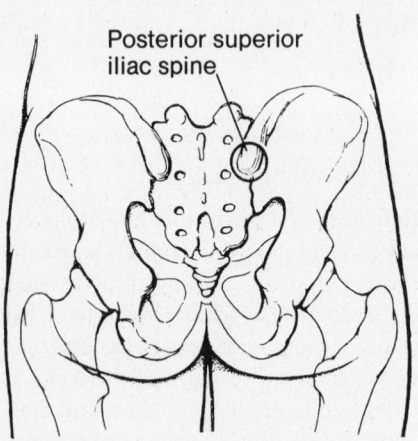

Posterior superior iliac spine

Figure 32-2. Site of bone marrow biopsy.

COMMON HEMATOLOGIC LABORATORY TESTS

TEST	DEFINITION
COMPLETE BLOOD COUNT	Includes enumeration of number of white cells, red cells, and platelets per cubic mm. of venous blood, as well as a differential count, percentage of each type of nucleated cell in the blood (i.e., percent polymorphonuclears, percent lymphocytes, etc.).
RETICULOCYTE COUNT	Percentage of young (1-2 days old) non-nucleated erythrocytes in peripheral blood; they are recognized in special stains of blood smears as cells with lacy inclusions, which consist of RNA.
HEMOGLOBIN ELECTROPHORESIS	A drop of blood placed on a solid medium (paper, starch block, gel, or cellulose acetate) is exposed to a current of electricity while being bathed by a buffer solution. The different hemoglobins (e.g., A, A-2, F, S) travel at varying speeds, depending on their charge. At the end of the procedure, the paper or gel is stained, and the hemoglobins in each sample can be identified.
SICKLING TEST	A drop of blood is mixed with a drop of a reducing agent (sodium metabisulfite). This substance deprives the red cells of oxygen and induces sickling if S hemoglobin is present. Sickling of red cells is observed under the microscope in 30 minutes if the blood was obtained from a person with either sickle trait or sickle cell anemia. Normal blood does not undergo any change.
LEUKOCYTE ALKALINE PHOSPHATASE	An enzyme present in high concentrations in granules of neutrophils. A special stain of peripheral blood smears is used to estimate the amount of LAP present per cell. The normal score is 20-130. Untreated chronic myelogenous leukemia patients have scores of less than 20, and the test is useful to help diagnose CML. High scores are seen in infection and steroid induced leukocytosis.
COOMBS' TEST	Determines the presence of gamma globulin (hence, antibodies) on the surface of erythrocytes (direct Coombs' test) or in the plasma (indirect Coombs' test).
BLEEDING TIME	A screening test for disorders of platelet function. It is the time taken for bleeding to cease after a standardized skin wound is produced, usually on the volar surface of the forearm. When it is prolonged, this suggests an inherited or acquired platelet defect, for example, von Willebrand's disease or aspirin ingestion.
PLATELET AGGREGATION	A measure of the time and completeness of the formation of platelet aggregates in a sample of plasma, after the addition of an agent such as epinephrine or ADP.
PROTHROMBIN TIME TEST	Measures the coagulant activity of the "extrinsic" system, including fibrinogen, prothrombin, and factors V, VII, and X. It is used to monitor Coumadin therapy, as well as for a screening test for liver disease.
PARTIAL THROMBOPLASTIN TIME TEST	A screening test for deficiencies of all plasma coagulation factors except VII and XIII. Is usually abnormally prolonged if levels of factors are less than 30 percent of normal.

stream, hemoglobin itself appears in the plasma (hemoglobinemia) and, if its concentration there exceeds the capacity of the plasma haptoglobin to bind it all, i.e., if the amount is more than about 100 mg./100 ml., then this pigment is free to diffuse through the renal glomeruli and into the urine (hemoglobinuria). Thus, the presence or absence of hemoglobinemia and hemoglobinuria provides information about the location of abnormal blood destruction in a patient with hemolysis and can be a clue to the nature of the hemolytic process.

A conclusion as to whether the anemia in a particular patient is caused by hemolysis or by inadequate erythropoiesis usually can be reached on the basis of (1) the reticulocyte count in the circulating blood, (2) the degree to which young red cells are proliferating in the bone marrow and the manner in which they are maturing as observed on biopsy, and (3) the presence or absence of hyperbilirubinemia and hemoglobinemia. Moreover, one can actually quantitate erythropoiesis by measuring the rate at which injected radioactive iron is incorporated into circulating erythrocytes, and one can measure the life span of the patient's red cells (ergo, the hemolytic rate) by tagging a portion of these with radioactive chromium, reinjecting them and following their disap-

COMMON PROBLEMS OF PATIENTS WITH BLOOD DISORDERS

THE PROBLEM	NURSING MANAGEMENT
Fatigue and weakness	Plan nursing care to conserve the patient's strength. Give frequent rest periods. Encourge ambulation activities as tolerated. Avoid disturbing activities and noise. Encourge optimal nutrition.
Hemorrhagic tendencies	Keep the patient at rest during the bleeding episodes. Apply gentle pressure to the bleeding sites. Apply cold compresses to the bleeding sites when indicated. Do not disturb clots. Use small gauge needles when administering medications by injection. Support the patient during transfusion therapy. Observe for symptoms of internal bleeding. Have a tracheostomy set available for the patient who is bleeding from the mouth or the throat.
Ulcerative lesions of the tongue, gums, and/or mucous membranes	Avoid irritating foods and beverages. Give frequent oral hygiene with mild, cool mouthwash solutions. Use applicators or soft-bristled toothbrush. Keep the lips lubricated. Give mouth care both before and after meals.
Dyspnea	Elevate the head of the bed. Use pillows to support the patient in the orthopneic position. Administer oxygen when indicated. Prevent unnecessary exertion. Avoid gas-forming foods.
Bone and joint pains	Relieve pressure of bedding by using a cradle. Administer either hot or cold compresses as prescribed. Provide for joint immobilization when prescribed.
Fever	Administer cool sponges. Give antipyretic drugs as prescribed. Encourage fluid intake unless contraindicated. Maintain a cool environmental temperature.
Pruritus and/or skin eruptions	Keep the patient's fingernails short. Use soap sparingly. Apply emollient lotions in skin care.
Anxiety of the patient and his family	Explain the nature, the discomforts, and the limitations of activity associated with the diagnostic procedures and treatments. Offer the patient the service of listening. Have an empathetic attitude. Promote the patient's relaxation and comfort. Remember the patient's individual preferences. Encourage the family to participate in the patient's care (as desired). Create a comfortable atmosphere for the family to visit with the patient.

pearance from the circulating blood over the course of the ensuing days or weeks. Methods by which one particular type of marrow failure can be distinguished from another type, and one hemolytic disease from another, are specified in relation to each of the conditions discussed.

Clinical Manifestations

Aside from the severity of the anemia, several factors affect the anemic patient, and tend to influence the severity and even the presence of his symptoms: (1) the speed with which the anemia has developed, (2) its prior dura-

tion, i.e., its chronicity, (3) the metabolic requirements of the particular patient, (4) any other disorders or disabilities with which the patient is currently afflicted, and (5) special complications or concomitant features of the condition that has produced this anemia.

The more rapidly an anemia develops, the more severe its symptoms. An otherwise normal individual can tolerate as much as a 50 percent gradual reduction in hemoglobin, red count, or hematocrit without pronounced symptomatology or significant incapacity, whereas the rapid loss of as little as 30 percent may precipitate profound vascular collapse in the same individual. A person who has been anemic for a very long period of time, with hemoglobin levels between 9 and 11 gm./100 ml., experiences few or no symptoms other than slight tachycardia on exertion; exertional dyspnea is likely to occur below, but not above 7.5 gm./100 ml.; weakness, only below 6.0 gm./100 ml.; dyspnea at rest, below 3.0 gm./100 ml.; and cardiac failure, only at the profoundly low level of 2.0 to 2.5 gm./100 ml.!

Patients who customarily are very active are more likely to experience symptoms, and symptoms that are more pronounced, than a more sedentary individual. A hypothyroid patient, requiring, as he does, less than the usual amount of oxygen, may be perfectly asymptomatic, without tachycardia or increased cardiac output, at a hemoglobin level of 10 gm./100 ml. Contrariwise, at any given level of anemia, patients with underlying heart disease are far more apt to experience angina or symptoms of congestive failure than someone without heart disease.

Finally, as will emerge in the discussions that follow, many anemic disorders are complicated by various other abnormalities—abnormalities that do not depend on the anemia but that are inherently associated with these particular diseases. These abnormalities may give rise to symptoms that completely overshadow those of the anemia, as is exemplified by the painful crises of sickle cell anemia (page 663).

There are a number of hematologic disorders in which anemia is the presenting problem, or the problem of paramount concern, and which, as a group, exemplify all of the etiologic factors that have been discussed and all of the pathogenic mechanisms that have been formulated to date with respect to anemia.

Classification of Anemias

There are several ways to classify the anemias; the physiologic approach is to determine whether the deficiency in red cells is due to a defect in production of red cells (hypoproliferative anemia) or in survival of the red cells (hemolytic anemia).

In the hypoproliferative anemias, red cells usually survive normally, but the marrow is unable to produce adequate numbers of cells: thus, the reticulocyte count is depressed. This situation can be a result of marrow damage by drugs or chemicals (e.g., chloramphenicol, benzene) or may be due to lack of erythropoietin (as in renal disease) or to lack of iron, vitamin B_{12}, or folic acid.

When hemolysis is the major cause of anemia, the abnormality is usually within the red cell itself (as in sickle cell anemia or G-6-PD [glucose-6-phosphate dehydrogenase] deficiency), in the plasma (as in the immune hemolytic anemias), or in the circulation (as in heart valve hemolysis). In all of these hemolytic anemias, the reticulocyte count is elevated and the indirect bilirubin is high, often enough to cause clinical jaundice.

HYPOPROLIFERATIVE ANEMIAS

Aplastic Anemia

Pathophysiology. *Aplastic anemia* is anemia caused by a decrease in precursor cells in the bone marrow. The type encountered in adults usually proves to be the expression of a toxic myelopathy, that is, bone marrow depression or destruction by a drug or chemical, or as a result of radiation damage. Agents that regularly produce marrow aplasia in sufficient dosage include benzene and benzene derivatives, antitumor agents such as nitrogen mustard and its congeners the periwinkle alkaloids, etc., the antimetabolites, including methotrexate and 6-mercaptopurine, and certain toxic materials, such as inorganic arsenic. Other agents occasionally responsible for aplasia or hypoplasia include certain antimicrobials, anticonvulsants, antithyroid drugs, antidiabetic agents, antihistamines, analgesics, sedatives, phenothiazines, insecticides, and heavy metals. The most common offenders in this respect are the antimicrobials chloramphenicol and the organic arsenicals, the anticonvulsants Mesantoin and Tridione, the anti-inflammatory analgesic drug phenylbutazone, and gold compounds.

Only a relatively small minority of persons who have received these drugs in their recommended dosage have developed a blood dyscrasia. The cases we are describing, therefore, may be considered a type of idiosyncratic drug reaction in persons who are hypersusceptible for reasons as yet unknown. Provided that their exposure is terminated early (i.e., on the first appearance of reticulocytopenia, anemia, granulocytopenia or thrombocytopenia), a prompt and complete recovery may be anticipated. (Unfortunately, one cannot be so optimistic in the case of chloramphenicol recipients. Reactions in individuals hypersusceptible to this drug may be completely unrelated to dosage; they may develop without premonitory changes in the hemogram long after the drug has been discontinued and can progress to a complete and fatal aplasia despite all available therapy.)

Whatever the offending drug, if exposure is allowed to continue after signs of hypoplasia have appeared, bone marrow depression almost certainly progresses to the point of complete and irreversible failure—hence the importance of frequent complete blood counts for every patient receiving a drug or exposed regularly to any chemical that has been implicated in the production of aplastic anemia.

Clinical Manifestations. Since the bone marrow is hypocellular, attempts at marrow aspiration frequently yield only a few drops of blood. A biopsy is usually necessary to demonstrate a severe decrease in normal marrow elements and replacement by fat. The abnormality is probably in the stem cell, the precursor of both myeloid and erythroid cells. As a result, pancytopenia (deficiency in all of the cellular elements of the blood) occurs.

The onset of aplastic anemia characteristically is a gradual one, marked by weakness, pallor, breathlessness on exertion, and other manifestations of anemia. A presenting symptom in about a third of the patients is abnormal bleeding due to thrombocytopenia. When the granulocytic series is involved as well, the patient is likely to present with fever, acute pharyngitis, or some other form of sepsis, in addition to bleeding. Physical signs, save for pallor and skin hemorrhages, are unremarkable. The blood count is marked by variable degrees of pancytopenia, with normocytic normochromic red cells.

Frequently, patients have no characteristic physical findings: adenopathy and hepatosplenomegaly are lacking. The peripheral smear shows normocytic normochromic red cells.

Treatment. There is no specific therapy for aplastic anemia. The therapeutic objective is to bring the patient to a remission. Any offending drug is discontinued. The patient is supported with transfusions of red cells and platelets as necessary to prevent symptoms. Eventually such patients may develop antibodies to minor red cell antigens and to platelet antigens, so that the transfusions no longer raise the counts sufficiently. Death is usually caused by hemorrhage or infection, although modern antibiotics, especially those active against gram-negative bacilli, have been a major advance for these patients. Reverse isolation techniques are used for the patient with pronounced leukopenia. Antibiotics should not be used prophylactically in neutropenic patients, since this favors the emergence of resistant bacteria and fungi. Corticosteroids and androgenic hormones have been used in an attempt to stimulate the marrow. However the responses are so rare that they may be due to spontaneous recovery. It is not certain that these agents really influence the course of the disease. Bone marrow transplantation (page 678) is now the most successful form of therapy. The prognosis for patients with aplastic anemia is very poor; about 60 percent die of the complications, many within several months of diagnosis.

Nursing Management. The nurse can help to prevent minor infections in these very susceptible patients. Any wound, abrasion, or ulcer of mucous membrane or skin is a potential site of infection and should be guarded against. Oral hygiene also is very important. Regular atraumatic bowel movements are important in bedridden patients, since hemorrhoids can develop and easily become infected. When thrombocytopenia is present, minor trauma including subcutaneous and intramuscular injection must be avoided.

Red Cell Aplasia

Red cell aplasia is an isolated anemia due to lack of red cell formation in the marrow. This is a rare disorder in which only the erythroid cells are affected. The marrow is cellular, but the erythroid element is almost absent.

There is a severe anemia without granulocytopenia or thrombocytopenia. The condition is sometimes associated with tumors of the thymus or certain drugs such as phenytoin (Dilantin). Some patients can be shown to produce an antibody to immature red cells, and this may be the cause of the disease. It is occasionally treated successfully with immunosuppressive drugs, such as azathioprine or cyclophosphamide.

Myelophthisic Anemias

Myelophthisic anemias are a varied group of anemias which differ as to cause but are similar in that all show partial replacement of normal marrow space by abnormal tissue. This tissue may be fibrous (in myelofibrosis) or it may consist of plasma cells (in multiple myeloma) or metastatic carcinoma cells. A marrow biopsy is often necessary to make the diagnosis. Pancytopenia is present, although usually less severe than in aplastic anemia, but there are also young marrow cells circulating, apparently because there is abnormal release from the damaged marrow. Myeloblasts and nucleated red cells are seen in small numbers. The treatment is that of the primary disease. Androgens occasionally improve the patient's condition.

Anemias in Renal Disease

There is a great deal of variability in the degree of anemia seen in kidney disorders, but in general, patients with a BUN greater than 100 mg./100 ml. blood are anemic. The symptoms of anemia often constitute the patient's major problems. The hematocrit usually falls between 20 and 30 percent and is lower for more severe uremia, although it rarely falls below 15 percent. The red cells appear normal on peripheral smear.

This anemia is due to both a mild shortening of red cell survival and a deficiency of erythropoietin. Some erythropoietin is evidently produced outside the kidney, since some erythropoiesis does continue, even in anephric patients (those whose kidneys have been removed), and developing red cells can be seen in the bone marrow.

- Patients undergoing chronic hemodialysis lose blood into the artificial kidney and may thus become iron deficient. Folic acid deficiency develops because this vitamin passes into the dialysate.
- Dialysis patients should be treated with iron and folic acid and occasional transfusions.

Androgens have been shown to stimulate enough erythropoiesis to obviate the need for transfusions in some patients. Most patients with uremia can tolerate moderate anemia with few symptoms and should not be transfused unless symptoms are present.

Anemias in Chronic Diseases

Many chronic inflammatory diseases are associated with anemia of a normochromic normocytic type. These include rheumatoid arthritis, lung abscesses, osteomyelitis, tuberculosis, and many malignancies. The hemoglobin rarely falls below 9 gm./100 ml. and the bone marrow has normal cellularity with increased stores of iron. Erythropoietin levels are low, perhaps because of decreased production, and there is a block in the utilization of iron by erythroid cells. Most of these patients are comfortable and do not require treatment for the anemia. With amelioration of the underlying disorder, the marrow iron is used to make red cells, and the hemoglobin rises.

Iron Deficiency Anemia

Iron deficiency anemia is the most common type of anemia in all age groups. It is a condition in which the total body iron content is decreased below a normal level.

Etiology. The common cause of iron deficiency in men or postmenopausal women is bleeding (e.g., from ulcers, gastritis, or gastrointestinal tumors) or malabsorption, especially after gastric resection. Rarely, iron can be lost in the urine during intravascular hemolysis, as in paroxysmal nocturnal hemoglobinuria or heart valve hemolysis.

Clinical and Laboratory Manifestations. In individuals who are iron deficient, the blood hemoglobin and the red blood cell count are reduced. The hemoglobin is reduced more than is the number of red cells, and for this reason the latter tend to be small and relatively devoid of pigment, i.e., "hypochromic." Hypochromia is the hallmark of iron deficiency. The cause of this deficiency is the failure of the patient to ingest, or absorb, sufficient dietary iron to compensate for the iron requirements associated with body growth or for the loss of iron that attends bleeding, whether the bleeding is physiologic (e.g., menstrual) or pathologic.

The patient with iron deficiency presents primarily with the symptoms of anemia. If the deficiency is severe, he may also have a smooth, sore tongue, thin, spoon-shaped fingernails, and pica (a craving to eat unusual substances such as clay, laundry starch, or ice). All of these symptoms subside after therapy.

The laboratory studies show a hemoglobin which is proportionately lower than the hematocrit and red count, because of the small, poorly hemoglobinized red cells (microcytosis and hypochromia). White count and platelets are usually normal, but the latter may be elevated. Serum iron is low, and the iron-binding capacity is high. The marrow has no visible iron on special stain.

Management. It is always important to search for a cause of iron deficiency. This may be a sign of a curable gastrointestinal malignancy or of uterine fibroids or cancer. Except in pregnancy, when the cause is obvious, stool specimens should be tested for occult blood. Several oral iron preparations are available: ferrous sulfate, gluconate, or fumarate are equally effective, but the enteric forms may be poorly absorbed and should be avoided. Usually three or four doses a day are necessary. Iron preparations are best absorbed if taken 1 hour before meals. Iron salts may cause some gastric distress, constipation, or diarrhea. However, patients usually can tolerate the therapy if the dose is started at one tablet daily and then raised. Patients should be warned that iron salts often change the stools to a darker color.

Patient education is important, since iron therapy usually has to be continued for many months to replenish iron stores. In rare cases, intramuscular administration of iron may be necessary; i.e., when oral iron is not absorbed or is poorly tolerated or when iron is needed in large amounts. The injection causes some local pain, and can stain the skin.

A method for parenteral administration of iron preparations follows:
1. Discard needle used to draw medication into syringe; use fresh needle for injection.
2. Use a needle 5 cm. (2 inches) long — medication is injected deep into muscle.
3. Retract skin over muscle *laterally* before inserting needle — to prevent leakage and staining of skin.

Occasional febrile or allergic reactions are seen.

Megaloblastic Anemias

The anemias caused by deficiencies of the vitamins B_{12} and folic acid show identical bone marrow and peripheral blood changes. This is because both vitamins are essential for normal DNA synthesis. In each case, the marrow is hyperplastic and the precursor erythroid and myeloid cells are large and bizarre; some are multinucleated. But many of these cells die within the marrow, so that the mature cells which leave the marrow are decreased in number. Thus a pancytopenia develops. In a far advanced situation, the hemoglobin may be as low as 4-5 gm./100 ml., the white blood count 2,000-3,000 per cu. mm., and platelets less than 50,000 per cu. mm. The red cells are large and the polymorphonuclears are hypersegmented.

Pernicious Anemia

Pernicious anemia is a megaloblastic anemia caused by vitamin B_{12} deficiency due to lack of the intrinsic factor in the gastric juice. This is primarily a disorder of elderly persons and has a familial tendency. The abnormality is in the gastric mucosa: the stomach wall becomes atrophic and fails to secrete intrinsic factor. This substance ordinarily binds with the dietary vitamin B_{12} and travels with it to the ileum, where the vitamin is absorbed. Without intrinsic factor, no orally administered B_{12} can enter the body. Therefore, after the body stores of B_{12} are used up, the patient begins to show signs of the anemia.

Clinical Manifestations. The patient gradually becomes weak, listless, and pale. The hematologic effects of deficiency are accompanied by effects on other organ systems, particularly the gastrointestinal tract and nervous system. Patients with pernicious anemia develop a smooth, sore, red tongue and mild diarrhea. They may become confused, but more often have paresthesias in the extremities and difficulty keeping their balance because of damage to the spinal cord: they lose position sense. These symptoms are progressive, though the course may be marked by spontaneous partial remissions and exacerbations. Without treatment, patients die after several years, usually from congestive failure secondary to anemia.

Diagnostic Evaluation. The diagnostic laboratory studies are gastric analysis and the Schilling test. All pernicious anemia patients have gastric achlorhydria (absence of hydrochloric acid), even after histamine stimulation. However, older people can also lack gastric acid without lacking intrinsic factor, so the Schilling test is essential. The purpose of this test is to prove that the patient cannot absorb oral vitamin B_{12} unless intrinsic factor is added.

The patient is given a small dose of radioactive B_{12} in water to drink, followed by a large nonradioactive intramuscular dose. When the oral vitamin is absorbed, it will be excreted in the urine; the IM dose helps to flush it into the urine. A 24-hour specimen is collected and measured for radioactivity. If very little has been excreted, the test is repeated several days later (the "second stage"), with a capsule of oral intrinsic factor added to the oral B_{12}. If the patient has pernicious anemia, this time much more radioactivity will be found in the 24-hour urine.

It is also possible to measure the B_{12} level in the serum. This test usually requires several weeks to perform but can be very helpful if one of the newer, faster methods is used. However, a low B_{12} level could be due not only to pernicious anemia but also to other less common causes of the vitamin deficiency: strict vegetarian diets, total gastric resection, inflammatory disease of the ileum, blind-loop syndrome, and infestation with fish tapeworm.

Treatment. The treatment of pernicious anemia is intramuscular injections of vitamin B_{12}. At first, B_{12} is given daily, but eventually most patients are managed with 100 μgm. IM monthly. This can produce dramatic recoveries in desperately ill patients. The reticulocyte count rises within a week, and in several weeks the blood counts are all normal. The tongue improves in several days. The neurologic manifestations require more time for recovery, and if there is severe neuropathy, paralysis, or incontinence, the patient may never recover fully.

- Vitamin B_{12} therapy must be continued for the life of the patient who has had pernicious anemia in order to prevent recurrence of the anemia.

Nursing Management. These patients may need support during the diagnostic tests and nursing care for several aspects of their disease: anemia, congestive failure, neuropathy. When they are incontinent or paralyzed, care must be taken to prevent pressure sores and contracture deformities. The Schilling test can be useful only if the urine collections are complete; here, the nurse's assistance is essential. The patients must be taught about the chronicity of their disorder and the necessity for monthly injections, even when they are asymptomatic.

Folic Acid Deficiency

Folic acid is another vitamin which is necessary for normal red blood cell production. It is stored as different compounds referred to as folates. The folate stores in the body are much smaller than those of vitamin B_{12}, so it is much more common to see dietary folate deficiency. This occurs in patients who rarely eat uncooked vegetables or fruits, i.e., primarily elderly people living alone or alcoholics. Folic acid requirements are increased in chronic hemolytic anemias and in pregnancy, hence these patients may develop the anemia while ingesting an adequate diet.

- Patients on prolonged intravenous feeding or hyperalimentation may become folate deficient after several months, unless the vitamin is given intramuscularly. Some patients with small bowel diseases may not absorb it normally.

Clinical Manifestations and Laboratory Tests. All of these patients have the characteristic findings of megaloblastic anemia along with a sore tongue, but they lack any of the neurological manifestations of pernicious anemia. The diagnosis is made by assay of serum folic acid.

Management. Treatment is good diet and 1 mg. of folic acid a day. This should be given intramuscularly only in patients with malabsorption. With the exception of the vitamins given during pregnancy, most proprietary vitamin preparations do not contain folic acid, hence it must be given as a separate tablet.

HEMOLYTIC ANEMIAS

In hemolytic anemias, the erythrocytes have a shortened life span. The bone marrow is usually able to compensate partially by producing new red cells at three or more times the normal rate. Consequently, all of these anemias have certain laboratory features in common: the reticulocyte count is elevated, the fraction of indirect bilirubin is increased, the haptoglobin (a binding protein for free hemoglobin) is often low. The bone marrow is hypercellular, with erythroid proliferation. The only truly diagnostic test for hemolysis is the red cell survival study. This is usually only necessary for difficult diagnostic problems. About 20 to 30 ml. of the patient's blood is removed, incubated with radioactive chromium-51, and then reinjected. The chromium-51 labels the red cells exclusively. After these cells have equilibrated with the circulating blood, small samples are taken at intervals over the next days and weeks, and the radioactivity is measured. A normal chromium-51 survival time is 28 to 35 days. Red cells of patients with severe hemolysis (such as sickle cell anemia) have survivals of 10 days or less.

INHERITED HEMOLYTIC ANEMIAS

Hereditary Spherocytosis

Hereditary spherocytosis is a hemolytic anemia characterized by small, sphere-shaped red cells and splenomegaly. This is an uncommon disorder inherited in a dominant fashion.

Clinical Manifestation and Diagnosis. An abnormality of the erythrocyte membrane causes cells to lose membrane as they pass through the spleen and to become spherical in shape. These spheres are relatively rigid and easily destroyed. The peripheral blood contains many of the characteristic small spherical cells, and the patient has an anemia which may be exacerbated during infections, even minor viral illnesses. In addition, the spleen is enlarged. The disorder is usually diagnosed in childhood, but may be missed until adult life, since there are few symptoms.

Management. Splenectomy is the treatment; it does not change the erythrocyte defect but removes the site of membrane loss and hemolysis. After splenectomy (page 674), the patients have normal hemoglobin levels, only slight shortening of red cell survival, and few spherical cells in the peripheral smear. Patients have a normal life expectancy. The major complications are all prevented by splenectomy: (1) aplastic crises after infection, often with severe anemia, (2) nonhealing leg and ankle ulceration, and (3) gallstones.

Sickle Cell Anemia

Sickle cell anemia is a severe hemolytic anemia resulting from a defective hemoglobin molecule and associated with attacks of pain. This disabling disease is found predominantly in Africans and in black Americans, but it also occurs in people from Mediterranean and Arab countries.

Pathophysiology. The defect is a single amino acid substitution in the β chain of hemoglobin. Since normal hemoglobin A contains two α and two β chains, there are two genes for synthesis of each chain. A person with sickle cell trait has inherited only one abnormal gene, hence his red cells can synthesize both normal β chains and β^s chains; thus, he has A and S hemoglobin. If two people with sickle trait marry, some of their children may inherit two abnormal genes and will then have only β^s chains and only S hemoglobin; these children have sickle cell anemia.

Clinical Manifestations. The sickle hemoglobin has the unfortunate property of acquiring a crystal-like for-

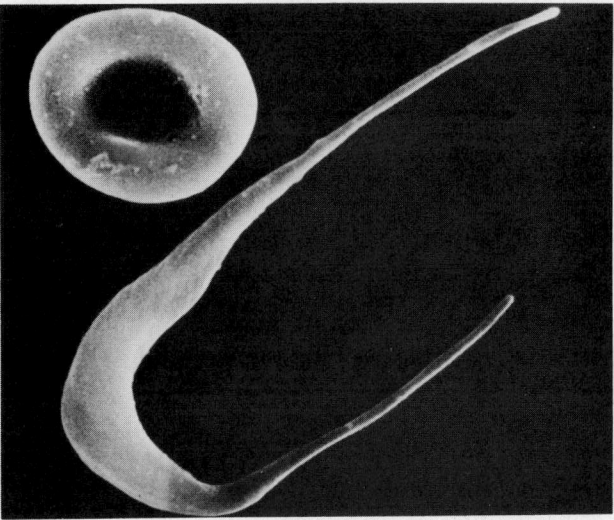

Figure 32-3. Unusual photo of a sickled and a normal red blood cell was taken under the auspices of the Comprehensive Sickle Cell Center, University of Miami. Photo by Dr. Bruce R. Cameron.

mation when exposed to low oxygen tension. The oxygen in venous blood is low enough to cause this change; consequently, the cell containing S hemoglobin becomes deformed, rigid and sickle-shaped, when in the venous circulation (Fig. 32-3). These long, rigid cells can become lodged in small vessels, and when they pile up against each other, blood flow to a region or an organ may be slowed. When ischemia or infarction results, the patient may experience pain, swelling, and fever. Such a chain of events is presumed to explain the painful crises of this disease, but what triggers the chain or how to prevent it is not understood.

Diagnostic Evaluation. The diagnosis can be made by hemoglobin electrophoresis, a costly procedure, or by "sickle prep," in which a drop of blood is mixed with sodium metabisulfite and watched under the microscope for sickling. Sickling in this test occurs whether the patient has sickle trait or sickle cell anemia; only the electrophoresis can make the distinction. The patient with sickle trait has a normal hemoglobin and hematocrit level as well as a normal blood smear; however, the "sickler" has a low hematocrit and sickled cells on smear.

SICKLE TRAIT. The patient with sickle trait is protected from crises because the hemoglobin A in his cells prevents them from sickling under ordinary circumstances. He has no anemia and looks and feels well. About 5 percent of black Americans have sickle trait.

SICKLE CELL ANEMIA. Patients with sickle cell anemia are usually diagnosed in childhood, since they are anemic in infancy and begin to have crises at 1 or 2 years of age. Many die in the first years of life, but antibiotics and patient and physician education about this disease have probably improved the outlook in the last 10 or 20 years, and some patients live into the sixth decade. All siblings of a patient with sickle cell anemia should be tested for the disease.

Symptoms. Symptoms are secondary to hemolysis and thrombosis. Patients are always anemic, with hemoglobin values in the 7-10 gm./100 ml. range. Jaundice is characteristic and is usually obvious in the sclerae. The bone marrow expands in childhood in a compensatory effort, sometimes leading to enlargement of the bones of the face and skull. As a result, patients may have prominent foreheads and high cheekbones. The chronic anemia is associated with tachycardia, flow murmurs, and often cardiomegaly. Arrhythmias and heart failure may occur in older patients.

Like patients with spherocytosis, sicklers may develop aplastic crises when infected and may have gallstones and leg ulcers. The latter may be chronic and painful and require grafting. These patients are unusually susceptible to infection, particularly pneumonias and osteomyelitis. Infection has been one of the most common causes of death.

All of the patient's tissues and organs are constantly vulnerable to microcirculatory interruptions by the sickling process and therefore are susceptible to hypoxic damage or true ischemic necrosis at any time. Thrombotic episodes may result in minor pain in an extremity, in severe pain and swelling in a hand or knee, in pain simulating an acute abdominal crisis, or in the sudden appearance of a "stroke," with hemiplegia. These crises are completely unpredictable; they can occur monthly or very rarely and may last for hours, days, or weeks. Certain effects of infarction are permanent, such as hemiplegia, aseptic necrosis of the femoral head, and renal concentrating defects.

Treatment. There is no specific treatment for the hemoglobin abnormality. The disease could be prevented only by intensive genetic counseling of the population at risk, a difficult and controversial task. Crises cannot now be prevented although researchers are evaluating several chemicals with antisickling properties. However, these are still in the experimental stage. Since infection seems to predispose to crises in children, all infections should be promptly treated or prevented when possible. Since dehydration and hypoxia promote sickling, patients are instructed to avoid high altitudes, anesthesia, or fluid loss. Because of the renal defect, these patients easily become dehydrated. Folic acid therapy is given continuously, since the marrow has an increased requirement.

When sickle crisis occurs, the mainstays of therapy are hydration and analgesia. Increased fluid intake helps to dilute the blood and reverse the agglutination of sickled cells within the small blood vessels. Patients and families can learn to handle minor crises at home, but if there is no relief after several hours, hospital admission may be necessary. The patients often have fever and leukocytosis with crisis, so that infection or appendicitis or cho-

lecystitis may be suspected and must be ruled out. Intravenous fluids (3-5 L./day for adults) are essential. Narcotic analgesics are often necessary because of the severity of pain and should be given in adequate doses. They should never be used chronically, however, for some patients do become addicted.

Transfusions are reserved for particular situations: (1) aplastic crisis, when the patient's hemoglobin falls rapidly, (2) severe painful crisis not responding to any other therapy after several days, (3) as a preoperative measure, to dilute the amount of sickle blood, (4) sometimes during the latter half of pregnancy in an attempt to prevent crises.

Management. The nurse can help the patient and family to adjust to this chronic disease and to understand the importance of hydration and prevention of infection. When leg ulcers are present, they require careful dressing and protection from trauma. If they fail to heal, grafting may be necessary. Cardiac disease is managed in the same way as for the nonsickler. During crisis, the patient should be kept quiet and allowed to rest undisturbed; swollen limbs should not be exercised. The community health nurse should be a case finder for this disease. Ideally, every black child should be tested for sickle cell anemia before entering school.

Other Hemoglobinopathies

C Hemoglobin. C hemoglobin is less common among American blacks than S hemoglobin. The C trait is asymptomatic, and homozygous C disease is a mild hemolytic anemia with splenomegaly but no serious complications.

Thalassemia. Thalassemia occurs primarily in people of Greek and Italian extraction. In this disease, A hemoglobin is made in smaller than normal amounts, but there is no abnormal hemoglobin. Thalassemia minor (or trait) has few symptoms. Thalassemia major (Cooley's anemia) is a very severe hemolytic disease, often fatal in childhood. It is rarely encountered in adults.

Glucose-6-Phosphate Dehydrogenase Deficiency

The abnormality in this disorder is in G-6-PD, an enzyme within the red cell which is essential for membrane stability. A few patients have inherited an enzyme so defective that they have a chronic hemolytic anemia. But the most common type of defect results in hemolysis only when the red cells are stressed by certain situations, such as fever or the presence of certain drugs. The disorder came to the attention of researchers during the Second World War, when some soldiers developed hemolysis while taking primaquine, an antimalarial drug. Drugs that are hemolytic for G-6-PD-deficient individuals are antimalarial drugs, sulfonamides, nitrofurantoin, the common coal tar analgesics (including aspirin), the thiazide diuretics, the oral hypoglycemic agents, chloramphenicol, para-aminosalicylic acid (PAS), vitamin K, and, for certain individuals subject to "favism," the fava bean. Primarily blacks and peoples of Greek or Italian origin are affected. The type of deficiency found in the Mediterranean group is more severe than that in the black group, resulting in greater hemolysis and sometimes in life-threatening anemias. All types are inherited as X-linked defects; thus, many more males are at risk than are females. In this country, about 15 percent of black males are affected.

Clinical Manifestations. The patients are asymptomatic and have normal hemoglobin levels and reticulocyte counts most of the time. Several days after exposure to an offending drug, they may develop pallor and jaundice, and the hemoglobinuria and the reticulocyte count will rise. Special strains of the peripheral blood may then show Heinz bodies (degraded hemoglobin). Hemolysis continues for a week, and then spontaneously the counts begin to improve, since the new young red cells are resistant to lysis. In the Mediterranean type, this recovery does not occur.

Diagnosis and Management. The diagnosis is made by a screening test or a quantitative assay of G-6-PD. The treatment is removal of the drug. Transfusion is only necessary in the Mediterranean variety. The patient should be educated about his disease and given a list of drugs to avoid. These include: sulfonamides, hypoglycemic agents, antimalarials, nitrofurantoin, phenacetin, aspirin (in high doses) and para-aminosalicylic acid.

ACQUIRED HEMOLYTIC ANEMIAS (TABLE 32-2)

Immune Hemolytic Anemia

When antibodies combine with red cells they can be either isoantibodies, reacting with foreign cells, as in transfusion reactions or erythroblastosis fetalis, or autoantibodies, which react with the cells of the host. The immune hemolysis which results may be very severe. Antibodies coat the red cells, producing a positive Coombs' test. These cells are then removed by the spleen and the rest of the reticuloendothelial system. Many cells are destroyed, and others return to the circulation as spherocytes with reduced membrane and a shortened survival rate.

In *idiopathic autoimmune hemolytic states,* it is not known what induces the immune system to produce the antibodies. The disease usually begins suddenly, often in persons over 40 years of age. In some cases, the hemolysis is associated with systemic disease (especially systemic lupus erythematosus, chronic lymphatic leukemia, or lymphoma). Other patients, with identical clinical pictures, can be shown to be producing antibodies to a drug (especially penicillin, cephalosporins, or Quinidine). The antibodies or the drug-antibody complexes then attach to red cells, resulting in hemolysis. Patients taking large

TABLE 32-2. ACQUIRED HEMOLYTIC ANEMIAS

NAME	CAUSE	MANIFESTATIONS AND TREATMENT
Paroxysmal nocturnal hemoglobinuria	Unknown—sometimes occurs after aplastic anemia.	Dark urine (hemoglobinuria) especially in morning Sometimes pancytopenia Multiple venous thrombosis No treatment known
Immune hemolytic anemia	Antibodies produced, sometimes secondary to drug (methyldopa [Aldomet], penicillin)	Jaundice, spherocytes Responds to steroids
Microangiopathic hemolytic anemia	RBC damaged during flow through abnormal small blood vessels, as in malignant hypertension.	Fragmented RBC seen on smears Treat primary disease
Heart valve hemolysis	RBC damaged by regurgitant flow through incompetent valve prosthesis	Fragmented RBC Treatment: replace valve
Spur cell anemia	Severe liver disease, usually portal hypertension Increased lipid in RBC membrane	Spur-shaped RBC No treatment
Infections	Malaria, *Clostridium welchii,* especially after septic abortion	Hemoglobinuria possible Treat the infection
Hypersplenism	Large spleen from any cause: cirrhosis, lymphomas	Sometimes pancytopenia Treatment: splenectomy

doses of methyldopa may develop antibodies to their own red cells; only a few of these patients have a significant hemolytic anemia.

Clinical Manifestations. The disease is characterized by fatigue, dyspnea, palpitations, and jaundice which develop over several weeks. The spleen may be slightly enlarged, or the patient may show evidence of one of the diseases mentioned above. Older patients can present with heart failure. The hemoglobin is usually 6-9 gm. per 100 ml. at diagnosis, but can be much lower; the reticulocyte count is very high, and the Coombs' test is strongly positive.

Management. Any possibly offending drug should be discontinued. Since the antibody may react with all possible donor cells, transfusion is often impossible. The treatment consists of high doses of corticosteroids (60-100 mg. of Prednisone daily) until hemolysis decreases. Usually after several weeks, the hemoglobin has returned toward normal and the steroid dose can be lowered; in some patients it can be discontinued entirely.

Splenectomy removes a major site of red cell destruction, hence this operation is often performed if steroids do not produce a remission. Recurrences of the idiopathic type of autoimmune hemolytic anemia are common.

POLYCYTHEMIA

Polycythemia refers to an increased concentration of red cells; it is a term used when the red cell count is greater than 6 million/cu. mm. or the hemoglobin exceeds 18 gm./100 ml. True polycythemia is present when the total body red cell mass is increased. "Relative" polycythemia occurs when the red cell mass is normal but the plasma volume is reduced; this may be produced by diuretic therapy or by unknown factors. Red cell mass can be measured accurately by an isotopic technique.

Secondary Polycythemia. Secondary polycythemia is due to excessive production or erythropoietin. This may occur in response to a hypoxic stimulus, as in chronic obstructive pulmonary disease or cyanotic heart disease, or in certain hemoglobinopathies in which the hemoglobin has an abnormally high affinity for oxygen (e.g., hemoglobin$_{Chesapeake}$). In some cases of secondary polycythemia, the production of erythropoietin is inappropriate, since there is no hypoxemia: this is the situation in a few patients with renal carcinoma, renal cysts, cerebellar hemangioblastoma, hepatoma, or uterine fibroids.

Polycythemia Vera. Polycythemia vera, or primary polycythemia, is a proliferative disorder in which all the marrow cells seem to have escaped from the normal control mechanisms. The bone marrow is intensely cellular, and in the peripheral blood, the red count, white count, and platelets are often all elevated. Patients typically have a ruddy complexion and hepatosplenomegaly. The symptoms are referable to the increased blood volume (headache, dizziness, fatigue, and blurred vision) or to decreased blood flow (angina, claudication, thrombophlebitis). Bleeding is also a complication, perhaps because of the engorged capillaries.

Management. The objective of management is to reduce the high blood viscosity by administering radioactive phosphorus or an alkylating agent such as busulfan or by doing repeated phlebotomies. In addition, when the patient has an elevated uric acid level, allopurinol is often used to prevent gouty attacks. The average survival is 10 to 15 years. Some patients develop acute leukemia; others develop myelofibrosis and myeloid metaplasia.

LEUKOPENIA AND AGRANULOCYTOSIS

Leukopenia is a condition in which the white cells number fewer than normal. *Agranulocytosis* is a condition in which there is almost complete absence of polymorphonuclear cells. A leukocyte count of fewer than 5,000/cu. mm. or a granulocyte count of fewer than 2,000/cu. mm. is abnormal and may be a signal of a generalized bone marrow disorder, such as megaloblastic anemia, aplasia, metastatic tumor, myelofibrosis, or acute leukemia. Viral infections and overwhelming bacterial sepsis can also cause leukopenia. Most commonly, the etiology is drug toxicity: phenothiazines are implicated most frequently; antithyroid drugs, sulfonamides, phenylbutazone, and chloramphenicol are also contributing factors. The patient is not symptomatic unless infection develops, which usually occurs when the granulocytes are fewer than 1,000/cu. mm. Fever and severe sore throat with ulcerations are common complaints. Bacteremia may follow soon after.

Management. Any possibly offending drugs are withdrawn. If the granulocyte count is very low the patient is isolated from hospital personnel and visitors by strict precautions. Cultures of all orifices and blood are essential, and when fever occurs it is treated with broad spectrum antibiotics until the specific organism is known. Good oral hygiene is helpful.

Hot saline irrigations of the throat are employed to keep it clear of necrotic detritus and exudate. Comfort is provided by supplying an ice collar and whatever analgesic, antipyretic, and sedative drugs may be indicated. The essence of treatment, apart from eradicating the infection, is to eliminate, if possible, the factor responsible for the bone marrow depression. Spontaneous restoration of marrow function, except in the case of neoplastic diseases, often occurs in time, i.e., within 2 or 3 weeks, if death from infection can be averted.

LEUKEMIA

The leukemias are neoplastic disorders of the blood-forming tissues (spleen, lymphatic system, and bone marrow). The common feature of the leukemias is an unregulated proliferation or accumulation of white cells in the bone marrow, with replacement of normal marrow elements. There is also proliferation in the liver, spleen, and lymph nodes, and invasion of non-hematologic organs such as the meninges, gastrointestinal tract, kidney, and skin. The leukemias are classified according to the cell line involved, as either lymphocytic, granulocytic, or monocytic, and according to the maturity of the malignant cells, as either acute (immature cells) or chronic (differentiated cells). The etiology is unknown, but there is some evidence that genetic influence and viral pathogenesis may be involved. Bone marrow damage with radiation (as in the atomic bomb survivors) or chemicals (benzene) can cause leukemia.

Acute Leukemia

Acute leukemia may be lymphocytic, granulocytic, or monocytic. Acute lymphocytic leukemia is a disease of young children and is uncommon after the age of 20 years. Acute granulocytic (or myelocytic) leukemia affects all age groups but is most common in adults. Monocytic leukemia is rare, but resembles the myelocytic type in most respects. The clinical course of the acute leukemias is similar for all types.

Clinical Manifestations. Symptoms reflect one of the following characteristics of the disease: (1) organ infiltration or (2) bone marrow failure. Organ infiltration results in a variety of symptoms: pain from enlarged liver or spleen; lymphadenopathy; headache or vomiting secondary to meningeal leukemia (most common in lymphocytic leukemia); and bone pain from expansion of marrow. Bone marrow failure leads to weakness and pallor from anemia; fever or infection secondary to granulocytopenia; and skin and mucous membrane bleeding due to thrombocytopenia.

The onset may be insidious, occurring over several weeks, or it may occur suddenly with high fever and hemorrhage. The patient is often treated for what appears to be a routine infection, and only when blood counts are performed is the diagnosis suspected. The peripheral blood usually shows anemia and thrombocytopenia as well as an elevated white count (10,000–100,000/cu. mm.) with a predominance of immature blast cells. Occasionally the white count is low and few leukemic cells are seen: this is referred to as "aleukemic leukemia." However, in all cases, a bone marrow specimen is diagnostic.

Management. Before chemotherapy was available, almost all patients with acute leukemia died within weeks or months. Now children with acute lymphocytic leukemia often live 3 to 5 years, and some are cured. Adults with acute myelocytic leukemia still generally die in a year.

Chemotherapy destroys abnormal leukemic cells, causes bone marrow depression, and depresses the patient's immunological defense mechanism. Drugs most useful in acute lymphocytic leukemia are vincristine, corticosteroids (often used together as the first treatment), methotrexate, 6-mercaptopurine and cyclophosphamide. The drugs are used in combination at high dose levels to produce greater leukemic cell damage. Newer drugs are asparaginase, daunorubicin, and cytosine arabinoside. After a patient achieves a remission (bone marrow is no longer leukemic) he is put on a combination of drugs for maintenance. Often he can live a completely normal life during a remission. In acute myelocytic leukemia, cytosine arabinoside, thioguanine, and daunorubicin are the best drugs at present, though all of those mentioned above are useful.

Transfusions of platelets and red cells are essential in management, as are antibiotics. Since many of the drugs are toxic to normal marrow cells, a period of marrow aplasia is common during treatment, especially for acute myelocytic leukemia. During this period, severe infections often occur: patients should not be treated prophylactically with antibiotics, but the appropriate drugs should be used whenever positive cultures are obtained. Frequent cultures are necessary. The major causes of death in acute leukemia are infection (often gram-negative sepsis) and bleeding.

Chronic Myelocytic Leukemia

Chronic myelocytic leukemia is primarily a disorder of young adults. The onset is usually insidious; the disease is usually discovered accidentally or as a result of the patient's complaining of weakness, unusual bleeding, or pain or a mass in the left abdomen, due to splenomegaly.

Clinical Manifestations. Patients look well initially, and the examination may reveal only a large spleen. Late in the disease, patients are pale, febrile, and wasted, with bone tenderness and a huge spleen extending into the pelvis. The white count is often greater than 100,000/cu. mm., and mature granulocytes and metamyelocytes predominate. Increases in basophils and eosinophils are found, and some myelocytes and blasts are usually seen. Thrombocytopenia occurs late in the disease.

Management. Symptoms can be managed well with busulfan (Myleran), but therapy has to be monitored closely, since profound marrow toxicity can occur with this drug and a serious late complication is pulmonary fibrosis. Radiation to the spleen is also sometimes helpful. The final event in most patients is a transformation into an acute myelocytic leukemia which is usually resistant to all therapy. Overall, patients live for about 3 years.

Chronic Lymphocytic Leukemia

Most patients with chronic lymphocytic leukemia are over 50 years of age. The disorder is often found accidentally during a physical examination or blood count studies.

Clinical Manifestations. Patients may be troubled by enlarged nodes or by symptoms of anemia, but they usually do not appear ill. The spleen and liver are only slightly enlarged. The white cell count may be 20,000–200,000/cu. mm. with 80–90 percent of small mature lymphocytes. These patients may develop thrombocytopenia or autoimmune hemolytic anemia at any time during their course; these conditions are best managed with corticosteroids. Once nonhemolytic anemia develops, it is generally progressive, despite chemotherapy. Bacterial infections plague these patients because their impaired ability to synthesize antibodies results in hypogammaglobulinemia. Pneumonias and ear and sinus infections are common. Occasionally, leukemic infiltrations of the skin are seen. Pleural or peritoneal effusions occur.

Management. Treatment is usually with one of the alkylating agents, such as cyclophosphamide or chlorambucil.

Nursing Management of the Patient with Leukemia

Like other patients with malignant diseases, patients with leukemia are often depressed, frightened, and lonely. A well-informed and sympathetic nurse can contribute immeasurably to their comfort by explaining procedures, anticipating side effects of drugs, and encouraging patients to participate in the therapeutic regimen. The therapy can become very complex, and too often the patient feels that more is being done "to him" than "for him." The nurse can be a sympathetic listener and help him to mobilize his defenses to cope with his emotional and physical stresses. When a patient is placed in reverse isolation because of granulocytopenia, his sense of rejection is intensified, and nursing personnel must be sensitive to this.

These patients should be approached in the same manner as those with aplastic anemia (see page 659), since they are usually thrombocytopenic, granulocytopenic, and anemic. The bleeding tendencies should be recognized, and undue trauma or intramuscular injections must be avoided. Acetaminophen rather than aspirin should be used for analgesia since aspirin increases bleeding in thrombocytopenic patients. Any increase in petechiae, any melena, hematuria, or nosebleeds should be reported. Hemorrhage is treated by bed rest and transfusions of red cells and platelets. All transfusions carry certain hazards (see page 677).

Because of the lack of mature and normal granulocytes, these patients are always threatened by infection, the major cause of death in leukemia. Antibacterial soap (pHisoHex) is used on the skin to reduce bacterial flora. Any evidences of infection (fever, chills, phlebitis, or abscesses) must be reported promptly. Rectal abscesses are not unusual, hence it is important to ensure normal elimination and avoid rectal thermometers, enemas, or rectal trauma. Intravenous sites must be kept meticulously clean and must be checked frequently for signs of phlebitis. Some of these patients must receive intravenous therapy for weeks at a time, hence the status of veins becomes a major concern.

The chemotherapeutic agents may be associated with many unpleasant side effects. Mucosal ulcerations are common; these can be treated with sodium carboxymethylcellulose (Orabase) or lidocaine (Xylocaine) solution to reduce pain. Antiemetics are helpful if given before the administration of certain of the more nauseating drugs. Dietary planning has to be reevaluated frequently since the patient's status changes rapidly. But a good fluid intake is important for all of these patients, since they tend to form uric acid deposits in the kidney due to massive turnover of cells with excretion of uric acid. Since vincristine causes constipation, patients are given laxatives routinely for prophylaxis. Paresthesias and footdrop, which may occur after treatment with vincristine, should be reported. Cyclophosphamide and other drugs produce alopecia; this hair loss is not permanent but is often very distressing to patients. Cyclophosphamide administration is sometimes followed by painless hematuria, a complication which can be avoided by good hydration.

When the patient no longer responds to therapy, he may be hospitalized for supportive care. He has often experienced remissions and exacerbations of his disease, and he has known hope and despair. He is very tired and ill and requires knowledgeable nursing assessment, support, and expert physical care. (See also chapter on patients with advanced carcinoma, page 275.)

MALIGNANT LYMPHOMA

The lymphomas are neoplasms of the cells of the lymphoid system: the lymphocytes and histiocytes. They are classified according to the predominant malignant cell, as lymphocytic lymphoma (previously called lymphosarcoma), histiocytic lymphoma (previously called reticulum cell sarcoma), or Hodgkin's disease. These tumors usually start in lymph nodes, but can involve lymphoid tissue in the spleen, the gastrointestinal tract (for example, the tonsils or the wall of the stomach), the liver, or bone marrow. They often spread to all of these areas and to extralymphatic tissues (lungs, kidneys, skin) by the time of death. The etiology of these tumors is unknown.

HODGKIN'S DISEASE

Hodgkin's disease, like other lymphomas, is a malignant disease of unknown etiology that originates in the lymphatic system and involves predominantly the lymph nodes. It occurs at all ages and in both sexes equally.

The malignant cell of Hodgkin's disease, its pathologic hallmark and its essential diagnostic criterion, is the "Reed-Sternberg cell," a gigantic atypical tumor cell, morphologically unique and of uncertain lineage, which many regard as an aberrant histiocyte.

Patients with Hodgkin's disease are customarily classified into subgroups based on pathologic criteria that reflect the grade of malignancy and suggest the prognosis. *Hodgkin's paragranuloma,* for example, with fewest Reed-Sternberg cells and least disturbance of nodal architecture, carries a much more favorable prognosis than *Hodgkin's sarcoma,* in which the lymph nodes are virtually replaced by tumor cells of the most primitive type. The majority of patients, with so-called *Hodgkin's granuloma* (which includes two conditions currently designated "nodular sclerosis" and "mixed cellularity") are in an intermediate position with respect to the density and destructiveness of tumor cells, therapeutic responsiveness, and overall outlook.

Clinical Manifestations

Hodgkin's disease usually begins as a painless enlargement of the lymph nodes on one side of the neck, which becomes increasingly conspicuous. However, for months generalized pruritus may be the first and only symptom and later is often a most distressing one. The individual nodes remain firm and discrete (that is, they do not soften and do not fuse) and they are seldom tender and painful. Soon the lymph nodes of other regions, usually the other side of the neck, also enlarge in the same manner. The mediastinal and retroperitoneal lymph nodes may also enlarge, causing severe pressure symptoms: pressure against the trachea results in dyspnea; pressure against the esophagus causes dysphagia; pressure on the nerves causes laryngeal paralysis, and brachial, lumbar, or sacral neuralgias; pressure on the veins results in edema of one or both extremities and effusions into the pleura or peritoneum; and pressure on the bile duct causes obstructive jaundice. Later the spleen may become palpable, and the liver may enlarge. In some patients the first nodes to enlarge are those of one axilla or of one groin. Occasionally, the disease starts in mediastinal or peritoneal nodes and may remain limited to them. In still other cases the enlargement of the spleen is the only conspicuous lesion.

Sooner or later a progressive anemia develops. A leukocytosis often is observed with an abnormally high polymorphonuclear count and an elevated eosinophil count. About half of the patients have a slight fever, the temperature seldom rising above 38.3° C. (101° F.). However, the patients with mediastinal and abdominal involvement present a remarkable intermittent fever. The temperature goes as high as 40.0° C. (104° F.) for periods of 3 to 14 days, returning to normal within a few weeks. Untreated, this disease is progressive in its course; the patient loses weight and becomes cachectic, the anemia becomes marked, anasarca appears, the blood pressure falls, and in 1 to 3 years death is likely to ensue.

Diagnosis

The diagnosis of Hodgkin's disease hinges on the identification of its characteristic histologic features in an excised lymph node. A diagnosis having been firmly established on the basis of the requisite criteria, it becomes necessary to assess as accurately as possible the total extent of tumor involvement and to define the manner in which it is distributed. In other words, one attempts to pinpoint the location of every tumor lesion inside and outside the lymphatic system and to exclude the presence of a tumor in organs and tissues that are not yet involved. This is a difficult, expensive, and uncertain undertaking but an extremely important one, since these are the very considerations on which treatment is to be based.

Management

Current concepts of treatment stem from the following observations and premises:

1. Hodgkin's disease spreads from its original location (usually a single node) by way of the lymphatic channels to contiguous lymph nodes, which in turn become the sites of tumor growth; it rarely skips lymph nodes en route to more distant sites of metastasis.
2. Rarely does Hodgkin's disease spread beyond the lymphatic system to involve other organs and tissues until late in the disease.
3. Hodgkin's disease is completely and permanently eradicated from any site that has received a radiation dose of 4,000 to 4,500 rads within the space of about 4 weeks. Megavoltage radiation techniques permit the delivery of such a dose to one or more entire lymph node chains.
4. Areas of the body in which the lymph node chains are located can tolerate doses of this magnitude without serious damage (as can the area of the spleen and the oronasopharynx, both of which may become involved in Hodgkin's disease), provided that vital structures such as the lungs, liver, gastrointestinal tract, kidneys and bone marrow are protected by carefully shaped lead shields.

From the foregoing it is postulated that Hodgkin's disease is potentially curable by radiotherapy, provided it has not extended beyond the lymph node chains, spleen, and oronasopharynx. Failing signs of such extension, patients with this disease should have the benefit of "curative" radiotherapy in which tumoricidal doses are delivered not only to obvious tumor nodes but to all adjacent nodes and lymph node chains as well. Conversely, any sign of spread beyond the treatable areas automatically disqualifies the Hodgkin's patient from such a program, in which case a combination of chemotherapy and palliative radiotherapy would be indicated.

Radiation therapy often requires many weeks of daily trips to the hospital. At least 3,500 R (rads) must be given to the tumor and adjacent lymph node areas. Patients develop dysphagia, dry mouth, nausea, skin rashes, and some hair loss. They are helped by such measures as skin creams, oral lidocaine, and antiemetics. The drugs used in Hodgkin's disease include nitrogen mustard, chlorambucil, prednisone, vincristine (Velban), procarbazine, carmustine (BCNU), bleomycin and adriamycin. They are often used in combinations of three or four drugs, in monthly courses. Since patients may have a complicated dosage schedule to remember, it is helpful if the physician or nurse writes out the schedule. Encourage the patient to continue the therapy. The side effects of most of these drugs are covered in the section on leukemia (pages 666–668).

It may be necessary to give laxatives and stool softeners to control constipation that accompanies chemotherapy. Surgery may be performed to alleviate complications caused by pressure or obstruction due to tumor masses.

Staging of Hodgkin's Disease. For the sake of simplicity, uniformity, and convenience in categorizing Hodgkin's patients with respect to the extent and activity of their disease, and hence their eligibility for curative radiotherapy, the disease generally is classified, or "staged," as follows:

Stage I: disease limited to a single node and contiguous structures;

Stage II: disease involves more than a single node or group of contiguous nodes, but is confined to one side of the diaphragm only;

Stage III: disease is present both above and below the diaphragm, but does not extend beyond the lymph node chains, spleen, or oronasopharynx;

Stage IV: disease has extended to the bone marrow, lung parenchyma, pleura, skin, gastrointestinal tract or liver.

Stage II and stage III patients are further subdivided on the basis of the presence or absence of constitutional symptoms: those without are designated IIA or IIIA; those with, IIB or IIIB. Therapeutic programs vary in different instititions, but most would agree that all stage I and stage II patients should receive "curative" radiotherapy. Some would also include stage IIIA patients in this program, whereas others would be inclined to substitute a combination of chemotherapy and palliative radiation. For stages IIIB and IV the use of cytostatic and antimetabolite drugs generally is regarded as the therapeutic mainstay, radiation being reserved for the palliative treatment of local lesions that are especially damaging or painful.

NON-HODGKIN'S LYMPHOMAS

Lymphocytic lymphomas are more indolent and have a better prognosis than histiocytic lymphomas. In its mildest form, lymphocytic lymphoma is very similar to chronic lymphatic leukemia, but bone marrow infiltration occurs late or not at all. Patients with these disorders are likely to have generalized lymph node disease or extranodal disease when first discovered. Therefore, radiation is not often curative. Nevertheless, radiation can be very helpful in palliation. Chemotherapy can produce remissions which last from several months to a year. In unusual cases, the lymphomas can present as isolated tumors of the stomach, small intestine, or spleen, and these are sometimes curable.

The chemotherapeutic agents are the same as for Hodgkin's disease, but cyclophosphamide and vincristine are especially effective.

MYCOSIS FUNGOIDES

This is a rare lymphoma of the skin. It usually begins as a pruritic, red rash, and months or years later the skin becomes infiltrated with plaques and tumors of lymphoma. The body may be covered with mushroom-like growths varying in size from 1 to 5 cm. (0.4-6 inches). Eventually the malignant process reaches nodes, liver, and spleen. Patients are very uncomfortable with the itching and disfigurement of this disease. Treatment with nitrogen mustard (which may be used topically) or irradiation can achieve palliation.

The patient with painful ulcerative lesions will require skilled nursing. A bed cradle should be placed over him to remove the weight of bedding from his painful skin lesions. Bacteriostatic ointment may be prescribed as a preventive measure against secondary infection and to seal off air from open nerve endings. Other aspects of management are similar to those for the patient with Hodgkin's disease.

MULTIPLE MYELOMA

Multiple myeloma is a malignant disease of plasma cells that infiltrate bone and soft tissues. This is not classified as a lymphoma. The malignant cell is the plasma cell, the neoplastic proliferation taking place mainly in the bone marrow. Lymph nodes are not involved.

Patients generally present with a normochromic normocytic anemia, bone pain, and sometimes leukopenia or thrombocytopenia, due to marrow infiltration by malignant plasma cells. Reticulocyte counts are low or normal. The blood smear shows "rouleau" formation: the red cells are aligned in aggregates resembling stacks of coins; this is caused by the presence in plasma of high concentrations of proteins produced by the plasma cells. The diagnosis of myeloma can be made by aspiration or biopsy of the bone marrow. X-rays showing destructive lesions of many bones are suggestive but not diagnostic for this disease. Bone fractures are common, especially in the vertebrae or ribs.

Patients may be incapacitated by constant bone pain. Plasma cell tumors can appear in many sites in these patients, including skin, mouth, and pleura; these are often painless. The osteolytic lesions are often associated with hypercalcemia; nausea, vomiting, constipation, and lethargy are the symptoms. The malignant plasma cells produce large quantities of abnormal globulins, which appear in the serum electrophoresis as a paraprotein "spike." Fragments of these globulins are excreted in urine as Bence Jones proteins. These proteins can contribute to renal failure, which is common in myeloma.

Management. Phenylalanine mustard (Alkeran), cyclophosphamide, and steroids are the drugs used to decrease the tumor mass and relieve bone pain. They can prolong life from 1 year to 2 or 3 years. Radiation is very useful for palliation of bone pain and for reducing the size of extraskeletal plasma cell tumors. Good hydration is essential in order to prevent renal damage from precipitation of Bence Jones protein in the renal tubules, hypercalcemia, and hyperuricemia. Thus it is important to assess these patients for signs and symptoms of renal insufficiency. When the patients have severe pain, they need narcotic analgesics and local irradiation, and sometimes back braces to relieve pressure. Pathological fractures are also possible. It is important to keep the patients as active as possible, since bed rest only increases the likelihood of hypercalcemia. Bacterial infections, especially pneumonia, are common in these patients, since they have impaired capacity for antibody production. Patients with multiple myeloma should not be put on fasting regimens for diagnostic tests since dehydrating procedures can precipitate acute renal failure.

BLEEDING DISORDERS

Pathophysiology. Protection of the body against excessive and lethal blood loss is afforded by several mechanisms. Thus, hemorrhage from a large lacerated vessel is retarded as a result of an abrupt lowering of the arterial blood pressure, i.e., "shock," which reduces the rate of blood flow throughout the body and therefore reduces the rate of its escape. Further protection also may be furnished by compression of the leaking vessel by the swelling mass of blood (hematoma) surrounding the vessel. Complete and permanent sealing of the latter, however, is accomplished through the clotting of the blood, which results in the production of an adherent gel-like mass that effectively controls most types of hemorrhage.

As was indicated in Figure 32-1, the normal blood-clotting mechanism is fairly complex. When a small blood vessel is injured, the first line of protection is the platelet. These tiny cells are rapidly attracted to the damaged endothelium and form loose plugs. More platelets gather, and eventually these fuse together and contract, forming stable plugs. A lipid substance on the platelet surface (platelet factor 3) stimulates a series of chemical reactions involving proteins in the blood plasma, the result of which is the conversion of prothrombin to thrombin. This is a very active enzyme which has several functions: one is to encourage further platelet aggregation; another is to convert fibrinogen to fibrin. Therefore, strands of fibrin begin to form in the vicinity of the platelet plug, reinforcing the plug and producing a larger clot. The fibrin clot is then further stabilized by the formation of bonds between the molecules, catalyzed by another plasma protein, factor XIII. The result is that the damaged vessel is sealed, and blood flow in the area is slowed. Then, tissue repair of the vessel endothelium can proceed. Eventually, much of the fibrin clot will be lysed by another plasma protein system—the plasmin system, which produces fibrinolysis.

A final factor of great importance in the prevention of bleeding is the normal resistance of blood vessels to mechanical rupture, whether by the pressure of blood exerted from within the vessel or traumatic pressures exerted from the outside.

Abnormalities which predispose to hemorrhagic diseases can affect vessels, platelets, any of the plasma coagulation factors, fibrin, or plasmin. Some patients can have defects at several sites simultaneously. Bleeding may be a manifestation of a primary coagulation defect (as in hemophilia), may occur secondary to another disease (as in cirrhosis, uremia, or leukemia), or may even be due to drugs (overdose of coumadin).

Clinical Manifestations

The symptoms and signs of bleeding disorders vary, depending on the type of defect. A careful history can often give clues to the diagnosis. Since platelets are primarily responsible for the cessation of bleeding from small vessels, patients with thrombocytopenia will have petechiae—small red or purple spots, often in clusters, seen on the skin and mucous membranes. Trauma results in excessive bruising but not large uncontrolled hematomas. After cuts or skin puncture, bleeding stops promptly with local pressure and does not recur when pressure is released. In contrast, in hemophilia and abnormalities of other coagulation factors, the platelets function normally so that there are no petechial or superficial hemorrhages. Instead, deep bleeding occurs after minor trauma, such as intramuscular hematomas and hemorrhage into joint spaces. External bleeding recurs several hours after pressure is removed—as, for example, severe bleeding starting several hours after a tooth extraction. Abnormalities of the vascular system give rise to local bleeding, usually into the skin.

Vascular Defects

Based on a disturbance of one or another of the mechanisms operating to prevent bleeding—the clotting properties of the blood, the availability of platelets, and the stamina of the blood vessels—a variety of disorders are encountered that are characterized by an abnormal tendency to bleed. These will be discussed in three major categories: those classed as vascular purpura, marked by the spontaneous rupture of small vessels that presumably are defective or injured; those attributable to a deficiency of platelets; and those related to the existence of a clotting defect.

VASCULAR PURPURAS

Purpura is the term applied to small hemorrhages in the skin and the mucous membranes that occur spontaneously as an isolated phenomenon or as an accompaniment of obvious disease. The smallest hemorrhages, pinhead in size, are called "petechiae," whereas larger hemorrhagic lesions are described as "ecchymoses." Both types occur as the result of vascular rupture, permitting the leakage of blood into the subcutaneous tissue of the mucous membranes. In one type, called "symptomatic" or "secondary" purpura, this bleeding is quite unrelated to any intrinsic defect of the blood vessels; certain types of bloodstream infections (e.g., meningococcemia and subacute bacterial endocarditis) exhibit this phenomenon due to direct damage to the vascular walls by the infectious agent.

Another group of patients exhibiting this type of purpura are those with severe arterial hypertension and "easy bruising," perhaps due to an abnormal degree of pressure in the fragile capillary circuits when the blood flow within these vessels is increased, as may occur as a result of a blow, exposure to heat, or following the release of a tourniquet on an extremity. Other examples of vascular purpura, the mechanism of which is even more obscure, are found in cachectic individuals and in patients with uremia.

Anaphylactoid Purpura

Anaphylactoid purpura represents yet another type of vascular purpura, the clinical features of which are somewhat more complex and comprise a distinct entity. Among its numerous manifestations are various skin lesions, purpuric and otherwise, and episodes of arthritis, abdominal pain, hematuria, gastrointestinal hemorrhages, and fever. These attacks recur for years, and each attack lasts for several weeks. The leakage of blood vessels at localized points throughout the system apparently is responsible for the principal complications of anaphylactoid purpura, the basic cause of which, however, is obscure. Generally it has been regarded as an allergic disorder. Steroid therapy often is effective.

Familial Hemorrhagic Telangiectasia

This is a hereditary disorder manifested by an abnormal tendency to bleed and become bruised. Localized aggregations of dilated capillaries may be observed in the skin and in the mucous membranes of the nose or the mouth. They also may be present in the gastric mucosa, explaining certain cases of gastrointestinal bleeding. Whether the characteristic lesions are present or absent, there may be a generalized decrease in capillary "resistance," as is evidenced by the abnormal ease with which the vessels are ruptured by minor traumas. However, the precise nature of the defect is obscure, and the condition does not respond to any proved method of treatment.

Toxic Purpura

This condition has been observed after exposure to certain drugs and poisons, including aniline, certain arsenicals, and snake venom. Some of these toxic cases present the features of thrombocytopenic purpura, but others are explained more readily on the basis of blood vessel damage.

PLATELET DEFECTS

The sudden onset of petechiae, purpura, or excessive bruising or bleeding from the nose or gums should stimulate a search for a platelet defect. Deficiencies of platelet number, or thrombocytopenias, are most common, but there are also some rare disorders of platelet function, in which the platelet count is normal but the clinical picture is identical to that in thrombocytopenia. The platelet function disorders can be diagnosed by special tests for platelet factor 3 and platelet adhesiveness and aggregation. The most important functional disorder to remember is that induced by aspirin: even small amounts of aspirin prevent normal platelet aggregation, and the bleeding time test is prolonged for several days after aspirin ingestion. Although this defect does not cause bleeding in most normal people, patients with another coagulation disorder (such as thrombocytopenia or hemophilia) can experience life-threatening hemorrhage after taking aspirin.

Thrombocytopenia

Thrombocytopenia can result either from decreased production of platelets by the marrow or from increased peripheral destruction. Some of the causes are listed in

TABLE 32-3. THROMBOCYTOPENIAS

CAUSE	TREATMENT
I. Failure of Production	
Leukemia	Treat the leukemia
Tumor invasion of marrow	
Aplastic anemia	Androgens and steroids
Megaloblastic anemia	B_{12} or folic acid
Hereditary types (rare)	
Toxins: especially alcohol	Discontinue alcohol
Drugs: thiazides	Discontinue drug
II. Increased Destruction	
Due to antibodies	
ITP	Steroids, splenectomy
Lupus erythematosus	Steroids
Malignant lymphoma	Steroids
Drugs: quinine, sulfonamides	Discontinue drug
Due to entrapment in large spleen	Splenectomy
Cirrhosis of the liver	
Gaucher's disease	
Myelofibrosis and myeloid metaplasia	
Infections	
Septicemia	
Postviral (rubella, infectious mononucleosis)	
Disseminated intravascular coagulation	Heparin

Table 32-3. If the platelet deficiency is secondary to an underlying disease, this can usually be diagnosed from the examination of the patient or the bone marrow. When peripheral destruction is the cause of thrombocytopenia, the marrow is cellular, with increased megakaryocytes, and the Chromium-51 platelet survival is very short (several hours or days instead of the normal 7-10 days). Bleeding and petechiae usually do not occur with platelet counts above 50,000/cu. mm., although excessive bleeding can follow surgery.

When the platelet count drops below 20,000/cu. mm., petechiae appear and there is excessive menstrual bleeding, nosebleeds, and hemorrhage after surgery or dental extractions. When the platelet count is less than 5,000/cu. mm., spontaneous fatal central nervous system hemorrhage or gastrointestinal hemorrhage can occur.

Management. The management for secondary thrombocytopenia is usually that of the underlying disease. If platelet production is impaired, platelet transfusions may help to raise platelet counts and stop bleeding or prevent intracranial hemorrhage. If excessive destruction is the problem, transfused platelets will also be destroyed and will not raise the count.

Idiopathic Thrombocytopenic Purpura (ITP)

ITP is a disease of all ages but commonly affects children and young women. Antiplatelet antibodies are produced for unknown reasons, so that platelet life span is markedly shortened. Occasionally the antibodies can be demonstrated in vitro, but usually the diagnosis is made from the platelet survival data and the lack of any underlying disease. Symptoms begin suddenly, with petechiae and mucosal bleeding. The platelet count is generally below 20,000/cu. mm. Death may result from intracranial bleeding. There are no physical findings of note other than the hemorrhages.

Management. Corticosteroids are the treatment of choice: the bleeding ceases in 1 to 2 days, and platelet counts rise in a week or so. About three quarters of patients respond to steroids, but many have a relapse when the drug is withdrawn. These patients, as well as the nonresponders, are subjected to splenectomy. Splenectomy produces a lasting remission in most patients, though transient recurrences of thrombocytopenia sometimes occur months or years later. The rare patients who do not respond to splenectomy are sometimes treated with the immunosuppressive drugs azathioprine or cyclophosphamide.

CLOTTING FACTOR DEFECTS

Hemophilia

There are two hereditary bleeding disorders which are indistinguishable clinically, but which can be separated by laboratory tests—hemophilia A and hemophilia B. Hemophilia A is due to a deficiency of factor VIII, whereas hemophilia B stems from a deficiency of factor IX. Factor VIII deficiency is about five times more common. Both types of hemophilia are inherited as X-linked traits, so that almost all affected individuals are males; their mothers and some of their sisters are carriers but are asymptomatic.

Symptoms. The disease, which may be very severe, is manifested by large spreading bruises and bleeding into muscles and joints, even after minimal trauma. Patients often note pain in a joint before swelling and limitation of motion are apparent. Recurrent joint hemorrhages can result in damage so severe that chronic pain or ankylosis (fixation) of the joint occurs. Many of the patients are crippled by the joint damage before they become adults. The disease is recognized in early childhood, usually in the toddler age group.

Prior to the availability of factor VIII concentrates, many patients died of the complications before reaching adulthood. Some hemophiliacs have a milder deficiency, having between 5 to 25 percent of the normal level of factor VIII or IX. These patients do not experience the painful and disabling muscle and joint hemorrhages, but bleed only after dental extractions or surgery. Nevertheless, such hemorrhages can prove fatal if the cause is not recognized quickly.

Management. In the past, the only treatment was fresh frozen plasma, which had to be given in such large quantities that the patients became volume overloaded. Now factor VIII and IX concentrates are available to all blood banks. Patients are given concentrates when they are actively bleeding or as a prophylactic measure before dental extractions or surgery. Some families are taught how to administer the concentrate at home, at the first sign of bleeding. The objective is to raise the factor level to more than 30 percent. The infusions must be repeated every 8 to 12 hours to maintain the desired level.

A few patients eventually develop antibodies to the concentrates, so that their factor levels cannot be elevated. Treatment of this problem is extremely difficult and often unsuccessful. Epsilon aminocaproic acid (EACA) is an inhibitor of fibrinolytic enzymes. This drug can slow the dissolution of blood clots which do form, and is sometimes used after oral surgery in hemophiliacs.

In terms of general care, patients with hemophilia should never be given aspirin or intramuscular injections. Dental hygiene is very important as a preventive measure, since dental extractions are so hazardous. Splints and other orthopedic devices may be very useful in patients who have suffered joint or muscle hemorrhages.

Von Willebrand's Disease

This is a common bleeding disorder, inherited as a dominant character and affecting males and females equally. It is due to a mild deficiency of factor VIII (15-50 percent of normal) associated with an impairment of platelet function. The laboratory tests show normal platelet count, prolonged bleeding time, and slightly prolonged partial thromboplastin time. Patients commonly have nosebleeds, excessively heavy menses, bleeding from cuts, and postoperative bleeding. They do not suffer from massive soft tissue or joint hemorrhages. Both of the defects can be corrected by the administration of cryoprecipitate (any precipitate that results from cooling). (See page 677.)

Hypoprothrombinemia

Prothrombin, as was previously noted, is essential for the clotting process.

This protein is produced in the liver by a vitamin K dependent chemical process. Vitamin K enters the body from food sources as well as from synthesis by bacteria that reside in the intestine. Normal prothrombin activity in the blood depends on adequate absorption of this vitamin from the gastrointestinal tract and on adequate liver function. Therefore, prothrombin deficiency may arise as a result of diarrhea, from a lack of bile in the gastrointestinal tract (necessary for absorption of fat-soluble vitamin K) due to biliary tract obstruction, from surgical removal or mucosal damage of a large part of the small intestine, from prolonged antibiotic therapy, or as the result of liver disease.

The principal manifestation of prothrombin deficiency, as observed in patients with hemophilia, is prolonged hemorrhage from blood vessels that are damaged by trauma or disease, which explains the characteristic occurrence of ecchymoses, hematuria, gastrointestinal bleeding, and postoperative hemorrhages.

Dicumarol Toxicity. Dicumarol is a drug that is often employed medically for the express purpose of inducing a partial depression of prothrombin activity, since the drug interferes with the action of vitamin K in the liver. Dicumarol therapy is usually calculated to prolong the prothrombin time by 2 to 2½ times the normal time. In this range, thrombosis is inhibited and thrombophlebitis is prevented. However, if Dicumarol is taken in excessive dosages, whether intentionally or mistakenly, or if certain other drugs are administered simultaneously which interfere with the metabolism of Dicumarol, the complete picture of prothrombin deficiency, with a severe hemorrhagic disorder, may be produced.

Management. Hypoprothrombinemia, if due to vitamin K deficiency, responds to treatment with any of several preparations that are available for oral or parenteral administration. However, when corrective measures are urgently required, particularly in patients with liver disease or Dicumarol toxicity, the effective treatment requires the direct replacement of prothrombin by means of transfusion, since purified preparations of prothrombin are not yet available.

Liver Disease. The liver cell makes all the plasma coagulation factors except factor VIII. Therefore, in severe hepatic disease of any sort, deficiencies of these factors may occur. The prothrombin time and partial thromboplastin time will both be prolonged. If the spleen is enlarged as well (as in cirrhosis), the platelet count may also be depressed. These patients frequently bruise easily and may have life-threatening hemorrhage from peptic ulcers or esophageal varices. Treatment includes fresh frozen plasma, fresh blood, and factor IX complex (Konyne). Vitamin K does not improve the disorder.

Disseminated Intravascular Coagulation (DIC)

Occasionally, widespread clotting in small vessels of the body occurs, leading to consumption of the clotting factors and platelets, so that paradoxically the patient presents with a bleeding disorder characterized by low fibrinogen, prolonged prothrombin time and partial thromboplastin time, low factor VIII, and thrombocytopenia. Such patients may bleed from mucous membranes, venipuncture sites, and the gastrointestinal and urinary tracts. They may also develop renal failure due to fibrin deposition in small vessels of the kidney. Many serious illnesses may predispose to DIC, including septicemia, premature separation of the placenta in a pregnant woman, metastatic malignancies, hemolytic transfusion reactions, and massive tissue trauma. The best treatment is correction of the underlying disease, but in the meantime intravenous heparin may retard the coagulation process and permit normalization of clotting tests and a decrease in the hemorrhagic manifestations.

THERAPEUTIC MEASURES IN BLOOD DISORDERS

SPLENECTOMY

The surgical removal of the spleen is sometimes necessary following trauma to the abdomen. Since the spleen is very vascular, severe hemorrhage can result after splenic rupture. Under such circumstances, splenectomy becomes an emergency procedure.

Splenectomy is also often performed as a treatment for a number of hematologic disorders. An enlarged spleen may be the site of excessive destruction of blood cells, and when this destruction is life-threatening, the operation may prove palliative. This is the case in autoimmune hemolytic anemia or idiopathic thrombocytopenic purpura when these disorders do not respond to corticosteroids. Some patients with severe anemia due to inherited red cell defects (such as thalassemia or pyruvate kinase deficiency) may benefit from splenectomy. Patients with rheumatoid arthritis may develop splenomegaly with destruction of granulocytes and granulocytopenia; removal of the spleen may improve the blood count and reduce the tendency toward infection.

Very large, bulky, and painful spleens (as may occur in myelofibrosis or chronic myelogenous leukemia) usually do not need to be removed, but when symptoms and blood counts do not respond to drugs, splenectomy can be helpful. Most patients with hereditary spherocytosis are essentially cured of their hemolytic process by splenectomy.

When the spleen is large, the operation can be difficult, but generally there is a very low mortality. Morbidity may result from postoperative atelectasis, pneumonia, abdominal distention, and subphrenic abscess formation. Young patients are at increased risk of pneumococcal infections for several years after splenectomy. Patients with high platelet counts (such as those with myelofibrosis) often are found to have even higher counts after splenectomy—greater than a million—and this can predispose the patient to serious thrombotic or hemorrhagic problems.

BLOOD TRANSFUSION

Blood Donation

Since blood and blood components are used so frequently, nearly all hospitals now have blood banks, and most large hospitals also have facilities for removal of blood from donors. These donor clinics are often the responsibility of nurses, who must screen prospective donors, supervise the phlebotomies, and care for the health and safety of the donors.

Donor Interviewing

Each prospective donor is examined and interviewed before the donation for his own protection and that of the recipient. The questioning must be tactful but complete, and an experienced interviewer will learn how to ask each question in several ways in order to obtain the most complete answers.

Donors should appear to be in good health and should be free of any of the following disqualifying factors:
1. A history of viral hepatitis, recently or at any time in the past, or a history of close contact with a hepatitis patient within 6 months. For safety, any history of jaundice should be a reason for exclusion, whatever the cause of jaundice.
2. A history of receiving a blood transfusion or injection of any fraction of blood other than serum albumin or gamma globulin, within 6 months.
3. A history of untreated syphilis or malaria, since these can be transmitted by transfusion even years later. If an individual has been free of symptoms and off therapy for 3 years after malaria, he may be a donor.
4. A history of evidence of alcoholism or narcotic addiction (since addicts have a high hepatitis carrier rate).
5. A skin infection, because of the possibility of contamination of the phlebotomy needle.
6. A history of recent allergy to drugs, asthma, or urticaria, because hypersensitivity can be passively transferred to the recipient.
7. Pregnancy within 6 months, because of the nutritional demands of pregnancy on the mother.
8. A history of oral surgery within 72 hours, since such procedures are frequently associated with transient bacteremia.

Blood donors who pass this screen are then examined with regard to blood pressure, pulse, oral temperature, weight, and hemoglobin level. The latter is often checked via a screening test that only estimates the hemoglobin. Individuals over 65 years of age are usually disqualified.

Donors are expected to meet the following minimal requirements:
1. The body weight should exceed 50 kg. (110 pounds) for a standard 450-ml. donation. Donors weighing less than 50 kg. (110 pounds) may be bled proportionally less.
2. The oral temperature should not exceed 37.5° C. (99.6° F.).
3. The pulse rate should be regular and between 60 and 120 beats per minute.
4. The systolic arterial pressure should be between 100 and 200 mm. Hg, and the diastolic between 50 and 100 mm. Hg.
5. The hemoglobin level in the case of a female should be at least 12.5 gm./100 ml.; in the case of a male, 13.5 gm./100 ml.

Phlebotomy

The donor is first given a full glass of water or juice to make sure he is not dehydrated. He is placed in a semi-recumbent position. The skin over the antecubital fossa is cleansed with iodine, a blood pressure cuff is inflated to around 100 mm. Hg (between systolic and diastolic pressures), and venipuncture is performed. The volume of blood collected into a plastic donor set is measured by weighing the bag, and this weight is watched closely so that no more than 450 ml. is drawn. The donor tube is doubly clamped and cut, the cuff deflated, and the needle withdrawn. The labels on the blood bag and tubes are checked carefully before and after donation, to avoid any error which could prove fatal to a recipient. The donor is asked to remain recumbent for 5 minutes and then sits up. If weakness or faintness are experienced, he should rest for a longer period. He should always remain in the donor area for 20 to 30 minutes for observation for any reaction.

Complications

Excessive bleeding at the site of venipuncture is sometimes due to a bleeding disorder in the donor, but more often is the result of a technical error: laceration of the vein, failure to release the blood pressure cuff before withdrawal of the needle, or failure to apply pressure to the venipuncture site for 5 minutes.

Fainting is relatively common and may be related to emotional factors, vasovagal reaction, or prolonged fasting before donation. Sometimes, because of the loss of blood volume, hypotension and syncope occur when the donor assumes an erect posture.

• If the donor appears pale or complains of faintness, he should immediately lie down or sit with his head lowered below his knees. The nurse should observe him for another 30 minutes.

Anginal chest pain may be precipitated in patients with unsuspected coronary artery disease.

Convulsions may occur in epileptic patients. Both angina and convulsions require further medical evaluation.

Blood and Blood Components

A unit of blood which has been drawn from a donor consists of approximately 450 ml. of whole blood and 60 to 70 ml. of acid-citrate-dextrose (ACD) solution. The latter serves as the anticoagulant and also provides the red cells with a sugar for metabolism. This blood can be maintained at 4° C. (39.2° F.) in the blood bank for 21 days, but after that it is discarded because too many of the red cells are unable to survive in vivo. Samples of the unit are always taken immediately after donation so that the blood can be typed and tested for the presence of syphilis and hepatitis-associated antigen (HAA). A label on the unit thereafter states the blood type and certifies that the unit is negative for syphilis serology and HAA.

Whole blood is a complex tissue, with both cellular and many noncellular plasma components. Recently it has been recognized that whole blood is necessary only in certain clinical situations; many times, component therapy can replace the particular deficiency without subjecting the patient to unnecessary risks such as circulatory overload. In addition, use of components is more economical, since it makes it possible to meet the needs of more than one patient from a single blood donation. Many blood banks are able to separate whole blood into these fractions, and all of the components are available from the American Red Cross.

Whole Blood. Whole blood is the treatment of choice for acute, active hemorrhage or hypovolemic shock due to hemorrhage. It is not indicated for the correction of anemia. Fresh whole blood is needed very rarely and only under certain conditions. If a patient undergoes massive transfusion, receiving 10 or more units of stored blood in 24 hours, he may become thrombocytopenic because platelets are labile in stored blood. He also may develop deficiencies of factors V and VIII, which remain active in storage only for several days. These deficiencies can be prevented if he receives some units of blood that are less than 24 hours old. Exchange transfusions always require blood less than 5 days old.

Packed Red Cells. Red cells are separated from whole blood by centrifugation or sedimentation; about 80 percent of the plasma is removed, leaving a hematocrit of 60 to 70 percent. Packed red cells are indicated for transfusions in all anemic patients and in surgical patients before and after operation. The use of packed cells instead of whole blood reduces the volume load. Thus this method is safer for patients with incipient congestive failure and reduces the incidence of transfusion reactions due to plasma factors.

Frozen Red Cells. The method of freezing red cells allows storage for long periods of time—even years—but is expensive. Hence, frozen cells are used only under unusual circumstances, such as for patients with very rare blood types or with antibodies to the common minor antigens.

Platelets. Patients with thrombocytopenia and hemorrhage often require transfusions of large numbers of platelets. Platelets taken from 5 to 10 units of blood are necessary to raise the count of a severely thrombocytopenic patient to a hemostatic level. Therefore, "platelet rich plasma" with a small volume is used rather than whole blood. Several methods are available for harvesting fresh platelets: (1) Plasma can be removed after centrifugation of a unit of freshly collected whole blood; the plasma is then centrifuged again slowly to separate the platelets. Several such platelet "units" can then be pooled and given to the recipient, who thus receives platelets from several different donors. The red cells are kept in the blood bank for future use. (2) A single donor can undergo *plasmapheresis,* in which 2 units of blood are donated, the red cells are separated and returned to the donor immediately, and the plasma is spun down to obtain platelets in a volume of only 10 to 20 ml. A closed system of interconnected plastic bags allows for safe phlebotomy and reinfusion. A single donor can give four units of platelets at one time in this way. (3) A more recent method of plasmapheresis involves centrifugation using the continuous or discontinuous "Haemonetics" system. The donor's red cells are returned faster, since the blood goes directly from vein to centrifuge, and in a period of one to two hours he can donate 6 units of platelets safely. Platelet concentrates are generally kept at room temperature with agitation, and are administered within 48 hours of collection to ensure viability. Each unit of platelets will raise the recipient's platelet count by about 5,000 per cu. ml. Single donor platelet transfusions are especially valuable for patients who have received many transfusions and have developed antibodies to all except HLA (transplantation antigen) matched blood products.

Granulocytes. Severely granulocytopenic patients with infection can sometimes benefit from transfusions of normal white cells. Large numbers of granulocytes (equivalent to 20 units of blood) less than 24 hours old must be administered. The methods utilized are either (1) continuous flow centrifugation or (2) filtration leukopheresis, a process in which the blood passes through nylon fiber filters which remove granulocytes; later the filters are separated and the cells are eluted in plasma and saline. In both methods, the donor's white cells are continuously removed as blood is drawn from one vein and constantly returned to another vein. The process requires about 4 hours of donor time and the donor must be anticoagulated during the procedure.

Plasma. Whole plasma was originally used in the treatment of hypovolemic shock, but now other colloids (such as albumin) or electrolyte solutions (like Ringer's lactate) are usually preferred. Plasma can be used to replace deficient coagulation factors in acquired or inherited bleeding disorders. Only fresh frozen plasma (which can be stored for 12 months) contains all the coagulation factors, including V and VIII. However, fractions of plasma have now been prepared which can replace all the factors, except V, in small volume concentrates. Thus, there is little use for whole plasma, except in patients with severe liver disease.

Albumin. Plasma albumin comprises 50 to 60 percent of the protein and therefore accounts for most of the oncotic pressure of the plasma. It is the chief determinant of plasma volume. This material is used to expand the blood volume of patients in hypovolemic shock and to elevate the level of circulating albumin in patients with hypoalbuminemia. These preparations, in contrast to all other fractions of human blood, cellular or soluble, are subjected to heating at 60° C. (140° F.) for 10 hours, and therefore can be certified unequivocally as free of all viral contaminants, including the hepatitis virus. Whereas the risk of hepatitis transmission is an important consideration in connection with every other type of transfusion therapy (except gamma globulin), no such complication has ever been known to follow the use of albumin.

Fibrinogen. This material is used primarily in congenital hypofibrinogenemia associated with bleeding and sometimes in the acquired defibrination syndromes. Its use is associated with a very high incidence of serum hepatitis, and this complication must be carefully considered whenever fibrinogen therapy is contemplated.

Factor VIII Fractions. These components have brought about a revolution in the treatment of patients with classical hemophilia. Whereas previously large volumes of plasma were necessary to treat bleeding episodes in this disease, now the volumes are so small that circulatory overload cannot occur. Cryoprecipitate is made from fresh frozen plasma, and the method of preparation is simple enough for use in most blood banks. Once the precipitate is separated, the rest of the plasma can be used for other purposes. The cryoprecipitate is redissolved in plasma or saline for use in patients who are deficient in fibrinogen, factor VIII, and factor XIII or have von Willebrand's disease. A glycine precipitate is available commercially, as Hemofil.

Prothrombin Complex. This fraction, commercially marketed as Konyne and Proplex, contains prothrombin and factors VII, IX, and X and some factor XI. It is useful for the treatment of bleeding in congenital or acquired deficiencies of these factors. However, the hepatitis hazard is significant with this material.

Transfusion Technique

Most aspects of the administration of transfusions are now within the province of the nurse. The nurse is the first to receive the unit from the blood bank, at which time it is necessary to refrigerate the blood if it is not to be used in the next half hour or so. Perhaps the most important function of the nurse is to check the labels on the donor blood and to make sure that the appropriate patient receives it.

Blood is generally administered through a large needle in an antecubital vein. The tubing should always include a filter so that any small clots are prevented from entering the patient. The nurse records the time at which the blood is started and discontinued, monitors pulse and temperature during the transfusion, and is alert to any *changes* or any *complaints* of dyspnea, nausea, vomiting, urticaria, or other symptoms which might indicate a reaction. It is important to stay with the patient for the first 10 minutes of the transfusion, since it is during this period that major reactions occur. During this time, the rate of infusion should not exceed 20 drops per minute, but it can be speeded up later unless the patient is in incipient congestive failure. The flow should be continuous; if it stops, either the nurse or physician must correct it immediately.

- If any sign of a transfusion reaction appears, the blood should be stopped and the physician should be notified without delay.

Transfusion Complications

Much has been learned about the cause of transfusion reactions in recent years; hence, many of the adverse effects can be prevented. Nevertheless, transfusion is never without certain risks, and these must be considered before the therapy is initiated.

Circulatory Overloading. In patients with normal blood volume (as in chronic anemia) or increased blood volume (as in renal failure or heart failure), the addition of whole blood or packed cells can precipitate pulmonary edema. Packed red cells are safer to use, and if the rate of administration is sufficiently slow, circulatory overloading may be prevented.

- The signs to look for are dyspnea, orthopnea, cyanosis, or sudden anxiety. If the transfusion is continued, severe dyspnea and coughing of pink, frothy sputum can occur.
- The patient should be placed in an upright position, the blood should be discontinued, and rotating tourniquets applied. Phlebotomy may be necessary if improvement does not occur rapidly.

Febrile Reactions. Patients may develop a fever during transfusion because of the presence of bacterial pyrogens, sensitivity to leukocytes or platelets, hemolytic episodes, or unknown factors. Due to the widespread use of disposable transfusion equipment, bacterial pyrogens are rarely a cause. Infrequently, blood can be grossly contaminated with large numbers of microorganisms which survive in the 4° C. (39.2° F.) storage. If such blood is infused, the patient develops fever and shaking chills within 30 minutes, and shock soon follows. Even when the cause of this reaction is recognized early (by gram stain of the donor blood), the mortality rate is high. Sensitivity to leukocyte or platelet antigens is much more common, especially in previously-transfused patients or women who have borne children. The temperature rises during the administration of blood or shortly afterward, and is rarely associated with chills, hypotension, or nausea. This type of reaction has a good prognosis, and the treatment is aspirin. Subsequent transfusions should utilize leukocyte-poor blood.

Allergic Reactions. Some patients may develop urticaria (hives) or generalized itching or, rarely, wheezing or anaphylaxis. The cause of these reactions is thought to be sensitivity to a plasma protein in the transfused blood, or passive transfer of antibodies from the donor which react with some antigen (for example, in a drug or food) to which the recipient is exposed. To avoid this, allergic individuals are disqualified as donors. The reactions are usually mild and respond to antihistamines. If severe, parenteral epinephrine is used.

Hemolytic Reactions. The most dangerous type of transfusion reaction occurs when the donor blood is incompatible with that of the recipient. Antibodies in the recipient's plasma rapidly combine with donor erythrocytes, and the cells are hemolyzed either in the circulation or in the reticuloendothelial system. The most rapid hemolysis occurs in ABO incompatibility, i.e., if the donor is group A and the recipient is group O (and therefore has anti-A and anti-B antibodies).

- Symptoms consist of chills, low back pain, headache, nausea, or chest tightness, followed by fever and hypotension and vascular collapse. Severe reactions usually start within 10 minutes after the transfusion is begun. Hemoglobinuria (red urine) appears at the next voiding.
- The reaction must be recognized promptly and the transfusion discontinued immediately; the chances of a fatal episode are much reduced if less than 100 ml. of incompatible blood are infused.

Treatment is directed toward correcting the hypotension and preventing the renal damage which can follow hemoglobinuria. The patient is supported with intravenous colloid and given mannitol as an osmotic diuretic to maintain a good urine flow. An indwelling catheter may be necessary for accurate measurement of output. If, after 24 hours, urine flow cannot be maintained, mannitol is contraindicated since it can be assumed that acute tubular necrosis has occurred. The management henceforth will be that of the renal disorder and will include

fluid restriction and possibly dialysis until spontaneous healing takes place.

Delayed Reactions. Delayed hemolytic reactions occur at about 1 to 2 weeks and are recognized by a gradual fall in hemoglobin level and a positive Coombs' test. There is no hemoglobinuria, and these reactions are not dangerous.

Serum Hepatitis. Serum hepatitis is an important risk of transfusion therapy, both for whole blood and for most components (see above). Blood obtained from "skid row" paid donors carries a higher risk than that from volunteer donors. Some of the hepatitis carriers can be screened out by use of the new tests for hepatitis-associated antigen, but even these methods give negative results for more than 50 percent of units which do transmit hepatitis. The recipient begins to have the symptoms of the disease (fever, lethargy, and jaundice) from 2 to 6 months after transfusion (see page 814).

Malaria. Malaria is sometimes transmitted in blood donated by asymptomatic individuals who have been exposed to the disease in Southeast Asia. Recipients develop high fever and headache several weeks after the transfusion.

Syphilis. Syphilis is rarely transmitted now because of the serologic tests required on all units of blood and because the organism does not survive refrigeration.

Nursing Responsibilities in Transfusion Reaction

If it is suspected that a transfusion reaction is occurring because of any of the symptoms mentioned above, the nurse should stop the transfusion and call the physician immediately.

The following steps are taken in order that a diagnosis may be made regarding the type and severity of the reaction:

- The transfusion set is disconnected, but the intravenous line is kept open with a dextrose or saline solution in case intravenous medication should be needed rapidly.
- *The blood bag and tubing are saved, not thrown away.* They should be sent to the blood bank for repeat typing and culture.
- The patient's blood is drawn for plasma hemoglobin, culture, and retyping.
- A urine sample is collected as soon as possible and sent to the laboratory for a hemoglobin determination. Subsequent voidings of urine should be observed.
- The blood bank is notified that a suspected transfusion reaction has occurred.

BONE MARROW TRANSPLANTATION

This is an exciting addition to the therapeutic possibilities for hematologic disease. Bone marrow can be aspirated by needle from multiple sites of an anesthesized normal donor and easily transfused intravenously into the recipient. The marrow cells immediately travel to the marrow spaces which have been emptied by disease (i.e., aplastic anemia), or by chemotherapy.

The major barrier to the success of bone marrow transplantation is the antigenic difference between donor and recipient. Thus, transplants between identical twins are almost always successful, and sibling transplants are often successful. If the donor and the patient are not identical in HLA (transplantation antigen) types, pretreatment of the patient with immunosuppression is necessary. Many recipients succumb to graft vs. host disease or severe infections while awaiting the recovery of the transplanted marrow. However, methods of immunosuppression and supportive care have improved greatly over the last few years, and this is currently the best treatment for severe aplastic anemia. In the future, it may be applicable to leukemia also.

BIBLIOGRAPHY

BOOKS

Boone, D. C.: Comprehensive Management of Hemophilia. Philadelphia, F. A. Davis, 1976.

Dougherty, W. M.: Introduction to Hematology, 2nd ed. St. Louis, C. V. Mosby, 1976.

Leavell, B. S., and Thorup, O. A.: Fundamentals of Clinical Hematology, 4th ed. Philadelphia, W. B. Saunders, 1976.

Miller, W. V., ed.: Technical Manual of the American Association of Blood Banks, 7th ed. Philadelphia, J. B. Lippincott, 1977.

Ogston, D., and Bennett, B.: Haemostasis: Biochemistry, Physiology and Pathology. New York, John Wiley and Sons, 1977.

Thompson, R. B.: Disorders of the Blood. New York, Churchill Livingstone, 1977.

Williams, W. J., et al.: Hematology, 2d ed. New York, McGraw-Hill, 1977.

Wintrobe, M. M., et al.: Clinical Hematology, 7th ed. Philadelphia, Lea and Febiger, 1974.

ARTICLES

Blood Transfusion

Buickus, B. A.: Administering blood components. AJN, 79:937-941, May 1979.

Cullins, L. C.: Preventing and treating transfusion reactions. AJN, 79:935-936, May 1979.

McCullough, J., and Scharr, J. B.: Blood: Which fraction? When? Why? Patient Care, 11:20-45, Dec. 15, 1977.

Parker, A. L.: Massive transfusions. AJN, 79:944-948, May 1979.

Scarlato, M.: Blood transfusions today: What you should know and should do. Nursing '78, 8:68-72, Feb. 1978.

Selleck, C.: Primary nursing in a hematology unit. NLN Pub., 52-1716:73-76, 1978.

Thomas, S. F.: Transfusing granulocytes. AJN, 79:942-944, May 1979.

Disseminated Intravascular Coagulation

Collins, G. J., et al.: Pitfalls in peripheral vascular surgery. Disseminated intravascular coagulation. Am. J. Surg., 134:375-380, Sept. 1977.

Eagle, M.: Nursing care study. Septicaemia proceeding to disseminated intravascular coagulation. Nurs. Times, 74:17-21, Jan. 5, 1978.

Ryan, F. P., et al.: Cerebral involvement with disseminated intravascular coagulation in intestinal disease. J. Clin. Pathol., 30:551-555, June 1977.

Schipper, H. G., et al.: Antithrombin-III transfusion in disseminated intravascular coagulation. Lancet, 1:854-856, Apr. 22, 1978.

Leukemia/Lymphoma

Desotell, S.: A brighter future for leukemia patients. Nursing '77, 7:18-24, Jan. 1977.

Gadsby, J. G.: Nursing care study: Acute myelomonocytic leukaemia. Nurs. Times, 74:1680-1683, Oct. 1978.

Hovenden, A. L.: Hodgkin's disease. Nurs. Times, 73: 1520-1522, Sept. 1977.

LeBlanc, D. H.: People with Hodgkin's disease. The nursing challenge. Nurs. Clin. N. Am., 13:281-300, June 1978.

Rossman, M., Slavin, R., and Taft, E. G.: Pheresis therapy. Patient care. AJN, 77:1135-1141, July 1977.

Varricchio, C. G.: Nursing care during total body irradiation. AJN, 77:1314-1315, Aug. 1977.

Walker, P.: Bone marrow transplant: A second chance for life. Nursing '77, 7:24-25, Jan. 1977.

Wallace, J., and Freeman, P. A.: Mouth care in patients with blood dyscrasias. Nurs. Times, 74:921-922, June 1, 1978.

Zimmerman, S., et al.: Bone marrow transplantation. AJN, 77:1311-1313, Aug. 1977.

Thrombocytopenia

Ahn, Y. S., et al.: The treatment of idiopathic thrombocytopenia with vinblastine-loaded platelets. New Eng. J. Med., 298:1101-1107, May 18, 1978.

Ayromlooi, J.: A new approach to the management of immunologic thrombocytopenic purpura in pregnancy. Am. J. Obstet. Gynecol., 130:235-236, Jan. 1978.

Branda, R. I., et al.: Plasma exchange in the treatment of fulminant idiopathic (autoimmune) thrombocytopenic purpura. Lancet, 1:688-690, Apr. 1, 1978.

Homan, W. P., and Dineen, P.: The role of splenectomy in the treatment of thrombocytopenic purpura due to systemic lupus erythematosus. Ann. Surg., 187:52-56, Jan. 1978.

McMillan, R.: The pathogenesis of immune thrombocytopenic purpura. CRC Crit. Rev. Clin. Lab. Sci., 8:303-332, Dec. 1977.

Nagasue, N., et al.: Platelet aggregability after splenectomy in patients with normosplenism and hypersplenism. Am. J. Surg., *136*:260–264, Aug. 1978.

Verheyden, C. N., et al.: Accessory splenectomy in management of recurrent idiopathic thrombocytopenic purpura. Mayo Clin. Proc., *53*:442–446, July 1978.

Zeluff, G. W., Natelson, E. A., and Jackson D.: Thrombocytopenic purpura—idiopathic and thrombotic. Heart Lung, 7:327–333, Mar.-Apr. 1978.

AGENCIES

Governmental

National Heart, Lung and Blood Institute, National Institutes of Health, Bethesda, Md. 20205

Voluntary

American Red Cross, 18th and E sts., N.W., Washington, D.C. 20006

Center for Sickle Cell Disease, Howard University, 2121 Georgia Ave., N.W., Washington, D.C. 20060

Leukemia Society of America, 211 East 43rd St., New York, N.Y. 10017

National Hemophilia Foundation, 25 West 39th St., New York, N.Y. 10018

American Cancer Society, 777 Third Ave., New York, N.Y. 10017

Digestive and Gastrointestinal Problems

UNIT EIGHT

33

ASSESSMENT AND MANAGEMENT OF PATIENTS WITH INGESTIVE PROBLEMS AND UPPER GASTROINTESTINAL DISORDERS

Since the process of ingestion begins with the mastication of food in the mouth, adequate nutrition is related to good dental health and the general condition of the mouth. The status of the teeth can have a direct bearing on nutritional well-being by influencing the type of food ingested and the degree to which food particles are properly mixed with salivary enzymes. Any discomfort in the mouth, due to lip lesions, inflammation of the buccal mucosa, or other conditions, can have a deleterious effect on food intake. Esophageal problems related to the apparently simple act of swallowing can also adversely affect food and fluid intake, thereby jeopardizing general health and well-being.

Given the close interrelationship between adequate nutritional intake and all of the structures of the upper gastrointestinal tract (lips, mouth, teeth, esophagus), it goes without saying that preventive health teaching should place heavy emphasis on helping people to avoid the common discomfort and disorders associated with any of these structures.

DENTAL CONDITIONS AND CARE OF THE TEETH

Care of the Teeth

The nurse, as a proponent of sound health practices, is in a unique position to teach and emphasize the importance of regular, periodic dental examinations. By supporting community dental health programs, by demonstrating proper dental techniques, and by supervising appropriate dental practices, the nurse can facilitate the dental therapeutic plan and encourage patient cooperation, and persistence with periodontal programs.

Healthy teeth require conscientious and effective daily cleaning. The purpose of toothbrushing is to mechanically break up the bacterial plaque that collects around teeth. Proper brushing requires a soft, rounded-tip bristle brush. The bristles of the brush are directed into the gingival sulcus in a horizontal scrubbing motion. Ten strokes are recommended for each surface. Dental floss should also be used every 24 hours to reach those areas

683

between the teeth not accessible to the brush. The floss is inserted between the teeth and moved back and forth in a gentle sawing motion until it reaches under the gum line. Of course, the normal movement of the muscles of mastication and the normal flow of saliva also aid greatly in keeping the teeth clean. Even so, it is necessary to disorganize plaque once during each 24-hour period, preferably before bedtime. This practice prevents decay and periodontal disease.

Nursing Intervention. Since many ill patients do not eat and salivate normally, the natural cleaning process of the teeth is reduced. If the patient is unable to clean his teeth adequately, he must be taught to do so. If a patient is absolutely unable to brush his teeth, as in the case of patients with cerebrovascular disease or those disabled by trauma, then it becomes a nursing responsibility. In any case, merely swabbing the patient's mouth and teeth with glycerine and lemon juice is inadequate, since all it does is coat collections of bacteria without removing them. The *most effective method is,* again, *mechanical cleansing.* It is better to wipe the patient's teeth with a washcloth than to have him swish an antiseptic mouthwash several times and then emit it into the emesis basin. If a toothbrush is used, an electric brush is more effective in cleansing someone else's teeth than the conventional hand toothbrush. While the left hand of the nurse retracts the lips and cheeks, the right hand can direct the electric brush to all surfaces of the patient's teeth. Even the tongue may receive a beneficial light brushing. Once any toothbrush is used, it should be cleaned thoroughly with soap and water and allowed to dry.

Dental Plaque and Caries

At least 95 percent of Americans sooner or later experience tooth decay. This is an erosive process that results from the action of bacteria on fermentable carbohydrates in the mouth, which in turn produces acids that dissolve tooth enamel. The extent of damage to the teeth depends on several factors, the most significant of which are (1) the presence of dental plaque; (2) the strength of the acids and the ability of the saliva to neutralize them; (3) the length of time the acids are in contact with the teeth; and (4) susceptibility of the teeth to decay. Dental plaque is a gluey, gelatinlike substance that adheres to the teeth and affords protection for the bacteria. The initial action that causes damage to a tooth occurs under dental plaque.

Dental decay begins with a small hole, usually in a fissure or flaw of the enamel, or in an area that is hard to clean. Left unchecked, it penetrates the enamel into the dentin. Because the dentin is not as hard as the enamel, decay progresses somewhat more rapidly and in time reaches the pulp. When the blood, lymph vessels, and nerves are exposed, they become infected, and an abscess may form, either within the tooth or at the tip of the root.

Soreness and pain usually accompany the abscess. As the infection increases, the face may become swollen, and there may be pulsating pain. The dentist can determine by x-ray pictures the extent of damage, and the type of treatment needed. It may be necessary to extract the tooth.

Measures used in the prevention and control of dental caries include reducing the intake of *sugars* (refined carbohydrates), practicing effective mouth care (as described), and applying fluoride to the teeth, or drinking fluoridated water.

Fluoridation. Adjusting the fluoride level in the drinking water to an optimal healthful level of one part per million can help to prevent up to two-thirds of tooth decay. Such a concentration of fluoride makes tooth enamel more resistant to the acids that are formed in the mouth. When ingested from birth to about ten years of age, fluoridated water can give permanent protection. Some sections of the western United States have natural fluoridation; other areas of the country have enacted legislation for controlled fluoridation of public water supplies. In these areas, studies have demonstrated a reduction in dental decay. Fluoridation also lessens the possibility of malocclusion and gingival disease.

Most areas of this country, however, do not have fluoridated water, and people must find other ways of receiving the benefits of fluoride. Four other methods are possible: (1) Vitamin preparations can include fluoride. Treatment must start early in life and continue until the age of ten. (2) A concentrated solution can be applied directly to the teeth. This procedure is done by the dentist and has the advantage of providing professional control and also encouraging regular check-ups. (3) Sodium fluoride can be added to the water in the home; however, home fluoridators that operate automatically are expensive and may do little good, since children drink most of their daily water supply in school. (4) Sodium fluoride can be provided in tablet or liquid drops as a dietary additive; this, too, is expensive and often impractical.

Technological Advances. Technological advances in recent years have produced several new coatings that bond to the enamel of the tooth and protect it from decay. These composite dental resins consist of an epoxy resin product and a form of acrylic acid, plus reinforcing fillers such as glass beads or quartz fillers. Dentists can use the new materials to seal pits and fissures when the teeth first grow in, thus preventing decay. The new materials can also be used to restore teeth eroded near the gum, a common site of periodontal disease.

A new translucent tooth-filling material, made by mixing a special aluminosilicate glass powder with a solution of polyacrylic acid, has several advantages over conventional enamel fillings made with phosphoric acid. The polyacrylic acid is much milder than phosphoric acid (which can damage the tooth, if the cavity is not lined before it is filled). Also, the new filling is adhesive, which eliminates the need for extensive drilling to secure the filling.

Dentoalveolar Abscess or Periapical Abscess

This type of abscess results from a suppurative process involving the apical dental periosteum and the alveolar process in the periapical region. It may appear in two forms. The acute form is usually secondary to a suppurative pulpitis that arises from an infection extending from dental caries. The infection of the dental pulp extends through the apical foramen of the tooth to form an abscess about the apex, at its site of implantation in the alveolar bone. The abscess produces a dull, gnawing, continuous pain, often with a surrounding cellulitis and edema of the adjacent facial structures. The gum opposite the apex of the tooth is usually swollen on the cheek side, where the abscess is prone to point. The swelling and cellulitis of the facial structures may make it difficult to open the mouth. In well-developed abscesses there may be a systemic reaction, fever, and malaise.

Management.   In the early stages of the infection, an opening may be drilled into the pulp chamber to relieve tension and pain and to provide drainage. Usually the infection has progressed to periapical abscess, and drainage must be provided by an incision through the gingivae down to the jaw bone. A foul pus escapes under pressure.

The postoperative care consists of hot saline mouthwashes given at least every 2 hours, except when the patient is asleep. He should be encouraged to expectorate the foul pus that escapes, and a basin should be within easy reach. External heat, in the form of hot compresses or a heating pad, hastens the subsidence of the inflammatory swelling and soreness. In patients with a high fever, an antibiotic (penicillin) is usually administered.

It goes without saying that bed rest and a soft diet are necessary during the acute stage. Analgesic drugs are used as necessary, to relieve pain. The nurse must recognize that the pain and swelling may interfere with an adequate fluid intake, and a special effort must be made to overcome any deficit. After the inflammatory reaction has subsided, the tooth may have to be extracted, or appropriate root canal therapy given.

Chronic dentoalveolar abscess is a slowly progressive infection, with the same mode as the acute form. It differs from the acute form in that the process may progress to a fully formed abscess without the patient's knowing it. The infection eventually leads to a "blind dental abscess" that is really a periapical granuloma. It may enlarge to as much as 1 cm. in diameter. It is often discovered in x-ray examination and is treated by extraction or root canal therapy, often with apicoectomy.

Periodontal Disease

Periodontal disease (pyorrhea) is a condition affecting the gums (gingivae) and other supporting structures (bone, cementum, and periodontal membrane). At the onset, there is little discomfort and few other signs of the condition. Later there may be bleeding, infection, gum recession, and loosening of the teeth. As a result, the teeth may fall out or may need to be extracted. It is estimated that one in four persons have the disease at some stage of its development, and up to 90 percent of all persons in their 40s are affected. Dental authorities suggest that the principal reason why most people, after age 50, require dentures is the effect of this increasingly prevalent disease.

Malocclusion, poor fillings, and inadequate diet are suspected causes of periodontal disease; in addition, improper cleaning and poor mouth hygiene contribute to the problem. Tartar or calculus that cannot be brushed from the teeth tends to build up and requires professional removal twice a year. If this is not done, gums become swollen and tender, infection progresses, and pockets that collect pus and bacteria are formed between the gums and teeth. The protective layer that normally covers the gums is destroyed, exposing the blood vessels, which bleed easily. Bacteria thrive on the nutrients in the blood and tissues which fill and line the space. The bone supporting the teeth is destroyed, and the tooth becomes loose.

Some authorities believe that this condition is frequently associated with other systemic diseases, such as diabetes and certain skin and blood disorders; however, conclusive evidence is lacking. At present, the best advice is to brush the teeth and floss carefully, at least once a day, and to have the teeth cleaned professionally twice a year. Such a cleaning should include the area below the gum line. Poor occlusion should be corrected, crooked teeth straightened, and missing teeth replaced with bridgework or another form of splinting. Not too long ago, such work by an orthodontist was considered a luxury and done only for cosmetic reasons. Today the value of such treatment is seen in the prevention of periodontal disease and other mouth problems. In the near future, perhaps, three-dimensional photography will assist periodontists in measuring the changes in the shape or elevation of the gum, signs that allow early detection of periodontal disease.

Orthodontal Correction for Malocclusion

Malocclusion is a faulty relationship between the teeth when the jaws are closed. Correction of malocclusion requires three factors: an orthodontist who has special training, a patient who cooperates, and adequate time. Most treatments begin when the patient has shed his last primary tooth and the last permanent successor has erupted, usually around 12 or 13 years of age.

In order to realign the teeth, the orthodontist gradually forces the teeth into a new location, by the use of wires or bands. This therapy is commonly known as teeth-straightening. Although the patient may object to the effect of these devices on his appearance, this psychological burden must be overcome, if good results are to be achieved in the future. During this time, it is essential that the patient keep his mouth meticulously clean. In the final phase of treatment, a retaining device is worn for several hours each day to support the tissues as they adjust to the new location of the teeth. Encouragement is often necessary for the individual to persist in this most important part of the treatment. When an adolescent undergoing orthodontal correction is admitted to the hospital for some other problem, it may be necessary to remind him to continue wearing the retainer, if it does not interfere with the problem requiring hospitalization.

Dental Implants and Transplantation

Successful research is being done involving the transplantation of teeth and the possible "storage" of teeth in a bank. Some researchers have restricted their transplants to undeveloped or "bud" teeth, whereas others are trying to transplant teeth at many stages of development. However, at present, homotransplants (transplanting teeth from one person to another) will have to await additional research to combat the rejection process. Successful autotransplants (using the patient's own teeth) have been reported. For example, a defective first molar has been replaced successfully by the patient's own third molar.

Teeth made from acrylic and other plastics have been implanted successfully, in several instances. In 1972, Neff, of Georgetown University, reported on an artificial plastic tooth made of Vacalon which, when implanted in baboons, functioned much like a natural tooth. New tissue grew around the implant, and bone grew through vents in the implant roots, as would occur with natural teeth. Neff's research may lead to the development of similar implants for humans. Also under study is the use of ceramic tooth roots made of high-density alumina (with metallic post and a conventional gold crown).

Implants are not to be considered as fully acceptable alternatives to other forms of dental treatment. Rather they are to be used only when other forms of treatment do not suffice to restore the mouth to its masticatory function. There is, and always will be an element of unpredictability in the field of oral implants. Therefore their use should be regarded as a last approach to sound dentistry.

Dental Extraction

A tooth is extracted because it is defective, damaged, or in the path of future orthodontic correction.

Extraction wounds usually heal quickly and without

complications, if simple precautions are taken. Lessened activity reduces the likelihood of bleeding. Cold applications soon after extraction, such as an ice bag or cold, moist cloth applied to the side of the face for about 15 minutes of every hour for several hours, will relieve discomfort and swelling. Rinsing the mouth is not done the first day, so that the clot will not be disturbed. Thereafter, rinsing and cleansing of the teeth is resumed.

Oozing of blood may be apparent the first day, but if heavier bleeding occurs, place a clean, folded gauze pad directly on the bleeding spot. Instruct the patient to close his teeth tightly over the pad, to apply pressure for about 30 minutes. Repeat, if necessary. If there is prolonged or severe pain, swelling, or bleeding, the dentist should be notified.

Impacted Third Molars. It may be desirable to hospitalize the patient when all four molars are to be extracted at one time. Using endotracheal general anesthesia, the oral surgeon inserts a mouth retractor to provide exposure. Incisions are made laterally in the mandible to approach the impacted tooth. The jaw eventually regenerates bone that has been removed. Closure of the mucous membrane is accomplished with black silk sutures.

Postoperatively, soreness and edema are noticeable, but can be relieved by analgesics and ice packs. Liquids may be offered from a spouted container if the facial muscles are too sensitive to allow the patient to suck from a straw. After the fifth day, stitches are removed and mouthwashes can proceed from saline to sodium peroxyborate monohydrate (Amosan). Brushing of the teeth is resumed when the gums have healed. Any pain or swelling after 1 week should be reported; infection is common, but can be easily treated with drainage, packing, and antibiotics.

Artificial Dentures

It is common practice for people to postpone indefinitely the final decision to obtain artificial dentures, even though there is no possibility of having the few remaining teeth repaired. Hesitant patients may be encouraged to pursue this health need by pointing out to them the positive aspects of obtaining dentures: improved appearance, better nutrition, and reduced likelihood of infection. When dentures have been obtained, patience is required in learning to use them effectively.

Dentures require careful scrubbing, using a good denture brush, mild soap and water, salt and sodium bicarbonate. The addition of a drop of household chlorine acts as a deodorant and gives a fresher taste. Most dentists recommend that dentures be removed at night, scrubbed, and allowed to soak in a proprietary cleaner. Sodium hypochlorite-phosphate (Mersene) has been shown to be most effective.

Pressure or irritation caused by dentures should be

reported to the dentist, who can make the proper adjustment. Uncorrected pressure areas may cause lesions, that in turn may become malignant.

Many persons now prefer to have "immediate dentures." Usually the back teeth are extracted first, which allows the tissues time to heal. Meanwhile, the artificial teeth are made and are ready for placement immediately after the front teeth have been extracted.

Partial dentures should not be left in place for prolonged periods without being removed for a good cleaning. They are held in place with metal clasps that encircle the teeth. These clasps can be spread: using gentle force with two index fingers, one side can be loosened, and then the other. When reapplied, the cleaned partial dentures usually can be pressed into place.

LESIONS OF THE LIPS

Actinic Cheilitis. Actinic cheilitis results from the cumulative effect of exposure to sun radiation and may lead to squamous cell carcinoma. It is manifested by whitish hyperkeratosis, fissuring, and erythema. Treatment consists of protecting the lips with a good sunscreen ointment; in some instances, electrosurgery or cryosurgery may be required. Periodic check-ups are mandatory to detect possible malignancy.

Contact Dermatitis. Lipsticks, cosmetics, ointments to prevent chapping, and even toothpaste and chewing gum may be the source of allergens that cause erythema, vesiculation, burning, and itching of the lip. These conditions are treated by eliminating the suspected contactant, applying topical corticosteroid ointment, and using hypoallergenic cosmetics.

MOUTH CONDITIONS

Herpes Simplex Infection

The herpes simplex virus most commonly produces the familiar *herpes labialis* (cold sore, fever blister, or canker). The infection may take the form of an acute herpetic gingivostomatitis. The patient frequently experiences a burning sensation, 24 to 48 hours before blisters appear. Small vesicles, single or clustered, may erupt on the lips, the tongue, the cheeks, and the pharynx. These soon rupture, forming sore, shallow ulcers that are covered with a gray membrane. Herpes infections appear often in association with other febrile infections, such as pneumococcus pneumonia, meningococcic meningitis, and malaria. The herpes virus does not yield in the slightest to any of the chemotherapeutic agents that have become available to date. Some relief is experienced with the application of topical analgesics. Other common therapies include (1) applying spirits of camphor twice a

day; (2) applying a moistened styptic stick to the vesicles several times a day; (3) dusting the lesions with bismuth-formic-iodide (BFI) antiseptic powder twice daily.

Some patients may associate herpes simplex with hearsay stories relating this herpes virus to cancer. Although herpes virus 2 has been associated with carcinoma of the cervix in women, there is no documented evidence to show the exact relationship between the two.

Gingivitis

Gingivitis (inflammation of the gums) is the most common disease of oral tissues. At first there is inflammation and slight swelling of the superficial gingivae and interdental papillae. Slight bleeding may occur and prompt the patient to refrain from adequately cleaning his teeth. Such neglect compounds the problem, in that food debris, bacterial plaque, and calculus (tartar) can result in chronic degenerative gingivitis, and, later, in periodontal disease. Good conscientious mouth hygiene and periodic professional teeth-cleaning can prevent the problem.

Necrotizing Gingivitis (Vincent's Gingivitis, "Trench Mouth")

Necrotizing gingivitis is a pseudomembranous ulceration affecting the edges of the gums, the mucosa of the mouth, the tonsils, and the pharynx. It is thought to be caused by a combination of two organisms, a spirochete and a fusiform bacillus. Smears made from the ulcerations are found to be teeming with the characteristic organisms, and establish the diagnosis. However, the condition may also be due to poor oral hygiene, low tissue resistance, and infection produced by a complex of microorganisms.

The chief symptom is painful, bleeding gums. Swallowing and talking are also painful, especially when infection has spread to the tonsils and pharynx. There may be a mild fever and swelling of the lymph nodes in the neck.

Management. Objectives of care are directed toward controlling and treating the infection, reducing fetid breath, making the patient comfortable, and maintaining nutrition. The plan of care includes washing and irrigating the mouth hourly with fluids rich in free oxygen, such as dilute hydrogen peroxide or sodium perborate in a 2 percent solution, to combat the anaerobic spirochete. Procaine penicillin, given intramuscularly, or potassium phenoxymethyl penicillin (penicillin V), given orally, is effective. Definitive measures such as dental prophylaxis and gingival massage are postponed until the acute inflammation has subsided.

Food should be of liquid or soft consistency to reduce trauma to the gums. Highly seasoned or strongly acid foods should not be served; it is also desirable to avoid smoking and alcohol.

Adolescents are often afflicted with this problem because of poor eating habits, irregularity, and insufficient rest. Patient education is directed toward correcting mouth problems and emphasizing proper oral hygiene to prevent a recurrence.

White Lesions of the Mouth

White lesions of the mouth may be keratotic or nonkeratotic.

White Keratotic Lesions. These lesions are elevated, have an uneven surface, and are firmly adherent and slow to change.

FOCAL KERATOSIS. These lesions are white patches or plaques that do not fit a disease entity and seem to be caused by irritation. Treatment consists of eliminating the irritant, such as smoking, chewing tobacco, jagged teeth, malocclusions, and biting the cheek or lip. Biopsy may be necessary if the lesion persists.

LICHEN PLANUS. Lichen planus is a mucocutaneous disease recognized as white papules at the intersection of a network of interlacing lesions. Often the lesions are ulcerated and painful. If asymptomatic, reassurance may be all that is needed. If painful, the diet is limited to soft, bland foods. Small amounts of viscous lidocaine (Xylocaine viscous 2 percent) held in the mouth for 2 to 3 minutes may relieve soreness while eating. Direct application of triamcinolone acetonide (Kenalog in Orabase) after meals or at bedtime may promote healing. Corticosteroids given systemically or injected intralesionally have been effective. Periodic examinations of chronic lesions are necessary, because of their malignancy potential.

White Nonkeratotic Lesions. These lesions are due to exudative or ulcerative processes, are of short duration, and are fairly easy to remove.

APHTHOUS STOMATITIS (APHTHOUS ULCERS, CANKER SORES). Among the most common lesions of the mouth are recurrent aphthous ulcers (canker sores). Aphthous ulcers are shallow ulcers found in the mucous membrane of the mouth, most often on the inner side of the lips and cheeks, and in the sulcus between the lips and gums. However, they may appear anywhere in the mouth, including on the tongue. The lesions begin with a burning, tingling sensation and slight swelling of the mucous membrane, which soon becomes a shallow ulcer with a whitish center surrounded by a red border. These ulcers are especially painful when eating, and are particularly aggravated by acid or spicy foods. Since these ulcers are tender to pressure, any abrasion of, or movement of, the skin around the ulcer makes it painful to speak or move any of the facial muscles. The ulcers may be single or multiple, and they often tend to heal at one site and recur elsewhere. The sores may appear at any time in life; most often they begin in childhood or adolescence and may appear as frequently as once a month. In most cases, however, they do not occur more than once a year or so. These ulcers last only a short time—from 10 to 14 days—and eventually heal spontaneously, leaving no scar.

In spite of intense studies, no definite cause can be found for canker sores. An L-form of alpha hemolytic streptococcus has been proposed as the microbial cause. There seem to be definite predisposing factors, such as emotional or mental stress, related to their occurrence. In females, they seem to appear at the time of menstrual periods, and they occur much more frequently among women than men. Fatigue, change in a life situation, and anxiety are other predisposing factors.

Because these studies have uncovered no specific cause, there is no specific treatment for canker sores. Where anxiety is an obvious etiologic factor, tranquilizing drugs may be beneficial. A soft, bland diet may reduce pain. Various antibiotic and steroid preparations applied locally, or injected systemically, offer some relief. Fortunately these ulcers eventually heal spontaneously in a relatively short time.

Oral Candidiasis (Moniliasis, Thrush). This condition produces white, cheesy plaques that can be rubbed off to leave an erythematous and, often, bleeding base. Predisposing factors may include diabetes mellitus, lymphoma, or other debilitating conditions, corticosteroids, and antibiotics. Treating the basic cause may improve the condition. In addition, nystatin (Mycostatin), taken orally or as an oral suspension, is effective. The suspension is a medicated fluid that should be swished about the mouth vigorously for at least one minute. If the condition becomes chronic, it is more difficult to treat and requires persistent attention to basic care.

DISORDERS OF THE SALIVARY GLANDS

Acute Inflammation—Parotitis

The most common inflammation of the salivary glands is *parotitis* (inflammation of the parotid gland); however, infection can occur in the other glands as well. The essential lesion of mumps (epidemic parotitis) is an inflammation of the salivary gland (usually the parotid) and is primarily a pediatric communicable disease.

Elderly, acutely ill, and debilitated individuals whose salivary glands fail to secrete sufficiently because of general dehydration often develop parotitis. The infecting organisms travel from the mouth through the salivary duct. Because older people tend to have parched mouths and do not chew solid foods adequately, they offer poor defense against invasion of the parotid ducts by pathogenic organisms.

The offending organism usually is the staphylococcus (except in mumps). The onset of this complication is sudden, with an exacerbation of the fever and of the symptoms of the primary condition. The gland swells and becomes tense and tender. Pain is felt in the ear, and there is interference with swallowing. The swelling rapidly increases, and the overlying skin soon becomes red and shiny.

Postoperative Prevention. In order to prevent parotitis in the postoperative patient, any necessary dental work should be done before surgery. In addition, optimal patient preparation includes maintaining an adequate nutritional and fluid intake along with good mouth hygiene. After surgery, having the patient chew gum or suck hard candy may prevent obstruction of the salivary gland ducts.

Management. At the onset of the swelling, an icebag may be applied over the affected gland, and chemotherapy may be instituted with penicillin or one of the sulfonamides. A suppurating gland may require incision and drainage.

Salivary Calculus (Sialolithiasis)

Salivary stones may develop in the submaxillary gland, following glandular infection or ductal stricture due to trauma or inflammation. Sialograms (x-ray pictures taken with a radiopaque substance injected into the duct) may be required to show obstruction of the duct by stenosis. Salivary stones are composed mainly of calcium oxalate. If located within the gland, they are irregularly lobulated and vary in diameter from 3 to 30 mm. Stones in the duct are small and oval.

Calculi within the salivary gland cause no symptoms unless infection arises; but a calculus that obstructs the gland's duct causes sudden, local, and often colicky pain, which is suddenly relieved by a gush of saliva. Where this condition exists, the gland is swollen and quite tender, the stone itself often is palpable, and its shadow may be seen on roentgenograms. The calculus can be extracted fairly easily from the duct in the mouth; sometimes enlarging the orifice permits the stone to pass spontaneously. It may be necessary to remove the gland if there are repeated recurrences of symptoms and calculi in the gland itself.

Tumors of the Salivary Glands

Neoplasms of almost any type develop in salivary glands, but the majority of them are malignant. In 75 percent of all these patients, tumors develop in one parotid gland. The tumors remain small and quiescent for years, then suddenly begin to increase in size. Neoplasms are diagnosed on the basis of history and physical examination; tests such as needle biopsy are contraindicated. Encouraging results in detection of neoplasms have been reported with radiosialography (scanning with Tc-99m).

The best treatment of parotid tumor is the early and complete excision of the mass. Fortunately, most of these growths occur superficially, rather than in the deep retro-

mandibular lobe. Partial excision of the gland, along with all of the tumor, combined with careful dissection to preserve the vulnerable facial (7th) nerve, is the common procedure. For more involved tumors, it may be necessary to sacrifice the nerve when a parotidectomy is done. If the tumor is malignant or mixed, irradiation therapy follows surgery. Local recurrences are common; the recurrent growth usually is more malignant than the original one.

In the postoperative period, the nurse should be aware that the patient may have some facial paralysis (if the nerve was not excised), due to tissue trauma and edema. This will gradually subside.

FRACTURE OF THE MANDIBLE, JAW REPOSITIONING OR RECONSTRUCTION

Fractures of the mandible may consist of simple fractures without displacement, resulting from a blow on the chin, or they may be very complicated, involving loss of tissue and bone from a severe accident. Mandibular fractures are usually compound. In simple fractures, without loss of teeth, the lower jaw is immobilized by wiring it to the upper jaw. The wires are placed around the teeth in both the upper and lower jaw, on each side of the fracture line. The lower jaw is held tight against the upper jaw by cross-wires or rubber bands placed around the wires about the teeth (Fig. 33-1). This simple form of fixation is used when there are teeth that can be used in the wire fixation. In other cases, in which teeth are missing or bone displacement has occurred, various other forms of fixation can be used. Some of these, such as metal arch bars, are applied in the mouth; other methods are more involved, requiring pins inserted into the bone, with fixation to a plaster head piece. The nursing problem

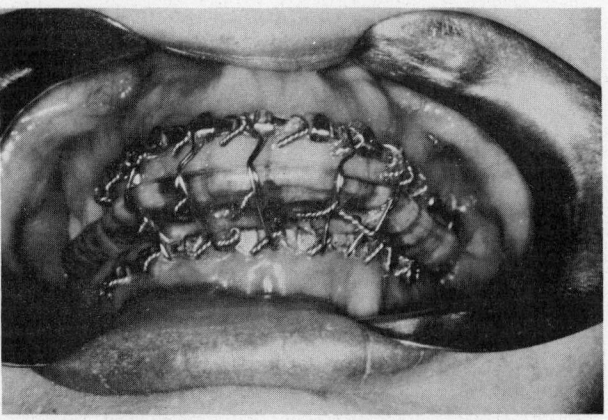

Figure 33-1. For this patient's intermaxillary fixation, arch bars were placed about the maxillary and mandibular arches of teeth. The intermaxillary wires are the vertical ones between the arch bars. It is these wires that must be cut in an emergency. (Marsh Robinson, D.D.S., M.D.)

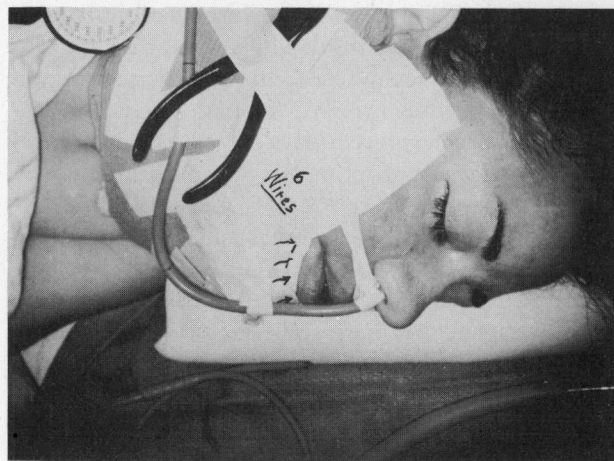

Figure 33-2. This patient, shown in the lateral position in the recovery room, had surgery for mandibular prognathism, necessitating intermaxillary fixation. Note the wire cutter attached to the collar bandage, the bandage marked with the location and number of intermaxillary wires, the Levin tube in place, and a nasopharyngeal tube and suction catheter readily available. Also note the manometer available to ascertain blood pressure. (Marsh Robinson, D.D.S., M.D.)

then is one of treating a fracture in the mouth in a patient who cannot open his jaws.

Management. Immediately following surgery, the patient should be placed on his side, with his head slightly elevated. The nasogastric suction tube inserted during surgery is connected to low pressure suction; this removes stomach contents and lessens the danger of aspiration (Fig. 33-2). Antiemetic drugs are also administered. Prevention of vomiting is most desirable. If the patient does vomit, and the wires are cut, surgery and rewiring have to be repeated later. A plier-type of wire cutter (or scissors, if rubber bands are used) should be taped to the head of the bed for emergency use.

Clearing of the nasopharyngeal area can be done with a small catheter inserted through the nasal orifice. The oral cavity can be aspirated by first inserting a tongue blade to

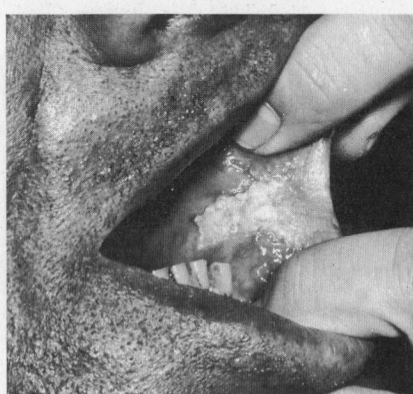

Figure 33-3. Leukoplakia. Note the white patches above and to the right of the teeth.

move the cheek away from the teeth; the catheter is inserted in an area where teeth are not in close position or where a tooth is missing, or in the space behind the third molar.

Constant attention by the nurse in the postsurgery recovery time is necessary. As the patient regains consciousness, he needs to be reminded again that his jaw is wired but that he can breathe and swallow. As he emerges from anesthesia, his head may be elevated. If an extraoral appliance is used to immobilize the mandible, the patient needs instruction on positioning himself so that he does not roll onto the device. To prevent dry and cracking lips, a lubricant is applied.

Careful attention to the hygiene of the mouth must be insisted upon, using warm alkaline mouthwashes or oxygenating rinses at least every 2 hours, and after each feeding. In addition, the mouth should be inspected at least once or twice daily to ensure thorough cleansing. A flashlight and a tongue blade to retract the cheeks are essential equipment. If permissible, a small, soft toothbrush can be used carefully.

The diet must necessarily be liquid, but sufficient caloric and fluid intake can be given easily to these patients. They can be fed through a straw without much difficulty, and occasionally soft foods may be given with a spoon. Water should be given after each liquid feeding, followed by a mouthwash.

Usually the patient is out of bed the first postoperative day, and the length of time for ambulation is gradually increased each day.

Patient Education and Convalescent Care. Depending on conditions, including age and the patient's stability, most patients are able to leave the hospital before the wiring is removed. Of prime importance is the proper functioning of the fixation appliance. To ensure this, the patient has to see his physician at certain intervals. At these examinations, the patient's mouth and device are checked for cleanliness, and his general nutritional condition is assessed. This means that he needs to know how to give himself mouth care, how to feed himself, and what kinds of foods to take. If there are any sites of irritation, these need to be reported. Instruction on these matters is given to the patient before he is discharged.

PRECANCEROUS LESIONS

Leukoplakia buccalis (also called "smoker's patch") and the related *keratosis labialis* are seen in middle-aged adults, more than 80 percent of whom are men. These conditions are characterized in the early stages by the appearance of one or two small, thin, often crinkled, pearly patches on the mucous membrane of the tongue, the mouth, or both, due to keratinization of the mucosa and sclerosis of its underlying tissue (Fig. 33-3). In time, most of the tongue and the mouth may become covered by a creamy, white, thick, fissured or papillomatous mucous membrane that desquamates occasionally, leaving a beefy-red base. This condition results from chronic irritation by carious, infected, or poorly repaired teeth, by tobacco, and by highly spiced foods. It will disappear in time after cessation of smoking. Occasionally it is due to syphilis. Not infrequently, cancers start in the keratinized patches.

ORAL CANCER

Cancer in the oral cavity, which may occur in any part of the mouth, including the pharynx, is highly curable, if discovered early. However, it accounts for 3 percent of all cancer deaths in this country. Males are afflicted three and a half times more than females.

Of the 8,000 oral cancer deaths annually, the distribution by site is estimated as follows:

Lips	3%
Tongue	24%
Salivary gland	8%
Floor of mouth	6%
Other and unspecified sites in mouth	15%
Pharynx	44%

Squamous cell (epidermoid) carcinoma constitutes over 90 percent of all mouth cancer. The next most common type, adenocarcinoma, arises from the submucous glands. The third grouping includes malignancy of the jaw bone. The cure rate for these cancers is below 30 percent. However, most oral cancers can be prevented by good dental care and avoidance of smoking. In tobacco chewers, the mucous membrane of the cheek is the most common site of cancer. A jagged tooth and poor dental hygiene may be the cause. Betel and areca nut, mixed with tobacco, used widely for chewing in South India, is believed to be related to that country's high incidence of oral cancer (40 percent of all cancers).

Cancer of the Lip

This tumor, usually called an epithelioma, occurs most frequently as a chronic ulcer on the lower lip in men. Predisposing factors may be chronic irritation of a warm pipe stem or prolonged exposure to the sun and wind. More significant, however, is the tendency for leukoplakia to progress to an epidermoid lip cancer. A typical lesion is a painless indurated ulcer with raised edges. Any wart or ulcer of the lip that does not heal in 3 weeks should be biopsied.

Small lesions usually are excised liberally; larger le-

sions involving more than one third of the lip may be treated best by radiotherapy, because of superior cosmetic results. The choice depends upon the extent of the lesion, the skill of the surgeon or radiologist, and what is necessary to cure the patient while preserving the best appearance. Fortunately only about 10 to 15 percent of lip cancers mestastasize. When lymph nodes appear to be involved, a neck dissection is indicated.

Cancer of the Tongue

The tongue is a muscular and highly vascular organ with abundant lymphatic drainage. If cancer of the tongue develops, the constant expansion and contraction of the tongue can easily force small tumor cells into the lymphatic channels and eventually into the regional lymph nodes, where they become embedded. This cancer is most common in men in their later decades of life.

Clinical Manifestations. The early stage of cancer of the anterior undersurface of the lateral aspects of the tongue usually is detected as a small ulcer that has not healed in 3 weeks, or as an area of thickening. After several months, the cancer invades the underlying muscle body of the tongue. Pain or soreness of the tongue on eating hot or highly seasoned foods, and limitation of motion, are noticeable. As the growth spreads to neighboring structures, other symptoms develop, such as excessive salivation, slurred speech, blood-tinged sputum, trismus, and pain on swallowing liquids. If untreated, the patient is unable to swallow, and earache, faceache, and toothache become almost constant. Unable to eat or sleep, the patient finally succumbs to hemorrhage (lingual artery), cervical lymph node metastasis, or general debilitation.

Management. Radiation and surgery are the treatments of choice. Often preoperative irradiation is followed by surgery 4 to 6 weeks later. Enlargement of lymph nodes indicates metastases, necessitating more extensive surgical dissection, combined with radium and x-ray therapy. When the tongue is involved, it is often necessary to perform a *hemiglossectomy* (removal of a lateral segment of the tongue).

Malignancy at the base of the tongue (posterior) produces less obvious symptoms: slight dysphagia, sore throat, salivation, and some blood-tinged sputum. This is a difficult site for effective irradiation, and because of the mutilating effects of total glossectomy, and the likelihood of metastasis, the cure rate of posterior tongue cancer is very low. (For nursing management, see Cancer of the Mouth.)

Cancer of the Mouth

Clinical Manifestations. Because the mouth is such an accessible and observable site, more intensive professional and patient educational programs are needed for early detection of mouth lesions. Any patient with a white patchy area, sore spot, or ulceration of lips, gums, or mouth that fails to heal in 3 weeks should be urged to see a physician.

Most oral cancers cause no symptoms in the early stages. Often the individual feels a roughened area with his tongue. Since pain is often one of the last symptoms to appear, a painless condition should not prevent further professional examination; swelling, numbness, or loss of feeling in any part of the mouth may also be symptoms.

The patient's first complaint may be the appearance of a lump in the neck, indicating metastatic spread. Pain usually occurs when there is secondary infection or tumor invasion of adjacent tissues. Occasionally, the first complaints are difficulty in chewing, swallowing, or speaking.

Assessment. Oral exfoliative cytology is a means of screening intraoral lesions. As the first step in the screening process, the patient's mouth is examined carefully. Then the tongue is grasped with a 4 × 4 gauze square and moved gently to expose the suspicious area. With a moistened tongue blade, the lesion is then scraped. If a hyperkeratotic lesion is present, the surface keratin is scraped off so that the deeper epithelial cells are available for the specimen, since these cells are usually involved in early malignant change. The cells are smeared on a glass slide, immersed carefully in alcohol, and sent to the laboratory for cytologic examination.

Adequate examination of the oral cavity requires good lighting, including a head mirror. The use of a wooden tongue blade is helpful in retracting the cheek and holding back the tongue. A finger cot or rubber glove is helpful to the examiner in palpation (see page 59). Look for white areas (leukoplakia), fissures, ulcers, red areas (erythroplakia), masses, or unusual pigmentation. Biopsy is essential for definitive diagnosis. Exfoliative cytology is an adjunct to biopsy, as are staining techniques (e.g., toluidine blue test).

Management. Management varies with the nature of the lesion and preference of the physician. Electrocoagulation, radiotherapy, resectional surgery, or combinations of therapy are effective. In more extensive ablative procedures it may be necessary to graft tissue by flap or pedicle grafts (page 1072). For even more advanced lesions involving the tongue, mandible, larynx, and neck, the trend is away from extremely radical surgery (which only ends in cosmetic and functional disaster) and toward combining chemotherapy and radiation.

Surgical Intervention. General preparation for surgery is similar to that described on page 311. Depending upon the nature of the operation, the anesthesia may be local or general. The surgery may be confined to the lip, may involve only the tongue, or may include resection of facial tissue and the mandible, with possible dental extraction. If there is metastasis to the lymph nodes of the neck, neck dissection may be necessary.

- In the postoperative period, the chief objective is to maintain a patent airway. The patient is placed in a supine position, with the head turned to the side, or in the lateral position, with special emphasis on facilitating drainage from the mouth.
- If suctioning is required, precautions are necessary to avoid injury to the suture line and sensitive tissues, such as exist in a hemiglossectomy. Perhaps a dental suction tip may be required until such time as the patient is able to take care of his own secretions.

Mouth Hygiene. To reduce the number of bacteria and to keep the mouth clean are important objectives before, as well as after, surgery or radiation. If the patient is conscious and able to help himself, the nurse can teach him effective mouth care. He may need reminding and proper supplies, including an effective toothbrush or gauze-padded applicator stick, as well as oxygen-releasing and antimicrobial mouth-rinsing solutions. If the patient is a mouth-breather, he needs more mouth attention than the average person. The use of swabs of mineral oil with lemon juice, or milk of magnesia and mineral oil, is refreshing. Lanolin applied to dry and cracking lips is also soothing.

Dentures must be removed frequently and cleaned. Before they are replaced, the mouth also should be cleaned. Frequently care is given to the teeth, but the "furred" or coated tongue is neglected, resulting in bad breath.

Mouth irrigations are given to keep the mouth clean, provide comfort, and assist in the healing process. The prescribed solutions may be normal saline, diluted hydrogen peroxide, sodium bicarbonate solution, or alkaline mouthwash. Gentle lavaging with a catheter inserted between the cheek and teeth loosens mucus and is refreshing. A power spray has the advantage of getting the solution into inaccessible areas.

In the unconscious patient, the nurse is wholly responsible for maintaining good mouth hygiene. The use of a special mouth tray with all necessary applicator sticks, padded tongue depressors, mouthwashes, lubricants, and so forth, encourages frequent mouth attention.

Dry Mouth (Xerostomia) or Excessive Salivation. Dryness of the mouth is a frequent sequela of oral cancer, particularly when the salivary glands have been exposed to radiation or major surgery. It also is noted in patients who are receiving psychopharmacologic agents or in those who are unable to close the mouth, and who become mouth-breathers.

To minimize this problem, the patient is advised to avoid dry, bulky, and irritating fluids and foods as well as alcohol and tobacco. He should also be encouraged to increase his intake of fluids, if not contraindicated. Some degree of relief is obtained through the lubricating action of such substances as petrolatum, mineral oil, and glycerine (cough drops with glycerine). Salivary flow can be stimulated with sugar-free lemon lozenges or sugar-free chewing gum. In a dry environment, the use of humidifiers may also help.

Drooling or excessive salivation may be an annoying problem to the patient in the pre- or postoperative period. The measures taken to control drooling depend upon the cause, severity, and relative permanence of the dysfunction. If the problem is moderate to severe but temporary, as may be the case following surgery, mechanical suction devices used with a soft catheter are effective. If drooling is mild, management may be obtained by training the patient to swallow more frequently, by providing emotional reassurance and support, and by using anticholinergic agents (antisialogogues), such as those containing atropine or belladonna (Banthine, Robinul). For more severe drooling, it may be necessary to resort to plastic reconstruction of the oral structures.

Mouth wipes, as well as a paper bag attached to the bed or the bedside stand to receive soiled tissues, always should be on hand. An effective way of holding dressings of the mouth or the lower jaw in place is by the use of a face mask. The strings can be tied at the top of the head.

To combat odors, the physician may prescribe oxidizing agents for a mouthwash, such as potassium permanganate 1:10,000, hydrogen peroxide in half strength, sodium perborate, and so forth. In extensive mouth sores, a power spray can clean wounds effectively, and necrotic tissue can be removed more easily.

Nutritional Needs. The general physical condition of a person often is reflected in his mouth. Therefore, good nutritional levels must be maintained. If the breath has a foul odor, the nurse must encourage and assist the patient with his oral hygiene before and after each feeding. A bad taste in the mouth spoils the taste of food and limits the intake of nourishment.

Individuals with mouth lesions may have feeding problems. The use of a plastic straw or a teaspoon may be effective. The type of feeders employed with children may be of use. Food should be soft or liquid, and nonirritating; i.e., not too hot or too cold, and not highly seasoned. It should be served attractively, to tempt the patient to take it. Small, frequent feedings are more desirable than large, less frequent ones. The desires as well as the nutritional needs of the patient should be taken into consideration. If he is not able to take anything by mouth, it may be necessary to feed him parenterally to maintain fluid and electrolyte balance and to prevent starvation and negative nitrogen balance. Such feeding may be by way of parenteral hyperalimentation (page 728), a lateral pharyngostomy stab wound (to prevent nasal discomfort), or nasogastric intubation. The position of the tube can be checked by injecting slowly, drop by drop, 1 or 2 ml. of saline. If the tube is in the esophagus, as it should be, the patient should have no reaction. If it is in the trachea, he will cough violently. The care of this tube is similar to that of a gastrostomy tube (see page 727). As the patient progresses to the point where he can insert his own feeding catheter, he should be given time, privacy, assistance, and encouragement. Perhaps a mirror will help.

Psychosocial Concerns. The patient with a mouth or facial problem requires patience and understanding. Quite naturally he tends to withdraw from people, is self-conscious about mouth odors, and is sensitive about his appearance. The nurse is challenged to get through to him, encourage his expression of fears and concerns, and offer him support and explanations as necessary. The immediate family needs to be aware of their supporting role and, in turn, should be informed of the plan of therapy for the patient.

Particular areas of patient concern are fear of pain, drooling, and difficulty in communicating, feeding, and swallowing. In addition, he may express a strong desire for solitude and be self-conscious about his appearance. (The need to remove, temporarily, any large mirrors in the room should be considered by the nurse.) The results of surgery or radiation concern him, especially the fear of disfigurement; if the resection is extensive, the possibility of prosthetics (fitting an artificial part) may be explained.

Environmental Considerations. A therapeutic environment must be maintained by good room ventilation, particularly with the patient who has a malodorous cancer lesion. A room deodorant may be advisable.

Speech Rehabilitation. Surgery for mouth cancer often interferes with speech. Providing the patient with a pad of paper and a pencil or "magic slate," so that he can express his needs and thoughts, may make a tremendous difference in his depressed condition. Often these patients are reluctant to associate with other patients, and prefer to be alone. If there are two or more patients with a similar condition, they can help each other. It is easier for them, and for others, if they have their meals apart from other patients.

The patient's family and friends should be encouraged to visit so that he is aware that others care about and for him. He can be helped to care for his appearance. With speech training and adjustment to a prosthesis, he will become increasingly aware that the future holds promise for him.

Radium. If radium implants are used, the usual radium precautions are observed. When radium needles are implanted, a thread is attached to each needle. The patient should know upon waking from surgery that these needles will be present and that they are not to be removed. Mouth care in this instance can be given with a power spray. Radium may be implanted in a moulage (molded dental compound) which may be applied to some part of the mouth for a specific length of time. It is usually permissible to remove the mold for meals and at night. When it is reinserted, it is important for the nurse to note that it is in its proper position. (For care of radium, see page 291.)

Convalescent and Extended Care in the Home. The posthospital objectives of patient care are similar to those in the hospital. The individual who is recovering from treatment for a mouth condition needs to breathe, to secure nourishment, to avoid infection, and to be alert for adverse signs. The patient, members of his family or the person responsible for his home care, the nurse, and whoever else may be involved, such as a speech therapist, dietitian, psychologist, and so forth, need to prepare an individualized plan. If suctioning the mouth or a tracheostomy tube is required, it is important to determine what equipment is needed and how to use it, as well as where it can be obtained. Consideration should be given to the humidification and aeration of the room, as well as to measures to control odors. How to prepare foods that are nutritious, properly seasoned, and of the right temperature can be explained. Perhaps it may be more feasible to use commercial baby food than to prepare liquid and soft diets in a blender. The use and care of prostheses must be understood. The importance of cleanliness with dressings and mouth care is reviewed. The person caring for the patient needs to know the signs of obstruction, hemorrhage, infection, depression, and withdrawal, as well as what to do about these problems. Follow-up visits to the clinic or physician are important, to determine progression or regression and to receive any modifications in medication or general care.

Over 90 percent of recurrences will appear within the first 18 months; therefore, meticulous inspection by the physician every 4 to 6 weeks is essential. Early detection of local recurrences or metastasis, followed by aggressive treatment, can cure as many as 50 percent of these patients. Follow-up visits become less frequent after 2 years but must be continued for life, because of the frequency of other primary carcinomas. One important part of continuing care is the elimination of alcohol consumption and smoking.

Palliative Patient Care. Because of further extension of a malignancy by metastasis and necrosis, it may not be possible medically to halt the spread of disease. All efforts are then directed toward comfort measures — physical, psychological, and spiritual. With the family's help this may be continued in the hospital, a nursing home, a hospice setting, or the patient's own home.

NURSING MANAGEMENT OF THE PATIENT WITH ORAL CANCER
Objectives, principles, and rationale of care

PREOPERATIVE CARE

A. To provide psychosocial support to the patient with mouth cancer.
　1. Recognize that the patient is unusually concerned about appearance and possible disfigurement following surgery.
　2. Respect his feelings, accept him as a person, and support him as he faces his selected treatment.
　3. Encourage family support; explain that the patient needs encouragement and understanding.
　4. Anticipate the patient's concerns about cancer, effectiveness of treatment, and likelihood of cancer spread.
B. To promote optimum cleanliness of the involved area, in order to minimize postoperative complications due to infection:
　1. Solicit patient participation in conscientious mouth hygiene.
　2. Provide materials suitable to the condition; if a soft-bristled toothbrush cannot be used, because "it hurts," suggest a turkish washcloth wrapped around a finger.
　3. Utilize Water-pik or a power spray to loosen adhering particles in the mouth.
　4. Select mouth rinses that are effective, noninjurious, and soothing; Cepacol may be too stringent, whereas half-strength hydrogen peroxide may be more bland.
　5. Use oxidizing mouth rinses if the bubbling action can assist in removing necrotic material.
　6. Clean mouth before cleaned dentures are replaced.
C. To promote optimum nutritional condition:
　1. Encourage adequate intake of food and fluids; if anorexia is noted, try to overcome it by serving attractive, small servings frequently.
　2. Provide an environment conducive to relaxation during mealtime.
　3. Supplement the diet with vitamins (particularly vitamin C, to assist in wound healing) and other dietary requirements as needed by the particular patient.
　4. Avoid irritating foods or beverages: too hot, too cold, too bitter, too rough.
D. To prepare patient physically and psychologically for the treatment and its possible after-effects:
　1. If the treatment is radiation, explain what form. *Example:* cobalt exposure, moulage implant, radium needle insertion.
　2. Answer questions regarding effects of radiation. *Example:* loss of hair, visitors permitted during treatment, affect on sterility, skin irritation.
　3. If surgery is the mode of treatment, check with physician as to anticipated surgery and determine what information has been given to the patient. Support this therapeutic plan.

(Continued)

PREOPERATIVE CARE (CONTINUED)

4. Acquaint patient with what to expect after the operation.
5. Teach him how he can help himself and those caring for him:
   a. Anticipate voice and communication problems: use of magic slate and other means of communication.
   b. Types of dressings and drainage equipment.
   c. How pain can be relieved.
   d. How long he will be in the recovery room.
   e. Where his family will be.

POSTOPERATIVE MANAGEMENT

A. To avoid respiratory and circulatory complications:
   1. Maintain a functioning airway by placing patient in a supine position with head turned to side (or lateral position with facilitation of drainage from mouth).
   2. Suction carefully to avoid injury to freshly sutured areas.
   3. Initiate conscientious monitoring of vital signs and patient responses.
   4. Anticipate physical activity on emergence from anesthesia and be prepared to protect patient and operative site.
      a. Use sedation, as judgment dictates.
      b. Prevent patient's hands from pulling out tubes.
      c. Quietly explain where he is and what he can or cannot do.
B. To maintain cleanliness of mouth during healing phases:
   1. Practice those oral hygienic measures used prior to treatment.
   2. Apply lubricant to dry lips.
   3. Provide increased humidity with humidifier, if environment is dry.
   4. Increase fluid intake, if dry mouth (xerostomia) is a problem.
   5. Suction for drooling or make a gauze wick which can be placed in the corner of patient's mouth to direct excessive salivation to an emesis basin.
   6. Practice asepsis in changing dressings; be gentle, and remember that the patient can see your facial expressions.
C. To provide adequate nutrition for systemic needs and wound healing:
   1. Utilize parenteral or nasogastric tube feedings as recommended.
   2. Maintain proper fluid intake; monitor fluid output.
   3. Encourage range of motion and other exercises, so that appetite is enhanced and body circulation is stimulated.
   4. Offer small, attractive servings when patient begins oral feedings.
   5. Promote a pleasant environment for eating: radio, clean surroundings, conversation, and perhaps the presence of other similar patients.
D. To encourage optimism by a carefully planned psychosocial program:
   1. Prepare spouse or family for their role in helping the patient.
   2. Stress the positive, and compliment the patient on each step of progress.
   3. Involve the patient in his own care; gradually increase this activity until he can use a mirror and care for himself.
   4. Answer his queries honestly; encourage his questions.
E. To prepare patient for convalescence (speech rehabilitation, extended care, and use of prosthesis):
   1. Explain the objectives of convalescent care:
      a. Maintain nutrition.
      b. Be fastidious with cleanliness.
      c. Emphasize positive accomplishments.
      d. Develop hobby-like activities.
      e. Encourage seeing friends.
      f. Look forward to getting back to usual work.
      g. Be aware of signs of complications and what to do about them.
      h. Keep follow-up appointments.
   2. Learn how to use and maintain a prosthesis.
   3. Practice the art of communication if speech has been disturbed.
   4. Recognize limitations, and how to adjust by using alternative measures.
   5. Return to the physician for annual or semiannual check-ups.

RADICAL NECK DISSECTION

Malignancies of the head and neck, including cancers of the lips, tongue, gums, palate, tonsils, and of the mucosa of the mouth, pharynx, and larynx, may be treated early by surgery, irradiation, or chemotherapy, with good results. These cancers (stages I and II) are in an area that can be easily seen and early diagnosis and treatment given. Most observers agree that such patients do not die from recurrence at the site of the primary growth, but rather from metastasis to the cervical lymph nodes in the neck, which often takes place by way of the lymphatics before the primary lesion has been treated. Only the nodes on one side of the neck are involved, unless the tumor is located at or near the midline, in which case the nodes of both sides of the neck may contain metastatic tumor.

Because radiation does not by itself give good results in controlling the metastatic cancer in the lymph nodes in the neck, an operation called a "radical neck dissection" is performed. This operation attempts to remove all of the lymph-node bearing tissue on one side of the neck. It may be done at the time of the treatment of the primary tumor or carried out independently at a later date.

The operation is radical, as the name implies, and involves removal of all the tissue under the skin, from the ramus of the jaw down to the clavicle, and from the midline back to the angle of the jaw, in one mass. This includes removing the sternomastoid muscle and other smaller muscles, as well as the jugular vein in the neck, because the lymphatic nodes are found widely distributed throughout these tissues (Fig. 33-4A). For stages III and IV (more advanced malignancy) a combination of treatment modalities may be used.

During or after the procedure a tracheostomy is often performed. Because there may be profuse drainage of serum and lymph after such an extensive procedure, drainage tubes or portable wound suction are often used in the wound (Fig. 33-4B).

Psychosocial Concerns. Before the operation, the patient should be informed about the impending surgery, what is to be done in the operating room (amplification of surgeon's explanation), and what the postoperative period will be like. At the same time, the patient can be given an opportunity to express concerns about the upcoming surgery. During this exchange, the nurse has an opportunity to assess the patient's coping abilities, encourage questions, and develop a plan for offering assistance. A sense of mutual understanding and rapport will make the postoperative experience less troublesome for the patient. After the operation, any expressions of concern on the patient's part can guide the nurse in providing additional support.

Postoperative Nursing Management

The principles of nursing care described on pages 347–355 can be applied to the patient who has extensive neck surgery. In addition, the special needs of the patient must be recognized, including emotional support to help him cope with his concern about (1) the ability to breathe normally, (2) the ability to swallow, (3) the ability to speak, (4) his appearance, and (5) the prognosis.

After the endotracheal tube or airway has been removed and the effects of the anesthesia have worn off, the patient may be placed in a Fowler position to facilitate breathing and promote comfort. This position also increases lymphatic and venous drainage, facilitates swallowing, and decreases venous pressure on the skin flaps.

Signs of respiratory distress, such as dyspnea, cyanosis, and changes in vital signs, must be watched for, since they may suggest edema, throat irritation from the endotracheal tube, hemorrhage, or inadequate drainage. Temperature is usually taken rectally.

In the immediate postoperative period, the nurse may be able to detect the presence of stridor (coarse, high-pitched sound on inspiration) by listening frequently at the trachea with a stethoscope. In this situation, the physician should be summoned.

Coughing is encouraged, to remove secretions. The patient should assume a sitting position, with the nurse supporting the neck with her hands, so that he may be able to bring up bothersome secretions. If this technique fails, the patient may have to be suctioned. Care must be exerted to protect the suture lines during suctioning. If a tracheostomy tube is in place, suctioning is done through this tube.

With portable wound suction drainage, there is no need for pressure dressings, because the skin flaps are drawn down tightly; approximately 80–120 ml. of serosanguineous secretions are drawn off by a portable suction unit the first day. This amount diminishes thereafter. If portable wound suction is not used, drains may be placed in the wound and pressure dressings applied, to obliterate dead spaces and to provide immobilization. These may need to be reinforced from time to time. Dressings are observed for evidence of hemorrhage and constriction, which may affect respiration. Drains may be removed before the massive dressings are changed in about 5 days. Lighter dressings permit greater freedom of movement. Aeroplast or other antiseptic plastic sprays protect the wound. The patient usually is allowed out of bed the first postoperative day.

Mouth hygiene is necessary and welcomed by this patient. It is done frequently and helps to enhance the appetite. A nasogastric tube may be inserted for feeding purposes or to help decompress the stomach.

Psychosocial Support. The person who has had extensive neck surgery often is sensitive about his appearance, either when the operative area is covered by bulky dressings or when an incision line is exposed, as with portable drainage. If the nurse conveys acceptance of the patient and his appearance, and expresses a positive, optimistic attitude, the patient is more likely to be encouraged. In spite of the wide removal of tissue, the cosmetic and functional defects are less than might be

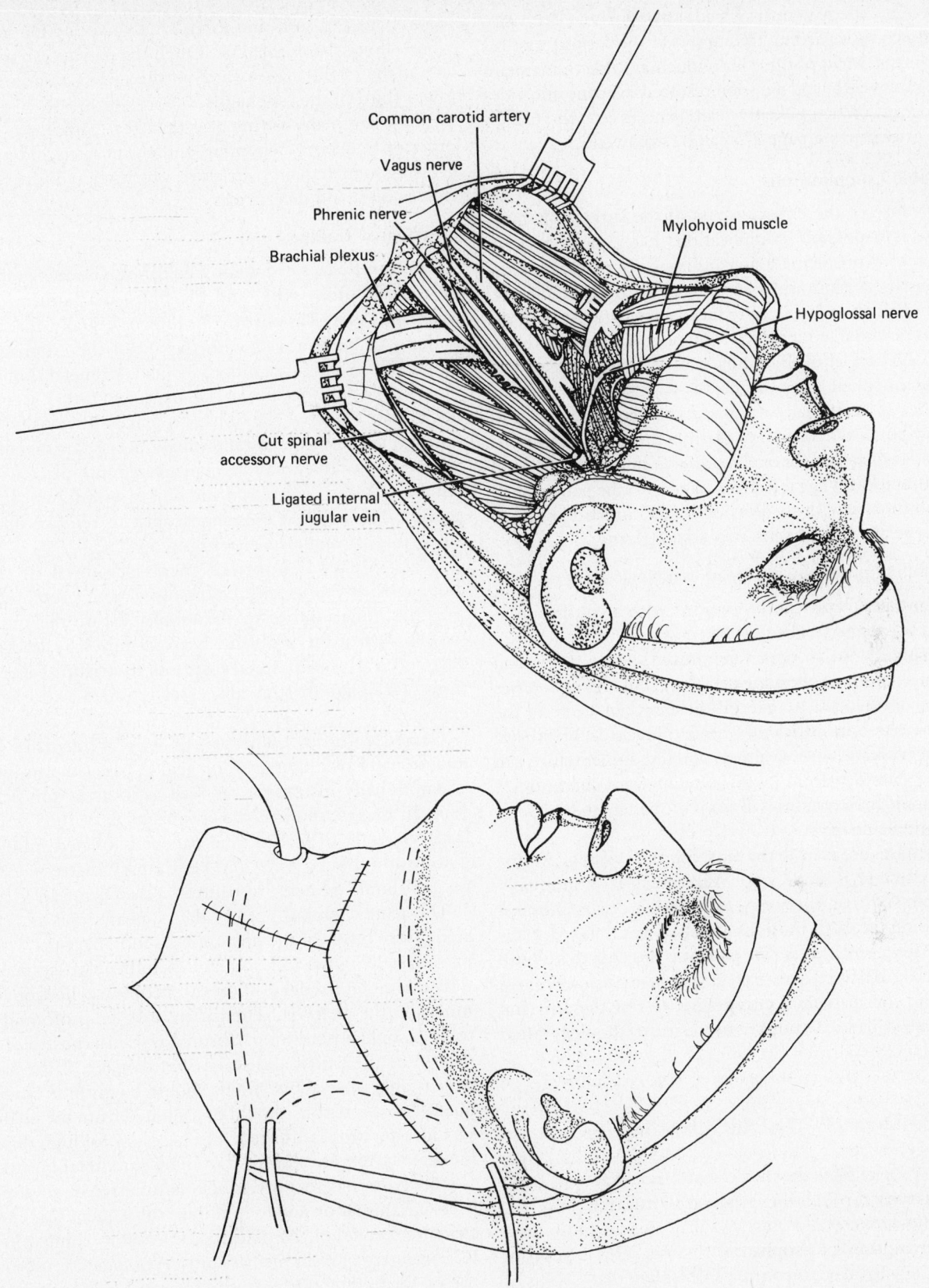

Common carotid artery

Vagus nerve

Phrenic nerve

Brachial plexus

Mylohyoid muscle

Hypoglossal nerve

Cut spinal
accessory nerve

Ligated internal
jugular vein

Figure 33-4. Radical neck dissection is indicated in the presence of enlarged malignant lesions of the tongue, pharynx, and nasopharynx, or gross metastasis in the neck. (*top*) Skin flaps are raised to expose the superficial structures of the neck. The surgeon then removes all lymph nodes, fat, muscles, areola tissue, and nerves. *Note:* Postoperative deficits are: (1) neck is sunk in to a certain degree, is somewhat stiff, and has a large external scar; (2) the spinal accessory nerve is usually removed, causing the shoulder to drop 1-2 cm. Rehabilitation efforts gradually minimize the crippling effect. (*bottom*) This view shows wound closure with portable suction drainage tubes in place. (Redrawn from Conley, J. J.: Radical neck dissection. 5:65, Contemporary Surgery, Sept. 1974)

expected. The patient also needs an opportunity to voice his concerns regarding the success of the surgery and his prognosis. Most of these individuals are able to maintain and gain weight and are soon restored to economic independence. (When palliative care is necessary, the principles presented on page 275 can be followed.)

Possible Complications

Because of the extensiveness of the surgery, hemorrhage is a possible complication. Later, postoperative respiratory problems may cause pneumonia, unless the patient is turned and encouraged to breathe deeply. Wound infection has been reduced considerably, with the use of portable wound suction in place of pressure dressings. Neural complications can occur if the cervical plexus or spinal accessory nerves were severed.

Since lower facial paralysis may occur as a result of injury to the facial nerve during the dissection, this should be watched for, and reported if noted. Likewise, if the superior laryngeal nerve is damaged, the patient may have difficulty with swallowing liquids and food because of the partial lack of sensation of the glottis.

Rehabilitation Following Head and Neck Surgery

Many problems can be avoided with a conscientious exercise program. The purpose of the exercises depicted in Figure 33-5 is to regain maximum shoulder function and neck motion following neck surgery. These exercises are recommended by the physician when he feels the neck incision is sufficiently healed. Excision of muscle and nerve results in a weakness of the shoulder which can cause "shoulder drop," with some forward curvature of the shoulder. Exercises will assist the patient in returning to normal activity.

Exercises are done in the morning and evening. At first each exercise is done once; thereafter, it is gradually increased by one, every day, until each is done ten times. Sweeping, smooth motions are used, in a relaxed manner. After each exercise the patient is directed to go limp and relax. Between exercises and when not using the arm or hand, the patient is encouraged to rest the arm and hand on a padded support to keep the shoulder lifted slightly.

CONDITIONS OF THE ESOPHAGUS

The esophagus is the mucus-lined tube that leads from the pharynx through the chest to the stomach.

Difficulty in swallowing (dysphagia) is the most common symptom of esophageal disease. This symptom may range from an uncomfortable feeling that a bolus of food is "caught" in the upper esophagus (before it eventually passes into the stomach) to acute pain on swallowing (odynophagia). Obstruction to the passage of food (both solid and soft) and even liquids may be felt anywhere along the esophagus. Often the patient can indicate if the problem is located in the upper, middle, or lower third of the esophagus.

There are many forms of esophageal pathology, the order of frequency beginning with esophagitis and progressing to malignancy, stricture, obstruction due to foreign bodies, and diverticula.

Esophageal Trauma

Foreign Bodies. Swallowed foreign bodies — dentures, fishbones, pins, and the like — may injure the esophagus as well as obstruct its lumen. Usually, foreign bodies can be removed with the aid of the esophagoscope. When the foreign body is made of metal (bobby pins, safety pins, needles, jacks, nails, and tacks), it may not be safe to allow the object to make its way slowly through the stomach and intestinal tract. A bar magnet, fastened to a cable, may be maneuvered into place with the aid of fluoroscopy, and the object withdrawn. It is possible for a skilled esophagoscopist to remove open safety pins through the esophagoscope.

If an impacted bolus of meat is lodged in the esophagus, it can usually be dissolved with proteolytic enzymes. The injuries to the esophagus are the more serious part of the problem, because they may lead to deep cervical or mediastinal abscess or to stricture formations. Drainage of such abscesses requires a thoracic exposure.

Chemical Burns. The patient who accidentally or intentionally swallows a strong acid or base (such as lye) is emotionally distraught, as well as in acute physical pain. In these instances, the esophagus is washed with large volumes of water. The patient is treated immediately for shock, pain, and respiratory distress. Attempts should be made to neutralize the chemical.

The acute chemical burn of the esophagus has associated severe burns of the lips, mouth, and pharynx, with pain on swallowing and, sometimes, difficulty in respiration, due either to edema of the throat or to a collection of mucus in the pharynx. The patient may be profoundly toxic. Esophagoscopy is performed as soon as possible to determine the extent and severity of damage. If the patient is able to swallow, fluids should be given in small quantities. Secretions should be aspirated from the pharynx if respiration is affected. The necessity for high fluid intake may require administration by parenteral means.

Corticosteroid therapy is also administered, to suppress inflammation and to minimize subsequent scar and stricture formation. Antibiotics are given to combat infection and to prevent mediastinitis. A nasogastric tube is passed for feeding purposes and to ensure patency of the esophageal lumen.

About a week after chemical ingestion, passage of a dilating bougie (*bouginage*) may be done daily, beginning

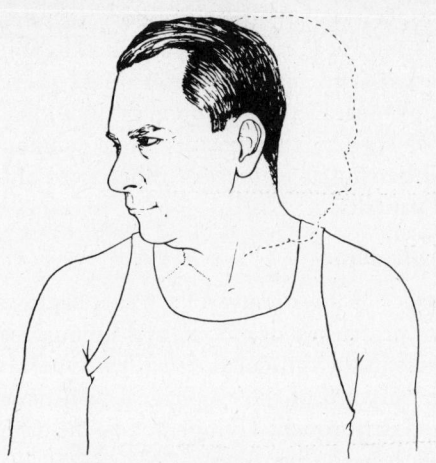

1a. Gently turn head to each side and look as far as possible.

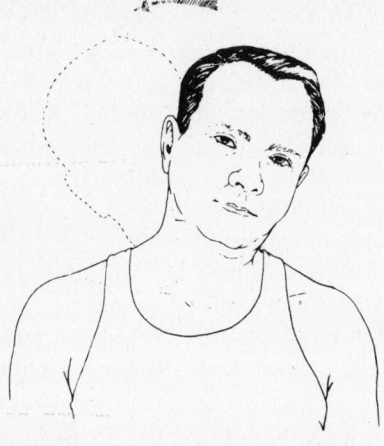

1b. Gently tip right ear toward right shoulder as far as possible. Repeat on left side.

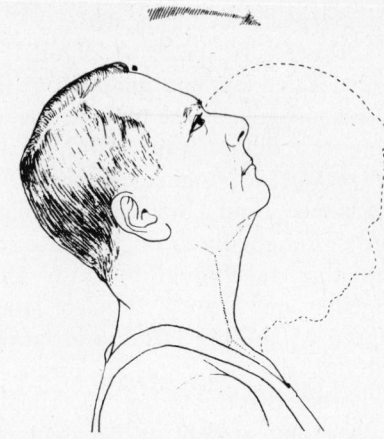

1c. Move chin to chest and then lift head up and back.

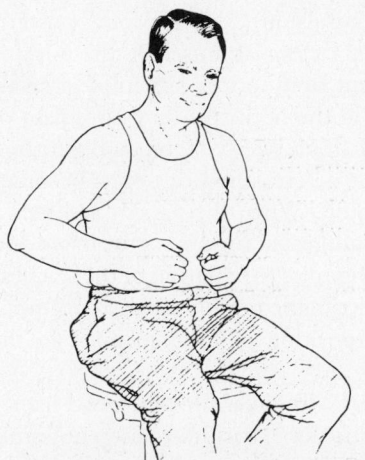

2a. Place hands in front with elbows at right angles away from body.

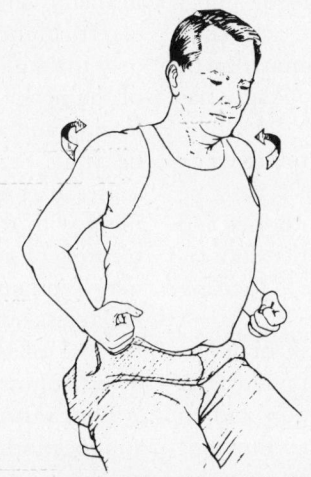

2b. Rotate shoulders back, bringing elbows to side.

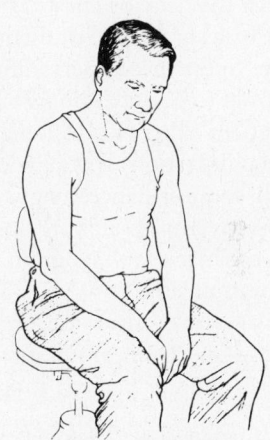

2c. Relax whole body.

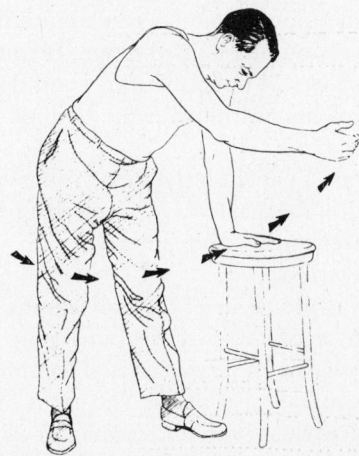

3a. Lean or hold onto low table or chair with hand on the unoperated side. Bend body slightly at waist and swing shoulder and arm from left to right.

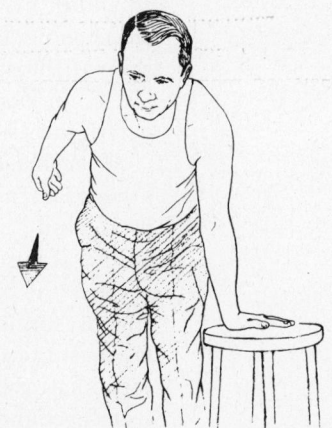

3b. Swing shoulder and arm from front to back.

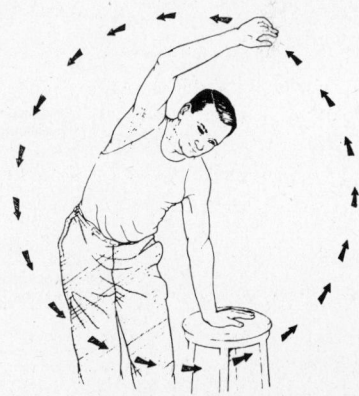

3c. Swing shoulder and arm in a wide circle, gradually bringing arm above head.

Figure 33-5. Rehabilitation exercises following head and neck surgery. The objective is to regain maximum shoulder function and neck motion following neck surgery. (From Exercise for Radical Neck Surgery Patients. Published by Head and Neck Service Department of Surgery, Memorial Hospital, New York, N.Y.)

with a No. 28 Fr. bougie. When the lumen is "stable," bouginage can be terminated.

Occasionally a patient is admitted after the acute phase has subsided, but multiple stricture levels have formed in the esophagus. These may be dilated by peroral use of bougies; if this is not successful, it may be necessary to try the retrograde bouginage method. A gastrostomy opening is made, and a braided silk string is swallowed. One end is brought out through the gastrostomy opening and the other end through the nose. The two ends are tied together and form a complete loop. Dilatation is obtained by pulling larger and larger bougies upward through the esophagus by means of the string. It is important that this string be left in place at all times. The gastrostomy is kept open by means of a gastrostomy tube, through which feedings may be given if necessary.

Perforation. The esophagus is not an uncommon site of injury. Perforation may result from stab or bullet wounds of the neck or chest, as well as from accidental puncture by a surgical instrument during examination or dilatation. Spontaneous perforation of the esophagus has been known to occur during vomiting.

The patient experiences spontaneous pain followed by dysphagia. Infection, fever, and leukocytosis may be noted. In some instances, signs of pneumothorax and subcutaneous emphysema are observed. X-ray examination and possible esophagogram are effective in locating the perforation site.

MANAGEMENT. Because of the high risk of infection, broad-spectrum antibiotic therapy is initiated. A nasogastric tube is passed, to provide suction and to reduce the amount of gastric juice which can reflux into the esophagus and mediastinum. Nothing is given by mouth, but nutritional needs are met by intravenous hyperalimentation. Surgery is performed to close the

wound, and postoperative nutritional support then becomes a primary concern. Parenteral hyperalimentation is preferred to gastrostomy since the latter might cause reflux into the esophagus. Depending upon the incisional site and nature of surgery, the postoperative nursing management will be similar to that for thoracic or abdominal surgical patients.

Esophageal Diverticulum

Pathophysiology. A *diverticulum* of the esophagus is an outpouching or protrusion of mucosa and submucosa through a weakness in the musculature (*pulsion* type). If there is a pulling outward of the esophageal wall from inflamed or scarred peribronchial lymph nodes, the term *traction diverticulum* is used (Fig. 33-6).

Pharyngoesophageal Diverticulum. The most common type of diverticulum, which occurs more frequently in men than in women, is pharyngoesophageal pulsion diverticulum (Zenker's pulsion), which occurs posteriorly through the cricopharyngeal muscle in the midline of the neck. The patient first notices difficulty in swallowing and a fullness in the neck. He may complain of belching, regurgitation of undigested food, and gurgling noises after eating. The diverticulum or pouch becomes filled with food or liquid. When the patient assumes a recumbent position, undigested food is regurgitated and may also cause coughing, due to irritation of the trachea. Halitosis and a sour taste in the mouth are also common, because of the decomposition of food retained in the diverticulum.

Diagnostic Measures. To determine the exact nature and location of a diverticulum, barium roentgenograms are done. Esophagoscopy usually is contraindicated, because of the danger of perforating the diverticulum, with resulting mediastinitis. The blind passing of a nasal tube should be avoided. The tube should be guided into the stomach under direct vision of a lighted scope. Because this patient is often a victim of unbalanced diet and fluid levels, an evaluation of his nutritional state is done to determine dietary needs.

Management. When a patient has difficulty in swallowing, it is usual to limit the diet to those foods that pass more easily. Blenderized meals supplemented with vitamins are usually prescribed.

Since the condition is progressive, the only means of cure is surgical removal of the diverticulum. Care is taken, surgically, to avoid undue trauma to the common carotid artery and internal jugular veins. The sac is dissected free and amputated flush with the esophageal wall. In addition to a diverticulectomy, a myotomy of the cricopharyngeal muscle is often done, in order to relieve spasticity of the musculature, which otherwise seems to contribute to a continuation of the previous symptoms.

Midesophageal and Epiphrenic Diverticula. The occurrence of diverticula in the mid-tubular

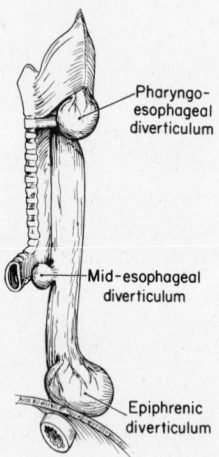

Pharyngo-esophageal diverticulum

Mid-esophageal diverticulum

Epiphrenic diverticulum

Figure 33-6. Illustration shows possible sites for the occurrence of esophageal diverticula. The site will determine the location of the surgical incision to correct the problem. (Hardy: Rhoads Surgery, Philadelphia, J. B. Lippincott, 1977)

esophagus is less common; symptoms are less acute and usually the condition does not require surgery.

Epiphrenic diverticula are usually larger pulsion diverticula occurring in the lower esophagus just above the diaphragm, and occasionally higher. They are thought to be related to the improper functioning of the lower esophageal sphincter. Surgery is indicated only if the symptoms are troublesome and growing progressively worse. A transthoracic (thoracotomy) approach is used, which means that pre- and postoperative nursing management is similar to that for chest surgical patients (pages 559–564).

After operation, the patient is fed through a nasogastric tube that usually is inserted at the time of operation. The feedings may include any liquid, but a careful record of their kind, amount, and character must be kept. After each feeding, the tube should be irrigated carefully with water. The wound also must be observed for evidences of leakage from the esophagus and a developing fistula.

If the operative risk is prohibitive, medical and nursing management is similar to that advocated for the peptic ulcer patient: antacids, anticholinergics, and abstinence from coffee, alcohol, and smoking (see page 741). In addition, reflux is avoided by (1) keeping the head elevated, (2) remaining upright for 2 hours in the postprandial period, (3) avoiding abdominal compression from garments and posture, (4) eating small meals, and (5) reducing, if overweight.

Esophageal Achalasia

Achalasia is the term used to designate functional esophageal obstruction, with a marked dilatation of the esophagus. This is usually associated with a lack of peristaltic activity in the esophagus itself and with a failure of the esophageal sphincter to relax in response to swallowing. Narrowing of the esophagus just above the stomach results in a gradually increasing dilatation of the esophagus in the upper chest, and the symptoms produced are those of difficulty in swallowing, both liquids and solids. The patient has a sensation of food sticking in the lower portion of the esophagus. As the condition progresses, regurgitation of the food is common; this may occur spontaneously or may be brought about by the patient to relieve the discomfort that is produced by the prolonged distention of the esophagus by food that will not pass into the stomach. There may be secondary pulmonary complications due to spillover of esophageal contents (aspiration pneumonia). The cause of this condition is believed to be a degeneration of the nerves that go to the involuntary muscles of the esophagus. Emotional upsets may aggravate the problem. Achalasia is diagnosed by cineroentgenograms using barium, which show the marked dilatation of the upper esophagus and

the narrowing of its lower end. Esophagoscopy is done to rule out carcinoma.

Management. There are differences of opinion as to the best method of treating esophageal achalasia. The conservative approach to treating early achalasia involves stretching the narrowed area of the esophagus via the distention of a bag (Mosher pneumatic) placed in this area through the mouth (Fig. 33-7). Vigorous dilatation produces subxiphoid pain; therefore an analgesic or tranquilizer is prescribed before the treatment.

Other dilating agents (bouginage), such as French bougies or mercury-weighted dilators, are not effective, since achalasia is not a stricture, but a failure of the inferior esophageal sphincter to relax. Hydrostatic dilatation usually gives good results, but the dilatation required may result in a rupture of the esophagus, in a small number of patients.

In late achalasia or the more resistant lesions, an *esophagomyotomy* is performed, which is the division of the muscular fibers that enclose the narrowed area of the esophagus, allowing the mucosa to pouch out through the divided area in the muscle layer (Fig. 33-7). This permits food to be swallowed without obstruction, and the operation is used with very good results. A disadvantage of esophagomyotomy is that about a third of the patients develop reflux of gastric contents into the esophagus. When the above operation is extended to include the cardiac end of the stomach, it is referred to as a *cardiomyotomy*.

It has been claimed by Ellis that surgery is preferred for early achalasia. His study indicates that dilatation is painful, traumatic, and involves a definite risk of rupture of the distal esophagus. In addition, when surgery follows dilatation which has failed, the scarring of the thin esophageal wall caused by the initial procedure makes it difficult to create a relaxed esophageal sphincter.

Diffuse Esophageal Spasm

Diffuse esophageal spasm is a motor disorder of the esophagus diagnosed by esophageal pressure examination. It is usually manifested in old age and may be an early stage of achalasia. There is pain on swallowing (odynophagia), dysphagia, and chest or back pain.

Conservative therapy is to administer sedatives for pain, avoid food and fluids that precipitate symptoms, and eliminate sources of tension. Nitroglycerin or long-acting nitrites sublingually will relieve substernal pain in some patients. Later, it may be necessary to utilize pneumatic dilatation, if manometric studies reveal increased lower esophageal sphincter pressure.

Hiatus Hernia and Reflux Esophagitis

Pathophysiology and Clinical Manifestations. The esophagus enters the abdomen through an opening in the diaphragm, to empty, at its lower end, into the upper part

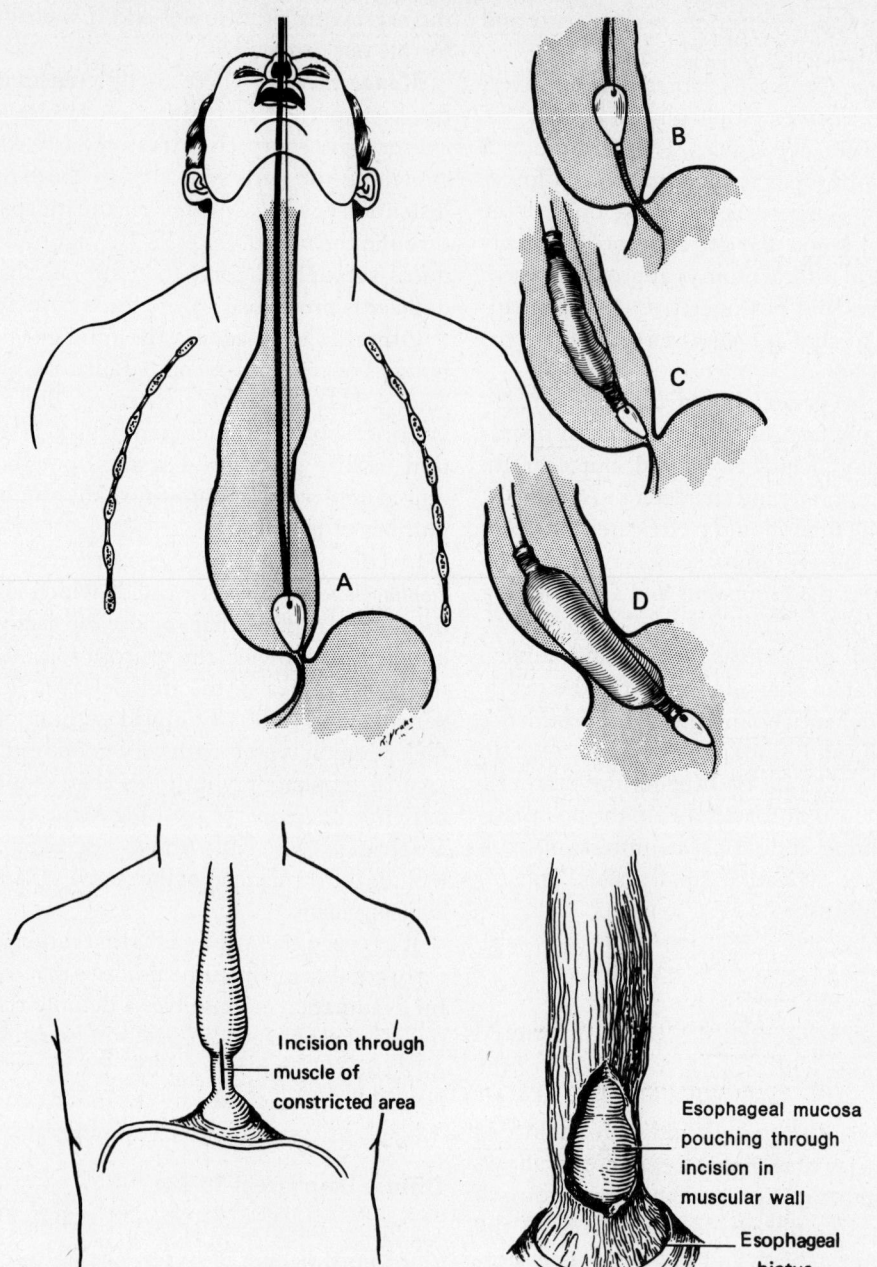

Figure 33-7. (*top*) Minor surgical approach. Dilatation of the lower esophagus with rubber balloon technique in cases of cardiospasm (achalasia). The dilator is passed, guided by a previously swallowed thread, into the upper stomach. When the balloon is in proper position, it is distended by pressure sufficient to dilate the narrowed area of the esophagus. (Olsen, Ellis and Creamer: Achalasia of the cardia. Amer. J. Surg., 93:299-307.)

(*bottom*) Major surgical approach. Treatment of achalasia. The esophagus is approached from in front, on the left side. An incision is made through the muscularis of the esophagus sufficiently to allow a pouching of the esophageal mucosa. Separation of the muscular fibers relieves the narrowing at the lower end of the esophagus and permits the patient to swallow normally again.

of the stomach. The opening in the diaphragm normally encircles the esophagus tightly; therefore, the stomach lies completely within the abdomen. In a condition known as *hiatus* (or *hiatal*) *hernia*, the opening in the diaphragm through which the esophagus passes becomes enlarged, and part of the upper stomach tends to come up into the lower portion of the thorax. This complication may be present in many patients without any signs or symptoms. It is only when the sphincter of the lower end of the esophagus becomes incompetent and reflux occurs that symptoms develop.

Assessment may include the following queries:
When does the pain start?
How long does it last?
Where is it?
How frequently does it occur?
What kind is it? (Radiating?)
How severe is it?
What aggravates or relieves the discomfort?
What food seems to irritate or aggravate the problem?
Is the pain related to changes in position?

Often there is a feeling of fullness in the lower chest and a splashing sound noted in the substernal area, in patients in whom the hiatal hernia is large. In addition, the gastric juice produced by the stomach mucosa tends to be retained in the portion of the stomach above the diaphragm, and for this reason, ulcerations and bleeding may occur. Finally, the erosive action of the gastric juice on the stomach and the lower esophagus may produce a condition known as *esophagitis,* which causes pain and discomfort in the substernal area.

All of these symptoms produce an uncomfortable, and often very ill patient, if bleeding is a factor.

MANAGEMENT. In those hernias that are found incidentally on x-ray examination and do not produce symptoms, no treatment is necessary. Many of these hernias are of the *sliding* type (axial, esophagogastric), in which the stomach tends to extend into the chest when the patient is lying down but slides back into the abdomen when the patient is erect. For this type of hernia, the patient is placed on a strict medical regimen of antacids and advised to avoid lying down after meals (or, the head of the bed should be elevated). He should also avoid tight garments and heavy lifting. Weight reduction is adequate treatment for about 90 percent of patients. For severe heartburn and pain, an oral mucilage preparation (such as Oxaine-M) which contains both an antacid and local anesthetic may be effective. Some physicians prescribe diazepam (Valium) to be taken several minutes before meals.

When the hernia is of the *rolling* type (concentric, paraesophageal), it is a constant problem and must be corrected surgically. The same is true of sliding hernias in which symptoms occur. To correct the main problem caused by reflux, modern surgical treatment involves wrapping the upper end of the stomach around the esophagus (fundoplication) in order to restore an effective high-pressure barrier to reflux. Other techniques (valvuloplasties) are available, depending upon the preference of the surgeon.

Postoperative Nursing Management. The immediate postoperative care of these patients is that used for any thoracotomy or laparotomy. In patients with thora-

cotomy, a chest tube is often introduced and placed in closed suction. The drain is usually taken out in a day or two, after the lung has completely expanded. The patient is given fluids and food on the second or third day after operation, and gradually increasing amounts of food are given as tolerated. In some individuals, edema at the site where the esophagus passes through the diaphragmatic hiatus may interfere with food intake for a time, but usually this subsides without incidence in 2 or 3 days.

Esophageal Varices

Varices of the lower esophagus are really a secondary manifestation of cirrhosis of the liver. This subject is discussed on page 819.

Cancer of the Esophagus

Incidence and Etiology. About 1 percent of all cancer deaths in the United States are due to cancer of the esophagus; more than twice as many men as women acquire this condition, usually between the ages of 50 and 70. Chronic trauma such as that produced by the frequent use of alcohol, tobacco, spicy food, and poor mouth hygiene, appear to be underlying factors. In the Orient, the drinking of large quantities of very hot tea is suspected of contributing to the high incidence of esophageal malignancy.

Pathophysiology. Unfortunately, the patient may have an advanced ulcerated lesion of the esophagus before symptoms present. Malignancy, usually of the squamous cell epidermoid type, may spread beneath the esophageal mucosa, or it may spread directly into, through, and beyond the muscle layers into the lymphatics. In the latter stages, obstruction of the esophagus is noted, with possible perforation into the mediastinum and erosion into the great vessels.

Assessment and Clinical Manifestations. The patient is first aware of intermittent and increasing difficulty in swallowing. At first only solid food gives trouble, but as the growth progresses and the obstruction becomes more complete, even liquids cannot pass into the stomach. Regurgitation of food and saliva occurs, hemorrhage may take place, and there is a progressive loss of weight and strength, due to starvation. Later symptoms include substernal pain, hiccough, respiratory difficulty, and foul breath. *The delay between onset of early symptoms and the time when the patient seeks medical advice is often 12 to 18 months.* Herein lies a clue for the nurse to insist that any person with swallowing difficulties be encouraged to see a physician immediately.

The diagnosis is confirmed by esophagogram, cytologic examination of esophageal washings, barium x-ray studies, and esophagoscopy. Bronchoscopy usually is performed, especially in tumors of the middle and the upper third of the esophagus, to determine whether the trachea has been involved by the tumor and to help in determining whether the lesion can be removed. Mediastinoscopy is used to determine involvement of nodes and other mediastinal structures. Cancer of the lower end of the esophagus may be due to adenocarcinoma of the stomach, extending upward into the esophagus.

Management. The patient may be treated by surgical excision of the lesion, radiation, or a combination of both modalities. Usually surgery is preferred for lower esophageal tumors, whereas radiation is favored for upper esophageal lesions. With radiation, the lesion may shrink, thereby expanding the lumen and permitting the patient to swallow. Relatively few patients are cured; hence palliative therapy may be required, including combinations of treatment such as gastrostomy, jejunostomy, cervical esophagostomy, dilatation of the stricture, insertion of an intraluminal prosthetic tube, and chemotherapy.

The surgical approach may be through the thorax, or through the abdomen and thorax, depending upon the location of the tumor. A common approach for lesions of the lower esophagus is to remove the involved portion of the esophagus and reform the continuity of the gastrointestinal tract by bringing the stomach into the chest and implanting the proximal end of the esophagus into it (esophago-gastrostomy, Fig. 33-8). The chest is closed, after a drain is inserted into the pleural cavity and connected to closed suction.

Lesions in the middle and upper thirds of the esophagus, particularly, are often not suitable for surgical excision and, fortunately, occur less frequently. However, some success has been reported with a method in which a tunnel is created beneath the sternum and a resected segment of either jejunum or colon replaces the diseased esophagus (Fig. 33-8). A palliative procedure in which a plastic tube is introduced through a cervical incision has been done with resultant symptomatic relief, improvement in nutrition, and amelioration of psychological symptoms.

Radiation is used before surgery, in some clinics; in others, it is used after surgery. The ideal method of treating this problem has not yet been found; each patient is approached in a way that appears best for him. If the growth is found to be inoperable, either before or at operation, a gastrostomy is performed as a palliative procedure to permit the administration of food and fluids (see page 727).

Preoperative Nursing Management. The major nursing problems of the patients with an esophageal carcinoma are difficulty in swallowing (dysphagia), malnutrition, and psychological concern and awareness of the seriousness of the condition. Another annoying problem is excess saliva (drooling and spitting). Nursing planning and intervention are directed toward improving the patient's nutritional and physical condition in prepa-

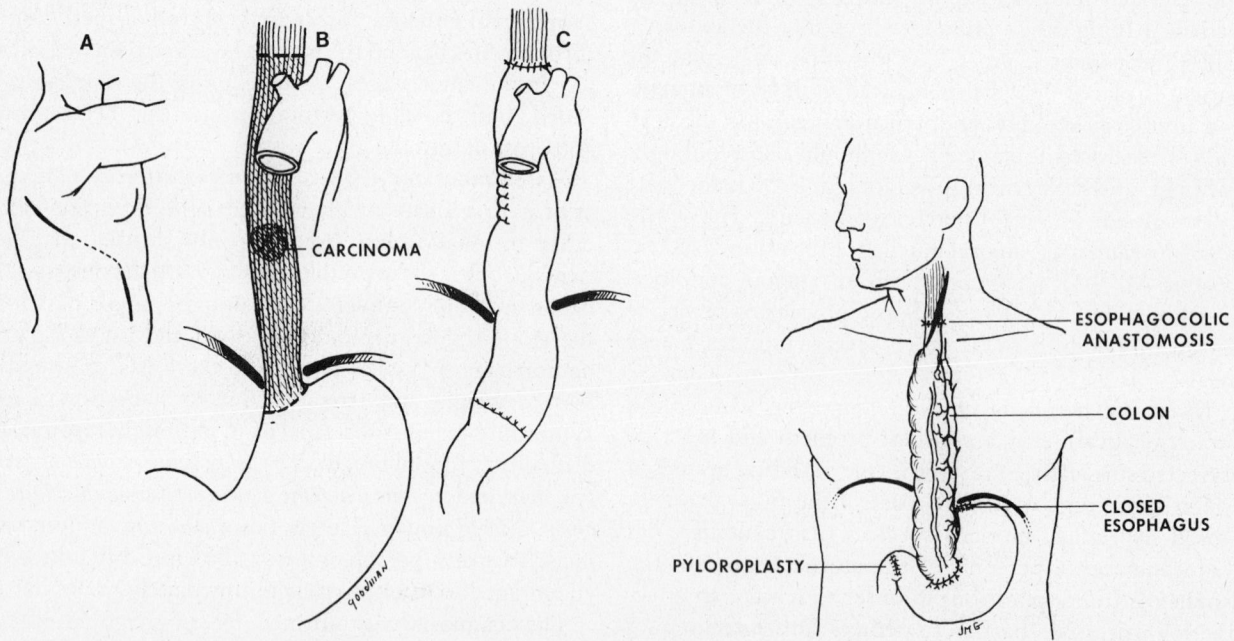

Figure 33-8. (*left*) A. The initial portion of the operation is performed through an upper abdominal incision (lower incision), with the gastroesophageal anastomosis completed through a right thoracotomy incision (upper incision). B. The shaded area is the esophagus; a carcinoma is shown in the middle third. (*B*) shows the tumor location and the esophagus to be removed. C. The stomach is pulled up through the diaphragm (blackened heavy lines) and anastomosed to the upper remaining esophagus (esophagogastric anastomosis and pyloroplasty). (*right*) Cancer of the esophagus has been removed and esophagus has been replaced with colon. The colon may be brought through the right or left hemithorax or it may be brought up through the anterior mediastinum, as shown. The small intestine may also be used. (Hardy: Rhoads Surgery, Philadelphia, J. B. Lippincott, 1977)

ration for surgery and/or radiation therapy. A weight-gaining program based on a high caloric and high protein diet, in liquid or soft form, is advocated, if it can be managed by mouth. If not, then intravenous or parenteral hyperalimentation is initiated.

Since the most common postoperative complication is aspiration pneumonia, the preoperative teaching program must emphasize postanesthetic turning, deep breathing, coughing, and exercises. As part of the effort to prevent pulmonary complications, expectorants and bronchodilators may be prescribed. Good oral hygiene is also encouraged, since regurgitation leaves an unpleasant taste in the mouth.

This patient should be acquainted with the nature of the postoperative equipment which will be used, including closed chest drainage, nasogastric suction, parenteral fluids, and perhaps a gastrostomy tube.

Postoperative Nursing Management. Immediate postoperative care is similar to that provided for patients undergoing thoracic surgery (page 423). Following emergence from anesthesia, the patient is placed in a semi-Fowler, and later a Fowler position, to assist in preventing reflux of gastric secretions. He is observed carefully for regurgitation and dyspnea. Temperature is monitored to detect any elevation which may indicate seepage of fluid through the operative site into the mediastinum.

If a prosthetic tube has been inserted or an anastomosis has been done, the patient will have a functioning continuum between the throat and the stomach. He will need encouragement and patience as he begins to swallow small sips of water and, later, pureed small feedings. When he is able to increase food intake to a significant amount, intravenous and parenteral findings are discontinued. If a prosthetic tube (such as a pliable latex tube held open with fine wire coils) is used, it may easily become obstructed if food is not chewed sufficiently. After each meal, he is to remain upright for at least two hours to assist in movement of food. The nurse is challenged to encourage this patient to eat, since his appetite is usually poor. Family involvement and home-cooked favorite foods may help the patient to eat. If he complains of gastric distress, antacids may help. When radiation is part of the therapy, the patient's appetite is further depressed.

Often, in either the pre- or postoperative period, an obstructed or nearly obstructed esophagus causes difficulty with excess saliva, so that drooling becomes a problem. This is of concern in an esophagostomy, also. In this situation, the use of small plastic bags fastened to the stoma are helpful in collecting secretions. Or, a wick-type piece of gauze may be placed at the corner of the mouth to direct secretions to a dressing or emesis basin. Of more concern is the possibility of aspiration of saliva into the tracheobronchial tree, with the danger of pneumonia.

When the patient is ready to go home, the family is instructed in how to give nutritional care; what to observe; how to handle signs of complications; and how to keep the patient comfortable.

Prognosis. If the malignancy is detected early, removal is simplified, and the continuity of the digestive system is easily maintained. However, the mortality rate among patients with cancer of the esophagus is high, due to three factors: (1) Usually the patients are older persons, in whom the incidence of pulmonary and cardiovascular disorders is high. (2) Before significant symptoms occur, the tumor has already invaded surrounding structures. It is impossible to excise a liberal area of tissue because of the proximity of vital structures. (3) The malignancy tends to spread to nearby lymph nodes, and the unique relation of the esophagus to the heart and lungs makes these organs easily accessible to the extension of the tumor. In several series of operative cases, 45 to 80 percent showed evidence of metastasis when examined in the operating room.

BIBLIOGRAPHY

ARTICLES

Mouth

Checchio, A. L., and Dowd, G. T.: Oral lesions — which ones may be cancer. Today's Clinician, 2:32-35, June 1978.

DeSanto, L. W.: Cancer of the posterior oral cavity. Surg. Clin. N. Am., 57:597-609, June 1977.

Johnston, W. D., and Ballantyne, A. J.: Prognostic effect of tobacco and alcohol use in patients with oral tongue cancer. Am. J. Surg., 134:444-447, Oct. 1977.

Kirkis, E. J.: This oral care technique gets results. RN, 41:82, Oct. 1978.

Krull, E. A., et al.: White lesions of the mouth. Clin. Symposia, 25:2-32, No. 2, 1973.

Maurer, J.: Providing optimal oral health. Nurs. Clin. of N. Am., 12:671-685, Dec. 1977.

Mendelson, B. C., et al.: Cancer of the oral cavity. Surg. Clin. N. Am., 57:585-596, June 1977.

Myers, J. D., et al.: Failure of neutral-red photodynamic inactivation in recurrent herpes simplex virus infections. New Eng. J. Med., 293:945-949, Nov. 1975.

Potter, B. E., et al.: Management of intraoral lesions. Am. Fam. Phys., 18:96-102, Nov. 1978.

Reitz, M., and Pope, W.: Mouth care. AJN, 73:1728-1730, Oct. 1973.

Sabin, A. D.: Misery of recurrent herpes, What to do? (Editorial) New Eng. J. Med., 293:986-988, Nov. 1975.

Turner, S. L.: Orthodontia for an adult. AJN, 78:2091-2093, Dec. 1978.

West, D. W.: Social adaptation patterns among cancer patients with facial disfigurements resulting from surgery. Arch. Phys. Med. Rehabil., 58:473-479, Nov. 1977.

Woods, J. E., and Masson, J. K.: Indications and techniques for resection of intraoral squamous cell carcinoma. Surg. Clin. N. Am., 57:515-521, June 1977.

Esophagus

Arvanitakis, C.: Achalasia of the esophagus: a reappraisal of esophagomyotomy vs. forceful pneumatic dilatation. Am. J. Dig. Dis., *20*:841-846, Sept. 1975.

Boyce, H. W.: Symposium on cancer of the esophagus: the case for palliation. Hosp. Pract., *11*:73-75, Oct. 1976.

Buckley, J. E., et al.: Feeding patients with dysphagia. Nurs. Forum, *15*:69-85, No. 1, 1976.

Campbell, G. S., et al.: Treatment of corrosive burns of the esophagus. Arch. Surg., *112*:495-500, Apr. 1977.

Carcinoma of the esophagus. Contemp. Surg., *12*:50-65, Apr. 1978.

Cohen, S.: Esophageal reflux: new concepts in medical management. Hosp. Pract., *11*:131-137, May 1976.

Ellis, F. H., Jr.: Esophagomyotomy for esophageal achalasia. Surg. Clin. N. Am., *53*:319-325, Apr. 1973.

————: Symposium on cancer of the esophagus — the case for surgery. Hosp. Pract., *11*:64-68, Oct. 1976.

Gallagher, E. G., et al.: Celestin tube intubation for advanced esophageal carcinoma. Am. J. Surg., *136*:405-407, Sept. 1978.

Lane, F. W., Jr.: Symposium on cancer of the esophagus — the case for irradiation. Hosp. Pract., *11*:68-73, Oct. 1976.

Machety, C. J.: Esophageal endoprosthesis. RN, *40*:51-53, Oct. 1977.

Price, S. P., and Castell, D. O.: Esophageal mythology. JAMA, *240*:44-46, July 1978.

Rayan, R. K.: Esophageal diverticula. Amer. Fam. Physic., *19*:119-122, Mar. 1979.

Sotus, P. C., et al.: Carcinoma in situ of the esophagus. JAMA, *239*:335-336, Jan. 1978.

Head and Neck

Beahrs, O. H.: The surgical anatomy and technique of parotidectomy. Surg. Clin. N. Am., *57*:477-493, June 1977.

Conley, J. J.: Radical neck dissection. Contemp. Surg., *5*:65-73, Sept. 1974.

Noone, R. B., and Graham, W. P., III: Nutritional care after head and neck surgery. Postgrad. Med., *53*:80-86, June 1973.

Schneider, W. R.: Nutrition in head and neck cancer: Nursing implications. Oncol. Nurs. Forum, *6*:5-11, Jan. 1979.

Stuart, M. S.: Skin flaps and grafts after head and neck surgery. AJN, *78*:1368-1374, Aug. 1978.

AGENCIES

American Dental Association, 211 East Chicago Ave., Chicago, Ill. 60611

34

ASSESSMENT OF DIGESTIVE AND GASTROINTESTINAL FUNCTION

PHYSIOLOGIC OVERVIEW

Anatomy of the Gastrointestinal Tract

The gastrointestinal tract is a tube that is continuous with the external environment at both ends. The pathway extends from the mouth through the esophagus, stomach, and intestines to the anus. The esophagus is located in the mediastinum in the thoracic cavity, anterior to the spine and posterior to the trachea and heart. It is a collapsible tube that becomes distended when food passes through it.

The stomach is situated in the upper portion of the abdomen to the left of the midline, just under the left diaphragm. It is a distensible pouch with a capacity of approximately 1500 ml. The inlet to the stomach is called the esophagogastric junction. It is surrounded by a ring of smooth muscle, called the lower esophageal sphincter, which, on contraction, closes the stomach off from the esophagus. The outlet from the stomach is called the pylorus. Circular smooth muscle in the wall of the pylorus forms the pyloric sphincter and controls the size of the opening between the stomach and small intestine.

The small intestine is the longest segment of the gastrointestinal tract and accounts for about two thirds of the total length. It is folded back and forth upon itself and occupies a major portion of the abdominal cavity. It is divided into three parts: an upper part called the *duodenum*, the middle part called the *jejunum*, and the lower part called the *ileum*. The common bile duct, the conduit for both bile and pancreatic secretions, empties into the duodenum.

The junction between the small and large intestines usually lies in the right lower portion of the abdomen. It is in this area that the vermiform appendix is located. At the junction of the small and large intestines is a valve (ileocecal valve) that functions in a similar fashion to the pyloric and esophagogastric sphincters, mentioned previously. The large intestine consists of an ascending segment on the right side of the abdomen, a transverse segment that extends from right to left in the upper abdomen, and a descending segment on the left side of the abdomen. The terminal portion of the large intestine is the rectum, which is continuous with the anus. The anal outlet is surrounded by the external anal sphincter, which, unlike the other sphincters of the gastrointestinal tract, is composed of striated muscle and is under voluntary control.

Blood Supply to the Gastrointestinal Tract. Since the gastrointestinal tract is so long, its blood supply is from arteries that originate along the entire length of the thoracic and abdominal aorta. Of particular importance are the vessels to the large and small intestines—the superior and inferior mesenteric arteries. These two arteries form small loops, or arcades, which encircle the intestine, supplying its wall with oxygen and nutrients. Blood in the veins that drain the intestine is enriched by nutrients absorbed from the lumen of the gastrointestinal tract. These veins merge with others in the abdomen to

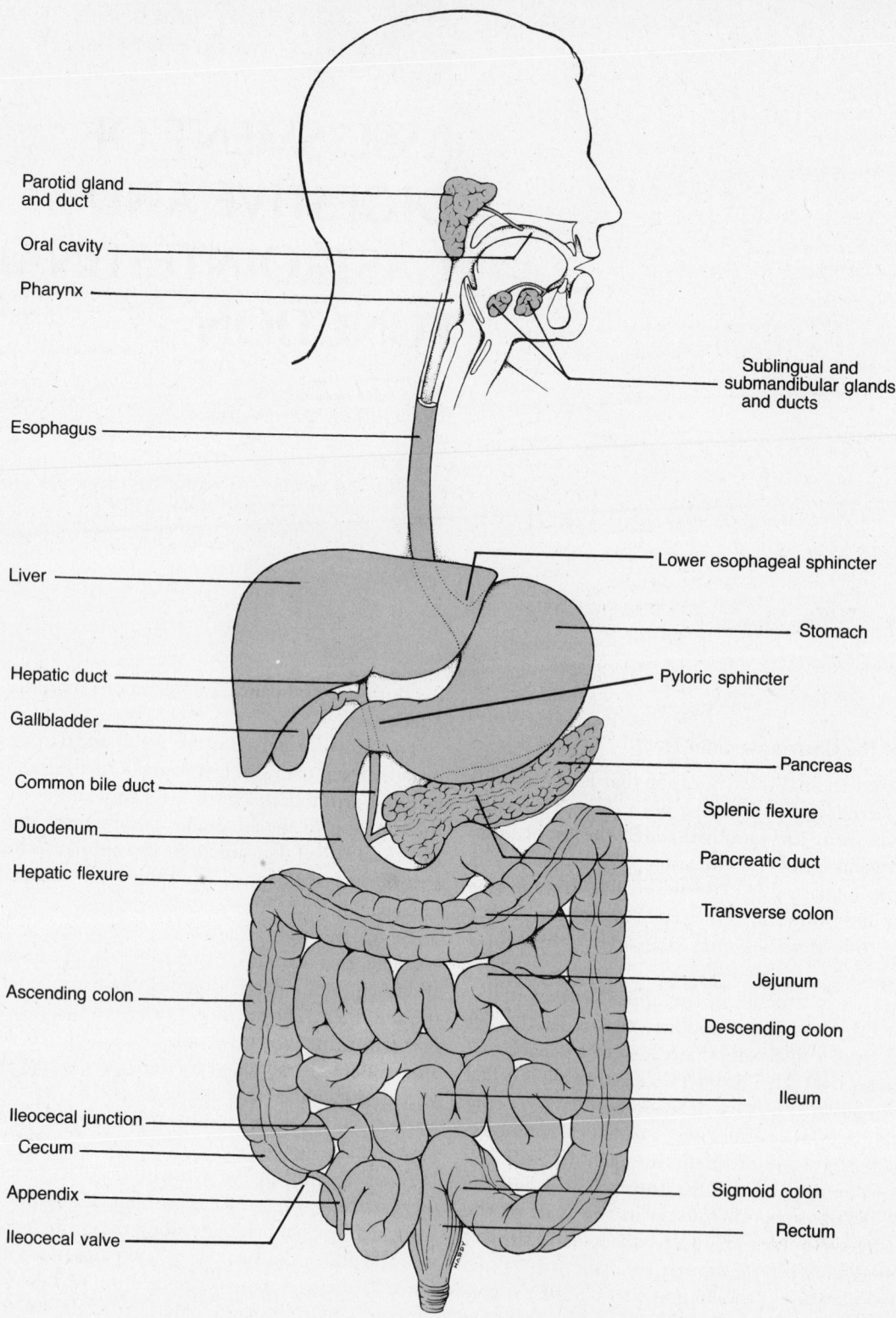

Figure 34-1. Diagram of the digestive system, showing the digestive or alimentary canal and sphincters. (Chaffee and Greisheimer: Basic Physiology and Anatomy. Philadelphia, J. B. Lippincott, 1974)

708

form a large vessel called the portal vein, which carries the nutrient-rich blood to the liver. The blood flow to the entire gastrointestinal tract is about 20 percent of the total cardiac output, and it is significantly increased after eating.

Innervation. The gastrointestinal tract is innervated by both the sympathetic and parasympathetic parts of the autonomic nervous system. The parasympathetic fibers travel in the vagus nerve and in nerves that arise from the sacral segment of the spinal cord. In addition, the upper esophagus and the external anal sphincter are under voluntary control, and are supplied by somatic nerves that arise from the cervical spinal cord and from the sacral spinal cord, respectively.

The Digestive Process

In order to perform their functions, all cells of the body require nutrients, which must be derived from the intake of food that contains protein, fat, carbohydrates, vitamins, and minerals, as well as cellulose fibers and other vegetable matter without nutritional value. This diet provides the energy needs of the body and maintains body weight at approximately constant levels.

The intake of food is a voluntary act that is controlled by conscious sensations of hunger and satiety, modified by learned behavior. These sensations originate in the higher centers of the brain, probably in the hypothalamus. The hypothalamus itself is influenced by visual and olfactory sensations, nervous and hormonal signals originating in the digestive tract, and behavioral patterns.

The primary functions of the gastrointestinal tract are:
1. To break down food particles into their small constituent molecules, for digestion;
2. To absorb the small molecules produced by digestion into the bloodstream;
3. To eliminate undigested and unabsorbed foodstuffs and other waste products from the body.

The pathway that foodstuffs take in the digestive tract begins at the mouth, where they are chewed and swallowed. The bolus of food is then conveyed down through the esophagus into the stomach, where it remains for a variable length of time. It then enters the small intestine, where much of the digestion and absorption of nutrients takes place. The unabsorbed food passes from the small intestine into the colon (also called the large intestine) for further modification and storage prior to elimination (defecation). A schematic diagram of the structures of the gastrointestinal tract is shown in Fig. 34-1. The total length of the gastrointestinal pathway, from mouth to anus, is approximately 400-500 cm.

Large volumes of fluid containing hormones and enzymes are secreted into the gastrointestinal tract in order to aid in the processes of digestion, absorption, and elimination. The total secretion into the lumen of the gastrointestinal tract is about 8 liters per day, but less than 200 ml. per day of liquid is excreted in the feces. This illustrates the massive absorptive capacity of the gastrointestinal tract.

- Derangements of the absorption function of the digestive system can lead to serious alterations of body fluids.

Gastrointestinal Motility and Secretions

Motility refers to the coordinated contractions of the muscles in the walls of the gastrointestinal tract that propel food and secretions from the mouth toward the anus. These sequential rhythmic contractions are referred to as *peristalsis*. At the same time that the food is being propelled through the gastrointestinal tract, it comes into contact with a wide variety of secretions that aid in breaking down and digesting the food particles (Fig. 34-2).

Oral Digestion. The first secretion encountered is saliva, which is secreted in the mouth by the salivary glands at the rate of about 1.5 liters daily. Saliva contains

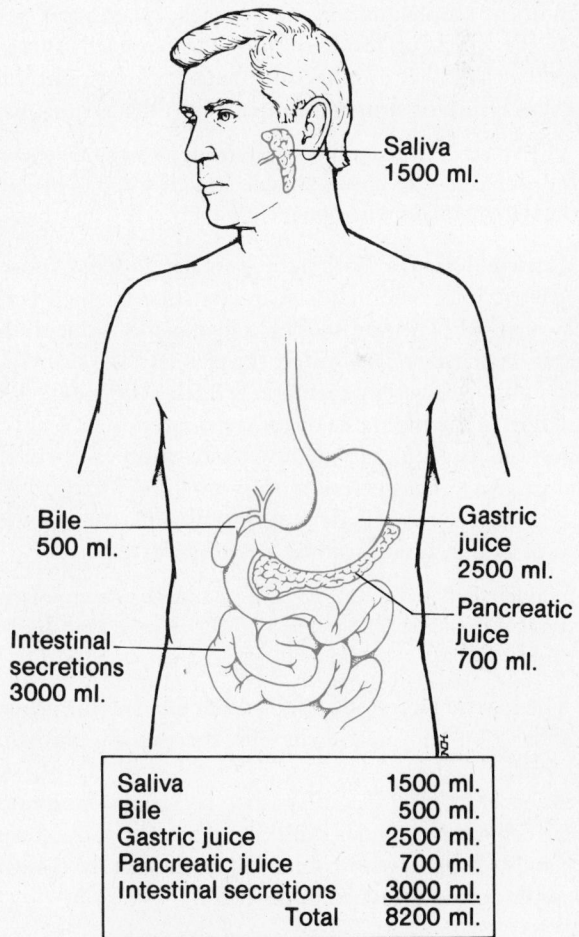

Saliva
1500 ml.

Bile
500 ml.

Gastric
juice
2500 ml.

Pancreatic
juice
700 ml.

Intestinal
secretions
3000 ml.

Saliva	1500 ml.
Bile	500 ml.
Gastric juice	2500 ml.
Pancreatic juice	700 ml.
Intestinal secretions	3000 ml.
Total	8200 ml.

Figure 34-2. Total volume of digestive secretions produced in 24 hours. (Adapted from Bowen, Arthur: Intravenous alimentation in surgical patients. Mod. Med.)

an enzyme, *ptyalin*, or salivary amylase, which helps in the digestion of starches. It also serves as a solvent for the molecules in the food that stimulate the taste buds. Eating, or even the sight, smell, or thought of food can cause reflex salivation. The major function of saliva is to lubricate the food as it is chewed, thereby facilitating swallowing.

Swallowing. Swallowing, the initial act in the propulsion of food, is under voluntary control. It is regulated by a swallowing center in the medulla oblongata of the central nervous system. Voluntary efforts to initiate swallowing are ineffective unless there is something to swallow, such as air, saliva, or food. As the food is swallowed, the epiglottis moves to cover the tracheal opening and thus prevents aspiration of food into the lungs. Swallowing results in the propulsion of the bolus of food into the upper esophagus. The smooth muscle in the wall of the esophagus undergoes rhythmic contractions which move sequentially from above to below and help to propel the bolus of food from the upper esophagus toward the stomach. During this process of esophageal peristalsis, the lower esophageal sphincter, at the junction of the esophagus and the stomach, relaxes and permits the bolus of food to enter the stomach. Subsequently, the lower esophageal sphincter closes tightly to prevent reflux of stomach contents into the esophagus.

- When there is reflux of the acid contents of the stomach into the esophagus, an uncomfortable sensation occurs beneath the sternum. This sensation is commonly called heartburn.

Gastric Action. Within the stomach, food is exposed to gastric juice, the major characteristic of which is its very acid pH. The acidity (pH as low as 1.0) is due to the secretion of *hydrochloric acid* by the glands of the stomach. The volume of gastric secretion is 2.5 liters per day. The function of the highly acid stomach secretion is to aid in digestion, breaking food down into more absorbable components. The secretion of hydrochloric acid occurs in response to a meal. Between meals, the rate of secretion of acid into the stomach is low.

- Individuals who chronically secrete excessive amounts of gastric acid are susceptible to development of gastric and duodenal ulcers.

The gastric secretions also contain the enzyme *pepsin*, which is an important enzyme for the digestion of proteins.

Another component of gastric secretions is *intrinsic factor*. This compound is synthesized by cells of the stomach and combines with vitamin B_{12} in the diet, so that the vitamin can be absorbed in the ileum.

- In the absence of intrinsic factor, vitamin B_{12} cannot be absorbed, resulting in pernicious anemia. Research studies have shown that the death of an animal after its stomach is removed is caused by the loss of intrinsic factor.

Peristaltic contractions in the stomach propel its contents towards the pylorus. Large food particles cannot pass through the pyloric sphincter and are churned back into the body of the stomach. In this way, food in the stomach is mechanically agitated and is broken down into smaller particles. Therefore, different types of meals remain in the stomach for times varying from one-half to several hours, depending upon the size of food particles, composition of the meal, and other factors.

Peristalsis in the stomach and contractions of the pyloric sphincter allow the partially digested food to enter the small intestine at a rate that permits efficient absorption of nutrients.

Intestinal Secretions. Secretions in the *duodenum* come from the pancreas, the liver and the glands in the wall of the intestine itself. The major characteristic of these secretions is their high content of digestive enzymes.

The pancreatic secretion has an alkaline pH, due to a high *bicarbonate* concentration. This serves to neutralize the acid entering the duodenum from the stomach. The pancreas also secretes digestive enzymes, including: *trypsin*, which aids in the digestion of protein, *amylase*, which aids in the digestion of starch, and *lipase*, which aids in the digestion of fats.

Bile (secreted by the liver and stored in the gallbladder) contains bile salts, *cholesterol*, and *lecithin*, which emulsify the ingested fats and make them more accessible to digestion and absorption. The bile salts themselves are reabsorbed into the portal blood when they reach the ileum.

Secretions from the intestinal glands consist of mucus, which coats the cells and protects the duodenum from attack by hydrochloric acid; hormones; electrolytes; and enzymes. The total amount of intestinal secretions is approximately 1 liter per day of pancreatic juice, 0.5 liters per day of bile, and 3 liters per day from the glands of the small intestine.

Gastrointestinal Hormones and Bacteria

Hormones. Three major hormones have been found to control the rate of secretion of the gastrointestinal fluids and gastrointestinal motility.

Gastrin is secreted by the cells of the stomach. It partially regulates the secretion of gastric acid and influences contraction of the lower esophageal and pyloric sphincters. The stimulus to gastrin release is distention of the stomach.

Secretin, secreted by the mucosa in the upper portion of the small intestine, stimulates the secretion of *bicarbonate* in pancreatic juice and inhibits the secretion of gastric acid. The stimulus to the release of secretin is acid entering the small intestine from the stomach.

Cholecystokinin-pancreozymin (CCK-PZ), also released from the cells in the upper small intestine, acts on both the gallbladder and the pancreas. It causes contraction of the gallbladder and release of digestive enzymes from the pancreas. The stimulus to the release of CCK-PZ is the presence of fatty acids and amino acids in the small intestine.

Bacteria.   Bacteria are normal components of the contents of the gastrointestinal tract. Their presence is essential for normal gastrointestinal function. Few bacteria are present in the stomach or upper small intestine, probably because they are killed by the acid secretions in the stomach. However, the bacterial population increases in the ileum and becomes a major component of the contents of the large intestine. Bacteria function as an aid to digestion, and also synthesize essential nutrients that otherwise might not be available for absorption. The bacterial mass comprises about 10 percent of the dry weight of the stool.

Digestion and Absorption of Nutrients

Food, ingested in the form of fats, protein, and carbohydrates, is broken down into its constituent nutrients by the process of digestion.

Carbohydrate digestion begins in the mouth with the breakdown of starches by the action of *salivary amylase.* It continues in the esophagus, but is inhibited in the stomach by gastric acid. Continuation of carbohydrate digestion occurs in the duodenum by the action of *pancreatic amylase.* The end result of this process is the liberation of small sugar molecules known as *disaccharides* (e.g., sucrose, maltose, galactose). Enzymes attached to the mucosal cells of the intestine convert the disaccharides into *monosaccharides* such as glucose and fructose, which are then absorbed into the blood.

• Glucose is the major carbohydrate that the tissue cells utilize as fuel.

Proteins are long chains of amino acids linked together chemically. The hydrochloric acid in the stomach aids in breaking down proteins into smaller particles that are more easily attacked by the digestive enzymes. The process of protein digestion begins in the stomach by the action of pepsin and continues in the duodenum by the action of pancreatic enzymes, such as trypsin. When the proteins are broken down into their constituent amino acids, they are actively absorbed through the mucosal cells of the small intestine into the blood. The tissues utilize amino acids in synthesizing their constituent proteins.

Ingested fats must be dispersed into small droplets (emulsified) so that they can be attacked by digestive enzymes. Emulsification of fats takes place as the result of the churning action in the stomach and duodenum and contact with bile salts. Pancreatic lipase then breaks down the emulsified fats into monoglycerides and fatty acids. These are solubilized as *micelles,* which move to the mucosal surface of the intestine where they are absorbed.

Within the mucosal cells, the fatty acids are recombined into fats, which then enter the lacteals (part of the lymphatic system) and eventually enter the bloodstream. The tissues utilize fats as a fuel; excess fat is stored in the fat cells that are widely distributed throughout the body.

Vitamins in the diet are absorbed essentially unchanged from the gastrointestinal tract. The fat-soluble vitamins A, D, E, and K are absorbed by a mechanism similar to that described above for fats. Vitamin B_{12} is absorbed after combination with intrinsic factor, as previously described.

Minerals in the diet, such as calcium and iron, are absorbed in the small intestine. Calcium absorption requires the presence of vitamin D and is modified by the action of parathyroid hormone.

• Iron in the diet is needed to replace small amounts of iron normally lost by the body, but only a limited fraction of the ingested iron can be absorbed. Therefore, repletion of iron stores of the body by oral therapy, in a patient with iron deficiency, is a long-term process.

Little of the *water and electrolytes* in the diet, and in the 8 liters per day of gastrointestinal secretions, are excreted in the stool.

Intestinal Peristalsis

Peristalsis propels the contents of the small intestine toward the colon. Intense peristaltic waves may be responsible for the gurgling sounds emanating from the gastrointestinal tract at various times. Segmental contractions of the intestinal smooth muscle occur, in addition to its peristaltic contractions. These segmental contractions do not propel contents towards the colon, but rather churn it back and forth, to permit more efficient digestion and absorption. Food leaving the small intestine must pass through the ileocecal valve to enter the colon. This valve is normally closed, and helps prevent colonic contents from refluxing back into the small intestine. However, with each peristaltic wave of the small intestine, the valve opens briefly and permits some of the contents to pass through. The first part of a meal usually reaches the ileocecal valve in about 4 hours, and all of the unabsorbed food has entered the colon by 8 or 9 hours after eating.

Motility of the colon consists of relatively weak peristaltic activity that moves the colonic contents slowly, and strong peristaltic rushes that propel the contents for considerable distances. When the contents reach and distend the rectum, an urge to defecate is experienced. Eating stimulates the peristaltic rushes in the colon, resulting in desire to defecate, shortly after a meal. This gastrocolic reflex is the reason that defecation after meals is the rule in children. However, in adults, habit and cultural factors are more important in determining the time for elimination of fecal contents. The first part of a meal reaches the rectum about 12 hours after eating. From the rectum to the anus, transport is much slower, and as much as one-fourth of the meal may still be in the rectum three days after ingestion. This slow transport of colonic contents allows efficient reabsorption of water and electrolytes.

Defecation

Distention of the rectum reflexly initiates contractions of its musculature and relaxation of the internal anal sphincter, which is ordinarily closed. When the desire to defecate is felt, the external anal sphincter voluntarily relaxes, permitting expulsion of colonic contents. Normally, the external anal sphincter is maintained in a state of tonic contraction. Thus, defecation is seen to be a spinal reflex which can be voluntarily inhibited by keeping the external anal sphincter closed. In this regard, it is similar to micturition. Contraction of abdominal muscles (straining) facilitates emptying of the colon.

- The presence of neurologic lesions which disrupt the innervation of the rectum lessens the effectiveness of reflex evacuation and can lead to abnormal retention of fecal material (fecal impaction).

The average frequency of defecation in humans is once daily, but the range is extremely variable. It is commonly observed that some people defecate several times daily, while others may defecate only a few times per week. More importantly, changes in bowel habits may signify colonic disease. An increase in frequency of defecation is called *diarrhea,* whereas decreased frequency is called *constipation.*

FECES AND FLATUS. The feces consist of undigested foodstuffs, inorganic materials, water, and bacteria. Their composition is relatively unaffected by alterations of diet, since a large fraction of the fecal mass is of nondietary origin, derived from the gastrointestinal tract. This is why appreciable amounts of feces continue to be passed despite prolonged starvation. The brown color of the feces is due to breakdown of bile by the intestinal bacteria. With obstruction of the bile ducts, bile is absent from the intestine, and the stools become white (acholic stools). Formation of chemicals, especially indole and skatole, by the intestinal bacteria are responsible in large part for the fecal odor.

The gastrointestinal tract normally contains approximately 150 ml. of gas. Gas expelled from the upper gastrointestinal tract (belching) has its origin as swallowed air. Gas expelled from the lower gastrointestinal tract (flatulence) consists of swallowed air, as well as gas produced by bacteria in the colon. The gas in the colon contains methane, hydrogen sulphide, ammonia, and other potentially harmful gases. These gases can be absorbed into the portal circulation and are detoxified by the liver.

- Patients with liver disease are frequently treated with antibiotics to reduce the number of colonic bacteria and thereby inhibit the production of toxic gases.

PATHOPHYSIOLOGIC OVERVIEW

Abnormalities of the gastrointestinal tract are numerous and exemplify every type of major pathology that can affect other organ systems. Figure 34-3 presents a composite view of the various types of gastrointestinal disorders which may occur. Congenital, inflammatory, infectious, traumatic, and neoplastic lesions have been encountered in every portion, and at every site, along its 7.5-meter (25-foot) length. In common with many other organ systems, it is subject to circulatory disturbances, faulty nervous control, and senescence.

Obstruction of the Gastrointestinal Tract. Various degrees of obstruction to the passage of intestinal contents in the gastrointestinal tract may result from tumors growing into the lumen, twisting or kinking of the intestine, infarction of tissue due to interruption of the blood supply, aspirated foreign bodies, or other reasons. As a consequence of obstruction, the force of the intestinal contractions is increased, the intestine becomes distended above the point of obstruction, and abdominal pain and bloating result. The peristaltic waves may actually reverse their direction, leading to vomiting. Excessive vomiting may result in the loss of large volumes of fluid from the body, causing *dehydration,* and loss of large amounts of hydrochloric acid, causing *systemic alkalosis.* If the obstruction in the gastrointestinal tract occurs at, or below, the duodenum, biliary material will be in the vomitus, giving the characteristic green color. If the colon is obstructed, the ileocecal valve may become stretched and incompetent, colonic contents can reflux, and the patient may vomit fecal material.

Diarrhea. Diarrhea, defined as the presence of more than the usual number of daily bowel movements, or an increase in volume of stool, is another major abnormality of gastrointestinal function. A common mechanism for diarrhea is an increased rate of movement of the contents through the intestine and colon, so that inadequate time is available for absorption of the gastrointestinal secretions, resulting in an increased fluid content of the stool. Inflammation or other diseases of the colonic mucosa can also lead to diarrhea. When these occur, water and electrolytes are not sufficiently reabsorbed and increased amounts of fluids or liquid reach the rectum, resulting in increased stool volume. *Steatorrhea,* defined as a large amount of fat in the stools, is commonly due to pancreatic disease. The decreased activity of pancreatic enzymes is responsible for decreased fat digestion. Disease of the biliary tract can also cause steatorrhea, due to the absence of bile salts. The consequences of diarrhea are loss of potassium, causing electrolyte imbalance; loss of bicarbonate, leading to acidosis; and loss of nutrients, leading to malnutrition.

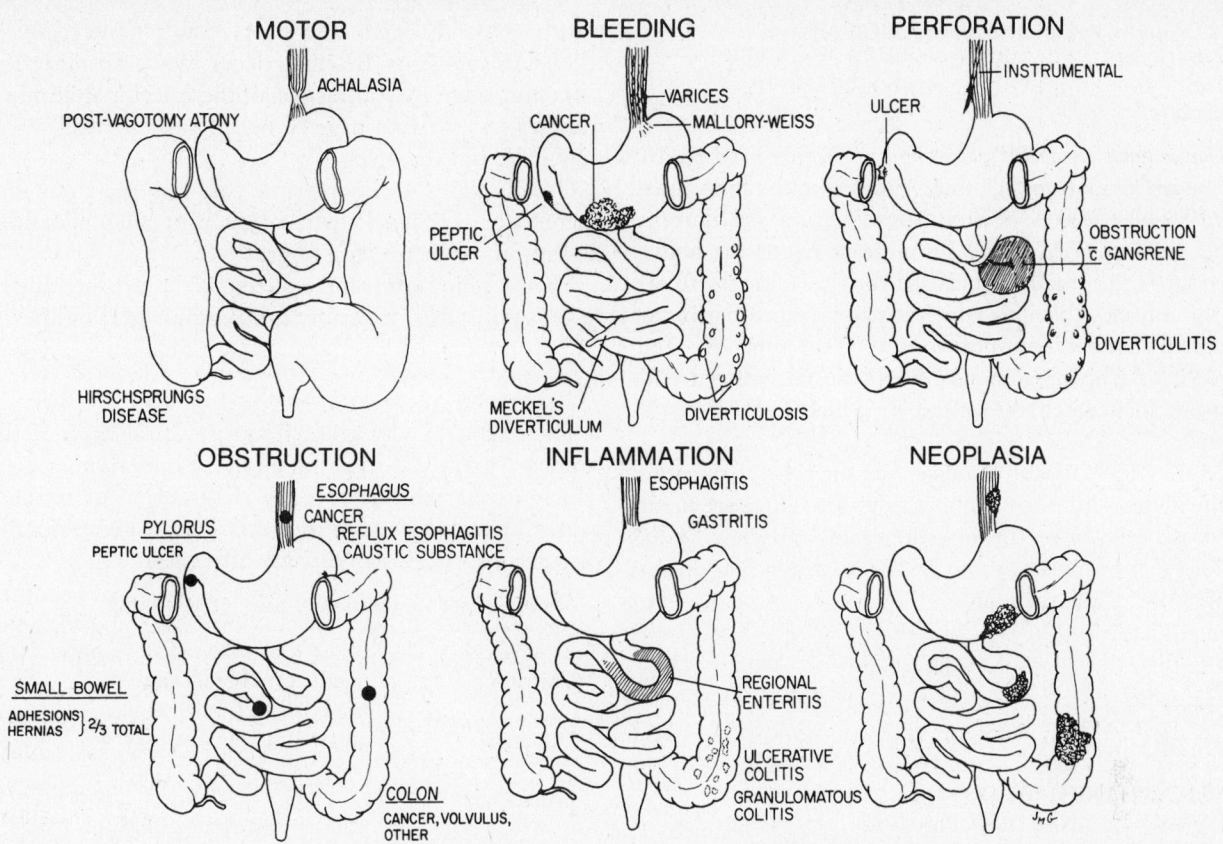

Figure 34-3. Pathophysiology of the gastrointestinal tract can be classified in many ways. The above illustration vividly shows the many conditions which can occur under the six classifications. (From Hardy: Rhoads Surgery, Philadelphia, J. B. Lippincott, 1977)

Psychosocial Considerations in Gastrointestinal Disorders

Quite apart from the multiplicity of organic diseases to which the gastrointestinal tract is heir, there are many extrinsic factors—some related to disease, others not—which can interfere with its normal functions and produce symptoms duplicating those of intrinsic gastrointestinal disease. An anxiety state, for example, often finds its chief expression in the syndrome of functional indigestion, or motor disturbance of the intestine. Moreover, certain organic diseases have been ascribed to emotional imbalances. Stress ulcer, for example, has been explained by many observers on a psychogenic basis. Such diseases are commonly referred to as "psychosomatic" disorders, a term that underlines, so to speak, the importance of the mind-body relationship in the pathogenesis. Regarding the importance of this relationship there can be no doubt, because regardless of the fundamental etiology involved, the severity, course, and outcome of these conditions are influenced greatly by the mental health of the patient.

The nurse should be thoroughly cognizant of the relation between the level of the patient's mood and his appetite and bowel function, and between his sensory awareness and the manner in which he interprets sensations. It is also important to recognize that the nurse's own attitude toward the patient and his complaints is an influential factor, capable of modifying his symptoms in either direction. A display of genuine tolerance and sympathetic interest toward the patient is often the key to cooperation, and if that is obtained, the major obstacle to therapeutic success has been removed.

SURGICAL CONSIDERATIONS

ABDOMINAL TOPOGRAPHY

For purposes of convenience in description, the abdomen has been divided into nine regions by imaginary lines, as illustrated in the chart on page 715.

The abdominal cavity normally contains a small amount of fluid that lubricates the peritoneal surfaces. This cavity is lined with a thin, glistening membrane called the *peritoneum,* which covers most of the abdominal organs, forming folds between which the coils of intestine are located. Some organs (such as the liver, pancreas, kidney, and urinary bladder) are not covered completely by peritoneum; hence inflammations of these structures may not always involve the general abdominal cavity but may develop into retroperitoneal extensions or abscesses.

ABDOMINAL INCISIONS AND SURGICAL PROCEDURES

Incisions

Laparotomy or *abdominal section* are terms used to describe any operation that involves opening the abdominal cavity. The gridiron, or McBurney, incision (see figure in chart on page 715) is the simplest. It opens the abdomen through a small wound made by spreading the fibers of the muscles through which it passes. This incision is especially suitable for operations upon the appendix, and since it has the advantage of being closed without tension, it makes a firm wound in which hernias rarely form.

More widely useful, however, are the vertical incisions made in the midline or to either side of it. These are made to pass between or through the rectus muscles. Many other types of incisions may be made, depending on the preference of the surgeon.

ASSESSMENT OF GASTROINTESTINAL FUNCTION

CLINICAL MANIFESTATIONS OF GASTROINTESTINAL DISTURBANCES

Indigestion

As a result of disturbed nervous control of the stomach, or of disease elsewhere in the body, many persons suffer intensely from "indigestion," although their stomachs appear normal. Abdominal pain is the most common complaint of these patients. This pain is usually in the upper abdomen and is frequently associated with eating, occurring during, or immediately after, a meal. Its character may be described as crampy, or a feeling of fullness, distention, or burning. Fatty foods are apt to cause the most discomfort, probably because they remain in the stomach longest, and because these patients commonly have an abnormal aversion to fatty foods. Coarse vegetables and highly seasoned foods likewise cause considerable distress. Alkalies such as sodium bicarbonate afford only partial relief, or perhaps none at all. The basis for the abdominal distress is obviously the patient's own gastric peristaltic movements. Bowel movements may or may not relieve the pain.

Intestinal "Gas"—Belching and Flatulence

The accumulation of gas in the gastrointestinal tract may result in *belching,* the expulsion of gas from the stomach through the mouth, or *flatulence,* the expulsion of gas from the rectum.

Air that reaches the stomach is quickly expelled, but not necessarily by belching. Periodically, stomach gas moves into the lower esophagus (simple reflux) and then returns to the stomach, due to a peristaltic contraction of the distal esophagus. Belching occurs when simple reflux is accompanied by contraction of the anterior abdominal muscles. At the first urge to belch, simply swallowing may interrupt the belch.

Usually gases in the intestine pass into the colon and are released as flatus. Patients often complain of bloating, distention, or being "full of gas."

The so-called *heartburn, acid eructation,* etc., are due to reverse peristalsis, probably gastroesophageal reflux.

Pain

The character, duration, frequency, and time of the pain vary greatly, depending upon the underlying cause, which affects the location and distribution of referred pain. Other factors such as meals, rest, defecation, and vascular disorders may directly affect pain.

Major sites of localization of pain are as follows:

Esophageal:	Retrosternal; may radiate to back
Gastric:	Epigastric; may radiate to back, especially left subscapular
Duodenal:	Epigastric; may radiate to back, especially right subscapular
Gallbladder:	Right upper quadrant or epigastric; may radiate to back or right subscapular
Pancreatic:	Epigastric; may radiate to back or left lumbar
Appendicular:	Periumbilical, later to right lower quadrant
Colonic:	Hypogastrium, right or left lower quadrant
Rectal:	Pelvic area

Vomiting

This is an involuntary act in which violent contractions of the abdominal muscles forcefully expel gastric contents up through the esophagus. It is preceded by closure of the glottis and pylorus, together with relaxation of the gastric wall and cardiac orifice. *Retching* involves these same movements, except that the cardiac orifice remains closed, so that gastric contents are not expelled. Vomiting is usually preceded by *nausea,* an unpleasant sensation suggesting that vomiting is imminent. Such symptoms are associated with gastrointestinal disturbances. Assessment includes determining from the patient any aggravating factors, frequency of vomiting, time of occurrence, and the quantity, odor, color, and taste of the eructed material.

Hematemesis is the vomiting of blood. When this happens soon after hemorrhage, the vomitus is bright red. If blood has been retained in the stomach, digestive processes change the hemoglobin to a brown pigment which gives the vomitus a coffee-ground appearance. Occasionally the patient has difficulty in differentiating be-

ABDOMINAL INCISIONS AND SURGICAL PROCEDURES

Before studying about patients with specific gastrointestinal problems and operations, the nurse should be familiar with the prefixes denoting abdominal organs and the suffixes used to denote the diseases of or operations on these organs.

Suffixes used to denote the names of diseases and operations are:

itis—inflammation of—as *appendicitis,* an inflammation of the appendix.

otomy—to make a cut into—as *gastrotomy,* to make an opening into the stomach.

ostomy—to make a mouth or opening into—as *cystostomy,* to insert a tube into the urinary bladder.

ectomy—to cut or remove—as *salpingectomy,* to remove the fallopian tube.

pexy—to sew up in position—as *nephropexy,* to sew the kidney up in position.

orrhaphy—to repair a defect—as *herniorrhaphy,* to repair a hernial defect.

plasty—to improve by changing the position of the tissue—as *pyloroplasty,* an operation to enlarge the pyloric opening of the stomach.

Organs	Prefix	
Stomach	*Gastr*	*Gastritis*—inflammation of stomach
Pylorus	*Pylor*	*Pylorectomy*—removal of pyloric end of stomach
Liver	*Hepa*	*Hepatitis*—inflammation of liver
Gallbladder	*Cholecyst*	*Cholecystitis*—inflammation of gallbladder
Common bile duct	*Choledoch*	*Choledochitis*—inflammation of common bile duct
Small intestine	*Enter*	*Enteritis*—inflammation of intestine
Colon	*Col*	*Colitis*—inflammation of large colon
Appendix	*Appendic*	*Appendicitis*—inflammation of appendix
Rupture	*Herni*	*Herniorrhaphy*—repair of hernia
Loin or abdomen	*Lapar*	*Laparotomy*—incision in the abdomen
Urinary bladder	*Cyst*	*Cystitis*—inflammation of urinary bladder
Fallopian tube	*Salping*	*Salpingitis*—inflammation of fallopian tube
Ovary	*Oophor*	*Oophoritis*—inflammation of ovary
Pelvis of kidney	*Pyel*	*Pyelitis*—inflammation of pelvis of kidney
Kidney	*Nephr*	*Nephritis*—inflammation of kidney

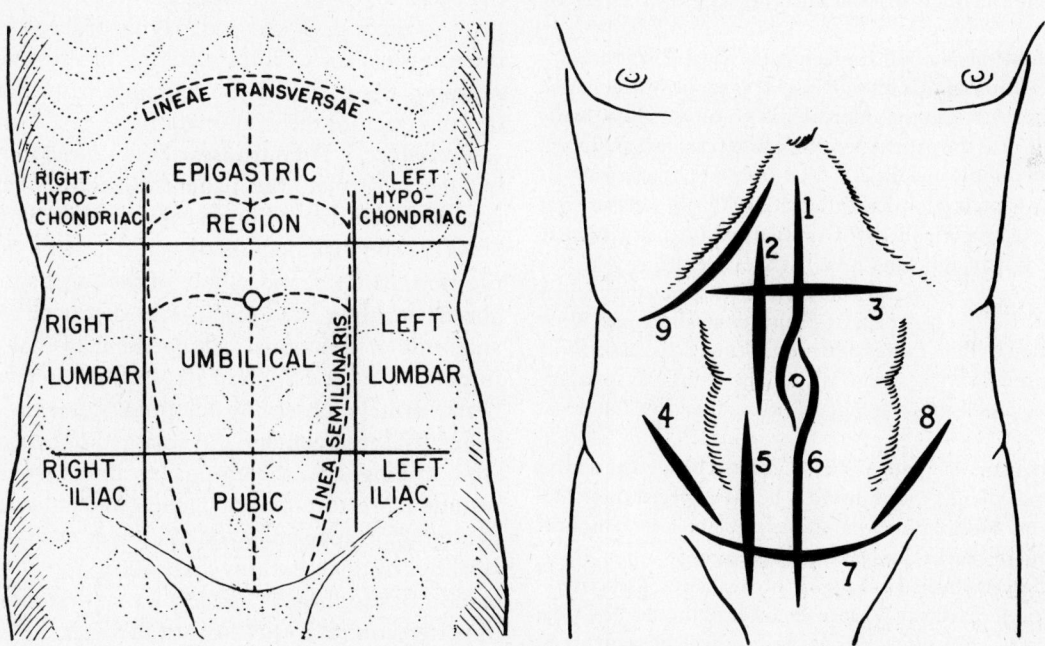

(*Left*) Regions of the abdomen. (*right*) Diagram to show the various abdominal incisions which are used: (1) upper midline incision, (2) upper right rectus incision, (3) transverse incision in the upper abdomen, (4) gridiron incision on the right, (5) lower right rectus incision, (6) lower midline incision, (7) Pfannenstiel incision, (8) left gridiron incision, (9) subcostal incision.

tween hematemesis and hemoptysis (expectoration of blood-tinged sputum), particular if a coughing paroxysm has preceded it.

Anorexia, Dysphagia, and Polyphagia

Anorexia is the lack of appetite for food. *Dysphagia* refers to swallowing difficulty, while *odynophagia* indicates pain on swallowing. *Polyphagia* means excessive eating, or voracious appetite. These are descriptive signs which alone may mean little, but in combination with other symptoms are important.

Changes in Bowel Patterns

Diarrhea, constipation, and flatulence constitute the major changes in bowel patterns. (See page 755.)

NURSING ASSESSMENT

Nursing assessment of a patient with a gastrointestinal problem aids in establishing a diagnosis, contributes to the medical plan of care, and provides a basis for a plan of patient care and nursing intervention. Such information is pertinent in determining the needs of the patient and evaluating his progress.

The following considerations and related questions provide the basis for patient assessment.

- *The Patient's Chief Complaint:* Is this different from anything he has experienced before? Is it related to a past history of such difficulty? Has there been previous surgery?
- *Appearance of the Patient:* Is there pallor, cyanosis, jaundice? Is the patient clutching his abdomen? Is there any effect on ambulation?
- *Nausea and Vomiting:* What precipitates nausea? Is it accompanied by vomiting? Is blood present? If so, how much, and what kind? What is the odor of the vomitus? How many times today has the patient vomited? What can be kept down? Does the vomitus include any food from previous meal?
- *Abdominal Pain:* Is it localized? Radiating? Quality of Pain: Is it constant? Crampy (colicky)? Duration and Intensity: Nature of onset? What aggravates it? What alleviates it?
- *Swallowing and Food Intake:* When and what has the patient eaten last? Is there any pain or difficulty swallowing? What kind of food or fluid causes difficulty? When does discomfort occur in relation to eating? Is there belching, dysphagia, flatulence, distention, a feeling of fullness, or any abnormal taste?
- *Nutrition:* Have the patient's food habits changed recently? What foods disagree with him? Is he on a special diet? Describe. Has his weight been stable? weight loss? amount? What kind of snacks does he eat? How often?
- *Elimination:* Has he had a change in bowel habits? Describe — constipation? diarrhea? What is the color of the stool? Odor? Consistency? How often does he have a bowel movement? At a regular time? Does he take laxatives? Why? What kind? Frequency? Does he take enemas? Why? What kind? Frequency? Has he noticed blood in his stool? Is there pain with bowel movements? Describe.

- *Quality of Vital Signs:* Is there any evidence of fever? of hemorrhage?
- *Examination of Abdomen:* Have patient identify area of pain. Is abdomen rigid? Tight? Tender to gentle pressure? Does the patient guard the area with voluntary muscle contractions? Is there rebound tenderness (when gentle pressure is suddenly released, pain is more intense). NOTE: Such examination should be limited to as few examiners as possible, since it may be very uncomfortable for the patient. Assess for frequency of peristaltic sounds. Use stethoscope. Is abdomen distended?
- *Associated Symptoms:* Has the patient been around anyone who had the same trouble recently? Is he urinating more than usual? Does he have any allergy to any medications?
- Patient's Own Reaction: Ascertain in the patient's own words his reaction to his problem.

DIAGNOSTIC ASSESSMENT

Roentgenography of the Upper Gastrointestinal Tract

The entire gastrointestinal tract can be delineated by x-rays, following the introduction of barium sulfate or a similar radiopaque liquid as the contrast medium. This material, a tasteless, odorless, nongranular, and completely insoluble (hence, not absorbable) powder, is ingested in the form of a thick or thin aqueous suspension for purposes of upper gastrointestinal tract study ("upper G.I. series") and is instilled rectally for visualization of the colon ("barium enema").

Patient Preparation. In preparation for a G.I. series, the patient is to receive nothing by mouth after midnight prior to the test. A laxative may be ordered to clean out the intestinal tract. Since smoking can stimulate gastric motility, the patient is discouraged from smoking the morning before the examination.

Procedure. For purposes of examining the upper gastrointestinal tract, the patient is required to swallow barium under direct fluoroscopic examination.

As the contrast medium descends into the stomach, the position, patency, and caliber of the esophagus are visualized, enabling the examiner to detect or exclude any anatomic or functional derangement of that organ. An important observation can also be made in relation to the heart, namely, observing the presence or the absence of right atrial enlargement. An enlarged right atrium invariably impinges on the esophagus and is revealed by the resulting pressure defect in the esophagus. The roentgenographic appearance of the lower esophagus after a swallow of thick barium suspension also allows for detection of esophageal varices, a manifestation of portal hypertension, as in cirrhosis of the liver.

Fluoroscopic examination extends next to the stomach, as its lumen fills with barium. The motility and the thickness of the gastric wall, and the mucosal pattern are observed for evidence of spasms, ulcerations, malignant infiltrates, and other anatomic abnormalities, including pressure defects from without. The patency of the pyloric valve and the anatomy of the duodenum are also observed, with particular reference to possible ulceration of the mucosa, spasm of the wall, or displacement of the structure as a whole by a tumor in the adjacent area.

During the fluoroscopic examination, roentgenograms are exposed in order to obtain a permanent record of the findings. Additional roentgenograms are taken at intervals, for as long as 24 hours thereafter, as a means of estimating the rate of gastric emptying and the degree of small bowel motility.

Double Contrast Studies. The double contrast method of examining the upper gastrointestinal tract involves administering a thick barium suspension medium to outline the stomach and esophageal wall. Next, tablets that release carbon dioxide in the presence of water are given. (To reduce these bubbles, simethicone is given.) The primary advantage of this technique is the finer detail that can be shown within the esophagus and stomach, permitting signs of early superficial neoplasms to be noted.

Continuous Infusion Method. A truly detailed study of the small intestine involves the continuous infusion, through a duodenal tube, of 500-1000 ml. of a thin barium sulfate suspension. This is carried out as a separate procedure. The barium column fills the intestinal loops and is observed continuously by fluoroscope and filmed at frequent intervals as it progresses through the jejunum and the ileum.

Roentgenography of the Colon (Barium Enema)

The purpose of a barium enema is to reveal the presence of polyps, tumors, and other lesions of the large intestine and to demonstrate any abnormal anatomy or malfunction of the bowel.

Patient Preparation. The preparation of the patient includes those measures necessary to produce an empty and clean lower bowel. Usually this includes taking nothing by mouth after midnight, cleansing enemas until returns are clear, and perhaps a laxative by mouth and/or a rectal suppository.

- If the patient has active inflammatory disease of the colon, only gentle enemas should be used.

Procedure. In the x-ray department, the radiopaque substance is instilled rectally; it is viewed in the fluoroscope and then filmed. If the patient has been prepared satisfactorily and the colonic contents have been evacuated completely by enemas, the contour of the entire colon, including cecum and appendix (if patent), is clearly visible, and the motility of each portion readily observed. The procedure takes about 15 minutes and is followed by an evacuating enema or laxative to facilitate barium removal.

Gastric Analysis

Examination of the gastric juice offers a means of estimating the secretory activity of the gastric mucosa and of ascertaining the presence, or the degree, of gastric retention in patients suspected of having pyloric or duodenal obstruction.

- A diagnosis of pernicious anemia is excluded by the finding of acid.
- A diagnosis of gastric carcinoma may be established by the discovery of cancer cells in the gastric juice.

The fasting patient is intubated through a nostril with a Levin duodenal tube, a small rubber tube with catheter tip marked at points 45, 55, 65, and 75 cm. from the distal end. (See page 724 for nursing management during intubation.)

When the second marker of the Levin tube is at the point of entering the nares, the tip of the tube, 55 cm. distant, should be within the stomach. Once in place, the tube is secured to the patient's cheek by means of a small strip of adhesive tape, and the patient is placed in a semireclining position. If he exhibits any tendency to gag, he is instructed to pant gently with his mouth wide open, the effect of which is to minimize contact between the tube and the soft palate. The entire stomach contents are aspirated by gentle suction into a syringe.

Pentagastrin, histamine, or betazole hydrochloride (Histalog) may be given to stimulate gastric secretions. Pentagastrin is preferred because of the lack of side effects. If histamine or Histalog is used, the patient is told that he may experience a flushed feeling after the injection of this medication. Also, blood pressure and pulse are frequently monitored to detect hypotension. Emergency medications such as epinephrine and diphenhydramine hydrochloride (Benadryl) are to be kept nearby if required. Specimens are labeled to indicate time before and after histamine injections.

The acidity of the specimen is determined by means of an indicator dye, such as Töpfer's reagent, by indicator paper, or by a pH meter. Other examinations, in special instances, may include cytologic study by the Papanicolaou technique for the presence or absence of carcinoma cells. Enzyme analysis of the gastric juice is sometimes indicated.

One of the most important items of information to be gained from gastric analysis relates to the ability of the mucosa to secrete hydrochloric acid.
- Patients with pernicious anemia secrete no acid under basal conditions or after stimulation.
- Patients with severe chronic atrophic gastritis secrete little or no acid. Some patients with gastric cancer secrete little or no acid.
- Patients with peptic ulcer invariably secrete some acid; patients with duodenal ulcers usually secrete an excess amount.

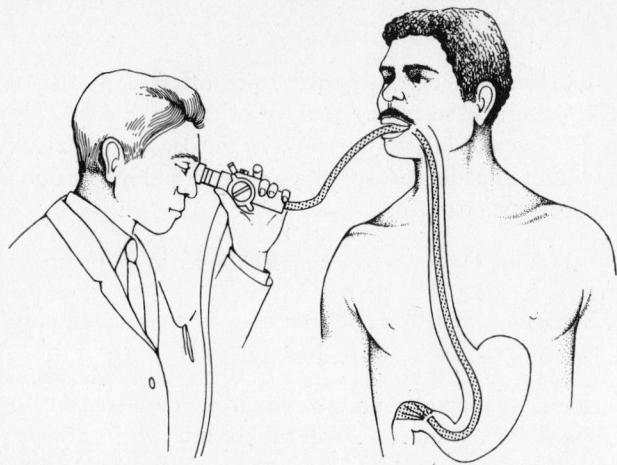

Figure 34-4. Patient undergoing gastroscopy. Note the extreme flexibility of the tube with the patient in the sitting position.

Upper Gastrointestinal Fiberoscopy

This procedure allows for direct visualization of the gastric mucosa through a lighted endoscope (gastroscope) and is especially valuable when gastric neoplasm is suspected (Fig. 34-4). Fiberscopes are flexible scopes equipped with fiberoptic lenses. Colored photographs or motion pictures can be taken through them. However, precautions must be taken to protect the scope, since the fiberoptic bundles may be broken if the scope is bent acutely. To prevent the patient from biting the scope, mouth guards are essential.

Patient Preparation. The patient is placed in a fasting state for 6 to 8 hours before the examination. One half hour before the procedure he is given meperidine hydrochloride (Demerol). Usually gargling with a local anesthetic, along with the administration of intravenous Valium just before the scope is introduced, will suffice. Sometimes atropine may be helpful in reducing secretions. Glucagon may be given to relax smooth muscle.

Procedure. The patient's lips, oral cavity, and pharynx are sprayed with tetracaine hydrochloride (Pontocaine) or a liquid gargle of ethyl aminobenzoate (Hurricane), after which the gastroscope is passed smoothly and slowly. The fiber gastroscope is almost completely flexible and gives the physician an opportunity to view a large part of the gastric wall. Experienced gastroscopists may recognize a cancer and remove a piece of tissue for microscopic examination. Ulcers may be identified and their healing in response to treatment documented.

Follow-up Care. Following a gastroscopy the patient is instructed not to eat or drink until the gag reflex returns in about 3 or 4 hours; this is done to prevent aspiration into the lungs. Postgastroscopy assessment by the nurse includes observation for signs of perforation, such as pain, unusual discomfort, and an elevated temperature. Minor throat discomfort can be relieved with lozenges, cool saline gargle, and oral analgesic medications.

Fiberoptic Colonoscopy

Direct visual inspection of the colon is possible by means of a flexible colonoscope. This procedure is used as a diagnostic aid and the instrument may be used to remove foreign bodies, polyps, or tissue for biopsy (Fig. 34-5).

Patient Preparation. The patient is informed about the procedure and requested to cooperate and relax during the examination. In addition, the intestinal tract is emptied by limiting the patient's intake to liquids and cleansing the tract with a laxative and a saline enema. Before the examination, Demerol may be administered. During the examination, Valium may be useful in relieving anxiety.

Stool Examination

The basic examination of the stool includes an inspection of the specimen for its amount, consistency, and color, and a screening test for occult blood. Special tests indicated in specific cases may include tests for fecal urobilinogen, fat, nitrogen, parasites, food residues, and other substances.

Stool Color. The color of stools varies from light to dark brown. (Milk-fed infants pass stools that are golden-yellow in color, due to unchanged bilirubin.) Various foods and medications affect stool color as follows: meat protein produces a dark brown coloration; spinach, a green hue; carrots and beets, red; cocoa, dark red or brown; senna and santonin, a yellowish hue; calomel, green; bismuth, iron, licorice, and charcoal, black; and barium, a milky white appearance.

- Blood in sufficient quantities, if shed into the upper gastrointestinal tract, produces a tarry black color (melena).
- Blood entering the lower portion of the gastrointestinal tract or passing rapidly through it will appear bright or dark red.
- Lower rectal or anal bleeding can be suspected if there is streaking of blood on the surface of the stool or if blood is noted on toilet tissue.

Even considerable quantities of hemoglobin may fail to produce a distinctive color, in which event it is termed "occult blood."

Tests for Occult Blood or to Confirm Melena. The most common stool tests are based on the benzidine, gum guaiac or the orthotolidin reaction. A form of the guaiac test is the Hemoccult test. A dry paper slide is used, on which the stool specimen is smeared. The slide comes in an envelope that can be mailed, if needed, and examined later.

Stool Consistency and Appearance. In various disorders the stool assumes a typical appearance:

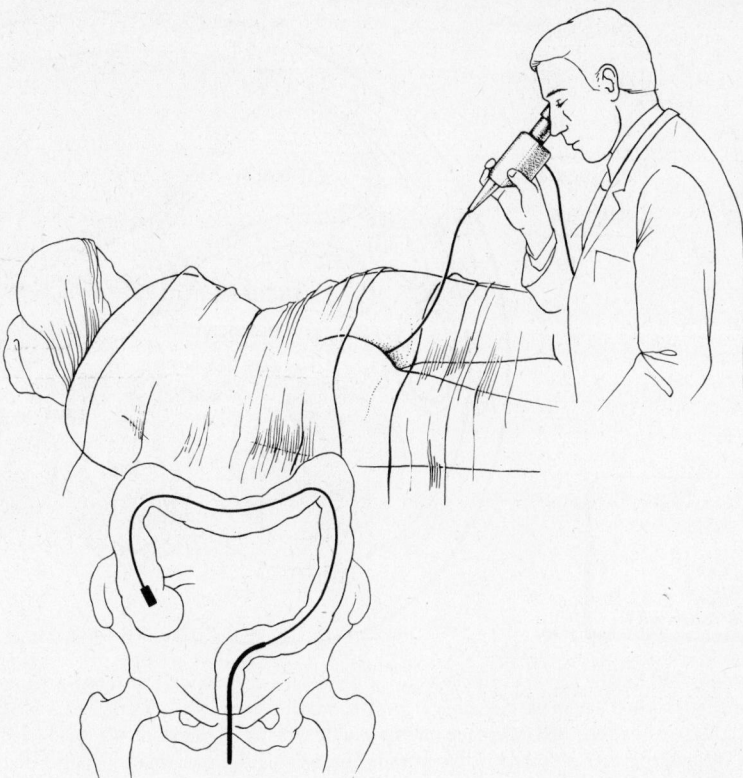

Figure 34-5. Technique of colonoscopy. The patient is turned from one side to the other to take advantage of gravity as the scope is being advanced. Insert shows path of flexible scope from rectum through sigmoid colon and descending, transverse, and ascending colon. If the physician desires to check scope position with fluoroscopy, a lead apron should be donned.

In *steatorrhea,* the stools are generally bulky, greasy, foamy, and foul in odor; stool color is gray, with a silvery sheen.

With *biliary obstruction,* the stool becomes "acholic" and is light gray or "clay colored," due to the absence of urobilin.

In *chronic ulcerative colitis,* mucus or pus may be visible on gross inspection of the stool.

Constipation, obstipation, or *fecal impaction* may result in the passage of small, dry, rocky-hard masses called *scybala.* This type of stool may traumatize the rectal mucosa sufficiently to cause hemorrhage, in which case the fecal masses are streaked with red blood.

Ultrasonography

Ultrasonography is a noninvasive diagnostic technique in which sound waves are passed into internal body structures; varying deflections of these sound waves are bounced back, much like a reflection. Reflections, in turn, are displayed on an oscilloscope. Vertical deflections from a horizontal baseline represent the depth of the reflected tissues. When scans are taken from several angles, and a computer is added to the system, a two-dimensional image of the abdominal organs can be pro-

duced. Usually, for abdominal examination, a transducer is placed on the abdomen after a coating of lubricant jelly has been applied to the skin.

The chief advantage of ultrasonography is the spatial reproduction of masses in transverse and longitudinal directions. There is no ionizing radiation or any noticeable biologic side effects, in the energy range used for diagnostic purposes. It is relatively inexpensive. This type of diagnostic procedure is useful in studying the liver, pancreas, spleen, gallbaldder, and retroperitoneal tissues.

Disadvantages include the following: (1) A high degree of skill is required of the operator. (2) This technique cannot be used when a structure to be examined lies behind bony tissue which prevents passage of sound waves to deeper structures. (3) Gas in the abdomen or air in the lungs present a problem, since ultrasound is not well transmitted through gas or air.

Computed Body Tomography (CBT Scanning)

CBT is a diagnostic method in which a very narrow beam of x-ray is used to detect the density differences from very small cubes of tissue. This data is computerized and then reconstructed so that transverse cross-

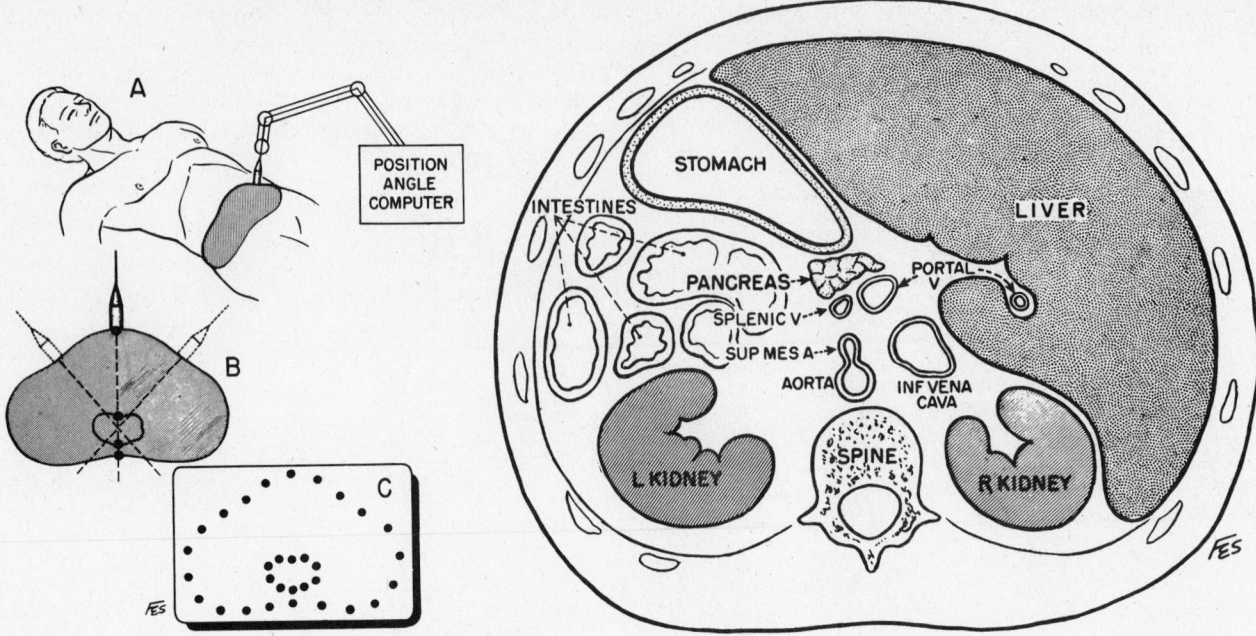

Figure 34-6.   Ultrasonic scanning. (*left*) Panel *A* shows the transducer mounted on a mechanical arm. The transducer is moved across the patient's body, and a position-angle computer (housed within the mechanical arm) records the spatial relationship and angle of the transducer. As the latter is moved across the body, reflected echoes are recorded from each interface within the plane perpendicular to the transducer (faded area in panel *B*). These echoes are stored on an oscilloscope and are shown schematically as a two-dimensional image of panel *C*. (*right*) A schematic diagram of a cross section through the abdomen 2 cm. below the xiphoid process. *SUP MES A* = superior mesenteric artery; *INF VENA CAVA* = inferior vena cava. (From Naggar, C. Z., and McDonald, D. G.: Ultrasound in medical diagnosis. Part II. Neurologic and abdominal applications. Heart & Lung, 6:829-837, 1977)

sections of the body can be shown on a television monitor.

The indications for CBT scanning are diseases of the liver, spleen, kidney, pancreas, and pelvic organs (Fig. 34-6). However, good detail depends upon the presence of fat, which means that this diagnostic tool is not useful for very thin, cachectic individuals. Also, since a scanning time of 5 seconds is required, it is impossible to maintain complete stillness (e.g., heartbeat) during the procedure. Therefore, motion artifacts are produced and the results are a less than clear picture. Finally, radiation doses are appreciable.

BIBLIOGRAPHY

BOOKS

Bates, B.: A Guide to Physical Examination, 2nd ed. Philadelphia, J. B. Lippincott, 1979.

Bockus, H. L., et al.: Gastroenterology. Philadelphia, W. B. Saunders, 1976.

Given, B. A., and Simmons, S. J.: Gastroenterology in Clinical Nursing, 3rd ed. St. Louis, C. V. Mosby, 1979.

Hill, R. B., and Kern, F., Jr.: The Gastrointestinal Tract. Baltimore, Williams and Wilkins, 1977.

Sleisenger, M. H., and Fordtran, J. S.: Gastrointestinal Disease (Pathophysiology, Diagnosis, Management). Philadelphia, W. B. Saunders, 1978.

Spiro, H. M.: Gastroenterology, 2nd ed. New York, Macmillan Co., 1977.

(See also Bibliography for Chapter 5, page 89.)

ARTICLES

Alfidi, R. J., and Haaga, J. R.: Computed tomography of the body. Postgrad. Med., 60:133-136, Aug. 1976.

Abramson, D. J.: Sigmoidoscopy in women: comparison with breast and gynecologic examinations in 1,000 patients. CA-A Cancer J. for Clinic., 28:202-210, July-Aug. 1978.

Castell, D. O., and Frank, B. B.: Abdominal examination, role of percussion and auscultation. Postgrad. Med., 62:131-132, Dec. 1977.

Long, G. D.: G.I. bleeding. Nursing '78, 8:44-50, Mar. 1978.

Marshall, C. H.: Principles of computed tomography. Postgrad. Med., 60:105-109, Aug. 1976.

Matsishe, J. W., and Phillips, S. F.: Chronic diarrhea. Med. Clin. N. Am., 62:141-154, Jan. 1978.

Morton, P. C.: Proctosigmoidoscopy in asymptomatic men: a 24-month study. CA-A Cancer J. for Clinic, *28*:211-217, July-Aug. 1978.

Ryan, A. J.: Validation of appendectomy, can it be done? Postgrad. Med., *65*:19-21, Jan. 1979.

Sackler, J. P., and Passalaqua, A. M.: Diagnostic uses of ultrasound. Postgrad. Med., *60*:95-101, Aug. 1976.

Sheridan, J. L.: Obstructions of the intestinal tract. Nurs. Clin. N. Am., *10*:147-155, Mar. 1975.

Silverstein, F. E., and Rubin, C. E.: The new *look* into the gastrointestinal tract. Disease-a-Month, Vol. *22,* Feb. 1976.

Stahlgren, L., and Morris, N. W.: Intestinal obstruction. AJN, 77:999-1002, June 1977.

Stroup, P.: Recognition and management of G.I. bleeds. J. Emerg. Nsg., *4*:19-25, Sept.-Oct. 1978.

Wichern, W. A.: The surgical abdomen. Postgrad. Med., *62*:145-148, Nov. 1977.

AGENCY

National Institute of Arthritis, Metabolism and Digestive Diseases, National Institutes of Health, Bethesda, Md. 20205

35

GASTROINTESTINAL INTUBATION AND SPECIAL NUTRITIONAL MANAGEMENT

GASTROINTESTINAL INTUBATION

Gastrointestinal intubation is the insertion of a short or long flexible rubber or plastic tube into the stomach or intestine via the mouth or nose. The purpose may be diagnostic, preventive, or therapeutic. Aspiration (suctioning) through this tube is achieved by various means: suction from a syringe, suction from an electric suction machine, or suction from a built-in wall suction outlet.

Short Tubes

A *nasogastric catheter,* or so-called short tube, is introduced through the nose or the mouth into the stomach. Two such short tubes are the Levin tube and the Salem sump tube.

Levin Tube. The Levin tube (14 F.), is a single-lumen tube made of plastic or rubber, with holes near its tip. The tube is used to remove fluid and gas from the upper gastrointestinal system or to obtain a specimen of gastric contents for laboratory studies. It may also be the means of administering medications or feeding (gavage) directly into the gastrointestinal tract (Fig. 35-1).

The Levin tube usually has circular marks on the tubing; when the tube has been inserted in the stomach, the section at the patient's nostril is located between the second and third marks. Gas, and the fluids that collect in the stomach, may be removed by aspiration through the tube.

Gastric Sump Tube (Salem, Ventrol) is a radiopaque, clear plastic, double-lumen nasogastric tube (Fig. 35-2). It is used to decompress the stomach and keep it empty. The inner, smaller tube vents the larger suction-drainage tube to the atmosphere by means of an opening at the distal end of the tube. It is passed the same way as the Levin tube. It can protect gastric suture lines because, when used properly, the sump pump never allows the force of suction at the drainage "eyes," or outlets, to exceed 25 mm. Hg, the level of capillary fragility. This action is controlled by a small vent tube (blue pigtail). Continuous suction is set at a low of 30 mm. Hg with the pigtail (usually blue) outlet kept open. If available suction is intermittent, rather than continuous, it may be set at 80-120 mm. Hg. Because of its cyclic setting, by the time suction reaches the gastric mucosa, it will be reduced to about 25 mm. Hg.

To prevent reflux of gastric contents through the vent lumen (blue pigtail), the vent lumen is kept above the patient's midline; otherwise it will act as a siphon. Irrigation may be done through either the main lumen or the vent lumen; if the vent lumen is used, irrigation is followed with 10 ml. of air, to clear the lumen.

Long Tubes

The *long tubes, or nasoenteric tubes,* are introduced through the nose, esophagus, and stomach into the intestinal tract. They are used to aspirate the intestinal con-

722

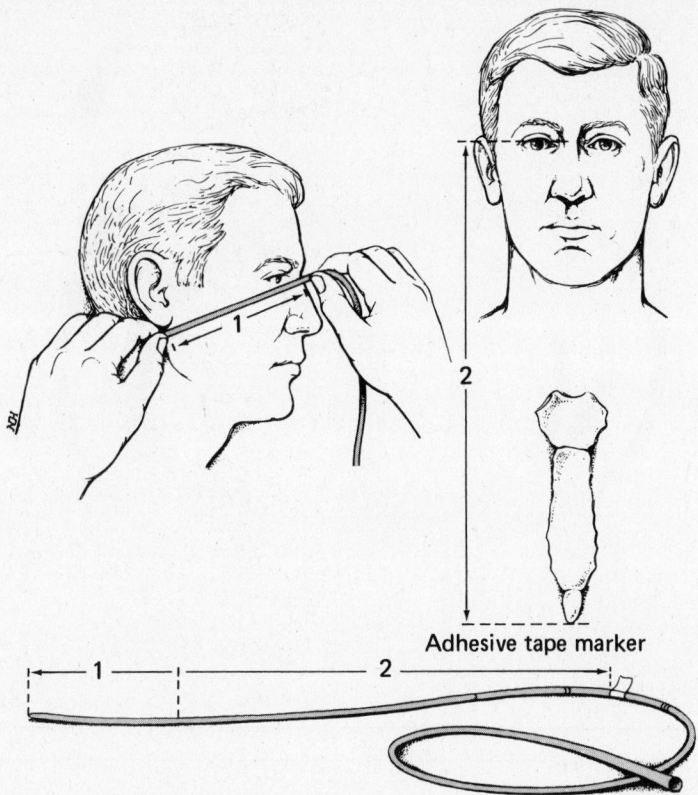

Adhesive tape marker

Figure 35-1. To measure the distance a Levin tube is to be passed in a patient to insure passage into the stomach: (1) Measure the distance on the tube from the patient's tragus (ear lobe) to bridge of nose, plus (2) the distance from the bridge of the nose to the bottom of the xiphoid process. Mark this distance with a piece of adhesive tape. Note that the Levin tube usually has circular marks on the tubing; when it is in the patient's stomach, it is between the second and third marks.

tents to prevent gas and fluid distention of the coils of intestine (decompression).

The long tubes are the Miller-Abbott, the Harris, and the Cantor tubes. These are used in the active treatment of intestinal obstruction of the small intestine. They also are used prophylactically, being inserted the night before an abdominal operation to prevent obstruction after the operation. The intestine is threaded on the tube and so shortened, and held together compactly, making it relatively easier to pack off the intestine at the time of operation on the colon.

Because peristalsis either decreases or stops for 24 to 48 hours after an operation, due to the effects of anesthesia and of visceral manipulation, nasogastric or nasoenteric suction prevents certain sequelae from developing. Fluids and flatus are evacuated, so that vomiting is prevented and tension reduced along the incision line. Edema, which can cause obstruction, is also reduced. Blood supply to the suture line is enhanced, thereby providing nutrition to the site. Usually, the tubes are allowed to remain in place after operation until peristalsis is resumed, as shown by the passage of gas by rectum.

Miller-Abbott Tube. This is a double-lumen, No. 16 F., 3 meter- (10-foot) tube, one lumen of which is used to introduce mercury or to inflate the balloon at the end of the tube; the other lumen, entirely independent, is used for aspiration. Before the tube is inserted, the balloon should be tested and its capacity measured; it is then deflated completely. The tube should be lubricated sparingly, and chilled well, before the tip is inserted through the patient's nose. Markings on the tube indicate the distance it has been passed.

Harris Tube. This is a single-lumen mercury-weighted tube of about 1.8 meters (6 feet), with a lumen of 14 F. This tube has a metal tip that is introduced first, into the nostril, after having been lubricated. The mercury-weighted bag follows. The weight of the mercury carries the bag by gravity. Since this is a single-lumen tube that is used wholly for suction and irrigation, there is no difficulty in irrigating it. Usually a Y tube is attached to the end of the tube, so that the suction apparatus is attached to one side, and an outlet with a clamp is available on the other side for irrigating purposes.

Cantor Tube. The Cantor tube is 3 meters (10 feet)

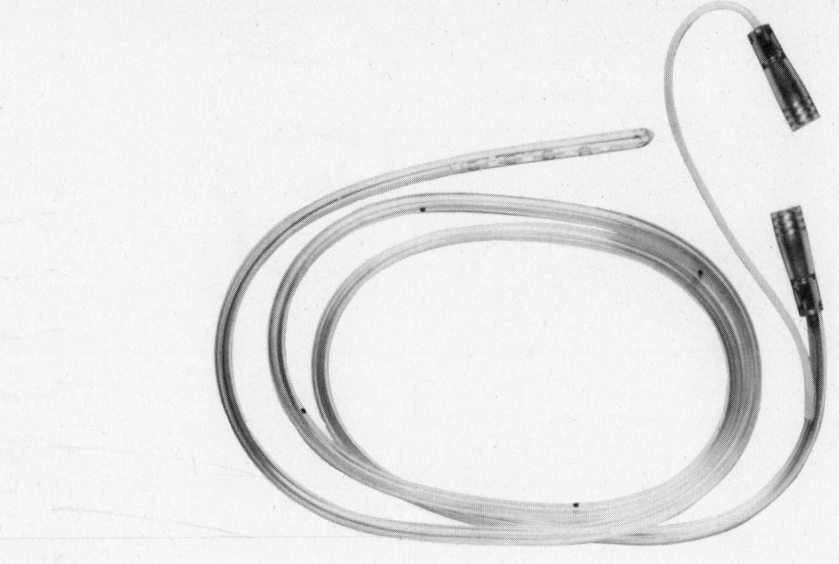

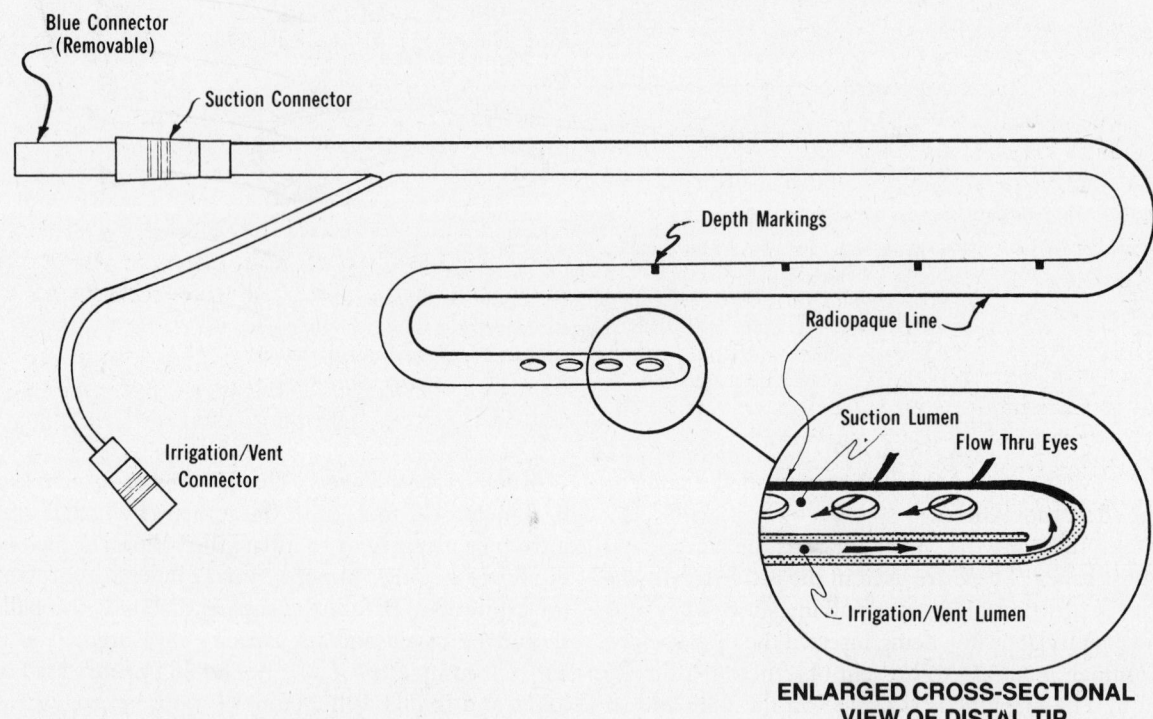

Figure 35-2.   The photograph and line drawing are of the VENTROL® Levin (Sump) tube. Note the blown-up version showing the direction of flow for suction and irrigation. (National Catheter Co., Argyle, New York)

long, and No. 18 F. Its distinguishing feature is that it is larger than the other long tubes, and has 4 or 5 ml. of mercury in the bag at the extreme end of the rubber tubing. Prior to insertion, the bag is wrapped about the tube. After the tube is lubricated, it is passed through the nostril and advanced to the esophagus (Fig. 35-3). The patient is in a sitting position, and is offered sips of water to facilitate passage of the tube. Fluoroscopy is helpful in passing the tube into the duodenum.

Ewald Tube.   This is a large-lumen gastric tube which can be passed through the mouth and into the stomach for the purpose of washing out poisons or aspirating large clots, or other substances, from the stomach.

Nursing Management

Insertion of Nasogastric or Nasoenteric Tube.   Before the patient is intubated, the nurse explains the treatment and its purpose. A cooperative patient adds much to the success of the procedure. He may be allowed to sit up, with a towel spread bib-fashion over his chest. Tissue wipes should be available. The patient is screened from other patients, and adequate light is provided. Occasionally the physician will swab the nostril and spray the oropharynx with tetracaine hydrochloride (Pontocaine) to dull the nasal passage and the gag reflex and make the procedure more tolerable. Gargling with a liquid anesthetic or holding ice chips in the mouth for a few minutes will have the same effect. Encouraging the patient to breathe through his mouth or pant often helps, as does swallowing water, if permitted.

A rubber nasogastric tube is sterilized and placed in a basin containing cracked ice for about 5 minutes before use, to make the tubing firm, rather than limp. (A plastic tube may need to be warmed to make it more pliable.)

After the end of the tube is lubricated with water-soluble jelly, the patient is instructed to hyperextend his neck while the tube is introduced through the nostril. When the tip is positioned in the stomach, the nasogastric tube is secured to the nose, forehead, or above the upper lip (Fig. 35-4). In the case of nasoenteric intubation, the tube is not taped immediately.

After the tube has passed through the pyloric sphincter, it may be advanced 5-7.5 cm. (2-3 inches) every hour, so that gravity and peristalsis will aid in the passage of the tube. If it is advanced too rapidly, it will curl and kink in the stomach. If the position of the tube must be verified, the diaphragm of a stethoscope may be placed over the xiphoid process, while 5-10 ml. of air are injected into the lumen of the tube, at which time a "whooshing" sound is heard. Another method is to aspirate the tube and check secretions with pH paper. If the pH is above 7 (alkaline), the tube is in the intestine; if below 7 (acid), the tube is still in the stomach. When the tube has been inserted the required distance, it is secured.

The nasogastric catheter is attached to the tube leading to the trap bottle, usually by a Y tube. The other end of the Y tube is attached to a small piece of rubber tubing closed by a clamp. Through this tube, irrigations of the nasogastric catheter may be done to insure its patency. Otherwise, fluid or gas may accumulate, which can result in discomfort, vomiting, or abdominal distention. Repositioning the patient is another way of facilitating drainage. When double-lumen tubes are used, it is wise to note which tube is for irrigation and which for suction. To avoid tension on the tube, the tube line from the nose to the trap bottle is fixed in position on the bed, either with a safety pin threaded through the bed sheet or with adhesive-tape loops, tied or pinned to the bed.

Mouth and Nostril Hygiene.
Regular and conscientious mouth and nostril hygiene is a vital part of patient care, since the tube may be in place for several days. Applicator sticks dipped in water can be used to clean the nose. This can be followed by cleansing with water-soluble oil. Frequent mouth attention is comforting. If the nasal and pharyngeal mucosa is excessively

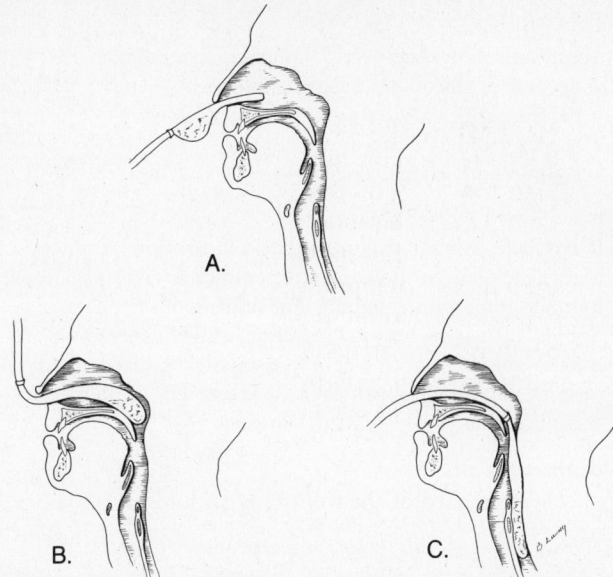

Figure 35-3. Passage of Cantor tube. (A) Tube with weighted mercury bag is introduced into the nostril. Note the natural tilt of the tubing. (B) After the mercury bag has entered the nostril, the catheter is tilted upward (head can also be tilted slightly upward) to facilitate gravity pull on the weighted bag. (C) The weight of the mercury pulls the bag downward. (Hardy: Rhoads Textbook of Surgery. Philadelphia, J. B. Lippincott, 1977)

dry, steam or cool vapor inhalations may be beneficial. Throat lozenges, an ice collar, chewing gum (if permitted), and frequent movement also assist in relieving discomfort.

Nursing Evaluation.
Patients undergoing suction decompression are susceptible to water and electrolyte imbalance such as fluid volume deficit.

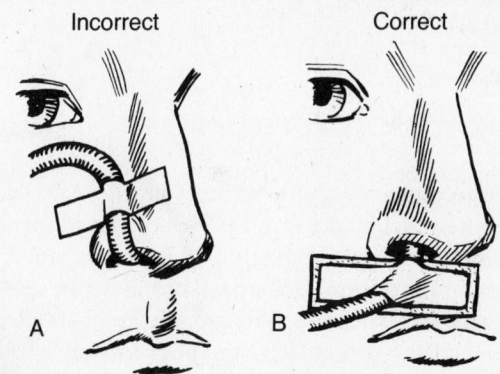

Figure 35-4. Nasogastric tube attachment. (A) Excessive pressure by the tube on the ala nasi should be avoided. (B) Satisfactory method for securing the tube which will prevent injury to the nasopharyngeal passages. Method of tube fixation: apply a thin coat of tincture of benzoin to the area under the nose and place a strip of nonallergenic tape on the prepared area. The nasogastric tube is fixed in position by anchoring it on top of the tape. By using this method, the nares may be cleaned frequently and the tube reanchored, without causing undue discomfort to the patient. (Adapted from Artz, C. P., and Hardy, J. P.: Complications in Surgery and their Management. Philadelphia, W. B. Saunders)

Fluid Volume Deficit

- Symptoms indicating a fluid volume deficit include:
  dryness of skin and mucous membranes
  decreasing urinary output
  lethargy and exhaustion
  drop in body temperature

Pulmonary Complications

- It has been shown that nasogastric intubation produces a higher incidence of postoperative pulmonary complications by interfering with coughing and clearing of the pharynx.
- Should such signs become manifest, it may be necessary to make a judgment as to whether nasogastric intubation does, or does not, take priority over the possibility of pulmonary complications.

Documentation

Accurate record of the following should be kept:

1. Drainage—amount, color, and type, every 8 hours.
2. Amount of fluid instilled by irrigation of the nasogastric catheter, and the amount of water taken by mouth.
3. Amount and character of vomitus, if any.
4. Duration of any period in which the suction apparatus did not appear to function.
5. Effects produced by the treatment.

Removal of Tube. When it is desirable to remove the tube, it is necessary to deflate the balloon and withdraw it, gently and slowly, for about 15-20 cm. (6-8 inches), at intervals of 10 minutes, until the tip reaches the esophagus, when the remainder is withdrawn rapidly from nostril. If the tube does not come out easily, force should not be used—notify the physician.

As it is withdrawn, the tube is concealed in a towel, because the sight of it may cause the patient to vomit. After its removal the patient will be grateful for good mouth care.

NASOGASTRIC TUBE FEEDINGS

Tube feedings are given to meet nutritional requirements when oral intake is not possible. Liquid formulas are designed to improve nutritional intake by either oral or tube administration. In the past, hospital tube feedings were based on various combinations of milk and cream. However, many patients showed poor tolerance of such feedings by displaying symptoms of diarrhea, flatulence, fullness, borborygmi, and even nausea and vomiting. This intolerance may be directly related to lactase deficiency. Such a deficiency has been demonstrated in 6 to 20 percent of white Americans and 60 percent of black Americans. The result has been modifications in formulas, and reliance on commercially prepared synthetic liquid diets. Such products vary greatly in cost and composition, completeness of nutritional content, presence of "residue," lactose, amino acids, and other nutrients.

Commercial formulas frequently present problems because the composition is "fixed." Some patients may not be able to tolerate certain ingredients, such as sodium, protein, or potassium. "Modular" diets can be prepared commercially, and the critical constituents sodium, potassium, or fat can be added by the dietitian. Attention should be given to including all essential minerals and vitamins. Total intake of calories and nutrients needs to be assessed when there is a reduction in total intake, or excessive dilution, of feedings.

Dehydration and azotemia (an excess of urea and other nitrogenous wastes in the blood) may occur from high protein mixtures or from those lacking fat. Additional fluid should be given, so that the desired urinary output is maintained and waste products are excreted. Fat, in the form of highly unsaturated vegetable oils, may be added.

Diarrhea may occur if feedings are administered cold or too rapidly, or if the formula is high in osmolality (due to excessive amounts of sugars, free amino acids, and electrolytes), or if there is bacterial contamination. A point to remember regarding contamination is that adding raw eggs to the mixture may carry a danger of introducing *Salmonella* contaminants.

Many patients are highly resistant to tube feedings, particularly those feedings administered via nasogastric intubation. Often a medium or fine bore Silastic tube is tolerated better than a plastic or rubber tube. The finer bore tube, however, requires a finely dispersed formula, to prevent the tube from clogging.

Gormican and Liddy suggest the following characteristics of an ideal tube feeding formula: (1) low cost; (2) bacteriologic safety; (3) relatively low osmolality; (4) caloric density equivalent to 1 calorie per milliliter; (5) adequate but not excessive nutrient intake, with nutrients present in nontoxic ratios and amounts; (6) balanced nutrient composition, including electrolyte composition, proper balance of amino acids, and well-utilized supplementary sources of nutrients; (7) nutritional adequacy for short-term use, or, when indicated, for long-term feeding; (8) convenience and ease of administration; and (9) suitable viscosity and homogenization.

Preliminary assessment of an individual patient should answer the following questions:

1. What is his nutritional status?
2. Is his fluid and electroyte balance in order?
3. Is his digestive tract functioning? Does it have good absorptive capacity?
4. Are his kidneys and urinary system adequate?
5. What medications is he on, and what other therapy is he receiving which may affect his digestive intake and digestive system?
6. Does the dietary prescription fulfill his needs?

Nutritionists must work closely with physicians and nurses in determining the best formula for the individual patient. Factors to consider are the route of administration, flow rate, and composition (osmolality, type and amounts of carbohydrates, amino acids, fats). Some formulas may be given by the slow-drip method, with no adverse effects, whereas more rapid rates may be disastrous. Some feedings are given as supplements, and others are provided to meet the patient's total nutritional needs.

Nursing Evaluation

Continuous monitoring of the tube-feeding regimen is necessary to determine its effectiveness.

- Assess placement of tubing, position of patient, and flow rate.
- Observe patient's ability to tolerate the formula (assess for feeling of fullness, bloating, urticaria, nausea, vomiting, diarrhea, constipation).
- Check clinical responses, as noted in laboratory findings: blood urea nitrogen, hemoglobin, serum protein, and hematocrit.
- In assessing the patient's general condition, note condition of skin (turgor, dryness, color) and mucous membranes; urinary output; state of hydration.
- Determine psychosocial adjustment to nasogastric feedings: Is the patient comfortable, tolerant, annoyed, relaxed or tense, troubled—and so forth?

GASTROSTOMY

This operation is performed to create an opening into the stomach for the purpose of administering food and fluids. In some instances, it may be used for prolonged nutrition, as in the elderly or debilitated patient. Gastrostomy is preferred to nasogastric feedings in the comatose patient because the cardioesophageal sphincter remains intact. Also, regurgitation may occur in nasogastric feedings, but is less likely in gastrostomy.

When an impermeable stricture of the esophagus exists, the gastrostomy opening may be permanent. The esophageal stricture may be due to scar-tissue contracture. In children, it occurs often as a result of lye burns, and in older people it is usually due to a carcinomatous growth.

Preoperative Preparation

The purpose of the operative procedure should be explained to the patient so that he will have a better understanding of his postoperative course. He needs to know that liquid feedings will be administered directly into the stomach, by means of a rubber or plastic tube (Fig. 35-5). Psychologically, this is often difficult for the

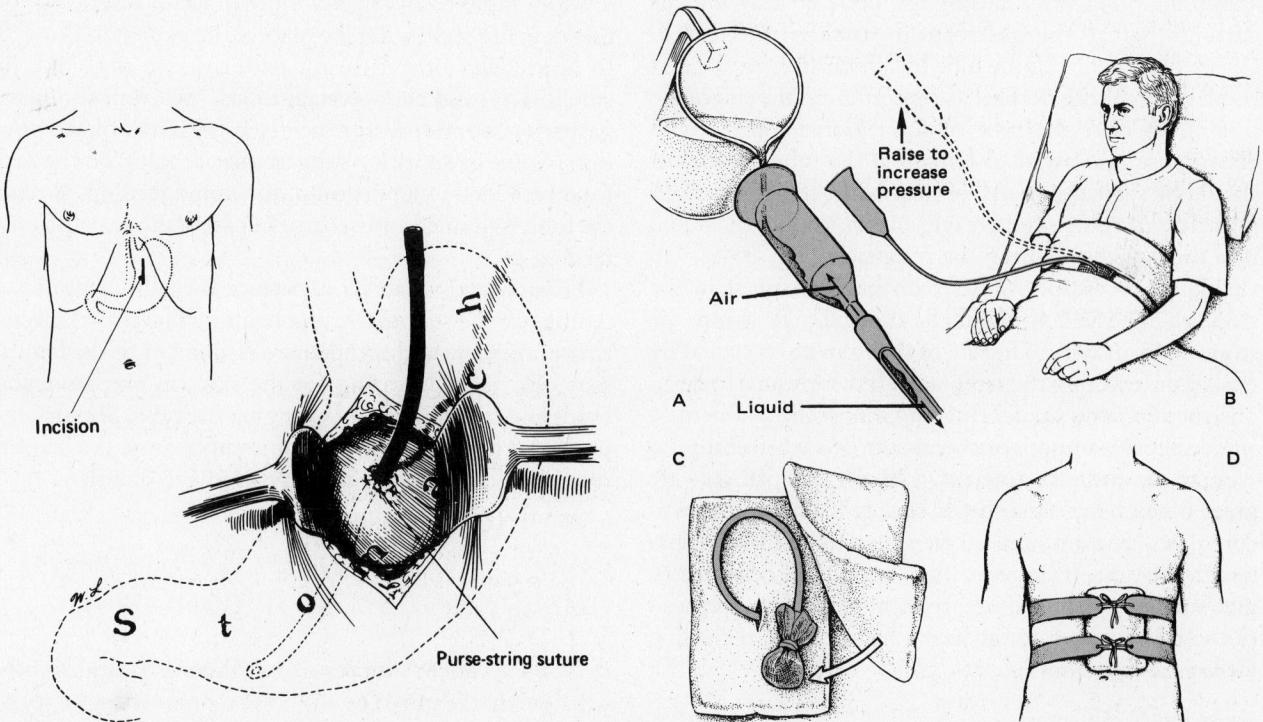

Figure 35-5. The patient with a gastrostomy. (*left*) The drawing at the top shows the site of incision. A tube is inserted into the anterior gastric wall and held in place with several purse-string sutures, as shown below. (*right*) Gastrostomy feeding. (A) indicates the proper method of tilting the receptacle to permit air to escape. (B) shows that raising the receptacle increases the pressure. (C) After the feeding, opening of tube is covered with sterile gauze square held by rubber bands, and tubing is coiled on dressing. (D) Tubing is covered with dressing or abdominal pad held with Montgomery straps.

patient to accept; however, when the procedure is being done to relieve discomfort, prolonged vomiting, and inability to eat, it is more acceptable.

Postoperative Nursing Management

The first fluid nourishment is given by the surgeon soon after surgery. This is usually tap water and 10 percent glucose. At first only 30-60 ml. (1-2 oz.) are given at a time, but the amount is gradually increased. By the second day, from 180-240 ml. (6-8 oz.) may be given at one time, provided it is tolerated. In some clinics, in the early postoperative period the nurse aspirates gastric secretions and reinstills them, after adding enough feeding to bring the volume to the desired total. By this method, gastric dilatation is avoided.

Blended foods are gradually added to clear liquids until a full diet is reached. Powdered feedings that are easily liquefied are commercially available. However, a food blender can be used to liquefy a normal diet, which can then be fed through the tube. Blenderized tube feedings allow the patient to follow his usual diet pattern, which proves to be psychologically more acceptable. In addition, good bowel function is promoted, since the fiber and residue are similar to that of a normal diet. Excessive intake of milk is to be avoided in patients with lactase deficiency.

In preparing the patient for his gastrostomy feeding, assure his privacy by closing the door or drawing the curtains before the gastrostomy tube is uncovered. Check the patency of the tube by administering water at room temperature. Repeat the procedure at the end of the feeding to clear the tube of food particles that could decompose if allowed to remain in the tube. The meal should be served at room, or near body, temperature. A funnel or barrel of a syringe is used to introduce the liquid into the catheter. Tilting the receptacle (Fig. 35-5) will enable air to escape, rather than being trapped in the stomach. The feeding should be allowed to flow into the stomach by gravity. The rate of flow can be regulated by raising or lowering the receptacle. If there seems to be an obstruction, stop the feeding and report the problem.

Record the amount and contents of each feeding, as well as the patient's reaction. Usually 300-500 ml. are given for each meal and should require 10 or 15 minutes to complete. The amount is often determined by the patient's reaction. If he feels "full" it may be desirable to give smaller amounts more frequently. Keeping the head of the bed elevated for at least a half-hour after feeding facilitates digestion.

Tube and Skin Care

After 5 or 6 days, the tube may be removed, if loose, and a fresh one inserted after being lubricated with a thin coating of petrolatum. The tube is held in place by a thin strip of adhesive that is first twisted about the tube and then firmly attached to the abdomen. A catheter plug or rubber-tipped hemostat may close the outlet of the tube immediately following a feeding, to prevent leakage. This can also be facilitated by having the patient relax for a short time after his feeding. A small dressing is applied over the tube outlet; the tube is coiled on a dressing and is held in place by Montgomery straps or a firm abdominal binder. Thereafter the tube should be changed every 2 or 3 days and the patient taught how to do this for himself. Once the opening into the stomach has been established, there is no need for sterile technique in changing and introducing a gastrostomy tube. However, items are to be thoroughly clean. The patient can learn how to feed himself and what foods may be taken.

The skin about a gastrostomy opening requires special care. It may become irritated, due to the enzymatic action of gastric juices that leak around the tube. If uncared for, the skin becomes macerated, red, raw, and painful. Daily washing with soap and water around the tube, and the application of a bland ointment such as zinc oxide or petrolatum, are protective measures.

After several weeks, the tube may be removed and reinserted 10-15 cm. (4-6 inches) for feedings. Between times, the gastrostomy opening may be protected by a small gauze pad, held in place by adhesive.

Psychosocial Considerations

More rapid recovery and more graceful acceptance of this new life style will take place if the patient is allowed to approach normal eating patterns. He may like to smell, taste, and chew certain foods. This will stimulate gastric secretion and more nearly approach normal digestion. Some authorities suggest that a bolus of chewed food be added to a portion of the liquid feeding, so that the food is thinned and becomes a part of the gastrostomy feeding.

Privacy, and whatever assistance is required from the family, can be supportive and helpful. The patient needs encouragement and acceptance. A member of the family may also assist in caring for the skin, in preparing the food, and in cleaning and changing the tube. Should any problems need solving, the community nurse is a helpful resource person, as are the physician and dietitian.

PARENTERAL HYPERALIMENTATION THERAPY (TOTAL PARENTERAL NUTRITION—TPN)

When a patient's intake of nutriments is significantly less than that required by the body to meet energy expenditures, a state of *negative nitrogen balance* results. This means that protein utilization is greater than protein intake. Many hospitalized patients (postsurgical, cancer, burns, renal failure) exhibit nutritional deficits, particularly protein depletion; this can delay wound healing and increase the likelihood of infection, shock, and other pathophysiologic conditions. A successful way of correcting nutritional problems and nitrogen imbalance in carefully selected patients is parenteral hyperalimentation.

Parenteral hyperalimentation is a method of supplying nutrients to the body by the intravenous route, when it is unwise or impossible to supply these needs by way of the normal digestive tract. Heretofore, intravenous feeding has not provided sufficient calories or nitrogen to meet the daily requirements of the patient. Therefore, the body begins to convert protein to carbohydrate by the process of *gluconeogenesis.*

The average adult postoperative patient requires approximately 1,500 calories a day to spare body protein. If this patient has complications, such as fever, trauma, or hypermetabolic disease, he will require up to 10,000 additional calories daily. The amount of volume necessary to provide these calories would surpass fluid tolerance and lead to pulmonary edema or congestive heart failure. To provide the required calories in small volume, it is necessary to increase the concentration and use an avenue of administration which will rapidly dilute incoming nutrients to the proper levels of body tolerance.

When hypertonic glucose is administered, it satisfies caloric requirements and allows amino acids to be released for protein synthesis, rather than being utilized for energy. Additional potassium is added, to provide proper electrolyte balance and to transport glucose and amino acids across the cell membranes. In order to prevent deficiencies and fulfill requrements for tissue synthesis, other elements, such as calcium, phosphorus, magnesium, and sodium chloride, are added.

The pharmacy department may prepare the prescribed nutritional intravenous solutions. These are mixed, utilizing strict aseptic precautions, under a filtered air laminar flow hood. Basically the solution consists of 25 percent glucose and synthetic amino acids (FreAmine); this provides the patient with 1,000 calories and 6 gm. of nitrogen per liter. Electrolytes are added as determined by the serum electrolyte needs of the individual patient. Solutions delivered to the unit are refrigerated until needed and then allowed to warm to room temperature. Formulas for local hospital use can be made for individual patients. Commercial preparations (Amigen, Aminosol, FreAmine, Hyprotigen C, and others) are available but also must be modified to meet individual needs.

Clinical Applications

Parenteral nutrition is indicated when oral or nasogastric intubation is either ineffective, impossible, or hazardous. When oral feedings are contraindicated, as in central nervous system dysfunction, such as may be caused by cerebral vascular accident or neurosurgery, or when the patient refuses to eat, as in anorexia nervosa,

hyperalimentation is recommen... must be met before a patient recei... nutrition (example: a 10 percent deficit i... an inability to take oral food or fluids within ... tive days, and hypercatabolic situations, such a... infection with fever).

Parenteral hyperalimentation is desirable in patient... experiencing nitrogen loss (gastrointestinal); it provides an intake of protein nitrogen that exceeds the nitrogen lost in metabolism and excretion. It is recommended also for patients with gastrointestinal fistula. Hyperalimentation allows the intestinal tract to rest and helps reduce secretions of the gallbladder, pancreas, and small intestine. The rest factor, plus improved nutritional balance, promotes closure of the fistula without surgery. Should surgery still be required, the patient is in far better physiological condition.

Intravenous nutritional support may also be used following major intestinal resection and in the instance of inflammatory bowel disease, such as regional enteritis and ulcerative colitis. Some surgeons prescribe hyperalimentation following abdominal and retroperitoneal surgery.

Patients who are receiving radiation or chemotherapy for metastatic cancer may suffer such side effects as anorexia and weight loss and may therefore benefit from hyperalimentation. Patients who have suffered a major burn would also benefit from parenteral nutritional feeding, since wound healing and the formation of granulation tissue are hastened with adequate nutrition. In addition, grafts appear to take better. This patient, of course, requires the ultimate in nursing care, so that sepsis and metabolic imbalance are under control.

Method of Administration and Nursing Management

Because hyperalimentary solutions have about five or six times the solute concentration of blood (and exert an osmotic pressure of about 2,000 mOsm. per liter) they are injurious to the intima of peripheral veins. Therefore, to prevent phlebitis and other venous complications, these solutions are administered into the circulatory system by means of a large-bore needle or catheter inserted into a high-flow large blood vessel. Concentrated solutions are then diluted in this vessel, very rapidly, to isotonic levels.

The preferred route is the subclavian vein, which leads into the superior vena cava. An alternate route is the internal jugular to the superior vena cava. With longterm use, an indwelling catheter is a constant source of potential infection.

Nursing objectives are: (1) to maintain the integrity of the system; (2) avoid contamination, and maintain sterility and patency of the indwelling catheter; (3) administer the prescribed infusion at a constant rate over the 24-

balance; (5) carefully ... tiate preventive mea- ... eutic nurse-patient

... ocedure is explained to ... the importance of not ... theter is inserted and is ... ambulatory during the ... he procedure, the patient ... burg position (to produce ... der vessels, which makes ... embolus). A rolled sheet is plac... ...vertebral column, from the neck to the end o... ...age, in order to hyperextend the shoulders. The area is shaved, if necessary, and the skin prepared with acetone or ether to remove surface oils. Final skin preparation includes scrubbing with tincture of iodine or povidone-iodine solution. The patient is instructed to turn his head facing to the side opposite from the site of venipuncture; he is to remain motionless while the catheter is inserted and the wound dressed, so as to afford maximum accuracy in the placement of the tube.

Insertion of the Catheter. Sterile drapes are applied. Procaine or lidocaine is injected for local anesthesia into the skin and underlying tissues. The target area is the inferior border at midpoint of the clavicle (Fig. 35-6). A No. 14, 5-cm. (2-inch) needle on a syringe is inserted and moved parallel to and beneath the clavicle until it enters the subclavian vein. The syringe is then detached and a 20-cm. (8-inch), 16-gauge radiopaque catheter is inserted through the needle into the vein; the needle is withdrawn. Until the syringe is detached from the needle and the catheter inserted, the patient may be asked to perform the Valsalva maneuver. (To do this, he is instructed to bear down with his mouth closed. Compression of the abdomen may also accomplish the maneuver.) The Valsalva maneuver is done to produce a positive phase in the central venous pressure in order to lessen the possibility of air being drawn into the circulatory system.

The intracath is attached to tubing from a 250-ml. flask of 5 percent dextrose in water. The catheter is usually sutured to the skin. The position of the tip of the catheter may be checked at this point by x-ray to confirm its location before the hyperalimentation solution is administered. Following this, the area is again swabbed with germicide solution, and antibiotic ointment is applied directly to the insertion site. A spray of tincture of benzoin to a liberal area precedes the application of a 5-cm. (2-inch) adhesive strip to provide an occlusive dressing.

Continuing Fluid Flow and Nursing Care. The insertion site is to be kept dry under an air-occlusive dressing. Dressings or adhesive are not to be removed for 48 hours. The patient is encouraged to move from side to side or to ambulate as desired. However, he must be reminded not to touch the dressings. If they bother him or cause itching, he is to report this.

The infusion rate is calculated on the basis of amount of fluids ordered over a 24-hour period. This rate must be maintained *consistently*: (example: 3,000 ml. for 24 hours = 125 ml. per hour). The rate is checked every 30 minutes. Intravenous alarm controllers may be used. If the rate increases or decreases, the infusion rate may be speeded up or slowed down by not more than 10 percent of the original rate (unless otherwise ordered by physician) in order to compensate.

- If the rate is too rapid, hyperosmolar diuresis occurs (excess sugar will be excreted), and if severe enough may cause intractable seizures, coma, and death. (Fractional urine determinations, using Clinitest tablets or test tapes, may be done every 6 hours, to monitor excess secretion of sugar.)
- If the flow goes too slowly, the patient does not get the maximum benefit of calories and nitrogen.

The patient is weighed daily at the same time, under the same conditions, for accurate comparison. Under this regimen, 0.11-0.45 kg. (¼-1 lb.) per day weight gain of lean body tissue can be expected. Accurate input and output records are kept, and if the patient also receives oral nutrients, this is recorded according to caloric count.

Vital signs are checked every 4 hours and temperature elevations are reported. Special care is given to draining wounds, fistulas, and pressure areas. Ambulation and activity, both physical and psychological, are encouraged and occupational or diversional therapy suggested, since hyperalimentation could be a restricting therapy—but ought not to be.

Procedure for Dressing Change

Inform the patient that his dressings are to be changed every other day and have him lie in a low Fowler's position. The nurse and patient may reduce the possibility of airborne contamination by wearing masks. Remove old dressings very carefully, to prevent the catheter from becoming dislodged. Check the area for leakage, kinked catheter, and skin reactions, such as inflammation, pain, or purulence. Using sterile gloves, cleanse area with acetone, followed by tincture of iodine or thimerosal (Merthiolate), with the aid of a sponge holder and 3 × 3 gauze pledgets. Clean from the center, moving outward. Alcohol may be used in the same manner, to remove iodine. Apply antibiotic ointment to insertion site and cover with a small dressing, slit to fit around catheter. Remove gloves and apply tincture of benzoin to skin area around sterile dressing to protect skin and to facilitate application of an adhesive tape (elastoplast) occlusive dressing. Rapidly replace intravenous tubing, including piggyback lines, to prevent buildup of organisms along the lumen of the inner tubing. Replace filter, if required.

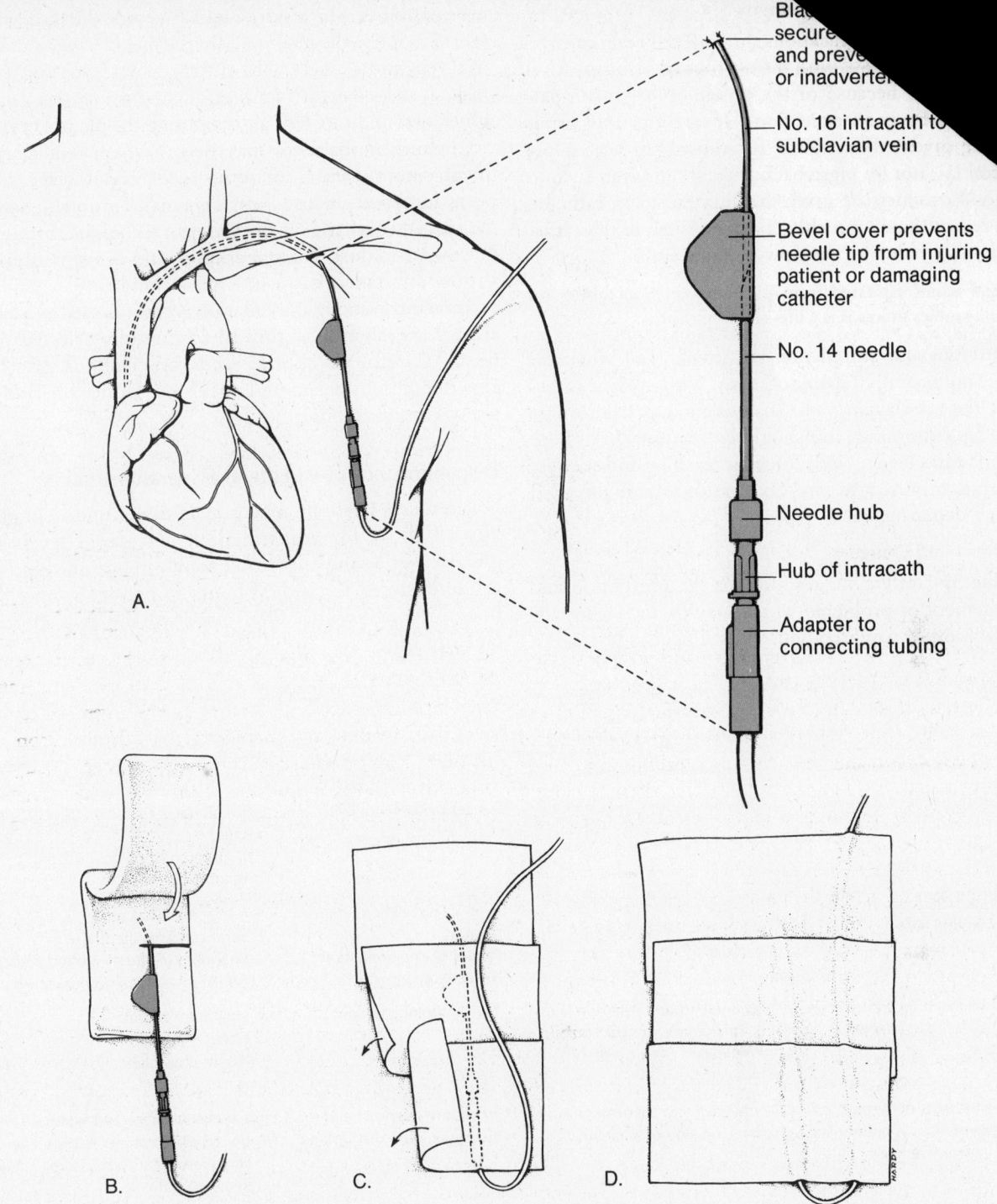

Bla...
secure...
and preve...
or inadverte...

No. 16 intracath to...
subclavian vein

Bevel cover prevents
needle tip from injuring
patient or damaging
catheter

No. 14 needle

Needle hub

Hub of intracath

Adapter to
connecting tubing

A.

B.

C.

D.

Figure 35-6.   Hyperalimentation. (A) Note insertion of needle into subclavian vein. (B) A split sterile dressing accommodates intracath. Covering this split dressing is another sterile dressing. (C) Adhesive dressings complete the occlusive dressing. (D) Completed dressing.

Cover union of catheter and tubing to prevent separation and to avoid exposure to air. Secure with adhesive tape.

If the patient has a draining wound, such as a tracheostomy, in the nearby area, additional precautions are taken to keep the wound dry by applying transparent plastic operating-room adhesive drape over the dressings, to insure waterproofing. Use allergenic adhesive tape if the patient complains of itching from conventional tape. Record the dressing change and report condition of local area as well as patient reaction.

h the main catheter
ional solution is not
ibility of incompat-
incompatible drugs
fused through a pe-
or should transfusions
ugh the main catheter,
the lumen of the cathe-
f solution.

peralimentation tubing for
aving measure.

Activities a̲n̲... are encouraged when the patient is physically capabl̲e̲ of them. With a plastic catheter in the subclavian vein, the patient has freedom to move his extremities and should be encouraged to keep up good muscle tone. Reinforce the teaching and exercise program initiated in the occupational and physical therapy departments.

Problems and Dangers

Table 35-1 offers suggestions for the prevention and management of problems which may occur during administration of parenteral nutrients. Pneumothorax is a rare possibility which can occur at the time the catheter is inserted, due to the proximity of the pleura to the subclavian vein and clavicle. The patient is observed for dyspnea, decreased breath sounds, or chest pain or back pain which may indicate that air is entering the pleural cavity.

Chemical imbalances may occur, which require frequent determinations of serum electrolytes (especially potassium) and glucose. Sepsis is a major problem; hence the special emphasis on strict aseptic technique throughout the procedure. Incompatibility and deterioration of various substances must be kept in mind.

Total intravenous alimentation is complicated and hazardous and should be limited to carefully selected patients. Careful monitoring and conscientious care by experienced physicians and nurses can reduce the risk of many complications.

Discontinuance of Parenteral Hyperalimentation

Parenteral hyperalimentation is discontinued gradually to allow for adjustment to decreased levels of glucose. Following hypertonic solution, isotonic glucose is administered for several hours to protect against rebound hypoglycemia. Oral carbohydrates will shorten tapering time.

TABLE 35-1 PREVENTION AND MANAGEMENT OF PROBLEMS IN PARENTERAL HYPERALIMENTATION

PREVENTIVE MEASURES	PROBLEM SITUATION	IMPLICATION	NURSING ACTION
Insure occlusiveness of dressing. Assess status of dressing frequently.	*Dressing loosens* or comes off.	Danger of contamination → infection.	Reinforce with 5-cm. (2-inch) tape. If question of contamination, reapply dressing.
Inspect each flask before using; note expiration date.	*Possible contamination* of solution; cloudy, floating particles.	Solution is excellent culture medium. Danger of contamination → infection, emboli.	Replace flask at once. Send contaminated flask to pharmacy. Cultures are required. Adjust intake and output records.
Frequently examine tissues near insertion site; note patient complaints.	*Swelling* around insertion site; edema of face or neck; pain in shoulder or arm on side of intracath.	Fluid infiltrating tissues.	Slow infusion rate. Check vital signs. Notify physician.
Observe for signs of dyspnea, respiratory difficulty, pulmonary edema, congestive heart failure.	*Engorged veins* of neck, arm, hand, on side of intracath.	Circulatory overload and inadequate fluid distribution.	Check vital signs and report all signs and symptoms to physician. Have resuscitative measures ready. Reassure patient.
Monitor the flow rate frequently (every half-hour), so that it is constant.	*Fluid running too rapidly:* nausea, headache, lassitude.	Hyperglycemia with glucosuria → cellular osmotic diuresis and extensive dehydration.	Check vital signs. Notify physician. Slow infusion to newly calculated flow rate.
Make fractional urine determinations every 6 hours. Observe for signs of hyperglycemia: nausea, headache, lassitude.	Test tapes show glucosuria. Patient symptoms: agitation, twitching, convulsions, mental lethargy, semicoma, coma → death.	Hypertonic overload → dehydration.	Administer insulin, if prescribed (very small doses). Administer IV fluid (isotonic) relatively rapidly.

PREVENTIVE MEASURES	PROBLEM SITUATION	IMPLICATION	NURSING ACTION
Check tubing for kinks. Monitor the flow rate frequently (every half-hour). Observe for signs of hypoglycemia: general muscular weakness, restlessness, perspiration, vertigo, pallor, trembling, hunger pangs in epigastrium.	*Fluid running too slowly.*	Hypoglycemia; patient not receiving adequate nutrition.	Recalculate flow rate so that adjustment compensates for slowdown (not to exceed 10% without physician's direction). Avoid too rapid flow rate. Assess patient for symptoms of hypoglycemia.
Monitor flow rate regularly. Assess patient status frequently.	*Infusion runs dry.*	Deficient nutrition. Possibility of air embolus during flask replacement. Backflow of blood into catheter, with possible clot formation and occlusion.	Replace with next bottle. Remove air from tubing aseptically or change administration tubing completely.
Change catheter dressing with patient in low Fowler's to recumbent position. Change administration tubing rapidly and secure snugly, while patient performs Valsalva maneuver.	*Air embolus.*	Segment of vascular system may be blocked, causing circulation cutoff. Signs and symptoms: cyanosis, hypotension, rapid, weak pulse, elevated venous pressure, change in heart sounds → coma.	Be alert for chest pain or fainting. Listen for air being sucked into catheter during change of tubing. Replace tubing immediately. Place patient on left side in Trendelenburg position. Keep him quiet and reassure him. Take vital signs; notify physician.
Monitor vital signs every 4 hours. Maintain strict aseptic practice at all times.	*Chills and/or fever.*	Allergic reaction. Sepsis: wound infection, caused by catheter, tubing, or solution. Infection from patient's disease.	Notify physician; be prepared to replace nutrient solution with 5% glucose in water. Check temperature every half-hour until normal. Be prepared for possible discontinuance of hyperalimentation.
Record daily intake and output, as well as weight.	*No weight gain* and possibly a weight loss.	There must be a reason for this negative outcome; cancer?	Check daily weighing procedure for consistency in conditions.
Change position frequently. Observe for signs of redness over bony areas. Provide good skin care.	*Pressure sores.*	Lying in one position too long.	Institute appropriate nursing measures to treat reddened area.
Promote active and passive exercises to improve muscle strength.	*Loss of muscle strength.*	Lack of exercise.	Encourage range of motion exercises at least 3 times daily.
Encourage patient to verbalize feelings.	*Discouraged patient.*	Inadequate understanding; lack of support.	Provide psychosocial support and encouragement. Explain all aspects of therapy.
Be alert for signs of scaly skin, poor wound healing, increased capillary fragility, alopecia.	*Serum essential fatty acid deficiency.*	Fatty acids are not available to transport metabolites.	After recognizing the deficiency, alert the physician to need. If patient is able to absorb minimal amounts of food, safflower oil may be given daily. Folic acid and vitamin B_{12} may be required intramuscularly.
Assess patient's electrolyte levels.	*Deficiency or excess of nutritional essentials:* calcium, phosphate, sodium, potassium, magnesium, iron, copper, folic acid, vitamin A, vitamin D.	Nutritional imbalance.	Alert physician to initiate corrective measures.

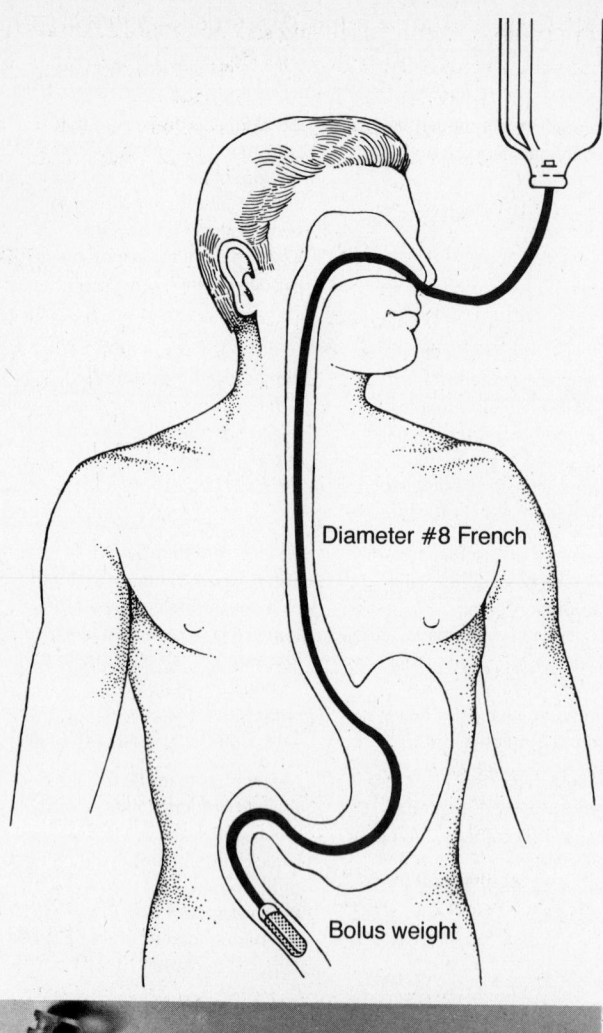

Diameter #8 French

Bolus weight

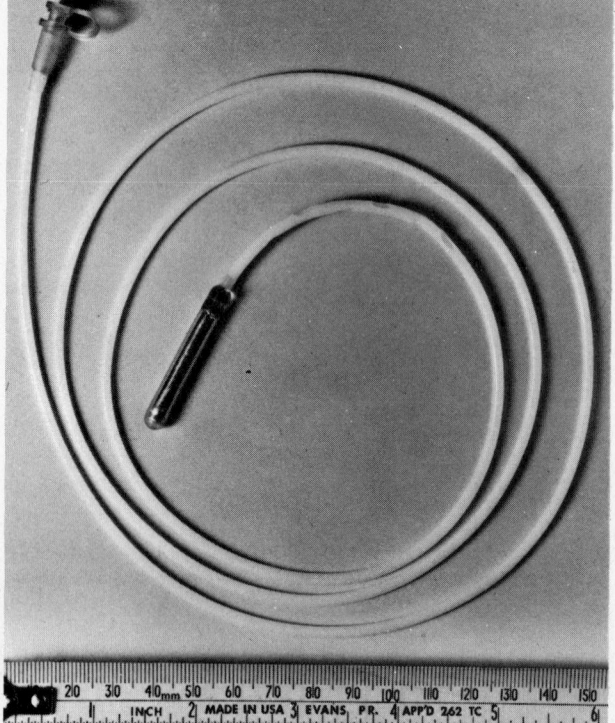

ENTERAL THERAPY (CONTINUOUS PUMP/TUBE ENTERIC HYPERALIMENTATION)

Enteral hyperalimentation is a form of nutritional feeding whereby the patient receives a complete liquid diet by means of a small feeding tube passed transnasally into the stomach and distal to the pylorus (Fig. 35-7). It is the recommended method of providing nutritional support when the gastrointestinal tract is functioning, in the following instances: severe trauma and major burns, gastrointestinal diseases of malabsorption syndrome, fistulas, acute ulcerative colitis, and chronic and partial obstruction, inborn errors of metabolism, renal failure, and many other conditions where the patient is unable to ingest, digest, and absorb food.

The choice of liquid formula for enteral feeding often depends on the patient's ability to digest and absorb certain nutrients: various types of carbohydrate, such as lactose; various types (and level) of electrolytes, in cases of cardiac, renal, or hepatic disease; and larger or smaller amounts of protein.

The route of administration may be nasogastric, or via esophagostomy, gastrostomy, or jejunostomy.

Osmosis and Osmolality. Solutions that are highly concentrated and foods that have certain characteristics can upset the normal water balance within the body. Fluid balance is maintained by the process of *osmosis*. It is accomplished within the body by moving water through membranes from a dilute solution of lower osmolality to a more concentrated one of higher osmolality until the solutions are nearly of equal osmolality. The osmolality of normal body fluids is approximately 300 mOsm. per kg. The body attempts to keep the osmolality of the contents of the stomach and intestines at approximately this level.

The proteins are extremely large particles and therefore have little or no osmotic effect. However, individual amino acids and carbohydrates are smaller particles and therefore have greater osmotic effect. Fats are not water soluble and do not form a solution in water; thus they have no osmotic effect. Since electrolytes such as sodium and potassium are comparatively small particles, they have a great effect on osmolality, and consequently on tolerance.

When a concentrated solution of high osmolality is taken in large amounts, water will move to the stomach and intestines from fluid surrounding the organs and the

Figure 35-7. The enteric feeding tube is small in diameter (No. 8 Fr.) and radiopaque, with mercury-filled bolus weight. It is passed easily through the nostril into the stomach and through the pylorus to allow continuous pump tube feeding in the distal duodenum or proximal jejunum. Made of polyurethane, it is sterilized with ethylene oxide. (The above Dubbhoff™ Enteric Feeding tube is a product of Biosearch Medical Products, Inc., Raritan, New Jersey)

vascular compartment. The patient experiences a feeling of fullness, nausea, and diarrhea which can bring about dehydration, resulting, in some cases, in hypotension and tachycardia. Collectively, these symptoms have been given the name of "dumping syndrome."

There is a wide range of tolerance among patients as to the effects of osmolality. Usually, debilitated patients are more sensitive to such disorders. Therefore the nurse should be knowledgeable about the osmolality of formulas and should observe and prevent such disorders.

Patient Preparation. Before administering an enteral feeding it is necessary to gain the patient's confidence and cooperation. Explaining the procedure and its purpose will help to overcome the patient's fears and perhaps his resistance. He should know that he will be asked to take sips of water while swallowing the tube and to give a proper signal if the procedure becomes painful. Letting the patient handle and feel the softness of the tube may also be helpful.

Management

When preparing and administering a tube feeding, it is essential that all measures of cleanliness be observed. Temperature of the feeding, volume of the feeding, flow rate, and adequate fluid intake are critically important.

The newer polyurethane or silicone rubber feeding tubes are of small diameter, No. 6 or 8, and have a mercury tip (rather than a weighted mercury-filled bag). A variety of tubes are available (Dobbhoff, Keofeed, MedPro), and each has instructions for ease of passage. Since they are softer, more pliable, and much thinner than the conventional nasogastric tube, they provide greater patient comfort. However, kinking of tubing may present a problem. A guide or other means of stiffening the tube may be recommended to ease its passage. Essentially, such a tube is passed in the same way as a nasogastric tube—that is, with the patient in high Fowler's position. If this is not feasible, place the patient on his side.

Feedings are administered either by gravity (drip) or by continuous controlled pump that is either volumetric (ml./hr.) or peristaltic (drops/hr.). The pump, preferably, is a small, simple finger-action pump* which has a rechargeable battery and permits patient ambulation. Feedings are lactose-free, with an osmolality of only 300 mOsm./kg.; a feeding may be given undiluted, and provides 1 calorie/ml. Feeding rates of about 100–150 ml./hr. (2,400–3,600 calories/day) are effective in inducing positive nitrogen balance and progressive weight gain, without producing abdominal cramps and diarrhea. If the feeding is intermittent, 200–350 ml. are given in 10–15 minutes. Additional water after feeding is important to prevent hypertonic dehydration. At the beginning

*IVAC pump Model 530, IVAC Corp., LaJolla, Cal.

of administration, the feeding should be diluted to at least half the strength, and not more than 50–100 ml. given at a time, or 40–60 ml./hour in continuous drip administration. This gradual administration helps the patient to develop tolerance, especially for hyperosmolar solutions.

Nursing Assessment

The patient is carefully monitored to detect initial signs of complications so that they can be minimized. Intake and output are carefully documented. Periodic laboratory studies are done to determine renal, hepatic, and hematologic status. Elevated blood glucose (hypergly-

TABLE 35-2.   COMPLICATIONS OF ENTERAL HYPERALIMENTATION AND THEIR MANAGEMENT

TYPE OF COMPLICATION	FREQUENCY %	THERAPY
Mechanical		
Tube lumen clogged by solution	Infrequent (<10)	Flush with water; replace tube if unsuccessful
Pulmonary aspiration of stomach contents	Rare (<1)	Unlikely, with head of bed elevated; discontinue if aspiration occurs
Esophageal erosion	Rare (<1)	Discontinue tube
Gastrointestinal symptoms		
Vomiting and bloating	10-15	Reduce flow rate and add peripheral hyperalimentation if needed
Diarrhea and cramping	10-20	Reduce flow, dilute solution, consider different type of solution, add anti-diarrheal drug
Metabolic, fluid, and electrolyte abnormalities		
Hyperglycemia and glucosuria	10-15	Reduce flow, administer insulin
Hyperosmolar coma	Rare (<1)	Discontinue therapy
Edema	20-25	Usually none; may reduce Na content or slow hyper-alimentation rate; rarely use diuretics
Congestive heart failure	1-5	Slow hyperalimentation, administer diuretics and digoxin
Hypernatremia, hypercalcemia	<5	Adjust electrolyte content of hyper-alimentation
Essential fatty acid deficiency	Common*	Linoleic acid supplement orally or Intralipid† intravenously

*If enteral feeding mixture lacks linoleic acid.
†Cutter Laboratories, Berkeley, California.
(Heymsfield, S. B., et al.: Enteral hyperalimentation: An alternative to central venous hyperalimentation. Ann. Intern. Med., 90:69, Jan. 1979.)

cemia) or glucosuria may indicate an excess of carbohydrates. If unchecked, this may lead to nonketotic dehydration and coma. If the patient has diarrhea, the infusion should be slowed, although it may not be desirable to do so because the amount of needed nutrients will be reduced. It may be necessary to administer antidiarrheal medications, such as tincture of opium, paregoric, or Lomotil. If vomiting or aspiration occur, the infusion should be stopped; if the patient is nauseated, the infusion should be slowed. These signs suggest delayed stomach emptying; gastric residual may have to be measured. If it is more than 150 ml., the physician is notified.

Guidelines for the nurse monitoring the management of tube-fed patients include:
• Watch for sudden gain in weight.
• Observe for signs of edema.
• Observe for signs of dehydration.
• Record the actual formula intake by the patient, including incidents of vomiting and diarrhea.
• Note any signs of inability of the patient to communicate.
• Test for urine glucose concentration.
• Consult daily laboratory tests for blood urea nitrogen and serum electrolytes.
• Check the proper positioning of the tube.
• Watch for possible complications (Table 35-2).

If the patient is ambulatory, he should be encouraged to walk, since movement facilitates absorption of the feeding. A portable pump and movable infusion standard can be managed easily. Prior to discharge, the patient should receive nutritional counselling for adequate food intake. Frequent outpatient follow-up visits are necessary to reassess and evaluate the patient's nutritional status and the progress of his recovery.

BIBLIOGRAPHY

BOOKS

Ballinger, W. F., et al. (eds.): Committee on Pre- and Postoperative Care, Manual of Surgical Nutrition, by the Committee on Pre- and Postoperative Care, American College of Surgeons. Philadelphia, W. B. Saunders, 1975.

Davenport, H. W.: Physiology of the Digestive Tract, 4th ed. Chicago, Year Book Medical Pub., 1977.

Dickerson, J. W. T., and Lee, H. A.: Nutrition in the Clinical Management of Disease. Year Book Medical Pub., 1978.

Given, B. A., and Simmons, S. J.: Gastroenterology in Clinical Nursing, 3rd ed. St. Louis, C. V. Mosby, 1979.

Hodges, R. E.: Nutrition in Medical Practice. Philadelphia, W. B. Saunders, 1979.

Mead Johnson: Nutritional Perspectives. Evansville, Ind., Mead Johnson & Co., 1978.

Schneider, H. A., et al. (eds.): Nutritional Support of Medical Practice. Hagerstown, Md., Harper & Row, 1977.

Sleisenger, M. H., and Fordtran, J. S.: Gastrointestinal Disease (Pathophysiology, Diagnosis, Management). Philadelphia, W. B. Saunders, 1978.

Spiro, H. M.: Gastroenterology, 2nd ed. New York, Macmillan Co., 1977.

Taylor, K. B.: Gastroenterology. *In* Schneider, H. A., et al.: Nutritional Support of Medical Practice. Hagerstown, Md., Harper and Row, 1977.

ARTICLES

General

Bass, L.: More fiber — less constipation. AJN, 77:254-255, Feb. 1977.

Fischer, J. E.: Parenteral and enteral nutrition. Disease-a-Month, 24:1-84, June 1978.

Hongladarom, G. C., and Russell, M.: An ethnic difference — lactose intolerance. Nurs. Outlook, 24:764-765, Dec. 1976.

Mendeloff, A. I.: Dietary fiber and gastrointestinal diseases. Med. Clin. N. Am., 62:165-171, Jan. 1978.

Welling, P. G.: How food and fluid affect drug absorption. Postgrad. Med., 62:73-82, July 1977.

Intubation/Tube Feeding

Bedine, M., and Bayless, T.: Intolerance of small amounts of lactose by individuals with low lactase levels. Gastroenterol., 65:735-743, Nov. 1973.

Bayless, T. M.: Recognition of lactose intolerance. Hosp. Pract., 11:97-102, Oct. 1976.

Bush, J.: Cervical esophagostomy to provide nutrition. AJN, 79:107-109, Jan. 1979.

Feldtman, Maj. R. W., and Andrassy, Maj., R. J.: Meeting exceptional nutritional needs, 1. Total parenteral nutrition. Postgrad. Med., 64:64-77, Aug. 1978.

Fricke, F. J., and Niewodowski, M. A.: Hazardous gaseous distention of intestinal balloons. JAMA, 235:2611-2613, June 1976.

Gormican, A., and Liddy, E.: Nasogastric tube feedings. Postgrad. Med., 53:71-76, June 1973.

Johnson, F. W., et al.: Rapid long-tube intubation of the jejunum by a new endoscopic device. Am. J. Surg., 131:91-93, Jan. 1976.

McConnell, E.: Gastrointestinal intubation. Critical Care Update, 4:5-15, Apr. 1977.

————: Stomach suctioning with the Salem sump tube. Nursing '77, 7:54-57, Sept. 1977.

————: Ten problems with nasogastric tubes . . . and how to solve them. Nursing '79, 9:78-81, Apr. 1979.

McCormick, P. W.: Immediate care after aspiration of vomit. Anesthesia, 30:658-665, Sept. 1975.

Moss, G.: Postsurgical decompression and immediate elemental feeding. Hosp. Pract., 12:73-82, May 1977.

Rosenberg, F. H.: Lactose intolerance. AJN, 77:823-824, May 1977.

Rosenberg, H.: The difficult nasogastric intubation: tips and techniques. Emerg. Med., 9:235-237, Mar. 1977.

Shils, M. E., et al.: Liquid formulas for oral and tube feeding. Clin. Bull., 6:151-158, no. 4, 1976.

Walike, B. C., and Walike, J. W.: Relative lactose intolerance. JAMA, *238*:948–951, Aug. 1977.

Welsh, J. D., Klotz, A. P., and Lubos, M. C.: Gastrointestinal symptoms and intestinal lactase deficiencies: a word of caution (discussion). Am. J. Dig. Dis., *12*:424–425, Apr. 1967.

Parenteral Hyperalimentation and Gastrostomy

Borgen, L.: Total parenteral nutrition in adults. AJN, *78*:224–228, Feb. 1978.

Buselmeier, T. J., et al.: Peripheral blood access for hyperalimentation. JAMA, *238*:2399–2400, Nov. 1977.

Copeland, E. M., III, et al.: Intravenous hyperalimentation as an adjunct to cancer chemotherapy. Am. J. Surg., *129*:167–173, Feb. 1975.

———: Effects of intravenous hyperalimentation on established delayed hypersensitivity in the cancer patient. Ann. Surg., *184*:60–64, July 1976.

Dobbie, R. P., and Butterick, O. D.: Continuous pump/enteric hyperalimentation—use in esophageal disease. J. Parenteral and Enteral Nutr., *1*:100–104, no. 2, 1977.

Driscoll, R. H., and Rosenberg, I. H.: Total parenteral nutrition in inflammatory bowel disease. Med. Clin. of N. Am., *62*:185–201, Jan. 1978.

Duke, J. H., Jr., and Dudrick, S. J.: Parenteral feeding. *In* American College of Surgeons, Manual of Surgical Nutrition. Philadelphia, W. B. Saunders, 1975, pages 285–317.

Englert, D. M., and Dudrick, S. J.: Principles of intravenous hyperalimentation. AORN J., *25*:1253–1267, June 1977.

Fischer, J. E.: Parenteral and enteral nutrition. Disease-A-Month, *24*:no. 9, June 1978.

Griggs, B. A., and Hoppe, M. C.: Update—nasogastric tube feeding. AJN, *79*:481–485, Mar. 1979.

Heymsfield, S. D., et al.: Enteral hyperalimentation; an alternative to central venous hyperalimentation. Ann. Int. Med., *90*:63–71, Jan. 1979.

Hodges, R. E.: Total parenteral nutrition. Postgrad. Med., *65*:171–180, Mar. 1979.

Johnston, D. W. B., and Prasad, J. K.: A simplified technique for gastrostomy. Surg. Gynecol. Obstet., *144*:84–85, Jan. 1977.

Kaminski, M. V., Jr., and Burke, W. A.: Parenteral hyperalimentation, prevention and treatment of complications. Surgical Team; Part I, *5*:18–25, Nov.–Dec. 1976; Part II, *6*:30–36, Jan.–Feb. 1977.

Sanders, R. A., et al.: Septic complications of total parenteral nutrition. Am. J. Surg., *132*:214–220, Aug. 1976.

TPN control needed (edit.): Arch. Intern. Med., *137*:1671, Dec. 1977.

White, P. L., and Nagy, M. D.: Total Parenteral Nutrition. Acton, Mass., Pub. Sciences Group, Inc., 1974.

AGENCIES

National Institute of Arthritis, Metabolism and Digestive Diseases, National Institutes of Health, Bethesda, Md. 20205

American Dietetic Association, 430 N. Michigan Ave., Chicago, Ill. 60611

American Institute of Nutrition, 9650 Rockville Pike, Bethesda, Md. 20014

American Society for Clinical Nutrition, 9650 Rockville Pike, Bethesda, Md. 20014

36

MANAGEMENT OF PATIENTS WITH GASTRIC (AND DUODENAL) DISORDERS

GASTRITIS

Acute Gastritis

Gastritis (inflammation of the stomach) is most often due to a dietary indiscretion. The individual eats too much or too rapidly or eats food that is noxious because it is too highly seasoned or is infected. Other causes of acute gastritis include alcohol, aspirin, uremia, or radiotherapy. Gastritis may also be the first sign of an acute systemic infection.

Pathophysiology and Clinical Manifestations. The gastric mucous membrane becomes edematous and hyperemic and undergoes superficial erosion; it secretes a paucity of gastric juice, containing very little acid but much mucus. The patient may have uncomfortable feelings in his abdomen, with headache, lassitude, nausea, and anorexia, often accompanied by vomiting and hiccupping. Some patients, however, are asymptomatic.

The gastric mucosa is capable of repairing itself after a bout of gastritis. Occasionally hemorrhage occurs; it may be severe and may require surgical intervention. If the irritating food is not vomited, but reaches the bowel, colic and diarrhea may result. As a rule, the patient is well in about a day, although he may not have much appetite for the next 2 or 3 days.

Management and Nursing Intervention. Management consists of permitting the patient nothing by mouth until acute symptoms subside. When the patient is able to take nourishment by mouth, a bland diet, perhaps supplemented by alkalies, is offered. If the symptoms persist, parenteral administration of fluids may become necessary.

Corrosive Gastritis. A more severe form of acute gastritis is caused by the ingestion of strong acids or alkalies (corrosive gastritis).

Immediate treatment consists of diluting and neutralizing the offender.
- To neutralize acids, use common antacids (milk, aluminum hydroxide, etc.); to neutralize an alkali, use lemon juice or dilute vinegar.
- If corrosion is extensive and severe, avoid emetics and lavage, because of the danger of perforation.

Therapy thereafter is supportive, including nasogastric intubation, analgesics and sedatives, antacids, intravenous fluids, and electrolytes.

It may be necessary to evaluate the situation by fiberoptic endoscopy. Emergency surgery may be required, to take care of gangrenous or perforated tissue. Corrosive gastritis can result in scarring and cause pyloric obstruction, which may require gastrojejunostomy or resection.

Chronic Gastritis

Pathophysiology. In patients with chronic gastritis, the mucous membrane of the stomach becomes thickened and its rugae are prominent. As time passes, both the lining and the walls become thinned and secretion lessens in quantity and in quality, eventually consisting almost entirely of mucus and water.

Causes. One of the important causes of chronic gastritis is chronic uremia. Among the local causes of gastritis are benign and malignant ulcers of the stomach and cirrhosis of the liver complicated by portal hypertension, the latter causing chronic congestion of the stomach wall.

738

Clinical Manifestations. Symptoms of chronic gastritis vary greatly. The appetite may be poor (anorexia) or too good (bulimia); there is usually some distress ("heartburn") after eating, and often there are eructations of gas. The taste in the mouth is unpleasant; there is usually considerable nausea, and perhaps some vomiting, especially early in the morning. The diagnosis is determined by gastroscopy, upper gastrointestinal x-ray series, and histologic examination.

Management. Treatment is similar to the medical regimen recommended for the patient with peptic ulcer. Patients with diffuse atrophic gastritis may require supplementary vitamin B_{12}.

PEPTIC ULCER

A *peptic ulcer* is an excavation formed in the mucosal wall of the stomach, the pylorus, the duodenum, or the esophagus (Fig. 36-1). It is caused by the erosion of a circumscribed area of mucous membrane. This erosion may extend as deeply as the muscle layers or through the muscle to the peritoneum. Peptic ulcers are more apt to be in the duodenum than in the stomach. As a rule, they occur singly, but there may be a number of them present at one time.

Etiology and Incidence. The etiology of peptic ulcer is poorly understood. It is known that peptic ulcers occur only in the areas of the gastrointestinal tract that are exposed to hydrochloric acid and pepsin. The disease occurs with the greatest frequency between the ages of 30 and 50, but is relatively uncommon in women of childbearing age, although it has been observed in childhood, and even in infancy. More males than females are affected, but after the menopause, the incidence of peptic ulcer in women is almost equal to that in men. Since peptic ulcers in the body of the stomach occur without excessive acid secretion, an attempt should be made to differentiate gastric from duodenal ulcers.

It is estimated that 5 to 15 percent of the population in the United States have ulcers, but only about half of these are recognized. Duodenal ulcer was first recognized around 1900, and the incidence increased until the 1950s. Since then there has been a steady decrease in the United States, but the reason is unclear.

Predisposition. Attempts continue to be made to delineate the "ulcer personality." Psychoanalysts claim that an ulcer results from repression of strong dependency needs. Others claim that occupational stress, with no opportunity to express hostility, is another strong factor. It seems to develop in persons who are emotionally tense, but whether this is the cause or the effect of the condition is uncertain. Familial tendency also appears as a significant predisposing factor, revealing that three times as many ulcer patients have relatives with the same diagnosis. A further hereditary link is noted in the find-

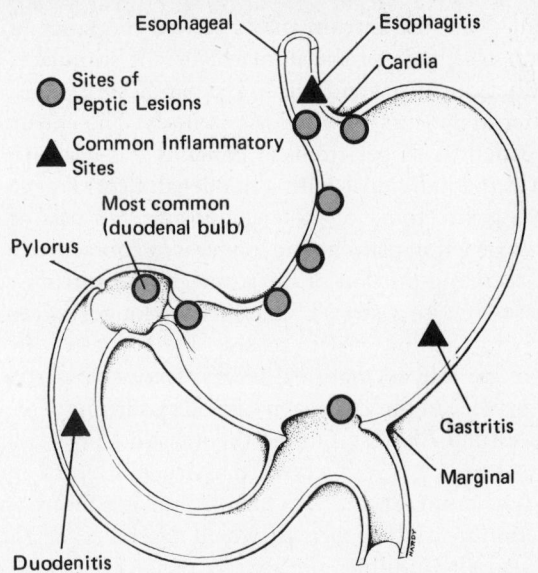

Figure 36-1. "Peptic" lesions may occur in the esophagus (esophagitis), stomach (gastritis), or duodenum (duodenitis). Note peptic ulcer sites and common inflammatory sites.

ing that individuals in blood-group O are 35 percent more susceptible than persons in groups A, B, and AB. Other predisposing factors associated with peptic ulcer include emotional stress, eating hurriedly and irregularly, and smoking excessively. Rarely, ulcers are due to excessive amounts of the hormone gastrin, produced by tumors (gastrinomas—Zollinger-Ellison syndrome).

Pathophysiology

Peptic ulcer occurs in gastroduodenal mucosa because such tissue is unable to withstand the digestive action of gastric acid and pepsin. The erosion is due to an increase in concentration or activity of acid-pepsin, and/or to a decrease in the normal resistance of the mucosa.

Gastric secretion occurs in three phases: (1) cephalic, (2) gastric, (3) intestinal. Since these phases are interactive and not independent of one another, a disturbance in any one phase may be ulcerogenic.

Cephalic (Psychic) Phase. The first phase is initiated by stimuli such as the sight, smell, or taste of food, acting upon cerebral cortical receptors which, in turn, stimulate the vagal nerves. Essentially, an unappetizing meal has little effect on gastric secretion, whereas a more tasty, appealing meal evokes a high secretion. This accounts for the traditional emphasis on serving a bland meal to the peptic ulcer patient. Today many gastroenterologists agree that the bland diet has no significant effect on gastric acidity or ulcer healing. However, excessive vagal activity during the night, when the stomach is empty, is significant.

Gastric Phase. The gastric phase of gastric secretion is mediated by the hormone *gastrin*. Gastrin, which can be measured by a radioimmunoassay, enters the bloodstream from the antrum and is carried to glands in the fundus and body of the stomach; here it stimulates the production of gastric juice. Gastrin activity may be greater in patients with pyloric stenosis. The antrum of the patient with gastric ulcer contains less gastrin than that of the individual with a duodenal ulcer. Following partial gastrectomy or gastrojejunostomy, if part of the antrum is left in place but no longer is in contact with the acid-secreting portion of the stomach, the antrum continues to release gastrin, because acid no longer bathes the mucosa to inhibit gastrin release. Excess gastrin in the blood can lead to marginal ulcers. Excessive gastrin is also present in the Zollinger-Ellison syndrome.

Intestinal Phase. During the intestinal phase a hormone, secretin, is secreted when hydrochloric acid enters the duodenum. Secretin, in turn, stimulates bicarbonate secretion from the pancreas, which neutralizes the acid. Secretin also inhibits the gastric phase of gastric secretion.

Gastric Mucosal Barrier. In man, gastric secretion is a mixture of mucopolysaccharides and mucoproteins se-

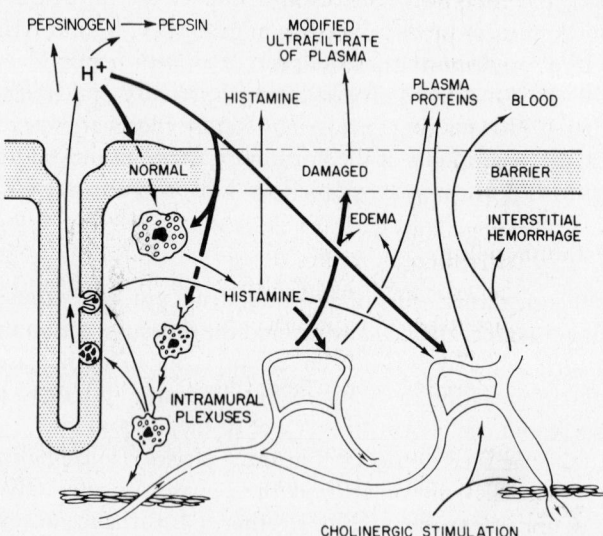

Figure 36-2. Pathophysiological consequences of the back-diffusion of acid through the broken gastric mucosal barrier. Acid, which diffuses slowly through the normal mucosa, rapidly enters one whose barrier has been broken. Acid destroys mucosal cells and liberates histamine. Histamine stimulates acid secretion, causes vasodilatation, and increases capillary permeability to proteins. The mucosa become edematous, and fluid derived from interstitial fluid is forced through the mucosa. This fluid may contain a large amount of plasma proteins. Acid stimulates the intramural plexuses, and motility of the stomach is increased. It also stimulates pepsin secretion, perhaps by way of histamine liberation and perhaps through its effect on the plexuses. Mucosal capillaries may be destroyed by acid, so that interstitial hemorrhage and frank bleeding occur. Bleeding is more frequent and copious when there is concurrent cholinergic stimulation, probably because contraction of gastric muscle increases venous and capillary pressures. (Davenport, H. W.: Physiology of the Digestive Tract, 3rd ed., Copyright © 1971 by Year Book Medical Publishers, Inc., Chicago. Used by permission.)

creted continuously by the mucosal glands. This mucus adsorbs pepsin and protects it against acid. Hydrochloric acid is secreted continuously, but secretions increase due to neurogenic and hormonal mechanisms which are initiated by gastric and intestinal stimuli. If hydrochloric acid were not buffered and neutralized, and if the outer layer of mucosa did not offer protection, hydrochloric acid, along with pepsin, would destroy the stomach. Hydrochloric acid comes into contact with only a small gastric mucosal surface (oxyntic glandular mucosa): it diffuses into it with amazing slowness. This impenetrability of the mucosa is called the *gastric mucosal barrier*. It is the chief defense of the stomach against being digested by its secretions. Other factors which influence mucosal resistance are the blood supply, acid-base balance, integrity of mucosal cells, and epithelial regeneration (Fig. 36-2).

Note then, that a person is likely to develop a peptic ulcer from one of two causes: hypersecretion of acid-pepsin, or a weakened gastric mucosal barrier. Anything which decreases the production of gastric mucus or damages gastric mucosa is ulcerogenic: salicylates, alcohol, and indomethacin fall into this category.

Clinical Manifestations

Symptoms of duodenal ulcer (the most common form of peptic ulcer), may last for a few days, weeks, or months and may even disappear only to reappear, often without an identifiable cause. Exacerbations seem to occur in the spring or fall, but even this pattern is inconsistent. Many individuals have symptomless ulcers, and in 20-30 percent, perforation or hemorrhage may occur without any preceding manifestations.

Pain. As a rule, the patient with duodenal ulcer complains of pain, or a burning, sharply localized sensation in the midepigastrium or in the back. It is believed that the pain occurs when the increased acid content of the stomach and duodenum erodes the lesion and stimulates the exposed nerve endings. Another theory suggests that contact of the lesion with acid stimulates a local reflex mechanism that initiates contraction of the adjacent smooth muscle.

Pain precedes meals from 1-3 hours and becomes progressively more severe toward the end of the day. It may also waken the individual between 12 and 3 A.M. However, there is no pain when the patient awakens in the morning because the flow of gastric acid is at its lowest at this time.

Pain typically is relieved quite promptly by food or alkalies, either of which neutralizes the free acid in contact with the ulcer. If the patient takes neither food nor alkali, the pain gradually wears off as the secretion of acid stops and it empties into the intestine. The character of the pain may be described as a dull, burning sensation, a feeling of emptiness, or a gnawing pain so severe that the patient is in agony. When the ulcer has begun to penetrate into the pancreas, pain in the back may become notice-able.

Some relief is obtained by local pressure on the epigastrium. Sharply localized tenderness can be elicited by gentle pressure in the epigastrium at, or slightly to the right of, the midline.

In assessing the patient's pain, the nurse observes and records in the nursing history the following responses: Where is the pain located? Does it radiate? How long does it last? At what time does it occur? Is it relieved by food or alkalies? How does the patient describe the pain? (Quality is usually not well described.)

Pyrosis. (Water brash, hypersialorrhea, heartburn.) Some patients experience a burning sensation in the esophagus and stomach, which moves up to the mouth, occasionally with sour eructation.

Vomiting. Although rare in uncomplicated duodenal ulcer, vomiting may be a symptom of peptic ulcer. It is due to gastric outlet obstruction caused by either muscular spasm of the pylorus or mechanical obstruction. The latter may be due to scarring or to acute swelling of the inflamed mucous membrane adjacent to the acute ulcer. Vomiting may or may not be preceded by nausea; usually it follows a bout of severe pain, which is relieved by ejection of the acid gastric contents. The vomitus may contain food particles from the previous day.

Constipation and Bleeding. Constipation may be apparent in the patient with duodenal ulcer, probably as a result of diet and medications.

About 20 percent of individuals who bleed from an acute duodenal ulcer have had no previous digestive complaints; however, they develop symptoms thereafter.

Assessment

The history of the patient serves as an important base for diagnosis (see chart on "risk factors"). The presence of pain that is relieved by food or antacids, and the absence of pain upon arising are highly suggestive of duodenal ulcer. The appearance of blood in the stools is an important diagnostic finding, suggestive of hemorrhage. Stools should be collected daily until the laboratory reports are negative for occult blood.

Diagnosis of duodenal ulcer is most easily made by barium studies of the upper gastrointestinal tract. Gastric secretory studies may be of some value in determining the type of treatment and to check for the possibility of Zollinger-Ellison syndrome. An analysis of the gastric juice, obtained by aspiration of the juice through a tube, is described on page 717. Often, production of acid for the sample is stimulated by injecting pentagastrin. However, gastric secretory studies have largely been replaced by fiberoptic endoscopy, for diagnosis, and for determining the healing of duodenal ulcer. This is a procedure which augments radiographic studies and permits direct visualization of the duodenal mucosa (page 718).

RISK FACTORS FOR DUODENAL ULCER

FAMILY HISTORY OF PEPTIC ULCER

EMOTIONAL STRESS:
   Anxiety
   Anger
   Resentment

CAFFEINE-CONTAINING BEVERAGES:
   Coffee
   Tea
   Cola

CERTAIN DRUGS:
   Salicylates
   Indomethacin

Management and Nursing Implementation

The major objectives of therapy are: (1) to control gastric acidity, (2) to reduce emotional stress, (3) to heal the ulcer, and (4) to instruct the patient concerning his future life style. From the beginning, once the diagnosis is established, the patient should be informed that he cannot expect a cure for peptic ulcer. He can learn how to keep his problem under control to some extent, but he can expect both remissions and recurrences.

Gastric acidity is controlled by appropriate sedation and by neutralization of the gastric juice, at frequent and regular intervals, with bland foods and antacids. Sometimes antispasmodics are given, to reduce pylorospasm and intestinal motility. Anticholinergic agents may be prescribed to inhibit gastric secretion. Recently, drugs which block the acid-secreting action of histamine (H_2 blockers) — cimetidine, for example — have been shown to be effective in healing duodenal ulcers.

Hospitalization, if required at all, can be limited to 2 or 3 days, unless bleeding, obstruction, perforation, or severe nocturnal pain are present.

To reduce environmental stress, the patient should, ideally, be on bed rest until he is free of pain and eating normally. Sedatives and tranquilizers are given according to the individual patient's needs. These may be prescribed on a regular schedule. The surroundings of the patient should provide an optimal milieu for healing.

The patient may become quite drowsy, in which event he will require close supervision when ambulatory, as well as protective rails on his bed, in order to avoid injury.

Diet. Since there is little evidence to support the theory that bland diets are more beneficial than regular meals, patients have been encouraged to eat whatever agrees with them. However, there are a few precautions to consider in the early stages of healing. *The objective of the diet for peptic ulcers is to avoid over-secretion and hypermotility in the gastrointestinal tract.* These can be minimized by avoiding extremes of temperature, overstimulation by meat extractives, coffee, alcohol, and seasonings, especially pepper and mustard. In addition, an effort should be made to neutralize the acid by the use of buffering foods such as milk, and by the use of antacids. At first, small, frequent feedings also will be beneficial.

Diet compatibility becomes an individual matter. If the patient tolerates a particular food, he may eat it. If it produces pain, he will avoid it. Milk and cream are no longer considered central to therapy. In fact, diets rich in milk and cream are potentially harmful, over a long period, because they increase serum lipids, a contributing factor in producing atherosclerosis. Skim milk stimulates secretion to some extent; the more effective the neutralization, the more enhanced is the stimulus to new acid secretion. As the patient approaches alkalinity, gastrin release is stimulated and acid secretion is increased.

Unless there are unusual problems, current therapy permits meals of normal size three times a day, eaten at the same time each day, with no evening snack—rather than six small meals a day.

Antacids. Antacids continue to be a mainstay of peptic ulcer treatment. The objective is to select the antacid which provides the safest and longest period of acid neutralization. Usually, antacids leave the stomach rapidly, so that frequent doses are required.

Sodium bicarbonate is probably the best neutralizer of acid contents in the stomach, but is not recommended, because it is emptied from the stomach too rapidly, and over a period of time can easily lead to alkalosis. The next most effective antacids are calcium-containing compounds; however, they are unpleasant-tasting, and constipating. They are in disfavor because calcium produces an increase in serum gastrin and in acid secretion. Taken over a period of time, they can lead to hypercalcemia and impaired renal function. Less effective are the aluminum hydroxide and magnesium hydroxide preparations. However, they are the most effective antacids available.

Most antacids contain mixtures of aluminum and magnesium hydroxide, or magnesium hydroxide, aluminum hydroxide, and calcium carbonate in various combinations and suspensions. Magnesium hydroxide is a good buffering antacid, but used alone may cause diarrhea. Therefore a preferable combination is magnesium hydroxide with magnesium trisilicate (which has less laxative effect) or aluminum hydroxide (more constipating). Aluminum hydroxide gels can bring on hypophosphatemia.

Although no antacid presently available is capable of maintaining a pH of 3.5 or above (required to keep pepsinogen inactive) for longer than 30–45 minutes, antacids are capable of preventing rebound hyperacidity and systemic alkalosis.

In the early phase, liquid antacids are taken hourly, 15–30 ml. (1 or 2 tablespoons), beginning 1 hour after breakfast until bedtime (examples: Gelusil, Mylanta, Maalox, Creamalin, Amphojel). If the patient is awakened at night with epigastric pain, he notes the time,

and thereafter sets his alarm clock for an hour earlier, to take the antacid (see "Duration of Regimen" for continued pattern of antacid therapy).

• For patients who have an associated heart problem requiring sodium restriction, magaldrate (Riopan) is an antacid of choice, since it contains practically no sodium. This is especially recommended for elderly patients.

COMPOSITION OF COMMON ANTACIDS	
Antacid	**Contents**
Aludrox	Aluminum hydroxide gel, magnesium hydroxide
Amphojel	Aluminum hydroxide gel
A-M-T	Magnesium trisilicate, aluminum hydroxide gel
Camalox	Aluminum and magnesium hydroxide, calcium carbonate
Creamalin	Hexitol stabilized, aluminum hydroxide gel, magnesium hydroxide
Di-Gel	Aluminum hydroxide and magnesium hydroxide, simethicone
Ducon	Aluminum hydroxide and magnesium hydroxide, calcium carbonate
Delcid	Aluminum hydroxide, magnesium hydroxide
Gelusil	Magnesium hydroxide, aluminum hydroxide, simethicone
Gelusil-M	Magnesium trisilicate, aluminum and magnesium hydroxide
Kolantyl Gel	Aluminum hydroxide, magnesium hydroxide
Maalox	Magnesium hydroxide and aluminum hydroxide, simethicone
Malcogel	Magnesium trisilicate, aluminum hydroxide gel
Marblen	Magnesium and calcium carbonates, aluminum hydroxide
Mylanta	Aluminum hydroxide gel, magnesium hydroxide, simethicone
Mylanta-II	Aluminum hydroxide gel, magnesium hydroxide, simethicone
Phosphaljel	Aluminum phosphate gel
Riopan	Magaldrate and simethicone
Robalate	Dihydroxyaluminum aminoacetate
Silain-Gel	Aluminum and magnesium hydroxide, simethicone
Titralac	Calcium carbonate, glycine
Trisogel	Magnesium trisilicate, aluminum hydroxide gel
Wingel	Aluminum and magnesium hydroxide, hexitol stabilized

Anticholinergics. As an adjunct to the antacid compounds, an anticholinergic drug is usually given. Anticholinergics are given to block vagal stimulation of parietal cells, so as to reduce acid secretion. Anticholinergics also decrease gastric motor activity, which allows the antacid to remain in the stomach longer.

Among the antisecretory drugs are atropine, propantheline bromide (Pro-Banthine), methantheline bromide (Banthine), oxyphencyclimine (Daricon), methscopolamine (Pamine), and others. These are usually only recommended for a short period of time, when pain has not been relieved with antacids. They are occasionally used at nighttime with a double dose of antacid, for persistent night pain.

Side effects of anticholinergic drugs include: dryness of the mouth and throat, excessive thirst, difficulty in swallowing, flushed dry skin, rapid pulse and respiration, dilated pupils, and emotional excitement.

- Anticholinergic medications should not be used by patients with glaucoma, urinary retention, or pyloric obstruction.

Physicians vary in their preference for prescribing anticholinergic drugs. At times such drugs are in favor, and at other times they are not. While these drugs are suggested for patients who suffer from severe, persistent nocturnal pain, they are not recommended for long-term use.

H_2 Receptor Antagonist – Cimetidine (Tagamet). Histamine has two receptors for its action: H_1 receptor is located on bronchial and nasal mucosa, cardiac tissue, and blood vessels; H_2 receptor is found primarily in the stomach. Common antihistamines block the action of H_1 receptors but have no effect on H_2 receptors in the stomach. Cimetidine, a H_2 receptor antagonist, has a dramatic effect on lowering acid secretion in the stomach. A very high dose of the drug reduces acid secretion to an almost unmeasurable level.

Cimetidine is given orally with each meal and at bedtime. It relieves ulcer pain, but how effective it is in healing an ulcer is not yet known. When the drug is stopped, the ulcer tends to recur. Low-dose maintenance therapy may prevent recurrence. Even though H_2 receptors are distributed in body tissue, only gastric receptors appear to be affected by this drug. No serious toxicity has been reported; it appears to be a valuable medication.

Duration of Regimen. The patient should stay on the drug program to ensure complete healing of the ulcer. Since most patients become symptom-free in a week, it becomes a nursing objective to emphasize the importance of following the prescribed regimen so that the breakdown of the healing process and the return of chronic ulcer symptoms are averted. Rest, sedatives, and tranquilizers add to the comfort of the individual and are used as needed.

After the first week, the purpose of using antacids switches from that of relieving symptoms to preventing symptoms. If antacid is taken on a fasting stomach, its buffering action is effective for only about 30 minutes, but when taken an hour after a meal, the buffering effect may last 2-3 hours. For the 2nd through the 6th weeks, the best plan appears to be to have the patient on regular meals. One hour after each meal, he takes 30 ml. of antacid; 3 hours after each meal, he takes another 30 ml. of antacid. This medication is also recommended at bedtime. This pattern of therapy concentrates antacid in the stomach and duodenum at those times when the gastric secretion otherwise would be highest, achieving the desired neutralizing effect. The goal is to keep the pH of gastric contents above 4, between meals. At this pH, pepsin becomes relatively inactive.

From the 6th or 7th week to 6 months, antacid is taken about an hour after meals and at bedtime. Thereafter, antacid therapy is usually dropped. If the person experiences a stressful situation or has been indiscrete in his diet and symptoms recur, he may resume antacid therapy until he is symptom-free.

Prognosis

Recurrence of an ulcer is possible and may happen within 2 years in about one-third of all patients. The likelihood is lessened if the individual avoids tea, coffee, alcohol, tobacco, and ulcerogenic drugs. If symptoms recur, he is to resume antacid medications hourly. (Antacid tablets may be taken when required during a normal day's activities; however, it is necessary to chew them thoroughly and to recognize that three or four tablets are equal in potency to one tablespoon of liquid antacid.) If relief is not obtained, medical advice should be sought.

Psychosocial Evaluation and Patient Education

In communicating with the patient with a peptic ulcer, the nurse may learn what kind of person he is by referring to the nursing history and the initial patient assessment data. The patient's reactions to daily events can be ascertained through conversation and observation. The clinically oriented nurse can readily relate the patient's frustrations, ambitions, annoyances, impatience, etc. to his medical problem. When these overt manifestations do not offer clues to the patient's current situation, it may be necessary to pay special attention to his reactions to questions, to his family and visitors, and the kind of activities and interests he pursues.

A patient with a peptic ulcer is often irritable, anxious, and very sensitive, taking offense easily. The patient may be preoccupied with some concrete problems as a conscious basis for his anxiety. Usually he is eager to discuss them with the nurse during unhurried contacts, and such discussions afford satisfaction and relief.

Indeed, the very presence of the nurse brings relief. This relationship with the patient can be significant in providing an atmosphere conducive to effective education of the patient regarding his future life style.

Life Style Adjustments.   Many patients with acute ulcer symptoms (due to the proved presence of an ulcer), derive complete temporary relief merely by severing all connections with those environmental factors that produce anxiety—unfavorable diet and hygienic conditions notwithstanding. Such a solution is rarely practicable, however, for environments, particularly internal emotional environments, are not easily shed.

Freedom from ulcer recurrences is favored by adherence to a sound hygienic routine of living, which implies the following:
- regularity of habits, in general
- moderation in all pursuits
- adequate daily rest
- ample relaxation
- good diet discipline
- abstinence from caffeine, alcohol, and drugs which have acid-producing potential
- avoiding cigarettes, since nicotine decreases pancreatic alkaline secretions

Beneficial alterations of stress situations frequently are possible through wise counseling (in some cases aided by a psychiatrist) of the patient and the patient's family. The nurse's observations may provide the basis for this counsel. Ulcers are apt to recur despite medical and surgical measures if the patient must return to his former environment to face the same problems that earlier had helped to produce the condition.

For an overall coverage of medical and nursing management of the patient with a peptic ulcer see the chart that appears below.

Complications and Therapeutic Management

There are four major complications of a peptic ulcer: hemorrhage, perforation, pyloric obstruction, and intractable ulcer.

Hemorrhage.   Manifested by hematemesis, melena, or both, hemorrhage is the common complication of peptic ulcer. Occasionally this appears without any ante-

---

PRINCIPLES OF MEDICAL AND NURSING MANAGEMENT OF THE PATIENT WITH A PEPTIC ULCER

MAJOR PROBLEMS
1. Pain and dyspepsia
2. Anxiety and emotional distress
3. Promotion of physical and emotional rest
4. Prevention of complications

OBJECTIVES
A. To assure mental and physical rest:
   1. Bed rest, to remove patient from stressful environment
   2. Written nursing-care plan to provide for optimal coordinated care
   3. Sedatives and soporific medications to promote relaxation and sleep
   4. Medications and dietary feedings, given on time

B. To rest the motor and secretory activities of the stomach through a therapeutic diet:
   1. Small feedings, to rest the gastrointestinal tract
   2. Frequent feedings, to absorb excess acid
   3. Bland protein and fat foods, to neutralize acidity
   4. Nonstimulating foods, to avoid irritation of the gastric mucosa
   5. Progression to nutritionally adequate diet as rapidly as possible

C. To relieve pain and discomfort and to promote healing:
   1. Antacid drugs given to neutralize gastric secretions and afford symptomatic relief
   2. Anticholinergic drugs given to decrease gastric motility and reduce volume of gastric secretions
   3. Adequate hydration, to relieve side effects of anticholinergic drugs
   4. H_2 receptor antagonist, to reduce acid secretion

D. To assist the patient to accept and follow his therapeutic program:
   1. Demonstrate interest in patient, and eliminate factors producing anxiety.
   2. Teach importance of taking prescribed medication and diet on time.
   3. Assist patient to develop insight into causes of his tension and frustration.
   4. Implement and reinforce instructions issued by the physician.
   5. Teach the importance of moderation in all activities.
   6. Encourage the elimination of smoking.
   7. Stress the value of psychiatric interviews, if prescribed.

E. To recognize the complications of peptic ulcer:
   1. Hemorrhage:
      a. Prepare for prompt and rapid transfusion for blood replacement.
      b. Administer sedatives, to allay anxiety and keep patient at rest.
      c. Assist with gastric intubation for aspiration of stomach contents.
      d. Evaluate clinical response to blood replacement.
      e. Observe continuously, to maintain blood pressure at physiologic level.
      f. Observe urinary volume.
      g. Observe stools for blood; collect stool specimens daily for laboratory analysis.
      h. Prepare for surgical intervention, if indicated.
   2. Perforation:
      a. Assist with transfusion, to treat shock.
      b. Prepare to institute nasogastric suction to remove gastrointestinal secretions.
      c. Give drugs to control pain.
      d. Prepare patient for immediate surgery.

cedent history of dyspepsia. Early symptoms may be giddiness and faintness; nausea may precede or accompany bleeding. A large amount of blood, even 2,000 to 3,000 ml., may be vomited. The patient may become almost exsanguinated, and rapid blood replacement may be required to save his life. When the hemorrhage is of large proportions, most of the blood is vomited; when small, much or all of the blood may be passed in the stools, which will appear tarry black, due to the digested hemoglobin.

Nursing Intervention. Since hemorrhage can be massive and fatal, bleeding must be stopped quickly, and the blood replaced.

- Immediate nursing evaluation will include assessment of vital signs. If vital signs are unstable, preparation should be made for a *peripheral line* intravenous infusion (saline, and later blood or blood component) and a *central line* for infusion and measurement of central venous pressure (arterial line optional).
- The laboratory is notified to type and crossmatch 6 units of blood.
- Additional laboratory tests are requested, including hemoglobin and hematocrit evaluations, and chemical tests such as benzidine, guaiac, or orthotoluidine, to detect occult blood that does not alter the gross appearance of the stools, since this type of melena is decidedly more common than gross hemorrhages from the bowel.
- An indwelling urinary catheter is inserted to monitor urinary output. Special diagnostic studies, such as endoscopy (to locate the exact bleeding site), arteriography, and barium studies, may be called for.
- A nasogastric tube may be placed in the stomach to determine the presence of fresh blood or "coffee-ground" material, which can then be removed by suction.
- Some clinics use normal iced saline for lavage to remove blood and clots. Often the No. 18 French tube is too small, and a No. 22 French size is used. The normal saline solution may be taken by mouth and the fluid withdrawn through the tube by suction. Usually the nasogastric tube is left in place during the cooling procedure. This removes acid, prevents nausea and vomiting, and provides a means of monitoring for further bleeding.
- Whole-blood and/or plasma transfusions are employed to keep the circulating blood volume at a safe level. One does not wait for a drop in blood pressure before embarking on transfusion therapy, if there are signs of tachycardia, sweating, and coldness of the extremities.
- The blood pressure and pulse rates are monitored at half-hourly intervals when bleeding is suspected, and hemoglobin and hematocrit are frequently checked.
- It is important to observe and record the color, consistency, and the volume of stools and vomitus.
- All of the aforementioned symptoms must be monitored and reported immediately.
- In the event of hypovolemic shock, the procedures outlined on page 368 are carried out.
- When bleeding ceases, hourly antacids and diet as tolerated are given. Anticholinergic medications are postponed, because of masking effects on pulse rate.

Indications for Surgery. If bleeding recurs in 48 hours after medical therapy has begun, or if more than 5 units of blood are required in 24 hours to maintain blood volume, the patient is likely to be scheduled for surgery. Some clinics have a policy that if a patient with peptic ulcer hemorrhages three times, surgery is indicated.

Other determining factors for surgery are: the patient's age; if he is over 60, massive hemorrhaging is 3 times more likely to be fatal; a history of chronic duodenal ulcer; and a coincidental gastric ulcer.

The ulcer-bearing area is removed, or the bleeding vessels are ligated. In many patients a procedure is included which is aimed at controlling the underlying ulcer diathesis, e.g., vagotomy and pylorectomy, or gastrectomy.

Perforation. Perforation of a peptic ulcer may occur unexpectedly, without much evidence of preceding indigestion. Perforation into the free peritoneal cavity is an abdominal catastrophe, and an indication that surgery may be needed.

The typical history consists of:
- Sudden, severe upper abdominal pain (persisting and increasing in intensity).
- Pain may be referred to the shoulders, especially the right shoulder, due to irritation of the phrenic nerve in the diaphragm.
- Vomiting and collapse.
- Abdomen extremely tender, and boardlike in rigidity.
- Signs of shock.

Immediate surgical intervention is indicated, because chemical peritonitis develops within a few hours following perforation and is followed by a bacterial peritonitis. Therefore, the perforation must be closed as quickly as possible. In a few patients, it may be deemed safe and advisable that a definitive operation be performed for the ulcer disease, in addition to the perforation being sutured.

Pyloric Obstruction. Pyloric obstruction occurs when the area distal to the pyloric sphincter becomes scarred and stenosed from spasm or edema, or from scar tissue that is formed when the ulcer alternately heals and breaks down. The patient has symptoms of nausea and vomiting, constipation, epigastric fullness, anorexia, and (later) weight loss.

In treating the patient, the first consideration is the relief of the obstruction by gastric decompression. At the same time, attempts are made to confirm that obstruction is the cause of discomfort. This is done by checking the amount of fluid aspirated from the nasogastric tube. A residual of over 200 ml. is strongly suggestive of obstruction. Some physicians also utilize the load test, which involves infusing 750 ml. of normal saline via the nasogastric tube into the mid-antrum of the stomach. The patient is rotated, to permit normal gastric emptying; 20 minutes later, aspiration is done, and if more than 400 ml. is retrieved, obstruction is confirmed.

Before surgery is undertaken, decompression continues, and extracellular fluid volume, as well as electrolyte and metabolic derangements, are corrected. Conscientious daily fluid monitoring is continued. With supportive measures, the patient's condition may improve. It may be feasible to repeat the load test; if negative, medical treatment continues. If positive, surgery, in the form of a vagotomy and antrectomy, may be required. If the patient is severely malnourished during this time, parenteral hyperalimentation may be utilized.

Intractability. An intractable ulcer is one that continues to give problems and is resistant to all forms of treatment. A careful history of the patient includes a thorough review of dietary and drug habits, which could reveal long-term use of caffeine-containing drinks or aspirin-containing medications. The entire gastrointestinal tract is carefully assessed to determine other possible problems, such as hiatus hernia, gallbladder disease, or diverticulitis.

The patient and spouse are informed of the fact that surgery is no guarantee that an ulcer will not return. The possible postoperative sequelae, such as intolerance to dairy products and sweet foods, are also discussed. Surgery is done only if medical therapy is unsuccessful.

Duodenal vs. Gastric Ulcers

Whereas most patients with duodenal ulcer can be treated successfully on a medical regimen, unless complications require surgical intervention, gastric ulcer is considered a surgical problem. There is a high recurrence rate with gastric ulcer. For a comparison between duodenal and gastric ulcers, see Table 36-1.

Surgical Treatment

Preoperative Assessment and Nursing Intervention. Often the cause of the ulcer is not removed by surgical intervention alone. Constant fear or worry may be disturbing the individual. Only when this factor is eliminated can the best results be expected. Since the "psyche" has much influence over the "soma," all efforts to allay the apprehension and fears of the patient should be employed. Because these patients have a long illness, they are frequently discouraged and often are helped by spiritual therapy. Economic and social factors may have influenced the patient to such an extent that long hours of work, lack of recreation, tension, fatigue, etc., have contributed in good measure to his illness.

Through a careful nursing history and assessment of the patient, these factors can be elicited and used in developing specific nursing goals. By collaborating with other members of the health team and seeking input from them, the nurse can develop a therapeutic plan of care to assist in resolving the patient's problem and to reduce the chances of recurrences.

1. *Preparing the patient for diagnostic tests.*

   The patient undergoes laboratory analyses, roentgenologic series, and a general physical examination before surgery is attempted. The nurse prepares the patient for each of these diagnostic measures by explaining their nature and significance to him.

2. *Attending to the patient's fluid and nutritional needs.*

   The nutritional and fluid needs of the patient are of major importance. In those patients with pyloric obstruction, there usually is prolonged vomiting, with resultant weight and fluid loss. Every effort is made to restore an adequate nutritional level and to maintain an optimal fluid and electrolyte balance.

3. *Clearing and emptying the gastrointestinal tract.*

   Nasogastric suction often is required to empty the stom-

TABLE 36-1. COMPARISON BETWEEN DUODENAL AND GASTRIC ULCER

	CHRONIC DUODENAL ULCER	CHRONIC GASTRIC ULCER
Age	Usually 50	Usually age 45 and over
Sex	Male-female; 4:1	Male-female; 2:1
Blood group	Most frequently—O	No differentiation
Social class	More frequently in those subjected to stress and responsibility: executives, leaders in competitive fields	More common among laboring persons
General nourishment	Usually well-nourished	Often malnourished
Acid production: stomach	Hypersecretion	Normal—hyposecretion
Pain	2-3 hours after a meal. Nighttime: often awakened between 1-2 A.M. Ingestion of food relieves pain	Occurs ½-1 hour after a meal. Nighttime: rarely. Relieved by vomiting. Ingestion of food does not help; sometimes pain is increased
Vomiting	Uncommon	Common
Hemorrhage	Melena more common than hematemesis	Hematemesis more common than melena
Malignancy possibility	Never	Perhaps in less than 10%

ach, especially in patients with pyloric obstruction. The tube is inserted before the operation and left in place for operative and postoperative use.

It is important that the colon be empty when the patient comes to surgery; this is ensured by an enema the day before operation. If gastrointestinal roentgenograms have been made shortly before the day of operation, it is most important that enemas be given to remove the barium that may remain in the colon completely.

4. *Limiting fluid intake.*

The patient usually is limited to fluids during the 24-hour period preceding surgery.

5. *Shaving and preparing the skin.*

The abdomen should be prepared, from the nipple line to the symphysis, although the incision usually is made in the upper right quadrant or the midline.

Intraoperative Care. When there is recurrence of ulcer symptoms for several years, and conservative therapy is unsuccessful, surgery is recommended. This occurs in about 10-15 percent of ulcer patients. Surgery is also recommended when complications such as hemorrhage, perforation, pyloric obstruction, and intractability occur. The purpose of operation is to relieve complications and treat the tendency to ulcer formation.

Vagotomy and Gastroenterostomy or Pyloroplasty. A popular method of treating the patient with a peptic ulcer involves cutting the vagus nerves (vagotomy) and establishing gastric drainage. The drainage operation is

necessary because vagotomy is often followed by gastric retention. Since the vagus nerves provide the motor impulses to the gastric musculature, severing the nerves often leads to gastric atony. The drainage operations may be in the form of a gastroenterostomy or a pyloroplasty. The vagotomy divides the nerves that are known to stimulate gastric acid hypersecretion in most cases of duodenal ulcer. The gastric drainage operation not only drains the atonic stomach produced by the vagotomy but also reduces the stimulation of gastric acid, by reducing the formation of gastrin produced in the antral area of the stomach.

Vagotomy and Antrectomy. Since the ulcers are believed to result from the acid pepsin of the stomach, vagotomy and antrectomy are designed to lower the production of acid by the stomach to a point at which further ulcerations will not occur. This may be done by removing the acid-stimulating mechanism of the stomach, i.e., dividing the vagus nerves and removing the antral portion of the stomach (vagotomy and antrectomy).

Partial Gastrectomy and Possible Vagotomy. A third method is partial gastrectomy, with or without vagotomy. The remaining segment of stomach is anastomosed to the duodenum (Billroth I procedure), or more extensive excision of the stomach may be performed and the remaining segment anastomosed to the jejunum (Billroth II procedure). (See Table 36-2.)

TABLE 36-2. GASTRIC OPERATIONS FOR PEPTIC ULCERS

OPERATION	DESCRIPTION	MORTALITY	RECURRENCE	ADVANTAGES	SEQUELAE
Vagotomy with drainage: pyloroplasty or gastroenterostomy.	Vagotomy may be total or partial (preserving hepatic branch of anterior nerves and celiac branch of posterior nerve)	Under 1%	10-15%	Fairly simple. Clinical results: 75% excellent 10% fair 10% poor	Some patients experience problems of fullness after eating (33%), dumping syndrome (10%), diarrhea (10%)
Vagotomy with antrectomy	Resection of vagus nerves and removal of antrum	3.9%	3.3%	Marginal ulceration rate lowest	In some patients, fullness after eating, dumping syndrome, diarrhea, anemia, malabsorption.
Partial gastrectomy Billroth I (gastroduodenostomy; anastomosis after resection)	Removal of distal ⅓-½ of stomach; anastomosis with duodenum	2%		Restores normal continuity	Dumping syndrome, anemia, malabsorption, and weight loss. Billroth I has a 4% marginal ulceration rate.
Billroth II (Gastrojejunostomy; anastomosis after resection)	Removal of distal segment of stomach and antrum; anastomosis with jejunum				Billroth II has a 2% marginal ulceration rate.
Proximal gastric vagotomy without drainage	Denervation of acid-secreting parietal cells but preserving vagal innervation to gastric antrum and extragastric abdominal visera.	Under 1%	1-9%	No dumping, reflex gastritis, or diarrhea. No need for antibiotics, since gastrointestinal tract is not open.	Appears to be a safe procedure. Needs long-term assessment.

Proximal Gastric Vagotomy without Drainage. A relatively new procedure in the United States (widely done in Great Britain and Europe) is the denervation of the acid-secreting parietal cell mass of the stomach, while preserving vagal innervation to the gastric antrum and extragastric abdominal viscera. This procedure (also referred to as highly selective or parietal cell vagotomy) is safe, with few side effects such as dumping syndrome. However, it is too early to assess the effect of this operation on long-term recurrence of duodenal ulcers.

Postoperative Care. Postoperative care is the same as for gastric surgery. See page 753.

Zollinger-Ellison Syndrome (Gastrinoma)

Zollinger-Ellison syndrome should be considered a possibility when a patient presents with several peptic ulcers; it is identified by a triad of findings: hypersecretion of gastric juice, multiple duodenal ulcers (second and third portions), and gastrinomas (islet cell tumors) in the pancreas. The incidence of malignancy is approximately 65 percent. The huge amounts of secreted hydrochloric acid almost has the effect of the stomach's trying to digest itself. The serum gastrin level is increased. Steatorrhea (unabsorbed fat in the stool) may be evident, because excessive gastric acid inactivates lipase in the intestine, thereby precipitating bile salts and decreasing fat digestion. The result is steatorrhea and diarrhea. Gastrin also decreases water and salt absorption, which in turn leads to diarrhea.

Patient Assessment. Diarrrhea and hypercalcemia are common problems. A nursing assessment frequently reveals that the patient's symptoms are often refractory (unyielding) to large amounts of antacids. He may disclose taking several pints of milk a day with no apparent relief from pain.

Management. Hypersecretion of acid can be controlled with H$_2$ receptor blocking agents (cimetidine) while the patient is prepared for surgery. (Long-term use of cimetidine in these patients has not been evaluated yet.) The patient's weight needs to be monitored, and fluid and electrolyte balance must be brought under control. Surgery that is necessary usually includes a gastrectomy (to remove acid-secreting surface) and possibly partial pancreatectomy (to remove tumors). In the postoperative period, dietary instruction is necessary; vitamin B$_{12}$ is given monthly. Careful follow-up monitoring is done to detect metastasis.

Stress Ulcer

Stress ulcer is the term given to a group of duodenal or gastric ulcers which occur following physiologically disturbing conditions.

Pathophysiology and Etiology. Stressful conditions such as burns, shock, severe sepsis, and multiple organ trauma can initiate the development of such ulcers. Fiberoptic endoscopy within 24 hours of injury reveals shallow erosions of the stomach wall; by 72 hours, multiple gastric erosions are observed. As the stressful condition continues, the ulcers spread. When the patient recovers, the lesions are reversed. This is typical of stress ulceration.

Differences of opinion exist as to the actual causation of mucosal ulceration. Usually it is preceded by shock; this leads to a decrease in gastric mucosal blood-flow and a reflux of duodenal content into the stomach. In addition, large quantities of pepsin are released. The combination of ischemia, acid, and pepsin creates an ideal climate to produce ulceration. When acute stress ulceration is combined with central nervous system trauma, stress ulcers (Cushing's ulcers) are often deeper and more penetrating. Gastric erosions are frequently observed about 72 hours after extensive burns (Curling's ulcers).

Prophylactic Therapy. Antacids are the basis of this mode of treatment. If the patient is acutely ill, antacids may be given through the nasogastric tube. Frequent gastric aspiration is done to check pH, in an attempt to get it to, or above, 3.5. Antacid therapy can also inhibit the activity of proteolytic enzyme pepsin.

Management. Stress ulcers are treated aggressively with antacid therapy. Conn and his associates advocate selective intra-arterial infusion of Vasopressin to treat patients who are bleeding extensively from stress ulcers. However, this method of management is still controversial, as is surgical intervention. If at all possible, the best treatment is prevention.

GASTRIC CANCER

Cancer of the stomach continues to decrease in the United States, for some unexplained reason (a 40 percent decline in the United States in the past 25 years). However, it is still a serious problem, accounting for 15,000 deaths annually, mostly in persons over 40, and occasionally in younger people. The incidence is 4 times greater in Japan, which has led to mass surveys for earlier diagnosis. Heredity appears to be a factor, as does chronic inflammation of the stomach.

Pathophysiology and Clinical Assessment

The early symptoms of this disease are often indefinite, since most of these tumors start on the lesser curvature, where they cause little disturbance to the gastric functions. Later, after they have spread to the cardiac orifice, or especially to the pylorus, the suffering may be distressing; this is due not to the cancer as such, but to disturbance in gastric motility. Weight loss, weakness, anemia, and sometimes icterus appear late in the disease. Pain, in gastric cancer, as in cancer in almost all other parts of the body, is a late symptom. Whereas pain is a sensitive indicator of disturbed physiology or disease, it is ironic that pain rarely warns the individual who has cancer while there is still an opportunity of curing it.

The most important early symptoms of gastric cancer are:
- a progressive loss of appetite
- the appearance of, or change in, gastrointestinal symptoms that have been increasingly apparent for a matter of weeks or months only
- the appearance of blood in the stools
- vomiting. (If the tumor causes obstruction at the cardiac orifice, vomiting or a feeling of fullness will immediately follow a meal. If the tumor is near the pylorus, it eventually obstructs this channel, and vomiting becomes a prominent symptom.)
- occasional vomiting of coffee-ground vomitus, or signs of blood in the stool

The blood that leaks slowly from the cancer (large hemorrhages are rare in patients with gastric cancer) is altered chemically and forms small clots or precipitates. The patient may not vomit but traces of blood may be found in the stools when examined in the laboratory.

When gastric juice, obtained by aspiration, reveals no free hydrochloric acid, gastric neoplasm is suspected. Biopsies through the gastroscope are most helpful. Cytologic studies verify the diagnosis. Occasionally the tumor is palpable, especially if it is located near the pylorus. Since metastasis frequently occurs before warning signs are experienced, roentgenograms, fluoroscopy, and gastroscopy are most valuable in determining the extent of the problem.

Dyspepsia of more than 4 weeks' duration in any person over 40 calls for complete roentgenographic examination of the gastrointestinal tract.

Surgical Management

There is no successful treatment of gastric carcinoma except removal of the tumor. If the tumor can be removed while it is still localized to the stomach, the patient can be cured. If the tumor has spread beyond the area that can be excised surgically, cure cannot be effected. However, in many of these patients, effective palliation may be obtained by resection of the tumor (see page 753, "Nursing Care Following Gastric Surgery"). If a *radical subtotal gastrectomy* has been performed, the stump of the stomach is anastomosed to the jejunum, as in the gastrectomy for ulcer. When *total gastrectomy* is performed, gastrointestinal continuity is restored by an anastomosis between the ends of the esophagus and jejunum. Palliative, rather than radical, surgery is done if there is metastasis to other vital organs, such as the liver.

NURSING MANAGEMENT OF PATIENTS UNDERGOING GASTRIC SURGERY

Part of the preoperative nursing plan involves preparing the patient for what to expect after the operation, such as nasogastric intubation and the giving of fluids intravenously. However, if the operation is an emergency, because of hemorrhage, perforation, or acute obstruction, adequate psychological preparation may not be possible. In this event, the nurse caring for the patient in the postoperative period should anticipate his concerns, fears, and queries, and be available for support and explanation.

Nursing Care Following Partial Resection

1. *Positioning the patient*
When recovery from anesthesia is complete, the patient is placed in a modified Fowler's position, for comfort and for easy drainage of the stomach.
2. *Avoiding pulmonary complications*
Pain medications are administered as prescribed, so that deep breathing and productive coughing may be effective in preventing pulmonary complications. This will overcome the patient's tendency to take shallow breaths in fear of incisional pain.
3. *Checking nasogastric tube drainage*
Drainage from the nasogastric tube may contain some blood for the first 12 hours, but excessive bleeding should be reported. Since a nasogastric tube is in place and peristalsis has not yet recommenced, fluids by mouth are withheld.
4. *Giving nose and mouth care*
The nostrils can be cleaned with an applicator stick moistened with water, followed by swabbing with another applicator stick dipped in mineral oil. To relieve dryness of the mouth, mouthwashes may be given frequently. Cool water sponges to the lips are preferred to cracked ice chips, since ice often intensifies thirst.
5. *Attending to fluid needs*
Parenteral fluids are given to meet fluid and nutritional needs, as well as to compensate for fluid lost in drainage and vomitus. Fluid input as well as output is recorded.

Following the return of peristalsis and the removal of the nasogastric tube, fluids by mouth may be restricted for several hours, then begun sparingly. Small amounts of water are used at first, after which the amount is gradually increased as tolerated. Cold fluids usually cause distress. Therefore warm, weak tea with sugar and lemon is preferred.
6. *Providing dietary intake*
Bland foods are gradually added until the patient is able to eat six small meals a day and drink 120 ml. of fluid between meals. The key to increasing the dietary content is to offer increments gradually as tolerated and to recog-

nize that each person is different. If regurgitation occurs, the patient may be eating too fast or too much. It also may indicate that edema along the suture line is preventing fluids and food from moving into the intestinal tract. If gastric retention does occur, it may be necessary to reinstitute naogastric suction.

7. *Encouraging ambulation*

Usually on the first postoperative day, the patient is encouraged to get out of bed. Ambulation is then increased daily.

8. *Providing wound care*

Wound dressings may have serosanguineous drainage because of drainage tubes left in the wound. Dressings are reinforced if necessary; however, undue drainage saturation is reported.

Total Resection

Nursing management of the patient having a total gastric resection will include that care described on page 350 ("Postoperative Abdominal Surgical Care") and page 423 ("Postoperative Chest Surgical Care"), since the chest cavity is usually entered. Nasogastric suction will not involve as much drainage, since the stomach is no longer present to produce secretions or to act as a receptacle. The nasogastric tube is removed as soon as normal bowel sounds are heard. Clear fluids are given hourly and small feedings offered after 2 or 3 days, providing there is no evidence of anastomosis leakage (temperature elevation), edema, or obstruction (regurgitation). If there is regurgitation or an increase in temperature, report it immediately.

For an outline of overall nursing management following gastric resection, see page 753.

Nutritional Management after Gastric Surgery

Often a patient who has had gastric surgery has been undernourished before the operation because of food intolerance or preoperative diagnostic testing. There may be significant protein deficiency, which may require parenteral nutritional support (page 728) for the first 5 or 6 postoperative days. Mouth feeding is resumed as soon as the patient feels hungry and bowel sounds are elicited.

Dysphagia may be noticed in those patients who have had truncal vagotomy, which causes trauma to the lower esophagus. This patient may be more comfortable on a soft diet for the first 10 days to 2 weeks. To encourage the patient to eat, attractive dishes and appetizing food should be served in a pleasant atmosphere. With regard to long-term management of this patient, weight loss is a common problem due to diminished food intake, since the patient experiences early fullness which, in turn, curbs his appetite. Anorexia may also be due to the "dumping syndrome," which occurs in about one-fifth

of individuals, following partial gastrectomy (see "Dumping Syndrome," page 752).

Appropriate nursing intervention is to suggest the following patient teaching points:

- Fluids should be taken before or between meals, rather than with meals.
- Smaller but more frequent meals should be eaten.
- Meal composition should be more dry than fluid-filled.
- Diets with small-molecule carbohydrates, such as sucrose and glucose, should be avoided, but fat may be consumed to tolerable levels.
- It may be advisable to supplement diet with vitamins and medium-chain triglycerides.

Other dietary deficiencies which the nurse should be cognizant of include (1) malabsorption of organic iron, which may have to be supplemented with oral or parenteral iron; (2) low serum level of vitamin B_{12}, which may require supplementation by the intramuscular route.

Postoperative Complications

(For an overall outline of the complications following gastric resection and the related nursing management, see chart on page 753.)

Shock. Shock has been mentioned as a complication, especially in very ill patients. The restoration of normal temperature and the administration of fluids are the prophylactic measures necessary. For symptoms and treatment of shock, see pages 364–370.

Hemorrhage. Hemorrhage is occasionally a complication after gastric operations. The patient exhibits the usual signs (page 370) and may vomit bright red blood in considerable amounts. Since this experience can prove upsetting to the patient, diazepam (Valium) or phenobarbital is effective in lessening patient apprehension. Nasogastric drainage and/or lavage is also helpful. Adrenalin hydrochloride solution may be given to produce vasoconstriction.

- When hemorrhage occurs, it is important to initiate antishock measures and notify the physician. Blood, blood substitutes, and intravenous equipment are made available.
- Nursing support of the patient is given concurrently with emergency therapy.

Pulmonary Complications. Pulmonary complications frequently follow upper abdominal incisions because of the tendency to shallow respirations. Therefore, the nurse utilizes foresight and initiates appropriate preventive measures to promote optimum oxygen-carbon dioxide exchange and adequate circulation.

Steatorrhea. Steatorrhea (unabsorbed fat in stool) is partially the result of rapid gastric emptying, which prevents adequate mixing with pancreatic and biliary secretions. In mild cases, steatorrhea can be controlled by reducing the intake of fat and taking an antimotility drug.

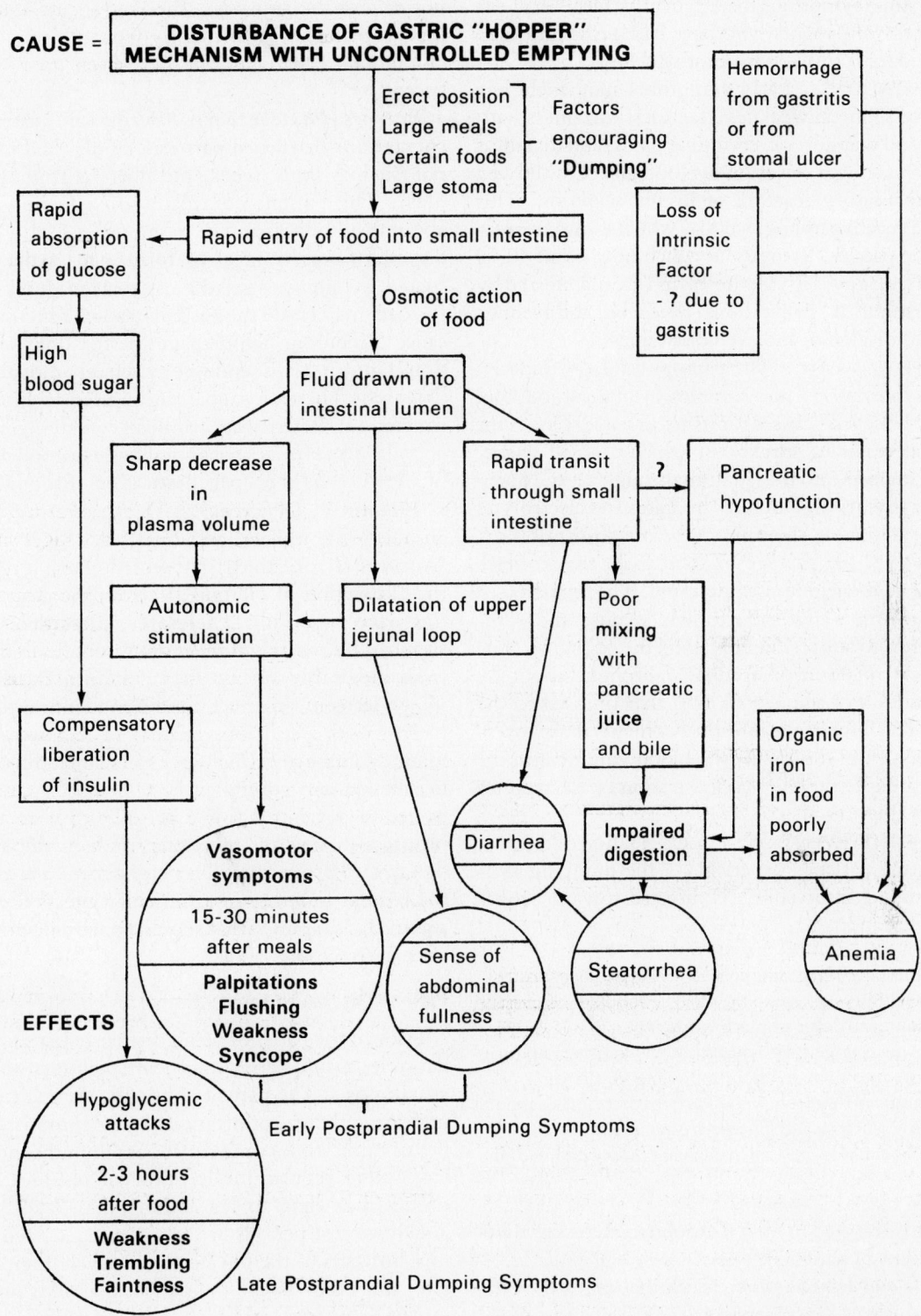

Figure 36-3. Mechanisms underlying some of the complications of partial gastrectomy and gastroenterostomy—"Dumping Syndrome" (Truelove, S., and Reynell, P.: Diseases of the Digestive System, 2nd ed. London, Blackwell Scientific Pub.)

The Dumping Syndrome. The term *dumping syndrome* designates an unpleasant set of vasomotor and gastrointestinal symptoms that occur after meals in about 10-50 percent of patients who have had gastrointestinal surgery and/or a form of vagotomy.

MANIFESTATIONS. Early symptoms may include a sensation of fullness, weakness, faintness, dizziness, palpitations, and diaphoresis, cramping pains, and diarrhea. Later, there is a rapid elevation of blood glucose followed by a compensatory reaction of insulin secretion. This results in a reactive hypoglycemia, which is also unpleasant for the patient. Symptoms which may occur 10-90 minutes after eating are vasomotor and are manifested by pallor, perspiration, palpitations, headache, and feelings of warmth, dizziness, and even drowsiness.

PATHOPHYSIOLOGY. The pathophysiology underlying this syndrome is not completely understood, but there may be several causes for its occurrence. One is the mechanical result of surgery in which a small gastric remnant connects into the jejunum through a large opening. Foods that are high in carbohydrates and electrolytes have to be diluted in the jejunum before absorption can take place, yet the passage of food from the stomach remnant into the jejunum is too rapid. The ingestion of fluid at mealtime is another factor which causes the stomach contents to empty rapidly into the jejunum. The symptoms that occur are probably brought about by rapid distention of the jejunal loop anastomosed to the stomach. The hypertonic intestinal contents draw extracellular fluid from the circulating blood volume into the jejunum to dilute the high concentration of electrolytes and sugars (Fig. 36-3).

NURSING INTERVENTION. In anticipation of the possibility of the patient's experiencing the dumping syndrome, nursing intervention is directed toward proper dietary instruction.

- The patient should be positioned in a semirecumbent position during mealtime. Following the meal he should lie down for 20-30 minutes to delay stomach emptying.
- Fluids are discouraged with meals but may be given up to an hour before mealtime or 1 hour following mealtime.
- Fat may be given to tolerance, but carbohydrate intake should be kept low (sucrose and glucose are avoided).
- Antispasmodics also may aid in delaying the emptying of the stomach.

Surgery is resorted to only if absolutely necessary (less than 1 percent of patients).

Gastritis and Esophagitis. With the removal of the pylorus, which acted as a barrier to the reflux of duodenal contents, a bile reflux gastritis and esophagitis may occur. This is manifested by burning epigastric pain and the vomiting of bilious material. Eating or vomiting does not relieve the situation. Binding agents such as cholestyramine, aluminum hydroxide gel, or Metoclopramide Hydrochloride have been used with some success.

Bezoars (Phytobezoar). Bezoars are gastrointestinal concretions (hardened particles) of digested plant material (such as skins, seeds, and fibers of fruit and vegetables). The patient complains of a feeling of upper abdominal fullness and a "dragging" sensation. The undigested fibers congeal to form a mass that becomes coated by mucous secretions; this produces a *bezoar*. Bezoars may erode the gastrointestinal mucosa and may cause ulceration, hemorrhage, perforation, or obstruction. Upon x-ray or endoscopy, a freely movable mass is observed. The endoscope can be used to break up the concretion. Restricting cellulose-containing foods (especially citrus fruits such as oranges) is a good prophylactic measure, as is proper mastication of food.

Vitamin B$_{12}$ Deficiency. Total gastrectomy brings to an abrupt, complete, and final halt the production of "intrinsic factor," the gastric secretion that is required for the absorption of vitamin B$_{12}$ from the gastrointestinal tract (see page 710). Therefore, unless this vitamin is supplied by parenteral injection throughout life, the patient inevitably suffers from vitamin B$_{12}$ deficiency, which leads in time to a condition identical to that of a patient with pernicious anemia in relapse. All of the manifestations of pernicious anemia, including macrocytic anemia and combined system disease, may be expected to develop within a period of 5 years or less, to progress in severity thereafter, and, in the absence of therapy, to prove fatal. This complication is avoided by the regular monthly intramuscular injection of 100-200 μg. of B$_{12}$, a regimen that should be started without delay after gastrectomy.

Patient Discharge Instructions

Prior to the patient's being discharged, a gastrointestinal series may be done to observe the functioning of the anastomosis. The patient is usually advised to continue increasing the size of his meals and to diminish the number of eating times until, in about 6 months, he is able to have three regular meals. Gradual resumption of activities according to his abilities may take 3 months. Adequate rest periods are recommended each day. Follow-up visits to the physician are psychologically effective, since they assure the patient that all is progressing satisfactorily and that his questions will be answered. Dietary consultation may be required.

PRINCIPLES OF NURSING MANAGEMENT OF A PATIENT FOLLOWING A GASTRIC RESECTION

MAJOR PROBLEMS
1. Postoperative pain and discomfort
2. Maintenance of adequate nutrition
3. Prevention of complications

OBJECTIVES
I. To relieve the patient of pain and discomfort:
   A. Frequent turning for comfort and for the prevention of pulmonary and vascular complications.
   B. Meticulous oral hygiene to counteract mouth dryness.
   C. Analgesics or narcotics for pain control.
   D. Parenteral antibiotics for prevention of infection.
   E. Oral fluids withheld until prescribed (to allow sealing of suture line).
   F. Gastric suction to remove liquids, blood, and gas from stomach.

II. To promote adequate nutrition:
   A. Intravenous fluids to prevent shock and maintain optimal fluid and electrolyte balance.
   B. Oral fluids when audible bowel sounds are present.
   C. Fluids to be increased according to patient's tolerance.
   D. Bland diet with vitamin supplements as indicated by patient's condition.
   E. Supplementary iron-vitamin therapy to ensure adequate intake.
   F. Avoidance of foods that may initiate development of "dumping syndrome." (III. F.)

III. To develop an awareness of complications that may follow gastric surgery:
   A. Shock
      1. Evaluate drainage from dressing and drainage bottle.
      2. Evaluate blood pressure, pulse, and respiratory rates.
      3. Give blood and fluid replacement at time prescribed.
   B. Hemorrhage
      1. Watch gastric aspirate in drainage bottle for evidence of blood.
      2. Observe the suture line for bleeding.
      3. Evaluate blood pressure, pulse, and respiratory rates.
      4. Prepare patient for blood transfusion, and start replacement if indicated.
      5. If bleeding continues, prepare patient for surgical intervention.
   C. Pulmonary complications
      1. Encourage deep breathing and coughing to counteract voluntary diaphragm splinting.
      2. Promote frequent turning and moving to mobilize bronchial secretions.
      3. Ambulate, when prescribed, to increase respiratory exchange.
   D. Thrombosis and embolism
      1. Encourage participation in self-care activities to increase circulation.

2. Encourage early ambulation to minimize stasis of venous blood.
3. Use elastic stockings as indicated to prevent venous stasis.
4. Check dressing and binders for tightness that impairs circulation.

E. Wound evisceration
   1. Use abdominal binders if prescribed for support.
   2. Prevent distention and wound infection.
   3. Support incision when coughing.
   4. Promote good nutrition.
   5. Inspect dressing frequently.

F. "Dumping syndrome"
   1. Teach patient to avoid eating large meals.
   2. Avoid salty, or highly concentrated carbohydrate foods.
   3. Take fluids between meals.
   4. Avoid liquids with meals.
   5. Eliminate sweets from the diet.
   6. Eat regularly, slowly, and in a relaxed environment.
   7. Lie down after meals.
   8. Take anticholinergic drugs before meals (as directed) to lessen gastrointestinal activity.

G. Leakage from duodenal stump (disruption of duodenum)
   1. Evaluate for pain, elevation of temperature, accelerated pulse rate, abdominal rigidity, and deteriorating clinical course.
   2. Observe for appearance of bile-stained drainage.
   3. Prepare for surgical drainage.
      a. Obtain drainage equipment.
      b. Prepare for intravenous infusions and blood transfusions.
      c. Institute nasogastric suction.
      d. Protect skin from irritating drainage.

H. Pancreatitis
   1. Assess for abdominal pain, rapid pulse, and temperature elevation.
      a. Establish continuous gastric suction.
      b. Maintain fluid and blood volume and electrolyte balance.
      c. Control pain.
      d. Give medications and antibiotics as prescribed.

IV. To promote the rehabilitation of the patient:
   A. Help him to modify his environmental stresses.
   B. Encourage him to remain under medical supervision.
   C. Advise adequate caloric intake after discharge from the hospital.
   D. Weigh regularly.
   E. Have yearly hematologic study and medical evaluation for evidences of pernicious anemia.

BIBLIOGRAPHY

BOOKS

Bockus, H. L., et al.: Gastroenterology. Philadelphia, W. B. Saunders, 1976.

Brooks, F. P. (ed.): Gastrointestinal Pathophysiology, 2nd ed. New York, Oxford Univ. Press, 1978.

Given, B. A., and Simmons, S. J.: Gastroenterology in Clinical Nursing, 3rd ed. St. Louis, C. V. Mosby, 1979.

Hill, R. B., and Kern, F., Jr.: The Gastrointestinal Tract. Baltimore, Williams and Wilkins, 1977.

Sleisenger, M. H., and Fordtran, J. S.: Gastrointestinal Disease (Pathophysiology, Diagnosis, Management). Philadelphia, W. B. Saunders, 1978.

Spiro, H. M.: Gastroenterology, 2nd ed. New York, Macmillan Co., 1977.

ARTICLES

General

Breu, C., and Dracup, K.: Helping the spouses of critically ill patients. AJN, 78:50-53, Jan. 1978.

Black, C. D., et al.: Drug interactions in the gastrointestinal tract. AJN, 77:1426-1429, Sept. 1977.

Long, G. D.: G.I. bleeding. Nursing '78, 8:44-50, Mar. 1978.

Stroup, P.: Recognition and management of G.I. bleeds. J. Emerg. Nsg., 4:19-25, Sept.-Oct. 1978.

Welling, P. G.: How food and fluid affect drug absorption. Postgrad. Med., 62:73-82, July 1977.

Wichern, W. A.: The surgical abdomen. Postgrad. Med., 62:145-148, Nov. 1977.

Peptic Ulcer and Gastric Conditions

Acetaminophen hepatotoxicity. Med. Letter, 20:61, July 1978.

Baron, J. H., and Spencer, J.: Facts and heresies about vagotomy. Surg. Clin. N. Am., 56:1297-1312, Nov. 1976.

Bodemar, G., et al.: Diminished absorption of cimetidine caused by antacids. Lancet, 1:444-445, Feb. 24, 1979.

Borland, J. L.: Rational management of peptic ulcer disease. Hosp. Pract., 11:33-38, July 1976.

Brunner, L. S.: What to do (and what to teach your patient) about peptic ulcer. Nursing '76, 6:27-34, Nov. 1976.

Chapman, M. L.: Peptic ulcer, a medical perspective. Med. Clin. N. Am., 62:39-51, Jan. 1978.

Cimetidine (Tagamet): update on adverse effects. Med. Letter, 20:77-78, Sept. 1978.

Clayman, C. B.: Evaluation of cimetidine (Tagamet). JAMA, 238:1289-1290, Sept. 1977.

Conn, H. O., and Blitzer, B. L.: Nonassociation of adrenocorticosteroid therapy and peptic ulcer. New Eng. J. Med., 294:473-479, Feb. 1976.

Conn, H. O., et al.: Selective intraarterial vasopressin in the treatment of upper gastrointestinal hemorrhage. Gastroenterol., 63:634-635, Oct. 1972.

Cohen, S., and Uooth, G. H., Jr.: Gastric acid secretion and lower-esophageal sphincter pressure in response to coffee and caffeine. New Eng. J. Med., 293:897-899, Oct. 1975.

Finkelstein, W., and Isselbacher, K. J.: Cimetidine. New Eng. J. Med., 299:992-996, Nov. 1978.

Fisher, R. S., and Cohen, S.: Gastroesophageal reflux. Med. Clin. N. Am., 62:3-20, Jan. 1978.

Fordtran, J. S.: Placebos, antacids and cimetidine for duodenal ulcer. New Eng. J. Med., 298:1081-1083, May 1978.

Gold, M. H., Jr., et al.: Cellulose bezoar injection: A new endoscopic technique. Gastroint. Endosc., 22:200-202, May 1976.

Grossman, M. I.: Elevated serum pepsinogen I: a genetic marker for duodenal disease (edit). New Eng. J. Med., 300:89, Jan. 1979.

Harris, A. I., and Janowitz, H. D.: Medical management of problems following peptic ulcer surgery. Postgrad. Med., 63:127-132, Apr. 1978.

Hedberg, S. E.: Endoscopy in gastrointestinal bleeding, Surg. Clin. N. Am., 54:549-559, June 1974.

Hines, J. R.: Duodenal ulcer: selecting patients for surgical treatment. Mod. Med., 46:36-39, Mar. 1978.

MacGregor, I., et al.: Gastric emptying of liquid meals and pancreatic and biliary secretion after subtotal gastrectomy or truncal vagotomy and pyloroplasty in man. Gastroenterol., 72:195-205, Feb. 1977.

Menguy, R.: Gastric mucosal injury from common drugs. Postgrad. Med., 63:82-86, Apr. 1978.

Meredith, P. S.: Decline in duodenal ulcer surgery. JAMA, 237:987-988, March 1977.

More on Tagamet: some not so good. Nurses' Drug Alert, 2:16, Feb. 1978.

Over-the-counter antacid preparations can have adverse effects on bone. JAMA, 238:1018, Sept. 1977.

Page, C. P.: Continual catheter administration of elemental diets. Contemp. Surg., 12:29-32, June 1978.

Passaro, E., and Stabile, B. E.: Late complications of vagotomy. Postgrad. Med., 63:135-141, Apr. 1978.

Penn, I.: Management of the perforated duodenal ulcer. Heart & Lung, 7:111-117, Jan.-Feb. 1978.

Peptic Ulcer. *In* Thorn, G. W. (ed.): Harrison's Principles of Internal Medicine, 8th ed. New York, McGraw-Hill, 1977.

Rotter, J. T.: Duodenal-ulcer disease associated with elevated serum pepsinogen I. New Eng. J. Med., 300:63-65, Jan. 1979.

Rudick, J.: Peptic ulcer, surgical alternatives. Med. Clin. N. Am., 62:53-57, Jan. 1978.

Sawyers, J. L.: Proximal gastric vagotomy without drainage. Postgrad. Med., 63:115-121, Apr. 1978.

Spiro, H. M.: Duodenal ulcer, (Chap. 14); Gastric Ulcer, (Chap. 15); Complications (Chap. 16). *In* Spiro: Clinical Gastroenterology. New York, Macmillan, 1977.

Sturdevant, R. A. L., et al.: Antacid and placebo produce similar pain relief in duodenal ulcer patients. Gastroenterol., 72:1-5, Jan. 1977.

Symposium on peptic ulcer (entire issue). Surg. Clin. N. Am., 56:Dec. 1976.

Timms, D.: M.I. scare to total gastrectomy — in one incredible patient. RN, 41:63-69, Oct. 1978.

Wyllie, J. H.: Histamine H_2-receptor antagonist. Postgrad. Med., 63:91-97, Apr. 1978.

Zollinger, R. M.: Preoperative evaluation of patients with duodenal ulcer. Postgrad. Med., 63:105-111, Apr. 1978.

AGENCY

National Institute of Arthritis, Metabolism, and Digestive Diseases, National Institutes of Health, Bethesda, Md. 20205

37

MANAGEMENT OF PATIENTS WITH INTESTINAL DISORDERS

CONSTIPATION

Constipation is a term which describes an abnormal infrequency of defecation, and also abnormal dryness of the stools.

Obstipation (no bowel movements) is indicative of bowel obstruction or adynamic ileus.

Chronic Constipation

Most normal persons have one bowel movement a day. Some, however, go 2, 3, or 4 days without a movement; their stools are normally moist, and they suffer no discomfort. On the other hand, some constipated persons at times have a diarrhea of liquid stools, due to the irritation caused by the presence in the colon of hard, dry fecal masses. Such stools contain a good deal of mucus, secreted by glands in the colon in response to these irritating masses. In severe constipation, the rectum may become impacted, that is, filled with masses of hard feces that must be removed by the fingers or first softened by instillations of oil before they can be washed out by an enema.

Assessment

To establish a data base for assessing the patient, the following information should be elicited.
1. Do you have a sense of fullness or distention? Is this discomfort relieved by defecating?
2. Do you have pain or discomfort in your anus or rectum?
3. How would you describe your stool? Hard, dry, small, large, pelletlike, sticky, bulky?
4. Can you get to the bathroom when you have the urge to defecate?
5. Are you worried about your stool habits?
6. Do you use laxatives or enemas? Can you have a movement with these?
7. Have you noticed mucus, blood, pus, or undigested food particles in your stool?
8. Is this a new problem for you, or have you had it before?
9. Have you traveled recently? Out of the country?

Pathophysiology. There are few organic causes of chronic constipation. The most important of these are morphine addiction, lead poisoning, and cancer of the large bowel, a condition in which constipation usually alternates with diarrhea. Painful hemorrhoids and anal fissures, by inducing rectal spasm, also may lead to temporary constipation. Other factors that predispose to its development include limitation of muscular exercise, unfamiliar diet, weakness, debility, and fatigue.

By far the most common type of constipation is functional, rather than organic. Many patients develop a constipation habit because of the careless or neurotic habit of delaying each bowel movement as long as possible. The rectal mucous membrane and musculature become insensitive to the presence of fecal masses, and consequently the stimulus required to produce the necessary peristaltic rush for defecation becomes increasingly greater. The initial effect of this fecal retention, or hoarding, is to produce irritability of the colon, which, at this

755

stage, goes frequently into spasm, especially after meals, giving rise to colicky midabdominal or low abdominal pains. Eventually, after several years, the colon loses muscular tone; it is essentially unresponsive to normal stimuli. At this point, the patient may be said to have *atonic constipation,* whereas in the earlier stage the condition is sometimes referred to as *spastic constipation,* although neither type should be regarded as a separate entity.

Patient Education. In simple or functional constipation, the role of the nurse is to assist with the reeducation of the patient. The physiology of defecation should be explained carefully, with particular emphasis on the importance of heeding promptly the urge to defecate. Instruct the patient to have a regular time for defecation, preferably after a meal. Thinking about the act of defecation, i.e., "autosuggestion," may be an aid in initiating the reflex. A small footstool to promote flexion of the thighs ensures an optimal posture during defecation.

Patients who worry about having a *daily* bowel movement need reassurance. Carefully explain that some healthy persons have a bowel movement three times daily while others do so only two or three times a week. Knowing that some of the food eaten may normally remain in the intestinal tract 48 hours after ingestion will help the patient to understand and accept the fact that a daily bowel evacuation is not always necessary. The use of laxatives should be discontinued. If the feces remain in the rectum too long and become dehydrated and hardened, the patient may be instructed to instill 60-90 ml. (2-3 oz.) of warm oil into the rectum at bedtime. A small enema of physiologic saline the next morning should help to alleviate this condition.

Measures helpful in breaking the constipation habit include:
1. Establishing a regular time to go to stool each day.
2. Drinking a large glass of prune juice or lemon juice in warm water each morning.
3. Taking a bulk-forming laxative that does not irritate the bowel, such as Metamucil: one heaping teaspoonful in a glass of water, followed by a second glass of water, once or twice daily.
4. Assuring a plentiful daily fluid intake.

The patient must know what constitutes a normal diet and should be aware of the similarities between his prescribed diet and the normal diet. In general, a high-residue, high-fiber diet is prescribed for atonic constipation; a bland or low-residue diet is indicated for the patient with an irritable colon (see Table 37-1). Approximately the same amount of food should be eaten at each meal, and 2 liters of fluid ingested daily (or more, if the patient perspires freely).

Acute Constipation

Acute constipation, in contrast with the chronic variety, always indicates an acute and, frequently, a serious disorder. The symptom may prompt one to think in terms of a laxative, but it must be remembered that acute constipation may be an early symptom of acute appendicitis, and that a purge given in this condition may well produce perforation of the inflamed appendix. In general, a cathartic should not be given for fever, nausea, or pain merely because the bowels fail to move; and, before such medication is offered, it must be quite clear that no inflammatory disease of the intestinal tract is present.

Enemas are relatively safe as regards the possible perforation of an inflammatory lesion of the bowel, provided that they are administered with extreme caution. Saline solutions, or water alone, may be instilled, but nothing more irritating should be used, and the nurse should be prepared to halt the irrigation at once if pain is induced or increased in the slightest degree.

Complications of Constipation

The maintenance of elimination is basic to the care of every patient. The mechanical difficulties and the physical discomforts associated with defecation and micturition that harass the bed patient are widely known. The effort entailed in defecation is considerable. With the use of a bedpan the muscular strain is inevitably greater, and when constipation is imposed in addition, the performance of this function can be extremely fatiguing, if not altogether exhausting. This is a serious consideration in the management of patients with congestive heart failure, those who have suffered a recent myocardial infarction and are susceptible to cardiac rupture, and those with arterial hypertension.

Straining at stool has a striking effect on the arterial blood pressure (Valsalva maneuver). During the period

TABLE 37-1. A SUGGESTED RELATIONSHIP BETWEEN DIET AND EFFECT ON INTESTINE

DIET	MOVEMENT	BULK	CONSISTENCY	INTRALUMEN PRESSURE	SUSCEPTIBILITY TO DISEASE
High-residue Bulky Unrefined	Rapid	Large	Soft	Low	Low
Low residue Concentrated Refined	Slow	Small	Hard	High	High

of active straining, the flow of venous blood in the chest is temporarily impeded, due to an increase in intrathoracic pressure that tends to collapse the large veins in the chest. The atria and the ventricles receive less blood, and consequently less is delivered by the systolic contractions of the left ventricle; the cardiac output is decreased, and there is a transient drop in arterial pressure. Almost immediately after this period of hypotension, a rise in arterial pressure occurs; the pressure is elevated momentarily to a point far exceeding the original level (the "rebound" phenomenon). In patients with arterial hypertension, this compensatory reaction may be exaggerated greatly, and the peaks of pressure attained may be dangerously high — sufficient, indeed, to rupture a major artery in the brain or elsewhere.

It is not possible to make more than a rough estimate of the frequency with which the act of defecation is the terminal event and brings on death due to vascular accidents that result from straining at stool. The danger is not sufficiently appreciated, however, particularly in patients with vascular diseases of the type described. Inasmuch as straining is promoted by constipation, the latter cannot be dismissed as altogether inconsequential; on the contrary, it must be concluded that the regularity and the consistency of the stools, as well as the mechanical aspects of defecation, are matters of primary concern.

To facilitate elimination, the patient should assume the normal position for defecation. In most instances there is less strain if the patient is assisted to a bedside commode. Or the patient may be seated on the bedpan at the side of the bed, with his feet supported on a chair. If he cannot sit up, a small support should be placed under the lumbosacral curve to minimize strain and increase his comfort while using the bedpan.

DIARRHEA

Diarrhea is one of the cardinal symptoms of small-bowel disease. It is a condition in which there is unusual frequency of bowel movements, as well as changes in the amount, the character, and the consistency of the stools. It is best defined, quantitatively, as more than 200 gm. of stool per day.

Clinical Manifestations. In acute cases the stools are grayish-brown, foul smelling, and filled with undigested particles of food and mucus. The patient complains of abdominal cramps, distention, intestinal rumbling (borborygmus), anorexia, and thirst. Painful spasms (tenesmus) of the anus may attend each defecation.

Nursing Assessment. Diarrhea and its associated symptoms occur in a variety of disorders. The nurse will facilitate the diagnosis in each case by recording discerning observations, including the patient's symptoms, behavior, and remarks. Watery stools are characteristic of small-bowel disease, whereas loose, semisolid stools are associated more often with disorders of the colon. Voluminous, greasy stools suggest intestinal malabsorption, and the presence of mucus and pus in the stools denotes inflammatory enteritis or colitis. Oil droplets in the toilet water are almost always diagnostic of pancreatic insufficiency. Nocturnal diarrhea may be a manifestation of diabetic neuropathy.

Questions to ask the patient include:
- Do you have loose stools or more frequent stools? How frequent?
- What do they look like?
- How long have you had this problem? Is this the first time?
- Does this occur during the day only? Just in the morning? Nightly too?
- Is there an urgency about your movements? Signs of incontinency?
- Have you noticed mucus mixed with your stool? Blood, pus, or undigested food?
- Have you traveled recently? Out of the country?

Acute Diarrhea

Pathophysiology. Most acute diarrheas are due to increased secretion of water and electrolytes by the intestinal mucosa. The irritant stimulating the diarrhea may arise from a localized infection or ulceration in the intestinal wall, due, for example, to a carcinoma, a diverticulitis, or a tuberculous lesion. The irritant may be chemical. Castor oil, after it has been acted upon by the digestive juice, is an example of a mild intestinal irritant, as are most of the vegetable cathartics. Certain unripe fruits, which cause crampy diarrhea, likewise belong in this category.

The inflammatory response to these mild irritants is slight; little or no mucous membrane lining is destroyed on exposure to them unless their concentration in the intestinal fluid is excessive. Their chief effect is to produce hyperemia (vascular dilatation, with local increase in blood flow) of the intestinal mucosa and increase in mucous secretion. There also occurs a motor response of hyperperistalsis, which persists until the irritant is excreted. This explains the symptoms of crampy diarrhea.

Infectious. By far the most common intestinal irritants are the products of certain bacteria, whether their growth occurred in the intestine or in the food before it was eaten. In the case of the enteric pathogens, the organisms causing bacillary dysentery, bacterial growth with release of the irritating toxins takes place in the intestine. On the other hand, practically all cases of food poisoning, or ptomaine poisoning, are due to the ingestion of food heavily contaminated and already containing the toxin. *Staphylococcus aureus,* for example, if given an opportunity to grow in food, produces an exotoxin that is extremely irritating to the intestinal tract.

Whether the gastrointestinal tract is exposed to toxins introduced in food or produced by bacteria growing within the intestine, an infectious enterocolitis is produced. The inflammatory response may vary from mild hyperemia and hypermotility of the gastrointestinal tract to severe inflammation of the intestine, depending on the virulence of the infecting organism and the amount of toxin liberated.

Clinically, except for the presence of diarrhea, there is little similarity between a case of food poisoning due to the ingestion of food containing bacterial toxins and a case of bacillary dysentery. The diarrhea in food poisoning is explosive in onset, develops within a very few hours following the toxic meal and, except in severe cases, subsides within 1 or 2 days—as soon as the toxin is excreted and the inflammatory response subsides. There is little or no fever, and usually the only associated symptoms are those directly attributable to the diarrhea, namely, dehydration and weakness.

Dysentery due to the growth of gastrointestinal pathogens within the gastrointestinal tract, on the other hand, develops with a more gradual onset, persists for several days or weeks, with striking constitutional symptoms in addition to the diarrhea.

These clinical differences are quite understandable when it is realized that in the infectious diarrheas, a bacterial invasion of the intestinal mucosa is involved. Then, not only must the bacterial toxins be excreted or destroyed, but also the bacteria themselves must be eradicated, and this takes considerably longer.

Assessment. The diagnosis of an acute diarrhea is based on the course of the disease: the type of onset and progression, the presence or absence of fever, and a study of the stools, which are examined for bacteria as well as for blood and pus. In cases of possible infection, the suspected food is tested by bacteriologic cultures. It is very important to remember that diarrhea often is present in various systemic infections. It may be the initial misleading complaint in certain of the exanthemata before the appearance of the rash, or it may appear as an early symptom of hepatitis. It may complicate or mask such conditions as pneumonia and pyelitis.

Management and Nursing Intervention. Patients with acute diarrhea are placed on bed rest until the episode has terminated. Fluid and electrolyte replacement, orally or parenterally, is an extremely important measure, symptomatically as well as supportively. During the acute stages the gastrointestinal tract is kept at rest by administering only liquids and foods low in bulk or by withholding oral feeding entirely. Glucose can be absorbed normally in many diarrheas and will reduce water loss.

The following antidiarrheal agents are given to delay the passage of food through the intestine: Kaopectate (hydrated aluminum silicate kaolin with pectin) as an adsorbent, and diphenoxylate hydrochloride (Lomotil); narcotics, such as paregoric (camphorated tincture of opium) and codeine, which delay transit through the intestine.

Preventive Health Measures. All cases of acute diarrhea should be treated as potentially infective until they are proved otherwise. If the diarrhea is of infectious origin, those caring for the patient should determine whether there is any diarrhea among the family and neighbors. Ask the patient about recent sources of food and water. By reporting a larger than usual number of cases of diarrhea, the nurse assists in determining whether an epidemic is starting in the community.

Proper precautions to avoid the spread of the disease through contamination of the hands, the clothing, the bed linen, etc., with feces or vomitus, must be taken.

Diarrhea always should be regarded as a potential risk under conditions of crowding; outbreaks occur with particular frequency in institutions such as prisons, boarding schools, army camps, trailer camps, and even hospitals, unless sanitary precautions are observed rigidly and constantly.

Precautions include ensuring that proper storage and refrigeration facilities are available and are used for the handling of all fresh fruits and meats. Meat products should be cooked thoroughly, and all cooked meats should be refrigerated immediately unless they are consumed promptly. Milk and milk products should be refrigerated constantly and protected against exposure. Food items that are particularly prone to infection and provide the best environment for bacterial growth include custards and cream fillings, such as are prepared in éclairs, cream pies, layer cakes, cream puffs, etc. Such materials should be cooked thoroughly and should then be brought to refrigerator temperature immediately, unless they are to be eaten within a very few hours after cooking.

Proper housekeeping, especially in kitchen maintenance, is obviously very important in the prevention of epidemic diarrhea. All materials used in the preparation and the serving of food must be cleansed rigorously and kept in immaculate condition. All food handlers should receive detailed instructions in hygienic principles and practices and, upon the development of any illness that is potentially infectious, should be relieved of their duties immediately.

DISEASES OF MALABSORPTION

Digestion is the process whereby nutrients are reduced to appropriate form for intestinal absorption. Intestinal absorption transports nutrients across the mucosa to the portal blood system.

Besides nutrients, the intestinal tract is the recipient of

a large volume of fluid and electrolytes. Of about 1,500 ml. of ingested liquid, plus about 7,000 ml. from the gastrointestinal tract (salivary, gastric, biliary, pancreatic, and intestinal sources), all but 500 ml. is absorbed proximal to the ileocecal valve. Thus the intestine continually shifts the volume and composition of its contents to fulfill its major function of absorption.

Interruptions in the complex digestive process may occur anywhere to cause *malabsorption*. The chief result of malabsorption is malnutrition manifested by weight loss. Diarrhea is a prominent symptom. Steatorrhea is of more specific value in diagnosis.

Malabsorption diseases may be grouped according to the following three classifications: (1) maldigestion, (2) decreased absorption by intestinal mucosa, (3) a combination of causes (see Table 37-2). In addition, certain

TABLE 37-2.   CLINICAL AND PATHOPHYSIOLOGIC ASPECTS OF DISEASES OF MALABSORPTION AND MALDIGESTION

DISEASES OF MALDIGESTION	PHYSIOLOGIC PATHOLOGY	CLINICAL FEATURES
Gastric resection with gastrojejunostomy	Decreased pancreatic stimulation because of duodenal bypass; poor mixing of food, bile, pancreatic enzymes; decreased intrinsic factor; bacterial stasis in afferent loop	Weight loss, moderate steatorrhea, anemia (combination of iron, vitamin B_{12} malabsorption, folate deficiency)
Pancreatic insufficiency (chronic pancreatitis, pancreatic carcinoma, pancreatic resection, cystic fibrosis)	Reduced intraluminal pancreatic enzyme activity, with maldigestion of lipid and protein	History of abdominal pain followed by weight loss; marked steatorrhea, azotorrhea; also frequent glucose intolerance (70 percent in pancreatic insufficiency)
Ileal dysfunction (resection or disease)	Loss of ileal absorbing surface leads to reduced bile-salt pool size and reduced vitamin B_{12} absorption; bile in colon inhibits fluid absorption	Diarrhea, weight loss with steatorrhea, especially when greater than 100 cm. resection, decreased vitamin B_{12} absorption
Stasis syndromes (surgical strictures, blind loops, enteric fistulas, multiple jejunal diverticula, scleroderma)	Overgrowth of intraluminal intestinal bacteria, especially anaerobic organisms, to greater than 10^6 per ml., results in deconjugation of bile salts, resulting in decreased effective bile-salt pool size, also bacterial utilization of vitamin B_{12}	Weight loss, steatorrhea; low vitamin B_{12} absorption; may have low D-xylose absorption
Zollinger-Ellison syndrome	Hyperacidity in duodenum inactivates pancreatic enzymes	Ulcer diathesis, steatorrhea
Lactose intolerance	Deficiency of intestinal lactase results in high concentration of intraluminal lactose with osmotic diarrhea	Affects 70 percent of U.S. blacks and probably all other non-Caucasian races; varied degrees of diarrhea and cramps after ingestion of lactose-containing foods; positive lactose tolerance test, decreased intestinal lactase
Celiac disease (gluten enteropathy)	Toxic response to a gluten fraction by surface epithelium results in destruction of absorbing surface	Weight loss, diarrhea, bloating, anemia (low iron, folate), osteomalacia, steatorrhea, azotorrhea, low D-xylose absorption; folate and iron malabsorption; diagnostic biopsy change
Tropical sprue	Unknown toxic factor results in mucosal inflammation, partial villous atrophy	Weight loss, diarrhea, anemia (low folate, vitamin B_{12}); steatorrhea; low D-xylose absorption, low vitamin B_{12} absorption; typical but nonspecific biopsy change
Whipple's disease	Bacterial invasion of intestinal mucosa	Arthritis, hyperpigmentation, lymphadenopathy, serous effusions, fever, weight loss; steatorrhea, azotorrhea, diagnostic biopsy change
Certain parasitic diseases (giardiasis strongyloidiasis, coccidiosis, capillariasis)	Damage to, or invasion of, surface mucosa	Diarrhea, weight loss; steatorrhea; organism may be seen on jejunal biopsy or recovered in stool
Immunoglobulinopathy	Decreased local gut defenses, lymphoid hyperplasia, lymphopenia	Frequent association with *Giardia*; hypogammaglobulinemia or isolated IgA deficiency; diagnostic or typical biopsy changes

(From: Halsted, J. A.: The Laboratory in Clinical Medicine. Philadelphia, W. B. Saunders, 1976, page 379)

inflammatory bowel disorders, such as ulcerative colitis and Crohn's disease, cause increased protein breakdown (catabolism) in the small intestine, with resulting loss of protein into the lumen of the intestine (protein-losing enteropathy).

The Primary Malabsorption States

The above term is applied to three closely related conditions: (1) *tropical sprue,* (2) idiopathic steatorrhea (nontropical sprue), and (3) *celiac disease.*

Pathophysiology and Clinical Manifestations. Tropical and nontropical sprue are diseases of adults; in clinical manifestations and pathologic changes, the two conditions are very similar. However, their geographic incidence and their causes differ, and they respond to different treatments. Celiac disease is limited to childhood but resembles idiopathic steatorrhea in all other respects, and probably represents the juvenile phase of that disease. Other causes are extensive resection of the small bowel and tumor infiltration of the small bowel wall.

The pathologic defect is similar in all three conditions. The principal lesion involves the mucosa of the small intestine, especially the intestinal villae, which become severely blunted or are lost altogether. As a result, the absorptive surface within the small bowel is substantially reduced in area, and food absorption is correspondingly impaired.

The hallmarks of the *malabsorption syndrome,* of whatever cause, are diarrhea or frequent loose, bulky, foul stools which have increased fat content and are often greyish in color; associated weakness, weight loss, and lack of well-being round out the picture.

Patients with the malabsorption syndrome, if neglected, become weak and emaciated, due to starvation. Failure to absorb the fat-soluble vitamins A, D, and K causes these patients to develop the corresponding avitaminoses. Manifestations of abnormal bleeding are likely to appear as a result of K deficiency and hypoprothrombinemia (page 674). Anemia develops, which is of the macrocytic type characteristic of folic-acid deficiency (page 662). Impaired absorption of calcium may be responsible for gradual demineralization of the skeleton and, in the case of children with celiac disease, for the stunting of growth. Moreover, calcium deficiency may lead to extreme neuromuscular hyperirritability, including attacks of hypocalcemic tetany.

Management. Dietary considerations are preeminent, as the basic factor in the pathogenesis of idiopathic steatorrhea and celiac disease is a specific and profound intolerance to a protein substance (gluten) contained in wheat, rye, and barley. A constituent of gluten, *gliadin,* for reasons that are not clear, exerts toxic effects on the mucosa of the small intestine, damaging or destroying its villi and crippling its function. The increased familial incidence of these disorders suggests that a hereditary factor, i.e., an inborn error of metabolism, may be involved, and that enzymatic activities governing the digestion of gliadin may be affected. In any case, the elimination of gluten from the patient's diet is followed by striking clinical improvement. His diarrhea ceases and his nutritional status is restored to normal. This gratifying remission may be expected to last as long as the patient remains on a gluten-free diet, and no longer. Unfortunately, the total exclusion of gluten is difficult to accomplish, since this substance is incorporated into many foods as a binder and filler. It is contained in almost every bakery product, "wheat-free" or otherwise, and is an ingredient of other foodstuffs as well, including some brands of ice cream.

The factors primarily responsible for the onset and the progression of tropical sprue have not as yet been clarified. Its clinical course appears to be unaffected by the presence or the absence of gliadin in the diet; hence gliadin intolerance seemingly plays no role in its pathogenesis. Of greatest benefit in this condition is the administration of folic acid, which usually is prescribed until a remission is established, and daily thereafter for a period of 4 to 6 months. Broad-spectrum antibiotics are equally important. The beneficial effects of folic acid in patients with tropical sprue appear with such regularity and on occasion are so striking as to suggest that this particular malabsorption syndrome may be attributable to, as well as productive of, folic-acid deficiency.

APPENDICITIS

The appendix is a small, fingerlike appendage about 10 cm. (4 inches) long, attached to the cecum just below the ileocecal valve. No definite function can be assigned to it in man. It fills with food and empties as regularly as does the cecum, of which it is a part. It empties inefficiently, however, and its lumen is very small, so that it is prone to become obstructed and is particularly vulnerable to infection (appendicitis).

Appendicitis is the most common cause of acute inflammation in the right lower quadrant of the abdominal cavity. About 6 percent of the population will have appendicitis at some time in their lives; males are affected more than females, and teenagers more than adults.

Clinical Manifestations

Acute appendicitis starts typically with a progressively severe generalized or upper abdominal pain, which, within a few hours, becomes localized in the right lower quadrant of the abdomen. This pain usually is accompanied by a low-grade fever, and often by vomiting. At McBurney's point, located halfway between the umbilicus and the anterior spine of the ilium, local tenderness is noted when pressure is applied and there is some rigidity of the lower portion of the right rectus muscle. A moderate leukocytosis is often present. Loss of appetite is common.

Just how much tenderness there will be, how much muscle spasm, whether or not there is constipation or diarrhea, etc., depend not so much on the severity of the appendiceal infection as on the location of the appendix. If the appendix curls around behind the cecum (retrocecal appendix), pain and tenderness may be felt in the lumbar region; if its tip is in the pelvis, these signs may be elicited only on rectal examination. Pain on defecation suggests that its tip is against the rectum; pain on micturition, that it is near the bladder or impinges on the ureter. Eventually, the inflamed appendix fills with pus and then is apt to perforate. Once it has ruptured, the pain becomes more diffuse; abdominal distention develops, due to paralytic ileus, and the condition of the patient worsens.

Assessment

When these symptoms occur in the male, they may be strongly suggestive of acute appendicitis. In the female between 10 and 40 years of age, these manifestations may also suggest a problem with an ovarian cyst, ruptured ovarian follicle or corpus luteum, ruptured ectopic pregnancy, or mittelschmerz (intermenstrual pain).

Upon physical examination, common findings include local and rebound tenderness. Early gentle palpation of the abdomen reveals diffuse tenderness around the umbilicus and midepigastrium. As the condition progresses, pain shifts to the lower right quadrant. If the patient coughs or the anterior abdominal wall is percussed, pain is enhanced. An interesting Rovsing's sign may be elicited by palpating the left lower quadrant (Fig. 37-1), which, paradoxically, causes pain to be felt by the patient in the right lower quadrant.

The more severe the pain, the more the patient will guard and protect the abdomen, and the greater will be muscular rigidity.

A posture of right hip flexion is a protective maneuver by the patient, suggesting irritation of the psoas muscle (positive psoas sign) by the inflamed appendix. Application of an ice pack (*never of heat*) may provide comfort.

Management and Nursing Intervention

Operation is always indicated if acute appendicitis is suspected, unless there is good evidence that perforation has occurred recently and that a generalized peritonitis has developed. Many surgeons believe that with free peritonitis, removal of the cause, along with copious irrigation, is effective. When the patient is treated conservatively, he is given parenteral electrolyte and amino acid solutions, gastric suction, and antibiotics, in the expectation that the infection will localize and be suscep-

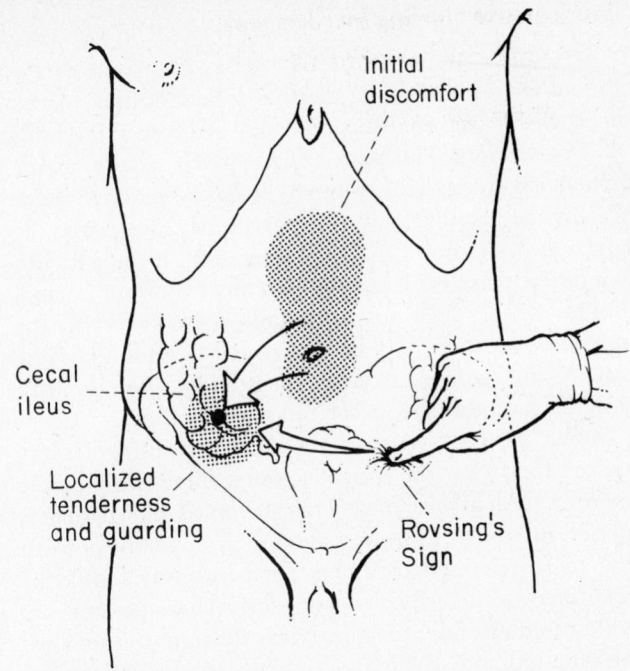

Figure 37-1. This illustrates the area of initial discomfort in appendicitis. As the inflammation progresses, discomfort shifts to the lower right segment of the abdomen. To elicit Rovsing's sign, pressure in the left lower quadrant will intensify pain in the right lower quadrant. (Gelin, L. E., et al.: Abdominal Pain: A Guide to Rapid Diagnosis. Philadelphia, J. B. Lippincott, 1969)

tible to surgical drainage. As long as the question of operation is undecided, morphine is withheld, even in the face of moderate suffering, because it may mask the patient's symptoms. After the decision has been made, the patient may be sedated comfortably.

Preparation for Operation

If an operation is necessary, the patient is carefully prepared; an intravenous infusion is started, to establish good urinary output and replace existing fluid loss. Acetylsalicylic acid may be prescribed to lower the elevated temperature. Antibiotic therapy is often instituted as a preventive measure against infection. If there is evidence or likelihood of paralytic ileus, a nasogastric tube may be passed. The patient is asked to void, the abdomen is shaved, and the prescribed preoperative medications are given. Usually an enema is not given, but, if one is requested, it is given low and slowly. Chemotherapy and/ or antibiotics are administered before and after surgery.

If the patient has been suffering from acute abdominal pain, he accepts the operation as a means of relief. This acceptance of surgery makes his anesthetic and postanesthetic course a relatively easy one. The operation may be performed under general or spinal anesthesia. The usual incisions are the McBurney, the muscle-splitting or the gridiron, and the Rockey-Davis (transverse).

Postoperative Nursing Management

APPENDECTOMY WITHOUT DRAINAGE. As soon as the patient recovers from the anesthesia, he should be placed in Fowler's position. Morphine may be given at intervals of 3 or 4 hours. Fluids are usually given as soon as the patient can tolerate them, unless he has been dehydrated. In this case they are given intravenously. Food may be given as desired on the day of operation, if the patient's condition permits. If his temperature is within normal limits and he does not have undue discomfort in the operative area, he may be discharged in 48 hours. The stitches are removed from the incision between the fifth and the seventh days, in the physician's office.

APPENDECTOMY WITH DRAINAGE. If drainage is required following the appendectomy, there is a possible complication of local or general peritonitis. The patient is placed in Fowler's position as soon as he recovers from the anesthetic, and treatment for peritonitis should be instituted, as described on page 764. These patients are monitored carefully for many days for signs of intestinal obstruction and secondary hemorrhage. Secondary abscesses may form in the pelvis, under the diaphragm, or in the liver. These cause an elevation of temperature and pulse rate, with an increase in the leukocyte count. A fecal fistula, with the discharge of feces through the drainage tract, develops at times. This complication arises most often after the drainage of an appendiceal abscess. Any sign of feces on the dressing should be brought to the attention of the surgeon.

Complications

If the appendix can be removed before inflammation has progressed to the point of perforation, there is no further trouble. The abdomen can be closed at once, and the patient can be out of the hospital in a few days. However, if perforation has occurred, the patient may develop generalized peritonitis, or an appendiceal abscess may result, in which case the surrounding loops of bowel become adherent and wall off the spreading peritonitis. For an explanation of nursing management in these instances, see Table 37-3.

MECKEL'S DIVERTICULUM

Meckel's diverticulum is a congenital abnormality consisting of a blind tube, comparable with the appendix, that usually opens into the distal ileum near the ileocecal valve. A portion of this duct persists as a diverticulum in approximately 2 percent of the population. It is more common in men than in women.

The importance of Meckel's diverticulum lies in the fact that its mucosal lining not infrequently may become inflamed and may lead to intestinal obstruction, or it may perforate, causing peritonitis.

The most common symptoms of a diseased Meckel's diverticulum are abdominal pain, typically umbilical in location, or the passage of stools containing blood. The blood is a dark crimson color. (A slowly bleeding gastric or upper intestinal lesion is tarry black; a colonic hemorrhage usually produces bright red bleeding.) The treatment is surgical excision of the diverticulum.

PERITONITIS

Peritonitis is inflammation of a part or all of the parietal and visceral surfaces of the abdominal cavity. Usually it is due to bacterial infection, the organisms coming from disease of the gastrointestinal tract, the internal genital organs of the female, and, less often, from outside, by injury or by extension of inflammation from an extraperitoneal organ such as the kidney. *Inflammation* and *ileus* are the direct effects of this infection. Common causes of peritonitis are presented in Figure 37-2.

Pathophysiology. Peritonitis is caused by leakage of contents from abdominal organs into the abdominal cavity, usually as a result of inflammation, ischemia, trauma,

TABLE 37-3.   POTENTIAL COMPLICATIONS FOLLOWING APPENDECTOMY
Prompt recognition by the nurse and effective management of treatment can prevent prolonged disability for the patient.

COMPLICATION	NURSING ASSESSMENT AND INTERVENTION
Peritonitis	Observe for abdominal tenderness, fever, vomiting, abdominal rigidity, and tachycardia. Employ constant nasogastric suction. Correct dehydration. Give antibiotic agents.
Pelvic or lumbar abscess	Evaluate for anorexia, chills, fever, and diaphoresis. Watch for "diarrhea," which may indicate pelvic abscess. Prepare patient for rectal examination. Prepare patient for operative drainage procedure.
Subphrenic abscess (abscess under the diaphragm)	Assess patient for chills, fever, and sweats. Prepare for x-ray examination. Prepare for surgical drainage of abscess.
Ileus: Paralytic ileus Mechanical ileus	Employ nasogastric intubation and suction. Replace fluids and electrolytes by intravenous route. Prepare for operation, if diagnosis of mechanical ileus is established.

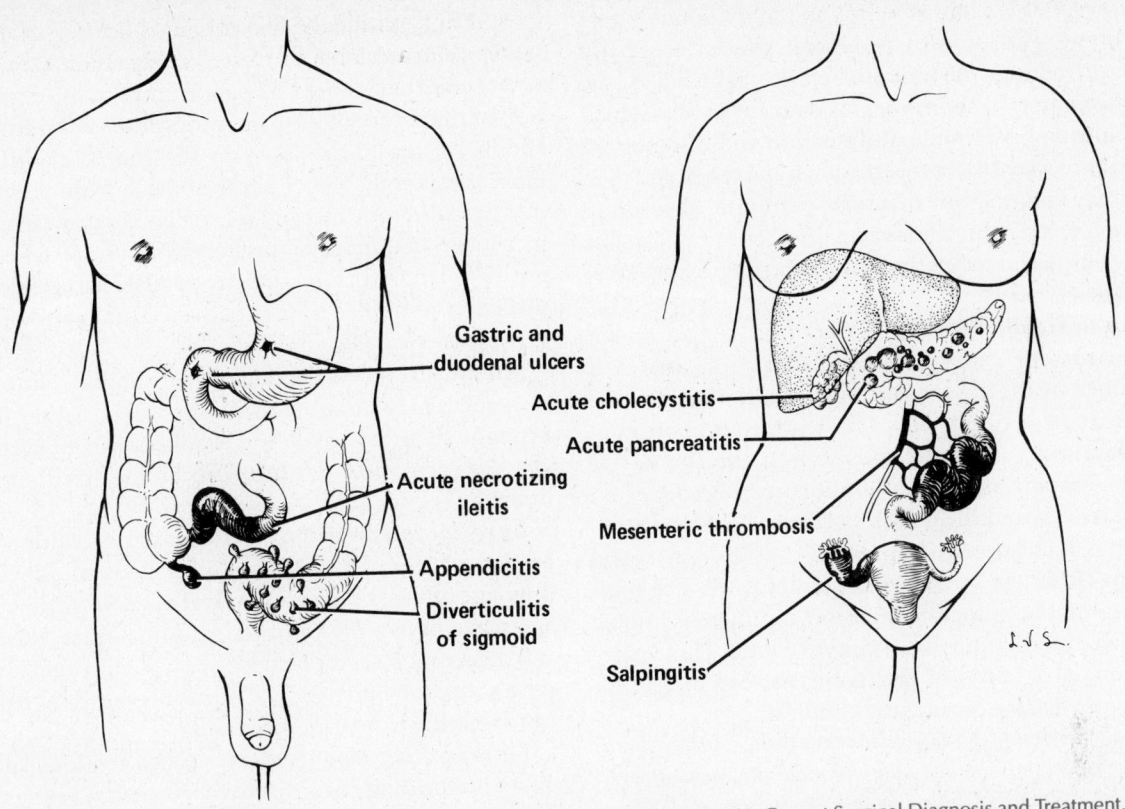

Figure 37-2. Common primary causes of peritonitis. (Dunphy, J. E., and Way, L. W.: Current Surgical Diagnosis and Treatment. Los Altos, Calif., Lange Medical Publishers, 1977)

or tumor perforation. Initially the material that spills into the abdominal cavity is sterile, but within hours bacterial contamination occurs. Edema of tissues results, and in a short while exudation develops. Fluid in the peritoneal cavity becomes turbid with increasing amounts of pro-

tein, white cells, cellular debris, and blood. The immediate response of the intestinal tract is hypermotility, but this is soon followed by paralytic ileus, with an accumulation of air and fluid in the bowel.

Figure 37–3 (left side of the chart) shows that the

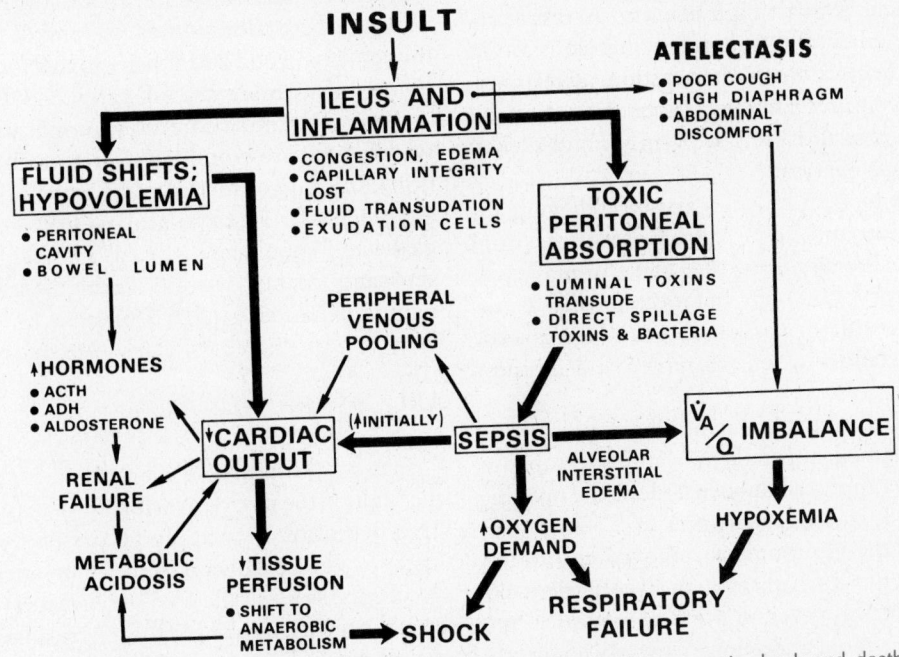

Figure 37-3. Sequential pathophysiology of peritoneal insult leading to septic shock and death. Surgical intervention occurring early in this sequence of events may prevent the more serious later complications. (Hardy: Rhoads Textbook of Surgery, 5th ed. Philadelphia, J. B. Lippincott, 1977)

cardiac response is hypovolemia and a lowering of cardiac output. Perfusion of peripheral tissues, especially muscle, is reduced. As indicated on the right side of the chart, respiratory response begins with atelectasis, which is brought on by abdominal distention and discomfort. This leads to a ventilatory-perfusion hypoxemia and then respiratory failure. Note that toxic peritoneal absorption produces sepsis, which leads to a number of undesirable results. Surgical intervention may interrupt the progressive chain of events.

Clinical Manifestations.

Symptoms depend on the location and the extent of the inflammation, which is determined by the disease causing the peritonitis. At first a diffuse type of pain is felt. This tends to become constant, localized, and more intense near the site of the process. The affected area of the abdomen becomes extremely tender, and the muscles become rigid. Rebound tenderness and ileus may be present. Usually, nausea and vomiting occur, and peristalsis is diminished. The temperature and the pulse rate increase, and there is almost always an elevation of the leukocyte count. These early clinical manifestations of peritonitis also are the symptoms of the disease causing the condition.

Management and Nursing Intervention.

Objectives of management are to establish and eliminate the cause of peritonitis, correct fluid and electrolyte imbalance, combat infection, and make the patient as comfortable as possible.

Because there often is an outpouring of fluids and electrolytes, it is necessary to prevent hypovolemia, shock, and impaired renal function. In addition to these potential threats, fluid accumulates in the abdominal cavity, exerting pressure against the diaphragm, which, in turn, restricts proper ventilatory function. To avert these life-threatening complications, fluid, colloid, and electrolyte replacement is given high priority. Accurate recording of input and output, including vomitus, assists in calculating fluid replacements. In addition, determination of central venous pressure (page 516) may be helpful. A rise in pressure levels to 15 cm. or higher may indicate circulatory overload.

Intestinal intubation and suction assist in relieving abdominal distention and help in promoting intestinal function. Oxygen therapy by nasal catheter or mask will promote ventilatory function, but occasionally a tracheostomy, and ventilatory assistance may be required. Urinary catheterization is done to record and monitor urinary output.

Treatment is directed toward removing the cause: if it is an acutely inflamed appendix, an appendectomy is performed; if it is a ruptured duodenal ulcer, the opening in the duodenum is closed; and so on.

If the cause of the peritonitis is removed at an early stage, the inflammation subsides and the patient recovers. Frequently, however, the inflammation is not localized, and the whole abdominal cavity becomes involved, in which case, the patient is acutely ill. He has severe pain and must be treated compassionately.

Accurate assessment of pain is important. A description of the nature of the pain, its location and shifts in the abdomen, may help ascertain the source of difficulty. Since sepsis is the major cause of death from peritonitis, massive antibiotic therapy is usually initiated early in the treatment. Cultures of peritoneal fluid are taken, but until the laboratory reports are available, large doses of penicillin combined with broad-spectrum antibiotics are given intravenously.

Eventually, unless the cause of peritonitis is eliminated, the patient may succumb to intestinal obstruction. This is brought about by small bowel adhesions and even local abscess formation. If these can be localized, surgical drainage is effective.

Surgical Intervention.

"Refunctionalization" may be done surgically. This requires lysis of adhesions, drainage of the abscesses, removal of necrotic tissue, and assurance of continuity of the intestinal tract. Resection and anastomosis may be necessary. Such surgery, along with proper maintenance of nutrition and fluid balance, can assist the patient in recovering.

Postoperative Management.

Conscientious and frequent monitoring of cardiac activity, central venous pressure, ventilation, fluid input, and urine output is essential.

Drains are inserted frequently during the operation, and it is essential that the nurse observe and record the character of the drainage. Care must be taken in moving and turning the patient to prevent the drain from being dislodged accidentally.

Signs that the peritonitis is subsiding include: a fall in temperature and pulse rate, a softening of the abdomen, a return of peristaltic sounds, passing of flatus, and bowel movements. Food and fluids can then be given by mouth in increasing amounts, and parenteral fluids are reduced.

Two of the most common complications that must be watched for are wound evisceration and abscess formation. Any suggestion from the patient that an area of the abdomen is tender or painful or "feels as if something just gave way" should be reported. The sudden occurrence of serosanguineous wound drainage strongly suggests wound dehiscence (page 376).

ABDOMINAL HERNIA

A *hernia* ("rupture") is a protrusion of a viscus through the wall of the cavity in which it is naturally contained. This definition may apply to any part of the body; for instance, the protrusion of the brain after a subtemporal decompression is called *cerebral hernia*. However, in general, the term is applied to the protrusion of an abdominal viscus through an opening in the abdominal wall.

Indirect inguinal hernia is the most common type of hernia (see Table 37-4). This hernia is due to a weakness of the abdominal wall at the point through which the spermatic cord emerges in the male, and the round ligament in the female. Through this opening the hernia extends down the inguinal canal and often into the scrotum or the labia (Fig. 37-4). It is common in the male, and it may appear at any age.

Inguinal hernia is a major cause of hospitalization, especially among men, in whom it occurs three times more frequently than in women. Most hernias result from congenital or acquired weakness of the abdominal wall, coupled with sustained increased intra-abdominal pressure from coughing or straining, or from an enlarging lesion within the abdomen. Once the hernia occurs, it has a tendency to increase in size.

The hernial sac is formed by an outpouching of the peritoneum and may contain the large or small intestine, omentum, and, occasionally, the bladder. When the hernia first is formed, the sac is filled only when the patient is on his feet, the contents returning to the abdominal cavity as soon as he lies down.

Direct inguinal hernia passes through the posterior inguinal wall. It also is most common in males, more difficult to repair than indirect inguinal hernia, and often recurs after surgery.

Umbilical hernia results from failure of the umbilical orifice to close. It is most common in obese women and in children, as a protrusion at the umbilicus. This hernia is also seen in patients with cirrhosis and ascites.

Ventral or incisional hernias occur due to a weakness of the abdominal wall. They are due most frequently to previous operations in which drainage was necessary, complete closure of the tissues being impossible. Weakened by infection, only a slight bulge results at first, but this increases gradually in size until a definite hernial sac is produced.

Femoral hernia appears below the inguinal (Poupart's) ligament (i.e., below the groin) as a round bulge. It is more frequent in women.

A hernia is referred to as *reducible* when the protruding mass can be placed back into the abdominal cavity. This can occur naturally when the patient lies down, or it may require manual reduction (the mass is pushed back into the cavity). As time goes on, adhesions form between the

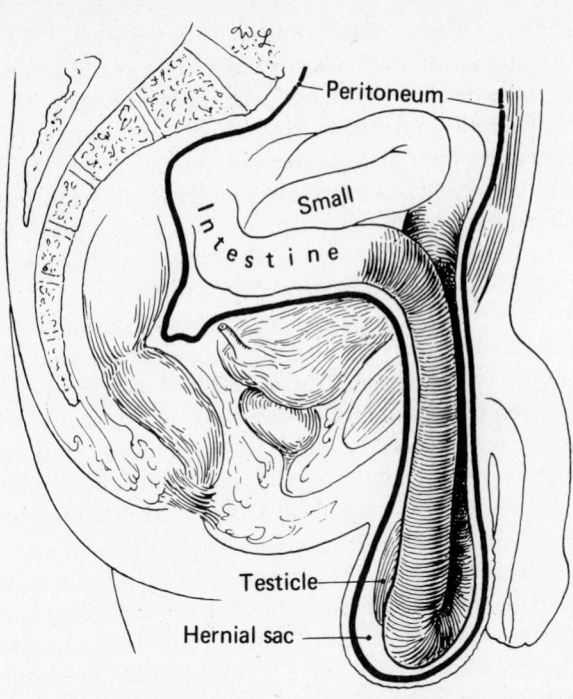

Figure 37-4. Inguinal hernia. Note that the sac of the hernia is a continuation of the peritoneum of the abdomen and that the hernial contents are intestine, omentum, or other abdominal contents that pass through the hernial opening into the hernial sac.

sac and its contents, so that the hernia becomes *irreducible* or *incarcerated*. Such a hernia is one which cannot be reduced and in which the intestinal flow may be obstructed completely.

In a *strangulated hernia* the contents not only are irreducible, but the blood and intestinal flow through the intestine in the hernia is stopped completely. This condition develops when the loop of intestine in the sac becomes twisted or swollen and a constriction is produced at the neck of the sac. The result then is an acute intestinal obstruction, plus the added danger of gangrene of the bowel. The symptoms are pain at the site of strangulation, followed by colicky abdominal pain, vomiting, and swelling of the hernial sac.

Management

In most instances, the hernia should be repaired by operation; otherwise, it is in continual danger of strangulation. When strangulation occurs, operation becomes imperative and is attended invariably by considerable risk.

Mechanical Reduction. Very often the patient can reduce his own hernia. In order to keep the mass from protruding when a standing position is assumed, a *truss* (a pad made of firm material which is placed over the hernia and held in place with a belt) may be worn. Most authorities agree that a truss creates more problems than it can solve. It may cause skin irritation and lesions, due to

TABLE 37-4. INCIDENCE OF HERNIA

TYPE	FREQUENCY (APPROXIMATE %)
Inguinal, indirect	70
Inguinal, direct	15
Umbilical	5-10
Incisional	5-10
Femoral	5 or less
Others	2 or less

constant rubbing. When improperly fitted it may cause strangulation of the hernia. However, a truss may be recommended (1) for infants, when there is need to wait for a weight gain before surgery or for remission of another problem, such as bronchitis or diaper rash; (2) for adults who have an underlying problem that needs to be resolved first; or (3) when a patient has worn a truss for years, is terrified of the hospital, and will not part with the truss. In this latter instance, the proper fitting of the truss must be done by a physician. The Valsalva maneuver can also be used to check for the effectiveness of the truss. Daily bathing and the use of corn starch powder can lessen the possibility of skin irritation. Usually, the truss is worn directly over the hernia and not over clothing, which could cause slipping. It must be emphasized that a *truss does not cure a hernia;* it simply prevents the abdominal contents from entering the hernial sac.

Surgical Repair. The operation involves removal of the hernial sac after it has been dissected free from surrounding structures and the contents have been replaced in the abdominal cavity, and the neck ligated. The muscle and the fascial layers then are sewed together firmly over the hernial orifice to prevent a recurrence. When the tissues are not sufficiently strong, reinforcement can be obtained by overlaying the suture line with synthetic sutures or mesh, which is also sutured in place (hernioplasty). The presence of the mesh stimulates more than the usual amount of fibroblastic activity and thereby enhances the strength of the repair. When a strangulation has occurred, the operation is complicated by an intestinal obstruction and injury to the bowel.

Preoperative Care. In emergency conditions of strangulated or incarcerated hernia, the nurse prepares the patient as in any other acute surgical problem. However, most patients are in good physical condition and are having a herniorrhaphy as elective surgery. The patient may be prompted by the knowledge that an unrepaired hernia may become a serious emergency, or that he may have difficulty securing employment because of this condition.

An important nursing checkpoint is to determine whether the patient has an upper respiratory infection, chronic cough from excessive smoking, or sneezing due to an allergy. It may be necessary to postpone the operation until a more preferable time, since coughing or sneezing could weaken the postoperative wound, thereby negating the purpose of surgery.

Postoperative Care. The patient may be allowed out of bed the day of, or the day after surgery. Diet is determined by the desires of the patient, following local or spinal anesthesia. However, if a general anesthesia was used, fluid and food are restricted until peristalsis returns.

Urinary retention is common in the postoperative period; if the patient can get out of bed to void, there usually is no difficulty. In any case, it is necessary to prevent bladder distention; this may require catheterization, if other nursing measures fail.

Following repair of an inguinal hernia, swelling of the scrotum may occur. Because this is extremely painful, the patient is reluctant to move. Elevating the scrotum on a rolled towel and applying small ice bags intermittently are helpful. A narcotic may be given for pain, and antibiotics to prevent epididymitis. A suspensory bandage or jock strap may give support and comfort.

Infection which interferes with healing occurs occasionally. Soreness in the operative region and temperature elevation may suggest such a problem. Systemic antibiotics or local wound treatment with heat application, followed by incision and drainage, may be required.

Should the patient cough or sneeze after the operation, he should be instructed to splint the incision site with his hand, to lessen the pain and also protect the incision site.

For more extensive hernia repair such as may be required following umbilical or large incisional hernia, nasogastric suction may be used to prevent distention, vomiting, and straining. Mild cathartics may be prescribed to prevent straining during defecation.

Patient Education. Once the hernia is repaired, some surgeons permit the patient to do whatever he wishes, on the premise that he will not engage in painful activity, thereby preventing injury to the incision. If the patient has had local anesthesia, he is allowed more liberties than one who has had general anesthesia.

Usually the stay in the hospital lasts about 5 or 6 days. There may be restrictions on heavy lifting for 2 months; however, some surgeons believe that activities of everyday life help to strengthen the hernia repair. In any event, the nurse may review good body mechanics with the patient before his discharge.

CROHN'S DISEASE

Crohn's disease (granulomatous colitis, regional enteritis, granulomatous ileocolitis) is a chronic transmural inflammatory disease of unknown etiology, that may involve any portion of the intestinal tract.

This disease is characterized by inflammatory involvement of segments of the intestine separated by normal intervening areas. Other pathology may include a thickened mesentery and bowel wall and enlarged lymph nodes.

Clinical Manifestations. Symptom onset is usually insidious, but abdominal pain and diarrhea are prominent, and unrelieved by defecation. Scar tissue and formation of granulomas interfere with the ability of the intestine to transport products of the upper intestinal digestion through the constricted lumen, resulting in crampy abdominal pains. Since intestinal peristalsis is stimulated by the eating of food, the crampy pains occur after meals. To avoid these bouts of crampy pain, the patient avoids food or takes it only in amounts and types inadequate for normal nutritional requirements, so that weight loss, malnutrition, and secondary or macrocytic anemia occur. In addition, ulcers form in the lining membrane of the intestine, and other inflammatory changes take place, resulting in a constant irritating discharge that is emptied into the colon from the weeping, swollen intestine. This causes a chronic diarrhea. The end result is a very uncomfortable person who is thin and emaciated from inadequate food intake and constant fluid loss. In some cases, the inflamed intestine may perforate and form intra-abdominal and anal abscesses. Melena may occur, along with malabsorption syndrome. Fever is not a prominent symptom, except when abscesses are present.

Common complications are stricture and fistula formation. Fistulae may extend to the skin or to other loops of bowel; they are apt to occur when a patient has had an unrecognized regional enteritis and undergone an appendectomy.

This disease affects both sexes equally and appears more often in those of Jewish origin. There is a definite familial occurrence. Regional enteritis may occur in any decade of life, but it reaches its highest incidence between the ages of 15 and 35.

Assessment. The most conclusive diagnostic aid is a barium study of the upper gastrointestinal tract which reveals the classic "string sign" on x-ray of the terminal ileum, indicating the constriction of a segment of intestine.

Management. In mild episodes, conservative treatment consists of a low-residue, bland diet, with vitamin supplements to improve nutrition. Iron may be prescribed for concomitant anemia. Diarrhea is treated symptomatically. Sedatives may help, and steroids are useful in the treatment of acute attacks but have not been shown to prevent recurrences.

When the symptoms do not respond to these conservative measures, or when massive bleeding occurs, surgical treatment is necessary. This will be determined by the individual case. If the lesion can be delineated to a particular area, it may be resected. Unfortunately, even with surgery, recurrences are common.

ULCERATIVE COLITIS

Ulcerative colitis is an ulcerative and inflammatory disease of the colon and rectum, with rare involvement of the distal ileum.

Pathophysiology

Ulcerative colitis is characterized by multiple ulcerations, diffuse inflammations, and desquamation of the colonic epithelium, with alternating periods of exacerbations and remissions. Most commonly the disease begins in the rectum and sigmoid and spreads upward, ultimately involving the entire colon. The complications of ulcerative colitis may be local or systemic. Local complications include perforation, hemorrhage, abscess, stricture, and carcinomatous degeneration. Systemic complications include arthritis, erythema nodosum, and nephrolithiasis.

The cause of the disease is unknown. In some patients, an autoimmune mechanism may be responsible. Some authorities consider ulcerative colitis an example of psychosomatic disease, but to date this has not been substantiated. There may be several precipitating factors, the net effect of which is a self-perpetuating destructive infection of the mucosal lining of the large intestine. It is a serious disease, accompanied by systemic complications and a high mortality rate. Eventually, 10-15 percent of the patients develop carcinoma of the colon.

Clinical Manifestations and Assessment

Diarrhea, abdominal pain, and rectal bleeding are the usual symptoms of this condition. In addition, there may be evidence of weight loss, fever and tenesmus, and possibly vomiting. There often is cramping, and the feeling of an urgent need to defecate. Hypocalcemia and iron deficiency frequently develop.

In the diagnosis of chronic ulcerative colitis, dysentery due to the common intestinal organisms, and especially *Entamoeba histolytica* infection, must be ruled out by careful stool examination. Sigmoidoscopy and barium enema x-ray examination are of value in distinguishing this condition from other diseases of the colon with similar symptoms.

- In acute ulcerative colitis, cathartics are contraindicated when the patient is being prepared for barium enema, since they may cause severe exacerbation of the condition, which may lead to megacolon (excessive dilatation of the colon), perforation, and death. If the patient is required to have this diagnostic test, perhaps a liquid diet for a few days before the x-ray, followed by a gentle tap water enema on the day of examination, is sufficient.

Management

Treatment for chronic ulcerative colitis may be pursued in three areas: medical, surgical, and psychotherapeutic. The objectives of medical therapy are to reduce inflammation and suppress inappropriate immune responses, and also to provide rest for a diseased bowel, so that it may heal. Surgical treatment is designed to remove the source of symptoms, that is, to remove the diseased segments of the intestine and maintain intestinal function through a permanent ileostomy. Psychotherapy is aimed at determining the environmental factors which distress the patient, dealing with these factors, and attempting to resolve conflicts, so that they no longer aggravate the patient.

Years ago, the psychosomatic factor in the disease was emphasized. This emphasis has waned, recently, for several reasons: surgical management has improved considerably, and improved knowledge of how to care for the patient with an ileostomy has made this approach a reasonably optimistic one. In addition, steroid therapy has alleviated distressing physical symptoms, producing a marked decrease in anxiety and depression in this patient.

There are several objectives in the treatment of the patient with ulcerative colitis: to promote rest and relaxation of the intestinal tract, to combat infection, to meet the nutritional and fluid needs of the body, and to correct, if possible, any psychosocial problems.

The patient with ulcerative colitis is encouraged to rest after meals, but usually he is not confined to bed unless absolutely necessary. Activity within the limit of his physical capacity is desirable, so that he will not regard himself as an invalid. Toilet facilities and privacy should be available nearby.

Well-balanced, low-residue, high-protein diets with supplemental vitamin therapy and iron replacement are effective in meeting nutritional needs. Fluid and electrolyte imbalance due to dehydration caused by diarrhea is corrected by intravenous therapy. Any foods which exacerbate diarrhea should be avoided, including bovine milk products. Milk may contribute to diarrhea if lactose intolerance is present. In addition, cold foods are to be avoided, along with smoking, since both increase intestinal motility.

Sedation and antidiarrheal medications are given to reduce to a minimum the colonic peristalsis, in order to rest the inflamed bowel. Constipation must be watched for, since it may lead to megacolon, with impending perforation. The nurse can be on guard for this possibility by measuring abdominal girth.

Antidiarrheal medications and sedation are continued until the patient's stools approach normal frequency and consistency. Sulfonamides such as nonabsorbable salicylazo-sulfapyridine (Azulfidine) or sulfisoxazole (Gantrisin) are often effective in mild or moderate colitis. Antibiotics are used for secondary infections, particularly for purulent complications such as abscesses, perforation, and peritonitis.

ACTH and corticosteroids are most effective early in the course of an acute inflammatory phase of this disease, rather than in the chronic phase. A clinical remission is noted in 5–10 days, in four-fifths of patients treated, as indicated by improved appetite, better mood, a decrease in fever, and an absence of bloody diarrhea. When steroids are reduced or stopped, the symptoms of the disease are likely to return. If steroids are continued, adverse sequelae such as hypertension, fluid retention, subcapsular cataracts, and hirsutism may develop. Azulfidine is helpful in preventing recurrences.

Careful assessment and recording of the clinical manifestations as the patient responds to various medications is of high priority among the nurse's responsibilities. It requires an understanding of drug action and potential side effects.

Education of the patient to accept and learn to live with a chronic disease is an important aspect of treatment. Recognition of the fact that disability is lessened following surgery for ulcerative colitis is an optimistic aspect in treating this patient surgically.

Psychosocial Concerns

Authorities agree that it is unwise to sterotype the patient with ulcerative colitis. While emotional factors may play a role in this ailment, they need not overshadow its physical basis. It is possible that the disease may be associated with a wide range of psychological symptoms, including emotional immaturity, dependency, ambitiousness, perfectionism, or a combination of these traits. The patient may display evidence of excessive dependency, mood swings, depression, extreme sensitivity, anxiety, and outbursts of aggressive behavior. If this is so, it is important that the nurse recognize that this behavior is not directed at any one individual, but is a means of expressing a need. Obviously, a patient who is suffering a severe debilitating disease such as ulcerative colitis will not have the control or stamina of other patients. Therefore, his moods will vary, and his symptoms will fluctuate as his condition improves or deteriorates.

The nurse needs to recognize that the patient's behavior may be affected by innumerable factors aside from any inherent emotional characteristic. Any patient who is suffering from the discomforts of frequent bowel movements and rectal soreness is anxious, discouraged, and depressed. Thus it is important to develop a relationship with the patient that gives him a feeling that he is receiving support in his attempts to deal with the stresses that have plagued him. Let him know that his complaints are understood, encourage him to talk and ventilate his feelings, and listen to matters that are disturbing to him, even if they seem trite. Try to direct his attention to himself, and not his intestinal tract.

Surgical Treatment and Nursing Management

Approximately 15–20 percent of patients with ulcerative colitis require surgical intervention. Indications for surgery include: no improvement and continued deterioration, profuse bleeding, perforation, stricture formation, and indications that carcinoma has developed. The operation of choice is usually a total colectomy (removal of the colon) and ileostomy; any procedure more limited will prove to be of only temporary benefit in most patients.

Preoperative Care.   A prolonged period of preparation, with intensive fluid, blood, and protein replacement, is necessary before operation is attempted. Chemotherapy and antibiotics are useful adjuncts. If the patient has been on steroids for a long period of time, steroids will probably be continued during the surgical phase, before being gradually tapered. Meanwhile, assess the patient for adrenal insufficiency by observing and recording pulse, blood pressure, urinary output, general appearance, and reaction.

Usually, the patient is on a low-residue diet offered frequently in small feedings. All other preoperative measures are similar to general abdominal surgery. The abdomen is marked for the proper placement of the stoma by the surgeon. Information about an ileostomy is presented to the patient by means of literature, models, and discussion. The patient should have a fairly good idea of what his surgery is all about and what to expect postoperatively. He may even be encouraged to wear an ileostomy appliance for a day or two before surgery. This will facilitate his adjustment to it after the operation.

Since it is rather difficult to accept an ileostomy, the patient deserves all the support possible. It is necessary to help him to develop an outlook that views an ileostomy as a challenge; if accepted with courage, he can master it and proceed to live normally and effectively. Such an outlook is difficult to accept; thus the task of developing a proper attitude in the patient becomes a major objective for the nurse, who also must have a positive attitude if an optimistic outlook is to be transmitted to the patient. Other patients who have had ileostomies are an excellent source of help to this patient, as are especially trained enterostomal therapists.

Postoperative Care.   The opening of the small intestine on the abdomen (ileostomy) continuously discharges the liquid contents of the small intestine, because the stoma does not have a controlling sphincter. As soon as the operation is completed, a temporary plastic bag with an adhesive facing is placed over the ileostomy and firmly pressed onto surrounding skin. The contents draining from the ileostomy are thus kept from coming into contact with skin and are collected and measured as the bag becomes full. After the ileostomy has had a chance to heal, a permanent appliance is obtained and held in place on the skin with a special cement. This should be rechecked in 3 weeks, when edema has subsided. The final size and type may be selected in 3 months, after the patient's weight has stabilized and the stoma shrinks to a stable shape.

Because these patients lose much fluid and food in the early postoperative period, an accurate record of fluid intake, urinary output, and fecal discharges is necessary, to help the surgeon to gauge the fluid needs of the patient. Fluids, blood, and a low-residue, high-calorie diet are given in large amounts until the patient becomes accustomed to the new digestive arrangement.

COMPARISON OF CROHN'S DISEASE AND ULCERATIVE COLITIS

	CROHN'S DISEASE Granulomatous (Transmural) Colitis	ULCERATIVE COLITIS (Mucosal)
I. *Pathology:*		
Early	Transmural thickening	Mucosal ulceration
Late	Deep, penetrating granulomas	Mucosal minute ulceration
II. *Clinical Manifestations:*		
Location	Ileum, right colon (usually)	Rectum, left colon
Bleeding	Usually not, but may occur	Common—severe
Perianal involvement	Common	Rare—mild
Fistulas	Common	Rare
Rectal involvement	About 20%	Almost 100%
Diarrhea	Less severe	Severe
III. *Diagnostic Studies*		
X-ray	Reveals skip areas Shortening of colon	Diffuse involvement No shortening of colon
IV. *Therapeutic Management*	Steroids, Azulfidine Intravenous alimentation Partial or complete colectomy, with ileostomy or anastomosis Rectum can be preserved in some patients Recurrence common	Steroids, Azulfidine Azulfidine is useful in preventing recurrence Proctocolectomy, with ileostomy Rectum can be preserved in only a few patients "Cured" by colectomy
V. *History*	Crippling; indolent	Exacerbations, remissions; may be lethal Toxic megacolon

ILEOSTOMY

Psychosocial Implications

In an ileostomy, the excretory orifice is located on the lower abdomen and must be attended to several times each day. Because of this, the patient understandably may think that everyone is aware of the ileostomy. He may consider the stoma as mutilative, when compared with other abdominal incisions which heal and are hidden. Because there is loss of a body part, or a major change in anatomy, the ileostomy patient often goes through the various phases of grieving. The nurse can expect the patient to experience shock, disbelief, denial, rejection, anger, and restitution. Nursing support through these phases is important, and understanding of the patient's emotional outlook in each instance should determine the nurse's approach. For example, any form of teaching is of no avail until the patient has reached the stage of restitution.

Concern over body image may lead to questions related to family relationships, sexual function, and the ability to become pregnant and to deliver normally.

Finally, this patient needs to know that someone understands and cares about him. Sincere friendliness and a nonjudgmental attitude must be exhibited by the nurse. This evident interest will aid in gaining the patient's confidence, so important to medical therapy and preoperative preparation. Dependency needs are satisfied through good nurse-patient relationships.

Such patients probably are the most challenging of all to nurse. Their prolonged illness makes them irritable, anxious, and depressed. The nurse can coordinate patient care through nursing conferences attended by consultants such as the physician, psychologist, psychiatrist, social worker, and dietitian. The team approach lends support in approaching a complex nursing problem.

On the other hand, an operation establishing an ileostomy can produce dramatic changes in a patient who has suffered from colitis for several years. Once the misery of the disease is lifted and the patient learns how to take care of the ileostomy, he becomes a normal, affable person. But until the patient has progressed to this phase, an empathetic and tolerant approach by the nurse will play an important part in the patient's recovery.

The camaraderie of other ostomates is also a help. A nonprofit health service agency which is dedicated to the rehabilitation of ostomates is the United Ostomy Association, Inc.* This organization gives patients useful knowledge of living with an ostomy, through an educational program of literature, lectures, and exhibits. Local associations provide visiting services by qualified members and give hope, and rehabilitation services, to new ostomy patients. Local hospitals may have an enterostomal therapist on the staff; this is a valuable resource person for the ileostomy patient.

Rehabilitation and Patient Education Following an Ileostomy

There are certain rehabilitation problems unique to the ileostomy patient, one of which is irregularity of bowel evacuation. The patient with an ileostomy cannot establish regular bowel habits, because the contents of the ileum are fluid and are discharging continuously. Therefore, the patient must wear an appliance (a vinyl or plastic bag) day and night. The appliance is regarded, then, as an intestinal prosthesis.

Several days after the operation, the ileostomy diameter is carefully measured with a stoma-measuring card (various apertures indicate various sizes) so that a suitable opening in the mounting ring will be available in the permanent appliance. The ring is sealed to the skin with an adhesive disk and permits the patient to carry on normal activities without fear of leakage or odor.

The location and length of the stoma is significant in the management of the ileostomy by the patient. Today's surgeon is considerate in placing the stoma as close to the midline as possible and in a position where even an obese patient with a protruding abdomen can care for himself easily. Usually the ileostomy stoma is about 2.5 cm. (1 inch) long, which makes it convenient to attach the appliance.

The ileostomy may be noisy at first, due to edema caused by slight obstruction of tissues. Eventually it will become silent. A low-roughage diet is followed at first, with strained fruits and vegetables. These foods are important for vitamins A and C. Later there are few dietary restrictions, except for avoiding foods that are high in fiber, or hard-to-digest kernels such as celery, popcorn, corn-on-the-cob, poppy seed or caraway seeds, and coconut. Fluids may be a problem during the summer, when they are lost during perspiration as well as through the ileostomy. Drinks such as Gatorade are helpful in maintaining electrolyte balance. If the fecal discharge (called the *effluent*) is too watery, fibrous foods (such as whole grain cereals, fresh fruit skins, beans, corn, and nuts) are restricted. If the effluent is excessively dry, salt intake is increased. An increased intake of water or fluid will not increase the effluent, since excess water is excreted in the urine.

Another possible problem is skin excoriation around the stoma. Not only does the ileostomy drainage contain enzymes that rapidly excoriate the skin, but if cement is used in putting the appliance on, the skin may be irritated when the appliance is removed. To avoid these problems,

*1111 Wilshire Blvd., Los Angeles, California 90017.

PHASES OF THE REHABILITATION PROCESS OF THE ILEOSTOMY PATIENT

I. PREOPERATIVE PHASE: THE PERIOD BEFORE SURGERY
Objective: To reduce fear as much as possible.
Approach:
1. Present precise factual explanations regarding nature of surgery and creation of an ileostomy.
2. Plan to be repetitive in presenting facts.
3. Provide ample opportunity for patient to ask questions of a professional person.
4. Use diagrams, photographs, and appliances, to acquaint the patient with an ileostomy.
5. Allow sufficient time to assimilate the prospect of an ileostomy.
6. Recognize the psychological value of having the patient converse with a successful ileostomate.
7. Include the family in spelling out patient needs and in answering his questions.
8. Explore vocational possibilities through the state vocational rehabilitation service, to allow time for processing.

II. CRISIS PHASE: IMMEDIATE POSTOPERATIVE PERIOD
Objective: To offer support, hope and a sense of security.
Approach:
1. Provide consistent, effective care, to instill confidence in the patient.
2. Exert vigilance in skin care to prevent the discomfort and pain of excoriation.
3. Utilize several approaches in odor control: (a) small doses of bismuth subcarbonate by mouth, (b) adequate appliance hygiene, (c) ventilation and deodorizers in room.
4. Avoid appliance management near mealtime.
5. Accept the patient's feelings (depression, silence, uncooperativeness, and refusal to eat) with understanding.
6. Acquaint the family with the possibility of the patient's exhibiting anxiety by his being demanding or abusive.
7. Avoid having the patient experience an emotional and intellectual vacuum by providing opportunities for verbalization.
8. Provide opportunity for gradual but steady involvement of the patient in handling the appliance.

III. RECUPERATIVE PHASE: INCREASED RESPONSIBILITY FOR SELF-CARE
Objective: To assist patient in accepting self, expressing doubts, and adapting to his total situation.
Approach:
1. Reassure the patient (to offset his doubts) by letting him know that progress is being made toward the goal of making him self-dependent in managing his ileostomy.
2. Encourage the patient to talk about his self-acceptance with a sympathetic social worker or a psychiatrist.
3. Develop a united expression of patient-acceptance among nurses, family, and friends.
4. Repeat explanations of the surgery performed (if required) and reassure patient that he does not have cancer (if this is the case).

5. Suggest that it is normal, in recovery, to have occasional pains and upsets.
6. Obtain literature for him from ileostomy groups.
7. Encourage visits by the dietitian so that he will know when and how to resume a normal diet.
8. Involve him further in self-care so that he continues to move toward independence of others with regard to bowel function.

IV. TRANSITION PHASE: RETURN TO COMMUNITY
Objective: To shift patient's concern from himself to that of himself-in-relation-to-others.
Approach:
1. Assist the patient in previewing the home situation and seeking out fears and concerns.
2. Suggest discrimination in revealing or concealing his ileostomy from friends and work-associates: tell those who would understand but do not tell those whom he suspects would not understand.
3. Encourage the patient to do more and more for himself, but refrain from letting him feel abandoned.
4. Acquaint the patient thoroughly with his permanent appliance, and plan a routine that can be transferred to his own bathroom.
5. Provide instruction and literature in anticipation of skin problems: prophylaxis is easier than treatment.
6. Plan one or two outings away from the hospital for short times to offset the possible fears of the appliance's falling off, or of people staring.
7. Initiate referrals to community nursing agency, an ileostomy patient, and social or vocational agencies, as needed.

V. POSTHOSPITAL PHASE: THE FIRST POSTOPERATIVE YEAR
Objectives: To recover physical well-being and offset physical disability.
To perfect self-care, to negate any handicap.
To resume social role and complete rehabilitation.
Approach:
1. Instruct patient in the detection of serious difficulties and whom to contact for assistance.
2. Direct the patient on how to avoid fluid and electrolyte imbalance, which can be initiated by partial obstruction, a bout of flu, or an accident.
   Report diarrhea of more than 12 hours' duration to the physician.
3. Have patient carry an ID card on which is included: a brief description of the method of removing the appliance and giving skin care; the name and phone of surgeon or hospital to contact in case of emergency.

(Adapted from Lenneberg, E., and Rowbotham, J. L.: The Ileostomy Patient. Springfield, Charles C Thomas, 1970)

nystatin powder (Mycostatin) is dusted lightly on the peristomal skin, to prevent irritation and yeast growth.

A regular schedule for changing the appliance before leakage occurs is established. In teaching the patient to use and care for his appliance, stress the following essential points:

To remove the appliance:
1. Sit or stand in a comfortable position.
2. Fill a container with the prescribed solvent. Apply a few drops of solvent with a medicine dropper between the disk of the appliance and the skin. *Do not pull off the appliance.* As the solvent works, the pouch loosens, and pulling is unnecessary.

To cleanse the skin:
1. Use a cotton ball soaked in solvent. Wet the skin around the stoma. During the time the skin is being cleansed, a gauze dressing may cover the stoma, or a vaginal tampon can be inserted gently to absorb excess drainage. Avoid rubbing, because solvents are irritating.
2. Wash the skin with a soft cloth moistened with *tepid* water and mild soap, or permit the patient to shower or bathe before putting on the clean appliance. If the patient prefers, he may shower before removing the bag. Micropore tape

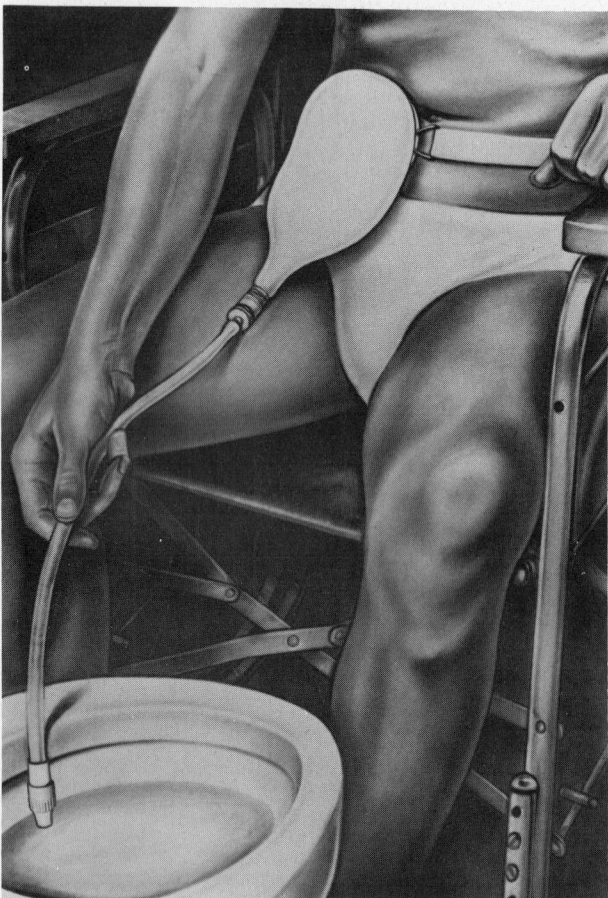

Figure 37-5. Patient has attached an extension of plastic tubing to an adaptor on his ostomy pouch. This is convenient to use in public washrooms, by persons in wheelchairs, bed, and by the elderly as well as children. (Marlen Manufacturing & Development Co.)

applied to the sides of the disk will keep it secure during bathing.

To put on the appliance:
1. When there is no irritation, a disposable plastic bag can be applied directly to the skin, after the cover has been removed from the adherent surface of the bag. Press firmly in place for 30 seconds.
2. When there is skin irritation, after skin cleansing, apply Kenalog spray (antibiotic); blot excess moisture with a cotton pledget and dust lightly with nystatin (Mycostatin) powder.
3. Moisten a Karaya gum washer and apply when it is tacky.
4. Press the adhesive disk on the faceplate of the pouch against the washer. This will allow skin to heal while the appliance is in place.

The amount of time that a person can keep the appliance sealed to his body depends on the location of the stoma and on body structure. Usually the normal wearing time is 2–4 days. The appliance is emptied every 4–6 hours, or at the same time the patient empties his bladder. The pouch has an emptying spout at the bottom (Fig. 37-5) that is closed with a rubber band or special clip made for this purpose.

The appliance is cleaned and aired according to the manufacturer's directions. Usually thorough washing with soap and water, using a soft nylon brush, is effective. There are many deodorizers and cleaning aids available that the patient can use. Full-strength distilled vinegar, rather than strong bleaches, is effective for soaking the bag. Commercial liquid deodorizers are also available, and preferred by some patients. Other deodorants which are inexpensive are pieces of charcoal, or two aspirin tablets crushed and dropped into the bag. Foods such as spinach and parsley act on the intestinal tract as deodorizers, whereas foods that cause odors are cabbage, onions, and fish. Most patients alternate bags and allow the cleaned bag to be exposed to moving fresh air, out of direct sunlight. Bismuth subcarbonate tablets taken by mouth three or four times a day are effective in reducing odor. Some physicians prescribe a stool-thickener, such as diphenoxylate (Lomotil) (by mouth) to assist in odor control.

Finally, the person with an ileostomy is able to resume any activity, sport, or occupation he desires. There are no restrictions on sexual activity or bearing children. The only limitation is the person himself. Most patients do very well in adjusting because of feeling better and being free of pain.

CONTINENT ILEOSTOMY (Kock Pouch)

An interesting variation from the traditional incontinent ileostomy is the continent ileostomy introduced in the late 1960s by Nils Kock, a Swedish surgeon. Although thousands of patients have learned to adapt to the usual ileostomy, there is great appeal in the idea of an ileostomy device that gives patients voluntary control

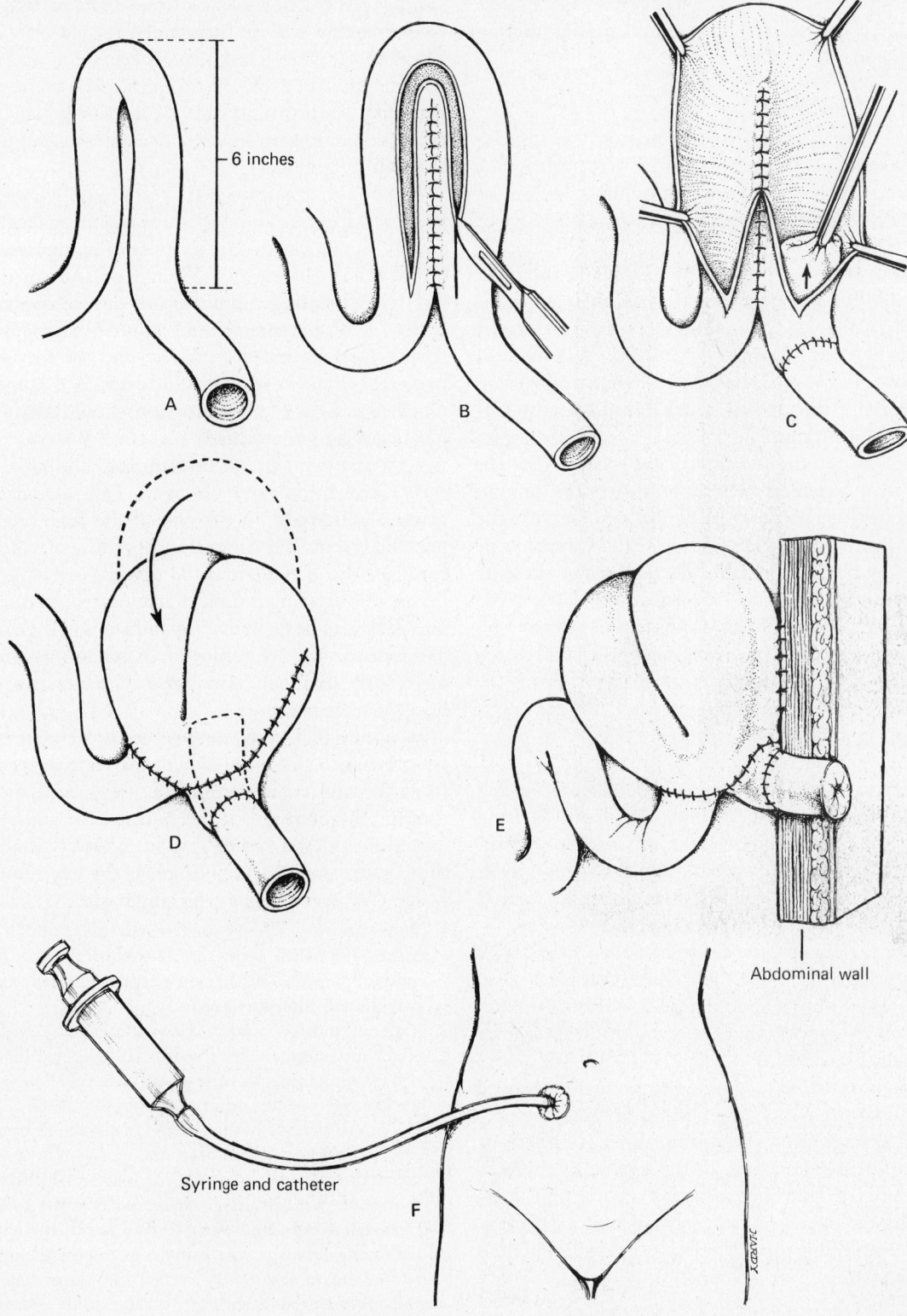

6 inches

Abdominal wall

Syringe and catheter

Figure 37-6. Continent ileostomy.

over the emptying from an ileostomy, without the cumbersome "bag." Not all patients requiring an ileostomy can benefit from the continent (Kock pouch) type. Patients with Crohn's disease are not suitable candidates, because the condition affects the terminal ileum, which is the section used to create the pouch. Eligible candidates are those with chronic ulcerative colitis and multiple or familial polyposis, or patients who have the traditional ileostomy for ulcerative colitis. This procedure cannot be performed in every hospital but requires special training for the surgeon.

Physiological Adaptation

The amount of effluent from an ileostomy is approximately 1,000 ml. per 24 hours. In order to accommodate this volume, a receptacle capable of holding 500 ml. of fluid would have to be constructed, with the objective of emptying about 3 times daily. Consideration also needs to be given to reducing pressure at the outlet to prevent the receptable contents from backing up into the proximal small intestine. Kock's method was to split an intestinal segment at its antimesenteric border and fold the split segment twice in a special way; thus the motor activity in different parts of the created pouch counteracted itself, and no raise in intraluminal pressure occurred, despite vigorous motor activity. A nipple valve is constructed at the outlet from the receptacle by purposely creating an intussusception of a part of the terminal segment into the receptacle (Fig. 37-6C). The creation of this receptacle or reservoir may be done initially when a patient presents for an ileostomy, or it may be constructed from the conventional ileostomy if sufficient ileum is present.

After the diseased colon and terminal ileum have been resected, the continent pouch is constructed. From the resected end, about 45 cm. (18 in.) of ileum are freed. The initial 15 cm. (6 inches) will eventually be used to create the nipple, which will emerge on the abdomen (about ¼ inch). The next 30 cm. (12 inches) are folded in a loop and stitched together (Fig. 37-6A). Then a *U*-shaped incision is made along the full length of the stitched loop (Fig. 37-6B). The remaining septum (initial suture line) is resutured to bring the raw edges together to form a smooth internal surface for the reservoir.

To create the nipple, the ileum is pulled in on itself (intussuscepted) (Fig. 37-6C) and stitched in place as an opening (stoma) on the abdomen. The edges of the exposed pouch are approximated to form the ileal receptacle or pouch (Fig. 37-6D).

The "valve" is forced to close when pressure is created by feces filling the pouch; the closing of the valve prevents fecal leakage from the stoma. When a catheter is inserted, effluent is released. In the operating room, a catheter is inserted through the nipple valve and is attached, after the operation, to gentle suction, to prevent the pouch from filling until all incision and stitching lines heal (about 10 days).

Nursing Management and Patient Education

Preoperative preparation is similar to that for the patient having a traditional ileostomy. Teaching before surgery will relate to managing the drains from the outlet, the nature of drainage, need for nasogastric intubation, parenteral fluids, and perineal packing and care.

After the operation, a catheter will extend from the stoma and will be attached to a closed suction system. This drainage will be maintained for close to 2 weeks. The catheter is irrigated, usually every 2 hours, to assure its patency. About 20-30 ml. of normal saline or sterile water may be introduced gently into the pouch by means of a syringe. Return flow is not aspirated, but permitted to drain by gravity.

Nasogastric suction also is a part of immediate postoperative care, with the tube requiring frequent irrigation, as requested. The purpose of nasogastric suction is to facilitate healing and to relieve pressure on the suture line by preventing a build-up of gastric contents. The patient is on parenteral fluids for 4-5 days. Thereafter, sips of clear liquids are offered, and the diet gradually progressed. Nausea and abdominal distention are watched as signs of an obstruction; should they occur, the physician is to be notified.

As with other patients undergoing abdominal surgery, early ambulation is encouraged. Pain medications are given if required. By the end of the first week, rectal packing is removed. Since this procedure may be uncomfortable, the patient may be given a sedative an hour before this dressing is done. Changing the perineal dressings may also be facilitated by moistening the dressings a day before they are removed. After the packing is removed, the perineum is irrigated 2-3 times daily until full healing takes place.

In about 10-14 days, when the healing process has progressed to the point where the catheter is removed from the stoma, it is time for the patient to learn to manage the drainage of the pouch. The equipment required includes: a catheter, tissues, water-soluble lubricant, gauze squares, a syringe, irrigating solution in a bowl, and an emesis or receiving basin.

1. Lubricate the catheter and gently insert about 5 cm. (2 inches), at which point some resistance may be felt at the valve or "nipple." When gentle pressure is used, the catheter usually will enter the pouch.
2. If there is much resistance, fill a syringe with 20 ml. of air or water and inject the air or water through the catheter, while still exerting some pressure on the catheter. This will permit the catheter to enter into the pouch (Fig. 37-6F).
3. Place the other end of the catheter in a drainage basin, which is placed below the level of stoma, so that gravity will facilitate drainage. Later, of course, drainage can be carried out at the toilet, with drainage delivered into the toilet bowl. Drainage may include flatus as well as effluent.
4. Following drainage, the catheter is removed, and the area around the stoma is gently washed with warm water. Pat dry and apply an absorbent pad over the stoma. Fasten the pad with hypoallergenic tape.

The whole procedure should not require more than 5-10 minutes and is done at first every 3 hours. The time between irrigations is gradually lengthened so that it is done about 3 times daily.

When discharge is thick, water can be injected via the catheter to loosen and soften it. Effluent consistency is affected by food intake. As time goes on, the pouch will stretch, and whereas at first drainage is only about 60-80 ml., it will eventually increase to accommodate 500-1,000 ml. The gauge to determine frequency of drainage is the sensation of pressure in the pouch.

Continued Patient Education for Home Care

The spouse or family should be familiar with the adjustment that will be necessary when the patient returns home. They need to know why it is necessary for the ileostomate to occupy the bathroom for 10 minutes at certain times of the day, and why he needs certain equipment. Their understanding is necessary to reduce tension—a relaxed patient tends to have fewer problems.

Psychosocial needs of the patient are stressed. For the most part, he is particularly pleased that he will not need to wear an ileostomy bag, and this encourages him to master control over his own pouch.

A successful cover for the stoma for home use has been described by Cox and Wentworth: the stoma is covered with a dressing that is absorbent on one side and plasticized on the other. (High-quality disposable diapers can be cut into 7.5 × 7.5 cm. (3 × 3) squares; this makes an ideal dressing.) The dressing is held in place with tape. To reduce skin excoriation, the tape is placed differently with each application, so that it does not contact the same area of skin each time.

A water-soluble lubricant, rather than petrolatum, should be used. The latter has a tendency to clog the catheter and is difficult to wash from it.

The position to assume in the bathroom is one of individual preference and convenience. The patient may sit on the toilet seat, stand in front of the toilet, or sit on a chair in front of toilet. It is suggested that an adaptor and a length of tubing be available to attach to the catheter so that effluent does not splatter, but drains easily into the toilet bowl.

Encourage experimentation when there are problems with drainage. If the catheter meets resistance when attempts are made to insert it, the patient should be encouraged to relax before draining the pouch and to be sure to lubricate the catheter well. It may be easier for the patient to lie down when the catheter is inserted and then stand up for drainage purposes.

Injection of air or water may help in passing the catheter through the stoma into the pouch. (Skin care, odor, diet, activities, and so forth, are similar to that recommended for other ostomy patients; see page 770.)

DIVERTICULOSIS AND DIVERTICULITIS

A *diverticulum* is a saccular dilatation, a blind passage, so to speak, leading from the lumen of the bowel. (An example of abnormality is Meckel's diverticulum, an outpocketing of the ileum.) Diverticula, in fact, may occur anywhere along the course of the gastrointestinal tract, from the esophagus to the rectum. Congenital predisposition is likely. They may be the result of local degeneration and weakening of the muscular wall, or they may be due to increased mechanical pressure from abnormal, high-pressure contractions of the sigmoid colon in response to neurohumoral stimuli. An individual who possesses diverticula is said to have *diverticulosis*. An obstruction of a diverticulum leads to infection and inflammation. This is referred to as *diverticulitis*.

Incidence and Pathophysiology

Diverticulitis usually occurs in patients over 40 years of age. It is by no means rare. It has been estimated that approximately a third of the patients with diverticulosis at one time or another experience diverticulitis. Diverticulitis is most common in the sigmoid colon. This condition may occur in acute attacks, or it may persist as a long-continued, smoldering infection. Inflammation of a diverticulum, if its obstruction continues, tends to spread to the surrounding bowel wall, giving rise to irritability and spasticity of the colon. An abscess may develop, leading to peritonitis, and erosion of the blood vessels (arterial) may produce bleeding.

Clinical Manifestation and Diagnostic Evaluation

Constipation from spastic colon syndrome often precedes the development of diverticulosis by many years. Other signs of diverticulosis are bowel irregularity and diarrhea. A moderately severe acute diverticulitis has as its most common symptom crampy pain in the left lower quadrant of the abdomen, and a low grade fever. Following local inflammation of the diverticula, there may be a narrowing of the large bowel, with fibrotic stricture, leading to cramps, narrow stools, and increased constipation. With the development of granulation tissue, occult bleeding may occur, producing iron-deficiency anemia. In addition, weakness and fatigue are evident. If an abscess develops, there is tenderness, a palpable mass, fever, and leukocytosis. If an inflamed diverticulum perforates, abdominal pain results that is localized over the involved segment—usually the sigmoid; local abscess or peritonitis results. With the development of peritonitis, the symptoms of rigidity, abdominal pain, loss of bowel sounds, and shock, develop. Uninflamed or slightly inflamed diverticula may erode areas adjacent to arterial branches, thus causing massive rectal bleeding.

Diagnosis is made on the basis of sigmoidoscopy (direct visualization) and fluoroscopic and x-ray findings with a barium enema.

Management and Patient Education

The patient should understand the nature of his problem and recognize that the objective is to rest the intestinal tract and alleviate constipation. Heretofore, diverticulosis of the colon was considered relatively harmless, but because of the potential for developing complex problems, prevention is now given major emphasis.

There are differences of opinion regarding the proper type of diet for these patients. Some recommend refined, low-roughage foods, to avoid irritation. Others suggest a fibrous diet to avoid collection of feces in pouches, with resulting infection. At present, there is a fair amount of

clinical evidence that increased dietary fiber appears to improve diverticular disease; however, even though this evidence is persuasive, the value of fiber still has not been demonstrated.

If mastication is a problem, foods should be puréed. For spastic pain, antispasmodics such as propantheline bromide (Pro-Banthine) and oxyphencyclimine (Daricon) are taken before meals and at bedtime. Sedatives and tranquilizers, as well as bowel antimicrobials, may also be required. Stool normalization can be achieved by the use of one or more of the following: a lubricant such as mineral oil, nightly; bulk preparation, such as Metamucil, stool softener, such as dioctyl sodium sulfosuccinate (Colace); instillation of warm oil into the rectum; and an evacuant suppository, such as Dulcolax. Such a prophylactic plan will reduce the bacterial flora of the bowel, diminish the bulk of the stool, and soften the fecal mass, so that it traverses more easily the area of inflammatory obstruction. During therapy, fluid and nutritional requirements may be met intravenously.

Acute Diverticulitis without Obstruction

The patient is placed on bed rest and a low-residue diet, supplemented with intravenous fluids and electrolytes. If there is distention, nasogastric suction may be initiated. Antibiotics, analgesics, and antispasmodics are usually given. Upon subsidence, the above prophylactic regime may be followed.

Surgical Treatment

Surgery is considered if obstruction is untreatable medically or if there is perforation or bleeding. There are two types of surgery: (1) one-stage resection of the involved sigmoid section, for recurrent attacks, or (2) multiple-staged procedures for complications (obstruction, perforation, fistulae) (Fig. 37-7). Surgery is preceded by barium studies. In preparing the patient for surgery, it is important to avoid irritating the colon, which is already terribly sensitive and susceptible to perforation. A mild saline laxative and carefully administered cleansing enemas may be sufficient.

The surgery performed varies with the operative findings. When possible, the area of diverticulitis is resected and the remaining bowel joined end to end (primary resection and end-to-end anastomosis). A two-stage resection is sometimes done in which the diseased colon is resected, as with a one-stage operation, but no anastomosis is performed, and both ends of the bowel are brought out onto the abdomen as stomata. The "double-barrel" colostomy is then anastomosed at a later procedure (Fig. 37-7). In some patients, such an operation may appear impossible or inadvisable, in which case a colostomy is performed in the right transverse colon. Diverting the fecal flow from the area of diverticulitis allows the inflammatory process to subside, and a later

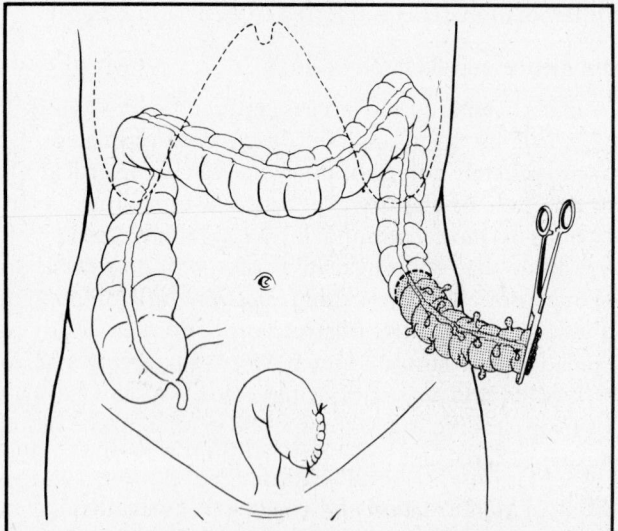

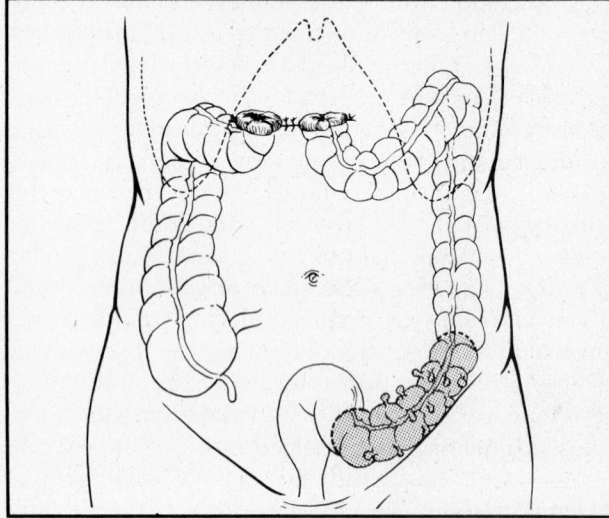

Figure 37-7.   (*Top*) Two-stage (Hartmann) resection for diverticulitis of the colon. *Stage I:* The affected segment (shaded) has been divided at its distal end and brought out through the abdominal wall. It will then be removed by transection at its proximal margin (dotted line), leaving a healthy colostomy stoma on the surface of the abdomen. The upper end of the rectosigmoid stump has been sutured closed. Alternatively, it could have been exteriorized without closing it. *Stage II:* The divided ends of the bowel will be mobilized and anastomosed. (*Bottom*) Three-stage procedure for resection of a segment of the colon involved by diverticulitis. *Stage I:* Transverse colostomy. *Stage II:* Resection of the involved segment (shaded) (lines of resection indicated by dotted lines) and anastomosis of healthy ends. *Stage III:* Closure of transverse colostomy. (Dunphy, J. E., and Way, L. W. (eds.): Current Surgical Diagnosis & Treatment, ed. 3. Los Altos, Calif., Lange Med. Pub., 1977)

operation removing the colon containing the diverticulitis is done, followed by an anastomosis. When this method of treatment is chosen, the colostomy is only temporary, and after the area of diverticulitis has been removed and the intestinal continuity established by the anastomosis, the colostomy is closed. Thus, this is a 3-stage procedure, requiring the care for a colostomy during part of the treatment (see page 780). This colostomy, on the right side of the transverse colon (Fig. 37-10), drains liquid or mushy feces and requires that a bag be worn constantly. Irrigations are rarely of value in this type of colostomy, but ordinary cleanliness is obtained by baths or showers, using soap and water to cleanse the skin about the colostomy stoma. (The nursing management of the patient with a colostomy is discussed on page 780.)

POLYPS

Benign polyps are much more common in the large intestine than in the small intestine. If there are numerous growths, the condition is referred to as *polyposis* — often, apparently, a congenital abnormality. These polyps frequently become cancerous; invariably, in familial polyposis, simple benign polyps infrequently become malignant.

CANCER OF THE COLON

Tumors of the small intestine are rare; on the other hand, tumors of the colon are relatively common. In fact, cancer of the colon and rectum is now the most common type of internal cancer in the United States. Over 100,000 Americans are afflicted annually; about half that number die of it annually — although almost three out of four patients might be saved by early diagnosis and prompt treatment.

Pathophysiology and Clinical Manifestations

Cancer of the colon and the rectum always arises from the epithelium lining the intestine. The effects produced depend largely on the location of the cancer.

As in the case of cancer elsewhere in the gastrointestinal tract, the chief symptoms are the passage of blood in the stools, anemia, obstruction, and perforation. A suddenly developing obstruction may be the first symptom of cancer involving the colon anywhere between the cecum and the sigmoid, for in this region, where the bowel contents are liquid, a slowly developing obstruction will not become evident until the lumen is practically closed. Cancer of the sigmoid and the rectum causes earlier symptoms of partial obstruction, with constipation, alternating with diarrhea, lower-abdominal crampy pains, and distention.

• Any patient with a history of unexplained change in bowel habit and the passage of blood in the stools should be studied carefully to rule out cancer of the large bowel.

The possibility that a rectal carcinoma exists — detectable, but still asymptomatic and still operable — is one important reason for the inclusion of a rectal examination as part of every routine physical examination. Additional symptoms, often present, are those of progressive weakness, anorexia, weight loss, anemia, and lower-abdominal pain.

Assessment

The most important diagnostic procedures are the abdominal and rectal examinations, sigmoidoscopy, repeated examination of the stools for the presence of blood, determination of the blood-hemoglobin concentration for anemia, CEA monitoring, and, usually the most conclusive of all, biopsy with colonoscopy (page 718).

CEA Monitoring. Carcinoembryonic antigen (CEA) is a complex protein found in serum or plasma that is readily detected by specific radioimmunoassay. CEA is present on the cell wall of certain tumors. With increasing growth or cell activity, CEA is released into circulation. (*Note:* Some tumors do not produce CEA.)

The plasma CEA level increases quantitatively as the tumor cell population increases.

Under 5 ng./ml. — Clinically normal.
5-10 ng./ml. — May be clinically indicative of a benign inflammatory condition.
10-20 ng./ml. — May reflect tumor, but false-positive from benign disease may occur.
Over 20 ng./ml. — Direct correlation with tumor volume.

(Example: patient with colon carcinoma and metastasis reached CEA level of 1,500 ng./ml.)

CEA monitoring appears to be a useful means of prognosticating early recurrent disease. Guidelines will be developed when more specific data regarding reliability is determined.

RISK FACTORS FOR CANCER OF THE COLON

Age—over 40
Blood in stool
History of rectal polyps
Presence of adenomatous polyps or villous adenomas
Family history of colon cancer or polyposis
Personal history of chronic inflammatory bowel disease

Management and Nursing Intervention

Preparation for Operation.   Usually a high calorie, low-residue diet is given for several days before operation, if time and the patient's condition permit. If an emergency does not exist, these patients are prepared for several days by being given intestinal antiseptics of the sulfa group (succinylsulfathiazole or phthalylsulfathiazole [Sulfathalidine]) and neomycin. These are given by mouth to reduce the bacterial content of the colon and to soften and decrease the bulk of the contents of the colon. In addition, mechanical cleansing of the bowel may be done by laxatives, enemas, or colonic irrigations.

Careful attention is given to complaints of pain, which are assessed and described as to their nature, location, and duration. The nurse also records fluid losses such as occur with vomiting and diarrhea. This will aid in regulating the fluid intake and maintaining adequate balance. If the hemoglobin is below 12 gm., a blood transfusion may be given, since anemia is common. Preoperative nasogastric intubation facilitates the performance of intestinal surgery and minimizes postoperative distention. An indwelling catheter is inserted to ensure that the bladder is empty during surgery. This will aid in keeping postoperative perineal dressings dry. The abdomen and perineum are shaved as described on page 315.

In the event that there is any possibility of a *colostomy* (a temporary or permanent opening of the colon through the abdominal wall), the patient should be informed by the surgeon. This is a life saving arrangement that is compatible with active participation in social and business life. The nurse is in a position to assist the patient in accepting a colostomy; with courage, optimism, and

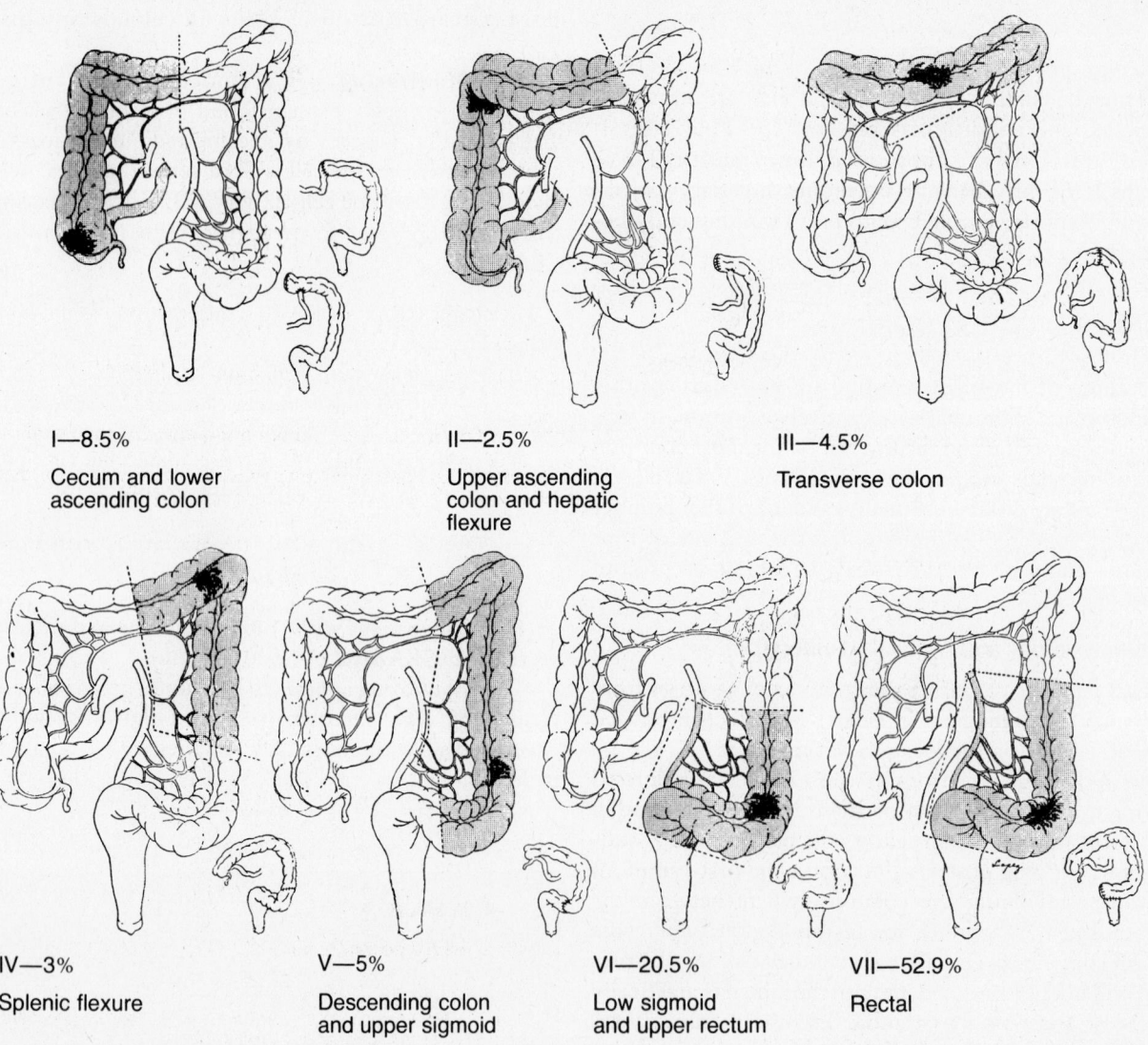

I—8.5%

Cecum and lower ascending colon

II—2.5%

Upper ascending colon and hepatic flexure

III—4.5%

Transverse colon

IV—3%

Splenic flexure

V—5%

Descending colon and upper sigmoid

VI—20.5%

Low sigmoid and upper rectum

VII—52.9%

Rectal

Figure 37-8.   This indicates an approximate incidence of cancer of the colon, Also shown are areas where cancer can occur, what area is removed and (in the very small diagram), how the anastomosis is done. For rectal cancer, an abdominoperineal resection is done with colostomy. (Adapted from American Cancer Society)

determination, the patient can adjust to a new life style, with daily improvement until he has established his individual pattern of management. Members of the health team, the enterostomal therapist, his family, and other ostomates are available to assist and support him.

Operative Treatment. This will depend on the position and the extent of the cancer. When the tumor can be removed, the involved colon is excised for some distance on each side of the growth to remove the tumor and the area of its lymphatic spread (Fig. 37-8). If distant (liver) metastasis has occurred, the tumor may be excised for palliation, but without benefit of cure. The intestine may be reunited by an end-to-end anastomosis of the colon. When the growth is situated low in the sigmoid or the

rectum, the colon is cut above the growth and brought out through the abdominal wall, forming thus an abdominal anus, called a *colostomy*. The growth then is removed from below by a perineal incision (*abdominoperineal resection,* Fig. 37-9).

In the event that the tumor has spread and involves surrounding vital structures, it is considered to be inoperable. When the growth in the rectum or the sigmoid is inoperable, and especially when symptoms of partial or complete obstruction are present, a colostomy may be performed. A loop of the colon, near the junction of the descending colon and the sigmoid, is brought out of the abdomen through a lower left rectus incision and maintained in place by a plastic rod or rubber tube inserted

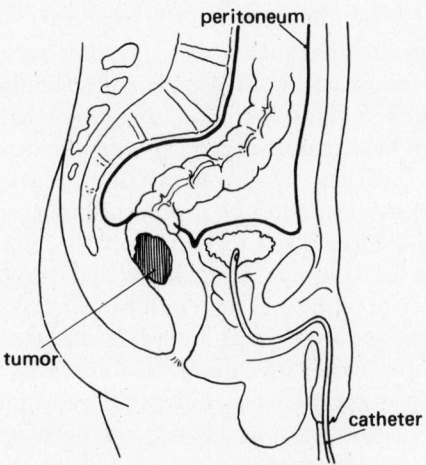

1. Presurgical patient. Note tumor in rectum.

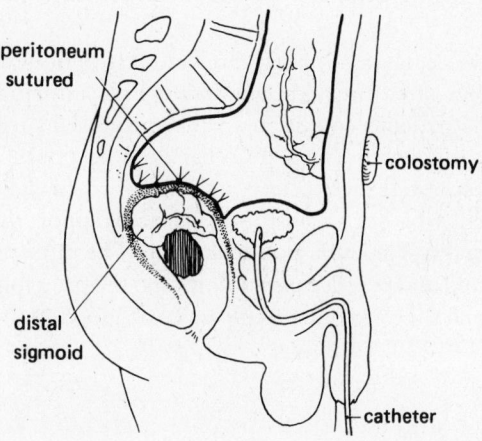

2. At operation, sigmoid is removed and colostomy established. The distal bowel has been dissected free to a point below pelvic peritoneum, which is sutured over the closed end of the distal sigmoid and rectum.

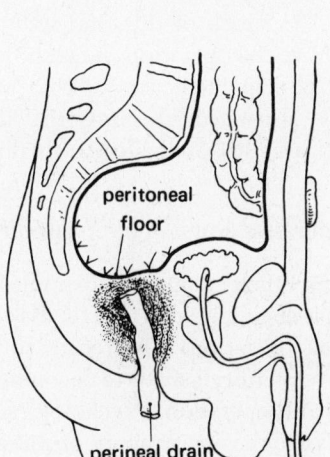

3. Perineal resection includes removal of the rectum and free portion of the sigmoid from below. A drain is inserted in this void.

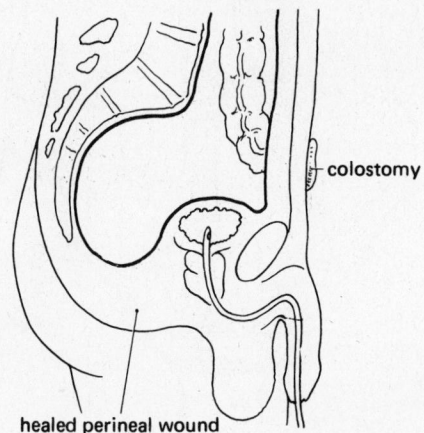

4. The final result after healing. Note healed perineal wound and the permanent colostomy.

Figure 37-9. Abdominoperineal resection for carcinoma of rectum.

underneath the loop (Fig. 37-10). If the obstruction is complete, the loop may be drained by the insertion of a rubber tube or by the use of a right-angled tube, which is held in the intestine by a purse-string suture. When the obstruction is incomplete, the colostomy loop is allowed to remain unopened for several days to permit the peritoneal cavity to become thoroughly sealed off. During this time the patient is given a liquid diet. The intestine is opened by electrocautery, as hemorrhage is slight after its use. (See Table 37-5 to compare differences and similarities between a colostomy and an ileostomy.)

CARE OF THE PATIENT WITH A COLOSTOMY

Nursing Assessment

To give adequate support, care, and instruction to this patient, the nurse must know not only basic information about the patient's condition and the proposed surgery, but also the patient himself. What does he think, feel, express, suppress, desire, fear, etc.? In daily contacts with the patient who has a colostomy, valuable rapport can be established to facilitate his adjustment. The nurse must understand and practice psychology and the principles of learning as they apply to each particular individual.

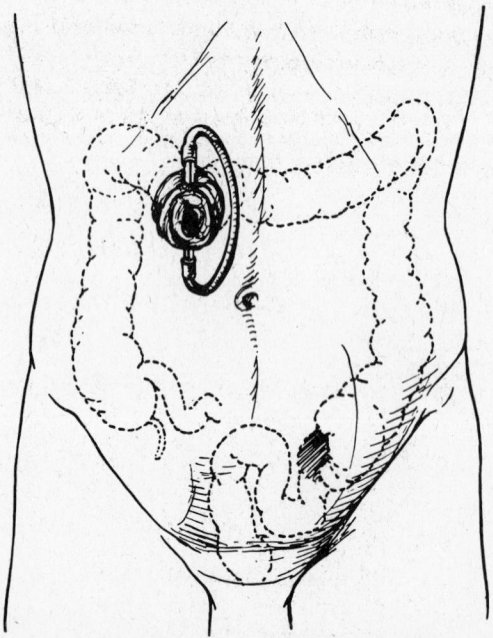

Figure 37-10. Transverse colostomy through a right paramedian incision about 5 cm. (2 inches) above the umbilicus. A rod is carried under the transverse colon and is used as a temporary support to hold the loop of colon outside the abdomen. This location of colostomy is best suited to patients whose obstructions are in the splenic flexure and distally. (From Rhoads, et al.: Surgery. Philadelphia, J. B. Lippincott, 1970)

Psychosocial Preparation

Thousands of people who have colostomies are engaged actively in business today. With the improvement of surgical and nursing procedures, and the assistance of patients who have "lived" with their colostomies, it is now possible to give intelligent assistance to the person about to have a colostomy or an ileostomy. (See Table 37-5 for a comparison of ileostomy and colostomy.)

The support and the teaching of a patient must be individualized. Therefore, the same approach may not be appropriate for all patients. Before operation, some may find that a simple line drawing illustrating the nature and the function of the lower intestinal tract is helpful. By this means the deviations necessary for the particular situation can be explained. For others, having another patient who has had a colostomy talk to them presents a comfortable opportunity for the expression of fears and doubts. In still other situations, some surgeons believe that a minimal amount of explanation should be given the patient before the operation; simply telling a patient that he will have major surgery in order to correct his problem is sufficient. In other words, the extent of psychological preparation must be approached on a personal basis.

The patient needs to know what a colostomy is and how it functions; he should know that it need not hamper his way of living and that with patience, as well as some trial-and-error methods, he will be able to manage, control, and master it. During the interval of preoperative care the nurse should encourage the patient to talk out his concerns and fears; in this way the nurse will be able to direct and help him.

It is well to remember that this is a strange and new experience for the patient. Most likely he has never seen an incision under surgical dressings and, less likely, a colostomy. The shock of this first sight may be minimized if, before the operation, he is shown drawings, a model, and perhaps a picture or two of the anatomy involved. He also needs to know that the reddish appearance and large size of the stoma will diminish in time.

Early Postoperative Nursing Intervention

The patient is helped out of bed on the first postoperative day and is encouraged to care for his colostomy from the very first irrigation. The return to normal diet is rapid, and every effort is made to encourage him to live as he did before his operation. Psychologically, this appears to de-emphasize the abnormality of the situation.

The colostomy is opened on the second or the third postoperative day by the surgeon, at which time there is often an evacuation of loose stools. In anticipation of this the nurse will have protected the bedding with a plastic sheet covered with a towel and will have an emesis basin positioned at the patient's side.

TABLE 37-5.   COMPARISON OF COLOSTOMY AND ILEOSTOMY*

CATEGORIES	COLOSTOMY	ILEOSTOMY
Definition	A portion of the colon is brought through the abdominal wall, thereby creating a temporary or permanent opening.	A portion of the ileum is brought through the abdominal wall, thereby creating a permanent opening.
Indications	Pathological conditions involving large bowel, e.g.: (1) Inflammatory or obstructive processes of the lower intestinal tract. (2) Congenital or traumatic disruption of the intestinal tract. (3) Cancer of the rectum or sigmoid flexure, where anastomosis is not possible.	Pathological conditions involving small bowel, e.g.: (1) Ulcerative colitis, in the vast majority of cases. (2) Crohn's disease (regional ileitis).
Purpose	To provide an outlet for intestinal waste products.	To serve as an exit for waste products when colon has been removed.
Location	Colon	Ileum
Reservoir	Limited	None
Incidence of Evacuation	24-48 hours with control measures	Constant
Consistency of Discharge	Liquid to formed stool	Yellow, green, or brown liquid
Means of Control	No voluntary control. Potential control with diet and/or irrigation.	No voluntary control. Adherent appliance necessary.

*(From American Cancer Society: Colostomy and Ileostomy Care. A Guide of Practical Information for Nurses, 1971)

Regulating the Colostomy

Colostomy Irrigations.   Regulation is effected either by irrigation or by training the bowel to evacuate naturally without irrigations. The choice often depends on the individual and the nature of the colostomy. An ascending colostomy is difficult to control and usually requires daily irrigation. Sigmoidostomy may require irrigation only every 2 or 3 days, if at all.

The stoma on the abdomen does not have voluntary muscular control and may empty at irregular intervals. The time of irrigation should be selected with regard to the schedule the person will pursue after leaving the hospital.

The purpose of irrigating a colostomy is to empty the colon of gas, mucus, and feces so that the patient can go about his social and business activities without fear of fecal drainage. By irrigating the stoma at a *regular* time, there is less gas and retention of irrigating fluids. It is best to irrigate after a meal, since ingestion of food stimulates peristalsis and defecation.

The initial irrigation is usually done on the fourth or fifth postoperative day. There are two methods of irrigating a colostomy: the conventional one, using an enema irrigation procedure, and a second method utilizing a bulb syringe.

Irrigation by Enema.   The following equipment is used:

Irrigating set (2-liter [quart] can or bag, tubing, adapter); catheter, clamp, colostomy irrigator
Solution at 40.5° C. (105° F.)

Petrolatum to lubricate catheter
Toilet tissue to clean around colostomy before and after irrigation
Newspaper or paper bag to receive soiled dressings
A place to set or hang the irrigating container
Dressings for colostomy following irrigation

The patient may sit in a chair before the toilet in the bathroom. A rubber or plastic sheet can be used as a trough leading to the toilet bowl. Encourage the patient to watch the procedure, and explain each step as it is performed. The catheter, lubricated with petrolatum to reduce friction, is inserted 5-7.5 cm. (2-3 inches) at first, and the solution is allowed to run into the colon. (A Laird or wide cone tip, when plugged into the stoma about 1.2 cm. (½ inch), permits irrigation without leakage or the danger of perforation.)

The catheter then can be inserted gently up to 15-20 cm. (6-8 inches). If resistance is met, digital examination may reveal muscle spasm or a mass of stool. *Force is contraindicated, since it is possible to perforate the bowel.*

At first, only about 500 ml. of solution is given, after which the amount may be increased gradually every day up to 1,500 ml. The temperature of the solution is about 40.5° C. (105° F.), and the irrigating can is placed about 45-60 cm. (18-24 inches) above the level of the colostomy opening. Since distention of the colon is an effective stimulus for bowel evacuation, the irrigating solution should be introduced in such amount, and with such pressure, as to distend the bowel and give the patient a feeling of fullness. If the patient complains of cramps, the

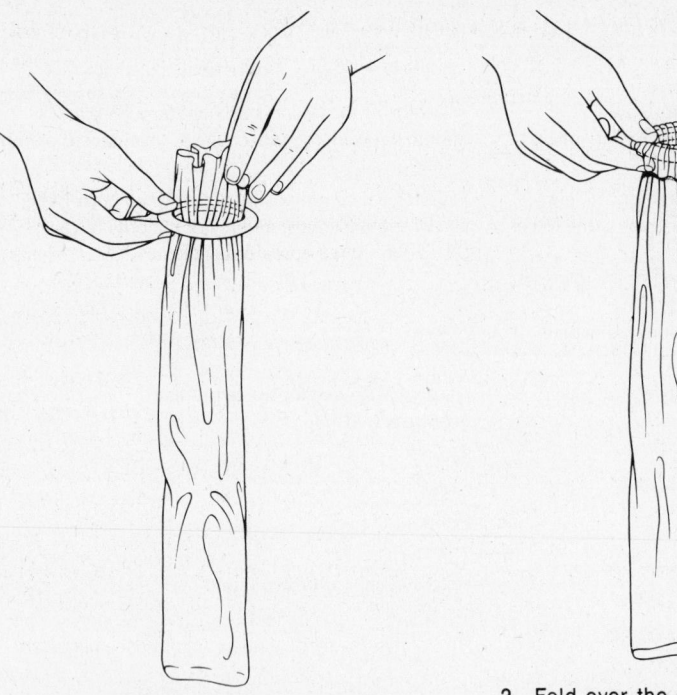

1. Insert one end of drainage sheath through the plastic ring.

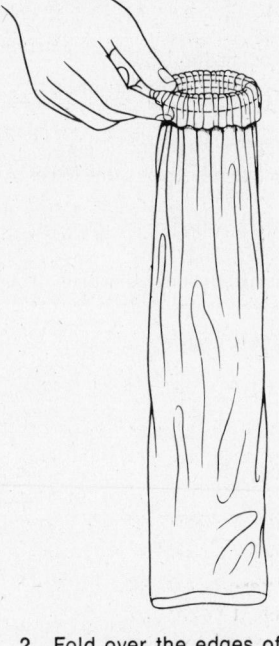

2. Fold over the edges of the sheath and roll around ring securely and evenly.

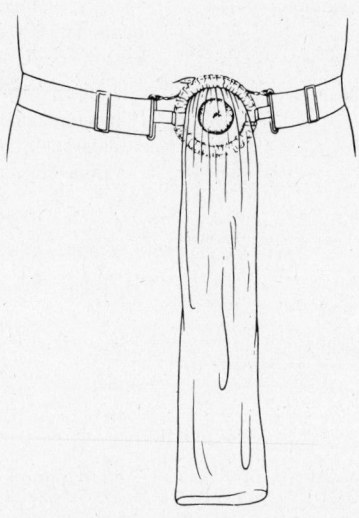

3. The ring with sheath is placed over the stoma, and the belt clips hooked onto the ring. This holds the appliance securely over the opening.

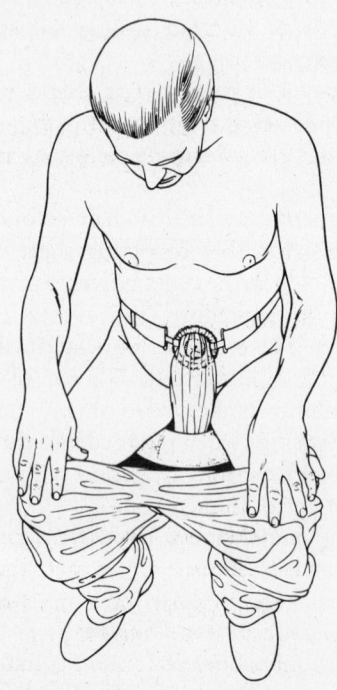

4. After cutting a small hole in the sheath above and to one side of the stoma, the sheath is tucked between the legs so that it leads directly into the toilet.

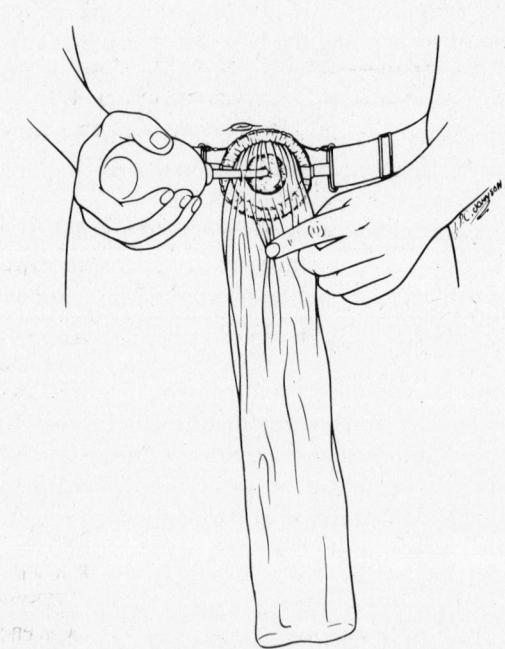

5. Moisten the tip of the syringe with a standard lubricating jelly. Insert the lubricated syringe tip through the hole of the drainage sheath and gently into the stoma about 7.5–12.5 cm. (3–5 inches).

Figure 37-11. The bulb syringe method of colostomy irrigation. (From Postel, A. H., Grier, W. R. N., and Localio, S. A.: Training the Patient in the Bulb Syringe Method of Colostomy Irrigation. New York, New York University Medical Center)

level of the can may be lowered to lessen the force of flow. The patient should be taught that the rate of flow of solution varies with the pressure and the caliber of tube. Pressure depends on height; therefore, when increased pressure is desired, the container of solution may be raised, and vice versa. Solutions may be soapy solution, plain water, or saline. The irrigation may be given daily, every other day, or every 3 days, according to the need and preference of the patient. Some patients prefer to take a warm bath after an irrigation. This promotes a feeling of cleanliness and relaxation. During the irrigation, when done at home, it may be pleasant and diverting to have a radio nearby. While waiting for the return flow, it may be an opportune time to read. (The entire procedure usually takes between 45 minutes and 1 hour.) Nothing but flatus and a slight amount of mucus should escape from the colostomy between irrigations.

Irrigation by Bulb Syringe. The second method of colostomy irrigation is the *bulb syringe* method. This type of irrigation stimulates fecal return, rather than washing the feces out. There is no prolonged trapping of water in the colon and no spillage or accidents during the day.

The patient is seated on the toilet. A 250-ml. (8-oz.) soft rubber bulb syringe is used. The hard nozzle is cut off, and a No. 24 French catheter is attached to the end of the bulb syringe. *No more than 750 ml. (24 oz.) of water is used.* The bulb syringe method is shown in Figure 37-11.

The patient may massage the lower part of the abdomen to ensure adequate return. The bag is left in place for 15 minutes, after which the stoma is covered with a piece of gauze and held in place by a girdle, elasticized shorts, or an elastic belt. The patient completes the procedure by washing the pitcher and bulb syringe with soapy water.

Other Types of Colostomies

"Wet" Colostomy. "Wet" colostomies are those through which both urine and feces are excreted, because of transplantation of ureters into the colon. These colostomies are never irrigated, because of the danger that contaminated material will be forced into the ureters and produce infection.

Double-barrel Colostomy. In a double-barrel colostomy, there are two openings, the proximal and distal segments of colon. The proximal portion is the functioning colon, whereas the distal end is irrigated only to keep it clean and free of mucus. If there is an obstruction in this section, it may be necessary to siphon the fluid. In case the cancer has not been removed, it is well to irrigate the lower loop, from anus to colostomy, every 2 or 3 days, to remove the irritating mucus that collects.

Care of Perineal Wound

If the malignancy has been removed by the perineal route, the wound is observed carefully for signs of hemorrhage. This wound usually contains a drain or packing that is removed gradually, so that about the seventh day all drains are out. There usually are sloughing bits of tissue that must come away for the following week or 10 days. This process is hastened by mechanical irrigation of the wound. It is appreciated by the patient if the pre-

COMMON INTESTINAL OSTOMIES

	ILEOSTOMY	ILEAL LOOP (URINARY CONDUIT)	TRANSVERSE COLOSTOMY	DESCENDING OR SIGMOID COLOSTOMY
1. Intestinal segment involved:	End of ileum	Loop of ileum is made into a pouch into which transplanted ureters drain urine	Transverse colon	Descending or sigmoid colon
2. Effluent	Liquid, semi-liquid, soft	Urine only	Soft and, at occasional intervals, fairly firm; softer toward ileum	Descending—fairly firm stool; Sigmoid—even more solid
3. Odor	Slightly odorous	Nonodorous	Very malodorous	Usually malodorous
4. Skin effect	Enzymes highly irritating	Rarely irritating, unless infection present	Irritating, with continuous discharge	Fairly irritating
5. Types of appliance	Open-ended pouch worn at all times; if Kock pouch, no appliance is worn	Open-ended pouch worn at all times	Pouch worn at all times. (Either a large stoma with 2 openings, or 2 separate stomas; fecal discharge from one and mucus from the other)	Depends upon patient and his control. Some wear no appliance, and irrigate regularly. Others wear closed pouch, if effluent is firm; open-ended, if discharge is more liquid continuously

scribed medication for pain is administered before the procedure is begun. An irrigating container with normal saline or hydrogen peroxide is effective, particularly since the latter effervesces, thereby promoting mechanical removal of tissue debris. Enzymes (streptokinase or streptodornase) are also effective in liquefying necrotic tissue. This may be done two or three times a day and then gradually less frequently. Observe and record the condition of the perineal wound; note any bleeding, infection, or necrosis. During the procedure it is important to protect the bed with an extra waterproof sheet and absorbent pads, and it may be well to plan the irrigation so that it can be performed before the patient receives morning care.

Changing the patient's position from one side to the other every 2-4 hours is desirable, since not only is it uncomfortable to lie in a dorsal recumbent position, but such a position may also interfere with healing by causing wound separation. By the beginning of the second postoperative week, sitz baths may be prescribed, to improve circulation and promote healing and cleanliness. A half-inflated rubber ring is comfortable to sit on.

An indwelling catheter remains in place for several days, to prevent urinary retention and pressure on the perineal area. Continuing assessment of the patient's urinary status is maintained, to control infection and maintain hydration.

Choice and Care of Equipment

Early in the postoperative care of the colostomy or ileostomy patient, the use of a plastic stoma bag is effective in preventing skin irritation and reducing offensive odors. Such protection is relatively inexpensive, since the bags are disposable. Various types of irrigating sets are available from surgical supply houses.*

Colostomy bags may be worn immediately after irri-

*Public Law HR-1, Oct. 30, 1972, specifically has included "colostomy bags and supplies directly related to colostomy care" as being covered under Medicare.

gation; then a change to a simple dressing may be effective. Patients are instructed in the care and the cleaning of equipment to prolong its life and keep it free of odors. Cleaning by soap or a detergent and water, and exposure to fresh air, usually is sufficient; however, it may still be necessary to deodorize the appliance; liquid deodorizers are available to use in washing and soaking equipment. The other aspect of the problem is the control of odors arising from the body excreta as they collect in the appliance. Inserting readily soluble deodorizing tablets in plastic or rubber bags or putting a few drops of chlorophyll solution into the bag will help in the control of odors. Powdered charcoal, two crushed aspirin tablets, or a teaspoon of baking soda may be sprinkled into the bag to absorb odors. Also effective is commercially available colostomy deodorant.

As a rule, colostomy bags are not necessary. As soon as the patient has learned a routine for his evacuation, bags may be dispensed with, and a simple dressing of disposable tissue (often covered with Saran wrap) is used, held in place by an elastic belt or girdle. Except for the escape of gas and a slight amount of mucus, nothing comes from the colostomy opening between irrigations; therefore, the inconvenience of a colostomy bag is unnecessary.

Hygienic Measures

Thorough drying after washing with soap and water may be all that is necessary for good skin care. If the skin around the stoma appears red or irritated, the following may be applied, after cleaning and drying the area: triamcinolone acetonide (Kenalog) spray followed by a light dusting of nystatin powder (Mycostatin). Milk of magnesia paste, Maalox, or Gelusil are also soothing and facilitate healing.

Diarrhea and constipation are controlled as described on page 785.

In general, the patient needs to be reminded that good health practices will materially aid his feeling of well-being and his positive adjustment to his colostomy. Diet should be adequate and well-balanced; laxatives are

TABLE 37-6. DIETARY SUPPORT OF COMMON COMPLICATIONS IN SURGICAL TREATMENT FOR CANCER

PROCEDURE	COMPLICATIONS	DIETARY SUPPORT
Small bowel resection	Poor absorption Weight loss Absorptive capacity improves with time	Immediate support after surgery: long-term parenteral nutrition Later: Oral intake of high protein, high calorie, low-fat diet Medium-chain triglycerides
Ileostomy Colostomy	Initial loss of water and electrolytes	Daily replacement of electrolytes, full liquid diet, high in protein
By-pass surgery	For relief of pain and obstruction Malabsorption syndrome Maldigestion, diarrhea	Feedings by natural route High protein, high vitamin C Adequate vitamins and minerals

(Valassi, K.: Nutritional management of cancer patients in a variety of therapeutic regimens. Arch. Phys. Med. Rehabil., *58*: Sept. 1977)

rarely used. Lastly, it is valuable to observe a usual time for doing certain activities, e.g., mealtime, irrigation time, bedtime, and so forth.

Selection of Appropriate Diet

Diet is individualized as long as it is well–balanced and does not cause diarrhea or constipation. Since certain foods will produce odors or gas, the patient may wish to avoid them: beans, cabbage, cucumbers, fish, radishes, or onions.

If the patient has problems with diarrhea, the use of pectin (Kaopectate), paregoric, bismuth subgallate, bismuth subcarbonate, or diphenoxylate with atropine (Lomotil) will control it. For constipation, prune or apple juice or a mild laxative is effective. For dietary support of complications, see Table 37-6.

GUIDELINES TO NURSING MANAGEMENT OF A PATIENT HAVING A COLOSTOMY

Objectives/Nursing Action	Rationale/Amplification
PREOPERATIVE	
To reduce intestinal flora to as low a level as possible.	
1. Administer intestinal antiseptics as prescribed—usually given several days before surgery.	1. Usually sulfa drugs are most effective. Not only is bacterial count reduced, but there is a softening and reduction of colon contents.
2. Give laxatives, enema, or colonic irrigations as prescribed.	2. Promotes intestinal cleansing.
To promote patient physical and psychosocial comfort.	
1. Assess patient's complaints.	1. Assists in pinpointing source of problem.
2. Support patient's coping mechanism.	2. Permits patient to verbalize feelings and allows nurse to anticipate his concerns. Respect for patient's privacy must be granted.
3. Ascertain whether a temporary or permanent colostomy is to be performed, and whether surgeon has instructed the patient regarding this plan.	3. An informed patient greatly assists in optimum postoperative care. Patient preparation and acceptance are necessary for successful adjustment to new life style.
To maintain optimum physiological levels of all bodily functions.	
1. Record in descriptive form all intake and output.	1. Fluid losses may occur, due to vomiting and diarrhea; electrolytes such as potassium, sodium, and chloride need to be replaced.
2. Note hematocrit and hemoglobin levels.	2. If hemoglobin is below 12 gm., it may be necessary to transfuse patient.
To prevent postoperative discomfort and complications.	
1. Insert a nasogastric tube, as recommended by the physician.	1. Minimizes abdominal distention, and eliminates the discomfort of vomiting.
2. Insert indwelling catheter, if so prescribed.	2. Keeps bladder "flat" during intestinal surgery, and helps to avoid accidental injury.
3. Perform usual activities related to the immediate preoperative nursing care of this patient.	3. Systematic preparation enhances psychological acceptance of surgery.
POSTOPERATIVE	
To provide skilled nursing care through the immediate postoperative, postanesthetic stage.	
Follow usual nursing management of patient having abdominal surgery.	See page 350.
To assess normal and healthy status of colostomy, so that any deviation is easily detected.	
1. Recognize nature of colostomy, so that type and frequency of effluent can be anticipated.	1. Ascending colostomy—fluid feces. Colostomy near hepatic flexure—semi-fluid feces. Transverse colostomy—mushy feces. Splenic flexure colostomy—semi-mushy feces. Descending colostomy—solid feces.

(Continued)

Objectives/Nursing Action	Rationale/Amplification

POSTOPERATIVE (CONTINUED)

2. Observe stoma and surrounding tissue for adequacy of viability.

2. Mature stoma is deep pink or red; will be moist with mucus. Stoma will feel soft to firm.
The nonmature stoma will be friable.
Skin margins should approximate to the stoma completely, circumferentially.
Peristomal skin should look healthy, and similar to that of entire abdomen.

To anticipate problems in caring for the colostomy–psychosocial and physical.
See page 770, Phases of the Rehabilitation Process of the Ileostomy Patient.

Note the similarities in the care of "ostomy" patients.

To plan for colostomy care based on the needs of the particular individual.

1. Select a method of taking care of the colostomy and adhere to this method.

1. Consistency is effective in maintaining optimal functioning of colostomy.
Patient is less likely to be confused if the method is clearly spelled out.

2. Use available agents which have proven their effectiveness.

2. Karaya comes in various forms and is effective in keeping skin healthy and free from enzymatic action of stomal drainage. Stomahesive (Squibb) is effective when excoriation is present.

3. Soap and water is sometimes irritating to the skin and stoma.

3. May be particularly true of the elderly patient. Oil-base soaps could be used, but may prevent adherence of Stomahesive or Karaya ring.

To review and stress information needed when patient with a colostomy goes home.
See Regulating the Colostomy, page 781; Choice and Care of Equipment, page 784; Hygienic Measures, page 784; and Selection of Appropriate Diet, page 785. Also review Phases of the Rehabilitation of the Ileostomy Patient, pages 770-772.

SUMMARY OF THE PRINCIPLES AND OBJECTIVES OF MEDICAL, SURGICAL, AND NURSING MANAGEMENT OF THE PATIENT UNDERGOING INTESTINAL SURGERY

PREOPERATIVE OBJECTIVES:

I. To ensure optimal patient condition for surgery:
  A. Give whole blood or packed red cells as prescribed to patient debilitated by bleeding, infection, or a malignant neoplasm.
  B. Correct fluid and electrolyte deficiencies before operation.
    1. Give intravenous infusions of lactated Ringer's solution, etc., as prescribed prior to surgery, to prevent electrolyte imbalance and diminished renal function during surgery.
  C. Promote the nutrition of the patient.
    1. Correct existing protein deficiencies before operation.
    2. Encourage between-meal feedings.
    3. Give intravenous protein hydrolysates or albumin, if indicated.
  D. Assist in diagnostic examinations to evaluate the patient's pulmonary, cardiac, hepatic, and renal functions.
    1. Evaluate T.P.R. and B.P. at prescribed intervals.
    2. Give medications and treatments indicated, when heart failure is present.
    3. Support the patient undergoing diagnostic bowel studies.
  E. Insert indwelling catheter immediately before surgery to prevent manipulation and trauma to the bladder.

II. To reduce bacteria in the intestinal tract to prevent postoperative infection:
  A. Employ effective measures to empty the colon.
    1. Give laxatives as prescribed, to cleanse the bowel by catharsis.
    2. Administer enemas and colonic irrigations to rid the bowel of feces and gas.

PREOPERATIVE OBJECTIVES (CONTINUED):

3. Offer a low-residue diet, to reduce fecal content in lower bowel.
4. Place patient on liquid diet at the prescribed interval before surgery.

B. Give antibacterial agents (intestinal antiseptics) to control the bacterial flora of the gastrointestinal tract.
   1. Give drug combinations (usually sulfathalidine and neomycin) as prescribed.
   2. Observe patient for symptoms of pseudomembranous enterocolitis.
      a. tender distended abdomen
      b. vomiting, diarrhea
      c. fever

III. To decompress gastrointestinal tract through an indwelling tube to minimize vomiting and distention:
   A. Use a Levin tube for stomach and upper small bowel decompression.
   B. Use a Miller-Abbott tube or other prescribed tube for intestinal decompression.

POSTOPERATIVE OBJECTIVES:

IV. To supply fluids and electrolytes and body nutrients to the patient in the immediate postoperative period:
   A. Use an intravenous catheter if IV therapy is to be carried out for more than a few days.
      1. Use arm for placement of intravenous catheter, to permit greater patient mobility.
      2. Examine needle site for evidences of thrombophlebitis or chemical phlebitis.
      3. Elevate patient's head and back (after he regains consciousness) while he is receiving intravenous infusions.
   B. Record type of intravenous fluid, starting time, finishing time, amount absorbed, and any untoward reactions.
   C. Employ meticulous oral hygiene measures when patient is not taking fluids by the oral route.

V. To ensure continuing function of the nasogastric or nasoenteric tube so that postoperative aspiration, distention, and ileus are minimized:

A. Record amount and type of gastrointestinal aspirate.
B. Watch for symptoms of fluid volume deficit.
   1. Skin dryness
   2. Lethargy
C. Promote comfort of intubated patient.
   1. Lubricate nares with water-soluble ointment.
   2. Turn the patient frequently.
   3. Humidify the room, to decrease dryness of mucous membranes.
   4. Apply cold compresses to neck periodically, if patient complains of sore throat.
D. Remove tube when peristalsis is reestablished (indicated by auscultation, the passage of flatus by rectum, and the clinical symptoms of the patient). (This done at request of the physician.)

VI. To promote the comfort and safety of the patient:
   A. Give analgesic agent according to clinical symptoms and needs of the individual patient.
      1. Assess the patient for hypotension and restlessness.
      2. Use special caution in giving narcotics to elderly patients.
   B. Combat sleeplessness with appropriate nursing measures and prescribed sedative and hypnotics.
   C. Encourage the patient to turn, breathe deeply, and cough, at specified intervals.
   D. Change the dressing, when indicated, if patient has a draining wound, ileostomy, or colostomy.
   E. Encourage the patient to ventilate his feelings and anxieties about his condition.

VII. To observe the patient for complications (see chart below):

VIII. To encourage the patient to have follow-up examinations following surgery:
   A. Inform the patient to expect periodic x-ray examinations of the colon, chest, lumbar spine (especially if patient has cancer).
   B. Reinforce the physician's instructions concerning regular follow-up examinations.
   C. Advise the patient to report any unexplained symptoms or recurring symptoms immediately to his physician.

SUMMARY OF POTENTIAL COMPLICATIONS FOLLOWING SURGERY OF SMALL AND LARGE INTESTINE

Anticipation of and vigilance for complications have first priority in caring for postoperative patients. Prompt recognition and management of these complications can prevent prolonged disability and, in some instances, death.

Complication	Nursing Assessment and Action
Paralytic ileus	Initiate or continue nasogastric intubation. Prepare patient for x-ray study. Ensure adequate fluid and electrolyte replacement. Give antibiotics if patient has symptoms of peritonitis.
Mechanical obstruction	Evaluate patient for intermittent colicky pain, nausea, and vomiting. Prepare for intestinal intubation, electrolyte replacement, and reoperation, if patient does not respond to conservative treatment.

(Continued)

SUMMARY OF POTENTIAL COMPLICATIONS FOLLOWING SURGERY OF SMALL AND LARGE INTESTINE (CONTINUED)

Complication	Nursing Assessment and Action

Infection:
  Intraperitoneal infections
  Abdominal wound infection
	Assess for evidence of constant or generalized abdominal pain, rapid pulse, and elevation of temperature.
	Prepare for tube decompression of bowel.
	Restore fluid and electrolytes by IV route.
	Give antibiotics as directed.

Intra-abdominal septic conditions:
  Peritonitis
	Evaluate patient for nausea, hiccuping, chills, spiking fever, tachycardia.
	  Give antibiotics as prescribed.
	  Prepare patients for drainage procedure.
	  Institute intravenous fluid and electrolyte therapy.
	  Prepare patient for reoperation if his condition deteriorates.

Abscess formation	Administer antibotics as directed. Apply hot compresses as prescribed. Prepare for surgical drainaage.
Wound complications: Infection	Watch temperature graph for evidences of spiking fever. Observe for redness, tenderness, and pain around wound. Assist in establishing local drainage. Obtain specimen of drainage material for culture and sensitivity studies.

Wound disruption	Watch for sudden appearance of profuse serous drainage from wound.
	  Cover wound area with sterile towels held in place with binder.
	  Prepare patient immediately for surgery.

Anastomotic complications: Dehiscence of anastomosis	Prepare patient for surgery.
Fistulas	Employ bowel decompression. Give parenteral fluids to correct fluid and electrolyte defects.

INTESTINAL OBSTRUCTION

An intestinal obstruction is inability of the intestinal contents to flow normally along the intestinal tract, due to some hindrance.

There are two types of intestinal obstruction:
1. Mechanical (dynamic ileus, organic ileus, spastic ileus), in which there is an intraluminal obstruction or a mural obstruction from pressure on the intestinal walls, and
2. Paralytic ileus (adynamic ileus) in which the intestinal musculature is unable to propel the contents along the bowel. (Stimuli which inhibit intestinal peristalsis are: laparotomy, trauma, infection, mesenteric ischemia, and metabolic disorders.)

An obstruction may be partial or complete. Its seriousness depends on the region of bowel that is affected, the degree to which the lumen is occluded, and, especially, the degree to which the blood circulation in the bowel wall is disturbed. Small bowel obstruction is always serious, because, as a consequence of persistent vomiting, it leads to profound disturbances in the electrolyte balance of the body: first, to alkalosis, from the loss of the gastric hydrochloric acid; then, to profound dehydration and acidosis, due to the loss of water and sodium from the small intestine. If the obstruction is only partial and develops slowly, the symptoms are relatively mild. Large bowel obstruction, even if complete, is also comparatively undramatic, provided that the blood supply to the colon is not disturbed. However, if the blood supply is cut off, intestinal strangulation (tissue death) occurs, and the patient's life is in jeopardy.

Causes and Pathophysiology. Proximal to the intestinal obstruction there is an accumulation of intestinal contents, fluid, and gas. In the small intestine, distention reduces the absorption of fluids and stimulates gastric secretion. As a result, fluids and electrolytes are lost. With increasing distention, pressure within the intestinal lumen causes a decrease in venous and arteriolar capillary pressure. This, in turn, causes edema, congestion, necrosis, and eventual rupture or perforation of the intestinal wall.

With vomiting, there is a loss of hydrogen ions and potassium from the stomach, producing hypochloremia, hypokalemia, and metabolic acidosis. When there are acute fluid losses, hypovolemic shock may occur. In the large intestine, dehydration occurs more slowly because there is less fluid loss, due, primarily, to less fluid intake.

One of every three cases of acute colonic obstruction is due to cancer of the large bowel (see page 777). Intestinal obstruction very occasionally results from a foreign body lodged in the bowel, i.e., jewelry, a large fruit stone, a gallstone, a mass of parasitic worms, etc. In other patients, a stricture of the bowel may result from the contracting scar of an ulcer in its wall, due, for example, to tuberculosis.

The intestine may also become pinched in a peritoneal pocket (hernia) or linked by peritoneal adhesions (prime cause of small bowel obstruction), or a loop of intestine may become twisted about itself *(volvulus)*.

Volvulus (Fig. 37-12) is a life-threatening obstruction, because the intestinal lumen is obstructed both proximally and distally. The accumulation of gas and fluid in the trapped bowel leads to necrosis, perforation, and peritonitis.

Hernia (pages 764–766) is one of the most common and important causes of intestinal obstruction (second to small bowel obstruction), and, if strangulated, is a surgery emergency.

Paralytic Ileus

A paralytic ileus is a paralysis of peristaltic movement due to the effect of trauma or toxins on the nerves that regulate intestinal movement. Functional paralytic ileus following abdominal surgery may last 12–36 hours. Because of this, food and fluids are withheld until normal peristalsis returns, as indicated by bowel sounds (heard with the stethoscope) or the passing of flatus. Paralytic ileus may also happen after back injuries, after operation on the kidney, and frequently with peritonitis.

The lack of peristalsis results in a distention of the intestine with gas produced by decomposition of the intestinal contents or by the swallowing of air. Few or no peristaltic sounds can be heard, and the patient may be extremely uncomfortable, if not in marked pain. Relief of the distention associated with paralytic ileus often is obtained by intestinal intubation (see page 722).

Intussusception

Intussusception is another cause of intestinal obstruction. In this condition, the bowel above a certain point pushes itself into the bowel below that point, much as a telescope is shortened by pushing one section into the next. This occurs through peristalsis. The point at which intussusception most commonly develops is at or near the ileocecal valve. The telescoping, or invagination, also may start at the point of attachment of a tumor in the colon — particularly a pedunculated tumor — as a result of its becoming engaged by a peristaltic wave and propelled along the colon, dragging into the lumen that portion of the wall to which its pedicle is attached.

Postoperative Adhesions

After abdominal operations, there are many areas within the abdomen that may not be completely healed, and loops of intestine may become adherent to these areas. Such inflammatory adhesions usually are only temporary and of no particular importance. However,

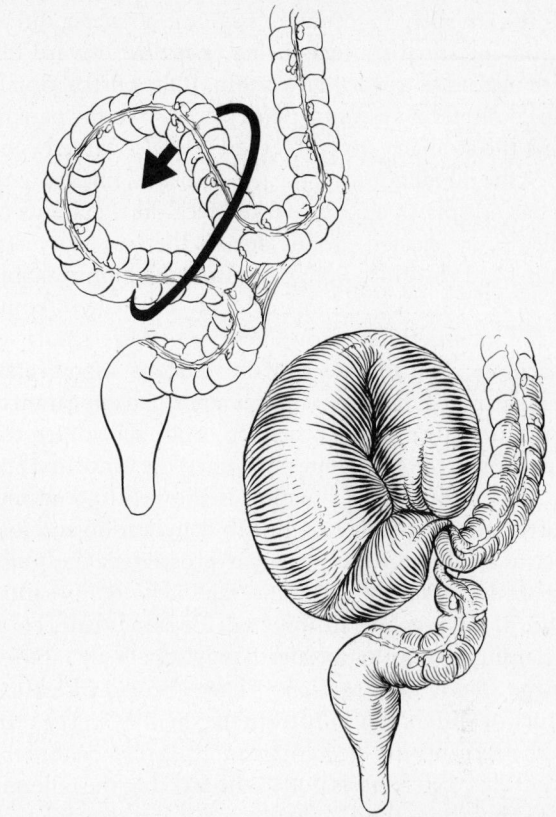

Figure 37-12. Volvulus of the sigmoid colon. The twist is counterclockwise in most cases of sigmoid volvulus. Note the edematous bowel. (Dunphy, J. E., and Way, L. W. (eds.): Current Surgical Diagnosis and Treatment. Los Altos, Calif., Lange Medical Publishers, 1977)

occasionally these adhesions may produce a kinking of an intestinal loop, which causes obstruction of the intestinal flow. This obstruction usually appears on the third or fourth day after operation, when peristalsis normally is resumed and when food and fluids are being given to the patient for the first time. The symptoms are typical of any intestinal obstruction — crampy abdominal pain, distention, vomiting, etc.

The difficulty usually is relieved by nasoenteric suction. Decompressing the bowel above the site of the obstruction allows the inflammation to subside and relieves the obstruction. When the obstruction cannot be relieved by this conservative means, a reoperation may be necessary to free the adherent intestine and to permit the intestinal flow to be resumed.

Clinical Manifestations of Intestinal Obstruction

The symptoms of intestinal obstruction depend on what part of the bowel is obstructed.

Small Bowel Obstruction. The initial symptom is usually pain which is wavelike in character. The patient may pass blood and mucus, but no fecal matter and no flatus. Vomiting occurs. This pattern is often characteristic. If the obstruction is complete, the peristaltic waves become extremely vigorous and assume a reverse direction, the intestinal contents being propelled toward the mouth instead of toward the rectum. If the obstruction is in the ileum, fecal vomiting takes place. First, the patient vomits the stomach contents, then the bile-stained contents of the duodenum and the jejunum and, finally, with each paroxysm of pain, the darker, fecal-like contents of the ileum are ejected. Soon, due to the loss of water, sodium, and chlorides in the vomitus, the unmistakable signs of dehydration become evident. The patient complains of intense thirst, drowsiness, generalized malaise, and aching. The tongue and the mucous membranes become parched; the face acquires a pinched appearance. The abdomen becomes distended, and, the lower the obstruction in the gastrointestinal tract, the more marked is the distention. If the situation is allowed to continue uncorrected, shock appears, due to dehydration and loss of plasma volume. The patient is prostrated; the pulse becomes increasingly weak and rapid; the temperature and the blood pressure are lowered; the skin is pale, cold, and clammy. At this point, death may supervene rapidly.

Large Bowel Obstruction. Large bowel intestinal obstruction differs clinically from the small bowel type in that the symptoms develop and progress relatively slowly. This difference is due to the fact that the colon is able to absorb its fluid contents and it can distend to a

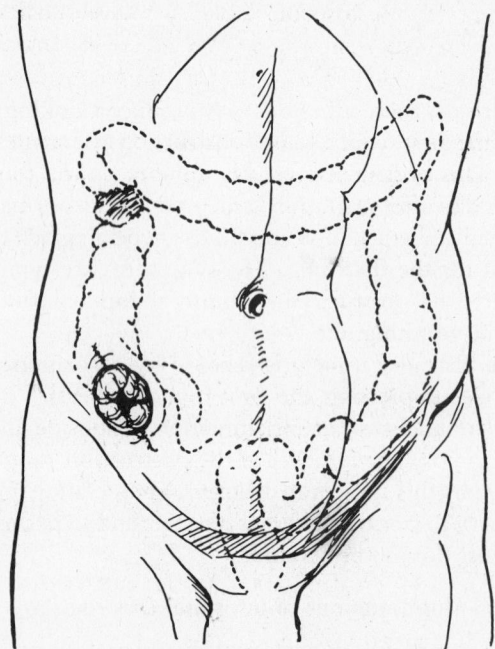

Figure 37-13. Cecostomy drainage for decompression of the colon with lesion lying at hepatic flexure. Cecostomy here is a temporary one, and bowel resection is planned within 2-3 weeks. Location of the cecostomy site is too low in this illustration for a colostomy appliance, but in this instance it is purposely placed low, as incision for the second operation will be largely above the present cecostomy. (From Rhoads, et al.: Surgery. Philadelphia, J. B. Lippincott, 1970)

considerable degree beyond its normal full capacity. In patients with an obstruction in the sigmoid or the rectum, constipation may be the only symptom for days. Eventually the abdomen becomes markedly distended; loops of large bowel become visibly outlined through the abdominal wall, and the patient suffers from crampy lower-abdominal pain. Finally, fecal vomiting develops. The terminal features are essentially those of ileum obstruction. In patients with fecal impaction, there is no shock.

Nursing Assessment and Intervention

The nurse obtains a patient history relative to the function of the gastrointestinal tract, including descriptive information related to stool passage (constipation, obstipation, diarrhea — and frequency). The patient's appetite is assessed to see if it is normal or if there have been signs of anorexia. The patient is queried with regard to weight gain or loss, vomiting (frequency, amount, and description) and pain (location and description).

The abdomen should be assessed with a stethoscope in order to auscultate audible peristalsis (bowel sounds) and gas movement. Whereas bowel sounds are normally gurgling and swishing in nature, obstructions are reflected in high-pitched peristaltic rushes (sudden intense sounds that reach a crescendo peak and then collapse readily). The girth of the abdomen is also noted. Although it may be flat at first, as the obstruction continues distention is noted. For purposes of comparison, the abdomen should be measured with a tape at the same time each day, by the same person. When infection and necrosis are progressing, there is evidence of temperature and pulse elevation and a white blood cell count rapidly rising to 15,000 or 20,000. Tenderness is usually a symptom of strangulation.

Any stool that is passed is to be saved, so that it can be inspected directly and tested for the presence of occult blood.

If the disorder is an incarcerated external hernia, an attempt may be made to reduce it, not by applying pressure to the extruded mass, but simply by having the patient lie flat on his back with knees flexed and an ice compress placed continuously over the mass. This position, and the cold, may cause the edema and swelling of the incarcerated bowel to subside, allowing the loop to escape back through the ring or opening into which it has worked itself.

Fluid, electrolyte, and nutritional needs are evaluated, and met by parenteral therapy. Decompression of the small intestine is accomplished by nasoenteric suction. X-rays, especially survey films of the abdomen and possibly barium studies, in selected instances, may be done to confirm the diagnosis. Preoperative nursing attentions are similar to those followed for major abdominal surgery (page 307).

Surgical Intervention

The surgical treatment of intestinal obstruction depends largely on the cause of the obstruction. In the most common causes of obstruction, such as strangulated hernia, obstruction by adhesions, and so forth, the operation consists of repair of the hernia or division of the adhesion to which the intestine is attached. In some hernias, it may be necessary to remove the strangulated portion of bowel and perform an anastomosis. Operation for intestinal obstruction may be simple or complicated, depending on the duration of the obstruction and the condition of the intestine found at operation.

When the large intestine becomes obstructed, usually by cancer, it is frequently necessary to relieve the colonic obstruction before it is possible to resect the cancer itself. This is done by inserting a large tube into the cecum (cecostomy) (Fig. 37-13) or by making an opening in the colon above the site of the obstruction, by bringing a loop of colon up to the skin surface. When this is opened, the obstruction is relieved, and the tumor can be treated at a later time. This operation is called a *loop colostomy* (see page 779).

ANORECTAL CONDITIONS

Patients with anorectal disorders seek medical help primarily because of pain and rectal bleeding. Other frequent complaints are protrusion of hemorrhoids, anal discharge, itching, and swelling.

Bleeding is frequently seen in anorectal disease. (The most common cause of rectal bleeding is hemorrhoids.) The patient's description of the bleeding, as well as the nurse's assessment, assists in establishing the diagnosis.

The bleeding may be bright red, but occasionally it is a darker color, due to its remaining in the rectal ampulla before expulsion, and also from admixture with feces. Bleeding from the anal canal usually has a bright red appearance.

Nursing Assessment

In assessing the patient's symptoms, the nurse should investigate the following:

1. Is there blood coating the stool or is it mixed with the feces?
2. Is there pain during evacuation? Is there associated abdominal pain?
3. How long does the pain last after evacuation?
4. How does the *patient* describe the pain?
5. Is any protrusion noted from the anus?
6. Is a discharge evident? Mucoid? Purulent? Bloody?

The Rectal Examination and Patient Preparation

Visual inspection and digital examination of the anus and the rectum are indispensable for detecting and identifying lesions involving these structures. Moreover, rectal examination is extremely useful in diagnosing or excluding many intra-abdominal and pelvic conditions, including appendicitis, diverticulitis, salpingitis, tumors of the ovary, the uterus, and the colon, and prostatic lesions of various types.

Rectal examinations may be done with the patient in the knee-chest, Sims's lateral, or in the inverted position, on a special proctoscopic table. Whatever position is used, the patient is informed of the procedure and how it is to be done. He is draped so that only the rectal area is exposed.

As the first step, the buttocks are spread apart with gauze pads or tissue wipes, and the anus and the parianal area are surveyed for fistulas, hemorrhoids, abscesses,

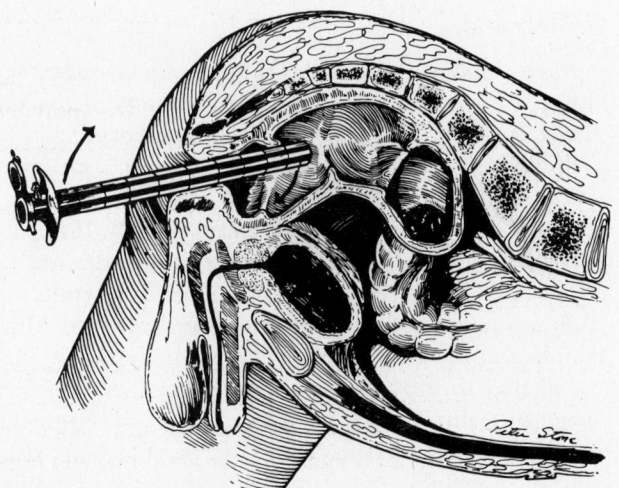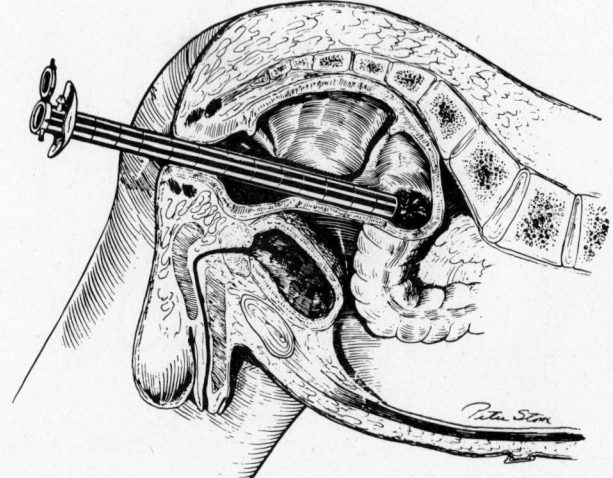

Figure 37-14. Sigmoidoscopy. (*Left*) Direction of motion as the sigmoidoscope, with obturator in place, enters the rectum. (*Right*) The sigmoidoscope reaches the rectosigmoid junction. At this point, the obturator is removed, light carrier is inserted, and a magnifying lens is attached to aid in visualization.

fissures, and other abnormalities. Next, the examiner palpates the anal orifice and rectum, using the index finger, covered with a glove or a finger cot. The nurse should ensure that the requisite items are at hand, including a nonsterile glove or finger cot, lubricant, tissue wipes, and a light source. The nurse also offers support and reassurance and helps the patient to assume the positions necessary for this examination.

Anoscopy, Proctoscopy, Sigmoidoscopy, and Colonofiberoscopy. By means of tubular instruments that incorporate small electric lights, the lumen of the lower bowel may be viewed directly. The anoscope is employed to examine the anal canal; proctoscopes and sigmoidoscopes to inspect the rectum and the sigmoid, respectively, for evidence of ulceration, tumors, polyps, or other pathology.

The flexible fiberoptic colonoscope (Fig. 37-14) has a lens connected by thousands of fiberglass threads to the distal lens at the tip of the colonoscope. Transmission of an image through the threads affords viewing of any adequately illuminated field at a distance of from 1 cm. to several meters away. Hence in the hands of an experienced endoscopist, the splenic and hepatic flexures can be viewed, as can the ileocecal valve. Such an examination requires that the lower bowel be clean; therefore, a warm tap-water enema is given. It may be necessary for the patient to be on clear liquids the day before the examination and to receive a cathartic the evening before it.

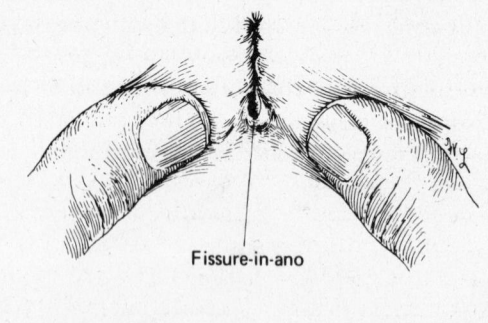

Fissure-in-ano

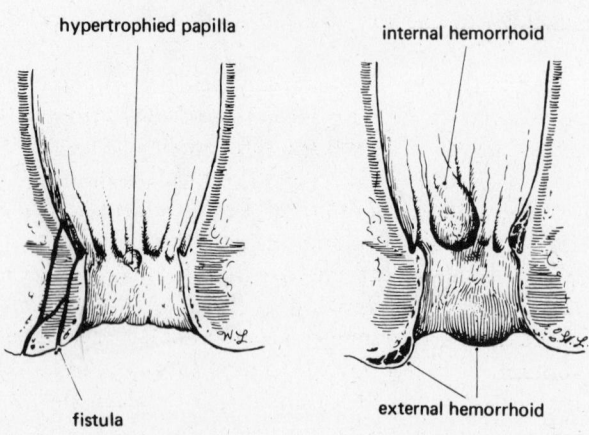

Figure 37-15. Various types of anal lesions.

The patient assumes the knee-chest position, resting on his knees, feet extending over the edge of the bed or the examining table. With knees spread apart to give steady support, the patient leans over and rests the side of his face on the bed or the table, with his forearms on either side of the head and his hands placed, one on top of the other, above the head. His back is now inclined at about a 45-degree angle, and he is in proper position for the introduction of an anoscope, proctoscope, or sigmoidoscope. Maximal convenience and comfort are afforded by a table that has been especially designed for rectal endoscopy—the so-called proctoscopic table, which tilts the patient into the optimal position.

- The patient undergoing a proctosigmoidoscopic examination should be kept informed as to the progress of the examination, and praised for his cooperation. Let him know that he will experience a feeling of pressure and will feel as though he is going to have a bowel movement. Explain that this is from the pressure of the instrument and will last only a brief period of time. It may be necessary to attach suction equipment through the scope to remove any secretion, exudate, blood, or excreta that might be obstructing the area of observation. After each use these tubes must be cleansed thoroughly and the collecting bottles emptied and cleaned likewise. Disposable sigmoidoscopes are now available. While they eliminate the need for cleaning, they must be disposed of safely.

As part of the endoscopic examination, one or more small pieces of tissue may be removed for histologic study, a procedure referred to as a *biopsy*. This is done with small biting forceps introduced through the instrument. Rectal and sigmoidal polyps, if present, may be removed by means of a wire snare which is used to grasp the pedicle or stalk, and an electrocoagulating current used to sever it and to prevent bleeding. It is extremely important that all tissue that is excised by the endoscopist be placed immediately in moist gauze or in an appropriate receptacle, labeled correctly and legibly, and then delivered without delay to the pathology laboratory.

Anorectal Abscess

Anorectal abscess is located in the pararectal spaces. Usually it is caused by infection of pathogenic microorganisms. Incidence is higher in men than women.

Management. An abscess may occur in a variety of spaces in and around the rectum. Often it contains a quantity of foul-smelling pus, and is painful. If the abscess is superficial, swelling, redness, and tenderness are observed. A deeper abscess may result in toxic symptoms and even lower abdominal pain, as well as fever. More than half of rectal abscesses will result in fistulas.

Palliative therapy consists of sitz baths and analgesics. Surgical treatment consists of incision and drainage; this may be all that is necessary. When deeper infection exists, with the possibility of a fistula, it is necessary to remove the fistulous tract. This may be done initially, or it may require a second operation. Often no packing is used; if packing is used, usually the wound is lined with petrolatum gauze. Later, when it is necessary to remove the packing, soaking it first with peroxide of hydrogen is helpful.

These wounds are allowed to heal by granulation. Bowel movements should be formed, rather than liquid or soft. Cathartics or mineral oil are not usually used.

Fistula in Ano

Fistula in ano is a tiny tubular tract that extends into the anal canal from an opening located beside the anus (Fig. 37-15). Pus and/or stool leak constantly from the cutaneous opening, making it necessary for the patient to wear a protective pad. This condition may be an early sign of Crohn's disease.

Management. Three or 4 hours before operation, the perineum should be shaved and the lower bowel evacuated thoroughly with several warm soapsuds enemas. The patient should be allowed to evacuate the enemas on a commode. The last enema should return clear and should be evacuated entirely.

For operation, the patient usually is placed in the lithotomy position, and the sinus tract is identified by inserting a probe into it or by injecting the tract with methylene blue solution. The fistula then may be dissected out or laid open by an incision from its rectal opening to its outlet. The wound is packed with gauze.

Postoperative treatment and complications are the same as those described under "Nursing Management of Patients Having Rectal Surgery" (pages 794-795).

Fissure in Ano

Fissure in ano is a longitudinal ulcer in the anal canal (Fig. 37-15). It is associated frequently with constipation, and its most pronounced symptom is excruciating pain during defecation.

Management. Over half of these fissures will heal if treated by conservative measures, and the remainder will require minor surgery. A bland laxative will prevent constipation. A suppository combining an anesthetic with a steroid is comforting. Anal dilatation may be required, under anesthesia.

In surgical management the same preoperative preparation as for fistula in ano is indicated. Several types of operations may be performed: in some cases, the anal sphincter is dilated and the fissure is excised; in others, a part of the external sphincter is divided. This establishes a paralysis of the external sphincter, with consequent relief of spasm, and permits the ulcer to heal. When there is a large overhanging sentinel hemorrhoid, excision of the ulcer and of the hemorrhoid is performed.

Hemorrhoids

Hemorrhoids are simply varicose veins in the anal canal. They may come and go, and almost everyone has them at some time. They are very common in pregnancy. When they fade away, they may leave a telltale skin tag. They occur in two locations. Those occurring above the internal sphincter are called *internal hemorrhoids,* and those appearing outside the external sphincter are called *external hermorrhoids* (Fig. 37-15). They cause itching, bleeding at stool, and pain. Internal hemorrhoids prolapse frequently through the sphincter and cause considerable discomfort. If the blood within them clots and becomes infected, they grow painful and are said to be *thrombosed.*

Management. Hemorrhoid symptoms and discomfort can be relieved by good personal hygiene and by avoiding excessive straining during defecation. A diet that contains fruit and bran may be all the treatment that is necessary; failing this, perhaps a hydrophilic laxative will help.

Another conservative treatment is that of injecting sterile arachis oil with 5 percent phenol or a mixture of quinine and urea. Many physicians have their preferred medications, which, when injected above the sensitive squamous mucosa through an anoscope have no direct effect on thrombosed veins, per se, but induce a fibrous reaction. This reaction in submucosal tissues of the upper anal canal and lower rectum tends to draw tissue upward toward its normal site. This method has little effect on advanced hemorrhoids.

A recently innovated conservative measure is the rubber-band treatment. As the hemorrhoid is visualized through the proctoscope, the upper part above the mucocutaneous line is grasped with an instrument and a small rubber band is slipped over it. Tissue distal to the rubber band becomes necrotic and is removed. Because of fibrosis, lower anal mucosa is drawn up and adheres to the underlying muscle. While this treatment has been satisfactory in some patients, it has proved painful in others and may cause some secondary hemorrhage.

The most recent treatment is cryosurgical hemorrhoidectomy, which is currently being evaluated for its effectiveness. By freezing the tissues of the hemorrhoid for a sufficient time to cause necrosis, this method acts similarly to the rubber-band method. However, it is painless.

The methods of treating hemorrhoids just described are not effective for advanced thrombosed veins, which are usually treated by surgical hemorrhoidectomy.

The operation usually involves digital dilatation of the rectal sphincter and removal of the hemorrhoids by the use of a clamp and cautery or by ligation and excision. After completion of the operative procedures, a small tube, often covered with petrolatum gauze, may be inserted through the sphincter to permit the escape of flatus and also of blood, if there should be any hemorrhage. Instead of the tube, some surgeons place pieces of Gelfoam or Oxycel gauze over the anal wounds. Dressings, in such cases, are held in place by a T-binder.

Pilonidal Cyst

A *pilonidal cyst* is found in the intergluteal cleft on the posterior surface of the lower sacrum. It is thought by some to be formed by an infolding of epithelial tissue beneath the skin, which may communicate with the skin surface through one or several small sinus openings. Hair frequently is seen protruding from these openings, and this gives the cyst its name—*pilonidal*—a nest of hair. The cysts rarely give symptoms until adolescence or early adult life, when infection produces an irritating drainage or an abscess. This area is easily irritated by perspiration and friction.

Trauma appears to play a part in producing the inflammatory reaction in these cysts.

Management. In the early stages of the inflammation, the infection may be controlled by antibiotic therapy. Once an abscess has formed, as in cases of a hair-containing sinus, surgery is indicated. When an abscess is present, incision and drainage are performed. Usually, however, because the abscesses tend to recur or form secondary sinuses that cause irritating drainage, radical excision of the cyst is necessary. In patients with hair-containing sinuses without marked inflammatory reaction, operation is necessary, for the same reason. The entire cyst and the secondary sinus tracts are excised. In many patients the resulting defect may be sutured, but in some the defect may be so large that it cannot be closed entirely, and it is allowed to heal by granulation.

The *nursing care* of these patients is relatively simple. In those with abscess, hot, moist applications are used frequently. After excision of the cyst, the care is that of any superficial wound. For the first few days, this patient often is more comfortable lying on his abdomen or side with a pillow between his legs. Most patients may be allowed out of bed soon after operation, and their postoperative care is managed at home.

Preoperative Nursing Management of Patients Having Rectal Surgery

Patients facing rectal surgery are ordinarily upset and irritable. The nursing approach should focus on the special psychological problems involved. This patient has a special need for privacy. The perineum often is shaved carefully before surgery. This may vary with the nature of the operation. Usually a lower bowel irrigation is prescribed, which should be given at least 2 hours prior to surgery. The skin area is cleaned as thoroughly as possible.

Postoperative Nursing Management

The first 24 hours after rectal surgery there may be painful spasms of the sphincter and muscles. Therefore, control of pain is of prime consideration. Liberal use of analgesics during this time may be necessary. After 24 hours have elapsed, topical anesthetic agents may be beneficial for relief of local irritation and soreness.

Voiding may be a problem, due to a reflex spasm of the sphincter at the outlet of the bladder and a certain amount of muscle-guarding, from apprehension and pain. All methods to encourage voluntary micturition should be tried before resorting to catheterization. After rectal operations, patients are usually allowed out of bed to void.

- After hemorrhoidectomy, hemorrhage may occur from the veins that were cut. If a tube has been inserted through the sphincter after operation, evidence of bleeding should be apparent on the dressings. If, however, the patient feels faint, restless, and anxious, and the pulse rate increases, the nurse should recognize internal or concealed hemorrhage and give appropriate treatment until the surgeon arrives.

Hygiene of the perianal area is important for patient comfort. This is accomplished by gentle cleansing with warm water and *drying* with absorbent cotton wipes. The patient should be instructed to avoid rubbing the area with toilet tissue.

To relieve soreness and pain, moist heat is employed in the form of warm compresses and sitz baths three or four times daily, and especially after each bowel movement. Moist heat is soothing and relaxes sphincter spasm. An icecap to the head or over the heart helps to prevent the faint feeling experienced by many patients during sitz baths. Wet dressings saturated with equal parts of cold water and witch hazel help relieve edema. Petrolatum should be applied around the anal area when wet compresses are being used continuously, to prevent skin maceration. Instruct the patient to assume a prone position at intervals, since this position promotes dependent drainage of edema fluid.

Medications prescribed may include *suppositories* which contain anesthetics, astringents, antiseptics, tranquilizers, antinauseants, and even bronchodilators. Patients will be more compliant, and less apprehensive and uncomfortable, if the suppository is inserted properly. The most effective position for the patient to assume while the suppository is being inserted is side-lying, with the uppermost leg flexed. The suppository is unwrapped; the buttocks are spread apart with one hand and the suppository inserted with the other. If the suppository was stored in the refrigerator (to prevent melting), it may be warmed to room temperature to lessen irritation of rectal mucosa. Water-soluble suppositories may be lubricated with water or lubricating jelly; however, cocoa butter suppositories are self-lubricating.

The patient may be so fearful of pain that he fails to respond to the signal for defecation and thus develops constipation. Usually cathartics are avoided. It is better to have a formed stool rather than many liquid or soft ones. The painful sphincter spasm can be relieved at once by a hot sitz bath or hot compresses. Mineral oil may be prescribed. Some surgeons prefer that a warm oil retention enema be given when the patient feels a desire to defecate; a soapsuds enema given through a well-lubricated catheter may be prescribed if there has been no bowel movement by the third day after operation. The food preferred by the patient is usually given.

The patient may assume any position that is comfortable. The prone position or side-lying position, with a pillow between the knees, is quite comfortable for these patients. A foam cushion or air ring will greatly increase the patient's sitting comfort. Early ambulation is generally encouraged.

Patient Education

When it is time for the patient to be discharged from the hospital, he should know how to take sitz baths and how to test the temperature of the water. Sitz baths may be given in a bathtub three or four times a day. If this tends to make some postoperative patients weak, sitz baths may be given by employing a dishpan or some large container with enough water to cover the perineum.

The patient is informed about his diet and made aware of the significance of proper eating habits. Also, he ought to know what laxatives he can take safely and why exercise is important. The surgeon usually outlines a schedule in detail to cover the daily routine. This can be reviewed with the patient by the nurse.

BIBLIOGRAPHY

BOOKS

Bockus, H. L., et al.: Gastroenterology, Philadelphia, W. B. Saunders, 1976.

Brooks, F. P. (ed.): Gastrointestinal Pathophysiology, 2nd ed. New York, Oxford Univ. Press, 1978.

Davenport, H. W.: Physiology of the Digestive Tract, 4th ed. Chicago, Year Book Medical Pub., 1977.

Gross, L., and Bailey, Z.: Enterostomal Therapy: Developing Institutional and Community Programs. Wakefield, Mass., Nursing Resources, Inc., 1979.

Hill, R. B., and Kern, F., Jr.: The Gastrointestinal Tract. Baltimore, Williams and Wilkins, 1977.

Mahoney, J. M.: Guide to Ostomy Care. Boston, Little Brown & Co., 1976.

Nyhus, L. N., and Condon, R. E. (eds.): Hernia. Philadelphia, J. B. Lippincott, 1978.

Sleisenger, M. H., and Fordtran, J. S.: Gastrointestinal Disease (Pathophysiology, Diagnosis, Management). Philadelphia, W. B. Saunders, 1978.

Spiro, H. M.: Gastroenterology, 2nd ed. New York, Macmillan Co., 1977.

ARTICLES

General

Bass, L.: More fiber—less constipation. AJN, 77:254-255, Feb. 1977.

Budd, D. C., and Fouty, W. F., Jr.: Familial retrocecal appendicitis. Am. J. Surg., 133:670-671, June 1977.

Breu, C., and Dracup, K.: Helping the spouses of critically ill patients. AJN, 78:50-53, Jan. 1978.

Black, C. D., et al.: Drug interactions in the gastrointestinal tract. AJN, 77:1426-1429, Sept. 1977.

Hongladarom, G. C., and Russell, M.: An ethnic difference—lactose intolerance. Nurs. Outlook, 24:764-765, Dec. 1976.

Hogstel, M.: How to give a safe and successful cleansing enema. AJN, 77:816-817, May 1977.

Literte, J. W.: Nursing care of patients with intestinal obstruction. AJN, 77:1003-1006, June 1977.

Long, G. D.: G.I. bleeding. Nursing '78, 8:44-50, Mar. 1978.

Matsishe, J. W., and Phillips, S. F.: Chronic diarrhea. Med. Clin. N. Am., 62:141-154, Jan. 1978.

Mendeloff, A. I.: Dietary fiber and gastrointestinal diseases. Med. Clin N. Am., 62:165-171, Jan. 1978.

Ryan, A. J.: Validation of appendectomy, can it be done? Postgrad. Med., 65:19-21, Jan. 1979.

Sack, D. A., et al.: Prophylactic doxycycline for travelers diarrhea. New Eng. J. Med., 298:758-763, Apr. 1978.

Sheridan, J. L.: Obstructions of the intestinal tract. Nurs. Clin. N. Am., 10:147-155, Mar. 1975.

Stahlgren, L., and Morris, N. W.: Intestinal obstruction. AJN, 77:999-1002, June 1977.

Stroup, P.: Recognition and management of G.I. bleeds. J. Emerg. Nsg., 4:19-25, Sept.-Oct. 1978.

Sweet, K.: Hiatal hernia. Nursing '77, 7:36-43, Aug. 1977.

Welling, P. G.: How food and fluid affect drug absorption. Postgrad. Med., 62:73-82, July 1977.

Wichern, W. A.: The surgical abdomen. Postgrad. Med., 62:145-148, Nov. 1977.

Ileostomy

Alpers, D.: Inflammatory bowel disease (ulcerative colitis). Arch. Int. Med., 138:286-291, Feb. 1978.

Baum, M., and Fletcher, J. C.: Porcine dressing for ileostomy retraction. AJN, 76:760-761, May 1976.

Cotton, C.: Phillip was saved but not by the rule book (Crohn's disease). RN, 41:77-82, Jan. 1978.

Cox, B. G., and Wentworth, A. A.: The Ileal Pouch Procedure, 2nd ed. (booklet). Rochester, Minn., Mayo Foundation, 1977.

Geels, W., et al.: The enterocutaneous fistula. Nursing '78, 8:52-55, Apr. 1978.

Grubb, R. D., and Blake, R.: Emotional trauma in ostomy patients, AORN J., 23:52-55, Jan. 1976.

Hill, G. L.: Ileostomy: surgery, physiology, and management. New York, Grune and Stratton, 1976.

Heyman, E., et al.: The pouch ileostomy. Nursing '77, 7:44-47, Sept. 1977.

Isler, C.: If the ileostomy is continent, the benefits are obvious. RN, 40:39-45, Apr. 1977.

Kock, N. G.: A new look at ileostomy. In Nyhus, L. M.: Surgery Annual, 8:241-256, 1976.

Lamanske, J.: Helping the ileostomy patient to help himself. Nursing, '77, 7:34-39, Jan. 1977.

Lenneberg, E. S., and Sohn, N.: Modern concepts in the management of patients with intestinal and urinary stomas. Clin. Obstet. Gynecol., 15:542-579, June 1972.

Sachar, D. B., and Present, D. H.: Immunotherapy in inflammatory bowel disease. Med. Clin. N. Am., 62:173-183, Jan. 1978.

Watson, P. G.: A family centered ostomy rehabilitation program. Crit. Care Update, 4:5–17, Sept. 1977.

Watson, P. G., et al.: Comprehensive care of the ileostomy patient. Nurs. Clin. N. Am., 11:427–444, Sept. 1976.

Watt, R. C.: Ostomies: why, how and where, an overview. Nurs. Clin. N. Am., 11:393–404, Sept. 1976.

Watt, R. C., and Traverso, C. J.: Patients with abdominal stomas: critical care nursing considerations. Crit. Care Update, 4:5–16, Nov. 1977.

Wentworth, A., and Cox, B.: Nursing the patient with a continent ileostomy. AJN, 76:1424–1428, Sept. 1976.

Colon, Colostomy, Intestinal Obstruction

Auld, L. S.: Pseudo-ostomy. AJN, 78:1525, Sept. 1978.

Broadwell, D. C., and Sorrells, S. L.: Loop transverse colostomy. AJN, 78:1029–1031, June 1978.

Castro, A. F., and Tuxen, P.: Inflammatory bowel disease. Surg. Clin. N. Am., 58:573–580, June 1978.

Clarke, J. S., et al.: Preoperative oral antibiotics reduce septic complications of colon operations. Ann. Surg., 186:251–259, July 1977.

Connell, A. M.: Dietary fiber and diverticular disease. Hosp. Pract., 11:119–124, Mar. 1976.

Dericks, V. C.: The ostomy patient really needs you. Nursing '76, 6:9, 30–33, Sept. 1976.

Gallagher, D. M., and Russell, T. R.: Surgical management of diverticular disease. Surg. Clin. N. Am., 58:563–572, June 1978.

Heindel, M.: How to protect your ostomy patients from post-op skin problems. RN, 41:43–46, Jan. 1978.

Herrero, A. F.: Medical therapy of colonic diverticular disease. Postgrad. Med., 60:107–109, Dec. 1976.

Hilkemeyer, R., and Rodriguez, D.: Development of an enterostomal therapy education program, Nurs. Clin. N. Am., 11:469–478, Sept. 1976.

Jackson, B. S.: Colostomates reactions to hospitalization and colostomy surgery. Nurs. Clin. N. Am., 11:417–425, Sept. 1976.

Jeter, K. F.: Reality therapy: a realistic approach to enterostomy rehabilitation. Nurs. Forum, 17:72–83, no. 1, 1978.

Kodner, I. J.: Colostomy and ileostomy. Clin. Sympos., 30:2–36, no. 5, 1978.

Lindensmith, S.: Body image and the crisis of enterostomy. Canad. Nurse, 73:24–27, Nov. 1977.

Literte, J. W.: Nursing care of patients with intestinal obstruction. AJN, 77:1003–1006, June 1977.

McCloskey, J. C.: How to make the most of body image theory in nursing practice. Nursing '76, 6:5, 68–72, May 1976.

Miller, S. F.: The detection of asymptomatic colorectal cancer. Am. Fam. Phys., 18:89–92, Sept. 1978.

Painter, N. S.: Diverticular disease of the colon: a bane of the elderly. Geriatrics, 31:89–94, Feb. 1976.

Rush, A.: Cancer and the ostomy patient. Nurs. Clin. N. Am., 11:405–415, Sept. 1976.

Sheridan, J. L.: Obstructions of the intestinal tract. Nurs. Clin. N. Am., 10:147–155, Mar. 1975.

Stahlgran, L. H., and Morris, N. W.: Intestinal obstruction. AJN, 77:999–1002, June 1977.

Stevens, L. W.: Surgical management of colonic diverticulitis and complicated diverticulosis. Postgrad. Med., 85:122–125, Dec. 1976.

Shinya, H., and Wolff, W. I.: Colonoscopy. *In* Nyhus, L. M., Surgery Annual, 8:257–295, 1976.

Sredl, D. R.: Another look at the ostomy patient. J. Pract. Nurs., part 1, Jan. 1977; part 2, Feb. 1977; part 3, Mar. 1977.

Talbott, T. M., and MacKeigan, J. M.: Colonic endoscopy in perspective. Surg. Clin. N. Am., 58:459–468, June 1978.

Visintainer, M., and Wolfer, J.: Sex and the colostomy. RN, 42:61–62, Jan. 1979.

Watt, R. C.: Colostomy irrigation — yes or no? AJN, 77:442–444, Mar. 1977.

————: Ostomies: why, how and where, an overview. Nurs. Clin. N. Am., 11:393–404, Sept. 1976.

Waye, J. D.: Colitis, cancer, and colonoscopy. Med. Clin. N. Am., 62:211–224, Jan. 1978.

Winawer, S. J., and Sherlock, P.: Detecting early colon cancer. Hosp. Pract., 12:49–56, Mar. 1977.

Wood, R. Y., and Watson, P. G.: People with temporary colostomies. Canad. Nurse, 73:28–30, Nov. 1977.

Wayle, M.: An ostomy information clinic. Nurs. Clin. N. Am., 11:457–476, Sept. 1976.

Rectal Conditions

Breitung, J.: Have we frozen out the Walters of the world? (rectal cancer). RN, 40:65–68, Aug. 1977.

Buls, J. G., and Goldberg, S. M.: Modern management of hemorrhoids. Surg. Clin. N. Am., 58:469, June 1978.

Downs, G. E.: Rectal suppositories. Am. Fam. Phys., 15:152–154, Apr. 1977.

Fay, M. R., and Snider, W. R.: Nonoperative therapy for hemorrhoids. AORN J., 24:448–452, Sept. 1976.

Goldberg, et al.: Symposium on anal surgery. Contemp. Surg., 11:39–55, Nov. 1977.

Hoexter, B.: Use of Water Pik lavage in pilonidal wound care. Dis. Colon, Rectum, 19:470–471, 1976.

Lewis, M. D.: Cryosurgical hemorrhoidectomy. Dis. Colon, Rectum. 15:128–134, Mar.–Apr. 1972.

Lord, P. H.: Approach to the treatment of anorectal disease, with special reference to hemorrhoids. *In* Surgery Annual. New York, Appleton-Century-Crofts, 9:195–211, 1977.

Mazier, W. P., et al.: Anal fissure and anal ulcers. Surg. Clin. N. Am., 58:479–485, June 1978.

Pietsch, J., et al.: Injury by hypertonic phosphate enema. Canad. Med. Assoc. J., 116:1169–1170, May 1977.

Reeder, G. D., and McGehee, R. N.: Office management of pilondal disease and common anorectal lesions. Am. Fam. Phys., 8:178–189, Sept. 1973.

Sullivan, E. S., and Garnjobst, W. M.: Pruritus ani: a practical approach. Surg. Clin. N. Am., 58:505–512, June 1978.

Stearns, M. W.: Benign and malignant neoplasms of colon and rectum. Surg. Clin. N. Am., 58:605–618, June 1978.

AGENCIES

Canadian Foundation for Ileitis and Colitis, 294 Spadina Ave., Toronto, Ontario M5T 2E7, Canada

National Foundation for Ileitis and Colitis Inc., 295 Madison Ave., New York, N.Y. 10017

National Institute of Arthritis, Metabolism and Digestive Diseases, National Institutes of Health, Bethesda, Md. 20205

United Ostomy Association, 1111 Wilshire Blvd., Los Angeles, Calif. 90017

Metabolic and Endocrine Problems

UNIT NINE

38

ASSESSMENT AND MANAGEMENT OF PATIENTS WITH HEPATIC AND BILIARY DISORDERS

PHYSIOLOGIC OVERVIEW

The liver, the largest organ of the body, can be considered a chemical factory whose job is to manufacture, accumulate, alter, and excrete a large number of substances involved in metabolism. The location of the liver is essential in this function, since it receives nutrient-rich blood directly from the gastrointestinal tract, and then either stores or transforms these nutrients into chemicals that are used elsewhere in the body for metabolic needs. The liver's role is especially important in the regulation of glucose and protein metabolism. The liver manufactures and secretes bile, which has a major role in the digestion and absorption of fats in the gastrointestinal tract. The liver functions as an organ of excretion by removing waste products from the bloodstream and secreting them into the bile. The bile produced by the liver is stored temporarily in the gallbladder until it is needed for the process of digestion, at which time the gallbladder empties and bile enters the intestine.

Anatomy

The liver is located behind the ribs in the upper right portion of the abdominal cavity. It weighs about 1,500 gm. and is divided into four lobes. Each lobe is sur-rounded by a thin layer of connective tissue, which extends into the lobe itself and divides the liver mass into small units, called *lobules*. A schematic diagram of the liver and its anatomic relationships is shown in Figure 38-1.

The circulation of the blood into and out of the liver is of major importance in its function. The blood that perfuses the liver is derived from two sources. Approximately 75 percent of the blood supply comes from the portal vein, which drains the gastrointestinal tract and is rich in nutrients. The remainder of the blood supply enters by way of the hepatic artery and is rich in oxygen. Terminal branches of these two blood supplies join to form common capillary beds which constitute the sinusoids of the liver. Liver cells (hepatocytes) are thus bathed by a mixture of venous and arterial blood. The sinusoids empty into a venule which occupies the center of each liver lobule and is called the *central vein*. The central veins join to form the hepatic vein, which constitutes the venous drainage from the liver and empties into the inferior vena cava, close to the diaphragm. Note that there are two sources of blood flowing into the liver, but there is only one exit pathway.

In addition to hepatocytes, phagocytic cells belonging to the reticuloendothelial system are present in the liver.

799

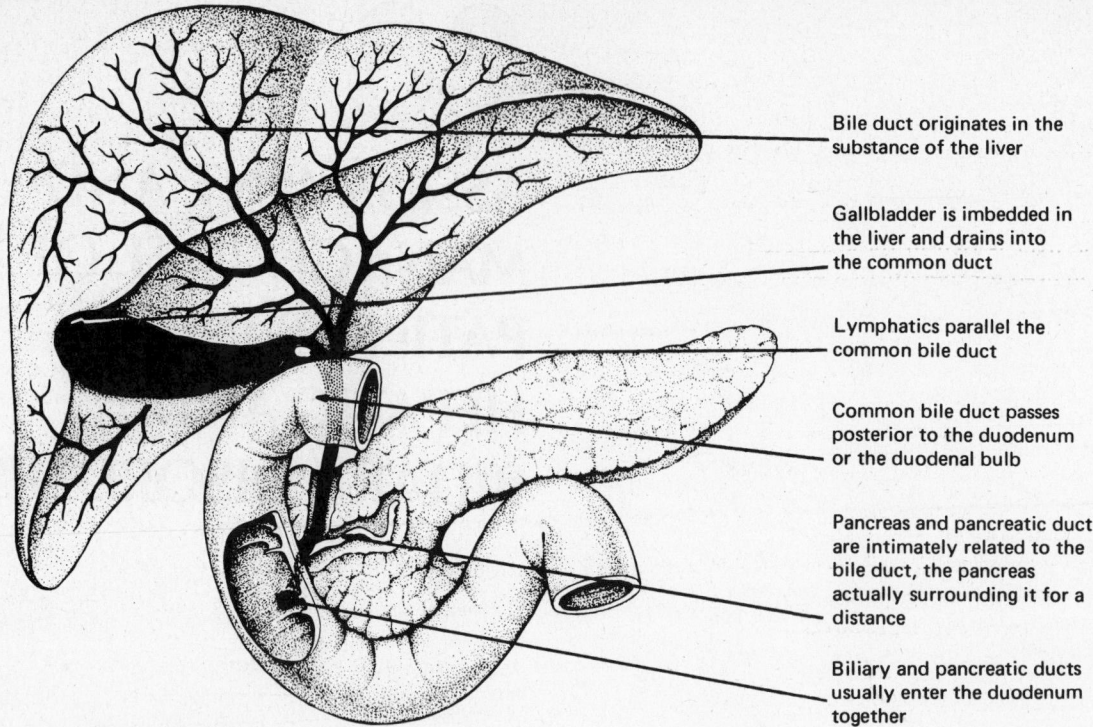

Figure 38-1. Anatomical relationships of the biliary tract. (From Iber, F. L.: Hospital Medicine 4:no. 6, June 1968)

Labels:

Bile duct originates in the substance of the liver

Gallbladder is imbedded in the liver and drains into the common duct

Lymphatics parallel the common bile duct

Common bile duct passes posterior to the duodenum or the duodenal bulb

Pancreas and pancreatic duct are intimately related to the bile duct, the pancreas actually surrounding it for a distance

Biliary and pancreatic ducts usually enter the duodenum together

Other organs that contain reticuloendothelial cells are the spleen, the bone marrow, lymph nodes, and lungs. In the liver, these cells are called *Kupffer cells.* Their main function is to engulf particulate matter in the blood.

The smallest bile ducts, called *canaliculi,* are located between the lobules of the liver. These canaliculi receive secretions from the hepatocytes and carry them to larger bile ducts, which eventually form the *hepatic duct.* The hepatic duct from the liver and the cystic duct from the gallbladder join to form the *common bile duct,* which empties into the small intestine. The flow of bile into the intestine is controlled by the sphincter of Oddi, located at the junction where the common bile duct enters the duodenum.

The gallbladder, a pear-shaped, hollow, saclike organ, about 7.5-10 cm. (3-4 inches) long, lies in a shallow depression on the inferior surface of the liver, to which it is attached by loose connective tissue. The capacity of the gallbladder is 30-50 ml. of bile. Its wall is composed largely of smooth muscle. The gallbladder is connected to the common bile duct by the cystic duct.

Metabolic Functions of the Liver

The liver plays a major role in the regulation of blood glucose concentration. After a meal, glucose is taken up from the portal venous blood by the liver and converted into glycogen, which is stored within the hepatocytes. Subsequently, the glycogen is converted back to glucose and released as needed into the bloodstream, in order to maintain normal levels of blood sugar. Additional

glucose can be synthesized by the liver through a process called *gluconeogenesis.* For this process, the liver can utilize amino acids from protein breakdown, or lactate produced by exercising muscles.

Utilization of amino acids for gluconeogenesis results in the formation of ammonia as a by-product. The liver converts this metabolically generated ammonia into urea. Ammonia produced by bacteria in the intestines is also removed from portal blood for urea synthesis. In this way, the liver converts ammonia, a potential toxin, into urea, a harmless compound that can be excreted in the urine.

The liver also plays an important role in protein metabolism. The liver synthesizes almost all of the plasma proteins (except gamma globulin) including albumin, alpha and beta globulins, blood-clotting factors, specific transport proteins, and most of the plasma lipoproteins. Vitamin K is required by the liver for synthesis of prothrombin and some of the other clotting factors. Amino acids serve as the building blocks for protein synthesis.

The liver is also active in fat metabolism. Fatty acids can be broken down for the production of energy and production of ketone bodies (acetoacetic acid, beta-hydroxybutyric acid, and acetone). Ketone bodies are small compounds which can enter the bloodstream and provide a source of energy for muscles and other tissues. Breakdown of fatty acids into ketone bodies occurs predominantly when the availability of glucose for metabolism is limited, as during starvation or in diabetic patients. Fatty acids and their metabolic products are also used for the synthesis of cholesterol, lecithin, lipoproteins, and other complex lipids. Under some conditions, lipids may accumulate in the hepatocytes and result in the abnormal condition called fatty liver.

Vitamins A, B₁₂, D, and several of the B complex are stored in large amounts in the liver. Certain metals, such as iron and copper, are also stored within the liver. Because the liver is rich in these substances, liver extracts have been used for therapy of a wide range of nutritional disorders.

DRUG METABOLISM. Many drugs, such as barbiturates and amphetamines, are metabolized by the liver. Metabolism generally results in loss of activity of the drug, although in some cases activation may occur. One of the important pathways for drug metabolism involves alteration of the drug by the cytochrome P-450 system. Another pathway of importance involves conjugation (binding) of the drug with a variety of compounds, such as glucuronic or acetic acid, to form more soluble substances. The conjugated products may be excreted in the feces or urine, similar to bilirubin excretion.

Bile

Bile is continuously formed by the hepatocytes and collected in the canaliculi and bile ducts. It is composed mainly of water and electrolytes such as sodium, potassium, calcium, chloride, and bicarbonate, and also contains significant amounts of lecithin, fatty acids, cholesterol, bilirubin, and bile salts. Bile is collected and stored in the gallbladder and is emptied into the intestine when needed for digestion. The functions of bile are excretory, as in the excretion of bilirubin, and as an aid to digestion through the emulsification of fats by bile salts.

BILE SALTS. Bile salts are made by the hepatocytes from cholesterol. After conjugation with amino acids (taurine and glycine), they are excreted into the bile. The bile salts, together with cholesterol and lecithin, are required for emulsification of fats in the intestine. This process is necessary for efficient digestion and absorption. Bile salts are then reabsorbed, primarily in the distal ileum, into portal blood for return to the liver and are again excreted into the bile. This pathway from hepatocytes to bile to intestine and back to the hepatocytes is called the *enterohepatic circulation*. Because of the enterohepatic circulation, only a small fraction of the bile salts that enter the intestine is excreted in the feces. This decreases the demand for active synthesis of bile salts by the liver cells.

Bilirubin Excretion

Bilirubin is a pigment derived from the breakdown of hemoglobin by cells of the reticuloendothelial system, including the Kupffer cells of the liver. Hepatocytes remove bilirubin from the blood and chemically modify it through conjugation to glucuronic acid, which makes the bilirubin more soluble in aqueous solutions. The conjugated bilirubin is secreted by the hepatocytes into the adjacent bile canaliculi and is eventually carried in the bile into the duodenum. In the small intestine, bilirubin is converted into urobilinogen, which is in part excreted in the feces and in part absorbed through the intestinal mucosa into the portal blood. Much of this reabsorbed urobilinogen is removed by the hepatocytes and is secreted into the bile once again (enterohepatic circulation). Some of the urobilinogen enters the systemic circulation and is secreted by the kidneys in the urine. Elimination of bilirubin in the bile represents the major route of excretion for this compound. The bilirubin concentration in the blood may be increased either in the presence of liver disease or when the flow of bile is impeded (e.g., with gallstones in the bile ducts). If bilirubin does not enter the intestine (e.g., with bile duct obstruction), urobilinogen will be absent from the urine.

Gallbladder

The gallbladder functions as a storage depot for bile. Between meals, when the sphincter of Oddi is closed, bile produced by the hepatocytes enters the gallbladder. During storage, a large portion of the water in bile is absorbed through the walls of the gallbladder, so that gallbladder bile is five to ten times more concentrated than that originally secreted by the liver. When food enters the duodenum, the gallbladder contracts, and the sphincter of Oddi relaxes, allowing the bile to enter the intestine. This response is mediated by secretion of the hormone cholecystokinin-pancreozymin (CCK-PZ) from the intestinal wall.

Pathophysiology (Fig. 38-2)

Disease processes that may lead to hepatocellular dysfunction include viral infections and the effects of toxins. Chronic alcohol ingestion resulting in cirrhosis is a common example of toxic liver damage. Hepatocellular dysfunction is manifested by alteration of the metabolic and excretory functions of the liver. Serum bilirubin concentration rises, leading to jaundice (yellowing of skin). Abnormalities of the glucose tolerance test result. Gynecomastia (enlarged breasts) and other manifestations of feminization may occur, due to failure of the liver to normally inactivate estrogens. Serum albumin concentration decreases and edema may result. Ammonia absorbed from the gastrointestinal tract may not be converted to urea and may be responsible for central nervous system impairment. Vascular architecture of the liver may be disturbed, causing elevation of portal-vein blood-pressure, resulting in ascites (leakage of fluid into abdominal space) and esophageal varices. The lack of normal production of various blood-clotting factors can lead to bleeding from any site, but the patients become particularly prone to gastrointestinal bleeding.

Impairment of liver function may also occur when the flow of bile into the intestine is impeded. This most commonly is due to obstruction of the biliary tract by

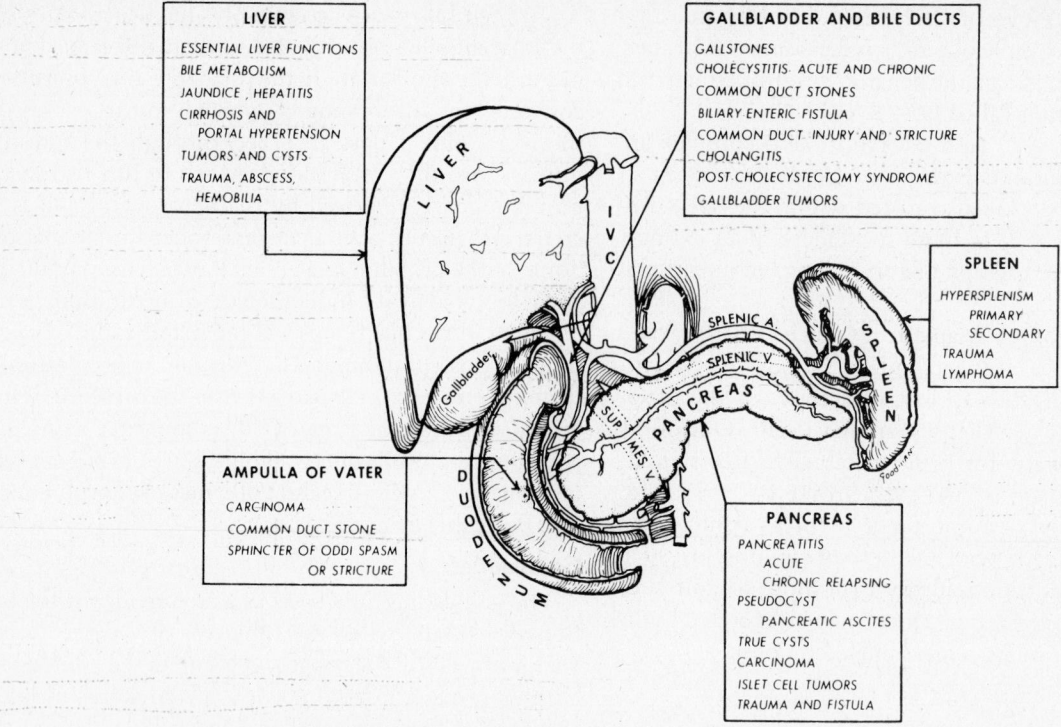

Figure 38-2. Some surgical disorders of the liver, extrahepatic biliary tract, pancreas, and spleen. (Hardy: Rhoads Textbook of Surgery. Philadelphia, J. B. Lippincott, 1977, p. 928)

gallstones or a tumor. The major manifestations are related to impaired bilirubin excretion, with resulting jaundice, dark urine, and clay-colored stools.

Liver Failure

Liver failure is present when the ability of the liver to carry out its excretory and metabolic functions falls below the needs of the body. It results from damage to the liver parenchymal cells, either directly, from primary liver parenchymal diseases, or secondary to obstruction to bile flow or to derangements of hepatic circulation. Acute liver damage may cause acute liver failure, may be completely reversible, or may progress to chronic disease. The end result of chronic liver damage is cirrhosis, characterized by replacement of parenchymal cells with fibrotic tissue. In the usual patient with cirrhosis, areas of regenerating liver coexist with areas of fibrosis during the course of progression to chronic liver failure.

Disease of the liver parenchyma may be caused by infectious agents such as bacteria and viruses, and by anoxia, metabolic disorders, toxins and drugs, nutritional deficiencies, and states of hypersensitivity. Probably the most common cause of parenchymatous damage is malnutrition, especially in alcoholism. The response of the parenchymal cells is much the same for most noxious agents: replacement of glycogen by lipids (fatty infiltration), with or without cell death (necrosis). This is commonly associated with inflammatory cell infiltration and growth of fibrous tissue. Cell regeneration can occur if the disease process is not too toxic to the cells. The end result of chronic parenchymatous disease is a shrunken and fibrotic liver (cirrhosis). Portal hypertension due to intrahepatic obstruction to portal blood flow, or jaundice due to intrahepatic obstruction of bile channels may result.

Biliary disease generally is associated with obstruction of biliary channels, either of the small bile canaliculi (cholangioles) inside the liver (intrahepatic) or of the bile ducts outside the liver (extrahepatic). Extrahepatic biliary obstruction may be due to neoplasm or to benign causes such as gallstones or strictures, while intrahepatic disease is usually due to viral hepatitis or drug reactions. The result of biliary disease is accumulation of bile pigments in the liver and blood to produce jaundice. These conditions are often associated with proliferation of the cholangioles and cellular infiltration resulting in parenchymal liver damage. Scarring may result, which in this case is called *biliary cirrhosis*. In mild cases of biliary disease, however, the liver architecture is not appreciably altered.

The most common circulatory problem involving the liver is hepatic congestion due to increased blood pressure in the inferior vena cava. Chronic congestive heart failure is the usual underlying etiology. Hepatic vascular congestion results in a large edematous liver that may pulsate. If the process is prolonged, parenchymal cells may be damaged and cirrhosis ("cardiac cirrhosis") may result.

DIAGNOSTIC ASSESSMENT OF HEPATIC FUNCTION

LIVER FUNCTION TESTS. Over 70 percent of the parenchyma of the liver may be damaged before liver function tests become abnormal. Function is generally measured in terms of serum enzyme activity (e.g., alkaline phosphatase, transaminases, lactic dehydrogenase), clearance of sulfobromophthalein (Bromsulphalein or BSP), and serum concentrations of proteins, bilirubin, ammonia, clotting factors, and lipids. A list of the commonly used liver-function tests is shown in Table 38-1; further details for some studies are described in Figure 38-3.

LIVER BIOPSY. A procedure that greatly facilitates the diagnosis of most hepatic disorders is the liver biopsy, i.e., the sampling of liver tissue by needle aspiration for the purpose of histologic study. Nursing responsibilities in relation to liver biopsy and the rationale of the nurse's participation in this procedure are summarized on page 804. A graphic presentation is found in Figure 38-4.

TABLE 38-1. LIVER-FUNCTION STUDIES

TEST	NORMAL	CLINICAL FUNCTIONS
I. *Pigment Studies*		
A. Serum bilirubin, direct (Fig. 38-3)	0.-0.3 mg. %	These are measures of ability of liver to conjugate and excrete bilirubin. They are abnormal in liver and biliary tract disease, causing jaundice, clinically.
B. Serum bilirubin, total	0.-0.9 mg. %	
C. Urine bilirubin	0	
D. Urine urobilinogen	0-1.16 mg./24 hrs.	
E. Fecal urobilinogen (infrequently used)	40-280 mg./24 hrs.	
II. *Dye Clearances*		
A. Bromosulphalein excretion (BSP test)	<5% retention 45 minutes after dye injection of 5 mg./kg. body weight	BSP binds to albumin in blood. Liver cells unbind BSP, conjugate it, and excrete it in bile. Normal clearance depends on hepatic blood flow, functioning liver cell mass, and lack of obstruction. Retention is increased in liver cell damage or decreased liver blood flow.
B. Indocyanine green	500-800 ml./sq. m. body surface/min.	Extracted from blood and excreted by liver. Depends on hepatic blood flow, functioning liver cells, and lack of obstruction.
III. *Protein Studies*		
A. Total serum protein	7.0-7.5 gm. %	Proteins are manufactured by the liver. Their levels may be affected in a variety of liver impairments.
B. Serum albumin	3.5-5.5 gm. %	
C. Serum globulin	1.5-3.0 gm. %	Albumin Cirrhosis
D. Serum protein electrophoresis	Albumin 63-69% of total	Chronic hepatitis
	Alpha 1 glob. 3.9-7.3%	Edema, ascites
	Alpha 2 glob. 3.9-7.3%	Globulin Cirrhosis
	Alpha 2 glob. 6.9-11.8%	Liver disease
	Beta glob. 6.9-11.8%	Chronic obstructive jaundice
	Gamma glob. 9.8-20%	Viral hepatitis
IV. *Prothrombin Time*		
Response of prothrombin time to vitamin K	100% return to normal	Prothrombin time may be prolonged in liver disease. It will not return to normal with vitamin K in severe liver-cell damage.
V. *Serum Alkaline Phosphatase* (Fig. 38-3)	Varies with method. 2-5 Bodansky units	Manufactured in bones, liver, kidneys, intestine. Excreted through biliary tract. In absence of bone disease, it is a sensitive measure of biliary tract obstruction.
VI. *Serum Transaminase Studies*		
A. SGOT	10-40 units	Based on release of enzymes from damaged liver cells. These enzymes are elevated in liver cell damage.
B. SGPT	5-35 units	
C. LDH	165-400 units	
VII. *Blood Ammonia* (arterial)	20-50 mg. %/100 ml.	Liver converts ammonia to urea. Ammonia level rises in liver failure.
VIII. *Flocculation Tests*		
A. Cephalin flocculation	0-1+	Depend on ability of serum proteins to stabilize colloidal suspension. Abnormal in liver and other diseases. Positive thymol turbidity also produced by elevated gamma globulin levels.
B. Thymol turbidity	0-5 units	
(These protein reactions are too nonspecific to be of great value.)		
IX. *Cholesterol*	150-250 mg. %	Elevated in biliary obstruction. Decreased in parenchymal liver disease.
Ester	60% of total	

(Continued)

TABLE 38-1. LIVER-FUNCTION STUDIES (CONTINUED)

TEST	NORMAL	CLINICAL FUNCTIONS
X. *Radiologic Studies*		
A. Barium study of esophagus		For varices. Varices in esophagus indicate increased portal pressure.
B. Plain film of abdomen		To determine gross liver size.
C. Liver scan with radio-tagged iodinated rose bengal, gold, or technetium		To show size, shape of liver. To show replacement of liver tissue with scars, cysts, or tumor.
D. Cholectystogram and cholangiogram		For gallbladder and bile duct visualization.
E. Celiac axis arteriography (Fig. 38-3)		For liver and pancreas visualization.
F. Splenoportogram (splenic portal venography—Fig. 38-3)		To determine adequacy of portal blood flow.
XI. *Peritoneoscopy* (Fig. 38-3)		Direct visualization of anterior surface of liver, gallbladder, and mesentery.
XII. *Liver Biopsy* (page 803 and Fig. 38-4)		To determine anatomic changes in liver tissue.
XIII. *Measurement of Portal Pressure*		Elevated in cirrhosis of the liver.
XIV. *Esophagoscopy*		To search for esophageal varices and abnormalities.
XV. *Electroencephalogram*		Abnormal in hepatic coma and impending hepatic coma.

LIVER BIOPSY AND THE ROLE OF THE NURSE

Nursing Activities

1. Ascertain in advance that hemostasis tests have been requisitioned, completed, and reported and that compatible donor blood is available.

2. Measure and record the patient's pulse, respirations, and arterial pressure immediately prior to biopsy.

3. Describe to the patient in advance:
   a. Steps contemplated
   b. Sensations expected
   c. Aftereffects anticipated
   d. Restrictions of activity to be imposed afterward

4. Give support to the patient during the procedure.

5. Expose the right side of the patient's upper abdomen (rt. hypochondriac).

6. Instruct the patient to inhale and exhale deeply several times, finally to exhale and to hold his breath at the end of expiration (Fig. 38-4).

   The physician promptly introduces the biopsy needle by way of the transthoracic (intercostal) or transabdominal (subcostal) route, penetrates the liver, aspirates and withdraws. The entire procedure is completed within 5-10 seconds.

7. Instruct the patient to resume breathing.

8. Immediately following the biopsy, assist the patient to turn on his right side; place a pillow under his costal margin, and caution him to remain in this position, recumbent and immobile, for several hours.

9. Measure and record the patient's pulse and respiratory rates and his arterial pressure at 10- to 20-minute intervals for the prescribed period of time, or until his status proves to be stable, and his condition has been pronounced to be satisfactory. Be alert to detect and to report promptly any increase in pulse rate or any decrease in arterial pressure, any complaint of pain or manifestations of apprehension.

Rationale

1. Many patients with liver disease have clotting defects and are prone to bleed abnormally.

2. Prebiopsy values provide a basis on which to compare the patient's vital signs and evaluate his status following the procedure.

3. Explanations serve to allay his fears, to ensure his cooperation, and to reinforce his instruction.

4. The proximity of an understanding nurse enhances comfort and promotes a sense of security.

5. The skin at the site of penetration will be cleansed and infiltrated with local anesthetic.

6. Holding the breath immobilizes the chest wall and the diaphragm; penetration of the diaphragm thereby is avoided, and the risk of lacerating the liver is minimized.

8. In this position, the liver capsule at the site of penetration is compressed against the chest wall, and the escape of blood or bile through the perforation is impeded.

9. These signs may indicate the presence and the progress of hepatic bleeding or bile peritonitis, the most frequent complications of liver biopsy.

SERUM BILIRUBIN

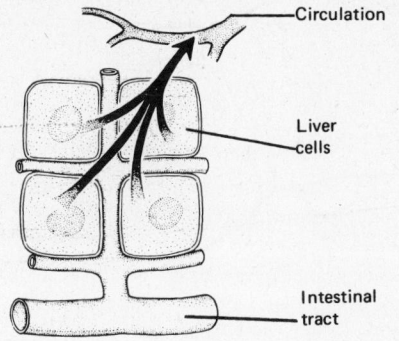

Circulation

Liver cells

Intestinal tract

RATIONALE

Interruption of the normal bile pathways to the intestinal tract (red arrow) results in increased serum bilirubin levels (large arrow).

QUESTION ANSWERED

Is there jaundice?

ALKALINE PHOSPHATASE

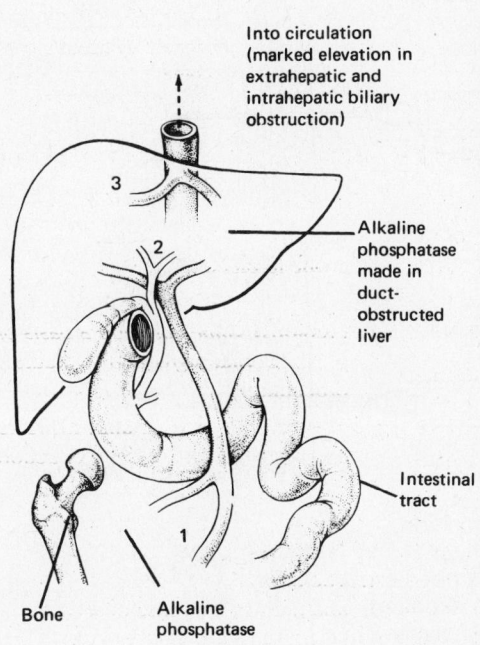

Into circulation (marked elevation in extrahepatic and intrahepatic biliary obstruction)

Alkaline phosphatase made in duct-obstructed liver

Intestinal tract

Bone

Alkaline phosphatase

RATIONALE

Alkaline phosphatase delivered to the liver (1) is excreted in the bile, as indicated by red arrows (2). In the event of biliary obstruction, serum alkaline phosphatase increases by virtue of impaired bile flow pathways and increased hepatic manufacture, as indicated by black dotted arrow (3).

QUESTIONS ANSWERED

Is the biliary tract blocked? Has it been blocked recently?

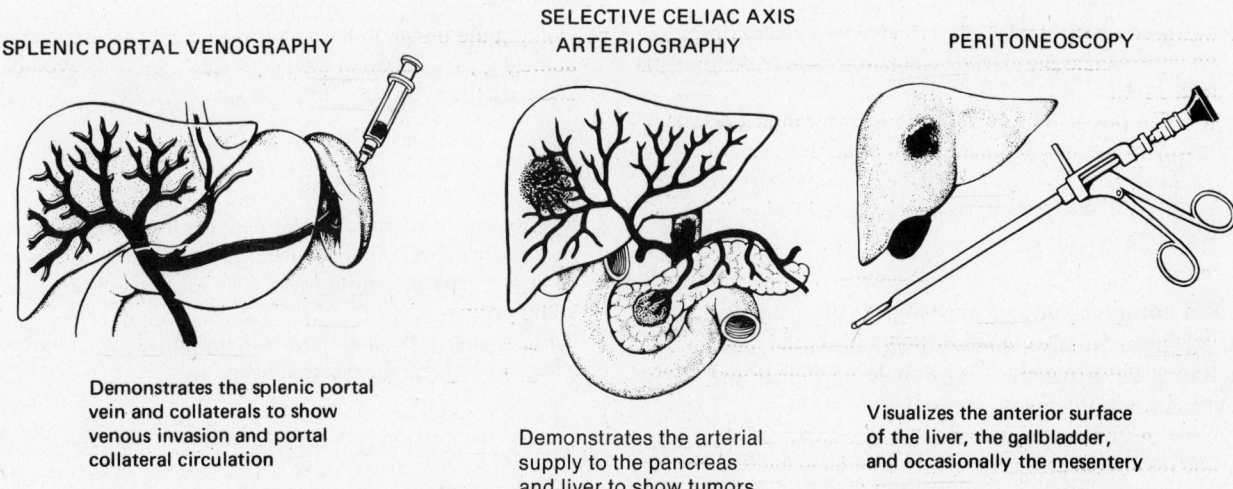

SPLENIC PORTAL VENOGRAPHY

Demonstrates the splenic portal vein and collaterals to show venous invasion and portal collateral circulation

SELECTIVE CELIAC AXIS ARTERIOGRAPHY

Demonstrates the arterial supply to the pancreas and liver to show tumors

PERITONEOSCOPY

Visualizes the anterior surface of the liver, the gallbladder, and occasionally the mesentery

Figure 38-3.   Amplification of some liver function studies. (From Iber, F. L.: Hospital Medicine, 4:no. 6, June 1968)

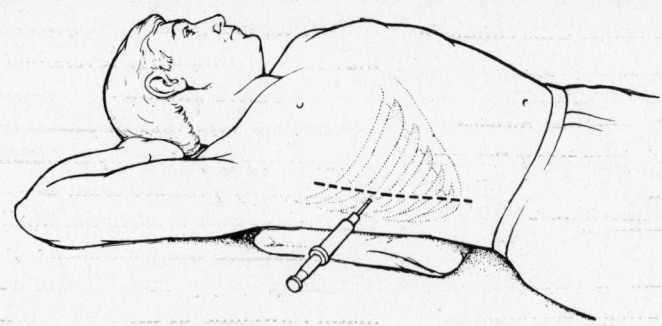

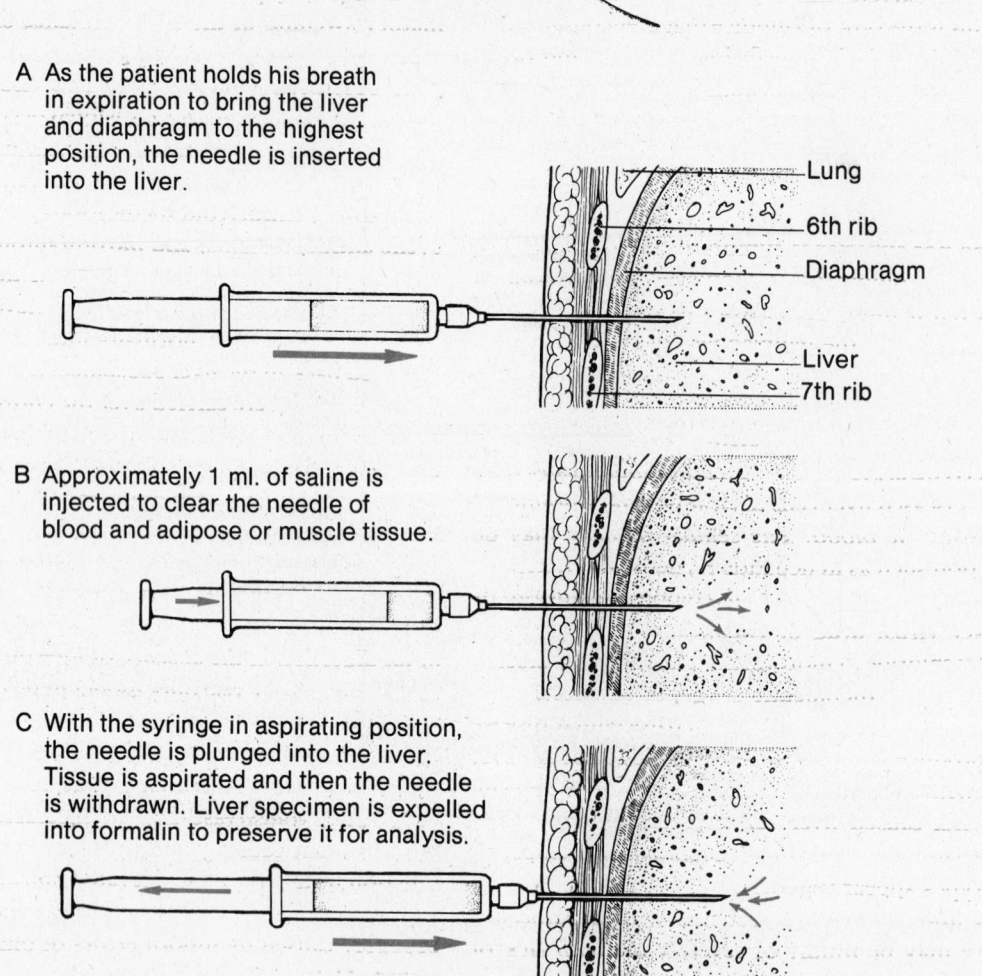

A As the patient holds his breath in expiration to bring the liver and diaphragm to the highest position, the needle is inserted into the liver.

B Approximately 1 ml. of saline is injected to clear the needle of blood and adipose or muscle tissue.

C With the syringe in aspirating position, the needle is plunged into the liver. Tissue is aspirated and then the needle is withdrawn. Liver specimen is expelled into formalin to preserve it for analysis.

Lung
6th rib
Diaphragm
Liver
7th rib

Figure 38-4. Liver biopsy.

CLINICAL MANIFESTATIONS OF HEPATIC DYSFUNCTION

The complications of liver disease are numerous and varied. In many instances their ultimate effects are incapacitating or lethal; their advent is ominous, and their treatment is notoriously difficult.

Among the most important of these complications are:
1. severe gastrointestinal hemorrhages, and excessive salt and water retention with ascites and edema, the result of circulatory changes within the diseased liver leading to portal hypertension;
2. impairment of the central and peripheral nervous systems and abnormal bleeding tendencies, attributable to the inability of malfunctioning liver cells to metabolize certain vitamins;
3. hepatic coma, reflecting the incomplete metabolism of protein fragments by the diseased liver.

JAUNDICE

When, for any reason, the bilirubin concentration in the blood becomes abnormally increased, all the body tissue, including the sclerae and the skin, become tinged with a yellow or a greenish-yellow color. This condition is called *jaundice*. There are three types of jaundice: (1) hemolytic, (2) hepatocellular, and (3) obstructive. Only the latter two types are associated with liver disease.

HEMOLYTIC JAUNDICE. Hemolytic jaundice is the result of an increased destruction of the red blood cells, the effect of which is to flood the plasma with bilirubin so rapidly that the liver, although functioning perfectly normally, cannot excrete this pigment as rapidly as it is formed. This is the type of jaundice that is encountered in patients with hemolytic transfusion reactions and other hemolytic disorders. The bilirubin in the blood of these patients is predominantly of the unconjugated, or "free," type. Fecal and urine urobilinogen are increased; on the other hand, the urine is free of bilirubin. Patients with this type of jaundice, unless their hyperbilirubinemia is extreme, do not experience symptoms or complications as a result of the jaundice *per se*. However, very prolonged jaundice, even if mild, predisposes to the formation of "pigment stones" in the gallbladder, and extremely severe jaundice—e.g., in patients with levels of free bilirubin above 20 to 25 mg. per 100 ml.—is attended by a definite risk of possible brain-stem damage.

HEPATOCELLULAR JAUNDICE. This is jaundice caused by inability of diseased liver cells to clear normal amounts of bilirubin from the blood. The cellular damage may be from infection such as in hepatitis A, hepatitis B, hepatitis nonA nonB (from virus-infected blood transfusion) or yellow fever virus, drug or chemical toxicity (such as carbon tetrachloride, chloroform, phosphorus, arsenicals, certain psychotherapeutic drugs, or ethanol).

Cirrhosis of the liver is a form of hepatocellular disease that may produce jaundice; it is usually, but not always, associated with excessive alcoholic intake. It may be a late result of viral-caused liver cell necrosis. In prolonged obstructive jaundice, cell damage eventually develops, so that both types appear together.

Clinical Manifestations. Patients with hepatocellular jaundice may be mildly or severely ill, with lack of appetite, nausea, loss of vigor and strength, and possible weight loss. In some instances of hepatocellular disease, there may be no jaundice clinically. The SGOT (serum glutamic oxaloacetic transaminase) and the SGPT (serum glutamic pyruvic transaminase) are two intracellular enzymes of the liver that are liberated with cellular necrosis and rise in the bloodstream. Measurements of the levels of these substances are excellent tests for liver cell damage. The cardiogreen test and bile acids radioimmunoassay are replacing the BSP (bromosulphalein excretion) test. In addition, bilirubin and alkaline phosphatase may be elevated, as well as the urine urobilinogen. In long-standing cases, the serum proteins are abnormal and the prothrombin time prolonged. At onset there may be complaints of headache, chills, and fever, if the cause is infectious. Depending on the cause and extent of the liver cell damage, hepatocellular jaundice may or may not be completely reversible.

OBSTRUCTIVE JAUNDICE. Obstructive jaundice of the extrahepatic type may be caused by the bile duct's being plugged by a gallstone, by an inflammatory process, by a tumor, or by pressure from an enlarged gland. Or the obstruction may involve the small bile ducts within the liver substance (i.e., intrahepatic obstruction), caused, for example, by pressure on these channels from inflammatory swelling of the liver substance or by an inflammatory exudate within the ducts themselves. Intrahepatic obstruction due to stasis and inspissation of bile within the canaliculi is an occasional occurrence, following the ingestion of certain drugs, which accordingly are referred to as "cholestatic" agents. These include phenothiazines, antithyroid medications, sulfonylureas, tricyclic antidepressants, and nitrofurantoin.

Clinical Manifestations. Whether the obstruction is intrahepatic or extrahepatic, and whatever its cause may be, if bile cannot flow normally into the intestine, but is dammed back in the liver substance, it is reabsorbed into the blood and there carried over the entire body, staining the skin and the sclerae. It is excreted in the urine, which becomes a deep orange color and foamy in appearance. Because of the decreased amount of bile in the intestinal tract, the stools become white or clay-colored. The skin may itch intensely, requiring repeated starch baths and oil inunctions. Dyspepsia, and especially an intolerance to fatty foods, may develop temporarily, due to impairment of fat digestion in the absence of intestinal bile. Here the SGOT and SGPT rise only moderately, but the bilirubin and alkaline phosphatase are elevated.

HEREDITARY HYPERBILIRUBINEMIA. *Gilbert's syndrome* is a familial disorder which is due to a diminution of glucuronyl transferase and an increased unconjugated bilirubin that causes jaundice. Liver histology and liver function tests (other than elevated bilirubin) are normal, and there is no hemolysis. Other conditions that are probably caused by inborn errors of biliary metabolism include *Dubin-Johnson syndrome* (chronic idiopathic jaundice, with pigment in the liver) and *Rotor's syndrome* (chronic familial conjugated hyperbilirubinemia without pigment in the liver); "benign" cholestatic jaundice of pregnancy, with retention of conjugated bilirubin, probably secondary to unusual sensitivity to the hormones of pregnancy; and probably also benign recurrent intrahepatic cholestasis.

PORTAL HYPERTENSION AND ASCITES

One set of problems largely limited to patients with hepatic cirrhosis arises as a result of obstruction to the flow of portal venous blood through the liver, the effect of which is to elevate the blood pressure throughout the entire portal venous system. Portal hypertension may be

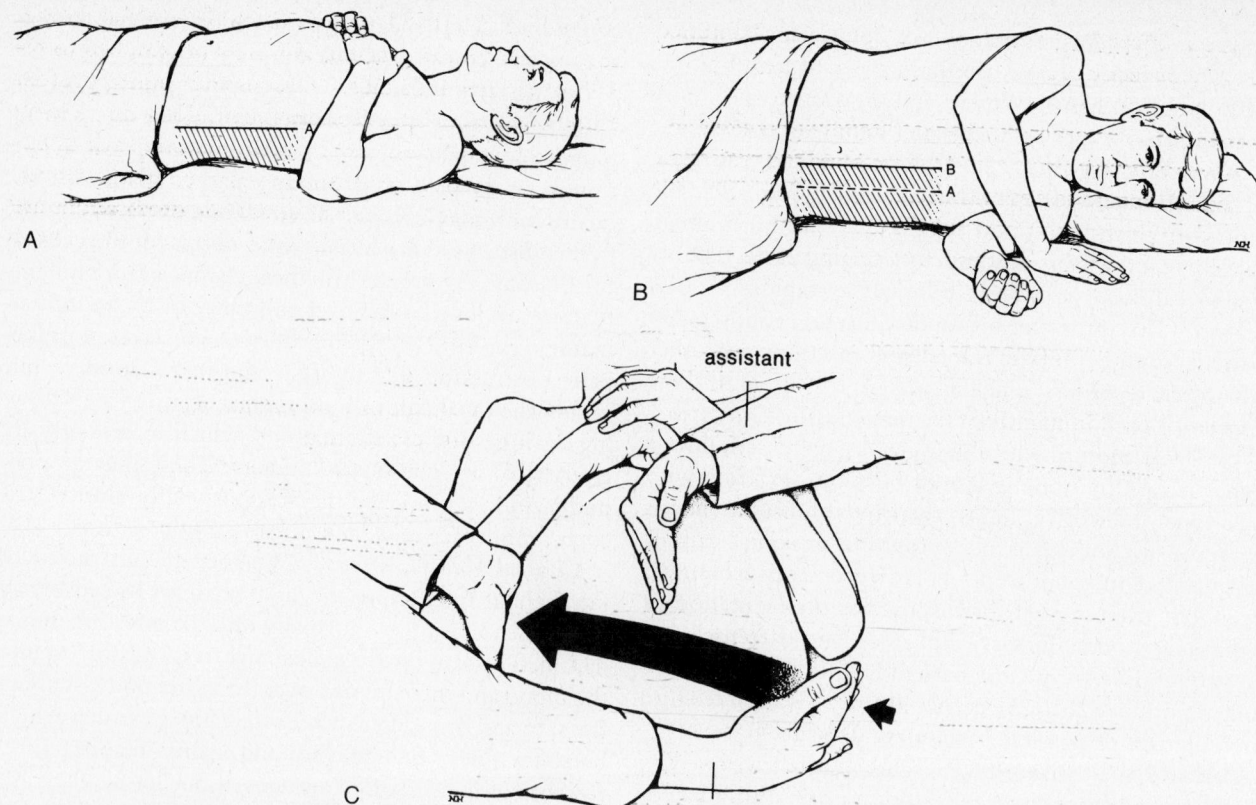

Figure 38-5. Assessing for ascites. *A.* To percuss for shifting dullness, each flank is percussed, with the patient in a supine position. If fluid is present, dullness will be noted at each flank. The most medial limits of the dullness should be marked as indicated in *A.* The patient should then be shifted to his side. *B.* shows what happens to the area of dullness if fluid is present. *C.* To detect the presence of a fluid wave, the examiner places one hand alongside each flank. A second person then places a hand, ulnar side down, along the patient's midline, and applies light pressure. The examiner then strikes one flank sharply with one hand, while the other hand remains in place to detect any signs of a fluid impulse. The assistant's hand dampens any wave impulses traveling through the abdominal wall. (Copyright © 1974, American Journal of Nursing Company. Reproduced with permission from American Journal of Nursing, *74:*no. 9, Sept. 1974)

classified as presinusoidal or postsinusoidal, depending upon the location of the intrahepatic sinusoids that are blocked, but the effects are the same.

There are two major sequelae of portal hypertension:
1. The formation of esophageal, gastric, and hemorrhoidal varicosities, which are prone to rupture and often are the source of massive hemorrhages from the upper gastrointestinal tract and the rectum (see page 819). The likelihood of bleeding may be increased by the blood-clotting abnormalities frequently present in patients with cirrhosis. The varicosities form because of the elevated pressures transmitted to all of the veins which drain into the portal system.
2. The second important manifestation of portal hypertension is accumulation of fluid (ascites) in the abdominal cavity. As ascites develops, intravascular volume tends to fall, and renin is released by the kidneys. This results in secretion of increased quantities of the hormone aldosterone by the adrenal glands, which, in turn, causes the kidneys to retain sodium and water in an attempt to return intravascular volume to normal. Unfortunately, if portal hypertension continues, fluid retention will contribute to the formation of even more ascites.

Assessment. Ascites can be determined by percussing the abdomen. When fluid has accumulated in the peritoneal cavity, the flanks will bulge when the patient assumes a supine position. Fluid can be confirmed either by percussing for shifting dullness (Fig. 38-5A, B) or by detecting a fluid wave (Fig. 38-5C). A fluid wave is likely to be found only when there is a large amount of fluid present.

Controlling Fluid Retention

NUTRITIONAL CONTROL. The objective of care is to achieve a negative sodium balance. Table salt, salty foods, salted butter and margarine, and all the ordinary canned and frozen foods should be avoided. The taste of unsalted foods can be improved by using salt substitutes such as lemon juice, oregano, and thyme. Commercial substitutes need to be cleared with the physician; for example, those containing ammonia could precipitate hepatic coma. Liberal use should be made of powdered, low-sodium milk and milk products. If water accumulation is not controlled on this regimen, the salt restriction must be more stringent; i.e., the daily sodium allowance should be reduced to 200 mg., and diuretics administered.

DIURETICS. Another method of reducing edema and ascites is to induce diuresis. This involves the reduction of sodium intake to approximately 9-22 mEq. (200-500 mg.) daily; restriction of fluids, if the serum sodium is low; and administration of an oral diuretic drug such as chlorothiazide (Diuril). Spironolactone (Aldactone), an aldosterone-blocking agent, also may be supplied to reinforce the action of these diuretics and to help prevent undue potassium loss. If these medications fail, it may be necessary to use a more potent diuretic such as furosemide (Lasix). Beyond this, ethacrynic acid (Edecrin) may be prescribed. These latter diuretic medications are used cautiously, since with long-term use, they may

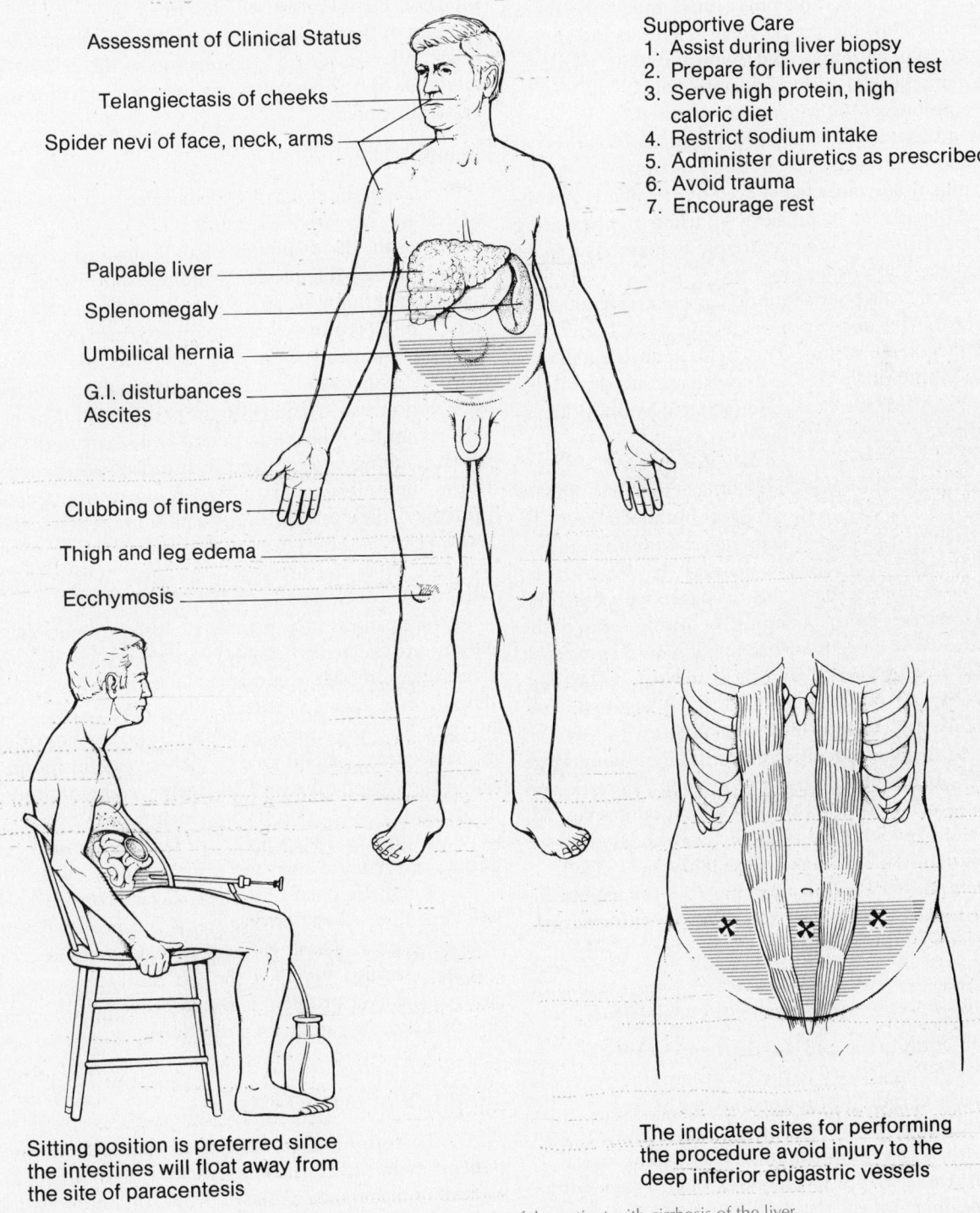

Assessment of Clinical Status

Telangiectasis of cheeks

Spider nevi of face, neck, arms

Palpable liver

Splenomegaly

Umbilical hernia

G.I. disturbances
Ascites

Clubbing of fingers

Thigh and leg edema

Ecchymosis

Supportive Care
1. Assist during liver biopsy
2. Prepare for liver function test
3. Serve high protein, high caloric diet
4. Restrict sodium intake
5. Administer diuretics as prescribed
6. Avoid trauma
7. Encourage rest

Sitting position is preferred since the intestines will float away from the site of paracentesis

The indicated sites for performing the procedure avoid injury to the deep inferior epigastric vessels

Figure 38-6. Nursing management of the patient with cirrhosis of the liver.

induce severe sodium depletion (hyponatremia). Ammonium chloride and acetazolamide (Diamox) are contraindicated, because of the possibility of precipitating hepatic coma. Daily weight loss should not exceed 0.227 kg. (or less than ½ lb.) daily.

Diuretic therapy should be carefully monitored by the nurse to detect possible complications: encephalopathy and electrolyte disturbances. When potassium stores are depleted, the amount of renal ammonia in the systemic circulation increases, which may cause impaired cerebral functioning. Possible electrolyte problems include hypokalemia, hyponatremia, and hypochloremic alkalosis. Careful intake and output documentation, as well as daily weighing of the patient, are required.

Skin integrity will be affected if meticulous care is not carried out. Pressure over bony prominences and edematous tissue must be relieved by frequently changing body position, or possibly by using an alternating pressure mattress. Lower extremities may have to be elevated and support hose worn.

Sometimes salt-poor albumin is given intravenously to temporarily elevate the serum albumin, which increases serum osmotic pressure. This helps reduce edema by causing the ascitic fluid to be drawn back into the bloodstream, from whence it can be eliminated by the kidneys.

Paracentesis

Accumulations of ascitic fluid often lessen or disappear in response to the diuresis program outlined above. To conserve the patient's body proteins, abdominal paracentesis is avoided for as long as possible. However, if the abdomen of the patient is tightly distended with fluid which interferes with breathing or eating, and if the ascites shows no evidence of becoming reduced as a result of a low sodium intake, diuretics, and spironolactone, the mechanical removal of the fluid is justified (Fig. 38-6). Each aspiration is limited to the slow removal of 2-3 liters, to relieve acute symptoms. Removing large amounts of fluid may cause hypotension, oliguria, and hyponatremia. If fluid in excess of this amount is tapped, ascitic fluid tends to form again, drawing fluid from extracellular tissue throughout the body.

NURSING ACTION. The nurse prepares the patient for the treatment by supplying the necessary information, instructions, and reassurance.

• *Have the patient void as completely as possible just prior to paracentesis, to lessen danger of inadvertently piercing the bladder.*

Sterile equipment and appropriate receptacles are made ready. Preparatory to the procedure, the patient is placed in the upright position on the edge of the bed, fully supported, with his feet resting on a stool and one arm fitted with a sphygmomanometer cuff. The trocar is introduced with aseptic technique through a stab wound in the midline below the umbilicus, and the fluid is drained through an effluent tube into a container.

During the procedure the nurse helps the patient to maintain the proper posture.

• Observe the patient closely for evidence of vascular collapse, such as the appearance of pallor, increase in pulse rate, or decline in blood pressure, the latter having been recorded at frequent intervals from the beginning of the procedure.

When the procedure is concluded, the patient is again placed in his original recumbent position. The amount of fluid collected is measured, described, and recorded, and samples of the fluid, properly labeled, are sent to appropriate laboratories for examination of the cellular sediment, its specific gravity, protein concentration, and bacterial content.

Shunts

Portacaval shunt may be tried in attempting to control ascites, but operative mortality is high.

One of the disadvantages of abdominal paracentesis is the loss of valuable plasma proteins; some clinics return such tapped fluid, via an infusion, to the general circulation. A more recent development is the use of the LeVeen (peritoneo-jugular) shunt (Fig. 38-7). In this method, a perforated silicone tube is directed through a small transverse abdominal incision into the peritoneum. The proximal end of the tube is attached to a valve; from the valve another tubing emerges and is threaded subcutaneously to the superior vena cava. According to the operating principle, when pressure in the abdominal cavity rises to 3 cm. H_2O or above, the valve opens, and excess fluid is transported to the superior vena cava. When pressure falls, the valve closes.

In the postoperative period, the patient is monitored closely and the hematocrit is measured every four hours. Excessive hemodilution may be interrupted by placing the patient in a sitting position. Usually a diuretic such as furosemide is prescribed to avoid the possibility of pulmonary edema. Blood studies include careful monitoring of the coagulation profile. Body weight, abdominal girth, and urinary output are documented every two hours. Ordinarily, the hematocrit falls, abdominal girth decreases, weight drops, and urinary output rises.

Following the relief of ascites, dietary considerations will depend upon the cardiac status and presence of peripheral edema. These patients require continued care and monitoring, for even though the ascites may be cleared, the liver problem is not improved by the insertion of a shunting drainage procedure.

NUTRITIONAL DEFICIENCIES

Another group of complications that is common to patients with severe chronic liver disease of all types is caused by inadequate intake of proper vitamins. Among the specific deficiency states that occur on this basis are (1) vitamin A deficiency, beriberi, polyneuritis, and

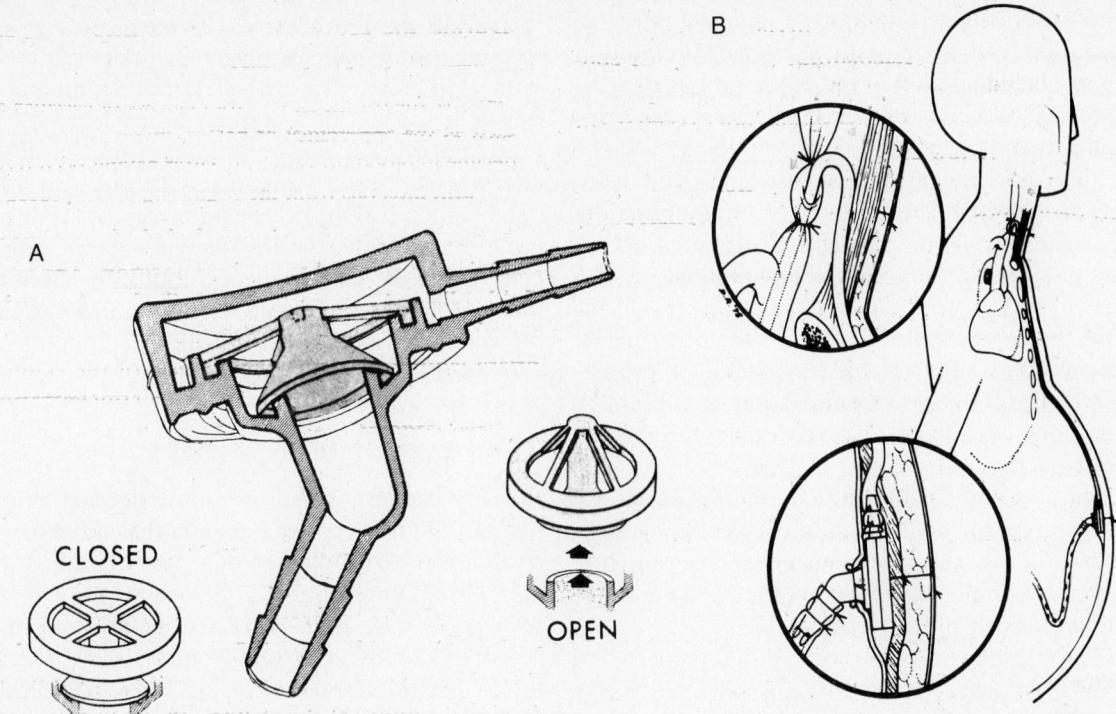

Figure 38-7. LeVeen peritoneo-jugular shunt for ascites. *A*. This shows the pressure-activated valve. The diaphragm and struts are made of silicone rubber and remain in the closed (*left*) position unless a force of greater than 3-4 cm. of water opens the valve (*right*). *B*. This indicates how the valve is placed. The lower section (and blown-up version) shows the valve under the muscles and fascia of the abdomen. The collecting tube extends into the peritoneal cavity. The tube then extends subcutaneously from the valve in the abdomen up to the jugular vein (see also upper blown-up version). (LeVeen, H. H.: Peritoneo-jugular shunt for ascites. Resident & Staff Physician, Feb. 1978, pp. 97-98)

Wernicke-Korsakoff psychosis, all attributable to a deficiency of thiamine; (2) skin and mucous membrane lesions characteristic of riboflavin deficiency; (3) "rum fits," which probably are due to pyridoxine deficiency; hypoprothrombinemia (page 674), characterized by spontaneous bleeding and ecchymoses, due to vitamin K deficiency; (4) the hemorrhagic lesions of scurvy, i.e., vitamin C deficiency; and (5) the macrocytic anemia of folic acid deficiency.

• The threat of these avitaminoses provides the rationale for supplementing the diet of every patient with chronic liver disease (especially when alcoholism is involved) with ample quantities of vitamins A, B complex, C, K, and folic acid.

HEPATIC COMA

Hepatic coma, one of the dreaded complications of liver disease, occurs with profound liver failure due to brain dysfunction and damage (hepatic encephalopathy) caused by accumulation in the blood of ammonia and other unidentified toxic metabolites. Ammonia accumulates because damaged liver cells fail to detoxify (by converting to urea) the ammonia that constantly is entering the bloodstream as a result of its absorption from the gastrointestinal tract, its production by metabolizing kidney tissue, and its liberation from contracting muscle cells.

Clinical Manifestations. The earliest symptoms of hepatic coma, i.e., the manifestations of impending coma, include minor mental aberrations and motor disturbances. The patient appears to be slightly confused; he becomes untidy; there is a faraway look in his eye; he tends to drowse during the day and to wander at night; and he may exhibit a coarse, or "flapping" tremor (asterixis), especially of the hands. (A unique way of measuring this involuntary unclenching and reclenching of the fingers is to have the patient grasp a blood pressure bulb attached to a recording system. In this way it is possible to record and measure the degree of asterixis which appears to be due to lack of oxygen.) Electroencephalogram (EEG) shows generalized slowing and an increase in amplitude of brain waves, and the appearance of characteristic tri-phasic waves. Except for the tri-phasic waves, all of the other manifestations noted are also observable in other conditions. Occasionally, fetor hepaticus, a characteristic odor something like fresh mowed grass, acetone, or old wine, may be noticed. In a more advanced stage there are gross disturbances of consciousness, and the patient is completely disoriented with respect to time and place. With further progression of the disorder he lapses into frank coma and is likely to succumb.

Aggravating and Precipitating Factors. Circumstances that increase blood ammonia content tend to aggravate or precipitate hepatic coma. The largest source of blood ammonia is the enzymatic and bacterial digestion of proteins (including dietary and blood proteins) in the gastrointestinal tract. Ammonia from this source is *increased* as a result of gastrointestinal bleeding, a high-protein diet, bacterial growth in the small and large intestines and uremia. The ingestion of ammonium salts will also increase blood ammonia. In the presence of alkalosis or hypokalemia, increased amounts of ammonia are absorbed from the gastrointestinal tract (and also from the renal tubular fluid). On the other hand, blood ammonia is *decreased* by elimination of protein from the diet and by the administration of antibiotics (such as neomycin sulfate) that reduce the number of intestinal bacteria.

Other factors unrelated to increased blood ammonia which may induce hepatic coma in susceptible patients include overdiuresis, dehydration, infections, surgery, and administration of consciousness-altering drugs (sedatives, tranquilizers, and narcotics).

Management

- The patient with impending hepatic coma is observed and assessed several times each day from the standpoint of neurologic status. A daily record is kept of handwriting and performance in arithmetic.
- Fluid intake and output and, if feasible, body weight, are recorded each day.
- Vital signs are measured and recorded every 4 hours.
- Evidence suggesting pulmonary or other infection is sought frequently and reported promptly if observed.
- If it becomes apparent that liver coma is indeed impending, the patient's protein intake is reduced sharply or eliminated altogether, for the time being.
- To reduce ammonia absorption from the gastrointestinal tract, a high cleansing enema may be prescribed.
- In addition, an antibiotic drug such as neomycin is given as an intestinal antiseptic.
- Electrolyte status is carefully monitored, and corrected if abnormal.
- Sedative and analgesic drugs, if prescribed at all, are administered to this patient in very conservative doses and under very close observation.

Lactulose (Cephulac, Duphalac) is given to reduce blood ammonia, which probably acts by a combination of mechanisms that promote the excretion of ammonia in the stool: (1) ammonia is kept in the ionized state, resulting in a fall in colon pH — this reverses the normal passage of ammonia from the colon to the blood; (2) catharsis takes place, which decreases the ammonia absorbed from the colon; and (3) the fecal flora are changed to organisms that do not produce ammonia from urea.

Two or three soft stools per day are hoped for; this means lactulose is performing as intended. However, watery diarrheal stools indicate drug overdose. Possible side effects include intestinal bloating and cramps which usually disappear in a week. To overcome the sweet taste to which some patients object, lactulose can be diluted with fruit juice. The patient is closely monitored for hypokalemia and dehydration. Other laxatives are not given during lactulose administration, because their effects would disturb dosage regulation.

Levodopa (L-Dopa) is being investigated for possible use in the treatment of hepatic coma. Some researchers believe that the displacement of dopamine accounts for the neurologic dysfunction noted in portal systemic encephalopathy, indicating that administration of L-Dopa may correct this.

OTHER MANIFESTATIONS OF LIVER FAILURE

Many patients with liver failure develop generalized edema, due to hypoalbuminemia that results from decreased hepatic production of serum albumin. The production of blood-clotting factors by the liver is also reduced, leading to an increased incidence of bruising, nosebleeds, bleeding from wounds, and, as described above, gastrointestinal bleeding. Decreased production of several clotting factors may be due, in part, to deficient absorption of vitamin K from the gastrointestinal tract. This probably is caused by the inability of liver cells to use vitamin K to make prothrombin. Absorption of the other fat-soluble vitamins (vitamins A, D, and E), as well as dietary fats may also be impaired, due to decreased secretion of bile salts into the intestine.

Abnormalities of glucose metabolism also occur; the blood sugar may be abnormally high shortly after a meal (i.e., a diabetic-type glucose tolerance test) but hypoglycemia may occur during fasting, because of decreased hepatic glycogen reserves and decreased gluconeogenesis.

- Because of decreased ability to metabolize drugs, usual drug dosages must be reduced for the patient with liver failure.

Decreased metabolism of estrogens can lead to gynecomastia, testicular atrophy, loss of pubic hair in the male, and menstrual irregularities in the female, as well as spider angiomata and reddened palms ("liver palms"). Splenomegaly (enlarged spleen) with possible hypersplenism occurs commonly as a manifestation of portal hypertension. Patients with liver failure due to biliary obstruction commonly develop severe itching (pruritus) due to retention of bile salts.

LIVER DISORDERS

VIRAL HEPATITIS

Of increasing importance to those concerned with public health is the increasing incidence of viral hepatitis. Peaks of maximal incidence occurred in 1954 and 1961 in the United States, which led some authorities to suggest a cyclical pattern. Although the mortality rate is low, the disease is important because of its ease of transmission, morbidity, and the prolonged loss of time from school or employment which it can cause.

Breakthroughs in better understanding of viral hepatitis in the recent past have been due to recognition in 1968, by Blumberg, that Australian, or Au antigen, was a specific immunologic marker for hepatitis B infection. This led to a series of new designations, and Australian antigen now is referred to as hepatitis B surface antigen: HB_sAg. More recently, a specific antigen for hepatitis A has been identified (HA Ag). Also, tests have been developed to detect anti-HA, HB_s, and HB_c antibodies, as well as the E-antigen and anti-E-antibody associated with hepatitis B. This means that diagnostic tests are available for recognizing hepatitis A and hepatitis B (complement fixation, immune adherence, and radio-immunoassay).

The existence of one or more agents capable of producing viral hepatitis (nonA nonB) infection has also been recognized.

NURSING CONSIDERATIONS. The nurse is especially concerned with four major problem areas of viral hepatitis: (1) the care of the patient so afflicted, (2) the increased risks in hemodialysis units and in individuals using illicit drugs, (3) the fact that many individuals who have the disease are asymptomatic, which may present serious epidemiological problems, and (4) the apparent health needs of the community required for its elimination.

The last category includes the following considerations:
- proper community and home sanitation
- conscientious individual hygiene at all times
- safe practices of food preparation and dispensation
- effective health supervision in schools, dormitories, barracks, camps
- continuous health education programs

For a comparison of the many aspects of the major forms of viral hepatitis, see Table 39-2.

Hepatitis A Virus (HAV)

Hepatitis A is probably an RNA virus of the enterovirus family. The mode of transmission of this disease is fecal-oral contact (e.g., the ingestion of food or liquids infected by the virus), although a respiratory mode of transmission has not been excluded. The virus has been found in the stool of infected patients prior to the onset of symptoms, and during the first few days of illness. Typically, a young adult acquires the infection at school and brings it home, where haphazard sanitary habits spread it through the family. It is more prevalent in underprivileged countries or in instances of overcrowding and poor sanitation. An infected person who handles food in a restaurant can spread the disease, or people may drink sewage-contaminated water or eat shellfish from sewage-polluted shoreland. It is rarely, if ever, transmitted by blood transfusions. There is no evidence of a chronic carrier state. Nonhuman primates may be infected transiently and may serve as a source of contact and infection for humans.

The incubation period is estimated to be from 1 to 7 weeks (usually 30 days). The course of the illness may be prolonged (usually shorter in the young, and more serious in those above age 40), lasting from 4 to 8 weeks.

Assessment. Most patients are anicteric (without jaundice) and symptomless. When symptoms appear, they are of a mild, flulike upper respiratory infection, with low-grade fever. Later, jaundice and dark urine may become apparent. Indigestion is present, in varying degrees, marked by vague epigastric distress, anorexia, nausea, heartburn, and flatulence. These symptoms tend to clear as soon as the jaundice reaches its peak—perhaps 10 days after its original appearance. Anti-HA appears in the serum; this finding indicates prior hepatitis A and suggests immunity to reinfection. The liver and the spleen are often moderately enlarged for a few days after onset; otherwise, apart from jaundice, there are few physical signs to be elicited.

Management. Bed rest during the acute stage and the provision of a diet that is both acceptable and nutritious are part of the treatment and nursing care. During the period of anorexia, the patient should receive frequent small feedings, supplemented, as needed, by intravenous infusions of glucose. Since this patient would rather not look at food, or eat, it requires gentle persistence and ingenuity to whet his appetite. Optimal food and fluid levels need to be maintained to counteract probable weight loss and unduly prolonged recovery. Even before the icteric phase, however, many patients recover their appetites and thereafter need no reminders to maintain a good diet.

Prognosis. Recovery from Type A hepatitis is the rule; a rare case progresses to acute liver necrosis (fulminant hepatitis), terminating in cirrhosis of the liver, or even death. Infectious hepatitis confers immunity against itself; however, the person may acquire other forms of hepatitis.

Prevention, Control, and Community Concern. Ways to reduce the risk of contracting infectious hepatitis are:

- Good personal hygiene, stressing careful handwashing (after bowel movement and before eating).
- Environmental sanitation—safe food and water supply, as well as effective sewage disposal.
- Administration of Immune Serum Globulin, Human (ISG)—Type A hepatitis can be prevented by the administration of globulin intramuscularly during the period of incubation, if this treatment is instituted within a period of 2 to 7 days following exposure. This bolsters the person's own antibody production and provides about 6 to 8 weeks of immunity.

HEPATITIS GLOSSARY

HAV	Hepatitis A virus
HBV	Hepatitis B virus
NANBH	Hepatitis nonA nonB
(nA, nB)	Hepatitis nonA nonB
HB_sAg	Hepatitis B surface antigen; Australian antigen
HB_cAg	Hepatitis B core antigen
Anti-HA	Antibody to hepatitis A virus
Anti-HB_s	Antibody to hepatitis B surface antigen
Anti-HB_c	Antibody to hepatitis B core antigen
Anti-HB_e	Antibody to hepatitis e-antigen
HBIG	Hepatitis B immunoglobulin
ISG	Immune serum globulin
HB_eAg	Hepatitis B e-antigen

Hepatitis B Virus (HBV)

Hepatitis B virus is a double-shelled particle containing DNA. This particle is composed of:

Antigenic material in an outer coat—hepatitis B surface antigen (HB_sAg).

Antigenic material in an inner core—hepatitis B core antigen (HB_cAg).

An independent protein circulating in the blood—HB_eAg.

Each antigen elicits its specific antibody:
anti-HB_s (develops early after hepatitis B infection)
anti-HB_c (may not be detected until late in convalescence)
anti-HB_e (may not be detected until late in convalescence)

HB_sAg can be detected transiently circulating in the blood in 80 to 90 percent of infected patients. HB_cAg cannot be detected in blood. HB_sAg may be noted in the blood for months and years, which suggests that these individuals may be asymptomatic carriers, if HB_eAg is absent. If it is present, these patients may have chronic hepatitis and may be more infectious.

From the community health point of view, about 15 percent of American adults are positive for anti-HB_s, which indicates that they have had hepatitis B. Among drug addicts, anti-HB_s may be positive in as many as two-thirds.

Spread may be oral–oral via saliva, and even by breast feeding. Particularly susceptible individuals are the general surgeon, clinical laboratory worker, oral surgeon and orthodontist, nurse, and respiratory therapist. Mandatory screening of blood donors for HB_sAg has greatly reduced the occurrence of posttransfusion hepatitis, Type B.

Assessment. Clinically, the disease closely resembles Type A hepatitis. However, the incubation period is relatively much longer: between 2 and 5 months. The mortality is appreciable, ranging from 1 to 10 percent, depending on the infective dose and the condition of the patient. Symptoms and signs of hepatitis B may be insidious and variable. Fever and respiratory symptoms are rare: some patients have arthralgias and rashes. The patient may lose his appetite, have dyspepsia, abdominal pain, generalized aching, malaise, and weakness. Jaundice may or may not be evident.

Management. It is important that bed rest be continued until the hepatitis has definitely subsided. Subsequently, the patient's activities should be restricted until the hepatic enlargement and the elevation of serum bilirubin have disappeared. Adequate nutrition should be maintained; proteins are restricted when the liver has a decreased ability to metabolize protein by-products, as demonstrated by symptoms. Other therapeutic measures employed to control the dyspeptic symptoms and general malaise include the use of alkalies, belladonna, and antiemetics. However, all medications should be avoided if emesis is a problem. This patient should be hospitalized and treated with fluid therapy.

Convalescence may be prolonged, complete symptomatic recovery sometimes requiring 3 to 4 months or longer. During this stage, gradual restoration of physical activity is permitted and encouraged, following complete clearing of the jaundice.

Psychosocial considerations are recognized by the nurse, particularly as they apply to isolation and separation procedures. Special planning is required to minimize any alterations in sensory perception. The family must be included in such planning.

Control and Prevention. The objectives at present, since a vaccine is not yet available, are (1) to interrupt the chain of transmission, and (2) to use passive immunization.

A reduction in the number of persons acquiring hepatitis B could occur if paid blood donors could be replaced by an all-volunteer donor population. Washed red blood cells appear to reduce the risk of hepatitis transmission. The use of disposable syringes, needles, and lancets reduces the risk of spreading this infection from one patient to another in the process of collecting blood samples or administering parenteral therapy. Good personal hygiene practices are fundamental to infection control. In the laboratory, work areas should be disinfected daily. Gloves are to be worn when handling HB_sAg positive specimens. Eating is prohibited in the laboratory.

Administering medication by individual-dose ampules is essential and is the prescribed policy of most hospitals. Where a group of narcotic addicts share the same needle, serious outbreaks of hepatitis have occurred.

Hepatitis B immunoglobulin (HBIG) is given for postexposure prophylaxis ("needle stick," splashing from pipetting accidents, or eye contamination). Vaccines for hepatitis B are being evaluated.

Hepatitis nonA nonB

Those varieties of hepatitis that are not identified as hepatitis A or B are classified as nonA nonB hepatitis. Continued research may result in a further division of this classification. The cause for this kind of hepatitis has not been identified. However, it is blood-borne, and the possibility of a carrier state is likely. This form of hepatitis is now the major cause of transfusion-related viral hepatitis and is often observed in parenteral drug abusers.

Hepatitis nonA nonB occurs not only in patients, following blood transfusion, and among drug addicts, but in personnel associated with renal transplantation units and in residents in homes for the mentally retarded. Another community-health related implication is that whereas only about 10 to 20 percent of posttransfusion hepatitis is type B, 80 to 90 percent is nonA nonB hepatitis. Commercial blood appears to transmit hepatitis virus much more than blood from volunteer donors.

Incubation time is variable, and severity covers a wide spectrum that most resembles hepatitis B. Most manifestations are anicteric (without jaundice). Illness may be prolonged, lasting several months, and resulting in chronic hepatitis.

Immune Serum Globulin

Hepatitis B Immune Globulin, Human (HBIG) is prepared from pooled venous plasma of donors with a high titer of anti-HB$_s$ antibodies. The United States Public Health Service Advisory Committee on Immunization Practices recommends HBIG for one particular circumstance: a single exposure to blood containing hepatitis B virus, either by accidental inoculation (needle stick) or by splashing contaminated material on mucous membranes, such as might occur while pipetting blood or fluid. HBIG is given intramuscularly as soon as possible, but no later than 7 days after exposure. A second dose is given in 25 to 30 days after the first.

Immune Serum Globulin (ISG) is given within 2 to 7 days after exposure to hepatitis A; it is 80 to 90 percent effective. If an outbreak occurs in a school or institution, ISG is indicated to prevent infection or reduce infection to subclinical levels, permitting the development of a natural immunity.

It is possible that ISG may offer limited protection against nonA nonB hepatitis, but this cannot be assessed.

PRECAUTION WHEN TAKING IMMUNE SERUM GLOBULIN. The most common adverse effect is pain and tenderness at the injection site.

- Caution is required when anyone who has previously had angioedema, hives, or other allergic reaction is treated with any human immune globulin. Epinephrine should be available for use during systemic or anaphylactic reactions.

TOXIC HEPATITIS AND DRUG-INDUCED HEPATITIS

Certain chemicals have poisonous effects on the liver, and when taken by mouth or injected parenterally produce acute liver cell necrosis, or *toxic hepatitis*. The chemicals most commonly implicated in this disease are carbon tetrachloride, phosphorus, chloroform, and gold compounds. These are true hepatotoxins.

Many drugs may induce hepatitis, but are sensitizing, rather than toxic. The liver disorder, in this instance (*drug-induced hepatitis*) is similar to acute viral hepatitis; however parenchymal destruction tends to be more extensive. Some examples of drugs which can lead to hepatitis are cinchophen, isoniazid, and halothane.

Clinical Manifestations and Management. Toxic hepatitis resembles viral hepatitis in onset. Anorexia, nausea, and vomiting are the usual symptoms; jaundice and hepatomegaly are noted on physical assessment. Symptoms are more intense for the more severely poisoned patient.

Recovery from acute toxic hepatitis is rapid if the hepatotoxin is identified early and removed. It usually is not, however, due to the long period between exposure and manifestation of symptoms, and so, in general, recovery is unlikely. There are no effective antidotes. The fever mounts; the patient becomes deeply toxic and prostrated. Vomiting may be persistent, with the vomitus containing blood. Hemorrhages appear under the skin. Delirium, coma, and convulsions develop, and within a few days the patient usually dies.

There is little to be done by way of treatment, except to provide comfort measures, blood, fluids, and electrolytes. A few patients recover, only to develop cirrhosis.

Drug-induced hepatitis may progress to hepatic failure. In the event that the liver heals, there may be scarring, followed by postnecrotic cirrhosis. Manifestations of sensitivity to a drug may occur on the first day of its use or not until several months later, depending upon the drug. Usually the onset is abrupt, with chills, fever, rash, pruritus, arthralgia, anorexia, and nausea. Later, there may be jaundice and dark urine, and an enlarged and tender liver. When the offending drug is withdrawn, symptoms may gradually subside. However, once provoked, reactions may be severe and even fatal, even though the drug is stopped. If fever, rash, or pruritus occur from any medication, it should be stopped immediately.

Concern has been expressed regarding the effect of

TABLE 38-2. HEPATITIS

	HEPATITIS A VIRUS (HAV)	HEPATITIS B VIRUS (HBV)	nonA/nonB HEPATITIS VIRUS (NANBH)
Other Names	Type A hepatitis, infectious or epidemic hepatitis; IH virus	Type B hepatitis, serum hepatitis, SH virus, Dane particle	Hepatitis "C", "D"; Type C
Epidemiology			
Cause	Hepatitis A virus	Hepatitis B virus	Another virus
Method of transmission	Fecal-oral; poor sanitation Person to person Waterborne, foodborne—shellfish Rarely, if at all, by blood transfusion	Parenterally, or by intimate contact with carriers or those with acute disease; male homosexuals. Vertical transmission from mothers to babies. Contaminated instruments, syringes, needles; renal dialysis*	Transfusion association Personnel in renal transplant and dialysis units Parenteral drug abusers Blood transfusion products Institutions with long-term residents*
Source of virus/antigen	Blood, feces; saliva, occasionally; urine suspected	Blood Saliva Semen, vaginal secretions	Appears to be blood-borne
Distribution by age	Young adults (15-29) and middle-aged who have escaped childhood infection	Affects all ages, but mostly young adults	Same as HBV
Incubation period	3-5 weeks Mean: 30 days	2-5 months Mean: 90 days	Variable: 14-115 days Mean: 50 days
Occurrence	Worldwide	Worldwide	Worldwide Accounts for 20% of sporadic cases
Antibody	Anti-HAV Present in convalescent sera and immune serumglobulin (ISB)	Anti-HB$_c$ (core antigen) Anti-HB$_s$ (surface antigen)	— — —
Immunity	Homologous	Homologous	— — —
Severity	Most anicteric and asymptomatic	More severe than HA*	Wide spectrum of severity, resembling HA or HB. Often prolonged illness—months. May progress to chronic hepatitis.*
Nature of Disease			
Signs and Symptoms	May occur with or without symptoms: flulike illness Preicteric phase: Headache, malaise, fatigue, anorexia, lassitude, fever Icteric phase: Dark urine, scleral icterus, jaundice, liver tenderness, and perhaps enlargement	May occur without symptoms 1,000 IU/liter-serum transaminase level May develop antibodies to virus Similar to HAV, but more severe Fever and respiratory symptoms rare, but may have arthralgias, rash	Similar to HBV Less severe and anicteric
Diagnosis and method	Elevated serum transaminase Complement fixation rate Radioimmunoassay	Check serum for HB$_s$Ag, HB$_e$Ag, anti-HB$_c$, in absence of anti-HB$_s$ Elevated serum transaminase Radioimmunoassay— hemagglutination	(Obtainable as a panel)
Severity	Usually mild Fatality rate 0-1%	Variable, may be severe Fatality rate varies: 1-10%	— — —
Specific treatment	Adequate fluids, rest, nutrition	Same as HAV In research: vaccine antiviral chemotherapy to eliminate chronic HBV carrier state (being tested)	— — —
Prevention	Good sanitation Proper personal hygiene Effective sterilization procedures Careful screening of food handlers Immune Serum Globulin (ISG) given within a few days of exposure	Specific hepatitis B immune globulin (HBIG) probably useful after exposure by ingestion, inoculation, or splash involving hepatitis B surface antigen (HB$_s$Ag)	Mandatory screening of blood donors: 1) for HB$_s$Ag, 20% 2) for NonA NonB, 80%

*Probably the same, for HBV and NANBH, recent intensive research suggests.

halothane (Fluothane)—a popular nonexplosive inhalation anesthetic—on the liver. Since there is some suspicion that it may cause serious, and sometimes fatal, liver damage, precautions should preclude its use in (1) persons with known liver disease, (2) repeated instances, particularly in patients who have had a fever of unknown cause after the first administration of halothane, and (3) patients with evidence of prior sensitization. Such sensitization would have been in evidence during the second postoperative week, with such manifestations as fever, rash, eosinophilia, arthralgia, or jaundice.

HEPATIC CIRRHOSIS

Cirrhosis of the liver refers to scarring of the liver. Three kinds are generally considered:

1. *Laennec's portal cirrhosis* (alcoholic; nutritional), in which the scar tissue characteristically surrounds the portal areas. This is most commonly due to chronic alcoholism and will be discussed below.
2. *Postnecrotic cirrhosis,* in which there are broad bands of scar tissue, as a late result of a previous acute viral hepatitis.
3. *Biliary cirrhosis,* in which there is pericholangitic, perilobular scarring. This type usually is the result of chronic biliary obstruction and infection (cholangitis) and is much more rare and more serious than Laennec's and postnecrotic cirrhosis.

Etiology and Incidence

The basic mechanism responsible for the development of cirrhosis is yet to be described. Cirrhosis occurs with greatest frequency among alcoholics. However, many explain the role of alcohol in the production of cirrhosis on the basis of nutritional deficiency with reduced protein intake, rather than on alcohol toxicity, and certainly some cases of cirrhosis are observed among people who do not drink alcoholic beverages. Nonetheless, several investigators have shown that although nutritional factors are undoubtedly involved, alcohol itself has to be incriminated in the pathogenesis of the alcoholic fatty liver and the associated effects.

Some individuals appear to be more susceptible than others to this disease, whether they are alcoholics, malnourished, or not. Other factors may play a role, such as exposure to certain chemicals (carbon tetrachloride, chlorinated naphthalene, arsenic, or phosphorus) or infectious schistosomiasis. Twice as many men as women are affected, and the majority of patients are between 40 and 60 years of age.

Pathophysiology and Clinical Manifestations

Laennec's cirrhosis is a disease characterized by episodes of necrosis involving the liver cells, sometimes occurring repeatedly throughout the course of the disease. The destroyed liver cells are replaced by scar tissue, the amount of which, in time, may exceed that of the functioning liver tissue. The disease usually has a particularly insidious onset and a very protracted course, occasionally proceeding over a period of 30 or more years.

Early in the disease, the liver is apt to be large and its cells loaded with fat; later, as the replacing scar tissue contracts, the liver becomes small. Also, its surface often becomes rough, because the scar tissue within it is disposed in coarse bundles, which contract and pull in the capsule at certain points and cause the islands of residual normal tissue and of new regenerating liver tissue to project in little lumps. Hence arose the term *hobnail liver.*

The late manifestations are due partly to chronic failure of liver function and partly to *obstruction of the portal circulation.* Practically all the blood from the digestive organs is collected in the portal veins and carried to the liver. Since a cirrhotic liver does not allow the blood free passage, it is dammed back into the spleen and the gastrointestinal tract, with the result that these organs become the seat of chronic passive congestion; that is, they are stagnant with blood, and so cannot function properly. Such patients are apt to have chronic dyspepsia and changes in bowel habit, with constipation or diarrhea. There is a gradual weight loss. Fluid may accumulate in the peritoneal cavity (ascites), in which event diuresis is induced.

At certain points in the abdomen the portal circulation anastomoses with the general circulation, and through these channels some portal blood can flow to the heart without first passing through the liver. One of the points of collateral circulation is at the cardiac orifice of the stomach. The blood from the esophagus flows directly to the heart; that from the stomach flows to the liver. Veins always anastomose, so that blood here can choose between these two routes. When there is obstruction to the portal circulation, as in cirrhosis, portal hypertension develops, and, because of its increased pressure, a portion of the blood in the gastric veins escapes through the esophageal veins. Unfortunately, however, these veins become distended, forming esophageal varices, the thin walls of which often rupture. Thus, about 25 percent of patients with cirrhosis experience small hatemeses, while some have profuse hemorrhages from the stomach and esophagus.

Within the lower rectum there is a point at which the portal and the general circulations meet. In cirrhosis of the liver, venous varices form here, also. These are known as hemorrhoids and may rupture and cause severe hemorrhages. Of course, hemorrhoids are common, and usually are due to simple constipation, and involve the external hemorrhoidal veins (external hemorrhoids), which usually thrombose before they bleed. However, in cirrhosis, the internal hemorrhoidal veins dilate, and because blood is less apt to clot in them, they bleed severely when they rupture.

A third anastomosis is around the umbilicus; when varicosities appear here, the condition is called *caput medusae.*

Other late symptoms of cirrhosis are attributable to chronic failure of liver function. The concentration of plasma albumin is lowered, predisposing to the formation of edema. Overproduction of aldosterone probably occurs in cirrhosis, causing sodium and water retention and potassium excretion. Because of inadequate formation, utilization, and storage of certain vitamins, notably vitamins A, C, and K, signs of their deficiency frequently are encountered—particularly hemorrhagic phenomena associated with vitamin-K deficiency. Chronic gastritis and poor gastrointestinal function, together with the factors of poor diet and impaired liver function, account for a deficiency type of anemia likewise often associated with this disease.

Therefore, the *chief signs of liver cirrhosis* are, in the early stages, fever, jaundice, gastrointestinal disturbances, and enlargement of the liver. Later in the disease this organ becomes smaller and nodular, the spleen enlarges, ascites appears, jaundice recurs, distended veins develop at the anastomotic points described previously, and spider telangiectases (dilated superficial arterioles resembling little bluish-red spiders) appear in the skin of the face and the trunk. As the condition progresses, edema, anemia, purpura, and signs of polyavitaminosis are likely to appear. The patient may die in liver failure, experiencing increasing weakness, wasting, and depression, and finally delirium, coma, and convulsions.

Assessment

The extent of liver disease and the kind of treatment are determined after studying the laboratory findings. Because the liver is a complex, functioning organ, the tests are many (see Table 39-1). The patient needs to know why these tests are being done, why they are important, and how he can assist.

Parenchymal liver-cell function can be evaluated with cephalin flocculation tests and thymol turbidity (increased). Serum albumin tends to fall, and serum globulin rises. Enzyme tests indicate liver-cell damage: serum alkaline phosphate rises, serum cholinesterase may decrease, and SGOT increases. Excretory function is tested by the liver's ability to eliminate sulfobromophthalein (Bromsulphalein) and cardiogreen dye. In cirrhosis, the sulfobromophthalein and cardiogreen are retained. Bilirubin tests are done to measure bile excretion or bile retention. Photolaparoscopy, in conjunction with biopsy, may be done to permit direct visualization of the liver. A scintillation scan can be done and will reveal an inability of the liver to take up radioactive materials homogenously in cirrhosis.

Ultrasound scanning will measure the difference in density of parenchymal cells and scar tissue. Palpation will indicate the presence of ascites.

Additional nursing assessment includes documentation of the patient's general behavior, his reliability in describing his illness, cognitive abilities, orientation to time and place, and speech patterns. Neurological assessment is in order with this patient, because of the possibility of hepato-encephalopathy. Fine motor coordination may be observed in the manner in which he writes his name, while cognitive abilities can be assessed through a device known as the Number Connection Test. The test consists of a printed form on which a series of circled numbers are scattered at random. The patient is asked to draw a connecting line between the numbers, beginning with number 1 and proceeding in sequence through 25.

Management

Rest. The patient with active liver disease requires rest and other supportive measures to permit the liver to reestablish its functional ability. The patient's weight and the volume of his fluid intake and output are measured and recorded daily. His position in bed is adjusted for maximal respiratory efficiency, which is especially important if ascites is marked. Skin care is observed meticulously, because of the presence of subcutaneous edema and the relative immobility of the patient. Oxygen therapy may be required, in liver failure, to oxygenate the weakened cells, lest more die.

Rest permits the liver to restore itself by limiting the demands of the body and increasing the liver's blood supply. Since the patient is more susceptible to infection, efforts to prevent respiratory, circulatory, and vascular disturbances need to be initiated. These measures may help prevent such problems as pneumonia, thrombophlebitis, and pressure sores.

Hepatotoxic Drugs. During initial assessment, it is important to note any unusual or persistent eating, working, or personal habits that may disclose exposure to poisonous drugs. Thus any medications taken by the patient in the past several months should be recorded, and a check made for hepatotoxicity. It is also important to recognize that recent surgery with exposure to general anesthetics may have been harmful to the liver.

Bleeding Tendencies. Because of decreased production of prothrombin and the diseased liver's decreased synthesis of substances used in blood coagulation, hemorrhaging is possible. Precautionary measures include protecting the patient with padded side rails, applying pressure to an injection site, and avoiding injury from sharp objects. Observe for melena and check stools for blood, as signs of possible internal bleeding.

Meeting Nutritional Needs. The cirrhotic patient who has no ascites or edema and exhibits no signs of impending coma should receive a nutritious, high-protein diet supplemented by vitamins of the B complex and others as indicated (including vitamins A, C, and K, and folic acid). Since proper nutrition is so important, every effort must be made to encourage the patient to eat.

This is as important as any medication. Often, small frequent meals can be accepted better than three large meals. Patient preferences are to be considered. Patients with prolonged or severe anorexia, or those who are vomiting or eating poorly for any reason, can be fed by tube.

Patients with fatty stools (steatorrhea) should receive water-soluble forms of fat-soluble vitamins — A, D, and E (Aquasol A, D, and E). Folic acid and iron are prescribed, to prevent anemia. If the patient shows signs of impending or advancing coma, a low-protein diet should be given temporarily; too much protein from meats may produce portal systemic encephalopathy (PSE), and too little may cause negative nitrogen and wasting. Suggested protein foods are dairy products (eggs, skim milk), cereal (wheat germ, white rice), and fish (shellfish, salmon, sardines). A high caloric intake should be maintained, and supplementary vitamins and minerals should be supplied (e.g., oral potassium, if the serum potassium is normal or low, and if renal function is normal). As soon as the situation permits, the protein intake should be restored to normal, or above. Diet therapy is determined on an individualized basis.

Portal Systemic Encephalopathy (PSE). PSE is a possible neurologic syndrome that may display various combinations of myelopathy, chorea-athetosis, dysarthria, and even dementia. It has occurred in postshunt patients and those with advanced cirrhosis. PSE is mainly caused by ammonia and its effect on cerebral metabolism. Many factors predispose the patient with cirrhosis to PSE; some are unforseeable, but many are avoidable. The nurse is in a position to observe early evidence of this condition.

Patient Education and Posthospital Care

At the time of discharge, the patient receives detailed instructions, in part from the nurse, principally relating to dietary habits. Of utmost importance is the exclusion of alcohol from the diet. If this presents a problem, the patient may need the assistance of a skilled psychiatrist, trusted religious adviser, or of Alcoholics Anonymous.

Sodium restriction will have to continue for a considerable period of time, if not permanently; if this diet is to be followed correctly, the patient will require written instructions.

The success of treatment depends upon convincing the patient of the need to adhere willingly and wholeheartedly to the therapeutic plan. This includes rest, probably a change in life style, an adequate, well-balanced diet, and the elimination of alcohol. The patient is also instructed as to the symptoms of impending encephalopathy, and the possibility of bleeding tendencies and easy susceptibility to infection. Recovery is neither rapid nor easy; there are frequent setbacks and apparent lack of improvement. For many persons, the loss of support given by

alcohol is discouraging. The understanding nurse can play a significant role in offering support and encouragement to this patient.

SUMMARY. For an overall view of the nursing management of the patient with cirrhosis, refer to pages 820–821.

Postnecrotic Cirrhosis

Other types of cirrhosis include those of healed subacute yellow atrophy and hemochromatosis. In the latter type there occurs a pigment deposition with associated scarring not only of the liver but also of the pancreas and other organs.

Biliary Cirrhosis

A less common cause of cirrhosis is ascending infection of the biliary tract (cholangitis), with spread of the infection from the gallbladder by way of the hepatic duct to the small bile ducts in the liver substance. Prolonged obstructive jaundice may cause biliary cirrhosis. That portion of the liver chiefly involved, therefore, consists of the portal and the periportal spaces, where the bile canaliculi of each lobule communicate to form the liver bile ducts. These areas become the site of inflammation, and the bile ducts become occluded with inspissated bile and pus. An attempt is made by the liver to form new bile channels; hence, there is an overgrowth of tissue made up largely of disconnected, newly formed bile ducts and surrounded by scar tissue.

Clinical manifestations of this disease include intermittent jaundice and fever and the finding of an enlarged, hard, irregular liver, which eventually becomes atrophic. The treatment is the same as that described for portal cirrhosis, i.e., the treatment of any form of chronic liver insufficiency and, when indicated, surgical treatment designed to eradicate the biliary tract infection.

BLEEDING ESOPHAGEAL VARICES

Signs of jaundice, ascites, and portal hypertension are manifestations of advanced liver disease. Usually the patient is a potential bleeder and requires careful monitoring of laboratory blood studies, hematemesis, and melena.

Pathophysiology and Symptoms

Esophageal varices are dilated tortuous veins usually found in the submucosa of the lower esophagus; however, they may extend well up into the esophagus and into the stomach. Such a condition nearly always is caused by portal hypertension, which, in turn, is due to obstruction of the portal venous circulation within the substance of a cirrhotic liver (see page 807). Because of increased obstruction of the portal vein, venous blood from the intestinal tract and spleen seeks an outlet through collateral circulation (new avenues of return to

THE PATIENT WITH LAENNEC'S CIRRHOSIS

Problems	Nursing Implications
Anorexia	Encourage patient to eat meals and supplementary feedings. Offer frequent small feedings. Give attention to esthetic factors and attractive trays at mealtime. Eliminate alcohol.
Nausea and vomiting	Provide oral hygiene before meals. Use an ice collar for nausea. Give tube feedings, as required.
Weight loss and fatigue	Offer continuous encouragement of intake of high-protein, high-calorie diet. Give supplementary vitamins (A, B complex, C, and K). Give parenteral fluids as prescribed. Conserve patient's energy.
Abdominal pain	Assure bed rest to protect liver. Administer antispasmodics and mild sedatives. Encourage patient to eat slowly and chew thoroughly. Observe, record, and report presence and character of pain.
Hematemesis	Be alert for symptoms of anxiety, epigastric fullness, weakness, and restlessness. Observe for presence of bleeding and shock. Record vital signs at frequent intervals. Keep patient quiet and limit activity. Observe during blood transfusions. Assist physician in passage of tube for esophageal balloon tamponade. Measure and record nature, time, and amount of vomitus. Give meticulous oral hygiene. Maintain patient in fasting state, if indicated. Administer vitamin K as prescribed. Stay in constant attendance during episodes of bleeding. Offer cold liquids by mouth when bleeding stops (if prescribed).
Melena	Observe each stool for color, consistency, and amount.
Constipation	Ensure adequate fluid and food intake. Encourage exercises.
Diarrhea	Increase fluid intake. Give medications as prescribed.
Jaundice	Note and record varying degrees of jaundice of the skin and the sclerae. Relieve pruritus with good skin care, bathing without soap, and massage with emollient lotions. Keep patient's fingernails short to prevent skin excoriation from scratching. Give empathetic attention to patient's complaints and problems.
Edema of extremities	Restrict sodium. Administer diuretics as prescribed. Give careful attention and care to skin. Turn and change position frequently. Elevate extremities at intervals. Weigh patient daily. Record intake and output. Carry out passive range-of-motion exercises. Provide small foam-rubber supports under heels, malleoli, etc. Carefully control rate of flow of intravenous infusions.
Ascites	Restrict sodium. Give diuretics, potassium, and protein supplements as prescribed. Record intake and output. Give careful attention to skin. Elevate head of bed, to facilitate breathing. Give pillow support under costal margin when in side-lying positions. If above measures fail, a paracentesis may be required.

THE PATIENT WITH LAENNEC'S CIRRHOSIS (CONTINUED)

Problems	Nursing Implications
Ascites (*Continued*)	Assist patient during paracentesis: 1. Have him void before procedure. 2. Position correctly and use pillow support. 3. Record both the amount and the character of fluid aspirated. 4. Protect puncture site with dry dressings. 5. Check dressing for fluid seepage and evidence of wound infections. Observe for symptoms of impending coma.
Hydrothorax and dyspnea	Elevate head of bed. Conserve patient's strength. Change position at intervals. Assist patient during thoracentesis: 1. Support and maintain position during procedure. 2. Record both the amount and the character of fluid aspirated. 3. Observe for evidence of coughing, increasing dyspnea, and/or pulse rate.
Fever	Record temperature regularly. Encourage fluid intake. Give cool sponges for elevated temperature. Supply icecap to head as prescribed. Give antibiotics as prescribed. Avoid exposure to infections. Keep patient at rest. Note urinary volume and concentration.
Hemorrhagic manifestations: ecchymosis, epistaxis, petechiae, and bleeding gums	Avoid trauma. Maintain safe environment. Avoid forceful blowing of nose. Prevent trauma to gums from toothbrushing. Encourage intake of foods with high content of vitamin C. Apply cold compresses where indicated. Record location of bleeding sites. Avoid constrictive clothing. Use small-gauge needles for injections.
Increasing stupor: mental changes, lethargy, hallucinations, and hepatic coma	Restrict dietary protein. Give small, frequent feeding of carbohydrates. Protect from infection. Keep environment warm and draft-free. Pad the side-rails of the bed. Limit visitors. Provide careful nursing surveillance to ensure patient's safety. Avoid narcotics and barbiturates. Arouse at intervals. Give sensitive nursing care during terminal phase. Check for adequately fitting nasal tubings when nasal oxygen therapy is prescribed.

the right atrium). The pathophysiological effect is increased strain, particularly on the vessels in the submucosal layer of the lower esophagus and upper part of the stomach. These collateral vessels are not very elastic, but rather are tortuous, fragile, and bleed easily. Other lesser causes of varices are abnormalities of the circulation in the splenic vein or superior vena cava, and hepatic venothrombosis.

Bleeding esophageal varices are life-threatening and should be suspected in the presence of hematemesis and melena, especially in the patient who has been addicted to alcohol. Usually the dilated veins cause no symptoms unless the mucosa over them becomes ulcerated. Then massive hemorrhage takes place. Factors that contribute to rupture and hemorrhage are muscular strain from lifting heavy objects, straining at stool, sneezing, coughing or vomiting, esophagitis, or irritation of vessels by poorly chewed foods or irritating fluids. Salicylates and any drug that erodes esophageal mucosa or interferes with cell replication may also cause bleeding.

Assessment

The patient's history and physical examination serve as a basis for ascertaining the problem. Neurologic assessment will assist in identifying possible hepatic encephalopathy. Manifestations may range from sleepiness to coma. Portal hypertension may be suspected if dilated abdominal veins and rectal hemorrhoids are detected. Also apparent may be a palpable enlarged spleen (splenomegaly) and ascites. Laboratory tests that may be required are various liver function tests, such as Bromsulphalein retention, serum transaminase, bilirubin, alkaline phosphatase, and serum proteins. Esophagoscopy most clearly clinches the diagnosis, because even the site of hemorrhage may be seen. Nursing support before and during this examination can be effective in relieving a stressful experience (see page 404). Careful monitoring can detect early signs of cardiac arrhythmias, perforation, and hemorrhage. A flexible fiberscope will also permit endoscopic visualization of varices before they rupture. After the examination, fluids are not given until the gag reflex returns. Lozenges and gargles may be offered to relieve throat discomfort.

Portal vein pressure can be measured in the operating room by introducing a needle into the spleen; a manometer reading above 20 ml. saline is abnormal. Combined umbilical-portal and hepatic vein catheterization is the most practical method for measuring portal pressure and at the same time permits radiologic study of the hepatic vascular bed. Blood flow studies may also be done, which assists in determining cardiac output.

Splenoportography using iodopyracet (Diodrast) is studied in serial or segmental roentgenograms to detect extensive collateral circulation in esophageal vessels, which would be indicative of varices. Other tests are hepatoportography and celiac angiography. These are usually done in the operating room or x-ray department.

Overall nursing assessment includes an evaluation of the emotional concerns of the patient and any physical problems, such as abnormal body discharges. Vital signs are taken, and the nutritional needs are determined. If the patient was admitted for hemorrhage, the situation becomes an emergency.

Management

The patient with bleeding varices is critically ill, requiring continuous nursing attention. Nursing assessment requires that the extent of bleeding be evaluated and

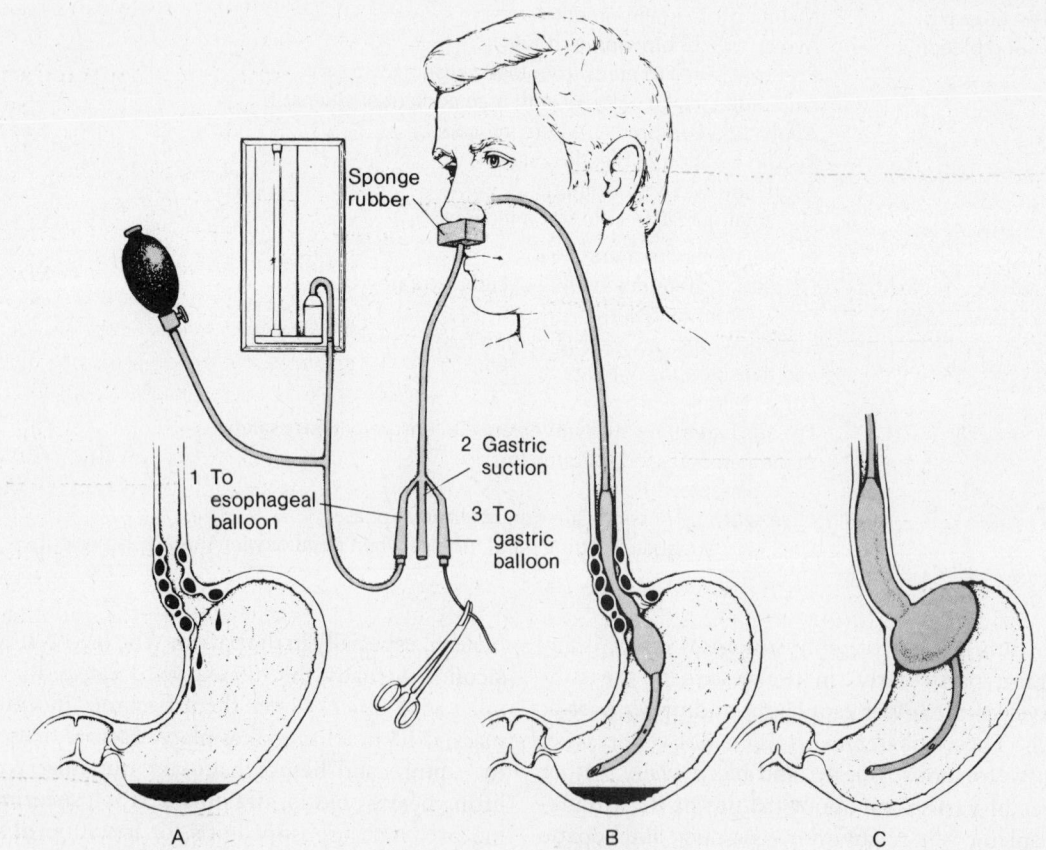

Figure 38-8. Diagram showing esophageal varices and their treatment by a compressing balloon tube (Sengstaken-Blakemore). (*A*) Dilated veins of the lower esophagus. (*B*) The tube is in place in the stomach and the lower esophagus, but is not inflated. (*C*) Inflation of the tube and the compression of the veins which can be obtained by inflation of the balloon.

vital signs monitored at least every 15 minutes, when hematemesis and melena are present. Signs of potential hypovolemia are to be noted, such as cold clammy skin, tachycardia, blood pressure drop, restlessness, increased or shallow peripheral pulse. Blood volume monitoring is accomplished with a central venous pressure (CVP) catheter. Oxygen is required, to prevent hypoxia and to maintain adequate blood oxygenation. Blood transfusion also may be needed.

Since patients with bleeding esophageal varices are subject to electrolyte imbalance, intravenous fluids are prescribed to restore fluid volume and replace deficient electrolytes. Urinary output is carefully monitored; an indwelling catheter may be indicated.

Drug Therapy. Before resorting to tamponade, some internists administer vasopressin Pituitrin (S) or Pitressin, because of its portal hypotensive action brought about by constriction of the splanchnic arterial bed. It may be given intravenously or by intra-arterial infusion. Either method requires monitoring by the nurse. Gastric aspiration and vital signs offer indices of the effectiveness of vasopressin.

• Coronary artery disease in this patient would be a contraindication to the use of vasopressin, since coronary vasoconstriction may promote a myocardial infarction.

Electrolyte evaluation and monitoring of fluid intake and output are necessary, since hyponatremia may occur and vasopressin may have an antidiuretic effect.

Sengstaken-Blakemore Tube. To control the hemorrhage in certain patients, pressure is exerted on the cardiac portion of the stomach and against the bleeding varices by a double balloon tamponade (Sengstaken-Blakemore tube, S.B.T.) (Fig. 38-8). The three openings are for specific purposes: gastric aspiration, inflation of the gastric balloon, and inflation of the esophageal balloon.

The balloon in the stomach is inflated, and the tube is pulled gently to exert a force against the cardia. Irrigation of the tubing is performed, to detect bleeding; if returns are clear, the esophageal balloon is not inflated, and vice versa—if bleeding continues, the esophageal balloon is inflated. The desired pressure in both balloons is 25 to 30 mm.Hg, as measured by the manometer. After the balloon is inflated, there is a possibility of injury or rupture of the esophagus. Constant nursing surveillance is necessary at this time. Traction is placed on the tube at the point where it enters the patient. A nasogastric tube may be inserted through the other nostril to aspirate esophagopharyngeal secretions. This is not necessary in the "Minnesota tube" (Fig. 38-9), because a fourth lumen is included in the outlets to the tamponade tube, to provide a direct route for esophageal aspiration.

Usually a cathartic such as magnesium sulfate is introduced through the tube. This, plus enemas, will elimi-

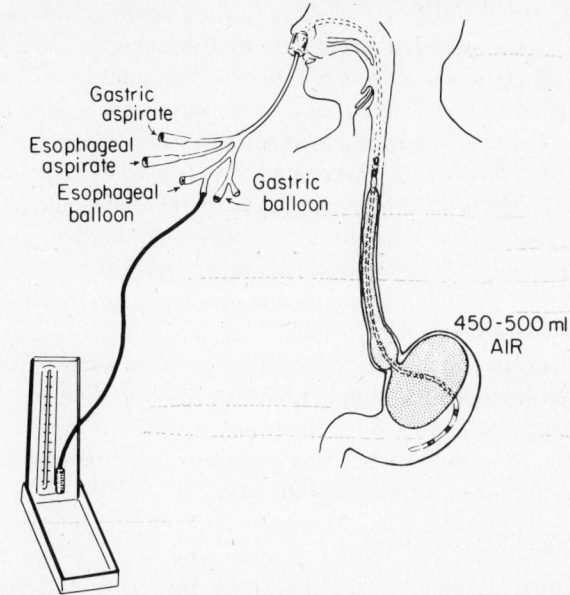

Figure 38-9.   This is the Minnesota Four-lumen Esophagogastric Tamponade Tube for the control of bleeding from esophageal varices. Note that this tube has an additional outlet for aspiration of the esophagus. This safety feature prevents the aspiration of regurgitated gastric juice, blood, and saliva during inflation of the gastric balloon. (Davol, Inc., Cranston, R.I.)

nate blood in the gastrointestinal tract; otherwise ammonia absorption could occur, which may lead to hepatic coma and death. Thereafter, neomycin is administered to reduce intestinal bacterial flora, which are a source of ammonia-forming enzymes.

Gastric suction can be provided by connecting the proper catheter outlet to suction. The tubing is irrigated hourly, and drainage will indicate whether bleeding has been controlled. Some physicians circulate ice water in and out of the stomach balloon in order to constrict the gastric vessels. In such instances, the nurse will anticipate possible chilling of the patient and provide comfort measures. The pressures on the tubes and traction are released periodically, as prescribed. Balloon tamponade is continued for several days and then cautiously released, followed by removal of the tube if no bleeding recurs.

Although this method has been fairly successful, it is well to note some inherent dangers. If the tube is left in place too long, ulcers can develop in the stomach. If the tube suddenly ruptures, the result is disastrous—(airway obstruction and aspiration of gastric contents into the lungs). Using a brand-new tested tube that is less than a year old may prevent this calamity. Asphyxiation is another problem, caused by the counterweight pulling the tube into the oropharynx. These potential dangers suggest the need for intensive and intelligent care. The balloon may be deflated for 5 minutes at 8- to 12-hour intervals to prevent erosion and necrosis of the stomach and esophagus.

Nursing comfort measures include frequent mouth and nasal care. For secretions that accumulate in the mouth, tissues should be within easy reach of the patient. The patient is more relaxed if he knows that the nurse is nearby and will respond immediately to his call.

Other Measures. Bleeding also is treated by sedation and complete rest of the esophagus (parenteral feedings). Straining and vomiting must be prevented. Gastric suction usually is employed to keep the stomach as empty as possible. The patient complains of severe thirst, which may be relieved by frequent oral hygiene and moist sponges to the lips, if permitted. The nurse keeps close surveillance on the patient's blood pressure. Vitamin K therapy and multiple blood transfusions often are indicated. A quiet environment and calm reassurance will help to relieve the patient's anxiety.

Surgical Management

Surgical procedures that may be employed for esophageal varices are (1) injection of sclerosing drugs, by way of the esophagoscope, (2) direct surgical ligation of varices, and (3) portacaval and splenorenal venous shunt operations.

Surgical By-Pass Procedures. The most common procedure is to create an anastomosis between the portal vein and the inferior vena cava, which is spoken of as a *portacaval anastomosis* (Fig. 38-10). When portal blood is shunted into the vena cava, the pressure in the portal system is decreased, and consequently the danger of hemorrhage from esophageal and gastric varices is reduced. When the portal vein cannot be used because of thrombosis, or for other reasons, a shunt may be made between the splenic vein and the left renal vein (*splenorenal shunt*), following splenectomy. Some surgeons prefer this shunt to the portacaval shunt, even when the portal vein can be used.

A *mesocaval* shunt is a third type of by-pass procedure, in which the inferior vena cava is severed and the proximal end of the cava is anastomosed to the side of the superior mesenteric vein.

These operations are rather extensive procedures and are not always successful, because of secondary clotting in the veins used for the shunt. Nevertheless, a shunt is the only method by which a lowering of pressure in the portal system may be brought about, and since hemorrhages from the esophageal varices are often fatal, many of these relatively poor-risk patients must be subjected to these attempts to save their lives.

Postoperative Nursing Management. Bleeding anywhere in the body is likely to be upsetting and anxiety-provoking, resulting in a crisis situation for the patient and his family when fears are manifested. If the patient is an alcoholic, behavioral problems can further complicate the situation. The nurse provides support and pertinent explanations regarding medical and nursing interventions. Monitoring the patient closely will help in preventing and managing complications.

Postoperative care is similar to that for any abdominal operation, but complications may arise, including hemodynamic shock, hepatic encephalopathy, electrolyte imbalance, metabolic and respiratory alkalosis, delirium tremens, and seizures.

HEPATIC TUMORS

Hepatic tumors generally are cancerous in nature. It has only been in recent years that benign liver tumors have gained any significance, since their incidence has increased with the use of oral contraceptives.

As for cancerous tumors, few cancers originate in the liver. Those that are primary tumors ordinarily occur in patients with cirrhosis, especially of the postnecrotic type. Such a *hepatoma* is generally inoperable, because of rapid extension and metastasis elsewhere. *Cholangiocarcinoma* is a primary malignant tumor, usually arising in normal liver. If found early, there may be cure; however, the likelihood is small.

Metastases are found in the liver in about one-half of all late cancer cases. The primary growth may be almost anywhere, and since the bloodstream and the lymphatics from the body cavities nearly all reach the liver, malignant tumors anywhere in the trunk are likely to reach this organ eventually. Moreover, the liver apparently is an ideal place for these malignant cells to take root and to grow. Often the first evidence of a cancer in an abdominal organ is the appearance of liver metastases, and, unless exploratory operation or necropsy is performed, the primary growth may never be discovered.

Diagnosis of malignant disease of the liver is made, regardless of the location of the primary tumor, when there is a recent loss of weight, loss of strength, and anemia (the last being the most common early symptoms of any cancer that interferes with nutrition), together with rapid enlargement of the liver, which on palpation presents an irregular surface. Jaundice is present only if the larger bile ducts are occluded by the pressure of malignant nodules in the hilum of the liver. Ascites occurs only if such nodules obstruct the portal veins, or if tumor tissue is seeded in the peritoneal cavity. The only treatment is palliative.

Surgical Management

Successful hepatic lobectomy for cancer can be done when the primary hepatic tumor is localized or when, in the case of metastasis, the primary site can be completely excised and the metastasis is limited. Capitalizing on the regenerative capacity of the liver cells, some surgeons have successfully removed 90 percent of the liver.

Preoperative Evaluation and Preparation. As the patient is being prepared for surgery, his nutritional,

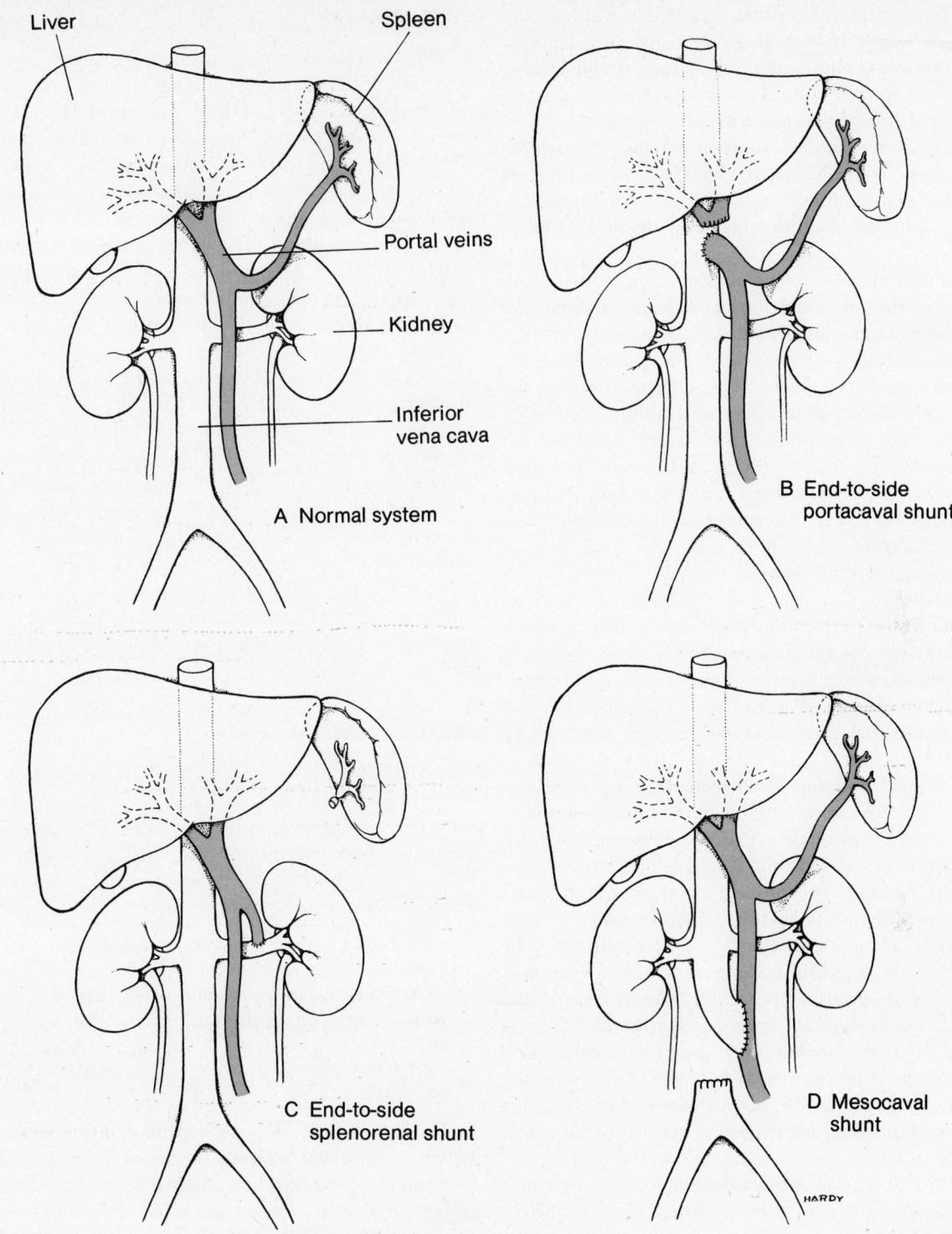

Figure 38-10. Types of portal-systemic venous shunts.

fluid, emotional, and physical needs are evaluated and met. Meanwhile, he may be undergoing extensive laboratory and roentgen studies. The support, explanation, and encouragement by the nurse will help him to achieve the most desirable level for surgery. Optimism is automatically generated for this patient, because not too long ago, liver surgery was unheard of. It may be necessary to prepare the intestinal tract by way of cathartic, colonic irrigation, and intestinal antibiotics to minimize any possibility of ammonium intoxification and to anticipate any possibility of the intestines being opened at surgery. Specific studies may include liver scanning, liver biopsy, cholangiography, selective hepatic angiography, percutaneous needle biopsy, peritoneoscopy, and laparoscopy, ultrasound and computerized tomography scans, and blood tests, particularly serum alkaline phosphatase and serum glutamic oxaloacetic acid.

Surgical Intervention. If it is necessary to restrict blood flow from the hepatic artery and portal vein beyond 15 minutes (under normothermic conditions, 15-minute occlusion is permissible), it is likely that hypothermia will be used.

The nurse needs to be cognizant of the anatomy referred to by the surgeon in the care of these patients. The usual true (functional) division of the liver is into two lobes, the larger (by 6 times) right lobe and the left lobe, with two smaller segments sandwiched between, the caudate and the quadrate (refer to anatomy textbook). Most surgeons prefer the anatomic (surgical) division of the lobes. Here the liver is divided into a right and a left lobe by a lobar fissure that is almost in line with the gallbladder bed and the inferior vena cava on the visceral surface. According to this division, the branching of hepatic vessels and the portal vein lend themselves to a more even segmentation. Obviously, a right-liver lobectomy according to the surgical division is less extensive than it would be in the functional division.

For a right-liver lobectomy or an extended right lobectomy (including medial left lobe), a thoracoabdominal incision is used. A generous abdominal incision is made for a left lobectomy.

Postsurgical Nursing Management. There are potential problems related to cardiopulmonary involvement, portal and general circulation, and respiratory and liver dysfunction. Metabolic abnormalities require meticulous correction. A constant infusion of 10 percent glucose may be required in the first 48 hours to prevent a precipitous fall in blood sugar. Since there is impairment of protein synthesis and derangement of lipid metabolism, these all need careful medical supervision. The patient requires constant attention for the first 2 or 3 days, as described for abdominal and thoracic postsurgical nursing care (pages 350 and 423). Liver regeneration is rapid; in one patient who had a 90 percent resection of the liver, a normal liver mass was restored in 6 months.

Early ambulation is encouraged under the knowledgeable supervision of the nurse, who is able to translate untoward signs into desired action.

For more extensive malignancy of the liver, percutaneous infusions of antitumor drugs or radioactive gold (^{198}Au) may make the patient more comfortable.

Irradiation. In most instances this form of treatment is considered to be palliative for metastasis to the liver. Such control has resulted in longer survival and improved quality of life.

LIVER ABSCESSES

Whenever an infection develops anywhere along the gastrointestinal tract, there is danger that an embolus will be transported by way of the portal venous system to the liver. Secondary abscess formation may take place in that organ. Morever, in patients with bacteremia, organisms may be carried through the hepatic artery to the liver. Most bacteria are promptly destroyed, but occasionally some gain a foothold. The bacterial toxins destroy the neighboring liver cells, and the necrotic tissue produced serves as a protective wall for the organisms. Meanwhile, leukocytes migrate into the infected area. The result is an abscess cavity full of a liquid containing living and dead leukocytes, liquefied liver cells, and bacteria. Pyogenic abscesses of this type are usually multiple and small, but may be single. The result is an extremely serious disease, manifested by high fever, chills alternating with sweats, jaundice, painful enlargement of the liver, anemia, toxemia, and usually death. Specific chemotherapy is given, depending on the identity of the infective agent. (The student is referred to a text on pharmacology.)

Liver abscesses may be due to several kinds of bacteria and to a fungus. The most common agent, however, is a protozoan, *Entamoeba histolytica,* one of the most important causes of dysentery.

HEPATIC TRANSPLANTATION

Human liver transplantation has in most instances been done for life-threatening liver disease for which no other form of treatment was available. This includes nonresectable malignant liver tumor (moratorium put into effect because of high incidence of tumor recurrence), biliary atresia, liver cirrhosis, and chronic aggressive hepatitis.

Transplants are divided into two classifications:
1. *Orthotopic* — total replacement of the liver, with anatomic reconstruction of the vasculature, or replacement of the liver with a transplant in the same area of the right upper quadrant.
2. *Heterotopic* — placing an auxiliary or second liver in the groin or pelvis.

The main difficulties in hepatic transplantation are technical problems causing obstruction, drug toxicity, immunochemical rejection, hepatic arterial thrombosis, or hepatic abscess. The patient is maintained in as germ-free an environment as possible, because immunosuppressive drugs reduce the body's natural defense.

Postoperative Nursing Management. In the postoperative period the patient is monitored constantly for all cardiovascular parameters, as well as arterial blood gases and pH. Respiratory assistance is provided via a volume-cycled ventilator, with the patient in a semi-Fowler position. The patient is suctioned as required and sterile humidification is provided. Rejection signs are monitored through such liver function tests as SGOT, liver scans, bilirubin, and cholangiogram. Coagulation studies indicate the functioning of the donor liver. Cultures of urine and blood, and throat swabs are taken frequently.

Intravenous fluids are prescribed, along with antibiotics and immunosuppressive drugs. Constant emotional support is needed to assist this patient to accept the fact that he has endured surgery and is slowly recovering with a new liver. Hourly progress determines when he is weaned from the ventilator, when he may take oral fluids, and when physical activity may gradually be resumed. The incidence of long-term survival is still low.

BILIARY CONDITIONS

Estimates indicate that approximately 500,000 persons a year in the United States are hospitalized for gallbladder disease and that about two-thirds of these are treated surgically. More women than men (4 to 1) acquire this disease; they are usually past 40, multiparous, and overweight. By way of prevention, it is suggested that steps be taken to lose weight and to avoid fatty foods.

The Boston Collaborative Drug Surveillance Program has shown that postmenopausal women on estrogen therapy are 2½ times at greater risk of gallbladder disease; also, women on birth control pills are at 2 times greater risk of gallbladder disease than nonusers.

Most (90 percent) of the problems of patients with gallbladder disease are related to gallstones (cholelithiasis). Infection (cholecystitis) is also a common problem, that may or may not be related to calculi. Only 1 percent of patients with biliary tract disease have neoplasms.

CHOLECYSTITIS

At times the gallbladder may be the seat of an acute infection (*cholecystitis*) that causes acute pain, tenderness, and rigidity of the upper right abdomen, associated with nausea and vomiting and the usual signs of an acute inflammation. This condition is spoken of as *acute cholecystitis*. If the gallbladder is found to be filled with pus, there is said to be an *empyema* of the gallbladder.

CHOLELITHIASIS

Cholelithiasis (calculi) usually form in the gallbladder from the solid constituents of bile and vary greatly in size, shape, and consistency.

Gallstones are uncommon in children and young adults but become increasingly prevalent after age 40.

The incidence of cholelithiasis increases thereafter to such an extent that it has been estimated that by the age of 75, one of every three persons will have gallstones.

Pathophysiology. Upon analysis, gallstones are found to be made of cholesterol, calcium combined with bilirubin, and inorganic salts. Those gallstones composed predominantly of pigment are treated only by surgical removal. Those that are predominantly cholesterol (i.e., over 70 percent cholesterol), are the most common, comprising about three-quarters of all gallstones found in patients in this country.

Research has indicated that the formation of cholesterol gallstones is probably due to secretion by the liver cells of bile abnormally high in cholesterol and lacking the proper concentration and proportion of bile salts. It appears that cholesterol exists in the bile in a highly supersaturated state, so that it will later precipitate out in the gallbladder, if it is not kept in solution by the right mixture of bile salts. This would indicate that the liver is the origin of the disease, rather than the gallbladder itself. Cholesterol is insoluble in water, its solubility depending upon bile acids and lecithin (phospholipids). Saturated bile is a prerequisite to gallstone formation (lithogenesis). Since the liver produces saturated bile, evidence suggests there is decreased bile acid synthesis and increased cholesterol synthesis in the liver of gallstone-prone patients. This probably accounts for the increase in biliary cholesterol secretion and the lowered level of bile acids which are necessary to solubilize (dissolve) cholesterol. The role of the gallbladder is less well understood. However, it is known that gallbladder bile is never more saturated than hepatic bile.

Clinical Manifestations. The presence of stones indicates some dysfunction of the gallbladder, and the disease is spoken of as *chronic gallbladder disease*. The patient may notice two types of symptoms: those due to disease of the gallbladder itself—epigastric distress, such as fullness and chronic pain in the upper right abdomen; and those due to obstruction of the bile passages (especially the cystic duct) by a gallstone—excruciating upper right abdominal pain that radiates to the back or right shoulder, usually associated with nausea and vomiting. These symptoms are more noticeable several hours after a heavy meal that included fried or fatty foods. Such a bout of *biliary colic* is caused by contracture of the gallbladder, which has been stimulated by fat and is having difficulty releasing bile because of obstruction which, in all likelihood, is due to calculi. These symptoms generally are so severe as to require morphine or meperidine hydrochloride. (Some physicians believe these drugs may increase the spasm of the sphincter of Oddi; to give the patient relief, a nitroglycerin tablet is given under the tongue.)

Pharmacotherapy. Chenodeoxycholic acid continues to undergo extensive testing as a means of dissolving gallstones (chenotherapy). It appears to be effective in dissolving about 60 percent of radiolucent gallstones. The mechanism of action seems to be the inhibition of liver synthesis and secretion of cholesterol, thereby desaturating bile. Existing stones can be decreased in size (small ones may even dissolve) and new stones prevented from forming. Ideal dose needs to be determined. The National Cooperative Gallstone Study has been conducting a clinical trial utilizing different dosages and placebo in 1,000 patients. Results of this study should give direction to effective dosage.

Certain other medications, such as estrogens, oral contraceptives, clofibrate, and dietary cholesterol may adversely affect the results of treatment with chenodeoxycholic acid. If the patient is taking these drugs, the physician should be made aware of this.

Cholesterol stones may recur in a small percentage of patients after chenodeoxycholic acid is terminated; whether a low dose of this drug should be continued to prevent recurrence needs to be investigated, since the long-term cost and safety of continuous chenotherapy are unknown. An alternative consideration would be surgical therapy.

The role of chenodeoxycholic acid in prophylaxis needs further study, as do other agents: ursodeoxycholic acid (UDCA) and Zanchol, which are being tested for their gallstone-dissolving potential.

Nutritional Management. The diet, immediately after an attack, is usually limited to low-fat liquids. Powdered supplements high in protein and carbohydrate can be stirred into skim milk. The following may then be added as tolerated: cooked fruits, rice or tapioca, lean meats, mashed potatoes, non-gas-forming vegetables, bread, coffee, or tea. Avoid eggs, cream, pork, fried foods, cheese and rich dressings, gas-forming vegetables, and alcohol. The patient needs to be reminded that fatty foods may bring on an attack. Rest is a vital part of recovery from an attack.

BILIARY OBSTRUCTION

Pathophysiology. Not infrequently a gallstone may pass from the gallbladder through the cystic duct and lodge in the common bile duct; or the head of the pancreas, through which the common duct passes, may be the seat of a carcinoma. Either condition may obstruct the flow of bile into the duodenum and result in the following characteristic symptoms: the bile, no longer carried to the duodenum, is absorbed by the blood and gives the skin and the tissues a yellow color known as *jaundice*. There frequently is marked itching of the skin. The excretion of the bile pigments in some measure from the blood by the kidneys gives the urine a very dark color. The feces, no longer colored with bile pigments, are grayish, like putty, and usually are spoken of as "clay-colored." Nausea occurs after fatty foods are eaten, because there is a marked disturbance of the digestion and absorption of fats when bile does not flow into the duodenum. Various laboratory tests of the blood (icteric index, serum bilirubin, etc.) indicate the degree of pigment retention, and therefore the depth of jaundice.

Management. Operations on patients with obstructive jaundice are technically complex, and the patients are usually quite sick, because of extensive bile duct exploration. Therefore, these patients should receive special preparation. The diet should be low in fats and high in protein and carbohydrate. Frequently protein hydrolysates are administered intravenously for a day or two before operation.

It is well known that the hemorrhagic tendency in jaundice is due to a deficient formation of prothrombin. Prothrombin is an important factor in the clotting of blood, which becomes deficient when the patient becomes jaundiced because of inadequate absorption of the fat-soluble vitamin K. Often the blood prothrombin may be raised adequately by administration of vitamin K parenterally. Carbohydrates are given in large amounts by mouth, and intravenously, to build up the glycogen stores in the liver. The nurse notes the color of the urine and the stools and sends specimens of these excreta to be examined for bile pigments. The operations performed depend on the cause of the biliary obstruction.

ROENTGENOGRAPHY OF THE BILIARY SYSTEM

CHOLECYSTOGRAPHY. Radiologic examination of the gallbladder is carried out for the detection of gallstones and to estimate the ability of the gallbladder to fill, concentrate its contents, contract, and empty in normal fashion. Very few gallstones are sufficiently radiopaque to be visualized by ordinary roentgenographic technique; they must be demonstrated as negative shadows in a gallbladder filled with a radiopaque substance. To this end an iodide-containing dye that is excreted into the bile by the liver and concentrated in the gallbladder is administered to the patient, either by mouth or by intravenous injection.

Note: Oral or intravenous cholecystography in the obviously jaundiced patient is a waste of time, since the liver cells will not transport dye to the biliary tract in a jaundiced individual. This is important to the nurse, since the physician's orders may be written before obvious jaundice develops; if jaundice occurs, the nurse can inform the physician of this fact.

Drugs* given as contrast media include Telepaque, Cholografin, and Oragrafin. These preparations are

---

*Telepaque = iopanoic acid; Cholografin methylmeglumine = iodipamide methylglucamine; Oragrafin = sodium ipodate.

given in oral doses of 2 to 3 gm., 10 to 12 hours before x-ray study. Intravenous cholecystography involves the injection of an iodide approximately 10 minutes prior to roentgenography. During the interval between the administration of the iodide and the x-ray study, the patient is permitted nothing by mouth, lest the gallbladder be stimulated to contract and thereby expel the contrast medium.

Nursing Considerations. Instructions to patients who are scheduled for x-ray studies of the gallbladder (cholecystogram; gallbladder series) include:

1. One hour or more after the evening meal, and approximately 10 hours before roentgenography, the patient receives tablets or capsules of contrast medium by mouth.
2. These tablets are to be ingested as per directions, together with a volume of water totaling at least 8 oz.
3. The patient then is to receive nothing by mouth, excepting water, until bedtime. Thereafter, until the roentgenogram is taken, not even water is permitted. If the patient vomits after the ingestion of the dye, the physician may suggest that the medication be given after nausea subsides, or the test may be postponed.
4. Laxatives are not to be given during this preparation period.
5. A saline enema may be administered early in the morning of the test.
6. Breakfast is omitted.

Procedure. The right upper abdominal quadrant then is photographed by x-ray. If the gallbladder has filled and concentrated the dye normally, it is seen as a pear-shaped shadow from 5-7.5 cm. (2-3 inches) long, under the right costal margin. If stones are present, there are mottled densities within this shadow corresponding to their outlines. Next, to test the contractility of the gallbladder, the patient is fed a fatty meal containing cream, butter, or eggs, and the x-ray examination is repeated at intervals until the gallbladder has expelled the dye and becomes invisible (Graham-Cole test). If the gallbladder is found to fill and empty normally and to contain no stones, it is concluded that no gallbladder disease is present.

PERCUTANEOUS TRANSHEPATIC CHOLANGIOGRAPHY. The oral and the intravenous radiographic techniques just described permit the visualization of the gallbladder (and occasionally the larger ducts) only if the liver cells are functioning properly and are capable of excreting the radiopaque dye into the bile. Percutaneous transhepatic cholangiography, which involves the injection of dye directly into the biliary tree itself, is effective, regardless of the state of liver function. Moreover, because of the relatively large concentration of dye that is introduced into the biliary system, all components of the latter, including the hepatic ducts within the liver, the common hepatic duct throughout its length, the cystic duct, and the gallbladder, are delineated with clarity.

This procedure is useful in distinguishing jaundice caused by liver disease (hepatocellular jaundice) from that due to biliary obstruction; for investigating the gastrointestinal symptoms of patients whose gallbladders have been removed; for locating stones within the bile ducts; and in diagnosing cancer involving the biliary system.

Procedure. The patient, fasting and well sedated, lies supine on the x-ray table. The injection site, usually in the midclavicular line immediately beneath the right costal margin, is disinfected and anesthetized with lidocaine (Xylocaine). A small incision is made at this point and a thin flexible needle with stylet is inserted cephalad, posteriorly at a 45-degree angle and parallel to the midline. When the needle has penetrated to a depth of approximately 10 cm. (4 inches), the stylet is removed and replaced by a plastic connector tube with 50-ml. syringe attached. Gentle suction is applied while the needle is slowly withdrawn, until bile appears in the syringe. As much bile as possible is withdrawn, a radiopaque dye is injected, and an x-ray picture taken. Before the needle is removed, as much dye and bile as possible are aspirated, in order to forestall subsequent leakage into the needle tract and eventually into the peritoneal cavity, thus avoiding the possibility of bile peritonitis.

SURGICAL MANAGEMENT OF BILIARY DISORDERS

Surgical treatment is necessary for the relief of long-continued symptoms, for the removal of the cause of biliary colic, and for treatment of acute cholecystitis.

Preoperative Management. In addition to x-ray studies of the gallbladder, chest x-rays and electrocardiogram will probably be done, and possibly liver function tests (Table 39-1). Vitamin K preparations for a low prothrombin level may be given. If the level is unusually low, a fresh blood transfusion may be given before surgery is done to supply ingredients necessary for blood-clotting.

Nutritional requirements are respected; if the patient is not eating properly, it may be necessary to provide intravenous glucose with protein hydrolysate supplements. This will aid wound healing and help prevent liver damage.

Preparation for a simple gallbladder operation is the same as for any upper abdominal laparotomy. Instruction and explanation is given the day before surgery with regard to turning and deep breathing. Because the abdominal incision is high on the abdomen (subcostal), the patient is often reluctant to move and turn; pneumonia is a possible postoperative complication which is to be avoided by breathing deeply, and turning. Since drainage tubes are usually required after operation, the patient should be informed of this, so that he knows what to expect.

Surgical Intervention. Patients usually are placed on the operating table with the upper abdomen raised some-

---

TERMINOLOGY

Cholecystitis—inflammation of the gallbladder

Cholelithiasis—calculi in the gallbladder

Cholecystectomy—removal of the gallbladder

Cholecystostomy—opening and drainage of gallbladder

Choledochotomy—opening into the common duct, usually to remove duct stones

Choledocholithiasis—stones in the common duct

Choledocholithotomy—removal of stones in the common duct

Choledochoduodenostomy—anastomosis of common duct to duodenum

Choledochojejunostomy—anastomosis of common duct to jejunum

---

what by an air pillow or sandbag to make the biliary area more accessible.

Cholecystostomy. This operation is performed for the relief of certain patients with acute cholecystitis and chronic gallbladder disease. The gallbladder is opened, the stones and the bile or the pus are removed, and a tube is sutured in the opening for drainage. As soon as the patient is returned to bed, the nurse should connect this tube to a drainage bottle placed at the side of the bed. Failure to do this may result in the leakage of bile around the tube, and its escape into the peritoneal cavity.

Cholecystectomy. In this operation, the gallbladder is removed after ligation of the cystic duct and artery. The operation is performed in most cases of acute and chronic cholecystitis.

Choledochostomy. In this operation, an incision is made into the common duct for removal of stones. After the stones have been evacuated, a tube usually is inserted into the duct for drainage. The gallbladder also contains stones, as a rule. A cholecystectomy is performed.

Postoperative Nursing Management. As soon as the patient has recovered from anesthesia, he is placed in the low Fowler's position. Fluids may be given by vein, and nasogastric suction (tube probably inserted immediately prior to surgery) instituted to relieve distention. Water and other fluids may be given in about 24 hours, and a soft diet started later, after bowel sounds are elicited.

The location of the subcostal incision is likely to cause the patient to splint the operative site by inadvertently taking shallow breaths, to prevent pain. Since full aeration of the lungs is necessary to prevent respiratory complications, analgesics should be given as prescribed and the patient encouraged to turn, cough, and breathe deeply at frequent intervals.

Drainage. As mentioned before, in patients who have undergone a cholecystostomy or choledochostomy, the drainge tubes must be connected immediately to a drainage receptacle. In addition, tubing should be fastened to the dressings or to the bottom sheet, with enough leeway for the patient to move without dislodging it. The patient must know why he cannot roll onto the tube and that it must remain patent at all times.

Following a cholecystectomy, a drain (Penrose) is placed in the gallbladder bed and brought out through a stab wound. Drainage of blood, serosanguineous fluids, and bile are absorbed by dressings which are changed as required. Montgomery straps are helpful in maintaining a comfortable dressing.

After a cholecystostomy, a tube is placed in the gallbladder and fixed in position by a purse-string suture. This is connected to a gravity drainage tube and a receptable.

In a choledochostomy, after the bile duct has been explored, dilated, and probably relieved of stones, a T-tube is positioned in the common duct to permit drainage of bile until edema subsides. This tube is connected to gravity drainage tubing.

In order to prevent total loss of bile, the drainage tube or collecting receptacle may be elevated above the level of the abdomen, so that bile drains through the apparatus only if pressure develops in the duct system. The bile collected should be measured and recorded every 24 hours, its color and character being documented. After several days of drainage, the tubes may be clamped for an hour before and after each meal, the purpose being to deliver bile to the duodenum to aid in digestion. Within 7 to 14 days, the drainage tubes are removed from the gallbladder or common bile duct.

If bile is not draining properly, an obstruction is probably causing bile to be forced back into the liver and bloodstream. Since jaundice may result, the nurse should be particularly observant of the color of the sclerae.

Bile may continue to drain from the drainage tract in considerable quantities for a time, necessitating frequent changes of the outer dressings and protection of the skin from irritation. Skin pastes of zinc oxide, aluminum, or petrolatum prevent the bile from literally digesting the skin. In chronic biliary drainage, where there is excessive loss of bile, the drainage may be collected and readministered to the patient through the nasogastric tube, or orally. It is preferable not to tell the patient that he is receiving his own bile, since this may be psychologically upsetting. A simple statement to the effect that this is a special preparation to help the appetite may be sufficient. The bile should be chilled, strained, and diluted with grape or apple juice.

Careful Monitoring. In all patients with biliary drainage, the stools should be observed daily and their color recorded. At frequent intervals, specimens of both urine and feces should be sent to the laboratory for examination for bile pigments. In this way, it is possible to determine that the bile pigment is disappearing from the blood and is draining again into the duodenum. A careful record of fluid intake and output is kept and totaled for each 24 hours.

Nutritional Needs.   The diet of these patients is low in fats and high in carbohydrates and proteins. The patients themselves usually refuse to eat fatty foods because of the nausea that follows. Vitamin K administration is continued after operation.

Preventing Complications.   These patients are especially prone to pulmonary complications, as are all patients with upper abdominal incisions. Thus, they should be taught to take deep breaths every hour to aerate the lungs fully. Other complications such as thrombophlebitis and pulmonary atelectasis may be avoided by promoting early ambulation as soon as permissible. Such complications are more likely to occur in the more obese patient. An abdominal binder may help to make the patient comfortable when he first gets out of bed. Since a drainage receptacle is attached when the patient is ambulating, the collecting bag may be placed in a bathrobe pocket or fastened so that it is below the waist or common duct level.

Patient Education.   Ordinarily, barring complications, the patient may leave the hospital in 10 to 14 days. Usually there are no special dietary instructions, other than to maintain a nutritious diet and avoid excessive fats. Fat restriction usually is lifted in 4–6 weeks when biliary ducts dilate to accommodate volume of bile once held by the gallbladder, and when the ampulla of Vater again functions effectively. After this, when one eats fats, adequate bile will be released into the digestive tract to emulsify the fats and allow their digestion. Prior to this, fats would not be completely or adequately digested in some persons, and flatulence might occur. However, the purpose of gallbladder surgery is to allow for a normal diet, ultimately.

The patient should know what medications are required (vitamins, anticholinergics, and antispasmodics) and why they are given. He also should be aware of symptoms that are reportable to his physician—jaundice, dark urine, pale-colored stools, pruritus, or signs of inflammation, such as pain or fever.

Some patients note a "looseness of the bowels," consisting of one to three bowel movements a day—the reason being a continual trickle of bile through the choledochoduodenal junction following cholecystectomy. Usually such frequency diminishes over a period of a few weeks to several months. Follow-up visits are essential for this patient.

BIBLIOGRAPHY

BOOKS

Conn, H. A., and Lieberthal, M. M.: The Hepatic Coma Syndromes and Lactulose. Baltimore, Md., Williams & Wilkins, 1979.

Koff, R. S.: Viral Hepatitis. New York, John Wiley & Sons, 1978.

Schiff, L.: Diseases of the Liver, 4th ed., Philadelphia, J. B. Lippincott, 1975.

ARTICLES

General

Altshuler, A., and Hilden, D.: The patient with portal hypertension. Nurs. Clin. N. Am., 12:317–329, June 1977.

Babb, R. B.: Diagnosing ascites. Postgrad. Med., 63:219–223, May 1978.

Bossone, M. C. M.: The liver: a pharmacologic perspective. Nurs. Clin. N. Am., 12:291–303, June 1977.

Boyer, C. A., and Oehlberg, S. M.: Interpretation and clinical relevance of liver function tests. Nurs. Clin. N. Am., 12:275–290, June 1977.

Byrne, J.: Liver function studies: Pt. 1, Introduction and bilirubin. Nursing '77, 7:12–14, July 1977; Pt. 2, Conjugation and excretion test. Nursing '77, 7:88–90, Sept. 1977; Pt. 3, Tests that measure protein metabolism. Nursing '77, 7:13, Oct. 1977; Pt. 4, Using metabolism tests to investigate liver function. Nursing '77, 7:14, Dec. 1977; Pt. 5, Using enzyme levels to assess liver function. Nursing '78, 8:50–52, Jan. 1978.

Daniel, E.: Chronic problems in rehabilitation of patients with Laennec's cirrhosis. Nurs. Clin. N. Am., 12:345–356, June 1977.

Kaplowitz, N.: Cholestatic liver disease. Hosp. Pract., 13:83–92, Aug. 1978.

Localio, S. A.: Partial hepatectomy for metastatic carcinoma. Hosp. Pract., 11:60–68, Mar. 1976.

O'Brien, K. A.: Cross circulation for hepatic coma. AJN, 77:1459–1462, Sept. 1977.

Ostrow, J. D.: Jaundice in older children and adults. JAMA, 234:522–526, Nov. 1975.

Pierce, L.: Anatomy and physiology of the liver, in relation to clinical assessment. Nurs. Clin. N. Am., 12:259–273, June 1977.

Shahinpour, N.: The adult patient with bleeding esophageal varices. Nurs. Clin. N. Am., 12:331–343, June 1977.

Wittes, R. E., and Yeh, S. D. J.: Indications for liver and brain scans. JAMA, 238:506–507, Aug. 1977.

Hepatitis

Aach, R. D.: Viral hepatitis—A to E. Med. Clin. N. Am., 62:59–70, Jan. 1978.

Acute and chronic hepatitis revisited (review by an international group). Lancet, 2:914–919, Oct. 1977.

Alter, H. J.: Transmission of hepatitis B virus infection by transfusion of frozen deglycerolized red blood cells. New Eng. J. Med., 298:637–642, Mar. 23, 1978.

Blumberg, B. S.: The hepatitis B virus—new routes for an old traveler. Mod. Med., 45:34–40, Sept. 1977.

_____: Hepatitis: the plight of the carrier. Sciences, 18:10–11, 30, Mar. 1978.

Czaja, A. J., and Summerskill, W. H. J.: Chronic hepatitis. Med. Clin. N. Am., 62:71–85, Jan. 1978.

Dienstag, J. L.: Viral hepatitis: how far we have come, where are we going? Drug Ther., 3:31–33, Sept. 1978.

Feinstone, S. M., et al.: Transfusion-associated hepatitis not due to viral hepatitis type A or B. New Eng. J. Med., *292*:767-770, Apr. 1975.

Hepatitis B immune globulin (Human). Med. Letter, *20*:9-10, Jan. 27, 1978.

Hollinger, F. B., and Graham, D. Y.: Viral hepatitis: Types A, B, and nonA/nonB. Drug Ther., *3*:39-55, Sept. 1978.

Krugman, S., and Gocke, D. J.: Viral hepatitis. *In* Major Problems in Internal Medicine, vol. 15. Philadelphia, W. B. Saunders, 1978.

McElroy, D. B.: Nursing care of patients with viral hepatitis. Nurs. Clin. N. Am., *12*:305-315, June 1977.

Reed, J. S., and Boyer, J. L.: Viral hepatitis: epidemiologic, serologic, and clinical manifestations. Disease-A-Month, *25*: no. 4, Jan. 1979.

Sherlock, S.: Diagnosis and treatment of chronic active hepatitis. Med. Times, *105*:83-97, Apr. 1977.

World Health Organization Expert Committee on Viral Hepatitis: Terminology of hepatitis viruses and antigens. Intervirology, *8*:65-67, 1977.

Bleeding Esophageal Varices

Resnick, R. H.: Portal hypertension: inching ahead therapeutically. Heart & Lung, *6*:789-798, Sept.-Oct. 1977.

Shahinpour, N.: The adult patient with bleeding esophageal varices. Nurs. Clin. N. Am., *12*:331-343, June 1977.

Cirrhosis of the Liver

Altshuler, A., and Hilden, D.: The patient with portal hypertension. Nurs. Clin. N. Am., *12*:317-327, June 1977.

Ansley, J. D., et al.: Effect of peritoneovenous shunting with the LeVeen valve on ascites, renal function, and coagulation in six patients with intractable ascites. Surg., *83*:181-187, Feb. 1978.

Babb, R. R.: Diagnosing ascites. Postgrad. Med., *63*:214-222, May 1978.

Daniel, E.: Chronic problems in rehabilitation of patients with Laennec's cirrhosis. Nurs. Clin. N. Am., *12*:345-357, June 1977.

Dolan, P. O., and Greene, H. L., II: Conquering cirrhosis of the liver. Nursing '76, *6*:44-53, Nov. 1976.

LeVeen, H. H., et al.: Peritoneo-venous shunting for ascites. Ann. Surg., *180*:580-591, Oct. 1974.

Luke, B.: Your role in dietary therapy of cirrhosis. RN, *40*:49-50, Oct. 1977.

Lund, R. H., and Newkirk, J. B.: Peritoneo-venous shunting system for surgical management of ascites. Contemp. Surg., *14*:31-45, Feb. 1979.

O'Brien, K. A.: Cross circulation for hepatic coma. AJN, *77*:1459-1462, Sept. 1977.

Seybert, P. L., et al.: The LeVeen shunt: new hope for ascites patients. Nursing '79, *9*:24-31, Jan. 1979.

Sherman, D. W., et al.: Realistic nursing goals in terminal cirrhosis. Nursing '78, *8*:43-46, June 1978.

Steigmann, F.: Preventing portal systemic encephalopathy in the patient with cirrhosis. Postgrad. Med., *65*:118-126, Feb. 1979.

Liver Tumors and Transplantation

Advances in organ transplantation. AORN J., *25*:1146-1148, May 1977.

Calne, R. Y.: Orthotopic liver transplantation. Contemp. Surg., *13*:21-36, Oct. 1978.

Increased risk of hepatocellular adenoma in women with long-term use of oral contraception. Center for Disease Control, Morbidity and Mortality Weekly Report, U.S. Dept. HEW, PHS, *26*:293-294, Sept. 9, 1977.

Liver transplants: a realistic option at last. Med. World News, *18*:25-37, July 11, 1977.

Mazzola, P.: Nursing care of the liver-transplant patient. RN. *39*:34-37, May 1976.

Gallbladder

Boston Collaborative Drug Surveillance Program: Surgically confirmed gallbladder disease, venous thromboembolisms, and breast tumors in relation to postmenopausal estrogen therapy. New Eng. J. Med., *290*:15-19, Jan. 3, 1974.

Coyne, M. J., et al.: Treatment of gallstones with chenodeoxycholic acid and phenobarbital. New Eng. J. Med., *292*:604-607, Mar. 20, 1975.

Freeman, J. B., and Olson, C. M.: Refinements in the detection of gallbladder disorders. Contemp. Surg., *13*:9-33, Nov. 1978.

Glenn, F.: Acute cholecystitis. Surg. Gynecol. Obstet., *143*:56-60, July 1976.

Hofmann, A. F., et al.: Chenotherapy for gallstone dissolution, induced changes in bile composition and gallstone response. JAMA, *239*:1038-1046, Mar. 20, 1978.

Hutcheon, D. F., et al.: Postcholecystectomy diarrhea, JAMA, *241*:823-824, Feb. 23, 1979.

McAvoy, J. M., et al.: Role of ultrasonography in the primary diagnosis of cholelithiasis. Am. J. Surg., *136*:309-312, Sept. 1978.

Pearlman, B. J., and Schoenfield, L. J.: Gallstones, the present and future of medical dissolution. Med. Clin. N. Am., *62*:87-105, Jan. 1978.

Thistle, J. L., et al.: Chenotherapy for gallstone dissolution, 1. Efficacy and safety. JAMA, *239*:1041-1046, Mar. 13, 1978.

———: Chenotherapy for gallstone dissolution, 2. Induced changes in bile composition and gallstone response. JAMA, *239*:1138-1144, Mar. 20, 1978.

Watts, J. M., et al.: The effect of added bran to the diet on the saturation of bile in people without gallstones. Am. J. Surg., *135*:321-324, Mar. 1978.

39

ASSESSMENT AND MANAGEMENT OF PATIENTS WITH DIABETES MELLITUS

Diabetes mellitus is a chronic multisystem disorder characterized by hyperglycemia (abnormally high levels of blood glucose), insulin insufficiency due to failure of the beta cells of the islets of Langerhans or inadequate action of insulin in peripheral tissues. In essence it is a disorder in the metabolism of carbohydrate, fat, and protein. The disease is associated with abnormalities in a variety of tissues and organs and with a number of acute and long-term complications.

TYPES OF DIABETES

There are several distinct and broadly different types of diabetes: (1) *insulin-dependent diabetes* (juvenile onset, ketosis prone), which usually has its onset during childhood, but may develop at all ages; (2) *non-insulin-dependent diabetes* (maturity onset) which generally develops after age 40, but can also be seen in the young; (3) *diabetes secondary to other conditions and syndromes,* such as pancreatic disease, endocrine disorders, or administration of certain drugs. These forms differ in their clinical course, management, and complications.

In patients with insulin-dependent diabetes, there is inevitably a relative or total lack of insulin, due to failure of beta-cell function. This type of diabetes is correlated with various degrees of cell-mediated and antibody-related autoimmunity (see Chap. 10). Insulin-dependent diabetes represents about 5 to 10 percent of all cases of diabetes, and these patients require exogenous insulin to maintain life.

In the patient with non-insulin-dependent diabetes, the beta-cell function can be substantially, but not totally, impaired. There may be a defect in insulin release from the beta cells or a resistance to the effect of insulin in the peripheral tissues such as muscle, liver, and adipose tissue. About 80 percent of these individuals are overweight. In overweight diabetics there appears to be a significant decrease in the sensitivity of peripheral tissues to insulin, and there is a need for increased amounts of insulin to maintain normal blood glucose levels.

In diabetes secondary to other conditions, the need for exogenous insulin varies according to whether the pancreatic beta cells are severely affected (as in pancreatic disease) or whether there is interference with the action of insulin.

ETIOLOGY AND INCIDENCE

The etiology of the disease is not completely understood, and there are probably multiple etiologies within each type, varying from patient to patient. It is felt that both genetic and environmental factors are involved. There is evidence that viruses may have the potential to cause insulin-dependent (juvenile) diabetes. Mumps and

---

PERSONS AT RISK FOR DIABETES MELLITUS

1. Persons with a family history of diabetes
2. Obese individuals
3. Mother delivered of large babies or those who have had an abnormal obstetrical history
4. Persons with early onset of arteriosclerosis
   (a) Premenopausal women with myocardial infarction
   (b) Men having myocardial infarctions before the age of 40
5. Persons with frequent or chronic infections (gallbladder disease, pyelonephritis, pancreatitis, etc.)
6. Patients exhibiting temporary reduction of glucose tolerance during stress (myocardial infarction, infection, trauma, surgery)
7. Patients developing glucose intolerance during drug therapy (thiazides, glucocorticoids, ovulatory suppressants)
8. Persons with retinopathy, nephropathy, neuropathy, or other vascular manifestations

---

Coxsackie viruses have been mentioned as triggering agents of diabetes in children. An altered immune response has been implicated, in view of the fact that anti-islet-cell antibodies have been demonstrated in the sera of newly diagnosed insulin-dependent diabetics. Other possible causes in some instances include: hypersecretion of hormones that antagonize insulin action, insulin-receptor abnormalities, and insulin resistance.

Diabetes mellitus is a long-term illness that afflicts about 5 percent of Americans, occurring with greater prevalence after the age of 45. It is the 5th leading cause of death in the United States and a major cause of blindness in adults. In general, diabetics have a shorter life span than persons in the general population.

Although there is a family history of diabetes in one-third of all diabetics, the mechanism of inheritance has not been satisfactorily explained. Nonetheless, blood relatives of known diabetics should maintain life-long vigilance for this condition. Other people susceptible to diabetes include obese persons and mothers who have delivered large babies. These people and other high-risk individuals (see chart) should be examined regularly for evidences of diabetes.

PATHOPHYSIOLOGY

Diabetes mellitus is a disease resulting from a breakdown in the body's ability to produce or utilize insulin. Insulin is a powerful hormone secreted by the beta cells in the islets of Langerhans of the pancreas. It plays a major role in the metabolic processes of the body by controlling the storage and metabolism of ingested metabolic fuels. Following a meal, the secretion of insulin facilitates the uptake, utilization, and storage of glucose, amino acids,

and fat. It promotes the storage of glycogen in the liver, the utilization of glucose in the muscles, and the storage of fat in adipose tissues, by enhancing the transport of glucose across the cell membrane. Insulin regulates the level of blood glucose, which is formed from ingested carbohydrates, or from the conversion of amino acids and fatty acids to glucose by the liver (gluconeogenesis).

In the well person the rate at which insulin is released from the pancreas is proportional to the amount of glucose in the blood. Normally the beta cells in the pancreas stimulate or withhold insulin secretion minute by minute, according to changing blood glucose levels. In diabetes, insulin is not secreted in proportion to blood glucose levels because of several possible factors: deficiency in the production of insulin by the beta cells; insensitivity of the insulin secretory mechanism of the beta cells; delayed or insufficient release of insulin; or excessive inactivation by chemical inhibitors or "binders" in the circulation.

An elevated fasting blood glucose level in diabetes reflects decreased uptake of glucose by the tissues or increased gluconeogenesis. If the concentration of glucose in the blood is sufficiently high, the kidney may not reabsorb all of the filtered glucose; the glucose then appears in the urine (glucosuria).

With increased gluconeogenesis (which is in part under the control of the adrenocortical hormones), protein and fats are mobilized, rather than stored or deposited in the cells. When there is deficiency of insulin, muscles cannot utilize glucose. Free fatty acids are then mobilized from adipose tissue cells and broken down by the liver into ketone bodies for energy. Diabetic ketoacidosis is characterized by excessive amounts of ketone bodies in the blood. Patients with diabetic ketoacidosis exhibit hyperventilation, and loss of sodium, potassium, chloride, and water from the body. The net metabolic result of severe diabetes mellitus is loss of fat stores, liver glycogen, cellular protein, electrolytes, and water. The sequelae of long-term diabetes involves the large vessels in the brain, heart, kidneys, and extremities, and the small vessels in the eyes and kidneys, and leads to neuropathy. The mechanism is not precisely determined.

CLINICAL MANIFESTATIONS AND COURSE

Insulin-dependent diabetes usually begins in childhood, but may occur at any age and is not uncommon in adults. Measurable circulating insulin may occur early in the course of the disease, but it soon disappears. In most instances the onset is abrupt, with weight loss, weakness, polyuria (excessive excretion of urine), polydipsia (excessive thirst), and polyphagia (excessive ingestion of food). As insulin production decreases, hyperglycemia develops, as a result of the body's inability to use glucose. Hyperglycemia exceeds the renal threshold of glucose due to an exhaustion of the renal reabsorptive capacity. Fluid loss through the kidneys results, producing losses of water, sodium, magnesium, calcium, potassium chloride, and phosphate. Because the body is not able to utilize ingested calories, body tissues are broken down to supply carbohydrate. An increased appetite is seen at first, but the hearty appetite may soon disappear as the metabolism becomes more unbalanced. Protein and lipid catabolism produce loss of weight and muscular wasting. The patient is prone to develop ketosis (elevated level of ketone bodies in body tissues and fluids). Often the diagnosis is first made when the patient is brought to the hospital in a coma, due to ketoacidosis. Insulin is always required, and control may be difficult because of wide fluctuations in blood glucose.

Non-insulin-dependent, or maturity-onset diabetes, usually occurs after the age of 40, but it can occur in younger persons who do not require insulin and who are not ketotic. The majority (about 80 percent) of these patients are overweight when the condition is first discovered. The symptoms may be so minor that the disorder goes undetected for many years and the discovery is made as the result of a routine urinalysis. Often blood glucose tests are normal, with hyperglycemia being seen only postprandially or as a result of a glucose tolerance test. Frequently the diabetes is discovered when the patient presents for treatment because of complications or associated conditions: deteriorating vision, pain in the legs, impotence, etc.

The onset is insidious. Fatigue, tendency to drowse after a meal, irritability, nocturia, itching of the skin (especially about the vulva in the female), skin wounds that heal poorly, blurring of vision, loss of weight, and cramps in the muscles are all warning symptoms of diabetes.

The intensity of diabetes mellitus, as measured by blood glucose, tends to wax and wane, and depends on the patient's general health, stresses of life, dietary intake, weight control, activity, and other factors. Treatment is variable throughout the course of the disease and requires constant adjustment if good results are to be obtained. Poorly controlled diabetes is followed by the accelerated development of neuropathy, retinopathy, and generalized atherosclerosis. Decreased resistance to infection and the presence of hyperglycemia are common. On the other hand, meticulous control of diabetes postpones, but does not prevent, the development of these complications.

DIAGNOSTIC ASSESSMENT

Blood Glucose Tests

POSTPRANDIAL TEST. The presence of sugar in the urine is a signal of diabetes and calls for an immediate blood glucose test, principally a postprandial (following a meal) blood glucose test and/or a glucose tolerance test. If the blood glucose is normal, the patient may have a low renal threshold for sugar or may have some other non-diabetic melituria. A postprandial blood glucose test requires that a blood sample be taken 2 hours after the patient has eaten a high carbohydrate (75-100 gm.) meal. Values over 150 mg. per dl. of blood are diagnostic of diabetes, and values under 100 mg. per dl. rule out diabetes. Between this range a glucose tolerance test should be done.

GLUCOSE TOLERANCE TEST. The oral *glucose tolerance test* is the most sensitive test for diabetes. The patient ingests a high carbohydrate diet (150–300 gm.) for 3 days preceding the test. After an overnight fast, a blood sample is drawn. Then a 75-gm. carbohydrate load, usually in the form of a carbonated sugar beverage (Glucola), is given to the patient. The patient is instructed to sit quietly during the test and to avoid exercise, tobacco, or any oral intake except water.

Blood samples are drawn at 1-, 2-, and 3-hour intervals after glucose ingestion. The following glucose tolerance curve is considered within the upper limits of normal:

SERUM GLUCOSE	TRUE BLOOD GLUCOSE
Fasting value 125 mg./dl.	110 mg./dl.
1-hour value of 190 mg./dl.	170 mg./dl.
2-hour value of 140 mg./dl.	120 mg./dl.
3-hour value of 125 mg./dl.	110 mg./dl.

Since advancing age alters the glucose tolerance curve, higher values are permissible in people over 50. Interpretation of these tests must take into account the possibility that preexisting diet, activity, and concurrent medications may cause variation. Laboratory values also may vary according to the methodology used.

STRIP TESTS. The *Dextrostix* test is a quick method for approximating blood glucose. A drop of blood applied to a reagent strip and washed after 60 seconds will give a blue color; if the test is carefully done, the depth of the color will be proportional to the glucose concentration. This test does not substitute for a reliable laboratory. However, it is useful for differentiating between hyperglycemia and hypoglycemic states and is used to follow the progress of a patient in coma.

Urine Testing for Glucose and Acetone

In normal urine, small traces of glucose are present, but not enough to be detected by ordinary tests. The presence of glucose in the urine depends on the serum or plasma glucose level and the renal threshold. When the blood glucose level is higher than the renal threshold for glucose, glucose will be spilled in the urine and can be detected by a variety of tests. In diabetes, glucose may appear in the urine when the blood glucose rises above 160-180 mg. per dl. Glucosuria may appear in the diagnosed diabetic when the patient is not following the prescribed diet, when treatment is inadequate, when the patient is not getting enough exercise, or when infection is present.

The most reliable test results are obtained when the second-voided specimen is used. The patient is instructed to void and discard the urine. It is discarded because it was excreted by the kidneys over a period of time and retained in the bladder, resulting in a possible mixture of glucose-containing urine and glucose-free urine.) After the first specimen has been voided and discarded, the patient waits about 15–45 minutes before voiding into a clean container. The second specimen will be urine *recently* produced by the kidneys and will accurately reflect the blood sugar level.

There are several methods of testing urine for glucose and ketones. False tests may be obtained if deteriorated reagent tablets or strips are used or if the directions are not followed accurately. Certain drugs taken by the patient can also produce false test results.

COPPER REDUCTION TESTS. The *Clinitest* method of testing urine incorporates the idea of copper reduction in detecting glucose. The reagent tablet contains copper sulfate, which will yield an orange color if glucose is present in the urine.

Two-drop method: This method allows for an estimated concentration of sugar up to 5 percent and is more accurate at higher glucose concentrations.

1. Hold dropper vertically and place 2 drops (0.1 ml.) of urine in test tube.
2. Rinse the dropper. Add 10 drops (0.5 ml.) of water in test tube.
3. Add 1 Clinitest reagent tablet. Do not shake test tube.
4. Wait 15 seconds after boiling stops.
5. Compare color of urine with appropriate color chart. Use only the 2-drop method color scale, which has 7 colors, ranging in value from 0–5 percent.

Five-drop method:

1. Hold dropper vertically and place 5 drops of urine in the test tube.
2. Rinse dropper. Add 10 drops of water in test tube.
3. Add 1 Clinitest tablet in test tube.
   a. Watch while reaction takes place. Do not shake test tube during reaction or for 15 seconds after boiling inside test tube has stopped.
   b. Observe the solution in the test tube *while the reaction takes place and during the 15-second waiting period to detect pass-through color changes caused by glucosuria over 2 percent.*
      (1) If the solution passes through orange and dark shades of green-brown, it indicates that more than 2 percent (4+) urine sugar is present.
      (2) Record as such without reference to color scale.
4. After 15-second waiting period, shake test tube gently and compare with the color scale. Record the results.

ENZYME METHODS. The *Test-Tape, Clinistix,* and *Diastix* are enzyme-impregnated tapes/strips that are dip methods for testing the urine for glucose. The tape or strip is merely moistened with urine and subsequently indicates the presence or absence of glucose. The color on the tape/strip is compared to the closest matching color block on the color chart of the product being used.

Urine Tests for Ketone Bodies

Ketones in the urine signal that diabetic control is deteriorating and that the body has started to break down stored fat for energy. Mobilization of fat results in acetonemia and acetonuria and can be detected by testing the urine for acetone. Tests for ketone bodies are done when there is persistent glucosuria and/or the patient is not feeling well.

There are two tests that can be done by the patient to determine the presence of acetone (ketone bodies) in the urine. The *Acetest* uses a chemical reagent which reacts with ketone bodies in the urine to yield a colored product; the depth of color is roughly correlated to the ketone-body concentration.

The *Ketostix* test uses a reagent strip which is dipped in the urine. After the time specified on the product information sheet, a lavender color appears if the urine contains ketones. The depth of color is compared with the color chart.

Keto-Diastix is a combined reagent strip designed for the determination of ketones and glucose in urine.

MANAGEMENT

The objectives of management are to help the patient to live a comfortable and useful life and to attain and maintain optimal body weight, to correct biochemical and metabolic abnormalities, to prevent the progression of disease and complications, and to promote patient education.

Ideally, the well-controlled patient is (1) free of diabetic symptoms; (2) has normoglycemia, without episodes of hypoglycemia or hyperglycemia; (3) maintains optimum weight and, (4) has little or no glucosuria.

Management is based on dietary control, hypoglycemic agents, exercise, and patient education. Specific treatment depends on the type of diabetes being treated.

DIETARY SUPPORT IN DIABETES MELLITUS

Diet and weight control constitute the foundation of diabetic management. The basic nutritional requirements of the individual patient are satisfied by a diet that contains all of the essential food constituents and supplies enough calories to promote optimal body growth and maintenance of body weight.

The meals should be measured and spaced at regular intervals. The menu is varied, with emphasis placed on what the patient is allowed rather than on what is forbidden, as well as taking into consideration the patient's ethnic and cultural background in the daily selection of food.

Obesity is corrected as rapidly as possible, since obese people are more resistant to both endogenous and exogenous insulin. Many patients who are overweight may achieve normoglycemia through weight loss alone.

The first step in preparing the meal plan is to determine the patient's basic calorie requirements, taking into consideration age, sex, body weight, and degree of activity. There are several methods of assessing calorie needs. A simple method, for instance, in most weight-maintenance diets, is to multiply ideal weight by 30–35 cal./kg. For weight reduction, a 15–20 cal./kg. ideal weight is suitable. Long-term reduction diets can be achieved with caloric levels between 1,000 and 1,200 calories, for most people. The calorie requirement can be raised when the patient achieves the desired level.

The most important objective in dietary treatment of diabetic patients is control of total calorie intake to attain or maintain ideal weight. Success of this measure alone is often associated with reversal of the glucose intolerance. In the instance of a young, underweight patient with insulin-dependent diabetes, priority should be given to providing a diet with enough calories to maintain normal growth and development.

While sources of calories are also to be taken into consideration, there is less emphasis now upon strict carbohydrate control than in past years. This provides greater flexibility in diet and improves the ability of patients to adhere to an effective program of calorie restriction. Special consideration is also given to the fat content of diabetic diets. The Nutrition Committee of the American Diabetes Association issued a statement in 1971 pointing to the disadvantages of standard diabetic diets that are high in fat. Epidemiological evidence has been cited suggesting the favorable effects of high-starch, low-fat diabetic diets on both serum triglyceride levels and vascular disease.

The most preferred caloric distribution at present is as follows: 50 percent of calories deriving from carbohydrates, 30 percent from fat, and the remaining 20 percent from protein, for all caloric levels. Table 39-1 indicates the grams of carbohydrate, fat, and protein at various caloric levels, based on this distribution of calories. (A suggested meal distribution pattern for non-insulin-dependent diabetics, based on Table 39-1, is shown in Table 39-2.) Within the established calorie distribution, carbohydrates should be taken in the form of polysaccharides (complex sugars); this type of carbohydrate also contains fiber and pectins, from vegetables and fruits. Approximately 15 to 20 percent of the carbohydrate should also be derived from disaccharides and monosaccharides in the form of lactose and fructose, from foods such as milk and fruits, respectively. This type of carbohydrate seems to be more beneficial for the reduction of glucosuria, as indicated by the studies of Jenkins and others. The increase of carbohydrate has been made at the expense of fat, which is presently set at a level of 30 percent of caloric intake. The lowering of the proportion of dietary fat may

TABLE 39-1. GRAMS OF CARBOHYDRATE, FAT, AND PROTEIN OF DIABETIC DIETS BASED ON 50% CARBOHYDRATE, 30% FAT, 20% PROTEIN, AT SELECTED CALORIC LEVELS

FOODSTUFF	1,000-CALORIE DIET	1,200-CALORIE DIET	1,400-CALORIE DIET	1,600-CALORIE DIET	1,800-CALORIE DIET
Carbohydrate gm.	125	150	175	200	225
Fat gm.	33	43	47	53	60
Protein gm.	50	60	70	80	90

reduce factors predisposing to the development of coronary heart disease, the most important cause of death and debility in the diabetic. The protein level of 20 percent of calories is considered high, as compared to the 12 percent level in the customary American diet.

Adapting dietary therapy to specific needs of individual patients on the basis of diagnostic tests is essential. If, for instance, a diabetic patient is found to have Type IV hyperlipoproteinemia, a lower carbohydrate intake would be beneficial in controlling this type of lipid abnormality. Patients with high levels of triglycerides, however, will benefit from a lowered fat intake (less than 30 percent of the diet). Diabetics with high cholesterol levels may require even greater reductions of dietary cholesterol and saturated fat. Guidelines for the treatment of hyperlipoproteinemias in diabetes are available.

The 1976 revision of the "Exchange Lists for Meal Planning" reflects the most current thinking in the area of nutrition education. Many revisions and additions have been made to the Exchange Lists, based on concern for total caloric intake and modifications of fat and carbohydrate in the diet.

List 1   *Milk exchanges:* now include nonfat, low-fat, and whole milk.

List 2   *Vegetable exchanges:* includes all vegetables except starchy vegetables. Vegetables on list 2 average 25 calories per one-half cup serving. Starchy vegetables appear in the bread exchange.

List 3   *Fruit exchanges:* remain the same as in the old edition.

List 4   *Bread exchange:* has been expanded to include a wider variety of prepared foods. Those appearing in bold type are of low fat content.

List 5   *Meat exchanges:* include not only lean meat, but also medium-fat and high-fat meats, and other protein-rich foods.

List 6   *Fat exchanges:* have been revised to show differences in the kind of fat contained in them: saturated or polyunsaturated. Saturated fat has been associated with an increase in blood cholesterol (a possible risk factor in coronary heart disease). The physician may advise a reduction of foods high in this kind of fat. Polyunsaturated fat has been associated with a decrease in blood cholesterol. The physician may advise substituting foods containing this kind of fat whenever possible. A system of bold type is used in the booklet to indicate the low-fat concept.

Each list contains additional information on the vitamin and mineral content of the foods listed. The following foods should not be included in the meal plan without the permission of the diet counselor:

sugar, candy, honey, jam, jelly, cookies, syrup, condensed milk, chewing gum, soft drinks, pies, and cakes

The patient should become acquainted with foods which are advertized and labeled as "dietetic," "sugar free," and "fat free." The patient should also be counseled as to the use of alcoholic beverages and sugar substitutes.

The details of these exchange lists are widely available in hospitals, diet manuals, and books on nutrition and diabetes. Several cookbooks for diabetes are available and contain recipes which yield food portions with defined amounts of carbohydrate, fat, and protein, translated into food exchanges per portion.

To be practical and effective, a dietary program must be based on appropriate patient motivation coupled with careful dietary instruction and follow-up.

A number of sources of information show food exchanges. The H. J. Heinz Co. and the Campbell Soup Company have published lists showing the composition of their soups in terms of food exchanges. Kaufman has published a useful guide giving the amount of cholesterol and carbohydrate in various brand names. Books such as the one by Kay give a short review of the subject of diabetes and nutrition, with emphasis on recent progress in understanding the general principles, rather than details of clinical dietetics.

The nurse plays an important role in reinforcing the patient's knowledge and understanding of the importance of diet in diabetes, and the more effective use of the exchange lists. The effect of this counseling is to motivate the patient to follow the prescribed dietary regimen.

TABLE 39-2.   SUGGESTED MENU PATTERN FOR NON-INSULIN-DEPENDENT PATIENTS

	1,000-CALORIE DIET	1,200-CALORIE DIET	1,400-CALORIE DIET	1,600-CALORIE DIET	1,800-CALORIE DIET
Breakfast					
Fruit	1 serving	1 serving	1 serving	1 serving	2 servings
Egg	—	—	1 medium	1 medium	1 medium
Toast	—	—	2 slices	2 slices	2 slices
Cereal	1 serving	1 serving	—	—	—
Fat	1 teaspoon	1 teaspoon	2 teaspoons	2 teaspoons	2 teaspoons
Milk	1 cup	1 cup	1 cup	1 cup	1 cup
Beverage	1 cup	1 cup	1 cup	1 cup	1 cup
*Snack**				1 bread	1 fruit
Noon Meal					
Meat (lean)	2 ounces	2 ounces	2 ounces	2 ounces	2 ounces
Vegetable	—	—	—	1 serving	1 serving
Salad	As desired	As desired	As desired	As desired	As desired
Bread	2 slices	2 slices	2 slices	2 slices	2 slices
Fat	1 teaspoon	1 teaspoon	1 teaspoon	1 teaspoon	2 teaspoons
Fruit	1 fruit	1 serving	1 serving	1 fruit	1 fruit
Milk	1 cup	1 cup	1 cup	1 cup	1 cup
Beverage†	1 cup	1 cup	1 cup	1 cup	1 cup
*Snack**			1 fruit	1 fruit	1 fruit
Evening Meal					
Meat (lean)	2 ounces	3 ounces	3 ounces	4 ounces	5 ounces
Potato	1 serving	1 medium	1 serving	1 serving	1 serving
Vegetable	1 serving	1 serving	1 serving	1 serving	1 serving
Salad	1 serving	1 serving	1 serving	1 serving	1 serving
Bread	—	1 slice	1 slice	1 slice	2 slices
Fat	2 teaspoons	3 teaspoons	3 teaspoons	3 teaspoons	2 teaspoons
Fruit	1 serving	1 serving	1 serving	1 fruit	1 fruit
Milk	—	—	—	—	—
Beverage†	1 cup	1 cup	1 cup	1 cup	1 cup
*Snack**			1 fruit	1 fruit	1 fruit
					1 bread

*For insulin-dependent patients, certain food items can be used for between-meal snacks, taking into consideration the type of insulin the patient is receiving.
†Optional and noncaloric.

EXERCISE

Exercise is very important in managing the patient with diabetes, because it promotes metabolism and the utilization of carbohydrates and enhances the action of insulin, thereby reducing the insulin requirements of the body. There should be a regular pattern of exercise, done daily, which will improve the control of diabetes and the general well-being of the patient.

Insulin-treated patients may have a tendency to hypoglycemia during exercise, since exercise lowers the blood sugar. The insulin-treated patient should eat a rapidly absorbed carbohydrate in anticipation of increased physical exertion, and at intervals during an extended period of physical exercise. Extra food is required for extra activity, and this is not deducted from the regular diet.

INSULIN THERAPY

As stated earlier, insulin is secreted by the beta cells of the islets of Langerhans and works to lower the blood glucose by facilitating the uptake and utilization of glucose by muscle and fat cells and by decreasing the release of glucose from the liver. Since insulin is necessary for the normal metabolism of fat and protein, a lack of insulin causes a breakdown of these stores.

When the patient's body fails to produce enough insulin, and when diet cannot control the diabetes, then insulin must be administered. One or more insulin injections each day are usually taken by persons with insulin-dependent diabetes as well as by those with diabetes that is characterized by polydipsia, polyuria, weight loss, and ketonuria.

Not all diabetics require insulin. Obese diabetics who are not dependent on insulin injections and who have no complications, few symptoms, and no ketonuria, can usually control their diabetes by means of caloric restriction. However, these same patients, who are usually controlled by diet alone or by diet and an oral hypoglycemic agent, may require insulin during illness, infection, pregnancy, surgery, or during some other stressful event.

Insulin is extracted from both beef and pork pancreases obtained from animals going to slaughter. There are a number of insulin preparations available, each of which varies in onset of action, time of peak or maximum effect, and duration or length of action (see Table 39-3). These preparations are classified into three groups: (1) short-acting insulin (Regular or Semilente insulin); (2) intermediate-acting insulin (Globin, Isophane (NPH), and Lente) and (3) long-acting insulin (Protamine Zinc Insulin and Ultralente). In some patients, combinations of short-acting and an intermediate insulin are given to minimize the number of injections needed to maintain metabolic control. Other combinations are also used.

Insulin (which is prescribed in units) is available in three concentrations (strengths) which correspond to the number of units of insulin per milliliter of solution: U-40 (40 units per ml.), U-80 (80 units per ml.), and U-100 (100 units per ml.). In the United States, the aim is to have only one strength, U-100, available in all varieties of insulin. The insulin syringe must correlate with the strength of insulin used. For example, U-100 insulin is given with a U-100 syringe.

Regulation of Dosage

The dosage of insulin is adjusted according to the presence (or absence) of glucosuria, the degree to which glucosuria is present, and the time when glucosuria appears in relation to insulin administration and meals. Meals are distributed to conform to insulin peaks and the exercise patterns of the patient. Insulin curves vary from patient to patient, and the response of individual patients may be highly variable.

In the absence of complications, treatment may be started with 10 to 20 units of intermediate-acting insulin, given subcutaneously before breakfast. This dosage is increased gradually, as indicated by the patient's response to the previous dose, until glucosuria is absent and the blood glucose before each meal is not excessively elevated. If the diabetes is obviously severe, larger doses are employed at the onset. The meals must coincide with the action of the insulin. During initial regulation, and when insulin requirements are changing rapidly (during an acute illness), it is common practice to give supplemental injections of regular insulin before each meal, depending upon the results of a recent urine test and the previous response of the patient. If hypoglycemia occurs, the dose of insulin that had reached its peak at this time is reduced, or the diet is increased.

There is a narrow margin between the therapeutic and toxic (hypoglycemic) effects of insulin. It is important that the patient and the nurse know when hypoglycemia is most likely to occur with each type of insulin (Table 39-3). The patient is instructed to test his urine for sugar before each meal and at bedtime while insulin is being regulated or during periods of illness (see page 835). The patient keeps a record of the results in a notebook and takes it to the physician or clinic with each visit so that insulin adjustments can be made.

RESEARCH DEVELOPMENTS FOR INSULIN DELIVERY. Although the goal of treatment is to achieve levels of blood glucose as close as possible to those in the non-diabetic, this goal is very difficult to achieve in some patients who have significant levels of hyperglycemia, even with multiple insulin injections. Research is being conducted to find a more physiologic insulin-delivery system. Methods of insulin delivery under investigation include the implantation of insulin-producing islet tissue into the patient by dispersing it into the abdominal cavity

TABLE 39-3. INSULIN PREPARATIONS COMMERCIALLY AVAILABLE IN THE
UNITED STATES, CLASSIFIED ACCORDING TO APPROXIMATE DURATION OF ACTION

CLASSIFICATION	INSULIN PREPARATION*	ACTION		
		Onset	*Peak*	*Duration*
Rapid	Regular (neutral)	IV:† immediate	15-30 min.	1-2 hr.
		IM: 5-30 min.	30-60 min.	2-4 hr.
		SC: 30 min.	1-2 hr.	5-10 hr.
	Semilente (insulin zinc suspension prompt)	SC: 1 hr.	3-4 hr.	10-16 hr.
Intermediate	Globin zinc insulin	SC: 2 hr.	6-8 hr.	12-18 hr.
	NPH (isophane insulin suspension)	SC: 2 hr.	8-14 hr.	18-24 hr.
	Lente (insulin zinc suspension)	SC: 2 hr.	8-14 hr.	18-24 hr.
Slow	Protamine zinc insulin suspension	SC: 6 hr.	16-20 hr.	24-30 hr.
	Ultralente (insulin zinc suspension extended)	SC: 6 hr.	18-29 hr.	30-36 hr.
Combinations	Regular + NPH	SC: 30 min.	2-10 hr.	18-24 hr.
	Regular + Lente	SC: 1 hr.	2-10 hr.	18-24 hr.
	Semilente + Lente	SC: 1 hr.	4-10 hr.	18-24 hr.
	Semilente + Ultralente	SC: 1 hr.	2-24 hr.	30-36 hr.

*Preparations are available in concentrations of 40, 80, and 100 units/ml. in 10-ml. vials. Regular (concentrated) Iletin is also available in a concentration of 500 units/ml. in 20-ml. vials. Regular, NPH, and Lente insulins are available as beef-pork insulin mixtures and as special monospecies insulins made exclusively from beef or pork pancreas.
†IV, IM, and SC denote intravenous, intramuscular, and subcutaneous routes of administration.
(From Owen, O. E., Boden, G., and Shuman, C. R.: Managing insulin-dependent diabetic patients. Postgrad. Med., 59:128, Jan. 1976. Copyright, McGraw-Hill, Inc.)

or infusing it into the portal vein. Work also is being done on the development of a miniaturized implantable mechanical device (resembling a cardiac pacemaker) that will monitor blood glucose and release either insulin or glucose from reservoirs as needed. An artificial beta cell has been developed as a research tool, consisting of an on-line glucose analyzer. A built-in microcomputer for calculation and control of insulin or dextrose infusions; a multichannel infusion system; and a print-out recorder, showing on a minute-by-minute basis the glucose value measured, the insulin and/or dextrose rate, and the cumulative total of insulin given have also been developed.

Patient Teaching for Self-injection of Insulin

As soon as the need for insulin has been established, the patient should be instructed in the technique of self-injection. He should be persuaded to give his own injection as soon as possible. An optimistic but firm approach will offer the patient encouragement.

- The technique of filling the syringe is demonstrated to the patient, and the skin is wiped with alcohol.
- The patient is instructed to pull the skin taut on the anterior surface of the thigh or (if the patient is thin) to form a skin fold by picking up subcutaneous tissue between the thumb and forefinger. Either of these techniques ensures that the needle tip is inserted into subcutaneous tissue and outside the mus-

cle. The skin should not be pressed tightly together between the fingers, since this is a cause of local induration.

- The patient is assisted to insert the needle with a quick thrust into deep subcutaneous tissue (Fig. 39-1).
- The patient then pulls back slightly on the plunger of the syringe to assure that the needle is not in a blood vessel before the insulin is injected.
- After injecting the insulin, the patient holds the alcohol sponge against the needle, while gently withdrawing it, to prevent painful pulling of the skin while the needle is withdrawn.
- The syringe, barrel, plunger, and needle are rinsed under cold running water.

Rotation of Sites

The patient is then taught the technique for injecting insulin into the arm (Fig. 39-1). Systematic rotation of injection sites (Fig. 39-2) is necessary to prevent scar tissue from forming, to allow uniform absorption of insulin, and to keep the skin supple. To assure a definite rotation schedule, the patient should keep a record of each injection site. Areas with loose skin and a sufficient amount of subcutaneous fat are sites suitable for insulin injection; i.e., lateral surface of arms, anterior aspect of the thighs, anterior and lateral aspects of the abdominal wall, and lateral areas of the back, just above the buttock. Each injection should be separated from the previous injection by approximately 2.5 cm. (1 inch), and each site should be used no oftener than every 3 weeks.

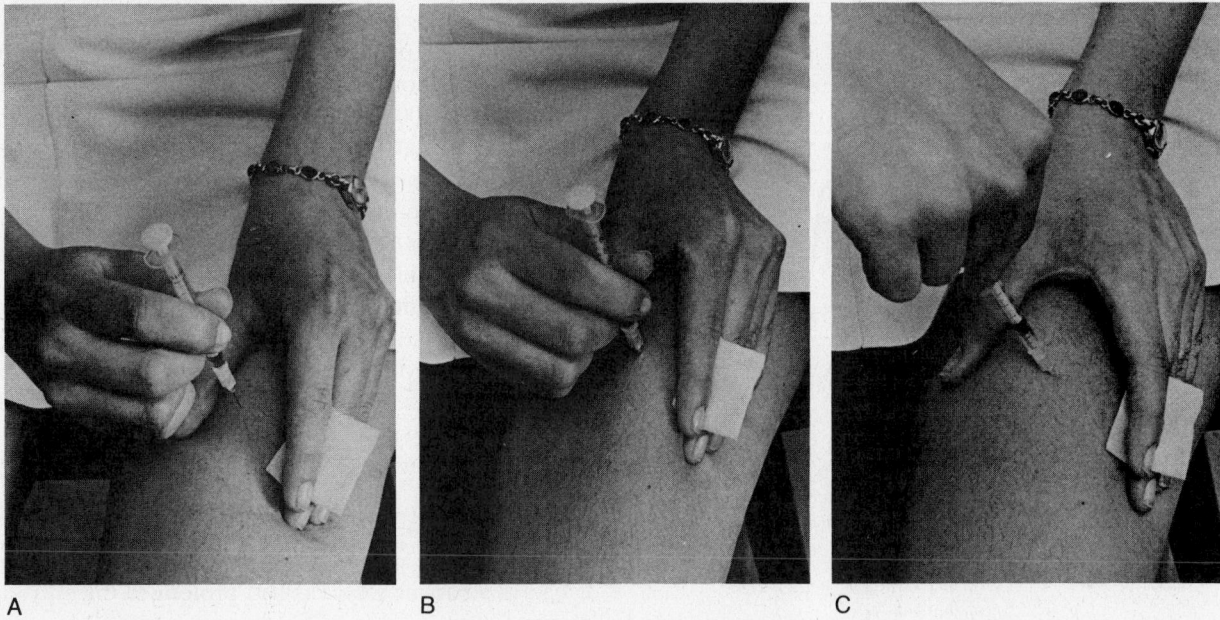

A   B   C

Figure 39-1.   (*Top*) Self-injection of insulin. (*A*) The insulin syringe is held perpendicular to the stretched skin before the needle is thrust into the subcutaneous tissues. (*B*) Alternate method: If the patient only has a thin layer of subcutaneous fat, a fold of skin is pinched between the fingers to keep the needle from penetrating into the muscle. (*C*) The patient pulls back slightly on the plunger before the insulin is injected. (*Bottom*) Self-injection of insulin into the arm. (*Left*) After cleansing the site, press down on the arm with the outer edge of the hand to stretch the skin. (*Right*) Alternate method: stabilize the arm against a wall and quickly insert the needle. Move the arm away from the wall to release the pressure before depressing the plunger to inject the insulin.

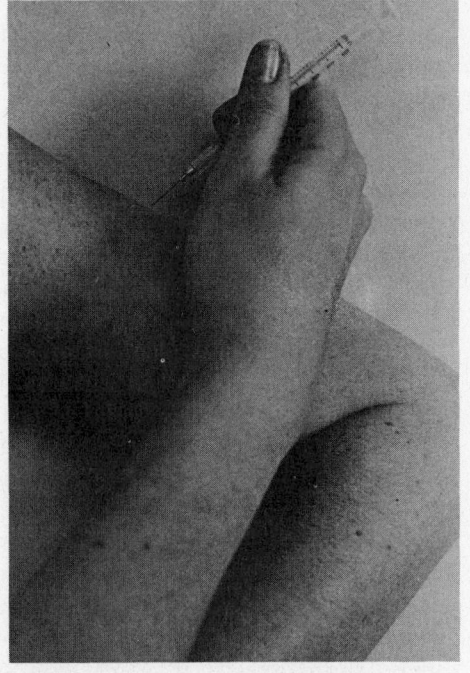 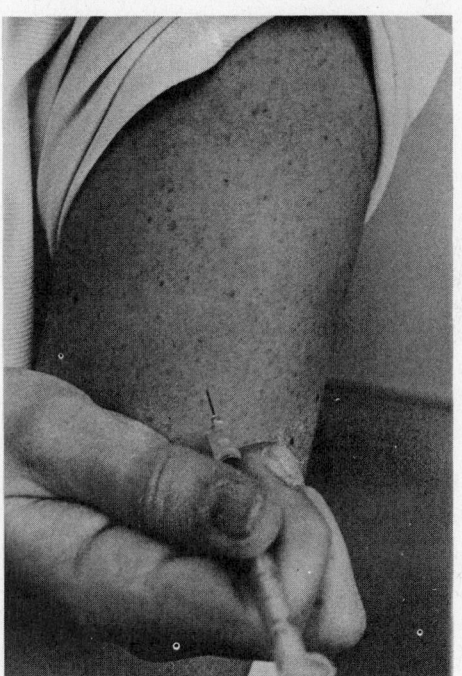

Care of Equipment

After the patient has mastered the technique of injection, he is taught to care for the equipment. To sterilize the glass syringe, the syringe is taken apart and placed in a medium-sized strainer, which is then placed in a saucepan covered by 5 cm. (2 inches) of water and boiled for ten minutes. Then the strainer is picked up, while the water is poured out of the pan. The strainer is placed back in the empty pan to allow the syringe to cool, and the syringe is then reassembled.

Patients who are physically frail or incapacitated, or

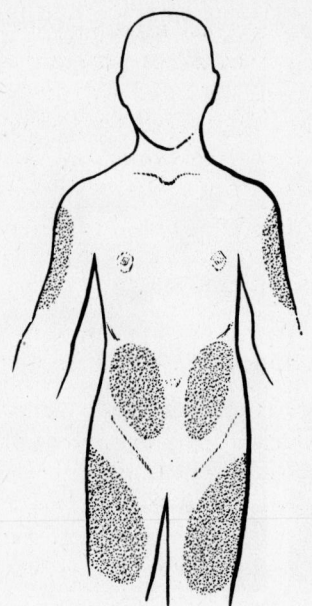

Figure 39-2. Sites for insulin injection. Absorption from arm sites is more rapid than from the thighs.

who suffer from tremors and visual difficulties, are unable to boil the syringe. They can be taught to immerse the syringe with needle attached in a 4-ounce bottle of alcohol with cotton at the bottom to protect the needle. (Ninety-one percent alcohol will not leave residue in barrel of syringe and does not cause rusting of the needle.) Before the syringe is loaded, all traces of alcohol are removed by pushing the plunger back and forth, as alcohol may alter the effect of insulin and is also irritating when introduced under the skin. The syringe and needle should be boiled at least one time weekly.

Disposable syringes are ideal, but rather costly. Insulin syringes that can be set for a predetermined dose are also available for patients with impaired vision. Not only the patient himself, but a member of the patient's family should also be instructed in insulin administration.

Reactions to Insulin

LOCAL REACTION.   A local reaction in the form of redness, swelling, tenderness and induration, or a wheal may appear at the site of injection. These reactions usually occur during the beginning stages of therapy and disappear with continued use of insulin. However, if local reactions persist, a pure strain of insulin (such as pure beef insulin) may be tried. The physician may prescribe an antihistamine to be taken one hour before the injection.

INSULIN LIPODYSTROPHY.   *Lipodystrophy* refers to a disturbance of fat metabolism, in the form of either lipoatrophy or lipohypertrophy. These reactions occur at the site of injection and may appear separately, in combination, or in succession, in the same patient. *Insulin-induced atrophy* is loss of subcutaneous fat and appears as slight dimpling or more serious pitting of subcutaneous fat. It occurs more commonly in women and children. The use of U-100 insulin, which is 99 percent pure, has almost eliminated this disfiguring complication. Lipoatrophy is sometimes treated by injection of a single-peak insulin into the periphery of the lipoatrophic area.

Lipohypertrophy is the development of fibrofatty masses at the injection site and occurs more often in children and adult men. It is caused by the prolonged use of the same injection site. If insulin is injected into scarred areas, the absorption is irregular and the action of the insulin unpredictable. This is one reason why the rotation of injection sites is so important. The patient should avoid injecting insulin into these areas until the hypertrophy disappears.

INSULIN EDEMA.   A generalized retention of fluid is sometimes seen after diabetic control is suddenly established in a patient who has had prolonged uncontrolled diabetes.

INSULIN RESISTANCE.   This term is applied to those patients who require in excess of 200 units of insulin per day to achieve normoglycemia. It may be due to the development of insulin antibodies, or it can be caused by infection.

SYSTEMIC ALLERGIC REACTIONS to insulin range from hives to angioedema and anaphylaxis. The treatment is desensitization, with small volumes of insulin given as desensitizing doses.

Hypoglycemic Reactions

Hypoglycemia (abnormally low blood glucose level) occurs when the blood glucose falls below 50 mg. per dl. It can be caused by too much insulin, too little food, or excessive physical activity. Hypoglycemia may occur 1 to 3 hours after regular insulin, 4 to 18 hours after NPH or Lente insulin, and 18 to 30 hours after protamine zinc or ultralente insulin. Most episodes occur before meals, but they may occur at any time of the day or night.

When the blood glucose falls rapidly, the sympathetic nervous system is stimulated to produce adrenalin, causing sweating, tremor, tachycardia, palpitation, and nervousness. When the blood glucose falls slowly, there is depression of the central nervous system, resulting in headache, light-headedness, confusion, emotional changes, memory lapses, numbness of the lips and tongue, slurred speech, incoordination, staggering gait, double vision, drowsiness, convulsions, and eventually, coma. Since the brain depends upon glucose for its energy supply, as hypoglycemia progresses, brain function deteriorates. Permanent central nervous system damage may result from prolonged hypoglycemia. In addition, renal insufficiency may develop from decreased renal gluconeogenesis, decreased renal insulinase, and diminished renal clearance.

The combination of symptoms varies considerably in different patients, and in the same patient at different times.

- Every patient taking insulin should be familiar with the warning symptoms so that he can take sugar promptly.
- Any abnormal behavior in a patient taking insulin should be considered to be hypoglycemia until proven otherwise.
- Hypoglycemia must be treated promptly, because sustained hypoglycemia can lead to convulsions and/or coma and death. When the first warning symptoms appear, the patient should take some form of simple, fast-acting sugar orally: orange juice, sugar, hard candy (Lifesavers), or a soft drink. If the symptoms persist for 10–15 minutes, the snack should be repeated.
- Every patient taking insulin should always carry a candy bar, a few lumps of sugar, or a tube of glucose jelly for the prompt relief of hypoglycemia.

If the patient is unconscious and unable to swallow, glucagon hydrochloride is administered subcutaneously or intramuscularly. This hormone, which is made in the alpha cells of the pancreas, causes glycogenolysis in the liver (if hepatic glycogen stores are not depleted). Glucagon raises the blood glucose high enough for most patients to wake up and take orange juice or ginger ale by mouth. This additional "sugar" intake is important, because the elevation of blood glucose following glucagon administration is only temporary, and a hypoglycemia relapse is a real and constant danger. Glucagon is packaged in 1-mg. vials and given in the same manner as insulin. It is useful in patients who receive little or no warning of their attacks and go into coma.

If the patient cannot swallow, the intravenous administration of 50 ml. of 50 percent glucose in water is the most effective treatment for hypoglycemia and is used when it is available or when glucagon is ineffective.

SOMOGYI PHENOMENON. The Somogyi phenomenon is a paradoxical situation in which sudden falls in blood sugar are followed by rebound hyperglycemia. This situation is usually caused by gradual excessive administration of insulin. The underlying mechanism is that the hormonal responses to hypoglycemia counteract the effect of insulin. The patient's condition becomes uncontrollable, because the effect of the administered insulin is antagonized. The situation remains out of control when more insulin is given, and the patient has periods of hyperglycemia interspersed with hypoglycemia. One is alerted to this possibility when there are symptoms of hypoglycemia (irritability, confusion, etc.), with urine tests showing frequent glucosuria. The treatment consists of gradually lowering the amount of insulin until the appropriate dosage is reached.

PREVENTION AND PATIENT EDUCATION. Hypoglycemia is prevented by following a regular pattern and timetable for eating, administering insulin, and engaging in daily exercise. Between-meals and bedtime snacks are often

needed to counteract the maximum insulin effect. In general, the patient should cover the time of peak activity of insulin by eating a snack and by taking additional food when engaging in an increased level of physical activity. Routine urine tests are performed so that changing insulin requirements may be anticipated.

Because unexpected coma may occur, any patient treated with insulin should wear an identification bracelet or card indicating that he is a diabetic.

ORAL HYPOGLYCEMIC AGENTS

Oral hypoglycemic agents may be effective for selected, stable, non-insulin-dependent, nonketotic diabetics who cannot be treated by diet alone or who otherwise require small doses of insulin or are unable or unwilling to take insulin. These drugs may be useful for the aged, those with poor vision, crippling arthritis of the fingers, and tremor of the hands, and for those who for some reason refuse to take insulin. (Insulin is preferable to oral hypoglycemic agents if dietary treatment fails to control diabetes.)

In the United States, the available oral hypoglycemic agents are the sulfonylureas (tolbutamide, chlorpropamide, acetohexamide, and tolazamide). They are thought to exert their primary action by direct stimulation of pancreatic insulin secretion. Therefore, a functioning pancreas is necessary for these drugs to be effective, and they cannot be used in the treatment of patients who are insulin-dependent and ketosis-prone. The sulfonylureas can be divided into short-, intermediate-, and long-acting agents with varying duration of action (Table 39-4). Side effects of these drugs are relatively rare and include hematologic, hepatic, and dermatologic reactions. Hypoglycemia may occur when an excessive dose of a sulfonylurea is used. The sulfonylureas also interact with various drugs: sulfonamides, salicylates, phenylbutazones, barbiturates, thiazides, alcohol, catecholamines, etc.

For successful treatment with oral agents, the diet must be restricted in total calories and carbohydrates, and the patient's urine and blood glucose values monitored.

TABLE 39-4. CHARACTERISTICS OF SULFONYLUREA COMPOUNDS

AGENT	DURATION OF ACTION (HRS.)	HOW GIVEN
Tolbutamide (Orinase)	6–10 hrs. (short)	Divided doses
Chlorpropamide (Diabinese)	20–60 hrs. (prolonged)	Single dose
Acetohexamide (Dymelor)	8–12 hrs. (medium)	Single or divided doses
Tolazamide (Tolinase)	8–12 hrs. (medium)	Single or divided doses

- Oral hypoglycemic drugs must be abandoned in favor of insulin if the patient develops an infection with fever, suffers trauma, or undergoes major surgery.

If, as time goes on, the patient's urine tests and blood glucose values are no longer responsive to oral hypoglycemic therapy, the patient is then treated with insulin.

A study by the University Group Diabetes Program has given rise to many questions concerning the safety and effectiveness of long-term oral hypoglycemic agents. This study group found a higher death rate from heart disease in their tolbutamide-treated patients than in those treated with a placebo. However, since the tolbutamide-treated patients were older and had more baseline cardiac disease than did the control patients, the conclusions may not be justified.

ACUTE COMPLICATIONS OF DIABETES

There are three conditions that can produce coma in the diabetic: hypoglycemia (as discussed earlier), diabetic ketoacidosis, and hyperosmolar coma.

DIABETIC KETOACIDOSIS AND COMA

Diabetic ketoacidosis is due to an absence or inadequate amount of insulin, which results in hyperglycemia and leads to a series of biochemical disorders. The pathophysiology is the result of insulin deficiency affecting many aspects of the metabolism of carbohydrate, protein, and fat. As a result, the amount of glucose entering the cells is reduced, and fat is metabolized instead of carbohydrate. Free fatty acids are mobilized from adipose tissue. Liver oxidases act upon these fatty acids to produce ketone bodies. The ketone bodies escape into the blood, and metabolic acidosis results, with lowering of serum bicarbonate, PCO_2, and pH. The overall clinical picture is one of hyperglycemia, water and electrolyte loss, acidemia, and coma.

Causes. Ketoacidosis may be precipitated by failure to take insulin, by insufficient insulin intake, or by resistance to insulin. It may be caused by infection (of the respiratory tract, urinary tract, gastrointestinal tract, or of the skin), or by physiological stresses such as acute illness, surgery, trauma, pregnancy, and emotional stresses which reduce the effectiveness of the available insulin. Anti-insulin factors (growth hormone, glucagon, cortisol) are released during stress and may play a part in the development of ketoacidosis. Ketoacidosis occurs more commonly in insulin-dependent diabetes. It is a serious complication, with a mortality rate ranging from 5 to 15 percent.

Clinical Manifestations. The clinical manifestations occur as a result of changes in body fluid, electrolytes, and acid base status. Early manifestations are polyuria (excessive urination), polyphagia (excessive appetite) and polydipsia (excessive thirst). Osmotic diuresis causes water loss (dehydration) and electrolyte depletion. As the patient becomes more dehydrated, oliguria (diminished urination) develops. Malaise and visual changes may be noted by the patient. Headache, muscle aches, and abdominal pain are frequent complaints, as are nausea, vomiting, and gastric stasis and ileus. If infection has precipitated the ketoacidosis, fever may be present. The patient's respiratory rate increases, to compensate for acidosis. Coma and severe acidosis are ushered in with Kussmaul breathing (very deep, but not labored, respirations) and a sweetish odor of the breath, due to acidemia.

The patient is drowsy and soon becomes comatose. The blood glucose is elevated, the serum bicarbonate and the blood pH are decreased, the blood urea is increased, and the plasma ketone is strongly positive. The urine is strongly positive for sugar and acetone. The patient's condition is serious at this stage, but recovery can be anticipated after prompt and vigorous treatment with insulin and intravenous fluids.

Management

The immediate objectives in the management of ketoacidosis are (1) to restore normal carbohydrate, protein, and fat metabolism; (2) to reverse hypovolemia, and (3) to correct electrolyte imbalance. A flow sheet is kept of vital signs, urine sugar, and acetone measurements, as well as of blood glucose and electrolytes, arterial blood gases, and the medications and treatment given. After blood and urine samples are collected, an indwelling catheter is usually inserted in the bladder, in order to obtain specimens at the prescribed times. A rapid physical examination is carried out, to detect evidence of infection, myocardial infarction, stroke, etc.

- An infusion of isotonic or hypotonic saline is started immediately to rehydrate the patient and improve tissue perfusion. The fluid deficit may range between 6 and 10 liters, and the rate of replacement depends on the patient's condition.
- Insulin is given to reduce blood glucose by promoting glucose utilization and to inhibit lipolysis (splitting up of fat), thereby preventing accumulation of ketones in the blood. The insulin regimens in current use are variable both in amounts and route of administration.

Until recently, high doses of insulin were given by intravenous boluses or by the intramuscular or subcutaneous routes, and repeated every four hours. It was difficult to maintain steady plasma levels by this protocol.

Low-dose insulin regimens are being used with increasing frequency. Continuous low-dose intravenous therapy with insulin may be given to obtain immediate insulin action and to maintain steady blood levels of insulin. Low-dose insulin is controllable and gives a more predictable response. A constant infusion pump or pediatric drip (with insulin placed in 250 ml. of half normal saline) may be used. Albumin or some other colloid may be added to the intravenous solution to prevent insulin from adhering to the infusion bottle and tubing. There are variations in the low-dose insulin regimens, including administration of insulin by intermittent intramuscular injection.

As the blood glucose level declines, glucose is added to the infusion, and the insulin concentration is reduced. There is now danger of hypoglycemia.

- Close monitoring of the patient is essential, since metabolic parameters change and call for continuing assessment of the patient and fluid and electrolyte status. Frequent laboratory determinations of blood glucose, serum ketones, serum bicarbonate, and serum potassium are needed.

At first the patient's serum potassium may be normal or raised, but when the blood glucose level begins to approach normal, hypokalemia threatens the patient. Hypokalemia occurs when serum potassium levels are reduced as a result of potassium "migrating" into the cells along with glucose, under the influence of insulin. Hypokalemia also results when extracellular potassium ions are exchanged for intracellular hydrogen ions, in the correction of acidosis.

- Frequent estimates of serum potassium and ECG monitoring are essential for early recognition of hypokalemia. Potassium replacement is usually started early. Tingling, paresthesia, decreased tendon reflexes, and respiratory depression are clinical manifestations of hypokalemia.

Hypotension that does not respond to intravenous fluids is treated with albumin, plasma, vasopressors, etc. Monitoring of central venous pressure is important, to achieve safe fluid balance, especially in elderly patients or those with myocardial disease. Nasogastric intubation and suctioning relieve vomiting and acute dilatation of the stomach and reduce the possibility of aspiration.

Consciousness should be restored and metabolic disturbances corrected within 12 to 24 hours. After the acute problem is corrected, the patient is regulated as described earlier. The precipitating cause of the coma should be determined, to prevent a recurrence.

Prevention. The patient should be taught and retaught the fundamentals of insulin administration, urine testing, and the management of diabetes to prevent recurrence of diabetic ketoacidosis.

HYPEROSMOLAR NONKETOTIC COMA

Hyperosmolar hyperglycemic coma is a syndrome in which hyperglycemia and hyperosmolarity predominate, with possible alterations of the sensorium (sense of awareness). At the same time, ketosis is minimal or absent. This condition occurs most frequently in older people (50 to 70 years) who have had no previous history of diabetes, or only mild maturity-onset diabetes. The acute development of the condition can be traced to some precipitating event such as an acute illness (pneumonia, myocardial infarction, stroke), ingestion of drugs known to provoke insulin insufficiency (thiazide diuretics, propranolol), and therapeutic procedures (peritoneal dialysis/hemodialysis, hyperalimentation). In the more chronic picture, there is a history of days to weeks of polyuria, with inadequate fluid intake. Upon admission to the hospital, the patient is found to have severe hyperglycemia ("syrupy blood"), profound dehydration, and variable neurologic signs ranging from sleepy confusion to coma.

The basic biochemical effect is lack of effective insulin. The patient's persistent hyperglycemia causes osmotic diuresis, resulting in losses of water and electrolytes. To maintain osmotic equilibrium, water shifts from the intracellular fluid space to the extracellular fluid space. With glucosuria and dehydration, hypernatremia and increasing hyperosmolality occur. The reasons why these patients show minimal ketosis is not clear.

The clinical picture is one of hypotension, dehydration (dry mucous membranes, poor skin turgor), fever, tachycardia, variable neurologic signs (alteration of sensorium, seizures, hemiparesis, etc.). This is a serious condition with a mortality rate ranging from 5 to 50 percent.

Management. The objective of management is to correct the volume depletion and hyperosmolar state. Then a search is made for the precipitating cause. Fluid therapy is started with hypotonic saline that is titrated by CVP monitoring. Insulin may be given either by highdose or low-dose regimen. Potassium chloride is added when the urinary output is adequate and is guided by ECG monitoring. Other therapeutic modalities are determined by the condition of the patient and the results of continuing clinical and laboratory evaluation.

LONG-TERM COMPLICATIONS OF DIABETES

There has been a steady decline in deaths due to diabetic ketoacidosis and infection, but an alarming rise in deaths due to cardiovascular and renal complications. Long-term complications are becoming more common as the average age of the population rises.

Atherosclerotic complications, with myocardial infarction, cerebrovascular accidents, uremia, and gangrene cause 70 percent of deaths among diabetic persons. There is no effective means of preventing or postponing the development of atherosclerosis in diabetics and nondiabetics. Even though much has been written on this subject, we do not know why it occurs earlier and progresses more rapidly in diabetics.

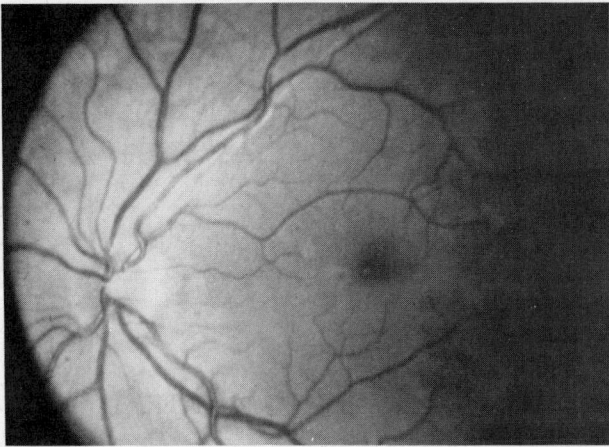

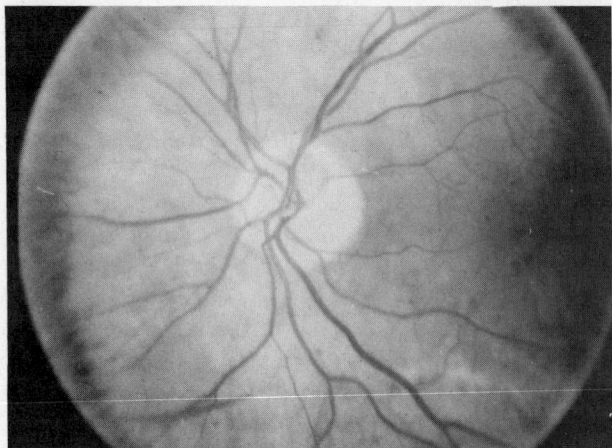

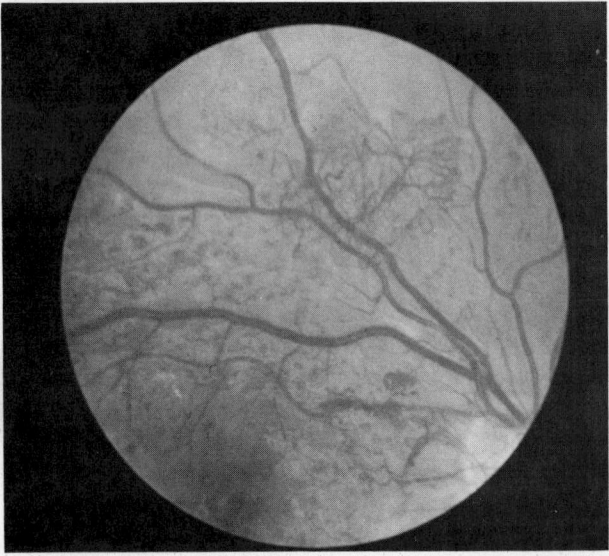

VASCULAR COMPLICATIONS

Diabetes mellitus is accompanied by changes in the entire vascular system. The changes occurring in the larger arteries appear to be the same atherosclerotic changes that occur in nondiabetics as a result of the aging process. However, the changes tend to occur at an earlier age in diabetics.

The specific pathological lesion (microangiopathy) of long-standing diabetes is characterized by thickening of the capillary basement membrane in every organ. The prevalence of microangiopathy parallels the duration of diabetes and its rate of progression.

Intracapillary glomerulosclerosis (Kimmelstiel-Wilson syndrome) is the specific renal disease of diabetes and is related to thickening of the capillary basement membrane in the glomerulus. It appears that a diabetic environment is injurious to the kidney. Renal failure is common in diabetics who develop the disease at an early age. (The pathophysiology and treatment of renal failure is discussed in Chapter 43.)

Involvement of the capillaries of the retina leads to blindness, due to diabetic retinopathy (page 847). Microangiopathy of the vessels supplying the skin, peripheral nerves, and walls of the large arteries may be a factor in skin diseases, diabetic neuropathy, and the increased prevalence of atherosclerosis. Occlusion of major vessels due to atherosclerosis causes strokes, myocardial infarction, intermittent claudication, and gangrene.

Advanced vascular disease in the large and small arteries of the legs is common in diabetes and is often severe enough to lead to gangrene of the affected extremity. In the large arteries, atheromas form in the subintimal tissues, and degenerative changes occur in the intima and media. The lipid-filled atheromas undergo progressive changes, such as fibrosis, calcification, and ulceration, and may eventually lead to thrombosis and occlusion of the artery. The smaller arteries of the lower extremities are often found to be affected by thickening of the intima, as a result of endothelial proliferation. Also prevalent is the occurrence of calcium deposits (primary calcinosis) of the media of the vessels, with or without atherosclerosis. Such calcinosis may be extensive enough to result in ossification of the wall of the artery. These changes in the smaller arteries present a serious problem, since an occlusion to one of the large arteries cannot be followed by the formation of adequate collateral circulation.

NURSING ASSESSMENT FOR IMPAIRED CIRCULATION. Clinical manifestations of impaired peripheral arterial

Figure 39-3. Diabetic retinopathy. *A.* In the fundus photograph of a normal eye, the light, circular area to the left, over which a number of blood vessels converge, is the optic disc, where the optic nerve meets the back of the eye. To the right of the optic disc is a smaller, dark spot on the photograph, the macula. The macula is the part of the retina on which images in the center of a person's visual field are focused. This part of the retina has a high concentration of light-sensitive cells, called *cones,* which provide sharp, clear color vision in bright light. *B.* The fundus photograph of a patient with diabetic retinopathy shows neovascularization—growth of a fine network of abnormal new vessels—directly on the optic disc. Small dots on the photograph are microaneurysms, while larger blotches are hemorrhages. One example of a hemorrhage in this photo is an almost horizontal streak on the lower left. *C.* This fundus photograph showing severe diabetic retinopathy reveals widespread neovascularization, microaneurysms, and hemorrhaging. (Photo: Courtesy National Eye Institute)

circulation include paleness of the lower extremities, reduced pulse volume in the arteries of the lower extremities, blanching and exaggerated pallor of the feet and legs after the legs are elevated for 60 seconds, delayed (greater than 10 seconds) return of color to the feet and legs after the lower extremities are moved from an elevated position to a dependent position, loss of hair over dorsal surface of the foot, thickened toenails, and brown spots on the skin of the lower extremities.

Diabetic patients who have impaired peripheral circulation are vulnerable to infection and/or gangrene, which commonly results from trauma. The patient may be unaware that he has somehow injured his leg. Such unawareness of injury is a result of peripheral neuropathy (page 848), which commonly accompanies diabetes.

DIABETIC RETINOPATHY

Diabetic retinopathy is a progressive impairment of retinal circulation that causes vitreous hemorrhage and loss of vision. It is now the leading cause of acquired blindness in adults under 60 (new adult blindness) in the United States. About 11 to 12 percent of all blind people in the United States are blind because of diabetes mellitus.

The basic cause of diabetic retinopathy is not known, although it frequently reflects the state of microangiopathy in the kidneys and other organs. The incidence and severity of retinopathy is generally proportional to the duration of the disease. It is less common in those patients who maintain meticulous diabetic control during the first 5 years of their disease. Half of the persons who have diabetes of more than 10 years' duration will show some

evidence of retinopathy, with initial vascular changes occurring in the capillary bed of the retina (Fig. 39-3). After 15 or more years, most patients will have retinal changes.

Diabetic retinopathy has two classifications, based on prognosis: background retinopathy and proliferative retinopathy. *Background retinopathy* is characterized by the development of microaneurysms on the retinal capillaries, with occasional thrombosis or rupture of the vessels, producing yellow spots (hard exudates) or red spots (deep hemorrhage). Background retinopathy may be present for many years with no deleterious effect on the vision. It does not usually require treatment unless it develops proliferative changes or the macula becomes involved (maculopathy).

Proliferative retinopathy is characterized by the growth of new blood vessels at the optic disk area and elsewhere in the retina. These vessels are very fragile, and their rupture leads to hemorrhage into the vitreous. Small hemorrhages may be completely absorbed, but larger hemorrhages become organized into fibrous bands that contract and lead to traction retinal detachment. Blindness results from repeated vitreous hemorrhages and retinal detachment.

Management. Diabetic retinopathy can be treated with photocoagulation, which is produced when an intensive, narrow beam of light is directed into the eye and focused on the retina (Fig. 39-4). The absorption of light produces heat, which coagulates the treated vessel and prevents it from bleeding. Photocoagulation of new vessels leads to their occlusion and fibrosis. The beam of

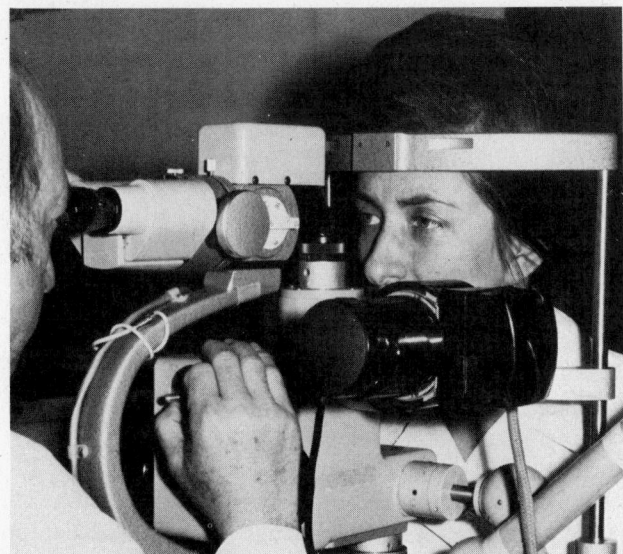
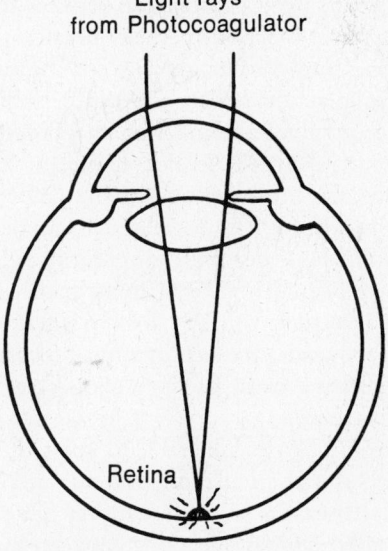

Light rays from Photocoagulator

Retina

Figure 39-4. Photocoagulation. (*Left*) The photograph shows a model receiving treatment with the argon laser, which generates a fine but intense blue-green beam of light. (Courtesy, Dr. Arnall Patz, Wilmer Eye Institute, Johns Hopkins Hospital, Baltimore, Md.) (*Right*) Principle underlying photocoagulation. (A) In this therapy an intense beam of light is directed into the eye and focused on a tiny spot in the retina. (B) The intense beam of light acts in much the same way as the sun's rays focused through a magnifying glass produce a small burn on a leaf. (Reproduced with permission from American Association of Workers for the Blind, Inc., Blindness Annual, 1969)

light acts in the same way that the sun's rays can burn a leaf when focused through a magnifying glass. The newer argon laser can be focused into a smaller point of light that will coagulate these tufts of new vessels. In order to be effective, this procedure must be carried out soon after neovascular proliferation appears, and before hemorrhage has occurred. Even a small group of new vessels may bleed and lead to permanent blindness. Photocoagulation impedes but does not cure retinopathy.

For those patients already blind as a result of vitreous hemorrhage, a vitrectomy may achieve some restoration of sight. This technique consists of simultaneously cutting cloudy vitreous and fibrous tissue, removing it from the eye by suction, and replacing it with a clear fluid which maintains the shape of the eye. This operation is not without risk, and may be accompanied by such complications as infection, an uncommon form of glaucoma, retinal detachment, or other problems. However, many ophthalmologists feel that the possible benefits of vitrectomy, when performed one year after a hemorrhage that has not cleared on its own, outweigh the risks. Others feel vitrectomy should be done sooner.

Patient Education. All diabetics should be examined by an ophthalmologist annually. Those with retinopathy should be seen at more frequent intervals. Also, diabetics should be urged not to smoke, since smoking is associated with a two-fold increase in proliferative retinopathy for patients with diabetes of 20 years' standing. Nonwhite female diabetic patients appear to have an especially high risk of blindness.

INFECTIONS

There appears to be a correlation between diabetes and susceptibility to infection, perhaps because of depleted host defenses and greater glucose concentration in the tissues. Insulin deficiency may impair the ability of granulocytes to carry out a number of vital functions, while hyperglycemia depresses leukocyte phagocytosis.

Infections are more serious in the diabetic because resistance to infection is decreased by hyperglycemia, and because diabetes becomes temporarily more severe in the presence of infection. Infections in the diabetic are exacerbated by dehydration, insulin antagonism, impaired phagocytosis, and neuropathy. Infection is a common precipitating cause of acute complications such as diabetic ketoacidosis.

The extremities are vulnerable to infection because of diminished arterial circulation, which lowers resistance to bacterial invasion and local injury. Cellulitis may spread rapidly. Fungal infections between the toes may produce fissures that provide further portals of entry for bacteria. Infections of the foot can lead to gangrene, with loss of toes, forefoot, or the foot and lower leg. A diabetic patient with an infected foot generally requires hospitalization. (The prevention of foot problems is discussed on page 849.)

Dermatologic problems abound in diabetes mellitus. Fungal infections, particularly monilia or candidiasis of the skin and vagina, are frequently found in poorly controlled diabetics. The presence of boils or carbuncles and severe pruritus should raise the suspicion of possible diabetes.

The increased prevalence of urinary-tract infections in diabetes is related to incomplete emptying of the bladder, due to poor bladder tone, a neurologic complication that may result from diabetic neuropathy—and possibly to an increased frequency of catheterization. Bladder infection produces ascending infections of the urinary tract. Serious complications from renal infection are more frequent in the diabetic.

Management. When the blood glucose is elevated, the leukocytes are unable to effectively destroy bacteria. All infections, and especially those associated with leukocytosis and a spreading infection, cause an increased need for insulin. Ketoacidosis may result if the insulin dose is not increased adequately. Testing the urine for sugar and acetone, and frequent blood glucose determinations are necessary to ascertain and compensate for rapidly changing insulin requirements. The cause of the infection should be determined by cultures, so that the appropriate antibiotic may be given.

THE DIABETIC NEUROPATHIES

Diabetic neuropathy (disorder of the nerves) of the peripheral and autonomic nervous system are common complications of diabetes. Diabetic neuropathy may affect the entire nervous system, but is more readily recognized in the peripheral nerves. The prevalence increases with the age of the patient and the duration of the disease.

Pathology. The causes for diabetic neuropathy are unknown. The pathogenesis may be due to either a vascular or a metabolic mechanism. There is support for the theory that metabolic aberrations of neurons or their myelin sheaths may be responsible for the nerve damage seen in diabetes. In the poorly controlled diabetic, an enzyme system (the sorbitol pathways) may become overactive during periods of insulin insufficiency, resulting in overproduction of fructose in the myelin sheath, which causes it to rupture, thereby disrupting nerve conduction.

Clinical Manifestations. Involvement of the autonomic nervous system covers a broad range of functions, including orthostatic hypotension, sexual impotency and retrograde ejaculation, pupillary changes, abnormal sweating, bladder paralysis, and nocturnal diarrhea.

Peripheral neuropathy most commonly manifests itself in the lower extremities. Pain and paresthesia are the outstanding manifestations. The pain has been described as dull or aching, cramping, burning, lancinating, or crushing. The pain is usually intensified at night and may be relieved by pacing the floor, which distinguishes this pain from the pain due to peripheral vascular insufficiency, which is intensified by walking.

The paresthesias have been described as sensations of tingling or burning, or of coldness and numbness. Because of these varied discomforts, it is quite common for the patient to be depressed and irritable and to suffer from anorexia.

Loss of sensation can lead to infection, gangrene, and amputation. The patient may be unaware of a blister, a protruding nail in his shoe, a burn from an electric blanket, etc. Instruction and reinforcement of previous learning about foot care is vital (see discussion below).

Nursing Assessment for Neuropathy of Extremities
- Place the patient in a supine position.
- Shield the patient's view of his feet with one hand, grasp the second toe on the sides with the thumb and forefinger, and move the toe back and forth several times.
- Stop the movement, and ask the patient in which direction the toe is pointed. If his proprioceptive senses (which provide information about position or movement of the body) are functioning adequately, the patient will respond correctly. An incorrect response may be an indication of neuropathy.
- Test also for response to pinprick and light touch, as well as knee and ankle reflexes. Absence of knee and/or ankle reflexes is significant.

Management. There is no evidence that treatment will reverse peripheral neuropathy, but some clinicians feel that careful diabetic control may halt or delay its progress.

FOOT CARE IN DIABETES

The feet of the diabetic patient are subject to sepsis and ischemia from deficient nerve function and poor circulation. Diabetic neuropathy may cause pain and paresthesia, but the greatest problem is loss of pain and temperature sensation in the feet.

Without pain perception, repeated trauma to the feet is tolerated until calluses and ulcers form, and the joints become damaged. Because of numbness of the feet, the patient may fail to notice a tack or a stone in his shoe. In addition, burns may occur when the patient is unable to recognize that a heating pad or a footbath is too hot. External heat is the most common single cause of gangrene. In view of these dangers, heat should not be applied below the knee of any diabetic patient.

Vascular involvement of the feet may lead to occlusion of large, medium, and small arteries and cause atrophic changes in the skin. The swelling that results from cellulitis may cause decreased circulation at a time when it needs to be increased. (Occlusive vascular disease can coexist with neuropathy.) If there is no response to antibiotics and debridement, the ischemia may cause gangrene

to start in the tips of the toes and then spread slowly up the leg.

Large-vessel insufficiency causes intermittent claudication (pain on walking, relieved by rest), blanching of the feet upon elevation, dusky redness of the feet when dependent, atrophic skin changes, cold feet, and finally pain at rest. Involvement of the autonomic nervous system may lead to an absence of sweating, which causes dry, cracked skin that permits bacteria to enter the foot.

Thus the triad of neuropathy, vascular disease, and infection leads to gangrene and amputation in older diabetics. In the presence of gangrene, amputation is done at the lowest level that has an adequate blood supply and is free of infection. The care of the patient undergoing amputation of an extremity is discussed on pages 1313–1319.

Management. Diabetic patients who have neuropathy and vascular problems should be under the supervision of a podiatrist. However, often the nurse is the only member of the health-care team who is available to provide direct care and guidance. The patient must be taught to wash and examine his feet every day. Unless the nails are thick, the vision poor, or the neuropathy severe, the patient should learn to trim his own nails. (See also patient education, page 850.)

Assessment by the Nurse
1. Ask the patient if he is a diabetic. Watch particularly for any lesion of the foot that does not heal.
2. Compare the skin color of the foot with the opposite foot and then with the other parts of the body (ankle, leg, hands).
3. Look for a mild cyanotic color in the digital or midtarsal area. This is caused by diminution of the arterial supply to the toes and sluggish venous return.
4. Change the position of the extremity and note the color changes. Pallor on elevation and dusky cyanosis on dependency indicate vascular insufficiency.
5. Feel the temperature of the feet. They should be about equal.
6. Examine the toenails. Thick, dry, and ridged nails may be a clue to circulatory impairment and diabetes.
7. Look for tinea pedis (fungal infection) between the toes and onchomycosis (fungal infection in the nails). Fungal infection of the feet is more serious in the diabetic.
8. Inspect for calluses, corns, blisters, cracks, and abrasions; look between the toes and on the soles of the feet.
9. Palpate the dorsalis pedis and posterior tibial arterial pulses; absence of a discernible pulse or diminution of pulses indicates atherosclerosis.

THE DIABETIC PATIENT UNDERGOING SURGERY

Because of generalized vascular disease, decreased resistance to infection, and changing insulin requirements due to stress, the diabetic patient must be followed very closely at the time of surgery. Surgical stress aggravates hyperglycemia because of an increased secretion of epinephrine and glucocorticoids. The metabolic stress of anesthesia also accentuates problems of hyperglycemia and ketosis. In addition, the patient's normal schedule of food intake, which is the foundation of diabetic treatment, is interrupted.

Preoperative Management. In the preoperative period, the aim is to have the diabetes well controlled and to correct any problems of hydration and electrolyte imbalance. The greatest danger is hypoglycemia, since the central nervous system is very sensitive to glucose deprivation and the clinical signs of hypoglycemia are difficult to interpret when the patient is unconscious from anesthesia.

If the patient has been on an oral hypoglycemic agent or long-acting insulin, then regular insulin is substituted a day or two before surgery. The preoperative medication is kept to a minimum, since these patients are susceptible to sedatives and narcotics.

There are a wide variety of protocols for the management of the patient's nutrient and insulin requirements before, during, and after surgery, depending on the degree of diabetes, nature of surgery, the degree and persistence of glucosuria, and whether or not ketonuria is present. The key to control is careful monitoring for potentially rapid changes that will affect the patient's metabolic state.

On the morning of surgery, a fasting blood sugar is drawn one hour before the operation. Usually the patient is given an intravenous infusion of 5 or 10 percent dextrose in water to provide necessary calories and carbohydrate, accompanied by the subcutaneous injection of insulin in a somewhat smaller dose than was required before surgery.

Postoperative Management. During the postoperative period, nutrition is maintained with intravenous dextrose until the patient is able to tolerate food by mouth. The insulin is adjusted on a sliding scale according to the results of the urine tests for glucose. Supplemental doses of regular insulin may be given as required.

It is desirable to give insulin subcutaneously, since insulin added to an intravenous solution may adhere to the walls of the bottle and tubing, and IV fluids may be given at different rates, making insulin dosages difficult to adjust.

Following surgery, the diabetes may intensify and become difficult to control. Healing is often delayed due to vascular disease, poor circulation, and altered metabolism. A higher incidence of vascular complications (myocardial infarction; stroke) may occur due to the increased incidence of atherosclerosis in diabetics.

PATIENT EDUCATION FOR DIABETES

Since the responsibility for the management of diabetes rests with the individual, each patient is taught to perform duties usually done by the physician, nurse, dietitian, and laboratory technician. The educational program is started at the time of diagnosis and must be continued throughout the life of the patient. Continuing education reinforces learning and is necessary for better control of the disease and for greater self-reliance of the patient. A responsible member of the patient's family should be included in the educational program. The community health nurse also has a role. Group instruction is an effective method of education in diabetic clinics, hospitals, and community health departments, and contributes to the security of these patients.

Realistic educational outcomes for the newly diagnosed patient include understanding of the (1) pathophysiology of diabetes; (2) basic concepts of dietary management; (3) administration of insulin; (4) urine testing; (5) recall of signs and symptoms of hypoglycemia and hyperglycemia, and (6) basic principles of foot care.

The reader is referred to Chapter 3 for discussion of the principles of health teaching and patient education. A summary of detailed information necessary for the education of diabetic patients is found below and on pages 851–852.

PATIENT EDUCATION FOR DIABETES MELLITUS

The person with diabetes mellitus must accept a major role in the management of his disease. His education must be amplified, reinforced, and updated continuously, since diabetes is a life-long disease.

Objective: to maintain the best possible control of diabetes.

PATIENT'S OBJECTIVES
A. *To become familiar with diabetes and how it affects the body.*
 1. Visit the physician on a regular basis.
 2. Study and review available literature from reputable sources.

 3. Secure booklets and pamphlets from the American Diabetes Association, Inc., 600 Fifth Ave., New York, N.Y. 10020.
 4. Attend available classes.

B. *To maintain health at an optimal level.*
 1. Maintain a consistent daily routine.
 2. Get adequate rest and sleep.
 3. Exercise regularly and consistently.
  a. Avoid "spurts" of arduous exercise before meals.
  b. Exercise 1½ hours after meals. *(Continued)*

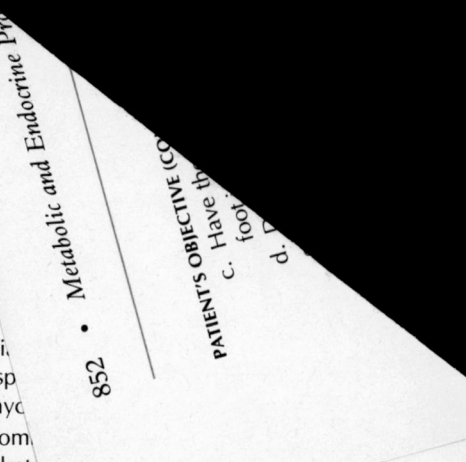
PATIENT EDUCATION FOR DIABETES MELLITUS (

PATIENT'S OBJECTIVE (CONTINUED)

   c. Keep some form of carbohydrate (sugar, candy, orange juice) available during exercise periods.

   d. Take extra food for extra physical activity.

4. Seek employment with regular hours.

5. Have an annual test for tuberculosis.

C. *To follow the prescribed dietary regimen.*

1. Eat three or more regularly spaced meals each day, timed to coincide with the action of insulin.

2. Become thoroughly familiar with the food exchange lists.

3. Learn how to follow a calculated diet.

4. Know the caloric value of foods frequently eaten.

5. Use household measures or a gram scale until serving sizes can be judged accurately.

6. Avoid concentrated carbohydrates.

7. Avoid periods of fasting and feasting.

8. Keep weight at optimal level; normalize body weight.

   a. Weigh weekly.

   b. Keep a weight record.

9. If taking insulin, eat extra calories when unusual physical activity is anticipated.

10. Eat a bedtime snack when taking insulin (if permissible).

11. Avoid foods high in cholesterol.

D. *To be aware of the degree of diabetic control.*

1. Test urine for both sugar and acetone at each testing.

2. Test urine before each meal and at bedtime while control is being attained or during periods of illness.

3. Test urine at least once daily.

4. Keep a daily record of urine sugar tests (date, hour, color reaction).

5. Test only freshly voided urine, using the second specimen (voided one half-hour after the first specimen).

6. Take the record of urine tests to physician at appointed times.

7. Know that acetone in the urine indicates need for *more insulin.*

8. Protect all urine testing equipment from light, moisture, and heat (to prevent false interpretation due to deterioration of test materials).

9. Monitor blood glucose with *Dextrostix* (capillary blood obtained by finger puncture is spread on enzyme strip) when insulin requirements vary and/or during illness.

E. *To become familiar with all aspects of insulin usage.*

1. Know when the prescribed insulin is having its peak action.

2. Adjust insulin dosage according to urine sugar tests, as prescribed.

3. Rotate the sites of insulin injections in a systematic manner.

4. Keep the syringe and needle in one particular place.

5. Keep a reserve supply of insulin in the refrigerator; be aware of expiration date on bottle.

   a. Keep bottle in current use at *room temperature.*

   b. Avoid injecting cold insulin, because it may contribute to tissue reaction.

6. Have an ex

7. Know the co

   a. Omission

   b. Unaccusto

   c. Too much i

8. Know the symp

   a. Any unfamili

   b. Hunger, persp

     pitation, tachyc

9. Know how to com

   a. Eat carbohydrate   en symptoms first oc

   b. Test urine.

   c. Carry extra carbohydrate at all times (sugar lumps, candy).

   d. Eat extra carbohydrate before strenuous exercise and during periods of prolonged exercise, or reduce insulin dosage.

   e. Eat a snack at bedtime.

10. Keep a check-off system, to ensure taking insulin.

11. Carry diabetic identification card or wear identification bracelet.

12. When traveling, carry diabetic supplies in hand luggage.

   a. Have letter from physician stating you are a diabetic.

   b. Keep your watch at the time-of-departure point until arrival at your destination; do not change diabetic regimen en route.

F. *To take prescribed oral hypoglycemic medication.*

1. Adhere faithfully to the prescribed diet.

2. Test urine daily.

3. Take the medication exactly as directed.

G. *To appreciate the importance of proper foot care to prevent infection.*

1. Inspect the feet carefully and routinely for calluses, corns, blisters, cracks, abrasions, redness, and nail abnormalities.

   a. Use a small mirror to check bottom of each foot.

   b. Use a magnifying glass under good light if eyesight is poor, or have someone else check feet.

2. Bathe the feet daily in warm (never hot) water.

   a. Do not soak the feet for prolonged periods.

   b. Dry feet carefully, especially between the toes.

3. Massage the feet with a lubricating lotion, except between the toes.

4. Prevent moisture between the toes, to avert maceration of the skin.

   a. Insert lamb's wool between overlapping toes.

   b. Use powder in the web spaces, especially if feet perspire.

5. Wear well-fitting, noncompressive shoes and socks— long enough, wide enough, soft, supple, and low-heeled.

   a. Buy shoes in the afternoon—feet are larger in the afternoon than in the morning.

   b. Have each foot measured before buying shoes—feet enlarge with age.

(Continued)

(...NTINUED)
...measurement taken while standing, since ...is larger in the standing position.
...Do not "break in" shoes all at one time.
  e. Check shoes repeatedly for protruding nails.
  f. Avoid rubber- or plastic-soled shoes, which cause feet to perspire and may lead to fungal infections.
  g. Avoid working in bedroom slippers or other casual foot attire.
6. Go to a podiatrist on a regular basis if corns, calluses, and ingrown toenails are present.
  a. Cut toenails straight across, to prevent ingrown toenails.
  b. See page 224 for instructions for cutting toenails.
7. Avoid heat, chemicals, and injuries to the feet—do not go barefoot or expose feet to hot water bottles, heating pads, caustic solutions, etc.
  a. Switch off electric blanket before going to bed; wear socks at night to keep feet warm, if necessary.
  b. Avoid overheated baths and sitting too close to the fire.
8. If an injury occurs to the foot:
  a. Wash the area with mild soap and water.
  b. Cover with a dry sterile dressing, *without* adhesive.
  c. Wear white socks; dye in colored socks and wool serve as irritants when skin is already irritated.
  d. Call the physician.
H. *To maintain diabetic control during periods of illness.*
  1. Call physician immediately when any unusual symptoms become evident; *do not allow diabetes to get out of control.*

2. Make dietary adjustments during illness according to physician's directions.
3. Continue taking insulin; physician may increase dosage during illness.
4. Test urine for sugar and acetone more frequently; keep records.
5. Monitor blood glucose with *Dextrostix.*
6. Know the conditions that bring about diabetic acidosis.
  a. Nausea and vomiting.
  b. Failure to increase insulin when urine sugar is increasing.
  c. Failure to take insulin.
  d. Dietary excesses.
  e. Infections.
7. Know how to combat impending diabetic acidosis.
  a. Examine urine for sugar and acetone, and report results to physician.
  b. Take additional insulin as advised by physician.
  c. Go to bed and keep warm.
  d. Alert someone to be in attendance.
  e. Drink a glass of liquid hourly, if possible.

I. *To follow other health directives.*
  1. Avoid tobacco—nicotine constricts blood vessels, causing reduction in blood flow to feet.
  2. Report excessive itching—may indicate elevated blood sugar.
  3. Take only medications prescribed by physician—many drugs enhance effect of insulin and oral antidiabetic agents.

BIBLIOGRAPHY

Diabetes Mellitus

BOOKS

General

Alsever, R. N., and Gotlin, R. W.: Handbook of Endocrine Tests, 2nd ed. Chicago, Year Book Med. Pub., Inc., 1978.

Bacchus, H.: Rational Management of Diabetes. Baltimore, University Park Press, 1977.

Bonar, J. R.: Diabetes. A Clinical Guide. Flushing, Medical Exam. Pub. Co., Inc., 1977.

Chaney, P. S. (ed.): Managing Diabetes Properly. Horsham, Pa., Intermed Communications, 1977.

Dolger, H., and Seeman, B.: How to Live with Diabetes. New York, W. W. Norton and Co., 1977.

Goldman, J. K.: The Diabetic Surgical Patient. *In* Siegel, J. H., and Chodoff, P.: The Aged and High Risk Surgical Patient: Medical, Surgical, and Anesthetic Management. New York, Grune and Stratton, 1976, pages 231-238.

Guthrie, D. W., and Guthrie, R. A. (eds.): Nursing Management of Diabetes Mellitus. St. Louis, C. V. Mosby Co., 1977.

Hershman, J. M.: Endocrine Pathophysiology: A Patient Oriented Approach. Philadelphia, Lea and Febiger, 1977.

Krall, L. P. (ed.). Joslin Diabetes Manual, 11th ed. Philadelphia, Lea and Febiger, 1978.

Levin, M. E., and O'Neal, L. W.: The Diabetic Foot, 2nd ed. St. Louis, C. V. Mosby, 1977.

Oakley, W. G., Pyke, D. A., and Taylor, K. W.: Diabetes and Its Management. Oxford, Blackwell Scientific Publications, 1978.

Report of the National Commission on Diabetes. Vol. 1: The Long-Range Plan to Combat Diabetes; vol. 3: Pt. 1, Scope and Impact of Diabetes (I); Pt. 2, Scope and Impact of Diabetes (II); Pt. 3, Etiology and Pathology of Diabetes; Pt. 4, Treatment of Diabetes; Pt. 5, Diabetes Education for Health Professionals, Patients and the Public. Washington, D.C., Public Health Service, 1976.

Steenrod, W. J. (ed.): Instructions for the Diabetic Patient. Seattle, The Mason Clinic, 1978.

Volk, B. W., and Wellman, K. I.: The Diabetic Pancreas. New York, Plenum Press, 1977.

Wilmore, D. W.: The Metabolic Management of the Critically Ill. New York, Plenum Publishing Corp., 1977.

Zoneraich, S.: Diabetes and the Heart. Springfield, Charles C Thomas, 1978.

Diet Therapy

Exchange Lists for Meal Planning, rev. ed. New York, American Diabetes Association, 1976.

Kaufman, W. I.: Brand Name Guide to Calories and Carbohydrates. New York, Pyramid, 1973.

West, K. M.: Diabetes Mellitus. *In* H. A. Schneider, C. E. Anderson, and D. B. Coursin (eds.): Nutritional Support of Medical Practice. Hagerstown, Md., Harper and Row, 1977, pages 278-296.

ARTICLES

Arky, R. A.: Diet and diabetes mellitus: concepts and objectives. Postgrad. Med., *63*:72-78, June 1978.

———: The engineering of blood sugar. New Engl. J. Med., *300*:618-619, Mar. 15, 1979.

Boyles, V. A.: Injection aids for blind diabetic patients. AJN, 77:1456-1458, Sept. 1977.

Bruhn, J. G.: Psychosocial influences in diabetes mellitus. Postgrad. Med., *56*:113-118, Aug. 1974.

Cahill, G. F., et al.: Blood glucose control in diabetes. Diabetes, *25*:237-239, Mar. 1976.

Cahill, G. F., Jr.: The diabetic pancreas (editorial). New Engl. J. Med., *299*:412-413, Aug. 24, 1978.

Eliopoulos, C. E.: Diagnosis and management of diabetes in the elderly. AJN, *78*:884-886, May 1978.

Fajas, S. S., Cloutier, M. C., and Crowther, R. L.: Clinical and etiologic heterogeneity of idiopathic diabetes mellitus. Diabetes, *27*:1112-1125, Nov. 1978.

Fonville, A. M.: Teaching patients to rotate injection sites. AJN, *78*:880-883, May 1978.

Isaf, J. J., and Alogna, M. T.: Better use of resources equals better health for diabetics. AJN, 77:1792-1795, Nov. 1977.

Kent, S.: Reevaluating the dietary treatment of diabetes. Geriatrics, *33*:99-107, May 1978.

Lawee, D.: Travel and the diabetic: How easy? Primary Care, *5*:615-624, Dec. 1978.

Lundin, D. V.: Reporting urine test results: switch from + to %. AJN, *78*:878-879, May 1978.

Manfredi, C., Cassidy, V., and Moffitt, D.: Developing a teaching program for diabetic patients. J. Contin. Educ. Nurs., *8*:46-52, Nov.-Dec. 1977.

McConnell, E. A.: Meeting the special needs of diabetics facing surgery. Nursing '76, *6*:30-37, June 1976.

Palumbo, P. J.: How to treat maturity-onset diabetes mellitus. Geriatrics, *32*:57-63, Dec. 1977.

Podolsky, D. (ed.): Symposium on diabetes mellitus. Med. Clin. N. Am., *62* (entire volume):627-866, July 1978.

Porter, A. L. (ed.): Symposium on Diabetes: Patient Education and Care. Nurs. Clin. N. Am., *12*:361-445, Sept. 1977.

Schumann, D.: Tips for improving urine-testing techniques. Nursing '76, *6*:23-27, Feb. 1976.

———: Assessing the diabetic. Nursing '76, *6*:62-67, Mar. 1976.

Small, D.: A patient education program. AJN, *78*:889-890, May 1978.

Sonksen, P. H., Judd, S. L., and Lowy, C.: Home monitoring of blood-glucose. Lancet, *1*:8067, 729-732, Apr. 8, 1978.

Ventura, E.: Foot care for diabetics. AJN, *78*:886-888, May 1978.

Yoon, J. W., et al.: Virus-induced diabetes mellitus. New Engl. J. Med., *300*:1173-1179, May 24, 1979.

Zinman, B.: Exercise and diabetic control. Primary Care, *4*:637-642, Dec. 1977.

Complications

Bienia, R., and Ripoll, K.: Diabetic ketoacidosis. JAMA, *241*:510-511, Feb. 2, 1979.

Bunick, E. M., and Lavine, R. L.: Potentially lethal complications of diabetes mellitus. Compr. Ther., *4*:40-48, June 1978.

Ellenberg, M.: The clinical aspects of diabetic peripheral neuropathy. Developments in Neurology: Peripheral Neuropathies, *1*:225-237, 1978.

Friedman, E. A.: Managing the diabetic with renal disease. Med. Times, *105*:46-54, May 1977.

Gonzalez-Villalpando, C., et al.: Low- and high-dose intravenous insulin therapy for diabetic ketoacidosis. JAMA, *241*:925-927, Mar. 2, 1979.

Kannel, W. B., and McGee, D. L.: Diabetes and cardiovascular risk factors: the Framingham study. Circulation, *59*:8-13, Jan. 1979.

Kohner, E. M. (ed.): Diabetic retinopathy. Int. Ophthal. Clin., *18*:1-207, Winter 1978.

Lavine, R. L.: How to recognize — and what to do about hypoglycemia. Nursing '79, *9*:52-55, Apr. 1979.

Leopold, I. H., and Mosier, M. A.: Four common ocular complaints of diabetes — and how to treat them. Geriatrics, *33*:33-41, Nov. 1978.

McCarthy, J.: Somogyi effect. Managing blood glucose rebound. Nursing '79, *9*:38-41, Feb. 1979.

McLaren, E. H.: Diabetic neuropathy. Compr. Ther., *4*:54-58, June 1978.

Miller, E. C.: Diabetic emergencies. Amer. Fam. Phys., *18*:115-121, Sept. 1978.

Palmberg, P. F.: Diabetic retinopathy. Diabetes, *26*:703-709, July 1977.

Patz, A.: Retinal vascular diseases. New Engl. J. Med., *298*:1451-1454, June 29, 1978.

Petrlik, J. C.: Diabetic peripheral neuropathy. AJN, *76*: 1794-1797, Nov. 1976.

Quayle, J. B.: Diabetic autonomic neuropathy in patients with vascular disease. Br. J. Surg., *65*:305-307, May 1978.

Slater, N. L.: Insulin reaction vs. ketoacidosis: guidelines for diagnosis and intervention. AJN, *78*:875-877, May 1978.

Walesky, M. E.: Diabetic ketoacidosis. AJN, *78*:872-874, May 1978.

Williamson, J. R., and Kilo, C.: Current status of capillary basement-membrane disease in diabetes mellitus. Diabetes, *26*:65-73, Jan. 1977.

Winegrad, A. I., and Greene, D. A.: The complications of diabetes mellitus (editorial). New Eng. J. Med., *298*: 1250-1252, June 1978.

Zimmerman, B. R.: Acute diabetic complications. Arch. Intern. Med., *138*:60-62, Jan. 1978.

Diet Therapy

Albrink, M. J.: Dietary and drug treatment of hyperlipidemia in diabetes. Diabetes, *23*:913-918, Nov. 1974.

Arky, R. A.: Current principles of dietary therapy of diabetes mellitus. Med. Clin. N. Am., *62*:655-662, July 1978.

Bierman, E. L., et al.: Special report: Principles of nutrition and dietary recommendations for patients with diabetes mellitus: 1971. Diabetes, *20*:633-634, Sept. 1971.

Jenkins, D. J. A., et al.: Decrease in postprandial insulin and glucose concentrations by guar and pectin. Ann. Intern. Med., *86*:20-23, Jan. 1977.

Kay, R. M.: Nutrition in the aetiology and treatment of diabetes mellitus. Nutrition, *28*:97-109, 1974.

Kiehm, T. G., Anderson, J. W., and Ward, K.: Beneficial effects of high carbohydrate, high fiber diet on hyperglycemic diabetic men. Am. J. Clin. Nutr., *29*:895-899, Aug. 1976.

Vitrectomy

Aiello, L. M., et al.: Retinopathy—eye care for your diabetic patients. Pat. Care, *12*:174-196, Apr. 15, 1978.

Effing, D. E.: Restore sight by microsurgery? Maybe (vitrectomy). Pat. Care. *13*:111-113, Jan. 15, 1979.

Insights into ophthalmic nursing through caring for a patient undergoing a vitrectomy. U.S. Dept. H.E.W., Pub. No. 77-1105, 1977.

Michels, R. G.: What role for vitrectomy in managing diabetic retinopathy? Hosp. Pract., *12*:73-78, Sept. 1977.

AGENCIES

Governmental

National Institutes of Arthritis, Metabolism and Digestive Diseases, National Institutes of Health, Bethesda, Md. 20205

Voluntary

American Diabetes Association, 600 Fifth Ave., New York, N.Y. 20205

American Dietetic Association, 620 N. Michigan Ave., Chicago, Ill. 60611

Joslin Diabetes Foundation, 15 Joslin Rd., Boston, Mass. 02215

Juvenile Diabetes Foundation, 23 East 26th St., New York, N.Y. 10010

40

ASSESSMENT AND MANAGEMENT OF PATIENTS WITH ENDOCRINE DISORDERS

PHYSIOLOGIC OVERVIEW

Endocrine glands, which secrete their products directly into the bloodstream, are clearly differentiated from exocrine glands, such as sweat glands, which secrete through ducts onto epithelial surfaces. The chemical substances secreted by the endocrine glands are called *hormones*. Hormones help to regulate organ function in concert with the nervous system. The dual regulatory system involving rapidly responding nervous activity with more slowly responding hormonal influences permits precise control of body function in the face of varied bodily and environmental changes.

Several different types of hormones are known to exist. These include steroid hormones such as hydrocortisone, peptide or protein hormones such as insulin, and amine hormones such as epinephrine. These different classes of hormones exert their actions on the target tissues by different mechanisms, as discussed below. A schematic diagram of the important endocrine glands is shown in Figure 40-1. Table 40-1 lists the important hormones, their target tissue, and some of their properties.

Certain anatomic features are common to the endocrine glands. The glands are composed of secretory cells arranged in minute clusters (acini). No ducts are present, but the glands are richly vascularized, so that the chemicals they produce can rapidly enter the bloodstream.

The concentration in the bloodstream of most hormones is maintained at a relatively constant level. If the hormone concentration rises, further production of that hormone is inhibited. When the hormone concentration falls, the rate of production of that hormone is stimulated. This mechanism for regulation of hormone concentration in the bloodstream is called *feedback control*. The principle of feedback control is important in the regulation of many biological processes.

MECHANISM OF HORMONE ACTION. Hormones can alter the function of the target tissue by interacting with chemicals (receptors) located either on the cell membrane or in the interior of the cell. Peptide and protein hormones interact with receptor sites on the cell surface which results in stimulation of the intracellular enzyme adenyl cyclase. This in turn results in increased production of cyclic 3':5'-adenosine monophosphate (cyclic AMP). The cyclic AMP inside the cell alters enzyme

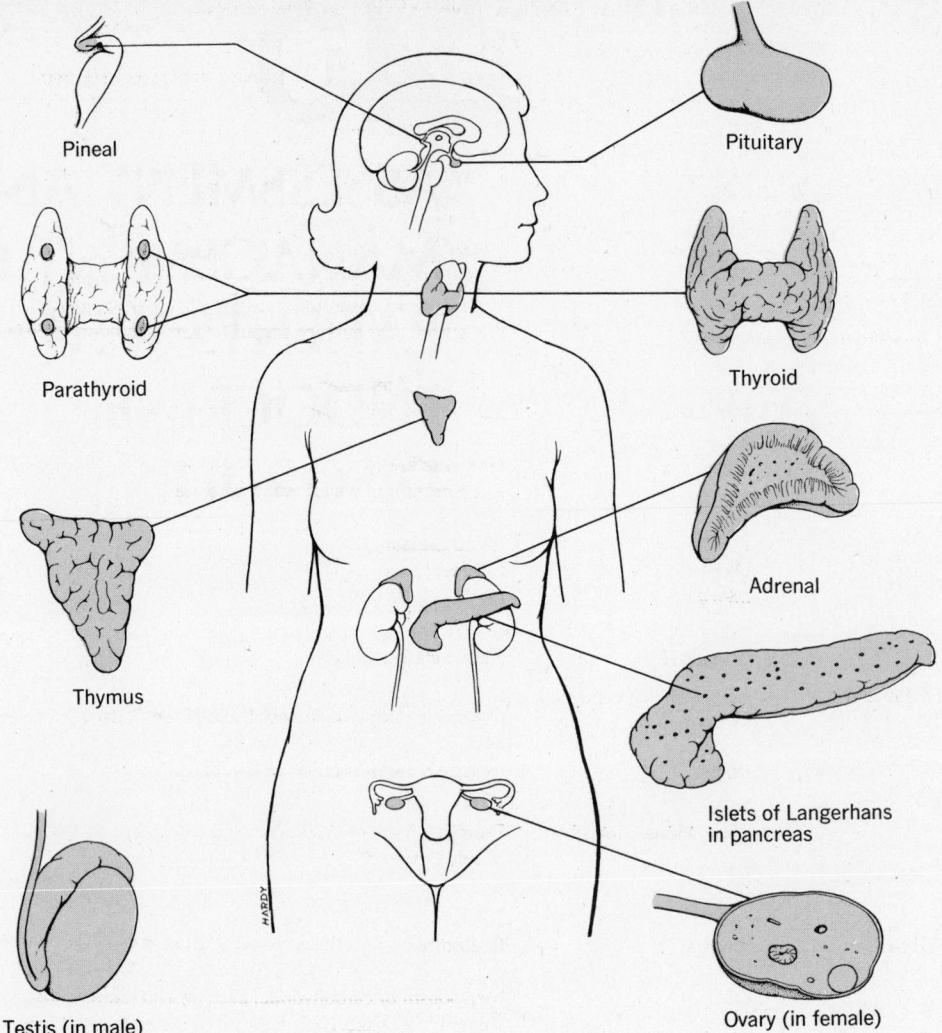

Pineal

Pituitary

Parathyroid

Thyroid

Thymus

Adrenal

Islets of Langerhans
in pancreas

Testis (in male)

Ovary (in female)

Figure 40-1.   General location of the major endocrine glands. (From Chaffee, R. N., and Greisheimer, E.: Basic Physiology and Anatomy, 3rd ed., Philadelphia, J. B. Lippincott, 1974)

activity. Thus, cyclic AMP is the "second messenger" that links the peptide hormone at the cell surface to a change in the intracellular environment. Some of the protein and peptide hormones may also act by inducing changes in membrane permeability. These hormones act relatively rapidly, within seconds or minutes. The mechanism of action for amine hormones is similar to that described above for peptide hormones.

Because of their smaller size and higher lipid solubility, steroid hormones penetrate through the cell membranes and interact with intracellular receptors. This steroid-receptor complex modifies cell metabolism by leading to the formation of messenger RNA from DNA. The messenger RNA then stimulates protein synthesis within the cell. Steroid hormones, because they exert their action by the modification of protein synthesis, require several hours in order to exert their effects.

The Pituitary Gland

The pituitary gland, or the hypophysis, has been referred to as the "master gland" of the endocrine system. It secretes hormones that, in turn, control the secretion of hormones by other endocrine glands. The pituitary itself is controlled in large part by the hypothalamus, an adjacent area of the brain. The pituitary gland is a round structure about 1.27 cm. (½ inch) in diameter located on the inferior aspect of the brain and connected to the hypothalamus by the pituitary stalk. The pituitary gland is divided into anterior, intermediate, and posterior lobes.

The important hormones secreted by the posterior lobe of the pituitary gland are *vasopressin* (antidiuretic hormone) and *oxytocin*. These hormones are synthesized in the hypothalamus and travel down the nerve cells that

TABLE 40-1. ENDOCRINE SYSTEM IN SUMMARY

ENDOCRINE GLAND AND HORMONE	PRINCIPAL SITE OF ACTION	PRINCIPAL PROCESSES AFFECTED
Pituitary gland		
(a) Anterior lobe		
Growth hormone (somatotropin)	General	Growth of bones, muscles, and other organs
Thyrotropin	Thyroid	Growth and secretory activity of thyroid gland
Adrenocorticotropin	Adrenal cortex	Growth and secretory activity of adrenal cortex
Follicle-stimulating	Ovaries	Development of follicles and secretion of estrogen
	Testes	Development of seminiferous tubules, spermatogenesis
Luteinizing or interstitial cell stimulating	Ovaries	Ovulation, formation of corpus luteum, secretion of progesterone
	Testes	Secretion of testosterone
Prolactin or lactogenic (luteotropin)	Mammary glands and ovaries	Secretion of milk; maintenance of corpus luteum
Melanocyte-stimulating	Skin	Pigmentation (?)
(b) Posterior lobe		
Antidiuretic (vasopressin)	Kidney	Reabsorption of water; water balance
	Arterioles	Blood pressure (?)
Oxytocin	Uterus	Contraction
	Breast	Expression of milk
Pineal gland		
Melatonin	Gonads (?)	Sexual maturation (?)
Thyroid gland		
Thyroxine and triiodothyronine	General	Metabolic rate; growth and development; intermediate metabolism
Thyrocalcitonin	Bone	Inhibits bone resorption; lowers blood level of calcium
Parathyroid glands		
Parathormone	Bone, kidney, intestine	Promotes bone resorption; increased absorption of calcium; raises blood calcium level
Adrenal glands		
(a) Cortex		
Mineralocorticoids (e.g. aldosterone)	Kidney	Reabsorption of sodium; elimination of potassium
Glucocorticoids (e.g. cortisol)	General	Metabolism of carbohydrate, protein, and fat; response to stress; anti-inflammatory
Sex hormones	General (?)	Preadolescent growth spurt (?)
(b) Medulla		
Epinephrine	Cardiac muscle, smooth muscle, glands	Emergency functions: same as stimulation of sympathetic system
Norepinephrine	Organs innervated by sympathetic system	Chemical transmitter substance; increases peripheral resistance
Islet cells of pancreas		
Insulin	General	Lowers blood sugar; utilization and storage of carbohydrate; decreased gluconeogenesis
Glucagon	Liver	Raises blood sugar; glycogenolysis
Testes		
Testosterone	General	Development of secondary sex characteristics
	Reproductive organs	Development and maintenance; normal function
Ovaries		
Estrogens	General	Development of secondary sex characteristics
	Mammary glands	Development of duct system
	Reproductive organs	Maturation and normal cyclic function
Progesterone	Mammary glands	Development of secretory tissue
	Uterus	Preparation for implantation; maintenance of pregnancy
Gastrointestinal tract		
Gastrin	Stomach	Production of gastric juice
Enterogastrone	Stomach	Inhibits secretion and motility
Secretin	Liver and pancreas	Production of bile; production of watery pancreatic juice (rich in $NaHCO_3$)
Pancreozymin	Pancreas	Production of pancreatic juice rich in enzymes
Cholecystokinin	Gallbladder	Contraction and emptying

(From Chaffee, R. N., and Greisheimer, E.: Basic Physiology and Anatomy, 3rd ed. Philadelphia, J. B. Lippincott, 1974)

connect the hypothalamus to the posterior pituitary gland where they are stored. Vasopressin secretion is stimulated by an increase in the osmolality of the blood or by a decrease in blood pressure. The primary function of vasopressin is to control the excretion of water by the kidney. Oxytocin secretion is stimulated during pregnancy and at the time of parturition (childbirth). The primary functions of oxytocin are to facilitate milk ejection during lactation and to increase the force of uterine contractions during parturition. Exogenous oxytocin can be used therapeutically to initiate labor.

The important hormones of the anterior pituitary gland are follicle-stimulating hormones (FSH), luteinizing hormone (LH), prolactin, adrenocorticotropic hormone (ACTH), thyroid-stimulating hormone (TSH), and growth hormone (GH). The secretion of each of these major hormones is controlled by releasing factors (RF) that are secreted by the hypothalamus. These releasing factors reach the anterior pituitary via the bloodstream in a special circulation called the pituitary portal blood system.

The hormones released by the anterior pituitary enter the systemic bloodstream and are transported to their target organs. TSH, ACTH, FSH, and LH have as their main function the release of hormones from other endocrine glands. Prolactin and growth hormone do not have as their primary effects the release of hormones from other endocrine glands. Prolactin acts on the breast to stimulate milk production. Growth hormone has widespread effects on many target tissues and is discussed below. The other trophic hormones will be discussed in conjunction with their target organs.

GROWTH HORMONE. Growth hormone, also referred to as somatotropin, is a protein hormone that increases protein synthesis in many tissues, increases the breakdown of fatty acids in adipose tissue, and increases the glucose levels in the blood. These actions of somatotropin are essential for normal growth, although other hormones such as thyroid hormone and insulin are required as well. The secretion of growth hormone is increased by stress, exercise, and low blood sugar. The half-time of growth hormone activity in the blood is about 20 to 30 minutes. It is largely inactivated in the liver. If secretion of growth hormone is insufficient during childhood, generalized limited growth and dwarfism result. Conversely, oversecretion during childhood results in gigantism, with individuals reaching 7 or even 8 feet in height. Excess growth hormone in adults results in deformities of bone and soft tissue and enlargement of viscera (acromegaly), but no increase in height.

ABNORMAL PITUITARY FUNCTION. Abnormalities of pituitary function are due to over- or undersecretion of any of the hormones produced and/or released by the gland. Abnormalities of the posterior and anterior portions of the gland may occur independently. Oversecre-

tion (hypersecretion) most commonly involves ACTH or growth hormone, resulting in the conditions known as Cushing's disease or acromegaly, respectively. Hyposecretion (undersecretion) commonly involves all of the anterior pituitary hormones and is termed panhypopituitarism. In this condition, the thyroid gland, the adrenal cortex, and the gonads atrophy due to loss of the trophic hormones. The most common disorder related to posterior lobe dysfunction is diabetes insipidus, a condition in which abnormally large volumes of dilute urine are excreted due to deficient production of antidiuretic hormone.

The Thyroid Gland

The thyroid gland is a butterfly-shaped organ located in the lower neck anterior to the trachea. It consists of two lateral lobes connected by an isthmus. The gland is approximately 5 cm. long and 3 cm. wide and weighs about 30 grams. The blood-flow to the thyroid, per gram of gland tissue, is very high (about 5 ml./min. per gram of thyroid), approximately five times the blood-flow to the liver. This indicates the high metabolic activity of the thyroid gland.

THYROID HORMONE. Two different hormones are made in the thyroid gland, thyroxine (T_4) and triiodothyronine (T_3). These hormones are amino acids which have the unique property of containing iodine molecules bound to the amino acid structure. T_4 contains four iodine atoms in each molecule, while T_3 contains only three. These hormones are synthesized and stored by the cells of the thyroid gland until needed for release into the bloodstream. The hormones are stored bound to a glycoprotein called thyroglobulin.

IODINE UPTAKE AND METABOLISM. Iodine is essential to the thyroid gland for synthesis of its hormones. In fact, the major use of iodine in the body is by the thyroid, and the major derangement in iodine deficiency is alteration of thyroid function. Iodine is ingested in the diet and absorbed into the blood in the gastrointestinal tract. The thyroid gland is extremely efficient in taking up iodide from the blood and concentrating it within the cells. There, iodide ions are converted to iodine molecules which react with tyrosine (one of the common amino acids) to form the thyroid hormones.

REGULATION OF THYROID FUNCTION. The secretion of thyroid stimulating hormone (TSH) by the pituitary gland controls the rate of thyroid hormone release. In turn, the release of TSH is determined by the level of thyroid hormones in the blood. If thyroid hormone concentration in the blood decreases, release of TSH increases, which causes increased output of T_3 and T_4. This is an example of feedback control. Thyroid releasing factor (TRF) secreted by the hypothalamus exerts a modulating influence on the release of TSH from the pituitary. Environmental factors, such as a fall in temperature, may lead to increased secretion of TRF and, thereby, result in elevated secretion of thyroid hormones.

FUNCTION OF THYROID HORMONES. The primary function of the thyroid hormones is to control the cellular metabolic activity. Thyroid hormone action can be evaluated through measurement of the basal metabolic rate (BMR) defined as milliliters of oxygen consumed by the body per minute at rest. In the absence of thyroid secretion, the BMR may decrease by 30 to 40 percent. Administration of exogenous thyroid hormones can return the BMR to normal. The presence of adequate thyroid hormone is also necessary for normal growth. The thyroid hormones, through their widespread effects on cellular metabolism, influence every major organ system.

THYROCALCITONIN. Thyrocalcitonin is another important hormone secreted by the thyroid gland. This hormone was only recently discovered and its effects are still not completely known. Its secretion is not controlled by thyroid-stimulating hormone but is stimulated by increased blood calcium concentration. The major action of thyrocalcitonin is to decrease calcium concentration in the blood.

ABNORMALITIES OF THYROID FUNCTION. During the formative years, inadequate secretion of thyroid hormone will result in stunted growth (cretinism), due to general depression of body metabolic activity. In the adult, hypothyroidism (myxedema) is manifested by lethargy, slow mentation, and generalized slowing of body functions. Oversecretion of thyroid hormones (hyperthyroidism) is manifested by greatly increased metabolic rate. Many of the other characteristics of hyperthyroid patients reflects the potentiation of circulating catecholamines (epinephrine and norepinephrine) by excess thyroid hormones. Oversecretion of thyroid hormones is usually associated with an enlarged thyroid gland (goiter). Goiter also commonly occurs in the presence of iodide deficiency. In this latter condition, lack of iodide results in low levels of circulating thyroid hormones, which causes increased release of TSH; the elevated TSH causes overproduction of thyroglobulin and hypertrophy of the thyroid gland.

The Adrenal Glands

There are two adrenal glands in the human, each attached to the upper portion of a kidney. Each adrenal gland is, in reality, two endocrine glands. The adrenal medulla at the center of the gland secretes catecholamines, while the outer portion of the gland, the adrenal cortex, secretes corticosteroids.

ADRENAL MEDULLA. The adrenal medulla functions as part of the autonomic nervous system. Stimulation of preganglionic sympathetic nerve fibers, which travel directly to the cells of the medulla, causes release of the catecholamine hormones, epinephrine or norepinephrine. About 90 percent of the secretion of the adrenal medulla in man is epinephrine (also called adrenalin). The major effects of epinephrine release are involved in preparation to meet a challenge (fight or flight response). Secretion of epinephrine causes decreased blood-flow to tissues such as the gastrointestinal tract, that are not needed in emergency situations, and causes increased blood-flow to those tissues such as cardiac and skeletal muscle, which are important for effective fight or flight. Catecholamines also induce release of free fatty acids, increase the basal metabolic rate, and elevate the level of blood sugar.

ADRENAL CORTEX. The three kinds of steroid hormones produced by the adrenal cortex are glucocorticoids, the prototype of which is hydrocortisone, mineralocorticoids, mainly aldosterone, and sex hormones, mainly androgens (male sex hormones).

Glucocorticoids. The glucocorticoids are given their name because they have an important influence on glucose metabolism; increased hydrocortisone secretion results in elevated blood sugar. However, the glucocorticoids have major effects on the metabolism of almost all organs of the body. Glucocorticoids are secreted from the adrenal cortex in response to the release of adrenocorticotrophic hormone (ACTH) from the anterior lobe of the pituitary gland. This system represents another typical example of negative feedback. The presence of glucocorticoids in the blood inhibits the release of corticotropin-releasing factor (CRF) from the hypothalamus, and also inhibits ACTH secretion from the pituitary. The resultant decrease in ACTH secretion causes diminished release of glucocorticoids from the adrenal cortex. A functioning adrenal cortex is necessary for life, although survival is possible by appropriate replacement with exogenous adrenal cortical hormones.

The glucocorticoids are frequently administered for their therapeutic effects. In pharmacological doses, they inhibit the inflammatory response to tissue injury and suppress allergic manifestations. Toxic effects of glucocorticoids include possible development of diabetes, osteoporosis, peptic ulcer, increased protein breakdown resulting in muscle wasting and poor wound healing, and redistribution of body fat. The presence of large amounts of exogenously administered glucocorticoids in the blood inhibits release of ACTH and endogenous glucocorticoids. Because of this, the adrenal cortex can atrophy. If exogenous glucocorticoid administration is suddenly discontinued, adrenal insufficiency results, due to inability of the atrophied cortex to adequately respond.

Mineralocorticoids. Mineralocorticoids exert their major effects on electrolyte metabolism. They act principally on renal tubular and gastrointestinal epithelium to cause increased sodium ion absorption in exchange for excretion of potassium or hydrogen ions. Aldosterone secretion is only minimally influenced by ACTH. It is primarily secreted in response to the presence of angiotensin II in the bloodstream. Angiotensin II concentration is increased when renin is released from the kidney in response to decreased perfusion pressure. The resultant increased aldosterone levels promote sodium reabsorption by the kidney and the gastrointestinal tract, which tends to restore blood pressure to normal. The release of aldosterone is also increased by hyperkalemia. Aldosterone is the primary hormone for the long-term regulation of salt balance.

Adrenal sex hormones (androgens). Androgens, the third major type of steroid hormones produced by the adrenal cortex, physiologically exert effects similar to male sex hormones. The adrenal gland may also secrete small amounts of some estrogens (female sex hormones). Secretion of adrenal androgens is controlled by ACTH. When secreted in normal amounts, the adrenal androgens probably have little effect, but when secreted excessively, as with certain inborn enzyme deficiencies, masculinization may result. This is called the *adrenogenital syndrome*.

The Parathyroid Gland

The parathyroid glands, normally four in number, are situated in the neck, embedded in the posterior aspect of the thyroid gland. These small glands are easily overlooked and can be removed at the time of thyroid surgery unless great care is exercised by the surgeon. Inadvertent surgical removal is the most common cause of hypoparathyroidism.

Parathormone, the protein hormone from the parathyroid glands, regulates calcium and phosphorus metabolism. Increased parathormone results in increased calcium absorption from the kidney, the intestine, and bones, thereby raising the blood-calcium level. Some actions of this hormone are potentiated by the presence of vitamin D. Parathormone also tends to lower the blood phosphorus. Excess parathormone can result in markedly elevated serum Ca^{++}, which constitutes a potentially life-threatening situation. When the product of serum calcium and serum phosphorus becomes high, calcium phosphate may precipitate in various organs of the body and cause tissue calcification.

The output of parathormone is regulated by the serum level of ionized calcium. Increased serum calcium results in decreased parathormone secretion, forming a feedback system.

The Pancreas

The pancreas, located in the upper abdomen, has both exocrine- (digestive enzymes) and endocrine-gland function. In contrast to endocrine glands, an exocrine gland is one whose secretions travel through a duct to their site of utilization and are not secreted into the bloodstream.

EXOCRINE PANCREAS. The secretions of the exocrine portion of the pancreas are collected in the pancreatic duct, which joins the common bile duct and enters the duodenum at the ampulla of Vater. Surrounding the ampulla is the sphincter of Oddi, which partially controls the rate at which the secretions from both the pancreas and gallbladder enter the duodenum.

The secretions of the exocrine pancreas are digestive enzymes and an electrolyte-rich fluid. The secretions are very alkaline because of their high concentration of sodium bicarbonate, and are capable of neutralizing the highly acid gastric juice that enters the duodenum. The enzyme secretions include *amylase,* which aids in the digestion of carbohydrates, *trypsin,* which aids in the digestion of proteins, and *lipase,* which aids in the digestion of fats. Other enzymes that aid in the breakdown of more complex foodstuffs are also secreted.

The stimulus for secretion of these exocrine pancreatic juices are hormones originating in the gastrointestinal tract. Secretin is the major stimulus for increased bicarbonate secretion from the pancreas, while the major stimulus for digestive enzyme secretion is the hormone cholecystokinin-pancreozymin (CCK-PZ). The vagus nerve also influences exocrine pancreatic secretion.

ENDOCRINE PANCREAS. The islets of Langerhans, the endocrine part of the pancreas, are collections of cells embedded in the pancreatic tissue. They are composed of two major cell types, alpha and beta. The hormone produced by the beta cells is called *insulin,* while the alpha cells secrete *glucagon.* A major action of insulin is to lower blood sugar by permitting entry of the sugar (glucose) into the cells of the liver, muscle, and other tissues where the glucose can be either stored as glycogen or burned for energy. Insulin is also instrumental in promoting the storage of fat in adipose tissue and in the synthesis of proteins in various body tissues. In the absence of insulin, glucose is not able to enter the cells and is excreted in the urine. This condition, called diabetes mellitus, can be diagnosed by high levels of glucose in the blood and urine. In diabetes mellitus, fats and protein can be utilized for energy instead of glucose, with consequent loss of body mass. The rate of insulin-secretion from the pancreas is regulated in normal people by the level of sugar in the blood.

The effects of glucagon are chiefly to raise the blood sugar (opposite to those of insulin), primarily by promoting the conversion of glycogen to glucose in the liver. Glucagon is secreted by the pancreas in response to a fall in the level of blood glucose.

ENDOCRINE CONTROL OF CARBOHYDRATE METABOLISM. Glucose for body energy needs is derived by metabolism of ingested carbohydrates and also from proteins by the process of gluconeogenesis. Glucose can be stored temporarily in the liver, muscles, and other tissues in the form of glycogen. The endocrine system controls the level of blood glucose by regulating the rate at which glucose is synthesized, stored, and removed into the bloodstream. Through the action of hormones, blood glucose is normally maintained at approximately 100 mg. per 100 ml. of blood. Insulin is the primary hormone that leads to a lowering of blood glucose. Hormones that act to raise the blood sugar are glucagon, epinephrine, adrenocorticosteroids, growth hormone, and thyroid hormone.

THE THYROID GLAND

ASSESSMENT: TESTS OF THYROID FUNCTION

The number of tests to determine thyroid function has increased steadily. No tests can be used to the exclusion of others; several may be required, to give a composite assessment of thyroid function. In addition, clinical signs and symptoms are evaluated before a diagnosis can be made.

The stimulating effect of the thyroid gland is exerted through the production and distribution of two hormones: levothyroxine (T_4), which maintains body metabolism in a steady state, and triiodothyronine (T_3), which is approximately five times as potent as thyroxine and has a more rapid metabolic action. In testing, reliance is placed on the measurement of the levels of thyroid hormones in the blood.

SERUM T_4. The most useful test is the determination of serum T_4 by radioimmunoassay or competitive binding techniques. A blood sample is not affected by exogenous iodine. The range of T_4 in serum is normally between 4.5 and 11.5 μg. per dl. T_4 is bound mainly to thyroxine-binding globulin and prealbumin; T_3 is bound less avidly.

Serum binding of thyroid hormone is clinically significant, since anything that interferes with binding may change the total concentration of the hormone measured in the serum.

RESIN T_3 UPTAKE. This test uses triiodothyronine labeled with ^{131}I in vitro (within a test tube and in the laboratory). The radioactivity taken up by the resin, compared to total radioactive T_3, is calculated as a percentage, commonly 25–35 percent. It detects alterations in T_4 and gives a reasonable estimate of the amount of free T_4 in the serum. (It does not measure T_3.) If binding sites are low (example, hyperthyroidism), the reading is high. If binding sites are high (example, hypothyroidism), the reading is low. The test is technically simple, but results may be altered if the patient has been taking estrogens, androgens, salicylates, or Dilantin.

THYROID-STIMULATING HORMONE. The secretion of T_3 and T_4 by the thyroid gland is under the control of thyroid-stimulating hormone (TSH, thyrotropin) from the pituitary gland.

Thyrotropin (TSH) Radioimmunoassay. Thyrotropin can be measured in the serum by radioimmunoassay; this method affords multiple determinations. In patients with primary hypothyroidism, TSH levels are elevated; low levels are seen in hyperthyroid patients.

Thyrotropin-releasing Hormone (TRH). The administration of synthesized TRH provides a direct means of testing pituitary reserve for TSH. The patient fasts overnight and then, 15 minutes prior to an injection of TRH, a blood specimen is drawn. TRH may be given orally or intravenously. If given intravenously, it may cause the patient to experience the following transient symptoms: nausea, or a desire to urinate.

PROTEIN-BOUND IODINE. Protein-bound iodine is a conjugated molecule formed when thyroxine becomes attached to certain plasma-protein components. Thyroid function may be assessed in relation to the concentration of protein-bound iodine (PBI) in the blood. In this test, serum proteins are precipitated, washed, and then measured for iodine content. Normal values range from 4 μg.-8 μg. per 100 ml. of plasma. Values above 8 μg. indicate thyroid overactivity; conversely, concentrations below 4 μg. are considered evidence of hypothyroidism.

A disadvantage of this test is the unreliable results which may occur if the patient has taken medications containing iodine.

When a patient is scheduled for thyroid function tests, it is necessary to know beforehand whether he has taken medications with iodine in them, since this will alter the results of some tests. Iodide-containing medications are divided into those containing inorganic iodide, and those containing organic iodide (Table 40-2).

Antiseptics, cough syrups, and nail strengtheners may also serve as sources of iodine. Other medications which may affect thyroid function test values are female hormones, salicylates, cortisone derivatives, antibiotics, and mercurial diuretics. The variety of interfering factors is one reason why this test is becoming outdated.

RADIOACTIVE IODINE UPTAKE (RAI). The patient is given a tracer dose of ^{131}I, and a count is made over the thyroid, usually within 24 hours. Thyroid activity, divided by the amount of administered activity (expressed as a percentage) is the uptake value. It is a simple test and provides reliable results. It is affected by the patient's intake of iodide or thyroid hormone; therefore, a careful preliminary clinical history is essential in evaluating results. Normal values vary from locality to locality with the

TABLE 40-2. INORGANIC AND ORGANIC IODIDES

EXAMPLES OF INORGANIC IODIDES	EXAMPLES OF ORGANIC IODIDES

Lugol's solution
Diiodohydroxyquin
  (Diodoquin)
Potassium iodide (Quadrinal)
Iodochlorhydroxyquin
  (Entero-Vioform)
Sodium iodothiouracil (Itrumil)
	X-ray contrast media: time required for elimination of contrast media from body:
	Gallbladder . . . . months
	Bronchographic . . . . years
	Myelogram . . . . life
	Pyelogram . . . . rapidly

intake of iodine (9-16 percent, 12-30 percent, etc.). Patients with hyperthyroidism accumulate a high proportion of the ^{131}I (in some patients up to 90 percent), whereas patients with hypothyroidism exhibit a very low uptake.

RADIOSCAN OR SCINTISCAN. In this test, a highly focused scintillation detector moves back and forth across the area to be studied in a series of parallel tracks which move progressively downward. At the same time, a printing device records a mark whenever a predetermined number of counts has been received. This produces a visual representation of the localization of radioactivity in the area being scanned. Although ^{131}I has been the most commonly used isotope, ^{125}I, and especially ^{99n}Tc (sodium pertechnetate), are being used, because of their physical and biochemical properties, which allows a lower radiation dose to be given to the patient.

Scanning is helpful in determining location, size, shape, and anatomical function of the thyroid gland, particularly when thyroid tissue is substernal or large. Discovery of decreased ^{131}I uptake in a localized area of the thyroid is construed as evidence of a malignancy. Scanning of the entire body, to obtain the total body profile, may be carried out in a search for a functioning thyroid metastasis.

HYPOTHYROIDISM AND MYXEDEMA

Hypothyroidism is a condition in which there is a slow progression of thyroid hypofunction, followed by symptoms indicating thyroid failure. This condition is usually referred to as primary hypothyroidism. When the thyroid dysfunction is due to failure of the pituitary gland, the condition is known as secondary hypothyroidism; when failure of the hypothalamus is the underlying cause, the term tertiary hypothyroidism is used. When thyroid deficiency is present at birth, the condition is known as cretinism. In such instances, the mother may also suffer from a thyroid deficiency.

The causes of hypothyroidism may be idiopathic; if the thyroid gland is removed surgically or treated by radioactive iodine, or is damaged by disease (Hashimoto's thyroiditis) the metabolism of the patient declines proportionately to the reduction in production of thyroid hormone.

Clinical Manifestations

Early symptoms of hypothyroidism are nonspecific, but tiredness makes it difficult for the person to complete a full day's work. Menstrual disturbances occur, as well as loss of libido. Complaints of hair loss, brittle nails, and dry skin are common, and numbness and tingling of the fingers may occur. On occasion, the voice may become husky.

With severer grades of hypothyroidism, the tempera-

ture and the pulse rate become subnormal and the patient begins to gain weight. (Severe hypothyroid patients may be cachectic.) The skin becomes thickened because of an accumulation of mucopolysaccharides in the subcutaneous tissues (the origin of the term *myxedema*). Menorrhagia is apt to develop; the hair thins and falls out; the expression of the face becomes stolid and masklike.

At first the patient may be irritable and may complain of fatigue, but as the condition progresses, an apathetic attitude prevails, the emotional responses are subdued, and the mental process becomes dulled. Speech is slow, the tongue enlarges, and hands and feet increase in size. Deafness also may occur. The advanced myxedematous state may produce personality changes similar to schizoid paranoia, which in the extreme may constitute myxedema madness.

Myxedema affects women five times as frequently as men and occurs most often between 30 and 60 years of age. It is not without its complications, because there is an associated tendency to the rapid development of arteriosclerosis, with all the undesirable features of that disease; also, anemia and poor reaction to anesthetic agents result.

Management

The prime objective is to restore a normal metabolic state by replacing the lost hormone. Synthetic levothyroxine (Synthroid) is the preferred preparation for treating hypothyroidism and suppressing nontoxic goiters. The dosage for hormone replacement is scheduled on the basis of the patient's normal or suppressed serum TSH concentration. Usually dosage varies from 0.1-0.2 mg. daily. Desiccated thyroid is used less frequently, since it often results in transient elevated serum concentrations of T_3, with occasional symptoms of hyperthyroidism. If replacement therapy is adequate, the symptoms of myxedema disappear, and normal metabolic activity is resumed.

Prevention of chilling is part of the nursing management of these patients, since a person with hypothyroidism cannot generate heat, and thus becomes hypothermic. Adequate hydration, a diet containing fruit and vegetables, and the use of stool softeners are usually necessary to prevent constipation and impaction. However, excess hydration is to be avoided, as the hypothyroid patient may not excrete a fluid load, even after diuretics, thus making hyponatremia a hazard.

Nursing judgment and selective action are required in caring for patients with myxedema, because of the possibility of several complications:

1. *Severe untreated hypothyroidism is attended by an increased susceptibility to all hypnotic and sedative drugs.* These agents, even in small doses, may induce profound somnolence, lasting far longer than anticipated. Moreover, they are prone to cause respiratory depression, which could easily prove fatal.

With this in mind, the dosage of any such drug is most conservative, e.g., no more than a half or one-third the dosage ordinarily employed in patients of similar age and weight who are not myxedematous. Drugs in this category are not used unless the indications are very specific, and, if they are given, the nurse must be unusually alert for signs of impending narcosis or respiratory failure.

2. *Myocardial ischemia or infarction may occur in response to therapy in patients with myxedema.* Any patient who has been myxedematous for a long period of time is almost certain to have coronary sclerosis to some degree. As long as metabolism is subnormal and the tissues, including the myocardium, require relatively little oxygen, a reduction in blood supply is tolerated very well. However, when thyroid hormone is given, the situation changes: the oxygen requirements are greater, but its delivery cannot be speeded up unless, or until, the arteriosclerosis improves, which will occur very slowly, if at all. The signal that the oxygen needs of the myocardium are outstripping its blood supply is angina pectoris.

The nurse must be alert for signs of angina, especially during the early phase of treatment, and if detected, it must be heeded at once, in order to avoid a fatal myocardial infarction. Obviously, the administration of thyroid hormone must be discontinued immediately, and later, when it can be resumed safely, substitution therapy should be given, with caution, at a lower level of dosage and under the close observation of the physician and the nurse.

Elderly arteriosclerotic patients may also become confused and agitated if their metabolic rates are raised too quickly in myxedema.

3. *Myxedema coma may be the final stage of severe, longstanding, untreated hypothyroidism.* Myxedema coma occurs mostly in the elderly, during winter months. Signs include: hypotension, bradycardia, hypothermia (even below 37° C., recorded on the average thermometer), and convulsions.

The treatment consists of maintaining vital functions by measuring arterial blood gases to determine carbon dioxide retention and to provide assisted ventilation to combat hypoventilation. Fluids are to be administered cautiously because of the danger of water intoxication. External heat application is discouraged, since it will increase oxygen requirements and may lead to vascular collapse. If hypoglycemia is evident, concentrated glucose may be given, to prevent fluid overload. Thyroid hormone (TH), usually sodium levothyroxine (Synthroid), is given intravenously until consciousness is restored. Then the patient is continued on oral thyroid hormone therapy. Because of an associated adrenocortical insufficiency, steroid therapy may be initiated.

Nursing measures appropriate to the unconscious patient (pages 1188-1195) apply, such as frequent turning, prevention of aspiration, and attention to constipation, fecal impaction, or urinary retention.

Marked clinical improvement follows the administration of hormone replacement; such medication must be continued for life, although signs of myxedema disappear over a 3- to 12-week period. The realization that the disorder has led to such severe consequences can cause the patient to feel depressed. In such a situation, conveying a sense of understanding and providing time to ventilate anger and frustration will help the patient adjust to the disorder.

GRAVES' DISEASE (HYPERTHYROIDISM)

Spontaneous hyperthyroidism constitutes a well-defined disease entity, variously designated as *Graves' disease, Basedow's disease,* and *exophthalmic goiter.* Its etiology is unknown, but immunoglobulin G (LATS [long-acting thyroid stimulator]) is found in significant concentration in the serum of many of these patients and may be related to a fault in the patient's immune surveillance system. The disorder, which affects women five times more frequently than men, may appear after an emotional shock, nervous strain, or an infection—but the exact significance of these relationships is not understood.

Assessment

Patients with well-developed hyperthyroidism exhibit a characteristic group of symptoms and signs. Their presenting symptom is often nervousness. They are emotionally hyperexcitable, their state of mind is apt to be irritable and apprehensive; they cannot sit quietly; they suffer from palpitation; and their pulse is abnormally rapid at rest as well as on exertion. They tolerate heat poorly and perspire unusually freely; the skin is flushed continuously, with a characteristic salmon color, and is likely to be warm, soft, and moist. A fine tremor of the hands may be observed. Many patients exhibit bulging eyes (exophthalmos), lending a startled expression to the countenance.

Other important symptoms include an increased appetite (unless gastrointestinal symptoms develop), progressive loss of weight, abnormal muscular fatigability and weakness, amenorrhea, and changes in bowel habit, either to constipation or diarrhea. The pulse rate of these patients ranges constantly between 90 and 160; the systolic, but characteristically not diastolic, blood pressure is elevated; atrial fibrillation may appear, and cardiac decompensation is common, especially in elderly patients.

The thyroid gland invariably is enlarged to some extent. It is soft and may pulsate; a thrill often can be felt over the thyroid arteries—a sign of greatly increased blood flow through the organ.

In the more advanced cases, the diagnosis is established readily on the basis of the symptoms and the tests described previously: an increase in serum thyroxine; and an increased ^{131}I uptake by the thyroid (in excess of 50 percent).

The course of the disease may be mild, characterized

by remissions and exacerbations and terminating with spontaneous recovery in the course of a few months or years. On the other hand, it may progress relentlessly, the untreated patient becoming emaciated, intensely nervous, delirious—even disoriented—and the heart eventually "racing itself to death."

Management

As yet, no treatment for hyperthyroidism has been discovered that combats its basic cause. However, reduction of thyroid hyperactivity provides effective symptomatic relief and removes the principal source of its most important complications.

Three forms of treatment are available for the control of excessive thyroid activity: (1) pharmacology, employing antithyroid drugs that interfere with the synthesis of thyroid hormones; (2) radiation, involving the administration of the radioisotope ^{131}I or ^{125}I for destructive effects on the thyroid gland; and (3) surgery, whereby most of the thyroid gland is removed.

In addition to the three primary methods of treatment, adjunctive therapy in the form of sympathetic antagonist drugs may be used. Examples are reserpine, propranolol, and guanethidine, which are useful in controlling nervousness, tachycardia, and tremor.

Pharmacotherapy. The objective of pharmacotherapy is to inhibit one or more stages in hormone synthesis or hormone release; another goal may be to reduce the amount of thyroid tissue, thereby reducing hormone production.

Antithyroid drugs (thiocarbamides, thioamides) effectively block the utilization of iodine by interfering with the iodination of thyrosine and the coupling of iodothyrosines in the synthesis of thyroid hormones. Since this prevents the synthesis of thyroid hormone, the patient with hyperthyroidism is greatly benefitted. The most commonly used medications are propylthiouracil (PTU) or methimazole (Tapazole), until the patient is euthyroid (i.e., neither hyper- nor hypo-thyroid). PTU blocks extrathyroidal conversion of thyroxine (T_4) to triiodothyronine (T_3). Stabilizing the patient usually takes from 3 to 6 weeks, at which time the maintenance dose is established, followed by a gradual withdrawal of the medication over the next several months.

Therapy is controlled on the basis of clinical criteria, including changes in pulse rate, pulse pressure, body weight, size of the goiter, and basal metabolic rate. Perhaps up to half of the patients experience prolonged remission of hyperthyroidism after thiocarbamide therapy is withdrawn. Toxic complications of thiocarbamides are relatively uncommon; nevertheless, periodic examinations cannot be neglected, in view of the possibility that drug sensitization, followed by fever, rash, urticaria, or even granulopenia, may develop. With any sign of infection, especially pharyngitis and fever, the patient is advised to stop the medication, call the physician, and probably have a blood examination. Patients on antithyroid drugs are instructed not to use decongestants for nasal stuffiness because they are poorly tolerated.

At times, thyroid hormone is given together with antithyroid drugs in an attempt to put the thyroid gland at rest. In this approach, hypothyroidism from excess antithyroid drug is avoided, as is stimulation of the thyroid gland by thyroid-stimulating hormone. Thyroid hormone is available as desiccated thyroid, thyroglobulin (Proloid), and sodium levothyroxine (Synthroid sodium). These are slow-acting preparations which take about 10 days to achieve their full effect. Sodium liothyronine (Cytomel) has a more rapid onset and lasts a short time.

Adjunctive Therapy. Lugol's solution (concentrated iodine solution) is a preparation of iodine rarely used as sole therapy in treating patients with hyperthyroidism. It acutely reduces the release of thyroid hormones from the thyroid (an effect lasting only a few weeks) and reduces the vascularity and size of the thyroid. It is used in preparing the patient for a subtotal thyroidectomy and for patients with thyrotoxic crisis. Reducing glandular vascularity prevents postoperative hemorrhage.

Lugol's solution is more palatable in milk or fruit juice and is taken through a straw, to prevent staining of the teeth. It reduces the metabolic rate more rapidly than antithyroid drugs, but its action is not as lasting.

Radioactive Iodine. Until recently, radioiodine was considered an ideal form of treatment for diffuse toxic goiter. The eventual occurrence of hypothyroidism, however, is one of the more prominent objections. Practically all of the iodine that enters and is retained in the body becomes concentrated within the thyroid gland. This applies to the radioactive isotopes of iodine as well, providing the basis for a very effective device for the selective inhibition of thyroid activity, namely, by the administration of radioiodine (^{131}I). The objective of this treatment is the irradiation of the gland, which is accomplished without jeopardizing other radiosensitive tissues. Radioactive iodine has been used in toxic adenomas or multinodular goiter, in most varieties of thyrotoxicosis (rarely permanently successful), and is especially preferred for the treatment of patients over 35 with diffuse toxic goiter.

As primary therapy, antithyroid drugs are given for 6 to 18 months. When drugs are given as temporary therapy for the purpose of reducing the production of hormones to normal, radiation or surgical therapy can then be undertaken safely.

Nursing supervision of this patient is primarily a teaching function. The patient is instructed as to what to expect of this tasteless, colorless radioiodine which is administered by the physician. No radiation precautions are necessary unless excretions are expelled on sheets or garments; decontamination would then be required. Usually the patient is discharged and followed by community nursing service until he returns to the euthyroid status.

A single dose of the drug is given by mouth (a radioactive "cocktail"), based on 80–160 microcuries per gram of estimated thyroid weight. The patient is watched for signs of thyroid storm (page 867).

In about 3 to 4 weeks, symptoms of hyperthyroidism subside. If remission is not achieved, the treatment is repeated after several months. Close supervision is required by periodic visits to the physician to ascertain normal rates of function. If hypothyroidism results from gland destruction, thyroid hormones will have to be taken by the patient.

Those caring for the patient need to give reassurance, since patients often overreact to such medications as radioactive drugs, which require special supervision.

Surgical Intervention. The surgical removal of about five-sixths of the thyroid tissue (subtotal thyroidectomy) practically assures a prolonged remission in most patients with exophthalmic goiter. Before surgery, the patient is given propylthiouracil until signs of hyperthyroidism have disappeared. Iodine also is prescribed, either before or after a full remission has been achieved with propylthiouracil. The effect of iodine is to reduce the size and the vascularity of the goiter. It may be given in the form of Lugol's solution, potassium iodide, or hydriodic acid.

- Patients receiving iodine medication must be watched for evidence of iodine toxicity (iodism), the appearance of which is the signal for immediate withdrawal of the drug. Symptoms of iodism include swelling of the buccal mucosa, excessive salivation, coryza, and skin eruptions.

Thyroidectomy usually is scheduled within a few days after the patient's basal metabolic rate has been reduced to normal.

In appraising the value of surgery, it is considered a less than ideal form of treatment, because there is a possibility of permanent postoperative hypothyroidism (there is a somewhat similar problem with radioiodine therapy), of hypoparathyroidism, and of damage to the recurrent laryngeal nerve. (See page 867 for pre- and postoperative management of the patient undergoing thyroidectomy.)

Overview of Nursing Management. The objectives of nursing management are to assist the patient in overcoming his symptoms and to help him return to a euthyroid condition. It is best to maintain a calm manner in approaching the patient, since much of his nervousness and anxiety is beyond his control. Added stress arises from a fear of cancer, which the patient may relate to the weight loss which is a characteristic feature of hyperthyroidism. In the initial nursing assessment, it is desirable to uncover such thoughts and to allay fears that are not justified.

Activities to lessen the irritability of the nervous system resulting from hyperthyroidism may include the following: protecting the patient from stressful experiences, such as upsetting visitors or the presence of annoying or very ill patients; providing a cool and uncluttered environment; and encouraging the patient to enjoy pleasant music, light television entertainment, and interesting and relaxing hobbies.

Hyperthyroidism also affects the gastrointestinal system. The appetite is increased but can be satisfied by providing several well-balanced meals of small size, even up to six meals a day. Proper foods and fluids are given to control diarrhea, which may result in weight loss and nutritional imbalance. Quiet and pleasant surroundings at mealtime will assist the digestive process. Highly seasoned foods, coffee (a stimulant), and alcohol in excess contribute to reflex diarrhea and are to be discouraged. Alcohol presents an additional problem; if the patient is sensitive to it, drinking without food may cause hypoglycemia.

Eye protection is afforded by instilling an ophthalmic medication such as methylcellulose. This is not only soothing, but protects the exposed cornea. The upward gaze increases prominence of the eyes and may provoke strabismus. Since exophthalmos is thought to be caused by excess fluid in the tissues, it may be helpful if salt and water intake are restricted. Tactfully moving the furniture in the room so that the patient does not see his reflection in a dresser mirror is a thoughtful maneuver. Friends and visitors are advised not to comment on the patient's protruding eyes.

THYROIDITIS

Subacute or granulomatous thyroiditis (deQuervain's thyroiditis), an inflammatory disorder of the thyroid gland which predominantly affects women in their 50s, presents as a painful swelling in the anterior neck that lasts 1 or 2 months, then disappears without residual effects. Evidence indicates that this disorder may be due to a viral infection. The thyroid enlarges symmetrically and occasionally is painful. The overlying skin is often reddened and warm. Swallowing may be difficult and uncomfortable. Irritability, nervousness, insomnia, and weight loss—manifestations of hyperthyroidism—are common, and many patients experience chills and fever as well.

The purpose of treatment is to control the inflammation. In general, acetylsalicylic acid (aspirin) controls symptoms in mild cases; in more severe infections, glucocorticoids (prednisone) are effective but do not necessarily influence the underlying cause.

Chronic Thyroiditis (Hashimoto's Thyroiditis).

Chronic thyroiditis, predominantly a disease of women from 30 to 50 years of age, has been classified as "Hashimoto's disease" depending on the histologic appearance of the inflamed gland. In contrast with acute thyroiditis, the chronic varieties are usually not accompanied by pain, pressure symptoms, or fever, and thyroid activity is apt to be normal or low, rather than increased.

There is evidence to suggest that cell-mediated immunity plays a significant role in the pathogenesis of thyroiditis. A genetic predisposition also seems to be significant in etiology. If untreated, the disease runs a slow progressive course leading eventually to myxedema.

The objective of treatment is to reduce the size of the thyroid gland and prevent myxedema. Thyroid hormone therapy is prescribed to reduce thyroid activity and the production of thyroglobulin. If hypothyroid symptoms are present, thyroid hormone is given. Thiocarbamide drugs may be given if an associated thyrotoxicosis exists. Surgery may be required if pressure symptoms persist.

THYROID TUMORS

Tumors of the thyroid gland are classified on the basis of being benign or malignant, as well as on the presence or absence of associated thyrotoxicosis, and the diffuse or irregular quality of the glandular enlargement. If the enlargement is sufficient to cause a visible swelling in the neck, the tumor is referred to as a "goiter."

All grades of goiter are encountered, from those that are barely visible to those producing an unsightly disfigurement. Some are symmetrical and diffuse, others nodular. Some are accompanied by hyperthyroidism, in which case they are described as "toxic"; others are associated with a euthyroid state and are called "nontoxic" goiters.

ENDEMIC (IODINE-DEFICIENT) GOITER.

The most common type of goiter, encountered chiefly in geographic regions where the natural supply of iodine is deficient (e.g., the Great Lakes area of the United States), is the so-called *simple* or *colloid goiter*. Aside from being caused by an iodine deficiency, simple goiter may also be caused by an intake of large quantities of goitrogenic substances in patients with unusually susceptible glands. These substances include excessive amounts of iodine or of lithium, which is currently in vogue in the treatment of manic-depressive states.

Simple goiter represents a compensatory hypertrophy on the part of the entire gland, presumably due to stimulation by the pituitary gland. The pituitary gland produces a hormone controlling thyroid growth, and this production is excessive if there is subnormal thyroid activity, as when insufficient iodine is available for production of the thyroid hormone. Such goiters usually cause no symptoms except for the swelling in the neck, which may result in tracheal compression, when excessive.

Management.

Many goiters of this type recede after iodine imbalance is corrected. Supplementary iodine such as saturated solution of potassium iodide (SSKI) is prescribed in order to depress the pituitary's thyroid-stimulating activity.

Surgery is recommended for certain patients with exophthalmic goiter when suggested criteria are met so that postoperative complications are minimized. Optimal conditions are (1) a relatively young person without the complications of concurrent medical illnesses such as diabetes, heart disease, drug allergies, (2) a preoperative euthyroid state resulting from treatment with antithyroid drugs, (3) proper preoperative iodide administration to reduce the size and vascularity of the goiter, and (4) an experienced surgeon in thyroid surgery.

Patient Teaching.

Simple goiter can be prevented by providing children in iodine-poor districts with iodine compounds. If the mean iodine intake is less than 40 μg. per day, the thyroid hypertrophies. The World Health Organization recommends that salt be iodized to a concentration of one part in 100,000, which is adequate for the prevention of endemic goiter. In the United States, salt is iodized to one part in 10,000.

NODULAR GOITER.

Certain thyroid glands are nodular because of the presence of one or several areas of *hyperplasia* (overgrowth) that appear to develop under conditions similar to those responsible for the colloid goiter. No symptoms may arise as a result of this condition, but, not uncommonly, these nodules slowly increase in size, some descending into the thorax, where they cause local pressure symptoms. Some nodules become malignant and some become associated with a hyperthyroid state. Thus, many nodular thyroids eventually require surgical attention.

THYROID CANCER

Cancer of the thyroid is much less prevalent than other forms of cancer. According to the American Cancer Society, approximately 1,000 patients die annually of this malignancy. The most common type is papillary adenocarcinoma, which accounts for over half of thyroid malignancy. This neoplasm starts in childhood or early adult life, remains localized, and eventually metastasizes along the lymphatics and lymph nodes. It appears as an asymptomatic nodule in a normal gland.

An association exists between external radiation of the head and neck in infancy and childhood and subsequent development of thyroid carcinoma. (Between 1940 to 1960 radiation therapy was usually given to shrink enlarged tonsillar and adenoid tissue, to treat acne, or to reduce an enlarged thymus.) Consequently, the American Thyroid Association emphasizes that people who underwent such treatment should consult a physician, request an isotope thyroid scan as part of the evaluation, either submit to surgical thyroidectomy or take thyroid hormones if prescribed for abnormalities of the gland, and continue with annual checkups if all is normal.

Follicular adenocarcinoma appears in later life, usually over age 40, and accounts for about 20 to 25 percent of thyroid neoplasms. It is encapsulated and feels elastic or rubbery on palpation. This tumor eventually spreads by hematogenous routes to bone, liver, and lung. The prognosis is not as favorable as for papillary adenocarcinoma.

Other types of cancer are medullary (5 percent), which present as solid, hard nodular tumors, and anaplastic (5 percent), which are hard, irregular masses that grow quickly and may be painful and tender.

Management. Proper management of thyroid carcinoma is surgical removal, the extensiveness of the resection varying from clinic to clinic. Total or near total thyroidectomy is performed when possible.

Modified neck dissection is done if there is lymph node involvement. Following surgery, ablation procedures are carried out with [131]radioactive iodine to eradicate residual thyroid tissue. Radioactive iodine also maximizes the chance of discovering thyroid metastasis at a later stage if total body scans are carried out.

Following surgery, thyroid hormone is administered in suppressive doses to lower the levels of thyroid-stimulating hormone (TSH) to an euthyroid state. Prior to planned total body scans, thyroid hormones are stopped for about a month preceding the tests.

Patient Teaching. Later follow-up includes clinical assessment for recurrence of nodules or masses in the neck, signs of hoarseness, dysphagia, or dyspnea. Chest x-rays are done as recommended. Total body scans are advised annually for the first 3 postoperative years and less frequently thereafter.

T_4, TSH levels, serum calcium and phosphorus are assessed to determine if the thyroid hormone supplementation is adequate and to note whether calcium balance is maintained.

While radiation sickness (page 293), neutropenia, or thrombocytopenia (page 672) may occur, these complications are rare when ^{131}I is used. Surgery combined with radioiodine produces a higher survival rate than does surgery alone.

THYROID CRISIS OR STORM

Thyroid storm or thyrotoxic crisis is a form of severe hyperthyroidism, usually of abrupt onset and characterized by hyperpyrexia, extreme tachycardia, and altered mental state (delirium). Thyroid storm is a life-threatening condition and is usually precipitated by stress such as injury, infection, nonthyroid surgery, thyroidectomy, tooth extraction, insulin reaction, diabetic acido-sis, digitalis intoxication, abrupt withdrawal of antithyroid drugs, or vigorous palpation of the thyroid. These factors will precipitate thyroid storm in the partially controlled or completely untreated hyperthyroid patient. Patients who are maintained in an euthyroid state through the proper adjustment of an antithyroid drug may go through many of these episodes without a crisis being precipitated.

While thyroid crisis may be difficult to identify, the following signs are suggestive: (1) tachycardia (over 130), (2) temperature above 37.7° C. (100° F.), (3) exaggerated symptoms of thyrotoxicosis, and (4) disturbances of a major system, e.g., gastrointestinal (weight loss, diarrhea, abdominal pain), neurological (psychosis, somnolence, coma), or cardiovascular (edema, chest pain, dyspnea, palpitations).

Untreated thyroid storm is almost always fatal, but with proper treatment, the mortality rate can be reduced to nearly 20 percent.

Management. The immediate objective is to reduce body temperature and heart rate. Measures to reduce the temperature include ice packs, fans, air-conditioned room, and hydrocortisone. Acetaminophen is preferred to aspirin (salicylates) because aspirin displaces T_4 and T_3 from thyroxine-binding globulin, thereby leading to an increase in free thyroid hormones. Oxygen is administered to improve tissue oxygenation, thereby meeting the high metabolic demand. Dextrose-containing intravenous fluids are administered to replace liver glycogen stores that have been decreased in the hyperthyroid patient.

Lugol's solution, intravenous sodium iodide, or saturated solution of potassium iodide (SSKI) orally may be given to decrease thyroxine output from the gland. Propylthiouracil (PTU) or methimazole are given to interrupt hormonogenesis. Hydrocortisone is prescribed to treat shock or adrenal insufficiency. For cardiac symptoms of an uncontrolled nature, sympatholytic agents are given. Guanethidine, reserpine, or propranolol may be effective in some patients.

When other efforts fail to reduce the level of serum thyroxine, it may be necessary to resort to exchange transfusion or peritoneal dialysis. Vitamin and mineral balance may indicate the need for the administration of vitamin B_{12}. Hyperthyroidism increases the requirement for thiamin.

THYROIDECTOMY

Preoperative Management. One important approach in the preoperative period is to gain the complete confidence of the patient and keep him free from worry and anxiety. Some forms of occupational therapy are recommended because they are quieting and relaxing.

The patient with hyperthyroidism often comes from a

home made tense and unhappy by his restlessness and nervousness. It is necessary to protect the patient from such unpleasantness and unhappiness. If there is any evidence of nervous upsets when family or friends visit, it may be advisable to limit the visiting privileges during the preoperative period.

Nutritional intake is to be regulated to include adequate carbohydrate and protein foods. A high daily caloric intake is necessary because of the increased metabolic activity and rapid depletion of glycogen reserves. Supplementary vitamins, particularly thiamine chloride and ascorbic acid, are to be provided. Tea and coffee are avoided because of their stimulating effects.

As with any diagnostic procedure, the patient is informed of the purpose of the test and the preoperative preparations in order to reduce anxiety. In addition, a special effort is made to ensure a good night's rest preceding surgery.

Preoperative teaching includes demonstrating to the patient how to support his neck with his hands to prevent stress on the incision, i.e., raising his elbows and placing his hands behind his neck will provide support and put much less strain and tension on the neck muscles.

Postoperative Management. The patient is moved with a great deal of care so as to support the head and avoid tension on the sutures. The most comfortable position is the semi-Fowler position with the head elevated and supported by pillows. The utmost quiet is observed, and narcotics are given as prescribed for pain. Occasionally the patient is given oxygen for the first few hours to facilitate breathing. The nurse should anticipate apprehension in the patient and inform him that oxygen will assist his breathing and help him to feel less tired. Fluid may be given by vein, but water may be given by mouth as soon as nausea ceases. Usually, there is a little difficulty in swallowing, and in this condition cold fluids and ice may be taken better than other fluids. Often patients prefer a soft diet to a liquid diet.

The dressings should be checked periodically and reinforced when necessary. It is important to remember that when the patient is in the dorsal position, evidences of bleeding should be looked for at the sides and the back of the neck as well as anteriorly. In addition to checking the pulse and the blood pressure for any indication of internal bleeding, it is also important to be on the alert for complaints from the patient of a sensation of pressure or fullness at the incision site. Such signs may indicate hemorrhage and should be reported.

Talking should be limited, but when the patient does speak, the nurse should note any voice changes which might indicate injury to the recurrent laryngeal nerve that lies just behind the thyroid next to the trachea.

Occasionally, difficulty in respiration occurs, with the development of cyanosis and noisy breathing, as a result of edema of the glottis or an injury to the recurrent laryngeal nerve. Since this complication requires that a tracheostomy tube be inserted, the surgeon is summoned at once.

When the nurse is not in constant attendance, an over-bed table may be used to afford easy access to those materials and items that are needed frequently, such as paper wipes, water pitcher and glass, small emesis basin, etc. These are kept within easy reach so that the patient will not need to turn his head in search of them. It is also convenient to use this table when inhalations are given for the relief of excessive mucous secretions.

The patient usually is permitted out of bed on the first postoperative day and has a choice of diet. A well-balanced high-caloric diet is prescribed to regain any weight loss. Sutures or skin clips usually are removed on the second day. By the fifth day, the average patient is ready for discharge from the hospital.

Complications. Hemorrhage, edema of the glottis, and injury to the recurrent laryngeal nerve are complications that have been reviewed previously. Occasionally, in thyroid operations, the parathyroid glands may be injured or removed, producing a disturbance of the calcium metabolism of the body. As the blood calcium falls, there appears a hyperirritability of the nerves, with spasms of the hands and feet and muscular twitchings; this group of symptoms is termed *tetany,* and its appearance should be reported at once. Tetany of this type usually is relieved by the administration of calcium in some form.

Patient Teaching. The patient should not be permitted to resume his former activities or responsibilities completely until thyrotoxicosis has been eliminated. The necessity for rest, relaxation, and nutrition is explained to both the patient and his family at the time of discharge. Specific instructions are issued regarding follow-up visits to the physician or the clinic, which are inevitably necessary and invariably important.

Responsibilities and factors relating to the home environment that engender emotional tension often have been implicated as precipitating causes of thyrotoxicosis. The patient's hospitalization affords an opportunity to evaluate these factors and possibly alter the environmental situation. This is the most favorable time for establishing a close rapport with the patient and for supplying whatever psychological support and assistance are needed to promote emotional readjustments.

THE PARATHYROID GLANDS

HYPERPARATHYROIDISM

Hyperparathyroidism, due to an overgrowth of the parathyroid glands, is characterized by bony calcification and the development of renal stones containing calcium in the kidneys. Parathyroid hyperactivity with similar manifestations also occurs in patients with chronic nephritis and so-called "renal rickets," presumably as a result of phosphorus retention and a secondary increase in parathyroid level.

Clinical Manifestations and Diagnosis. These patients experience symptoms of apathy, fatigue, muscular weakness, nausea, vomiting, constipation, and cardiac arrhythmias, all attributable to an increased concentration of calcium in the blood. Psychosocial manifestations may vary from emotional irritability and neurosis to psychoses due to the direct effect of calcium on the brain. Occasionally the patient may be misdiagnosed as "psychoneurotic." An increase in calcium actually produces an increase in the excitation potential of nerve and muscle tissue.

The formation of stones in one or both kidneys (usually one at a time), related to the increased urinary excretion of calcium and phosphorus, is one of the important complications of hyperparathyroidism. Renal damage results from the precipitation of calcium phosphate in the renal pelvis and parenchyma (nephrocalcinosis) often promoting pyelonephritis and uremia.

In the past, skeletal changes were the characteristic hallmark of hyperparathyroidism, whether as a primary disorder or as a secondary complication of calcium and phosphorus retention in patients with chronic renal disease. There are two aspects of this bony involvement to be considered: (1) demineralization of the bones, resulting in skeletal pain and tenderness, pain on weight-bearing, pathologic fractures, deformities, shortening of body structure, and the formation of bony cysts; (2) the development of bone tumors, composed of benign giant cells and representing an overgrowth of osteoclasts. This variety of neoplasm is encountered occasionally on dental examination and is manifested as a tumor of the jaw (referred to as an "epulis"). In the United States today, most cases of hyperparathyroidism are discovered through the recognition of hypercalcemia on a multichannel autoanalyzer before serious bone or renal pathology has occurred.

Further diagnosis is established by the clinical picture, by persistently elevated serum calcium, and by skeletal changes detected by x-ray pictures. Only occasionally can a parathyroid tumor be palpated. The Sulkowitch test* for calcium excretion in the urine is also a screening diagnostic aid.

Management. By being aware of the symptoms of hypersecretion of the parathyroid glands, the nurse is aware of the loosely related array of patient manifesta-

---

*Mix:
A 24-hour urine collection is made. Equal amounts of reagent (oxalic acid, ammonium oxalate, glacial acetic acid) and urine will produce a reaction.
Reaction:
Normal—fine white cloud of precipitated calcium, Hypercalcemia—heavy milky precipitate, Hypocalcemia—absence of precipitate.

tions, one of which is frustration because of the insidious and chronic nature of the problem.

In the preoperative period it must be recognized that kidney involvement is possible, since these patients are subject to renal calculi. Fluids to 2,000 ml. are encouraged to help prevent calculi formation. However, thiazide diuretics should not be used in the patient with hyperparathyroidism since they decrease the renal excretion of calcium, thereby causing hypercalcemia. Cranberry juice is suggested because it is effective in lowering urinary pH. It can be added to juices and ginger ale for variety. Because of the possibility of stone formation, urine is strained, and any evidence of calculi is saved for laboratory analysis. The patient is observed for other manifestations such as abdominal pain and hematuria.

Mobility of the patient (sitting in a rocking chair or walking) is encouraged as much as possible; bones under stress give up less calcium. Bed rest, on the other hand, increases calcium excretion.

Nutritional needs are met, but foods high in calcium and phosphorus, such as milk and milk products, are limited. Occasionally this patient may have a coexisting peptic ulcer which requires specifically prescribed antacids and protein feedings. Since anorexia is common, all efforts to encourage the patient's appetite are made. Prune juice, stool softeners, and physical activity, along with increased fluid intake, should offset constipation, a common postoperative problem for this patient.

The treatment of hyperparathyroidism is the surgical removal of abnormal parathyroid tissue. The nursing management is essentially the same as that for a thyroidectomy patient (page 867). The patient must be closely watched to detect symptoms of tetany, which may be an early postoperative occurrence.

HYPOPARATHYROIDISM

Hypoparathyroidism occurs when too much parathyroid tissue is removed surgically or in association with idiopathic atrophy.

Pathophysiology. Symptoms of hypoparathyroidism are due to a deficiency of parathormone which results in an elevation of blood phosphate (hyperphosphatemia) and a decrease in the concentration of blood calcium (hypocalcemia). Hypocalcemia results because the deficiency of parathormone causes a decrease in the intestinal absorption of dietary calcium and a decrease in the resorption of calcium from bone and through the renal tubules. Decreased renal excretion of phosphate causes hypophosphaturia, while low serum calcium results in hypocalciuria.

Clinical Manifestations. Hypocalcemia causes irritability of the neuromuscular system and contributes to the chief symptom of hypoparathyroidism, *tetany*—a general muscular hypertonia, with tremor and spasmodic or incoordinated contractions occurring with or without efforts to make voluntary movements. In latent tetany there is numbness, tingling, and cramps in the extremities, with the patient complaining of stiffness in the hands and feet. In overt tetany the signs include bronchospasm, laryngeal spasm, carpopedal spasm (flexion of the elbows and wrists and extension of the carpophalangeal joints—Fig. 40-2), dysphagia, photophobia, cardiac arrhythmias, and convulsions. Psychiatric symptoms include anxiety, irritability, depression, and even delirium.

Assessment. Latent tetany is suggested by a positive Trousseau's sign or a positive Chvostek's sign. *Trousseau's sign* is positive when carpopedal spasm is induced by occluding the blood flow to the arm for 3 minutes (using a blood pressure cuff). *Chvostek's sign* is usually positive when a sharp tapping over the facial nerve just in front of the parotid gland (anterior to the ear) causes the mouth, nose, and eye to twitch.

The diagnosis is often difficult because of vague symptoms of aches and pains, as well as neuroses. Therefore, laboratory studies are especially helpful. Serum calcium is at 5-6 mg./100 ml. when tetany develops. Serum phosphate increases, and x-ray studies of bone show increased density. Calcification is noticed on x-rays of subcutaneous or paraspinal basal ganglia of the brain.

Management. The objective of therapy is to elevate serum calcium to approximately 9-10 mg./100 ml. and to render the patient free of symptoms. When hypoparathyroidism occurs with tetany, following a thyroidectomy, the immediate treatment is to administer calcium gluconate intravenously. If this does not control convulsive tendencies immediately, it may be necessary to give chloral hydrate, paraldehyde, or pentobarbital.

Therapy for the patient with chronic hypoparathyroidism is determined after serum calcium levels are studied. The prescribed diet is high in calcium and low in phosphorus. Although milk, milk products, and egg yolk are high in calcium, they are restricted because they also contain high levels of phosphorus. Spinach is also avoided because it contains oxalate which would form insoluble calcium substances. Oral tablets of calcium gluconate may supplement the diet. Aluminum hydroxide gel or aluminum carbonate (Gelusil, Amphojel) is also given after meals to bind phosphate in the intestine.

Variable dosages of a vitamin D preparation, dihydrotachysterol (DHT) (A.T.10 or Hytakerol) or calciferol (vitamin D_2) or cholecalciferol (vitamin D_3) are usually required.

Nursing management encompasses the following actions:
- The attention of the nurse in the care of postoperative thyroidectomy and parathyroidectomy patients is directed toward anticipating signs of tetany, convulsions, and respiratory difficulties.
- Calcium gluconate is kept at the bedside with equipment necessary for intravenous administration. If the patient has cardiac problems, is subject to arrhythmias, or is receiving digitalis, then calcium gluconate is administered by slow infusion.
- Calcium and digitalis increase systolic contraction, and furthermore, they potentiate each other. This may produce potentially fatal arrhythmias. Consequently, the cardiac patient requires constant vigilance and undoubtedly should be on continuous cardiac monitoring.

Because of neuromuscular irritability, the patient requires an environment which is free of noise, sudden drafts, bright lights, or sudden movement. If the patient requires assistance in overcoming respiratory problems, bronchodilating medications, a tracheostomy, or positive pressure apparatus may be necessary.

The convalescent phase of patient care is the time to instruct the patient in drug and diet therapy. He needs to know why he must maintain a high calcium and low phosphate intake, and what the symptoms of hypo- and hypercalcemia are so that he may immediately contact his physician should these symptoms occur.

THE ADRENAL GLAND

Pheochromocytoma

A *pheochromocytoma* is a tumor originating from the adrenal medulla, and in particular, from the chromaffin cells. In 90 percent of patients, the tumor arises in the medulla, whereas in about 10 percent it occurs in the extra-adrenal chromaffin tissue (aorta, ovaries, spleen, or wherever these cells are located). It affects people between the ages of 25 and 50 and is equally divided between males and females. The patient's family should also be screened for this tumor.

Clinical Manifestations. Functioning tumors of the

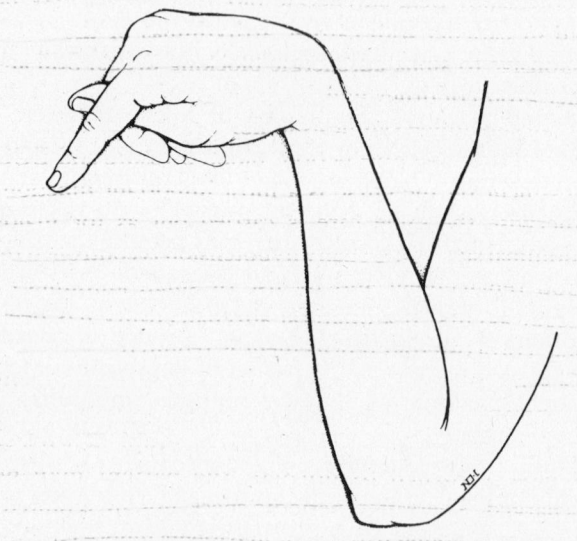

Figure 40-2. Carpopedal spasm.

adrenal medulla cause arterial hypertension and other cardiovascular disturbances. The nature and severity depend on the relative proportions of epinephrine and norepinephrine in its secretions.

The hypertension may be intermittent or persistent. If it is of the sustained type, it may be difficult to distinguish from so-called "essential hypertension." In addition to hypertension, the symptoms are essentially the same as those encountered after the administration of epinephrine in large doses, namely, tachycardia, excessive perspiration, tremor, nervousness, and hyperglycemia. Pharmacological doses of epinephrine stimulate the conversion of liver and muscle glycogen to glucose (hyperglycemia).

The clinical picture in the paroxysmal case of pheochromocytoma usually is characterized by acute, unpredictable attacks, lasting several hours or only a few seconds, during which the patient feels excessively anxious, tremulous, and weak, and suffers from headache, vertigo, blurring of vision, tinnitus, air hunger, and dyspnea. Other symptoms include polyuria, nausea, vomiting, diarrhea, abdominal pain, and fear of death.

Assessment. Because of mass educational programs stressing the importance of periodic blood pressure determination, the nurse is frequently involved in evaluating patients with hypertension. Of particular concern is the patient who experiences attacks of paroxysmal hypertension. (Under 1 percent of hypertensive patients have pheochromocytoma.) These occurrences, along with the precipitating factor, are to be carefully documented. Since paroxysmal hypertension is a frightening experience, the patient should not be left alone.

The diagnosis of pheochromocytoma is suspected if signs of sympathetic overactivity occur in association with marked elevation of blood pressure. Determination of the catecholamines in urine and blood offers the most direct and conclusive test for overactivity of the adrenal medulla. VMA (vanillylmandelic acid) determination in particular is preferable (normal urinary values: 2 to 6 mg./24 hours). In addition, urine collected over a 2- to 3-hour period after a spontaneous or induced attack of hypertension should be assayed for catecholamine content. After a definitive diagnosis of pheochromocytoma is made, the ratio of norepinephrine to epinephrine in the urine may aid in locating the tumor.

Pharmacologic tests may be used for screening purposes, although they are less popular and rarely necessary. They depend on the reaction of the blood pressure to *provocative* drugs and to *adrenergic blocking* drugs. Provocative agents are those that stimulate a sharp rise in arterial pressure, while adrenergic blocking drugs precipitate a definite fall in arterial pressure in patients with this disease. The most commonly used provocative drug is histamine. The test is positive for pheochromocytoma if there is a marked increase in both systolic and diastolic blood pressures within 1 to 4 minutes after the intravenous injection of histamine. (Normotensive persons without pheochromocytoma experience a headache, flush, and often a slight fall in blood pressure.)

The testing agent of choice among the adrenergic blocking agents is phentolamine (Regitine), which neutralizes the action of epinephrine. Injections of this material in patients with epinephrine-secreting tumors cause a precipitous fall in the arterial blood pressure. Norepinephrine (Levophed) should be available if required.

The tyramine test depends on direct release of catecholamines from nerve endings. Rapid intravenous administration of tyramine in graded doses up to 2 mg. will produce an increase in blood pressure within 45 to 60 seconds and will reach a peak in 1 to 1½ minutes. The response lasts less than 3 minutes. If systolic pressure rises 20 to 80 mm. Hg and diastolic pressure rises about 40 mm., it is considered positive. (If the increase in blood pressure is unusually high or prolonged, phentolamine will reverse it rapidly.)

In summary, about 90 percent of patients with pheochromocytoma can be diagnosed by a single test for urinary norepinephrine and epinephrine or VMA levels. Pharmacologic tests are dangerous but may aid in diagnosing the other 10 percent of patients with this condition. Histamine and tyramine tests are performed with caution and not in patients with a blood pressure over 170/100. Adrenergic blocking agents should be used only when the blood pressure is high.

Management. The treatment of pheochromocytoma is surgical removal of the tumor. Preliminary patient preparation includes effective control of blood pressure and blood volumes. Usually this is spread out over 10 days to 2 weeks. Alpha-adrenergic blocking agents such as phentolamine or phenoxybenzamine hydrochloride (Dibenzyline) may be used safely without causing undue hypotension. Beta adrenergic blocking agents may be used in patients with cardiac arrhythmias or those not responsive to alpha-adrenergic blocking drugs. Still another group of drugs which may be used preoperatively are catecholamine synthesis inhibitors.

In the postoperative period, blood pressure and ECG assessment by the nurse is a most important function. Otherwise the same care is carried out as for major abdominal surgery. Usually hypotension is controlled by blood replacement and by use of small amounts of pressor agents. If a bilateral adrenalectomy has been done, corticosteroid replacement is required.

Several days after surgery, 24-hour urine excretion of catecholamines and their metabolites is measured to determine whether surgery has been successful. When levels have returned to normal, the patient may be discharged. Thereafter, periodic check-ups are required, especially in young patients or in patients whose families have a history of pheochromocytoma.

ADRENAL CORTEX

For the most part, the adrenal cortex is considered necessary for life. Adrenocortical secretions make it easier for the body to adapt to stress of all kinds. How well one adapts varies from individual to individual, although severe shock will cause peripheral circulatory failure and prostration. Without the adrenal cortex, life can be maintained with nutritional and electrolyte replacement and with replacement of adrenocortical hormones.

Adrenocortical hormones are classified into three groups: mineralocorticoids, glucocorticoids, and sex hormones. *Mineralocorticoids* are concerned with sodium and water retention and potassium excretion. Examples are aldosterone (secreted by the adrenal cortex) and desoxycorticosterone, a natural precursor of aldosterone. *Glucocorticoids* are concerned with metabolic effects, including carbohydrate metabolism. Examples are cortisol and corticosterone. Glucocorticoids enhance the metabolic breakdown of body proteins and fat to provide fuel during periods of fasting. They antagonize the action of insulin, enhance protein catabolism, and inhibit protein synthesis. They affect defense mechanisms of the body and influence emotional functioning either directly or indirectly. In high concentrations, they suppress inflammation and inhibit scar tissue formation. In adrenal insufficiency, patients may be depressed and upset, whereas with excessive replacement they tend to become optimistic, happy, and euphoric. The *sex hormones* secreted by the adrenal cortex are androgens and estrogens.

Disorders of the adrenal cortex develop as a result of hypo- or hypersecretion of the adrenocortical hormones. Adrenal insufficiency may result from disease, atrophy, hemorrhage, or surgical removal of the adrenal gland or glands.

Addison's Disease (Chronic Primary Adrenocortical Insufficiency)

Pathophysiology and Clinical Manifestations. Addison's disease, caused by a deficiency of cortical hormones, results when the adrenal cortex is destroyed, often as a result of idiopathic atrophy or infections such as tuberculosis or histoplasmosis. This hormonal deficiency gives rise to a characteristic clinical picture. The chief clinical manifestations include muscular weakness, anorexia, gastrointestinal symptoms, fatigue, emaciation, generalized dark pigmentation of the skin, hypotension, low blood sugar, low blood sodium, and high serum potassium. In severe cases the disturbance of sodium and potassium metabolism may be marked with depletion of the sodium and water through the urine and severe chronic dehydration.

Assessment. Although the clinical manifestations presented appear specific, the onset of Addison's disease usually occurs with nonspecific symptoms. The community nurse might very well think of Addison's disease when a patient displays vague signs and is referred to as "psychoneurotic." The eventual diagnosis of Addison's disease depends on the proper laboratory tests. Suggested laboratory findings include a decrease in the concentrations of blood sugar and sodium (hypoglycemia and hyponatremia), an increased concentration of blood potassium (hyperkalemia), and relative lymphocytosis.

The definitive diagnosis depends on the demonstration of low levels of adrenocorticol hormones in the blood or urine. If the adrenal cortex is destroyed, baseline values are low, and ACTH injection fails to cause the normal rise in plasma cortisol and urinary 17-hydroxycorticosteroids. If the adrenal gland is normal but not stimulated properly by the pituitary, a response to repeated dosages of exogenous ACTH is seen, but no response follows the administration of metyrapone (which stimulates endogenous ACTH).

As the disease progresses, with acute hypotension developing due to hypocorticism, the patient moves into Addisonian crisis, which is a medical emergency marked by cyanosis, fever, and the classic signs of shock: pallor, apprehension, rapid weak pulse, rapid respirations, and low blood pressure. In addition, the patient may complain of headache, nausea, abdominal pain, and diarrhea, and show signs of confusion and restlessness. Even slight overexertion, exposure to cold, acute infections, a decrease in the salt intake, or diarrhea from overenthusiastic purgation may lead to circulatory collapse.

Management. Immediate treatment is directed toward combating shock: restoring blood circulation, administering fluids, monitoring vital signs, and positioning the patient in a recumbent position with legs elevated. Emotional support is provided the patient concurrently with physical care. Hydrocortisone is given intravenously and followed with 5 percent dextrose in normal saline. Vasopressor amines may be required if hypotension persists.

When the patient's condition is stabilized, precautions are taken to avoid stressful conditions, since this could precipitate another hypotensive experience. Attempts are made to detect signs of infection which may have triggered the crisis in the first place.

By the second or third day, oral intake may be initiated. Fruit juice and broth (salted) are given to supply sodium in an effort to correct electrolyte imbalance. Gradually, intravenous fluids are decreased as oral fluids are accepted.

During hospital convalescence, the nurse watches for symptoms of sodium or potassium imbalance. Vital signs continue to be monitored, and the patient's physical energy and emotional state are assessed. Cortisol (hydrocortisone) continues to be administered to simulate the diurnal pattern of normal secretion (highest levels between 4 and 6 A.M., and lowest in the evening).

When the patient is discharged from the hospital, the

basal dosage of cortisol is established; however, the patient is instructed to supplement this dosage during stressful conditions. He needs to know the signs of excessive or insufficient amounts, since he will be managing his own intake. He probably should get professional guidance in dosage changes.

Cushing's Syndrome

Cushing's syndrome is the antithesis of Addison's disease, its clinical characteristics reflecting excessive, rather than deficient, adrenocortical activity. The syndrome may result from excessive administration of cortisone or ACTH, or hyperplasia of the adrenal cortex.

The basic lesion responsible for Cushing's syndrome may be a tumor arising in the cortex of one of the adrenal glands or a basophilic adenoma of the pituitary glands (page 1225) involving an overgrowth of pituitary cells producing the adrenocorticotrophic hormone (ACTH).

Assessment and Clinical Manifestations. Diagnostic evaluation of this syndrome includes an increase in blood sodium and blood sugar and a decreased concentration of potassium, a reduction in the number of blood eosinophils, and a disappearance of lymphoid tissue.

Levels of 17-hydroxycorticoids and 17-ketosteroids in the urine are elevated, as is plasma cortisol. Plasma ACTH is elevated in those cases caused by pituitary tumor.

When overproduction of the adrenal cortical hormone occurs, growth arrest, obesity, and increased bone age occur. In females of all ages, osteoporosis, typical facies, and variable elements of virilization are produced. Excess androgens also cause virilism, which is characterized by the appearance of masculine traits and the recession of feminine physical and mental traits. There is an excessive growth of hair on the face (hirsutism), the breasts atrophy, menses cease, the clitoris enlarges, and the patient's voice and habits approach the masculine.

The classical picture of Cushing's syndrome in the adult shows a characteristic "central type obesity," with a fatty "buffalo hump" in the neck and supraclavicular areas, a heavy trunk, and relatively thin extremities (Fig. 40-3). The skin is thinned and fragile; ecchymoses and striae develop. The face is rounded, plethoric, oily, and hirsute. The patient complains of weakness and lassitude. Menses become irregular and scanty, and libido is lost. Muscles are wasted because of excessive protein catabolism, and the patient is susceptible to infections. Osteoporosis occurs, resulting in the characteristic kyphosis, backache, and sometimes compression fractures of the vertebrae. Hypertension commonly develops, and congestive heart failure may occur. Changes occur in mood and mental activity, with the patient occasionally developing a psychosis. If a pituitary tumor is the cause, visual disturbances may exist on rare occasions. These tumors are all small.

Management. Many of the aforementioned man-

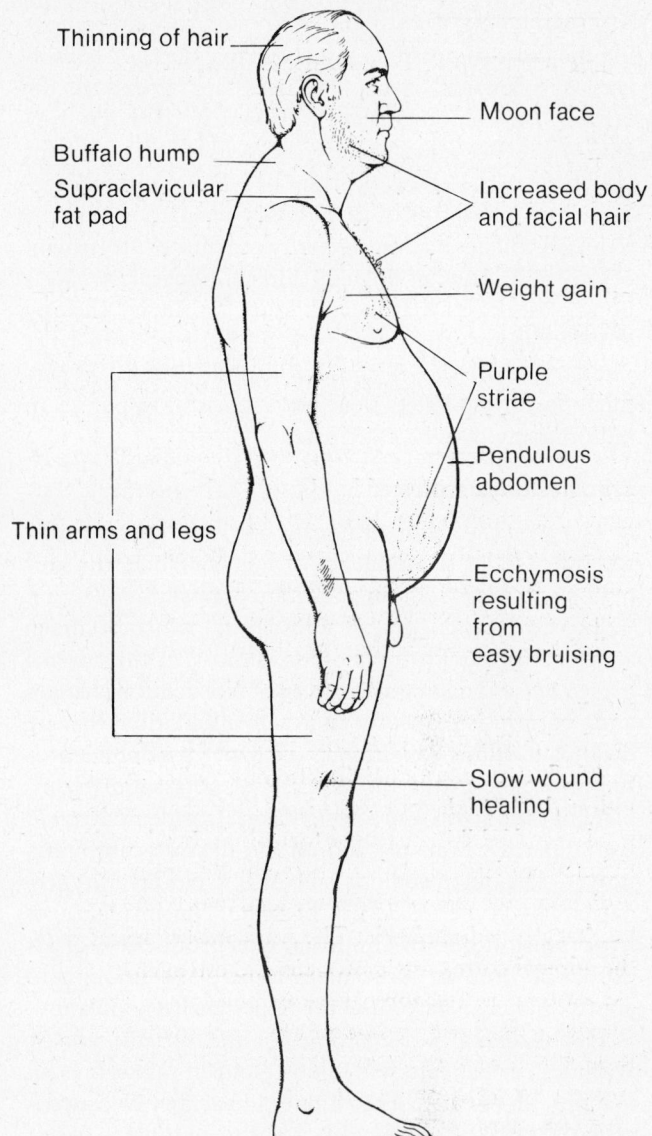

Figure 40-3. Features of Cushing's syndrome invariably include truncal obesity; thin extremities, moon face, buffalo hump, and supraclavicular fullness. Broad purple striae appear at stretch points such as the abdomen, hips, and shoulders. Body and facial hair is increased, and thinning of scalp hair may be noted only if androgens are increased.

Labels on figure: Thinning of hair; Moon face; Buffalo hump; Supraclavicular fat pad; Increased body and facial hair; Weight gain; Purple striae; Pendulous abdomen; Thin arms and legs; Ecchymosis resulting from easy bruising; Slow wound healing

ifestations are due to excessive protein catabolism. Thus, symptoms may be minimized by providing a high-protein, low-carbohydrate, low-sodium diet with supplements of potassium.

Diagnostic evaluation usually involves a total 24-hour urine collection. It is most important that no specimens be missed. Psychosocial concerns of this patient are intense, since the change in physical appearance and altered sex functions give rise to anxiety. The effects on the patient may be manifested in altered behavior, such as anxiety, depression, hostility, and guilt. Learning more about the patient and his responses to stress situations provides a groundwork for appraising the situation and planning the proper approach.

Treatment. Treatment is directed toward removing the cause, if possible. If it is due to externally administered corticoids, it may be necessary to reduce the dosage. On the other hand, this course of action may have to be weighed against the original disorder for which the corticoids were prescribed. For pituitary disorders, hypophysectomy or pituitary irradiation may be required. Bilateral adrenalectomy remains the treatment of choice in cases of bilateral adrenal hyperplasia. Rare hyperplasia cases may benefit from a primary therapy directed against the pituitary, e.g., patients with large pituitary adenomas or those with mild adrenal hyperfunction. In the latter, slow but successful responses to radiotherapy may be anticipated.

Primary Aldosteronism

The principal action of aldosterone is to conserve body sodium. Under the influence of this hormone, the kidneys excrete less sodium and more potassium.

Excessive production of aldosterone, which occurs in some patients with functioning tumors of the adrenal gland, causes a distinctive pattern of biochemical changes and a corresponding set of clinical manifestations that are diagnostic of this condition. Such patients exhibit a profound decline in the blood levels of potassium (hypokalemia) and hydrogen ions (alkalosis), as demonstrated by an increase in its pH and carbon-dioxide-combining power. The blood sodium is normal to elevated (hypernatremia). Hypertension is present. The incidence of hypertension due to abnormal overproduction of aldosterone from an adenoma or hyperplasia amounts to approximately 3 percent of the hypertensive population.

Hypokalemia is responsible for the variable muscle weakness in patients with aldosteronism, as well as an inability on the part of the kidneys to acidify or concentrate the urine. Accordingly, the urine volume is excessive, leading to complaints of polyuria. Blood serum, by contrast, becomes abnormally concentrated, contributing to excessive thirst (polydipsia) and arterial hypertension. A secondary increase in blood volume and possible direct effects of aldosterone on nerve receptors like the carotid sinus are other factors producing the hypertension. Tetany and paresthesias are to be expected in such patients, as complications of alkalosis. Cure usually follows surgical removal of the adrenal tumor.

ADRENALECTOMY

Adrenalectomy, aside from being performed in Cushing's syndrome and primary aldosteronism, is also used for adrenal tumors and for malignancy of the breast and prostate.

For Adrenal Tumors. All of the endocrine disturbances associated with a functioning tumor of the adrenal cortex or medulla can be relieved completely, and the patient improved dramatically, by surgical removal of the involved gland. Adrenalectomy is performed through an incision in the loin or the abdomen. In general, the postoperative care resembles that given for any abdominal operation. Following surgery for adrenal cortical tumors, some patients may require the temporary administration of a steroid hormone, such as hydrocortisone.

As for any surgery, the patient is prepared in the best possible manner before the operation. Hyperglycemia may have to be corrected by diet and insulin; protein deficiency also may have to be ameliorated.

Nursing management in the postoperative period includes frequent blood pressure determination and an assessment of the quality of the pulse, so that early indications of hemorrhage and possible adrenal crisis may be detected. The nurse continues to be aware of replacement therapy in order to avoid acute adrenal insufficiency. Glucocorticoids will be administered until the desired maintenance level is reached. Avoiding stressful situations can be achieved by explaining the treatments, promoting comfort measures, establishing priorities of care, and providing rest periods. Conscientious measures are taken to avoid cardiovascular postoperative complications, since these would require increased glucocorticoids.

For Malignancy of Breasts or Prostate. (See also pages 1008 and 1037.)

Certain malignancies, notably those of the breast and the prostate, are affected by the hormones produced by endocrine glands. Thus the ovary is known to have an effect on carcinoma of the breast, and the testes on carcinoma of the prostate. In some patients, even after suppression of endocrine stimulation, the hormones are still present, and they have been found to arise from adrenal glands. For this reason, bilateral adrenalectomy may be performed in an effort to control or benefit recurrent carcinoma of the breast or the prostate. The adrenals are approached either transabdominally or through the bed of the 12th rib, from behind.

Postoperatively, adrenal cortical hormone must be administered in appropriate dosage to overcome the sudden deprivation of those hormones by the operation. The dosage of adrenal cortical hormone may be reduced gradually as the body adjusts itself to its new plane of hormone production.

CORTICOSTEROID THERAPY

While corticosteroids are used extensively for adrenal insufficiency, they are also widely used in suppressing inflammation and controlling allergic reactions. Such *anti-inflammatory* and *antiallergy* actions make corticosteroids effective in treating collagen diseases such as rheumatoid arthritis, systemic lupus erythematosus, and pemphigus. High doses seem to permit individuals to tolerate higher degrees of stress. Such *anti-stress* action may be due to the ability of corticosteroids to aid circulating vasopressor substances in keeping the blood pressure elevated, or it may be due to other effects, such as the maintenance of plasma glucose.

Although the synthetic steroids are safer for some patients because of relative freedom from mineralocorticoid activity, most natural and synthetic corticosteroids (Table 40-3) produce similar kinds of chronic toxicity. The size of the dose required to bring about desired antiinflammatory and antiallergy effects also causes metabolic toxicity, pituitary gland suppression, and changes in the function of the central nervous system. Such changes may be disabling and even dangerous.

In view of the above, it is obvious that while adrenocorticosteroids are highly effective therapeutically, they may also be very dangerous. Dosages of these medications are frequently altered to allow high concentrations when absolutely necessary and then tapered in an attempt to avoid undesirable effects. This requires that patients be closely observed for side effects and discouraged from depending on these potent drugs when high doses are no longer required.

Problems Encountered in Clinical Use

Dosage of corticosteroids is determined by the nature and chronicity of the illness as well as by any other medical problem the patient has. Rheumatoid arthritis and bronchial asthma are chronic disorders which corticosteroids do not cure; however, these drugs may be useful when other measures no longer provide adequate control. In such a situation, the adverse effects of steroids are weighed against the current problems of the patient. These drugs may be used for a period of time but then should be gradually discontinued as the patient's symptoms subside. The nurse plays an important role in providing encouragement and understanding during the times the patient may feel less comfortable while taking smaller doses.

Acute flare-ups and crises are treated with massive doses of corticosteroids, as in emergency treatment for bronchial obstruction in status asthmaticus, systemic toxicity of an acute rheumatic fever attack, and shock from septicemia caused by gram-negative bacteria. Of course other measures are utilized as required, such as anti-infective agents or drugs, and measures to treat shock.

At times corticosteroids are continued past the acute flare-up stage for the purpose of combating possible complications which are deemed worse than the side effects of steroids. Such conditions may be pemphigus and systemic lupus erythematosus.

A different problem exists when glucocorticosteroids are used in treating eye infections. Outer eye infection

TABLE 40-3. COMMONLY USED STEROID PREPARATIONS

COMMONLY USED NAME	OTHER NAMES
Hydrocortisone	Cortisol, Hydrocortone, Compound F
Cortisone	Cortone, Compound E, Cortogen
DOC	Percorten
Aldosterone	Electrocortin, Aldocorten
Prednisolone	Meticortelone, 1-2 Dehydrocortisol
Prednisone	Meticorten, 1-2 Dehydrocortisone
Methyl prednisolone	Medrol
Triamcinolone	Aristocort, Kenacort
Dexamethasone	Decadron, Hexadrol, 9a-Fluoro-16a-methyl-prednisolone
Fludrocortisone	Florinet, F-Cortef, 9a-Fluoro-hydrocortisone

can be treated by topical application of eye drops, since these do not cause systemic toxicity. However, long-term application may cause an increase in intraocular pressure which may lead to glaucoma in some patients. In other individuals, prolonged use of steroids may lead to cataract formation.

Topical administration of steroids in the form of creams, ointments, lotions, and aerosols are especially effective in many dermatologic disorders. It may be more effective in some conditions to use occlusive dressings around the affected part so that maximum penetration of the drug is achieved. Occasionally intralesional injections are required; however, the adverse effect of the underlying tissues becoming atrophied may occur. Fortunately such dimpling or atrophy is only temporary.

Undesirable Effects of Corticosteroid Therapy

The likelihood of adverse effects is more likely when steroid therapy is used for long periods of time. In general, such effects are classified as follows:

1. Metabolic Effects. Changes in the metabolism may occur following large doses of glucocosteroids or mineralocorticoids. Excessive glucocorticoid activity (hypercorticism) causes clinical manifestations that resemble those noted in Cushing's syndrome (page 873), including the characteristic rounding of the face and an abnormal distribution of body fat.

Because of changes which the steroids make in the metabolism of carbohydrate, protein, and fat, certain other complications may occur. For example, some patients may develop peptic ulcer, diabetes mellitus, or osteoporosis. This does not mean that steroid therapy is to be avoided. It does mean that supportive therapy is required to minimize the threat of these other conditions. For example, it is necessary for the patient with a history of peptic ulcer to continue with antacids and perhaps antispasmodic medications, at the same time recognizing that peptic ulcer pain may not be present as a warning sign during the administration of corticosteroids. For the patient with diabetes, oral hypoglycemia agents should be continued or insulin dosages adjusted as needed. For the patient with osteoporosis, it is helpful to adhere to a high-protein diet and to take calcium salt (a vitamin D supplement), looking out for a possible hypercalciuria. Special efforts are made to prevent an injury that may result in a fracture.

Infection may spread with minimal symptoms, because the patient's defense against invading organisms is lowered by the metabolic effects of the steroid. Viral and fungal infections create further problems because of the difficulty in treating these conditions.

2. Central Nervous System Toxicity. A euphoric effect of happiness and talkativeness results from the action of corticosteroids on the central nervous system. Since such reaction often creates psychological dependency upon steroids, the patient may resist being removed from these drugs. With prolonged use of corticosteroids, the patient may experience mood swings that include excitement, restlessness, depression, and sleeplessness. Nursing support and understanding are required as the patient moves through these experiences. Any tendency to emotional, psychological, or psychotic difficulties needs to be brought to the attention of the physician before steroids are prescribed.

3. Endocrine Toxicity. Prolonged steroid therapy has a tendency to suppress certain functions of the anterior portion of the pituitary gland. Hence, growth in children may be halted following long-term treatment

---

THE PATIENT ON STEROID THERAPY

Acceptable and Expected Side Effects

Nature of Effect	Action
Facial mooning (Cushing's syndrome)	May be minimized by restricted caloric intake.
Weight gain	Restrict caloric intake; may require a switch in steroid medication.
	May require diuretics and potassium.
Edema	Prescribe diuretics and potassium.
Potassium loss	May require switch to a fluorinated synthetic.
	Administer potassium supplement.
Acne	Treat with topical medications.
Increased urinary frequency and nocturia	Check for evidence of genitourinary infection or diabetes mellitus; urinalysis.
Insomnia, headache, fatigue	Treat symptomatically.

Undesirable and Unacceptable Side Effects

Nature of Effect	Action (Report to Physician)
Allergic reaction to bovine ACTH or steroid	Withdraw drug promptly.
	Substitute synthetic ACTH or steroid.
Cardiovascular system effect:	
Hypertension	Suggest reduction in dosage of steroids.
Thromboembolic complications	
Arteritis	
Infection	Suggest antimicrobial medications as indicated.
	Suggest local treatment and cleanliness.
Eye complications:	
Glaucoma	Refer to ophthalmologist.
Corneal lesions	
Musculoskeletal effects	Suggest sex hormones—synthetic estrogens and/or androgens.
	Suggest calcium supplement and vitamin D.
Adrenal insufficiency (after prolonged use) as manifested by peripheral circulatory collapse—in upright position.	Administer hydrocortisone promptly (intravenously) and saline intravenously.
	The following day, give steroid replacement.

Advice and Admonitions for Patients on Long-term Steroids

1. Recognize that steroids are valuable and useful medications but if taken longer than 2 weeks, certain side effects may be noticed.
2. "Acceptable" side effects may include weight gain (perhaps due to water retention), acne, headaches, fatigue, and increased urinary frequency.
3. "Unacceptable" side effects which are to be reported to the physician include: dizziness when rising from chair or bed (postural hypotension indicative of adrenal insufficiency), nausea, vomiting, thirst, abdominal pain, or pain of any type.
4. Additional side effects which are reportable are: feelings of depression or nervousness or development of an infection.
5. If the patient has a fall or is in an auto accident, his condition may precipitate adrenal failure. He requires an immediate injection of hydrocortisone phosphate. (Long-term patients should wear a Medic Alert tag and have a kit with hydrocortisone.)

with steroids, not from the suppression of hormones but from protein depletion. The effect is to cause partial adrenal atrophy and suppression of the pituitary's capacity to release ACTH, and although this effect may not be apparent under ordinary circumstances, it is obvious during times of unusual stress. During these periods of acute adrenal insufficiency, massive doses of corticosteroids are required to prevent adrenal collapse.

Dosage Schedule

Experiments have been conducted in an attempt to determine the best time to administer pharmacological doses of steroids. Once the patient's symptoms have been controlled on a 6-hour or 8-hour program, a switch is made to a once daily or every-other-day schedule. In keeping with the natural secretion of cortisol, the best time of the day for total steroid dose is in the early morning from 7 to 8 A.M. Large-dose therapy at 8 A.M., when the gland is most active, produces maximal suppression of the gland. A large 8 A.M.-dosage is more physiological, as it allows the body to escape effects of the steroids from 4 P.M. to 6 A.M. when serum levels are normally low — hence minimizing Cushingoid effects. If symptoms of the disease being treated are successfully suppressed, alternative-day therapy is helpful in preventing pituitary-adrenal suppression in patients requiring chronic therapy. Taking the total steroid dose every other day presents some problems in that patients complain of discomfort on the second day. It may be necessary for the nurse to explain to the patient that this regime may be necessary to prevent toxic reactions.

Withdrawal of Steroids. Corticosteroid dosages are reduced gradually to prevent steroid-induced adrenal insufficiency. Authorities differ as to the benefits of administering injections of adrenal-stimulating pituitary hormone corticotropin to assist in increasing the rates at which the adrenal glands recover their function.

THE PANCREAS

ACUTE PANCREATITIS

Pathophysiology and Etiology

Acute pancreatitis (inflammation of the pancreas) is brought about by the digestion of this organ by the very enzymes it produces, principally trypsin. Exactly how this autodigestion gets started is not known with certainty. However, in view of the frequent association of pancreatitis with gallbladder disease, it is believed that gallstones entering the common bile duct and lodging at the ampulla of Vater may obstruct the flow of pancreatic juice or cause a reflux of bile from the common duct into the pancreatic duct, thus activating the powerful pancreatic enzymes within the gland. (Normally, these remain in an inactive form until the pancreatic juice reaches the lumen of the duodenum.) Spasm and edema of the ampulla of Vater, resulting from duodenitis, can probably produce pancreatitis. Infectious pancreatitis may occur as a complication of mumps or a bacterial disease. The excessive ingestion of alcohol appears to be another etiologic factor in this disease: a definite relationship can be established between alcoholic intake and the onset of symptoms in many patients with acute pancreatitis.

CLASSIFICATION OF ACUTE PANCREATITIS. There are three types of acute pancreatitis, depending on the pathologic changes that occur: mild acute (interstitial) pancreatitis, acute hemorrhagic pancreatitis, and necrotic hemorrhagic pancreatitis.

Mild Acute (Interstitial) Pancreatitis. This type of pancreatitis is also known as acute pancreatic edema, characterized by an edematous swelling of the gland and the escape of its enzymes into the surrounding tissues and the peritoneal cavity. Pancreatic lipase produces fat necrosis of the omentum, and the amount of peritoneal fluid increases because of the irritating effect of these digestive enzymes. Symptoms of the disease, caused by this irritation and the edema and swelling of the inflamed gland, include abdominal and back pain, nausea, vomiting, and tenderness across the upper abdomen. Enzyme changes occur in the patient's blood, urine, and peritoneal fluid.

Acute Hemorrhagic Pancreatitis. This kind of pancreatitis may represent a more advanced form of acute interstitial pancreatitis. Enzymatic digestion of the gland is more widespread and complete. The tissue becomes necrotic, and the damage extends to its vascular radicles, so that blood escapes into the substance of the pancreas and beyond into the retroperitoneal tissues. Symptoms are severe, consisting of pain in the upper abdomen and back, nausea, vomiting, and the development of shock with hypotension, tachycardia, cold, clammy skin, and cyanosis.

Necrotic Hemorrhagic Pancreatitis. This is the most severe form of acute pancreatitis and has a 30 percent mortality; survivors may suffer from chronic pancreatic insufficiency. Late complications consist of pancreatic cysts or calculi. If the patient survives the initial shock, pancreatic necrosis often leads to the formation of secondary abscesses in the region of the gland, which are manifested clinically by mounting fever and leukocytosis.

Assessment of Patients with Pancreatic Disease

STOOLS. Usually the stools of patients suffering with pancreatic disease are bulky, pale, and foul-smelling. Fat content varies between 50 and 90 percent (normal, 20 percent).

BLOOD STUDIES. Amylase is the most important aid in diagnosing acute pancreatitis. Peak levels are reached in

GUIDELINES FOR NURSING AND MEDICAL MANAGEMENT OF THE PATIENT WITH ACUTE PANCREATITIS

Major Goals of Therapy: To treat the present affliction and prevent recurrence and progression of the disease.

Nursing Actions	**Rationale**
A. Relieve pain and discomfort.	A. The agonizing pain is probably due to edema and distention of the capsule, and peritoneal irritation.
1. Give meperidine (Demerol) in fairly high dosages, as indicated by the amount of pain present (unless patient is hypotensive).	1. Meperidine acts by depressing the CNS and thereby increasing the patient's pain threshold. Morphine is not usually given because it has a tendency to produce spasm of the sphincter of Oddi. Control of pain is important because restlessness increases body metabolism, which stimulates the secretion of pancreatic and gastric enzymes. The vagal stimulation to pancreatic secretion is stimulated by pain and anxiety.
2. Assist the patient to assume positions of comfort. Encourage the patient to turn at regularly scheduled intervals. Use pillow supports and foam-rubber pads, as necessary.	2. Frequent turning relieves pressure and aids in preventing pulmonary and vascular complications.
B. Minimize pancreatic secretion.	
1. Give antispasmodic drugs as prescribed.	1. Antispasmodic drugs reduce gastric and pancreatic secretion.
2. Withhold oral intake.	2. The intestinal stimulus to pancreatic secretion is influenced by food and fluid intake.
3. Keep the patient on bed rest.	3. Bed rest decreases body metabolism and thus reduces pancreatic and gastric secretions.
4. Employ continuous nasogastric suction. a. Measure gastric secretions at specified intervals. b. Observe and chart color and viscosity of gastric secretions. c. Ensure that the nasogastric tube is patent, to permit free drainage.	4. Nasogastric suction removes gastric contents and prevents gastric secretions from entering the duodenum and stimulating the secretin mechanism. Decompression of the intestines (if intestinal intubation is used) also assists in relieving respiratory distress.
C. Promote the comfort of the intubated patient.	
1. Use water-soluble lubricant around external nares.	1. To prevent irritation.
2. Turn patient at intervals.	2. To relieve pressure of tube on esophageal and gastric mucosa.
3. Give oral hygiene and gargling solutions.	3. To relieve dryness and irritation of oropharynx.
4. Utilize semi-Fowler's position frequently.	4. To decrease pressure on diaphragm and allow greater lung expansion.
D. Give medications as directed.	
1. Give antibiotic drugs only for coexisting infections.	1. Edema, necrosis, hemorrhage, and suppuration are present in varying degrees in acute pancreatitis. These conditions are the results of secondary infection. Pancreatic abscess and bacteremia may also be present.
2. Give insulin as prescribed.	2. To combat hyperglycemia, if present.
E. Prevent serum calcium deficiency.	E. Keep a supply of intravenous calcium gluconate readily available to prevent tetany.
F. Replace blood and fluid and electrolyte loss.	F. Electrolyte losses occur from nasogastric suctioning, severe diaphoresis, emesis and as a result of the patient's being in a fasting state.
1. Give plasma albumin and blood as prescribed.	1. During acute pancreatitis, plasma may be lost into the abdominal cavity, which diminishes the blood volume.
2. Give intravenous electrolytes (sodium, potassium, chlorides) as prescribed.	2. The amount and type of fluid and electrolyte replacement is determined by the status of the blood pressure, the laboratory evaluations of serum electrolyte and blood urea nitrogen levels, the urinary volume, and the assessment of the patient's condition.

GUIDELINES FOR NURSING AND MEDICAL MANAGEMENT OF THE PATIENT WITH ACUTE PANCREATITIS (CONTINUED)

Nursing Actions	Rationale

G. Combat shock if present.
  1. Administer adrenocorticol steroids to those who do not respond to conventional treatment.
  2. Evaluate the amount of urinary output. Attempt to maintain this at 50 ml./hr.
	G. Extensive acute pancreatitis may cause peripheral vascular collapse and shock. Blood and plasma may be lost into the abdominal cavity, and therefore there is a decreased blood and plasma volume. The toxins from the bacteria of a necrotic pancreas may cause shock.

H. Support patient's heart and lungs, to prevent complications.
  1. Maintain blood volume with blood transfusions, plasma, albumin, dextran.
  2. Guard the patient's cardiopulmonary reserve.
    a. Evaluate the pulse, respiratory rate, and blood pressure at indicated intervals.
    b. Give digitalis as prescribed.
	1. Patients with hemorrhagic pancreatitis lose large amounts of blood and plasma, which decreases effective circulation and blood volume. Replacement by blood, plasma, albumin, or dextran assists in ensuring effective circulating blood volume.
	
	Acute pancreatitis produces retroperitoneal edema, elevation of the diaphragm, pleural effusion, and inadequate lung ventilation. Intra-abdominal infection and labored breathing increase the body's metabolic demand, which further decreases pulmonary reserve and leads to respiratory failure.

I. Reduce the excessive metabolism of the body.
  1. Give antibiotics as prescribed.
  2. Place patient in an air-conditioned room.
  3. Administer nasal oxygen as required for hypoxia.
  4. Utilize a hypothermia blanket if necessary.
	I. Pancreatitis produces a severe peritoneal and retroperitoneal reaction that causes fever, tachycardia, and accelerated respirations. Placing the patient in an air-conditioned room and supporting him with oxygen therapy decreases the work load of the respiratory system and the tissue utilization of oxygen. Reduction of fever and pulse rate decrease the metabolic demands of the body.

J. Educate the patient to try to prevent further attacks of pancreatitis.
  1. Keep appointments with physician (or clinic) at specified times.
  2. Refrain from alcoholic beverages and avoid excessive use of coffee.
  3. Avoid heavy meals. Abstain from eating when nervous or tense.
	1. Known causes of pancreatitis (gallbladder disease, gastric or duodenal ulcer, etc.) should be searched for and treated.
	2. Alcohol and coffee increase pancreatic secretion.
	
	3 Spicy foods and heavy meals are strong gastric stimulants.

Mnemonic device for acute pancreatitis
P—pain
A—antispasmodics
N—nasogastric suction
C—calcium
R—replacement of fluids/electrolytes
E—endocrines
A—antibiotics
S—steroids
   (after Kaplan, N.H.)

---

24 hours, with a rapid fall to normal levels within 48 to 72 hours. Blood lipase also becomes elevated and remains this way longer than amylase.

DUODENAL INTUBATION AND ASPIRATION. These procedures (under fluoroscope) may be done to assay pancreatic juices.

Management. Since the pathologic process responsible for this disease is autodigestion of the pancreas, the objective of therapy is *to decrease the production of these enzymes.* Oral feedings are interrupted to control the formation of secretin; the patient is maintained on parenteral fluids and electrolytes. Anticholinergic drugs are administered to block the nerve impulses that stimulate pancreatic secretion, and nasogastric suction is employed. Demerol is given to relieve pain. Most attacks of acute interstitial pancreatitis are self-limited and may be expected to subside in 3 or 4 days.

Treatment of hemorrhagic and necrotic pancreatitis consists of the measures recommended for acute interstitial pancreatitis plus those indicated for shock (page 366). They include intravenous fluid and plasma therapy, blood transfusion, antibiotics, and nasogastric suction.

As indicated earlier, pancreatic necrosis often leads to

the formation of secondary abscesses. Such abscesses must be drained surgically, during the later stages of the disease. Drainage is likely to be profuse and long-standing, so that these patients are certain to require close observation and constant care for a considerable period of time.

Careful nursing observation is extremely important, since this condition has a high mortality rate. Between acute attacks, the patient receives a diet high in carbohydrates and low in fat and proteins. Heavy meals are to be avoided, as are alcoholic beverages. A summary of the nursing management of patients with acute pancreatitis is found on page 878.

CHRONIC PANCREATITIS

After repeated attacks of acute interstitial pancreatitis, or, in some instances, after the prolonged use of alcohol in large amounts, patients may develop a chronic fibrosis of the pancreatic gland itself, with obstruction of its ducts and destruction of its secreting cells. This type of pancreatitis is prone to appear in adult men and is characterized by recurring attacks of severe upper abdominal and back pain, accompanied by vomiting. Attacks often are so painful that morphine, even in large doses, does not provide relief. As the disease progresses, these patients may become addicted to opiates. Because of the destruction of the gland by fibrosis, the pancreatic secretions may be deficient in amount, or obstruction of the ducts by fibrosis may prevent the pancreatic juice from entering the duodenum and playing its role in digestion. As a result, the digestion of foodstuffs, especially proteins and fats, is disrupted. The stools become frequent, frothy (or soaplike), and foul-smelling, due to the impairment of fat digestion, which results in a stool with a high fat content. This condition is referred to as *steatorrhea*. As the disease progresses, calcifications of the gland may occur, and calcium stones may form within the ducts.

Management. The management of chronic pancreatitis depends on its probable cause in each particular patient. When it develops in association with gallbladder disease, efforts are made to relieve the difficulty by operating on the biliary tract, exploring the common duct, and removing the stones; usually, the gallbladder is removed at the same time. In addition, an attempt is made to improve the drainage of the common bile duct and the pancreatic duct by dividing the sphincter of Oddi, a muscle that is located at the ampulla of Vater (this operation is known as a *sphincterotomy*). Nursing management after such an operation is the same as that indicated for all patients undergoing biliary tract surgery. A T-tube usually is placed in the common bile duct, requiring a drainage bottle to collect the bile after the operation.

In the absence of evidence indicating biliary tract disease, the most common cause of chronic pancreatitis is chronic alcoholism. In such patients, the pancreas becomes markedly fibrotic, to the extent that the pancreatic ducts may be obstructed. In some patients the obstruction may be relieved by sphincterotomy, but in others, the obstruction is located within the confines of the gland itself and therefore not amenable to this procedure. Other possible approaches include opening the pancreatic duct and placing the entire gland inside a loop of jejunum; or the tail of the pancreas may be removed and the remaining stump sutured into the end of a loop of jejunum. These somewhat complicated operations are performed with the object of draining the pancreatic juice by way of a route that by-passes the obstruction in the ductal system.

Despite these operative procedures the patient is likely to continue having pain and digestive difficulties from the pancreatitis unless he abstains completely from the use of alcohol. This point should be emphasized by the nurse in the course of instructing the patient and the family.

PANCREATIC CYSTS

As a result of the local necrosis that occurs at the time of acute pancreatitis, collections of fluid may form in the vicinity of the pancreas. These become walled off by fibrous tissue and are called *pancreatic cysts*. They are the most common type of pancreatic cyst, most other types developing as a result of congenital anomalies.

Pancreatic cysts may attain considerable size. Because of their location behind the posterior peritoneum, when they enlarge, they impinge on and displace the stomach or the colon, which are adjacent. Eventually, through pressure or secondary infection, they produce symptoms, requiring that they be drained.

Management. Drainage may be established into the gastrointestinal tract or through the skin surface. In the latter instance, the drainage is likely to be profuse and damaging to tissue because of the enzyme contents. Hence, steps must be taken to protect the skin in areas adjacent to the drainage site to prevent excoriation. Ointments protect the skin, provided that they are applied before excoriation takes place. Another method involves the constant aspiration of juice from the drainage tract by means of a suction apparatus, so that enzyme contact is avoided. This method demands a great deal of nursing attention to be sure that the suction tube does not become dislodged from the drainage tract and that the entire apparatus functions properly without interruption.

PANCREATIC TUMORS

Carcinoma of the Pancreas

Cancer may arise in any portion of the pancreas: in the head, the body, or the tail, producing clinical manifestations that vary, depending on the location of the lesion and whether or not functioning, insulin-secreting pancreatic islet cells are involved. Tumors that originate in the head of the pancreas—decidedly the most common location—give rise to a distinctive clinical picture and will be discussed separately. Functioning islet cell tumors, whether benign (adenoma) or malignant (carcinoma) are responsible for the syndrome of hyperinsulinism, and are described on page 882. With these exceptions, carcinoma of the pancreas is notoriously lacking in clear-cut, characteristic symptomatology, and because of its rather nondescript features, patients with this form of cancer often are denied the advantages of an early diagnosis.

Assessment. Common to all types of pancreatic carcinoma are symptoms of rapid, profound, progressive, and inexplicable weight loss; vague, ill-defined, upper or midabdominal discomfort which is totally unrelated to any gastrointestinal function and difficult to describe, and which radiates as a boring pain in the midback that is unrelated to posture or activity. People with pancreatic carcinoma often find that they get some relief from pain by sitting hunched foward. Since pain is often accentuated by lying supine, a full-length foam rubber pad placed under the patient has proven beneficial. A very important clue, when present, is an indication of insulin deficiency—glucosuria, hyperglycemia, and abnormal glucose tolerance. Diabetes is sometimes an early sign of carcinoma of the pancreas. Eating often aggravates epigastric pain; this usually occurs weeks before jaundice and pruritus. A helpful tool in diagnosis is a gastrointestinal roentgenography series which may demonstrate deformities in adjacent viscera caused by the impinging pancreatic mass.

Management. Therapy usually is limited to palliative measures. Definitive surgical treatment, i.e., total excision of the lesion, often is not feasible because of the extensive growth when the lesion is finally diagnosed and the probable widespread metastases—especially to the liver, the lungs, and the bones.

Tumors of the Head of the Pancreas

Assessment. Tumors in this region of the pancreas are detected by the fact that they obstruct the common bile duct where it passes through the head of the pancreas to join the pancreatic duct and empty at the ampulla of Vater into the duodenum. Obstruction to the flow of bile produces jaundice, clay-colored stools, and dark urine. There may be some degree of abdominal discomfort or pain, and pruritus may be noted. Nonspecific symptoms such as anorexia, insensible weight loss, and malaise may or may not be present. If present, suspicion of visceral cancer is heightened.

This disease usually occurs in older, thin men. It must be differentiated from the jaundice due to a biliary obstruction caused by a gallstone in the common duct, which usually is intermittent and appears typically in obese individuals, most often women, who have had previous symptoms of gallbladder disease. The tumors producing the obstruction may arise from the pancreas, from the common bile duct, or from the ampulla of Vater.

Management. When these patients come to the hospital, they are in such a poor nutritional and physical state that a fairly long period of preparation is necessary before operation can be attempted. Various liver and pancreatic function studies are carried out, vitamin K is given to restore the blood prothrombin activity, and diets high in protein often are given, with pancreatic enzymes. Blood transfusions frequently are used as well.

Following conventional blood and roentgen studies, more sophisticated diagnostic aids may be used, including duodenography, angiography by the hepatic or celiac artery, catheterization, pancreatic scanning, and per-

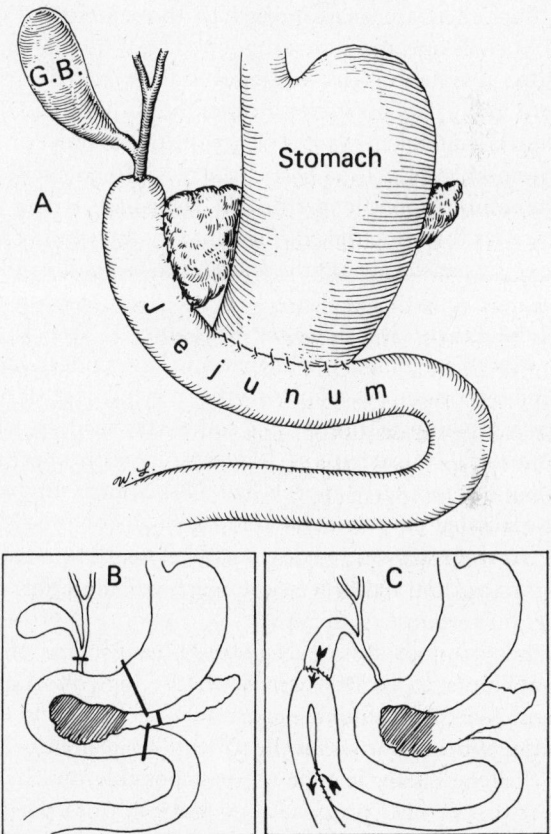

Figure 40-4.   Pancreatoduodenectomy (after Whipple). (*B*) Shows lines which indicate removal of head of pancreas, duodenum, and adjacent stomach, and distal segment of common bile duct. (*A*) Indicates the end result for resection of the carcinoma of the head of the pancreas or the ampulla of Vater. The common duct is sutured to the end of the jejunum, and the remaining portion of the pancreas and the end of the stomach are sutured to the side of the jejunum. (*C*) An alternate method of treatment when an inoperable tumor of the head of the pancreas has been found. In such cases the bile may be permitted to flow again into the intestine by anastomosing the jejunum to the gallbladder. In addition, an accessory operation between the loops of jejunum has been performed.

cutaneous transhepatic cholangiography. However, undoubtedly the most valuable aid is laparotomy with biopsy of the pancreas.

Surgical Management. Many surgeons perform only a biliary-enteric shunt, to relieve the jaundice. This will give some relief and, perhaps, time for a suspicious lesion to eventually prove nonmalignant. Others believe that pancreatoduodenectomy should be performed.

Preoperative preparation includes adequate hydration and nutrition, correction of prothrombin deficiency with vitamin K, and treatment of anemia to minimize postoperative complications.

In the operating room, if a tumor is found, it may be removed if it has not invaded many of the important structures adjacent to it (portal vein, superior mesenteric artery). The operation entails removal of the head of the pancreas, the duodenum, and adjacent stomach, and the distal part of the common bile duct (Fig. 40-4B). The stomach, the cut end of the pancreas, and the common bile duct then are anastomosed to the jejunum (Fig. 40-4A). This operation, first suggested by Whipple, may be done in either one or two stages. It has resulted in the cure of many patients with cancer of the ampulla and the bile ducts, but unhappily it is only palliative in most cases of carcinoma of the head of the pancreas. When excision of the tumor cannot be performed, the jaundice may be relieved by diverting the bile flow into the jejunum. This is done by anastomosing the jejunum to the gallbladder (cholecystojejunostomy).

Management for Whipple Procedure. The postoperative management of patients who have undergone a Whipple procedure is similar to the management of patients following gastrointestinal and biliary surgery. The psychosocial considerations, however, are more specific, and must be properly approached by the nurse. In view of the fact that the patient has undergone major and risky surgery and is severely ill, he most likely will experience bouts of anxiety and depression which will undoubtedly affect his response to therapy.

While many professionals question the justification of the Whipple procedure because of the high mortality rate, this negative thinking must not affect the attitudes of those who are caring for the patient. As in all nursing, the challenge is to provide the best possible care in an effort to prevent complications and promote patient comfort.

Pancreatic Islet Tumors

In the pancreas are located the islets (islands) of Langerhans—small nests of cells that secrete directly into the bloodstream and, therefore, are part of the glands of internal secretion (endocrines). The secretion, insulin, is involved in the metabolism of sugar. A deficient secretion of insulin produces diabetes mellitus. On the other hand, tumors of these cells produce a hypersecretion of

insulin, so that the body sugar is metabolized too rapidly. The fall of the blood sugar level (hypoglycemia) produces symptoms of weakness, mental confusion, and even convulsions. These may be relieved almost immediately by taking sugar by mouth or by intravenous glucose. The 5-hour glucose tolerance test is helpful in diagnosing insulinoma and in distinguishing it from the more common functional hypoglycemia.

Once the diagnosis of a tumor of the islet cells has been made, surgical treatment with removal of the tumor usually is recommended. The tumors may be benign adenomas or they may be malignant. Complete removal usually results in a most dramatic cure. In some patients, such symptoms may not be produced by an actual tumor of the islet cells, but by a simple hypertrophy of this tissue. In such cases a partial *pancreatectomy*—removal of the tail and part of the body of the pancreas—is performed.

Management. In preparing these patients for operation, the nurse must be alert for symptoms of hypoglycemia and be ready to give sugar, usually with orange juice, should they appear. After operation, the nursing mangement is the same as that following any upperabdominal operation.

Ulcerogenic (Zollinger-Ellison) Tumors

Some tumors of the islets of Langerhans are associated with a hypersecretion of gastric acid that produces ulcers in the stomach, the duodenum, and even the jejunum. The hypersecretion is so great that even after partial gastric resection, enough acid to produce further ulceration may remain. When a marked tendency to develop gastric and duodenal ulcers is noted, an ulcerogenic tumor of the islets of Langerhans is suspected.

These tumors, which may be benign or malignant, are treated, when possible, by excision. Frequently, however, because of extension beyond the pancreas, removal is not possible. In many patients, a total gastrectomy may be necessary to reduce the secretion of gastric acid sufficiently to prevent further ulceration.

HYPERINSULINISM

This disorder results from the overproduction of insulin by the pancreatic islets. Symptoms resemble those of excessive doses of insulin and are attributable to the same mechanism—an abnormal reduction in the concentration of blood sugar. Clinically, it is characterized by episodes during which the patient experiences unusual hunger, nervousness, sweating, headache, and faintness; in severe cases, convulsive seizures and episodes of unconsciousness may occur. The findings at operation or postmortem examination may indicate hyperplasia (overgrowth) of the islets of Langerhans, or a benign or malignant tumor involving the islets and capable of pro-

THE PATIENT UNDERGOING A WHIPPLE PROCEDURE*

Objectives of Care	Nursing Action
To facilitate respiratory exchange following prolonged surgery.	1. Maintain on ventilator until fully reacted. 2. Give oxygen and monitor arterial pO_2 and pH. 3. Administer IPPB as required. 4. Attend the tracheostomy which is often performed at the time of the operation.
To detect adverse signs indicating peripheral vascular collapse, hemorrhage, or other complications.	1. Monitor vital signs intensively for the first 48-72 hours: temperature, pulse, respiration, blood pressure, and C.V.P. 2. For hypotension, assist in administration of whole blood and albumin; recognize signs of incompatibility, such as sudden chilling, hives, headache, nausea, vomiting. If these occur, discontinue the transfusion and notify surgeon.
To assess kidney function; renal failure is a common postoperative complication.	1. Maintain an hourly record of urinary output. 2. Keep running account of input.
To relieve pain and discomfort of patient.	1. Administer meperidine hydrochloride (Demerol) to increase patient's pain threshold. Morphine is used sparingly because it depresses respiration. 2. Assist the patient in assuming positions of comfort; frequent turning relieves pressure areas and aids in preventing pulmonary and vascular complications.
To overcome prothrombin deficiency and to assist in prevention of postoperative hemorrhage—renal failure.	Continue administration of vitamin K as prescribed (begun preoperatively) until oral feedings are resumed.
To prevent chest complications and assist abdominal drainage.	Have patient sitting on first postoperative day; offer steam inhalations and encourage leg exercises.
To detect untoward signs, as revealed in laboratory reports: 1. Hemoconcentration	1. Note increase in hematocrit, such as $45\% \rightarrow 50\% \rightarrow 55\% \rightarrow 60\%$ This would indicate a significant loss of plasma; be prepared to administer serum albumin.
2. Falling serum calcium level	2. Recognize variations in serum calcium levels; if they are falling, have calcium gluconate available for daily administration with IV therapy.
To provide for adequate decompression of afferent jejunal segment.	Check for adequate drainage from T-tube; prevent kinking of tube.
To prevent dilatation of jejunum (which would exert pressure against anastomoses) and to prevent subdiaphragmatic pressure.	Provide suction to the Levin tube; keep nasogastric tube in place until gastrointestinal function is resumed.
To maintain comfort of intubated patient and prevent mucous membrane and skin irritation.	1. Assist him in receiving cleansing and refreshing mouth care. 2. Apply lubricant to external nares. Provide vapor-mist therapy to increase humidity.
To minimize the possibility of infection or abscess formation.	1. Administer antibiotics as prescribed. 2. Maintain aseptic technique in handling wound dressings and drainage, and tracheostomy aspiration.
To sustain nutritional requirements of the body and to maintain homeostasis.	Assist in replacing fluids and electrolytes when assessment indicates these are lost.
To prevent major gastrointestinal complications: 1. Partial intestinal obstruction; this may cause increased intraluminal pressure, which may disrupt a weak point in the pancreaticojejunal anastomosis. 2. Pancreatic leakage, which in turn may promote paralytic ileus and eventually produce a partial intestinal obstruction.	Withhold oral intake until gastrointestinal function is resumed.
To assess the patient's need for insulin.	Note any symptoms suggestive of diabetes mellitus (rare unless pancreas is removed): irritability, skin-itching, blurring of vision, hyperglycemia. *(Continued)*

*Brunner, L.: Whipple procedure, reprinted with permission from December 1973 issue of Nursing '73. Copyright © 1973 by Intermed Communications, Inc., Jenkintown, Pa. 19046.

THE PATIENT UNDERGOING A WHIPPLE PROCEDURE (CONTINUED)

Objectives of Care	Nursing Action
To detect early signs of other complications:	
1. Infection: subdiaphragmatic abscess, wound abscess, peritonitis.	1. Continue monitoring vital signs until sufficient time for healing has elapsed and until it is determined that all anastomoses are secure and patent.
2. Hemorrhage: due to leakage of activated pancreatic juice and digestion of neighboring arteries.	2. Check stools for blood. Recognize variations in vital signs indicative of hemorrhage.
3. Jaundice	3. Observe color of sclera; recognize that patient may scratch skin because of itchiness.
4. Undigested fat	4. Observe stools; if frothy and light-colored, it may indicate undigested fat. This may require tablets of pancreatic enzyme to aid in fat digestion.
To prepare patient for convalescence and understanding of posthospital activities, including the importance of consistent follow-up visits.	1. Discuss role of pancreas regarding insulin and intestinal digestion and the possible need for continued treatment.
	2. If chemotherapy (cancer) is to be used after the operation, stress its need and effects.
	3. Remind patient to eat small, frequent meals initially.
	4. Encourage family support of the patient.
	5. Instruct family in recognizing untoward signs which need to be reported should they occur.

---

ducing large amounts of insulin. Occasionally, tumors of nonpancreatic origin produce an insulinlike material that can cause hypoglycemia. This condition occasionally is responsible for convulsions coinciding with decreases in the blood glucose to levels which are inadequate to sustain normal brain function (i.e., below 30 mg./100 ml.).

All of the symptoms that accompany spontaneous hypoglycemia are relieved by the oral or parenteral administration of glucose. Surgical extirpation of the hyperplastic or neoplastic tissue from the pancreas offers the only successful method of treatment. About 15 percent of people with spontaneous (functional) hypoglycemia eventually develop diabetes mellitus.

DIABETES INSIPIDUS

Diabetes insipidus is a disorder of the pituitary gland due to a deficiency of vasopressin, the antidiuretic hormone (ADH). It is characterized by great thirst (polydipsia) and large volumes of dilute urine. The cause is unknown, although it may be secondary to head trauma, brain neoplasm, or surgical ablation or irradiation of the pituitary gland. When the action of ADH on the distal nephron of the kidney is absent, an enormous daily output of very dilute, waterlike urine with a specific gravity of 1.001 to 1.005 occurs. The urine contains no abnormal substances such as sugar and albumin. Because of the intense thirst, the patient tends to drink 4 to 40 liters of fluid daily, with a special craving for cold water.

The primary symptoms may begin at birth. When it occurs in adults, the polyuria may have an insidious onset, although sometimes it occurs suddenly and may be related to an injury.

The disease cannot be controlled by limiting the intake of fluids. Attempts to do this causes the patient to suffer extremely from an insatiable craving for fluid. Great embarrassment, inconvenience, and interference with daily activities are occasioned by the urgent need to allay thirst and pass urine.

Assessment. The fluid deprivation test is carried out, in which fluids are deprived for 8 to 12 hours or until 3 percent of the body weight is lost. The patient is weighed frequently during the time fluid is withheld. Plasma and urine osmolality studies are done at the beginning and end of the test. Inability to increase specific gravity and osmolality of the urine are characteristic of diabetes insipidus.

Management. The objectives of therapy are (1) to replace vasopressin (which is usually a life-long therapeutic program) and (2) to search for and correct the underlying intracranial pathology.

Desmopressin (DDAVP) is a new synthetic drug for the treatment of diabetes insipidus and is particularly valuable because its action lasts longer and it has fewer adverse effects than other preparations previously used to treat the disease. It is administered intranasally with the patient blowing the solution into his nose through a flexible plastic tube. Two administrations daily appear to control the symptoms.

Another form of therapy is the intramuscular administration of antidiuretic hormone, vasopressin tannate in oil, which is given at intervals of 36 to 48 hours, or longer. The effect is a reduction in urinary volume for 24 to 48 hours. The vial of medication should be warmed to make it easier to administer the oil preparation. The injection is given in the evening so that maximum results are obtained during sleep. Abdominal cramps may be a problem with this type of therapy.

The drug, lypressin (Diapid nasal spray) is absorbed through the nasal mucosa into the blood and is another method of administering vasopressin. Its duration may be too short for patients with severe disease. The patient should be observed for chronic rhinopharyngitis if this modality of treatment is used.

Recently clofibrate, a hypolipidemic agent, has been found to have an antidiuretic effect on patients with diabetes insipidus who have some residual hypothalamic vasopressin. Chlorpropamide (Diabinese) is another drug used as an antidiuretic in mild forms of the disease. However, the patient should be warned of a possible hypoglycemic reaction when this drug is used. Thiazide diuretics are also used adjunctively.

The patient will require encouragement and support if he is undergoing studies of a possible cranial lesion.

THE PITUITARY GLAND

HYPOPITUITARISM

Hypopituitarism is pituitary insufficiency resulting from destruction of the anterior lobe of the pituitary gland. *Panhypopituitarism* (Simmonds' disease) is total absence of all pituitary secretions.

The total destruction of the pituitary gland by trauma, tumor, or a vascular lesion removes every stimulus that is normally received by the thyroid, the gonads, and the adrenal glands. The resulting endocrinopathy is characterized by extreme weight loss, emaciation, atrophy of all organs, hair loss, impotence, amenorrhea, hypometabolism, hypoglycemia, eventual coma, and death.

PITUITARY TUMORS

Tumors of the pituitary gland are of three principal types, representing an overgrowth of (1) eosinophilic cells, (2) basophilic cells, or (3) chromophobic cells (i.e., cells with no affinity for either eosinophilic or basophilic stains).

Eosinophilic tumors, if they develop early enough in life, result in gigantism. The individual thus affected may be over 7 feet tall and large in all proportions, yet so feeble that he can hardly stand. If the disorder begins during adult life, the excessive skeletal growth occurs only in the feet, the hands, the superciliary ridges, the molar eminences, the nose, and the chin, giving rise to the clinical picture called *acromegaly.* Enlargement, moreover, is not confined to the skeleton, but involves every tissue and

organ of the body. Many of these patients suffer from severe headaches and become partially blind, because the tumors exert pressure on the optic nerves. Decalcification of the skeleton, muscular weakness, and endocrine disturbances, similar to those occurring in patients with hyperthyroidism, also are associated with tumors of this type.

Basophilic tumors give rise to the so-called *Cushing syndrome* (see page 873), with features largely attributable to hyperadrenalism, including masculinization and amenorrhea in females, girdle obesity, hypertension, osteoporosis, and polycythemia.

Chromophobic tumors, which comprise 90 percent of pituitary tumors, produce no hormones, but destroy the rest of the pituitary gland, causing hypopituitarism. Patients with this disease are inclined to be obese and somnolent, exhibiting fine, scanty hair, dry soft skin, pasty complexion, and small bones. They also experience headaches, loss of libido, and visual defects progressing to blindness. Other symptoms include polyuria, polyphagia, a lowering of the basal metabolic rate, and a subnormal body temperature.

See page 1209 for the transsphenoidal approach to the removal of a pituitary tumor and page 1206 for the nursing management of a patient undergoing cranial surgery.

HYPOPHYSECTOMY

Hypophysectomy, or removal of the pituitary gland, may be done for several reasons, especially to remove primary tumors of the pituitary gland. In diabetic retinopathy (page 847) it is used to halt the progress of hemorrhagic retinopathy and avoid blindness. Hypophysectomy is also done as a palliative measure to relieve bone pain secondary to metastasis of malignant lesions of the breast and prostate. Pituitary hormones influence the growth of the normal breast and stimulate the function of the ovaries and the adrenal glands. Hypophysectomy removes the hormonal influences of these glands. The procedure creates a hormonal environment that is hostile to the continued growth of the neoplasm.

There are several methods of pituitary ablation (removal). It can be done surgically through the transfrontal, subcranial, or oronasal-transsphenoidal approaches (page 1209). The pituitary can also be destroyed by implantation of radioactive yttrium or x-ray radiation. Destruction may also be accomplished by localized radio frequency (heat) or cryosurgery (freezing).

The absence of the pituitary gland alters the function of many parts of the body. Substitution therapy with adrenal steroids (hydrocortisone) and thyroid hormone may be necessary. Menstruation ceases and infertility occurs almost always, after total or nearly total ablation of the pituitary gland.

DISORDER OF PURINE METABOLISM: GOUT

Gout is a disease manifested by an acute inflammation of a joint and is caused by the deposit of uric acid crystals in joints and connective tissues. Uric acid is the end product of purine metabolism. Hyperuricemia, the persistent elevation of urates in the blood, is usually found in gout and is caused by *overproduction* or *underexcretion* of uric acid.

Primary gout may be due to a genetic defect of purine metabolism or a renal defect resulting in decreased excretion of uric acid. This disorder occurs most frequently in male patients, usually in their 40's.

In secondary gout (an acquired disease), hyperuricemia occurs in conditions in which there is an increase in cell turnover (leukemia, multiple myeloma, psoriasis) and an increase in cell breakdown. Or it may occur because renal excretion of uric acid is somehow blocked. Other causes of hyperuricemia and gout include: prolonged ingestion of certain diuretic agents (thiazides) and aspirin, trauma, or the treatment of myeloproliferative disease.

Because of its low solubility, uric acid tends to precipitate and form deposits at various sites where blood flow

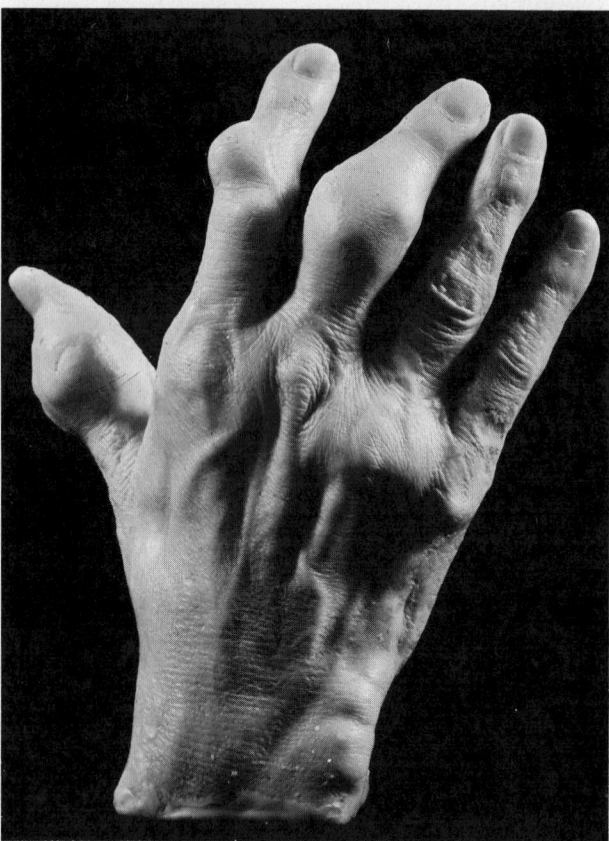

Figure 40-5. Accumulation of uric acid crystals on the knuckles of a patient with gout. (Photo courtesy of National Institute of Arthritis, Metabolism and Digestive Diseases)

is least active, including cartilaginous tissue. These masses of sodium urate crystals, called *tophi,* are deposited in the vicinity of the joints, particularly the great toe, on the knuckles (Fig. 40-5), and in the ears. Tophi may cause pressure symptoms, deformity, or ulceration of overlying skin and are generally considered to be a late sign.

In some patients, renal urate lithiasis (kidney stones) may be the earliest manifestation of gout. Chronic renal disease secondary to urate deposition may develop.

Clinical Manifestations. An attack of acute gout usually begins with sudden onset of severe pain in one or more of the peripheral joints which may be accompanied by intense inflammation, swelling, and tenderness. The first joint of the great toe is most often affected. Other joints (ankle, knee, and, less commonly, the wrist and elbow) may also be affected. Sometimes fever is present. An untreated attack of gout subsides in about one week, with the joint returning to normal.

The attacks usually recur at irregular intervals. After repeated acute attacks, gout may become chronic, leaving certain joints (particularly those of the hands) permanently disabled, deformed, and painful. Diagnosis is based on the presence of urate crystals noted in fluid aspirated from a joint cavity. Subcutaneous deposits of urates (tophi) are considered to be positive signs of gout. Roentgenograms of the joints reveal tophi and urate deposits. The serum urate levels may exceed 8 mg./100 ml. in men and 6.5 mg./100 ml. in women.

Management

The objectives of management are to relieve the acute discomfort and prevent the development of chronic gouty arthritis, renal calculi, and renal damage. The treatment of gout falls into two categories: the acute attack and long-term management.

TREATMENT OF ACUTE ATTACK. The treatment of the acute attack is directed towards relieving pain and inflammation by means of anti-inflammatory drugs. Those drugs in current use include indomethacin, phenylbutazone, oxyphenbutazone, and the new nonsteroidal anti-inflammatory agents, ibuprofen, naproxen, and fenoprofen (see pages 1328-1329).

Colchicine, given early in the attack, will provide dramatic relief. A response to colchicine is regarded as diagnostic evidence of the disorder. Colchicine has no effect on uric acid metabolism. An initial dose of colchicine is given and followed by doses every 1 to 2 hours until the pain is relieved or the patient develops symptoms of gastrointestinal irritability: diarrhea, nausea and vomiting. The drug is then stopped temporarily. Joint pain and swelling start to subside in 6 to 12 hours after therapy is started.

Narcotics or analgesics may be needed for severe pain

until specific therapy is effective. The patient is encouraged to rest in bed or a chair, with the affected limb protected (by a bed cradle), and elevated. Weight-bearing is avoided until the attack subsides, since early ambulation may precipitate a recurrence. If joints in the hand, wrist, or elbow are involved, a splint may be worn to immobilize the hot and tender joint. Cold applications to the joint may be helpful. The patient is advised to increase fluid intake.

LONG-TERM MANAGEMENT OF GOUT. Once the acute attack subsides, the objective of management is to lower the serum uric acid levels to a normal range. Therefore the therapy may involve inhibiting production of uric acid or increasing urinary excretion of uric acid.

Uricosuric Drugs. Agents that lower uric acid are used for long-term management to prevent complications (destructive joint disease, nephropathy) and to reduce the occurrence of acute attacks. Such a drug inhibits the reabsorption of uric acid by the renal tubules, thus resulting in increased excretion of uric acid, thereby lowering the serum urate level. In time, the size of tophi are reduced, and the formation of new tophi is prevented.

One such drug is probenecid (Benemid), which apparently has no more significant side-reaction than an occasional mild gastrointestinal upset and a tendency to constipation. However, this drug is not to be given in conjunction with aspirin or any other salicylate, because each tends to offset the action of the other. Another useful uricosuric drug is sulfinpyrazone (Anturane), which acts similarly to probenecid. Anturane and salicylates are also mutually antagonistic and should not be administered together. Once uricosuric drug therapy is initiated, the urinary concentration of urates may rise to such heights that crystals may precipitate out of solution, causing urolithiasis and renal complications. To avoid this complication, a large fluid intake (at least 8 glasses) is encouraged, to assure a high 24-hour urinary volume. Sodium bicarbonate or citrate solutions may be given to maintain an alkaline urine in patients with a history of stone-formation.

Xanthine-Oxidase Inhibitors. For patients in whom there is an overproduction of uric acid or those who have nephrolithiasis or renal impairment, allopurinol (Zyloprim) may be given. Allopurinol is a xanthine-oxidase inhibitor that interferes with the conversion of the products of purine metabolism to uric acid. Thus it inhibits uric acid synthesis. The administration of allopurinol generally produces a prompt fall in both serum and urinary uric acid. It is also used prophylactically during chemotherapy for myeloproliferative disorders.

Many persons with chronic gout have been relieved of their joint pain and have experienced increased joint mobility. Tophaceous deposits cease to form and draining urate sinuses tend to heal on this regimen. The dosage is based on serum urate determinations.

Patient Education

The patient should be asked to remember how he felt during an acute attack. These symptoms then are warnings of an impending attack, and therapy should be started promptly in order to abort an attack. Colchicine may be prescribed as a prophylactic measure against an acute attack. Uricosuric agents or allopurinol may be prescribed to prevent further deposition of uric acid in the joints. Aspirin is to be avoided, because it counteracts the uricosuric effect. A high fluid intake to maintain a high urinary volume minimizes urate precipitation in the urinary tract. Fasting, either to lose weight or during an alcoholic spree, is to be avoided, since fasting has been found to increase the serum uric acid level. However, obese patients should lose weight *slowly* to avoid strain on involved joints.

Specific foods known to precipitate an attack should be avoided. Purines are derived from ingested food and from breakdown of body proteins. Purines are also synthesized in the liver. Although a low-purine diet is seldom used, it is usually recommended that patients with high blood uric acid levels avoid foods rich in purine content, including organ meats, liver, shellfish, anchovies, and sardines. A moderate-protein diet may reduce the amount of uric acid present. Restriction of dietary fat is also recommended, if the patient has hyperlipidemia, which is commonly associated with gout.

BIBLIOGRAPHY

BOOKS

Azarnoff, D. L.: Steroid Therapy. Philadelphia, W. B. Saunders, 1975.

Dillon, R. S.: Handbook of Endocrinology. Philadelphia, Lea & Febiger, 1973.

Rose, L., and Lavine, R. L.: New Concepts in Endocrinology and Metabolism. New York, Grune & Stratton, 1977.

Schwartz, T. B., and Ryan, W. G.: 1978 Year Book of Endocrinology. Chicago, Year Book Med. Pub., 1978.

Turner, C., and Bagnara, J. T.: General Endocrinology. Philadelphia, W. B. Saunders, 1976.

Werner, S. C., and Ingbar, S. H.: The Thyroid. Hagerstown, Md., Harper & Row, 1978.

ARTICLES

Adrenal—Corticosteroids

Bissada, N. K.: Surgical diseases of the adrenal gland. Am. Fam. Phys., *15*:130-135, June 1977.

Davis, P. J.: Endocrine and aging. Hospital Pract., *12*:113-128, Sept. 1977.

Hartley, B.: Now you're on cortisone. Canad. Nurse, *74*:21-27, Feb. 1978.

Melick, M. E.: Nursing intervention for patients receiving corticosteroid therapy. *In* Kintzel, K. C. (ed.): Advanced Concepts in Clinical Nursing, 2nd ed. Chap. 18. Philadelphia, J. B. Lippincott, 1977.

Newton, D. W., et al.: You can minimize the hazards of corticosteroids. Nursing '77, 7:26-33, June 1977.

One more topical corticosteroid. Med. Letter, *20*:112, Dec. 15, 1978.

Ricciatti, D., and Lester, R. S.: A primer on topical corticosteroid therapy. Mod. Med., *45*:42-47, Dec. 15, 1977.

Rose, L. I.: Choosing corticosteroid preparations. Am. Fam. Phys., *17*:198-204, Mar. 1978.

Schteingart, D. E.: Cushing's disease: an update. Drug Ther., *8*:125-135, Feb. 1978.

Tzagournis, M.: Acute adrenal insufficiency. Heart & Lung, 7:603-609, July/Aug. 1978.

Thyroid and Parathyroid

Acute adrenocortical insufficiency. Nurses' Drug Alert, 2:150-151, Dec. 1978.

Bain, J., and Walfish, P. G.: The assessment of thyroid function and structure. Otolaryngol. Clin. N. Amer., *11*:419-443, June 1978.

Barzel, V. S.: The changing face of hyperparathyroidism. Hosp. Pract., *12*:89-94, Nov. 1977.

Braverman, L. B.: Treatment of hypothyroidism, a practical guide. Thyroid Today, 2:1-6, Jan. 1979.

Bunner, D. L.: Thyroid hormone replacement therapy, 1891-1977. Arch. Int. Med., *138*:978-979, June 1978.

Check, W.: High marks for hyperthyroid therapies. JAMA, *240*:1832-1833, Oct. 20, 1978.

Chopra, I. J.: Laboratory aids in the diagnosis of hyperthyroidism. Thyroid Today, 1:1-6, Apr.-May 1978.

Edis, A. J.: Surgical anatomy and technique of neck exploration for primary hyperparathyroidism. Surg. Clin. N. Am., *57*:495-503, June 1977.

Feldman, J. M.: The practical use of thyroid function tests. Am. Fam. Phys., *16*:159-165, Sept. 1977.

Gorman, C. A.: Management of the patient with Graves' ophthalmopathy. Thyroid Today, 1:1-6, Oct.-Nov. 1977.

Greenfield, L. D., et al.: Radiation safety precautions with [131]iodine therapy. Cancer Nurs., 1:379-384, Oct. 1978.

Halbertstam, M. J.: The thyroid and me (can clinical assessment be improved?). Mod. Med., *47*:13-18, Mar. 15-30, 1979.

Hyperthyroidism — thyroid storm (thyrotoxicosis). Nurses' Drug Alert, 2:148-149, Dec. 1978.

Hypothyroidism — myxedema coma. Nurses' Drug Alert, 2:149-150, Dec. 1978.

Karo, J. T., et al.: Ultrasonography and parathyroid adenomas. JAMA, *239*:2163-2164, May 19, 1978.

Mazzaferri, E. L.: Thyroid cancer: an overview. Thyroid Today, 1:1-6, Sept. 1978.

Merimee, T. J.: Thyroid function tests. Postgrad. Med., *63*:113-117, June 1978.

Potteiger, W. R.: The care of the patient having a thyroidectomy. Point of View, *15*:14-15, Jan. 1978.

ReMine, W. H., and McConahey, W. M.: Management of thyroid nodules. Surg. Clin. N. Am., *57*:523-531, June 1977.

Schlaff, S.: Thyrotoxicosis: a synopsis of diagnosis and clinical management. Today's Clinician, 2:13-29, June 1978.

Schottenfeld, D., and Gershman, G. T.: Epidemiology of thyroid cancer. CA-A Cancer J. for Clinic., *28*:66-86, Mar.-Apr. 1978.

Surks, M. I.: Laboratory aids in the diagnosis of hypothyroidism. Thyroid Today, 1:1-6, Dec. 1977.

Thompson, N. W., et al.: Thyroid carcinoma: current controversies. Current Prob. in Surg., *15*:5-67, Nov. 1978.

Thyroid replacement therapy. Med. Letter, *19*:50-51, June 17, 1977.

Thyroid storm from radioiodine. Nurses' Drug Alert, 3:50-51, May 1979.

Ultrasonic detection of parathyroid adenomas. JAMA, *240*:2163, May 19, 1978.

Urbanic, R. C., and Mazzaferri, E. L.: Thyrotoxic crisis and myxedema coma. Heart & Lung, 7:435-447, May-June 1978.

Van Heerden, J. A.: The pathology and surgical management of primary hyperparathyroidism. Surg. Clin. N. Amer., *57*:557-563, June 1977.

Volpe, R.: Treatment of Graves' disease: an overview. Thyroid Today, 1:1-6, Aug. 1977.

Wong, E. T., and Schultz, A. L.: Changing values for the normal thyroid radioactive iodine uptake test. JAMA, *238*:1741-1744, Oct. 17, 1977.

Pancreas

Arvanitakis, C., et al.: Laboratory aids in the diagnosis of pancreatitis. Med. Clin. N. Am., *62*:107-128, Jan. 1978.

Burke, M. D.: Clinical enzymology [section or acute pancreatitis], Postgrad. Med., *64*:151-152, Aug. 1978.

Cameron, J. L.: Lipid abnormalities and acute pancreatitis. Hosp. Pract., *12*:95-101, Apr. 1977.

Farrar, W. H., and Calkins, W. G.: Sensitivity of the amylase-creatinine clearance ration in acute pancreatitis. Arch. Int. Med., *138*:958-962, June 1978.

Gilsanz, V., et al.: Glucagon vs. anticholinergics in the treatment of acute pancreatitis. Arch. Int. Med., *138*:535-538, Apr. 1978.

Go, V. L., and Sheedy, P. F.: Ultrasonography, computed tomography, endoscopic retrograde cholangiography and angiography in the diagnosis of pancreatic cancer. Med. Clin. N. Am., *62*:129-140, Jan. 1978.

Meeting the challenge of pancreatitis. Patient Care, *11*:71-117, Sept. 15, 1977.

Snape, W. J., Jr.: Medical management of acute pancreatitis. Drug Ther., 2:19-27, Apr. 1977.

Stillman, M. J.: Nursing intervention in acute pancreatitis. RN, *41*:67-73, Dec. 1978.

Weir, G. C., and Novelline, R. A.: The glucagonoma syndrome. Am. Fam. Phys., *16*:83-84, July 1977.

Pheochromocytoma

Macaron, C., and Yuk-pui, L.: What not to do in pheochromocytoma. Am. Fam. Phys., *17*:120-122, Apr. 1978.

Wallace, J. M., and Gill, D. P.: Prazosin in the diagnosis and treatment of pheochromocytoma. JAMA, *240*:2752-2753, Dec. 15, 1978.

Diabetes Insipidus

Desmopressin for diabetes insipidus. Med. Lett. Drugs Ther., *20*:26–27, March 10, 1978.

Thompson, P., Earll, J. M., and Schaaf, M.: Comparison of clofibrate and chlorpropamide in vasopressin-responsive diabetes insipidus. Metabolism, *26*:749–762, Jan. 1977.

Gout

Emmerson, B. T.: Drug control of gout and hyperuricaemia. Drugs, *16*:158–166, Aug. 1978.

Gordon, G. V., and Schumacher, H. R.: Management of gout. Am. Fam. Phys., *19*:91–97, Jan. 1979.

Klinenberg, J. R.: Hyperuricemia and gout. Med. Clin. N. Am., *61*:299–312, Mar. 1977.

Scott, J. T.: Choice of treatment in gout. Practitioner, *219*:469–474, Oct. 1977.

Talbott, J. H. (ed.): Gout (symposium). Postgrad. Med., *63*:132–180, May 1978.

AGENCIES

American Thyroid Association, Inc., Mayo Clinic, Rochester, Minn. 55901

Renal and Urinary Problems

UNIT 10

41

ASSESSMENT OF RENAL AND URINARY FUNCTION

PHYSIOLOGIC OVERVIEW

The kidneys, ureters, bladder and urethra comprise the urinary system. The kidney's main responsibility is to extract unwanted substances, including water, from the blood. The extracted materials which comprise the urine are transported through the ureters for temporary storage in the urinary bladder. During the act of micturition (urination), the bladder contracts and the urine is expelled from the body through the urethra. The purpose of urine formation is to regulate the water content and electrolyte composition of the body fluids. Over a period of time, the amount of electrolytes and water excreted by the kidneys very nearly approximates the amount that is taken into the body orally. Although fluid and electrolytes can be lost by other means, such as in sweat or feces, it is the kidneys that have to precisely regulate the internal environment of the body. The renal excretory function is necessary for maintenance of life. However, unlike the cardiovascular and respiratory systems, complete malfunction of the kidneys may not cause death for several days. In addition, with modern medical management it is possible to completely substitute for renal function by means of an artificial kidney.

An important feature of the urinary system is its ability to adapt to wide variations in fluid load based on the personal habits of the individual. Basically, the kidney must be able to excrete that which is ingested into the diet, and not eliminated by other organs. This usually amounts to 1 to 1½ liters of water per day, 6 to 8 gm. of salt (sodium chloride) per day, 6 to 8 gm. of potassium chloride per day, and 70 mg. of acid equivalents per day.

In addition, protein is ingested and metabolized by the body into urea and other waste products that must also be excreted in the urine.

Anatomy of the Urinary System

The kidneys are paired organs, each weighing approximately 125 gm., located in a position lateral to the bodies of the lower thoracic vertebrae, a few centimeters to the right and left of the midline. They are surrounded by a thin fibrous tissue known as the capsule. Anteriorly, the kidneys are separated from the abdominal cavity and its contents by layers of peritoneum. Posteriorly, they are shielded by the lower thoracic wall. There is no anatomical difference between the two kidneys other than they are located on opposite sides of the body. The blood supply to each kidney is delivered through the renal artery and drained through the renal vein. The renal arteries arise from the abdominal aorta and the renal veins carry blood back into the inferior vena cava. The kidneys can efficiently clear the blood of waste materials in part because their total blood flow is great and represents 25 percent of cardiac output.

Urine is formed within the kidneys in functional units, known as nephrons. The urine formed within these nephrons passes into collecting ducts which join to form the pelvis of each kidney. Each kidney pelvis gives rise to a ureter. The ureter is a long tube (25 cm.) with a wall composed largely of smooth muscle. It connects each kidney to the bladder and functions as a conduit for urine.

The urinary bladder is a hollow organ that is situated anteriorly just behind the pubic bone. It acts as a temporary storage reservoir for the urine. The walls of the

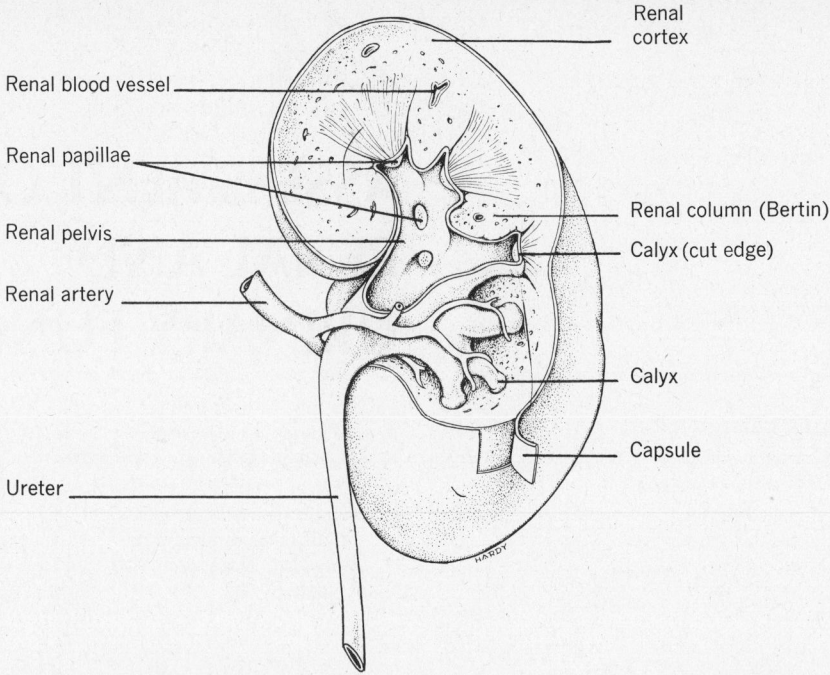

Renal cortex

Renal blood vessel

Renal papillae

Renal column (Bertin)

Renal pelvis

Calyx (cut edge)

Renal artery

Calyx

Capsule

Ureter

Figure 41-1. Diagram of internal structure of kidney, showing relations of renal pelvis and calyces to pyramids in medullary region. (From Chaffee, E. E., and Greisheimer, E. M.: Basic Physiology and Anatomy, 3rd ed., Philadelphia, J. B. Lippincott, 1974)

bladder consist largely of smooth muscle called the detrusor muscle. Contraction of this muscle is mainly responsible for emptying the bladder during urination. The urethra rises from the bladder and runs through the penis in the male and opens just above the vagina in the female. A short distance from its origin, the urethra is encircled by a small bundle of muscle fibers that is called the external urinary sphincter. This sphincter is the major site for control of the initiation of urination.

The Nephron. The kidney is divided into an outer portion called the cortex and an inner portion known as the medulla (Fig. 41-1). In the human, each kidney is composed of approximately 1 million nephrons, the functional unit of the kidney. Each nephron consists of a glomerulus and a tubule (Fig. 41-2) with the glomerulus measuring about 0.2 mm. in diameter and the tubule approximately 25 to 45 mm. in length. The glomerulus, the beginning of the nephron, is composed of tufts of capillaries that are fed by an afferent arteriole and drained by an efferent arteriole. The latter is a thick-walled muscular vessel (it is not a vein) which helps to maintain a high pressure in the glomerular capillaries. Like capillaries in general, the walls of the glomerular capillaries are composed of a layer of endothelial cells and a basement membrane. On the other side of the basement membrane are the epithelial cells that form the beginning of the tubule. The tubule itself is divided into three parts: a proximal tubule, the loop of Henle, and a distal tubule. The distal tubules coalesce to form collecting ducts which are about 20 mm. long and pass through the renal

cortex and the medulla to empty into the pelvis of the kidney. The total length of a typical nephron, including the collecting duct, ranges from 45 to 65 mm.

Function of the Nephron. The process of urine formation begins as blood flows through the glomerulus. Fluid is filtered through the walls of the glomerular capillary tufts into the proximal tubule. Under normal conditions, approximately 20 percent of the plasma passing through the glomerulus is filtered into the nephron, amounting to about 180 liters of filtrate per day. The filtrate, very similar to blood plasma without its proteins, consists essentially of water, electrolytes and other small molecules. Within the tubule and collecting ducts, some of these substances are selectively reabsorbed into the blood. Other substances may actually be secreted into the filtrate as it travels down the tubule. The urine is the remaining fluid (along with its contents) that reaches the pelvis of the kidney. Some substances such as glucose are usually completely reabsorbed in the tubule and do not appear in the urine. The processes of reabsorption and secretion in the tubule frequently involve active transport and require the utilization of metabolic energy. The amount of various substances normally filtered by the glomerulus, reabsorbed by the tubules, and excreted in the urine is shown in Table 41-1.

Urine Composition

The kidney functions as the main excretory organ of the body. It disposes of unwanted materials that are ingested as well as the byproducts of the body's metabo-

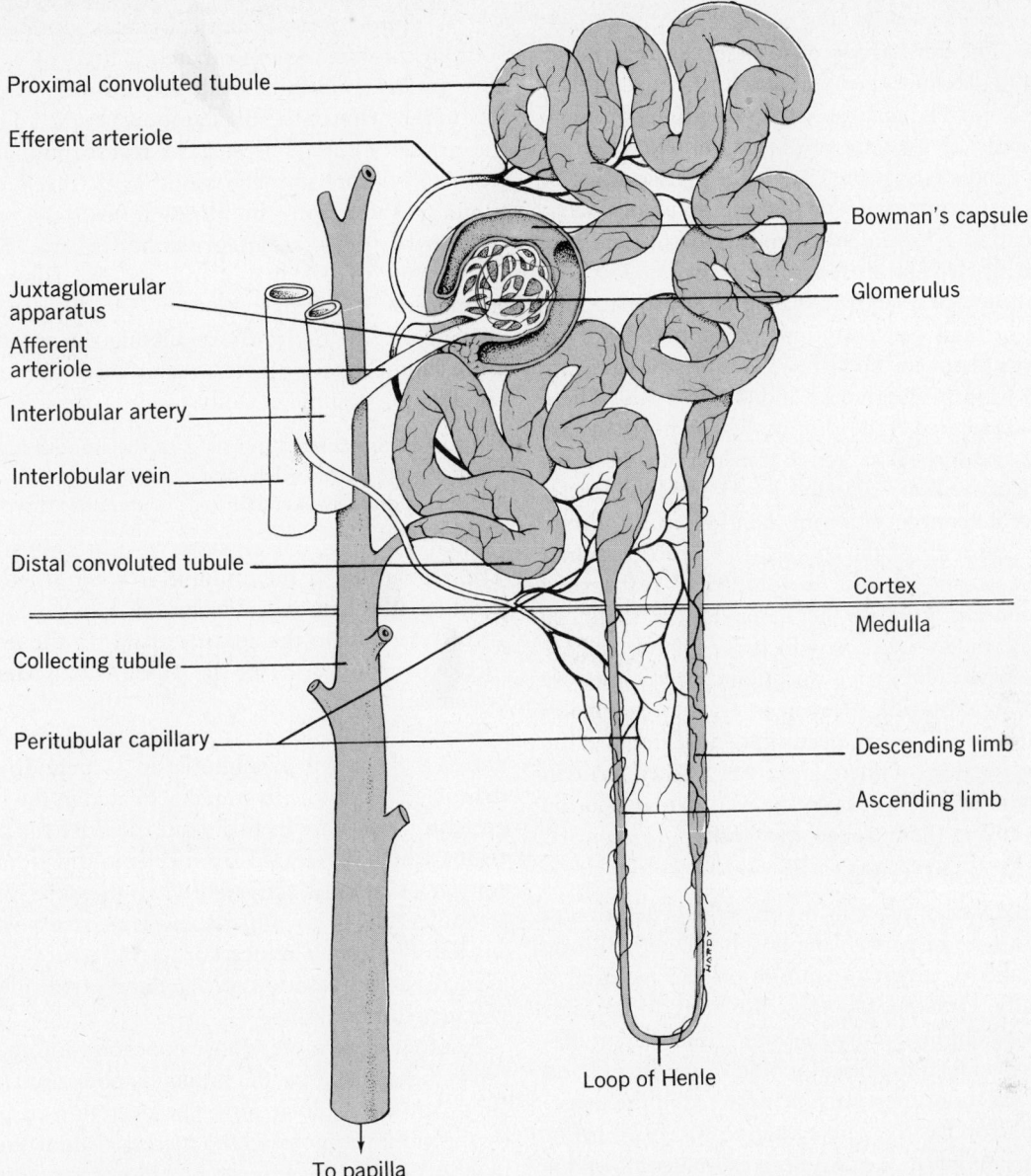

Proximal convoluted tubule

Efferent arteriole

Juxtaglomerular apparatus

Afferent arteriole

Interlobular artery

Interlobular vein

Distal convoluted tubule

Collecting tubule

Peritubular capillary

Bowman's capsule

Glomerulus

Cortex

Medulla

Descending limb

Ascending limb

Loop of Henle

To papilla

Figure 41-2. Diagram of a nephron and its blood supply. Also shown is a collecting tubule that receives urine from neighboring nephron units. Note that the loop of Henle dips into the medullary layer of the kidney. (Chaffee and Greisheimer)

lism. In the normal individual, the amounts of these materials excreted per day are exactly equal to the amounts ingested and formed so that over a period of time, there is no net change in the total body composition.

Urine is composed primarily of water. A normal person ingests approximately 1 to 2 liters of water per day, and normally all but 400 to 500 ml. of this is excreted in the urine. The remainder is lost from the skin during breathing and in the feces. The second major class of substances excreted in the urine is the electrolytes, including sodium, potassium, chloride, bicarbonate and other less abundant ions. The normal person ingests about 6 to 8 gm. each of sodium chloride (salt) and

TABLE 41-1.   FILTRATION, REABSORPTION AND EXCRETION OF CERTAIN NORMAL CONSTITUENTS OF PLASMA

	FILTERED 24 HR.	REABSORBED 24 HR.	EXCRETED 24 HR.[1]
	g.	g.	g.
Sodium	540	537	3.3
Chloride	630	625	5.3
Bicarbonate	300	300	0.3
Potassium	28	24	3.9
Glucose	140	140	0
Urea	53	28	25
Creatinine	1.4	0	1.4
Uric acid	8.5	7.7	0.8

[1]These are typical normal values. Wide variation is found depending on diet.

potassium chloride per day, and nearly all of this appears in the urine. The third group of substances appearing in the urine is made up of the breakdown products of protein metabolism. The major breakdown product is urea, of which about 25 gm. are produced and excreted per day. Other products of protein metabolism that must be excreted are creatinine phosphates and sulphates. Uric acid, formed as a breakdown product of nucleic acid metabolism, is also eliminated in the urine.

It is important to recognize that some substances that are present in high concentrations in the blood are ordinarily not present in the urine. Examples of these are the normal foodstuffs, glucose and amino acids. These substances are filtered at the glomerulus and normally are completely reabsorbed by active transport in the renal tubule. Glucose will appear in the urine if its blood level is so high that its concentration in the glomerular filtrate exceeds the capacity of the tubules to reabsorb it. In a normal person, the glucose is completely reabsorbed when its concentration in the blood is less than 200 mg./100 ml. In diabetes, in which the blood glucose levels exceed the kidney's reabsorption capacity, glucose will appear in the urine. Protein is also not normally found in the urine. These molecules are not filtered at the glomerulus because of their large size. When protein appears in the urine, it usually signifies damage to the glomeruli causing them to become "leaky."

Regulation of Acid Excretion

The breakdown of proteins involves the generation of acid compounds, in particular phosphoric and sulfuric acids. In addition, a certain amount of acid material is ingested daily. Unlike CO_2, these are nonvolatile acids and cannot be eliminated by the lung. Since accumulation of these acids in the blood would lower its pH and inhibit cell function, they must be excreted in the urine. A normal person has to excrete approximately 70 mEq. of acid each day. The kidney is able to excrete some of this acid directly into the urine to the extent of lowering its pH to 4.5, one thousand times more acidic than blood.

More acid usually needs to be eliminated from the body than can be excreted directly as free acid in the urine. This is accomplished by the renal excretion of acid which is bound to chemical buffers. The acid (H^+) is secreted by the renal tubular cells into the filtrate where it is buffered chiefly by phosphate ions and ammonia (NH_3). Phosphate is present in the glomerular filtrate and ammonia is produced by the kidney cells and secreted into the tubular fluid. Through the buffering process, the kidney is able to excrete large quantities of acid in a bound form without further lowering the pH of the urine.

Regulation of Electrolyte Excretion

The amount of electrolytes and water that must be excreted by the kidney each day varies greatly, depending on the amounts ingested. The 180 liters of filtrate formed by the glomeruli each day contains about 1100 gm. of sodium chloride. Approximately 2 liters of water and 6 to 8 gm. of sodium chloride are normally excreted per day in the urine. The small amounts excreted relative to the amount filtered reflect active reabsorption of sodium from the filtrate into the blood as it travels down the tubules. Water from the filtrate follows the reabsorbed sodium in order to maintain osmotic balance. Thus, over 99 percent of the water and sodium filtered at the glomerulus is reabsorbed into the blood by the time the urine leaves the body. By regulating the amount of sodium (and therefore water) reabsorbed, the kidney can regulate the volume of body fluids.

- If sodium is excreted in excess of the amount ingested, the patient will become dehydrated.
- If less sodium is excreted than is ingested, the patient will retain fluid.

The regulation of the amount of sodium excreted depends on the hormone, aldosterone, which is synthesized and released from the adrenal gland. In the presence of increased aldosterone in the blood, less sodium is excreted in the urine.

Release of aldosterone from the adrenal gland is largely under the control of angiotensin, a peptide hormone manufactured in the liver and activated in the lung. Angiotensin levels are in turn controlled by the hormone, renin, which is released from cells in the kidneys. This complex system is activated when pressure in the renal arterioles falls below normal levels as occurs with shock and dehydration. The effect of activation of this system is to increase the retention of water and expansion of intravascular fluid volume.

Another electrolyte whose concentration in the body fluids is regulated by the kidney is potassium, the most abundant intracellular ion. The excretion of potassium by the kidney is increased by increased aldosterone levels in contrast to the effects of aldosterone on sodium excretion.

- Retention of potassium is the most life-threatening effect of renal failure.

Regulation of Water Excretion

Regulation of the amount of water excreted is also an important function of the kidney. With a large water intake, a large volume of dilute urine must be excreted. Conversely, with a low water intake, the urine that is excreted must be concentrated. The relative degree of dilution or concentration of the urine can be measured in terms of its *osmolality*. This term refers to the amount of solid material (electrolytes and other molecules) that is dissolved in the urine. The filtrate in the glomerular capillary normally has the same osmolality as the blood, with a value of approximately 300 mOsm./liter. As the filtrate passes through the tubules and collecting ducts, the osmolality may vary anywhere from 50 mOsm./liter to 1200 mOsm./liter, the maximal diluting and concentrating ability of the kidney.

The osmolality of the urine specimen can be measured, but, more commonly, it is estimated from its specific gravity. The *specific gravity* refers to the weight of a given volume of fluid. Pure water has a specific gravity of 1 gm./ml. If no electrolytes or other particles are suspended in the urine, the specific gravity would be 1.000 However, the presence of electrolytes or other materials raises the urinary specific gravity to as high as 1.030 when it is most concentrated.

How are water excretion and urine concentration regulated by the kidney? The glomerular filtrate has essentially the same electrolyte composition as the blood plasma without the proteins. Therefore, regulation of urine concentration is carried out in the tubule by varying the amount of water that is reabsorbed in relation to electrolyte reabsorption. The amount of water that is reabsorbed is under the control of antidiuretic hormones (ADH, vasopressin). ADH is a hormone that is secreted by the posterior part of the pituitary gland in response to changes in osmolality of the blood. With decreased water intake, blood osmolality tends to rise and stimulate ADH release. ADH then acts on the kidney in order to cause increased reabsorption of water, thereby restoring the osmolality of the blood back towards normal. With excess water intake, the secretion of ADH by the pituitary is depressed and, therefore, less water is reabsorbed by the kidney tubule. This latter situation leads to increased urine volume and is called diuresis.

• Loss of the ability to concentrate and dilute the urine is the most common early manifestation of kidney disease.

In this condition, the specific gravity of the urine cannot be altered from approximately 1.010, which is the specific gravity of the glomerular filtrate and the blood plasma.

Renal Clearance

The most commonly used test to evaluate how well the kidney performs its excretory function is termed *clearance*. Clearance of a substance A is given by the following equation: clearance equals (the urine concentration of A) times (the urine volume in a given time) divided by the plasma concentration of A.* For example, if the arterial plasma concentration of a substance is 0.1 mg./ml., the urine concentration of the same substance is 50 mg./ml., and the urine volume is 1.0 ml./min., the clearance of that substance according to the above equation is 500 ml./min. This means that 500 ml. of blood is completely cleared of that substance in one minute. In the body, few substances are actually completely cleared from the blood during a single passage through the

*Clearance =
$$\frac{\text{(urine concentration of A)} \times \text{(urine volume in a given time)}}{\text{plasma concentration of A}}$$

kidney. In the example given above, if the blood is cleared of only 50 percent of the substance, urine concentration of the substance would be 25 mg./ml. and the calculated renal clearance would be 250 ml./min. It is possible to measure the renal clearance of any substance, but the one that has proven particularly useful is the creatinine clearance. The amount of creatinine excreted is approximately the amount filtered at the glomerulus. Therefore, creatinine clearance is a good measure of the glomerular filtration rate (GFR). The normal adult GFR is about 100-120 ml./min. Urea clearance is sometimes used instead of creatinine clearance as a measure of GFR but generally gives a slightly lower number. Urea clearance gives its best indication of GFR when urine flow rate is high, above 2 ml./minute.

Storage of Urine and Micturition

Urine formed by the kidney is transported from the renal pelvis through the ureters and into the bladder. This movement is facilitated by peristaltic waves occurring about 1 to 5 times per minute and generated by the smooth muscle in the ureter wall. Urine flows into the bladder in spurts synchronous with the peristaltic contractions. There are no sphincters between the bladder and the ureters, although reflux of urine from the bladder in normal subjects is prevented by the unidirectional nature of the peristaltic waves and because each ureter enters the bladder at an oblique angle. However —

• with overdistention of the bladder due to disease, the elevated pressure in the bladder can be transmitted back through the ureters leading to ureteral distention and possible reflux of urine. This can lead to kidney infection (pyelonephritis) and damage from the elevated pressure (hydronephrosis).

The pressure in the bladder is normally very low, even as the urine accumulates because the bladder's smooth muscle adapts to the increased stretch as the bladder is slowly filled. The first sensations of bladder filling ordinarily occur when about 100 to 150 ml. of urine are present in the bladder. In most cases, there is a desire to void when the bladder contains approximately 200 to 300 ml. With 400 ml., a marked feeling of fullness is usually present.

Voiding of urine is prevented by contraction of the external urethral sphincter. This muscle is under voluntary control and is innervated by nerves from the sacral area of the spinal cord. Voluntary control is a learned behavoir that is not present at birth. When there is a desire to urinate, the external urethral sphincter is relaxed and the detrusor muscle (bladder smooth muscle) contracts and expels the urine from the bladder through the urethra. The pressure generated in the bladder during micturition (urination) is approximately 50 to 150 cm. of water. Residual urine in the urethra drains by gravity in the female and is expelled by voluntary muscle contractions in the male.

The contraction of the detrusor muscle is regulated by a reflex involving the parasympathetic nervous system. The reflex is integrated in the sacral portion of the spinal tract. The sympathetic nervous system plays no essential part in micturition, but does prevent semen from entering the bladder during ejaculation.

- If the pelvic nerves to the bladder and sphincter are destroyed, voluntary control and reflex urination are abolished and the bladder becomes overdistended with urine. If the spinal pathways from the brain to the urinary system are destroyed (for example, after a spinal cord transection), reflex contraction of the bladder is maintained, but voluntary control over the process is lost. In both of these types of loss of innervation, the muscle of the bladder can contract and expel urine, but the contractions are generally insufficient to empty the bladder completely, and residual urine is left behind.

The most common clinical method used to study bladder function is catheterization—passage of a catheter through the urethra into the bladder. With this technique, it is possible to measure the amount of urine left in the bladder after micturition (residual urine). Normally, this should be no more than 50 ml. However, catheterization is to be avoided whenever possible, because it increases the risk of infection. Another test for bladder dysfunction is to measure the pressure in the bladder after instillation of various volumes of saline. This latter procedure is called a *cystometrogram*.

RENAL PATHOPHYSIOLOGY

Diseases of the kidney can be classified according to the segment of the nephron that is primarily affected. Glomerulonephritis and the various etiologies of the nephrotic syndrome primarily affect the renal glomerulus. Vascular diseases, infections and toxins affect primarily the renal tubule, although some element of glomerular dysfunction may coexist. Obstruction to the outflow of urine due to calculi (stones), protein, or other material in the collecting ducts or ureters may eventually lead to damage of the entire nephron. When the degree of kidney damage is severe, renal failure occurs and may result in the condition called *uremia*.

Glomerular Diseases

Nephritic Syndrome. The nephritic syndrome occurs in response to a group of diseases in which inflammation of the glomerulus (glomerulonephritis) is predominant. The major manifestations are hematuria (red blood cells in the urine) and urinary red blood cell casts. These abnormalities are due to damage to the glomerular capillaries which permits leakage of red blood cells into the tubular lumen. Glomerulonephritis most commonly results from immune reactions. Common causes are the reaction to some streptococcal infections predominantly in children and the autoimmune diseases such as Goodpasture's syndrome and lupus erythematosus. Glomerulonephritis may resolve completely although in some patients renal failure may result.

Nephrotic Syndrome. The nephrotic syndrome results from a group of glomerular diseases associated with increased permeability of the glomerulus to proteins. Frequently, there are no observable alterations of kidney structure by light microscopy. The primary manifestation of the disease is the loss of plasma proteins, particularly albumin, in the urine. Although the liver is capable of increasing its production of albumin manyfold, it is unable to keep up with the daily loss of albumin through the kidney; thus hypoalbuminemia results. The resultant decreased oncotic pressure leads to generalized edema. A tendency to decreased circulating blood volume activates the renin-angiotensin system leading to retention of sodium, which also contributes to the development of edema. Figure 41-3 shows the pathways that may be involved in the development of edema in the nephrotic syndrome. Patients with nephrotic syndrome also exhibit an elevated lipid concentration in their blood (lipemia), the cause of which is not known. The nephrotic syndrome can occur with almost any intrinsic renal disease or systemic disease that affects the glomerulus. See page 935 for further discussion.

Renal Failure

Renal failure is present when the excretion of water, electrolytes and metabolic waste products is insufficient because of kidney damage which prevents the kidneys from maintaining the normal internal environment of the body. Acute renal failure has a sudden onset and is frequently reversible. Chronic renal failure usually develops gradually but can also occur as a consequence of a preceding acute episode. One normal kidney is generally sufficient for normal urinary function so that renal failure requires bilateral kidney damage. The signs and symptoms of renal failure are in large part a manifestation of the altered fluid and electrolyte balance of the body. The diagnosis is generally made by the finding of *azotemia,* defined as elevation of nitrogenous waste products in the blood. Uremia results when this condition is severe.

Pathogenesis of Renal Failure. Decreased excretion of metabolic waste products can occur as a result of kidney damage, a decrease in blood flow to the kidney, or acute obstruction to the flow of urine.

- Decreased urine output due to complete urinary obstruction can occur in patients who have an enlarged prostate, stones (calculi) in the ureters or urethra, or infiltrating tumors. Secondary damage to the kidneys and renal failure will result if the obstruction is not relieved promptly.
- Alterations of renal blood flow can occur with hypotension, congestive heart failure, dehydration, or thrombosis of renal

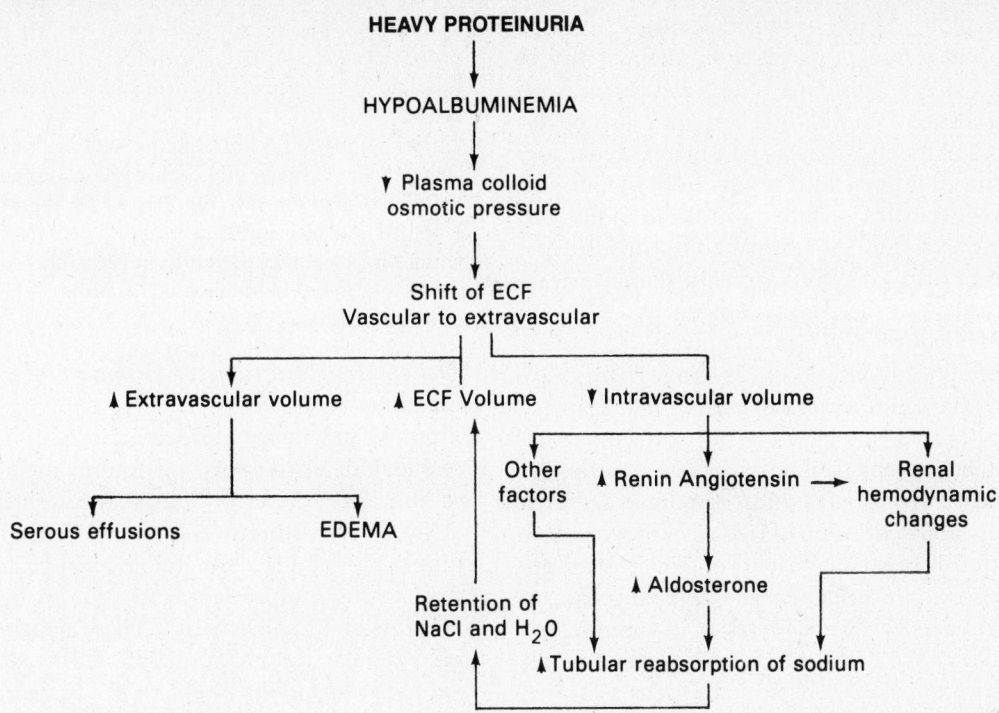

HEAVY PROTEINURIA

↓

HYPOALBUMINEMIA

↓

▼ Plasma colloid
osmotic pressure

↓

Shift of ECF
Vascular to extravascular

▲ Extravascular volume   ▲ ECF Volume   ▼ Intravascular volume

Other factors   ▲ Renin Angiotensin →   Renal hemodynamic changes

Serous effusions   EDEMA

▲ Aldosterone

Retention of NaCl and H₂O

▲ Tubular reabsorption of sodium

Figure 41-3.   Pathogenesis of edema in the nephrotic syndrome. From: *Harrison's Principles of Internal Medicine.* Edited by Thorn, Adam, Braunwald, Isselbacher and Petersdorf. McGraw-Hill, N.Y., 1977, p. 1420.

arteries. Acute decrease in renal blood flow may lead to secondary renal damage and renal failure. Decreased excretion of waste products due to decreased renal blood flow in the absence of kidney damage is called "prerenal azotemia."

- Acute renal failure due to kidney injury results from acute vasculitis, acute glomerulonephritis, severe ("malignant") hypertension, or, more commonly, acute damage to the renal tubules (acute tubular necrosis, ATN).
- The clinical conditions that may result in ATN include hypotension (shock), exposure to nephrotoxic chemicals, intravascular hemolysis with hemoglobinuria (e.g. due to transfusion reactions, extensive burns, or infusion of water intravenously), or crush injury of an extremity with myoglobinuria.

The etiologies of chronic renal failure include the causes for acute renal failure and include, in addition, chronic infection (pyelonephritis), nephrosclerosis, diabetic nephropathy, collagen diseases, and other chronic, progressive kidney diseases. See page 929 for further discussion.

Uremia

Uremia is a term used to designate the manifestations of chronic renal dysfunction. Uremia is a generalized condition that affects all organ systems of the body.

Fluids and Electrolytes.   The fluid and electrolyte abnormalities that occur in renal failure are the consequence of a decreased number of functional nephrons. The fundamental pathophysiological alteration in kidney func-

tion is a decreased overall glomerular filtration rate (GFR) due to a reduced number of filtering glomeruli, leading to decreased clearance of substances that depend on the rate of filtration for their excretion. Decreased glomerular filtration rate can be diagnosed by a decreased inulin, urea, or creatinine clearance. When more than 50 percent of the normal nephrons have been destroyed, the urea concentration in the blood (commonly measured as the blood urea nitrogen—BUN) begins to rise above normal. The degree of elevation of urea depends in part on the amount of protein in the diet, since urea is a normal end product of protein metabolism. In the presence of decreased GFR, plasma concentrations of creatinine and uric acid also rise.

In addition to decreased GFR, a decrease in the number of functional nephrons results in decreased modification of the glomerular filtrate by the tubules prior to its excretion as urine. As a result, the urine resembles a filtrate of plasma, having a fixed specific gravity of approximately 1.010. This inability to concentrate or dilute the urine prevents appropriate responses by the kidneys to fluctuations in daily intake of water and electrolytes. Decreased intake of fluid or salt can lead to dehydration or sodium depletion; excess salt or water intake may cause water intoxication or sodium overload. Decreased tubular function also results in inability to excrete increased loads of potassium (K^+) and acid (H^+). With advanced renal disease, the normal production of H^+ by body metabolism or release of K^+ from damaged cells of the body can themselves result in acidosis or hyperkalemia. Decreased excretion of acid results primarily from the inability of the tubules to secrete ammonia (NH_3) and to reabsorb sodium bicarbonate ($NaHCO_3$). There may also be decreased excretion of phosphates and organic acids. Decreased excretion of potassium results from inability of the tubules to secrete this ion into the urine. In addition to the inability to excrete these normal body constituents, the excretion of drugs may be markedly altered, necessitating adjustment of their usual dosages.

Calcium Metabolism and Bone Changes. Disorders of calcium metabolism with secondary bone changes are among the major manifestations of uremia. The primary finding is usually a decreased serum calcium concentration. The pathophysiologic processes leading to hypocalcemia are diverse. The most important factor is probably reciprocal depression of free calcium secondary to the elevation of serum phosphorous due to its decreased excretion in the urine. An additional mechanism for hypocalcemia is decreased conversion of vitamin D to its active form by the damaged kidneys, leading to diminished absorption of calcium from the gastrointestinal tract. Decreased serum calcium secondarily stimulates the parathyroid glands to produce increased parathormone, resulting in the condition called secondary hyperparathyroidism. This condition is manifested by demineralization of bone and formation of bone cysts. The bone changes are worsened as a result of decreased deposition of calcium due to decreased active vitamin D and increased resorption of calcium due to chronic acidosis. The demineralization of bone leads to frequent fractures and bone pain. The term *renal osteodystrophy* is frequently used to designate the complex bone changes that occur with uremia.

Anemia. Anemia, another common manifestation of uremia, is generally due to decreased rate of production of red blood cells by the bone marrow and increased rates of red blood cell destruction. Decreased erythropoiesis may be related to a decreased rate of production of erythropoietin by the kidneys. The red cells in the peripheral blood generally appear to be of normal size (normocytic) and of normal hemoglobin concentration (normochromic). Blood loss due to bleeding from the gastrointestinal tract or other sites may contribute to the anemia.

Cardiovascular Manifestations. Hypertension, frequently associated with chronic renal failure, may be either the cause or the result of renal damage. Primary hypertension leads to kidney damage as a result of atherosclerosis of the renal vasculature manifested by nephrosclerosis. Secondary hypertension occurs due to increased renin production by the diseased kidney leading to generalized vasoconstriction as well as salt retention with consequent expansion of the vascular volume.

- Patients with compromised excretory function are more prone than normal persons to volume overload since they are less able to compensate for acute increases in water and salt intake.
- Chronic congestive heart failure with pulmonary and peripheral edema frequently occurs as a consequence of hypertensive cardiac disease complicated by the effects of fluid overload and anemia.
- Congestive heart failure results in decreased renal blood flow with elevation of blood urea out of proportion to the degree of kidney damage.

Other Manifestations of Uremia. Among the diverse manifestations of uremia are: gastrointestinal symptoms including anorexia, nausea, vomiting, and hiccoughs; neuromuscular symptoms including mental clouding, inability to concentrate, drowsiness, lethargy, twitching, convulsions, and tetany (related to the low serum calcium); and dermatologic symptoms including severe itching and uremic frost (due to the high concentration of urea in sweat). These patients also have altered cellular immunity manifested by decreased delayed hypersensitivity and increased susceptibility to infection probably related to a decreased ability of leukocytes to kill bacteria. The precise mechanism for many of these diverse conditions has not been worked out. However, retention of products normally excreted in the urine, such as ammonia, phenols, and other organic and inorganic compounds, is the probable cause.

Course of Renal Failure

The basic mechanisms underlying the pathophysiologic changes of acute and chronic renal failure are similar. However, their clinical presentations are markedly different. There are two phases of acute renal failure: the oliguric phase and the polyuric phase.

Oliguric Phase. Acute renal failure occurs due to sudden insults to the kidney that result in a decreased rate of urine formation. This is called the oliguric phase of acute renal failure.

- During the oliguric phase, the potential life-threatening complications are related to fluid and electrolyte retention (in particular, hyperkalemia and acidosis).

Polyuric Phase. If the original insult is removed, the recovery process begins with gradually increasing glomerular filtration rate. At this stage, the renal tubular cells may still be unable to reabsorb the water and electrolytes in the increasing volume of glomerular filtrate. As a result, the volume of urine that is excreted is increased above normal, resulting in the polyuric phase of acute renal failure.

- The potential life-threatening complications of the polyuric phase are dehydration and electrolyte depletion.

Complete recovery from acute renal failure, if it occurs, may require several months. Some patients with acute renal failure, despite the removal of the initial insult, will not recover normal renal function and will develop chronic renal failure. More commonly, however, chronic renal failure develops gradually and insidiously. The disease is frequently not discovered until the patient develops symptoms related to the fluid and electrolyte abnormalities. At this stage, kidney function has generally decreased by more than 50 percent and the urea concentration in the blood has risen above normal.

ASSESSMENT OF URINARY FUNCTION

CLINICAL MANIFESTATIONS OF URINARY DYSFUNCTION

The following symptoms and signs are suggestive of urinary tract disease: pain, changes in micturition, and gastrointestinal symptoms.

Pain

Genitourinary pain is not always present in renal disease but is generally seen in the more acute conditions. Pain of renal disease is caused by sudden distention of the renal capsule. Its severity is related to how quickly the distention develops.

Kidney pain may be felt as a dull ache in the costovertebral angle and may spread to the umbilicus. Ureteral pain produces pain in the back radiating to the abdomen, upper thigh, testis, or labium. Pain in the flank (the side between the ribs and ilium) radiating to the lower abdomen or epigastrium and often associated with nausea, vomiting, and paralytic ileus may indicate renal colic. Bladder pain (low abdominal pain or pain over the suprapubic area) can be due to an overdistended bladder or bladder infection. Urgency, tenesmus (painful straining), and dysuria are usually present. Pain at the urethral meatus reveals irritation of the bladder neck or infection. Severe pain in the scrotal regions results from inflammatory swelling of the epididymis or testicle, while perineal and rectal fullness and pain signal acute prostatitis or prostatic abscess. Back and leg pain may be due to metastases of cancer of the prostate to the pelvic bones. Pain in the penile shaft may originate from urethral problems while pain in the glans penis is usually due to prostatitis.

Changes in Micturition (Voiding)

Normal micturition is a painless function occurring five to six times daily and occasionally once at night. The average person voids 1200 to 1500 ml. of urine in 24 hours. This of course is modified by fluid intake, sweating, outside temperature, vomiting or diarrhea.

Urinary frequency may stem from an acutely inflamed bladder while *urgency* (strong desire to void) may be due to irritation of the trigone and posterior urethra.

Burning on urination is seen in patients with urethral irritation. Urethritis frequently causes burning during the act of voiding, whereas trigonitis may produce burning both during and after urination.

Pneumaturia (passage of gas in the urine while voiding) raises the suspicion of a fistulous connection between the bowel and bladder, rectosigmoid cancer, regional enteritis, or the presence of gas-forming organisms.

Dysuria (painful or difficult voiding) stems from a wide variety of pathological conditions.

Hesitancy (undue delay and difficulty in initiating voiding) may indicate compression of the urethra.

Nocturia (excessive urination at night) suggests decreased renal concentrating ability or heart failure.

Urinary incontinence (inability of the bladder to retain urine) may result from injury of the external urinary sphincter, acquired neurogenic disease, and severe urgency from infection.

Stress incontinence (intermittent leakage of urine from sudden strain) is from weakness of the sphincteric mechanism.

Enuresis (involuntary voiding during sleep) is physiologic to the age of 3 years. After this it may be functional or symptomatic of disease of the lower urinary tract.

Polyuria (large volume of urine voided in a given time) may be due to diabetes mellitus, diabetes insipidus, chronic renal disease, diuretics, and excessive fluid intake.

Oliguria (small volume of urine; output between 100 to 500 ml./24 hours) and anuria (absence of urine in the bladder; output less than 50 ml./24 hours) indicates a serious renal dysfunction requiring immediate medical intervention. These conditions may occur from shock, trauma, incompatible blood transfusion, drug poisoning, etc.

Hematuria (red blood cells in the urine) is considered a serious sign since it may indicate cancer of the genitourinary tract, acute glomerulonephritis, or renal tuberculosis. The color of bloody urine is dependent upon the pH of the urine and the amount of blood present. Hematuria may also be due to systemic causes such as blood dyscrasias, anticoagulant therapy and neoplasms.

Gastrointestinal Symptoms

Gastrointestinal symptoms may occur with urological conditions because of renointestinal reflexes. The anatomic relation of the right kidney to the colon, duodenum, head of the pancreas, common bile duct, liver, and gallbladder may also cause gastrointestinal disturbances. The left kidney is also related to the colon (splenic flexure), stomach, pancreas, and spleen. Gastrointestinal symptoms related to urologic conditions include nausea, vomiting, diarrhea, abdominal discomfort, paralytic ileus, and gastrointestinal hemorrhage.

Appendicitis also may be accompanied by urinary symptoms.

HEALTH HISTORY AND ASSESSMENT

When reviewing a health history it is important to be sure that the patient understands the questions being asked. In discussing problems involving the genitalia, the patient may "forget" or deny symptoms because of anxiety.

The following information related to urinary function is sought:

- What is the patient's chief concern? Why is he seeking help?
- What is the patient's present and past occupation(s)? (Look for occupational hazards relevant to the urinary tract: contact with chemicals, plastics, pitch, tar, rubber.)
- What is the past history especially in relation to urinary problems?
- Are there any accounts of renal disease in the family history?
- What childhood diseases did the patient have?
- Is there a history of urinary infections?
- Did enuresis extend beyond the usual age (past 3 years old)?
- Is nocturia present or absent? Date of onset?
- Are there any disorders of voiding?

    Dysuria? When does it occur? Where is it felt? Initial or terminal dysuria?

    Hesitancy? Straining? Pain during or after urination?

    Changes in color of urine? Diminished urine output?

    Incontinence? Stress incontinence? Urge incontinence?

    Any history of hematuria?

- Is pain present?

    Location? Character? Radiation? Duration? Related to voiding? What brings it on? What relieves it?

- Has the patient had fever? Chills? Passage of stones?
- Any history of genital lesions or venereal disease?
- For the female patient:

    Number of children? Their ages?

    Forceps deliveries?

    Catheterized?

    Any signs of vaginal discharge? Vaginal/vulvar itch or irritation?

- Does the patient have diabetes mellitus? Hypertension? Allergies?
- Has the patient ever been hospitalized with urinary tract infection?

    Before the age of 12?

    Cystoscopy? Indwelling catheter? Kidney x-ray procedures?

PHYSICAL ASSESSMENT

By direct palpation it is frequently possible to determine the size and movability of the kidneys.

- Place one hand on the patient's back so that the fingers are clear of the lower ribs and the other hand (palm down) is located anterior to the kidney with the fingers just above the level of the umbilicus.
- Ask the patient to inhale deeply, then push the anterior hand forward.

It may be possible to feel the smooth rounded lower pole of the kidney; the right is more easily felt than the left because it is somewhat lower than the left.

Renal disease may produce tenderness over the costovertebral angle. (The costovertebral angle lies where the twelfth or bottom rib joins the spine.)

In a rectal examination in the male, the prostate gland may be palpated digitally as a part of the study of urinary difficulty that occurs when there is hyperplasia of the prostate in older men (see page 79).

The inguinal area is examined for enlarged nodes, inguinal or femoral hernia and a varicocele. In women the vulva, urethra and vagina are examined.

DIAGNOSTIC ASSESSMENT

Roentgenograms

Roentgenograms are used in a variety of ways to study the urinary tract. The examination usually begins with a plain film of the abdomen or KUB (kidney, ureters, and bladder) to determine the size and position of the kidneys, and to reveal any deviations such as calcifications (stones) in the kidneys or urinary tract, hydronephrosis, cysts, tumors, or kidney displacement by abnormalities in the surrounding tissues.

Infusion Drip Pyelography. Infusion drip pyelography is an intravenous infusion of a large volume of dilute solution of contrast material to produce opacification of the renal parenchyma and complete filling of the urinary tract. This method of examination is especially useful when regular urographic techniques fail to show the drainage structures satisfactorily (e.g., in a patient with an elevated blood urea nitrogen) or when prolonged opacification of the drainage structures is desired so that tomograms (body section radiography) can be made. The patient preparation is the same as for excretory urography except the patient is not dehydrated. (See below.) Films are obtained at specified intervals after the start of the infusion to demonstrate the filled and distended collecting system.

Excretory Urography (Intravenous Urogram or Intravenous Pyelogram). An excretory urogram or intravenous pyelogram (IVP) provides a means for evaluating kidney function and visualizing the urinary tract. A radiopaque contrast material is introduced intravenously to be cleared from the blood by the kidneys and excreted through the urinary tract. As the contrast material concentrates in the urine, the kidneys, ureters, and bladder can be visualized. A *nephrotomogram* (body section roentgenograms which bring into focus the different layers of the kidney and the diffuse structures within each layer) is done as part of the study.

Excretory urography is conducted as part of the initial assessment of any suspected urologic problem, especially in the diagnosis of lesions in the kidneys and ureters. It also provides a rough estimate of renal function. The contrast material, such as sodium diatrizoate (Hypaque sodium) or meglumine diatrizoate (Renografin-60) is given intravenously, after which multiple films are taken serially to visualize drainage structures.

Patient Preparation:

The patient may be prepared for the procedure as follows:

1. A laxative may be given the night before the scheduled examination to eliminate feces and gas in the intestinal tract.
2. Liquids may be restricted 8 to 10 hours before the test. However, elderly patients with poor renal reserve or patients with multiple myeloma may not tolerate dehydrating procedures and should be given water to drink. Persons with uncontrolled diabetes mellitus may also be sensitive to fluid restriction.
3. The patient should not be overhydrated since this may dilute the contrast material causing inadequate visualization.
4. The patient's history should be checked for any indications of allergies which might cause an adverse reaction to the contrast material.

If the patient has a positive allergic history, a test dose of the contrast material may be injected intradermally. If no skin reaction occurs in 15 minutes, the regular intravenous test dose of contrast material is given. Although rare, as with the administration of any intravenous drug, an anaphylactoid reaction may occur. This reaction may occur even though the skin sensitivity test has been negative.

- All IV urogram rooms should have emergency drugs (epinephrine hydrochloride, vasopressors, etc.), as well as oxygen, tracheostomy equipment, etc., ready for immediate therapy in case an anaphylactoid reaction occurs.

Retrograde Pyelography. In retrograde pyelography, ureteral catheters are passed up through the ureters into the renal pelvis by means of cystoscopic manipulation. A contrast material is then introduced into the catheters by gravity or syringe. Retrograde pyelography is usually done when a nonfunctioning kidney is suspected or when the patient is allergic to intravenous contrast material. It is being used less frequently because of improved techniques in intravenous pyelogram.

Cystogram. A catheter is inserted into the bladder and radiopaque material instilled to outline the bladder wall and to evaluate vesicoureteral reflux (backflow of urine from the bladder into one or both ureters).

Cystourethrogram. A cystourethrogram provides visualization of the urethra and bladder either by retrograde injection of the contrast material into the urethra and bladder or by roentgenograms taken while the patient voids the contrast material. In a *voiding cystourethrogram,* the bladder is filled with radiopaque material and the patient voids while rapid spot films are taken. This test is used to determine the presence of vesicoureteral reflux or congenital abnormalities of the lower urinary tract. It is also used to investigate problems of bladder emptying and incontinence.

Renal Angiography. The purpose of this procedure is to visualize the renal arterial supply. A special needle is used to pierce the femoral artery and a catheter is threaded up through the femoral and iliac arteries into the aorta. Contrast material is injected to opacify the renal arterial supply. Angiography evaluates blood flow dynamics, demonstrates abnormal vasculature and differentiates primarily renal cysts from renal tumors.

Nursing Implications. Before the procedure a cathartic may be prescribed to eliminate fecal material and gas from the colon so that unobstructed x-rays will be visualized. The proposed injection sites (groin for femoral approach or axilla for axillary approach) are shaved. The peripheral pulse sites (radial, femoral, dorsalis pedis) are marked for easy access in post-procedural assessment. The patient is informed that a transient feeling of heat may be sensed along the course of the vessel when the contrast material is injected.

Following the procedure, the vital signs are taken until they are stabilized. If the axillary artery was punctured, the blood pressure is taken on the opposite arm. The puncture site is examined for swelling and hematoma development. The peripheral pulses are palpated. The color and temperature of the involved extremity is noted and compared with the uninvolved extremity. Cold compresses may be applied to the puncture site to decrease edema and pain.

Computerized Tomography. Computerized tomography is a noninvasive technique that provides an excellent cross-sectional view of the kidneys' anatomy. A computer measures small changes in x-ray absorption and magnifies the differences from tissue to tissue so that a display can be made and read. It is an accurate means of differentiating a renal cyst from a neoplasm. No special patient preparation is needed. (See page 289 for a more complete discussion of computed tomography.)

Ultrasonic Scan (Echogram). Ultrasound is used in this scanning technique to investigate renal disease. Since the kidneys produce a characteristic ultrasonic pattern, any abnormalities can be identified. This is a noninvasive technique and no special patient preparation is required.

The Cystoscopic Examination

A direct method of bladder study and visualization is the cystoscopic examination. The cystoscope has a self-contained optical lens system that provides a magnified, illuminated view of the bladder. It also has a guide system that allows a ureteral catheter to be passed through the ureter and up into the kidney. The cystoscope can be manipulated to allow complete visualization of the entire bladder and urethra as well as the ureteral orifices and prostatic urethra. The cystoscope also permits the urologist to obtain a specimen from each kidney to evaluate renal function. Calculi may be removed from the urethra, bladder, and ureter via cystoscopy.

A cystoscope consists primarily of an obturator and a telescope. The obturator is designed so that the cystoscope can be inserted with the least amount of trauma. After the cystoscope is passed into the bladder, the obturator is removed. Sterile irrigating solution is run in and out of the bladder to distend the bladder and wash away blood clots, thereby allowing better visualization.

The *telescope* with a very small lens is then passed through the cystoscope, enabling the urologist to view the inside of the bladder (Fig. 41-4). The use of a high intensity light allows for a better view of the bladder and urethra and permits still and motion pictures to be taken of these structures.

Prior to the procedure, a sedative may be given. A local topical anesthetic is instilled into the urethra by the urologist before the cystoscope is inserted. Some patients are given intravenous diazepam (Valium) in combination with topical urethral anesthesia. It may be necessary to use spinal or general anesthesia.

Nursing Intervention.   As with many diagnostic procedures, the nurse explains the meaning of the examination in order to inform the patient and allay his fears.

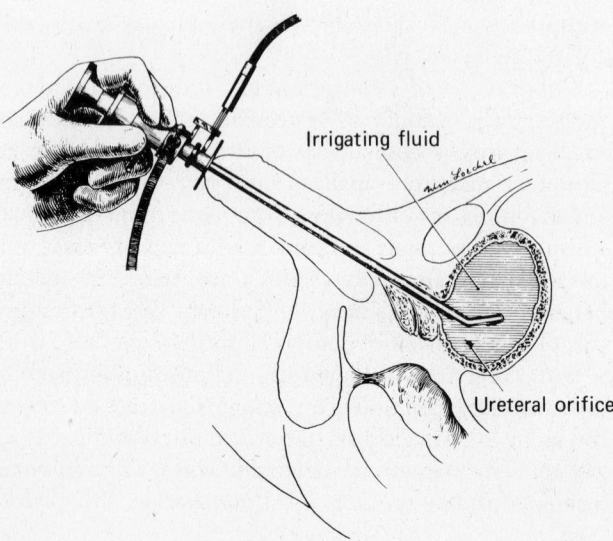

Irrigating fluid

Ureteral orifice

Figure 41-4.   A cystoscope being introduced into the bladder of the male. The upper cord is an electric line for the light at the distal end of the cystoscope. The lower tubing leads from a reservoir of sterile irrigating fluid that is used to inflate the bladder.

Additional preprocedure preparation usually includes having the patient drink one or two glasses of water before going to the examining department.

Postprocedure management is directed at relieving any possible discomfort resulting from the examination. Some burning upon voiding, blood-tinged urine, and urinary frequency from trauma to the mucous membrane may be expected after cystoscopic examination. Moist heat to the lower abdomen or hot sitz baths are helpful in relieving pain and promoting muscle relaxation. Occasionally following cystoscopic examination the patient with obstructive pathology may experience urinary retention as a result of edema caused by the instrumentation. The patient with prostatic hyperplasia should especially be watched for urinary retention. Hot sitz baths and relaxant medications are helpful for relieving retention, but an indwelling catheter may have to be inserted.

Renal and Ureteral Brush Biopsy

Brush biopsy techniques provide specific information when abnormal x-ray findings of the ureter or renal pelvis raise some uncertainty as to whether the defect is a tumor, a stone, a blood clot or an artifact. First a cystoscopic examination is conducted. Then a ureteral catheter is introduced, followed by a biopsy brush which is passed through the catheter. The suspected lesion is brushed back and forth in order to obtain cells and surface tissue fragments for histological analysis.

Following the procedure, the patient may be given an intravenous infusion to help clear the kidneys and prevent clot formation. Urine may show blood (usually clearing in 24 to 48 hours) from oozing at the brushing site. Postoperative renal colic occasionally occurs and responds to analgesics.

Needle Biopsy of the Kidney

Technical advances have made needle biopsy of the kidney a relatively safe procedure. Renal biopsy is useful in determining diagnostic and prognostic outcomes in patients with renal disease and in securing specimens for electron and immunofluorescent microscopy, particularly for glomerular disease. Before the biopsy is carried out an entire battery of coagulation studies are conducted to identify any patient at risk for postbiopsy bleeding.

The procedure is carried out as follows: The sedated patient is placed in a prone position with a sandbag under the abdomen. A local anesthetic agent is infiltrated into the skin at the biopsy site. The biopsy needle is introduced just inside the renal capsule of the outer quadrant of the kidney. The location of the needle may be identified through fluoroscopy or by ultrasound in which a special probe is used. Open biopsy may be done through a small flank incision.

Postbiopsy Nursing Management. After the specimen is obtained, pressure is applied to the kidney. To provide maximum quiet rest and to minimize bleeding, the patient may be kept in a prone position immediately following biopsy. The patient is usually kept flat for 24 hours.

The nurse must be watchful for hematuria, which may appear soon after biopsy. The kidney is a highly vascular organ and approximately one-fourth of the entire cardiac output passes through it in about 1 minute. The passage of the biopsy needle lacerates the kidney capsule and bleeding can occur in the perirenal space. Usually the bleeding subsides on its own, but a large amount of blood can accumulate in this space in a short period of time without noticeable signs until cardiovascular collapse is evident.

- To detect early signs of bleeding it is important that the vital signs be taken every 5 to 15 minutes for the first hour and then with decreasing frequency as indicated.
- Signs suggestive of bleeding include a rise or fall in blood pressure, anorexia, vomiting, and the development of a dull, aching discomfort in the abdomen. (Retroperitoneal hemorrhage acts as an irritant to the overlying posterior perineum.)
- Any signs of backache, shoulder pain, or dysuria are to be reported.

Flank pain may occur but usually represents bleeding into the muscle rather than around the kidney. Colicky pain similar to that of ureteral colic may develop when a clot is present in the ureter and cause excruciating sharp flank pain that radiates to the groin.

All urine voided by the patient is scrutinized for evidences of bleeding. If bleeding persists, as indicated by an enlarging hematoma which is palpable, surgical drainage is necessary. A hematocrit and hemoglobin study is done within 8 hours to assess for anemia. The nurse should keep in mind that a delayed hemorrhage can occur a number of days after biopsy.

Radioisotope Studies

Radioisotope studies are noninvasive procedures that do not interfere with normal physiologic processes and require no specific patient preparation. A radiopharmaceutical (^{99}Tc-labeled compound) is injected intravenously. Studies are obtained with a scintillation camera placed posterior to the kidney with the patient in a supine, prone or sitting position. The resultant image (called a scan) indicates the distribution of the radiopharmaceutical within the kidney. (It shows a dot image on film.) See also page 297.

This study provides information on kidney size and position and detects localized renal parenchymal defects or malfunction. If a lesion, such as a tumor or renal infarct, is contained within the kidney, it is readily detected by the absence of radioactivity within the involved area and the resultant defect in the scan.

Cystometrogram

A cystometrogram is the graphic recording of the pressures exerted at various phases of filling of the urinary bladder. Intermittent filling of the bladder can be recorded and compared with changes in intravesical (within the bladder) pressure. The patient voids while observation is made of the size, force, continuity of urinary stream, degree of straining, hesitancy and intermittency of urination and the presence of terminal dribbling. Then a retention catheter is placed into the bladder and the urinary volume measured. The catheter is connected to a water manometer, and water is allowed to flow into the bladder at a measured rate. The patient informs the examiner when he feels the first desire to void and again when the bladder feels full. The pressures and volumes within the bladder are plotted and recorded.

URINALYSIS

Urinalysis provides a wealth of important clinical information and is regarded as an indispensable part of every clinical study. (The more important urine tests are tabulated in the Appendix.)

Urine examination of every patient includes the observation and evaluation of:

1. urine color and clarity
2. measurement of urine acidity and specific gravity
3. tests for the presence of protein and sugar in the urine (proteinuria and glucosuria, respectively)
4. microscopic examination of the urine sediment after centrifuging for the detection of red blood cells (hematuria), white blood cells (pyuria), casts (cylindruria), crystals (crystalluria), and bacteria (bacteriuria).

Numerous additional tests are applicable in special situations.

Collection of Urine Samples

All urine tests are performed ideally on fresh specimens, preferably the first voiding of the day since this specimen is most concentrated and more likely to reveal abnormalities. Random specimens are satisfactory for most analyses provided that they have been collected in clean containers and have been adequately protected against bacterial and chemical deterioration. Urine should not be left standing at room temperature since it becomes alkaline due to contamination of urea-splitting bacteria from the environment. All specimens should be refrigerated as soon as possible after they are voided. Microscopic examination should be done within a half hour after collection, because allowing the specimen to stand causes dissolution of cellular elements and bacterial overgrowth unless the specimen is obtained by sterile methods. Urine cultures should be processed immediately. If this is not possible they should be stored at 4°C.

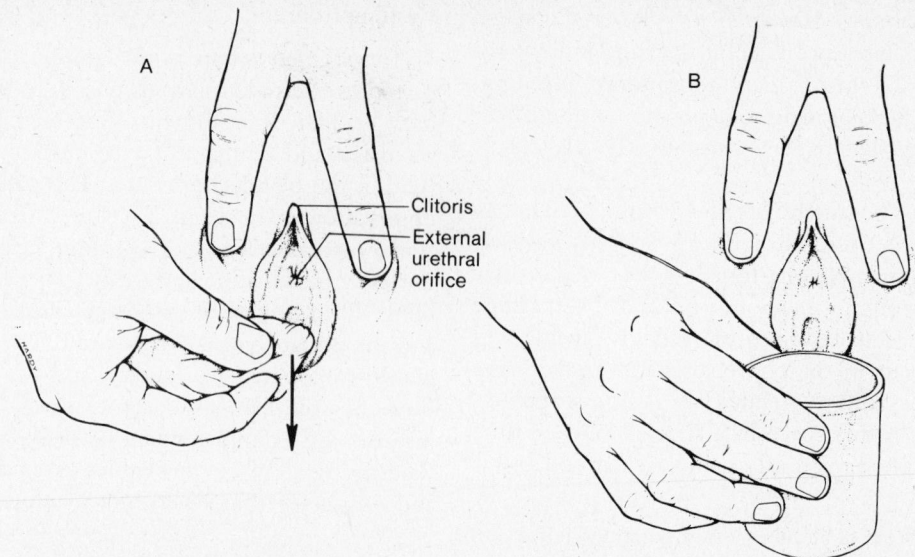

Figure 41-5. Obtaining a clean-catch midstream urine specimen in the female. *A.* Instruct the patient to hold the labia apart and wash from high up front toward the back with gauze soaked in soap. *B.* The collection cup is held so that it does not touch the body and the sample is obtained only while the patient is voiding with the labia held apart.

(39°F.). *Urine specimens should be collected from the patient by means of the clean-catch midstream technique using a wide-mouthed container* (see below, and Fig. 41-5).

24-Hour Urine Collections

Many quantitative analytic tests are carried out on specimens that represent the patient's urinary output over a 24-hour period. The procedure is as follows:

Instruct the patient to empty his bladder at a specified time (such as 8:00 A.M.). This urine is discarded. Collect all urine voided during the next 24 hours. The last specimen is collected and saved 24 hours after the collection was started (i.e., 8:00 A.M.).

The patient's bladder should be empty when the test starts and empty when it ends. The urine is collected in a clean container to which a preservative has been added and is kept in the refrigerator. Failure to transfer one specimen voided during the test period invalidates the test. A successful collection requires the complete understanding and cooperation on the part of the patient and all unit personnel concerned with the patient's care.

Clean-Catch Midstream Urine Specimens

Urine specimens voided in the usual manner are practically useless for bacteriologic study because of inevitable contamination by organisms residing in the vicinity of the urethral meatus. Such contamination can be avoided by catheterizing the urinary bladder. However, since the dangers of catheterization are known, especially the production of chronic pyelonephritis, this procedure is no longer recommended except for specific indications. Reliable bacteriologic studies are possible without catheterization, utilizing the so-called clean-catch midstream technique.

Instructions to the male patient:

- Expose the glans and cleanse the area around the meatus with soap and water using cotton pledgets or gauze squares.
- Do not collect the first portion of the voiding, but discard it.
- Collect the next portion by voiding into a sterile wide-mouthed bottle or large-caliber tube which is protected by a sterile closure.
- Do not collect the last few drops of urine since prostatic secretions may be introduced into the urine at the end of the urinary stream.

Instructions to the female patient:

- Separate the labia to expose the urethral orifice (Fig. 41-5).
- Cleanse around the urinary meatus with sponges soaked in soap and water.
- Wipe the perineum from the front to the back.
- Keep the labia separated and void forcibly, but do not collect the first portion of the voiding. (The distal portion of the urethral orifice is colonized by bacteria; the initial voiding washes away the urethral contaminants.)
- Collect the midstream portion of the urinary flow, making sure that the container does not come in contact with the genitalia.

Renal Function Tests

Renal function tests are used to evaluate the severity of kidney disease and to follow the patient's clinical progress. These tests also give information concerning the kidneys' effectiveness in carrying out their excretory function. Renal function may be within normal limits until about 50 percent of renal function has been lost. Best results are obtained by combining a number of clinical tests. Table 41-2 lists the more common tests of renal function.

EXAMINATION OF THE URINE

COMPOSITION OF URINE AFFECTED BY:

1. Nutritional status
2. Metabolic processes
3. Status of kidney function

VOLUME

1. Normal adult excretes between 1200-1500 ml./24 hours depending on intake; less than 500 ml. is considered oliguria.
2. Day volume is 2-3 times more than night volume.

ODOR

1. Normal urine has faint aromatic odor.
2. Characteristic odors are produced by ingestion of asparagus, thymol.
3. Cloudy urine with ammonia odor indicates urea-splitting bacteria such as *Proteus* causing urinary tract infections.
4. Offensive odor results from bacterial action in presence of pus.

APPEARANCE

1. Normal urine is clear.
2. Turbid (cloudy) urine is not always a sign of pathological condition. Normal urine may develop turbidity on refrigeration or from standing at room temperature; bacteria ferment urine quickly at room temperature.
3. Abnormally cloudy urine indicates presence of pus, blood, epithelial cells, bacteria, fat, colloidal particles, phosphates, urates.

COLOR

1. Color shows degree of concentration and depends on amount voided.
2. Normal urine is clear yellow or amber due to the pigment urochrome.
3. Color varies with the specific gravity:
   a. Dilute urine is straw-colored.
   b. Concentrated urine is highly colored.
4. Abnormally colored urine:
   a. Smoky-colored urine may be due to hematuria, spermatozoa, prostatic fluid, fat droplets, chyle.
   b. Red or red-brown urine is due to blood and blood pigments, porphyria, transfusion reaction, bleeding lesions in urogenital tract, beets, and some drugs.
   c. Yellow-brown or green-brown urine may indicate obstructive lesion of the bile duct system, obstructive jaundice.
   d. Orange-red or orange-brown urine is from urobilin or from phenazopyridine hydrochloride (Pyridium), a urinary antiseptic.
   e. Dark brown or black urine is seen in malignant melanoma and leukemia.

REACTION (pH) (HYDROGEN ION CONCENTRATION)

1. pH reflects the ability of the kidney to maintain normal hydrogen ion concentration in plasma and extracellular fluid; indicates *acidity* or *alkalinity* of urine.
2. Normal pH: 6 (acid); (may vary from pH 4.6 to pH 7.5); varies throughout the day.
3. Urine acidity or alkalinity has relatively little clinical significance unless the patient is on a special diet or a therapeutic program or is being treated for renal calculous disease.
4. Alkaline urine is often cloudy due to phosphate crystals.

SPECIFIC GRAVITY

1. Specific gravity measures the density of particles in urine; reflects concentrating and diluting power of kidneys.
2. Normal specific gravity ranges from 1.005-1.025.
3. Specific gravity fixed at 1.010 is seen in chronic renal failure.
4. In a person eating a normal diet inability to concentrate or dilute urine indicates disease.

OSMOLALITY

1. Osmolality is an indication of the amount of osmotically active particles in urine (specifically, it is the number of particles per unit volume of water). It is similar to specific gravity, but is considered a more precise test; it is also easy to do; only 1-2 ml. of urine are required.
2. The unit of osmotic measure is the osmole. Average values:
   Females: 300-1090 mOsm./kg.
   Males: 390-1090 mOsm./kg.

ABNORMAL URINE CONSTITUENTS

1. *Proteinuria* (albuminuria) is characteristically seen in all forms of acute and chronic renal disease.
   a. Normal urine does not have persistent protein in significant quantities.
   b. Proteinuria occurs in systemic diseases also where there are varying degrees of renal anoxia, cardiac decompensation, diabetic glomerulosclerosis, etc.
2. *Glucosuria*—glucose in the urine; seen most frequently in diabetes mellitus.
3. *Ketonuria*—presence of ketone bodies (acetone, acetoacetic acid and beta-hydroxybutyric acid). Ketonuria is indicative of incomplete fat metabolism (diabetic ketoacidosis) dehydration, starvation, after aspirin ingestion.
4. *Hematuria*—red blood cells in the urine; may be microscopic or gross. (See page 901.)
5. *Pyuria*—white blood cells in the urine.
6. *Bacteriuria*—bacteria in the urine.
7. *Crystalluria*—excretion of crystals in the urine.

TABLE 41-2.   TESTS OF RENAL FUNCTION

1. There is no single test of renal function; renal function is variable from time to time.
2. The rate of change of renal function is more important than the result of a single test.

TEST	PURPOSE/RATIONALE	TEST PROTOCOL

Renal Concentration Test
  Specific gravity
  Refractive index
  Qsmolality of urine
	Evaluates the ability to concentrate solutes in the urine
	Concentration ability is lost early in kidney disease; hence, this test detects early defects in renal function
		Fluids may be withheld 12 to 24 hours to evaluate the concentrating ability of the tubules under controlled conditions. Specific gravity measurements of urine are taken at specific times to determine urine concentration

Phenolsulfonphthalein Excretion Test (PSP)	A diagnostic agent (phenolsulfonphthalein) is given to determine the functional capacity of the kidney. (PSP test can also be used as a measure to assess residual urine.) Delayed excretion is seen in renal disease, cardiac failure, primary vascular disease.	Encourage fluids 1 to 1½ hours before the test. Phenolsulfonphthalein is given I.V.
		  1) Record exact time dye is administered
		  2) Collect urine in 15 minutes, 30 minutes, and 1 hour.

Creatinine Clearance* (Endogenous creatinine clearance)	Provides a reasonable approximation of rate of glomerular filtration. Measures volume of blood cleared of creatinine in 1 minute. Most sensitive indication of early renal disease. Useful to follow progress of patient's renal status.	Collect all urine over 24-hour period. Draw one sample of blood within the period.
Serum Creatinine	A test of renal function reflecting the balance between production and filtration by renal glomerulus. Amount of creatinine excreted varies and is dependent on muscle mass. Test results may be altered during exercise and in certain disease.	Do test on blood serum.
Serum Urea Nitrogen (Blood Urea Nitrogen—BUN)	Serves as index of renal excretory capacity. Serum urea nitrogen is dependent on the body's urea production and on urine flow. (Urea is the nitrogenous end-product of protein metabolism.)	Do test on blood serum.

*Clearance is the amount of blood cleansed of a constituent per unit of time. See Appendix for range of values.

BIBLIOGRAPHY

BOOKS

American Nurses Assoc. Division on Medical-Surgical Nursing Practice; Standards of Urologic Practice. Kansas City, Amer. Nurs. Assoc., 1977.

Blandy, J.: Lecture Notes on Urology. Oxford, Blackwell Scientific Pub., 1976.

Brenner, B. M., and Rector, F. C., Jr., eds.: The Kidney. Philadelphia, W. B. Saunders, 1976.

Brundage, D. J.: Nursing Management of Renal Problems. St. Louis, C. V. Mosby, 1976.

Cameron, J. S., Russell, A. M. E., and Sale, D. N. T.: Nephrology for Nurses, 2nd ed. Flushing, N.Y., Medical Examination Pub. Co., 1976.

Dunnill, M. S.: Pathological Basis of Renal Disease. Philadelphia, W. B. Saunders, 1976.

Free, A. H., and Free, H. M.: Urinalysis in Clinical Laboratory Practice. Cleveland, CRC Press, 1975.

Harrison, J. H. H., et al.: Campbell's Urology. Vols. 1 and 2, Philadelphia, W. B. Saunders, 1978.

Hekelman, F. P., and Ostendarp, C. A.: Nephrology Nursing. New York, McGraw-Hill, 1979.

International Committee for Nomenclature and Nosology of Renal Disease: A Handbook of Kidney Nomenclature and Nosology. Boston, Little, Brown, 1975.

Leaf, A., and Cotran, R. S.: Renal Pathophysiology. New York, Oxford University Press, 1976.

Massry, S. G., and Sellers, A. L.: Clinical Aspects of Uremia and Dialysis. Springfield, Ill., Charles C Thomas, 1976.

Maude, D. L.: Kidney Physiology and Kidney Disease: An Introduction to Nephrology. Philadelphia, J. B. Lippincott, 1977.

Muth, R. G.: Renal Medicine. Springfield, Ill., Charles C Thomas, 1978.

Schrier, R. W.: Renal and Electrolyte Disorders. Boston, Little, Brown, 1976.

Winter, C. C., and Morel, A.: Nursing Care of Patients With Urologic Disease, 4th ed. St. Louis, C. V. Mosby, 1977.

ARTICLES

Diagnosis

Brown, R. S., and Epstein, F. H.: Fluid and electrolyte disorders in urologic patients. Urol. Clin. N. Am., *3*:267-276, June 1976.

Crowe, L. R., and Hatch, F. E.: Evaluating renal function: Current status of clinical tests. Postgrad. Med., *62*:58-67, July 1977.

Gittes, R. R. S.: Retrograde renal and ureteral brush biopsy. AJN, *78*:410-412, Mar. 1978.

Hosten, A. O.: The early diagnosis of renal disease. J. Nat'l. Med. Assoc., *68*:172-176, May 1976.

Sagel, S. S., et al.: Computed tomography of the kidney. Radiology, *124*:359-370, Aug. 1977.

Townsend, R. M.: Enzyme tests in diseases of the prostate. Ann. Clin. Lab. Sci., 7:254-261, May-June, 1977.

Visel, J. M.: Clinical aspects of renal biopsy. Heart Lung, 4:900-902, Nov.-Dec. 1975.

AGENCIES

Governmental

National Institute of Arthritis, Metabolism and Digestive Diseases, National Institutes of Health, Bethesda, Md. 20205

Voluntary

National Kidney Foundation, 116 E. 27th St., New York, N.Y. 10016

United Ostomy Association, 1111 Wilshire Blvd., Los Angeles, Calif. 90017

42

MANAGEMENT OF PATIENTS WITH RENAL AND URINARY DYSFUNCTION

PSYCHOSOCIAL CONSIDERATIONS

Conditions of the genitourinary tract may precipitate emotional stresses and problems related to feelings of guilt and shame when the external genitalia are examined and treated. Problems of incontinence may cause disgust and feelings of helplessness. Some patients are constantly uneasy over the possibility of an "accident," although others appear careless and indifferent.

Operations on the male organs of reproduction can pose a threat to the masculinity of the patient, no matter what his age. Although many men may hide their fears of impotency by blaming "prostate trouble," many male sexual problems (difficulties in erection, premature ejaculation, etc.) are psychological in origin and related to a variety of causes—fear, guilt, aversion to partner, fatigue. Because of hidden fears, a male patient may react with anger and hostility to those caring for him, or his anger may turn inward and produce more than the usual amount of pain. Patients with urinary infections sometimes become depressed when they undergo prolonged periods of treatment. Anxiety in any stressful situation can produce urinary frequency and urgency.

The urologic patient, as any other patient, needs to feel respected as an individual and understood. He wants his questions answered, his fears allayed and his discomfort relieved. Reassurance is a part of nursing, and these patients may require more than the usual amount of reassurance, support, and acceptance.

FLUID AND ELECTROLYTE IMBALANCE

Assessment

A major problem for patients with renal disorders is the maintenance of fluid and electrolyte balance. The nurse must be skilled and conscientious in observing the clinical condition of the patient, and in recording the data gathered. Every patient with a urologic disorder has a fluid intake-output chart on which is recorded all fluid intake, whether by ingestion or by parenteral administration. The volume of urine excreted also is recorded. In addition, temperatures are charted every 4 hours, and the weight once daily. All these records provide invaluable assistance in determining how much fluid the patient should receive.

The nurse should also be alert to a host of signs and symptoms pertaining to body fluid disturbances (see Chapter 8 and also pages 896–897).

For example, the following symptoms are prone to occur in patients with renal disease:
1. Acute weight loss (in excess of 5 percent), a drop in body temperature, dryness of skin and mucous membranes, longitudinal wrinkles or furrows of tongue, and oliguria or anuria—could indicate volume deficit of extracellular fluid
2. Acute weight gain (in excess of 5 percent), edema, moist rales in lungs, puffy eyelids, and shortness of breath—could indicate volume excess of extracellular fluid
3. Abdominal cramps, apprehension, convulsions, fingerprinting on sternum, and oliguria or anuria—could indicate sodium deficit of extracellular fluid

4. Dry, sticky mucous membranes, flushed skin, oliguria or anuria, thirst, and rough and dry tongue—could indicate sodium excess of extracellular fluid

5. Anorexia, gaseous distention of intestines, silent intestinal ileus, weakness, and soft, flabby muscles—could indicate potassium deficit of extracellular fluid

6. Diarrhea, intestinal colic, irritability, and nausea—could indicate potassium excess of extracellular fluid.

7. Abdominal cramps, carpopedal spasm, muscle cramps, tetany, and tingling of ends of fingers—could indicate calcium deficit of extracellular fluid

8. Deep bony pain, flank pain, and muscle hypotonicity—could indicate calcium excess of extracellular fluid

9. Deep, rapid breathing (Kussmaul), shortness of breath on exertion, stupor, and weakness—could indicate primary base bicarbonate deficit of extracellular fluid

10. Depressed respiration, muscle hypertonicity, and tetany—could indicate primary base bicarbonate excess of extracellular fluid

11. Chronic weight loss, emotional depression, pallor, ready fatigue, and soft, flabby muscles—could indicate protein deficit of extracellular fluid

12. Positive Chvostek's sign, convulsions, disorientation, hyperactive deep reflexes, and tremor—could indicate magnesium deficit of extracellular fluid.

The nurse must possess a thorough understanding of the patient's gains and losses of body fluids and must share this information with other members of the team caring for the patient. When supervising intravenous therapy, the nurse adjusts the flow rate in accordance with the physician's request.

Repeated blood examinations are essential for maintaining surveillance of electrolyte balance. The nurse usually has the responsibility of preparing the patient for these somewhat unpleasant venipunctures by explaining that the studies are essential for the best possible medical care.

MAINTAINING ADEQUATE URINARY DRAINAGE

In the patient with urologic disease, as in any other patient (or any normal individual, for that matter) urinary excretion of waste materials is imperative. The composition of the body fluids is determined not so much by what the patient ingests as by what the kidneys keep. In health, the kidneys are amazingly efficient, excreting the materials that are not needed and retaining those that are. But in the patient with damaged kidneys, all therapeutic efforts are directed toward seeing that the homeostatic capabilities of the kidneys are not exceeded.

When drainage of the urinary system becomes necessary, catheters are inserted directly into the bladder, the ureters, or the kidney pelves. Catheters must be chosen for the purpose in mind. They come in various sizes and lengths and may have one or more openings placed in various positions near the tip. A catheter may be constructed of hard or soft rubber, woven fabric, silicone, metal, glass, or plastic. The tip may be opened or closed and may have a mushroom shape, such as the Pezzer catheter, a winged shape, such as the Malecot catheter, or may simply be round and blunt.

CATHETERIZATION

Principles of Catheter Management

There are times when the catheter is a lifesaving instrument, as is the case when the patient is unable to void. At other times, catheterization may be necessary to determine the amount of residual urine in the bladder after the patient has voided or to bypass an obstruction that blocks the flow or urine. However . . .

- No patient should be catheterized unless absolutely necessary since catheterization can lead to urinary tract infection.

To safeguard the patient, the following points of care are essential in urethral catheter management:

- Strict surgical asepsis should be employed.
- The urethra should be adequately cleansed.
- The catheter should be smaller than the external urinary meatus to help minimize trauma.
- The catheter should be well lubricated with an appropriate antimicrobial lubricant.
- The catheter should be passed gently and skillfully.

Management of an Indwelling Catheter and a Closed Urinary Drainage System

When an indwelling catheter is necessary, a closed drainage system is preferred. (A closed drainage system is one that is closed to outside air.) Such a system may consist of an indwelling catheter, a connecting tube and a collecting bag emptied by a drainage valve. Or it may consist of a triple-lumen indwelling urethral catheter attached to a closed sterile drainage system. The 3-way catheter allows urinary drainage through one channel, inflation of the bag with water or air through the second channel, and a continuous irrigation of the bladder with antibacterial solution through the third channel.

Certain principles of care should be followed when managing a closed urinary drainage system:
- In order to prevent contamination of a closed system, the tubing should not be disconnected nor should any part of the collecting bag or drainage tube be contaminated.
- The bag should not be raised above the level of the patient's bladder since this will cause reflux of contaminated urine into the patient's bladder from the bag. Urine flow must be downhill.
- Columns of urine should not be allowed to collect in the tubing since a free flow of urine must be maintained to prevent infection. Improper drainage occurs when the tubing is kinked or twisted, allowing pools of drainage to collect in the loops of the tubing.

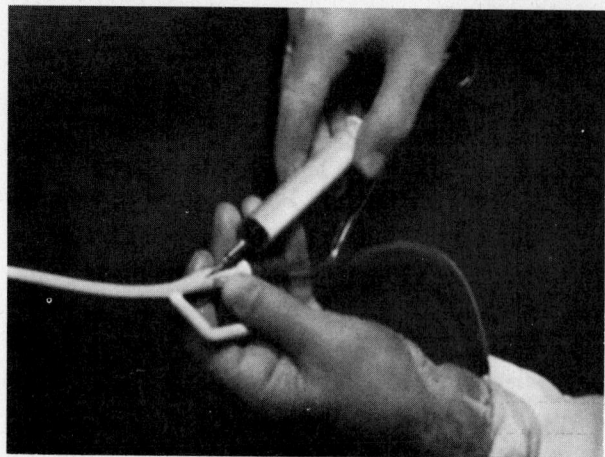

Figure 42-1.   The integrity of a closed urinary drainage system—whether urethral, suprapubic, ureteral, or for nephrostomy or pyelostomy—need not be interrupted to obtain urine for culture. The tube can be clamped distal to the catheter, the end of the rubber catheter can then be cleaned with an alcohol sponge, and a sterile syringe and fine bore needle (22-gauge) can be used to withdraw the urine. The needle should be inserted at an angle into the cleansed area of the catheter to avoid going through it. For a self-retaining catheter (*above*), the area between the balloon arm and the connecting tube should be used. (Courtesy, Joseph D. Schmidt, M.D., and Am. J. Nurs., Feb. 1973)

• The drainage bag should not be allowed to touch the floor. The bag and collecting tubing must be changed if contamination occurs.

• The bag should be drained at 8-hour intervals with care taken to see that the drainage tube (valve/spout) is not contaminated.

It is most important that the area around the urethral orifice be cleansed with soap and water or an antibacterial solution several times daily since bacteria can pass along the outside of the catheter from the urethral meatus and into the bladder. Suppurative drainage and encrustation occur at the exit of any tube. Encrustation arising from urinary salts may enter the bladder when the catheter is removed and may serve as a nuclei for stone formation. There appears to be significantly less encrustation associated with silicone catheters. The patient should be taught how to cleanse around the catheter if he is able.

A liberal fluid intake must be ensured in order to produce mechanical flushing and to dilute urinary elements producing encrustation. (The intake must be within limits of the patient's cardiac reserve.) Keeping the urine acid helps to prevent tube obstruction and encrustation of urinary sand and calculus deposits. Oral intake of ascorbic acid, potassium acid phosphate, and an acid ash diet help to acidify urine.

Urine cultures should be monitored daily or every other day as a means of surveying for infection. Many catheters have an aspiration port from which a specimen can be obtained.

The following is a method for securing a urine culture (Fig. 42-1):
1. Clamp the drainage tubing near the junction of the catheter to create a reservoir of urine.
2. Prepare the aspiration port or the hub of the catheter with alcohol or an iodine containing solution.
3. Insert a 25-gauge needle (attached to a syringe) into the hub of the catheter.
4. Aspirate a small volume of urine.
5. Avoid aspirating the shaft of the catheter as the balloon may be deflated.
6. Unclamp the catheter.

Measures must be taken to prevent cross contamination since many urinary tract infections are due to extrinsically acquired organisms transmitted by cross contamination.

• Catheterized patients with bacteria in the urine should not be in the same room with noninfected catheterized patients. It is best to assign only one patient with an indwelling catheter to a room.

Patients at risk are women, elderly debilitated patients, and those who are critically ill. Careful handwashing techniques are mandatory when going from one patient to another.

Anchoring the Indwelling Catheter.   In the male the catheter is taped horizontally to the thigh (Fig. 42-2) or to the lateral abdomen to prevent pressure on the urethra at the penoscrotal junction which can eventually lead to the formation of a urethrocutaneous fistula.

In the female patient, the drainage tubing attached to the catheter is taped to the thigh to prevent tension and traction on the bladder.

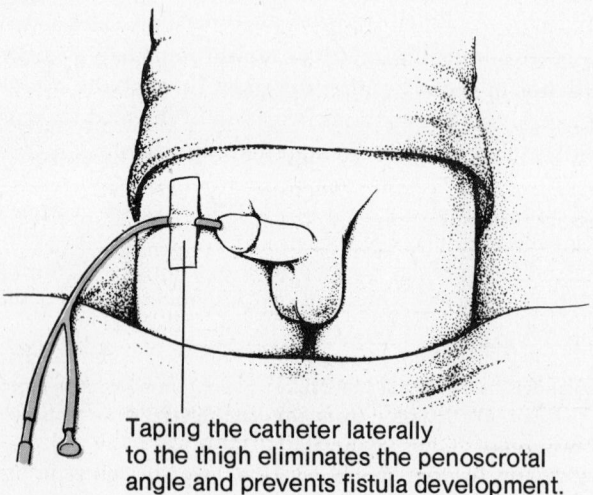

Taping the catheter laterally to the thigh eliminates the penoscrotal angle and prevents fistula development.

Figure 42-2.   The catheter is taped to the thigh in the male patient.

URINARY RETENTION

Urinary retention (both acute and chronic) refers to the inability to urinate despite a desire to do so. Chronic retention will often lead to overflow incontinence (due to pressure of retained urine in the bladder) or residual urine. *Residual urine* is the term applied to urine that remains in the bladder after voiding.

The problem of retention may arise in any postoperative patient, particularly those who have undergone surgery on the perineal or anal regions resulting in reflex spasm of the sphincters. It may also occur in the acutely ill, the elderly or the bedridden. Urinary retention may be due to prostatic enlargement, urethral pathology (infection, tumor, calculus), trauma, neurogenic bladder dysfunction and other conditions. Complications arising from retention include infection (which may readily develop as a result of overdistention of the bladder) or even impaired renal function, especially if obstructive uropathy (pathologic change in urinary tract due to obstruction) is present.

Nursing Assessment

The signs and symptoms of urinary retention may easily be overlooked unless there is a conscious effort to check their presence.

- Determine the time of the last voiding.
- Is the patient passing small amounts of urine frequently?
- Is the patient dribbling?
- Is the patient complaining of pain or discomfort in the lower abdomen? (Note, however, that discomfort may be relatively mild if the bladder distends slowly.)
- Check for signs of a rounded swelling arising out of the pelvis which could indicate retention.
- Palpate the suprapubic area for an oval-shaped mass.

Management

The objective of nursing management is to prevent overdistention of the bladder with resultant infection and to treat the underlying cause. Nursing measures to encourage voiding include helping the patient to the bathroom or commode in order to provide a more natural setting for voiding, or allowing the male patient to stand beside the bed while using the urinal, since most men find this position more comfortable and natural for urination. Additional measures include providing a source of warmth to relax the sphincters (i.e., sitz baths, warm compresses to the perineum, showers), giving the patient hot tea to drink, and offering psychological reassurance and support.

Following surgical procedures, the prescribed analgesic should be administered because pain in the incisional area can make voiding difficult. When the patient cannot void, careful catheterization is resorted to in order to decompress the bladder before overdistention occurs. In the case of prostatic obstruction, attempts at catheterization (by the urologist) may not be successful, requiring that a suprapubic cystostomy be done.

Urinary Incontinence

If urinary incontinence (involuntary loss of urine) results from an inflammatory condition (cystitis), it will probably be temporary in nature. However, if it results from a serious neurologic condition (paraplegia), it could easily be a permanent problem.

Stress incontinence is the involuntary loss of urine through an intact urethra as a result of a sudden increase in intraabdominal pressure. It is seen mostly in women and is due to congenital conditions (exstrophy of the bladder, ectopic ureter) or to obstetrical injury, lesions of the bladder neck, extrinsic pelvic disease, fistulae, detrusor dysfunction and a variety of other conditions. The therapy for this type of incontinence is usually surgical correction. However, a newer method of controlling stress incontinence is now under investigation and includes applying electronic stimulation to the pelvic floor by means of a miniature pulse generator with electrodes mounted on an intra-anal plug.

Management. Most patients with urinary incontinence can be conditioned to gain urinary control through systematic habit training or the establishment of an automatic bladder. Such a program requires more nursing time than changing the patient's wet bed, but it is most rewarding to see a patient lose his fear of embarrassment as progress is made in rehabilitation. The rehabilitation of the patient with urinary incontinence is discussed on page 202.

SUPRAPUBIC BLADDER DRAINAGE

Suprapubic bladder drainage is a method of establishing drainage from the bladder by inserting a catheter or tube through the suprapubic area into the bladder by either a stab incision or puncture with a needle or trocar. It is used as a temporary measure to divert the flow of urine from the urethra when the urethral route is impassable (urethral injuries; strictures; prostatic obstruction), following gynecological operations when bladder dysfunction is apt to occur (vaginal hysterectomy, vaginal repair surgery) and after pelvic fractures.

The patient lies supine. The bladder is distended with sterile saline solution via a urethral catheter (which is then removed), or the patient is given fluids before the procedure (oral or intravenous). Distention of the bladder makes the bladder easier to locate by the suprapubic route.

The suprapubic area is surgically prepared and the

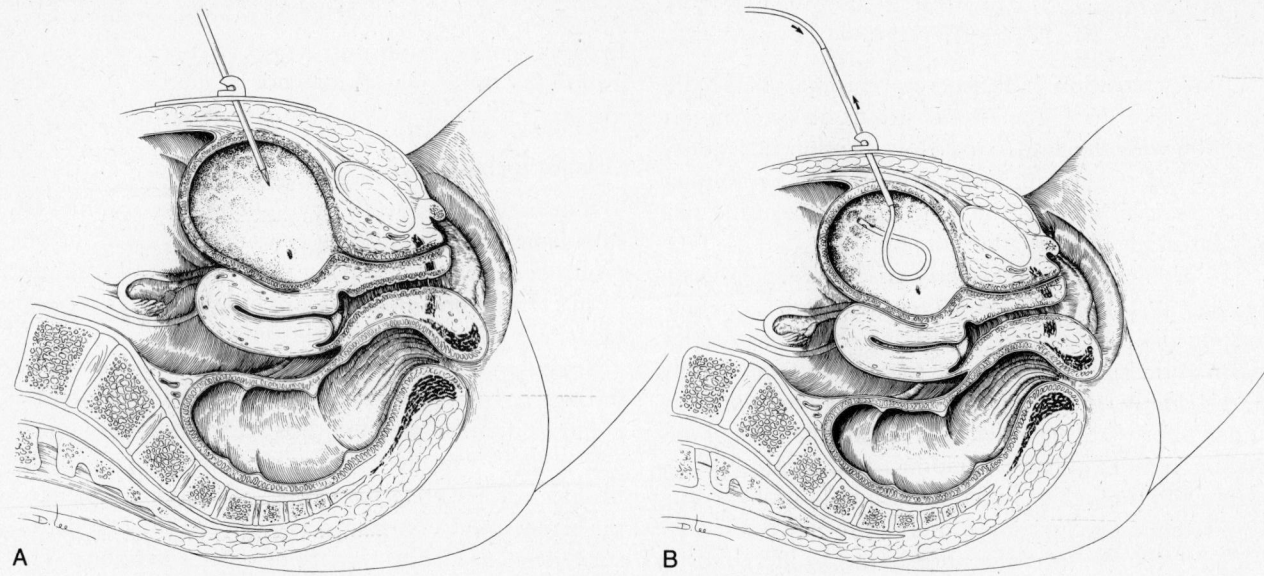

Figure 42-3. *A. Silastic® Cystocath®* suprapubic drainage system. Using steady pressure, the trocar-cannula is passed in a slightly caudal direction until entrance into the bladder is felt: The trocar-cannula is shown in its correct bladder entry position. The position can be verified by reflux of urine up through the trocar-cannula. *B.* The silicone drainage catheter is inserted through the cannula and well into the bladder. The catheter is inserted before the bladder is completely decompressed. When removing the cannula the catheter should be held fairly straight so that it will not accidentally get caught on the rim of the cannula as the cannula is withdrawn. This will prevent the inadvertent withdrawal of the catheter from the bladder while the cannula is removed. Courtesy Dow Corning Corporation.

puncture site located approximately 5 cm. above the symphysis. The procedure may be accomplished by open operation (incision of the bladder) or by puncture with a trocar/cannula assembly. The trocar/cannula is passed in a slightly caudal direction and entrance into the bladder is verified by reflux of urine through a hole in the trocar/cannula. A catheter is threaded through the cannula into the bladder (Fig. 42-3). The cannula is withdrawn leaving the catheter in place. The catheter is secured with sutures, tape or a body-seal system and the area around the catheter covered with a sterile dressing. The drainage tubing is attached to a closed sterile system and the tubing secured to the lateral abdomen with tape to prevent undue tension on the catheter.

Suprapubic bladder drainage may be maintained continuously for several weeks. If a trial of voiding is requested, the catheter is clamped for 4 hours during which time the patient attempts to void. After the patient voids, the catheter is unclamped and the residual urine measured. Usually if the amount of residual urine is less than 100 ml. on two separate occasions (morning and evening), the catheter may be removed. However if the patient complains of pain or discomfort, the catheter is usually left open.

Usually patients with suprapubic drainage are able to void sooner after surgery than those with urethral catheters. Suprapubic drainage is also considered to be more comfortable than an indwelling catheter, provides greater patient mobility, and presents less of a risk for bladder infection. The suprapubic catheter is removed upon request, and a sterile dressing placed over the site.

NEUROGENIC BLADDER

Neurogenic bladder refers to a bladder disturbance that results from a lesion of the nervous system. It may be caused by spinal cord injury or tumor, certain neurological diseases (multiple sclerosis), congenital anomalies (spina bifida, myelomeningocele), and infection.

There are two types of neurogenic bladders: spastic and flaccid. The spastic (reflex or automatic) bladder disorder is caused by any lesion of the cord above the voiding reflex arc (upper motor neuron lesion). The result is a loss of conscious sensation and cerebral motor control. There is reduced bladder capacity and marked hypertrophy of the bladder wall. As a result, the bladder behaves in a reflex fashion with minimal or no controlling influence to regulate its activity.

The flaccid (atonic, nonreflex or autonomous) neurogenic bladder is caused by a lower motor neuron lesion, most commonly due to trauma. The bladder continues to fill and becomes greatly distended. The bladder muscle does not contract forcefully at any time. Sensory loss may accompany a flaccid bladder, and the patient is unaware of discomfort. Overdistention causes damage to the bladder musculature, infection of stagnant urine, and infection of the kidneys by back pressure of urine.

The major complication of neurogenic bladder is infection which results from stasis of urine and subsequent catheterization. Hypertrophy of the bladder walls also results, ultimately leading to vesicoureteral reflux and hydronephrosis. Urolithiasis may develop from urinary stasis and infection and from demineralization of bone from the patient's being on prolonged bed rest. Renal failure is the major cause of death of patients with neurologic impairment of the bladder.

Management

The care of the patient with neurogenic bladder is a major challenge to the nurse. There are several long-term objectives to attain: (1) to prevent overdistention of the bladder, (2) to empty the bladder regularly and completely, (3) to maintain urine sterility with no stone formation, and (4) to maintain adequate bladder capacity without ureterovesical reflux.

The immediate management of the patient with a neurogenic bladder consists of catheterizing the patient intermittently or inserting a three-way catheter with closed drainage to avoid overdistention. In intermittent catheterization, the bladder is catheterized at designated intervals (4, 6, or 8 hours) with a small catheter. This intermittent emptying approximates physiological bladder function and circumvents complications usually encountered with an indwelling catheter; however, strict asepsis is necessary. An hourly fluid intake and output record is kept to assess individual output patterns. The patient may be taught self-catheterization (see page 916).

If continuous catheterization and drainage are used in a male patient, the catheter is taped to the abdomen to avoid the sharp angulation of the catheter and prevent pressure at the penoscrotal angle (Fig. 42-2).

With the use of either intermittent or continuous catheterization, a liberal fluid intake is encouraged to reduce the urinary bacterial count, reduce stasis, decrease the concentration of calcium in the urine and minimize the precipitation of urinary crystals and subsequent stone formation. The patient is kept as mobile as possible and is up on the tilt table or wheelchair or prepared for ambulation. The diet is low in calcium to prevent calculosis (presence of calculi).

As soon as the patient's condition permits, evaluation studies are performed to assess for bladder and bladder neck problems. The initial studies provide a baseline against which later changes can be measured. Serial studies of BUN, creatinine clearance and serum creatinine are done to determine the status of renal function. A cystogram determines the presence of vesicoureteral reflux. A urethrogram may be done to detect the presence of urethral complications. Pressure and flow studies as well as an IV urogram are also carried out. A cystoscopic examination may be requested to assess loss of muscle fibers and elastic tissues and to provide an opportunity for biopsy if necessary.

Treatment of Chronic Phase. The problems of patients with neurogenic bladder disease vary considerably from patient to patient. It is difficult to assess what the rehabilitation potential and eventual urological disability may be.

If possible the objective is to develop effective spontaneous reflex voiding which is accomplished in the following manner:

- Ask the patient to drink a measured amount of fluid from 8 A.M. to 10 P.M.; no fluids (except sips) are taken after 10 P.M. to avoid bladder overdistention.
- At a specific time(s) the patient attempts to void by applying pressure over the bladder, by tapping the abdomen, or by stretching the anal sphincter with a finger to trigger the bladder.
- Immediately following the voiding attempt, catheterize the patient to determine the amount of residual urine. Measure all urine voided and catheterized.
- Palpate the bladder at repeated intervals to determine whether the bladder is being emptied.
- Caution the patient to be alert for any signs that indicate a full bladder: perspiration, coldness of hands or feet, feelings of anxiety, etc.
- The intervals between catheterization are lengthened and the patient's program is moved forward as less and less residual urine is measured. Catheterization is usually discontinued when the volume of residual urine is at an acceptable level compatible with urine sterility and radiological normalcy of the upper urinary tract.

Flaccid Bladder

A patient with a flaccid bladder may be placed on the same type of bladder routine as outlined above. A 2-hour voiding schedule is established to prevent overdistention. Parasympathomimetic drugs (bethanechol [Urecholine]) may help to increase the contraction of the detrusor muscle. This approach may be very effective especially for a hypotonic bladder in which there is no significant obstruction of the bladder outlet.

Patients can also be taught self-catheterization at intervals until spontaneous complete emptying of the bladder is achieved. Although intermittent catheterization may have to be carried out for a prolonged period of time, it appears to be a safe and successful method of managing patients who have neurogenic bladders.

Sometimes it is not possible for the patient to achieve reflex bladder control or self-catheterization. The male patient then may use a condom-collecting device if the bladder empties well and no residual urine remains. The female patient may need to wear pads or waterproof pants. Surgical intervention may be carried out to correct bladder neck contractures or vesicoureteral reflux or to perform some type of urinary diversion procedure.

Intermittent Self-Catheterization

Intermittent self-catheterization provides periodic drainage of urine from the bladder. It is the treatment of choice following spinal cord injury. Aseptic techniques are required during the hospital training period, but the patient may use a "clean" (non-sterile) technique at home. Self-catheterization promotes independence, results in fewer complications and permits more normal sexual relations. The objectives are to decrease the morbidity associated with the long-term use of an indwelling catheter and to achieve a catheter-free status if possible.

The main teaching emphasis must be placed on the importance of frequent catheterization and the emptying of the bladder at the prescribed time irrespective of the circumstances. An overdistended bladder slows the circulation of blood through the bladder walls and weakens its resistance to infection.

The female patient will require a mirror to help locate the urinary meatus. She is taught to catheterize herself by inserting a catheter 7.5 cm. (3 inches) into the urethra in a downward and backward direction. The male patient is taught to lubricate the catheter, retract the foreskin of the penis with one hand while grasping the penis and holding it at a right angle to the body. (This maneuver straightens the urethra and makes it easier to insert the catheter.) The catheter is inserted 15 to 25 cm. (6 to 10 inches) until the urine begins to flow. After the catheter is removed, it is washed in soapy water (if available), rinsed and wrapped in a paper towel, plastic bag or case, depending on what is available. A patient following this routine should be seen by a urologist at regular intervals to prevent complications, such as reflux, hydronephrosis, and external sphincter spasm.

DIALYSIS

Dialysis refers to the diffusion of solute molecules through a semipermeable membrane, passing from the side of higher concentration to that of the lower. If the patient with renal failure does not respond to treatment, some method of dialysis is performed to remove the waste products. The purpose of dialysis is to maintain the life and well-being of the patient until kidney function is restored. Methods include *peritoneal dialysis* and *hemodialysis*. The main indication for dialysis is a high and rising level of serum potassium.

PERITONEAL DIALYSIS

Peritoneal dialysis is based on the principle of diffusion of substances across a semipermeable membrane. In this technique, an appropriate sterile dialyzing fluid is introduced into the peritoneal cavity at intervals. The surface area of the peritoneum, which amounts to approximately 22,000 sq. cm., acts as the diffusing surface. Urea is

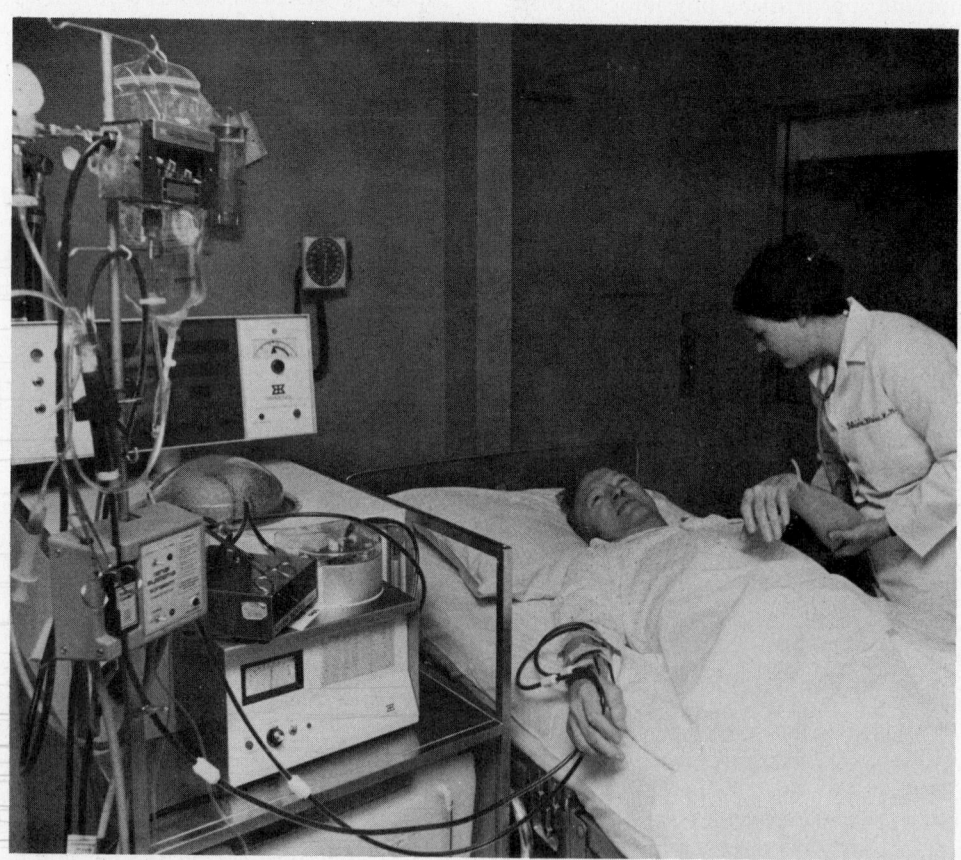

Figure 42-4.   Nurse monitoring the patient undergoing hemodialysis in the hospital. (Georgetown University Medical Center)

cleared at a rate of approximately 15-20 ml./minute. Creatinine is cleared somewhat more slowly. With the development of nonirritating silicone catheters and improvements in commercial dialyzing solution, peritoneal dialysis is fairly easy to perform.

Peritoneal dialysis is used in renal failure to remove toxic substances and body wastes normally excreted by healthy kidneys and in the management of patients with intractable edema, hepatic coma, hyperkalemia, azotemia, hypertension and uremia. Occasionally it is used as a means of therapy for peritonitis. The infected area is irrigated with added antibiotics that are able to come in direct contact with the infection. Peritoneal dialysis can be carried out a few days after abdominal surgery. It usually takes 36 to 48 hours to achieve with peritoneal dialysis what hemodialysis accomplishes in 6 hours. The procedure can be intermittent or continuous.

With the development of a permanent access device to the peritoneal cavity (implantable Tenkhoff catheter) and automated dialysis closed-cycle peritoneal dialysis machines, this procedure is being done in the home for long-term therapy of patients with chronic renal disorders.

(The role of the nurse in assisting the patient undergoing peritoneal dialysis is outlined on pages 918–920.)

HEMODIALYSIS

Hemodialysis is a process of cleansing the blood of accumulated waste products. It is used for patients in end-stage renal failure or for acutely ill patients who require short-term dialysis (Fig. 42-4). A synthetic semipermeable membrane (cellophane, cuprophan) replaces the renal glomeruli and tubules. For patients with chronic renal failure, hemodialysis provides reasonable rehabilitation and life expectancy. However, hemodialysis does not cure renal disease and is not able to compensate for losses of the kidneys' endocrine or metabolic activities. The patient must be given dialysis treatment for the rest of his life or until he receives a kidney transplant. Patients are selected for the program if they are free of irreversible complications, are psychologically stable and well-motivated and need dialysis therapy in order to live.

The requirements for hemodialysis for a patient with end-stage renal failure are (1) access to the circulation, (2) a dialyzer with a semipermeable membrane (artificial kidney) and (3) appropriate dialysate bath.

Access to Patient's Circulation. Access to the patient's circulation is achieved through a fistula (internal shunt—Fig. 42-5 or a surgically implanted prosthetic shunt (external arteriovenous shunt—Fig. 42-6).

A fistula is made surgically by the anastomosis of an artery to a vein (arteriovenous fistula, AVF). The shunt can be created wherever a vein and artery are close together. Usually the radial artery and adjacent vein are anastomosed but vessels in the leg may also be used. Following the procedure the superficial venous system of the arm dilates. By means of two large bore needles

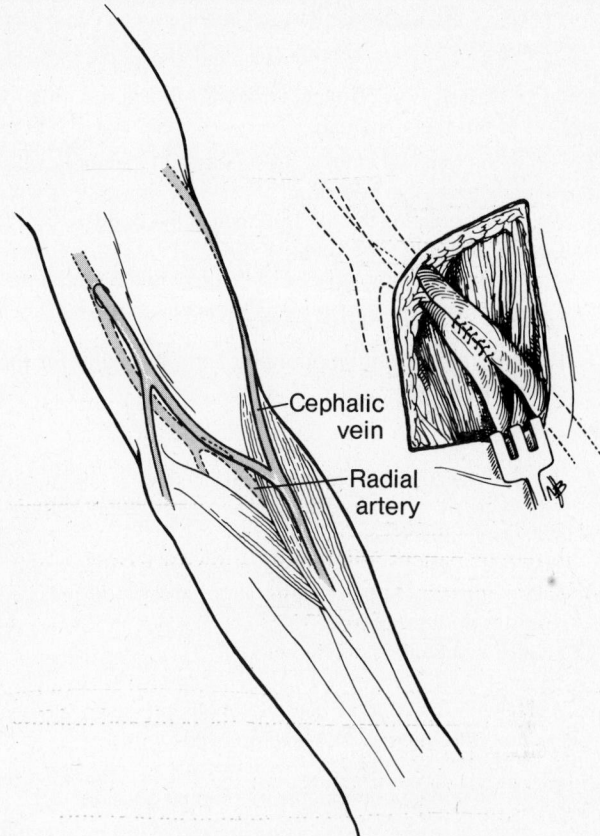

Figure 42-5. Fistula for hemodialysis.

inserted into the dilated venous system, blood can be obtained and passed through the dialyzer. The arterial end is used for arterial flow and the distal end for reinfusion of dialyzed blood. This technique has virtually eliminated the problems of infection and clotting. Most AVFs

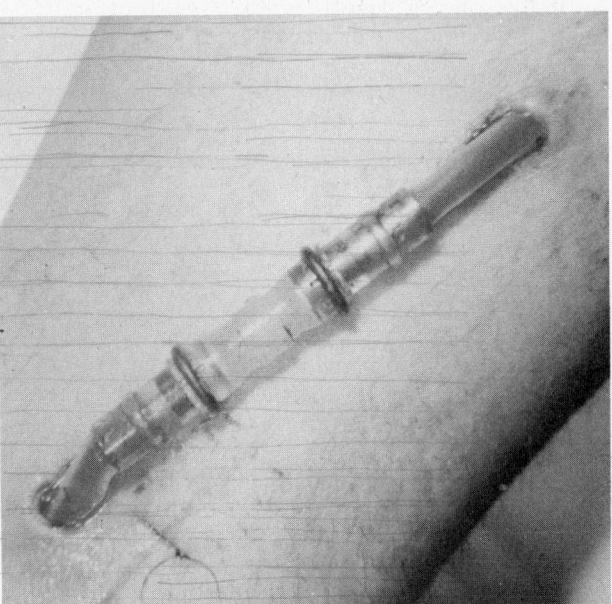

Figure 42-6. Arteriovenous shunt. (Photo Courtesy A. E. Parrish, M.D.)

Peritoneal dialysis is a substitute for kidney function during renal failure. The peritoneum is used as a dialyzing membrane. The purposes of this therapy are to:

1. Aid in the removal of toxic substances and metabolic wastes
2. Remove excessive body fluid
3. Assist in regulating the fluid balance of the body
4. Control the blood pressure
5. Control severe intractable heart failure when diuretics no longer promote elimination of water and sodium

Nursing Action	**Rationale**
1. Prepare the patient emotionally and physically for the procedure.	1. Nursing support is offered by explaining procedure mechanics, providing opportunities for the patient to ask questions, allowing him to verbalize his feelings, and giving expert physical care.
2. See that the consent form has been signed.	
3. Weigh the patient before dialysis and every 24 hours thereafter, preferably on an in-bed scale.	3. The weight at the beginning of the procedure serves as a baseline of information. Daily weight is helpful in assessing the state of hydration.
4. Take temperature, pulse, respiration, and blood pressure readings prior to dialysis.	4. A knowledge of vital signs at the beginning of dialysis is necessary for comparing subsequent changes in vital signs.
5. Have the patient empty his bladder.	5. If the bladder is empty there is less likelihood of perforating it when the trocar is introduced into the peritoneum.
6. Assist with insertion of central venous pressure catheter. ECG monitoring may also be employed.	6. CVP measurements may be carried out to assess fluid volume changes. Cardiac arrhythmias may occur due to serum potassium changes and vagal stimulation.
7. Make the patient comfortable in a supine position.	

The following is a brief résumé of the method of insertion of the peritoneal catheter (done under strict asepsis).

a. The abdomen is prepared surgically and the skin and subcutaneous tissues are infiltrated with a local anesthetic.	a. Surgical preparation of the skin minimizes or eliminates surface bacteria and decreases the possibility of wound contamination and infection.
b. A small midline stab wound is made 3–5 cm. below the umbilicus.	b. The midline area is relatively avascular.
c. The trocar is inserted through the incision with the stylet in place, or a thin stylet cannula may be inserted percutaneously.	
d. The patient is requested to raise his head from the pillow after the trocar is introduced.	d. This maneuver tightens the abdominal muscles and permits easier penetration of the trocar without danger of injury to the intraabdominal organs.
e. When the peritoneum is punctured, the trocar is directed toward the left side of the pelvis. The stylet is removed, and the catheter is inserted through the trocar and maneuvered into position. Dialysis fluid is allowed to run through the catheter while it is being positioned.	This prevents the omentum from adhering to the catheter, impeding its advancement or occluding its opening.
f. After the trocar is removed, the skin may be closed with a purse-string suture. (This is not always done.) A sterile dressing is placed around the catheter.	f. The catheter is attached to the skin to prevent loss of the catheter in the abdomen.
8. Flush the tubing with dialysis solution.	8. The tubing is flushed to prevent air from entering the peritoneal cavity. Air causes abdominal discomfort and drainage difficulties.
9. Attach the catheter connector to the administration set which has been previously connected to the container of dialysis solution (warmed to body temperature, 37° C.).	9. The solution is warmed to body temperature for patient comfort and to prevent abdominal pain. Heating also causes dilation of the peritoneal vessels and increases urea clearance.
10. Dry the dialysate bottles before inverting.	

*Automatic cyclers are available for peritoneal dialysis.

Nursing Action	Rationale
11. Drugs (heparin, etc.) are added in advance.	11. The addition of heparin prevents fibrin clots from occluding the catheter. Potassium chloride may be added on order unless the patient has hyperkalemia.
12. Permit the dialyzing solution to flow unrestricted into the peritoneal cavity (usually takes 5-10 minutes for completion).	12. The inflow solution should flow in a steady stream. If the fluid flows in too slowly the catheter may need to be repositioned since its tip may be buried in the omentum, or it may be occluded by a blood clot.
13. Allow the fluid to remain in the peritoneal cavity for the prescribed time period (15-30 minutes). Prepare the next exchange while the fluid is in the peritoneal cavity.	13. In order for potassium, urea, and other waste materials to be removed, the solution must remain in the peritoneal cavity for the prescribed time (dwell or equilibration time). The maximum concentration gradient takes place in the first 5-10 minutes and this is the most effective dwell time.
14. Unclamp the outflow tube. Drainage should take approximately 10 minutes or more, although the time varies with each patient.	14. The abdomen is drained by a siphon effect through the closed system. Gravity drainage should occur fairly rapidly, and steady streams of fluid should be observed entering the drainage container. The drainage is usually straw-colored.
15. If the fluid is not draining properly, move the patient from side to side to facilitate the removal of peritoneal drainage. The head of the bed may also be elevated. Ascertain if the catheter is patent.	15. If the drainage stops, or starts to drip before the dialyzing fluid has run out, it may indicate that the catheter tip is buried in the omentum. Rotating the patient may be helpful (or it may be necessary for the physician to reposition the catheter).
16. When the outflow drainage ceases to run, clamp off the drainage tube and infuse the next exchange, using strict aseptic technique.	
17. Take blood pressure and pulse every 15 minutes during the first exchange and every hour thereafter. Monitor the heart rate for signs of arrhythmia.	17. A drop in blood pressure may indicate excessive fluid loss from the glucose concentrations of the dialyzing solutions. Changes in the vital signs may indicate impending shock or overhydration.
18. Take patient's temperature every 4 hours (especially after catheter removal).	18. An infection is more apt to become evident after dialysis has been discontinued.
19. The procedure is repeated until the blood chemistry levels improve. The usual time is 12-36 hours; depending on the patient's condition, he will receive 24-48 exchanges.	19. The duration of dialysis depends on the severity of the condition and on the size and weight of the patient. Patients requiring only a few peritoneal dialysis treatments may have a plastic T-shaped button placed in the catheter tract between dialyses to avoid need to repuncture the abdomen for catheter insertion. Patients requiring prolonged peritoneal dialysis should have implanted silastic catheters used with closed automated dialysis systems.
20. Keep an exact record of the patient's fluid balance during the treatment. a. Know the status of the patient's loss or gain of fluid at the end of each exchange. b. The fluid balance should be about even or should show slight fluid loss.	20. Complications (circulatory overload, hypertension, congestive heart failure) may occur if most of the fluid is not recovered.
21. Promote patient comfort during dialysis. a. Frequent back care and massage of pressure areas. b. Rotate from side to side. c. Elevate head of bed at intervals. d. Allow patient to sit in chair for brief periods if condition permits.	21. The dialysis period is lengthy, and the patient becomes fatigued.
22. Observe for the following: a. Respiratory difficulty. (1) Slow the inflow rate. (2) Make sure tubing is not kinked.	22. a. This is caused by pressure from the fluid in the peritoneal cavity and the upward displacement of the diaphragm— producing shallow respirations.

(Continued)

THE ROLE OF THE NURSE IN ASSISTING THE PATIENT UNDERGOING PERITONEAL DIALYSIS
GUIDELINES FOR NURSING MANAGEMENT (CONTINUED)

Nursing Action	Rationale
(3) Prevent air from entering peritoneum by keeping drip chamber of tubing three-fourths full of fluid.	(3) In severe respiratory difficulty, the fluid from the peritoneal cavity should be drained immediately and the physician notified.
(4) Elevate head of bed; encourage coughing and breathing exercises.	
(5) Turn patient from side to side.	
b. Abdominal pain.	b. Pain may be caused by the dialyzing solution's not being at body temperature, incomplete drainage of the solution, chemical irritation, irritation by the catheter, peritonitis.
Encourage patient to move about.	
c. Leakage	c. Leakage around the catheter predisposes to peritonitis.
(1) Change the dressings frequently.	
(2) Use sterile plastic drapes to prevent contamination.	
23. Keep accurate records:	
a. Exact time of beginning and ending of each exchange; starting and finishing time of drainage	
b. Amount of solution infused and recovered	
c. Fluid balance	
d. Number of exchanges	
e. Medications added to dialyzing solution	
f. Pre- and postdialysis weight	
g. Level of responsiveness at beginning, throughout, and at end of treatment	
h. Assessment of vital signs and patient's condition	
Complications	
1. Peritonitis	1. Peritonitis is the most common complication. Antibiotics may be added to dialysate and also given systemically.
a. Watch for abdominal pain, tenderness, rigidity, cloudy dialysate return.	
b. Send specimen of dialysate for smear and culture.	
2. Bleeding	2. A small amount of bleeding around the catheter is not significant if it does not persist. During the first few exchanges, blood-tinged fluid from subcutaneous bleeding is not uncommon. Small amounts of heparin may be added to inflow solution to prevent the catheter from becoming clogged.

require several weeks for proper healing to take place. In the interim, an external shunt is used (see below). A disadvantage to this type of shunt is the need to "stick" the patient with large bore needles before each dialysis treatment.

External Arteriovenous Shunts. With this method, a teflon-silastic catheter is sewn into the radial artery and a forearm vein, with the two vessels connected by a teflon bridge. During dialysis, the bridge is removed and the arterial and venous ends are connected to the flow lines of the artificial kidney. Currently this type of shunt is used during the time the AVF is healing or for acutely ill persons who will require only short-term hemodialysis. The patient is taught to care for the cannula by cleaning the area around the cannula daily with an antiseptic solution, after which a dry sterile dressing is applied and secured with an elastic bandage. The patient is instructed to observe the shunt several times daily for evidence of

clotting and to avoid carrying packages or a handbag over the shunt arm. While the external AVF provides ready access to the patient's circulation, the shunt itself has a limited lifespan (surgical revision is necessary every few months) and may be subject to disruption, producing hemorrhage, clotting and infection. At the same time it is a visible reminder to the patient of his disability.

Alternative access to the circulation may be achieved by placing a bovine heterograph in the arm or femoral triangle or by a saphenous vein graft to make an arteriovenous fistula if no suitable veins are available in the forearm.

Dialyzers and Dialysate Bath. There have been unprecedented developments in dialyzers and technology for treatment of end-stage renal disease but most dialyzers conform to one of the following types: the coil dialyzer, the flat plate dialyzer and the hollow-fiber artificial kidney.

Underlying Principles of Dialysis

The objectives of hemodialysis are to extract toxic nitrogenous substances from the blood and to remove excess water. Heparinized blood passes down a concentration gradient through a semipermeable membrane by dialysis to the dialysate fluid. The dialysate is composed of all the important electrolytes in their ideal extracellular concentrations. Through the process of diffusion, the blood components equilibrate with those in the dialysate. Through appropriate adjustment of the composition of the dialysate bath, noxious substances (urea, creatinine, uric acid, phosphate and other metabolites) are transferred from the blood into the dialysate so that they can be discarded. Small pores of the membrane hold back desirable blood components, while excess water is removed from the blood (ultrafiltration). The body's buffer system is maintained by the addition of acetate which is diffused from the dialysate into the patient and metabolized to form bicarbonate. Purified blood is returned to the body through one of the patient's veins. At the end of the dialysis treatment the majority of poisonous wastes have been removed, electrolyte and water balances have been restored and the buffer system has been replenished.

During dialysis, the patient, the dialyzer and the dialysate bath require constant monitoring to detect the numerous complications that can arise during dialysis—hepatitis, air embolism, inadequate or excessive ultrafiltration, blood leaks, infection, shunt or fistula complications, etc. The nurse in the dialysis unit has an important role in monitoring and supporting the patient and carrying out a continuing program of patient assessment and education. The details of managing a patient on the dialyzer may be obtained from the written protocol of the machine being used.

Management of the Patient on Long-term Hemodialysis

An optimum dietary program is most important for patients on hemodialysis because of the effects of uremia (wasting, poor dietary intake), the reduced palatability of the restricted diet, the loss of nutrients during dialysis and any concurrent illnesses.

- The diet of the patient usually involves some adjustment or restriction of protein, sodium, potassium and/or fluid intake.

Protein intake must be of high biological quality consisting of complete amino acid composition (eggs, meat, milk, fish) to prevent poor protein utilization and to maintain positive nitrogen balance and replace amino acids lost during dialysis. If many water soluble nutrients and metabolites have been removed from the tissues as a result of the effects of dialysis, the patient may require additional vitamins and minerals. After dialysis procedures are initiated, the patient's clinical condition improves and there is a diminished need for stringent dietary restrictions.

Many drugs are excreted wholly or in part by the kidneys. Patients requiring drug therapy (cardiac glycosides, antibiotics, antiarrhythmic agents, hypertensive agents) are monitored closely to ensure that blood and tissue levels of these drugs are maintained without toxic accumulation. This type of information is kept in mind when the patient asks, "Is it all right to take this medicine for a headache?"

Complications

Although hemodialysis can prolong life indefinitely, it does not halt the natural course of the underlying kidney disease, nor does it completely control uremia. The patient is subject to a number of problems and complications. The leading cause of death among patients undergoing chronic hemodialysis is arteriosclerotic cardiovascular disease—an important factor in limiting survival. Disturbances of lipid metabolism (hypertriglyceridemia) appears to be accentuated by hemodialysis. Congestive heart failure, coronary heart disease with anginal pain, stroke and peripheral vascular insufficiency may incapacitate the patient. Anemia and fatigue contribute to diminished physical and emotional well-being with attendant lack of energy, drive, and loss of interest. Gastric ulcers and other gastrointestinal problems occur from the physiologic stress of chronic illness, medication, etc. Disordered calcium metabolism leads to renal osteodystrophy that produces bone pain and fractures. Other problems include fluid overload associated with congestive heart failure, malnutrition, and disequilibrium syndrome from rapid fluid and electrolyte changes. Patients with virtually no renal function have been maintained for a number of years by periodic hemodialysis. Their usual hope is to anticipate a kidney transplantation. Major problems yet to be solved include the heavy cost of securing trained personnel, facilities and equipment to carry out the dialysis.

Psychosocial Considerations

Persons undergoing long-term dialysis are concerned with very real problems. Unpalatable meals (from restrictions on sodium and potassium) and living with thirst imposed by a restricted fluid intake added to a regimented and complicated life style can be very demoralizing. Generally, the patient's medical status is unpredictable and his life is disrupted; he has serious financial problems, difficulty in holding a job, waning sexual desires and impotence, depression from living the life of a chronically ill person, and fear of dying. Younger persons worry about marriage, having children and the burden that they bring to their families.

Dialysis imposes on the family an altered life style. The amount of time required for dialysis decreases social activities and can create conflict, frustration, guilt, and depression in the family. Frequently the patient's family

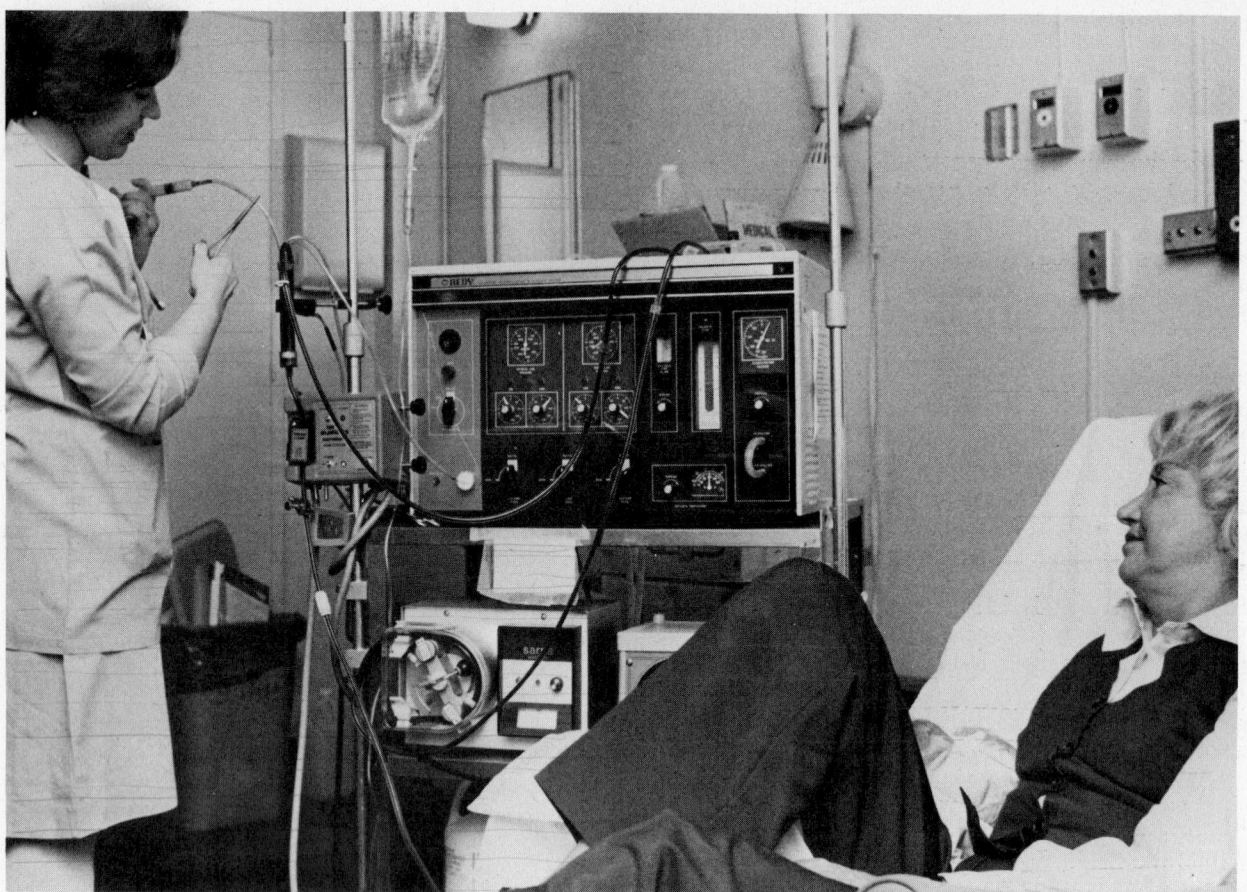

Figure 42-7. Patient receiving instruction for home dialysis. (Courtesy Georgetown University Medical Center)

and friends regard him as a "marginal person" with a limited life expectancy. It may be difficult for the patient, spouse and family to express anger and negative feelings.

The nurse can support the family by letting them know that feelings of anger and dismay are normal emotional reactions in this situation. It also helps to provide verbal and written instructions and to inform them of resources that are available for help. The family should be involved in treatment and decision making.

It is small wonder that the suicide rate among dialysis patients is high. To avoid such drastic outcomes and to provide an outlet for frustrations, the patient should be given a chance to express any feelings of anger and concern over the limitations imposed by the disease and treatment, as well as possible financial problems, job insecurity, pain, and discomfort.

If anger is not expressed there is always the danger that it will be directed inward and lead to depression. Or it can be projected outward to other people, thereby complicating an already tenuous family situation. The patient needs a close relationship with someone to whom he can turn in times of stress and discouragement. Some patients will use the mental mechanism of denial to deal with the overwhelming array of medical problems (in-

fections, hypertension, anemia, neuropathy, etc.). The nurse can help by doing everything possible to support the patient in coping with these ever-present problems and fears.

Home Dialysis

For selected patients, hemodialysis is carried out in the home with equipment similar to that used in the hospital (Fig. 42-7). However, not all people are candidates since this procedure requires a highly motivated patient who is willing to adhere to a prescribed dialysis schedule, a restricted diet, and limited intake of fluids to prevent fluid overload and consequent pulmonary edema.

The person and the family member who will act as helper must undergo a training program to learn how to prepare, operate and tear down the dialysis machine, maintain and clean the equipment, administer drugs (heparin) into the machine lines, and handle emergency problems (hemodialysis coil rupture, shock, convulsions). The home is surveyed to see if electrical outlets and plumbing facilities are adequate. The emphasis is on letting the patient assume primary responsibility for the treatment and to carry on with normal daily activities. When a home dialysis service is not feasible, the patient may be referred to a limited-care dialysis center outside the hospital.

Federal Assistance. In 1973 the Social Security Administration, through Medicare, became the third party payer for the dialysis and transplant costs of 95 percent of those patients on dialysis. In 1977 the Federal government spent over 594 million dollars in providing dialysis and transplantation for 33,000 patients. By 1981 it is estimated that a minimum of 1.25 billion will be spent for over 50,000 end-stage renal disease patients. In the meantime research is going forward to develop hemodialysis equipment that will be less cumbersome and easier to use (Fig. 42-8).

THE PATIENT UNDERGOING KIDNEY SURGERY

Preoperative Nursing Management

All operations on the kidney should be attempted only after a period of study and preparation. *Every effort is made to ensure that renal function is as good as possible.* This is the major preoperative objective. Fluids should be given in large amounts to promote increased excretion of waste products before the time of operation.

The general preoperative preparation is similar to that described on pages 309–317. Since the incision is usually made in the flank, the area to be shaved should extend past the spine posteriorly and beyond the midline anteriorly, above the rib margin and well below the iliac crest.

Patients facing kidney surgery are apprehensive and usually enter the hospital with pain, fever, hematuria, etc. Thus it is helpful to encourage the patient to recognize and express any feelings of anxiety. Confidence is reinforced by establishing a relationship of trust and by gentle and considerate care. A patient faced with the prospect of losing a kidney may think that he will be an invalid the rest of his life. This is not true in most instances, because normal function may be maintained by a single kidney.

The patient is placed on the operating table with a sand or air pillow under the loin of the unaffected side. The upper extremity corresponding to the side to be operated upon is extended to increase the size of the loin space. The lower extremity is flexed. The kidney is exposed by an oblique incision and the appropriate operation is performed. Other surgical approaches are also used.

Postoperative Nursing Management

The objective of postoperative care is to reduce factors that contribute to postoperative complications. The general nursing care after operation is much the same as that after a laparotomy. Deep breathing, coughing, and turning are especially essential for the patient who has had kidney surgery. However, these activities are very painful, because the incision is close to the diaphragm. Be-

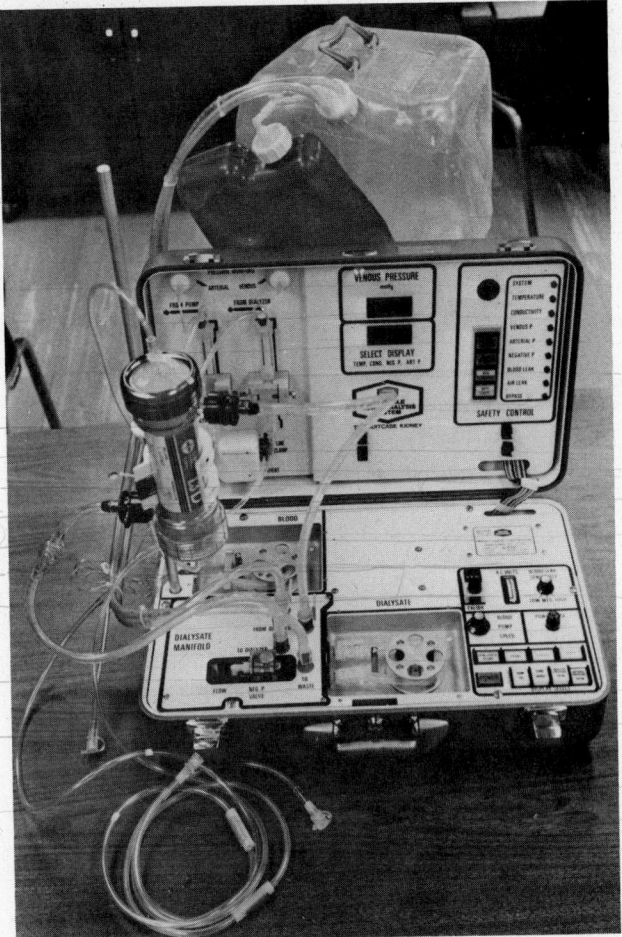

Figure 42-8. Small automated hemodialysis system controlled by a microprocessor for use in travel dialysis. Blood pumps and other components of this device are miniaturized, allowing patients to perform self-treatment in hotel rooms or on location without dependence on physicians or hospitals. This system is called the Friedman-Hutchisson Compact Suitcase Kidney.

cause of the pain, the patient will voluntarily tend to splint the chest while breathing. This in turn can lead to atelectasis and pneumonia. It is not wise to wait too long for pain control as the effect of the narcotic does not reach its peak for about 45 minutes after administration. Morphine sulfate or meperidine is usually given. If the narcotic is given at proper intervals, the patient will be able to perform the coughing and deep breathing exercises more effectively. The incentive spirometer may be used to help maximize lung inflation. The patient is encouraged to cough after each deep breath to loosen secretions.

The patient may complain of muscular aches and pains resulting from the position assumed on the operating table. Massage, moist heat, and analgesic medications provide relief.

Adequate fluids are given by vein and then by mouth when nausea ceases. An accurate intake and output chart should be kept. A normal diet may be given to these patients as soon as peristaltic activity is present. This is best indicated by passage of gas.

Drainage Tubes. Following operations, such as nephrotomy, pyelotomy, and ureterotomy, drainage tubes may be placed directly in the kidney, the pelvis, or the ureter, in order to divert the urine and keep the wound dry.

A nephrostomy tube is inserted directly into the kidney for temporary or permanent urinary diversion and is attached to closed gravity drainage. The patient and tubing are observed for signs of bleeding (immediate or delayed), urinary sand, stone formation, and fistulae.

- A primary nursing responsibility is to ensure that the nephrostomy catheter is draining freely. Any plugging of the tube causes pain, trauma, bursting of the suture lines, and infection. If the tube is inadvertently dislodged, it must be immediately replaced by the surgeon since the nephrostomy opening will contract, making it difficult to re-insert the tube.
- A *nephrostomy tube is not clamped* as such an action will precipitate acute pyelonephritis.

The nephrostomy tube is irrigated only upon order, but it is seldom necessary. Due to the small size of the renal pelvis, only 10 ml. of warm sterile saline is used for irrigation purposes (to avoid mechanical damage to the kidney or infection from pyelorenal backflow). Fluid intake is encouraged to produce good mechanical flushing and to dilute urinary elements that cause calculus formation. The urine is kept acid to prevent tube encrustation by urinary sediments. If the patient has a nephrostomy tube in each kidney, separate output records for each catheter are kept. The catheters are attached to leg urinals when the patient becomes ambulatory.

Sometimes a ureteral catheter(s) is inserted through a cystoscope and taped to an indwelling catheter to hold it in place. A notation is made on the nursing care plan that the catheter is a *ureteral* catheter.

- Do not irrigate a ureteral catheter; this is done by the urologist.

Clamps. Occasionally, clamps are left in the incision following nephrectomy, because it may be impossible to ligate the renal vessels. On examination of the operative site the nurse may see the handles of these instruments extending from the dressings over the wound.

- In no circumstances should the clamps be touched.

Obviously, such a patient is not permitted to lie on the operative side. Pillows placed strategically add to the comfort of this patient.

Drug Therapy. Antibiotics are given as necessary on the basis of culture identification of the causative organism. The toxic manifestations of these agents must be kept in mind when assessing the patient. Low doses of subcutaneous heparin therapy have been shown to prevent thromboembolism in urologic patients.

Complications

Hemorrhage. Hemorrhage (and shock) are the chief dangers following renal surgery. When the dressings are inspected it is important to recall that the seepage from the wound usually collects at the back and not on the anterior dressings. The constitutional signs of hemorrhage—an increasing pulse rate, restlessness, and sweating—should be watched for. Because of the large vessels ligated, hemorrhages may be rapidly fatal. Therefore, the nurse should not hesitate to call the surgeon should the slightest suspicion of this complication arise.

Abdominal Distention: Paralytic Ileus. This complication occurs at times following operations on the kidney and the ureter and is thought to be due to a reflex paralysis of intestinal peristalsis. In a weakened patient, the symptom may become very distressing, even causing respiratory or cardiac difficulties. Oral fluids should be avoided until active bowel sounds are heard (upon auscultation) or passage of flatus.

For relief of the abdominal distention, decompression via a nasogastric tube gives rapid relief. The tube may be removed as soon as normal peristalsis and passage of gas are apparent.

Pain. Pain similar to renal colic is often a distressing symptom after operations on the kidney and the ureter. It is caused commonly by the passage of clotted blood down the ureter. This symptom is usually of short duration but demands adequate doses of narcotics for relief.

Patient Education

Prior to discharge, the patient should be informed about the elements of posthospital care. If drainage tubes are still in place, the patient and a family member should be instructed about the care of the tubes and management of the dressings.

The patient is encouraged to continue a liberal intake of fluids. He is advised to take frequent short rest periods and to increase activity gradually in order to facilitate his return to strength.

BIBLIOGRAPHY

BOOKS

American Nurses Assoc. Division on Medical-Surgical Nursing Practice; Standards of Urologic Practice. Kansas City, Amer. Nurs. Assoc., 1977.

Blandy, J.: Lecture Notes on Urology. Oxford, Blackwell Scientific Pub., 1976.

———: Operative Urology. Oxford, Blackwell Scientific Pub., 1978.

———: Urology. Vols. 1 and 2. Philadelphia, J.B. Lippincott, 1976.

Brundage, D. J.: Nursing Management of Renal Problems. St. Louis, C. V. Mosby, 1976.

Caldwell, K. P. S.: Urinary Incontinence. New York, Grune and Stratton, 1975.

Cameron, E. M., and Kintzel, J. E.: Chronic Renal Failure. *In* Kintzel, K. C.: Advanced Concepts in Clinical Nursing. Philadelphia, J. B. Lippincott, 1977, pp. 535–582.

Cameron, J. S., Russell, A. M. E., and Sale, D. N. T.: Nephrology for Nurses, 2nd ed. Flushing, N.Y., Medical Examination Pub. Co., 1976.

Flocks, R. H., and Culp, D. A.: Surgical Urology, 4th ed. Chicago, Year Book Med. Pub., 1975.

Harrison, J. H. H., et al.: Campbell's Urology. Vols. 1 and 2, Philadelphia, W. B. Saunders, 1978.

Hekelman, F. P., and Ostendarp, C. A.: Nephrology Nursing. New York, McGraw-Hill, 1979.

International Committee for Nomenclature and Nosology of Renal Disease: A Handbook of Kidney Nomenclature and Nosology. Boston, Little, Brown, 1975.

Kolff, W. J.: Artificial Organs. New York, John Wiley and Sons, 1976.

Kuehnel, E., and Bennett, W.: Acute Renal Failure: Discussions in Patient Management. Flushing, N.Y., Medical Examination Pub. Co., 1976.

Lapides, J.: Fundamentals of Urology. Philadelphia, W. B. Saunders, 1976.

Libertino, J. A., and Zinman, L., eds.: Reconstructive Urologic Surgery. Baltimore, Williams and Wilkins, 1977.

Massry, S. G., and Sellers, A. L.: Clinical Aspects of Uremia and Dialysis. Springfield, Ill., Charles C Thomas, 1976.

Maude, D. L.: Kidney Physiology and Kidney Disease: An Introduction to Nephrology. Philadelphia, J. B. Lippincott, 1977.

Muth, R. G.: Renal Medicine. Springfield, Ill., Charles C Thomas, 1978.

Oberley, E. T., and Oberley, T. D.: Understanding Your New Life with Dialysis. Springfield, Ill., Charles C Thomas, 1979.

Rous, S. N.: Urology in Primary Care. St. Louis, C. V. Mosby, 1976.

Schrier, R. W.: Renal and Electrolyte Disorders. Boston, Little, Brown, 1976.

Smith, D. R.: General Urology. Los Altos, Lange Medical Publishers, 1978.

Smith, R. B., and Skinner, D. G.: Complications of Urologic Surgery. Philadelphia, W. B. Saunders, 1976.

Spitzer, M. E., Dickinson, B. B., and Rogers, P. W.: A Renal Failure Diet Manual Utilizing the Food Exchange System. Springfield, Ill., Charles C Thomas, 1976.

Stewart, B. H., ed.: Operative Urology. Baltimore, Williams and Wilkins, 1975.

Winter, C. C., and Morel, A.: Nursing Care of Patients With Urologic Disease, 4th ed. St. Louis, C. V. Mosby, 1977.

ARTICLES

Catheterization

Bodner, H.: Using the urinary catheter. Postgrad. Med., *58*:87–91, Nov. 1975.

Brown, R. S., and Epstein, F. H.: Fluid and electrolyte disorders in urologic patients. Urol. Clin. N. Am., *3*:267–276, June 1976.

Degroot, J., et al.: Indwelling catheters. AJN, *75*:448–449, Mar. 1975.

_____: Catheter-induced urinary tract infections. How can we prevent them? Nursing '76, *6*:34–37, Aug. 1976.

_____: Urethral catheterization. Nursing '76, *6*:51–55, Dec. 1976.

Desautels, R. E.: Managing the urinary catheter. Geriatrics, *29*:67–90, Sept. 1974.

Fincke, B. G., and Friedland, G.: Prevention and management of infection in the catheterized patient. Urol. Clin. N. Am., *3*:313–321, June 1976.

Garibaldi, R. A., et al.: Factors predisposing to bacteriuria during indwelling urethral catheterization. New Engl. J. Med., *291*:215–219, Aug. 1974.

Greene, W. R., et al.: Nonoperative suprapubic urinary drainage. Am. Fam. Phys., *16*:136–138, Oct. 1977.

Lapides, J.: Tips on self-catheterization. Urology Dig., *16*:11–13, July 1977.

Stamm, W. E.: Guidelines for prevention of catheter-associated urinary tract infections. Ann. Int. Med., *82*:386–390, Mar. 1975.

Whyte, J. F., and Thistle, N. A.: Male incontinence: The inside story of external catheterization. Nursing '76, *6*: 66–67, Sept. 1976.

Woodrow, M., Wilsey, G., and Wiley, N.: Suprapubic catheters: Part 1. A direct line to better drainage. Nursing '76, *6*:40–45, Oct. 1976.

Dialysis

Anger, D., et al.: Dialysis ambivalence: A matter of life and death. AJN, *76*:276–277, Feb. 1976.

D'Afflitti, J. G., et al.: Group sessions for the wives of home-hemodialysis patients. AJN, *75*:633–635, Apr. 1975.

Evans, D. B.: Diseases of the urinary system. Management of chronic renal failure by dialysis and transplantation. Brit. Med. J., *1*:No. 6076:1585–1588, 18 June 1977.

Ford, L.: A question of balance. The effects of chronic renal failure and long-term dialysis. Can. Nurse, *73*:19–24, Mar. 1977.

Garron, M. S.: The adjustment period: Coping with the diet. J. Am. Assoc. Nephrology Nurses & Technicians, *3*:42–45, 1976.

Gutierrez, L. F., and Kurtzmann, N. A.: Management of chronic renal failure. Surg. Ann., *8*:367–389, 1976.

Hamburger, R. J.: The management of uremia. Am. Fam. Phys., *16*:125–132, Sept. 1977.

Hickman, B. W.: All about sex—despite dialysis. AJN, *77*:606–607, Apr. 1977.

Jennrich, J. A.: Some aspects of the nursing care for patients on hemodialysis. Heart & Lung, *4*:885–889, Nov.-Dec. 1975.

Levy, N. B.: Psychological studies at Downstate Medical Center of patients on hemodialysis. Med. Clin. N. Am., *61*:759–769, July 1977.

Mazze, R. I.: Critical care of the patient with acute renal failure. Anesthesiol., *47*:138-148, Aug. 1977.

Moore, G. L.: Psychiatric aspects of chronic renal disease. Postgrad. Med., *60*:140-146, Nov. 1976.

Moya, C.: Mrs. Justice and I didn't get along—at all. Nursing '77, *7*:40-41, Jan. 1977.

Richard, C.: Nursing implications in prevention of complications in peritoneal dialysis. Heart & Lung, *4*:890-893, Nov.-Dec. 1975.

Smith, E. C., et al.: Dialysis—current status and future trends. Heart & Lung, *4*:879-884, Nov.-Dec. 1975.

Solomon, M. B.: The care and maintenance of A-V shunts. Dialysis and Transplantation, *3*:36-41, June-July 1974.

AGENCIES

Governmental

National Institute of Arthritis, Metabolism and Digestive Diseases, National Institutes of Health, Bethesda, Md. 20205

Voluntary

National Association of Patients on Hemodialysis and Transplantation, 505 Northern Blvd., Great Neck, N.Y. 11021

National Kidney Foundation, 116 E. 27th St., New York, N.Y. 10016

United Ostomy Association, 1111 Wilshire Blvd., Los Angeles, Calif. 90017

43

MANAGEMENT OF PATIENTS WITH RENAL AND URINARY DISORDERS

ACUTE RENAL FAILURE

Acute renal failure is a sudden and almost complete loss of kidney function caused by failure of the renal circulation or by glomerular or tubular damage. Renal failure results when the kidneys are unable to remove the body's metabolic wastes or perform their homeostatic function; e.g., the maintenance of a stable internal environment. The substances normally eliminated in the urine accumulate in the body fluids as a result of impaired renal excretion and lead to a disruption in homeostatic, endocrine, and metabolic functions. Renal failure is a total body disease and is a final common pathway of many different kidney and urinary tract diseases. Each year an estimated 42,000 Americans die of irreversible kidney failure.

Causes. Acute renal failure, which is manifested by sudden oliguria (less than 500 ml. of urine per day) or anuria (less than 50 ml. of urine per day) and also by the clinical condition of the patient, may be precipitated by a variety of insults. Any condition that causes reduction in renal blood flow, such as volume depletion, hypotension, or shock, leads to a reduction in glomerular filtration, renal ischemia, and tubular damage. Renal failure may also result from the adverse effects of burns, crushing injuries, and infection as well as from nephrotoxic agents that cause tubular necrosis and temporary cessation of renal function. Severe transfusion reactions may also cause renal failure as the hemoglobin which filters

through the kidney glomeruli becomes concentrated in the kidney tubules to such a degree that precipitation occurs, halting the excretion of urine. Following these events, the kidneys become swollen and edematous, and the epithelial cells in the tubules may undergo necrosis.

In many instances there is clear-cut underlying disease, mechanical blockage of the urinary tract by calculi or tumor, or renal artery obstruction.

In summary, risk factors for renal failure include hypovolemic hypotension (oligemic shock, hemorrhage, dehydration, burns), sepsis, nephrotoxic drugs, trauma, multiple blood transfusions, cardiopulmonary bypass, surgery of the aorta or renal vessels, obstructive jaundice, surgery of the biliary tree, and extensive surgery in the elderly.

Prevention. In caring for any patient, the nurse will be alerted by a careful history that reveals whether or not the patient has been taking potentially nephrotoxic antimicrobial agents. The kidneys are especially susceptible to the adverse effects of drugs because they receive such a large blood flow (25 percent of the cardiac output at rest). The nephrons are thus exposed to high concentrations of antimicrobials as a result of glomerular filtration and tubular secretion and reabsorption. Also, since the kidney is a major excretory pathway for many antimicrobials, it is more likely to suffer toxic effects from drugs. Therefore, in people taking potentially nephrotoxic drugs (aminoglycosides, gentamicin, tobramycin, colistimethate, polymyxin B, amphotericin

927

B, vancomycin, capreomycin) renal function should be monitored by BUN or serum creatinine evaluations within 24 hours following initiation of drug therapy and at least twice weekly while the patient is receiving therapy. Any agent that reduces renal blood flow (i.e., chronic analgesic abuse) may cause renal deterioration.

Other precautionary measures taken to avoid renal complications include the following:
- Adequate hydration procedures must be initiated before, during, and after operative procedures.
- Shock, in any clinical situation, must be prevented or treated promptly with blood and fluid replacement.
- Critically ill patients should be monitored by means of central venous pressure readings and hourly urinary output measurements to detect the onset of renal failure at the earliest possible moment.
- Hypertensive states require prompt therapy.
- Persons undergoing intensive diagnostic studies requiring dehydration (barium enema, intravenous pyelogram, etc.) should have "rest days," especially elderly patients who may not have adequate renal reserves.
- All precautions must be taken to ensure that the right person receives the right blood in order to avoid severe transfusion reactions which can precipitate renal complications.
- Infections, which may produce progressive renal damage, must be controlled and avoided.
- Special attention must be paid to draining wounds, burns, etc. which may lead to sepsis.
- Meticulous care must be given to patients with indwelling catheters to prevent ascending infections.

Clinical Manifestations

Almost every part of the body suffers when there is a failure of the normal renal regulatory mechanism. The patient appears critically ill, is lethargic with persistent nausea, vomiting, and diarrhea. The skin and mucous membranes are dry from dehydration, and the breath may have the odor of urine. Drowsiness, headache, muscle twitching and convulsions are the central nervous system manifestations that are present in varying degrees. The urinary output is scanty, may be bloody, and has a low specific gravity (1.010 compared to 1.025 normally). There is an increase in serum creatinine (equal to or greater than 1 mg./100 ml. daily).

There are three clinical phases of acute renal failure. The *period of oliguria* (urinary volume less than 400–600 ml./24 hours) is accompanied by a rise in the serum concentration of the elements usually excreted by the kidneys (urea, creatinine, uric acid, organic acids, and the intracellular cations, potassium and magnesium). In some patients there can be a decrease in renal function with increasing nitrogen retention, yet the patient is actually excreting 2 to 3 liters of urine daily. This is the so-called "high output failure" or nonoliguric form of renal failure and occurs predominantly after burns and traumatic injury. The oliguric phase lasts approximately 10 days.

In the second phase, *the period of diuresis,* the patient experiences a gradually increasing urinary output which signals that glomerular filtration has started to recover. Although the urinary output may reach normal levels, renal function is still markedly abnormal in the diuretic phase.

The *period of recovery* signals the improvement of renal function and may take from 3 to 12 months. There may be a permanent loss of some glomerular filtration rate and concentrating ability and a decreased ability to acidify urine.

Management

The kidney has a remarkable ability to recover from insult. Therefore, the objective of treatment of acute renal failure is to restore the normal homeostatic environment so that repair of renal tissue and restoration of renal function can take place. A search is made to remove and treat any possible cause.

Early dialysis is indicated to prevent metabolic deterioration and reduce catabolic response to acute uremia. Dialysis produces a more sustained correction of biochemical abnormalities, allows for liberalization of fluid, protein and sodium intake, helps wound healing, and diminishes bleeding tendencies and predisposition to infection. Peritoneal dialysis (page 916) or hemodialysis (page 917) may be carried out.

Maintenance of Fluid and Electrolyte Balance. Every effort is made to maintain fluid and electrolyte balance and prevent acidosis. Guides to establishing fluid balance include: daily body weight, serial measurements of central venous pressure, serum and urine concentrations, fluid losses, blood pressure, and the clinical status of the patient. These parameters should be kept on a flow chart to indicate the rate and trend of biochemical deterioration or improvement. Fluids are given to replace current daily (insensible) losses (usually 400 to 500 ml./24 hours) plus measured fluid losses during the oliguric phase. The input and output are measured, including urine, gastric suction, stools, wound drainage and perspiration. The patient is weighed daily and can be expected to lose 0.2 to 0.5 kg. (½ to 1 pound) daily. This weight loss represents obligatory tissue breakdown. If the patient fails to lose weight or develops hypertension, this indicates fluid retention. Fluid excesses can be evaluated by the clinical findings of dyspnea, tachycardia and distended neck veins. The lungs are auscultated for signs of moist rales. Since pulmonary edema may be precipitated by excessive administration of parenteral fluids, the presacral and pretibial areas must be examined for edema several times daily.

Sodium losses are measured (serum sodium levels) and replaced particularly if there are large losses from the gastrointestinal tract from diarrhea and vomiting. Patients with acute oliguria cannot eliminate the daily load of hydrogen ions produced by normal metabolic processes. This is reflected by a fall in the blood carbon dioxide combining power and blood pH. Thus, progressive acidosis accompanies renal failure. The arterial blood gases must be monitored and appropriate ventilatory measures instituted if respiratory problems develop. The patient may require sodium bicarbonate unless he is dialyzed.

Assessment and Control of Hyperkalemia.

A patient with renal disease in which the glomerular filtration rate is reduced has a decreased ability to excrete potassium. Protein catabolism (breakdown) results in the release of cellular potassium into the body fluids causing serious potassium intoxication. Sources of potassium are tissue breakdown, dietary intake, blood in the gastrointestinal tract, or blood transfusion and other sources (intravenous infusions, potassium penicillin and extracellular shift in response to metabolic acidosis). Thus a continuing patient assessment for hyperkalemia (potassium intoxication) is conducted by evaluating serum electrolyte (potassium) determinations (potassium value above 6.5 mEq./L.), ECG assessment (peaked T waves), and patient evaluation. The elevated potassium levels may be reduced by giving ion exchange resins (sodium polystyrene sulfonate — Kayexalate) orally or by retention enema. The drug's action depends upon the ability to move resin through the intestinal tract. Sorbitol induces water loss in the gastrointestinal tract and may be given orally or as an enema with Kayexalate. The patient should be watched for the development of fecal impaction. If a retention enema is given (the colon is the major site for potassium exchange), a catheter with a balloon may be used to facilitate retention if necessary. The patient should retain the resin 30 to 45 minutes to remove the potassium.

High serum potassium levels are dangerous and lead to cardiac arrhythmias and arrest.

- A patient with a high and rising level of serum potassium requires immediate peritoneal dialysis or hemodialysis.
- Intravenous glucose and insulin or calcium gluconate is sometimes used as an emergency and temporary measure for potassium intoxication to drive the potassium back into the cells.
- Sodium bicarbonate may be given to promote the elevation of plasma pH. When sodium ions are made available, there is a migration of potassium into the cell and a lowering of potassium in the plasma. This is short-term therapy and is used with other long-term measures.

There may be an increase in serum phosphate concentrations. This problem may be controlled with phosphate binding agents (aluminum hydroxide) to keep phosphate from being absorbed into the bloodstream and to help prevent a continuing rise in serum phosphate levels.

Serum calcium levels may be low in response to decreased absorption of calcium from the intestine and in association with an elevation in serum phosphate levels.

Adequate blood flow to the kidneys in some patients may be restored by intravenous fluids and medications. Mannitol or furosemide or ethacrynic acid may be prescribed to initiate a diuresis and prevent or minimize subsequent renal failure.

- Observe for signs of dehydration or hypovolemia during the diuretic phase. When hypovolemia is associated with hypoproteinemia, an infusion of albumin may be given. Shock, if present, is controlled and any infection is treated.

Dietary proteins are limited during the oliguric phase to minimize protein breakdown and to prevent accumulation of toxic end products. Caloric requirements are met with high carbohydrate feedings as carbohydrates have a protein-sparing power. Foods and fluids containing potassium and phosphorus (bananas, citrus fruits and juices, coffee) are restricted. The patient may require hyperalimentation. (See page 728.)

Anemia inevitably accompanies acute renal failure due to multiple causes: blood loss due to uremic gastrointestinal lesions, reduced red cell life span and reduced erythropoietin production.

The oliguric phase of acute renal failure may last from 10 to 20 days and is followed by the diuretic phase at which time urinary output begins to increase, signaling that glomerular filtration is taking place. Blood chemistry evaluations are made to determine the amounts of sodium, potassium and water needed for replacement along with assessment for over- or underhydration abnormalities.

- Be alert for urinary tract infection, which is common and potentially dangerous in the diuretic phase.

After the diuretic phase, the patient is placed on a high protein, high caloric diet and is encouraged to resume activities gradually since muscle weakness will be present from excessive catabolism.

CHRONIC RENAL FAILURE (UREMIA)

Chronic renal failure is a progressive deterioration in renal function in which the body's homeostatic mechanisms fail, resulting fatally in uremia (an excess of urea and other nitrogenous wastes in the blood) unless hemodialysis or a kidney transplantation is performed. It may be caused by chronic glomerulonephritis, pyelonephritis, uncontrolled hypertension, sodium and water depletion, vascular disorders, obstructive uropathy, renal disease secondary to systemic disease, renal disease secondary to drugs or toxic agents, infections, etc.

Pathophysiology

As renal function declines, the products of protein metabolism (which form the constituents of urine) accumulate in the blood. There are imbalances in the body chemistry and in the cardiovascular, hematological, gastrointestinal, neurological and skeletal systems. Skin and reproductive changes are also seen.

With the decrease in glomerular filtration there is a decrease in filtered phosphorus which will cause serum phosphate to rise. This results in a decrease in ionizable calcium. Consequently there is an increase in parathyroid release (secondary parathyroidism). The latter normally increases the excretion of phosphate and raises the serum calcium level, but in renal failure, phosphate excretion falls below normal and the major effect of parathyroid hormone is to remove calcium from the bone. Uremic bone disease (renal osteodystrophy) develops from changes in calcium, phosphate and parathyroid balance. Also, the active metabolite of vitamin D (1,25-dihydroxycholecalciferol) is manufactured by the kidney and the availability of this metabolite decreases with the progression of renal disease. In addition, the calcification process in the bone fails, resulting in osteomalacia. The serum magnesium may rise from the inability of the kidney to excrete magnesium and from losses through vomiting and diarrhea.

The patient may be unable to excrete sodium and water loads, causing both sodium and water to be retained. This is one factor that paves the way for fluid retention and congestive heart failure, pulmonary edema and hypertension. (Hypertension is also the consequence of the kidneys secreting increasing amounts of renin, which produces an increase in aldosterone secretion.)

Some patients have a tendency to lose salt and run the risk of hypotension and hypovolemia. Episodes of vomiting and diarrhea may produce sodium and water depletion which worsens the uremic state. Metabolic acidosis occurs due to the reduced ability of the kidney to excrete hydrogen ions, produce ammonia and conserve bicarbonate.

Anemia, which is considered inevitable, develops due to inadequate erythropoietin production, a decrease in red cell production, shortened life span of red cells and the uremic patient's tendency to bleed.

Neurological complications of renal failure may occur from severe hypertension, water intoxication and drug effects. Such manifestations include altered mental function, changes in personality and behavior and convulsions and coma.

Decrease in libido, impotence and amenorrhea are sexual and menstrual changes that occur. Skin changes include pruritus (in part from calcium/phosphate imbalance) which adds to the patient's distress.

Clinical Manifestations

Although at times the onset of chronic renal failure is sudden, in the majority of patients it begins with one or more of a group of symptoms—mild fatigue and lethargy, headache, general weakness, gastrointestinal symptoms (anorexia, nausea, vomiting, diarrhea) and bleeding tendencies. There is decreased salivary flow and dehydration which produces thirst, a metallic taste in the mouth, loss of smell and taste and parotitis or stomatitis. If active treatment is begun early, the symptoms may disappear. Otherwise these symptoms become more marked and others appear as the metabolic abnormalities of uremia affect virtually every body system.

The patient gradually or suddenly becomes increasingly more and more drowsy; the respiration becomes Kussmaul in character; a deep coma develops, often with convulsions, which may occur as mere muscle twitchings or severe spasms quite similar to those of epilepsy. A white powdery substance, "uremic frost," composed chiefly of urates, appears on the skin. Unless treatment is successful, death soon follows.

Management

The aim of management is to help the diseased kidneys to maintain homeostasis for as long as possible. All factors that contribute to the problem (obstructive uropathy, etc.) must be searched for and treated.

With the deterioration of renal function, dietary intervention is necessary with careful regulation of protein intake, fluid intake to balance fluid losses, and sodium intake to balance sodium losses, and some restriction of potassium and phosphate. At the same time, adequate caloric intake and vitamin supplementation must be ensured. There is some restriction of protein since urea, creatinine, uric acid and organic acids—the breakdown products of dietary and tissue proteins—will accumulate rapidly in the blood when there is impaired renal clearance. The allowed protein must be of high biologic value (dairy products, eggs, meat) to provide the essential amino acids. Usually the fluid allowance is 500 to 600 ml. of fluid more than the 24-hour urine output.

Sodium and potassium regulation is determined by measurements of these electrolytes in the serum and urine. If a patient has a tendency to lose sodium, sodium supplementation is given. Phosphate intake (accomplished by lowering protein intake) is lowered to halt secondary hyperparathyroidism. Aluminum hydroxide antacids are given because they bind phosphorus in the intestinal tract. Calories are supplied by carbohydrates and fat to prevent wasting. Vitamin supplementation is necessary as a protein restricted diet does not give the necessary complement of vitamins. (Also the patient on dialysis may lose all water-soluble vitamins from the blood during treatment.) Hyperkalemia is usually not a problem until profound oliguria (less than 250 ml.) develops.

Hypertension is managed by medications: hydralazine (Apresoline), propranolol (Inderal) or methyldopa (Aldomet). Usually the metabolic acidosis of chronic renal failure is asymptomatic, but it can be corrected by dialysis if need be.

Early evidences of cerebral irritation should be watched for. These may vary from slight twitching or headache to delirium. The patient must be protected from self-injury during involuntary movements; thus it is advisable to pad the side rails. The onset of convulsions is recorded as well as their duration, course, extent, and general effect on the patient. The physician is to be notified immediately. Intravenous diazepam (Valium) or phenytoin (Dilantin) is usually given to control convulsive seizures. (The nursing management of the patient having convulsions is discussed on page 1244.) Heart failure, infection and volume depletion are treated symptomatically.

Ideally, the patient is referred to a dialysis and transplantation center early in the course of progressive renal disease. (See page 916 and below for discussion of dialysis and transplantation.) Dialysis is usually begun when the patient cannot maintain a typical life style with conservative treatment. Unfortunately not all patients are candidates for dialysis or transplantation because of severe psychological problems, strokes, vascular complications of diabetes and advanced age.

Kidney Transplantation

Kidney transplantation involves transplanting a kidney from a living donor or human cadaver to a recipient who has end-stage renal failure and requires dialysis in order to maintain life. Transplantation is less expensive than dialysis and provides the patient with a more normal life style. Patients who have end-stage renal failure and are otherwise doomed to certain death may be considered for kidney transplantation. Kidney transplants from well matched living donors who are related to the patient (those with compatible ABO and HLA antigens) are more successful than those from cadaver donors.

Usually the patient's kidneys, which are nonfunctioning, are removed and a dialysis program instituted until a kidney from a suitable donor is obtained. The donor kidney is transplanted retroperitoneally in either iliac fossa. The ureter of the newly transplanted kidney is transplanted into the bladder or anastomosed to the ureter of the recipient (Fig. 43-1).

Preoperative Management. The preoperative objective is to bring the patient's metabolic state to a level as close to normal as possible. Tissue typing is done to determine histocompatibility of the donor and recipient. Antibody screening is also carried out. Immunosuppres-

Renal Homotransplantation

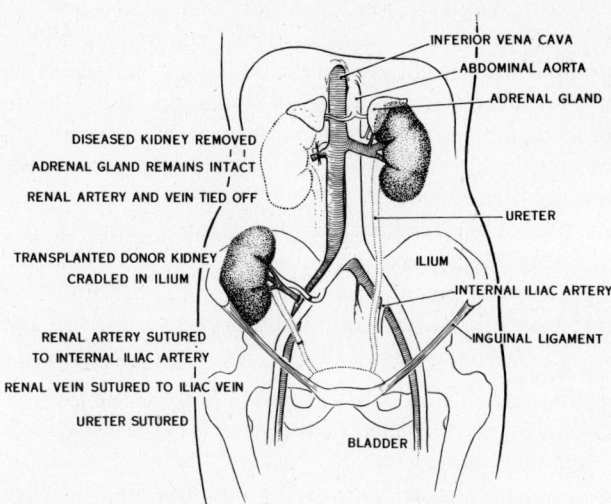

Figure 43-1. Renal homotransplantation.

sive drugs (azathioprine [Imuran] and Prednisone) are given to suppress or overcome the body's defense mechanism. Hemodialysis is usually done the day before the scheduled transplant, and any infection is treated. The lower urinary tract is studied to assess bladder neck function and to detect ureteral reflux. Other aspects of preoperative management are essentially the same as for patients undergoing renal and vascular surgery.

Postoperative Management. The goal of care is to maintain homeostasis until the kidney transplant is functioning well. The major limiting factor of this procedure is the body's immunologic response that leads to rejection of the transplanted kidney. The recipient's body recognizes the new kidney as a foreign protein and attempts to destroy it. The survival of a transplanted kidney depends upon the success of techniques that can suppress these immunologic reactions. In order to overcome or minimize the body's defense mechanism, immunosuppressive drugs (azathioprine [Imuran] and corticosteroids [Prednisone]) are given. Antilymphocytic globulin (ALG) and cyclophosphamide are other immunosuppressive agents that may be used. The doses are gradually tapered for a period of several weeks to maintain levels that depend upon the patient's immunologic response to the transplant. This therapy is continued indefinitely.

• Following a kidney transplant, the patient must be assessed for signs and symptoms of threatened graft rejection: oliguria, edema, fever, increasing blood pressure, apprehension, weight gain, swelling or tenderness over the graft. Blood chemistry tests are monitored for abnormalities, and leukocyte and platelet counts are scrutinized, since immunosuppression depresses the formation of leukocytes and resistance to infection is lowered.

Renal graft failure may occur early (24 to 72 hours) or within a few days (3 to 14 days) or later (after 3 weeks). Ultrasound may be used to detect edema around the graft, while renal biopsy and radiographic techniques are used to evaluate a failing renal transplant. When it appears that rejection is inevitable or when excessive immunosuppression is required to maintain the kidney, the transplanted kidney is removed (graft nephrectomy) and the patient is placed back on maintenance dialysis.

The patient is constantly monitored for infection since the kidney recipient is susceptible to faulty healing and infection due to both immunosuppressive therapy and complications of renal failure.

- A distinction must be made between infection and rejection since impaired renal function and fever are evidences of both infection and rejection.

Immunosuppressive drugs render the transplant patient more vulnerable to opportunistic infections (moniliasis, cytomegalic virus disease, *Pneumocystis carinii* pneumonia) and other relatively nonpathogenic viruses, fungi and protozoa which can be a major hazard. Protective isolation may be carried out with health team members wearing masks until immunosuppressive drug dosages are lowered. Septicemia (bacteremia or fungemia) in renal transplant patients causes high mortality.

- Clinical manifestations of septicemia include shaking chills, fever, tachycardia, tachypnea, and leukocytosis or leukopenia.

The portal of entry for septicemia may be the urinary tract, the lung, the operative site, and other sources. Urine cultures are done frequently in view of the high incidence of bacteriuria during both the early and late stages of transplant. Any type of wound drainage should be viewed as a potential source of infection since drainage is an excellent culture medium for bacteria. Catheter and drain tips are cultured on removal by cutting off the tip of the catheter or drain (using aseptic technique) and placing it in a sterile container for laboratory culture.

The vascular access to hemodialysis is monitored to ensure patency and to evaluate for evidences of infection. Hemodialysis may be necessary postoperatively to maintain homeostasis until the transplanted kidney is functioning well. A few donor kidneys function immediately after grafting and may produce large quantities of dilute urine. A cadaver kidney may or may not undergo tubular necrosis and not function for 2 or 3 weeks. Or the kidney may produce amounts of urine varying from extremes of no urine to large volumes of urine. The output from the urinary catheter (connected to a closed drainage system) is measured every 30 minutes to an hour. After the catheter is removed, the patient is instructed to void frequently to avoid stressing the bladder closure. Intravenous fluids are given in accordance with urine volume and serum electrolyte levels.

Gastrointestinal ulceration and bleeding (steroid induced) may occur. Fungal colonization of the gastrointestinal tract may occur secondarily to steroid and antibiotic administration.

Psychological Considerations

The rejection of a transplanted kidney remains a matter of concern to the patient, the patient's family, and the supporting health care team for many months. The fears of kidney rejection and the complications of immunosuppressive therapy (Cushingoid facies, diabetes, capillary fragility, osteoporosis, glaucoma, cataracts, acne) place tremendous psychological stresses on the patient. Additional problems include stricture or fistula from the grafted ureter and possible tumor growth since patients on long-term immunosuppressive therapy have been found to develop malignancies more frequently than the general population. This requires understanding and the expert management of emotional crises by all concerned with the person's care. (See page 163 for other aspects of psychological support.)

Patient Education

The patient is advised that follow-up care after transplantation is a lifelong necessity. He receives individual and written instruction concerning:

Diet
Medication
Fluids
Daily weight
Daily measurement of urine
Management of intake and output
Prevention of infection
Resumption of activity and avoidance of strenuous sports.

The patient is instructed to report to the physician immediately if any of the following occur: decrease in urinary output, weight gain, malaise, fever, respiratory distress, tenderness over graft, anxiety, depression, changes in eating, drinking or other habit patterns, and changes in blood pressure readings. The National Association of Patients on Hemodialysis and Transplantation, Inc.* is a nonprofit organization that serves the needs of kidney patients. Their quarterly publication, NAPHT NEWS, has many helpful suggestions.

ORGAN DONATION. For those interested in donating a kidney, the National Kidney Foundation* will provide a folder describing the organ donation program and a card specifying the organ to be donated in the event of death. The card is signed by the donor and two witnesses and is to be carried by the donor at all times. Procurement of kidneys for potential recipients is still a major problem.

Research is being devoted to solving the problem of rejection in kidney transplants. Tissue typing (identify-

*Address at end of chapter.

ing individuals with similar tissue characteristics) and drugs to suppress the body's natural defense mechanism are the major means of combating rejection.

ACUTE GLOMERULONEPHRITIS

Acute glomerulonephritis refers to a group of kidney diseases in which there is an inflammatory reaction in the glomeruli. It is not an infection of the kidney per se but rather the result of untoward side effects of the defense mechanism of the body. In most types of glomerulonephritis, IgG (the major immunoglobulin found in the serum of humans) is demonstrable in the glomerular capillary walls. As a result of an antigen-antibody reaction, aggregates of molecules (complexes) are formed and circulate throughout the body. Some of these complexes lodge in the glomeruli, the filtering bed of the kidney, and induce an inflammatory response.

In most cases, the stimulus of the reaction is Group A streptococcus infection of the throat which ordinarily precedes the onset of the nephritis by an interval of 2 to 3 weeks. The streptococcal product, acting as an antigen, generates circulating antibodies and results in an interaction capable of depositing the complexes in the glomeruli and injuring the kidney. Glomerulonephritis may also follow scarlet fever and impetigo.

Pathophysiology. Cellular proliferation, infiltration of the glomerulus by leukocytes and thickening of the glomerular filtration membrane (basement membrane) result in scarring and loss of filtering surface. In acute glomerulonephritis the kidneys become large, swollen, fatty and congested. All the renal tissues—glomeruli, tubules, blood vessels and stroma—are affected in every form of glomerulonephritis, but in each form the tissues are involved in varying degrees. In some patients, antigens outside the body (bacteria, viruses) initiate the process resulting in the complexes being deposited in the glomerulus. In other patients, the membrane tissue of the kidney becomes altered by disease and serves as the inciting antigen. With electronmicroscopy and immunofluorescent identification of the immune mechanism, the nature of the lesion can be studied.

Clinical Manifestations. The disease may be so mild that it is discovered accidently through a routine urinalysis, or the history may reveal a preceding incidence of pharyngitis or tonsillitis with fever. In the more severe form of the disease, the patient presents with headache, malaise, facial edema and flank pain. Mild hypertension is seen and tenderness over the costovertebral angle is common.

Acute glomerulonephritis is predominately a disease of youth. The cases that seem to have developed later are usually acute exacerbations of a quiescent glomerulonephritis already present.

Laboratory Assessment. The urine is scanty and bloody; there may even be no urine (anuria) for a day or two. Usually, however, the patient early in the disease passes from 50 to 200 ml. daily of a highly colored cloudy urine with a specific gravity between 1.020 and 1.025 (that is, low, considering the total amount) and with a thick sediment of red blood cells, leukocytes, and all kinds of casts. This urine contains large amounts of albumin. A large percentage of patients have an increased antistreptolysin titre owing to a reaction to the streptococcal organism. There are usually rising values in blood urea nitrogen and serum creatinine. The patient may be anemic because of loss of the red blood cells into the urine and changes in the hemopoietic mechanism of the body.

As the patient improves, the amount of urine increases, whereas the protein and the sediment diminish. Occasionally, perhaps oftener than we realize, the patient recovers entirely. Some patients become severely uremic and progress to a fatal termination within weeks or months, despite every form of therapy that can be offered; others, after a period of apparent recovery, insidiously develop chronic glomerulonephritis.

Management. The objectives of management are to protect the patient's poorly functioning kidneys and to recognize and treat complications promptly. If residual streptococcal infection is suspected, penicillin is given. Bed rest is encouraged during the acute phase until the urine clears and the BUN and blood pressure normalize. Rest also facilitates diuresis. The urine of the patient may serve as a guide to the duration of bed rest as increasing activity may increase proteinuria and hematuria.

Dietary protein is restricted when there is evidence of renal insufficiency and nitrogen retention (elevated BUN) since an accumulation of metabolic protein waste products in the body will occur in the patient with impaired renal clearance. Sodium is restricted if edema and congestive heart failure are present. Carbohydrates are given liberally to provide energy and reduce the catabolism of protein.

Fluids are given according to the patient's urinary output and daily body weight, plus additional amounts of insensible fluid loss through respiration and feces (approximately 500 to 1000 ml.). Therefore the intake and output are measured and recorded. Usually diuresis starts 1 to 2 weeks after the onset of symptoms. Edema decreases and hypertension lessens. However microscopic proteinuria or hematuria may persist for many months. Most persons with acute glomerulonephritis recover completely. In some, the disease may progress to chronic glomerulonephritis. Complications include hypertensive encephalopathy, congestive heart failure and pulmonary edema. Hypertensive encephalopathy is considered a medical emergency and therapy is directed toward reducing the blood pressure without impairing renal function. I.V. diazoxide may produce a rapid fall in blood pressure. Diuretics are usually given. Dialysis is considered if uremia and fluid retention cannot be controlled. (The treatment of congestive heart failure is discussed on page 578.)

Patient Education. Instructions to the patient include explanations and scheduling for follow-up evaluations of (1) blood pressure, (2) urinalysis for protein, and (3) blood for BUN studies to determine if there is exacerbation of disease activity. The patient is cautioned to call the physician if symptoms of renal failure occur (fatigue, nausea, vomiting, diminishing urinary output, etc.). Any infection must be treated promptly.

CHRONIC GLOMERULONEPHRITIS

Pathophysiology. Chronic glomerulonephritis is assumed to have its onset in the same manner as the acute form of the disease and to represent a milder type of antigen-antibody reaction, but one so mild that it can be overlooked easily. After repeated occurrences of these reactions, the kidneys are reduced to as little as one-fifth their normal size, consisting largely of fibrous tissue. Their cortex shrinks to a layer of 1 to 2 mm. in thickness, and in some areas it is gone entirely. The surface of the kidney is rough, because the renal tissue disappears in irregular patches, and bands of scar tissue distort the remaining cortex by contracting. The glomeruli suffer greatly. Many of them, and their convoluted tubes as well, disappear. The branches of the renal artery are thickened.

Clinical Manifestations. The symptoms of chronic glomerulonephritis are variable. Some patients with severe grades of this disease have no symptoms at all for a long time. They may discover their condition as the result of an application for life insurance, when the blood pressure is found to be elevated. Or it may be suggested during a routine eye examination, when vascular changes or hemorrhages are found. The first intimation others have is a sudden, severe nosebleed, a stroke, or uremic convulsion. Most patients merely notice that their feet are slightly swollen at night, but never markedly so, unless an acute exacerbation of the nephritis is in progress. The majority of all patients have also such general symptoms as loss of weight and strength, increasing irritability, and nocturia. Headaches, dizziness, and digestive disturbances are common.

If these patients are examined carefully, it is likely that the heart will be found to be considerably enlarged, the arteries sclerotic and tortuous, the blood pressure high, and the radial artery resistant because of the arteriosclerosis. Epistaxis and hemorrhages from the lungs and the kidneys and into the retina and the cerebrum are common.

Later in the disease these patients do not feel well; they lose weight and strength; they have severe headaches, shortness of breath, and dyspnea at night. Still later, Cheyne-Stokes respiration and the symptoms of chronic congestion of the gastrointestinal tract may appear. The heart dilates and fibrillates, and pulsus alternans and anginal pains appear, all of which indicate that the damaged heart cannot maintain an adequate output against such high arterial pressure. Various grades of edema develop, depending on the degree to which plasma albumin is decreased and on the severity of heart failure.

The examination of the eye grounds is most important. These patients complain of black spots before their eyes, flashes of light, dimness of vision, and transitory blindness. On examination, thickening of the retinal arteries is seen, also retinal hemorrhages and exudates, and edema of the disks. The skin is dry, with a tendency to eczema and pruritus. Cachexia, with secondary anemia, is common. Later, cardiac edema, often confused with renal edema, and the symptoms of renal failure may appear.

Among the common symptoms of chronic glomerulonephritis are polyuria, frequent micturition, particularly at night, and a fixation of a specific gravity of the urine, that is, the urine does not show the normal variability of concentration based on food and fluid intake or activity, but has the same composition regardless of these factors. It rarely contains more than a trace of protein, except during the occasional acute exacerbations, and this may be absent for weeks or be present only in the afternoon. The urine may contain fatty casts, and doubly refractile fat bodies help in diagnosis. Occasionally, red blood cells appear in the urine. In many patients the renal function tests indicate abnormal function early in the disease. Eventually, there is evidence of marked renal decompensation by even the most gross tests.

In the so-called *nephrotic stage* of chronic glomerulonephritis the picture is striking. The skin has a pale, pasty color; often the whole body is swollen with edema, and almost always the face, the lower extremities, and the dependent parts are so affected. The eyes are almost closed by the puffed lids, edema of the retina may interfere with vision, and the limbs appear to be twice their normal size. Often the finger can be pushed fully a quarter of an inch into the skin of the legs. This is referred to as *pitting edema.* Let an extremity hang down over the side of the bed, and more water accumulates, making it still larger. The fluid collects in the portion of the body that is in the lowest position. This is called *dependent edema.* These patients are truly "waterlogged." Fluid collects also in the abdominal cavity (ascites), which greatly distends the abdomen. It appears in one or both pleural cavities (hydrothorax, fluid in the chest); the patient is short of breath and must sit upright (orthopnea). Fluid may collect in the pericardial sac (pericarditis with effusion), and the patient is in consequence short of breath, and cyanotic and has a weak pulse, especially during inspiration (paradoxical pulse). Repeated chest taps may be necessary to relieve the dyspnea.

Prognosis. The prognosis at this stage of the disease is poor. A few patients will improve, and they may enjoy fair health for many years. However, the great majority fail progressively and die in 1 or 2 years, usually in renal failure.

Management. The treatment of the ambulatory patient with chronic nephritis is entirely nonspecific and symptomatic, depending on the situation that presents itself at any given time. Thus, if hypertension is present, treatment is directed toward sparing the cardiovascular system; if chronic uremia is developing, treatment is directed toward readjusting the diet and fluid intake in an effort to maintain as normal a metabolic situation as possible. Protein intake (of high biologic value) is adjusted according to the response of the patient with adequate calories to prevent protein being utilized for energy. If there is apparent chronic renal tract infection, a possible factor in producing further renal damage, steps should be taken to diagnose it and to treat it.

Treatment of patients with marked edema presents many difficulties. The patient is elevated in bed and made as comfortable as possible. Fluid intake is encouraged to promote elimination, the weight being carefully followed for evidence of increasing fluid retention. Sodium restriction, however, is extremely important. The nurse should watch for all symptoms that suggest renal failure. If exacerbations of the acute form of glomerulonephritis may appear from time to time, the treatment is the same as for acute glomerulonephritis.

NEPHROTIC SYNDROME

The *nephrotic syndrome* is a clinical disorder characterized by (1) marked proteinuria, (2) hypoalbuminemia, (3) edema and (4) hypercholesterolemia. It is seen in any condition that seriously damages the glomerular capillary membrane. Chronic glomerulonephritis, diabetes mellitus with intercapillary glomerulosclerosis, amyloidosis of the kidney, systemic lupus erythematosus and renal vein thrombosis are common causes. The pathophysiology of nephrotic syndrome is discussed on page 898.

Clinical Manifestations. There is an insidious onset of edema which progresses to pitting edema. The patient loses protein in the urine (proteinuria), leading to depletion of body proteins (hypoalbuminemia). In addition the blood cholesterol level is high. The diagnosis is made on assessment of the patient's signs and symptoms, the physical examination, renal function tests, and serum electrolye evaluations. Needle biopsy of the kidney is done for histologic examination of renal tissue to confirm the diagnosis. Urinary tests for microscopic hematuria and granular and epithelial cell casts are done rather frequently.

Management. The objective of management is to preserve renal function. It may be necessary to keep the patient on bed rest a few days to mobilize the edema. A high protein diet is given to replenish wasted tissues and restore body proteins. If the edema is severe, the patient is placed on a low sodium diet. Diuretics are given if renal insufficiency is not severe, and adrenocorticosteroids (Prednisone) may be used to reduce proteinuria.

In the early stages, the nursing management is similar to that of the patient with acute glomerulonephritis, but as the disease worsens, management is more in accordance with the care of the patient with chronic renal failure. (See preceding discussion.)

NEPHROSCLEROSIS

Nephrosclerosis is hardening or sclerosis of the arteries of the kidney and usually is seen as a result of renal hypertension. It is the renal manifestation of generalized arteriosclerosis.

Malignant nephrosclerosis, as opposed to benign nephrosclerosis, though different in degree, merely represents the situation presented in the section on Chronic Glomerulonephritis. Patients with the malignant type progress rapidly to a fatal termination through the stages of proteinuria, increasing hypertension, failing renal function, and eye-ground changes and die usually within a few months. The factor responsible for this termination may be uremia, congestive heart failure due to hypertensive heart disease, or a cerebral accident. It occurs most commonly among people from the third to the fifth decade of life. So far as one can state at the present time, it is a generalized vascular disease that starts in the kidney and finally involves the entire vascular tree. It is always difficult to decide to what extent the vascular damage is responsible for, and to what extent it is a result of, the hypertension.

Patients who develop benign nephrosclerosis are most apt to be found in older age groups. These individuals rarely complain of renal symptoms, although for years the urine has a low and fixed specific gravity and contains a small amount of protein and an occasional hyaline or granular cast. Only late in the disease does renal insufficiency appear. This type of renal disease is the result of a peculiar type of renal arteriosclerosis, which in a patchy manner produces wedge-shaped areas where glomeruli and tubules have largely disappeared, alternating with other areas where the renal units are practically intact— indeed, they are able to function more actively than normal. The diffuse glomerular changes and the evidences of inflammation seen in glomerulonephritis are absent.

HYDRONEPHROSIS

Hydronephrosis is dilatation of the pelvis and calyces of one or both kidneys from obstruction of urinary flow. Obstruction to the normal flow of urine cause the urine to "dam up" resulting in back pressure on the kidney. If the obstruction is in the urethra or the bladder, the back pressure affects both kidneys, but if the obstruction is in the ureter, due to a stone or kink, only one kidney is damaged.

The pelvis of the kidney (including the calyces) is the wide sac into which the urine is poured from the pyramids. As it narrows to a small tube it becomes the ureter. The pelvis has thin walls whose inner surface is lined with the same type of mucous membrane as the ureter and the bladder.

The pelvis of the kidney and its calyces are distended by the partly dammed-up urine when the ureter is somewhat obstructed. If in such a case no inflammation is present and the fluid is clear, the condition is called *hydronephrosis* (Fig. 43-2). In order to cause dilatation of the pelvis of the kidney, the obstruction of urine must be gradual, partial, or intermittent, but not sudden and total, for such would cause immediate anuria and therefore no distention at all of the pelvis.

Partial or intermittent obstruction may be caused by a renal stone that has formed in the renal pelvis but has dropped into the ureter and blocked it. Or the obstruction may be due to a tumor of some other abdominal or pelvic organ pressing on the ureter, or to bands of scar tissue resulting from an abscess or inflammation near the ureter that pinches it. The disorder may be due to an odd angle at which the ureter leaves the renal pelvis or to an unusual position of the kidney, favoring a ureteral twist or kink. In elderly males the most common cause is urethral obstruction at the bladder outlet by an enlarged prostate.

Whatever the cause, if the fluid accumulates intermittently in the renal pelvis, it distends the pelvis and its calyces. If the obstructions are frequent, and the pressure that develops is high, in time atrophy of the kidney results, which causes the kidney to spread out into a thin cyst-like shell. If, however, the pressure of the fluid is never very high, the kidney may not suffer much, although its dilated pelvis may almost fill the whole abdomen. In cases of hydronephrosis, the patient may scarcely be aware of the trouble or may have pains that are severe only when the fluid in the pelvis is under pressure.

Management.   The goal of management is to discover the cause of the obstruction and, if possible, to remove it. Sometimes the urine must be drained by catheter or by operation. Residual urine in the calyces may produce infection which must be treated. If the cause is a tumor or bands of adhesions, removal is indicated. If the cause is benign prostatic hyperplasia, the prostate may have to be extirpated, partially or wholly, depending on the patient's condition and the degree of obstruction. When one kidney only is involved, and its function is nil, nephrectomy may be performed.

NEPHROPTOSIS

Nephroptosis refers to the downward displacement of the kidney. It is found chiefly in thin, long-waisted women from 30 to 50 years of age. The pad of fat that normally surrounds the kidney is absent. The posture is usually poor and the abdominal muscles are relaxed, the result of which produces a weakness and a dragging pain in the loin. At times the kidney may sag so that it almost reaches the pelvis when the patient stands (floating kidney). This abnormal movability may produce torsion or kinks in the ureter. Acute pain, nausea and vomiting, and at times chills and fever may be produced by this obstruction to the ureter.

These attacks are known as *Dietl's crises*. The attack often may be relieved by having the patient lie down, with the hips elevated, or by manipulating the kidney.

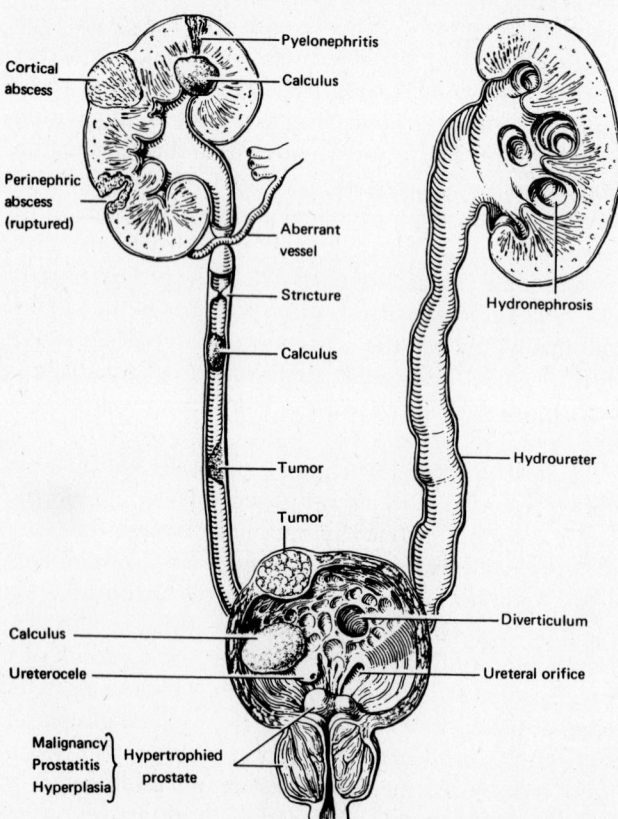

Cortical abscess

Perinephric abscess (ruptured)

Pyelonephritis

Calculus

Aberrant vessel

Stricture

Calculus

Tumor

Tumor

Hydronephrosis

Hydroureter

Calculus

Ureterocele

Diverticulum

Ureteral orifice

Malignancy
Prostatitis
Hyperplasia } Hypertrophied prostate

Figure 43-2.   Commonly encountered male urogenital problems.

Management. One attack of Dietl's crisis warrants a complete urologic study (cystoscopy, pyelography, urography). If obstruction, infection, or hydronephrosis is present from a ptotic kidney, surgical intervention may be necessary. The kidney is fixed in position by sutures in an operation called *nephropexy.* Exercises to improve the posture and strengthen the relaxed abdominal muscles are prescribed. Belts may be applied to give abdominal support. This is helpful to some patients but of questionable value to others. The belt should be adjusted with the patient lying down with the hips elevated. The belt is tightened from below and then upward.

INFECTIONS OF THE URINARY TRACT

A *urinary tract infection* (UTI) is caused by the presence of pathogenic microorganisms in the urinary tract, with or without signs and symptoms. Infection may predominate at the bladder (cystitis), urethra (urethritis), prostate (prostatitis), or kidney (pyelonephritis). The normal urinary tract is sterile except near the urethral orifice.

Bacteriuria refers to the presence of bacteria in the urine. A colony count of at least 100,000 colonies/ml. of urine on a clean-catch midstream or catheterized specimen implies infection. Unfortunately infections in any part of the urinary tract may persist for months or years without symptoms and eventually cause kidney damage.

The bacteria most commonly responsible for urinary tract infections are *Escherichia coli* (85 percent), one or more species of *Klebsiella, Enterobacter, Proteus,* and *Pseudomonas,* and the various enterococci. All these are normally found in the fecal flora.

Factors Contributing to Urinary Tract Infection. (Fig. 43-3). It is now believed that the majority of urinary infections *ascend from the urethra* and become established in the bladder (especially in the presence of residual urine) and then travel into the kidneys. Women

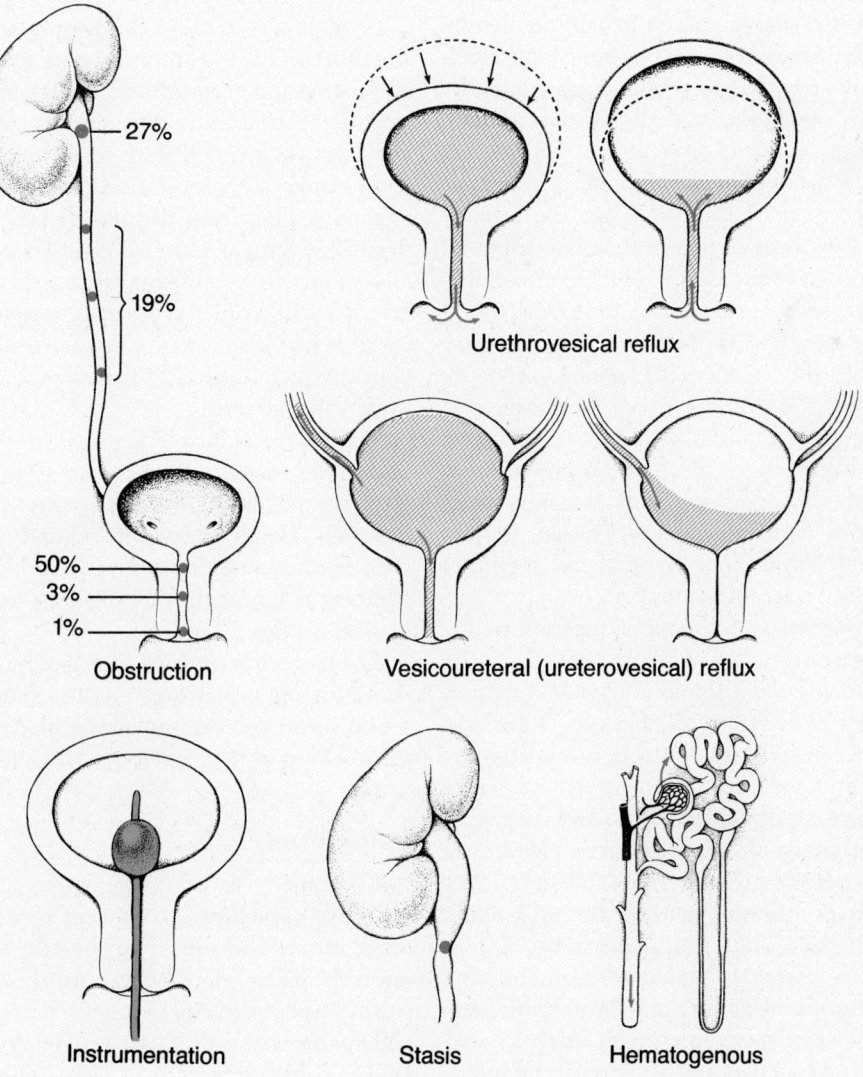

Figure 43-3. Causes of urinary tract and kidney infections.

are more prone to develop bladder infections because of the shortness of the female urethra and its anatomic proximity to the vagina, periurethral glands and rectum. In the male, the length of the urethra and the antibacterial properties of the prostatic secretions tend to ward off ascending urethral infections.

Urethrovesical reflux refers to the reflux (flowing back) of urine from the bladder into the urethra. It is caused by increase in intrabladder pressure (coughing, sneezing) which may squeeze the urine out of the bladder into the urethra. When the pressure returns to normal the urine flows back into the urethra bringing back into the bladder the bacteria from the anterior portions of the urethra. Urethrovesical reflux is also caused by dysfunction of the bladder neck or urethra.

Vesicoureteral reflux (or ureterovesical reflux) refers to the reflux (flowing back) of urine from the bladder into one or both ureters and is the most common cause of urinary tract infection. In the normal person the ureterovesical junction prevents urine from traveling back into the ureter, particularly at the time of voiding. When the ureterovesical valve is incompetent (congenital causes, ureteral abnormalities), the bacteria may reach the kidneys and there may be subsequent dilatation of the ureter, renal pelvis, and calyces with ultimate kidney destruction.

Fecal soiling of the urethral meatus is another common way in which bacteria are introduced into the urinary tract. *Instrumentation* (from catheterization, cystoscopic examinations) is also implicated in producing infections. *Stasis of urine in the bladder* leads to infection which will ultimately spread through the entire urinary system. Any *obstruction* to urinary flow renders the kidney more susceptible to infection. Common causes of urinary tract obstruction are congenital anomalies, urethral strictures, contracture of the bladder neck, bladder tumors, ureteral stones, and compression of the ureters. Urinary tract infection may also be from *hematogenous* (blood) or *lymphogenous* spread. *Metabolic disorders* (diabetes mellitus) predispose to urinary tract infections.

Clinical Manifestations. Signs and symptoms of urinary tract infections cover a broad range. Frequently the patient is asymptomatic and is found to have an infection while undergoing a periodic health checkup. Signs and symptoms of lower urinary tract infection (cystitis) include frequent painful and burning urination sometimes accompanied by bearing down sensations and spasms in the region of the bladder and suprapubic area. Hematuria and back pain may also be present. Signs and symptoms of upper urinary tract infection (pyelonephritis) include fever, chills, flank pain, and painful urination. Upon examination there is costovertebral angle pain and tenderness. Symptoms of renal failure may be present: nausea, vomiting, pruritus, weight loss, edema, and shortness of breath. Acute flareups of urinary tract infection may be silent.

Diagnostic Evaluation. The diagnosis is made from repeated systematic examinations of the urine. The urine is collected by a midstream clean-catch technique. As noted earlier, a bacterial count of 100,000 organisms (colonies) per ml. of urine indicates a urinary infection. Successive urine cultures are also used to find bacterial species present. In the male a culture is made of prostatic fluid or urine voided after prostatic massage. In all patients, the urine should be examined for tubercle bacilli. An intravenous urogram (IVP) detects abnormalities of function and shows any dilatations in the urinary system. Cystoscopic examination is also usually performed for patients with repeated infections.

Cystitis

Cystitis is an inflammation of the urinary bladder that is most often caused by an ascending infection from the urethra. It may be caused by urethrovesical reflux (flowing back of urine from the urethra into the bladder), fecal contamination, or the use of various instruments such as a catheter or cystoscope.

Cystitis is seen more commonly in women because of the shortness of the urethra and its anatomic proximity to the vagina and periurethral glands and rectum. The distal portion of the urethra is frequently colonized with bacterial flora. In women with recurrent urinary tract infections, bacterial colonization often occurs in the vaginal vestibule. There may be some defect of the mucosa of the urethra, vagina or external genitalia of these patients that allows enteric organisms to invade the bladder. Acute infections of women are usually caused by *Escherichia coli*. Cystitis may also occur in women following sexual intercourse which implicates the ascending urethral pathway in its pathogenesis.

Males have a much lower incidence of cystitis probably due to the longer length of the urethra and the antibacterial properties of prostatic secretion. Therefore cystitis in men is secondary to some other factor—infected prostate, epididymitis by reflux of urine along the vas or perivesical lymphatics as from an infected prostate, or bladder stones.

The patient complains of urgency, frequency, burning and pain on urination, nocturia, and a bearing down sensation in the region of the bladder and suprapubic area. There is pus, bacteria, and often red cells in the urine.

Management

The objectives of management are to eradicate the causative pathogens, to prevent recurrences and to preserve renal function. The specific treatment depends upon the cause. A urine culture is obtained for smears, culture and sensitivity studies to determine the pathogen and to prescribe the appropriate drug. The choice of antimicrobial is based on sensitivity studies. Urinary infections usually respond favorably to antimicrobials which are excreted in the urine in high concentration. A potentially effective drug should rapidly sterilize the urine and thus relieve the patient's symptoms. Urine cultures may be repeated several times during therapy and 7 to 10 days after completion of treatment to ensure elimination of infection. There is a propensity for these infections to recur. Recurrences are of two types: (1) reinfection with a new and different organism and (2) relapse with the original organism. Patients with recurring infections should undergo periodic urine cultures since most are from new infections with different organisms.

The effectiveness of certain antimicrobial drugs is affected by the reaction (pH) of the urine. Aminoglycoside antibiotics (streptomycin, kanamycin, neomycin and gentamicin) are more active with an alkaline pH. Sodium bicarbonate may be given to alkalize the urine. The tetracyclines, methenamine mandelate, and cycloserine are more active with an acid pH, and ascorbic acid may be given to acidify the urine.

Diagnostic studies are carried out to determine if the infection is secondary to a functional or structural disorder if there are recurring infections. Such studies include kidney and urinary bladder x-rays, intravenous urogram, and cystoscopy. In these studies, an obstruction is searched for—e.g., stricture, bladder calculus, etc.

The patient is encouraged to drink liberal amounts of fluids to promote renal blood flow and to flush the bacteria from the urinary tract. Frequent voiding (every 2 to 3 hours) is encouraged to empty the bladder completely since this enhances bacterial clearance, reduces urine stasis and prevents reinfection. Antispasmodic drugs may be useful in relieving bladder irritability and pain. Aspirin, heat to the perineum and hot tub baths help relieve urgency, discomfort and spasm.

Prevention and Patient Education. Since there is a marked tendency for infection to recur, follow-up urine studies are recommended for at least 2 years or more to determine if asymptomatic infection is present. It is especially important to have follow-up studies if urinary tract infections occurred during pregnancy.

Women who have repeated urinary tract infections should receive detailed instructions on the following points:
1. It is desirable to shower rather than bathe in a tub, since bacteria in the bath water may gain entrance into the urethra.
2. Cleanse around the perineum and urethral meatus (cleansing from the front to the back) after each bowel movement.
3. Drink liberal amounts of fluid all during the day to flush out bacteria. Void every 2 to 3 hours during the day and completely empty the bladder.
4. If sexual intercourse is the initiating event for development of bacteriuria:
   a. Void immediately after sexual intercourse
   b. Take the prescribed single dose of an oral antimicrobial agent following sexual intercourse.
5. If bacteria continue to appear in the urine, long-term anti-

microbial therapy may be required to prevent colonization of the periurethral area and recurrence of infection. The drug should be taken after emptying the bladder just before going to bed to ensure adequate concentration of the drug during the overnight period.

In addition the patient should be instructed to take all of the prescribed antimicrobial for the full time (10 days to 2 weeks) and not to stop taking the medication merely because there are no symptoms. A full glass of water may be taken with the medication. Noticeable improvement should be seen in 3 days. If burning on urination continues, the physician or clinic should be notified.

Pyelonephritis

Pyelonephritis is a bacterial infection (acute or chronic) of the renal pelvis, tubules and interstitial tissue of one or both kidneys. Bacteria may gain access to the bladder via the urethra and ascend to the kidney or may reach the kidney through the bloodstream. Pyelonephritis is frequently secondary to ureterovesical reflux in which an incompetent ureterovesical valve allows the urine to regurgitate into the ureters, usually at the time of voiding (Fig. 43-3). Urinary tract obstruction (which renders the kidneys more susceptible to infection) and renal diseases are among other causes.

Clinical Manifestations and Pathophysiology. Acute pyelonephritis is an active infection which presents with chills and fever, flank pain and tenderness, leukocytosis, bacteria and pus in the urine, and frequently with symptoms of lower urinary tract involvement such as dysuria and frequency.

There are areas of inflammation in the kidney with interstitial infiltrations of inflammatory cells which in time may produce tubular destruction and abscess formation. Low-grade interstitial inflammation may result in atrophy and destruction of tubules and in hyalinization of the glomeruli. Eventually when pyelonephritis becomes chronic, the kidneys become scarred, contracted and of little functional value.

Management. An intravenous urogram and other diagnostic tests are carried out to locate any obstruction in the urinary tract. The relief of obstruction is essential to save the kidney from destruction. The treatment is essentially the same as that of cystitis (preceding discussion). Culture and sensitivity tests are done on the urine since the choice of antimicrobial is determined by the causative organism. Acute pyelonephritis is often caused by *E. coli* which is sensitive to many antimicrobial drugs. The antimicrobial drug must be given for a long enough period to prevent re-seeding of a residual foci of infection.

A possible problem in treatment is chronic or recurring infections persisting for months or years without symptoms. After the initial antimicrobial regimen, the patient is kept on continuous antimicrobial treatment until there is no evidence of infection, all causative factors have been treated or controlled and kidney function is stabilized. Serial urine cultures and other evaluation studies must be continued indefinitely. The patient is also monitored with serum creatinine determinations and blood counts for the duration of the long-term therapy.

Chronic Pyelonephritis (Chronic Interstitial Nephritis)

Repeated bouts of acute pyelonephritis may lead to chronic pyelonephritis (chronic interstitial nephritis).

The patient with chronic pyelonephritis (persistent presence of bacteria in the urine) usually has no symptoms of infection unless an acute exacerbation occurs. Noticeable signs may include fatigue, headache, poor appetite, polyuria, excessive thirst, and weight loss. The persistent and recurring infection may produce progressive scarring of the kidney with ultimate kidney atrophy and failure.

Complications of chronic pyelonephritis include uremia (from progressive loss of nephrons secondary to chronic inflammation and scarring), hypertension and renal lithiasis (from chronic infection with urea-splitting organisms resulting in stone formation).

Management. The extent of the disease is determined by intravenous urogram and measurements of serum urea, creatinine levels and creatinine clearance. Sterilization of the urine is undertaken if significant bacteria is present. The choice of an antimicrobial is based on culture identification of the pathogen. If the urine cannot be made bacteria-free, nitrofurantoin, nalidixic acid, cephalosporin, or a combination of sulfamethoxazole and trimethoprim may be tried to suppress bacterial growth. The treatment of uremia is discussed on page 930. Hypertension is also carefully controlled.

Carbuncle of the Kidney

Carbuncle of the kidney is an infection of hematogenous origin that is caused usually by the staphylococcus. It usually follows a cutaneous boil or carbuncle and is characterized by fever, malaise, and dull pain in the region of the kidney. This type of infection, if recognized, usually subsides with chemotherapy and penicillin.

Perinephric Abscess

Perinephric abscess is an abscess in the fatty tissue about the kidney that may arise secondary to an infection of the kidney or as a hematogenous infection originating in foci elsewhere in the body. It may be secondary to a staphylococcal infection of the kidney or it is encountered as a complication of a chronic renal infection. The symptoms often are acute in onset, with chills, fever, high leukocytosis, and other signs of suppuration. Locally, there is tenderness posteriorly in the loin. The patient usually appears seriously ill.

Management. The treatment consists of administration of the appropriate antimicrobial agent and incision and drainage of the abscess. Drains are usually inserted and left in the perinephric space until all significant drainage has ceased. Because the drainage often is profuse, frequent changes of the outer dressings may be necessary. As in the treatment of an abscess in any site, the patient is monitored for sepsis, fluid input and output and for general response to treatment.

Tuberculosis of the Kidney and the Genitourinary Tract

Pathophysiology and Clinical Manifestations. Tuberculosis of the kidney and urinary tract is caused by the organism *Mycobacterium tuberculosis* and usually disseminates from the lungs via the bloodstream to the kidneys and to other organs of the genitourinary tract. At first the symptoms are mild, there is usually a slight afternoon fever and a loss of weight and appetite. The process of tuberculosis generally starts in one of the renal pyramids; ulceration into the kidney pelvis follows; the organisms are carried down with the urine into the bladder so that the bladder is likely to become infected, thereby presenting an opportunity for other ascending infections of the previously healthy kidney.

Tuberculosis of the lower genitourinary tract is almost always secondary to renal tuberculosis, the infection having been propagated downward. In the male, the prostate and epididymis may become infected.

Tuberculosis of the urinary bladder is practically never a primary infection but an extension of tuberculosis of a kidney. This disease gives rise to several small ulcers, the majority of them near the trigone. The symptoms of bladder tuberculosis are those of cystitis in general but with an unusual degree of bladder irritability. Suggestive early symptoms of this disease are an increased urinary output that contains considerable pus and yet is acid in reaction (in nearly all other pyurias the urine is alkaline), and hematuria (either microscopic or gross). The symptoms of pain, dysuria, and urinary frequency, when they occur, are due to bladder infection. Symptoms of bladder irritability (frequency of urination, nocturia) are a later manifestation of the disease.

Management. A search for tuberculosis elsewhere in the body must be conducted when tuberculosis of the kidney or urinary tract is found. Inquiry is made to determine if the patient has been in previous contact with tuberculosis. At least three clean-voided first morning urine specimens are concentrated and cultured for the diagnosis of urinary tract tuberculosis.

The objective of treatment is to eradicate the offending organism. A multiple-drug regimen appears to delay the emergence of resistant organisms. Combinations of ethambutol, isoniazid, cycloserine and, rifampin are among the drugs used. The multiple drug combinations are given for at least two years or longer.

Recent evidence indicates that it is more effective to

give all the medications together in a single daily dose. Since renal tuberculosis is a manifestation of a systemic disease, all measures to promote the general health of the person are used. Although emphasis is on medical treatment, surgical intervention may be necessary to prevent obstructive problems and to remove a severely infected organ. The patient must realize the need for follow-up examinations (urine cultures, excretory urograms) usually every 6 months for 5 years to detect reactivation of tuberculosis.

Treatment will need to be reinstituted if a relapse occurs and the tubercle bacilli again invade the genitourinary tract. Ureteral stenosis or bladder contractions are complications that may develop during the healing process.

UROLITHIASIS

Urolithiasis refers to the presence of stones in the urinary system. Stones are formed in the urinary tract by the deposit of crystalline substances (calcium phosphate, oxalate, uric acid) excreted in the urine. They may be found anywhere from the kidney to the bladder and vary in size from mere granular deposits, called sand or gravel, to bladder stones the size of an orange (Fig. 43-4).

Certain factors favor the formation of stones, including infection, urinary stasis, and periods of immobility (produces slowing of renal drainage and altered calcium metabolism). Hypercalcemia (abnormally high concentration of blood calcium compounds) and hypercalciuria (abnormally large amounts of calcium in the urine) may be caused by hyperparathyroidism, excessive intake of vitamin D, excessive intake of milk and alkali, and certain myeloproliferative diseases (leukemia, polycythemia vera) which produce an unusual proliferation of blood cells derived from bone marrow. Some stones are caused by an excessive excretion of uric acid. Vitamin A deficiency may be another cause. Heredity plays a part in the formation of calcium oxalate, cystine, and uric acid stones, while in many patients no cause may be found.

The problem occurs predominantly in the third to fifth decades, affecting men more than women. Persons who have had two stones tend to have recurrences. The majority of stones contain calcium or magnesium in combination with phosphorus or oxalate. Most stones are radiopaque and can be detected by roentgenography.

Clinical Manifestations. The clinical manifestations depend on the presence of obstruction, infection and edema. When the stones block the flow of urine, obstruction develops, and the constant irritation of the stone may be followed by a secondary infection that causes pyelonephritis and cystitis with chills, fever, and dysuria. Occasionally, stones in the kidney produce few symptoms; usually, however, there is an intense deep ache in

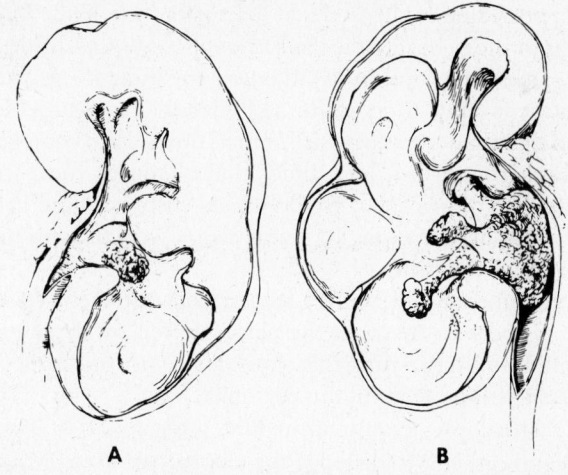

Figure 43-4. *A.* Single calculus obstructing and dilating the lower renal calyx. *B.* "Staghorn" calculus obstructing and dilating all the renal calyces. (From Flocks, R. H.: Urology. *In* Liechty, R. D., and Soper, R. T.: Synopsis of Surgery, 2nd ed. St. Louis, C. V. Mosby Co., 1972)

the loin and voiding of increased amounts of urine containing blood and pus cells. A renal stone produces an increase in hydrostatic pressure and distends the renal pelvis and proximal ureter. Thus painful afferent sensations are initiated. Pain originating in the renal area radiates anteriorly and downward toward the bladder in the female and toward the testicle in the male. If the pain suddenly becomes acute, the loin exquisitely tender, and nausea and vomiting appear, the patient has an attack of *renal colic.* Diarrhea and abdominal discomfort may accompany the attack. These gastrointestinal symptoms are due to reno-intestinal reflexes and the anatomical relation of the kidneys to the stomach, pancreas, colon, etc.

When stones lodge in the ureter, acute shocking colicky pain is experienced, referring down the thigh and to the genitalia. There is usually a frequent desire to void, but very little urine is passed, and it usually contains blood because of the abrasive action of the stone as urine is passed. This group of symptoms is called *ureteral colic.* In general the patient will spontaneously pass stones under 0.4 cm. Those over 1 cm. in diameter usually must be removed. The diagnosis is confirmed by intravenous urogram and/or retrograde pyelography.

Management

The basic objectives underlying the management of the patient are to eradicate the stone, to determine the stone type, to prevent nephron destruction, to control infection and to relieve any obstruction that may be present. Infection and back pressure of obstructed urine can destroy the renal parenchyma.

Active treatment must be instituted for renal and ureteral colic. The immediate objective of treatment is to relieve the pain until its cause can be removed; morphine or meperidine hydrochloride helps allay the pain. Hot baths or moist heat to the flank areas also is useful. Unless the patient is vomiting, fluids are encouraged, as this treatment tends to increase the hydrostatic pressure behind the stone and thus assists it in its downward passage. A high round-the-clock fluid intake reduces the concentration of urinary crystalloids and ensures a high urinary output. Encouraging fluids also lowers the specific gravity of the urine.

No time should be lost in carrying out these treatments, because at times the pain suffered by these patients is so excruciating that shock and syncope result. A patient will be grateful for any relief.

Cystoscopic examination and passage of a small ureteral catheter to dislodge the obstructive stone (when possible) immediately relieves back pressure upon the kidney and alleviates the intense pain.

The nursing care of patients with calculi requires constant observation to detect the spontaneous passage of a stone. All urine should be strained through gauze, since uric acid stones may crumble. Any blood clots passed in the urine should be crushed and the sides of the urinal and bedpan inspected for clinging stones. When stones are recovered crystallographic analysis is carried out to establish the type of stone formation, since treatment is based on the composition of the stone.

Diet Therapy. Diet therapy is most effective when stones are caused by metabolic abnormalities resulting in increased excretion of stone constituents (hypercalciuria) or altered physiochemical properties of the urine (urine acidity). Most stones contain calcium combined with phosphate or other substances. For these patients the diet selected is moderately reduced in calcium and phosphorus content (Table 43-1). The urine is acidified. Sometimes stones will cease growing simply by ensuring an adequate fluid intake and limiting certain foods in the diet that make up the main ingredient of the stone (e.g., calcium).

Patients who are inclined to develop phosphatic calculi should ingest only a limited amount of phosphorus. To offset excess phosphorus, aluminum hydroxide gel often is ordered, since it combines with the excess phosphorus, causing it to be excreted through the intestinal tract rather than the urinary system.

For uric acid stones the patient is placed on a low purine diet to reduce the output of uric acid in the urine. Allopurinol (Zyloprim) may be given to reduce serum uric acid and urinary uric acid excretion. The urine is alkalized. For cystine lithiasis, a low protein diet is given, the urine is alkalized, and penicillamine is given to reduce the amount of cystine in the urine.

Surgical Intervention. Surgical intervention is indicated if the stone is causing obstruction, unremitting pain, infection that does not respond to treatment or progressive renal damage. Surgical procedures are performed to remove the stone(s) with a minimum of trauma to the kidney or ureter.

If the stone is in the kidney, the operation performed may be a *nephrolithotomy* (incision into the kidney with removal of the stone), or *nephrectomy*, if the kidney is functionless due to infection or hydronephrosis. (See page 923 for the nursing management of the patient following kidney surgery.) Stones in the kidney pelvis are removed by a *pyelolithotomy,* or a *pyelotomy,* in the ureter by *ureterolithotomy;* and in the bladder by *cystotomy*. Sometimes an instrument is inserted through the urethra into the bladder, and the stone is crushed in the jaws of this instrument. Such an operation is called a *cystolitholapaxy.*

The lodgment of a stone in the ureter may at times cause complete suppression of urine, a condition termed *calculous anuria.* Unless this condition is relieved, renal failure develops, and death rapidly follows.

In prolonged operations for the removal of branched or multiple renal calculi, the kidney may be immersed in an iced saline slush solution during surgery to achieve kidney hypothermia. This surgical technique decreases the need for blood perfusion during surgery so that arterial blood flow to the kidney may be interrupted for longer periods during extended operative procedures.

Patient Education and Prevention of Urolithiasis. Because it is known that urinary calculi may recur after the first stone is found, the patient should be so informed and encouraged to follow a regimen of prophylaxis. One facet of prevention is to *maintain a high fluid intake* since stones form more readily in a concentrated urine. A patient who has shown a tendency to form stones, should drink at least 3000 ml. daily, should adhere to the prescribed diet and should avoid sudden increases in environmental temperatures which may cause a fall in urinary volume. Occupations and sports that produce excessive sweating can lead to severe temporary dehydration; fluid intake should be adjusted. Sufficient fluids should be taken in the evening to prevent urine from becoming too concentrated at night. Infections are to be avoided since toxins are eliminated by the kidney. Urine tests should be conducted every 3 or 4 months and urinary sediment evaluated for evidence of infection.

Since prolonged immobilization slows renal drainage and alters calcium metabolism, ambulation is to be encouraged whenever possible. In addition, excessive ingestion of vitamins (especially vitamin D) and minerals should be discouraged.

RENAL TUMORS

Renal tumors may arise from the renal capsule, parenchyma (renal cell carcinomas), connective tissue (sarcomas), or fatty tissue or may be neurogenic or vascular in origin. Adenocarcinomas constitute 75 percent of all

TABLE 43-1.   MODERATELY REDUCED CALCIUM AND PHOSPHORUS DIET
(This diet will contain from 500-700 mg. of calcium and from 1000-1200 mg. of phosphorus*)

FOODS ALLOWED	FOODS TO BE AVOIDED
Beverages Coffee, Postum, Sanka, tea, ginger ale.	*Beverages* Carbonated "soft" drinks; cocoa.
Milk Limited to 1 cup (½ pint) a day. Cream may be substituted for part of the milk.	
Cheese Pot or cottage cheese only. Limited to 2 ozs.	*Cheese* All except pot or cottage cheese.
Fats As desired.	
Eggs Limited to 1 a day; egg whites as desired.	
Meat, fish, fowl Limited to 4 ozs. daily of beef, lamb, pork, veal, chicken, turkey, fish. See those to be avoided.	*Meat, fish, fowl* Brains, heart, liver, kidney, sweetbreads. Game (pheasant, rabbit, deer, grouse). Sardines, fish roe.
Soups and broths All. Cream soups made with milk allowance only.	
Vegetables At least 3 servings besides potato. One or 2 servings of deep green or deep yellow vegetables to be included daily.	*Vegetables* Beet greens, chard, collards, mustard greens, spinach, turnip greens. Dried beans, peas, lentils, soybeans.
Fruits All except rhubarb. Include citrus fruit daily.	*Fruits* Rhubarb.
Breads, cereals, macaroni products White, enriched bread, rolls, and crackers except those made from self-rising white flour. Farina (not enriched), cornflakes, corn meal, hominy grits, rice, Rice Krispies, Puffed Rice. Macaroni, spaghetti, noodles.	*Breads, cereals, macaroni products* Whole-grain breads, cereals, and crackers. Rye bread. All breads made with self-rising flour. Oatmeal, brown and wild rice. Bran, Bran Flakes, wheat germ. All dry cereals except those allowed.
Desserts Fruit pies, fruit cobblers, fruit ices, gelatin. Puddings made with allowed milk and egg. Angel food cake. (Do not use packaged mixes.)	*Desserts* All except those allowed.
Condiments Sugar, jellies, honey, salt, pepper, spices.	*Miscellaneous* Nuts, peanut butter, chocolate, cocoa. Condiments having a calcium or a phosphate base. (Read labels.)

*Adapted from Mitchell, H. S., et al.: Nutrition in Health and Disease, 16th ed. Philadelphia, J. B. Lippincott, 1976.

renal tumors. These tumors occur more frequently in males and metastasize early to the lungs, brain, liver, and long bones.

Clinical Manifestations.   Many renal lesions produce no symptoms and are discovered on a routine physical as a palpable abdominal mass. *The usual sign that first calls attention to the tumor is painless hematuria.* There may be a dull pain in the back from back pressure produced by ureteral compression, perirenal extension, or hemorrhage into the substance of the kidney. Colicky pains occur if a clot or mass of tumor cells pass down the ureter. Symptoms from metastasis may be the first manifestation of renal tumor: unexplained weight loss, increasing weakness, anemia.

A battery of tests is useful in the diagnosis of renal neoplasms: selective renal angiography, excretion urography, sonography and drip infusion nephrotomography.

Management.   The objective of management is to eradicate the tumor before metastasis occurs. A radical nephrectomy is the preferred treatment if the tumor can be removed. (See page 923 for nursing management following renal surgery.) Radiation therapy may be carried out postoperatively.

There has been some evidence of patient response to single-agent chemotherapy (vinblastine), but the response rate for combination chemotherapy and hormonal therapy has not been encouraging. Immunotherapy may be helpful.

Follow-up and Health Teaching.   The patient who has had surgery for renal carcinoma should undergo a yearly physical and roentgen examination of the chest throughout life, since late metastases are not uncommon. All subsequent complaints should be evaluated with possible metastases in mind.

Renal Cysts

Cysts of the kidney may be multiple (polycystic) or single. Polycystic disease of the adult is inherited as an autosomal dominant trait and usually involves both kidneys. The patient presents with abdominal or lumbar pain, hematuria, hypertension, palpable renal masses and recurrent urinary tract infections. Renal insufficiency and failure usually develop in the terminal stages. Polycystic renal disease is also associated with cystic diseases of other organs (liver, pancreas, spleen) and aneurysms of the cerebral arteries. It is characteristically seen in midlife.

Management. As there is no specific treatment for polycystic renal disease, care of the patient is directed toward relief of symptoms and complications. Hypertension and urinary tract infections are treated aggressively. Hemodialysis appears to be effective when the patient reaches end-stage renal disease. Transplantation results have not been encouraging. Genetic counseling is part of patient education since polycystic kidney disease is a hereditary disease.

Simple cysts of the kidney usually occur unilaterally and differ clinically and pathophysiologically from polycystic kidney disease. The cyst is usually excised surgically.

CONGENITAL ANOMALIES

Congenital anomalies of the kidney are not uncommon. Occasionally, there is fusion of the two kidneys, forming what is called a *horseshoe kidney*. One kidney may be small and deformed and often is nonfunctioning.

Not infrequently there may be a double ureter or congenital stricture of the ureter. The treatment of these anomalies is necessary only if they cause symptoms, but it goes without saying that before renal surgery is attempted, it is important to know that the other kidney is present and functioning.

RENAL TRAUMA

Various types of injuries of the flank, back, or upper abdomen may result in bruising, lacerations or rupture of the kidney or pedicle injury (Fig. 43-5). The kidneys are protected by the musculature of the back posteriorly and a cushion of abdominal wall and viscera anteriorly. They are highly mobile and are "fixed" only at the renal pedicle. With traumatic injury, the kidney can be thrust against the lower ribs resulting in contusion and rupture. Rib fractures occurring with renal displacement and/or a fracture of the transverse process of the upper lumbar vertebrae may be associated with renal contusion or laceration. Injuries may be blunt (auto and motorcycle accidents, falls, athletic injuries) or penetrating (gunshot wounds, stabbings).

The most common renal injury is simple contusion or small internal laceration of the kidney. The kidneys receive half of the blood flow from the abdominal aorta; therefore, a fairly small renal laceration can produce massive bleeding.

PATHOPHYSIOLOGIC EFFECT OF RENAL TRAUMA

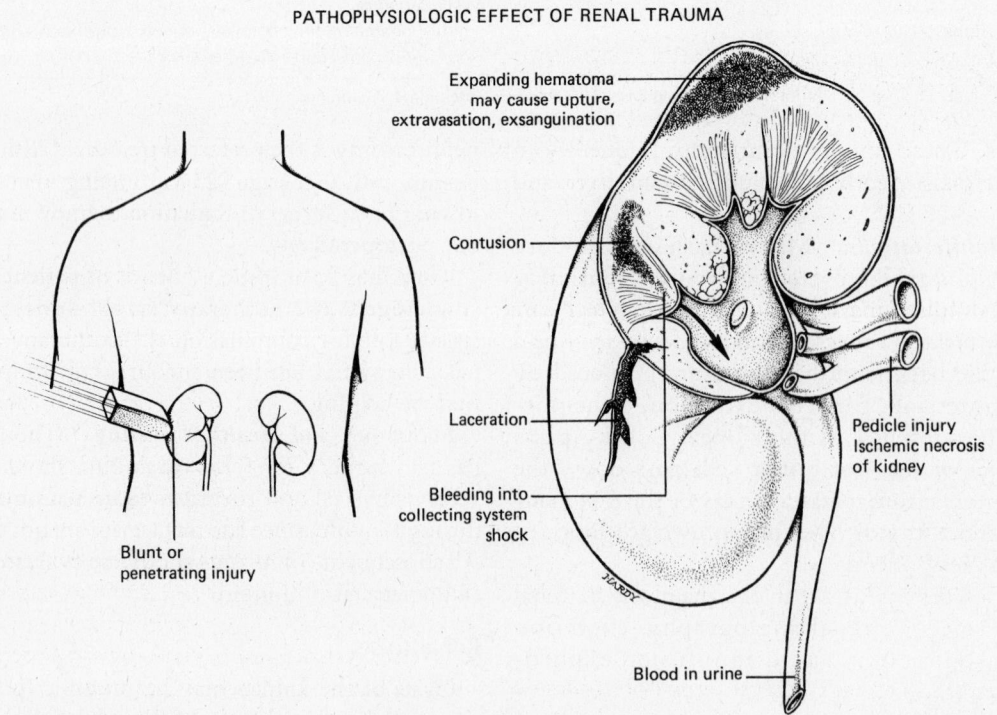

Expanding hematoma may cause rupture, extravasation, exsanguination

Contusion

Laceration

Bleeding into collecting system shock

Blunt or penetrating injury

Pedicle injury Ischemic necrosis of kidney

Blood in urine

Figure 43-5. Renal trauma.

Nursing Assessment and Patient Management.
Hematuria is the most common manifestation of renal trauma, therefore, the appearance of blood in the urine following an injury to the loin alerts to the possibility of renal injury. However, hematuria may be absent or noticeable only on microscopic examination. Therefore, all urine is saved and sent to the laboratory for analysis to detect the presence of red cells. The time the urine is voided and the volume should be recorded.

The patient is monitored for signs of oligemic shock since a pedicle injury or shattered kidney can lead to rapid exsanguination. An expanding hematoma may cause rupture of the kidney capsule. To detect the presence of hematoma, the area around the lower ribs, upper lumbar vertebrae, flank and abdomen is palpated for tenderness. A palpable flank or abdominal mass with local tenderness, swelling and ecchymosis suggests renal hemorrhage and extravasation. The area of the original mass can be outlined with a marking pencil so that the observer can evaluate the area for change. Skin abrasions, lacerations and entry and exit wounds in the muscles of the upper abdomen, flank and lower thoracic regions are important signs to check. Severe flank or costovertebral pain may signal a pedicle injury which can cause ischemic necrosis of the kidney. It is important to remember that renal trauma is associated with other injuries to the abdominal organs (liver, colon, small intestines).

Management. In minor injuries to the kidney, healing may take place with conservative measures. The patient is kept on strict bed rest. Intravenous infusions may be necessary, because retroperitoneal bleeding may produce a reflex ileus.

Serial hematocrits and hemoglobin determinations are done to assess the degree of anemia as progressive anemia indicates hemorrhage. Antimicrobials are given to discourage infection from perirenal hematoma or urinoma (a cyst containing urine). Patients with retroperitoneal hematomas will have a low grade fever as absorption of the clot takes place.

The patient should be evaluated frequently during the first few days following injury in order to detect flank and abdominal pain, muscle spasm, and swelling over the flank.

- Watch for any *sudden* change in the patient's condition which may indicate hemorrhage and require surgical intervention. The vital signs are monitored to detect evidences of bleeding. Narcotic analgesia is avoided as this may mask accompanying abdominal symptoms.
- Prepare for surgical exploration if the patient has an increasing pulse rate, hypotension and shock.

Most penetrating injuries require surgical exploration. The damaged kidney may have to be removed (nephrectomy) although on occasion it is possible to repair it.

Follow-up: Patient Education. Follow-up care includes monitoring the blood pressure to detect hypertension which may occur on a renovascular basis. Other complications include stone formation, infection, cysts, vascular aneurysms, and loss of renal function.

BLADDER INJURIES

Injury to the bladder may occur with a fracture of the symphysis pubic or from a blow to the lower abdomen when the bladder is full. Blunt trauma may result in contusion (an ecchymosis involving a segment of the bladder wall) or in rupture of the bladder, extraperitoneally, intraperitoneally or a combination of both. Complications from these injuries (hemorrhage, shock, sepsis, and extravasation) must be treated promptly.

A retrograde urethrogram is done first to evaluate for bladder rupture or urethral injury. The patient is catheterized after the urethrogram is done.

Management. Treatment for traumatic rupture of the bladder involves surgical exploration and repair of the laceration, with suprapubic drainage of the bladder and the perivesical space (around the bladder) along with insertion of an urethral indwelling catheter. In selected patients with extraperitoneal rupture, urethral catheter drainage alone may provide a satisfactory outcome as uninfected extravasated fluids are usually absorbed rapidly. (See page 923 for care of the patient following urological surgery.)

CANCER OF THE BLADDER

Cancer of the bladder is seen more frequently from the fifth decade onward and affects men more than women (3:1). Statistics indicate that these tumors make up approximately 3 to 4 percent of all cancers in the body and are on the increase.

Risk factors for cancer of the bladder include smoking, carcinogens in the environment such as dyes, chemicals, rubber, and ionizing radiation. There may be a relationship between coffee drinking and bladder cancer. Chronic schistosomiasis (parasitic infection that irritates the bladder) is also a risk factor. Cancer of the bladder may occur as a secondary metastasis from the prostate, colon and rectum in males and from the lower gynecologic tract in females.

Clinical Manifestations. These tumors usually arise at the base of the bladder and involve the ureteral orifices and bladder neck. *Gross, painless hematuria* is the most common symptom of bladder tumor, particularly cancer of the bladder. Infection of the urinary tract is a common complication producing frequency, urgency, and dysuria. However, any disturbance of micturition or change in the urine may indicate cancer of the bladder. Pelvic or back pain may be due to distant metastasis.

Cystourethroscopy, superficial and deep biopsies of the bladder, and bimanual examination are used to confirm the diagnosis. Other tests include cytologic staining of the urinary sediment and intravenous urography. Computed tomography and angiography of the pelvic vessels may be carried out to evaluate the stage of tumor invasion.

Management. Treatment of bladder cancer (Table 43-2) depends on the grade of the tumor (based on the degree of cellular differentiation), the stage of growth (the degree of local invasion and the presence or absence of metastasis) and the multicentricity (having many centers) of the tumor. The patient's age and physical, mental and emotional status are considered in determining treatment modalities.

Transurethral and transvesical electroexcision may be done for simple papillomas. Radiation may be tried for undifferentiated types of tumors and may be used preoperatively, in combination with surgical treatment or alone to control the disease in inoperative patients. A cystectomy (removal of the bladder) or a radical cystectomy is done for invasive and poorly differentiated tumors. Radical cystectomy in the male includes removal of the bladder, pelvic peritoneum, prostate, and seminal vesicles with regional node dissection and removal of the urethra to the meatus. In the female, radical cystectomy involves removal of the bladder, pelvic peritoneum, urethra, uterus, broad ligaments, vagina, tubes, ovaries, and regional iliac and pelvic lymph nodes. Removal of the bladder requires urinary diversion.

Palliative Therapy. If metastasis has occurred in the lymph nodes, doxorubicin (Adriamycin), methotrexate, 5-fluorouracil and cyclophosphamide seem to have

TABLE 43-2. METHODS OF TREATING CARCINOMA
OF THE BLADDER*

I SURGERY
  A. Transurethral resection and fulguration
  B. Transvesical resection and fulguration
  C. Segmental or partial cystectomy
  D. Simple cystectomy
  E. Radical cystectomy (anterior pelvic exenteration)
  F. Total pelvic exenteration

II RADIATION THERAPY
  A. Internal
    1. Interstitial
    2. Intracavitary
  B. External

III CHEMOTHERAPY
  A. Topical
  B. Regional
  C. Systemic

IV COMBINATIONS OF I, II, AND III

*From Maltry, E.: Benign and Malignant Tumors of the Urinary Bladder. Flushing, Medical Examination Publishing Co., Inc., 1971.

cytotoxic activity against bladder cancer when used as single agents. Bladder cancer may also be treated by direct infusion of the cytotoxic agent through the arterial supply of the involved organ. Thus a higher concentration of the chemotherapeutic agent can be achieved with lessened toxicity to the system. For more advanced bladder cancer or for patients with intractable hematuria (especially following radiation therapy) a water-filled balloon placed within the bladder produces tumor necrosis by reducing the blood circulating in the bladder wall. The instillation of formalin, phenol, or silver nitrate has achieved relief of hematuria and strangury (slow and painful discharge of urine) in some patients.

URINARY DIVERSION

Urinary diversion refers to a means of diverting the urinary stream from the bladder so that it exits via a new avenue. This is done primarily when a large or invasive bladder tumor requires that the entire bladder be removed. Other conditions requiring urinary diversion include pelvic malignancy, birth defects, strictures and trauma to ureters and urethra, neurogenic bladder and chronic infection causing severe ureteral and renal damage.

There is controversy concerning the best means of establishing permanent diversion of the urinary tract. The age of the patient, condition of the bladder, body build, degree of obesity, intelligence, degree of ureteral dilation, and state of renal function are all taken into consideration.

The most common methods of urinary diversion are:
1. *Ileal conduit:* transplanting the ureters to a section of the terminal ileum or loop of colon and bringing one end to the abdominal wall as an ileostomy (Fig. 43-6A).
2. *Ureterosigmoidostomy:* introducing the ureter into the sigmoid, thereby allowing urine to flow through the colon and out of the rectum (Fig. 43-6B).
3. *Cutaneous ureterostomy:* bringing the detached ureter through the abdominal wall and attaching it to an opening in the skin (Fig. 43-6C).
4. *Suprapubic cystostomy:* (or vesicostomy) draining the bladder through an abdominal wound (Fig. 43-6D).
5. *Nephrostomy:* inserting a catheter into the renal pelvis via an incision into the flank (Fig. 43-6E).

Management

Preoperative Management. A careful preoperative assessment of cardiopulmonary function is done since patients undergoing cystectomy are usually older people who may not fare well in a lengthy complex procedure. As part of preoperative management, the bowel is cleansed (to minimize fecal stasis and postoperative ileus), a low residue diet is prescribed and antimicrobial

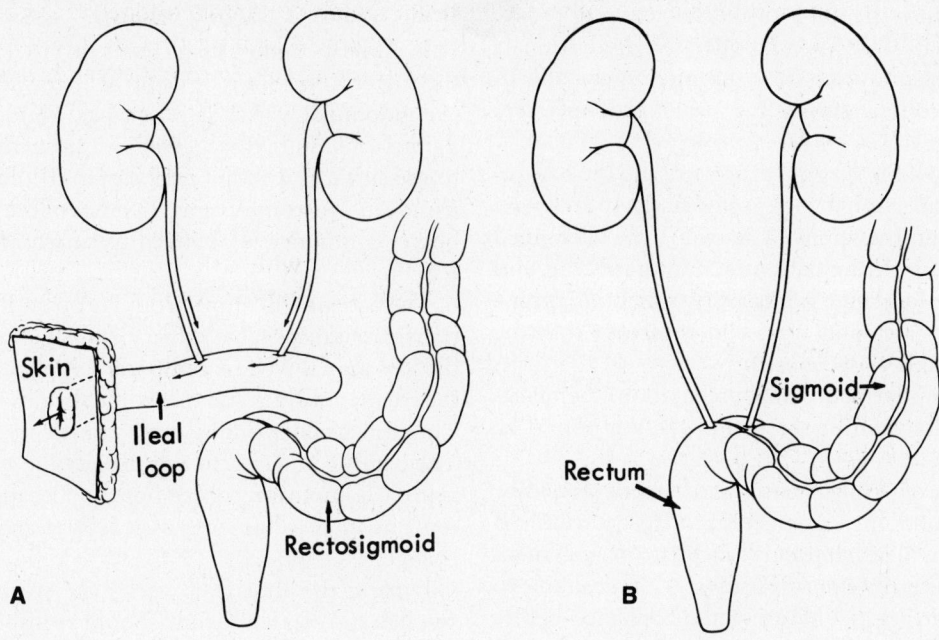

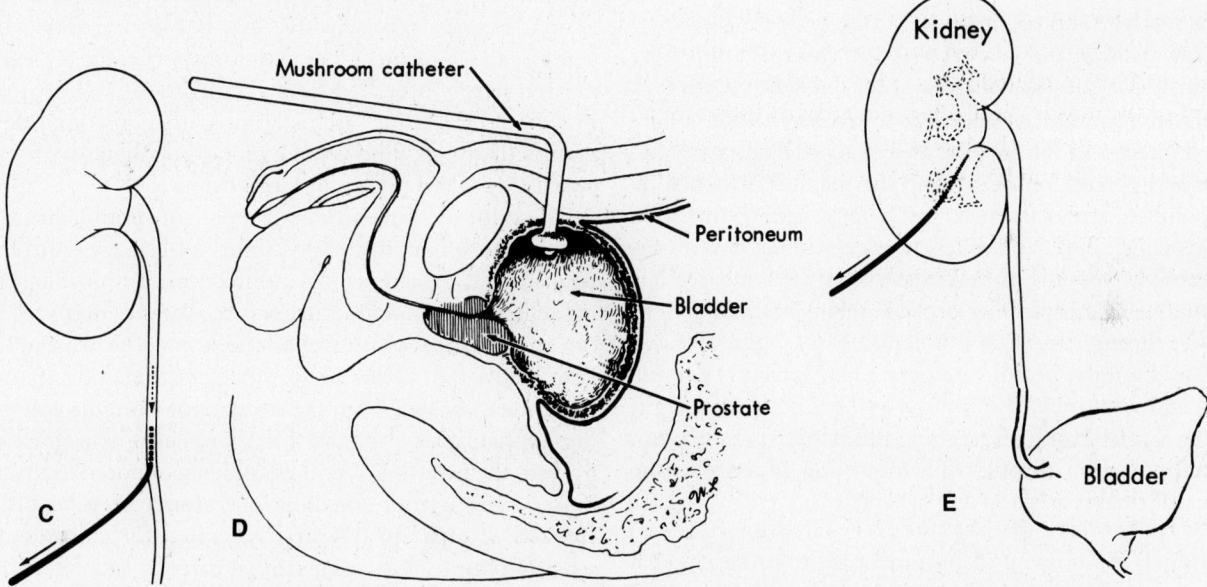

Figure 43-6. Methods of urinary diversion. *A.* Ileal conduit. Performed when the bladder is removed because of cancer of organs involving the bladder. In many instances the rectum also is removed, so that ureterosigmoidostomy could not be used. *Problems of the patient:* permanent ileostomy appliance must be worn; stricture development at the implant site. *B.* Ureterosigmoidostomy. Performed for congenital malformations of the bladder (exstrophy of the bladder) and in some patients with carcinoma of the bladder and pelvic organs not involving the rectum. *Problems of the patient:* chronic and recurring infection of the urinary tract; reabsorption of urinary electrolytes; malignancy at the site of ureter implantation. *C.* Ureterostomy. Performed for stricture of the ureter and inflammatory obstruction. *Problems of the patient:* obstruction of ureter; ureteral stricture; periureteral abscess; leakage around appliance. *D.* Cystostomy. Performed for obstruction of outlet of the bladder by prostatitis or prostatic carcinoma, following the removal of stones from the bladder, and in some cases of chronic cystitis. *Problems of the patient:* chronic infection of the bladder; stone formation. *E.* Nephrostomy. Indication for this is urinary obstruction in the lower urinary tract (prostate and prostatic obstructions, etc.) and in some cases of renal calculi in which the calculus is removed instead of a nephrectomy being performed. *Problems of the patient:* chronic urinary infection; chronic pyelonephritis; renal deterioration; accidental dislodgement of the tube. (*A, B, C,* and *E* from Bloom, J., and Merrill, J. P.: Review of methods of urinary diversion. G.P., 23:91-97)

drugs are administered (for bowel disinfection to reduce pathogenic flora). Adequate preoperative hydration is imperative to ensure urine flow during surgery and to prevent hypovolemia during the prolonged operative procedure.

Explanations of the surgical procedure and the reasons for wearing a collection device postoperatively are given to the patient and the family. The stoma site is planned preoperatively with the patient standing, sitting and lying in order to locate the stoma away from bony prominences, skin creases and scars and to assure that the patient will be able to see it easily.

In the preoperative abdominal preparation, the marks indicating the location of the stoma site are not to be washed off.

Several types of skin adhesives and cement should be applied to the abdomen preoperatively to determine if contact allergy will develop and to facilitate management of the ostomy appliance postoperatively. It is desirable to have the patient practice wearing the appliance before surgery. An enterostomal therapist can demonstrate the types of appliances and the methods for handling them.

Psychological Assessment and Support. The threat of cancer initiates fear related to losses—loss of love, body image, and security. In addition to problems of urinary leakage and adaptation to an external appliance, the male patient must also adapt to sexual impotency. A supportive approach is needed; it involves taking a personal interest in the patient, observing the patient's concept and perception of self and the manner in which he responds to stress and loss, and helping him to maintain his usual life style and independence with as few modifications as possible. If the disease progresses and death is inevitable, the mourning process begins and the patient moves through the phases of denial, loss, anger (directed towards family, health care personnel, society), depression and withdrawal. The nurse's role is not to lose sight of the human being undergoing this hard experience and to support him through the mourning process to the stage of final resolution and acceptance.

Postoperative Management. The objectives of postoperative nursing management are to preserve renal function and to assist the patient to adapt to an altered body image. The main focus of management is directed at the urinary and intestinal tract and ileal stoma as well as those elements of care given to a patient who has undergone intestinal surgery (page 786). Possible postoperative complications include: shock, cardiac decompensation or thrombosis. A nasogastric tube is inserted during surgery to allow for decompression and to relieve pressure on the intestinal anastomosis. As soon as bowel function resumes (as indicated by the passage of flatus), the patient may be given food and fluids by mouth, but until that time fluids and electrolytes are given intravenously. (The remainder of the postoperative management is discussed under the specific urinary diversion procedure.)

Ileal Conduit (Ureteroileostomy)

In an ileal conduit the urine is diverted by implanting the ureter into a loop of ileum which is led out through the abdominal wall as an ileostomy. This loop of ileum is a simple conduit (passageway) for urine from the ureters to the surface. A loop of the sigmoid colon may also be used. An ileostomy bag is used to collect the urine. The bowel continuity is obtained by anastomosis of the remaining ileum.

The patient will return from the operating room with a transparent disposable urinary drainage bag cemented to the abdominal wall. A temporary appliance is used until the edema subsides and the stoma shrinks to normal size. The ileal bladder drains urine constantly but not feces. The bag is connected to a drainage tube and bag and the urinary volume is recorded hourly. The appliance usually remains in place as long as it is watertight. Then it is changed.

During the first few weeks the stoma will appear swollen and edematous and should be inspected regularly for congestion and cyanosis. Low molecular weight dextran may be given to improve microcirculation and reduce mucosal slough if signs of congestion appear. The stoma is insensitive to touch, but the skin around the stoma is exquisitely sensitive if it becomes irritated by urine or the appliance. The skin is inspected for (1) signs of irritation, bleeding and friability of the stomal mucosa, (2) alkaline encrustation with peristomal dermatitis (from alkaline urine coming in contact with exposed skin), and (3) wound infections.

The odor of urine around the patient should alert the nursing personnel to the possibility of leakage from the appliance, the presence of an infection or a problem in hygienic management. Since severe alkaline encrustation can accumulate rapidly around the stoma, the urine pH is kept below 6.5. Urine pH can be determined by testing the urine dribbling from the stoma, not from the collecting appliance. A properly fitted appliance is a must to prevent the peristomal skin from being exposed to urine. If the urine is foul smelling, the stoma may be catheterized in order to obtain a specimen for culture and sensitivity or to determine stomal patency and detect the presence of residual urine. Scarring of the stoma can interfere with urine drainage.

A high fluid diet is encouraged, in order to flush the ileal conduit and prevent mucus from congealing. The patient may excrete a fairly large amount of mucus with the urine as a result of the urine irritating the intestine. To relieve anxiety in this regard, the patient should be reassured that this is a normal occurrence following an ileal conduit.

Patient Education and Rehabilitation

The urinary appliance may consist of one or two pieces and may be disposable, semi-disposable or reusable. The choice of appliance is determined by the location of the stoma and the patient's normal activity, body build, and economic status. A reusable appliance has a faceplate that is attached to the body with cement or adhesive. A semi-disposable appliance has a reusable faceplate to which disposable pouches are attached. Disposable appliances are discarded after each use.

Determining Stoma Size.   As the stoma shrinks with healing, the opening is re-calibrated every 3 to 6 weeks for the first few months postoperatively. The correct appliance size is determined by measuring the widest part of the stoma with a ruler. The permanent appliance should not be more than one-eighth of an inch larger than the diameter of the stoma.

Changing the Appliance; Skin Care

- The appliance should be changed at a time that will be most convenient to the patient. Early in the morning before taking fluids is the time chosen by many ostomates. Ideally the collecting appliance should not need to be changed more frequently than every 5 to 7 days.
- Moisten the edge of the faceplate with adhesive solvent or soap and water, and gently remove it. Adhesive solvent is not used if skin barriers are used.
- Instruct the patient to bend over quickly and remain in that position a minute to allow the conduit to empty before the skin is washed and dried.
- Clean all cement from the skin with adhesive solvent, using a soft cloth. Wash the skin with a non-cream-based soap and water. Pat dry. *The skin must be dry or the appliance will not adhere.*
  1. Insert a tampon or gauze or tissue wick over the stoma to absorb the urine while the appliance is being changed.
  2. Inspect the skin for signs of irritation. Keep the skin free from direct contact with urine.
  3. Apply a skin protector if required. If the patient has oily skin the peristomal skin area may be swabbed with alcohol before a new appliance is fitted.
- Prepare the appliance according to the manufacturer's directions. Center the appliance directly over the stoma and apply it carefully. Apply gentle pressure around the appliance so that it will adhere securely.
- Apply nonallergic tape in a picture-frame effect around the pouch. The skin under the appliance may be dusted with pure talcum powder and an appliance cover used to absorb perspiration and eliminate warmth from the pouch.
- The use of a belt is optional, but the manufacturer's directions should be followed, since a poorly fitting belt may cause abrasion of the stoma.

Since stomal protrusion is not the same in all patients, there are various accessories and custom-made appliances to solve individual problems. The advice and assistance of an enterostomal therapist is invaluable.

Odor Control.   The patient should be advised to avoid foods and medications that give the urine a strong odor. A few drops of liquid deodorizer or diluted white vinegar may be introduced through the drain spout into the bottom of the pouch with a syringe or eyedropper. Aspirin may be placed in the pouch to reduce uriniferous odor. Taking ascorbic acid by mouth helps acidify the urine and suppresses urine odor problems. Also the patient should be reminded that the pouch will develop an odor if it is worn too long and not cared for properly.

Managing the Ostomy Appliance.   The pouch is emptied by a drain valve when it is one-third to one-half full, since the weight of the urine may cause it to separate from the skin. Some patients prefer wearing a leg bag attached with an adapter to the drainage apparatus. To assure uninterrupted sleep, the outlet on the appliance is attached to a collecting bottle or bag with plastic tubing. The tubing may be threaded down the pajama leg to preventing kinking. At least 1.52 meters (5 feet) of tubing is necessary to allow the patient to turn in bed.

Cleaning and Deodorizing the Appliance.   Usually the reusable appliance is rinsed in warm water, soaked in a solution of detergent and white vinegar or a commercial deodorizing solution for 30 minutes. Then it is rinsed and air-dried away from direct sunlight. After drying, the appliance may be powdered with cornstarch and stored. Two appliances are necessary; one to be worn while the other is air-drying.

The patient should be encouraged to contact the local ostomy association* for visits, reassurance and practical information.

Ureterosigmoidostomy

Ureterosigmoidostomy is an implantation of the ureters into the sigmoid colon. In addition to the usual preoperative regimen, the patient may be placed on a liquid diet for several days preoperatively to keep the colon clean. Antimicrobial agents (neomycin; kanamycin) are administered for bowel disinfection. Ureterosigmoidostomy requires good anal sphincter control, adequate renal function and active ureteral peristalsis. The degree of anal sphincter control may be determined by assessing the patient's ability to retain enemas.

The patient will be informed that following surgery voiding will occur from the rectum for the rest of his life and that an adjustment in life style will be necessary because of urinary frequency (as often as every 2 hours) which will have a consistency equivalent to a watery diarrhea. There will be some degree of nocturia. Activities will have to be planned around the frequent need to urinate which in turn may restrict the patient's social life. However, the patient has the advantage of urinary control without having to wear an external appliance.

Postoperatively, a catheter is placed in the rectum to drain the urine and prevent reflux of urine into the ureters and kidneys. The tube is taped to the buttocks and special skin care given around the anus to prevent excoriation. Irrigations of the rectal tube may be requested but force should not be used because of the danger of introducing an infection into the newly implanted ureters.

*Address at end of chapter.

In this operation, larger areas of the bowel mucosa are exposed to urine and electrolyte reabsorption, so that electrolyte imbalance and acidosis may result. Potassium and magnesium imbalances may occur from the presence of urine in the bowel which simulates diarrhea. Fluid and electrolyte balance is maintained in the immediate postoperative period by serum chemical determinations and appropriate intravenous infusions. Acidosis may be prevented by placing the patient on a low-chloride diet supplemented with sodium potassium citrate. The patient should be instructed never to wait longer than 3 hours before emptying urine from the intestine in order to keep rectal pressure low and to minimize absorption of urinary constituents from the colon.

After the rectal catheter is removed, the patient learns to control the anal sphincter through special sphincteric exercises. At first urination is frequent. With reassurance and encouragement and the passage of time, the patient will gain greater control and will learn to differentiate between the need to void and the need to defecate.

Pyelonephritis (upper urinary tract infection due to reflux of bacteria from the colon) is fairly common in some patients who may have to take prophylactic antimicrobial therapy for the rest of their lives.

Specific diet instructions include avoidance of gas-forming foods since flatus can cause stress incontinence and socially embarrassing offensive odors. Other ways to avoid gas are to avoid chewing gum, smoking and any other activity that involves swallowing air. Salt intake may be restricted to prevent hyperchloremic acidosis. Potassium intake is increased through foods and medication since potassium may be lost in acidosis.

Cutaneous Ureterostomy (Cutaneous Urinary Conduit)

Urinary diversion may also be accomplished by connecting the divided end of the ureter to the skin or by intubating the ureter. When both kidneys require diversion, an anastomosis of the ureters and formation of a single cutaneous stoma (bilateral conjoined cutaneous ureterostomy) may be performed. Cutaneous ureterostomy is done when the ureters are dilated due to bladder obstruction or a tumor or vesicoureteric reflux. Bringing the ureters to the skin will prevent severe back pressure and damage to the kidneys.

A urinary appliance is fitted immediately following surgery. Since stenosis of the stoma can be a postoperative problem, periodic catheterizations and calibrations of the ureters are part of the follow-up examinations. The patient may be taught the sterile procedure involved in inserting a ureteral catheter.

The important point is to position the catheter properly: if the openings at the tip are inserted too far into the kidney pelvis, the catheter will go beyond the source of urine and will not drain. Likewise, if it is not inserted far enough, the openings of the catheter may be occluded by the wall of the ureter, and the catheter will not drain.

The management of the patient with a cutaneous ureterostomy is very similar to the care of the patient with an ileal conduit.

Cystostomy

An infrequently used method of urinary diversion is the suprapubic cystostomy, which is accomplished by inserting a special catheter through the abdomen into the bladder either through an incision in the lower abdominal wall or by a trochar punch technique. It is usually done under local anesthesia. Generally a cystostomy is done on the patient with an obstruction below the bladder (prostatic obstruction) when it is not possible to insert a urethral catheter. A cystostomy may be temporary (until corrective surgery can be done) or permanent.

The patient with a cystostomy requires liberal amounts of fluid to prevent encrustation around the catheter. Other problems encountered include the formation of bladder stones, acute and chronic infections, and problems in collecting urine. The advice and assistance of an enterostomal therapist is needed in choosing the most suitable urine collection bag and to instruct the patient in its use.

URETHRAL CONDITIONS

Caruncle

A caruncle is a small, red, extremely vascular polypoid growth situated just within, and protruding from, the external urethral meatus of women, probably the result of long-continued infection or irritation of the mucosa at this point. On rare occasions, it causes no subjective symptoms. However, it may be acutely sensitive, causing a local burning pain exaggerated by exertion and frequency of urination, which is exquisitely painful. Local excision of the caruncle will relieve the troublesome symptoms.

Urethritis

Urethritis, inflammation of the urethra, is usually an ascending infection. It may be caused by a bacterial or viral infection or by trauma from an indwelling catheter or repeated cystoscopic examinations.

The patient complains of itching and burning around the urethra, along with a possible urethral discharge, which varies in quantity from scanty to profuse and in character from thin and mucoid to thick and purulent.

Antimicrobial therapy may or may not be helpful. Associated prostatitis is treated. The patient is advised to temporarily discontinue sexual intercourse and ingestion of alcohol which prolongs the acute phase of urethritis.

Gonorrheal Urethritis.

Gonorrheal urethritis is caused by *Neisseria gonorrhoeae* and is transmitted by sexual contact. In the male, inflammation of the meatal orifice occurs with burning on urination. A purulent urethral discharge appears four to ten days (or longer) after sexual exposure. However, the disease may be asymptomatic. In the female there is not always a urethral discharge present, and the disease is often essentially asymptomatic. Therefore gonorrhea in the female is frequently not reported and diagnosed.

In the male the infection involves the tissues around the urethra causing periurethritis, prostatitis, epididymitis, and urethral stricture. Sterility may occur due to vaso-epididymal obstruction. Gonorrheal urethritis in the female tends to cause pelvic infection with abdominal pain, abscess of the greater vestibular glands (Bartholin's glands), and urethral stricture. It may spread to the bladder, causing cystitis, to the cervix of the uterus, to the fallopian tubes causing pelvic abscess, and to the peritoneal cavity giving rise to peritonitis. The gonococcus carried by the bloodstream causes one type of infectious arthritis, one form of acute infectious endocarditis, and certain skin diseases.

Treatment of gonorrhea is discussed on page 1374.

Patient Education.

Impress upon the patient the need to return for follow-up examination 7 to 14 days after completion of treatment. To avoid reinfection, sexual activity with untreated previous sexual partners is to be avoided until they have been treated and examined.

Urethral Strictures

A urethral stricture is a narrowing of the lumen of the urethra owing to scar tissue and contraction. Strictures result from urethral injury (urethral instrumentation for transurethral surgery, indwelling catheters, cystoscopic procedures), from straddle injuries and automobile accidents, from untreated gonorrheal urethritis, and from congenital abnormalities.

There is diminution in the force and size of the urinary stream, along with symptoms of urinary infection and retention. Stricture produces back pressure with resulting cystitis, prostatitis, and pyelonephritis. An important element of prevention is to treat all urethral infections promptly. Prolonged urethral catheter drainage is to be avoided and utmost care taken in any type of urethral instrumentation, including catheterization.

Management.

The treatment may be palliative (gradual dilatation of the narrowed area with metal sounds) or operative (incision of the stricture — urethrotomy). If the stricture has become so small as to prevent the passage of a catheter, the urologist uses several small filiform bougies in search of the opening. When one bougie passes beyond the stricture into the bladder, it is fixed in place, and urine will drain from the bladder. The stricture then can be dilated to larger size by the passage of a larger sound (a dilating instrument) following behind the filiform as a guide. Following dilatation, hot sitz baths and non-narcotic analgesics are given to control the pain. Antimicrobials are given for several days after dilatation to minimize the infectious reaction, thus lessening discomfort.

Surgical excision or urethroplasty may be necessary for severe cases. Sometimes a suprapubic cystostomy must be performed. The postoperative treatment for cystostomy is described on page 950.

BIBLIOGRAPHY

BOOKS

Blandy, J.: Lecture Notes on Urology. Oxford, Blackwell Scientific Pub., 1976.

_____: Operative Urology. Oxford, Blackwell Scientific Pub., 1978.

_____: Urology. Vols. 1 and 2. Philadelphia, J.B. Lippincott, 1976.

Brenner, B. M., and Rector, F. C., Jr., eds.: The Kidney. Philadelphia, W. B. Saunders, 1976.

Brundage, D. J.: Nursing Management of Renal Problems. St. Louis, C. V. Mosby, 1976.

Cameron, E. M., and Kintzel, J. E.: Chronic Renal Failure. *In* Kintzel, K. C.: Advanced Concepts in Clinical Nursing. Philadelphia, J. B. Lippincott, 1977, pp. 535-582.

Cameron, J. S., Russell, A. M. E., and Sale, D. N. T.: Nephrology for Nurses, 2nd ed. Flushing, N.Y., Medical Examination Pub. Co., 1976.

Cooper, E. H., and Williams, R. E.: The Biology and Clinical Management of Bladder Cancer. Oxford, Blackwell Scientific Pub., 1975.

Dunnill, M. S.: Pathological Basis of Renal Disease. Philadelphia, W. B. Saunders, 1976.

Harrison, J. H. H., et al.: Campbell's Urology. Vols. 1 and 2, Philadelphia, W. B. Saunders, 1978.

Hekelman, F. P., and Ostendarp, C. A.: Nephrology Nursing. New York, McGraw-Hill, 1979.

International Committee for Nomenclature and Nosology of Renal Disease: A Handbook of Kidney Nomenclature and Nosology. Boston, Little, Brown, 1975.

Johnson, D. E.: Testicular Tumors, 2nd ed. Flushing, N.Y., Medical Examination Pub. Co., 1976.

Kessler, R. J., and Anderson, R. U.: Handbook of Urologic Emergencies. Flushing, N.Y., Medical Examination Pub. Co., 1976.

Kolff, W. J.: Artificial Organs. New York, John Wiley and Sons, 1976.

Kuehnel, E., and Bennett, W.: Acute Renal Failure: Discussions in Patient Management. Flushing, N.Y., Medical Examination Pub. Co., 1976.

Lapides, J.: Fundamentals of Urology. Philadelphia, W. B. Saunders, 1976.

Leaf, A., and Cotran, R. S.: Renal Pathophysiology. New York, Oxford University Press, 1976.

Massry, S. G., and Sellers, A. L.: Clinical Aspects of Uremia and Dialysis. Springfield, Ill., Charles C Thomas, 1976.

Maude, D. L.: Kidney Physiology and Kidney Disease: An Introduction to Nephrology. Philadelphia, J. B. Lippincott, 1977.

Muth, R. G.: Renal Medicine. Springfield, Ill., Charles C Thomas, 1978.

Robertson, J. R.: Genitourinary Problems in Women. Springfield, Ill., Charles C Thomas, 1978.

Schrier, R. W.: Renal and Electrolyte Disorders. Boston, Little, Brown, 1976.

Smith, D. R.: General Urology. Los Altos, Lange Medical Publishers, 1978.

Spitzer, M. E., Dickinson, B. B., and Rogers, P. W.: A Renal Failure Diet Manual Utilizing the Food Exchange System. Springfield, Ill., Charles C Thomas, 1976.

Thomas, W. C.: Renal Calculi: A Guide to Management. Springfield, Ill., Charles C Thomas, 1976.

Walker, F. C., ed.: Modern Stoma Care. Edinburgh, Churchill Livingstone, 1976.

Winter, C. C., and Morel, A.: Nursing Care of Patients With Urologic Disease, 4th ed. St. Louis, C. V. Mosby, 1977.

ARTICLES

Bladder Cancer/Urinary Diversion

Barker, W. F., et al.: The creation and care of enterocutaneous stomas. Curr. Probl. Surg., *12*:3-62, Dec. 1975.

Chezen, J. L.: Urinary diversion: Select aspects of nursing management. Nurs. Clin. N. Am., *11*:445-456, Sept. 1976.

Friedell, G. H., ed.: National bladder cancer conference. Cancer Research, *37*:2743-2973 (entire vol.), Aug. 1977.

Gault, P. L.: Six patients with bladder cancer—and how they fared after surgery. Nursing '77, 7:48-55, Nov. 1977.

Kambouris, A. K., et al.: Ileal loop ureteroileostomy in patients with neurogenic bladder. Am. J. Surg., *131*:224-227, Feb. 1976.

Mahoney, J. M.: What you should know about ostomies: Guidelines for giving better postop. care. Nursing '78, 8:74-84, May 1978.

Miller, R. N.: The emotional problems of patients with bladder cancer. Cancer Res., *37*:2789-2791, Aug. 1977.

Remigailo, R. V., et al.: Ileal conduit urinary diversion. Ten-year review. Urology, 7:343-348, Apr. 1976.

Wood, R. Y.: Catheterizing the patient with an ileal conduit stoma. AJN, *76*:1592-1595, Oct. 1976.

Infection

Anderson, E. R.: Women and cystitis. Nursing '77, 7:50-53, Apr. 1977.

Cox, C. E. (ed.): Symposium on urinary tract infections. Urol. Clin. N. Am., *2*:407-567, Oct. 1975.

Craig, W.: Urinary tract infections: regimens to avoid recurrence. Medical Times, *105*:49-61, Sept. 1977.

Wechsler, H.: Ethambutol regimen in renal tuberculosis. J. Urol., *114*:498-499, Oct. 1975.

Other Renal Diseases

Baldwin, D. S.: Poststreptococcal glomerulonephritis: A progressive disease? Am. J. Med., *62*:1-11, Jan. 1977.

Bissada, N. K.: Renal carcinoma: Diagnostic and therapeutic aspects. Am. Fam. Phys., *16*:100-106, Aug. 1977.

Burton, B. T.: Nutritional implications of renal disease. J. Am. Diet. Assoc., *70*:479-482, May 1977.

Cameron, J. S.: Treatment of glomerulonephritis by drugs. Brit. Med. J., *1*:6074:1457-1459, 4 June 1977.

Carter, S. K., and Wasserman, T. H.: The chemotherapy of urologic cancer. Cancer, *36*:729-747, Aug. 1975.

Chester, A. C., Harris, J. P., and Schreiner, G. E.: Polycystic kidney disease. Am. Fam. Phys., *16*:94-101, Dec. 1977.

Grgicevic, D., et al.: Prevention of venous thromboembolism with low dose heparin in urologic patients. Urology, *9*:260-262, Mar. 1977.

Hayslett, J. P., et al.: Glomerulonephropathy. Adv. Intern. Med., *20*:215-248, 1975.

Luke, R. G., ed.: Symposium on renal diseases: Advances in diagnosis and treatment. Geriat., *31*:34-101, Aug. 1976.

Martinez-Maldonado, M.: Adult polycystic kidney disease. Kidney, *9*:1-4, Jan. 1976.

Salvatierra, O., et al.: End stage polycystic disease: Management by renal transplantation and selective use of preliminary nephrectomy. J. Urol., *115*:5-7, Jan. 1976.

Sterzel, R. B., Thomson, D., and Brod, J., eds.: Glomerulonephritis. Contributions to Nephrology, *2*:1-187 (entire vol.), 1976.

Swendseid, M. E.: Nutritional implications of renal disease. J. Am. Diet. Assoc., *70*:488-492, May 1977.

Vogel, C. H.: Keeping patients alive in spite of postobstructive diuresis. Nursing '79, *9*:50, 55-56, Mar. 1979.

Renal Failure/Transplantation

Appel, G. B., and Neu, H. C.: Nephrotoxicity of antimicrobial agents. New Eng. J. Med., *296*:663-670, Mar. 24, 1977.

Bennett, W. M., et al.: Guidelines for drug therapy in renal failure. Ann. Intern. Med., *86*:754-783, June 1977.

Cattell, W. R.: Acute renal failure. Recent Adv. Renal Dis., *1*:1-47, 1975.

Chatterjee, S. N.: Immunosuppressive drugs used in clinical renal transplantation. Urology (Suppl.), *9*:52-60, June 1977.

Dandy, W. E., Jr., and Sapir, D. G.: Acute renal failure. Crit. Care Med., *5*:146-149, May-June 1977.

Ehrlich, R. M., ed.: Renal transplantation. Surgical Aspects (Part II). Urology (Suppl.), *10*:5-63 (entire vol.), July 1977.

Evans, D. B.: Diseases of the urinary system. Management of chronic renal failure by dialysis and transplantation. Brit. Med. J., *1*:No. 6076:1585-1588, 18 June 1977.

Garron, M. S.: The adjustment period: Coping with the diet. J. Am. Assoc. Nephrology Nurses & Technicians, *3*:42-45, 1976.

Gutierrez, L. F., and Kurtzmann, N. A.: Management of chronic renal failure. Surg. Ann., *8*:367-389, 1976.

Hamburger, R. J.: The management of uremia. Am. Fam. Phys., *16*:125-132, Sept. 1977.

Juliani, L., and Reamer, B.: Kidney transplant: Your role in aftercare. Nursing '77, 7:46-53, Oct. 1977.

Kobrzycki, P.: Renal transplant complications. AJN, 77:641-643, Apr. 1977.

Mahony, J. F.: Treatment of acute renal failure. Drugs, *12*:381-387, Nov. 1976.

Mazze, R. I.: Critical care of the patient with acute renal failure. Anesthesiol., *47*:138-148, Aug. 1977.

Milne, J. E.: Psychosocial aspects of renal transplantation. Urology (Suppl.), *9*:82-88, June 1977.

Moore, G. L.: Psychiatric aspects of chronic renal disease. Postgrad. Med., *60*:140-146, Nov. 1976.

Murray, J. E., Tilney, N. L., and Wilson, R. E.: Renal transplantation: 25 year experience. Ann. Surg., *184*:565-573, Nov. 1976.

Straffon, R. A., ed.: Symposium on renal transplantation. Urol. Clin. N. Am., *3*:453-699 (entire vol.), Oct. 1976.

Trauma

Brosman, S. A., and Paul, J. G.: Trauma of the bladder. Surg. Gyn. Obstet., *143*:605-608, Oct. 1976.

Hai, M., Pontes, J. E., and Pierce, J. M., Jr.: Surgical management of major renal trauma: A review of 102 cases treated by conservative surgery. J. Urol., *118*:7-9, July 1977.

Mendez, R.: Renal trauma. J. Urol., *118*:698-703, Nov. 1977.

Thompson, I. M., and Carlton, C. E.: Symposium on genitourinary trauma. Urol. Clin. N. Am., *4*:3-162 (entire vol.), Feb. 1977.

Urolithiasis

Coe, F. L., Beck, J., and Norton, M. A.: The natural history of calcium urolithiasis. JAMA, *238*:1519-1523, Oct. 3, 1977.

Cook, J. H., and Lytton, B.: Intraoperative localization of renal calculi during nephrolithotomy by ultrasound scanning. J. Urol., *117*:543-546, May 1977.

McPherson, B. K., et al.: Nursing in slush surgery. AORN J., *25*:227-229, Feb. 1977.

Peirce, S. B., et al.: Slush technique in renal surgery. AORN J., *25*:223-226, Feb. 1977.

Williams, H. E.: The causes of kidney stones—their diagnosis and treatment. Med. Times, *105*:55-59, May 1977.

Rose, G. A.: The causes and medical treatment of renal calculi. Practitioner, *218*:74-80, Jan. 1977.

Yendt, E. R., and Cohanim, M.: The management of the patient with calcium stones. Br. J. Urol., *48*:507-514, 1976.

AGENCIES

Governmental

National Institute of Arthritis, Metabolism and Digestive Diseases, National Institutes of Health, Bethesda, Md. 20205

Voluntary

American Society for Artificial Internal Organs, P.O. Box 777, Boca Raton, Fla. 33432

Committee on Donor Enlistment, 2022 Lee Rd., Cleveland Heights, Ohio 44118

Medic-Alert Organ Donor Program, 1000 North Palm St., Turlock, Calif. 95380

National Association of Patients on Hemodialysis and Transplantation, 505 Northern Blvd., Great Neck, N.Y. 11021

National Kidney Foundation, 116 E. 27th St., New York, N.Y. 10016

United Ostomy Association, 1111 Wilshire Blvd., Los Angeles, Calif. 90017

Sexual and Reproductive Problems

UNIT ELEVEN

44

MANAGEMENT DURING THE REPRODUCTIVE CYCLE

HEALTH MAINTENANCE

Hygienic Features: Patient Education

The nurse is in a key position to teach and to advise girls and women regarding the principles of good health and personal hygiene, especially those principles dealing with feminine hygiene related to those parts of the female body concerned with reproduction. The reproductive system, like any other part of the anatomy, will function well if the body has adequate nutrition, exercise, rest, and elimination. Aside from teaching female patients about these general aspects of care, the nurse should provide instruction about venereal disease and prenatal and postnatal care.

It is important to recognize that concepts of feminine hygiene vary greatly with different cultures. What may be considered appropriate care for a European woman may be very different from that of an American or Japanese woman. An emphasis on cleanliness and neatness may be considered unnecessary by certain groups; climate and local customs may affect habits practiced. Even members of one family may have different opinions about personal tidiness.

Nurses need to understand the variations in attitudes and practices of hygiene and their relation to sexual function. Because many methods of feminine hygiene are empirical, it is necessary to apply a common-sense ap-proach. Douching of the vagina has come down from certain old cultures as a traditional practice of female hygiene. However, modern studies of vaginal physiology make clear that it has no health virtue; indeed, many douches which were once considered to be necessary, may irritate the vaginal mucosa or reduce the normal mechanisms of resistance to infection.

Contrary to popular opinion, genital odor rarely arises from the vagina, but is of external origin, arising from the interaction of oil secreted by the vulvar skin with surface bacteria. Occasionally, old menstrual blood or seminal fluid ejaculated in coitus will give some vaginal odor. A simple, low-pressure warm water irrigation or, at most, a douche of a solution of 30 ml. of white vinegar to a liter of water is appropriate. Really significant malodor from the vagina can result from a retained tampon or some other foreign body or a pathological condition indicating the need for examination. In general, a soap and water scrub and a sprinkle of a simple powder maintain cleanliness.

Sex Education

An awareness of the differences between boys and girls begins early with most children; often it is heralded by the arrival of a new baby in the family. The wise parent provides correct and simple answers to the questions raised by the growing child.

The nurse is often an advisor in these matters to patients, parents, and friends; or she may participate in sex education programs in school, church, or other groups. Filmstrips, movies, and informative literature are available. By being familiar with them, the nurse is able to be selective in meeting the needs of a particular group.

The Woman with a Gynecologic Problem

Complications of gynecologic disturbances can be prevented if proper medical care and supervision are available. The nurse is in a unique position to acquaint the lay person with the normal physiological processes of menstruation and menopause. Many difficulties encountered by the young girl or the middle-aged woman usually can be corrected quite easily; if allowed to go untreated, they may cause irreparable damage.

Danger signals that every woman should report to her physician are spotting, irregular or excessive bleeding, or any bleeding after menopause.

Persistent painful menstruation, leukorrhea, and urinary disturbances also ought to be investigated. Many of these early signs can be corrected simply and permanently. An annual pelvic examination is especially important for the woman who is past 30 years of age or for one who is actively engaged in sexual relations, regardless of age.

"Do it Yourself" kits, with which a woman may obtain her own cervical and vaginal smears and mail the slides to a laboratory, are being studied to determine their effectiveness. Such methods are inexpensive, but accuracy may be lower than desired; the danger is the possible oversight of other problems which could have been detected during a visit to a health professional.

Psychosocial Considerations

The gynecologic patient often calls for more understanding than other patients, because in addition to physical considerations, there are many emotional factors governing the situation. She may resent any reference to her genitourinary system, feeling that she is suspected of questionable social or sexual habits. Or she may have a real fear that venereal disease or cancer may exist. All or any of these thoughts may manifest themselves in her conversation with the nurse, who, by revealing an understanding attitude, can do much to dispel such anxieties.

Mixed emotional upsets can result from other fears. The suggestion of surgery as a means of treatment may raise a fear of disturbance of the reproductive process. Perhaps an explanation of the anatomy and the proposed treatment will clarify the situation. Any intention of sterilization must be explained carefully to the patient and her husband by the physician. Perhaps religious belief is more important to a patient than physical treatment. The decision rests with the patient, and, when it is made, it must be respected and supported.

Psychic factors may present themselves at the menopausal period. The loss of the reproductive capacity may cause disappointment, if the woman has had no children. For a woman with a grown family, it may mean that she feels there is no further need for her; leisure time may hang heavily on her hands. Circumstances affect the problems of each patient and must be considered on an individual basis.

Because gynecologic conditions often are of such a personal and private nature, the nurse is expected to keep knowledge of the patient's problems in confidence. This information is shared only with those directly involved in professional patient care.

Microbiologic Considerations

Because many gynecologic diseases may be caused by highly infective organisms, especially the gonococcus, it is absolutely imperative that all instruments and equipment (catheters, douche nozzles, bedpans, rectal tubes, and so forth) used in the treatment be sterilized, both before and after their use. The nurse may protect herself by the use of disposable sterile gloves. If the procedure does not require gloves, it is wise to scrub the hands thoroughly. When possible, dressings, perineal pads, and so forth should be handled with gloves or forceps, and the forceps should be sterilized after use.

ASSESSMENT

GYNECOLOGIC EXAMINATION

Preparation of the Patient

The patient who is to have a gynecologic examination often has many fears and worries. Not only does she dislike the thought of being exposed and examined, but being placed in an embarrassing position can make the experience an unpleasant one. In addition, the concern and worry about what may be found serves to influence her reaction to the examination. She needs reassurance, understanding, and tactful regard for her emotional as well as her physical problems.

Prior to the examination, the patient should be instructed to void and evacuate the lower bowel. Sufficient clothing should be removed to allow adequate exposure of the genitalia. All bands about the waist must be loosened, and the girdle should be removed to permit examination of the abdomen. In preparing for the examination and in placing the patient on the examining table, the nurse should take special precautions to avoid exposing the patient.

Positioning the Patient

The examination of the patient for a gynecologic condition is best made with the patient on the examining table. Three positions are employed commonly for these examinations (Fig. 44-1). The most common is the *lithot-*

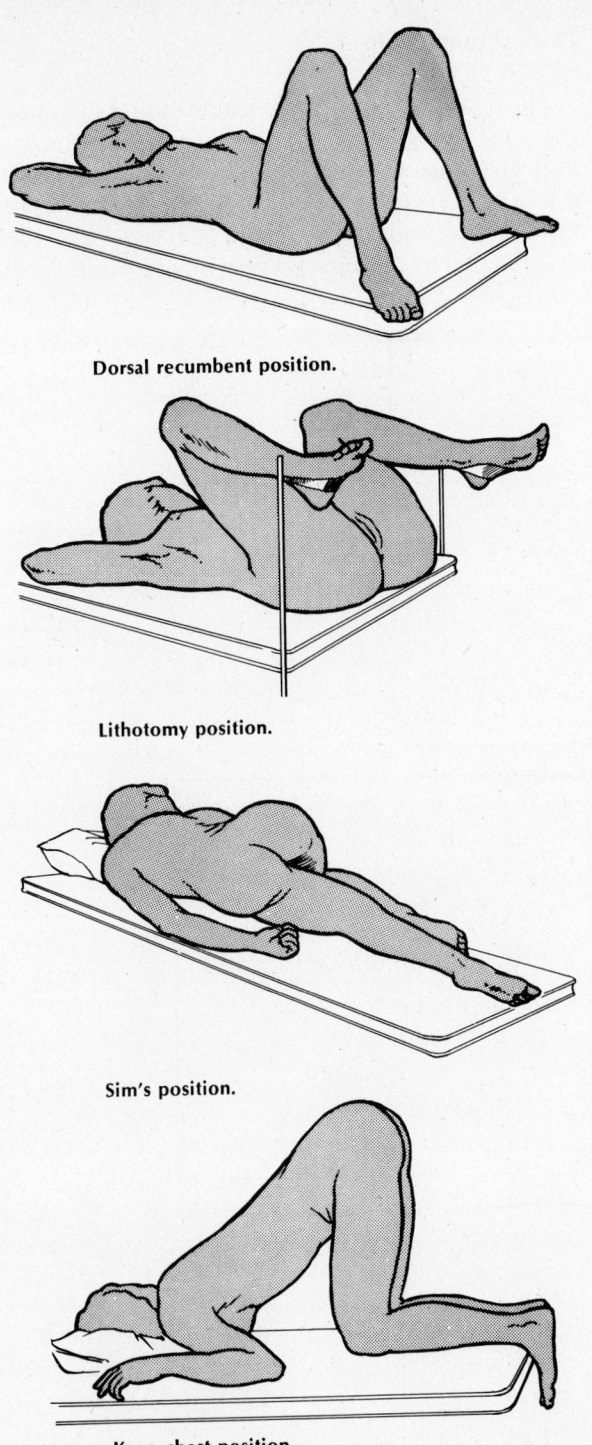

Dorsal recumbent position.

Lithotomy position.

Sim's position.

Knee-chest position.

Figure 44-1. Various positions for pelvic gynecologic examination. (From Fuerst and Wolff: Fundamentals of Nursing, 5th ed. Philadelphia, J. B. Lippincott)

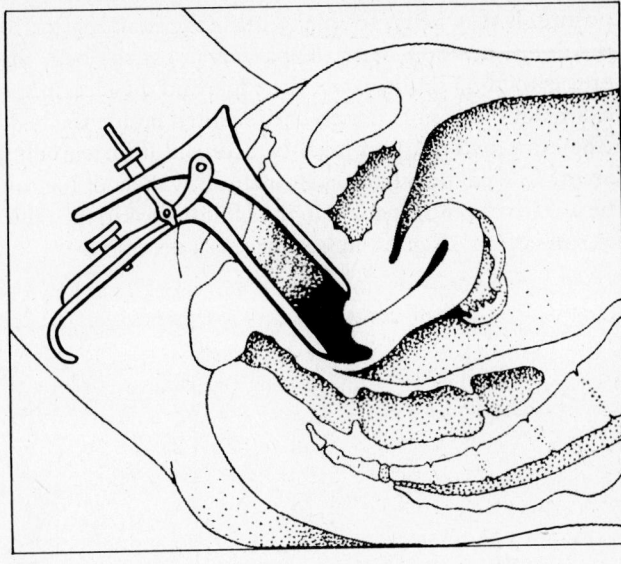

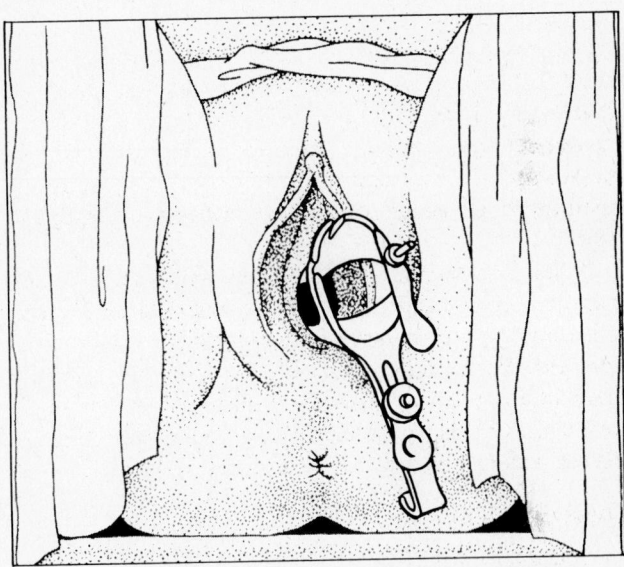

Figure 44-2. The speculum in position. (*Top*) lateral view; (*bottom*) anterior view. (Courtesy, Smith Kline & French Laboratories)

omy position, with the knees and the hips flexed, and the heels resting in foot rests. A sheet is draped diagonally over the patient, the lower corner being caught in the hands and gathered up so as to expose the vulva. A small towel then may be used to cover the exposed parts until the examiner is ready.

In *Sims's position*, the patient lies on one side, usually the left, with her arm behind her back. The right (uppermost) thigh and the knee are flexed as fully as possible, and the left leg is partly flexed. A sheet then is draped over the lower extremities and the hips in such a way as to expose the genitalia.

In the *knee-chest position*, the patient kneels on the table so that the feet extend over the end. The knees should be separated, and the thighs placed at right angles to the table. The head is turned to one side, and the arms grasp the sides of the table; the chest and the side of the face rest on a pillow.

If, for any reason, an examining table is not available, or the patient cannot be moved conveniently, these positions may be assumed in bed. Elevation of the buttocks on a covered, inverted bedpan may give adequate exposure. It may be preferable to make the examination in the dorsal position, with the patient across the bed, the hips extending slightly over the edge, and the feet on the examiner's knees or on two chairs placed beside the bed. The cross-bed position must be assumed if instruments are to be used during the examination. A sheet drape can be used to cover the patient in the same way as in the table examinations. A good light source is a necessity.

Pelvic Examination

The first step in the pelvic examination is an inspection of the external genitalia for signs of inflammation, swelling, bleeding, discharge, or local skin and epithelial changes. A speculum is inserted (Fig. 44-2) to examine visually the vagina and cervix (see page 961, vaginal examination by the nurse); a very small speculum may be

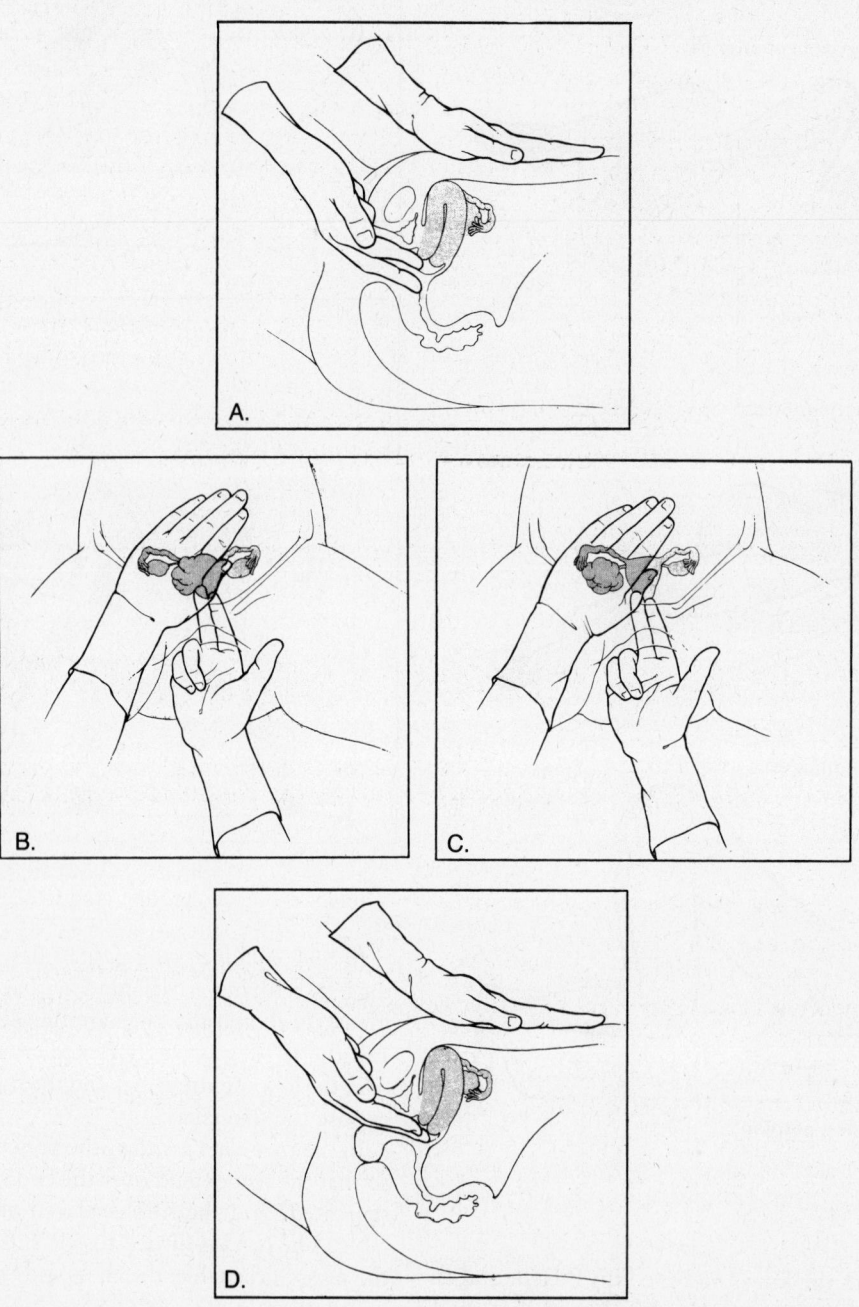

Figure 44-3. A bimanual pelvic examination. *A.* To palpate for the fundus, press gently down, with flattened palm and fingers. *B.* and *C.* To differentiate uterine and ovarian masses, press down, then forward and back. Cervical movement suggests a uterine fibroid (*B*); no movement, an ovarian mass (C). *D.* For rectovaginal exam, insert third finger in rectum and second in the vagina. (The feminine condition: The compleat pelvic. Emergency Med., 7:167-168, Oct. 1975)

used on a young virgin, or omitted altogether. The appearance of vaginal tissue and the nature of the cervix may be observed. The Papanicolaou smear and Schiller iodine test (below and page 963) can be done at this time.

A bimanual examination is the next step in the examination. It is important to proceed slowly, gently, and carefully. A relaxed patient will find the examination painless, whereas a tense person may experience discomfort. The index and third finger of the gloved hand are lubricated and held together extended with the index finger on top, while the introitus is penetrated. The hand is then rotated to the palm-up position, as fingers are advanced to the cervix.

When the fingers reach the cervix, gentle pressure is applied on the lower midabdomen with the flat palm and fingers of the other hand (Fig. 44-3A). Such pressure on the abdomen will be transmitted to the fundus, which, in turn, will be felt by the fingers against the cervix, if the uterus is in a normal position.

If the fundus cannot be located in this way, the uterus may be in a retroverted position. To differentiate between uterine and ovarian masses, pressure is applied, first downward, then forward and back. Cervical movement suggests a uterine fibroid (Fig. 44-3B); no movement, an ovarian mass (Fig. 44-3C). The detection of abnormal masses is reported.

Lastly, a bimanual rectovaginal examination is performed, by inserting the second finger into the vagina and the third into the rectum (Fig. 44-3D). The hand is then rotated so that the fingertips face somewhat anteriorly. With one hand on the abdomen, it is possible to palpate rectal and pelvic abnormalities if such are present.

During the examination, the nurse supports the patient, focuses the light, and assists the examiner. In primary care units, the nurse may do the pelvic examination. (See below.) At the conclusion of the examination, excess lubricating jelly or discharge should be wiped from the perineum before the patient is assisted from the table. Both legs are removed from the stirrups simultaneously, and the lower third of the table is brought to a horizontal position. The elderly patient should be encouraged to sit upright for a minute or two, and later should be assisted to the dressing room, where she may wish to rest before dressing. During this time, the nurse is available to answer questions or offer further explanations.

Cytologic Test for Cancer (Papanicolaou; "Pap Test"). This test is done for the purpose of diagnosing

---

VAGINAL EXAMINATION BY THE NURSE*

Purpose: To inspect the cervix and upper vagina.

Nature of Instrument: Graves' or duck-billed speculum is made of two blades: posterior (fixed) and anterior (movable). A thumbscrew on the handle holds the two blades together. This should be squeezed tight to allow blades to be together before speculum is inserted into vagina.

Patient Preparation: Have woman void before positioning her (Fig. 44-1). She should be as comfortable as possible, with a small pillow under the head, garments removed from the waist to the knees. Good lighting is essential. Explain to the patient what is being done, and proceed gently.

Examination and Inspection:
1. Be seated at proper elevation; visually examine external genitalia for indications of irritation, infection, or abnormalities.

2. Using sterile gloved hands, gently separate the labia.

3. Take a warmed speculum of appropriate size (moistened with warm water rather than lubricant) and gently insert vertically. By depressing the perineum and posterior vaginal wall with the speculum (avoids uncomfortable pressure against more sensitive anterior structures), easy entrance to the vagina is gained; the speculum is rotated to the horizontal position.

4. Slowly open the speculum; lock in open position. Speculum can be moved slightly to either side, up or down, permitting inspection of the vaginal walls and cervix. Normally, walls are pink and moist; a slightly milky secretion may be observed.

5. Note any different type of discharge, inflammation, irritation, or abnormality.

6. Inspect the cervix, which is about 2 cm. in diameter and 2-4 cm. long. The same pink color is normal; it may be darker pink to red, if the woman is taking the "pill," due to hormonal stimulation. The os may range from a mere indentation to the more noticeable slit in the woman who has had children. A string coming out of the os may indicate the placement of an IUD. Again, any variation from the normal pink smooth tissue, irregular or distorted contours, unusual discharge, should be noted and reported.

7. If the Pap test is to be done, follow procedure described on pages 961-962.

8. Unlock speculum and gently slide it out of the vagina, supporting speculum in open position so that it does not snap and pinch tissue on the way out.

9. Blot genitalia dry, and assist patient in getting out of the stirrups.

*Suggested reading—Magee, J.: The pelvic examination: A view from the other end of the table. Annals of Int. Med., *83*:536, 1975.

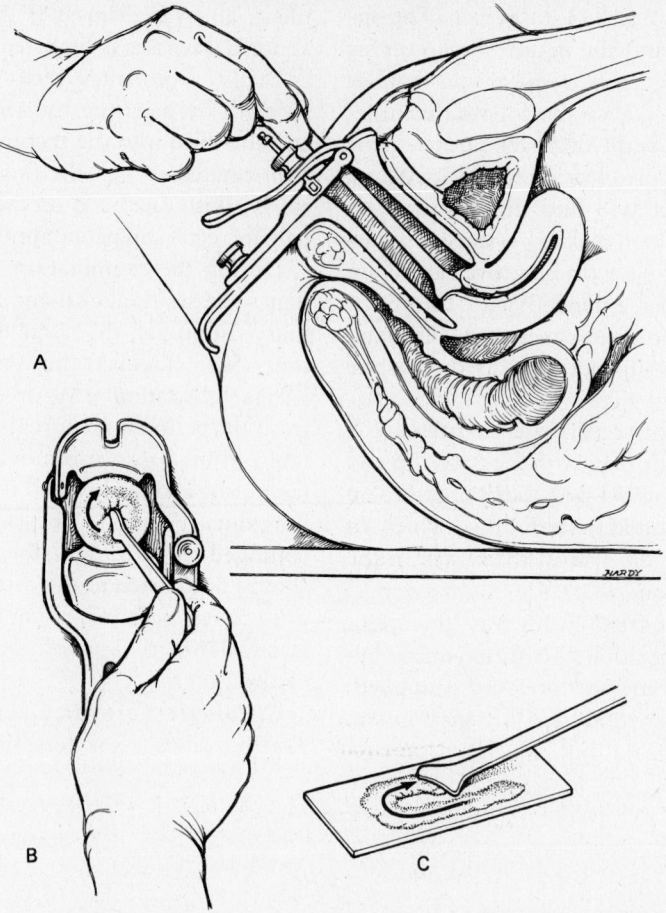

Figure 44-4. Method of using a wooden Ayre spatula to obtain cervical secretions for cytology. *A.* Shows the speculum in place and the Ayre spatula in position at the cervical os. *B.* By rotation of the spatula, a representative sample is obtained. *C.* Cervical secretions are transferred from wooden spatula to glass slide in a single circular motion.

cervical cancer. Vaginal secretions are aspirated or scraped from the posterior fornix and a smear transferred to a glass slide (Fig. 44-4). The secretion usually is "fixed" immediately by immersing the slide in equal parts of 95 percent alcohol and ether. The patient should be instructed not to take a douche before this examination, since such a treatment will wash away cellular deposits.

The pathologist examines and interprets the cytologic smear. The classification for cytologic findings as suggested by Papanicolaou is as follows:

Class 1. Absence of atypical or abnormal cells.
Class 2. Atypical cytology but no evidence of malignancy.
Class 3. Cytology suggestive of, but not conclusive for, malignancy.
Class 4. Cytology strongly suggestive of malignancy.
Class 5. Cytology conclusive for malignancy.

The finding of an abnormal smear (with the exception of Class 5) does not necessarily mean that the patient has cancer, but points out that additional procedures, such as biopsies or a dilatation and curettage, are indicated. The patient will be grateful for this explanation.

Endometrial (Aspiration) Smears. A smear obtained directly from the endometrium provides an even more accurate method of cytologic diagnosis. A cannula is inserted into the endometrial cavity, and tissue obtained by simple aspiration through a syringe. The *Gravlee Jet Washer* (Fig. 44-5) is a disposable examination unit that is safe, simple to use, and economical for screening patients for endometrial cancer. The unit consists of an intrauterine washing device that employs negative pressure to bathe the endometrium with isotonic solution, so as to dislodge cells and small tissue fragments. The use of negative pressure eliminates the possibility of flushing potentially malignant cells into the fallopian tubes.

Another similar diagnostic technique is that of *uterine aspiration* (suction curettage), in which a metal cannula 21 cm. long and 3 mm. in diameter is inserted through the cervical canal into the uterine cavity. The distal tip is

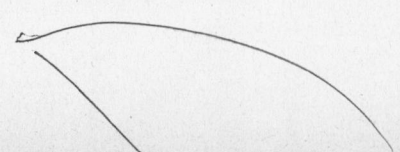

slightly curved, and open-ended on the concave surface. Pressure-equalizing holes are located near the proximal end of the cannula, enabling the examiner to maintain negative pressure by closing the holes with the fingertips. The proximal end is attached to a receptacle, in which aspirated tissue is gathered, and to a suction pump that generates negative pressure. Tissue is placed in a fixative solution and sent to the laboratory for histological analysis. This is a new diagnostic test designed to detect early endometrial malignancy.

Schiller Iodine Test. With the patient in lithotomy position (cervix exposed by speculum), a long cotton applicator is used to paint the cervix with Schiller's iodine solution.* The appearance of a mahogany-brown color covering the entire surface indicates a reaction between the iodine and the glycogen of normal cells. Such a reaction is considered negative. If abnormal, immature cells are present, tissues are not stained brown and the test is positive. The absence of staining directs attention to the sites requiring additional study, i.e., biopsy.

Cervical Biopsy

The type and extent of biopsy of the cervix will vary with the abnormality seen or the results of an abnormal Pap smear. When a lesion is clearly visible or can be seen with a magnifying instrument called a *colposcope,* one or more punch biopsies may be taken as an office procedure without anesthesia. However, when no lesion is visible, but the Pap smear is "suspicious," biopsy excision of an inverted cone of tissue is usually needed. This requires anesthesia and operating room facilities.

Cauterization. The application of a cautery is useful in controlling minor bleeding from small biopsies of the cervix and in treating superficial forms of chronic cervicitis.

Postbiopsy Patient Instruction. The patient is advised to rest for the next 24 hours and to leave the packing or tampon in place for the recommended time — usually 8 to 24 hours. Any excess bleeding is to be reported. Sexual intercourse is delayed until the physician indicates that it is permissible.

PELVIC ENDOSCOPY

Culdoscopy. With this procedure, it is possible to visualize directly the uterus, tubes, broad ligaments, uterosacral ligaments, rectal wall, and sigmoid and small intestine. This diagnostic procedure is done in the operating room with the patient in a knee-chest position. An incision is made in the posterior vaginal cul-de-sac to admit the culdoscope — a tubular lighted instrument.

*Aqueous iodine, 1 part; potassium iodide, 2 parts; water, 300 parts. This solution should be stored in a brown bottle to combat photosensitivity and rapid deterioration. The solution should be replaced every 4 to 6 weeks.

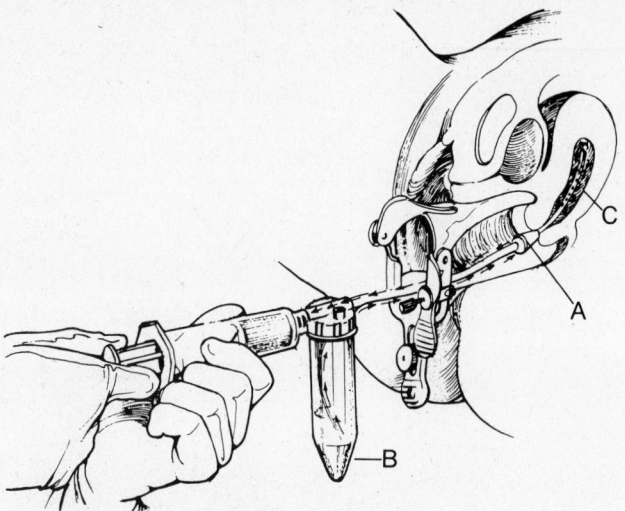

Figure 44-5. The Gravlee Jet Washer. To obtain a specimen, the distal tip of the cannula is inserted into the uterine cavity to a point where a preset rubber stopper (A) makes a firm seal with the cervical os. Isotonic saline is in the vertical reservoir (B) and is drawn into the uterus (C). The saline flows back to a connecting syringe. This fluid specimen is transferred into a vial with a fixative and sent to the laboratory for cytologic examination. (From Patient Care, January 1, 1973. Copyright © 1973, Miller and Fink Corporation, Darien, Conn. All rights reserved.)

The patient is prepared as for a vaginal operation, and anesthesia may be local, regional, or general.

Culdoscopy is indicated in suspected ectopic pregnancy, unexplained pelvic pain and in the presence of undetermined pelvic masses. Following this examination, the scope is withdrawn, and the patient is returned to her room. The incision through the posterior vaginal septum heals easily without sutures. Until healing takes place, the patient is instructed not to douche or have intercourse for about two weeks.

Laparoscopy (pelvic peritoneoscopy). A laparoscopy is carried out by inserting a scope into the peritoneal cavity through a 2-cm. (¾ inch) subumbilical incision (Fig. 44-6). Indications for laparoscopy are similar to those for culdoscopy. It is also possible to perform minor operative procedures such as tubal sterilization, ovarian biopsy, and lysis of peritubal adhesions by means of laparoscopy. A dilatation and curettage (D & C) precedes this procedure, not only because it affords additional information but also because a surgical instrument (intrauterine sound or cannula) may be positioned to permit manipulation of the uterus during laparoscopy, affording better visualization. A better view of the pelvis, lower abdomen, and visceral contents is also facilitated by the injection of a prescribed amount of carbon dioxide intraperitoneally into the cavity. This separates the intestines from the pelvic organs. The tubes are electrocoagulated, and a segment may be removed for histological verification. After the purpose of the laparoscopy has been accomplished, the scope is withdrawn, and carbon dioxide

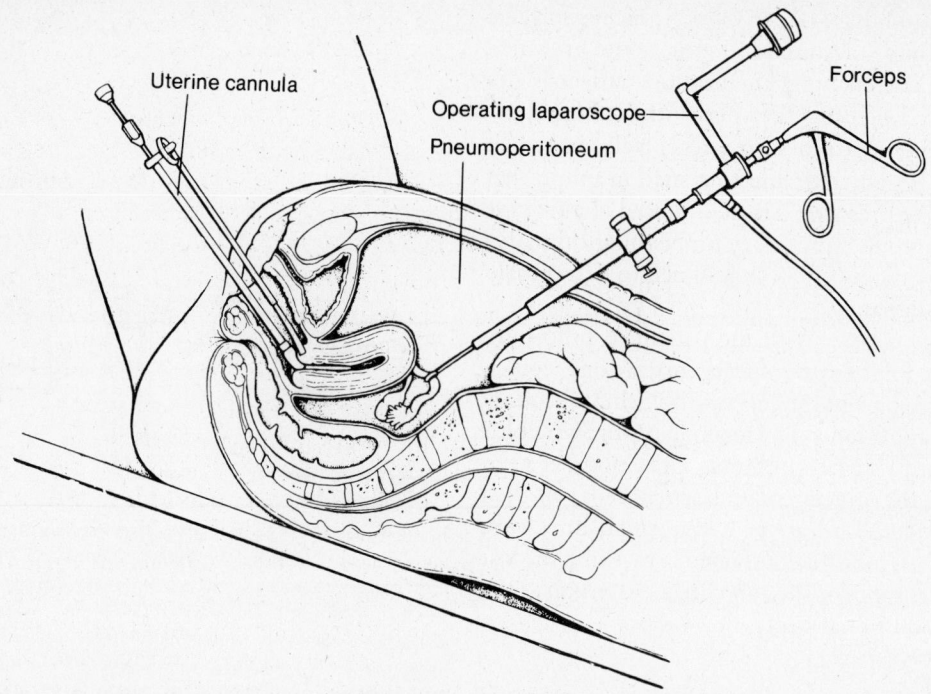

Figure 44-6. Laparoscopy.

is allowed to escape through the outer cannula. The skin incision is closed with stitches and covered with a Band-Aid.

The patient is carefully observed for several hours to detect any untoward signs indicating bleeding, injury, or burns from the coagulator. These rarely occur.

Hysteroscopy. This procedure allows direct visualization of all parts of the uterine cavity by means of a lighted optical instrument. Hysteroscopy is best performed about 5 days after completion of menstruation (estrogenic phase of menstrual cycle). The vagina and vulva are cleansed, and a pericervical anesthetic block is done. The instrument, a hysteroscope, is passed into the cervical canal and advanced under direct vision about 1 or 2 cm.; uterine-distending fluid (saline or 5% dextrose) is passed through the instrument to dilate the uterine cavity and provide better visualization.

Hysteroscopy is most commonly indicated as a diagnostic procedure in complex situations: infertility, unexplained bleeding, retained IUD. Hysteroscopy is contraindicated in patients with cervical or endometrial carcinoma.

Colposcopy and Colpomicroscopy. The colposcope (magnification, 10 to 25 times) and colpomicroscope (magnification to 400 times) are optical instruments designed to permit three-dimensional views of stained or unstained cervical epithelium in situ. These instruments provide visual access to suspicious tissue areas, but biopsy of the tissue is required for accurate diagnosis, in many instances.

ROENTGENOGRAM STUDIES

Hysterosalpingogram (Uterotubogram). A *uterotubogram* is an x-ray study of the uterus and the fallopian (uterine) tubes after the injection of a contrast media. The diagnostic procedure is done to study sterility problems, to evaluate tubal patency, and to determine the presence of pathology in the uterine cavity.

The patient is placed in the lithotomy position, and the cervix is exposed with a bivalved speculum. A cannula is inserted into the cervix, and radiopaque dye is injected into the uterine cavity and the tubes. X-ray films are taken to show the path and the distribution of the contrast materials.

In preparation for a salpingogram, the intestinal tract is prepared by a cathartic and an enema so that gas shadows do not distort the roentgenograms. An analgesic is prescribed for comfort, since some patients experience nausea, vomiting, cramps, and faintness. Following the test, it may be advisable for the patient to apply a perineal pad for several hours, because the radiopaque medium may stain clothing.

Arteriography, Venography, and Radioisotope Scanning. These procedures are also used as required. Since the uterus and adnexa are in close proximity to the kidneys, ureter, and bladder, urologic diagnostic aids, such as KUB (kidney, ureter, and bladder) and pyelogram, are frequently used.

Ultrasonography. Ultrasonography employs a simple procedure based on transmission of sound waves similar to the sonar detection used in submarines. Diagnostic ultrasonic scanning equipment uses pulsed ultrasound waves of a frequency exceeding 20,000 cycles per second; the pelvis and abdomen are scanned in linear fashion. The transducer, which is placed in contact with the abdomen, converts mechanical energy into electrical impulses, which in turn are amplified and recorded on an oscilloscope screen. (A photograph is taken of the pattern.) The entire procedure takes about ten minutes. The findings of this test, in combination with other diagnostic tools, provide useful adjuncts, particularly in the obstetric patient and the obese patient in whom pelvic examination and x-ray studies may have been unsatisfactory. A definite advantage of ultrasound scanning is that exposure to ionizing radiation is avoided. Patients will appreciate knowing this fact.

MENSTRUATION

Physiological Background

The *gonads* are the organs which produce either the egg cells (ova) or the sperm cells of an organism. In the human female, the gonads are called *ovaries* and are located in the abdomen. In the male, the gonads are the *testes* and are contained within the scrotum. In addition to their reproductive function, the gonads are important endocrine glands.

Ovarian hormones. The ovaries produce steroid hormones, predominantly estrogens and progesterone. Several different estrogens are produced by the ovarian follicle, which consists of the developing ovum and its surrounding cells. The most important of the ovarian estrogens is estradiol. Estrogens are responsible for the development and maintenance of the female reproductive organs and the secondary sexual characteristics associated with the adult female. Estrogens have an important role in breast development and in the cyclical changes of the uterus that occur monthly.

Progesterone is also important in regulation of the changes that occur in the uterus during the menstrual cycle. It is secreted by the corpus luteum, which consists of the ovarian follicle after the ovum has been released. Progesterone is the most important hormone for conditioning the lining of the uterus (endometrium) in preparation for implantation of the fertilized ovum. If pregnancy occurs, the secretion of progesterone becomes largely a function of the placenta. This secretion is important for the maintenance of normal pregnancy. In addition, progesterone, working in concert with estrogen, prepares the breast for production and secretion of milk.

Androgens are also produced by the ovaries, but only in very small amounts. Very little is known concerning the function of androgens in the female.

Regulation of Ovarian Hormone Secretion. Follicle-stimulating hormone (FSH) secreted by the pituitary is primarily responsible for stimulating estrogen secretion. Luteinizing hormone (LH) is primarily responsible for stimulating the production of progesterone. Feedback mechanisms in part regulate FSH and LH secretion. Increased estrogen levels in the blood inhibit FSH secretion, but promote LH secretion. Elevated progesterone levels inhibit secretion of LH. In addition, stimuli from the hypothalamus (releasing factors) affect the rate of gonadotropin (FHS and LH) release.

Menstrual Cycle. In the human female, secretion of ovarian hormones follows a cyclic pattern that result in changes of the uterine endometrium (the inner lining of the uterus), and in menstruation (Fig. 44-7). At the beginning of the cycle (just after menstruation), FSH output is increased and estrogen secretion is stimulated. This causes the endometrium to thicken and become more vascular. Near the middle portion of the cycle, LH output increases and progesterone secretion is stimulated. It is at this time that ovulation occurs. Under the combined stimulus of estrogen and progesterone, the endometrium reaches its peak of thickening and vascularization. If the ovum has been fertilized, estrogen and progesterone levels remain high, and the complex hormonal changes of pregnancy follow. If fertilization has not occurred, the output of FSH and LH diminishes, secretion of estrogen and progesterone falls rapidly, and the vascularized, thickened endometrium is sloughed, with resultant vaginal bleeding (menstruation). The cycle then begins again.

Psychosocial Considerations

The girl between the ages of 11 and 14 who is approaching the *menarche,* or onset of menstruation, should be instructed about this normal process. Psychologically, it is more healthy to refer to this event as "my period" rather than as "being sick" or "having the curse." With adequate nutrition, rest, exercise, and good posture, there will be little discomfort. Some girls do experience breast tenderness and a feeling of fullness a day or two before the onset of menstruation. There may be a greater tendency to fatigue and some discomfort of the lower back, legs, and pelvis on the first day; temperament and mood changes may be apparent. Slight deviations from the usual healthy pattern of daily living is permissible, but signs of excessive deviations may require investigation.

The perineal pad is the most widely used method of disposing of menstrual discharge; powder, cream, and spray deodorants for the pads are available. Tampons are also used extensively, and there is no significant evidence of untoward effects from their use, providing there is no difficulty in inserting them. Should the "tail" string break and difficulty be encountered in removing the tampon, the woman's physician should be consulted. A third type

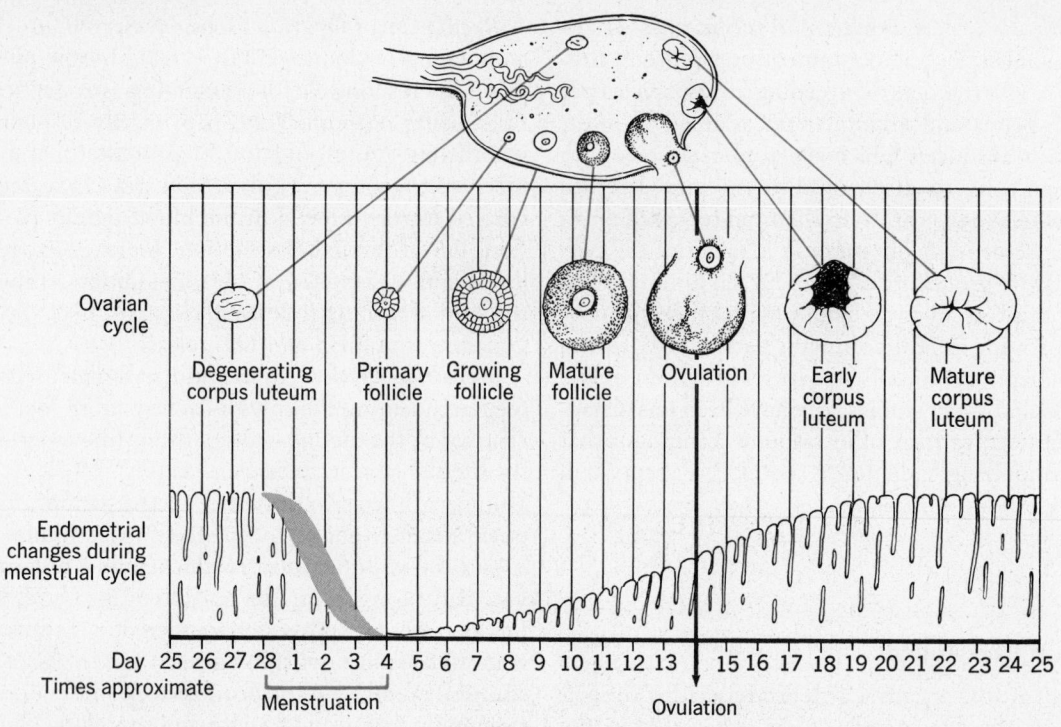

Phase	Menstrual	Follicular	Ovulation	Luteal	Premenstrual
DAYS	1 2 3 4 5 6 7 8 9 10	11 12 13 14	15 16 17 18 19	20 21 22 23 24 25	26 27 28 1 2
Ovary	Degenerating corpus luteum; Beginning follicular development	Growth and maturation of follicle	Ovulation	Active corpus luteum	Degenerating corpus luteum
Estrogen production	Low	Increasing	High	Declining, then a secondary rise	Decreasing
Progesterone production	None	None	Low	Increasing	Decreasing
FSH production	Increasing	High, then declining	Low	Low	Increasing
LH production	Low	Low, then increasing	High	High	Decreasing
Endometrium	Degeneration and shedding of superficial layer. Coiled arteries dilate, then constrict again	Reorganization and proliferation of superficial layer	Continued growth	Active secretion and glandular dilatation; highly vascular; edematous	Vasoconstriction of coiled arteries; beginning degeneration

Figure 44-7.   Correlation of hormonal activities with ovarian and uterine changes. (Adapted from Chaffee and Greisheimer, 3rd ed.: Basic Physiology and Anatomy. Philadelphia, J. B. Lippincott, 1974)

of protection is the internal rubber cup, but this is used less frequently.

As mentioned earlier, menstruation may be handled differently in different cultures. Some woman believe that it is detrimental to change a pad (or tampon) too frequently; they believe that by allowing the discharge to accumulate, an increased flow is stimulated, which is considered desirable. For the nurse to insist that a pad be changed before the time the patient believes proper may

cause conflict. These differences must be carefully reconciled so that proper understanding develops.

Other psychosocial aspects may need to be considered, such as vulnerability of the female to illness during menstruation. Many believe it is detrimental to swim, take a cold shower, receive a "permanent wave," get teeth filled, or eat certain foods during one's period. Such beliefs need to be recognized and corrected. Many other examples of misunderstanding could be listed; however, the objective is to alert the nurse to these unexpressed, deep-rooted beliefs. Aspects of gynecological problems cannot always be expressed easily. The nurse needs to convey confidence and trust, as well as offer sound advice, in order to set up a therapeutic environment.

DISTURBANCES OF MENSTRUATION

There is a definite interrelation between the hormonal secretions of the ovary, the thyroid, and the pituitary glands. A disturbance of this relationship by an increased or decreased function of one or more of these glands may influence the menstrual function.

Premenstrual Tension

Premenstrual tension is a combination of symptoms prior to the onset of menstruation: low back pain, engorged or painful breasts, feeling of abdominal fullness, and general irritability. Retained fluid, including cerebral edema and weight gain, is believed to account for these symptoms. While diuretics may be administered in extreme situations, the fact that this is a temporary condition makes it more tolerable for most women.

Dysmenorrhea (Primary or Essential)

Dysmenorrhea (painful menstruation) usually occurs within a few years of the menarche and, in the absence of any organic pelvic pathology, is a common condition, occurring in approximately 35 percent of all older adolescent girls, 25 percent of female college students, and 60 to 70 percent of older single females in their 30's. Primary dysmenorrhea accompanies ovulation, since the painful cramps are the result of the effects of progesterone, which causes increased myometrial contractility and arteriolar vasospasm. Psychologic factors, such as anxiety, tension, and dependency, may also contribute to dysmenorrhea.

The symptoms are mild cramps which begin 12 to 24 hours preceding onset of flow and become more acute with the flow, lasting an additional 12 to 24 hours. The pain is crampy, is located in the lower midabdomen, and may be associated with chills, nausea, vomiting, headache, irritability, and low backache.

Management. A complete physical examination is done to rule out possible abnormalities, such as strictures of the cervix or vagina or imperforate hymen. The reason for the discomfort is explained, and the patient is assured that it is a normal function of the reproductive tract. If the patient is a young girl and is accompanied by her mother, then the mother too can be reassured. Many daughters are conditioned to expect dysmenorrhea because their mothers experienced it. The pain, which is real, can be treated, once worry and concern over its possible significance are dispelled through accurate understanding. Symptoms subside in a few years and/or with normal sexual function and childbearing.

More specific methods of affording relief are as follows: urge the patient to carry on her usual activities, since mind-occupying functions and physical exercise provide a neurophysiologic basis for relief. Advise simple analgesics before cramps start, in anticipation of discomfort. Aspirin or Empirin may be taken at recommended doses every 4 hours. If necessary, antiemetics, antispasmodics, and mild tranquilizers may be effective. Some physicians recommend oral contraceptives to produce anovulatory cycles to relieve dysmenorrhea.

Dilatation and curettage is usually not indicated as a method of therapy. Psychiatric evaluation and therapy may be required if the problem appears to be psychosomatic or if a more serious psychiatric problem is suspected.

Amenorrhea (Absence of Menstrual Flow)

Primary amenorrhea (delayed menarche) refers to those instances when a young woman over age 17 has not yet begun to menstruate but otherwise shows evidence of sexual maturation. This may be of considerable concern to the person as well as to her mother, but is more than likely due to minor variations in body build, heredity, environment, as well as a general level of physical, mental, and emotional development.

The understanding nurse will provide an opportunity for the girl to express her concerns and anxiety about this problem, since she may feel that she is not like her peers and that she may not be able to fulfill her role as a woman. A complete physical examination, careful history, and simple laboratory studies will assist in excluding physiologic disorders, metabolic or endocrine difficulties, and other systemic diseases. Treatment is directed toward correction of any anomalies.

Secondary amenorrhea (at least 6 to 12 months in duration) occurs after a normal menarche and during pregnancy and lactation. In the adolescent the most common cause is a minor emotional upset related to being away from home, attending college, tension from school work, or interpersonal problems. Since the second most common cause is pregnancy, this possibility should always be investigated.

Secondary nutritional disturbances may also be apparent, such as weight loss or weight gain. This psychogenic or hypothalamic amenorrhea may last for a few years. On occasion there may be a pituitary or thyroid dysfunction that may be helped by appropriate measures. At any rate, consultation with a physician is necessary.

Menorrhagia, Metrorrhagia

Menorrhagia and metrorrhagia refer to abnormal uterine bleeding. In *menorrhagia,* the bleeding occurs at regular intervals, while in *metrorrhagia* the bleeding is irregular. For a more detailed discussion of these disorders see page 989.

MENOPAUSE

The *menopause* is described as the physiologic cessation of menses associated with failing ovarian function; it is often diagnosed in retrospect when a year has passed with no menses.

The *climacteric* is the transition period in the life of a woman during which the reproductive function gradually diminishes and is lost.

Physiological Overview

The menopausal period of a woman's life marks the end of her active reproductive life. It usually occurs between the ages of 49 and 52, but may occur in some women as early as 42 or as late as 55. Menstruation then ceases, and as a result of the complete cessation of activity on the part of the ovaries, the reproductive organs and the mammary glands atrophy. No more ova mature; therefore no ovarian hormones are produced. A similar situation prevails earlier if the ovaries are removed or destroyed by irradiation, producing an artificial menopause.

Menopause is not a pathologic phenomenon; in addition to estrogen deficiency, there are multifaceted psychological and physiological changes, including neuroendocrinological changes related to the aging process.

Usually, symptoms of menopause can be classified according to cause, as arising from (1) endocrine changes due to a lack of estrogen, or from (2) psychological changes. The process starts gradually and is recognized by the change in menstruation. The monthly flow becomes smaller in amount, then irregular, and finally ceases. Often, the time between periods gets longer — there may be a lapse of several months between them. Any prolonged menstrual flow or bleeding between periods should be reported promptly to the physician. Hot or warm flashes and other vascular disturbances are also endocrinologic in origin.

Additional physical manifestations may include atrophic changes, suggestion of stress incontinence, sagging structures, senile vaginitis, skin dryness, weight gain, and signs of calcium deficiency (shrinking in stature — osteoporosis).

Symptoms of a more psychological type may occur before or during these changes in the monthly periods, e.g., dizziness, weakness, nervousness, insomnia, headaches, inability to concentrate. This often is the time in a woman's life when the children have grown up and left home; thus, she may no longer feel needed. This realization, added to an acute awareness of the aging process, can have an effect on symptoms expressed. Fear of growing old may trigger feelings of depression. However, many women have very mild symptoms, and some have none. With a few, the discomfort is very severe.

The menopause is not a complete change of life. The normal sexual urges remain, and women retain their usual reaction to sex long after the menopause. There is nothing abnormal about the change of life, and nothing unusual about the continuation of happy marital relations afterward. Many women enjoy better health after the menopause than they have had for years. This is especially true with persons who have always suffered pain during their menstrual periods.

Management and Education of the Menopausal Woman

The majority of patients will respond to a program of education, reassurance, modification of their living habits, and an improved regimen of health. In some patients, mild sedatives and tranquilizers are necessary to control nervousness and to counteract mental depression, which is not at all unusual at this time. Sometimes even simple, everyday problems are too much to handle.

Persistent and severe hot flashes require treatment by estrogen therapy with diethylstilbestrol, Premarin, or ethynyl estradiol (Estinyl) given on a cyclic basis. The dosage is regulated by the physician according to a desired schedule, such as taking the medication each day except the first 5 days of every month. Close medical supervision is required, and any uterine bleeding is reported. Gradually, estrogen therapy is withdrawn.

Continued use of estrogen therapy to prevent widespread degenerative changes, including physical aging, is still controversial. Most authorities are conservative and prescribe estrogen replacement on an individual basis for acute estrogen deprivation or annoying signs of estrogen deficiency, such as atrophic vaginitis or osteoporosis. Restraint in prescribing estrogens for all menopausal women arises from concern that protracted treatment will induce neoplastic changes in estrogen-sensitive aging tissue. Unopposed long-term use of Premarin has recently been linked to carcinoma of the endometrium. It is believed that addition of progesterone may prevent these changes.

The physician and the nurse should take the time to explain to the patient that the cessation of the menses is a normal physiologic function that is not necessarily accompanied by extreme nervous symptoms and illness. Measures should be taken to promote her general health.

Since many patients are in the menopausal age-group, the following factors should be stressed in patient teaching:
1. The climacteric period is normal and self-limiting.
2. Overfatigue and environmental problems exaggerate the symptoms.
3. A nutritious diet and avoidance of overweight will improve the physical condition.
4. Interest and participation in outside activities help to absorb anxiety and to lessen tension.
5. Grown children should be treated as adults, since they are no longer children.

6. Old friendships should be revived, new friendships sought, and self-fulfillment provided.
7. This is an excellent time for intellectual growth and the stimulation of new ideas and experiences.
8. The menopause does not mean a termination of the sex life.
9. An annual physical examination is essential to the maintenance of continuing good health.

The current expected lifespan after menopause for the average woman is 30 to 35 years. This is an optimistic thought, since it encompasses as many years as the childbearing phase of her life.

Other effects of aging include a tendency to gain weight, particularly around hips, thighs, and abdomen. Paying increased attention to good grooming tends to give the woman a lift when it is most needed. The individual woman's evaluation of herself and her worth, now and in the future, certainly affects her emotional reaction to this change in her life.

CONCEPTION CONTROL

There is a growing attitude that conception control is not only of importance to the happiness and well-being of a family but to nations and the world as a whole. Since population control has extensive ramifications, the student is referred to other sources for background information.

Various forms of fertility control are available to individuals; it is their right to select the method most appropriate and acceptable to them. Of 100 women of proved fertility who are sexually active, 80 become pregnant within a year when no attempt is made to control conception.

With advanced scientific knowledge and greater dissemination of information about contraception, the traditional methods of contraception (withdrawal, household spermicides, rhythm method, and douches) have given way to proved methods of prevention. *Condoms, diaphragms, vaginal jellies,* and *foams* are all safe, with varying degrees of reliability (see Table 44-1). Great attention continues to be focused on oral ovulation-inhibiting steroids (the "Pill") and intrauterine devices. Other techniques being investigated are collagen sponges for vaginal insertion, and contraceptive pellets that can be implanted under the skin of men or women.

Rhythm Method

The rhythm method of contraception, to be sure, can be difficult to use because it is based on the woman's ability to determine her time of ovulation, and on the avoidance of intercourse during the fertile period The fertile phase (which requires sexual continence) is estimated to occur about 14 days before menstruation, although it may occur between the tenth and seventeenth

TABLE 44-1. PREGNANCY RATES BASED ON USE-EFFICACY*

(Pregnancy Rate—100 Women using technique for 1 year)	
Less than 1	Orals (combination)
2-5	Intrauterine devices
10-15	Diaphragm & jelly or cream
	Condom (rubber)
15-20	Aerosol vaginal foam
20-30	Jelly or cream alone
35	Rhythm
	Withdrawal
35-40	Suppositories
	Vaginal tablets
More than 40	Douche
80	Nothing

*Use-efficacy: a combination of both method-failure and patient failure.
(From Greenhill, J. P.: Office Gynecology, 9th ed. Chicago, Year Book Med. Pub., 1971. Used by permission.

day. It is assumed that spermatozoa can fertilize an ovum up to 72 hours after intercourse and that the ovum can be fertilized for about 24 hours after it leaves the ovary. Studies reveal that of 100 women practicing the rhythm method, 30 to 35 will conceive during a year.

If a woman carefully determines her "safe period," based on precise recording of her menstrual dates for at least one year, and follows a carefully worked out formula, some claim this method may achieve 90 to 95 percent protection. However, it requires a long period of abstinence during each cycle. New methods of detecting ovulation (ovulimeter, etc.) have improved statistics.

Diaphragm

The diaphragm is a ring made of flexible spring (approximately 7.5 cm. [3 inches] in diameter) which is covered with a domelike rubber cup. A spermicidal jelly or cream is used to coat the concavity of the diaphragm before it is inserted deep into the vagina. The combination of diaphragm and spermicide prevents spermatozoa from entering the cervical canal.

Each time the diaphragm is used, it must be examined carefully by holding it up to a bright light and making sure it has no pinpoint holes, cracks, or tears. Contraceptive jelly or cream is applied in a prescribed manner to the dome of the diaphragm. If it is applied more than two hours before intercourse, it must be reapplied. The diaphragm is then positioned to completely cover the cervix (see chart). Upon removal, the diaphragm is cleansed thoroughly with mild soap and water, rinsed, and dried before it is stored in its original container.

The diaphragm presents no discomfort, since it is lodged against the back wall of the vagina and anteriorly against the edge of the pubic bone. Since women vary in size, diaphragms are designed to fit the client; therefore it is necessary for the woman to be fitted for the proper size by a physician or a nurse practitioner.

INSTRUCTIONS FOR INSERTING A DIAPHRAGM*

I. PREPARING FOR INSERTION

1. Urinate and wash your hands before inserting the diaphragm.

2. Place one to two teaspoonful of contraceptive jelly or cream into the dome of the diaphragm (*A*). (Refer to package directions.) Spread the spermicide around the inner surface of the dome, and also a small amount around the rim. The spermicide on the rim makes the diaphragm easier to insert and helps seal the diaphragm in place. Too much jelly or cream can make the diaphragm too slippery to handle during insertion.

3. You can insert the diaphragm while you are standing with one leg up, squatting, or lying down (*B*). The position of the cervix and the walls of the vagina will be different, depending on your position. If you are used to one position and then change to another, take extra care in positioning the diaphragm to be sure the cervix is covered.

II. INSERTING THE DIAPHRAGM

1. Hold the diaphragm with the dome down (spermicide up) and press the opposite sides of the rim together between your thumb and third finger (*C*). The diaphragm can be held from above or below.

2. Spread the lips of your vagina with your free hand. Hold the compressed diaphragm dome down (spermicide up) and push it gently inward along the rear wall of the vagina as far as it can go. Your index finger, kept on the outer rim of the diaphragm, helps you guide the diaphragm into place (*D*).

3. With your index finger, push the front rim of the diaphragm up until it is locked into place just above the pubic bone (*E*).

4. Check with your index finger to be sure the diaphragm is in place and is holding the contraceptive jelly or cream over the cervix. It is important that the cervix be covered by the diaphragm and spermicide and that the diaphragm be locked in place between the upper edge of the pubic bone and the rear wall of the vagina. You should be able to feel your cervix through the rubber shield (*F*). You can feel the front rim of the diaphragm above the pubic bone, but you may not be able to follow the rim all the way around, since your fingers may not be long enough.

5. If, after some practice, you still find insertion awkward or difficult, vary your body and hand positions slightly until you can insert the diaphragm comfortably.

6. Some practitioners recommend that the diaphragm be inserted every night, to minimize unprotected intercourse.

III. REMOVING THE DIAPHRAGM

1. You should not remove the diaphragm, nor should you douche, for six or eight hours after intercourse.

2. You need not feel any urgency about removing the diaphragm; it is safe to let it remain in position for 24 hours. Should you forget to remove it for some hours, or should removal be inconvenient at any particular time, that is no cause for concern. Just bear in mind that if you desire to have intercourse again, you must first apply more spermicidal jelly or cream.

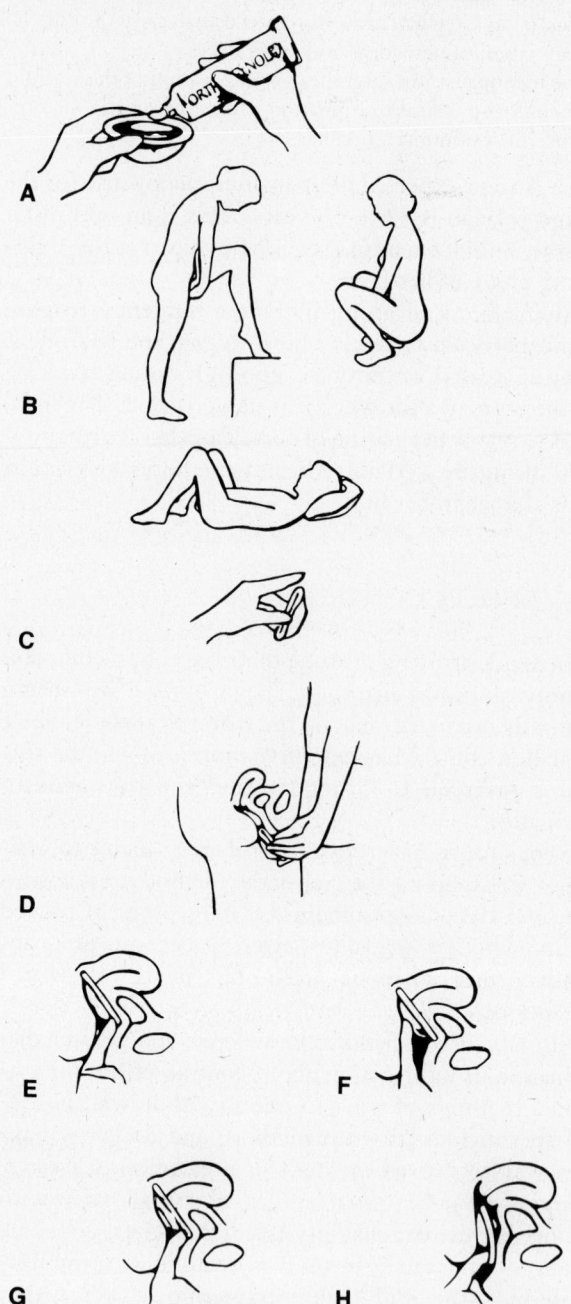

3. To remove the diaphragm, put your index finger behind the front rim (*G*) and pull the diaphragm down and out (*H*).

4. If you get up before it is time to remove the diaphragm and there is a discharge of cream or jelly, you may use a tampon or sanitary napkin.

*Material published by Ortho Pharmaceutical Corporation, used by permission.

Intrauterine Devices (IUD)

Intrauterine devices (IUD)* in principle are not new; however, the modern pioneer was a German physician, Ernst Graefenberg, who, around 1928, inserted silkworm gut and later silver or gold wire coils into the uterine cavity as a means of preventing conception.

In its current form, the intrauterine device is a plastic or metal piece which is inserted through the cervix into the endometrial cavity to prevent pregnancy. The method by which the IUD prevents conception is uncertain; however, one of several factors may be responsible: (1) increased tubal peristalsis may cause the fertilized ovum to be delivered to the uterus too early for implantation; (2) the endometrium may be changed, interfering with normal implantation; and (3) the zygote may be damaged by cytotoxic substances and phagocytosis.

A satisfactory IUD is easy to insert, remains in place, is an effective contraceptive device, causes no problems such as pain or bleeding, rarely needs to be removed, and is economical. Several types of intrauterine devices are currently in use; they are made of materials nonreactive with body tissues, usually polyethylene impregnated with barium to allow for visibility on x-ray. The most popular IUD is the double-S-shaped Lippes loop. Copper and some other metals enhance the effectiveness of an IUD; however, the long-term safety of copper IUDs has still not been established. The IUD is positioned in a narrow straight stylet that is introduced through the cervical os (Fig. 44-8). The device is then forced into the uterine cavity by means of a plunger. Most devices have nylon-thread tails that are used to remove the IUD and to help indicate that it is still in the uterus.

The advantage of this method is that it reduces the factor of patient error, which makes it suitable for large-scale use in lower socioeconomic groups. The disadvantages are that such a device may be expelled unnoticed (thereby accounting for a significant pregnancy rate) or, if it remains in place, may cause possible infection and perforation of the uterus. Because of these serious disadvantages, the IUD is a much less satisfactory method of preventing conception than either the diaphragm or the "Pill." Expulsion of an IUD, if it occurs at all, takes place during the first, second, or third menstrual period after insertion. If the device is retained beyond this time, it is likely to remain in position indefinitely. IUDs probably can remain in the uterus for several years without being changed (with exception of copper IUD); however, many American physicians prefer to replace the IUD every year or two and request annual check-ups.

Patient Education. In the United States, the Food and Drug Administration has established uniform pro-

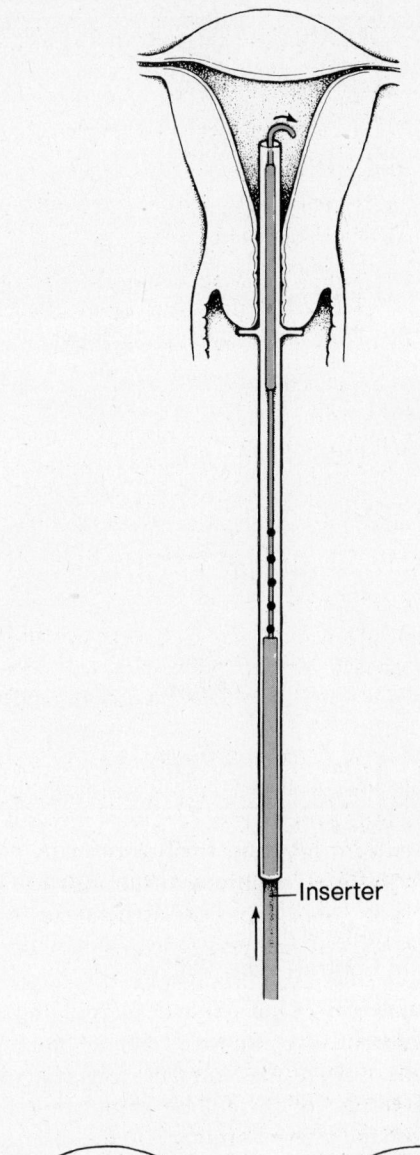

Inserter

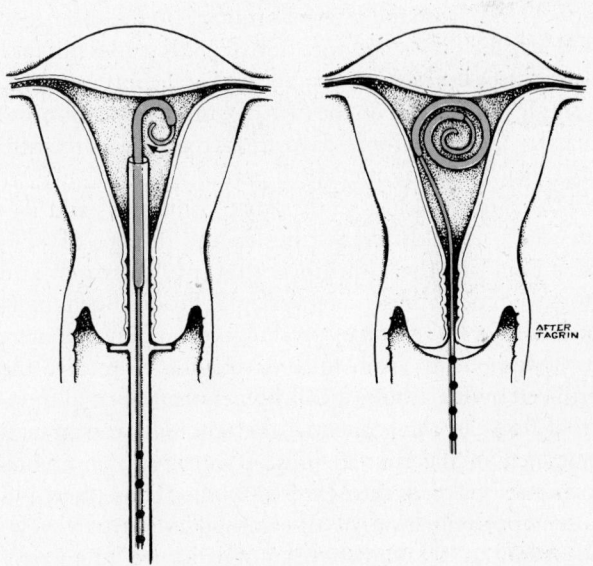

Figure 44-8.　An IUD. An intrauterine plastic ring as a contraceptive device.

---

*Sometimes referred to *IUCD*—intrauterine contraceptive device.

IUD INFORMATIONAL REQUIREMENTS

Professional Information

Description of the IUD (name, composition, etc.)

Mode of action or principles of IUD design

Indications and usage

Warnings (including pregnancy, ectopic pregnancy, pelvic infection, embedment, and perforation)

Precautions (include patient counselling, patient evaluation, clinical considerations)

Adverse reactions

Directions for use

Clinical studies (use-effectiveness data—i.e., pregnancy, expulsion rates)

Patient Information

Preinsertion

What you should know about the IUD

Use-effectiveness

What you should tell your physician

Adverse reactions

Postinsertion

Description of the IUD

Directions for use

Side effects

Warnings

Special warning about pregnancy with an IUD in place.

---

fessional and patient labeling for intrauterine contraceptive devices. These requirements are listed in the chart.

Oral Conception Control—The "Pill"

Physiological Basis. Oral synthetic steroid preparations of estrogen and progesterone tend to block the stimulation of the ovary by the central nervous system by preventing the release of the follicle-stimulating hormone (FSH) from the anterior pituitary. In the absence of FSH, a follicle does not ripen and ovulation does not take place; this is the basis of operation of oral contraceptives. A single pill is taken on the fifth day of menstruation and each day thereafter for 20 days; this is repeated on the fifth day of each ensuing menstrual period.

There are two kinds of therapy: "combined" and "sequential"—the difference lies in the dosage of progestogens. In the combined therapy, estrogen and progestogen are present in every pill. Progestogen interferes with cervical mucus production and prevents uterine endometrium from fully developing to receive the fertilized ovum, resulting in a lighter-than-normal menstrual flow. In the sequential therapy, only estrogen is contained in the first 15 pills, whereas the combined hormones make up the next 5 or 6 pills. Thus, there is a closer approximation of the normal menstrual cycle. According to 100 women-years of exposure, pregnancy control is greater with the combined steroid program than with the sequential method.

Side Effects. In a small percentage of patients, side effects may be noted, such as nausea, pelvic discomfort, backache, irritability, depression, headache, weight gain, leg cramps, breast soreness. Usually these disappear after 3 or 4 months. Because such symptoms are related to sodium and water retention caused by estrogen, a smaller dose of the hormone may alleviate the problem.

Other problems encountered are the occurrence of thromboembolic disorders, more rapid growth of uterine fibroids, and jaundice. Therefore these drugs should not be used by women who have had thromboembolic disorders, uterine fibroids, or liver or gallbladder disease. Noted also is an increased incidence of heart attack in smokers over the age of 35 who are on the Pill. Occasionally neuro-ocular complications arise, but any cause-and-effect relationship is unknown at present. Should visual disturbances occur, the drug should be terminated. An increased incidence of candidal vulvovaginitis has also been reported.

Certain nutritional side effects have been noted, such as folic acid deficiency and an increased need for vitamin C and vitamin B_{12}. However, the consequences of metabolic and nutritional effects of the Pill are not definitively established. Nutritional counseling must be done on an individual basis. Women with good dietary habits may be able to satisfy nutritional needs; however, women with depleted or limited nutritional resources may require vitamin and mineral supplements.

Women with scanty or irregular periods are strongly advised to use another method of contraception. If they use oral contraceptives, they may have difficulty becoming pregnant or may fail to have menstrual periods after discontinuing the Pill. With respect to how soon fertility returns after taking oral contraceptives, a study by Vessy and associates in England is significant. Of 17,000 women between the ages of 25 and 39 who discontinued various types of contraception with the object of becoming pregnant, no delay was experienced for those who used diaphragms, condoms, or IUDs. However, oral contraceptives consistently delayed fertility return. The fertility delay time became negligible after 30 months for

---

RISK FACTORS

Instances when the "Pill" should not be taken.

1. Women who have had:
   a. Blood-clotting disorders
   b. Cancer of the breast or sex organs
   c. Unexplained vaginal bleeding
   d. A stroke
   e. Heart attack
   f. Angina pectoris
   g. Suspected pregnancy
2. Cigarette smokers
3. Women with scanty or irregular periods

---

women who had previously conceived and after 42 months for women trying to become pregnant for the first time.

Insofar as potential long-term undesirable effects following prolonged use of oral contraceptives are concerned, it is generally accepted that no definite ill effects have been observed so far. Fetal anomalies do not appear to be a concern, and normal reproductive tract function and fertility are restored (although somewhat delayed, as was indicated above), following discontinuance of the Pill. Meanwhile, research and experimentation continue to develop a single monthly pill or injection that would be safe as well as effective.

Postcoital Conception Control

A properly timed administration of an adequate dosage of estrogen to a woman, following intercourse, will prevent pregnancy. Such a "morning after" pill is not applicable for use in long-term contraceptive control but is of real value in emergency situations such as rape, defective or torn condom or diaphragm, or other "accidental" intercourse. Such medication given immediately after fertilization and before the occurrence of implantation is effective. Usually the therapy is continued over 5 days using diethylstilbestrol or ethynylestradiol. Nausea can be minimized by taking the medication with meals and with an antiemetic drug. Other side effects may be experienced but are transient.

Permanent Conception Control

Permanent sterility may be achieved by hysterectomy or tubal ligation in the female and vasectomy in the male.

Tubal sterilization (ligation or electrocoagulation of fallopian tubes) terminates a woman's ability to have children without affecting her ovulatory or menstrual function. The number of tubal ligations is increasing each year, and the most common indications are hypertensive cardiovascular disease, two or more cesarean sections, and multiparity. Various surgical techniques have been developed utilizing the abdominal or vaginal approach.

Laparoscopy is a relatively new technique of sterilization (page 963).

For a discussion of vasectomy in male sterilization, see page 1031.

Investigational Conception Control

Antipregnancy Vaccine. The human chorionic gonadotropin molecule (HCG) is the hormone released by a freshly fertilized egg; it stimulates the release of progesterone, which halts menstruation. A vaccine has been produced which stimulates the formation of antibodies that are capable of neutralizing HCG, thereby blocking its signal. The next menses occurs as usual, thereby removing the ovum.

"Pill" for Males. A drug has been developed which cuts production of male hormones, thereby reducing sperm output. The drug is given with a monthly injection of testosterone (to insure normal sexual drive) and has shown encouraging results.

Patient Education

Much has been written about family planning and the availability and use of contraceptive devices. The nurse is in a strong position to help patients understand the options available. Religious groups have made clear their teaching and dogma regarding birth control, and these need to be respected and understood, as each couple makes its decision. Research is changing the methods used in fertility control, and more acceptable and longer-lasting types are sought. The nurse should be familiar with the information as it becomes available. A valuable source of information is the American College of Obstetricians and Gynecologists, 1 East Wacker, Chicago, Illinois 60601.

PREGNANCY TERMINATION

Interruption of pregnancy or expulsion of the contents of the pregnant uterus before the fetus is viable (up to 20 weeks) is called *abortion;* interruption between 20 to 28 weeks is commonly referred to as *miscarriage.* The viability of the fetus is usually considered to be probably any time after the sixth month of gestation; however, legal periods of viability vary in different states in the United States.

The aborted fetus weighs less than 1,000 gm.; beyond this weight, the fetus is usually viable, and the term *premature labor* is used, instead of *abortion,* to describe the situation. It is estimated that one out of every five or ten conceptions results in abortion. Most of these occur because of an abnormality in the fetus so that abortion is nature's method of rejecting a defective conception. Other causes may be due to systemic diseases, hormonal imbalance, or anatomic abnormalities.

Spontaneous Abortion

Spontaneous abortion occurs most commonly in the second or third month of gestation, probably due to a defective ovum and subsequent developmental defects of the fetus and placenta.

There are various kinds of spontaneous abortion, depending upon the nature of the process (threatened, inevitable, incomplete, and complete). Uterine bleeding and pain (uterine contractions) are suggestive of an abortion in a woman of child-bearing age. In such a *threatened abortion,* the cervix does not dilate; with bed rest and conservative treatment, it can be prevented. If it cannot be prevented, an *inevitable abortion* is imminent. If some of the tissue, but not all, is passed, the abortion is referred to as *incomplete;* however, if the fetus and all related tissue are expressed (removed), the abortion is *complete.*

Habitual Abortion

Habitual abortion is successive (three) repeated abortions of unknown cause; immunologic rejection is suspected. Ultraconservative measures are employed in an attempt to save the pregnancy, such as complete bed rest, administration of progesterone to prevent sloughing of the endometrium, thyroid extract therapy, and psychotherapy.

In the condition known as "incompetent cervical os," the cervix dilates painlessly in the second trimester of pregnancy, resulting in spontaneous abortion. A surgical procedure called the Shirodkar operation (cervical cerclage) is designed to prevent the cervix from dilating prematurely. A purse-string suture of fascia, polyethylene, or dermal graft strip obtained from the patient's lower abdominal skin is tied snugly around the cervix at the level of the internal os. It is most important that the patient and the nurses attending her, including those in community health agencies and industry, be informed that such a suture is in place. As soon as labor occurs, the physician should be notified immediately so that the suture can be cut and labor allowed to proceed; otherwise, the uterus may possibly rupture. Usually delivery is by cesarean section.

Therapeutic Abortion

Under certain circumstances, the physician may consider terminating a pregnancy; such a termination is called a *therapeutic abortion,* and is performed by skilled medical personnel. On January 22, 1973, the United States Supreme Court handed down its ruling, which in effect states the following:

1. In the first trimester of pregnancy, the abortion decision is to be left to the woman and her physician.
2. During the second trimester, the state may not prohibit abortion but may regulate its practice in the interest of protecting the woman's health. (Permissible regulations could determine who are qualified to do abortions and where they might be done.)
3. During the final weeks of pregnancy, the state may choose to protect the potential life of the fetus by prohibiting abortion, except where necessary to preserve the life or health of the woman.

Even though the liberalization of abortion laws makes many abortions legally permissible, the religious beliefs of the individual involved must be respected. Baptism of all stillborn and aborted fetuses is required by the Roman Catholic faith.

Management. Usually the opinions of two or more physicians are documented to identify the reasons for performing a therapeutic abortion. Appropriate informed permission is obtained from the patient.

Vacuum aspiration of uterine contents within 14 days of a missed menstrual period may be performed in a physician's office; this is called *menstrual regulation,* or *menstrual extraction.*

Therapeutic abortions may be carried out in the following ways, usually in the operating room:
1. Dilatation and curettage (page 990).
2. Dilatation and evacuation (suction curettage): the cervix is dilated, and a uterine aspirator is introduced. Suction from a pump is applied, and fetal tissue is removed from the uterus. This method is not used if the pregnancy has advanced beyond 12 weeks, since the fetus at this stage is supposedly too firm. More recently, some clinics have extended the period to 15 weeks and even beyond.
3. *Intra-amniotic injection of hypertonic saline:* This procedure is used beyond the fourteenth week of pregnancy. Under local anesthesia, a needle is inserted in the midabdomen, and an amniocentesis is performed. Over 200 ml. of fluid are withdrawn and replaced by hypertonic saline. In some clinics, after 6 hours, oxytocin is administered intravenously, with lactated Ringer's solution, to initiate labor. If no oxytocics are administered, labor will usually begin spontaneously within 8 to 20 hours, but may be delayed for several days. Subsequent curettage may be necessary to remove completely any remaining placental and residual tissue. The dangers of this procedure, such as accidental intravenous injection of saline, cerebral convulsion, and acute renal failure, need to be realized.
4. *Prostaglandins:* Intra-amniotic instillation of natural or synthetic prostaglandins produces strong uterine contractions, causing cervical dilatation and expulsion of fetus and placenta within 24 hours. This method appears safer than utilizing hypertonic saline, because it avoids the complication of DIC (disseminated intravascular coagulation) and hypernatremia.

Prostaglandins continue to be studied; side effects, such as nausea, vomiting, diarrhea, and painful uterine cramping may occur, although the incidence and frequency of such problems vary according to the medication, dosage, and technique of administration.
5. *Laminaria:* An age-old method of cervical dilatation is being revived in medical practice. Laminaria tents are made from a species of seaweed that grows in cold ocean waters; the stem is dried and cut into lengths of about 6-8 cm. (2.4-3.1 inches) and shaped into cylindrical (tampon-shaped) forms for sizing from 2-4, 4-6, 6-8, and 8-10 mm. in diameter. A string is looped through one end. When placed in a moist environment, the tent, which is highly hygroscopic, swells to three or five times its original diameter. The tent may be placed in the cervix in order to dilate it. The greatest amount of swelling occurs in 4 to 5 hours; however, additional dilatation may be expected over the next few hours.

Tents are used prior to the insertion of IUDs, for first- or second-trimester abortions, and for other medical procedures requiring dilatation.

Advantages of laminaria tents over metal-instrument dilators are many: tents cause limited cervical trauma, hold little risk of other serious complications, and are readily accepted and tolerated by patients. Disadvantages include the following: there is some discomfort and slight uterine cramping immediately after insertion, and mild-to-severe intermittent cramps may be experienced in some women for several hours. There is also risk of low-grade endometritis. Removal of the tent is difficult at times, and on occasion has resulted in the tent's slipping into the uterus. Tents are sterilized by gamma radiation or ethylene oxide gas.

When it is desirable to insert a tent overnight, hospitalization may be required. In such instances the nurse needs to know that a tent is in place (string will be noticed in the vagina). Many physicians, however, prefer to use laminaria for just 3 to 4 hours, followed by metal dilatation.

6. *Hysterotomy*—a "miniature" cesarean section: usually this method is reserved for women who also want to be sterilized at the same time. The patient remains in the hospital for 3 to 6 days; care is essentially the same as for an abdominal operation.

Septic Abortion

When unskilled attempts to end a pregnancy are made, the methods usually include administering large amounts of drugs (effects are toxic and never really evacuate the uterus) or performing a curettage, with an associated high risk of rupture of the uterus, hemorrhage, or infection.

Although this has been a major problem in the past, with the widespread dissemination of birth control information and the liberalization of abortion laws, a decline in septic abortion will be apparent.

If a woman who has had a simple, uncomplicated septic abortion receives proper medical attention early enough, the prognosis is excellent with treatment by broad-spectrum antibiotics. Fluid and blood replacement are required before very careful attempts are made to evacuate the uterus.

For the treatment of septic abortion complicated by impending shock, see the discussions of shock, page 364, and pelvic inflammatory disease, page 999.

Management of Abortion Patients

Signs of a threatening abortion are vaginal discharge or bleeding and abdominal cramps. The woman is encouraged to see a physician, who will probably recommend bed rest, light diet, and no straining on defecation. According to some estimates, when first seen, less than 30 percent of patients who are actually threatening to abort have viable fetuses, and 80 percent or more will proceed to abortion regardless of management.*

All tissue passed vaginally is saved for examination by the physician. Sedation or tranquilizers may be prescribed and if infection is suspected, antibiotics may be given. In the hospital, all personnel caring for the patient will be alerted to save the contents of the bedpan for

possible placenta tissue or fetus. If there is much bleeding, the patient may require transfusions and fluid replacement. An estimate of the amount of bleeding can be determined by recording the number of perineal pads and the nature of saturation per 24 hours. For an incomplete abortion, oxytocin may be prescribed to contract the fundus prior to the woman's having a dilatation and evacuation (D & E), or suctioning of the uterus. A patient with such an *evacuation of retained secretions* (ERS) requires the same nursing care as a person having a dilatation and curettage (see page 990).

Since this patient experiences a severe emotional reaction, the component of "caring" for her is an important aspect of nursing. The cause of the abortion colors the problem and the patient's reaction. The response of the woman who desperately wants the baby is quite different from that of the woman who does not want to be pregnant but may be frightened of the possible consequences

---

PATIENT EDUCATION: POST-THERAPEUTIC ABORTION*

1. Note that bleeding similar to menstruation will continue for seven days or less.
   - Report: If bleeding is heavier than usual menstrual flow.
     If followed by severe cramps, backache, nausea.

2. During bleeding:
   - Do not take tub baths; showers or sponge baths are permitted.
   - Do not douche or go swimming
   - Do not use tampons—use sanitary pads. (Tampons may be used during your next period.)
   - Do not have intercourse; preferably wait until you have one normal period.
   - Avoid strenuous exercise for at least one week, since it may cause further bleeding.

3. Medication for bleeding:
   - If medication has been prescribed to prevent bleeding, expect a few cramps or clots.

4. Take your temperature for 5 to 7 days.
   - Report: If it is elevated for 24 to 48 hours.
     If it is elevated and accompanied by symptoms mentioned in 1.

5. Normal expected signs due to hormonal changes (these will pass):
   - Some women experience depression.
   - Breasts may be sore and perhaps leak.
     To combat this, wear a supporting brassiere, and restrict fluids.

6. Follow-up
   - In about a month (or when requested), report to your physician or clinic for a checkup.

*Adapted from Easterbrook and Rust: Abortion counseling. Canadian Nurse, 73:30, Jan. 1977.

---

*Green, T. H., Jr.: Gynecology, 2nd ed. Boston, Little, Brown & Co., 1977.

of an abortion. In either event, providing opportunities for the patient to talk and vent her emotions will not only help her but will also provide clues for the nurse in planning more specific care.

INFERTILITY

Infertility is defined as the inability to conceive, and is usually designated as a problem when the couple fails to conceive after a year or more of normal marital contact. However, should the condition persist, it is referred to as *sterility*. In the United States, 15 percent of married couples (3.5 million couples) are childless because of infertility; it is a major medical and social problem. Both husband and wife are urged to seek medical attention for complete examinations and evaluation. Careful evaluation includes not only anatomic and endocrinologic investigation but also consideration of psychosocial factors. Often more than one factor may be responsible for the problem. Such tests may require the services of a urologist, gynecologist, endocrinologist, and internist.

Possible causative factors include: uterine displacement, tumors, congenital anomalies, and inflammation. For an ovum to become fertilized, the vagina, cervix, and uterus must be patent and the mucosal secretions must be receptive to the sperm. Semen is alkaline, as is cervical secretion; normal vaginal secretion is acid. Proceeding from this assumption, five types of factors are considered basic to the infertility: for the female, (1) ovarian, (2) tubal, (3) cervical, or (4) uterine conditions and for the male, (5) seminal. A composite estimate of the relative frequency of these factors as the major cause of infertility is as follows: ovarian, 20 percent; tubal, 30 percent; cervical, 18 percent; seminal, 30 percent.

Diagnostic Approach. A complete history, physical examination, and laboratory examination are done on both partners to rule out such causative factors as previous venereal disease, anomalies, injuries, tuberculosis, mumps orchitis, abortions, and psychosocial disorders.

1. *Ovarian Factor:* Tests are done to determine whether there is regular ovulation and a progestational endometrium adequate for implantation. This will include keeping a basal body temperature chart for at least four cycles, taking an endometrial biopsy, and performing other tests for ovulation and progesterone production.
2. *Tubal Factor:* Tubal insufflation or Rubin test: To determine tubal patency, carbon dioxide is introduced through a sterile cannula into the uterus and the tubes, and then into the peritoneal cavity. By listening with a stethoscope on the abdomen, the physician may hear gas swishing into the abdomen, indicating that the tubes are open. Another positive indication of tubal patency is the feeling by the patient of referred pain under the scapula or shoulder on the side of the patent tube. This suggests that the gas is under the diaphragm, exerting pressure on the phrenic nerve. If normal patency is present, there is a rise in pressure of 80 to 120 mm.,

with a sudden drop to 50 to 70 mm. as gas passes into the peritoneal cavity. If the gas pressure gauge reaches 200 mm., the test is considered negative, indicating an occlusion.

Hysterosalpingography (page 964) is an x-ray study which is useful when tubal occlusion is apparent, since other abnormalities may be found.

Culdoscopy or laparoscopy (page 963) permits direct visualization of the tubes and adnexa, including status of ovarian function.

3. *Cervical Factor:* Cervical mucus can be examined to determine whether proper changes occur at ovulation time which are favorable to sperm penetration, survival, and growth.

A postcoital cervical mucous test (Sims-Huhner or "PK" test) is done between 6 and 12 hours after intercourse. The physician aspirates cervical secretions, using a medicine dropper or special cannula. The woman has been instructed not to void, bathe, or douche between coitus and the examination; a perineal pad is worn until she is placed in a lithotomy position in the examining room. Aspirated material is placed on a slide and examined under the microscope for presence and viability of sperm cells.

4. *Uterine Factor:* Fibroids, polyps, and congenital malformations are possible problems in this category. Their presence may be determined by pelvic examination or by hysterosalpingography.

5. *Seminal Factor:* After 4 or 5 days of sexual abstinence, the sperm specimen is collected in a clean, dry glass container, kept at or below room temperature, and examined within 2 to 4 hours for volume, sperm motility, morphology, and cell count. About 3–5 ml. of viscid alkaline semen is normal; a normal count is 60–100 million per ml.

6. *Miscellaneous Factors, Including Immunologic Factors:* These are currently being investigated.

Management. Sterility may be difficult to treat, since it often is due to a combination of several factors. A total study program should be conducted, including a general physical as well as psychosocial evaluation of both mates. Statistics show that many couples undergoing study conceive without the cause of infertility coming to light; likewise, although some couples undergo all tests, the cause of the problem may remain undiscovered. Between these extremes, many problems, simple as well as complex, can be discovered and corrected, to the happy benefit of the couple. Between 25 and 50 percent of all infertile couples can be cured.

Therapy may require correction of faulty coital technique, surgery to correct a malfunction or anomaly, hormonal supplements, attention to proper timing, and recognition and correction of psychologic or emotional factors.

Note: Additional information may be obtained from the American Fertility Society, 1801 Ninth Ave., South, Birmingham, Ala. 35205.

Artificial Insemination

Artificial insemination is the deposition or introduction of semen into the female genital tract without sexual intercourse. If the sperm cannot penetrate the cervical canal normally, consideration may be given to *artificial insemination* using the husband's semen (A.I.H.). In the event of azospermia (lack of sperm in the semen), semen from carefully selected donors may be used (A.I.D.).

Two indications for using artificial insemination are (1) inability of the male to deposit semen in the vagina; this may be due to premature ejaculation, pronounced hypospadius, or dyspareunia (painful intercourse experienced by the female), and (2) inability of semen to be transported from the vagina to the uterine cavity; this is usually due to faulty chemical conditions such as may be produced with an abnormal cervical discharge. The latter may be corrected with chemotherapeutic agents.

Husband's Semen. Certain conditions need to be established before semen is transferred to the vagina. The wife must have no abnormalities of the genital system, the tubes must be patent, and ova must be available. In the husband, sperm need to be normal in shape, amount, motility, and endurance. The time of ovulation in the female should be determined as accurately as possible, so that the 2 or 3 days during which fertilization is possible each month can be utilized. Fertilization seldom occurs from a single insemination. Usually insemination is attempted between the tenth and seventeenth day of the cycle; three different attempts are made. Semen is collected in a wide-mouth, 2-ounce jar following masturbation.

Donor's Semen. A donor may be utilized when the husband's sperm is defective or absent, or when, for hereditary reasons, it is feared that an undesirable disease may be transmitted. Safeguards need to be set up to prevent legal, ethical, emotional, and religious problems. Written consent may protect the wife, donor, donor's wife, and legal status of the child.

The donor is selected on the basis of close resemblance to the husband, both physically and intellectually; there should be no family history of epilepsy, diabetes, or known genetic defects, and a negative Wasserman or Kahn reaction should be obtained.* Preferably, precautions should be taken so that the donor is not known by the recipient, and vice versa.

Procedure of Insemination. The recipient is placed in the lithotomy position on the examining table, a speculum is inserted, and the vagina and cervix are swabbed clean with a cotton applicator. Semen is drawn into a sterile syringe, and a cannula is attached. The semen is then directed to the external os. If this is contraindicated, the semen may be inserted directly into the cervical canal. Following the careful withdrawal of the syringe, the patient is to lie flat on the examining table for one-half hour. Thereafter there is no restriction on the activities of the woman.

*There are commercial firms which bank sperm in Chicago, New York City, Los Angeles, and St. Paul.

The success rate for artificial insemination is about 50 percent. About three to six inseminations are required over a 2- to 4-month period. Since this procedure is opposed by the Roman Catholic Church, this method should not be suggested to members of this faith.

ECTOPIC PREGNANCY

Ectopic pregnancy is a pregnancy in which the fertilized ovum does not reach the cavity of the uterus, but becomes caught and embedded in the fallopian tube or, occasionally, in the ovary or the abdomen (Fig. 44-9). As the fertilized ovum increases in size, the tube becomes more and more distended, until finally, about 4 to 6 weeks after conception, rupture takes place, and the ovum is discharged into the abdominal cavity.

Precipitating causes of ectopic pregnancy may be salpingitis, endometriosis, pelvic inflammatory disease, congenital anomalies of tubes, or spasm of tubes with muscular insufficiency. The Center for Disease Control reports that increasing use of fertility control measures such as tubal ligation and abortion has been directly associated with ectopic pregnancy.

Clinical Manifestations. The symptoms may start with attacks of colicky pain on the affected side, due to distention of the fallopian tube. When tubal rupture occurs, the patient experiences agonizing pain, faintness, shock, and air hunger. It is recognized at once that the patient is desperately ill; all the signs of hemorrhage— rapid, thready pulse, subnormal temperature, restlessness, pallor, sweating—are in evidence. Later the pain becomes generalized in the abdomen and radiates to the shoulder and neck because of irritation to the diaphragm. By vaginal examination the surgeon is able to feel a large mass of clotted blood that has collected in the pelvis behind the uterus.

Management. A history may be enough to confirm the diagnosis. However, some gynecologists do a culdoscopy and possibly a culdocentesis (aspiration of fluid from the cul-de-sac of Douglas); bloody, non-clotting fluid indicates intraperitoneal bleeding.

The treatment of ectopic pregnancy always is surgical. When the operation is performed early, practically all patients recover with remarkable rapidity, but without operation the mortality is 60 to 70 percent. The type of surgery is determined by the size and extent of local tubal damage; surgery ranges from conservative to more extensive. Very conservative surgery would include "milking" an ectopic pregnancy from the tube. Perhaps a resection of the involved tube with end-to-end anastomosis may be effective. Some surgeons today are doing a salpingostomy, which involves opening and evacuating the tube, controlling bleeding, and resuturing the tube to

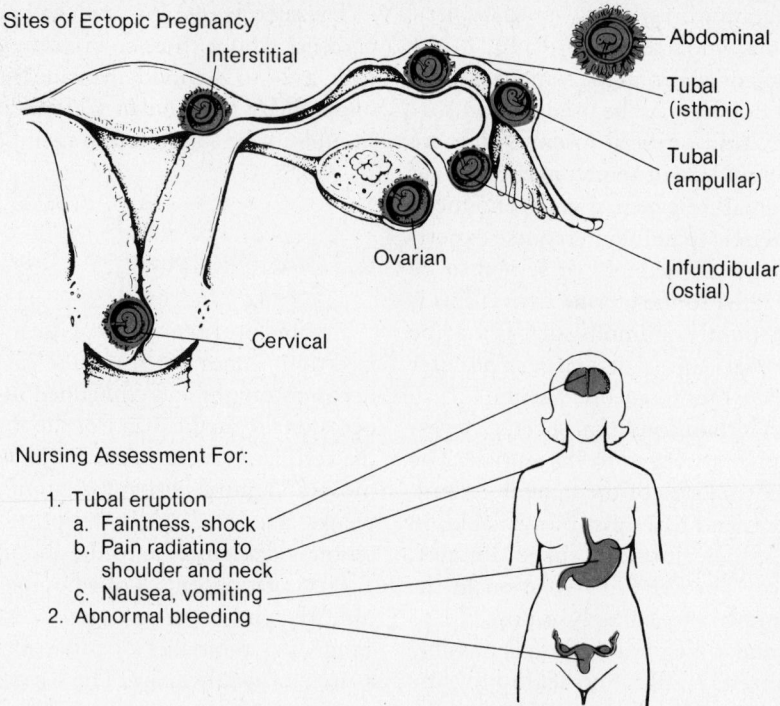

Sites of Ectopic Pregnancy

Interstitial

Abdominal

Tubal (isthmic)

Tubal (ampullar)

Ovarian

Infundibular (ostial)

Cervical

Nursing Assessment For:

1. Tubal eruption
   a. Faintness, shock
   b. Pain radiating to shoulder and neck
   c. Nausea, vomiting
2. Abnormal bleeding

Figure 44-9.   Ectopic pregnancy.

preserve it. More radical surgery includes salpingectomy or salpingo-oophorectomy. Depending upon the amount of blood lost, blood transfusions and treatment for shock may be necessary. Postoperative care is similar to that for any laparotomy.

BIBLIOGRAPHY

BOOKS

Anderson, B., et al.: The Menopause Book. New York, Hawthorn Books, 1977.

Borow, L. S., ed: Atlas of Gynecologic Laparoscopy and Hysteroscopy. Philadelphia, W. B. Saunders, 1977.

Boston Women's Health Book Collective: Our Bodies, 2nd ed. New York, Simon and Schuster, 1976.

DeAlvarez, R. R.: Textbook of Gynecology. Philadelphia, Lea and Febiger, 1977.

Danforth, D. N., ed.: Obstetrics and Gynecology, 3rd ed. New York, Harper and Row, 1977.

Green, T. H., Jr.: Gynecology, 3rd ed. Boston, Little, Brown, 1977.

Hatcher, R. A., et al.: Contraceptive Technology, 1978-1979, 9th ed. New York, Halsted Press, Div. John Wiley and Sons, 1978.

Ledger, W. J.: Infection in the Female. Philadelphia, Lea and Febiger, 1977.

Lytle, N. A.: Nursing of Women in the Age of Liberation. Dubuque, Brown, 1977.

Nichols, D. H., and Randall, C. U.: Vaginal Surgery. Baltimore, Williams and Wilkins, 1976.

Perlman, F., et al.: Urinary Tract Infection (UTI) Vaginitis Protocol. Boston, Beth Israel, Beth Israel Hosp. Assoc. and Mass. Institute of Technology, 1974.

Romney, S. L., et al.: Gynecology and Obstetrics, The Health Care of Women. New York, McGraw-Hill, 1975.

Shane, J. M., et al.: The Infertile Couple. Clinical Symposia. Summit, N. J., Ciba Pharmaceutical Co. 1976.

Taymor, M. L.: Infertility. New York, Grune and Stratton, 1978.

ARTICLES

Diagnostic Testing—Assessment

Cohen, S.: Patient assessment: Examination of the female pelvis, Part 1. AJN, 78:p1-p26, Oct. 1978.

Colon, V. F., and Schumann, G. B.: Gynecologic cytology. Am. Fam. Phys., 18:134-140, Nov. 1978.

Effer, S. B.: Gynecologic aspects of "routine" checkups. Postgrad. Med., 59:164-170, Mar. 1976.

Hebert, P., et al.: Colposcopy—what is it? JOGN, 5:29-32, May-June, 1976.

Homesley, H. D.: Evaluation of the abnormal Pap smear. Am. Fam. Phys., 16:190-194, Sept. 1977

Lindermann, H. J., and Mohr, J.: CO_2 hysteroscopy: Diagnosis and treatment. Am. J. Obstet. Gyn., 124:129-133, Jan. 15, 1976.

Magee, J.: The pelvic exam: A view from the other end of the table. Ann. Int. Med., 83:563-564, Oct. 1975.

Samuels, B. I., and Silver, T. M.: Diagnostic ultrasound in the evaluation of patients with gynecologic cancer. Surg. Clin. N. Am., 58:3-18, Feb. 1978.

Sargeant, E. J.: An aid to interpreting the abnormal Pap smear. Female Patient, *3*:59-62, Jan. 1978.

Tully, J. P.: The Pap test: Who needs it? Nursing '78, *8*:18-20, Mar. 1978.

Valle, R. F.: Intrauterine visualization by hysteroscopy. Female Patient, *3*:51-55, Jan. 1978.

Brueschke, E. E., et al.: Hysteroscopy. Am. Fam. Phys., *15*:126-130, Apr. 1977.

Fertility Control

A machine to predict ovulation time. Med. World News, *18*:40, June 13, 1977.

Balin, H.: Oral contraceptives, Am. Fam. Phys., *13*:109-116, Jan. 1976.

Connell, E. B.: A family planning expert comments on smoking and the pill. Female Patient, *3*:56-57, Feb. 1978.

Curtin, L. L., and Petrick, J. A.: Reproductive manipulation technical advances, options, and ethical ramifications. Nurs. Forum, *16 (1)*:6-25, 1977.

Deibel, P.: Natural family planning: Different methods, Am. J. Mat. Child Nurs., *3*:171-177, May-June 1978.

Easterbrook, B., and Rust, B.: A new role for nurses: Abortion counselling. Canad. Nurse, *73*:28-31, Jan. 1977.

Edgren, R. A., and Sturtevant, F. M.: Potencies of oral contraceptives. Am. J. Obstet. & Gyn., *125*:1029-1038, Aug. 15, 1976.

Freeman, W. S.: When patients "can't" take the pill. Am. Fam. Phys., *17*:143-149, Jan. 1978.

Heyman, A., and Hurlig, H.: Clinical complications of oral contraceptives. Disease-A-Month, Chicago, Year Book Med. Pub., Aug. 1975.

Hulka, J. F.: Spring clip sterilization: One year follow-up of 1,079 cases. Am. J. Obstet. & Gyn., *125*:1039-1043, Aug. 15, 1976.

Kilby-Kelberg, S., and Bradbury, B. A.: Diaphragm effectiveness depends largely on you: Patients practice what you teach. JOGN Nurs., *4*:24-32, Mar.-Apr. 1975.

Landesman, R.: Basic facts about contraception. Drug Ther. *8*:121-128; July 1978.

Manisoff, M.: Family planning democratized. AJN, *75*:1660-1665, Oct. 1975.

Pelvic inflammatory disease in IUD users. FDA Bulletin, *8*:19, May-July 1978.

Progestasert IUD and ectopic pregnancy. FDA Drug Bulletin, *8*:37, Dec. 1978-Jan. 1979.

Robbie, M. O.: Contraceptive counseling for the younger adolescent woman. JOGN Nurs., *7*:29-33, July-Aug. 1978.

Stern, M. P., et al.: Cardiovascular risk and use of estrogens or estrogen-progestagen combinations. JAMA, *235*:811-825, Feb. 23, 1976.

Taif, B.: The pill—how it affects your nutritional needs. J. Pract. Nurs., *27*:25- (+40), May 1977.

Tanz, A.: Barrier contraception. Female Patient, *3*:83-84, Jan. 1978.

Tyrer, L. B., and Hunt, R.: Counseling the patient on fertility control. Pract. Nurs., vol. 26, Part I, Nov. 1976, Part II, Dec. 1976; vol. 27, Part III, Jan. 1977, Part IV, Feb. 1977.

Tyrer, L. B., and Michaels, R. M.: Estrogens for contraception and menopause. Nurses' Drug Alert (special issue), *1*:169-180, Dec. 1977.

Vessy, M., et al.: Fertility after stopping different methods of contraception. Brit. Med. J., *1*:265-267, Feb. 4, 1978.

Zeitz, A. N.: Oral contraceptives: Women's rights, nurse's responsibilities. JOGN Nurs., *5*:54-55, May-June, 1976.

Human Sexuality

Burdette, J. A.: The routine sexual history. Am. Fam. Phys., *18*:145-148, Oct. 1978.

Lanahan, C. C.: Homosexuality: A different sexual orientation. Nurs. Forum, *15*:315-319, 1976.

Silverman, E. M., and Silverman, A. G.: Persistence of spermatozoa in the lower genital tracts of women. JAMA, *240*:1875-1877, Oct. 20, 1978.

Infertility

Gilbert, S.: Artificial insemination. AJN, *76*:259-261, Feb. 1976.

Marik, J. J.: Surgical management of secondary infertility. Female Patient, *3*:85-88, Feb. 1978.

Menning, B. E.: Resolve—a support group for infertile couples. AJN, *76*:258-259, Feb. 1976.

———: Infertility: Facts and feelings. Nurs. Dig., *4*:3-7, Summer, 1976.

Pakalnis, L., and Makoroto, J.: Reproduction and the test tube baby. Canad. Nurse, *73*:35-38, Feb. 1977.

Reckless, J., and Gieger, N.: Impotence as a practical problem. Disease-A-Month, Chicago, Year Book Med. Pub., May 1975.

Shane, J. M., et al.: The infertile couple. Clinical Symposia, *28 (5)*:2-40, 1976.

Winer, J. H.: The infertile male. Postgrad. Med., *38*:109-112, Nov. 1975.

Menopause

DeProsse, C. A., and Keetel, W. C.: The missed menstrual period. Postgrad. Med., *61*:251-256, Jan. 19, 1977.

Glowacki, G.: Postmenopausal gyn problems. Hosp. Pract., *12*:107-113, May 1977.

Gruis, M. L., and Wagner, N. N.: Sexuality during the climacteric. Postgrad. Med., *65*:197-207, May 1979.

Huffman, J. W.: Counseling the menopausal patient. Postgrad. Med., *65*:211-215, May 1979.

Seiler, J. C.: Estrogens for the menopause. Postgrad. Med., *62*:73-79, Sept. 1977.

The "new" estrogens: are they safer? Med. Letter, *18*:45-46, May 21, 1976.

Tyrer, L. B., and Michaels, R. M.: Estrogens for contraception and menopause. Nurses' Drug Alert (special issue), *1*:169-180, Dec. 1977.

Yen, S. S. C.: Estrogen and the menopause. Am. Fam. Phys., *16*:87-91, July 1977.

Menstruation

Yen, S. S. C.: Neuroendocrine regulation of the menstrual cycle. Hosp. Pract., *14*:83-97, Mar. 1979.

Pregnancy Termination

A vaginal suppository for abortion. Med. Letter, *19*:89-90, Nov. 4, 1977.

Barglow, P. D.: Abortion in 1975: The psychiatric perspective (with a discussion of abortion and contraception in adolescence). JOGN Nurs., 5:41-48, Jan.-Feb. 1976.

Cervical dilatation. Population Reports. George Washington University Medical Center, Series F., No. 6, Sept. 1977, F85-100.

Easterbrook, B., and Rust, B.: Abortion counselling. Canad. Nurse, 73:28-30, Jan. 1977.

Kopit, S., and Barnes, A. B.: Patients' response to tubal division. JAMA, 236:2761-2763, Dec. 13, 1976.

Progestasert (Progesterone-containing IUD). Med. Letter, 18:65-66, July 30, 1976.

Study shows D & E best midtrimester abortion. Med. World News, 18:71, Jan. 20, 1977.

Zeitz, A. N.: Oral contraceptives: Women's rights, nurse's responsibilities. JOGN Nurs., 5:54-55, May-June 1976.

Agency

American Association of Sex Educators and Counselors, 5010 Wisconsin Ave., N.W. Washington, D.C. 20016

45

MANAGEMENT OF PATIENTS WITH GYNECOLOGIC DISORDERS

CONDITIONS OF THE VULVA

The *vulva* (external female genitalia) is made up of the mons veneris, labia majora, labia minora, clitoris, vestibule, and accessory glands (Bartholin's, Skene's).

Inflammatory Conditions

Vulvitis, an inflammation of the vulva, usually occurs in conjunction with other local or systemic disorders, such as a dermatology problem, poor local hygiene, or venereal disease, or it may be secondary to a specific vaginitis. Hence, before therapy can be recommended, a complete physical examination is required, with pelvic evaluation as well as laboratory studies including vaginal smears, cultures, and blood studies to determine the possibility of diabetes. Symptoms may include complaints of itching and burning pain that is worse during urination and defecation. Genitalia may become red and edematous, and a discharge may be noticed.

Common related conditions include vulvovaginitis, e.g., moniliasis (candidiasis), trichomoniasis (page 984), venereal diseases (page 1372), neurodermatitis, and "idiopathic pruritus vulvae." This latter problem may be a psychosomatic disorder resulting from a precipitating factor, e.g., job frustration, marital difficulties. Other problems may include pyoderma, pediculosis, herpes, lichen sclerosus.

Management. Factors that may be involved should be assessed: (1) physical and chemical factors, such as increased perspiration plus decreased evaporation, antiperspirants, perfumes and powders, perineal soil, contraceptive jellies, vaginal discharges; (2) medical and endocrine factors, such as a predisposition for vulvar involvement in the diabetic, geriatric, or chronically ill patient; (3) anatomic factors, such as the nature of mucocutaneous tissue, nerve and secretory functions; and (4) psychogenic factors.

The patient should be instructed to avoid too frequent washing and scrubbing, particularly with detergent soaps, and to keep the area clean, dry, and free from irritation that may be caused by clothing that is too tight, perineal pads that may rub, and synthetic fabrics that may cause an allergic reaction.

Tight-fitting panty hose, pants suits, and slacks have caused an increase in vulvar and vaginal irritation due to fabric dyes, as well as restricted ventilation. Scratching should be avoided, since it compounds the problem. Talcum powder may be used sparingly to avoid irritation. Soothing compresses alternating with colloidal baths are helpful. Steroid cream may be prescribed; other medications are usually withheld until the specific cause has been determined. Then the medication is specifically directed to treating the cause.

Benign Cysts

A cyst of the greater vestibular gland is a cystic dilation of the duct of the Bartholin's gland resulting from obstruction. This is the most common of vulvar tumors and is located in the posterior third of the vulva, near the vestibule. A simple cyst may be asymptomatic. Infection may be due to the gonococcus organism, *Escherichia coli,* or *Staphylococcus aureus,* and can cause an abscess with or without inguinal adenopathy. Incision and drainage, plus antibiotics, are the best treatment.

A *Skene's duct cyst* is an obstruction of the ducts of the paraurethral glands, complicated with cyst formation and infection. Symptoms are pain, dysuria, and occasional dyspareunia (painful intercourse). Uninfected cysts may be excised; infected cysts are treated with appropriate antibiotics.

Potentially Premalignant Tumors

Lichen sclerosus et atrophicus, often mistaken for *leukoplakia,* is noted as very slightly raised whitish papules or macules of the vulvar dermis. Symptoms are usually mild or absent, in contrast to the intense pruritus of leukoplakia. It is believed that at least 10 percent of patients with cancer of the vulva have an associated lichen sclerosus, with or without leukoplakia. Biopsy and a careful follow-up program are definitely recommended. If cancer cells are detected on biopsy, a simple vulvectomy is performed, with continued follow-up.

Cancer of the Vulva

Preinvasive Cancer. Three types of intraepithelial varieties have been recognized: (1) Bowen's disease, (2) Paget's disease, and (3) squamous cell carcinoma in situ. The predominant symptom in at least two thirds of the patients is pruritus, but pain or soreness may be present. Diagnosis is made by biopsy. Treatment of in situ carcinoma of the vulva includes complete vulvectomy without lymphadenectomy. (With invasive carcinoma, the surgery is vulvectomy with lymphadenectomy.)

Invasive Cancer. Primary cancer of the vulva represents 3 to 4 percent of all gynecologic malignancies and is seen in elderly women. Long-standing pruritus is the most common symptom. Bleeding, foul-smelling discharge, and pain may also be present. The nurse is in a unique position to encourage a woman with this disease to seek help, since this is one of the most curable of all malignant conditions: it is visible, accessible, and relatively slow in growing. Although it begins on the skin surface and is easily noticed as a small ulcer that becomes infected and causes pain, women so affected seem reluctant to seek medical attention. Procrastination causes more extensive involvement, jeopardizing cure.

In addition to biopsy, which can verify the diagnosis, the Collin's test can assist in determining the extent of the lesion and whether other dystrophic lesions are present. This test is accomplished by staining the vulva with toluidine blue solution, allowing it to dry, and then washing the dye off with 1 percent acetic acid. Dystrophic and other abnormal lesions take up the stain and can be identified. Vulvectomy is preferred to radiation therapy.

The extensiveness of the vulvectomy depends upon the extent of the malignancy: For example, leukoplakic changes call for simple vulvectomy; carcinoma in situ requires a total vulvectomy; invasive carcinoma, a wide radical vulvectomy with pelvic and groin lymph-node dissection. Even with extensive surgery (pelvic exenteration) there have been encouraging recovery rates.

Management of the Patient Undergoing Vulvectomy

This patient must be allowed time to talk and ask questions. Fear of mutilation and loss of function is lessened when a woman of child-bearing age learns that the possibility of having sexual relations is good and that pregnancy is possible following a simple vulvectomy. Of course, the nurse must know what the physician has told the patient in this regard. Radical vulvectomy is more extensive and may require a second trip to the operating room for skin grafting.

In addition to the nursing care described on page 987, wide preparation of skin may include scrubbing the lower abdomen, inguinal areas, upper thighs, and vulva with a detergent germicide for several days prior to the operation. The extent of surgery is dependent upon the extent of the spread; more extensive lesions require deep pelvic node dissection. Occasionally even a part of the urethra, vagina, and rectum may have to be removed.

When the patient returns from the operating room, perineal dressings are more likely to remain in place and be comfortable for the patient if a T-binder is used. Groin wounds may be exposed, or covered with simple dressings. Pressure dressings may be placed over the wounds to aid in preventing the accumulation of lymph and serum. Many surgeons insert plastic tubes through the stab wounds in each inguinal area and attach them to portable suction. This arrangement facilitates apposition of tissue flaps and prevents accumulation of serum.

Since stitches may be taut because of the surgeon's attempt to approximate tissues, comfortable positioning is required. Perhaps a low Fowler's position, or occasionally a pillow placed under the knees, will relieve tension on the incision. Turning is important, and comfort may be achieved with a pillow placed strategically between the legs and against the lumbar region. Moving from one position to another requires time and patience on the part of both patient and nurse. Ambulation may be attempted on the second day.

Major nursing objectives are to prevent wound and bladder infection. The wound is cleansed daily with detergent soap solution, dilute hydrogen peroxide, or warm saline. After a *gentle* cleansing, a warm water spray is pleasant and nontraumatizing and enhances circulation. The wound should be exposed to the air at frequent intervals. While stitches are in, some physicians prefer dry heat from a heating lamp and, later, perineal packs or soaks. Plastic tubes are removed on the fifth to seventh day.

A low-residue diet helps to prevent straining on defecation, and wound contamination. Of particular concern is urethral and catheter care, inasmuch as an indwelling catheter is usually in place. The incidence of infection is high, which emphasizes the need for the best in nursing intervention. Many nursing researchers frown on the use of sitz baths for vulvectomy patients because of the likelihood of reinfecting the wound.

Analgesics are given as required for comfort. Since primary healing rarely occurs, debridement usually is done to provide satisfactory conditions for healing by secondary intention. Because the healing process is slow and the nature of the surgery disquieting to a female, this patient is apt to be discouraged. The nurse must be aware of the patient's uneasiness about being "caught" unduly exposed when visitors arrive or someone enters the room. She will tend to be sensitive and apologetic about odors. Thus cleanliness, deodorant sprays, immediate removal of soiled dressings, and adequate ventilation contribute to a more pleasant environment.

Posthospital care requires giving complete instructions to the community nurse or family member who will care for this patient at home. Gradual resumption of physical and social activities is to be encouraged. The cure rates of properly treated vulvar carcinoma are 50 to 60 percent. In the absence of lymph-node metastasis, cure rates are around 85 to 90 percent.

CONDITIONS OF THE VAGINA

Fistulas of the Vagina

A *fistula* is an abnormal, winding opening between two internal hollow organs or between an internal hollow organ and the exterior of the body. The name of the fistula indicates the two areas that are connected abnormally; a *ureterovaginal* fistula is an opening between the ureter and vagina; a *vesicovaginal* fistula, between the bladder and the vagina; and a *rectovaginal* fistula, between the rectum and the vagina. Fistulae may occur congenitally, but in the adult, breakdown often occurs because of tissue damage resulting from an invasive carcinoma.

Diagnostic Assessment. Methylene blue dye can be used to delineate the course of the fistula. In vesicovaginal fistula, the dye is instilled into the bladder and appears in the vagina; in a ureterovaginal fistula, the dye will not appear in the vagina. Following a negative methylene blue test, indigo carmine is injected intravenously; if the dye appears in the vagina, a ureterovaginal fistula is indicated.

Management. A fistula may develop inadvertently following vaginal surgery. It is not common, but the signs are important to detect. The immediate problem becomes one of infection and resulting excoriation. For example, the patient who has a vesicovaginal fistula has a continuous trickling of urine into the vagina. With a rectovaginal fistula, there is fecal incontinence, and flatus is discharged through the vagina. When such a discharge combines with a leukorrhea, a malodorous condition develops that is difficult to control.

Frequently, a fistula will heal without surgical intervention. Healing of the tissues is promoted by proper nutrition, with an increase in vitamin C and protein; by local cleanliness through douching and enemas; by rest; and by intestinal antibiotics. A rectovaginal fistula will heal faster if the patient is placed on a low-residue diet and if proper drainage of affected tissues is initiated. Perhaps a temporary colostomy may be required, to keep the site relatively clean; a surgical repair of the fistula may be performed, if necessary. If the person is older, more rest is required than in most postoperative patients, because of a higher incidence of debilitation, and the delicate as well as sensitive nature of the tissues. Warm perineal irrigations and controlled heat-lamp treatments are effective in stimulating the healing process.

For the patient who has had a repair of a vesicovaginal fistula, an indwelling catheter is usually inserted. Drainage from the catheter is observed carefully, and care is taken to assure that the catheter is functioning properly. If the catheter becomes clogged, urine may collect in the bladder, causing pressure that may damage the repaired tissue. Bladder irrigation and vaginal irrigations are done gently, with minimal pressure.

Effective measures to assist the woman whose fistula cannot be repaired must be planned on an individual basis. Cleanliness, frequent sitz baths, and deodorizing douches are required, as well as the use of perineal pads and rubber pants. Particular attention to skin care is necessary, to prevent excoriation. Bland creams or a light dusting of cornstarch may be soothing. Morale boosters and attention to the social and psychological needs of this patient are essential components of effective care.

Vaginal Infection (Table 45-1)

Leukorrhea and Simple Vaginitis. *Leukorrhea* is a whitish vaginal discharge, which in slight amount is considered normal at the time of ovulation, just prior to the menarche or onset of menstruation. The vagina is protected from infection by its acid secretion (pH 3.5 to 4.5) and the presence of Döderlein's bacilli. If the resistance of the patient is lowered and organisms such as *Escherichia coli,* staphylococci, and streptococci invade the vagina, a more profuse and yellowish mucoid discharge is present, and a simple *vaginitis* or inflammation of the lining of the vaginal wall develops. Often vaginitis is accompanied by an urethritis, because of the proximity of the urethra. The discharge may cause itching, redness, burning, and edema, which may be aggravated by voiding and defecation.

Treatment may be directed toward enhancing the natural flora of the vagina. This can be accomplished by a weak acid douche, 15 ml. of vinegar to 1 liter of warm water (1 tablespoon of white vinegar to 1 quart of warm

TABLE 45-1. VAGINAL INFECTIONS

CONDITION	CAUSE	CLINICAL MANIFESTATIONS	OBJECTIVES OF TREATMENT
Trichomoniasis	*Trichomonas vaginalis* (protozoan)	Inflammation of vaginal epithelium, producing burning and itching Frothy yellowish-white or yellowish-brown vaginal discharge	To remove exudate, relieve inflammation, restore acidity, and reestablish normal bacterial flora: Oral Flagyl For stubborn infections: oral plus vaginal Flagyl For recurrence: repeat treatment, and include sexual partner Some prefer vinegar douche followed by Floraquin vaginal tablets
Monilial infection	*Candida albicans* (fungus)	Inflammation of vaginal epithelium producing itching, reddish irritation White cheeselike discharge clinging to epithelium	To eradicate the fungus: local applications of gentian violet; Mycostatin vaginal suppositories To relieve other causative factors: stop antibiotic therapy; determine if diabetes or other systemic disease is present
Infection of Bartholin's gland (greater vestibular gland)	*Escherichia coli* *Trichomonas vaginalis* Staphylococcus Streptococcus Gonococcus	Erythema around Bartholin's gland Swelling and edema Development of Bartholin's abscess	To drain the abscess: antibiotic therapy; surgical drainage; excision of gland in patients with chronic bartholinitis
Cervicitis— acute and chronic	Gonorrhea Streptococcus Many pathogenic bacteria	Profuse purulent vaginal discharge Backache Urinary frequency and urgency	To determine the cause: cytologic examination of cervical smear To eradicate the gonococcus, if present: penicillin (as directed) or spectinomycin or tetracycline, if patient is allergic to penicillin To eradicate other causes: cervical cauterization
Postmenopausal vaginitis (atrophic vaginitis)	Lack of estrogen effects	Loss of redness, tissue folds, and epithelial covering of the vagina Itching and burning	To provide estrogen therapy for vaginal epithelialization: topical estrogen therapy; improve nutrition

water). In addition, beta lactose, a sugar, can be administered as a vaginal suppository. Upon insertion into the vagina, the suppository dissolves with body heat; the sugar then stimulates the growth of Döderlein's bacilli. An additional objective is to initiate chemotherapy. Local intravaginal applications may be dispensed from a tube with an applicator. The applicator is inserted into the vagina, and medication is expressed in the desired amount. Hydrocortisone vulvar ointment or cream may be applied locally after douching or sitz baths, as prescribed for symptomatic relief of itching. Cleanliness after voiding and defecation is stressed. During menstrual periods, tampons are preferred, since pads often cause chafing.

Trichomoniasis. *Trichomonas vaginalis* is a protozoan that is a common inhabitant of the vaginal tract. In some instances, however, when the normal pH, secretions, or mucosa are altered, an overgrowth of this organism occurs. If trichomoniasis is transferred venereally, the male may be the asymptomatic carrier who harbors the organisms in his urogenital tract and causes reinfection of his partner. The vaginal discharge is thin, frothy yellow to yellow-brown, malodorous, and very irritating. An accompanying vulvitis may result, with intense vulvovaginal burning and itching. In some women, the problem tends to become chronic. It is diagnosed by microscopic detection of the pear-shaped, mobile, flagellate organisms.

The most effective treatment appears to be metronidazole (Flagyl), given as a tablet orally 3 times a day with meals over a 10-day period. For stubborn infections, oral therapy is combined with a vaginal insert of the same medication. Some clinics suggest treating the patient and her sexual partner in a single-dose program (concentrated dose of Flagyl) under physician supervision. Some patients complain of an unpleasant but temporary metallic taste when taking Flagyl. Also, some note nausea and vomiting, as well as a hot and flushed feeling, when this medication is taken in combination with an alcoholic beverage. In view of these possible side effects, the patient should be advised not to take alcohol while on the drug.

Local treatment varies according to physician preference. Some prefer a thorough cleansing of the vaginal tract with a detergent soap solution, using cotton balls on a long Kelly clamp, to be followed by local use of suppositories, jellies, or powders containing appropriate medication.

Moniliasis (Candidiasis). Monilial vaginitis is a fungal infection caused by *Candida albicans.* It is seen commonly in patients with poorly controlled diabetes mellitus, which supports the fact that this fungus thrives in an environment rich in carbohydrate. Monilia is also found in patients who have been on antibiotic or steroid therapy for a while, since these medications probably reduce the number of natural protective organisms usually present in the vaginal tract.

In a recent study, Miles found that if *C. albicans* was cultured from the vagina, it was *always* found in the stool. Conversely, if it was not isolated from the stool, it was *never* found in the vagina. This strong correlation suggests that elimination of vaginitis cannot be achieved on a permanent basis unless special attention is directed to the gastrointestinal tract.

The vaginal discharge is irritating, watery, and tenacious, and may contain white, cheesy particles. The discharge causes itching and sometimes severe yeast vaginitis. White material may be noted adhering to the vaginal walls.

Management. Assessment of the patient includes identifying any underlying factors which may contribute to the overgrowth of monilial organisms, such as pregnancy, diabetes, or estrogenic or oral contraceptive medications. The patient should be informed that excessive moisture and chafing (such as may result from perspiration and tight garments, panty hose, etc.) may contribute to the problem.

Gentia-Jel is a convenient vaginal medication applied via prefilled disposable applicators each night for 12 to 24 nights. The medication of choice is nystatin (Mycostatin). Clotrimazole vaginal tablets are also effective. If vaginal tablets alone are not effective, oral nystatin, taken daily and concurrently, can control a possible intestinal source of infection. Antiseptic medications, such as Propion Gel, which contains calcium and sodium propionate, are also useful. Since clinical manifestations frequently disappear, early in the course of treatment, it is desirable to do a follow-up culture 4 to 6 weeks after treatment is discontinued. For the diabetic patient, efforts are directed toward controlling the diabetes.

Atrophic Vaginitis. A common postmenopausal occurrence is atrophy of the vaginal mucosa, which then becomes more prone to infection. An annoying vaginal discharge causes itching and burning. Treatment is similar to that of simple vaginitis. In addition, estrogenic hormones, taken orally or applied locally as an ointment, are effective in restoring epithelium.

Patient Education and Nursing Management. Douches are common therapeutic measures in the treatment of patients with gynecologic diseases. They are used both before and after operation and are of two types: vulvar and vaginal.

Vaginal irrigations are used therapeutically to cleanse or disinfect the vagina and adjacent parts, both before and after operation. They also serve to soothe inflamed tissues and to stimulate relaxed tissues. Occasionally, hot or cold douches are indicated in the treatment of oozing.

The patient is placed on the bedpan in dorsal position, with the knees apart and the labia separated. Prevent undue exposure of the patient. Protect the bed by placing a plastic sheet under the bedpan. Commonly used solutions include sterile water, normal saline, and antiseptic solutions.

Douches should be given at a temperature of 43.3° C. (110° F.) or as prescribed. To give the douche, the patient is placed in the dorsal position on the bedpan and covered, to prevent chilling. The tube leading from the douche bag is clamped, and the end of the tube with the douche nozzle is inserted into the reservoir, which then is hung not more than 60 cm. (2 feet) above the level of the patient's hips. The nurse then puts on sterile gloves, and, separating the labia with the thumb and the forefinger of the left hand, cleans the vaginal orifice and inserts the douche nozzle gently into the vagina for a distance of 5 cm. (2 inches), the tip being directed toward the hollow of the sacrum. The clamp then is removed from the tube, and the solution is allowed to flow. Pressure should be avoided, to prevent the douche fluid from refluxing through the uterus and the tubes. The solution can be allowed to flow intermittently until at least 1 liter of solution has been used.

The treatment should not be done hastily, if therapeutic benefits are to be achieved; it should take from 20 to 30 minutes. After the solution has been instilled, the nozzle may be removed, and the patient should be asked to strain, as if trying to move the bowels. This act tends to expel the fluid remaining in the vagina. The bedpan then is removed, and the parts are dried with cotton. The patient should be instructed to remain flat on her back for at least an hour after a hot douche.

After the douche has been completed, the apparatus should be cleansed and sterilized again (if not disposable), including the bedpan. When douching is done at home, the patient usually lies in the bathtub and follows the same principles just described.

Vulvar irrigations are indicated chiefly after operations on the perineum. They should be given after each urination or bowel movement, in an effort to keep the incision free from infection. The patient is prepared for a vulvar irrigation in the same manner as for a vaginal douche. Warmed sterile water then is poured gently over the vulva from a sterile container. The area is dried with sterile gauze or cotton, and a sterile dressing or pad is applied and held in place with a T-binder.

Vaginal antiseptic jellies are another form of medication which the patient can apply herself by means of an applicator. Creams or jellies can be used before and after operation, and in many instances they are substituted for the therapeutic and cleansing douche. It may be necessary for the patient to wear a perineal pad following application of medication.

The DES (Diethylstilbestrol) Syndrome

Prior to 1970, carcinoma of the vagina was considered to be a condition that occurred predominantly in the postmenopausal woman. However, in the early 1970s a research study revealed that seven adolescent women had developed adenocarcinoma of the vagina. Further investigation revealed that a common factor existed in such instances — maternal ingestion of diethylstilbestrol (DES). Subsequent studies of a large number of female offspring of women who had received DES during pregnancy showed that characteristic benign genital tract abnormalities had occurred in the majority of those young women who were exposed in utero. Follow-up studies continue in an effort to determine whether the benign changes noted represent premalignant lesions, and what percentage of such exposed young women are at risk for developing malignancies. As part of this ongoing research, daughters of women who took DES are encouraged to have regular gynecological examinations. In many instances, dysplasia noted in one examination had disappeared when the patient was examined subsequently.

Women who have taken DES should be encouraged to return for follow-up checks, even though they are asymptomatic. Such checkups include an annual pelvic examination, Pap smear, and breast examination. These women are to be advised to minimize their intake of estrogen preparations. Although oral contraceptives and DES preparations, taken as lactation suppressives or "morning-after" pills, are not contraindicated, a special task force of the United States Department of Health, Education and Welfare suggests that "the decision to use them should be made only after careful consideration of alternate methods of contraception, patient preference and medical judgment." The task force also recommended that administration of postmenopausal or perimenopausal replacement estrogens should be discouraged and that these substances should be given only to women who have "severe symptoms of the menopausal syndrome that cannot be controlled by other means, for the minimal duration necessary."*

RELAXATION OF PELVIC MUSCLES

Cystocele

Cystocele is a downward displacement of the bladder toward the vaginal orifice (Fig. 45-1). It is caused occasionally by tissue weakness, but most often it is a result of injuries received during childbirth. The condition appears some years later when genital atrophy associated with aging takes place. It occurs as a bulging downward of the anterior vaginal wall that causes a sense of pelvic pressure, easy fatigue, and often such urinary symptoms as incontinence, frequency, and urgency of urination.

The treatment of the condition is surgical, the operation for the repair of the anterior vaginal wall being termed *anterior colporrhaphy*. Perineal exercises sometimes are prescribed and help to strengthen the weakened muscles. These are more effective in the early stages of a cystocele. If surgery is refused or contraindicated, a pessary may be used (Fig. 45-4).

Rectocele and Lacerations of the Perineum

Injuries to the muscles and the tissues of the pelvic floor may occur at the time of childbirth. Because of tears in muscles below the vagina, the rectum may pouch upward, pushing the posterior wall of the vagina in front

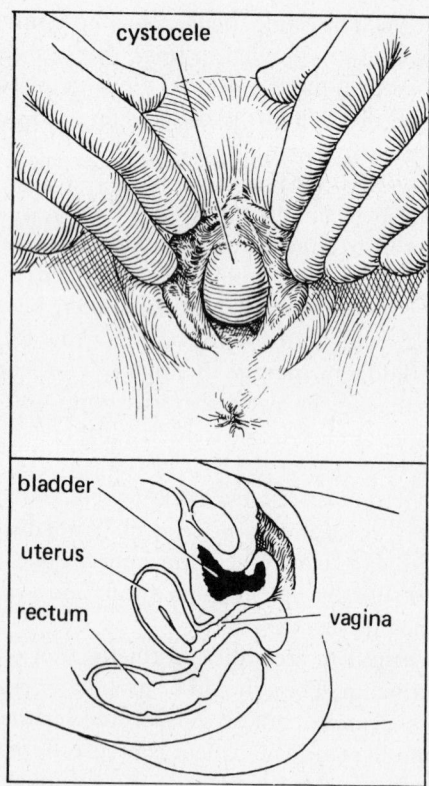

Figure 45-1. Cystocele. Relaxation of the anterior vaginal wall permits downward bulge of bladder, on straining.

*DHEW, FDA Drug Bulletin, 8:31, Oct.-Nov. 1978.

of it. This condition is termed a *rectocele* (Fig. 45-2). At times the lacerations may extend to such a degree as to sever completely the fibers of the anal sphincter (complete tear). The symptoms of this condition are similar to those given for cystocele, with the exception that instead of urinary symptoms, the patient experiences constipation and incontinence of gas and liquid feces when complete tears have occurred.

The operation for the repair of these conditions is called a *perineorrhaphy* or a *posterior colporrhaphy*.

The chief problem is to encourage women with these problems to see a gynecologist. There is a tendency to procrastinate, to feel embarrassed, to expect that in time the condition will take care of itself, or to even believe that this is a natural consequence of child-bearing that has to be accepted. Women need to know that the condition can become more restricting; it cannot cure itself, but can lead to complications such as infections, cervical ulceration, cystitis, hemorrhoids, and other problems.

Surgical Treatment

Preoperative Management. Before vaginal surgery, the patient needs to know the extent of the proposed surgery, the expectations for the postoperative period, and the effect of surgery on future sexual functions. Often, a clean voided specimen is required. If so, the patient is asked to clean her perineum, spread the labia, and void into a sterile bedpan. The specimen is then transferred to a sterile bottle.

In the operating room, special attention is given to placing both of the patient's legs in and out of stirrups simultaneously, in order to prevent muscular strain and excess pressure on the legs and thighs. Other preoperative details are similar to that described on page 307.

Postoperative Management. In the postoperative period, the objectives of care are to prevent infection and pressure on the suture line. This will require perineal care and may preclude the use of dressings. Voiding is to be encouraged. The patient always is urged to void within a few hours after operation, and every 4 to 8 hours thereafter. The bladder should not be allowed to accumulate more than 150 ml. of urine for the first few days, especially after operations for cystocele and complete tear. If the patient does not void within the above period, or if she feels uncomfortable, or has pain in the region of the bladder before 6 hours, catheterization should be performed. Some physicians prefer to have an indwelling catheter in place for 2 to 4 days. There are various other methods of bladder care.

After each urination or bowel movement, the perineum should be irrigated with warm sterile saline (see vulvar douche, page 985), and the area blotted dry with sterile cotton.

There are several methods used in caring for the sutures. In one method, the stitches are left alone until

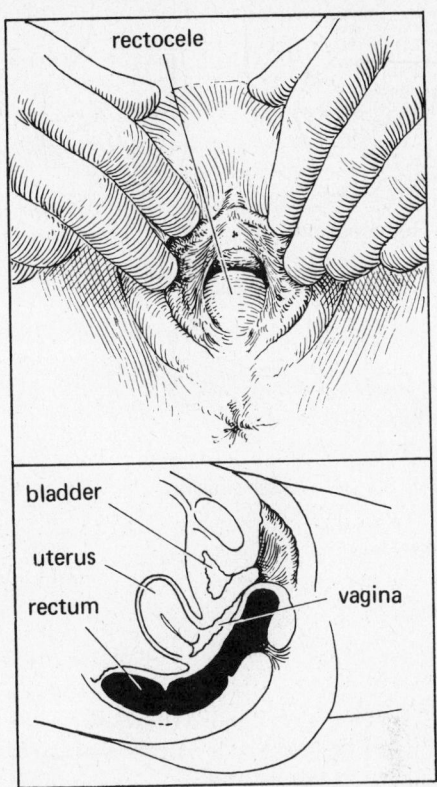

Figure 45-2. Rectocele. Relaxation of the posterior vaginal wall permits bulging of the rectum into the vagina, on straining.

healing occurs, i.e., for 5 to 10 days, and daily vaginal douches of sterile saline are given thereafter during the period of convalescence. In another method—the wet method—small douches of sterile saline are given twice daily, beginning on the day after operation and continuing throughout convalescence. Of course, the method to be used depends on the preference of the surgeon.

A heat lamp may be used to help dry the area and enhance the healing process. Commercially available sprays containing a combination of antiseptic and anesthetic solutions are soothing and effective. An ice pack applied locally may relieve discomfort. For effective relief of this type, a plastic bag can be filled with ice chips. However, the weight of the bag must rest on the bed, and not on the patient.

The routine postoperative care is much like that for an abdominal operation. The patient is placed in bed, with the head and the knees elevated slightly. A liquid diet (many surgeons omit milk) is given on the first day and then a full diet as soon as desired.

After an operation for a complete perineal laceration (through the rectal sphincter) special care and attention are required. The bladder should be emptied by catheterization if the patient is having discomfort. She should be kept flat in bed, with the head raised on a pillow. Most

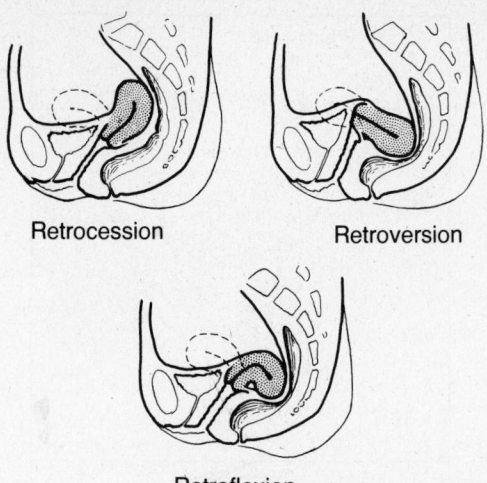

Retrocession   Retroversion

Retroflexion

Figure 45-3. Retrodisplacements of the uterus. (Hardy: Rhoads Textbook of Surgery. Philadelphia, J. B. Lippincott, 1977)

surgeons prefer that the patient have no bowel movements for 5 to 7 days, to prevent strain on the incision site. A rectal tube should not be introduced during this period, and enemas are restricted. Liquid diet without milk is given, and, in order to reduce peristalsis and inhibit bowel function, tincture of opium (paregoric) (15 minims) may be administered. On the sixth or the seventh day, 30 ml. (1 ounce) of mineral oil is given, followed, at the first inclination for a bowel movement, by a small oil enema, 90–120 ml. (3 or 4 ounces) that should be retained for a few minutes.

Throughout the convalescence of all patients who have had plastic surgery, liquid petrolatum or other stool-softening agent is given each night after the patient is permitted a soft diet. Instructions are given regarding douching and when to return to see the gynecologist.

Perineal exercises may be recommended to assist in strengthening muscles. The patient is instructed as follows: tense the perineal muscles by pressing the buttocks

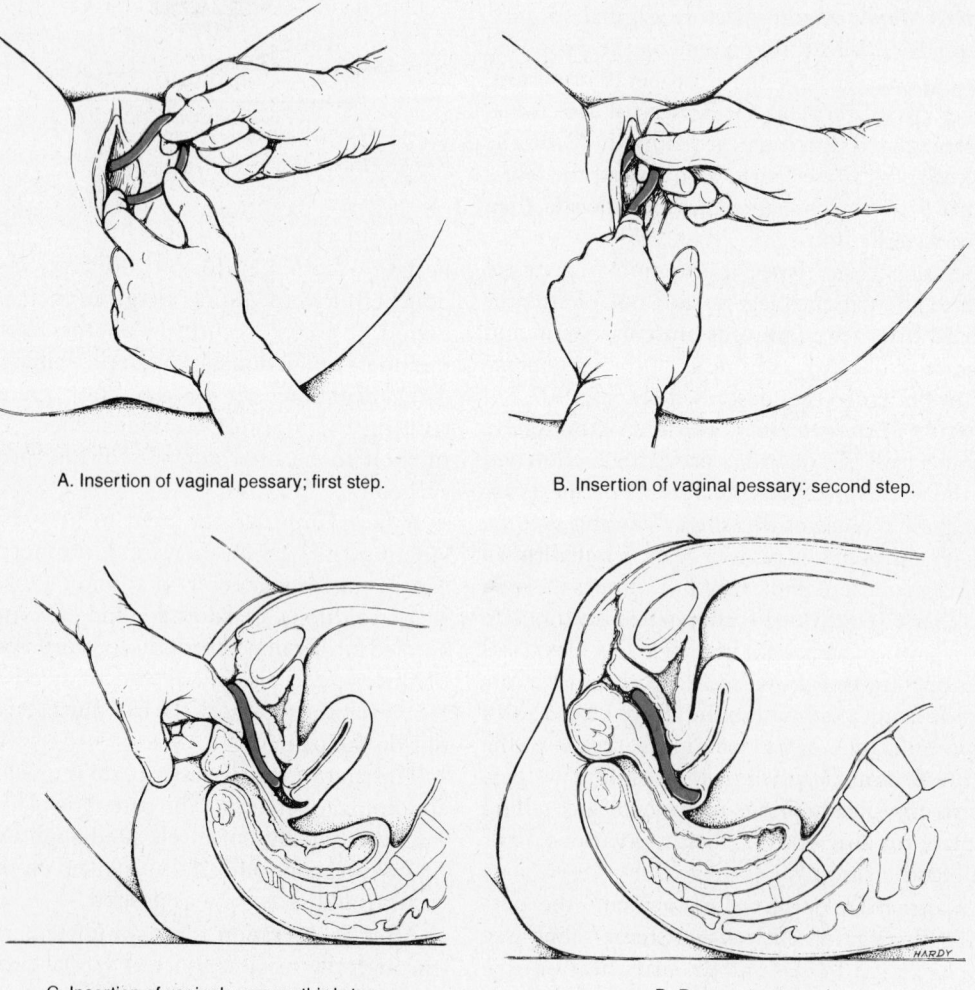

A. Insertion of vaginal pessary; first step.

B. Insertion of vaginal pessary; second step.

C. Insertion of vaginal pessary; third step.

D. Pessary in place.

Figure 45-4. Method of inserting a vaginal pessary. (Redrawn from Greenhill, J. B.: Office Gynecology, 9th ed. Chicago, Year Book Med. Pub., 1971. Used by permission.)

together; hold this position; relax. This exercise, done 10 to 20 times each hour, can be performed while the person is sitting or standing.

Displacements of the Uterus

The uterus lies normally with the cervix at right-angles to the long axis of the vagina and with the body inclined slightly forward. However, it is freely movable, owing to the requirements of pregnancy. The strain of this physiological function, the formation of adhesions, or a weakening of its natural supports may produce changes in the normal position of the uterus that usually cause no severe problems to the patient, but may give rise to many troublesome symptoms.

Backward Displacements (Fig. 45-3). Backward displacements (retroversion and retroflexion) of the uterus may give rise to such symptoms as backache, a sense of pelvic pressure, easy fatigue, and leukorrheal discharge. Most retrograde displacements are asymptomatic.

Surgery for backward displacements of the uterus is carried out only if the condition is incapacitating. An abdominal incision allows access to the uterus, which is brought forward into its normal position and is then maintained there by shortening its ligaments. Some patients with retroversion may be treated by the use of *pessaries.* These are instruments of hard rubber or crystal-clear Plexiglas that maintain the uterus in a forward position by exerting pressure on ligaments attached to the posterior wall of the cervix (Fig. 45-4). They are of great value as a test of the patient's symptoms, and often effect a cure. Pessaries must be removed and cleaned by the gynecologist at frequent intervals.

Prolapse and Procidentia (Fig. 45-5). Due to the weakening of the supports of the uterus, most often brought about by childbirth, the uterus may work its way down the vaginal canal (prolapse) and even appear outside the vaginal orifice (procidentia).

In its descent, the uterus pulls with it the vaginal walls and even the bladder and the rectum. The symptoms caused are similar to those mentioned for backward displacements, plus urinary symptoms (incontinence and retention) from displacement of the bladder. These symptoms are aggravated when the woman coughs, lifts a heavy object, or stands for a long while. Normal activities are troublesome tasks; even walking up the steps may aggravate the problem. Nurses can encourage women who have such difficulties to seek medical attention, because time is not likely to correct these conditions.

Patients with prolapse or procidentia should be kept flat in bed for 2 or 3 days, with a vaginal pack or a pessary in place. Since the best treatment is operative, this procedure serves to take the tension off the strained ligaments and allows the surgeon to proceed with greater

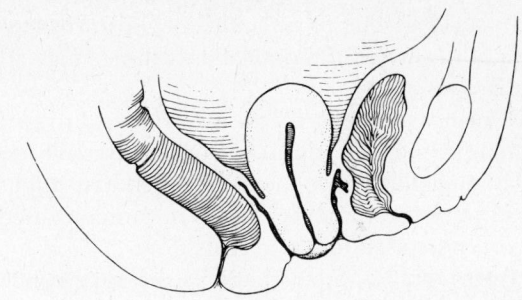

A. First-degree prolapse (cervix comes down to introitus)

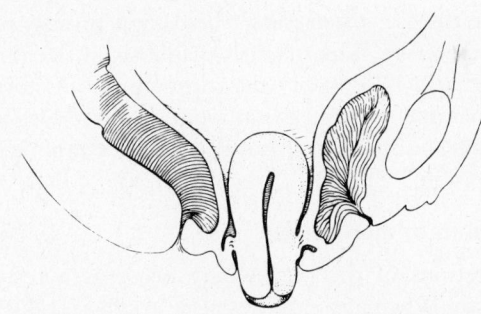

B. Second-degree prolapse (cervix protrudes through introitus)

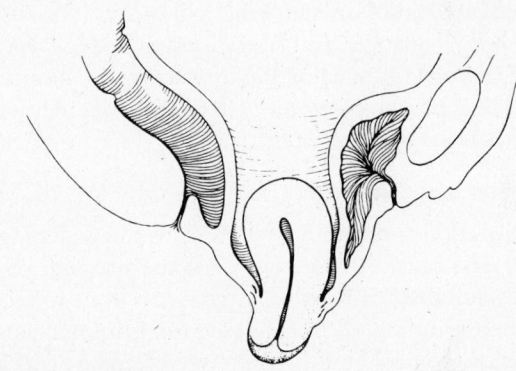

C. Third-degree prolapse—total procidentia (uterus protrudes through introitus)

Figure 45-5. Prolapse of the uterus and the vagina. (Adapted from Gray, L. A.: Postgrad. Med., *30*:209)

ease. The uterus is sutured back into place. In postmenopausal women, the uterus may be removed (hysterectomy). For elderly women or those who are too ill to stand the strain of surgery, pessaries may be the treatment of choice.

CONDITIONS OF THE UTERUS

Abnormal Uterine Bleeding

Menorrhagia. Menorrhagia is excessive bleeding at the time of the regular menstrual flow. In early life it may be due to endocrine disturbances, but with increase in duration of the menstrual periods in later life, menorrhagia usually is due to inflammatory disturbances or tumors of the uterus. Emotional disturbance may affect bleeding also.

A woman with menorrhagia is encouraged to see her gynecologist and relate the nature of the excessive bleeding. Although difficult to measure, an estimate might be given in terms of numbers of pads or tampons used in excess of those used for the regular flow.

Metrorrhagia. Metrorrhagia is the appearance of blood from the uterus between the regular menstrual periods or after the menopause. It is always the symptom of some disease, often cancer or benign tumors of the uterus; therefore, it merits early diagnosis and treatment. Metrorrhagia is probably the most significant form of menstrual dysfunction; the amount of blood loss is not important, but the fact that it occurred warrants further investigation.

Lacerations of the Cervix

Lacerations of the cervix may occur as a result of childbirth. When healing takes place, a considerable portion of the mucous membrane, which normally lies in the cervical canal, is everted. It practically always becomes infected and causes an annoying leukorrhea. Most surgeons believe that cervical lacerations predispose to cancer of the cervix, and for this reason these lacerations should be repaired, particularly in the fifth decade, when cancer is most likely to occur.

Dilatation and Curettage

A dilatation and curettage (D & C) is the widening of the cervical canal with a dilator and the scraping of the uterine endometrium with a curette. It is done to secure endometrial or endocervical tissue for cytologic examination, to control abnormal uterine bleeding, and as a therapeutic measure for incomplete abortion.

Since this procedure usually is carried out under anesthesia and requires surgical asepsis, it is performed in the operating room. Many gynecologists perform D & Cs under local anesthesia, supplemented with Valium or Demerol. Explanations as well as psychological and physical preparations are done by the nurse. The patient has a right to know what the procedure will involve (usually explained by her gynecologist) and what to expect in the way of postoperative discomfort, drainage, or incapacity. Many physicians do not require perineal shaving, but voiding and evacuation of the intestinal tract by small enema are usually desired.

In the operating room, the patient is placed in the lithotomy position, the cervix is dilated with an instrument, and scrapings of the endometrium are obtained by means of a curette. Tissue for biopsy also may be obtained with a electric needle or a punch biopsy forceps. A cone of tissue may be obtained with a cautery or scalpel.

Packing is placed in the cervical and vaginal canal, and a sterile perineal pad is placed over the perineum.

After the operation, a sanitary belt is used to hold the pad in place. When the pad must be changed while the packing is still in place (usually 24 hours), it must be replaced with a sterile pad. Evidence of excessive bleeding must be reported. Following the operation, the patient remains in bed for the remainder of the day, although she may get up to go to the bathroom if need be. No restrictions are placed on dietary intake. If pelvic discomfort or low back pain occurs, mild analgesics will usually suffice.

Endocervicitis

Endocervicitis is an inflammation of the mucosa and the glands of the cervix. It is a fairly common problem that may occur when organisms gain access to the cervical glands after abortion, intrauterine manipulation, or delivery. It is an infection which, if untreated, may extend into the uterus, tubes, and pelvic cavity. In the majority of cases the inflammation is caused by the ordinary pyogenic organisms, but gonorrheal infection of the glands can occur. Inflammation can cause erosion of the cervical tissue, resulting in spotting or bleeding. The chief symptom is leukorrheal discharge, at times associated with sacral backache, low abdominal pain, and urinary and menstrual disturbances.

Treatment should be preventive as well as curative. Prevention of gonorrhea will reduce the incidence of endocervicitis. Proper obstetric care can also prevent the occurrence of this condition. Delivery ought not to be attempted until the cervix completely dilates spontaneously; cervical lacerations should be repaired immediately.

Palliative treatment consists of douches and the application of antiseptics to the cervix, but often a cure is effected only after the cervical glands are destroyed with a cautery or the diseased tissue is excised. Anesthesia may or may not be required, since cauterization is a painless procedure. Following cauterization, the patient should rest more than usual for the next few days. The nature of vaginal discharge should be explained to the patient so that she can expect a grayish-green, malodorous discharge for up to 3 weeks, because of sloughing cervical tissue. A follow-up visit is recommended by the gynecologist in 2 to 3 weeks, when the cervix is checked for possible stenosis, which may require dilatation. Usually, 6 to 8 weeks are required for healing. Sexual relations are resumed upon recommendation of the physician.

For more severe chronic cervicitis, conization may be done, which may require overnight hospitalization. Anesthesia is optional. In the operating room, the tip of an electric instrument is inserted into the external os of the cervix and rotated to cut and coagulate a cone of tissue. After-care may require packing, but otherwise it is similar to that following electric cauterization. The patient should note any excess bleeding and report it to her physician.

Hysterectomy

Psychological Considerations and Physical Preparation. The psychosocial problems faced by women undergoing gynecologic surgery are similar to those discussed on page 958. Moreover, when hormonal balances are upset, as often occurs in disturbances of the reproductive system, the patient may exhibit depression and heightened emotional sensitivity to people and situations. Each patient must be understood in the light of such factors and approached and evaluated individually. This understanding must be shared by the family as well as the health care providers. The nurse who exhibits interest, concern, and willingness to listen to the patient's fears will add immeasurably to the patient's progress throughout the surgical experience, however temporary or prolonged that may be.

Physical preparation differs little from the details described for the preparation of a patient undergoing a laparotomy. The lower half of the abdomen, and the pubic and perineal regions should be carefully shaved and cleansed with soap and water. The intestinal tract and the bladder should be empty before the patient is sent to the operating room. This is most important.

Abdominal Hysterectomy. A hysterectomy is the surgical removal of the uterus. When the ovaries are removed along with the uterus, the procedure is referred to as a *total abdominal hysterectomy* and *bilateral salpingo-oophorectomy (TAH-BSO).*

POSTOPERATIVE MANAGEMENT. After operation, the principles of general postoperative care for abdominal surgery apply (page 347). In addition, because of the proximity of the surgical intervention to the bladder, problems of voiding may be expected; edema or nerve trauma may cause temporary atony, and an indwelling catheter may be used. If no catheter is in place, catheterization may be necessary if the patient has not voided after 8 hours. If the catheter is in place, it is usually removed on the third or fourth day. Bladder infection may result from the pooling of residual urine; therefore, the patient is catheterized after each voiding.

To combat the discomfort of abdominal distention, a nasogastric tube may be inserted before the patient leaves the operating room, especially if the surgeon realizes that excessive handling of viscera has taken place. If a large tumor was present, its excision could cause edema because of the sudden release of pressure. In the postoperative period, fluids and food may be restricted for a day or two. If there is abdominal flatus, a rectal tube may be prescribed, as well as heat to the abdomen. When peristalsis begins, the patient is served additional fluids and soft diet. Ambulation facilitates the return to normal.

Vascular disorders, such as phlebitis, thrombosis, or edema, must be guarded against. Frequent changes of position and avoidance of high Fowler's position and pressure under the knee will minimize stasis and pooling of blood. The nurse must be particularly alert if the patient has varicose veins in her legs. Special leg exercises to promote circulation and the application of elastic stockings or bandages can be helpful.

In patients who are anemic because of loss of blood due to a tumor, convalescence may be hastened by a high-protein diet supplemented by iron salts. If the tumor was large enough to produce marked relaxation of the abdominal walls, the patient may be advised to wear an abdominal support or a girdle for a time after the operation. In the immediate postoperative period, the surgeon may have applied an abdominal binder to be worn until the support is obtained.

In anticipation of posthospital care, the nurse provides opportunities for the patient to ask questions. The patient should be aware of the nature of her surgery and the immediate and long-range limitations, if any, imposed by it. Hormonal replacement may be prescribed by the physician. The patient needs to know when sexual relations and her usual physical activities can be resumed. Annual or more frequent physical examinations, including gynecologic evaluation, are imperative for maintaining peace of mind and detecting early evidence of pathology.

Vaginal Hysterectomy. In some women, and especially in women in whom prolapse has occurred, the uterus may be removed through the vagina. Entry via the abdomen is avoided, since in a vaginal hysterectomy, the entire procedure is carried out through the vagina. Either the uterus alone is removed or the uterus, the fallopian tubes, and the ovaries are taken out. Postoperative care of such patients is similar to that of patients who have undergone plastic surgical procedures (see page 987).

Physically, the patient recovers more quickly because there is no abdominal incision. However, she does require psychosocial support to help her adjust to the unnerving sensations triggered by occasional abdominal cramps which occur even though the uterus has been removed. There may also be a loss of vaginal sensation that can last for months. The patient should be assured that these paradoxical feelings will gradually disappear.

Tumors of the Uterus

Incidence and Patient Education. Malignant tumors of the female reproductive system (excluding the breast) rank as the second cause of death in the United States,

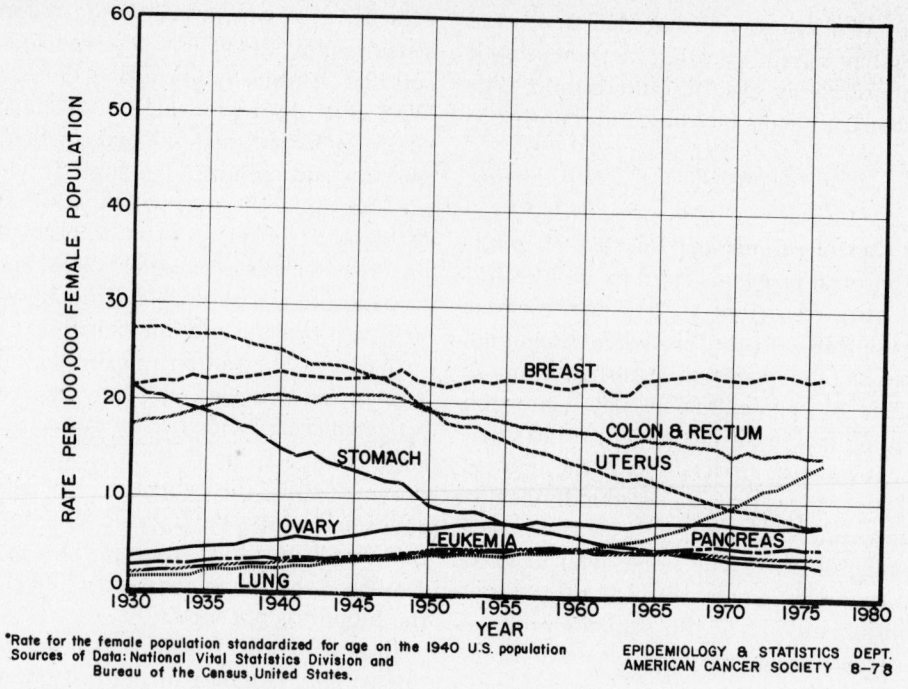

Figure 45-6. Female cancer death rates by site.

accounting for approximately 11,000 deaths yearly. However, the death rate for uterine cancer has shown a steady decline in recent years (Fig. 45-6), because more women are being educated to seek annual checkups that include the Papanicolaou test. However, when it is realized that only 53 percent of women over 20 have ever had a Pap test, it is obvious that much remains to be done.

Why a woman who knows about the Papanicolaou test does not have it done is a question to be explored by all those concerned with public health. Are women who feel and look healthy afraid to "look for trouble"? Is getting to the clinic or physician inconvenient, because of hours, transportation, or babysitting difficulties? Not only is the continued dissemination of information necessary, but it may be necessary for health personnel to "go more than halfway" in order to ensure the broadest possible application of this test. Perhaps a routine Papanicolaou test could be a required part of preemployment examinations, applications for marriage license, admissions to a hospital, and applications for insurance. Whatever measures are followed, an increase in the number of women having this simple, painless test will save lives that otherwise would be claimed by cancer.

There are two main types of primary uterine cancer — carcinoma of the cervix, which is predominantly epidermoid cancer, and carcinoma of the endometrium (corpus and body of the uterus). The incidence ratio of carcinoma of the cervix to carcinoma of the endometrium is 3 to 1.

Cancer of the Cervix

Cancer of the cervix is the most common cancer of the reproductive system in women. Although it rarely occurs before the age of 20, it is most common between the ages of 30 to 50. Statistics indicate that sexual activity has some relationship to the incidence of cancer of the cervix; before age 25, it is more prevalent in those who have had many sex partners and several pregnancies. Studies made on the incidence of cervical cancer among prostitutes also tend toward this conclusion.

Patient Education. Cervical cancer is almost always curable in its preinvasive state. Therefore, in an effort to discover the disease early, every woman over 20 years of age should have a complete gynecologic examination yearly. For the young woman under 20 who is sexually active, an annual Pap test is justified.

Although herpes simplex viral infection of the female genital tract has been tentatively linked to cervical carcinoma, this relationship has not been proven. Regular Pap smears will detect premalignant cervical dysplasia, so that women who have this type of infection and a positive Pap smear for premalignant cervical dysplasia should be advised to have a subsequent checkup within 6 months.

Clinical Manifestations. Early cancer of the cervix is usually asymptomatic. The two chief symptoms of early carcinoma of the cervix are leukorrhea and irregular vaginal bleeding or spotting. For a long time the leukorrhea may be the only abnormal symptom. The discharge increases gradually in amount, becomes watery and, finally, dark and foul-smelling because of necrosis and infection of the tumor mass. The bleeding occurs at irregular intervals, between periods (metrorrhagia) or after menopause. It may be very slight, just enough to spot the undergarments, and it is noted usually after some form of trauma (intercourse, douching, or defeca-

tion). As the disease continues, the bleeding may become constant and may increase in amount.

Chronic infections and erosions of the cervix seem to play a significant part in the development of cervical cancer. Such pathology becomes evident as a large cauliflowerlike growth or a deep, ulcerating crater before giving any symptoms of its presence.

As the cancer advances, the tissues outside the cervix may be invaded, including the lymph glands anterior to

TABLE 45-2. INTERNATIONAL CLASSIFICATION OF CARCINOMA OF THE UTERINE CERVIX

STAGE OF LESION	AREA	DESCRIPTION	POSSIBLE THERAPY	APPROXIMATE RECOVERY RATE
Stage 0	Carcinoma in situ	Cancer limited to epithelial layer; no evidence of invasion	Conization—fertility is preserved Hysterectomy, when fertility is not a consideration	95-100%
Stage I	Carcinoma strictly confined to cervix	Size is not a criterion		70-85%
Stage IA		Microinvasive	Radiation therapy or surgery (depending on depth of invasion)	
Stage IB		Clinically obvious Stage I	Radiation therapy or surgery (depending on depth of invasion) Wertheim abdominal hysterectomy and pelvic lymphadenectomy or radical Schauta vaginal hysterectomy	
Stage II	Vaginal cancer	Lesion has spread beyond cervix to involve vagina (not lower third) and/or paracervical region on one or both sides.		
Stage IIA		Vaginal extension only	Primary radiation therapy or primary radical therapy	65-75%
Stage IIB		Paracervical extension with or without vaginal involvement	Primary radiation therapy; if this fails, pelvic exenteration may be required	50-65%
Stage III	Cancer involves lower third of vagina or has extended to one or both pelvic walls.	Unequivocal palpable lymph node disease on the pelvic wall IV pyelogram shows one or both ureters obstructed by the tumor	Primary treatment by radiation If bilateral obstruction exists and renal function is compromised, preliminary nephrostomy may be required	20-30%
Stage IIIA		Extends to lower third of vagina only		
Stage IIIB		Isolated carcinomatous metastases are palpable on the pelvic wall		
Stage IV	Bladder extension	Evidence that carcinoma involves the bladder seen in cystoscopic examination or by presence of vesicovaginal fistula	Chance of cure by radiation is less than 5% Radical surgery (anterior, posterior, or total pelvic exenteration may achieve a cure rate of 20-25%	5-10%
	Rectal extension Distant spread	Carcinoma spreads outside true pelvis to other organs		

the sacrum. In one third of patients with invasive cervical cancer, the disease involves the fundus. The nerves in this region become involved, producing excruciating pain in the back and the legs that is relieved only by large doses of narcotics. The final picture is one of extreme emaciation and anemia, often with irregular fever due to secondary infection and abscesses in the ulcerating mass.

Surgical Management. Radiation is the most frequent form of treatment for invasive cervical cancer; however, radical pelvic surgical procedures may be required for the more advanced lesions. The method selected depends upon the stage of the lesion (Table 45-2) and on the judgment and skill of the physician. Radical surgery is advocated by some authorities, especially when a patient is unable to withstand the effects of radiation or has a radiation-resistant cancer.

Surgical procedures commonly carried out include the following:

Radical hysterectomy (Wertheim) — An abdominal incision is made, and the uterus, adnexa, proximal vaginal, and bilateral lymph nodes are removed en masse.

Radical vaginal hysterectomy (Schauta) — A vaginal approach is used to remove the uterus, adnexa, and proximal vagina.

"Radical" used before each of the above procedures means that an extensive area of the paravaginal, paracervical, parametrial, and uterosacral tissues is removed with the uterus.

Bilateral pelvic lymphadenectomy is accomplished by removing the common iliac, external iliac, hypogastric, and obturator lymphatics and nodes.

Pelvic exenteration (see this page).

Cancer of the Endometrium

Cancer of the endometrium (fundus or corpus) of the uterus has increased in incidence partly because of extended longevity and more accurate reporting. In the past, the ratio of cervical to endometrial cancer was about 8 to 1; now it is closer to 3 to 1. About 50 percent of all patients with postmenopausal bleeding have cancer of the fundus. Its progress is slow, metastasis occurs later, and the symptom of irregular vaginal bleeding often appears early enough in the disease to allow cure by removal of the uterus. In late metastasis, radium and roentgen rays are the usual therapeutic measures.

Heretofore, dilatation and curettage was the only means of early diagnosis. The Pap smear is inadequate because it alerts the physician only to about 25 percent of endometrial lesions; consequently diagnosis is made only after the development of overt symptoms. Endometrial smears (see page 962) are more accurate and relatively inexpensive.

Not all patients qualify for the use of these diagnostic aids because of complicating factors such as pelvic infection, stenosed cervix, or lack of cooperation on the part of the patient. However, they are helpful for those women who are unable to take the time to enter a hospital for a D & C, those for whom general anesthesia is not advisable, and those for whom D & C must be repeated or has been unsuccessful.

The major emphasis for the nurse is to encourage all women over age 20 to have annual check-ups that include a gynecological examination. More detailed nursing care following surgery or radiation therapy is found on pages 991 and 995.

Estrogen and Uterine Cancer. According to recent studies, menopausal and postmenopausal women who take estrogens have an increased risk of acquiring endometrial cancer. The Federal Drug Administration strongly supports warnings that advise health professionals and women patients that the risk is much lower if estrogens are taken in the lowest possible doses. The increased risk of endometrial cancer in estrogen users is proportional to the length of time during which the estrogens are taken (particularly 5 years or longer). It is recommended that estrogens not be given when they are not medically effective, such as in treating simple nervousness and depression during menopause or in helping women to feel and look younger. Estrogens are effective for the vasomotor symptoms of menopause if doses are kept low and treatment is limited to less than a year.

Pelvic Exenteration

Radical Pelvic Surgery. Pelvic exenteration, or evisceration, may be performed when other forms of therapy prove to be ineffective in checking the spread of cancer. When this therapy is contemplated, patients are selected carefully on the basis of their likelihood to survive the surgery as well as their ability to adjust to and accept the imposed limitations.

Anterior pelvic exenteration is the removal of the bladder and lower part of the ureters. In addition, in women the vagina, the adnexa, the pelvic lymph nodes, and the pelvic peritoneum are removed. The ureters are implanted in the colon or the small intestines.

Posterior pelvic exenteration is the removal of the colon and the rectum. In addition, in women the uterus, the vagina, and the adnexa are removed. The pelvic lymph nodes may or may not be excised.

Total pelvic exenteration is the removal of the rectum, the distal sigmoid colon, the urinary bladder, the distal portion of the ureters, and the internal iliac artery and vein. In addition, in the female all pelvic reproductive organs, lymph nodes, and the entire pelvic floor, including the pelvic peritoneum, levator muscles, and perineum are removed. Both urinary and fecal diversion are necessary in this procedure; hence, the patient will have a colostomy. A substitute bladder will be made from a segment of ileum.

Nursing Management. Although the following discussion considers pelvic exenteration from the perspective of the female patient, similar considerations apply to male patients who have undergone similar procedures. This patient has probably faced surgery before and is aware of most of the physical preparation required before going to the operating room. However, the most important preparation is psychological. This patient needs courage as she realizes what is about to happen and fortitude to be able to accept it. Consent to have the operation may have been given without question, since it may be clearly evident that this is a life-saving procedure.

The preoperative period is the time when a careful assessment of psychological, sociological, and economic needs is made. The patient's spouse or immediate family can be of valuable assistance in giving the patient hope and reason to live even with an altered body structure. Communication lines between the patient and professional staff must be open to be supportive. Strengths and weaknesses of the patient need to be identified, modified, and utilized so that the operation and postoperative phases will be approached in a positive way.

However, the full impact of adjustment may come several days after the operation. The patient may express feelings that will give direction to subsequent care. Usually, the patient's reaction takes one of three courses: (1) she may adjust very well without any abnormal complications; (2) she may become depressed and listless and may wish to die (this reaction may be altered with antidepressant medications; meanwhile, the nurse continues to emphasize the *positive* features of the patient's future); (3) there may be an insidious reaction in which the patient exalts her disfigurement, assuming an almost martyrlike pose. As she becomes preoccupied with herself and centers her attention on her disability, she may show pettiness, make selfish demands, and withdraw interest from her family. The nurse's hope in this instance is to try to turn the patient's thoughts from herself to others and to help the patient to see her body in its proper perspective, focusing attention on the intact parts.

This patient requires intensive care following the operation. Because satisfactory body function depends on adequate fluid balance, particular attention should be given to an accurate intake and output record. Proper functioning of the gastrointestinal tract may not return for several days. (See colostomy and ileostomy care on pages 780, 770.) Likewise, following radical surgery there is a greater risk of complications; therefore, the nurse must be aware of the signs and the symptoms of postoperative complications as well as the ways and means of avoiding such problems.

Teaching and rehabilitation are continuous in the care of the patient with a pelvic exenteration, moving gradu-ally from the simple to the complex. The family is included as the convalescence of the patient continues. The patient's reactions and day-by-day progress are observed carefully; encouragement and understanding go a long way in helping her to achieve as many goals as possible.

Leiomyomas ("Fibroids," Myomas, or Fibromyomas)

Myomatous or *fibroid tumors* of the uterus are benign tumors arising from the muscle tissue of the uterus. They are very common, occurring in about 20 to 30 percent of all women. They develop slowly between the ages of 25 and 40, and often become large in size after this period. There are instances in which such a tumor causes no symptoms. The most common symptom is menorrhagia. Other symptoms are due to pressure on the surrounding organs—pain, backache, constipation, and urinary symptoms. In addition, such tumors often cause metrorrhagia and even sterility.

Management. The treatment of uterine fibroids depends to a large extent on their size and location. The patient with minor symptoms is watched closely. If she wishes to have children, treatment is as conservative as possible. As a rule, large tumors that produce pressure symptoms should be removed. Usually, the uterus is removed (hysterectomy), while the ovaries are preserved, if possible. If the tumor is small, it may be removed (myomectomy); the wound in the uterus is then closed. This is the procedure of choice in young women. If the tumor is producing excessive bleeding, the uterus and the tumor are removed (hysteromyomectomy).

Principles of nursing management of the patient having a hysterectomy are on page 991.

RADIATION THERAPY

Radiation therapy plays a pivotal role in the treatment of gynecologic malignancy. In the treatment of squamous cell carcinoma of the cervix, it is frequently the procedure of choice. In the management of uterine and ovarian cancers, it is usually employed as an adjunct to surgery. In the definitive treatment of cervical disease by irradiation a combination of external pelvic irradiation and internal intracavitary irradiation is used. Only in the earliest microinvasive carcinomas of the cervix is internal (intracavitary) irradiation used alone. Cure rates of 85 percent or greater can be expected with cervical cancer that is limited to the cervix alone. As the disease extends into the parametria, the cure rate drops to approximately 65 percent. However, once the disease extends to the pelvic sidewalls, perhaps only one third of the patients will be cured, though many more will benefit from the palliative effects of irradiation as a result of the reduction in tumor bulk and the control of infection, pain, and bleeding.

External pelvic irradiation delivered by supervoltage equipment usually extends over 4 to 6 weeks. Thereafter, intracavitary radiation is performed. This sequence may be reversed, depending on anatomic considerations. The cervix and uterus lend themselves naturally to internal irradiation since they act as a receptacle for radioactive sources. Radium and cesium are two isotopes which are the mainstays of intracavitary irradiation.

External Beam Therapy. Betatrons, linear accelerators, and cobalt 60 units are capable of delivering high doses of well collimated irradiation deep within the pelvis to the site of the tumor. Radiation side effects are cumulative and tend to express themselves as the total dose exceeds the body's natural capacity to repair the radiation effect. A radiation enteritis expressed by diarrhea and abdominal cramping and a radiation cystitis manifested by frequency, urgency, and dysuria may ensue. This clearly does not indicate an overdosage. It is a natural manifestation of the normal tissues' response to the radiotherapy program. The radiation therapist and nurse inform the patient in advance of these possible side effects and employ a variety of measures to modify their impact when they occur. These measures include dietary control (by restricting the amount of fiber and roughage), the maintenance of fluid intake, and the use of antispasmodic drugs. On occasion, severe reactions will require that treatment be suspended briefly until the normal tissues repair themselves.

Internal (Intracavitary) Irradiation. In the operating room, an examination is performed under anesthesia, after which specially prepared applicators are inserted into the endometrial cavity and vagina. These devices are not loaded with radioactive material until the patient has returned to her room. X-rays are obtained to determine the precise relationship of the applicator to the normal pelvic anatomy and to the tumor. Only when this study is completed does the radiation therapist load the applicators with predetermined amounts of radioactive material. This is called *afterloading* and allows for precise control of the radiation exposure received by the patient, with minimal exposure of the physician and the nursing and health care team. A patient undergoing internal radiation treatment is placed in a private unit until the application is completed. (see Chart: Instructions for Nursing Care.)

Various applicators have been developed for intracavitary treatment. Some are inserted into the endometrial cavity and endocervical canal as multiple small irradiators (for example, Heyman's capsules). Others consist of a central tube (tandem or intrauterine "stem") placed through the dilated endocervical canal into the uterine cavity which remains in fixed relationship with irradiators placed in the upper vagina on each side of the cervix (vaginal ovoids) (Fig. 45-7). The Fletcher-Suit applicator is a well-known afterloading form of this classic tandem and ovoid pattern.

At the time of insertion of the applicator, an indwelling bladder catheter is inserted. The applicator is secured in place with vaginal packing. The objective of the internal treatment is to maintain the distribution of internal radiation at a fixed dosage throughout the application. Such applications usually last 24 to 72 hours, depending on dose calculations made by the radiation therapist and the radiation physicist.

Nursing Management During Radium Treatment

During the application, diligent nursing care must be given. The patient is carefully observed and attended, though the nursing staff must try to reduce as much as possible the radiation exposure to themselves. Nurses should stay in the immediate vicinity of the patient no longer than is necessary to give proper care and attention, and no nurse should attend the patient more than a half hour per day (see chart on page 997). Of course, a pregnant nurse should not be involved in the immediate care of such patients. Visits to the patient should not be aimless; nurse-patient contacts provide a good opportunity for the patient to talk about her anxiety and fear. To minimize radiation exposure, the nurse may stay at the foot of the bed or at the entrance to the room.

During the application, the patient will be on absolute bed rest. She may move from side to side with her back supported by a pillow, and the head of the bed may be raised to 45 degrees. The patient should be encouraged to

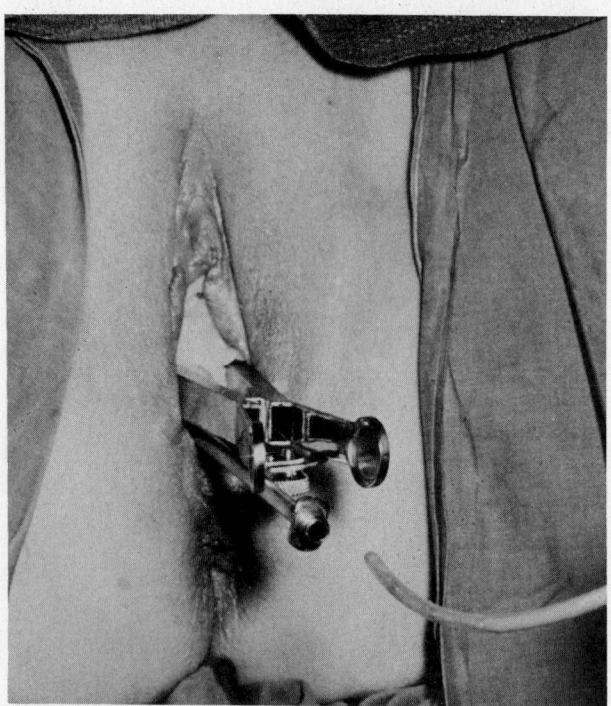

Figure 45-7. Applicator in position ready to be loaded. (From Hilkemeyer, N.: Nursing care in radium therapy. Nurs. Clin. N. Amer.)

Instructions for
NURSING CARE
of Patients Undergoing Treatment with Radioactive Materials*

_____ is being treated with _____ mgRa Eq of
        (name)

radioactive _____   _____ at
                (radium, radon seeds, Cs, etc.)   (date)

_____ M. The type of application or implantation is _____ .
        (time)

Precautions for hospital personnel to observe when handling patients who are undergoing treatment with encapsulated radioactive materials:

1. The PATIENT must be placed in a private room.
2. PREGNANT NURSES SHOULD NOT CARE FOR THESE PATIENTS.
3. NURSES should not stay in the immediate vicinity of the patient longer than is necessary (less than 1/2 hour per day) to give proper care and attention.
4. VISITORS should stay at least six feet from the bed and limit the visit to less than 3 hours per day. Children under age 14 and pregnant women may not visit.
5. If a radioactive source or applicator becomes dislodged from the patient, pick up the source with the long forceps provided and place in the lead container located in the patient's room. Notify the radiotherapist immediately. NEVER PICK UP A RADIOACTIVE SOURCE WITH YOUR HANDS.
6. Save all dressings, bed linens, etc. Do not vacuum the floor. Save floor sweepings in room. Dishes, trays, and eating utensils can leave the room. Do not save any of the patient's excreta or body fluids unless requested to do so by the radiotherapist.
7. After the patient is discharged, a radiation survey will be made to assure that no radiation hazard remains. The Radiation Therapy Department will then NOTIFY THE HEAD NURSE THAT USED LINENS AND DRESSINGS CAN BE REMOVED.

NOTIFY THE RADIOTHERAPY DEPARTMENT IMMEDIATELY:
In case of any doubt as to safe procedure.
In case of any emergency.
If any unexpected complications arise.
In case of death:
    before postmortem care is given,
    before an autopsy is performed,
    before the body is released,
During the day call Radiation Therapy Department, Ext. _____ .
During the night call Page Operator at _____ and ask for _____ .

*A form similar to one used at the Hospital of the University of Pennsylvania

---

practice deep breathing and cough exercises and to vigorously flex and extend the feet to stretch the calf muscles in order to promote venous return. Back care is much appreciated by the patient, but adequate care is given within the minimum amount of time at the bedside.

Usually the patient is on a low residue diet to prevent frequent bowel movements. One is less concerned here with dislodging the radium applicator than with the social and physical discomforts that the patient may experience. The nurse should inspect the catheter frequently to make sure that it is draining properly. The chief hazard of improper drainage is that the bladder may become distended. Although perineal care is omitted at this time, any profuse discharge should be reported immediately to the radiation therapist or gynecologic surgeon.

The patient is observed for evidence of temperature elevation, nausea, and vomiting. These symptoms should be reported, since they may be indicative of infection or perforation.

Finally, the radiation therapist takes steps to secure the internal applicator in place. Nursing personnel need not be preoccupied with the fear that the applicator will be prematurely extruded. However, one should check from time to time to see that the applicator or the radioactive sources have not been dislodged. Were this to happen, the radioactive source should be grasped with a long forceps and held at arm's length and returned to the lead container located in the patient's room. Radioactive sources should never be grasped with the bare hand. The radiotherapist should be notified immediately.

Radium Removal. The radiation therapist precisely calculates the radiation dose delivered. At the end of the prescribed period, the nurse may be requested to assist the physician in removing the applicator. As the sources are "afterloaded," they can be removed by the physician in the same manner as they were inserted. This does not require local or general anesthesia and is done in the patient's room. Medication with a mild sedative may be required before radium is removed.

Postinsertion Care. Slow, progressive ambulation is recommended after the period of enforced bed rest. The patient may shower as soon as she wishes; a vinegar or dilute saline douche may be prescribed. Diet may be advanced as tolerated.

CONDITIONS OF THE OVARIES AND THE PELVIC CAVITY

Ovarian Cysts and Tumors

Pathophysiology. The ovary is a frequent site for the development of cysts. These may be simply pathologic enlargements of normal ovarian constituents, the graafian follicle or corpus luteum, or they may arise from abnormal growth of ovarian epithelium. They are considered benign tumors with a possibility of becoming malignant.

Dermoid cysts are tumors that are believed to arise from parts of the ovum that disappear normally as ripening (maturation) takes place. Since their origin is undefined, all that can be said is that they are tumors made up of undifferentiated embryonal cells. They are slow-growing and at operation are found to contain a thick yellow sebaceous material arising from a skin lining. Hair, teeth, bone, brain, eyes, and many other tissues often are found in a rudimentary state within these cysts.

Clinically, cysts are manifested by their obvious presence as an ovarian mass. There may be lower abdominal pain that may be acute or chronic. Rupture may occur and simulate a variety of acute abdominal emergencies such as appendicitis or ectopic pregnancy. Larger cysts may produce abdominal swelling and pressure on adjacent abdominal organs.

Ovarian cancer carries a high mortality rate; therefore every effort should be made to diagnose this problem early. Because early signs and symptoms are similar to these of functional ovarian cysts or endometriosis, other means of differentiating benign from potentially malignant growths must be utilized. Manifestations include irregular menses, increasing premenstrual tension, menorrhagia with breast tenderness, and an early menopause. Before puberty and after menopause there may be precocious breast development and uterine bleeding. Virilization may be noted. Ovarian malignancy may be observed more frequently in women who are infertile, nulliparous, anovulatory, or habitual aborters. The identification of such a condition from information gathered in an initial assessment of the patient should alert the nurse to the possibility of early malignancy. Other high-risk signs include a progressively enlarging tumor or indications of a solid mass, as opposed to a cystlike growth.

Management. The treatment of ovarian cysts is surgical removal. However, if malignant degeneration has taken place, with invasion of the abdomen and general emaciation (general carcinomatosis), operation is of little benefit. The patient may be given roentgen therapy and testosterone. The abdomen may be tapped to relieve distention from ascites.

The postoperative nursing care after cystectomy is similar to that for abdominal surgery, except for one particular. The marked decrease in intra-abdominal pressure incidental to the removal of a large cyst often leads to considerable abdominal distention. This complication may be prevented to some extent by the application of a snug-fitting abdominal binder.

Endometriosis

Pathophysiology. Endometriosis is a benign lesion in which cells similar to those lining the uterus are found growing aberrantly in the pelvic cavity outside of the uterus. It is characteristically found in the young, nulliparous female. A similar condition affecting the uterine lining in older, multiparous patients is referred to as *adenomyosis*. At present these two conditions, which at one time were thought to be related, are now considered separate entities.

In order of frequency, pelvic endometriosis attacks the ovary, ureterosacral ligaments, the cul-de-sac, uterovesical peritoneum, cervix, umbilicus, laparotomy scars, hernial sacs, and appendix. The misplaced endometrium responds to ovarian hormonal stimulation and, indeed, depends on this for survival. When the uterus goes through the process of menstruation, this ectopic tissue bleeds — mostly into areas having no outlet — which then causes pain and adhesions. At surgery, these lesions are typically small, puckered, brown or blue-black, indicating concealed bleeding. If the endometrial tissue is within an ovarian cyst, there is no outlet for the bleeding and the formation is referred to as a *chocolate cyst*. Symptoms vary and may be misleading, since extensive endometriosis may cause few symptoms, whereas an isolated lesion may produce considerable symptomatology.

Incidence and Etiology. Endometriosis has been on the increase in the past several decades. There is a higher incidence among private patients who seem to marry later, bear children later, and have fewer children. In countries such as India, where tradition favors early marriage and early childbearing, endometriosis is rare.

Several theories have been advanced regarding the origin of these lesions: (1) reflux menstruation, or the backflow of menses, causes endometrial tissue to be transported to ectopic sites through the fallopian tubes;

(2) during surgery, endometrial tissue inadvertently may be transferred by way of instruments; (3) such tissue may possibly be spread by lymphatic or venous channels; and (4) tissue that covers the pelvic peritoneum and ovaries is a remnant of embryonic tissue. A combination of such factors may be responsible.

Pelvic endometriosis, rarely encountered in the black race, occurs in about 25 to 30 percent of women. It is thought to be the cause of 30 to 40 percent of all cases of infertility. Upon bimanual examination, fixed tender nodules may be detected and the uterus may be restricted in motility, indicating adhesion formation.

Clinical Manifestations. The chief symptom is a type of dysmenorrhea unlike typical uterine cramps. The patient complains of a deep-seated aching in the lower abdomen, vagina, posterior pelvis, and back that occurs a day or two before the menstrual cycle and lasts 2 or 3 days. Some patients, however, have no pain. Dispareunia (painful intercourse) may also be evident. Infertility is another possible effect.

Conservative Therapy and Nursing Considerations. Management depends upon the severity of the symptoms and the age group of the patient. Medical management is initiated with hormonal therapy that blocks ovulation. This relieves dysmenorrhea and postpones surgical intervention. When the function of childbearing is to be considered, conservative therapy is preferred, preserving as much of the reproductive tract as possible. Procedures of choice are resection of cysts and lysis (cutting) of adhesions. The likelihood of recurrence of endometriosis is high; however, the desire for and possibility of pregnancy takes priority. In women aged 35 to 45 years, ovarian tissue is saved when possible; after the menopause, atrophy occurs and the problem is solved.

Atrophy of the endometrium and subsequent amenorrhea may be produced by a synthetic androgen (Danazol, Danocrine) that is now available. However it is an expensive drug with unknown long-term effects. It probably acts by inhibiting release of gonadotropins from the pituitary gland, leading to atrophic changes in intrauterine and ectopic endometrial tissue. Endometriosis tends to recur when medication is stopped.

The nurse's role in patient education is to dispel false fears, such as a causative relation between the use of tampons and endometriosis—this is not true. In order to combat the upward statistical trend of endometriosis, women should be encouraged to have regular physical examinations. Unusual menstrual bleeding patterns should be reported and investigated.

Adenomyosis. In this condition, endometriosis involves the uterine wall; the incidence is highest in women from 40 to 50 years of age. Symptoms are hypermenorrhea (excessive and prolonged bleeding), acquired dysmenorrhea, polymenorrhea (abnormally frequent bleeding), and premenstrual staining. On physical examination, the uterus is felt to be enlarged, firm, and tender. Treatment depends upon severity of bleeding and pain; hysterectomy offers greater relief than more conservative forms of therapy.

Pelvic Infection (Pelvic Inflammatory Disease)

Pathophysiology. Pelvic infection is an inflammatory condition of the pelvic cavity that may involve the fallopian tubes (salpingitis), ovaries (oophoritis), pelvic peritoneum, or pelvic vascular system. This disease may be acute or chronic and may be caused by the gram-negative bacteria, staphylococcus, streptococcus, or venereal organisms.

Usually the site of infection and the method of spread serve to identify two types of infection: gonococcal and mixed infection. The gonococcal infection affects the urethra, cervix, and/or rectum. The disease can be self-limiting if it is properly treated and if reinfection is avoided. However, frequently the woman is reinfected and the secondary causative organisms (streptococcus, staphylococcus, *E. coli*) flourish, causing a chronic problem. This infection spreads by way of the uterine canal into the tube and fimbria.

The largest group of infections result from pelvic cellulitis, for instance, endometritis resulting from a complication of pregnancy or an intrauterine device. Pathogens spread by way of the lymphatics and blood vessels. Such a cellulitis tends to be unilateral, whereas gonorrheal infection is a bilateral infection. These pathogenic organisms usually are introduced from the outside and pass through the cervical canal and the uterus into the pelvis by way of lymphatic channels, uterine veins, or fallopian tubes. When pelvic infection is caused by the tubercle bacillus, it is usually conveyed by way of the bloodstream from the lungs.

Management. In order to give effective care, the nurse must know the cause, signs, and symptoms of pelvic infections, as well as methods of spread. The main objective of care is to keep the infection from spreading to other parts of the patient's system or to other people coming in contact with the patient. Spread of infection to others can be controlled in many ways: (1) perineal pads should be handled carefully with an instrument or gloves, and the soiled pad should be deposited in a paper bag for proper disposal; (2) hands should be washed carefully with a good germicidal soap; and (3) all items that come in contact with the patient (utensils, bedpans, toilet seats, and linens) should be properly disinfected by the correct procedure for controlling the specific organism responsible for the infection. The patient must be informed of the need for these precautions and encouraged to take part in plans to prevent contamination of others as well as protect herself from reinfection.

If reinfection or spread of infection occurs, symptoms

may include abdominal pain, nausea and vomiting, elevation of temperature, malaise, malodorous purulent vaginal discharge, and leukocytosis. The patient assumes the semi-Fowler position (dependent drainage). Catheterization and the use of tampons are avoided. In addition, the patient is supported nutritionally and with selective antibiotic therapy.

For comfort, heat can be applied to the abdomen externally and hot douches may be ordered to improve circulation. Proper recording of vital signs, the patient's physical and mental response to treatment, and the nature and amount of vaginal discharge are necessary to guide the physician in future therapy.

If untreated, pelvic inflammatory disease can lead to chronic pelvic discomfort. Scar tissue may close the fallopian tubes, resulting in sterility. Ectopic pregnancy could occur if a fertilized egg is unable to pass the stricture. Adhesions are a common development that eventually may require removal of the uterus, tubes, and ovaries.

The "caring" for the patient with pelvic infection is just as important as the "curing." This infection may be very distressing, both physically and mentally. Such a patient may feel well one day and develop vague symptoms and discomfort the next; she suffers from constipation and menstrual difficulties. These patients are frequently unjustly labeled "neurotic." The nurse must also keep in mind the social aspects of venereal diseases, which may cause pelvic inflammatory disease (see pages 1372 and 1392).

BIBLIOGRAPHY

BOOKS

Borow, L. S., (ed): Atlas of Gynecologic Laparoscopy and Hysteroscopy. Philadelphia, W. B. Saunders, 1977.

Boston Women's Health Book Collective: Our Bodies, 2nd ed. New York, Simon and Schuster, 1976.

DeAlvarez, R. R.: Textbook of Gynecology, Philadelphia, Lea and Febiger, 1977.

Danforth, D. N. (ed.): Obstetrics and Gynecology, 3rd ed. New York, Harper and Row, 1977.

Green, T. H., Jr.: Gynecology, 3rd ed. Boston, Little, Brown, 1977.

Ledger, W. J.: Infection in the Female. Philadelphia, Lea and Febiger, 1977.

Lytle, N. A.: Nursing of Women in the Age of Liberation. Dubuque, Brown, 1977.

Nichols, D. H., and Randall, C. U.: Vaginal Surgery, Baltimore, Williams and Wilkins, 1976.

Perlman, F., et al.: Urinary Tract Infection (UTI) Vaginitis Protocol. Boston, Beth Israel, Beth Israel Hospital Assoc. and Mass. Institute of Technology, 1974.

Romney, S. L., et al.: Gynecology and Obstetrics The Health Care of Women. New York, McGraw-Hill Book Co. 1975.

Shane, J. M., et al.: The Infertile Couple. Clinical Symposia. Summit, N.J. Ciba Pharmaceutical Co., 1976.

Taymor, M. L.: Infertility. New York, Grune and Stratton, 1978.

ARTICLES

Diethylstilbestrol (DES)

Bibbo, M., et al.: A 25-year follow-up study of women exposed to DES during pregnancy. New Eng. J. Med., *298*:763-767, Apr. 6, 1978.

Donahue, D.: DES: A case study. Cancer Nurs., *1*:207-210, June 1978.

Fuller, A. F., Jr.: The DES syndrome and clear cell adenocarcinoma in young women. Cancer Nurs., *1*:201-205, June 1978.

Hagg, S. N., and Herbst, A. L.: Evaluation and management of diethylstilbestrol-exposed offspring. Surg. Clin. N. Am., *58*:87-96, Feb. 1978.

Herbst, A. L., and Scully, R. E.: Adenocarcinoma of the vagina in adolescents. Cancer, *25*:745-757, Mar. 1970.

Herbst, A. L., et al: Clear cell adenocarcinoma of the genital tract in young females. Registry report. New Eng. J. Med., *287*:1259-1264, Dec. 21, 1972.

————: Clear cell adenocarcinoma of the vagina and cervix in girls: Analysis of 170 registry cases. Am. J. Obstet. & Gyn., *119*:713-724, July 1, 1974.

Ryan, K. J.: Diethylstilbestrol: Twenty-five years later. New Eng. J. Med., *298*:794-795, Apr. 6, 1978.

Schwartz, R. W., and Stewart, N. B.: Psychological effects of diethylstilbestrol exposure. JAMA, *237*:252-254, Jan. 17, 1977.

Radiation

Wharton, J. T., and Fletcher, G. H.: The principle of radiation therapy for malignant pelvic lesions. Surg. Clin. N. Am., *58*:181-199, Feb. 1978.

Uterus

Altchek, A.: Guidelines for hysterectomies. Female Patient, *1*:68-73, Mar. 1976.

Boutselis, J. G.: Endometrial carcinoma. Surg. Clin. N. Am., *58*:109-119, Feb. 1978.

Breeding, M. A., and Wollin, M.: Working safely around implanted radiation sources. Nursing '76, *6*:58-62, May 1976.

Cohen, M. H.: Estrogen therapy and endometrial carcinoma. Arch. Int. Med., *138*:526-527, Apr. 1978.

Cosper, B., et al.: Characteristics of posthospitalization recovery following hysterectomy. JOGN Nurs., *7*:7-11, May-June 1978.

Danazol—a new drug for treatment of endometriosis. Med. Letter, *19*:62-63, July 1977.

Gizynski, M. N.: Psychic trauma of gynecologic surgery. Female Patient, *3*:37, Feb. 1978.

Greiss, F. C.: Ovarian tumors, Am. Fam. Phys., *16*:170-175, Oct. 1977.

Hamilton, M. D., and Schlapper, N. B.: Pelvic exenteration. AJN, *76*:266-272, Feb. 1976.

Herpes simplex and cervical carcinoma. Med. Letter, *19*:52, July 1, 1977.

Hildebrand, B. F.: Nursing process and chemotherapy for the woman with cancer of the reproductive system. Nurs. Clin. N. Am., *13*:351-368, June 1978.

Jick, H., et al.: Replacement estrogens and endometrial cancer. New Eng. J. Med., *300*:218-222, Feb. 1, 1979.

Krantz, K., et al.: Quelling severe menstrual cramps. Patient Care, *12*:198-217, Apr. 15, 1978.

Lipsett, M. B.: Estrogen use and cancer risk. JAMA, *237*:1112-1115, Mar. 14, 1977.

Nagell, J. R., et al.: Evaluation and treatment of patients with invasive cervical cancer. Surg. Clin. N. Am., *58*:67-85, Feb. 1978.

Smith, J. P.: Chemotherapy in gynecologic cancer. Surg. Clin. N. Am., *58*:201-215, Feb. 1978.

Townsend, D. E.: Cryosurgery (gynecologic cancer) Surg. Cl. of N. Amer. *58*:97-108, Feb. 1978.

Update on estrogens and uterine cancer. FDA Drug Bulletin, *9*:2-3, Feb.-Mar. 1979.

Williams, M. A.: Earlier convalescence from hysterectomy. AJN, *76*:438-440, Mar. 1976.

Vagina—Vulva

Avery, W., et al: Vulvectomy. AJN, *74*:453-455, Mar. 1974.

Drugs for candida infections of the skin and vagina. Med. Letter, *21*:39, May 4, 1979.

Edwards, M. S.: Venereal herpes, a nursing overview. JOGN, *7*:7-14, Sept.-Oct. 1978.

Gizynski, M. N.: Psychic trauma of gynecologic surgery. Female Patient, *3*:37-39, Feb. 1978.

Gyne-lotrimin for vaginal infections. Med. Letter, *18*:66-67, July 30, 1976.

Huffman, J. W.: Office gynecology: Relieving dyspareunia. Postgrad. Med., *59*:223-226, Jan. 1976.

Hume, J. C.: Trichomoniasis—eight reasons why you should take it seriously. Med. Times, *106*:59-63, Aug. 1978.

Josey, W. E.: Vaginitis. Postgrad. Med., *62*:171-174, Sept. 1977.

Komaroff, A. L., et al.: Management strategies for urinary and vaginal infections. Arch. Intern. Med., *138*:1069-1074, July 1978.

Krupp, P. J.: Cancer of the vulva. Surg. Clin. N. Am., *58*:19-23, Feb. 1978.

Lukacs, J., and Corey, L.: Genital herpes simplex virus infection: An overview. Nurse Practitioner, *2*:7-9, May-June 1977.

McCormack, W. M.: Sexually transmissible diseases. Postgrad. Med., *58*:179-186, Sept. 1975.

Mead, P. B.: Management of herpetic vulvovaginitis. Female Patient, *3*:24-27, Feb. 1978.

Miles, M. R., et al.: Recurrent vaginal candidiasis. JAMA, *238*:1836-1837, Oct. 24, 1977.

National Cancer Institute: Important information about vaginal and cervical cancers. Med. Times, *114*:31d-36d, Nov. 1977.

Perlman, F., et al.: Urinary tract infection (UTI) vaginitis protocol. Boston, Beth Israel, Beth Israel Hospital Assoc. and Mass. Institute of Technology, 1974.

Rigg, L. A., et al.: Absorption of estrogens from vaginal creams. New Eng. J. Med., *298*:195-197, Jan. 26, 1978.

46
ASSESSMENT AND MANAGEMENT OF PATIENTS WITH BREAST DISORDERS

PHYSIOLOGY OF BREAST DEVELOPMENT

Up to the time of puberty it is impossible to find microscopically any difference in the breasts of the two sexes. At puberty, some slight swelling appears in the male breast. At the same time, a pronounced increase in size occurs in the female organ. This begins around the tenth year and increases rapidly up to the fourteenth and the sixteenth years. The development of the mammary gland is a result of hormonal action that begins with puberty in the female. At this time, the nipple takes on its natural protruding form. In the male, contrary to some statements, breast tissue always exists and may grow.

The breast is a glandular organ with many lobules; its secretion passes through collecting ducts to the nipple. In some women, there is a cyclic engorgement of the breasts, associated with tingling and tenderness; this is hormonal in origin. The symptoms begin usually in the latter part of the menstrual cycle and disappear when menstruation occurs. During pregnancy, about 8 weeks after a woman conceives, her breasts enlarge greatly, the nipples become more prominent and sensitive, and the breasts are prepared to nourish the infant. When pregnancy is over and lactation has ceased, the breasts shrink, lose their excessive fat, and often become flabby and flattened.

Psychosocial Implications

In Western cultures, the breast is considered a significant component of feminine beauty. Shapeliness is a quality much desired and is emphasized in a woman's choice of clothing. Particularly in the United States, the social value placed upon looking young has led to consumer demands for brassieres that further contribute to a trim, fit look. Thus, a woman's reaction to any actual or suspected disease or injury affecting her breast tends to reflect the prevailing societal view of the female breast. Not only do social values play a significant role in the rehabilitation of a patient who has undergone radical breast surgery, but the fear of disfigurement may prevent a woman from seeking immediate medical attention after she has detected suspicious signs or changes in her breast.

A major objective of the health professions is to spread sound advice regarding the prevention of illness and the detection of disease in its early stages. Every woman should be alerted to the early signs of breast pathology, and should be well informed about what to do about suspicious changes. The nurse has a major responsibility in the area of the prevention and early detection of breast diseases and in handling the concomitant psychosocial concerns of the patient. The nurse's associations with industry, diagnostic clinics, and community health agencies offer opportunities to teach and disseminate information, particularly concerning the value of breast self-examination.

INCIDENCE OF BREAST DISEASE

Although most of the disorders of the female breast are benign in character, the breast is one of the two female organs that are most frequently the primary site of cancer. The breast normally changes during menstruation, pregnancy, lactation, and menopause, and these variations must be differentiated from pathologic changes. Although the breast is fairly accessible to examination, the detection and accurate diagnosis of breast disease can be difficult.

About one fourth of all women have irregular areas in their breasts at some time. Just before menstruation, irregularities produced by hyperplasia and involution occur. These irregularities, which feel granular or finely nodular, usually occur in the upper outer quadrants. Some women have persistently irregular breast tissue that feels shotlike or plaquelike between periods. Such masses are not considered true masses because they usually are bilateral and neither increase in size nor consolidate. On the other hand, true masses do not fluctuate in size and are usually unilateral.

In both females and males, benign lesions of the breast occur more frequently than malignant lesions (70 percent benign vs. 30 percent malignant). Of the malignant tumors, 99 percent occur in females. Benign lesions occur frequently in premenopausal women.

The benign lesions, presented according to order of frequency and the common ages at which they occur, are: fibrocystic disease (20 to 45 years), fibroadenoma (20 to 39 years), and intraductal papilloma (35 to 45 years). By way of contrast, cancer of the breast is manifested chiefly in the menopausal and postmenopausal years, the incidence increasing progressively as the woman gets older. Approximately 75 percent of breast cancers occur in patients over the age of 40; less than 2 percent occur before the age of 30.

According to the latest statistics reported by the American Cancer Society, approximately 91,000 new cases of malignant breast tumors were discovered, and approximately 34,000 women died from the disease. The survival rate for all breast cancer patients, whether treated or untreated, is roughly 50 percent; the sooner women seek treatment and the lesions are recognized, the greater the possibility of survival.

ASSESSMENT

Breast Examination

Breast examination by palpation should be included in the annual complete physical examination of all women. (The examination procedure is described on page 66.) A breast examination should be done twice a year in women who have a family history of breast cancer.

Self-Examination of the Breast

Because 95 percent of breast cancers and 65 percent of early minimal breast cancers are detected by women themselves, top priority must be given to teaching all women how and when to examine their breasts. The nurse is in a unique position to offer this advice and to arrange for showings of the film *Breast Self-Examination,* available from local chapters of the American Cancer Society. The method of self-examination of breasts, which should be performed monthly, is shown in Figure 46-1.

The importance of this examination should be stressed, especially in the light of recent findings related to the occurrence of "interval cancers" (cancer that may develop after a negative screening visit and prior to the subsequent examination in the physician's office). Breast self-examination is essential in detecting these "interval cancers."

Some cancers grow very rapidly, whereas others grow very slowly. It has been reported that the course of a cancer from its inception to the death of the patient can be as short as 120 days; conversely, a chronic breast cancer has been known to last for 23 years without treatment.

Mammography

Mammography is a roentgenographic examination of the breast that does not require the injection of a contrast medium. The procedure takes about 20 minutes, can be done at most health centers, and is painless. (A balloon attachment may be used as a comfort measure when pressure is applied to flatten the breast while the pictures are being taken.) Usually two views are taken of each breast: a craniocaudal view, taken from above while the patient is seated, and a mediolateral view.

With mammography, breast cancer may be diagnosed before the appearance of any clinical manifestations. However, a skilled roentgenologist is required to interpret the findings. At the same time, it should be noted that this form of diagnostic examination has limitations since some carcinomas noted on clinical examination are not detectable by mammography. In addition, mammography is not as effective in studying very small breasts as it is for "fatty" breasts. More recently, certain architectural patterns of the breast have been distinguished, making it possible to identify patients who are at high risk for developing breast cancer.

At present there is evidence to suggest that a threshold dose level exists beyond which radiation could induce breast cancer. (Many authorities agree that a patient can have approximately 20 mammograms in her lifetime before the incidence increases from 1 in 13 to 1 in 12.)

Because of this, guidelines have been set up by the National Cancer Institute* to control exposure to x-rays in women, especially those under age 50.

1. Women over 50 should have mammography screening available to them.
2. Women between the ages of 40 and 49 who have a family

*National Cancer Institute and American Cancer Society Statement on X-ray Mammography in Screening for Breast Cancer. U.S. Dept. of Health, Education, and Welfare, Bethesda, Md. Aug. 23, 1976.

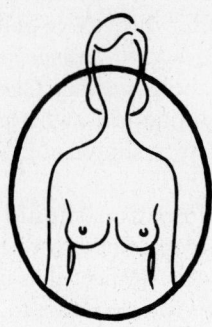 (1) Sit or stand in front of your mirror, with your arms relaxed at your sides, and examine your breasts carefully for any changes in size and shape. Look for any puckering or dimpling of the skin, and for any discharge or change in the nipples.

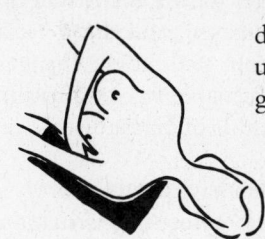 (5) Now bring your left arm down to your side, and still using the flat part of your fingers, feel under your armpit.

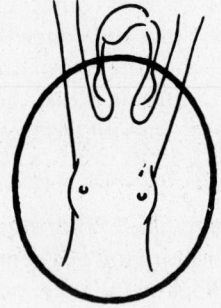 (2) Raise both arms over your head, and look for exactly the same things. See if there has been any change since you last examined your breasts.

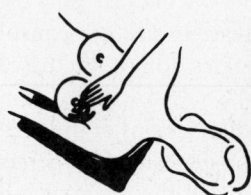 (6) Use the same gentle pressure to feel the upper, outer quarter of your breast from the nipple line to where your arm is resting.

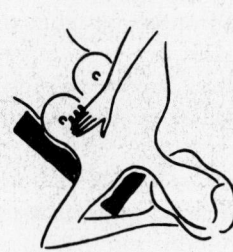 (3) Lie down on your bed, put a pillow or a bath towel under your left shoulder, and place your left hand under your head. (From this step through Step 8, you should feel for a lump or thickening.) Holding your right hand flat, with fingers together, press gently but firmly with small circular motions to feel the inner upper quarter of your left breast, starting at your breastbone and going outward toward the nipple line. Also feel the area around the nipple.

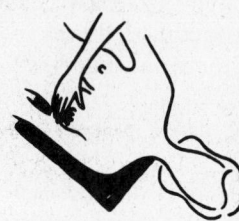 (7) Finally, feel the lower outer section of your breast, going from the outer part to the nipple.

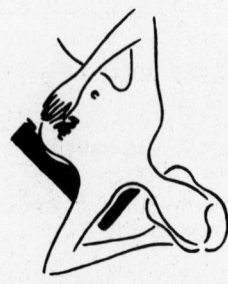 (4) With the same gentle pressure, feel the lower inner part of your breast. Incidentally, in this area you will feel a ridge of firm tissue or flesh. Don't be alarmed. This is perfectly normal.

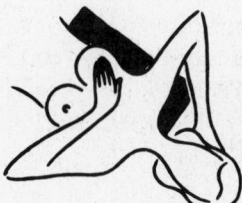 (8) Repeat the entire procedure, as described, on the right breast.

Figure 46-1. Self-examination of the breast. (Courtesy, American Cancer Society, Inc.)

BREAST EXAMINATION OF A WOMAN BY THE NURSE

Preparation: 1. By Examiner—Provide a good light.
Warm the hands under warm water (then dry) before touching the patient; if humidity is high, causing the hand to stick, dust hands with talcum powder.

2. By Examinee—Woman strips to the waist and sits in a comfortable position facing the examiner.

A. Woman sits with arms at her sides:
1. Compare contour of the two breasts; focus in a direct line from axillary crease to midline on each side.

    Observe for asymmetry, such as that caused by elevation of a nipple, dimpling, redness, bulging, orange-peel skin, flattening of normal contour.

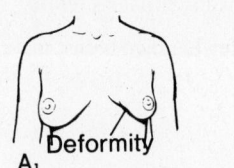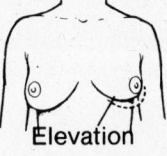

2. Palpate supraclavicular area.

    Note whether lymph nodes are enlarged, fixed, or movable.

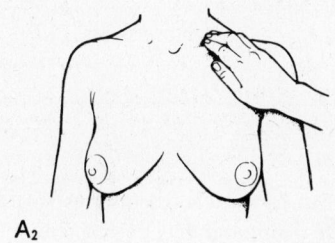

3. Examine axillary nodes.

    To relax pectoral muscles, support the woman's arm on one of your arms; with the palm of the other hand, use the fingertips to gently palpate the nodes lying against the thoracic wall. Gently rotate fingers downward. Note number, consistency, and mobility of nodes and whether they are fixed to underlying structures or overlying skin. (Fig. 46-2 shows lymph node distribution). Take the arm through the full range of motion, in order to discover any lesions that may be hidden under the pectoralis muscle or subcutaneous fat.

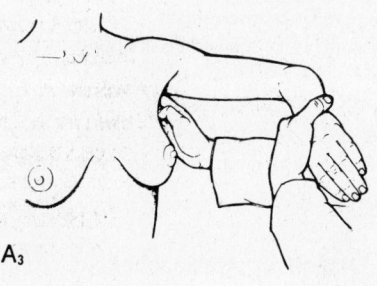

B. Woman is lying down with shoulder elevated on a small pillow on side to be examined (to balance breast on chest wall—otherwise, a mass may be missed in the thick tissue if breast is allowed to fall to the side).

1. Palpate *gently* and in an orderly fashion: begin at the upper segment and proceed clockwise; proceed over entire surface only once, unless a suspicious area is noted.

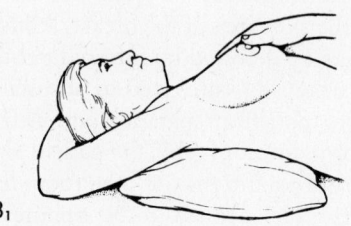

2. When palpating medial half, have the woman raise her arms above her head in order to tense pectoral muscles and provide a flatter surface (Figs. B₁ and B₂). When palpating lateral half, instruct woman to lower arm to the side (Figs. B₂ and B₃).

(Continued)

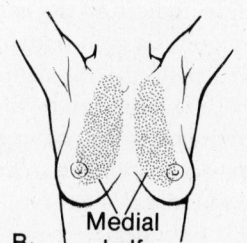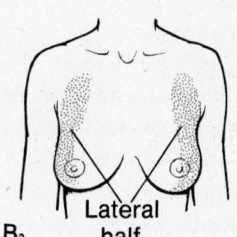

BREAST EXAMINATION OF A WOMAN BY THE NURSE (Continued)

C. A prolongation of the axillary extension of normal breast tissue may extend high into axilla and may be mistaken for pathology; if it is in evidence bilaterally and is symmetrical, it is normal.

D. Lastly, the areolar area should be gently compressed to determine whether there is any abnormal secretion.

E. Instruct the woman in doing her own breast self-examination (Fig. 46-1).

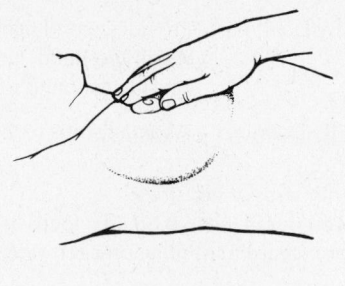

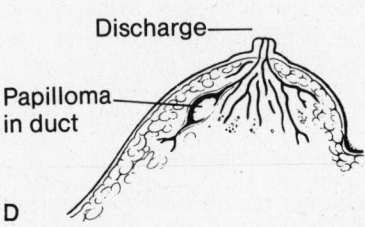

Discharge—

Papilloma in duct

D

---

history of cancer or who themselves have had the disease should have mammography performed.

3. Mammography should never be used to screen women under age 35.

4. Mammography should be used for any aged woman with a suspected breast neoplasm.

5. Thermography should be dropped from the program.

Nurses as health teachers should inform patients and women with whom they come in contact of the advantages and risks of mammography and the recent decisions about its use.

Other Diagnostic Approaches

Thermography. Thermography is a diagnostic procedure which provides a picture of the surface temperature of the skin area of the breast. Abnormal circulatory signs may be detected by infrared photography. Signals are electronically converted to an oscilloscopic display. Following patient preparation and instruction similar to those for mammography, the patient is placed in a room under basal conditions (i.e., the room has been cooled to 21° C. or 70° F.) for 20 to 30 minutes. By means of a sophisticated heat-sensing apparatus, it is possible to detect minute amounts of heat generated in and around areas of increased blood supply, indicating the existence of pathology. The method requires a well trained radiologist to interpret abnormal patterns. A diagnosis is made only within the context of a thorough history and complete physical examination. However, as was indicated previously, this procedure is no longer advocated as a diagnostic method for breast cancer.

Xerography. Xerography provides an x-ray of the soft tissue of the breast, using a very limited amount of radiation. In this procedure, a selenium-coated plate is subjected to an electrical charge, the x-ray exposure is made, and the plate is then developed by a special process under careful monitoring. The result is a xerogram in which all tissues of the breast, including skin, are portrayed in a bas-relief effect.

Most of the disadvantages that existed with regard to processing have been resolved, so that xerography appears to hold great promise in the detection of early cancers. However, it has not been established as a routine diagnostic procedure. Patient preparation and instruction are the same as for mammography.

Biopsy: Aspiration Cytology. This procedure, which involves obtaining tissue specimens for examination, can be done in the hospital outpatient department or the physician's office. Following the injection of a local anesthetic, a No. 22 needle is directed into the site to be sampled. Suction is applied to a syringe, and tissue is drawn into the needle. This material is spread on an albuminized glass slide and stained before being sent to the laboratory. Approximately 98 percent of lesions can be accurately diagnosed by this technique.

INCISIONAL VS. EXCISIONAL BIOPSY. Biopsies may be done in the operating room under general anesthesia or as an outpatient procedure under local anesthesia. A biopsy may comprise the entire lesion (*excisional*) or a piece of the specimen (*incisional*). Tissue may be sent to the laboratory to be frozen for subsequent study or it may be examined as quickly as possible if a 24-hour report is requested. Very thin slices containing a good cross section of tissue are stained with a dye to facilitate microscopic observation.

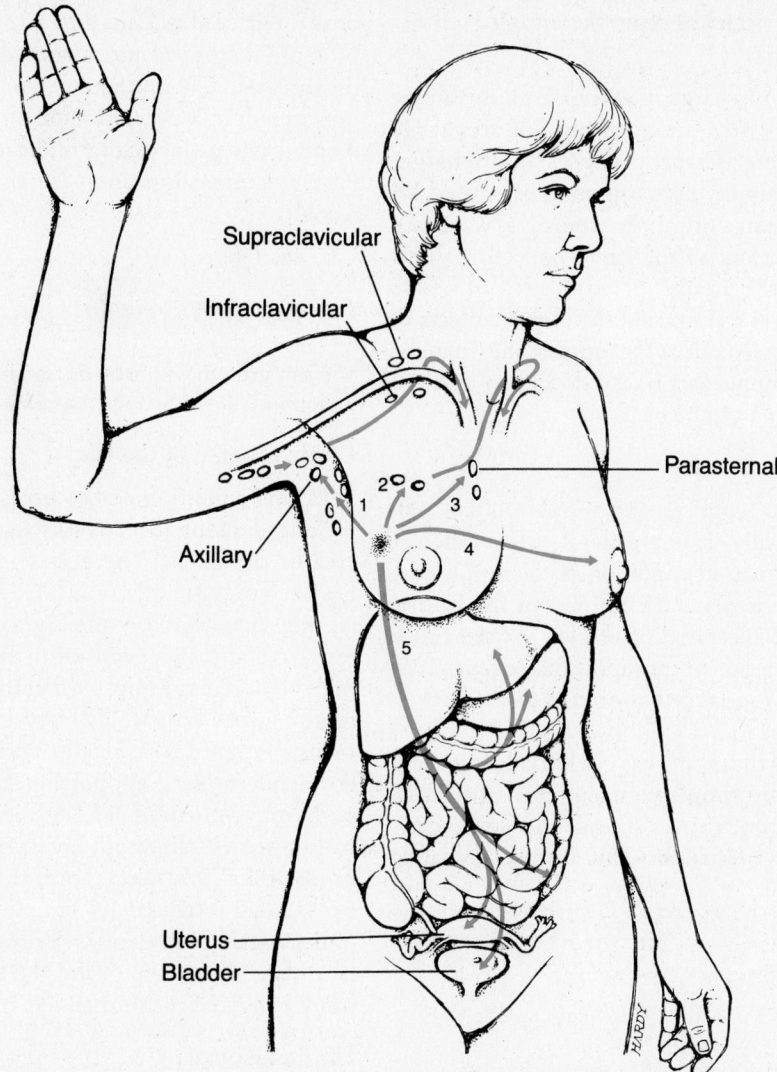

Supraclavicular

Infraclavicular

Parasternal

Axillary

Uterus
Bladder

Figure 46-2. Lymphatic drainage of the mammary gland. Metastases from cancer of the mammary gland may follow several lymphatic pathways: 1. Upper outer quadrant to axillary, infraclavicular, supraclavicular nodes, etc. 2. Upper inner quadrant to intercostal and parasternal nodes. 3. Upper inner quadrant directly to parasternal nodes. 4. Directly across midline to opposite breast. 5. Lower quadrants, particularly inner aspect, through pectoralis major, external oblique, and linea alba to subperitoneal lymphatic plexus, followed by abdominal and pelvic spread.

CONDITIONS AFFECTING THE NIPPLE

Fissure of the Nipple

A fissure of the nipple is a longitudinal ulcer that tends to develop in any woman who is nursing a baby. The ulcer is irritated constantly by the baby's suckling and causes the mother considerable pain, often associated with bleeding of the nipple. Prophylactic treatment, cleanliness, and washing and drying of the nipple after each nursing usually prevent the occurrence of this con-dition. In the prenatal period, the woman can wash, dry, and lubricate the nipples in preparation for nursing, in order to help prevent fissure development. If a fissure develops, it should be washed at frequent intervals with sterile saline solution, and nursing should continue only with the use of an artificial nipple. If healing does not occur promptly, or if the case is severe and painful, nursing should be stopped and a breast pump used in-stead. Persistent ulceration suggests carcinoma or a pri-mary syphilitic lesion.

Bleeding or Bloody Discharge from the Nipple (Intraductal Papilloma)

At times, a bloody discharge may seep from the nipple and stain the clothes. Often, there may be one area at the edge of the areola where pressure produces the discharge. Although a bloody nipple discharge may be caused by malignancy, it is most commonly due to a wart-like papilloma growing in one of the larger collecting ducts just at the edge of the areola, or in an area of cystic disease. This bleeds on trauma and the blood collects in the duct until it is pressed out at the nipple. The duct can be identified in the nipple and traced down, so that the duct and the papilloma can be excised.

Paget's Disease of the Breast

This disease of the nipple is seen most frequently in women over 45; usually, it is unilateral. Most often it begins as a mild eczematoid condition of the nipple that may spread over the areola and even part of the breast; later, it may become ulcerated or eroded. In the more advanced stages, retraction of the nipple may occur. This is a true carcinoma of the ducts of the breast that converge at the nipple.

When any lesion of the nipple has not healed after a few weeks of treatment by simple cleansing and protective measures, a suspicion of Paget's disease should be confirmed by biopsy examination. This disease demands early and total removal of the breast.

BREAST INFECTION

Lactational Mastitis

Lactational mastitis may occur at the beginning or the end of lactation. Mastitis may result from the transfer of microorganisms to the breast by the hands of the patient or those of the personnel caring for her. The baby with an oral, eye, or skin infection may be a source of infection. Mastitis may be caused by blood-borne organisms. An infection of the ducts results, causing stagnation of milk in one or more lobules. The breast becomes tough and doughy, and the patient complains of dull pain in the region affected. A nipple that is discharging pus, serum, or blood demands investigation.

Treatment consists of taking the baby off the breast temporarily. A broad-spectrum antibiotic may be given to the mother for 7 to 10 days. Progesterone has been found to reduce breast congestion, which in turn relieves the pain. The patient should wear a firm breast support and follow good habits of personal hygiene.

Lactational Mammary Abscess

A breast abscess usually develops as a sequela of an acute mastitis, although it may occur independently of lactation. The area affected becomes very tender and dusky red, and pus may be expressed from the nipple. Nursing is stopped and adequate support is provided for the breasts. Chemotherapy and antibiotic therapy are prescribed; however, incision and drainage may be performed when fluctuation indicates the presence of pus. Hot wet dressings increase the drainage and hasten resolution.

BENIGN CYSTS AND TUMORS OF THE BREAST

- Every growth within the breast should be viewed with suspicion and should be removed unless there is a contraindication.

Cystic Disease of the Breast

In this condition of the breast, many small cysts are produced owing to an overgrowth of fibrous tissue in the area of the ducts. The disease occurs most commonly between the ages of 30 and 50. These cysts are labile, that is, they may develop quickly to a considerable size in a few days and also decrease in size just as rapidly. They may be noted as lumps, which may be either painless or tender when palpated or pressed, particularly before menstruation. Occasionally, shooting pains may be felt. For tenderness, a supporting brassiere worn day and night may be helpful. The cyst itself rarely has any malignant potential, although breasts containing cysts may be more prone to develop cancer than normal breasts. Most cysts can be treated by simple aspiration of the fluid under local anesthesia. Usually the fluid will not reaccumulate. If, on aspiration the fluid is uncharacteristic, biopsy may be recommended.

Fibroadenomata

Fibroadenomata are firm, round, movable, benign tumors of the breast, usually appearing in the breasts of girls in their late teens and early twenties. They cause no pain and are not tender. They can be removed through a small incision and have no malignant potential.

BREAST CARCINOMA

Incidence. The incidence of breast cancer has continued to rise over the past 35 or 40 years, whereas the mortality rate has changed very little. This appears to be a hopeful sign in the battle against this disease and undoubtedly means that a higher proportion of women are being treated earlier and that the methods of treatment have improved. Mortality continues to increase with age except during the menopause at which time there is a slight decrease in incidence (the reason is unknown). The highest incidence is found in the unmarried female, and the lowest incidence occurs among those who have had multiple pregnancies or those who gave birth to their first child before the age of 27. Low incidence is also noted in women who have had an early artificial menopause. Racial differences have been noted, but no explanation is offered as to why, for example, the women of Japan have the lowest incidence. (See below: Women at High Risk for Breast Cancer.)

Etiology. The cause of breast carcinoma is not known; however, several factors appear to influence its occurrence. The strongest factor is genetic; women of succeeding generations are not only predisposed to develop breast cancer but they develop it 10 to 12 years earlier than women without a family history of breast cancer. Women who have more menstrual cycles are more prone to have breast cancer, whereas women with more children have a lower incidence of it. Obviously, bearing children reduces the number of menstrual periods. Breast feeding also appears to protect against breast cancer. The factor of a milk virus's being transmitted by nursing mothers has been noted with mice but studies are insufficient in humans at present.

The question continues regarding the effect of estrogens in promoting breast cancer. This uncertainty has a bearing on the use of the "pill" for contraceptive purposes. Although the long-range effects of using the "pill" are incomplete, there is reason to suggest that other means of contraception should be used by women who have a family history of breast cancer or those who have gross cystic disease, multiple breast papilloma, or cancer in one breast.

Pathophysiology. Basically, breast cancer is a disease of breast tissue. It begins as an atypical area, progresses to a carcinoma in situ (either ductal or lobular) and then enters a minimally invasive stage (up to 5 mm. [3/16 inch]). Once the carcinoma passes this stage, there is a higher likelihood of its invading the lymph nodes and the systemic circulation. Because the same factors affect both breasts, the opposite breast must be carefully watched for the development of a second carcinoma.

The tumor is located most frequently in the upper outer quadrant of the breast. As it grows, it becomes attached to the chest wall or the overlying skin. If no treatment is given, the tumor invades the surrounding

tissues and extends to the lymph glands of the adjacent axilla. When the tumor arises in the medial half of the breast, its extension may involve the lymph nodes within the chest along the internal mammary artery (see Fig. 46-2). Metastases may occur in the lungs, bone, brain, or liver. In untreated cases death usually results in 2 or 3 years.

Clinical Classification (Before Treatment)*

Symbols:

T — primary tumor
T_1 — up to 2 cm. (¾ inch), skin uninvolved
T_2 — 2 to 5 cm. (¾ inch to 2 inches), skin dimpled
T_3 } varies between International and American
T_4 } classifications

N — regional lymph nodes
N_0 — no palpable lymph nodes
N_1 — clinically palpable
N_2 } varies
N_3 }

M — distant metastasis
M_0 — no distant metastasis
M_1 — evidence of metastasis

Staging:

Classification by T, N, and M in a more precise grouping.
Ex. Stage I $T_1 N_0 M_0$
Stage III $T_3 N_2 M_0$
Stage IV Any TN symbol + M_1

Clinical Manifestations

The symptoms of the disease, unfortunately, are insidious. A nontender lump, which may be movable, appears in the breast, usually in the upper outer quadrant. Pain usually is absent, except in the very late stages. Eventually, dimpling or "orange peel" appearance of the skin may be observed. On examination in the mirror, the patient may note asymmetry and an elevation of the affected breast. Nipple retraction may be evident. Later, the breast becomes more or less fixed on the chest wall, and nodules appear in the axilla. Finally, ulceration occurs and cachexia (general ill health) becomes prominent.

Inflammatory carcinoma is a rare type of breast cancer (1-2 percent) which produces symptoms different from those of other breast cancers. The localized tumor is tender and painful; the breast is abnormally firm and enlarged. The skin over it is red and dusky in color. Often edema and nipple retraction occur. These symptoms rapidly increase in severity and usually prompt the woman to seek medical help sooner than the ordinary breast cancer patient.

WOMEN AT HIGH RISK FOR BREAST CANCER
High Risk Factors

Women over age 40 (North American, West European)
Familial history of breast cancer
Nulliparous women or those whose first parity occurred after age 30
Natural menopause occurring after age 50
Exposure to carcinogens
Chronic psychological stress
Presence of other cancer, such as endometrial, colon-rectum, salivary gland, ovarian

---

*International classification which is used most commonly in the United States.

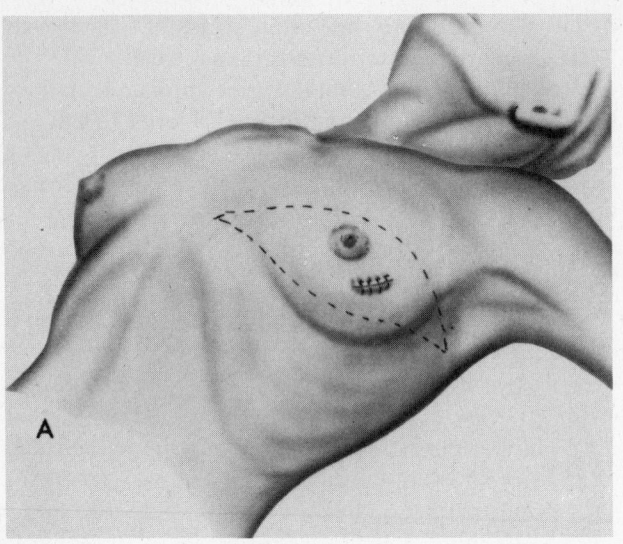

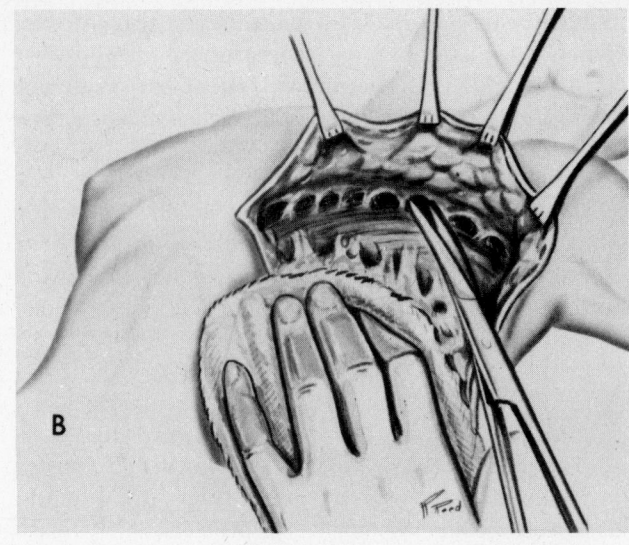

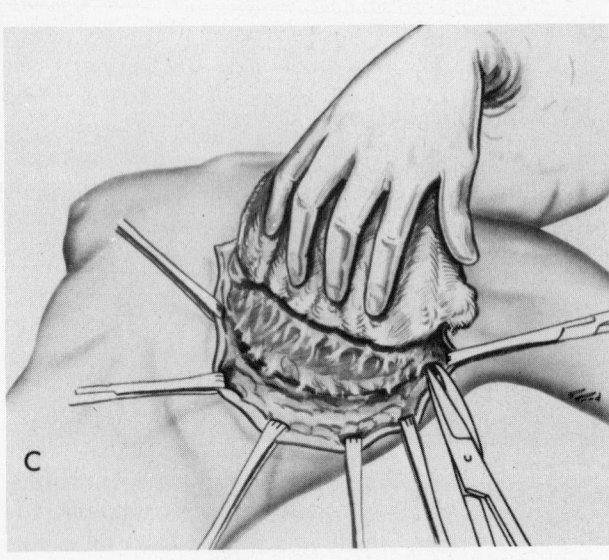

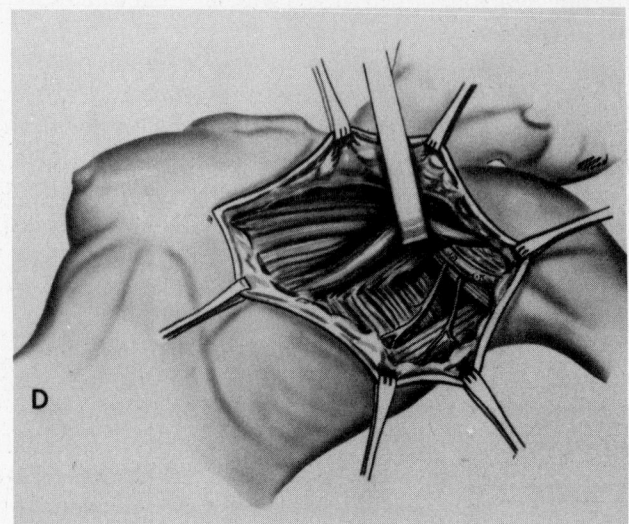

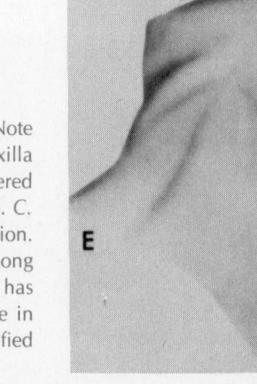

Figure 46-3.   *A.* Incision line for a modified radical mastectomy. Note the advantage of transverse incision—scar is kept below the axilla (lower border of axillary hairline) and remains within the area covered by a brassiere. *B.* Upper skin flap is dissected from breast tissue. *C.* Lower skin flap is dissected from breast tissue. *D.* Completed operation. Pectoralis major muscle is retracted to show the pectoralis minor. Long thoracic nerve and thoracodorsal nerve are depicted. *E.* Incision has been closed and suction catheters for postoperative drainage are in place. A light dressing will be placed. (Hermann and Steiger: Modified radical mastectomy. SCNA, *58*:743, Aug. 1978)

Prognosis. Breast cancer is more unpredictable than most other cancers because of hormone dependence, immune response, host resistance, and other variable factors. If the lymph nodes have not been involved, the prognosis is better than in those instances when cancer cells are found in the nodes. In clinical assessment, the absence of palpable nodes does not necessarily mean absence of malignancy (the growth may be microscopic). However, the presence of a palpable node, even a large node, may reflect an inflammation rather than a tumor. Tumor spread at the time of treatment appears to be more significant in prognosis than the type of treatment.

Management

The approach to treating breast cancer has altered during the last decade, reflecting the basic premise that *this disease is not local but systemic in nature*. Because of this assumption, not only is the local cancer treated, but the micrometastatic cancer, which may have disseminated throughout the body or may be present within the surrounding breast tissue, is also treated. More specifically, surgery combined with adjuvant chemotherapy is more effective than surgery alone for certain groups of patients. Studies are being conducted to determine the best strategy, correct combination of chemotherapeutic agents, and optimum timing in the multidisciplinary approach.

One of these approaches includes the use of hormonal manipulation, which is greatly influenced by the index of estrogen and progesterone receptors as determined by an assay done on 1 gm. of tumor taken at the original biopsy. Early studies suggest a 70 to 80 percent chance of favorable response to hormone manipulation if the receptor studies are positive.

More recently, combinations of drugs have become an important step in sequential chemotherapy as an adjuvant to surgery. Particularly useful is CMF (cytoxan, methotrexate, and fluorouracil). This may also be used with nonspecific immunotherapy, such as BCG (Bacillus Calmette-Guérin).

Surgical Management. The usual treatment of carcinoma of the breast is removal or destruction of the whole tumor. It is evident that complete removal of the tumor can be accomplished most surely when the cancer is still confined to the breast. This is borne out by clinical experience, which shows a rate of cure better than 80 percent if the tumor is confined to the breast. When cancer cells have spread to the nodes of the axilla, the cure rate falls to 40 percent.

Types of surgical intervention include the following:
1. Simple excision (lumpectomy or tumorectomy) followed by radiation of unremoved breast tissue and axillary nodes
2. Simple mastectomy followed by radiation of unremoved axillary nodes plus radiation boost to the scar area

3. Modified radical mastectomy: entire breast and axillary lymph nodes removed, with or without pectoral muscle (Fig. 46-3)
4. Radical mastectomy: entire breast, axillary lymph nodes, and both pectoral muscles removed
5. Extended radical mastectomy: same as radical mastectomy, plus other lymph nodes (parasternal) are removed

Some specialists recommend that unless distant metastasis is evident or the disease is highly malignant, radical or modified mastectomy produces the best therapeutic results. However, a great deal of controversy surrounds the choice of treatment.

Psychosocial Preparation (See Flow Chart, page 1021)

Emotional preparation of the patient begins at the moment when she is told that hospitalization and biopsy, and possibly other surgery, may be required. Actually, all women, when informed of possible breast disorders, should be prepared to follow through on suspicious findings. Upon admission to a hospital for a questionable tumor of the breast, most women have a real fear of cancer. Unfortunately, many times this fear has made them delay seeking treatment until the tumor has metastasized. Fear also stems from the emotional trauma of knowing that the breast may be removed.

It must be recognized that a mastectomy is a significant threat to a woman's feeling of femininity. Because of this, the nurse must be available to listen to and support the patient. One way to promote a positive attitude is to point out that loss of the breast, as against loss of life, is a small price to pay in a physical sense. The availability of well-fitted prostheses means that a woman can dress just as fashionably as she did prior to surgery. Even swimsuits can be worn in attractive styles by the postmastectomy patient.

However, deep-seated concerns may not only stem from problems of physical adjustment but may be related to other worries. "Will I be as attractive to my husband?" "Will he continue to love me?" "Will I be able to function as a wife?" "Will my children reject me?" These are the types of questions that plague many mastectomy patients. Because of such emotional concerns, the husband should be brought into those selected planning sessions intended to prepare the woman for surgery. If he is properly prepared, his support, devotion, and understanding can be of tremendous importance to his wife. A good relationship can soften the impact of surgery, lessen the possibilities of complications, and provide an easier adjustment to her altered image. The nurse is in a position to be most helpful in applying effective mental health principles as part of the patient's preparation for surgery.

Preoperative and Perioperative Management

After proper preoperative staging, nothing should delay the operation except the necessary check of the physical and nutritional needs of the patient. If radical surgery is anticipated, in which there may be fluid and blood loss, blood replacement must be available. The patient is told by the surgeon that there is a possibility of radical surgery, if it is indicated. No patient should go to the operating room anticipating a half-inch incision for a tumor excision and return having had a radical mastectomy. Because the emotional factor is a significant one, encouragement and reassurance must be given all along the way.

A hypnotic is administered and the usual physical preoperative preparation is carried out. Skin preparation should be extensive enough to meet the maximal possible surgery. If it is known that radical surgery, including a skin graft, is to be done, the donor skin area (usually the anterior aspect of the thigh) must be shaved and cleaned.

Surgical Procedure.   After receiving general anesthesia, the patient is placed in the supine position on the operating table. The arm of the affected side is positioned upward to expose the axilla. If a biopsy and frozen section are planned, the biopsy is done first. Then the entire field is redraped and a new set of instruments is used so that the possibility of transferring cancer cells from the biopsy site to the other areas of the wound is avoided. About 70,000 mastectomies are performed each year in the United States. A *simple mastectomy* involves removal of a breast without lymph node dissection or with removal of only a few low nodes. A *radical mastectomy* includes removal of the breast and the underlying muscles down to the chest wall after the breast lymphatics in the axilla have been removed. Such a radical operation removes the tumor and the areas of possible lymphatic spread.

Bleeding points are ligated and the skin is closed as well as possible over the chest wall. Skin grafting is done if the skin flaps are not of sufficient size to close the wound. Nonadhering dressing (Adaptic) permits serum and blood to escape between the strips. Pressure dressings may then be applied. Two drainage tubes usually are placed in the axilla and beneath the superior skin flap; portable suction may be preferred by some surgeons. Final dressings may be held in place by wide elastic bandages. A blood transfusion may be given during the operation to compensate for blood loss, if necessary.

Functional Considerations.   The objective in this regard is to restore normal function to the hand, arm, and shoulder girdle on the affected side. Before surgery is performed, the surgeon plans an incision which will provide maximum opportunity to excise the tumor and the affected nodes. At the same time, the patient's life style should be considered, and efforts should be made to avoid a scar that will be visible and restrictive. Skin flaps and tissue are handled meticulously to ensure proper viability, hemostasis, and drainage. A more recent and valuable technique involves injecting fluorescein dye into the peripheral vein at the time of surgical closure and actually inspecting the blood supply to the flaps with a Wood's lamp. When the light is turned off, the manner in which the blood has been distributed to the flaps can be assessed.

Postoperative Nursing Management

Postoperative nursing management is directed toward achieving proper drainage, avoiding injury, initiating an exercise plan, and meeting psychosocial needs.

Usually a general anesthetic is chosen for a simple mastectomy, a modified radical mastectomy, or a radical mastectomy. Postoperative care is given with special attention to pulse and blood pressure, since they are valuable indices in detecting shock and hemorrhage. Dressings must be inspected for bleeding, especially under the axilla and in the area on which the patient is lying. At the same time, tube drainage is monitored at close intervals.

After the patient has recovered from the anesthesia, analgesics are given for the relief of pain, and the patient is encouraged to turn and take deep breaths to avert pulmonary complications. The dressing usually is fairly snug; however, it should not be so tight that lung expansion is restricted. Some surgeons prefer to include the arm (flexed at the elbow) in the dressing to give added pressure. In other instances, gauze fluffs or foam rubber sponge may be added to the dressing within the binder to provide pressure.

In many patients a drainage catheter is inserted through a stab wound into the axilla; this catheter is then attached to a suction machine and drained into a trap bottle. By this means any serum and blood that collect are aspirated rapidly, and the skin flap is held tightly against the chest wall. Thus, collection of serum and formation of hematomas are avoided. Some surgeons eliminate pressure dressings early in the postoperative period and use portable suction instead. Dressings over incision and donor graft areas are changed according to the surgeon's preference.

Care of Incision Site.   When dressings are changed, the nature of the incision, the way it looks and feels now, and how it will gradually change are explained. The patient needs to know that sensation in the newly healed area may have lessened because nerves have been severed; however, the area should be bathed gently and blotted dry to avoid injury. Signs of irritation and possible infection should be described, so that if they occur, the patient will recognize them and report them to her physician. When talking about the incision, the nurse should use the term "incision" rather than "scar," since scarring connotes defect, deformity, and ugliness in the minds of many persons.

Gentle massage of the healed incision with cocoa butter helps to increase the elasticity of the skin and encourages circulation.

Positioning of the patient depends on the dressing;

semi-Fowler usually is desirable. The arm, if free, should be elevated with each joint positioned higher than the more proximal joint. Thus, gravity helps to remove the fluid via the lymphatic and the venous pathways. Whether the arm is flexed or extended depends on the preference of the physician. Elevation of the arm helps to prevent lymphedema, which may occur after surgery because of interference with the circulatory and the lymphatic systems (especially following true radical mastectomy). Whether or not there will be satisfactory postmastectomy lymph drainage depends upon how many collateral lymphatic avenues were not destroyed during surgery.

The patient usually is allowed out of bed on the first or the second day after operation; the arm on the affected side may be held in a sling for a time to prevent tension on the wound. Assistance is given only when it is needed; the nurse supports the patient from the unoperated side. A normal diet may be given unless nausea is a symptom. If a drainage tube has been inserted, it is removed usually when the drainage has decreased markedly or stopped.

Radiotherapy may be prescribed after the operation as a means of destroying any cancer cells that may have escaped removal at operation (if the tumor was central or medial, or if the tumor was very large or axillary nodes were involved). Radiation therapy usually is initiated three or four weeks after surgery. Anorexia, nausea, and vomiting can occur after irradiation; abstinence from eating and drinking for 3 hours before and after these treatments often helps. (See also Chapter 16.)

Psychosocial Considerations (See Flow Chart, page 1021). The full impact of the meaning of a mastectomy may not be felt by the patient until several days or even weeks after surgery. Meanwhile, it is frequently helpful if the nurse takes the time to talk or listen to the patient whenever the patient expresses the need for this kind of support. Frequently asked questions include: Is it normal to drain so much? Will the swelling of my arm go down? How will my husband react to my deformity? Will my appearance be changed? Will I be able to wear a regular swimsuit? Will I be able to swim, play tennis, drive a car? The nurse should be able to respond to these questions with empathy and in a way that will help the patient to find the answers she seeks. A personal, caring manner is imperative; this patient needs someone with whom she can share her troubled thoughts.

A real problem may arise if the patient is reluctant to look at the incision site. Although the presence of the scar must eventually be faced, the patient should not be forced at this time to look at her chest area. Her psychological defenses may require that she be spared this added shock at this moment. It is sometimes helpful to steer the patient to a point of acceptance by first drawing a picture of the incision line on a piece of paper. Then at a later time, when the dressings are being changed, the patient may show signs of being willing to look at her chest. However, the nurse must explore this area in a very gentle manner. Any resistance on the part of the patient must be sensed and respected. Each woman must work her way to acceptance on the basis of her own individual psychological needs.

Rehabilitation

A carefully orchestrated program for rehabilitation should be a part of the treatment plan for every woman who has breast cancer. Rehabilitation is a team effort that embraces psychosocial, physical, and functional (including vocational) considerations.

Some breast cancers grow and spread rapidly, whereas others may take years to extend. Some cancers may not be excised completely but can be controlled over long periods of time. Thus the rehabilitative management is geared to patients who have been cured and those whose disease is under control.

Clothing

HOSPITAL ATTIRE. Since bulky dressings and drainage equipment must be accommodated, the patient's usual attire is the hospital gown or an opaque, full-gathered nightgown with wide sleeves and probably a ribbon drawstring at the neck. The patient and her family should realize the need for this type of gown. Additional special clothing may include a temporary brassiere with an insert, which may be obtained through the hospital or the American Cancer Society's "Reach to Recovery" program, or from a local department store. Usually the garment can be laundered easily and has a pocket on the mastectomy side to accommodate a filler. (See below, Prosthesis.)

ATTIRE AT HOME. If dressings are still in place when the patient is discharged, loose-fitting clothing from the patient's wardrobe usually is satisfactory. The temporary "bra" is worn before the permanent prosthesis is prescribed. The incision must be healed before the surgeon's opinion is obtained regarding the kind of prosthesis needed and when it can be used. Garments that may present problems because of buttons or zippers should be avoided at first. Later, the exercise involved in manipulating buttons and zippers, especially for the arm on the affected side, is desirable. Zipper "pulls" are helpful when dresses with zippers in the back are worn.

Some surgeons use no dressings after the first day, and the patient is encouraged to wear her normal clothing as soon as possible. Cotton wads or a rolled-up stocking may be placed in the brassiere as a temporary prosthesis.

Literature from "Reach to Recovery" (American Cancer Society) offers suggestions for special clothing, such as night clothes, swimsuits, and evening wear. Most large department stores have mastectomy boutiques and personnel who can assist the woman who has had a mastectomy.

Prosthesis. When a prosthesis is prescribed, its effect on the incision site should be observed. To offset irritation, a layer of lamb's wool is effective when pressure is exerted. The kind of prosthesis suitable for the patient is suggested on an individual basis by the surgeon. Skilled fitters from reliable companies are available and they usually have many helpful suggestions, literature, and an optimistic, understanding approach that is most encouraging to postmastectomy patients.

In preparation for an individualized prosthesis, a temporary makeshift padded brassiere can be designed and stitched by the nurse with the patient's participation. Loose cotton covered with gauze can be stitched loosely into the patient's own brassiere; snaps can be used in making a pocket to fit the "falsie." Ingenuity and resourcefulness can fashion effective padding from sanitary pads, nylon stockings, and shredded foam rubber.

There are many types of breast prostheses available: foam rubber, air-filled, fluid-filled, fluffed cotton, lamb's wool, plastic, synthetic, and cloth, either ready-made or custom-made. A properly fitted brassiere is essential to a well-fitted prosthesis. Breasts readily follow the law of gravity and change their contour and position with every body motion. Therefore, the most satisfactory prostheses are those filled with a slow-flowing thick fluid. Often, when a patient knows that such appliances are available, her fear of disfigurement is greatly reduced.*

When the final prosthesis is to be obtained, consultants are available to assist the patient in selecting the one best suited for her with respect to specific need, cost, and use.

*A valuable guide that describes the various types of prostheses available may be found in the following consumer report article: After mastectomy: Finding the right prosthesis. Nov. 1975. Consumer's Union, Orangeburg, N.Y. 10962 ($0.40).

A. *Wall hand-climbing.* Stand facing the wall, with the toes as close to the wall as possible — feet apart. With elbows somewhat bent, place the palms on the wall at shoulder level. By flexing the fingers, work hands up the wall until arms are fully extended. Work hands down to starting point.

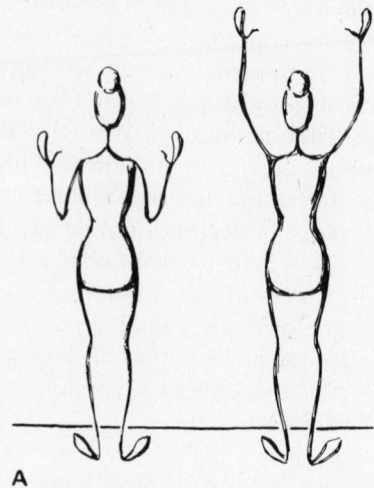

A

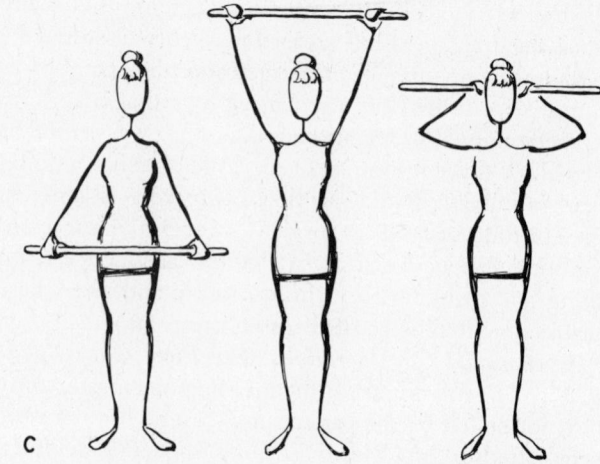

C

C. *Rod or Broom.* Grasp rod with both hands, held about 2 feet apart. With arms straight, raise rod over the head. Bend elbows, lowering rod behind the head. Reverse maneuver, raising rod above head, then to starting position.

B. *Rope turning.* Stand facing the door. Take free end of light rope in hand of the operated side. Place other hand on hip. With arm extended and held away from the body —nearly parallel with the floor—turn rope, making as wide swings as possible. Slow at first—speed up later.

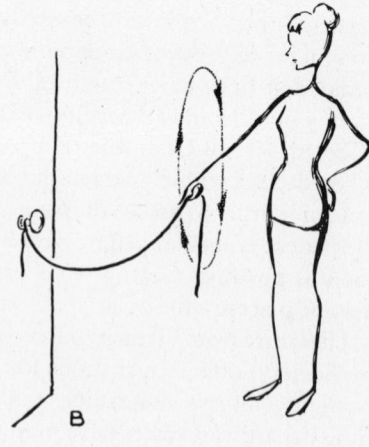

B

D. *Pulley.* Toss rope over shower curtain rod or doorway curtain rod. Stand as nearly under rope as possible. Grasp an end in each hand. Extend arms straight and away from body. Pull left arm up by tugging down with right arm, then right arm up and left down—like a seesaw.

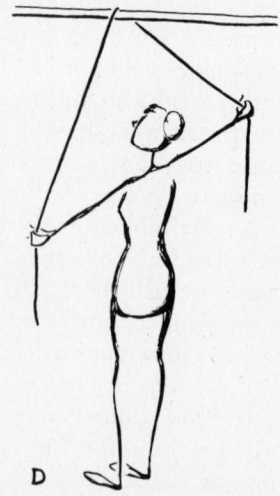

D

Figure 46-4. The purpose of the exercise program is to secure a complete range of motion of the affected shoulder joint. (Adapted from Radler: A Handbook for Your Recovery. New York, The Society of Memorial Center)

Suggestions are given to avoid imbalance, "riding up," and discomfort, along with hints on wearing short-sleeved or sleeveless garments, evening gowns, and swimsuits. With this guidance, the woman should find that she is able to regain a normal appearance with a fair degree of comfort.

For some patients, reconstruction with a permanent prosthesis may be an alternative, depending on a number of factors (see page 1020).

Arm Exercises

After 24 hours, the arm on the affected side should be engaged in active exercise. This activity can be increased each day, as the patient is encouraged to do more for herself—by brushing her teeth, washing her face, and combing her hair with the hand on the affected side. Failure to encourage such exercises as "climbing the wall with the fingers" may prolong the disuse of the arm and promote the development of a contracture. Exercise should not be accompanied by pain; if the patient has had a skin graft or if the incision was closed with considerable tension, such exercises are greatly limited and must be done very gradually.

Many hospitals promote classes for the postmastectomy patient; this provides encouragement for women who would otherwise remain passive and inactive in their own rooms. At the bedside, pulley-type ropes from the over-bed or curtain frame can be used for one kind of exercise. Turning a jump rope that is attached to the doorknob can be arranged easily (see muscle training exercises, Fig. 46-4). In all exercises, it is important to emphasize bilateral activity. Likewise, the value of proper posture must be emphasized; if the patient hunches over and favors the affected side as she combs her hair, the purpose of the exercise will be defeated.

Naturally, difficulty with arm movement is much greater in the patient who has undergone the classic radical mastectomy. Limitation of motion after simple and modified radical mastectomy is unusual, and the patient is encouraged to use the arm to the point of complete mobility almost immediately.

Lymphedema and Exercise. Edema of the arm is a complication that occasionally plagues a woman who has had a radical mastectomy. Although the cause of lymphedema is not known, it will result if the number of properly functioning lymphatic channels is insufficient to ensure a return flow of lymph into the general circulation. Though edema may affect only the upper arm, often the entire arm on the operated side is involved. Such swelling can occur immediately following operation (postoperative surgical edema) or may occur many months or years after surgery (secondary surgical edema). The immediate postoperative edema "can be avoided only by meticulous surgical technique which achieves perfect wound healing . . . a factor in achieving perfect wound healing is skin grafting of the operative

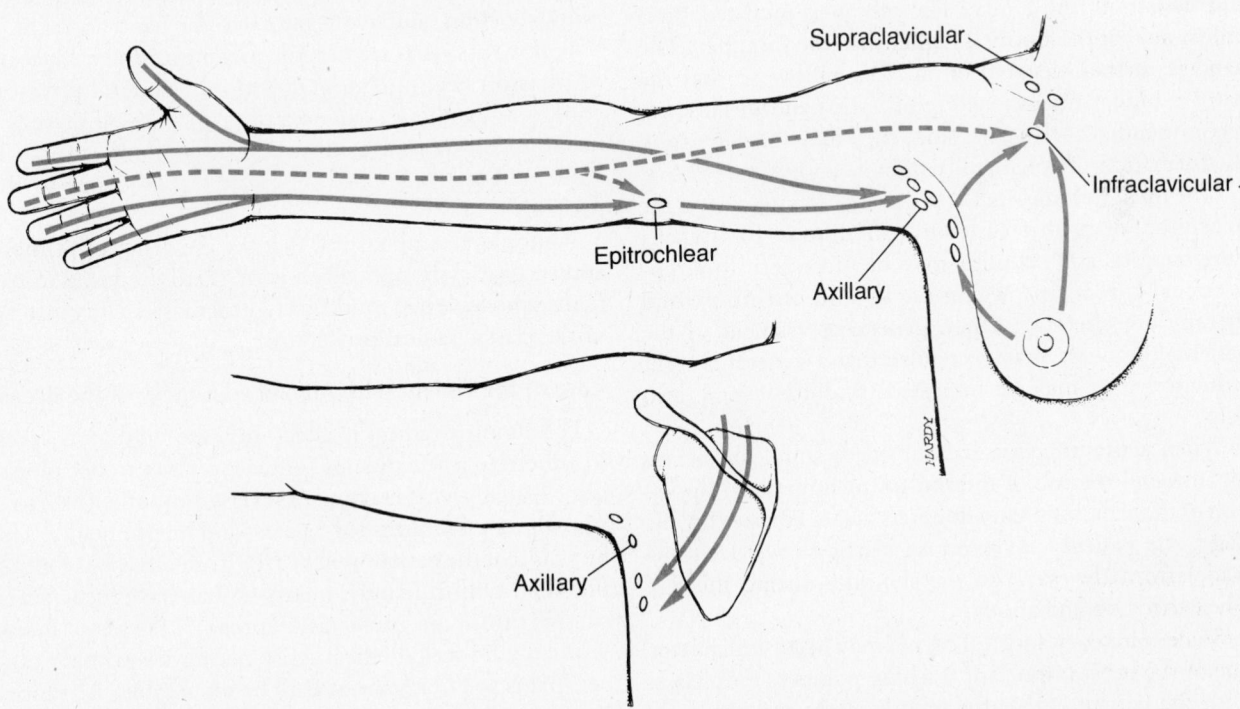

Figure 46-5. Lymphatic drainage of the upper extremity. The lymphatic vessels draining the fingers and the hand converge on the dorsum of the hand. From here the lymphatic drainage pursues three courses. The lymph vessels draining the ulnar aspect (little finger and ring finger) accompany the basilic vein and drain into the epitrochlear nodes and thence into the axillary nodes. The lymph vessels draining the thumb and the index fingers bypass the epitrochlear nodes and go directly to the axillary nodes. The lymph vessels draining the middle fingers may drain into the epitrochlear or the axillary, or may bypass both of these groups of nodes to drain directly into the infraclavicular, and thence into the supraclavicular, and finally into the bloodstream. The axillary nodes also receive lymph from the posterior scapular region (insert).

Special *HAND AND ARM CARE* on the Side of the Operation
For the Woman Who Has Had a Radical Mastectomy

AVOID	DO
Cuts, bruises, insect bites, burns	Protect the hand and arm on the operated side.
Injury to cuticles or hangnails	Apply lanolin hand cream several times daily.
Strong detergents	Use a thimble when sewing.
Working near thorny bushes	Stay out of the strong sun.
Digging in the garden	Wear a Medical-Alert tag engraved as follows: *Caution—*
Holding a cigarette	*lymphedema arm—no tests—no needle injections.*
Reaching into a hot oven	See physician if the arm gets red or swollen or becomes
Having blood drawn; injections	unusually hard.
Having a blood pressure cuff applied	
Wearing jewelry or a wrist watch	
Carrying heavy bags or purse	

---

wound to avoid the triad of tension on the skin flaps, necrosis and infection." * When axillary nodes and lymphatic system have been removed, a collateral system for lymphatic drainage from the hand and arm must be developed (Fig. 46-5). This is done within a month and is facilitated by exercise. Although 9 out of 10 postmastectomy patients escape massive lymphedema, this complication would occur even less frequently if nurses impressed upon their patients the importance of elevating, massaging, and exercising the affected arm for 3 or 4 months following the operation.

For marked lymphedema, the arm should be elevated *but not in adduction,* since this position is uncomfortable and constricts the axilla. The elbow is elevated on a pillow so that the elbow is higher than the shoulder. The hand is further elevated on another pillow so that the hand is higher than the elbow. Elastic bandages are not recommended at this time since they may interfere with the formation of collateral lymphatic pathways.

One must not rule out the possibility of infection in the presence of significant lymphedema. Recurrent lymphangitis and cellulitis may be secondary to streptococcal infection. Warm packs and antimicrobial therapy are effective. Upon general assessment of the patient, the nurse may recognize that a general weight reduction plan may be indicated. A diuretic may also help.

When acute infection has subsided, some physicians recommend the use of intermittnt pneumatic compression of the arm, but many doubt its value. For the chronic stage, the patient may wear an elastic sleeve (custom-made) from the wrist to the shoulder during the day when she is up and about.

Since secondary surgical edema may occur much later, one of the most important teaching points to emphasize with the patient is that for months and years she must

*Haagensen, C. D.: Diseases of the Breast, 2nd ed. Philadelphia, W. B. Saunders.

take extra precautions to avoid cuts, bruises, and infection of the hand and arm on the side of her operation. Even pushing the cuticles back and injuring finger tissue may provide the portal of entry for infection which in turn may trigger the development of lymphedema. Other precautions are listed in the chart above.

The exercises done in the hospital and illustrated in Figure 46-4 can be related to household activities. Putting dishes on a shelf, dusting window sashes, typing, and piano playing are activities that promote and maintain muscle tone. Other suggestions are to swing the arm while walking, wear loose or nonconstricting clothing, keep the mastectomy site, underarm, and arm scrupulously clean, and avoid injury to the hand and arm.

Follow-up visits are very important for the evaluation of incision healing, mental outlook, general physical condition, and any evidences of recurrence. If there is a need for consultation with a community nurse, the availability of such a service should be pointed out to the patient.

It should be emphasized that the incidence of primary and secondary lymphedema is markedly reduced in patients who have had modified radical mastectomy instead of the classic radical procedure.

Care of the Patient with Advanced Cancer of the Breast

Following a radical mastectomy, the woman is asked to adhere to a schedule of follow-up visits to her physician. Usually visits take place every 3 months for 2 to 3 years, every 6 months for 5 years, and then annually. The hope is that the patient will be free from disease as long as possible. Unfortunately, many woman have recurrences of the tumor or metastatic spread. Likewise, many woman who seek medical assistance have a primary cancer that is so far advanced as to be inoperable. Advanced breast cancer may indicate extensive spread within the breast or to adjacent tissues, or even metastasis to other parts of the body. The status of dissemination can be determined by metastatic x-ray series (chest, skull, long bones, and pelvis), liver chemistries, a mammogram of the other breast, and radioactive scans of the bone, liver, and brain.

Of the patients who have recurrences, almost half show evidences of recurrence locally and in regional lymph nodes, over a quarter have visceral involvement, and a similar percentage have bone involvement of the spine, rib, hips, or pelvis.

The nurse is challenged to utilize many skills in assessing the physical as well as the psychosocial condition of the patient. Information about changes in behavioral patterns can be elicited from the patient's family. The nurse can also assist the physician in determining the specific kind of palliation suitable for the individual patient. Such therapy is designed to keep the woman as comfortable as possible although it may not arrest the disease. Regression or abatement of symptoms for as long as possible is the goal, although individual differences make its attainment unpredictable. The emphasis is on improving the quality of survival.

A wide range of treatment is available depending on the specifics of the patient's condition. For a detailed outline of the various treatment modalities that are frequently used, see Table 46-1.

TABLE 46-1. CARE OF THE PATIENT WITH ADVANCED CANCER OF THE BREAST

PALLIATIVE THERAPY	OBJECTIVES OF THERAPY	CONCOMITANT EFFECTS	ESSENTIAL NURSING INTERVENTION
Radiation (See p. 291)	Effective in relieving pain. More effective in skeletal metastasis; less effective in visceral metastasis.	Depends on area affected: Chest: esophagitis, pneumonitis, shortness of breath, slight cough Abdomen: affects digestion Body: general lethargy	Administer pain-relieving medication as required until effects of radiation lessen the need for such drugs. Recognize that fatigue and weakness often result from radiation. When pain is controlled, instruct patient to take extra precautions in order to avoid pathologic fractures: avoid lifting heavy packages and children, and strenuous arm movements such as those used in sweeping. (see page 998 for surgical care)
Oophorectomy	Castration removes cyclic hormone stimulation of the tumor. Preferred for premenopausal women: 1. Surgical ⟶ Immediate estrogen withdrawal 2. Radiation ⟶ Estrogen withdrawal takes 4-6 weeks If breast cancer localized to breast, oophorectomy may or may not be advised.		
Hormonal Therapy	Androgens, fluoxymesterone (Halotestin) for premenopausal women Estrogens (diethylstilbestrol) for postmenopausal patients	Masculinization ⟶ Fluid retention Cholestatic jaundice Hypercalcemia ⟶	Watch for signs of increased libido, deepening voice, facial hirsutism. Note serum calcium levels. Observe for signs of: lethargy, insomnia, thirst, nausea, vomiting, thickened speech, fluid retention, collapse, coma. Assist with treatment: Moderately high doses of corticosteroids, vigorous hydration, low calcium diet.
Adrenalectomy, bilateral, posterior (flank), or anterior with oophorectomy	Removes another source of endogenous estrogens. Effective for metastasis to viscera or bone.	Removes a hormone essential to life ⟶	Replace cortisone daily for rest of patient's life. Otherwise adrenal crisis results. *(Continued)*

TABLE 46-1.   CARE OF THE PATIENT WITH ADVANCED CANCER OF THE BREAST *(Continued)*

PALLIATIVE THERAPY	OBJECTIVES OF THERAPY	CONCOMITANT EFFECTS	ESSENTIAL NURSING INTERVENTION
Adrenalectomy (Continued)			Symptoms: hypotension, diarrhea, nausea & vomiting, elevated temperature, weakness, abdominal pain

Hypophysectomy
  Method:
  1. Major craniotomy
  2. Transnasal implantation of radioactive Yttrium (Y⁹⁰)
  3. Transsphenoidal excision of pituitary
  4. Stereotactic cryohypophysectomy
  5. Stereotatic radio frequency to destroy pituitary.
	Removes source of adrenocorticotropic hormone (ACTH) as well as hormones that seem to stimulate the breast directly.	May cause salt wastage ——————→
		Following hypophysectomy, diabetes insipidus may occur (inability to conserve body water because of absence of posterior pituitary and its secretion, antidiuretic hormone, ADH).
		In 4-6 weeks, hypothalamus takes over function of antidiuretic hormone.
			Replace adrenal salt-regulating hormone fludrocortisone acetate (Florinef). Many patients do not require this.
			
			Recognize need for additional steroid replacement during stress periods, such as minor illness, infection, injury, serious vomiting, surgery.
			
			Otherwise, adrenal insufficiency results (symptoms similar to crises described above).
			
			For transsphenoidal hypophysectomy: Frequent oral care is required. Observe for hemorrhage, especially after nasal packing is removed. Clear nasal drip and patient swallowing constantly may indicate cerebrospinal leak. Keep patient in Fowler's position to facilitate cerebrospinal fluid drainage.
			
			Advise patient to wear Medic Alert bracelet with operation and the name of replacement medication.

Note: Medical adrenalectomy: When it is impossible to do an adrenalectomy or hypophysectomy (because of age, patient refusal, poor condition) administer high doses of cortisone to achieve adrenal suppression. This is combined with 5-Fluorouracil (5-FU).			

Chemotherapy
1. Antimetabolites
    5-Fluorouracil (5-FU) combined with adrenalectomy (See p. 264, chemotherapy)
	Permits a satisfactory mode of palliation and allows return to normal activity	Toxic effects:
		    stomatitis
		    nausea and vomiting
		    diarrhea, alopecia
		    burning sensation in mouth from acid foods
			Provide frequent mouth care.
			
			Use topical anesthesia for mouth before meals.
			
			Administer antiemetics.
			
			Change narcotics as tolerance for each develops.

2. Alkylating agents	When above no longer effective, switch to other chemotherapeutic agents: cyclophosphamide (Cytoxan); triethylene thiophosphoramide (Thiotepa).	Bone marrow depression
		    cystitis
		    alopecia
		    jaundice	

3. Corticosteroids (Prednisone)	Suppresses estrogen production by the adrenals and decreases urinary estrogenic metabolites.	Does not bring about hypercalcemia as does androgen or estrogen therapy. It is a good hormonal treatment for brain metastasis. Induces some degree of Cushing syndrome: fullness of face, gain in body weight and edema of lower extremities.	(See page 874, steroid therapy)

TABLE 46-1. CARE OF THE PATIENT WITH ADVANCED CANCER OF THE BREAST *(Continued)*

PALLIATIVE THERAPY	OBJECTIVES OF THERAPY	CONCOMITANT EFFECTS	ESSENTIAL NURSING INTERVENTION
4. Antibiotic (Doxorubicin hydrochloride) Adriamycin	Produces toxic effect by interfering with RNA and DNA synthesis.	Cardiac failure possible Leukopenia Depressed platelets	Urine will be red-tinged for 2-3 days after drug administration. Nausea and vomiting as well as diarrhea may occur. Loss of hair possible.
5. Antiestrogen (Tamoxifen citrate) Nolvadex	Effective in palliative treatment in postmenopausal women with positive assays for estrogen receptors. May permit delay or avoidance of adrenalectomy or hypophysectomy.	Adverse effects usually transient. Appears less toxic than other agents.	Expect hot flashes, nausea, vomiting. May cause anorexia, vaginal bleeding and discharge, skin rashes.

RECONSTRUCTIVE AND PLASTIC SURGERY OF THE BREAST

Hypertrophy of the Breast

The breasts are such an important part of the female figure that abnormalities often lead to requests for surgical management. The variations most often encountered are in size: breasts are too large or too small. Those that are too large are said to be hypertrophied; when the condition occurs in early life, it is called virginal breast hypertrophy. The condition is usually bilateral, but may occur on only one side. The hypertrophied breasts that occur in later life are always bilateral.

Symptoms of Breast Hypertrophy. These patients complain of tender breasts, diffuse pains, and fatigue. The tenderness and pain is particularly marked at the time of the menstrual period. The weight of the breasts causes a dragging sensation on the shoulders, and efforts to support these tremendous breasts with brassieres are futile. Most patients with virginal hypertrophy have deep grooves in the shoulder tissue caused by pressure from brassiere straps.

Not only are physical symptoms present, but psychological difficulties develop, especially in girls and younger women. They become too embarrassed to wear bathing suits, sweaters, or evening gowns. Their social life is restricted, and they become introverts, avoiding social contacts and even marriage. Because they think that they are unattractive, married women with this condition develop a sense of insecurity, fearing the loss of their husband's affection and, possibly, divorce. These are very real difficulties, which cause mental repercussions that may be very serious.

Mammoplasty. The operation performed to reduce the size of the breasts is termed a reduction mammoplasty. In this operation, the surgeon makes one incision beneath the breast and a similar curved incision in the skin of the anterior breast. The nipple is transplanted to a new location after the redundant tissue is cut away. The remaining skin edges are approximated with sutures and the nipple is sutured to its new location. Drains are placed in the incision and remain for only a day or two. Simple gauze dressings are used without pressure.

Postoperative care following mammoplasty is relatively basic. These patients sit up in bed the day after operation and may be out of bed and eating a normal diet thereafter. The results of these plastic operations are good for both relief of symptoms and appearance. There is no recurrence of the hypertrophy, and the operation is not a serious one. The newly transplanted nipple may turn black and be covered by a dry scab. This is to be expected, but the scab will come away after a week or two as the nipple regains a blood supply in its new location. It must be accepted that the breast cannot function for lactation after such an operation.

Usually, these patients are euphoric about the results, but it is not uncommon for some patients to experience negative psychological reactions related to the loss of a part of the body. The patient may feel anxious about this reaction, but it helps to let her know that these feelings occur frequently.

Operations to Enlarge or Uplift the Female Breast

Operations to enlarge or uplift the breast are requested fairly frequently. Although padded brassieres and other devices are available, they do not always give the desired result. The operations are performed through an incision along the undermargin of the breast (circumareolar). The breast is elevated and a pocket is formed between it and the chest wall into which are inserted various types of plastic and synthetic materials intended to enlarge and uplift the breast. This procedure is called an *augmentation mammoplasty* and may be done on an outpatient basis with local anesthesia by an experienced plastic surgeon. These operations are not serious, but complications do occur occasionally, in some instances requiring the removal of the inserted substance.

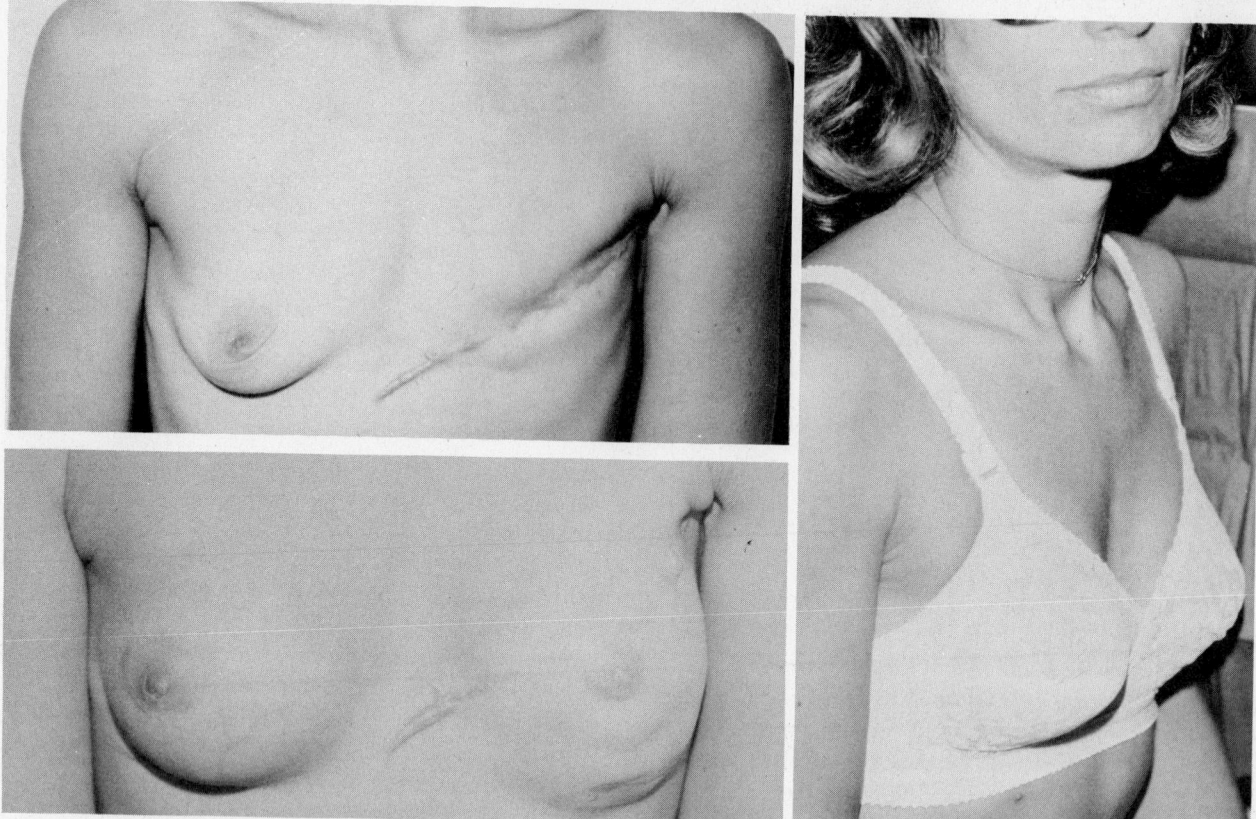

Figure 46-6.   Reconstruction of left breast and augmentation of right breast. (Guthrie, R. H., Jr.: The case for breast reconstruction after mastectomy. CA-A Cancer J. for Clinicians, July-Aug. 1978)

Following Mastectomy.   A more recent innovation is restoration of the female breast following mastectomy. Findings over the last decade indicate that the skin-sub-cutaneous complex is far looser and more supple than was previously thought and that the blood supply is usually sufficient to withstand wide undermining as well as the compromising effects of a tightly compressed prosthesis. The Ashley* implant, constructed of silicone gel in a molded shape buttressed by internal compart-mentalization, appears to be an effective device, as are the newer saline-filled prostheses.

A transverse incision is made in what will become the inframammary fold. Through this incision, the skin and subcutaneous fat of the chest wall are undermined and the implant is placed in the created pocket. The wound is drained via portable suction and is closed. A few months later, a nipple-areola complex may be reconstructed, the areola being created from a graft of the labia majora or minora, whereas the nipple is constructed from a trans-planted portion of the opposite nipple or a portion of earlobe (Fig. 46-6).

Postmastectomy patients are carefully selected by the surgeon in order to ensure effective results. Criteria for ineligibility include the need for large skin grafts, ex-posure to excessive radiation, and skin that is too tight or thin. The matter of tumor recurrence continues to be

*Ashley, F. L.: A new type of breast prosthesis: Preliminary report. Plastic Reconstructive Surgery, 45:421-424, 1970.

raised but does not appear to be too significant when compared with the psychological and physical advan-tages of this type of surgery.

After the operation, the patient is instructed to wear a brassiere during the day and night for at least a month. She is instructed to limit arm movement for a period of time to permit the tissues to heal. Usually this means keeping arms at the side with flexing at the elbows only. The patient should not sleep on her abdomen and should not lift anything weighing more than 13.6 kg. (30 lbs.) for the first 4 to 6 weeks.

With some very early tumors, there has been a great deal of interest in primary reconstruction at the time of initial surgery.

DISEASES OF THE MALE BREAST

In the male, *gynecomastia* (hypertrophy of the breast) is the lesion that most frequently affects the breast. Fibro-adenoma is rarely seen in the male. Ninety-nine percent of malignant lesions occur in the female. Gynecomastia may occur in the prepubertal or adolescent boy, is usually unilateral, and presents as a firm, circular, tender mass beneath the areola. In the adult male, diffuse gyne-comastia may occur and may be related to certain drugs the patient is taking, such as digitalis. Pain and tenderness are initial symptoms. The enlarged mammary gland is often removed through a small perioareolar incision.

PSYCHOSOCIAL PROBLEMS FACED BY THE PATIENT WITH BREAST CANCER*

This model is designed as a conceptual tool to assist in the development of a nursing care plan or in analyzing needs of individual patients with breast cancer. The diagrams reflect most of the major critical events and psychosocial problems associated with breast cancer as well as the usual kinds of responses of patients and their families to those problems and events. Each patient and each patient's family requires a unique assessment and intervention plan, since needs and experiences are as distinctive as they are individual. *This framework is designed to guide in the development of nursing interventions intended to alleviate stress, enhance coping abilities and improve the patient's and family's chances for emotional recovery.*

I. THE PRODROMAL PROFILE

By assessing the personal characteristics of the patient, the nurse can anticipate ways in which the patient will respond to or cope with illness.

How does she typically approach problems?

What are her attitudes toward her own health maintenance? towards physicians and seeking medical attention?

How flexible or rigid is she in making adjustments, accepting crisis situations?

What is her intellectual capability to make and accept decisions?

What is her physical condition?

What is her relation to her family? How supportive are they?

What has been the patient's personal experience with illness? with cancer?

How informed is she about breast cancer? about her own illness?

II. THE PREDIAGNOSTIC PERIOD

Usually shock is part of the reaction of discovering a sign or symptoms of a breast abnormality: a lump, dimpling of the skin, nipple discharge, or pronouncement by the physician of seeing a shadow on the mammogram. Then follow confusion and fear, withdrawal, and even avoidance of care (delay in seeking treatment). The family is usually unable to provide the hoped-for support, which finally forces the patient to seek medical attention and a clarification of the nature of the problem. Therefore, from a state of disorganization, the patient moves to seek more accurate information which in turn will affect the next step in her ability to cope.

III. THE DIAGNOSTIC PERIOD

The family is usually excluded during this time. The patient is likely to be fearful about test outcomes and even embarrassed in undergoing some of the procedures. Unless there is confirmation of a benign process, she is usually directed to a biopsy or other surgical treatment alternative.

*Adapted from Thomas, S. G.: Breast cancer; the psychosocial issues. Cancer Nursing, 1:53-60, Feb. 1978. Copyright by Masson Publishing USA, Inc., New York

---

I PRODROMAL PERIOD

Patient Experience

1. History of prior serious illness, especially cancer
2. Experience with health care system
3. Information about breast cancer
4. Relationship with breast or other cancer patient

Patient Variables	Family Variables
1. Personality	1. Stability
2. Coping patterns	2. Number and age of members
3. Health beliefs and practices	3. Proximity and intimacy
4. Affective state	4. Interdependence
5. Intellectual and cognitive abilities	5. Resources
6. Biographical data	6. Roles and responsibilities
7. Attitudes toward breast cancer	7. Cultural/ethnic background
8. Self-concept	

PURPOSE:
Help toward formulation of planned interventions as patient and family go through critical events

---

II PREDIAGNOSTIC PERIOD
(confusion, conflict)

Patient's Responses	Critical Events	Family's Responses
shock, disbelief	Discovery of symptom	shock, disbelief, uncertainty, fear
denial withdrawal avoidance of care	Delay in seeking treatment	supports denial discourages seeking treatment

---

III DIAGNOSTIC PERIOD
(coping)

Patient		Family
active problem solving	1. Seeks medical advice: x-rays	feels excluded
seeks reassurance when denial fails	2. referral to surgeon	encourages patient to seek information
fearful of outcome	3. needle biopsy	fearful of result
anxious about techniques, procedures		

IV. PREOPERATIVE PERIOD

This is a confused time for the patient and her family. The patient usually feels well but realizes she cannot obtain bona fide reassurance from those caring for her. Her care and control are slipping to others, causing her to feel confused. She may feel threatened because decisions are being made by others. The family reflects her confusion.

V. THE OPERATIVE PERIOD

The peak of anxiety is felt by the patient and her family. The mastectomy may either immediately follow the biopsy, or an interval of time may separate the two procedures. In some instances, the separation of time may permit the patient to develop coping mechanisms. For other women, this interval may be agonizing. If the patient is part of the decision-making process, her adjustment is improved.

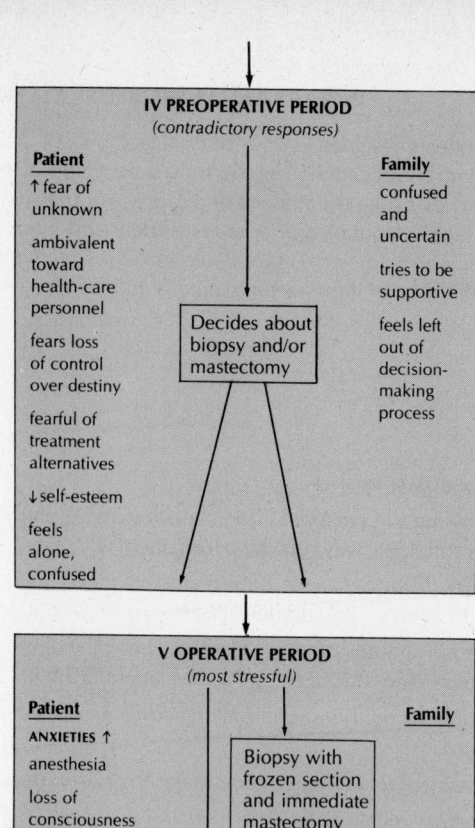

IV PREOPERATIVE PERIOD
(contradictory responses)

Patient
↑ fear of unknown

ambivalent toward health-care personnel

fears loss of control over destiny

fearful of treatment alternatives

↓ self-esteem

feels alone, confused

Decides about biopsy and/or mastectomy

Family
confused and uncertain

tries to be supportive

feels left out of decision-making process

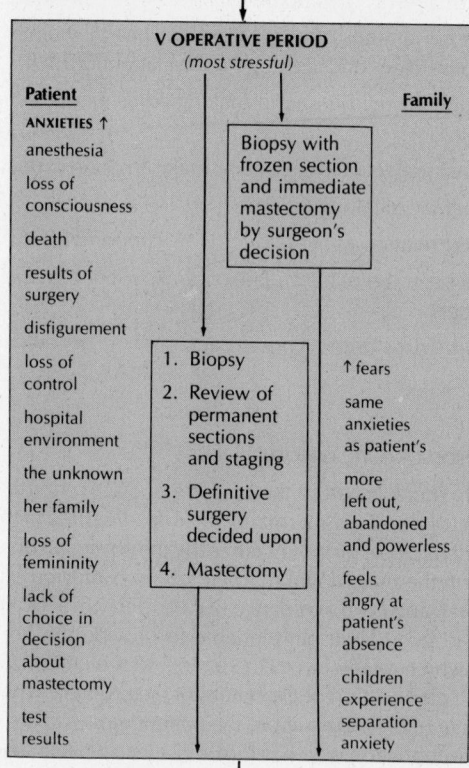

V OPERATIVE PERIOD
(most stressful)

Patient
ANXIETIES ↑
anesthesia

loss of consciousness

death

results of surgery

disfigurement

loss of control

hospital environment

the unknown

her family

loss of femininity

lack of choice in decision about mastectomy

test results

Biopsy with frozen section and immediate mastectomy by surgeon's decision

1. Biopsy
2. Review of permanent sections and staging
3. Definitive surgery decided upon
4. Mastectomy

Family
↑ fears

same anxieties as patient's

more left out, abandoned and powerless

feels angry at patient's absence

children experience separation anxiety

VI. THE IMMEDIATE POSTOPERATIVE PERIOD

Again the patient's feelings and responses may be ambivalent. On the one hand, there is relief that the operative phase is over and that she lived through it, but she may be angered about the loss of her breast. Even ambivalence toward herself may be apparent, as is indicated by self-blame for her delay in seeking treatment. This may result in sleeplessness and depression. Her thoughts drift to her family, her relationship with her husband or lover, her job, or her very future. Again, the family's reactions may parallel hers.

At home, the patient often feels lonely, isolated, and useless since she is unable to accept her former full role in the household or return to work, and other members of the family may express resentment over their extra work.

VII. EXTENDED POSTOPERATIVE PERIOD

The patient and her family are now moving into a period which they hope will bear some resemblance to the more normal time. There is less support and there are greater stresses. The family's responses appear no longer confused, and they may find it difficult to empathize with the patient during this period. Angers are often expressed.

The patient now faces the ordeal of being fitted for her prosthesis. This can be a trying time.

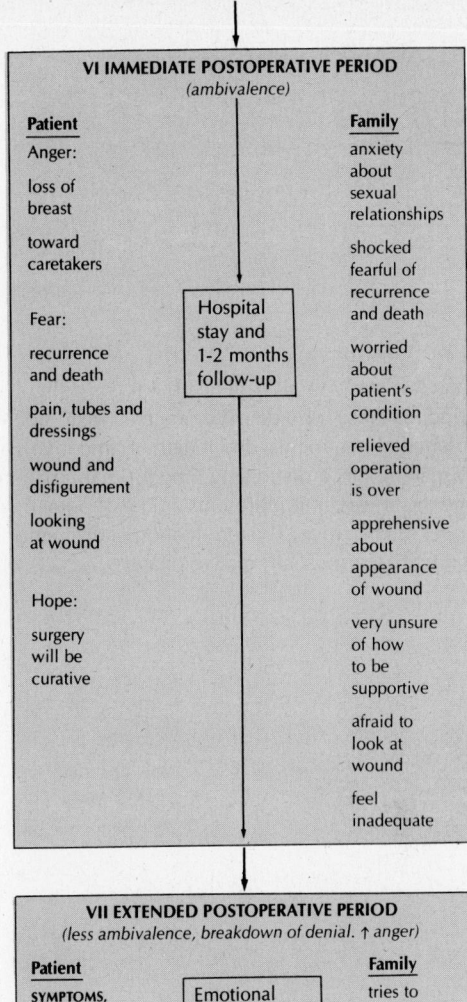

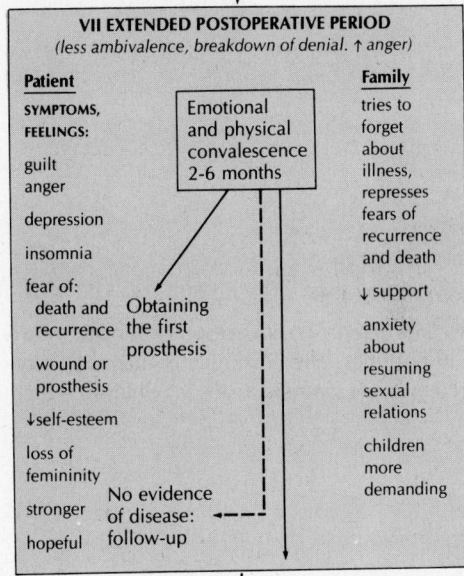

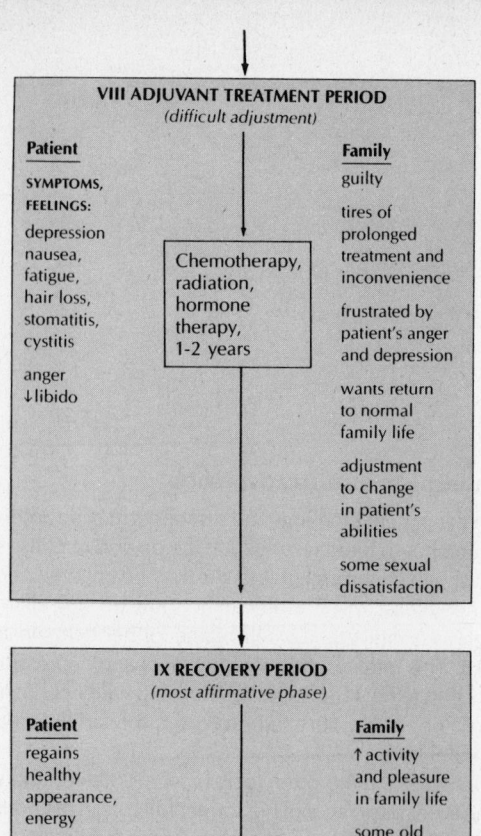

VIII ADJUVANT TREATMENT PERIOD
(difficult adjustment)

Patient

SYMPTOMS,
FEELINGS:

depression
nausea,
fatigue,
hair loss,
stomatitis,
cystitis

anger
↓libido

Chemotherapy,
radiation,
hormone
therapy,
1-2 years

Family

guilty

tires of
prolonged
treatment and
inconvenience

frustrated by
patient's anger
and depression

wants return
to normal
family life

adjustment
to change
in patient's
abilities

some sexual
dissatisfaction

VIII. ADJUVANT PERIOD

This may not apply to all patients, but it is a difficult adjustment period for those who do experience it. Toxic side effects, inconvenience of treatments, and length of time involved contribute to making this a distressing time for many patients. For some patients, however, it represents a time of potentiating the positive over the negative. The termination of this period marks the beginning of the most affirmative phase.

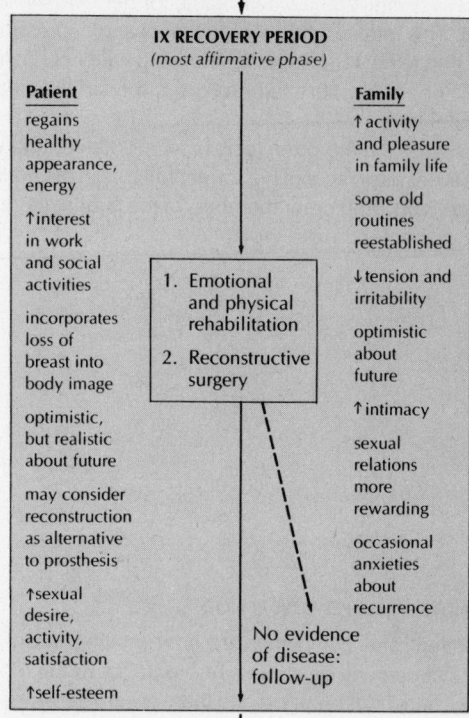

IX RECOVERY PERIOD
(most affirmative phase)

Patient

regains
healthy
appearance,
energy

↑interest
in work
and social
activities

incorporates
loss of
breast into
body image

optimistic,
but realistic
about future

may consider
reconstruction
as alternative
to prosthesis

↑sexual
desire,
activity,
satisfaction

↑self-esteem

1. Emotional
   and physical
   rehabilitation

2. Reconstructive
   surgery

Family

↑activity
and pleasure
in family life

some old
routines
reestablished

↓tension and
irritability

optimistic
about
future

↑intimacy

sexual
relations
more
rewarding

occasional
anxieties
about
recurrence

No evidence
of disease:
follow-up

IX. THE RECOVERY PERIOD

This is a time of more positive responses and the reordering of values and priorities. The possibility of mammoplasty may be considered by some women. Realistic optimism is increasingly evident.

```
                    X TERMINAL PERIOD
 Patient                                      Family
 worries                                      ↑anxiety,
 about                                        bitterness
 family
                                              confusion
 ↑fear,                                       hopelessness
 depression,      ┌──────────────┐
 anger           │ 1. Advanced  │            depression
                 │    disease   │
 bargaining      │              │            sleeplessness
                 │ 2. Metastasis│
 resignation     │              │            anorexia or
                 │ 3. Death     │            hyperphagia
 hopelessness    └──────────────┘
                                              abandoned
 possible
 acceptance                                   may feel
                                              relieved
 needs                                        when death
 family                                       occurs
 support
 ↑ or ↓                                       grieving

 withdrawal
```

X. THE TERMINAL PERIOD

For the person whose disease is terminal, the stages described by Kübler-Ross are usually experienced. The quality of life before death overtakes the actual fact of dying.

BIBLIOGRAPHY

BOOKS

Baker, R. R., ed.: Current Trends in the Management of Breast Cancer. Baltimore, Johns Hopkins University Press, 1977.

Brand, P. C., and Van Keep, P. A., eds.: Breast Cancer, Psychosocial Aspects of Early Detection and Treatment. Baltimore, University Park Press, 1978.

Gallagher, H. S.: Early Breast Cancer. New York, John Wiley and Sons, 1975.

Georgiade, N. G.: Reconstructive Breast Surgery. St. Louis, C. V. Mosby, 1976.

Goldwyn, R. M., ed.: Plastic and Reconstructive Surgery of the Breast. Boston, Little, Brown, 1976.

Haagensen, C. D.: Diseases of the Breast, 2nd ed. Philadelphia, W. B. Saunders, 1971.

Lasser, T., and Clarke, W. K.: Reach to Recovery. New York, Simon and Shuster, 1972.

Zalon, J., and Block, J. L.: I Am Whole Again: The Case for Reconstruction after Mastectomy. New York, Random House, 1978.

ARTICLES

Diagnostic Procedures and Assessment

Baker, R. R.: Preoperative assessment of the patient with breast cancer. Surg. Clin. N. Am., *58*:681-691, Aug. 1978.

Frazier, T. G., et al.: Aspiration cytology, the step before mammography. Today's Clinician, *2*:21-22, Oct. 1978.

Gorringe, R., et al.: The mammography controversy. J. Obstet. Gyn., & Neonat. Nurs.,*7*:7-12, July-Aug. 1978.

Leis, H. P.: The diagnosis of breast cancer. CA-A Cancer J. for Clinicians, *27*:209-232, July-Aug. 1977.

Logan, W. W.: Mammography in perspective. Contemp. Surg., *12*:33-46, June 1978.

Moore, F. D.: Breast self-examination (editorial). New Eng. J. Med., *299*:304-305, Aug. 10, 1978.

Moskowitz, M. L.: Mammography in medical practice. JAMA, *240*:1898-1899, Oct. 20, 1978.

Panaoussopoulos, D., et al.: Screening for breast cancer. Ann. Surg., *186*:356-362, Sept. 1977.

Strax, P.: Evaluation of screening programs for the early diagnosis of breast cancer. Surg. Clin. N. Am., *58*:667-679, Aug. 1978.

Turnbull, E.: Breast examination practices. AJN, 77:1450-1451, Sept. 1977.

_____: Effect of basic preventive health practices and mass media on the practice of breast self-examination. Nurs. Res., *27*:98-102, Mar.-Apr. 1978.

Breast Cancer

Albert, S., et al.: Recent trends in the treatment of primary breast cancer. Cancer, *41*:2399-2404, June 1978.

Becker, K. L.: Hypercalcemia of breast cancer. Female Patient, *3*:38-42, Jan. 1978.

Bernstein, T. C.: What are my chances of getting breast cancer? JAMA, *238*:345-346, July 25, 1977.

Bibbo, M., et al.: A twenty-five year follow-up study of women exposed to diethylstilbestrol during pregnancy. New Eng. J. Med., *298*:763-767, Apr. 6, 1978.

Bush, D. J.: Appraising current therapy for breast cancer. 2. Irradiation. Postgrad. Med., *80*:151-154, Aug. 1976.

del Regato, J. A.: Cancer of the breast. JAMA, *238*:2407-2408, Nov. 28, 1977.

Dixon, J. K., et al.: Breast cancer and weight gain. Oncol. Nurs. Forum, *5*:5-7, July 1978.

Fitzpatrick, G.: Caring for the patient with cancer of the breast. Nurs. Care, Part 1, *9*:9-15, Jan. 1976; Part 2, *9*:8-14, Feb. 1976; Part 3, *9*:16-20, Mar. 1976.

Fisher, B., and Wolmark, N.: New concepts in the management of primary breast cancer. Cancer, *36*:627-632, Aug. 1975.

Frazier, T. G., et al.: Prognosis and treatment in minimal breast cancer. Am. J. Surg., *133*:697-701, June 1977.

Haagensen, C. D.: The choice of treatment for operable carcinoma of the breast. Surgery, 76:685-714, Nov. 1974.

Holland, J. F.: Major advances in breast cancer therapy. New Eng. J. Med., *294*:440-441, Feb. 19, 1976.

Kennerle, S. L.: Breast cancer. AJN, 77:1430-1432, Sept. 1977.

Laatsch, N.: Nursing the woman receiving adjuvant chemotherapy for breast cancer. Nurs. Clin. N. Am., *13*:337-349, June 1978.

Levine, M. B.: A new role for radiation therapy. AJN, 77:1443-1444, Sept. 1977.

Mueller, C. B., and Jeffries, W.: Cancer of the breast: Its outcomes as measured by the rate of dying and causes of death. Ann. Surg., *182*:334-341, Sept. 1975.

Ochsner, A.: Appraising current therapy for breast cancer. 1. Surgery. Postgrad. Med., *60*:145-149, July 1976.

Packard, R. A., et al.: Selection of breast cancer patients for adjuvant chemotherapy. JAMA, *238*:1034-1036, Sept. 5, 1977.

Schnabel, F. M., Jr.: Concepts for systemic treatment of micrometastasis. Cancer, *35*:15-24, Jan. 1975.

Schwartz, M. K.: Hormone receptor assay. AJN, 77:1445-1446, Sept. 1977.

Segaloff, A.: Appraising current therapy for breast cancer. 3. Hormonal manipulation and chemotherapy. Postgrad. Med., *60*:191-193, Sept. 1976.

Teicher, I., ed.: The treatment of potentially curable breast cancer. Res. & Staff Phys., *24*:55-65, Sept. 1978.

Thomas, S. G.: Breast cancer: The psychosocial issues. Cancer Nurs., *1*:53-60, Feb. 1978.

Todd, A.: Prophylactic mastectomy. AJN, 77:1447-1449, Sept. 1977.

Tully, J. P., and Wagner, B.: Breast cancer. Nursing '78, *8*:18-25, Jan. 1978.

Woods, N. F., and Earp, J. L.: Women with cured breast cancer. Nurs. Res., *27*:279-285, Sept.-Oct. 1978.

Rehabilitation, Reconstructive Surgery, Breast Prostheses

Burdick, D.: Rehabilitation of the breast cancer patient. Cancer, *36*:645-648, Aug. 1975.

Deanesly, M.: Breast prostheses. JAMA, *236*:499, Aug. 2, 1976.

Dinner, M. I., and Peters, C. R.: Breast reconstruction following mastectomy. Surg. Clin. N. Am., *58*:851-868, Aug. 1978.

Dowden, R. V.: Advising the mastectomy patient about reconstruction. Am. Fam. Phys., *19*:103-106, May 1979.

Finn, K. L.: Augmentation mammoplasty. Nursing '79, *9*:60-63, Feb. 1979.

Grabois, M.: Rehabilitation of the postmastectomy patient with lymphedema. CA-A Cancer J. for Clinicians, *26*:75-80, Mar.-Apr. 1976.

Guthrie, R. H.: The case for breast reconstruction after mastectomy. CA-A Cancer J. for Clinicians, *28*:218-224, July-Aug. 1978.

Hazards of silicone injections (editorial). JAMA, *236*:959, Aug. 23, 1976.

Puhaty, H. D.: Two rehabilitative approaches. AJN, 77:1437, Sept. 1977.

Stallings, J. E., et al.: Reconstructing the breast after mastectomy. Female Patient, *3*:79-83, Feb. 1978.

Thomas, S. G., and Yates, M. M.: Breast reconstruction after mastectomy. AJN, 77:1438-1442, Sept. 1977.

Winkler, W. A.: Choosing the prosthesis and clothing. AJN, 77:1433-1436, Sept. 1977.

Woods, N. F., and Earp, J. L.: Women with cured breast cancer. Nurs. Res., *27*:279-285, Sept.-Oct. 1978.

AGENCY

American Cancer Society, 777 Third Ave., New York, N.Y. 10017

47

MANAGEMENT OF THE MALE PATIENT WITH DISORDERS RELATED TO THE REPRODUCTIVE SYSTEM

In the male, several organs serve as parts of both the urinary tract and the reproductive system. Disease of these organs may produce functional abnormalities of either or both systems. For this reason, diseases of the entire reproductive system in the male usually are treated by the urologist.

PHYSIOLOGIC OVERVIEW

The structures included in the male reproductive system are the testes, the vas deferens and the seminal vesicles, the penis, and certain accessory glands, such as the prostate gland and Cowper's gland (Fig. 47-1). The testes are formed in embryonal life within the abdominal cavity near the kidney. During the last month of fetal life, they descend posterior to the peritoneum, to pierce the abdominal wall in the groin. Later they progress along the inguinal canal into the scrotum. In this descent, they are accompanied by blood vessels, lymphatics, nerves, and ducts, which, along with supporting and investing tissue, make up the spermatic cord. This cord extends from the internal inguinal ring through the abdominal wall and the inguinal canal to the scrotum. As the testes descend into the scrotum, a tubular process of peritoneum accompanies them. This normally is obliterated, the only remaining portion being that which covers the testes, the *tunica vaginalis*. (When this peritoneal process

is not obliterated but remains open into the abdominal cavity, a potential sac remains, into which abdominal contents may enter to form an indirect inguinal hernia.)

The testes proper consist of numerous seminiferous tubules in which are formed the male reproductive elements, the spermatozoa. These are transmitted by a system of collecting tubules into the epididymis, which is a hoodlike structure lying on the testes and containing tortuous ducts that lead into the vas deferens. This firm tubular structure passes upward through the inguinal canal to enter the abdominal cavity behind the peritoneum and then extends downward toward the base of the bladder. An outpouching from this structure is the seminal vesicle, which acts as a reservoir for the secretion of the testes. The tract is continued as the ejaculatory duct, which then passes through the prostate gland to enter the urethra. The secretion of the testes is carried by this pathway to the end of the penis in the reproductive act.

The testes have a dual function. The primary function is reproduction—the formation of spermatozoa from the germinal cells of the seminiferous tubules. However, the testes are also important glands of internal secretion. This secretion is produced by the so-called interstitial cells and is called the male sex hormone, or testosterone, which induces and preserves the male sex qualities.

The prostate gland lies just below the neck of the bladder. It surrounds the urethra posteriorly and laterally and is traversed by the ejaculatory duct, the continuation

1027

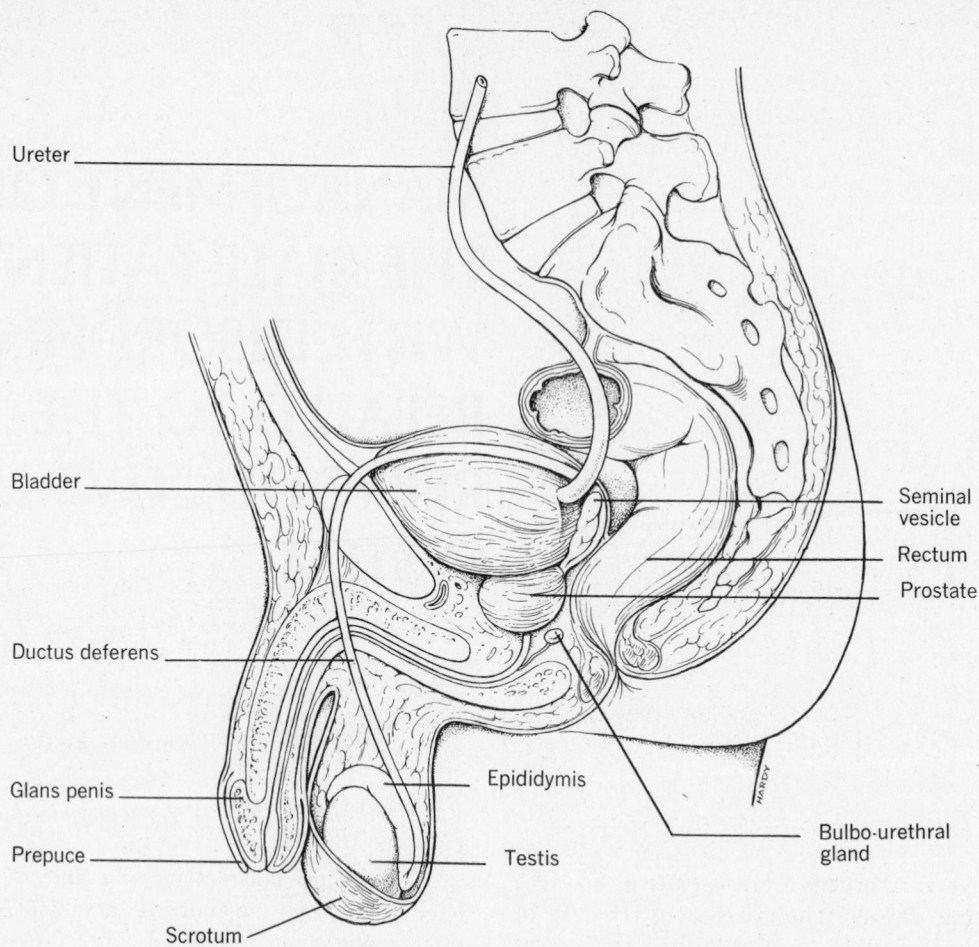

Ureter

Bladder

Ductus deferens

Glans penis

Prepuce

Scrotum

Seminal vesicle

Rectum

Prostate

Epididymis

Testis

Bulbo-urethral gland

Figure 47-1. Organs of the male reproductive system. (From Chaffee, E. E., and Greisheimer, E. M.: Basic Physiology and Anatomy, 3rd ed. Philadelphia, J. B. Lippincott, 1974)

of the vas deferens. This gland produces a secretion that is chemically and physiologically suitable to the needs of the spermatozoa in their passage from the genital glands.

The penis has a dual function of being the organ of copulation and of urination. Anatomically, it consists of a glans penis, a body, and a root. The glans penis is the soft rounded portion at the end that retains its soft structure even when erect. The urethra opens at the extremity of the glans. The glans normally is covered or protected by an elongation of the skin of the penis—the foreskin— which may be deflected to expose the glans. The body of the penis is composed of erectile tissues that contain numerous blood vessels that may become distended during sexual excitement. Through it passes the urethra, which extends from the bladder through the prostate to the end of the penis.

Congenital Malformations. Of the many disturbances of normal growth that may occur, the most common is a failure of the testes to descend into the scrotum. This condition is called *cryptorchidism.*

Failure of the urethra to form normally in the penis can result in hypospadias or epispadias. *Hypospadias* occurs

when the urethral opening is on the lower wall of the penis; when the urethral opening is a groove on its upper surface, the condition is called *epispadias*. These anatomical abnormalities may be repaired by various types of plastic operations. (The reader is referred to a pediatric textbook for a complete discussion of these conditions.)

CONDITIONS AFFECTING THE PENIS

Infections

Gonorrhea. Gonorrhea occurs as a result of an infection due to the gonococcus, which penetrates the tissues of the urethra as a result of sexual exposure. The time elapsing from the moment of infection until the development of disease may be from 4 to 10 days and sometimes longer. The infection produces a marked purulent, usually painful, urethral discharge.

However, some males may be asymptomatic, as seems to be indicated by the increased numbers of such carriers who are being identified.

At first the anterior portion of the urethra is invaded,

but not infrequently the infection extends posteriorly to involve the prostate and to extend along the vas deferens, producing infection in the seminal vesicles and in the epididymis. The disease is diagnosed by the examination of a stained smear of the pus from the urethra. The gonococci appear as bean-shaped organisms in pairs, lying within the pus cells and staining in a characteristic manner.

Early treatment of the infection is most likely to prevent development of the complications of gonorrhea (page 1373). It must not be forgotten that the transmission of the infection from the urethra to the eyes may produce a very marked ophthalmia. Therefore, secretion precautions (page 1366) must be followed, if drainage is present. Penicillin prophylaxis and therapy have given excellent results. (See page 1375 for treatment of gonorrhea.)

Penile Ulceration. Several types of penile ulcerations may occur, but because of the danger of chancre (syphilis), all lesions are considered to be syphilitic until proved otherwise. Diagnosis is made by a combination of history of the disease, a microscopic examination of a darkfield specimen removed from the lesions, and a blood serology examination. The treatment of penile ulceration varies greatly, depending on the cause of the ulceration. It is not started until the diagnosis is made.

Chancre is a venereal ulceration caused by *Treponema pallidum* and is the primary lesion of syphilis. It occurs as a result of sexual exposure. Local treatment usually is unnecessary, other than a mild antiseptic and a protective dressing, the main portion of the treatment being confined to systemic measures that usually result in a rapid healing of the local lesion. Penicillin produces a rapid cure.

Chancroid is an ulceration produced by a mixed infection, usually associated with marked lymphadenopathy in the groin. Treatment often necessitates circumcision, and cauterization of the ulceration.

Balanitis is an inflammation and ulceration of the glans penis produced by a spirochete and a gram-positive bacillus acting in symbiosis. These organisms are largely anaerobic; therefore, the infection always occurs under the foreskin. It is usually associated with phimosis (see below). Circumcision is the definitive treatment. The patient is instructed in proper hygiene of the foreskin to prevent recurrence.

Herpes of the glans penis begins as a small blister that produces secondary ulceration. This is not a venereal disease, and the ulcerations heal rapidly under protective dressing or with a mild antiseptic treatment.

Phimosis

Phimosis is a condition in which the foreskin is narrowed so that it cannot be retracted over the glans. It may be corrected by *circumcision*. The operation consists of removing the prepuce (foreskin) so that the glans penis is not covered. Since the adult male may experience a considerable amount of pain following circumcision, analgesia may be given as frequently as the patient's condition indicates. The patient is watched for bleeding, and the petrolatum (Vaseline) gauze dressing is changed as indicated. *Circumcision is an important preventive measure against carcinoma of the penis.*

Paraphimosis is a condition in which the foreskin is retracted behind the glans and, because of narrowness and subsequent edema, cannot be reduced back to its usual position (covering the glans). It is treated by manual reduction (compressing the glans firmly, to reduce its size, and then pushing the glans back as the prepuce is moved forward). Circumcision is usually indicated once the inflammation and edema subside.

Carcinoma

Cancer of the penis occurs in the skin of the penis and rarely in circumcised individuals. It appears as a painless, wartlike growth or ulcer on the glans or foreskin and represents about 3 percent of all skin cancer. Complete amputation of the penis with bilateral lymph-node dissections of the groin may be necessary. If there is nodal metastases, a partial penectomy is done, followed by palliative radiation for controlling ulceration.

Patient Education. Circumcision in infancy is considered by some to be a preventive measure, as chronic irritation and inflammation of the glans penis predisposes to penile tumors.

Priapism

Priapism is an uncontrolled persistent erection of the penis that causes the penis to become very large, hard, and, often, painful. It occurs from several causes, including sickle cell thrombosis, chronic irritation, and tumor invasion of the penis or its vessels. This condition may result in gangrene and often results in impotence, whether treated or not.

Initially, treatment is directed at relieving the erection, and includes bed rest, sedation, and application of ice packs. The corpora may be irrigated with an anticoagulant and a compression bandage applied. Surgical treatment may be carried out to provide venous drainage of the corpora cavernosa. This condition is considered a surgical emergency.

CONDITIONS AFFECTING THE TESTES AND ADJACENT STRUCTURES

Undescended Testis (Cryptorchidism)

Cryptorchidism is the absence of one or both testes from the scrotum. The testes may be located in the abdominal cavity or inguinal canal. If the testis does not descend, hormone therapy and/or surgery (*orchidopexy*) are employed to secure proper positioning.

In orchidopexy, an incision is made over the inguinal canal, and the testis is brought down and placed in the scrotum. To maintain proper position of the testis, traction may be applied to the thigh by means of a suture drawn from the lower end of the scrotum.

Epididymitis

Epididymitis is an infection of the epididymis which usually descends from an infected prostate or urinary tract. It may develop as a complication of gonorrhea or be of hematogenous origin. Postoperative epididymitis is a complication of prostatectomy and/or urethral catheterization. The infection passes upward through the urethra and the ejaculatory duct, and thence along the vas deferens to the epididymis.

The patient complains of pain and soreness in the inguinal canal along the course of the vas deferens and then develops pain and swelling in the scrotum and the groin. The epididymis becomes swollen and extremely painful; the temperature is elevated. The patient may experience pyuria and bacteriuria with resulting chills and fever.

Management. The patient is placed on bed rest with the scrotum elevated (scrotal support) to prevent tension on the spermatic cord and to improve venous drainage and relieve pain. Antimicrobials may be given until all evidence of the acute inflammatory reaction has subsided. If the patient is seen within the first 24 hours after onset, the spermatic cord may be infiltrated with a local anesthetic agent to relieve pain.

Intermittent cold compresses to the scrotum may help the pain. Local heat or sitz baths later in the infection may hasten resolution of the inflammatory process. Analgesics are given for pain relief. The patient is observed for abscess formation. An epididymectomy (excision of the epididymis from the testicle) may be performed for patients with recurrent incapacitating episodes or for those with chronic painful conditions. If no improvement occurs within two weeks, an underlying testis tumor should be considered.

Patient Education. The patient should avoid straining (lifting) and sexual excitement until the infection is under control. It may take four weeks or longer for the epididymis to return to normal.

Orchitis

Orchitis is an inflammation of the testis that may occur as a result of some systemic infection. Other causative factors include torsion of the spermatic cord or severe trauma. Mumps is the main cause of pure orchitis that is not secondary to epididymitis.

The symptoms are characteristic. The testicle becomes swollen, tense, and painful, and the condition often is accompanied by high temperature, nausea, and other systemic symptoms. The marked swelling inside the capsule of the testis may be sufficient to shut off the blood supply to the organ, so that gangrene of the testis may occur. The sudden cessation of pain is a symptom of this complication.

Rest, and the application of hot and cold compresses are the usual local measures. Support of the scrotum is very helpful. Antimicrobials are given to control some infections but are of no value in the treatment of mumps orchitis.

Bilateral mumps orchitis may lead to infertility. All susceptible children, over 1 year, especially boys, should receive mumps-attenuated virus vaccine to prevent mumps.

Tumors of the Testes (Cancer)

Testicular cancer accounts for only 1 percent of all malignant tumors, but it ranks first in cancer deaths among males in the 25 to 34 age group. The etiology of testicular tumors is unknown, but cryptorchidism, trauma, infections, and genetic and endocrine factors appear to play a part in their development. These tumors are almost always malignant and tend to metastasize early.

Clinical Manifestations. The symptoms appear very gradually with a painless enlargement of the testis accompanied by a feeling of heaviness in the scrotum. Backache (from metastatic deposits), pain in the abdomen, loss of weight, and general weakness may follow. Gynecomastia (enlargement of the breasts) due to elaboration of chorionic gonadotropins produced by the testicular tumor is considered a serious prognostic sign. The metastatic growth may be more marked than the local testicular one. The enlargement of the testicle without pain is a significant diagnostic finding.

Management. The objective of management is to control the spread of the tumor. The testicle is removed (orchiectomy) through an inguinal incision with a high ligation of the spermatic cord. The lumbar and iliac chains of lymph nodes may be resected, in certain histological types. Postoperative irradiation to the lymphatic drainage pathways is usually done.

Testicular carcinomas are highly responsive to drug therapy. Multiple chemotherapeutic agents (bleomycin, vinblastine, actinomycin D) or other combinations given according to the stage of the disease may be tried with disseminated testicular cancer. The program of therapy is probably best prescribed by those trained in oncology, since there are toxic effects from these drugs. Good results may be obtained by combining different types of treatment, including surgery, radiotherapy, and chemo-therapy. Disseminated testicular cancer is coming to be regarded as a treatable and probably curable disease.

Patient Education and Support. The patient may have difficulty in accepting his condition. He needs encouragement to maintain a positive attitude during what may be a long course of therapy. Radiotherapy does not necessarily prevent the patient from fathering children, nor will unilateral excision of a tumor necessarily lessen virility.

A patient with a history of one tumor of the testes has a greater chance of developing another. Follow-up evaluation includes chest x-rays, excretory urography, assay of urinary gonadotropins, and examination of lymph nodes to detect recurrence of malignancy.

Self-examination for testicular tumor may well be as important for men (especially those between 15 and 35 years, which are the tumor-prone years) as is self-examination for breast cancer by women.

The testis is easily accessible for self-examination, and most tumors are palpable. The patient should conduct the examination periodically, while showering or bathing.

The following are guidelines for self-examination for testicular tumor:
1. Use both hands to feel for any abnormalities. Examine the contents of the scrotum.
2. Locate the epididymis, which is the cordlike structure at the back of the testis. This is important in order to avoid confusing the epididymis with an abnormality.
3. Feel each testis between the thumb and first two fingers of each hand. The testes lie freely in the scrotum, are oval in shape, have a spongy, uniform texture, and measure 4 to 5 cm. in length, 3 cm. in width, and about 2 cm. in thickness.
4. Note the size and shape, and the presence, of any abnormal tenderness. An abnormality may be felt as a firm area on the front or on the side of the testis.
5. Stand in front of the mirror and look for changes in the size and shape of the scrotum. Tumors tend to involve only one side.

Hydrocele and Varicocele

Hydrocele. A hydrocele is a collection of fluid in the tunica vaginalis of the testicle or along the spermatic cord. It may be acute or chronic. The acute type occurs in association with acute infectious diseases of the epididymis or as a result of local trauma or of a systemic infectious disease, such as mumps. This type of hydrocele usually disappears spontaneously with improvement in the causative disease, and no local treatment is necessary.

Chronic hydrocele occurs as a result of a low-grade infection of the testes or the epididymis. It may occur also without any evident infection of these structures. The tunica vaginalis becomes widely distended with fluid; this lesion is differentiated from a hernia by the fact that it transmits light when transilluminated.

Usually therapy is not required. Treatment of the chronic type of hydrocele may be sought because of the inconvenience of the large scrotal mass, or for cosmetic reasons.

In the surgical treatment of hydrocele, an incision is made through the wall of the scrotum down to the distended tunica vaginalis. The sac is opened and excised or everted around the testicle. In the postoperative care of these patients, an athletic supporter is worn for comfort and support. The major complication is the formation of a hematoma in the loose tissues of the scrotum. The nursing management is the same as for a varicocele.

Varicocele. Varicocele is an abnormal dilation of the veins of the pampiniform venous plexus in the scrotum (a network of veins from the testicle and the epididymis, constituting part of the spermatic cord). Varicoceles occur most frequently in the veins on the left side in young adults. Very few, if any, subjective symptoms may be produced by the enlargement of the spermatic vein, and as a rule, no treatment is required. When pain, tenderness, and discomfort in the inguinal regions occur, therapy may be instituted. This usually consists of ligation of the enlarged veins. In the postoperative care of the patient, a scrotal support is worn for a time. An ice bag may be applied to the scrotum for the first few hours after operation to relieve edema.

Vasectomy

A *vasectomy* is the ligation and transection of a section of the vas deferens, with or without removal of a segment of the vas. The severed ends are occluded with ligatures or clips, or the lumen of each vas is coagulated. A bilateral vasectomy may be done as a sterilization procedure, since it interrupts the transportation of the sperm. (The sperm which are manufactured in the testicle are unable to travel up the vas deferens because of surgical interruption.) This procedure is also performed if the patient has recurrent acute epididymitis.

Seminal fluid is mostly manufactured in the seminal vesicles and prostate gland, which are unaffected by vasectomy. Thus there will be no noticeable decrease in the amount of ejaculated fluid, except that it contains no sperm. Because the sperm cells have no exit, they are reabsorbed into the body. The procedure has no effect on sexual potency, erection, ejaculation, or production of male hormones.

Psychological problems (impotency) have been noted in an occasional patient following this procedure. However, men reporting postvasectomy impotency had some problems with impotency before the operation. Some studies purport that vasectomy can lead to autoimmune disorders, in that antibodies which agglutinate the patient's own sperm may form after this procedure. However, an increased incidence of autoimmune disorders following vasectomy has not yet been clinically proven and the implications are not yet clear.

The patient is advised that he will be sterile, but that potency will not be altered following a bilateral vasectomy. The procedure does not prevent venereal disease. On rare occasions, a spontaneous reanastomosis of the vas deferens occurs, which may result in pregnancy of the partner. A legal consent form (usually signed by both the man and his partner) must be obtained before the procedure is carried out.

Postoperative Considerations. Ice bags are applied intermittently to the scrotum for several hours after surgery to reduce swelling and relieve discomfort. The patient is advised to wear an athletic supporter for added comfort and support. He may become greatly concerned about the discoloration of the scrotal skin and superficial swelling. This occurs frequently after vasectomy and responds to sitz baths. Complications of vasectomy include scrotal ecchymoses and swelling, superficial wound infection, vasitis (inflammation of the vas deferens), epididymitis or epididymo–orchitis, hematomas, and sperm granuloma. A sperm granuloma is an inflammatory response to the collection of sperm in the scrotum due to leakage from the severed end of the proximal vas. This can initiate recanalization of the vas, leading to possible pregnancy of the partner.

Patient Education. Sexual intercourse may be resumed as desired by the patient, although he should be informed that he will still be fertile for a varying length of time after vasectomy until the sperm that are stored distal to the point of interruption of the vas have been evacuated. Absence of sperm must be confirmed by two consecutive laboratory tests (taken one month apart) which demonstrate that no viable sperm are present in the seminal fluid. Contraceptives should be used until this is done, and for at least four months after operation.

Vasovasostomy (Sterilization Reversal). Microsurgical techniques are being used for vasectomy reversal (vasovasostomy) which restores patency to the vas deferens. However, the success rate of this procedure is still under investigation.

CONDITIONS OF THE PROSTATE

Benign Prostatic Hyperplasia

In many patients over 50 years of age, the prostate gland enlarges, extending upward into the bladder and obstructing the outflow of urine by encroaching on the vesical orifice. This condition is known as enlargement of the prostate. The etiology is uncertain, but the condition is related to endocrine changes that initiate hyperplasia of the supporting stromal tissue and of glandular elements in the prostate.

Since enlargement of the prostate gland produces an obstruction to flow of urine, a gradual dilatation of the ureters (hydroureter) and kidneys (hydronephrosis) results. The hypertrophied lobe extends upward into the bladder and forms a pouch that retains urine. This pouch is not emptied when voiding takes place, and the remaining urine (residual urine) decomposes and may produce calculi or a *cystitis*.

The symptoms (referred to as *prostatism*) include increasing frequency of urination, nocturia, hesitancy in starting urination, diminution in size and force of urinary stream, interruption of urinary stream, terminal dribbling, and/or acute urinary retention.

A battery of diagnostic examinations may be carried out to determine the degree of prostatic enlargement, the presence of any bladder wall changes, and the efficiency of renal function.

Management. The plan of treatment depends upon the cause, the severity of the obstruction, and the condition of the patient. If a patient is admitted as an emergency because he is unable to void, he is immediately catheterized. The ordinary catheter frequently will be too soft and pliable to pass through the urethra into the bladder. A thin wire, called a stylet, is introduced (by a urologist) into the catheter in order to prevent the catheter from collapsing when it encounters resistance. In severe cases, metal catheters with a pronounced *prostatic curve* may be used. Sometimes a suprapubic cystostomy is necessary to give adequate drainage.

Surgery is usually necessary when treatment is required because of obstruction. Complete removal of the hyperplastic prostatic tissue, without removal of the surgical capsule of the prostate, is usually done. (Nursing management following prostatic surgery is discussed on the page which follows.)

Prostatitis

Prostatitis is an inflammation of the prostatic gland. It may be caused by bacterial invasion, by other infectious agents (viruses, mycotic organisms, and those organisms intermediate between bacteria and viruses), or by a variety of other problems (urethral stricture, prostatic hyperplasia, etc.). Microorganisms usually are carried to the prostate from the urethra. The most common type of prostatitis is called *nonspecific prostatitis* or *prostatosis,* which produces symptoms of perineal discomfort, occasional burning, urgency, and frequency, but no pathogenic bacteria can be cultured from the urine or prostatic fluid.

Acute bacterial prostatitis may produce a sudden onset of fever and chills and perineal, rectal, or back pain. Urinary symptoms of burning, frequency, urgency, nocturia, and terminal dysuria may be evident. Some patients, however, are asymptomatic.

Diagnosis requires a careful history, culture of prostatic fluid or tissue, and, occasionally, a histological examination of tissue. In order to locate the source of the lower genitourinary infection, it is necessary to collect a divided urinary specimen. After the patient cleanses the glans penis and retracts the foreskin (if present), he voids 10 to 15 ml. of urine into the first container. This represents urethral urine. A second voiding of 50 to 75 ml. of urine is then collected in a second container without interruption; this represents bladder urine. If the patient does not have acute prostatitis, the physician immediately performs a prostatic massage, and any prostatic fluid which is expressed is collected by gravity drainage into a third container. If it is not possible to collect prostatic fluid, the patient voids a small quantity of urine. This specimen may contain the bacteria present in the prostatic fluid.

Management. The objective of management is to avoid the complications of abscess formation and septicemia. A broad-spectrum antimicrobial (to which the organism causing the infection is susceptible) is given for a period of 10 to 14 days. Intravenous administration of the drug may be necessary to achieve high serum and tissue levels. The patient is encouraged to remain on bed rest, and comfort is promoted with analgesics (pain relief), antispasmodics and bladder sedatives (relieves bladder irritability), sitz baths (relieves pain and spasm) and stool softeners (prevent straining at stool, which increases pain).

Swelling of the gland may produce urinary retention. Other complications include epididymitis, bacteremia or septicemia, and pyelonephritis.

Chronic bacterial prostatitis is a major source of relapsing urinary-tract infection in men. The treatment of chronic prostatitis is difficult, because of poor diffusion of most antimicrobials from the plasma into the prostatic fluid. A combination of trimethoprim and sulfamethoxazole (Bactrim; Septra) or a course of tetracycline has been advocated.

Patient Education. Alcohol and coffee may not be permitted and sexual intercourse is to be avoided during the period of chronic inflammation. Many patients secretly fear that the cause of prostatitis is venereal disease. Patients need to be reassured that this is not true. However, they should be followed medically for at least six months to a year, as recurrence of prostatitis caused by the same, or different, organisms can occur.

THE PATIENT UNDERGOING PROSTATECTOMY

Preoperative Considerations

The treatment of choice for prostatic hyperplasia is prostatectomy. *The preoperative objective is to establish optimum kidney function.* An indwelling catheter is introduced if the patient has continuing urinary retention, if residual urine amounts to more than 75 to 100 ml., or if there is evidence of azotemia (accumulation of nitrogenous waste products in the blood). It may be desirable to decompress the bladder gradually over a period of several days, especially if the patient is elderly and hypertensive and has diminished renal function or an excessive amount of urinary retention that has existed for many weeks. *The blood pressure may fluctuate and renal function declines the first few days after bladder drainage is instituted.* If the patient cannot tolerate a urethral catheter, cystostomy drainage is employed (page 913). Frequently the patient is dehydrated from self-limitation of fluids because of urinary frequency. If the patient's cardiac reserve is adequate, a liberal fluid intake (2500–3000 ml. daily) is encouraged to help overcome azotemia. The intake and output and daily weight are monitored.

Renal function studies are carried out to determine if there is renal impairment from prostatic back pressure and to evaluate renal reserve. All measures are taken to ensure that the patient is in the best possible condition for surgery, since older persons have diminishing reserves of vital-organ function. A complete hematologic investigation is done. Since hemorrhage is a major postoperative complication, all clotting defects must be corrected. A high percentage of these patients have cardiac or respiratory complications, or both. The patient's mode of life during the past few months should also be noted. Has he been reasonably active? Can he raise himself out of bed and return to bed without assistance? This assessment may help determine how quickly the patient will be returned to his normal activities following prostatectomy. He should stop smoking at least 2 days before surgery, especially if he has pulmonary emphysema.

Antiembolism stockings are applied before the operation and are particularly important if the patient is placed in a lithotomy position during surgery. The preoperative enema may prevent straining, which can induce postoperative bleeding.

Surgical Approach

Four different approaches are possible in removing the hypertrophied fibroadenomatous portion of the prostate gland (Table 47-1). In all four techniques, all hyperplastic tissue is removed, leaving behind the surgical capsule of the prostate.

Suprapubic prostatectomy is one method of removing the gland through an abdominal wound. An opening is made into the bladder, and the gland is removed from above (Fig. 47-2). Such an approach can be used for a gland of any size, and few complications occur, although blood loss may be greater than with other methods. Another disadvantage is the need for an abdominal incision with the concomitant hazards of any major surgical procedure.

TABLE 47-1   COMPARISON OF SURGICAL APPROACHES FOR PROSTATECTOMY

The operation of choice depends on (1) the size of the gland, (2) the severity of the obstruction, (3) the age of the patient, (4) the condition of patient, and (5) the presence of associated diseases.

	ADVANTAGES	DISADVANTAGES	NURSING IMPLICATIONS
Transurethral (removal of prostatic tissue by instrument introduced through urethra)	Safer for surgical-risk patient Shorter period of hospitalization and convalescence Useful for smaller gland Lower mortality rate Avoids abdominal incision Causes less pain	Requires highly skilled operator Not indicated for greatly enlarged prostate Recurrent obstruction, urethral trauma, and stricture may develop Delayed bleeding may occur	Watch for evidence of hemorrhage (drainage in bag). Observe for symptoms of urethral stricture (dysuria, straining, small urinary stream).
Open Surgical Removal			
Suprapubic	Technically simple Offers wider area of exploration Permits exploration for cancerous lymph nodes Allows more complete removal of obstructing gland Permits treatment of associated lesions in bladder	Requires surgical approach through the bladder Control of hemorrhage difficult Urinary leakage around suprapubic tube Convalescence more prolonged and uncomfortable	Watch for indications of hemorrhage and shock. Give meticulous aseptic attention to area around suprapubic tube.
Perineal	Offers direct anatomic approach Permits gravity drainage Particularly efficacious for radical cancer therapy Allows hemostasis under direct vision Low mortality rate Less incidence of shock Ideal for very old, feeble, and poor-risk patient with large prostate	Higher postoperative incidence of impotency and urinary incontinency Problem of damage to rectum and external sphincter Restricted operative field	Avoid rectal tubes, rectal thermometers, and enemas after perineal surgery. Use drainage pads to absorb excess urinary drainage. Secure foam-rubber ring for patient comfort. May be urinary leakage around wound for several days after catheter removal.
Retropubic	Most versatile procedure; affords direct visualization Avoids incision in the bladder Permits easier visualization and control of bleeders Shorter period of convalescence	Cannot treat associated pathology in bladder Increased incidence of hemorrhage from prostatic venous plexus; osteitis pubis	Watch for evidences of hemorrhage. Posturinary leakage may occur for several days after catheter is removed.

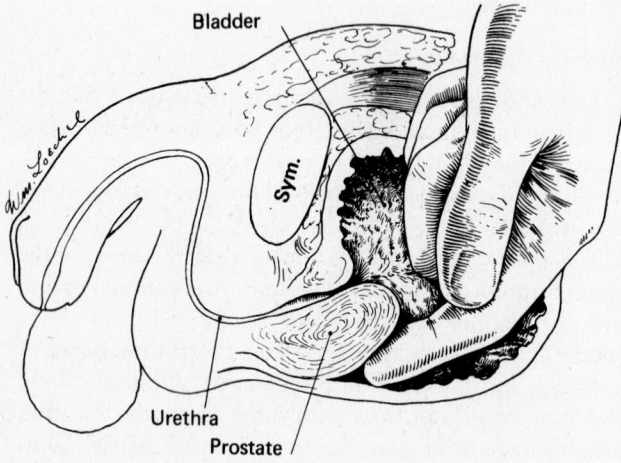

Figure 47-2. Suprapubic prostatectomy. Diagrammatic drawing shows how the prostate is shelled out of its bed with the finger.

In *perineal prostatectomy*, the gland is removed through an incision in the perineum (Fig. 47-3). This approach is practicable when other approaches are blocked. It is a useful procedure when open biopsy is needed. In the postoperative period, the wound may become contaminated rather easily because of the position of the incision. Incontinence, impotence, or rectal injury are more likely sequelae when this approach is used.

A *transurethral resection* of the prostate can be carried out by means of an endoscopic instrument that has an ocular and operating system. The instrument is introduced through the urethra to the prostate, which can be viewed directly. The gland is then removed piecemeal (Fig. 47-4). The real advantage of this method is the absence of an incision. It may be used for glands up to moderate size, and it is ideal for most poor-risk patients with small glands. This approach means a shorter hospital stay;

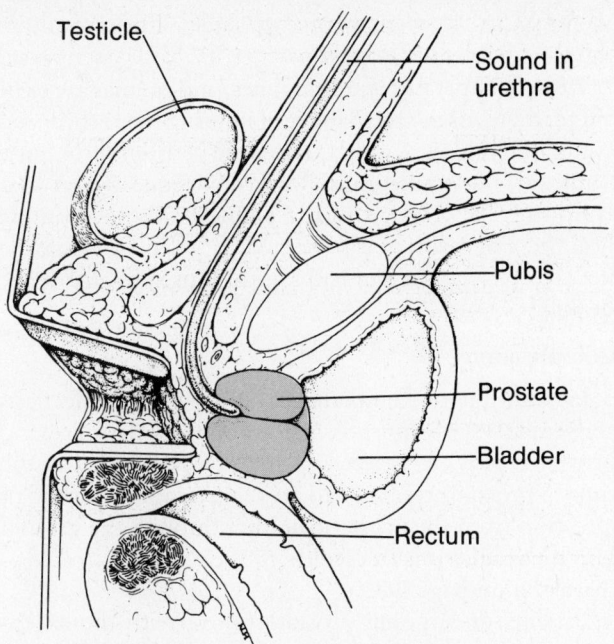

Figure 47-3.   Perineal prostatectomy.

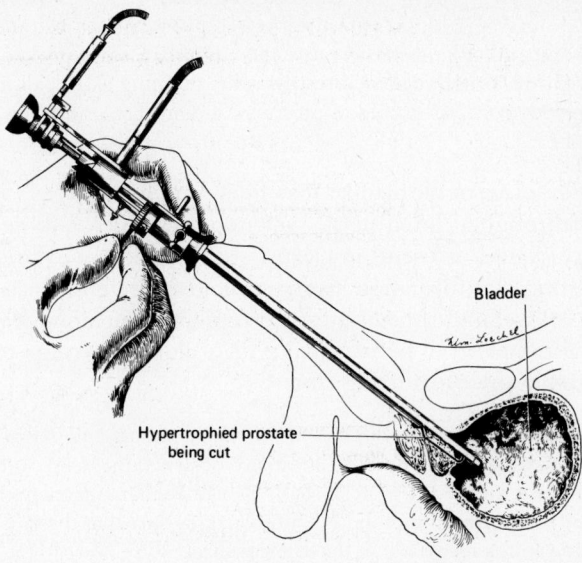

Figure 47-4.   Transurethral prostatectomy. A loop of wire connected with a cutting current is rotated in the cystoscope to remove shavings of prostate at the bladder orifice.

however, strictures are more frequent, and repeat operations may be necessary.

Another technique is *retropubic prostatectomy,* whereby a low abdominal incision is made and the prostate gland is approached between the pubic arch and the bladder (without entering the bladder) (Fig. 47-5). This procedure is suitable for large glands located high in the pelvis. Blood loss is controlled more easily; however, inflammation of the pubic bone (osteitis pubis) is more likely.

Cryosurgery may be performed on selected patients who have large prostatic adenomas or carcinomas and represent a high anesthetic or operative risk, due to compromised cardiopulmonary function. A probe is inserted transurethrally, and the prostate is frozen with liquid nitrogen. After the probe is removed, a urethral catheter is inserted. The tissue begins to slough off in several days. This sloughing-off process may continue for several weeks and may be troublesome.

Postoperative Nursing Management

Since a hyperplastic prostate gland is very vascular, the immediate dangers following a prostatectomy are bleeding and shock. Bleeding may occur from the bed of the prostate. Bleeding may also result in the formation of clots, which then obstruct the flow of urine. The drainage may be reddish-pink and begins to clear to a light pink within 24 hours after operation.

- Bright red bleeding with increased viscosity and numerous clots usually indicates arterial bleeding. Venous bleeding appears darker and less viscous.

- Arterial hemorrhage usually requires surgical intervention (e.g., suturing of bleeders or transurethral coagulation of bleeders), while venous bleeding may be controlled by applying traction to the catheter so that the balloon applies pressure to the prostatic fossa.

Following a transurethral prostatic resection, *the catheter must drain well;* a blocked catheter will produce distention of the prostatic capsule with resultant hemorrhage. Sometimes the patient is given furosemide to initiate postoperative diuresis, thereby helping to keep the catheter patent.

- Palpate the lower abdomen to see that no blockage of the catheter is occurring. An overdistended bladder presents a distinct rounded swelling above the pubis.
- Check the drainage bag, dressings, and incision site for evidence of bleeding.

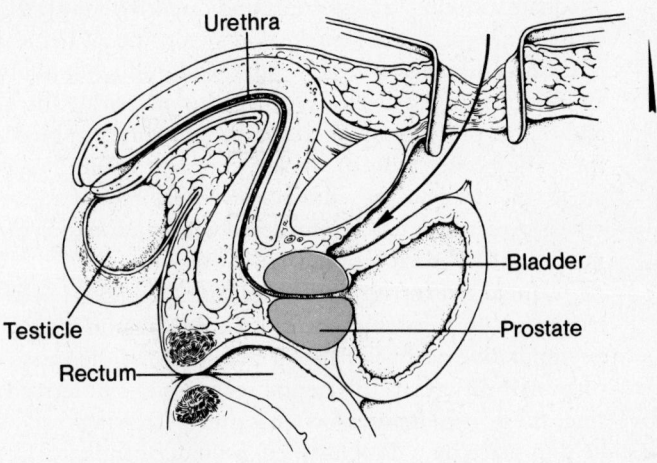

Figure 47-5.   Retropubic prostatectomy.

- Monitor the blood pressure, pulse, and respirations, and compare with the preoperative vital signs to assess for hypotension. Observe the patient for cold, sweating skin, pallor, restlessness, fall in blood pressure, and an increasing pulse rate.

Drainage of the bladder may be accomplished by gravity through a closed sterile system of drainage. A three-way system is useful in cleansing the bladder and preventing clot formation. Some urologists prefer to leave an indwelling catheter attached to dependent drainage. The catheter can be irrigated with a plunger syringe to remove any obstructing clots.

- If the patient complains of pain, check the tubing and irrigate the system, thereby correcting any obstruction, before administering an analgesic. Usually the catheter is irrigated with 50 ml. of irrigating fluid at a time, making sure that the same amount is recovered in the drainage bag.
- Avoid overdistending the bladder, which can produce secondary hemorrhage by stretching the coagulated vessels in the prostatic capsule.
- Maintain an input and output record, including the amount of fluid used for irrigation.

The drainage tube (not the catheter) is taped to the shaved inner thigh to prevent traction on the bladder If a cystostomy catheter is in place, it is taped to the lateral abdomen. Re-explain to the patient the purpose of the catheter. Assure him that the urge to void is from the presence of the catheter, and bladder spasms. Caution him not to pull on the catheter, since this causes bleeding, subsequent plugging of the tubing, and urinary retention.

Usually the patient is kept on bed rest for the first 24 hours following a prostatectomy. If pain occurs, the patient may strain from bladder irritability, causing an increase in venous pressure which can initiate bleeding and result in clot retention. Before the prescribed analgesic is given, the patient's blood pressure should be evaluated. Fluids (orally or intravenously) are given in adequate amounts unless contraindicated by congestive heart failure or water intoxication syndrome. When the patient is ambulatory he is encouraged to walk but not to sit for prolonged periods, since this increases intra-abdominal pressure and increases the possibility of bleeding. The bowel movements are kept soft (prune juice, stool softeners) to prevent excessive straining. If an enema is prescribed, it is administered with caution to avoid possible rectal perforation.

Perineal Prostatectomy. Following perineal prostatectomy, the urologist changes the dressing on the first postoperative day; after that it may become the nurse's responsibility. Careful aseptic technique is practiced, since the possibility of infection is great. Dressings can be held in place by a double-tailed T-binder bandage. The tails cross over the incision to give double thickness, and then each tail is drawn up on either side of the scrotum to the waistline, and fastened.

Rectal temperatures, rectal tubes, and enemas are to be avoided because of the danger of injuring the rectum and contaminating the wound. After the perineal sutures are removed, the perineum is cleansed as requested. A heat lamp may be directed to the perineal area to promote healing. The scrotum is protected with a towel while the heat lamp is in use. Sitz baths are also used to encourage healing.

Complications

In addition to hemorrhage, urinary-tract infections and epididymitis are possible complications following prostatectomy. A vasectomy may be performed at the time of prostatic resection to prevent retrograde spread of infection from the prostatic urethra through the vas and into the epididymis. If epididymitis occurs it is treated as discussed on page 1030.

Patients undergoing prostatectomy (with the exception of transurethral resection) have a high incidence of deep-vein thrombosis and pulmonary embolism. Low-dose heparin therapy may be given prophylactically.

Catheter Removal. After the catheter is removed (usually when the urine clears), urinary leakage may occur around the wound for several days in patients who have undergone perineal, suprapubic, and retropubic surgery. The cystostomy tube may be removed before or after the urethral catheter is removed. Some urinary incontinence may occur after the catheter is removed. Reassure the patient that this will probably disappear in time.

Rehabilitation and Patient Education

As the days pass and drainage tubes are removed, the patient often shows signs of discouragement and depression because he is not able to regain bladder control immediately. Urinary frequency and burning may occur after the catheter is removed.

The following exercises are helpful for regaining urinary control.
- Tense the perineal muscles by pressing the buttocks together; hold this position; relax. This exercise, done 10 to 20 times each hour, can be performed while sitting or standing.
- Try to shut off the urinary stream after starting to void; wait a few seconds and then continue to void.

Perineal exercises are continued until full urinary control is gained. The patient should be instructed to urinate as soon as the *first* desire to do so is felt. It is important for the patient to know that regaining urinary control is a gradual process, and that even though he may continue to "dribble" after being discharged from the hospital, the dribbling should gradually diminish (up to one year). The urine may be cloudy for several weeks but should clear as the prostate area heals.

While the prostatic fossa is healing (6 to 8 weeks) the patient should not engage in any Valsalva efforts (straining at stool, heavy lifting), since this increases venous pressure and may produce hematuria. He should avoid long automobile rides and strenuous exercise, which increase the tendency to bleed. The patient is cautioned to drink enough fluids to avoid dehydration which increases the tendency for a clot to form and obstruct the flow of urine. Any bleeding or decrease in size of the urinary stream is to be reported to the physician.

A prostatectomy does not usually cause impotence. In most instances, sexual activity may be resumed in 6 to 8 weeks, the time required for the prostatic fossa to heal. Following ejaculation, the seminal fluid will go into the bladder and is excreted with the urine.

After total prostatectomy (usually for cancer), impotence is almost always expected. For the younger patient who does not desire to give up sexual activity, a plastic insert may be used to make the penis rigid for sexual intercourse.

Cancer of the Prostate

Cancer of the prostate is the second most common cause of cancer and the third most common cause of cancer deaths in men. There appears to be an increased incidence of prostatic cancer, especially among black men.

Clinical Manifestations. Early cancer of the prostate does not usually produce symptoms. The obstructive symptoms occur late in the disease. This cancer tends to be variable in its course. If the neoplasm is large enough to encroach on the bladder neck or to cause obstruction of urine, there are symptoms and signs of obstruction, namely, difficulty and frequency of urination, urinary retention, and diminution in size and force of the urinary stream. Prostatic cancer commonly metastasizes to bone marrow (pelvis and lower spine), brain, and lungs. Symptoms due to metastases are backache, hip pain, perineal and rectal discomfort, anemia, weight loss, weakness, nausea, and oliguria. Hematuria may be present from urethral or bladder invasion, or both.

Early Detection. Every male over 40 should have a rectal examination as part of his annual health checkup. Earlier detection is the clue to a higher cure rate. Routine repeated rectal palpation of the gland (preferably by the same examiner) is important because early cancer may be felt as a nodule within the substance of the gland or as a diffuse induration in the posterior lobe.

Diagnostic Evaluation. On rectal examination, the prostate is usually found to be "stony hard" and fixed. A cystoscopy may be done to evaluate the local extent of the disease. A needle biopsy or an open perineal biopsy with frozen section is done to determine if a malignancy is present. The serum acid phosphatase is frequently increased when cancer extends outside the prostatic cap-

sule, while the serum alkaline phosphatase increases when there is bone metastases.

Other tests include bone scans to detect metastases, skeletal x-rays to reveal osteoblastic metastases, bone marrow aspiration to check for tumor cells, excretory urograms to demonstrate changes from ureteral obstruction, renal-function tests, and lymphangiography, to seek evidence of metastases to the pelvic nodes.

Management. A radical prostatectomy (removal of the prostate and seminal vesicles) still remains the standard operative procedure for patients who have potentially curable disease, and a life expectancy of 10 years or more. This procedure may be followed by bilateral orchiectomy or estrogen therapy. Sexual impotency follows this radical procedure, but urinary control is usually normal.

Since the majority of men do not have lesions that are amenable to cure by radical surgery, palliative measures are undertaken. Radiation therapy with high voltage is being used in the hope of cure in some stages of the disease, and for the purpose of palliation for patients in late stages. Radiation can decrease the tumor size, cause regression of obstructive lesions, and frequently relieve bone pain. Complications, which usually are transitory, include proctitis (inflammation of the rectum), diarrhea, and urinary frequency, due to radiation doses and the proximity of the bladder and rectum.

Hormonal Treatment (Antiandrogen Therapy). Hormonal treatment is a method of control rather than cure, since adenocarcinoma of the prostate is hormone-dependent. The rationale underlying hormonal treatment is that prostatic epithelium becomes atrophied when androgen hormones are greatly reduced or inactivated. Bilateral orchiectomy eliminates androgens of testicular origin. The administration of estrogen is thought to inhibit the gonadotropins (responsible for testicular androgenic activity), thus removing the androgenic hormone upon which the growth of the malignancy depends. Diethylstilbestrol is the most widely used estrogen at this time.

Diethylstilbestrol gives symptomatic control, lessens tumor size, lessens pain from metastatic nodules, and imparts an improved sense of well-being. However, there is now evidence that giving higher doses of diethylstilbestrol carries a significant risk of death from cardiovascular disease, especially from thromboembolic phenomena. Gynecomastia (enlargement of breasts in the male) is an annoying complication of estrogen therapy.

Orchiectomy (removal of testes) is performed as a complement to estrogen therapy, since 95 percent of circulating testosterone is of testicular origin. Prostatic atrophy occurs after this procedure. There is controversy concerning whether the most desirable treatment is estrogen therapy, orchiectomy, or both. Prostatic cryosurgery is done only for the poor-risk patient. Chemotherapy may also be tried.

To maintain patency of the urethral passage, repeated transurethral prostatectomies may have to be done until tumor growth is so rapid that surgical intervention becomes too frequent. When this is the case, catheter drainage is instituted by way of the suprapubic or transurethral route.

Patients with recurring symptoms are treated symptomatically. Corticosteroids may give relief but do not affect the tumor.

Blood transfusions are given to maintain adequate hemoglobin levels when bone marrow is replaced by tumor. External skeletal radiation is carried out to relieve the pain produced by the metastatic growth. Pain may be controlled by estrogens and narcotics and, if necessary, by severing spinal-cord pain fibers via neurosurgery. (See also page 240, the nursing management of the patient with pain, and page 275, the care of the patient with advanced cancer.)

BIBLIOGRAPHY

BOOKS

American Nurses Assoc. Division on Medical-Surgical Nursing Practice; Standards of Urologic Practice. Kansas City, Amer. Nurs. Assoc., 1977.

Blandy, J.: Lecture Notes on Urology. Oxford, Blackwell Scientific Pub., 1976.

———: Operative Urology. Oxford, Blackwell Scientific Pub., 1978.

———: Urology. Vols. 1 and 2. Philadelphia, J.B. Lippincott, 1976.

Blandy, J. B.: Transurethral Resection, 2nd ed. London, Pitman Medical, 1978.

Brundage, D. J.: Nursing Management of Renal Problems. St. Louis, C. V. Mosby, 1976.

Caldwell, K. P. S.: Urinary Incontinence. New York, Grune and Stratton, 1975.

Cameron, J. S., Russell, A. M. E., and Sale, D. N. T.: Nephrology for Nurses, 2nd ed. Flushing, N.Y., Medical Exam Pub. Co., 1976.

Flocks, R. H., and Culp, D. A.: Surgical Urology, 4th ed. Chicago, Year Book Med. Pub., 1975.

Harrison, J. H. H., et al.: Campbell's Urology. Vols. 1 and 2, Philadelphia, W. B. Saunders, 1978.

Johnson, D. E.: Testicular Tumors, 2nd ed. Flushing, N.Y., Medical Examination Pub. Co., 1976.

Kessler, R. J., and Anderson, R. U.: Handbook of Urologic Emergencies. Flushing, N.Y., Medical Examination Pub. Co., 1976.

Lapides, J.: Fundamentals of Urology. Philadelphia, W. B. Saunders, 1976.

Silber, S. J.: Transurethral Resection. New York, Appleton-Century-Crofts, 1977.

Smith, D. R.: General Urology. Los Altos, Lange Medical Publishers, 1978.

Smith, R. B., and Skinner, D. G.: Complications of Urologic Surgery. Philadelphia, W. B. Saunders, 1976.

Stewart, B. H., ed.: Operative Urology. Baltimore, Williams and Wilkins, 1975.

Tannenbaum, M.: Urologic Pathology: The Prostate. Philadelphia, Lea and Febiger, 1977.

Winter, C. C., and Morel, A.: Nursing Care of Patients With Urologic Disease, 4th ed. St. Louis, C. V. Mosby, 1977.

ARTICLES

Male Urologic Conditions

Bissada, N. K., Finkbeiner, A. E., and Redman, J. F.: Three common disorders of the prostate. Med. Times, *105*:48-54, Feb. 1977.

Boxer, R. J., Kaufman, J. J., and Goodwin, W. E.: Radical prostatectomy for carcinoma of the prostate: 1951-1976. A review of 329 patients. J. Urol., *117*:208-213, Feb. 1977.

Einhorn, L. H., and Donohue, J. P.: Improved chemotherapy in disseminated testicular cancer. J. Urol., *117*:65-69, Jan. 1977.

Finkbeiner, A. E., Bissada, N. K., and Redman, J. F.: Complications of vasectomies. Am. Fam. Phys., *15*:86-89, Mar. 1977.

Gault, P. L.: Coping with dangerous and distressing complications. Nursing '77, 7:34-38, Apr. 1977.

Gott, L. J.: Common scrotal pathology. Am. Fam. Phys., *15*:165-173, May 1977.

Grundmann, E., and Vahlensieck, W.: Tumors of the male genital system. Recent Results in Cancer Res., *60*:1-268 (entire vol.), 1977.

Hermanek, P.: Testicular cancer, histologic classification and staging, topography of lymph node metastases. Recent Results in Cancer Res., *60*:202-211, 1977.

Kline, T. S., Kelsey, D. M., and Kohler, F. P.: Prostatic carcinoma and needle aspiration biopsy. Am. J. Clin. Pathol., *67*:131-133, Feb. 1977.

Maier, J. G., and Mittemyer, B.: Carcinoma of the testis. Cancer, *39*: (suppl.) 981-986, Feb. 1977.

Murray, B. L. S., and Wilcox, L. J.: Testicular self-examination. AJN, *78*:2074-2075, Dec. 1978.

Moss, W. M.: Attitudes of patients one year after vasectomy. Urology, *6*:319-322, Sept. 1975.

Perrin, P., et al.: Forty years of transurethral prostatic resections. J. Urol., *116*:757-758, Dec. 1976.

Resnick, M. I., et al.: Radiation therapy for carcinoma of the prostate—5 year follow-up. J. Urol., *117*:214-215, Feb. 1977.

Silber, S. J., Galle, J., and Friend, D.: Microscopic vasovasostomy and spermatogenesis. J. Urol., *117*:299-309, Mar. 1977.

———: Microscopic technique for reversal of vasectomy. Surg. Gyn. Obstet., *143*:630-631, Oct. 1976.

Tobiason, S. J.: Benign prostatic hypertrophy. AJN, *79*: 286-290, Feb. 1979.

Wood, H. C., Jr.: Psychosocial aspects of sterilization. Curr. Psychiat. Ther., *16*:303-310, 1976.

Wood, R. Y., and Rose, K.: Penile implants for impotence. AJN, *78*:234-238, Feb. 1978.

Integumentary Problems and Disorders of Protective Function

UNIT TWELVE

48

MANAGEMENT OF PATIENTS WITH DERMATOLOGIC DISORDERS

PHYSIOLOGIC OVERVIEW

The skin is a structure that is indispensable for human life. It forms a barrier between the internal organs and the external environment and participates in many vital functions of the body. The skin is continuous with the mucous membrane at the external openings of the organs of the digestive, respiratory, and urogenital systems. Because disorders of the skin are readily visible, dermatologic complaints are frequently the primary reason for patient visits.

Anatomy of the Skin

The skin is composed of two layers of tissue, the *epidermis*, an outer layer, in contact with the environment, and a deeper layer called the *dermis*. The epidermis consists of live, continuously dividing epithelial cells covered on the surface by dead cells that were originally deeper and were pushed upward by newly developing cells underneath. The dead cells are constantly flaking off from the skin, frequently in irregular patches. These dead cells contain large amounts of *keratin*, a soluble, fibrous protein that forms the outer barrier of the skin. The epidermis is devoid of blood vessels and has few nerve endings. The superficial layers of the epidermis can be shaved from the body without pain or blood loss. The epidermis is modified in different areas of the body. Over the palms of the hands and the soles of the feet it is thickened and contains increased amounts of keratin, in contrast to the thin epidermis over most of the rest of the body. The thickness of the epidermis can increase with use, as is the case, for example, with the hands of a laborer.

The dermis is a broad layer of connective tissue that underlies the epidermal layer. It is composed of collagen and elastic fibers and contains blood and lymph vessels, nerves, sweat and sebaceous glands, and hair roots. Interdigitation between dermis and epidermis produces ripples on the surface of the skin. On the fingertips, these ripples are called *fingerprints*. They are perhaps a person's most individualistic characteristic and they almost never change. With aging, the number of elastic fibers in the dermis progressively decreases and the skin becomes wrinkled.

The color of the skin is determined by the pigment called *melanin,* which is produced by cells in the epidermis called *melanocytes.* The skin of black persons and the darker areas on the skin of white persons (for example, the nipple), contain large amounts of this pigment. Production of melanin by melanocytes is largely under the control of a hormone secreted from the hypothalamus of the brain, called melanocyte-stimulating hormone (MSH). Increased production of melanin occurs on exposure to ultraviolet light such as occurs with suntanning.

The skin is anchored to the muscles and bones underneath by subcutaneous tissue composed of connective tissue interlaced with fat. Fat is deposited and distributed according to the person's sex and in part accounts for the difference in body shape between men and women. Overeating results in increased deposition of fat beneath the skin.

HAIR. Hair is present over the entire body except for the palms of the hands and soles of the feet. The hair consists of a root formed in the dermis and a hair shaft which projects beyond the skin. It grows in a cavity called a *hair follicle.* The proliferation of cells in the bulb of the hair causes the hair to form. Hairs in different parts of the body serve different functions. The hairs of the eyes (eyebrows and lashes), nose, and ears screen dust, bugs, and airborne debris. Hair of the skin serves as thermal insulation in lower animals. This function is enhanced during cold or fright by piloerection (hairs "standing on end") caused by contraction of the tiny arrector muscles attached to the hair follicle. The piloerector response that occurs in humans is probably vestigial. The color of hair is due to the presence of varying amounts of melanin within the hair shaft. Gray or white hair is the result of loss of pigment. Growth of hair in certain locations on the body is under the control of sex hormones. The best examples are the hair on the face (beard and mustache) and on the body trunk that are controlled by the presence of the male hormones (androgens).

NAILS. On the dorsal surface of the fingers and toes, a hard, transparent plate of keratin, called the *nail,* overlies the skin. The nail grows from its root which lies under a thin fold of skin called the *cuticle.* The nail helps to protect the fingers and toes, in order to preserve their highly developed sensory function, and aids in the performance of certain fine functions of the fingers, such as picking up small objects.

GLANDS OF THE SKIN. Sebaceous glands are associated with hair follicles. The ducts of the sebaceous glands empty an oily secretion onto the space between the hair follicle and the hair shaft. For each hair there are at least two sebaceous glands, whose secretions oil the hair and render the skin soft and pliable.

Sweat glands are found in the skin over most of the body surface. They are heavily concentrated on the palms of the hands and soles of the feet. Only the glans penis, the margins of the lips, the external ear, and the nail bed are devoid of sweat glands. Sweat glands are subclassified into two categories: *eccrine* and *apocrine.* The eccrine sweat glands are found in all areas of the skin. Their ducts open directly onto the skin surface. The apocrine sweat glands are larger, and in contrast to that of the eccrine glands, their secretion contains parts of the secretory cells. They are located in the axillae, anal region, scrotum, and labia majora. Their ducts generally open onto hair follicles. The apocrine glands become active at the time of puberty. In the female, they enlarge and recede with each menstrual cycle.

The thin, watery secretion called *sweat* is produced in the basal coiled portion of the gland and is released into its narrow duct. Sweat is composed predominantly of water, and contains about half of the salt content of the blood plasma. Sweat is released from both apocrine and eccrine glands in response to elevated ambient temperature. The rate of sweat secretion is under the control of the sympathetic nervous system. Excessive sweating of the palms and soles, axillae, forehead, and other areas may occur in response to pain and stress. Specialized apocrine glands called *cerumenous glands* are found in the external ear where they produce wax (*cerumen*).

Functions of the Skin

PROTECTIVE FUNCTION. The skin protects the body against invasion by bacteria and foreign matter. The thickened skin of the palms and soles provides the tough covering necessary for the constant trauma occurring in these areas.

The epidermis is relatively impermeable to most chemical substances. It is this property of skin that allows it to be an effective barrier for protection. Some substances slowly pass through the skin, however, including gases such as oxygen, nitrogen, and carbon dioxide. Lipid soluble substances tend to move more easily through the skin than do electrolytes and other nonlipid soluble substances. Their route of penetration into the skin is probably through the follicular orifice and the sebaceous glands. The rate of absorption of a topical medication will depend upon how rapidly its suspending vehicle can penetrate the skin.

SENSORY FUNCTION. Stimulation of the receptor endings of nerves in the skin allows us to constantly monitor the conditions in our immediate environment. The primary functions of the receptors in the skin are to sense temperature, pain, light touch, and pressure (or heavy touch). Different nerve endings are responsible for responding to each of the different stimuli. Although the nerve endings are distributed over the entire body, they are more concentrated in some areas than in others. For example, the fingertips are much more densely innervated than the skin of the back.

WATER BALANCE. Skin forms a barrier that prevents loss of water and electrolytes from the internal environment and also prevents the subcutaneous tissues from drying out. When skin is damaged, such as occurs with a severe burn, for example, large quantities of fluids and electrolytes can be rapidly lost, possibly leading to circulatory collapse, shock, and death. On the other hand, the skin is not completely impermeable to water. Small amounts of water continuously evaporate from the skin surface. This evaporation, called *insensible perspiration,* amounts to approximately 500 ml. per day for a normal adult. Insensible water loss may vary with the body temperature, and in the presence of fever these losses can increase. During immersion in water, the skin can accumulate water up to approximately 3 or 4 times its normal weight. A common example of this is the swelling of the skin after prolonged bathing.

TEMPERATURE REGULATION. The body continuously produces heat as a result of the metabolism of foodstuffs to produce energy. This heat is dissipated primarily through the skin. Three major physical processes are involved in loss of heat from the body to the environment. The first process, *radiation,* is the ability of a body to give off its heat to another object of lower temperature situated at a distance. The second process, *conduction,* is the transfer of heat from the body to a cooler object in contact with it. Heat transferred by conduction to the air surrounding the body is removed by the third process, *convection,* which consists of bulk movement of warm air molecules away from the body. Evaporation from the skin aids the process of heat loss by conduction. Heat is conducted through the skin into water molecules on its surface, causing the water to evaporate. The source of the water on the skin surface may be insensible perspiration, sweat, or water from the environment. Normally, all of these mechanisms for heat loss are utilized. However, when the ambient temperature is very high, radiation and convection are not effective and evaporation from the skin constitutes the only means for heat loss.

Under normal conditions, metabolic heat production is exactly balanced by heat loss, and the internal temperature of the body is maintained constant at approximately 37° C. (98.6 F.). The rate of heat loss depends primarily upon the surface temperature of the skin, which is in turn a function of the skin blood flow. Skin is richly supplied with blood vessels that carry heat to the skin from the core of the body. Blood flow through these vessels is controlled primarily by the sympathetic nervous system. Increased blood flow to the skin results in delivery of more heat to the skin and a greater rate of heat loss from the body. On the other hand, decreased skin blood flow decreases the skin temperature and helps conserve heat for the body. When the temperature of the body begins to fall, such as occurs on a cold day, the blood vessels of the skin constrict and reduce heat loss from the body. This can be demonstrated by immersing the hand in cold water.

Sweating is another process by which the body can regulate the rate of heat loss. Sweating is increased when body temperature starts to rise. In extremely hot environments, the rate of sweat production may be as high as 1 liter per hour. Under some circumstances, for example, with emotional stress, sweating may occur on a reflex basis unrelated to the necessity to lose heat from the body.

WHEAL AND FLARE REACTION. Stroking the skin with sufficient firmness to cause local injury results in local reddening. This is followed within a few minutes by localized swelling and more diffuse redness around the injury site. The combination of the swelling (called a *wheal*) and the diffuse redness (called a *flare*) constitutes a normal reaction of the skin to injury. These responses are due to local edema secondary to increased capillary permeability and dilatation of the surrounding arterioles. The wheal and flare reaction is due to the action of locally released hormones such as histamine and kinins upon the local blood vessels.

PSYCHOSOCIAL ASPECTS OF DERMATOLOGIC PROBLEMS

Because patients with skin conditions (1 in 20 persons) can see and feel their problems, they are more apt to be disturbed by their ailments than are patients with other conditions. Skin conditions can lead to cosmetic disfigurement, social isolation, and economic hardship. In some instances, they are often erroneously associated with immorality and contagion. Some conditions can cost the patient his job, with devastating effects on the person's life. Others may subject the patient to a protracted course of illness, leading to feelings of depression, frustration, self-consciousness, and rejection. Itching and skin irritation may also be a constant annoyance—in fact, they are common features of most skin diseases. The result of these discomforts may be loss of sleep, anxiety, and depression, all of which reinforce the general distress and fatigue that so frequently accompany skin disorders.

Patients suffering from such physical and psychological discomforts require understanding, nursing support, unending patience, and continual encouragement. It takes time to help patients gain insight into their problems and work out their difficulties. It becomes imperative, therefore, to overcome any aversion that might be felt when caring for patients with unattractive skin disorders. There must be no sign of hesitancy when approaching these patients. Such behavior would only reinforce the psychological trauma of the disorder. Since very few skin conditions are contagious, there is no need to fear touching the patient. In fact, touching the patient reduces his sense of isolation.

Whenever possible, the patient should be given a chance to express any feelings of anger, ambivalence, and depression. An overall optimistic approach by the nursing personnel will help to alleviate these negative feelings and promote a sense of security and confidence.

ASSESSMENT

Many systemic conditions may be accompanied by dermatologic manifestations. In fact, any patient hospitalized with a medical or surgical condition may suddenly develop itching and a rash.

The data base that constitutes the basis of the nursing history may be obtained by asking the following questions:
- How long have you had this skin condition?
- Has it occurred previously?
- Are there any other symptoms besides the rash?
- What site was first affected?
- What did the rash/lesion look like when it first appeared?
- How did it spread?
- Are there itching, burning, tingling, or crawling sensations? loss of sensation?
- Is it worse at a particular time? season?
- Do you have any idea how it started?
- Do you have a history of hay fever, asthma, hives, eczema, allergies?
- Did the eruptions appear after certain foods were eaten?
- Was there a relationship between a specific event and the outbreak of the rash/lesion?
- What medications are you taking? What medication (ointment, cream, salve) have you put on the lesion? (Include over-the-counter medications.)
- What is your occupation?
- What in your immediate environment (plants, animals) might be precipitating this problem?
- Is there anything else you wish to talk about in regard to this problem?

Skin Lesions

Assessment of the skin involves the entire skin area including the mucous membranes, scalp, and nails. *Inspection,* along with *palpation,* constitutes the chief procedure used in examining the skin and requires that the room be well lighted, as well as warm. The patient should completely disrobe and should be adequately draped. A preliminary look at the eruption or lesion should help to identify the type of dermatosis (abnormal skin condition) and indicate whether the lesion is primary or secondary. At the same time, the anatomical distribution of the eruption should be noted since certain diseases tend to affect certain sites of the body and are distributed in characteristic patterns and shapes. To determine the extent of the distribution, the left and right sides of the body should be compared while the color and shape of the lesion are noted. Following observation, the lesions are palpated to determine their texture and to see if they are hard or soft or filled with fluid. A metric ruler is used to measure the size of the lesions so that any further extension can be compared with this initial baseline measurement. The dermatosis is then documented on the patient's record; it should be described clearly and in detail, using precise terminology.

Types of Skin Lesions. Skin lesions can be described as primary or secondary, depending on the stage of development, and are further divided according to type and appearance, as indicated in the following definitions:

Primary Lesions (initial lesions)

Macule—a nonelevated discoloration of the skin of various shapes and colors

Papule—a solid elevated lesion less than 1 cm. (0.4 inch) in diameter

Nodule—a raised, solid lesion that is larger and deeper than a papule

Vesicle—a small elevation of the skin that is filled with clear fluid

Bulla—a large vesicle or blister larger than 1 cm. (0.4 inch) in diameter

Pustule—an elevation of the skin that contains pus; may form as a result of purulent changes in a vesicle

Wheal—transient elevation of the skin caused by edema of the dermis and surrounding capillary dilatation

Plaque—a solid elevated lesion on the skin or mucous membrane, greater than 1 cm. (0.4 inch) in its largest diameter.

Secondary Lesions

As the term implies, these are the changes that take place in primary lesions and possibly modify them; they include:

Scales—heaped up horny layers of dead epidermis; may develop as a result of inflammatory changes

Crusts—a covering formed from serum, blood, or pus drying on the skin

Excoriations—linear scratch marks or traumatized area of skin

Fissure—a crack in the skin, usually from marked drying and long-standing inflammation

Ulcer—lesion formed by local destruction of the epidermis and part or all of the underlying dermis

After the characteristic distribution of the lesion has been determined, the following information should be obtained:
- What is (are) the color(s) of the lesion?
- Is there redness, heat, pain, or swelling?
- How large an area is involved? Where is it?
- Is the eruption macular, papular, scaling, oozing, discrete, confluent?
- What is the distribution of the lesion—symmetrical, linear, circular?

Definition of terms commonly used in dermatology*
Annular—ring-shaped
Arcuate—in the form of an arc
Circinate—circular
Confluent—lesions run together or join
Discoid—disc-shaped
Discrete—lesions remain separate
Eczematoid or eczematous—inflammation with a tendency to thicken, scale, vesiculate, crust, or weep
Erythema—red
Generalized—widespread eruption
Grouped—lesions clustered together
Guttate—drop-like
Gyrate—twisted spiral
Iris—circle within a circle
Keratosis—circumscribed horny thickening
Keratotic—horny thickening
Linear—in lines
Moniliform—beaded
Multiform—more than one kind of skin lesion
Polymorphous—more than one kind of skin lesion
Serpiginous—snake-like, creeping
Telangiectasia—relatively permanent dilatation of superficial vessels
Universal—entire skin affected
Zosteriform—linear arrangement along a nerve

*From Lewis, G. M., and Wheeler, C. E.: *Practical Dermatology*. Philadelphia, W. B. Saunders.

Assessing Patients with Dark or Black Skin

The gradations of color that occur in dark-skinned persons are largely determined by genetic transmission; they may be described as light, medium, or dark. In dark-skinned persons, melanin is produced at a faster rate and in larger quantities than in lighter-skinned persons. Healthy dark skin has a reddish base or undertone. The buccal mucosa, tongue, lips, and nails normally appear pink.

In examining the dark-skinned or black patient it is important to have good lighting and to look at the skin and the nail beds as well as in the mouth. All suspicious areas should be palpated.

ERYTHEMA. Because there is a tendency for black skin to assume a purplish-grayish cast when an inflammatory process is present, it may be difficult to detect erythema. To determine possible inflammation, the skin should be palpated for increased warmth or for signs of smoothness (edema) or hardness. The adjacent lymph nodes are also palpated.

RASH. In instances of itching, the patient should be asked to indicate what areas of the body are involved. The skin is then stretched gently to decrease the reddish tone and make the rash stand out. The differences in skin texture are then palpated by running the tips of the fingers lightly over the skin. Usually the borders of the rash can be felt. Included in the examination are the patient's mouth and ears. (Sometimes rubeola will cause a red cast to appear on the tip of the ears.) Finally, the patient's temperature is checked and the lymph nodes are palpated.

CYANOSIS. When a person with black skin goes into shock, the skin usually assumes a gray cast. To determine signs of cyanosis, the area around the mouth, lips, and over the cheekbones and earlobes should be checked. Other indicative signs to check include a cold, clammy skin, a rapid thready pulse, and rapid shallow respirations. When the palpebral conjunctiva are checked for petechiae, it is important to realize that deposits of melanin may normally appear in this area and should not be misinterpreted as petechiae.

SKIN PROBLEMS IN THE BLACK RACE. Because changes in skin color can occur in the black race, these changes are noticeable and cause great distress to the patient. For example, hypopigmentation (loss or decrease in skin color) which may be due to vitiligo (a condition characterized by destruction of melanocytes in small or large skin areas), may cause more concern in the dark-skinned person since it is so readily visible. Hyperpigmentation (increase in color) may occur after disease or injury to the skin. However, pigmented streaks in the nails are considered to be normal. On the other hand, a pigmented nasal crease may be an external sign of allergy.

In general, persons with black skin suffer from the same skin conditions as those with white skin, although they are less apt to have skin cancer. On the other hand, members of the black race and other dark-skinned persons have a greater propensity for keloid formation.

GENERAL MANAGEMENT IN DERMATOLOGIC DISORDERS

Since there is so much variation in the techniques prescribed, the following paragraphs will be concerned with general principles regarded as important in the nursing management of persons with skin diseases.

The major objectives of therapy are to (1) prevent damage to the healthy skin, (2) prevent secondary infection, (3) reverse the inflammatory process, and (4) relieve the symptoms.

Some skin problems are markedly aggravated by soap and water. Therefore bathing routines are modified according to the condition being treated.

Denuded skin, whether the area of desquamation is large or small, is excessively prone to damage by chemicals and trauma. The friction of a towel, if applied with vigor, is sufficient to excite a brisk inflammatory response that causes any existing lesion to flare up and increase in extent. Thus, the essence of skin care and protection in bathing a patient with abnormal skin is to use a mild superfatted soap or soap substitute and to ensure the complete removal of the soap when rinsing, before blotting the area dry with a soft cloth.

Pledgets saturated with oil will aid in loosening crusts, removing exudates, or freeing an adherent dry dressing. The dressing also may be saturated with sterile physiologic salt solution or dilute (3 percent) hydrogen peroxide, which softens it and permits it to be pulled away gently.

Potentially infectious skin lesions should be regarded strictly as such, and proper precautions should be observed until the diagnosis is established (see wound and skin precautions, page 1365). Some lesions with pus contain infectious material. Others, such as occur in acne, have no infectious material. Although some genital lesions are suspect, most are minor irritations.

- If the condition is infectious, disposable gloves are worn by the nurse and the physician. Dressings removed from infected skin should be wrapped in paper and burned as soon as possible.

The type of skin lesion (oozing, infected, or dry) usually dictates the local medication or treatment that is prescribed. As a rule if the skin is acutely inflamed (hot, red, and swollen) and is oozing, it is best to apply wet dressings and soothing lotions. In chronic conditions in which the skin surface is dry and scaly, water soluble emulsions, creams, ointments, and pastes are used. The therapy must be changed as the response indicates. Explain to the patient that he must contact the physician or clinic if the medication or compresses seem to irritate the dermatosis. Success or failure of skin therapy rests upon adequate instruction and motivation of the patient and the interest and support of the health personnel.

For a general outline of nursing management of the patient with a dermatosis see page 1048.

Wet Dressings

Wet dressings (wet compresses applied to areas of the skin) are employed for many types of lesions. They may be either sterile or unsterile depending on the condition being treated. The purposes of wet dressings are (1) to reduce inflammation by producing vasoconstriction (thus decreasing vasodilatation and the local blood flow in inflammation); (2) to cleanse the skin of exudates, crusts and scales, and (3) to maintain drainage of infected areas. Before these dressings are applied, the hands should be washed thoroughly.

Wet dressings are used for vesicular, bullous, pustular, and ulcerative disorders, as well as for acute inflammatory disorders, erosions, and exudative, crusted surfaces.

The solutions generally consist of cool tap water or physiologic saline. Other agents may be used to precipitate protein, thus acting as mild astringents and antibacterials. Medication may be applied before and/or after wet dressings.

Although some dressings must be covered to prevent evaporation, most are allowed to remain open. The *open dressing* requires frequent changes because evaporation is rapid. The *closed dressing* is changed less frequently. However, there is always a danger that it will cause not only softening but actual maceration of the underlying skin.

Areas of normal skin that may be exposed to moisture for any extended period should first be coated with petrolatum jelly, a silicone oil, or zinc oxide paste to avoid skin maceration.

Smooth muslin or cotton materials in the form of old bedding, diapers, etc. can be cut and folded to make dressings that are 2 to 4 layers thick. The dressing is saturated with the prescribed solution before it is applied. Usually, wet dressings are kept cool or at room temperature. Compresses are removed, wrung out of the solution, and reapplied every 5 to 10 minutes, since compresses reach body temperature in that period of time. Wet dressings are usually applied for 15- to 30-minute intervals every 2 to 3 hours unless otherwise prescribed. Medications applied to moist skin immediately after treatment with compresses are absorbed better than when applied to dry skin. If extensive areas are to be treated with wet compresses, the patient must be kept warm and not more than one third of the body treated at one time.

If warm compresses are prescribed, the area must be watched carefully, since the skin may be burned. If a closed dressing is used, it may be covered with sterile towels to hold the dressing in place and further protected with a plastic film. In this way the temperature can be maintained for a longer period.

Dressing materials should be laundered or discarded every 24 hours. Usually the acute stage of dermatitis subsides after 48 to 72 hours of treatment. Wet dressings continued beyond this point can lead to dryness.

Therapeutic Baths (Balneotherapy)

Baths are useful as a means of applying medications to large areas of the skin, removing crusts and scales and old medications, and relieving the inflammation and itching that accompany acute dermatoses. The temperature of the water should be comfortable, and the bath should last from 15 to 30 minutes, although the water should not be allowed to cool excessively. For the different types of therapeutic baths and their uses, see Table 48-1.

Topical Medications

Medications in the form of lotions, creams, ointments, and powders are frequently used to treat skin lesions. In general, wet dressings, with or without medication, are used in the acute stage; lotions and creams are reserved

TABLE 48-1. TYPES OF THERAPEUTIC BATHS

BATH SOLUTION AND MEDICATION	DESIRED EFFECT	NURSING ACTION
Water	Same effects as wet dressings	Fill the tub half full—94 L. (25 gallons)
Saline	Used for widely disseminated lesions	Keep the water at a comfortable temperature.
Colloidal—Oatmeal or Aveeno	Antipruritic and drying	
Sodium bicarbonate	Cooling	Do not allow the water to cool excessively.
Starch		Use a bath mat—*medications may cause tub to be slippery.*
Medicated tars (follow package directions) Alma-Tar, Balnetar	Tar baths are used for psoriasis and chronic eczematous conditions.	Apply a lubricating agent to wet skin after bath if emollient action is desired—increases hydration. Since tars are volatile, the bath area should be well ventilated.
		Dry by blotting with a towel.
Bath oils Alpha-Keri, Ar-Ex, Avenol, Domol, Lubath, Lubriderm	Bath oils are used for antipruritic and emollient actions.	Keep room warm to minimize temperature fluctuations.
	Used for acute and subacute eczematous eruptions.	Encourage patient to wear light, loose clothing after the bath.

for the subacute stage, whereas ointments and lubricating compounds are better suited for chronic inflammation.

Lotions exert a cooling action through water evaporation; they also have a protective effect, are antipruritic and drying, and may act as sunscreens. Lotions are applied easily with a soft paintbrush or cotton gauze and are not usually washed off between applications.

Powders usually have a talc, zinc oxide, bentonite, or cornstarch base and are dusted on the skin with a shaker or with cotton sponges. Although their medical action is brief, powders act as hygroscopic agents, absorbing moisture and reducing friction between skin surfaces and between the skin and bedding.

Creams are suspensions of oil and water, are easily applied, and usually are the most cosmetically acceptable to the patient. Creams are generally rubbed into the skin by hand.

Pastes are mixtures of powders and ointments and are used in inflammatory conditions. They adhere best to the skin and may need to be removed with mineral or olive oil.

Ointments retard water loss, lubricate and protect the skin, and are preferred in the more chronic or localized skin conditions. Both pastes and ointments are applied with a wooden tongue depressor or by hand, with gloves if necessary.

In all of the aforementioned types of topical medications, the patient should be taught to apply the medication gently but thoroughly. It may also be necessary to cover these medications with a dressing to prevent soiling of clothing. Other available topical medications include gels, which are greaseless and nonstaining jelly-like colloids. Gels generally contain propylene glycol and a jelling agent. Several new medications are being used in a gel form, including steroids. The gel seems to allow the steroid to penetrate more effectively than some of the other formulations.

Corticosteroids are being widely used in the treatment of many dermatologic conditions. Topical steroids frequently are used to suppress inflammation, thus relieving pain and itching. The patient should be instructed to use only small quantities of steroid cream and to rub it in thoroughly. Topical corticosteroids are frequently used with occlusive dressings to enhance skin penetration. When steroids are applied around the eyes, a great deal of caution is required.

Intralesional therapy consists of the injection of a sterile suspension of medication (usually a corticosteroid) into or just below a lesion. Although this treatment may have an anti-inflammatory effect, local atrophy may result if the injection is made into subcutaneous fat.

Systemic medications are also given for skin conditions. These include the adrenocorticosteroids, antibiotics, antihistamines, sedatives and tranquilizers, analgesics, and antineoplastics.

Dressings for Skin Conditions

Skin dressings are used to keep topical medication in place and to allay itching and pain. One very effective type of dressing is the occlusive dressing, which enhances the absorption of topically applied medications. Occlusive dressings also promote the retention of moisture, which keeps the medication from evaporating and reduces the expense of topical corticosteroid treatment. An airtight plastic film such as Saran Wrap is applied to cover the medicated skin. Plastic film is advantageous because it is thin and adapts itself readily to anatomical structures of all sizes and shapes. In a newer method of treatment, plastic surgical tape containing corticosteroid in the adhesive layer can be cut to size and applied to individual lesions. For areas that are difficult to cover, occlusive appliances of thin clear plastic can be constructed with dental materials. Plastic wrap should generally be used no more than 10 hours a day. The patient is given the following instructions: (1) wash the area; (2) rub the medication into the lesion while the skin is moist; (3) cover with plastic wrap (Saran Wrap, vinyl gloves, plastic bags, etc.); and (4) cover with an ace bandage, stocking, dressing, or paper tape to seal the edges.

It is important to remember that prolonged use of occlusive dressings may cause skin atrophy, striae, telangiectasia, folliculitis, nonhealing ulceration or erythema, and systemic absorption of corticosteroids.

There are other forms of dressings that can be used to cover topical medications. The best material is soft cotton cloth. Stretchable cotton dressings (Surgitube, Tubegauze) can be used for fingers, toes, and extremities. The hands can be covered with disposable polyethylene or vinyl gloves, sealed at the wrists, while the feet can be wrapped in plastic bags covered by cotton socks. When large areas of the body need to be covered, cotton cloth covered with tubular material can be used. Disposable diapers or cloth folded diaper-fashion are also useful as dressings for the groin and perineal areas. Axillary dressings can be made of cotton cloth taped in place or held by dress shields. A turban or plastic shower cap is useful for holding dressings on the scalp. A face mask may be made from gauze with holes cut out for the eyes, nose, and mouth and held in place with gauze ties looped through holes cut in the four corners of the mask. However, when strong (fluorinated) steroids are used on the face, precautions must be taken, because they may produce an acne-like dermatitis called *perioral dermatitis*.

PRURITUS

Pruritus (itching) is one of the most common complaints in dermatologic disorders. Although it is a symptom of many skin diseases such as eczema or contact dermatitis, it also occurs in the absence of any visible skin lesions. Thus it may be the first indication of an internal disease such as diabetes mellitus, blood disorders, or

---

THE PATIENT WITH A DERMATOSIS

Objectives and Principles of Nursing Management

A. To control itching and relieve pain:
   1. Examine area of involvement.
      a. Attempt to discover the cause of discomfort.
      b. Record observations in detail, using descriptive terminology.
   2. Encourage rest to reduce stimuli that cause pain and itching and to raise the threshold of discomfort.
   3. Advise patient to employ measures that produce vasoconstriction.
      a. Maintain cool environment.
      b. Remove excess clothing or bedding.
      c. Provide tepid, cooling baths.
      d. Apply cool wet dressings.
   4. Treat dryness (xerosis) with lubricating creams or lotions applied after bathing and before drying to enhance hydration.
   5. Apply prescribed lotions or ointments.
   6. Supply analgesic and antipruritic medications as indicated.
   7. Administer tranquilizing agents or sedative drugs, as necessary.
   8. Instruct patient to refrain from self-medication with salves or lotions that are commercially advertised.
   9. Assist the anxious patient to identify and cope with his problems.

B. To treat an inflammatory lesion:
   1. Apply continuous or intermittent wet dressings to reduce intensity of inflammation.
   2. Remove crusts and scales before applying topical medications.

3. Use topical applications containing corticosteroid drugs, as indicated.
      a. Rub topical medicaments well into skin to enhance penetration.
      b. Observe lesion periodically for changes in response to therapy.

C. To control oozing and prevent crust formation:
   1. Provide tub baths and wet dressings to loosen exudates and scales.
   2. Remove medications with mineral oil before reapplying.
   3. Use mildly astringent solutions to precipitate proteins and decrease oozing.
   4. Supply a high protein diet if oozing is voluminous and serum loss substantial.
   5. Administer antibiotics by topical application or by mouth, as indicated.

D. To avoid damage to skin:
   1. Protect healthy skin from maceration when applying wet dressings.
   2. Remove moisture from skin by blotting gently and avoiding friction.
   3. Guard carefully against risk of thermal trauma from excessively hot wet dressings.
   4. Advise patient to use sunscreening agents to prevent actinic damage (chemical changes from ultraviolet light).

E. To ensure efficacy of topical applications:
   1. Use occlusive dressings, as needed, to retain medication in constant contact with affected skin.
   2. Elicit the patient's cooperation in performing his own dermatologic treatments.
   3. Instruct patient clearly and in detail to ensure that treatments are carried out as prescribed.

cancer. Itching may also accompany renal, hepatic, and thyroid diseases. Pruritus may be caused by certain oral medications, by the external application of certain drugs, soaps, and chemicals, by prickly heat (miliaria), and by contact with woolen garments. It may also occur in the elderly as a result of dry skin.

Because pruritus usually leads to scratching, the secondary effects include excoriations, erythema, wheals, infections of the skin, and changes in pigmentation.

The cause of pruritus, if known, should be removed. In general, soap is avoided, and mineral oils (Lubath, Alpha-Keri bath oil) containing a surfactant that makes the oil mix with water in the bath may be sufficient for cleansing. (However, an elderly patient should not add oil to the bath because of the danger of slipping in the bathtub.) Soothing baths containing starch, camphor (½%), menthol (¼%) or water soluble tar derivatives may be prescribed. Tepid water is used for such baths. The patient can be instructed to shake off the excess water and to blot between intertriginous areas with a towel. Rubbing vigorously with the towel is avoided since this overstimulates the skin, causing more itching. It also removes water from the stratum corneum. Immediately after bathing, the skin should be lubricated with an ointment or cream that traps the moisture. Corticosteroids in cream form have proved to be effective for some patients. Inability to sleep causes an increased awareness of nighttime itching. Therefore, wearing cotton clothes next to the skin may be helpful. Excessive warmth should be avoided and the room should be kept cool and humidified. The fingernails can be trimmed to prevent injury from scratching while asleep.

Pruritus of the anal and the genital regions may be caused by poor hygiene, local irritants such as scabies and lice, local lesions such as hemorrhoids, infection with certain fungi and yeasts, and pinworm infestation. It occurs also in postmenopausal women and in conditions such as diabetes mellitus, the anemias, hyperthyroidism, and pregnancy. The treatment is removal of the local cause and use of the soothing applications mentioned above.

Patient Education. As part of health teaching, the patient is instructed to avoid both bathing in water that is too hot and using bubble baths, sodium bicarbonate, or detergent soaps, all of which aggravate dryness.

SECRETORY DISORDERS

The main secretory function of the skin is performed by the sweat glands, which help to regulate body temperature. These glands excrete a fluid, perspiration, which evaporates and thus cools the body. The sweat glands are located in various parts of the body and respond to different stimuli; those on the trunk generally respond to thermal stimulation; those on the palms and soles respond to nervous stimulation; and those in the axillae and forehead respond to both kinds of stimulation.

As a rule, moist skin is warm, and dry skin is apt to be cool. However, this is not a hard and fast rule. It is not unusual to observe cold sweats, warm, dry skin in a dehydrated patient, and very hot, dry skin peculiar to some febrile states.

HYPERHIDROSIS

Normally, temporary hyperhidrosis (excessive sweating) is associated with subcutaneous hyperemia. It may be due to exercise or to exposure to heat and certain light rays. However, a cold sweat often accompanies fright, shock, or very severe pain such as that of angina pectoris. Temporary hyperhidrosis is a response to the action of certain drugs, such as cholinergic agents and various coal-tar products (the so-called *antipyretics*). Hyperhidrosis is also a manifestation of hyperthyroidism or thyrotoxicosis.

Persisting hyperhidrosis, increased still more by hot weather and physical exertion, is natural to some persons. It affects the general body surface, but always is marked in those regions where sweating normally is most active.

In certain diseases of the central nervous system (irritative lesions of the hypothalamus), excessive sweating occurs over limited areas, such as half of the face or one side of the body. Profuse general sweating, most marked over the head, the face, and the neck, is one of the sequelae of epidemic encephalitis.

Hyperhidrosis of the palms and soles often is an indication of emotional stress. It may also be part of the symptom complex of a vasomotor disturbance such as Raynaud's phenomenon.

Management. The underlying disease should be diagnosed and treated. Temporary relief may be obtained by cooling baths, powders, the application of mild astringents, or the judicious use of tranquilizers.

SEBORRHEIC DERMATOSES

Seborrhea is excessive production of sebum (secretion of sebaceous glands) in those areas where glands are normally found in large numbers (face, scalp, eyebrows, eyelids, nasolabial folds, malar region, ears, axillae, under the breasts, groin, gluteal crease). *Seborrheic dermatitis* is a chronic inflammatory disease of the skin with a predilection for areas that are well supplied with sebaceous glands or lie between folds of the skin where the bacterial count is high.

The characteristic lesions are remarkably variable, but this is a dermatitis of the *seborrheic* areas. It may start in childhood with fine scaling of the scalp and may continue throughout life. The scales may be dry, moist, or greasy. There may be patches of sallow, greasy-appearing skin, with or without scaling, and slight erythema, predominantly on the forehead, nasolabial fold, and scalp.

The dry, flaky desquamation of the scalp with a profuse amount of fine, powdery scales is commonly called *dandruff*. The mild forms of the disease are asymptomatic. When scaling is present, it is often accompanied by pruritus that may lead to scratching and result in secondary complications such as infections and excoriations.

Seborrheic dermatitis has a genetic predisposition; hormones, nutritional status, infection, and emotional stress influence its course. There are remissions and exacerbations of this condition, which should be explained to the patient.

Management. Since there is no known cure for seborrhea, the objective of therapy is to control the disorder and allow the skin to repair itself. The person is advised to remove external irritants and avoid excess heat and perspiration, since rubbing and scratching the skin will prolong the disorder. Seborrheic dermatitis of the body and face may respond to a topically applied corticosteroid cream which allays the secondary inflammatory response. However, this medication should be used with extreme caution on the eyelids, since it can induce glaucoma in predisposed individuals. If exudation and crusting take place, an antibiotic (tetracycline) is given systemically, or antibiotic cream or ointment is applied. A secondary moniliasis (yeast infection) may occur in body creases or folds. To avoid this, patients should be advised to ensure maximum aeration of the skin and to cleanse intertriginous areas carefully. Patients with coincident moniliasis should be evaluated for diabetes.

For control of dandruff, the scalp may be shampooed with selenium sulfide suspension (Selsun, Exsel, Iosel) 2 to 3 times weekly for 5 to 10 minutes each time. The patient is advised to follow the directions on the container. There are many other good detergent shampoos on the market which may be beneficial. Brands which contain tar are also effective, especially in controlling itching.

Patient Education. Patients should also be encouraged to avoid systemically aggravating factors such as overwork, lack of sleep, infection, and emotional stress. Sunlight may be beneficial for this chronic dermatitis.

ACNE VULGARIS

Acne vulgaris is a common disorder of the sebaceous (oil) glands and their hair follicles (pilosebaceous follicles) characterized by the presence of comedones (whiteheads and blackheads), papules, pustules, nodules and cysts. The sebaceous follicles are more numerous on the face but are also found on the back and chest. Acne usually appears in the teenage years but may begin as early as 8 to 10 years of age. It becomes more marked at puberty and during adolescence, perhaps because at this age certain endocrine glands of the body which influence the secretion of the sebaceous glands are functioning at peak activity. The etiology of acne appears to be multiple, reflecting an interplay of genetic, hormonal, and bacterial factors.

Pathogenesis of Acne. During childhood the sebaceous glands are small and virtually nonfunctioning. However, during puberty the presence of androgen stimulates the sebaceous glands, causing them to secrete a natural oil, sebum, which rises to the top of the hair follicle and flows out onto the skin surface. In adolescents who develop acne, androgenic stimulation produces a heightened response in the sebaceous glands. Acne occurs when the pilosebaceous ducts through which the sebum flows become plugged.

The initial lesions of acne are comedones. Closed comedones ("whiteheads") are obstructive lesions formed from impacted lipids and keratin that plug the dilated follicle. Whiteheads are small, whitish papules with minute follicular openings that generally cannot be seen. These closed comedones may evolve into open comedones in which the contents of the ducts are in open communication with the external environment. Open comedones are termed "blackheads." The color of the blackhead is *not* due to dirt but to lipid with melanin pigment within the mass of horny cells.

Although the exact cause is not known, some comedones may rupture and result in an inflammatory reaction due to the leakage of follicular contents (sebum, keratin, bacteria) into the dermis. This inflammatory response may result from the action of certain skin bacteria, such as *Propionibacterium acnes* (formerly called *Corynebacterium acnes*) that live in the hair follicles and break down the triglycerides of the sebum into free fatty acids and glycerine. The resulting inflammation is seen clinically as papules, pustules, nodules, cysts, and/or abscesses.

Management. The objectives of management are to reduce colonization by the bacteria, prevent follicular obstruction, reduce inflammation, combat secondary infection, minimize scarring, and eliminate factors that may predispose to acne. The therapeutic regimen depends on the type of lesion (whether open or closed comedones or large cystic lesions). A combination of therapies may be tried.

Before treatment is initiated the adolescent is counseled and assured that the problem is not related to uncleanliness, dietary indiscretions, masturbation, etc., all of which are popular misconceptions. In general, over-the-counter preparations should be discouraged. When treatment is instituted, it usually takes 4 to 6 weeks or longer for results to be seen. The goal is to control the acne and keep scarring to a minimum. It is of great importance that the problems be taken seriously and that the teenager be given understanding, reassurance, and support. All facets of the emotional factors involved must be taken into account, including the possibility that acne can become a power struggle between teenager and parents.

The patient is instructed to wash his face with mild soap and water twice a day to remove the surface oils and prevent obstruction of the oil glands. Mild abrasive soaps and drying agents are prescribed to eliminate the oily feeling that troubles many patients. However, excessive abrasion is to be avoided since it only makes acne worse. Blackheads are removed manually with a comedone extractor to relieve the patient of unsightly lesions. (See this page.)

Topical Therapy. Benzoyl peroxide (PanOxyl, Desquam-X, Benzagel, Persa-Gel) are useful for inflammatory acne. They have both an antibacterial and a drying or peeling effect. Usually the patient applies a gel preparation of benzoyl peroxide once daily. In many instances this will be the only treatment needed.

For the patient with more severe involvement, topical agents are used to clear the keratin plugs from the pilosebaceous ducts. One such treatment calls for the application of topical vitamin A acid (tretinoin [Retin-A]) which acts by "unseating" the comedones. Thus, it is effective in the treatment of comedonal acne. However, the patient should be informed that symptoms may worsen during the early weeks of therapy, because the underlying noninflammatory lesions convert to inflammatory pustules prior to desquamation. Erythema and peeling are also a frequent result. Improvement may take 4 to 8 weeks. Vitamin A acid may be used alone or with other topical agents.

The following instructions are given to the patient when topical vitamin A acid is prescribed for acne:

1. Read the product information brochure.
2. Wash face with mild soap and water. Wait at least an hour to allow the skin to dry thoroughly to avoid unnecessary irritation.
3. Apply vitamin A acid as tolerated. The concentration of the preparation used and the frequency of its application are adjusted according to the reactivity of the skin to vitamin A acid.
4. Wash hands thoroughly after applying vitamin A acid.
5. Be cautious about exposure to the sun or to sunlamps, since susceptibility to sunburn is increased by the medication.
6. Avoid other irritants, such as strong soaps.
7. Do not apply vitamin A acid at the same time as benzoyl peroxide, since the Retin-A can be oxidized by the peroxide.

Topical Antibiotics. Topically applied antibiotics show promise as new therapeutic agents in the treatment of acne and are helpful when inflammatory lesions are present. Topical antibiotics penetrate the skin, diminish *P. acnes,* and do not have systemic side effects. Topi-

cycline is available by prescription. Clinda... erythromycin are usually mixed into specially p... formulas.

Systemic Antibiotics. Oral antibiotics given in s... doses over a long period are very effective in the trea... ment of patients with moderate and severe acne, especially when the acne is inflammatory and results in pustules, abscesses, and scarring. They appear to decrease the bacterial count of *Propionibacterium acnes* and to reduce fatty acids on the skin surface. Thus, inflammation is decreased. Tetracycline or erythromycin is given and adjusted according to the response of the patient. Therapy may be continued for months to years. The patient is advised to take tetracycline at least one hour before or two hours after meals, since the drug is poorly absorbed with food. Side effects of tetracyclines include photosensitivity, nausea, diarrhea, and moniliasis.

Hormone Therapy. Estrogen therapy (progesterone-estrogen preparations) has been found to suppress sebum production and reduce skin oiliness. It is usually reserved for young women when the acne begins somewhat later than usual and tends to flare at certain times in the menstrual cycle, which is often irregular. Estrogen in the form of estrogen dominant oral contraceptive compounds may be given on a prescribed cyclic regimen. Estrogen is not given to males because of undesirable side effects.

Surgical Treatment. Surgical treatment of acne consists of comedone extraction, injections of intralesional steroids into the cysts, and drainage of the cysts. Patients with deep scars may be treated with deep abrasive therapy (dermabrasion, page 1078) in which the epidermis and some superficial dermis are removed down to the level of the scars.

COMEDONE EXTRACTION. Comedones may be removed with comedone extractors. The site is first wiped with an alcohol sponge; the opening of the extractor is then placed over the lesion and direct pressure is applied to extract the contents of the lesion. Occasionally a sterile needle or scalpel blade is used to incise the follicular opening in order to widen the port and facilitate the removal of the comedone. Only noninflammatory comedones are so treated. The closed comedone (whitehead) may contain a cystic component which could rupture if excessive pressure were applied. Keratinous material would then be released into the dermis, producing an inflammatory reaction that could cause scarring.

Removal of comedones will leave areas of erythema which may take several weeks to subside. Recurrence of comedones after extraction is common. The procedure must be performed by a prepared person, although sometimes patients are taught to use the comedone extractor.

Patient Education. The patient is instructed to keep his hands away from his face and not to squeeze pimples

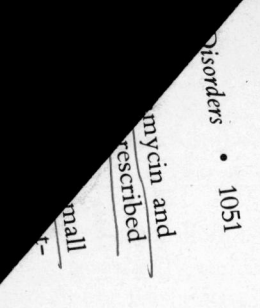

ng merely worsens the problem
ckhead is pushed down into the
ssibly causing the follicle to

autioned to avoid scrubbing the
e is not caused by dirt and
ll forms of friction and trauma
g the hands against the face,
ing tight collars and helmets.

cosmetics can aggravate acne, these are best avoided unless the patient is advised otherwise. Treatment is to be continued even though the skin clears. In general, a nutritious diet should be followed.

INFECTIONS AND INFESTATIONS OF THE SKIN

BACTERIAL INFECTIONS (PYODERMAS)

Bacterial infections of the skin may be primary, originating in previously normal-appearing skin and usually caused by a single organism, or secondary, arising from a preexisting skin disorder in which several microorganisms may be implicated. The most common primary bacterial skin infections are impetigo and folliculitis. Folliculitis may lead to furuncles or carbuncles.

Impetigo

Impetigo is a superficial infection of the skin caused by streptococci, staphylococci, or multiple bacteria. The lesions begin as small red macules which rapidly become discrete, thin-walled vesicles that soon rupture and become covered with a loosely adherent honey-yellow crust (Fig. 48-1). These crusts are easily removed and reveal smooth, red, moist surfaces on which new crusts soon develop. The exposed areas of the body, face, hands, neck, and extremities are most frequently involved. Impetigo is contagious and may spread to other parts of the patient's skin or to other members of the family who touch the patient or use towels which are soiled with the exudate of the lesions.

Although impetigo is seen at all ages, it is particularly common among undernourished children living in poor hygienic conditions. Often it appears secondary to pediculosis capitis, scabies, herpes simplex, insect bites, poison ivy, or eczema. In adults, ill health, poor hygiene, and malnutrition may predispose to impetigo.

Bullous impetigo, a superficial infection of the skin caused by *S. aureus,* is characterized by the formation of bullae from original vesicles. The bullae rupture, leaving a raw red area.

Management. A systemic antibiotic (benzathene penicillin, erythromycin, oral penicillin) is usually indicated, since a streptococcal infection of the skin can give rise to renal complications. Penicillinase-resistant penicillin (oxacillin; nafcillin) may be given for a staphylococcal infection that may be penicillin resistant.

The lesions are soaked or washed with soap solution to remove the crusts. After the crusts are removed, a topical medication (Betadine, neomycin, bacitracin, etc.) is applied. Gloves should be worn when care is given to these patients.

Patient Education. The patient and family should bathe at least once daily with bacteriostatic soap. Cleanliness and good hygienic practices help prevent the spread of the lesions from one skin area to another and from one person to another. Since impetigo is a contagious disorder, an infected child should be kept away from other children.

Folliculitis, Furuncles, and Carbuncles

Folliculitis refers to a staphylococcal infection which arises within the hair follicles. Lesions may be superficial or deep. Single or multiple papules or pustules appear close to the hair follicles. Folliculitis is commonly seen in the beard area of men who shave and on women's legs.

Pseudofolliculitis barbae ("shaving bumps") is an inflammatory reaction on the face of curly haired males caused by ingrowing hairs that pierce the skin and cause an irritative reaction. Curly hair has a curved root which grows at a more acute angle. This is a common problem in black males but may occur in others. The initial treatment is to avoid shaving and grow a beard. If this is not possible, a handbrush may be used over the facial area to mechanically dislodge the hairs. If the patient must shave, a depilatory cream may be useful.

A *furuncle* (boil) is an acute inflammation arising *deep* in one or more hair follicles and spreading into the sur-

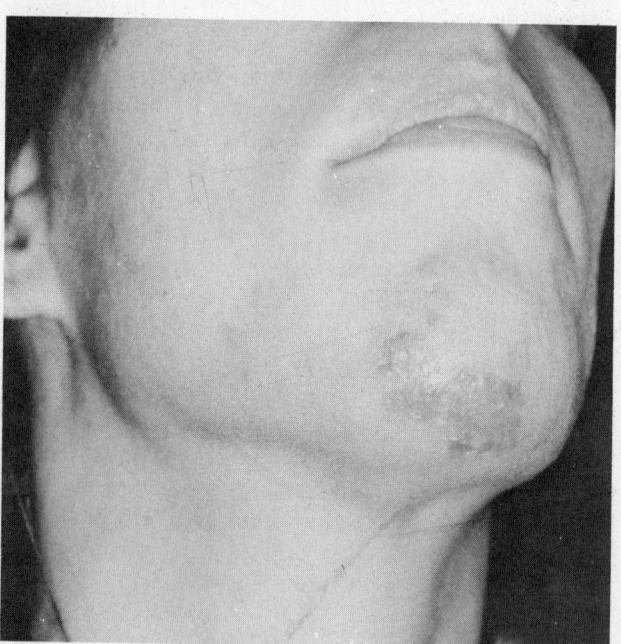

Figure 48-1. Impetigo of the chin. (Courtesy, Mervyn L. Elgart, M.D.)

rounding dermis. It is a deeper form of folliculitis. (*Furunculosis* refers to multiple or recurrent lesions.) Furuncles may occur anywhere on the body but are more prevalent in areas subjected to irritation, pressure, friction, and excessive perspiration, such as the back of the neck, the axillae, or the buttocks.

A furuncle may start as a small, red, raised, painful "pimple." Frequently the infection may progress and involve the skin and subcutaneous fatty tissue, causing tenderness, pain, and surrounding cellulitis. The area of redness and induration represents an effort of the body to keep the infection localized. The bacteria (usually staphylococcus) produce necrosis of the invaded tissues, followed in a few days by the characteristic pointing of a boil. When this occurs, the center becomes yellow or black, and the boil popularly is said to have "come to a head."

A *carbuncle* is an abscess of the skin and subcutaneous tissue representing an extension of a furuncle which has invaded several follicles and is larger and more deep-seated. It is usually caused by a staphylococcal infection. Carbuncles appear most commonly in areas in which the skin is thick and inelastic. The back of the neck and the buttocks are common sites. In carbuncles, the extensive inflammation frequently is not associated with a complete walling off of the infection, so that absorption occurs, resulting in high fever, pain, leukocytosis, and even extension of the infection to the bloodstream.

Furuncles and carbuncles are apt to occur in patients with underlying systemic diseases such as diabetes or hematologic malignancies and those receiving immunosuppressive therapy for other diseases.

Management. The follicular disorders (folliculitis, furuncles, carbuncles) are usually caused by staphylococci. If the immune system is impaired, the causative organisms may be gram-negative bacilli. Hot moist compresses increase vascularization and hasten the resolution of the furuncle or carbuncle.

In the conservative treatment of staphylococcal infections it is important not to rupture or destroy the protective wall of induration that has localized the infection. Therefore, the boil or pimple should never be squeezed.

When the pus has localized and is fluctuant (moving in palpable waves), a small incision with a scalpel will speed resolution by relieving the tension and ensuring a direct evacuation of the pus and slough. The patient is instructed to keep the draining lesion covered with a dressing. Soiled dressings should be wrapped in paper and burned. Nursing personnel should carefully follow isolation precautions in order to avoid becoming staphylococcus carriers. Disposable gloves should be worn when caring for these patients.

Systemic antibiotic therapy is generally indicated, and erythromycin, dicloxacillin, or another of the agents that are effective against staphylococcus may be prescribed.

The selection is determined by the results of sensitivity studies.

Special precautions must be taken with boils on the face, for the skin area drains directly into the cranial venous sinuses. Sinus thrombosis, with fatal pyemia, has been known to develop after manipulation of a boil in this location.

Bed rest is advised for patients who have boils on the perineum or about the anal region, and a course of systemic antibiotic therapy is indicated to control the spread of the infection.

Patient Education. To prevent and control staphylococcal skin infections (boils, carbuncles) the staphylococcus must be eliminated from the skin and environment. Efforts must be made to increase the patient's resistance and provide a hygienic environment. The mattress and pillow should be covered with plastic material and wiped off with alcohol daily; the bed linens, towels, and clothing should be laundered after each use; the patient should shower and shampoo with an antibacterial soap and shampoo for an indefinite period. The prescribed antibiotic should be taken for the full length of time as directed.

Infections of the Hand

SUPERFICIAL INFECTIONS. Trivial accidents in daily living often result in cuts, pricks, and abrasions of the skin, particularly of the hands and fingers. Although these wounds are potentially infected, they rarely become seats of infection if ordinary precautions are taken. Mechanical cleansing with soap and tap water and protection with a Band-Aid or other form of dressing are usually all that is required to permit healing without infection. Antiseptics may be used if desired, but their role in preventing infection is much less important than is ordinary washing with soap and water.

Infections of the fingers and the hand are of extreme importance to the nurse, not only because one must know how to take care of these lesions, but also because frequent accidents in nursing may lead to the development of such infections in the nurse. Therefore, it is important to know the cause and, especially, the prophylactic treatment of these infections, because they may lead to serious disability if not to fatal consequences.

Since almost all inflammations of the hand and finger are due to infection, it is important to identify the organism and to determine its sensitivity to antibiotics. In the treatment of these infections, the appropriate antibiotic properly administered will quickly alleviate the inflammatory process; it may abort the infection in some cases, and in well-established infections it hastens resolution of the infection.

PARONYCHIA. Paronychia ("runaround") is a common pyogenic infection involving the tissues around the fingernail. The infection extends between the soft tissues and the nail on the dorsum of the fingertip and forms a tense, painful, throbbing area of inflammation at the side of the nail. If the infection is allowed to go untreated, it may progress underneath the eponychium (cuticle) and then invade the space underneath the base of the nail. Hence the common name of the infection—runaround.

Cleanliness of the hands and careful care of the nails are the best prophylaxis against paronychia. If the infection does occur, it is treated by hot soaks and by lifting up the soft tissues from the edge of the nail with forceps to allow the pus to drain. A small gauze wick may be inserted into the cavity. Once the pus is evacuated, the inflammation usually subsides. The discharge is cultured, and appropriate antibiotics may be given. If the infection is due to monilia, amphotericin B (Fungizone) lotion or cream, miconazole (MicaTin), or clotrimazole (Lotrimin) is applied locally.

INFECTIONS OF THE PULP OF THE FINGERTIP. These infections usually are the result of a puncture wound or the stick of a pin or a needle, in which bacteria are carried into the layers of the skin or into the fatty tissues underlying it. This lesion is diagnosed easily, because it forms a small, tender, blister-like mound at the site of the pinprick. Puncture and removal of the overlying skin may be carried out without anesthesia, exposing the true skin below. In workmen and in others in whom the surface skin is thick, the infection may not progress to the surface so readily and, instead, may perforate through the true skin and invade the subcutaneous fatty tissues. This process is known as a *collar-button abscess,* one abscess cavity lying between layers of the skin connected by a narrow tract with a second abscess lying below the skin. In the treatment of such abscesses it is important that both the superficial and the deep collection be drained by incision.

FELON (DISTAL CLOSED SPACE INFECTION). The most common and serious type of infection of the fingertip occurs in the pulp of the finger and is caused by the streptococcus. There usually is a history of needleprick, pinprick, or some other form of puncture, followed several days later by throbbing pain, which may be intense enough to prevent sleep. The swelling and the edema produced by the infection may be sufficient to impair or shut off completely the arterial supply to the soft tissue, so that rapid necrosis and even invasion of the bone may occur. The resulting disability often is great because of the extreme importance of the fingertips in the use of the hand and fingers.

Management. Early incision and drainage prevent the necrosis from progressing; therefore, wide incision often is practiced for what may appear to be a relatively small area of infection. It is surprising to note that radical incision is the conservative therapy in dealing with infections of the pulp of the finger.

After incision, the wound is held open by a rubber dam or gauze drainage and immobilized by an appropriate splint. Warm moist dressings are used until the area of slough has separated entirely, after which time healing may be permitted to take place.

Prophylaxis. To prevent infection of the fingertip, any prick of the finger with a needle or pin should be reported. Occasionally, a slight enlargement of the incision or cauterization of the needle puncture with phenol may abort a serious infection. If throbbing pain becomes a prominent symptom, no time should be wasted before consulting a surgeon. The appropriate antibiotic must be administered.

INFECTIONS OF TENDON SHEATHS—TENOSYNOVITIS. Infections of the tendon sheaths on the palmar surface of the hand occur most frequently from puncture wounds. Most often they are caused by the streptococcus. They are serious, because they may lead to rapid destruction of the tendon itself and, therefore, to marked disability of the finger and hand. An infection may involve the sheaths of the tendons in the fingers and the thumb; it may invade the fascial spaces of the hand, or it may advance along the tendon sheaths of the thumb and the fifth finger, invading the bursal space through which the tendons pass at the wrist. It produces a tense swelling of the involved finger with extreme pain when motion is attempted.

Management. Early incision and drainage are necessary to prevent necrosis of the tendon. Petrolatum gauze usually is laid in the wound to provide drainage.

The specific antibiotic is administered. In the early phases of the infection, the antibiotic may prevent necrosis and the necessity for incision. After incision, it is used to prevent extension of the infection and to hasten healing.

Postoperative Nursing Management. Following surgical treatment, the part involved is generally bandaged and splinted in a position of function, usually by placing the hand on a padded volar splint from the fingertips to below the elbow.

Warm moist applications are applied either through the dressings directly or through tubes fastened in them. It is extremely important that sterile technique be observed when moistening the dressings because of the danger of producing a mixed infection, which usually is associated with the extension of the inflammatory process. Elevation of the part is necessary to reduce the inflammatory edema and to give comfort to the patient. This usually is accomplished by means of pillows covered with plastic.

After the acute inflammatory process has been controlled, the infected hand often may be treated in a warm saline bath two or three times daily. The basin and the solution should be sterilized and the solution placed in the basin at a temperature as warm as the patient can comfortably stand. The temperature is maintained as long as possible by adding more solution at intervals. The bath usually is continued for at least 30 minutes. Its purpose is to apply heat to aid in discharging the necrotic materials from the wound. After the hand is removed from the bath, it is placed in a sterile towel. In general, the infected hand is kept at rest.

VIRAL INFECTIONS

Herpes Zoster (Shingles)

Herpes zoster (shingles) is an inflammatory condition in which the virus produces a painful vesicular eruption along the distribution of the nerves from one or more posterior ganglia. It is caused by the varicella virus, commonly known as varicella-zoster virus, which is a member of a group of DNA viruses. (The viruses of chicken pox and zoster are indistinguishable, hence the name varicella-zoster). It is assumed that herpes zoster represents a reactivation of latent varicella (chicken pox) virus and reflects a lowered immunity. There is an increased frequency of herpes zoster in patients with certain malignancies, particularly Hodgkin's lymphoma. The activation of the latent infection results in the spread of the virus via the peripheral nerves to the skin. Here a localized vesicular eruption occurs.

The eruption is generally accompanied or preceded by itching, tenderness, and pain which may radiate over the entire region supplied by the nerves. Malaise and gastrointestinal disturbances may also precede the eruption.

The patches of grouped vesicles appear on the erythematous and edematous skin. The early vesicles contain serum and later become purulent, rupture, and form crusts. The inflammation is usually unilateral, involving the thoracic, cervical, or cranial nerves in a band-like configuration. The clinical course varies from 1 to 3 weeks. The healing time varies between 7 and 26 days. The disease is considered infectious only for the first 2 to 3 days and only to persons who are in a state of immunosuppression or those who have not previously had varicella.

Management. The objectives of management are to relieve the pain and to reduce or avoid complications. These include infection, scarring, and postherpetic neuralgia. The pain is controlled with analgesics, although postherpetic neuralgia does not respond well to analgesics and is a major problem in patient management. Antihistamines are given to control the itching.

Herpes zoster in healthy adults is usually localized and benign. However, in immunosuppressed patients the disease may be severe and the clinical course acutely disabling.

FUNGAL INFECTIONS

The fungi, tiny representatives of the plant kingdom which feed on organic matter, are responsible for a variety of common skin infections. In some cases they affect only the skin and its appendages (i.e., hair and nails), but in others, the internal organs are involved. In the latter instance fungal disease may be so serious as to constitute a threat to life. Superficial infections, on the other hand, rarely cause temporary disability and respond readily to treatment. To obtain material for diagnosis, the lesion is cleaned and a scalpel is used to remove scales from the margin of the lesion. The diagnosis is made by examining the infected scales microscopically and by isolating the organism in culture. Wood's light (a special ultraviolet light with maximum output in the 366 nm. range) may be helpful in diagnosing some cases of tinea capitis.

Tinea Pedis (Athlete's Foot)

Tinea pedis, the most common fungal infection, is a superficial infection that manifests itself as an acute, inflammatory, vesicular process, or as a chronic scaling, dusky erythematous rash involving the soles of the feet and the interdigital web spaces. The toenails may or may not be affected; if involved, they are apt to be discolored, brittle, and heaped-up. As a rule there is moderate to severe itching. Lymphangitis and cellulitis may be seen occasionally when bacterial superinfection occurs.

Management. During the acute (vesicular) phase, soaks of Burow's solution, saline, or potassium permanganate are used to remove the crusts, scales, and debris and to reduce the inflammation. Fungistatic cream or lotion, such as tolnaftate (Tinactin), haloprogin (Halotex), miconazole (MicaTin), or clotrimazole (Lotrimin), are applied to the involved areas. Topical therapy is continued for several weeks as there is a high rate of recurrence. An antifungal agent, griseofulvin, is given orally if there is an extension of the infection or resistance to topical therapy. If necessary, the patient is encouraged to rest in bed or elevate his feet frequently.

Preventive Measures and Patient Education. Since footwear provides a hospitable environment for fungi, the causative fungi may be in the shoes and socks. Because moisture encourages the growth of fungi, the patient is instructed to keep his feet as dry as possible, including the areas between the toes. Small pieces of cotton can be placed between the toes at night to absorb moisture. Socks should be made of absorbent cotton, and hosiery should have cotton feet, since synthetic material does not absorb perspiration as well as cotton. For individuals whose feet perspire excessively, perforated shoes permit better aeration of the feet. Plastic or rubber-soled footwear should be avoided. Talcum powder or antifungal powder (Tinactin) applied twice daily helps to keep the feet dry. The shoes should be alternated so that they may dry completely before they are worn again. Also, persons using swimming pools, club house showers, etc., should be instructed to wear clogs while in these places.

Tinea Capitis (Ringworm of the Scalp)

Ringworm of the scalp is a contagious fungal disease and a common cause of hair loss in children. Clinically, one or several round patches of redness and scaling are present. Small pustules or papules may be seen at the edges of such patches. As the hairs in the affected areas are invaded by the fungi, they become brittle and often break off at or near the surface of the scalp, resulting in areas of baldness. Most cases of tinea capitis heal wihout scarring, hence the hair loss is only temporary. Sometimes a boggy swelling resembling a furuncle occurs in an area of involvement; this lesion is known as a *kerion*.

In recent years, a second form of ringworm caused by *Trichophyton tonsurans* has become prominent in the inner city. It presents as a scaling dermatitis, similar to seborrhea, with scattered (not well-rounded) areas of hair loss. In this condition, diagnosis is made by examining the hair, since fluorescence is not present.

Management. Griseofulvin (Fulvicin-U/F), a fungistatic and fungicidal antibiotic, is given to patients with tinea capitis. It is taken with or just after a meal, since the presence of fat aids in the absorption of the drug. Topical agents are not effective as cure since the infection occurs within the hairshaft and below the surface of the scalp. However, topical agents are often used to inactivate organisms already on the hair. This diminishes contagiousness and eliminates the need to clip the hair, which is cosmetically unappealing and only adds to the patient's embarrassment. Infected hairs break off anyway, and noninfected ones may be left in place. The hair should be shampooed 2 to 3 times weekly and a topical antifungal preparation should be applied to reduce dissemination of the organisms.

Patient Education. Because the disease is contagious, the patient and family should be advised to set up a hygienic regimen for home use. Each person should have his own comb and brush and should avoid exchanging headgear. All infected members of the family and household pets must be examined since familial infections are relatively common.

Tinea Corporis

Tinea corporis or *tinea circinata* is ringworm of the body. Rings of vesicles with clear centers appear in clusters, usually on the exposed areas of the body: face, arms, shoulders, possibly extending to the scalp. As a rule there is an elevated border consisting of small papules or vesicles. Coalescence of individual rings may result in large patches with bizarre scalloped borders. A frequent cause of tinea circinata is the presence of an infected pet in the home.

Management. Topical antifungal medication (Tinactin, Holotex, MicaTin, Lotrimin) may be applied to small areas. Griseofulvin is used in extensive cases. Side effects of griseofulvin include photosensitivity, skin rashes, headache, and nausea.

Patient Education. The patient is instructed to use a clean towel and washcloth daily. All areas and skin folds that retain moisture must be dried thoroughly, since fungal infections are fostered by heat and moisture. Clean clothing should be worn next to the skin.

TINEA CRURIS. *Tinea cruris* ("jock itch") is ringworm infection of the groin, which may extend to the inner thighs and buttock area. It occurs more frequently in males. The infection starts with small, red, scaly patches and extends to form circinate (circular) plaques with elevated scaly or vesicular borders. Itching is usually present.

Mild infections may be treated with topical medication such as clotrimazole (Lotrimin cream), miconazole (MicaTin cream) or haloprogin (Halotex cream) for at least 3 to 4 weeks to ensure complete eradication of the infection. Oral griseofulvin may be required for more severe infections.

Patient Education. Heat, friction, and maceration (from sweating) predispose to the infection. The patient is instructed to avoid as far as possible excessive heat and humidity, nylon underwear, tight-fitting clothing, and the prolonged wearing of a wet bathing suit. The groin area should be cleansed, dried thoroughly, and dusted with a topical antifungal agent (tolnaftate [Tinactin]) as a preventive measure, since the infection is apt to recur.

Tinea Unguium (Onychomycosis)

Tinea unguium (ringworm of the nails) is a chronic fungal infection of the toenails or, less commonly, the fingernails and is usually caused by Trichophyton (*T. rubrum, T. mentagrophytes*) as well as *Candida albicans*. It is usually associated with long-standing fungal infections of the feet. The nails become thickened, friable (easily crumbled), and lusterless. In time, debris accumulates under the free edge of the nail, and ultimately the

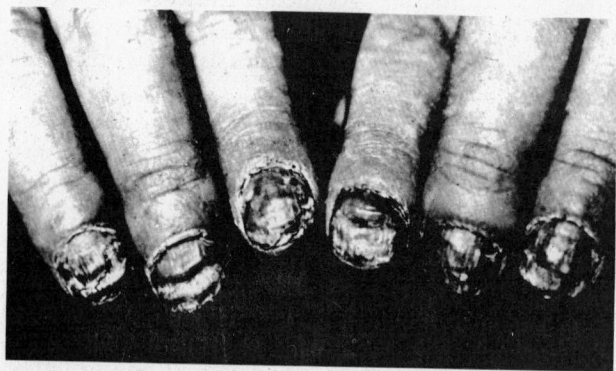

Figure 48-2. Fungal infection of the fingernails. Note that the disease has spread and involved the nail plate. The nails are hyperkeratotic and cracked. The patient may complain of discomfort from the pressure of the diseased nails. (Courtesy, Ralph E. McDonnell, M.D., New Haven)

nail plate becomes separated (Fig. 48-2). The nail may be destroyed.

Management. Griseofulvin is usually given orally for 6 months to a year when the fingernails are involved. Of course, griseofulvin is not of value in treating candidal infections; these infections must be treated topically with amphotericin B lotion, miconazole (MicaTin), clotrimazole (Lotrimin), nystatin (Mycostatin cream) or preparations such as thymol 4 percent in chloroform. These products penetrate poorly, and the infections are difficult to treat. Response to griseofulvin in fungal infections of the toenails is poor at best. Toenails are such slow-growing organs that the medication may have to be used for a year or more with only a 20 percent chance of cure. Frequently, when the treatment is stopped the infection quickly returns.

PARASITIC SKIN DISEASES

PEDICULOSIS (INFESTATION BY LICE)

Lice infestation affects persons of all ages. Three varieties of lice infest humans: *Pediculus humanus capitis* (head louse); *Pediculus humanus corporis* (body louse), and *Phthirus pubis* (pubic, or "crab," louse). Lice are termed ectoparasites because they live on the outside of the host's body. Thus they depend on another host for their nourishment, feeding on human blood approximately 5 times a day. They inject their digestive juices and excrement into the skin, which causes very itchy bites.

Pediculosis Capitis

Pediculosis capitis is an infestation of the scalp by the head louse, *Pediculus humanus capitis*. The female head louse lays her eggs (nits) close to the scalp. The nits become firmly attached to the hair shafts with a tenacious cement bond. The young lice hatch in about 10 days and reach maturity in 2 weeks. Head lice are found most commonly over the back of the head and behind the ears. The eggs are visible to the naked eye as silvery, glistening oval bodies that are difficult to remove from the hair. The bite of the insect causes *intense itching* and the resultant scratching often leads to secondary bacterial infection with pustules, crusts, matted hair, and impetigo and furunculosis. The infestation is more common in children and people with long hair. Head lice may be transmitted by direct physical contact or by the use of infested combs, brushes, wigs, hats, and bedding.

Management. Treatment involves washing the hair with a shampoo containing gamma benzene hexachloride (Kwell; Gamene). The patient should be instructed to shampoo the scalp and hair vigorously for at least 4 minutes. After the hair is rinsed thoroughly, it is combed with a fine-toothed comb that is dipped in vinegar to remove any remaining nits or nit shells freed from the hair shafts. All articles, clothing, towels, and bedding that might have lice or nits should be washed in hot, soapy water or dry-cleaned to prevent reinfestation. Combs and brushes are also disinfected with the shampoo. The regimen may be repeated in 24 hours (if unsuccessful) but not more than twice in one week. All family members and close contacts are treated.

Complications such as severe pruritus, pyoderma (pus-forming infection of the skin) and dermatitis are treated with antipruritics, systemic antibiotics, and topical corticosteroids.

Patient Education. The patient is reassured that head lice infestation may happen to anyone and is not a sign of uncleanliness. This condition spreads rapidly. Therefore, treatment must be started immediately. Control of school epidemics may be helped by having all of the students shampoo their hair on the same night.

Pediculosis Corporis

Pediculosis corporis is an infestation of the body by the body louse, *Pediculus humanus corporis*. The body louse lives chiefly in the seams of underwear and clothing, to which it clings as it pierces the skin with its proboscis. Its bites cause characteristic minute hemorrhagic points. Widespread excoriations may appear on the back and shoulders. Among the secondary lesions produced are hyperemia, parallel linear scratches, and a slight degree of eczema. In long-standing cases, the skin may become thickened, dry, and scaly, with dark pigmented areas. The areas of the skin chiefly involved are those that come in closest contact with the underclothing—i.e., the neck, trunk, and thighs. The lice may be seen in the seams of the clothing. Therefore the clothing and bedding must be laundered or dry-cleaned to destroy the parasite and its eggs. A shower should be taken and precautionary methods followed to prevent reinfestation.

Complications, such as severe pruritus, pyoderma (pus-informing infection of the skin), and dermatitis are treated with antipruritics, systemic antibiotics, and topical corticosteroids. One must keep in mind that body lice are vectors for rickettsial disease (epidemic typhus, relapsing fever, and trench fever). The causative organism may be in the gastrointestinal tract of the insect and may be excreted on the skin surface of the infested person.

Pediculosis pubis, infestation by *Phthirus pubis* ("crab louse") is an extremely common problem that is generally localized in the genital region and transmitted chiefly by sexual contact.

Reddish brown "dust" from the excretion of the insects may be found in underclothing. Lice may also infest the hairs of the chest, axillary hair, beard, and eyelashes. Gray-blue macules may sometimes be seen on the trunk, thighs, and axillae as a result either of the reaction of the insects' saliva with bilirubin (converting it to biliverdin) or an excretion produced by the salivary glands of the louse. Itching is the most common symptom, particularly at night. Infestation by pubic lice may coexist with other sexually transmitted diseases (gonorrhea, candidiasis, syphilis).

Management and Patient Education. The patient is instructed to bathe with soap and water. Then gamma benzene hexachloride (Kwell) cream or lotion is applied to affected areas of the skin and to hairy areas, according to the product information directives. Kwell is not applied to the eyebrows or eyelashes. Nits may be removed manually from the eyebrows and eyelashes with cotton-tipped applicators after yellow oxide of mercury or physostigmine ophthalmic ointment has been applied.

All sexual contacts and family members must be treated. The patient and his partner(s) must also be scheduled for a workup for coexisting venereal disease. All clothing and bedding should be machine washed or dry-cleaned.

Scabies

Scabies is an infestation of the skin by the itch mite, *Sarcoptes scabiei*. There has been a progressive increase in scabies during the past several years. The disease may be found in poor persons living under substandard hygienic conditions, but it is also common in very clean individuals. It is often found among the sexually active. However, infestations are not dependent on sexual activity since the mites frequently involve the fingers, and hand contact may produce infection. In children, overnight stays with friends or the exchange of clothes may be a source of infection. Health care personnel who have prolonged "hands on" physical contact with an infected patient may likewise become infected.

The adult female burrows into the superficial layer of the skin after fertilization has occurred on the skin surface. With her jaws and the sharp edges of the joints of her forelegs the mite extends the burrow, laying 3 to 4 eggs daily for up to 2 months. She then dies. The larvae hatch in about 6 days, go through several molts and then migrate to the skin surface where they reach maturity in 2 to 3 weeks. It takes approximately 4 weeks from the time of contact for symptoms to appear.

Nursing Assessment. During examination, the patient should be asked where the itch is most severe. A magnifying glass and a penlight are held at an oblique angle to the skin while a search is made for the small raised burrows. The burrows may be multiple straight or wavy brown or black threadlike lesions, most commonly observed between the fingers, the extensor surfaces of the elbows, knees, outer borders of feet, points of elbows, around the nipples, in axillary folds, under pendulous breasts, and in or near the groin or gluteal fold, penis, or scrotum. Red pruritic eruptions usually appear in intertriginous areas. The burrow, however, is not always seen. Any patient with a rash may have scabies.

One classic sign of scabies is the increased itching that occurs at night, perhaps because the increased warmth of the skin has a stimulating effect on the parasite. If the infection has spread, other members of the family and close friends will also complain of itching.

Secondary lesions are quite common and include vesicles, papules, pustules, excoriations, and crusts. Bacterial superinfection may result from constant excoriation of the burrows and papules.

A drop of oil is placed over a lesion to prevent the specimen from being lost. A sample of superficial epidermis is scraped off with a small scalpel blade. The scrapings are placed on a microscope slide and examined by low-powered microscope to demonstrate the presence of the mite and its products—eggs, fecal concretions.

Management and Patient Education. The patient is instructed to take a warm, soapy bath or shower to remove scaling debris from the crusts and then to thoroughly dry himself and allow the skin to cool. Then a scabicide, such as gamma benzene hexachloride (Kwell cream and lotion, Gamene) or crotamiton (Eurax cream and lotion) is applied in a thin layer and rubbed in thoroughly. The entire body is covered with the cream from the neck down. The medication is left on for 8 to 12 hours, after which the patient is instructed to wash thoroughly. One application is usually curative. The patient should wear clean clothing and sleep between freshly laundered bed linens. All bedding and clothing should be washed in very hot water.

After the treatment is completed, a bland ointment may be applied, because the solution may be irritating to the skin. The hypersensitivity state does not cease upon destruction of the mites. Itching may remain a troublesome problem for a few days or weeks. However, this is not a sign that the treatment has failed.

All family members and close contacts should be treated simultaneously to eliminate the mites. If scabies is sexually transmitted the patient may require treatment for coexisting venereal disease. Scabies may also coexist with pediculosis.

Bedbug Infestation

Two species of bedbugs, *Cimex lectularius* and *Cimex hemipterus* invade human habitations, particularly in older and poorer sections of cities. The female leaves eggs in the cracks of floors and furniture. After the nymphs hatch, they can survive for a month or two without food. Then the mature bug emerges at night to feed on the blood of a sleeping victim. The bites are grouped in a straight line and consist of hemorrhagic spots associated with papular or wheal-like lesions. There may be tiny red points marking the original size of the bites. The legs, particularly the ankles, are most frequently bitten, and the patient experiences variable degrees of itching, burning, pain, and urticaria, depending on the degree of previous sensitization. The patient may find his night clothing and bedding stained with blood. Secondary infection and pyoderma may occur.

Patient Education and Management. In general, lesions require no treatment. An antipruritic lotion (calomine with phenol) may be applied to local areas of bites. Antihistamines may be given for intense itching. The insects may be eliminated if all crevices in furniture, walls, floors, mattresses and beds are sprayed with an insecticide.

CONTACT DERMATITIS

Contact dermatitis (dermatitis venenata) is a common inflammatory, often eczematous, condition caused by a skin reaction to contact with a variety of irritating or allergenic materials. The epidermis is damaged by repeated physical and chemical insults. Contact dermatitis may be of the primary irritant type in which a nonallergic reaction results from exposure to an irritating substance, or it may be allergic in nature (allergic contact dermatitis) resulting from exposure of sensitized individuals to contact allergens. (Allergic dermatoses are discussed in Chapter 50.) Common causes of irritant contact dermatitis are soaps, detergents, scouring compounds, industrial chemicals, etc. Predisposing factors include extremes of heat and cold, frequent immersion in soap and water, and a preexisting skin disease.

Clinical Manifestations. The eruptions begin at the point at which the causative agent contacts the skin. The first reactions include itching, burning, and erythema, followed soon by edema, papules, vesicles, and oozing or weeping. In the subacute phase these vesicular changes are less marked and alternate with crusting, drying, fissuring, and peeling. If repeated reactions occur or if the patient continually scratches the skin, thickening of the skin (lichenification) and pigmentation (coloration) occur. Secondary bacterial invasion may follow.

Management. The objectives of management are to rest the involved skin and to protect it from further damage. The distribution pattern of the reaction is determined in order to differentiate between allergic contact dermatitis and the irritant type. A detailed history is obtained. Then the offending irritant is identified and removed. Local irritation should be avoided and soap is not generally used until healing occurs.

There are innumerable preparations advocated for the relief of dermatitis. In general, a bland unmedicated lotion is used for small patches of erythema. Cool wet dressings also are applied over small areas of vesicular dermatitis. Finely cracked ice added to the water often enhances its antipruritic affect. Wet dressings usually dry the oozing eczematous lesions. Then a thin layer of cream or ointment containing one of the steroids may be used. Medicated baths at room temperature are prescribed for larger areas of dermatitis. (See also, the patient with a dermatosis, page 1048.)

Systemic administration of sedatives and antihistamines may be required to relieve the intense burning and itching, whereas systemic antibiotics will be necessary if secondary bacterial infection is present.

In more widespread conditions, a short course of systemic steroids may be prescribed. This can diminish the course of a severe disease considerably.

Patient Education. The patient is instructed as follows:

1. Avoid heat, soap, and rubbing; all of these are external irritants.
2. Avoid topical medications except when specifically prescribed.
3. Wash the skin thoroughly immediately after exposure to irritants or antigens.
4. Do not touch uninvolved body areas with involved areas.
5. When gloves are used for washing dishes, use cotton-lined gloves, but do not wear them more than 15 to 20 minutes at a time.
6. The instructions given by the physician should be followed for at least 4 months after the skin appears to be completely healed, since the resistance of the skin is lowered.

NONINFECTIOUS INFLAMMATORY DERMATOSES

PSORIASIS

Psoriasis is a chronic inflammatory disease of the skin in which epidermal proliferation occurs. In psoriasis, the production of the epidermis occurs at a rate that is approximately 6 to 9 times faster than normal. The cells in the basal layer of the skin divide too quickly and the newly formed cells move so rapidly to the skin surface that they become evident as profuse scales. The psoriatic epidermal cell may travel from the basal cell layer of the epidermis to the stratum corneum (skin surface) and be cast off in 3 to 4 days which is in sharp contrast to the

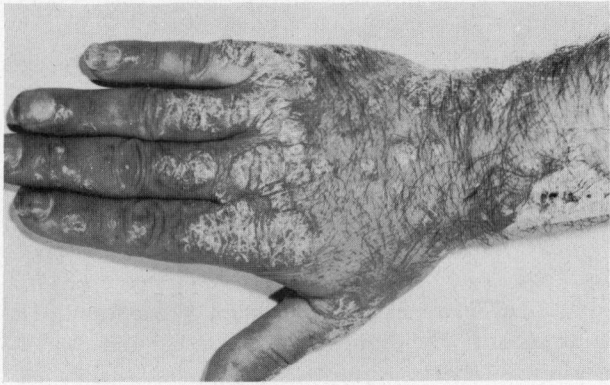

Figure 48-3. Psoriasis of the hand. (From Sauer: Manual of Skin Diseases. Philadelphia, J. B. Lippincott)

normal 26 to 28 days. As a result of the increased number of basal cells and rapid cell passage, the normal events of cell maturation and keratinization cannot take place. This abnormal process does not allow formation of the normal protective layers of the skin.

Appearance of Lesions. The lesions produced by epidermal hyperplasia and accelerated epidermal turnover appear as circular patches of all sizes that are sharply defined against the normal skin and covered with heavy, dry, silvery scales (Fig. 48-3). If the scales are scraped away, the dark red base of the lesion is exposed, producing multiple bleeding points. These patches are not moist and may or may not itch. The lesions may remain small, giving rise to the term "guttate psoriasis." Usually the lesions enlarge slowly, but after many months they coalesce, forming extensive irregularly shaped patches. Psoriasis may range from a cosmetic source of annoyance to a physically disabling and disfiguring affliction. Particular sites of the body tend to be affected by this ailment; they include the scalp, the area over the elbows and knees, and the lower part of the back.

Psoriasis appears most often on the extensor surfaces of the arms and legs, on the scalp and ears, and over the sacrum and intergluteal fold. Bilateral symmetry is a feature of psoriasis. In approximately one quarter to one half of the patients, the nails are involved, with pitting, discoloration, crumbling beneath the free edges, and separation of the nail plate. When psoriasis occurs on the palms and soles it can cause vesicular and pustular lesions. The disease may be associated with arthritis of multiple joints, causing a crippling disability. The relationship between arthritis and psoriasis is not understood.

Psoriasis is one of the most common skin diseases. There appears to be a hereditary biochemical defect that causes an overproduction of keratin. A combination of specific genetic makeup and environmental stimuli may trigger the onset of disease. Periods of emotional stress and anxiety aggravate the condition. The onset usually occurs before the age of 20, but all age groups are affected. Psoriasis has a tendency to improve and then recur throughout life.

Psychological Considerations. The "heartbreak of psoriasis" is the outcome of a chronic disease that leads to frustration and despair on the part of the patient and a tendency on the part of other people to stare, comment, ask embarrassing questions, or even avoid the person. The disease can eventually exhaust the patient's resources, interfere with his job, and make life miserable in general. Teenagers are especially vulnerable to the psychological effects of this ailment. Many a teenager's personality has been scarred by the occurrence of such a disfiguring disease at a stage of life when appearance is all-important. The family, too, is affected, since time-consuming treatments, messy salves, and constant shedding of scales disrupt home life and cause resentment. In many cases the patient's frustrations are expressed through hostility directed at the health care specialists.

The therapeutic approach should be one that the patient understands; it should be cosmetically acceptable and not too disruptive of life style, and it will involve the commitment of time and effort by the patient and those caring for him.

Management. The objective of management is to inhibit the rapid proliferation of the epidermis in order to reduce scaling and itching. The goal is limited to control of the problem, since there is no known cure.

First, any precipitating or aggravating factors are removed. Then an assessment is made of life style, since psoriasis is significantly affected by stress. The patient must also be advised that treatment is time-consuming, expensive, and esthetically unappealing at times.

Therapy may be divided into three types: topical, intralesional, and systemic.

TOPICAL THERAPY. Topically applied agents are the mainstay of the treatment of psoriasis. Such medications include tar preparations, anthralin, salicylic acid, corticosteroids, etc. These therapies seem to act by suppressing epidermopoiesis. Tar baths or tar preparations may retard and inhibit the rapid growth of psoriatic tissue. This aspect of therapy may be combined with carefully graded doses of ultraviolet radiation. However, the tar should be removed before the skin is exposed to ultraviolet light, since tar acts as a screening agent. During this phase of treatment, the patient is advised to wear goggles and to protect the eyes. Using a timer will prevent the danger of severe burns due to overexposure to the light rays. A daily tar shampoo followed by an application of steroid lotion may be used for scalp lesions. The patient is also taught to remove excess scales by scrubbing with a soft brush while bathing.

Anthralin preparations (a distillate of crude coal tar) are useful for thick and resistant psoriatic plaques. The patient is instructed to apply anthralin medication (Anthera, Anthra-Derm, Lasan Unguent) with a tongue blade or gloved fingers, taking special care not to cover normal skin. The hands must be washed after the medication is handled, because a chemical conjunctivitis can be produced if the patient touches his eyes while medication is still on his hands. Anthralin stains badly and should be covered in some way (gauze dressings, stockinette, old pajamas) when applied. The preparation is left on the skin for 8 to 12 hours.

TOPICAL STEROIDS. Topical steroids may be applied and covered with an occlusive plastic film dressing to enhance drug penetration and soften the scaly plaques. However, once the steroid treatment is stopped, the psoriasis may quickly reappear (rapid recurrence) and, in some instances, be more extensive than the original lesions.

OCCLUSIVE DRESSINGS. Some patients will require

occlusive dressings over the entire body. For the hospitalized patient, large plastic bags may be used—one for the upper body (with holes cut out for the head and arms) and one for the lower part (with holes for the legs). This leaves only the extremities to wrap. In some dermatological units, large rolls of tubular plastic are used (such as the kind that dry-cleaners place over clean clothes). However, when these substances are used, *it is important to check for flammability*. Some of these thin plastic films will burn slowly (if touched by a lighted cigarette), whereas others will burst rapidly into flame and may cause severe injury. The patient should be cautioned not to smoke while wrapped in these dressings. In patients being treated at home, a plastic vinyl jogging suit may be purchased. The medication is applied and the suit simply put over it. The hands can be wrapped in gloves, the feet in plastic bags, and the head in a shower cap. The suit can be machine washed, making a difficult task much easier.

INTRALESIONAL THERAPY. Intralesional injections of triamcinolone acetonide directly into highly visible patches of psoriasis have provided remissions for 6 to 12 months.

SYSTEMIC THERAPY. Systemic cytotoxic preparations such as methotrexate and hydroxyurea have been used in treating extensive psoriasis that fails to respond to other forms of therapy. Methotrexate (Amethopterin), a folic acid antagonist that prevents cell replication, may be prescribed. However, the drug can be very toxic, especially to the liver, which can suffer irreversible damage. Thus, laboratory studies must be monitored to ensure that the hepatic, hematopoietic, and renal systems are functioning adequately.

The patient should avoid drinking alcohol while on methotrexate, since this increases the possibility of liver damage.

Another drug currently being used is hydroxyurea (Hydrea) which inhibits cell replication by affecting DNA synthesis. The patient is monitored for signs and symptoms of bone marrow depression.

PHOTOCHEMOTHERAPY (PUVA THERAPY). A new and promising treatment for severely debilitating psoriasis is PUVA (psoralen, and ultraviolet A) therapy. However, it is still under investigation because of unanswered questions about the safety of long-term use. Photochemotherapy requires the combined effects of an orally administered phototoxic substance (8-methoxypsoralen [Methoxsalen]) and irradiation with a long-wave ultraviolet light. The 8-methoxypsoralen molecule absorbs the light energy and becomes an active molecule which binds to the DNA of the cell nucleus. This presumably leads to inhibition of epidermal DNA synthesis, thereby decreasing cellular proliferation.

PUVA therapy requires that psoralen be taken orally, followed in two hours by irradiation with high-intensity long-wave ultraviolet light (UVA). (Ultraviolet light is the portion of the electromagnetic spectrum containing wave lengths from 100 to 400 nm.) The PUVA unit consists of a light cabinet containing high-output blacklight lamps and an external reflectance system. The exposure time is calibrated according to the specific unit in use and the anticipated tolerance of the patient's skin. The patient is usually treated 2 to 3 times a week while the lesions are clearing. An interim period of 48 hours between treatments is necessary, because it takes this long for any PUVA burns to become evident. The patient is then placed on a maintenance program.

Patient Education. PUVA treatment produces photosensitization, which means that the patient is sensitive to the sun until Methoxsalen has been excreted from the body (about 8 to 10 hours). Therefore exposure to the sun must be avoided at this time. If exposure is unavoidable, the skin must be protected with sunscreen and clothing. Gray or green-tinted wraparound sunglasses may be recommended by the physician and should be worn to protect the eyes after treatment. Ophthalmologic examinations are carried out on a regular basis. Nausea, which may be a problem in some patients, is lessened when Methoxsalen is taken with food. Lubricants and bath oils may be used to help remove scales and prevent excess dryness. No other creams or oils are to be used except on areas that have been shielded from ultraviolet light. The patient must remain under constant and careful supervision.

EXFOLIATIVE DERMATITIS

Exfoliative dermatitis is a serious condition characterized by a progressive inflammation in which erythema and scaling often occur in a more or less generalized distribution. It may be associated with chills, fever, prostration, severe toxicity, and an itchy scaling of the skin. There is a profound loss of stratum corneum (outermost layer of the skin), which causes capillary leakage, hypoproteinemia, and negative nitrogen balance. The iron loss from the skin produces anemia. Thus, exfoliative dermatitis has a marked effect on the entire body.

It may develop as a primary condition, or it may arise secondary to other chronic skin diseases, such as eczema and psoriasis, particularly if these are treated with irritating ointments over a long period of time. Exfoliative dermatitis may appear as a part of the lymphoma group of diseases and may actually precede the appearance of lymphoma. It also appears as a severe reaction to a wide number of drugs, including penicillin and phenylbutazone. Thus, there are a multiplicity of causes.

This condition starts acutely as either a patchy or generalized erythematous eruption accompanied by fever, malaise, and, occasionally, gastrointestinal symptoms. The skin color changes from pink to dark red; then, after a week, the characteristic exfoliation (scaling) begins, usually in the form of thin flakes which leave the underlying skin smooth and red, new scales forming as the older ones exfoliate (cast off) (Fig. 48-4). Hair loss may accompany this disorder. Relapses are the rule. The systemic effects include high output congestive failure, enteropathy, gynecomastia, hyperuricemia, and thermoregulatory disturbances.

Management. The objectives of management are to maintain fluid and electrolyte balance and to prevent intercurrent or cutaneous infection. The treatment is individualized and supportive and depends on the cause. The patient is hospitalized and placed on bed rest. All drugs are stopped. However, oral or topical corticosteroids may be used. A comfortable room temperature should be maintained, since the patient does not have normal thermoregulatory control because of fluctuations in temperature due to vasodilatation and evaporative water loss. The fluid and electrolyte balance must be maintained since there is considerable water and protein loss from the skin surface. Plasma expanders may be indicated.

Continual nursing assessment is carried out to detect intercurrent and cutaneous infection. The erythematous moist skin is receptive to infection and becomes colonized with pathogenic organisms which produce more inflammation. Antibiotics are given if infection is present and are selected on the basis of culture and sensitivity.

- Watch for signs and symptoms of congestive heart failure, since hyperemia and increased cutaneous blood flow can produce a cardiac failure of high output origin.

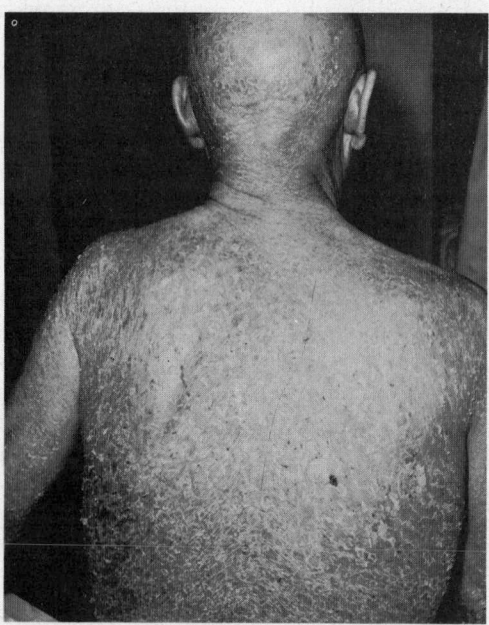

Figure 48-4. Exfoliative dermatitis secondary to leukemia. Note the generalized scaling. Itching in this patient was intense. (From Sauer: Manual of Skin Diseases. Philadelphia, J. B. Lippincott)

Hypothermia may also occur as increased skin blood flow, coupled with increases in water loss through the skin, leads to heat loss by radiation, conduction, and evaporation. Conversely, after a warm bath, hyperthermia may occur because of increased heat absorption.

As in any acute dermatitis, topical therapy is used to give symptomatic relief. Soothing baths, compresses, and lubrication with emollients are used to treat the extensive dermatitis. The patient is likely to be extremely irritable because of the severe itching. If the cause of exfoliative dermatitis is not known, steroids are given when the disease is not controlled by more conservative therapy.

Patient Education. The patient is advised to avoid all irritants in the future, particularly drugs.

PEMPHIGUS

Pemphigus is a serious disease of the skin characterized by the appearance of blisters of various sizes (bullae) on apparently normal skin (Fig. 48-5) and mucous membranes (mouth, vagina). The bullae enlarge, rupture, and leave eroded areas that eventually become crusted. The eroded skin heals slowly, so that eventually huge areas of the body are involved. Bacterial superinfection is common. In the mouth there are irregularly shaped erosions that are painful, bleed easily, and heal slowly.

Available evidence indicates that pemphigus is an autoimmune disease. (See Chapter 10.) Genetic factors may also play a role in its development. The disorder usually occurs in middle and late adult life.

Since patients with pemphigus are invariably hospitalized at one time or another during exacerbations of the disease, the nurse soon discovers that pemphigus is perhaps the most debilitating skin disease of all. The constant misery of the patient and the foul smell of the lesions makes good nursing a real challenge.

Management. The objectives of therapy are to bring the disease under control as rapidly as possible, to prevent loss of serum and the development of secondary infection, and to promote re-epithelialization of the skin.

Corticosteroids (prednisone) are administered in large doses to control the disease and keep the skin free of blisters. The high dosage level is maintained until remission is apparent. Prednisone is given with or immediately after a meal and may be accompanied by an antacid as prophylaxis against gastric complications. Essential to the patient's therapeutic management are daily evaluations of body weight, measurement of blood pressure, testing of urine for glucose, and recording of fluid balance. (High–dosage corticosteroid therapy has its own serious toxic effects.) Immunosuppressive agents (methotrexate or cyclophosphamide) may be given to help control the disease and reduce the maintenance dose of steroids.

The nursing management has been likened to that required for a patient with an extensive burn; particular attention is given to assessing the patient for signs of local and systemic infection, maintaining protein and electrolyte balance, and keeping the nutrition and hematologic status at physiologic levels. The patient is given a high protein, high calorie diet. There is a significant loss, through the skin, of tissue fluids and, therefore, of sodium chloride. This salt loss is responsible for many of the constitutional symptoms associated with the disease and is combated with administration of adequate saline, parenterally or otherwise.

A large amount of protein and blood is lost from the denuded skin areas. Blood or component therapy (packed red cells, plasma) may be used to maintain the blood volume as well as the hemoglobin and plasma protein concentrations. Systemic antibiotics may be given when cutaneous infection is present. Bullae are susceptible to infection, and septicemia may follow.

Cool wet dressings or baths are protective and soothing. Patients with large areas of blistering have a characteristic odor that is lessened when secondary infection is controlled. Tape should never be used on the skin since it may produce more blisters. Meticulous oral hygiene is important, since lesions in the mouth are common in pemphigus and add greatly to the patient's misery. Thus, mouthwashes should be offered frequently to soothe these ulcerative areas, and the patient should be encouraged to drink fluids. Since the patient is usually depressed, the nurse should strive to provide the small but important "extras" that serve to lift the morale.

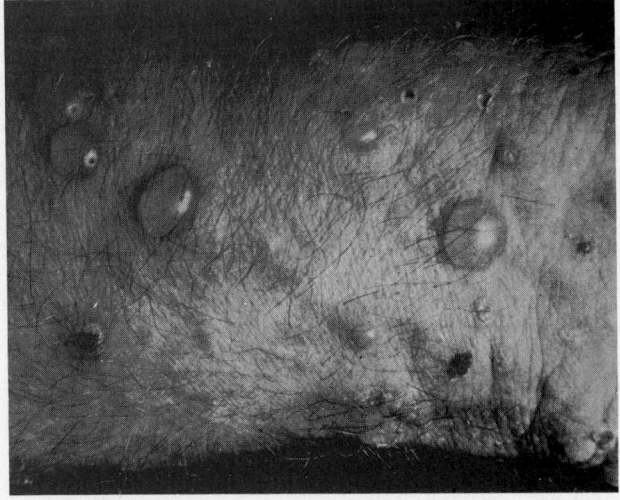

Figure 48-5. Pemphigus vulgaris bullae on the wrist. (From Sauer: Manual of Skin Diseases. Philadelphia, J. B. Lippincott)

SYSTEMIC DISEASES WITH DERMATOLOGIC MANIFESTATIONS

SYSTEMIC LUPUS ERYTHEMATOSUS (SLE)

Systemic lupus erythematosus (SLE) is an autoimmune collagen vascular disease involving multiple organ systems and producing widespread damage to connective tissues, blood vessels, serosal surfaces, and mucous membranes. The etiology is not understood, but evidence indicates that immune, genetic, and viral factors play a role. There is also a drug-induced form of SLE. Systemic lupus erythematosus, as an immune mediated disease, is discussed in detail in Chapter 10.

Approximately 50,000 new cases of SLE are diagnosed annually. It occurs most frequently in young women and peak incidence is seen between 20 and 40 years of age. It is more prevalent in black women.

Clinical Manifestations. The clinical manifestations are varied, since the disease can affect every organ system. The seemingly unrelated array of multiple organ involvement is explained by the deposit of antigen antibody complexes throughout the body. Antibodies, complement, and, in some cases, DNA, have been shown to be physically deposited on the kidneys, skin, brain, heart, and joints of SLE patients.

SLE has been termed the "new great imitator." The most common initial symptoms include arthritis and arthralgia, fever, skin rash, alopecia, and involvement of serosal surfaces (pleurisy and pericarditis). The skin signs are quite characteristic and may include a skin rash with a butterfly distribution over the bridge of the nose and malar prominences. Similar lesions occur over the neck, chest, upper and lower extremities, and possibly the mucous membranes. Alopecia is a frequent and recurring feature correlated closely with exacerbations of the disease.

There may be generalized lymphadenopathy, anemia, leukopenia and thrombocytopenia. Damage to connective tissue and thickening of the small vessels under the skin may obstruct the flow of blood and cause functional vasoconstriction of the toes (Raynaud's phenomenon). Mesenteric arteritis may produce ischemia and necrosis and perforation of the bowel. Cardiac manifestations include pericarditis, myocarditis, and endocarditis. Pleurisy is a common pulmonary manifestation, and renal involvement occurs in approximately half of the patients. Lupus nephritis, if untreated, progresses to end-stage renal failure requiring dialysis, etc. Central nervous system manifestations may occur as a result of changes in the connective tissues of the arterioles in the brain (lupus cerebritis), damage to nerve cells of the brain (organic brain syndrome), or other functional disorders. Other manifestations of central nervous system involvement include cranial neuropathies, peripheral neuropathies, seizures, and psychoses.

Numerous irregular laboratory findings reflect the immunologic abnormalities that exist in most patients with SLE, as evidenced by increases in antinuclear antibodies (ANA) and the presence of LE cells. A positive LE cell test is usually found. Hematologic abnormalities are evident during periods of active disease.

Course. SLE can be a chronically mild illness or it may be episodic, characterized by remissions and exacerbations. In some patients the disease may be protracted and life-threatening, whereas in others it may have an explosive onset and run a rapidly fatal course. Because of earlier recognition of the disease and improved diagnostic techniques and drug treatment, the survival rate in SLE is now more than 90 percent 5 years after diagnosis and more than 80 percent 10 years after diagnosis.

Management. Investigators emphasize that SLE must be considered a lifelong disease that can be controlled but not cured. The objective of management is to control the disease by suppressing inflammation and relieving symptoms. Since exacerbations of SLE may follow infection, drug administration, emotional stress, and surgical procedures, all intercurrent illnesses are treated.

The treatment methods depend on the nature and severity of the disease. For "mild" chronic disease characterized by arthritis, SLE may be controlled with salicylates. Just as with rheumatoid arthritis, the patient is advised to take salicylates on a regular schedule so that adequate blood levels can be maintained. Other nonsteroidal anti-inflammatory agents such as indomethacin or ibuprofen may be used. The antimalarials (chloroquine, hydroxychloroquine) may help control the discoid and rheumatic manifestations. However, since antimalarials can produce an irreversible retinitis, the patient must have careful ophthalmologic supervision. Skin problems are treated with topical steroid preparations. (See page 628 for treatment of Raynaud's phenomenon.)

Systemic corticosteroid therapy (prednisone) is given for active lupus, for life-threatening organ involvement (kidney, brain, heart) and for episodes of illness such as myocarditis, psychosis, and thrombocytopenic bleeding. Corticosteroids possess anti-inflammatory, antiproliferative and immunosuppressive properties. The improvement in symptoms may be quite dramatic or gradual or may not occur at all. Patients with chronically active disease require larger doses of steroids. The patient is monitored carefully during this therapy for the typical undesirable side effects frequently encountered with steroids (see page 875). The drug is tapered when remission has been achieved or a plateau in improvement is reached.

Occasionally, immunosuppressive agents (e.g., cyclophosphamide; azathioprine) are prescribed to suppress manifestations of SLE when a patient fails to respond to high doses of steroids. However, these agents have serious toxic side effects and their role in treatment is considered investigational.

There is always the possibility that disease will develop in a different organ system. Each problem is treated as it arises, depending on the organ system involved and its physiological consequences. Complications include infection, uremia, central nervous system disorders, acute abdominal catastrophes, and aseptic necrosis of the bone. Malignancies occur more frequently in lupus patients.

Patient Education. The patient should be encouraged to live as normal a life as possible. Undue exposure to the sun should be avoided because this can produce exacerbations and worsen dermal lesions. A sunscreen is used when exposure to the sun is necessary. The patient should avoid whatever situations or factors are known to aggravate the condition, especially sensitizing drugs (penicillin, etc.), cosmetics, and hair sprays. Another point of caution should be noted in the use of contraceptive pills, which may precipitate lupus syndrome in susceptible persons. If fatigue occurs, the patient should obtain more rest, nap during the day, and schedule activities to avoid precipitating undue fatigue. Since emotional turmoil can cause a flareup, coping mechanisms to deal with stress may be discussed with the patient. In addition, the patient should report to the physician *immediately* any worsening of symptoms such as fever, cough, skin rash, increasing joint pain, etc.

Discoid Lupus Erythematosus

Discoid lupus erythematosus is a chronic eruption of the skin, which although often disfiguring, does not pose a threat to life. It is essentially a cutaneous disorder which may appear anywhere on the body but most commonly affects the face, scalp, ears, upper part of the trunk, and arms.

At times the rash occurs on both upper cheeks and over the bridge of the nose, giving it a "butterfly" pattern. The process may involve the oral mucous membranes and lips. The individual lesions appear as erythematous, greasy, scaly plaques with follicular plugging and telangiectasis. These processes are sharply defined and discoid in appearance ranging from 1 mm. to several centimeters in diameter.

After persisting for a variable length of time, the lesions characteristically heal, leaving aftereffects of atrophy, scarring, and pigmentary changes. Scalp lesions usually result in permanent hair loss over the affected sites.

PERIARTERITIS NODOSA (POLYARTERITIS)

Periarteritis nodosa is a disease of unknown cause characterized by inflammation and necrosis of medium-sized and small arteries which result in altered function of the organ system in which the arterial supply has been impaired. It is probably a disease of altered immunity which causes antigen-antibody complexes to localize on blood vessel walls.

The walls of the small and medium-sized vessels are

affected by spotty inflammation, with resulting changes in circulation and tissue damage.

Clinical Manifestations. The clinical manifestations commonly encountered are quite similar to those enumerated in the foregoing description of systemic lupus erythematosus. They vary according to the organ(s) involved and the amount of necrosis produced by the obstructing vascular lesion.

Many patients with periarteritis nodosa have skin manifestations, usually in the form of painful nodules that may ulcerate. Subcutaneous nodules vary in size and may be located in any part of the body. The overlying skin may be reddened or ulcerated and purpuric macules may be present.

The patient is apt to exhibit signs of prolonged fever, weakness, myalgia, and arthralgia. Gastrointestinal manifestations (abdominal pain, nausea, vomiting, diarrhea) are also common. Coronary insufficiency and myocardial infarction result from arteritis of the coronary vessels, whereas arteritis of the renal artery or one of its branches may cause renal problems. When pulmonary lesions are present, the patient may present with pneumonia or bronchitis. Ocular manifestations (retinal exudates and hemorrhage) are fairly common.

Periarteritis is apt to run a course of several years' duration. Remissions may be induced with corticosteroids, although the disease is frequently fatal due to renal or heart failure.

Management. The objective of management is to give the patient symptomatic and supportive care. The treatment is similar to that given for systemic lupus erythematosus. A search is made for a possible offending drug. Corticosteroids (prednisone) are given to control symptoms and prevent progression of the disease. Large doses may be given initially and the patient is monitored for evidence that the disease has regressed. (See page 874 for management of the patient having steroid therapy.) Immunosuppressive drugs (cyclophosphamide; azathioprine) may be given in combination with corticosteroids. Intercurrent infection is treated with antibiotics.

Patient Education. It has been noted that the onset of the disease followed sensitivity reactions to drugs such as sulfonamides, iodides, and penicillin. This lends further emphasis to the importance of avoiding drugs that may exacerbate symptoms.

SCLERODERMA

Scleroderma (progressive systemic sclerosis) is a disease of unknown etiology in which there is chronic hardening and thickening of the connective tissues throughout the body. It is characterized by vascular abnormalities (sclerosis of blood vessels), fibrosis of the skin, atrophy of smooth muscle, and loss of visceral function.

The disease starts insidiously on the face and the hands, where the skin acquires a tense, wrinkle-free, bound-down appearance. The skin and the subcutaneous tissues become increasingly hard and rigid and cannot be pinched up from the underlying structures (hidebound). Wrinkles and lines are obliterated. The skin is dry since sweat secretion over the involved region is suppressed.

The face appears masklike, immobile, and expressionless, and the mouth becomes rigid. The buccal mucous membrane likewise may be affected. For years these changes may remain localized in the hands and the feet, but the condition spreads slowly. The extremities become stiff and immobile; the fingers semiflexed, immobile, and useless; the hands, clawlike.

The changes within the body, while not visible directly, are vastly more important than the visible changes. The heart muscle becomes fibrotic, causing dyspnea; the esophagus is hardened, interfering with swallowing; the lungs are scarred, impeding respiration; digestive disturbances occur due to hardening of the intestine; progressive renal failure may occur. A variety of other disturbances develop, including Raynaud's phenomenon (page 627) and arthritis.

Management. The treatment is largely symptomatic. The synovitis that often appears early in scleroderma may respond to anti-inflammatory drugs. However, adrenal corticosteroid therapy is often disappointing in its results. Aspirin is helpful in relieving joint stiffness, and physiotherapy is useful in preventing joint contractures. Since reflux esophagitis may cause the patient a great deal of discomfort, surgery (reconstruction of the esophagogastric junction) may be necessary. Cardiac, pulmonary, and renal involvement are treated symptomatically. Surgical procedures are used for arthritis to improve finger function of contracted joints. To relieve the skin condition, the taut, immobile skin should be kept lubricated with a bland cream.

Patient Education. When the hands are affected by the disease, warm hand baths and/or paraffin dips help to alleviate pain and prevent deformity. If esophageal reflux is a problem, the patient is taught to chew well and eat slowly to allow the bolus of food to descend the esophagus by means of gravity since normal esophageal peristalsis is disrupted. Antacids may be prescribed between meals and at bedtime. Elevating the head of the bed on blocks is also beneficial.

ULCERS AND TUMORS OF THE SKIN

ULCERATIONS

The superficial loss of surface tissue due to death of the cells is called an *ulceration*. A simple ulcer, such as is found in a small superficial second-degree burn, tends to heal by granulation if kept clean and protected from injury. If exposed to the air, the serum that escapes from it will dry and form a scab, under which the epithelial cells will grow and cover the surface completely. Certain diseases cause characteristic ulcers — tuberculous ulcers and syphilitic ulcers are examples.

Ulcers of the Skin. Skin ulcers usually arise from infection or interference with the blood supply. Infectious ulcers are not uncommon. They develop usually from an infection with anaerobic streptococci or from a combination of infections in which hemolytic anaerobic streptococci live in symbiosis with staphylococci. Ulcers of this type tend to progress peripherally and are seen often on the lower extremity or on the abdomen or chest after operation. They are characterized by an overhanging edge, and culture from them usually shows the type of organism causing the infection.

These ulcers tend to resist ordinary forms of treatment, but the application of zinc peroxide, which liberates oxygen over a long period of time, converts the anaerobic portions of the wound into an aerobic area. Penicillin administered locally or intramuscularly also is highly effective. Healing occurs rapidly owing to the inability of the anaerobic streptococci to live in an unfavorable environment.

Ulcers Due to a Deficient Arterial Circulation. These ulcers are seen in patients with peripheral vascular disease, arteriosclerosis, Raynaud's disease, and frostbite. In these patients, the treatment of the ulceration must be carried out in conjunction with the treatment of the arterial disease. The danger is from secondary infection. Frequently, amputation of the part is the only effective therapy.

Decubitus Ulcers. These skin ulcers, more commonly referred to as *pressure sores,* result from continuous pressure on a particular area of the skin. One of the main objectives in the nursing management of any bedridden patient is to avoid the development of pressure sores (see page 187).

TUMORS OF THE SKIN
Cysts

Cysts of the skin are epithelium-lined cavities containing fluid or solid material.

Epidermal cysts (epidermoid) occur frequently and may be described as slow growing, firm, elevated tumors found most frequently on the face, neck, upper chest, and back. Removal of the cysts provides cure.

Pilar cysts (originally called sebaceous cysts) are most frequently found on the scalp and are caused by the area of the skin involved in the formation of hair. Their lining corresponds to the isthmus of the hair follicle. The treatment is surgical removal.

Benign Tumors

Seborrheic Keratoses. These tumors are benign wartlike lesions of varying size and color ranging from light tan to black. They are usually located on the face,

shoulders, chest, and back and are the most common skin tumors seen in middle-aged and elderly persons. They may be cosmetically unacceptable to the patient, and a black keratosis may be erroneously diagnosed as malignant melanoma. The treatment is removal of the tumor tissue by excision, electrodesiccation and curettage, or the application of carbon dioxide or liquid nitrogen.

Verrucae (Warts). Warts are common benign skin tumors caused by infection with the human papilloma virus which belongs to the DNA virus group. All age groups may be affected, but the condition occurs most frequently between the ages of 12 and 16. Warts come in many varieties.

As a rule, warts are asymptomatic, except when they occur on weight-bearing areas such as the soles of the feet. They may be treated with locally applied liquid nitrogen, salicylic acid plasters, electrodesiccation, or the application of cantharidin.

Venereal Warts. Warts occurring on the genitalia and perianal areas are known as *condyloma acuminata* and have been shown to be sexually transmitted. These are treated with 25 percent podophyllin in tincture of benzoin, which is applied to the wart and washed off later. Other treatment modalities include liquid nitrogen cryosurgery, electrosurgery, and curettage.

Angiomas (Birthmarks). Birthmarks are benign vascular tumors involving the skin and the subcutaneous tissues. They may occur as flat, violet-red patches (portwine angiomas) or as raised, bright red nodular lesions (strawberry angiomas). The latter have a tendency to involute spontaneously. Port-wine angiomas, on the other hand, usually persist indefinitely and are not easily treated. Most patients use masking cosmetics (Covermark) to camouflage the defect.

Pigmented Nevi (Moles). Moles are common skin tumors of various sizes and shades ranging from yellowish to brown to black. They may be flat macular lesions or elevated papules or nodules that occasionally contain hair. The great majority of pigmented nevi are harmless lesions. However, in rare cases, malignant changes supervene and a melanoma develops at the site of the nevus. Therefore, some authorities recommend that nevi located at sites of repeated trauma should be removed. Nevi that show change in color or size or those that bleed should be removed to determine if malignant changes have occurred. Moles that occur in unusual places should be examined carefully for any irregularity and for notching of the border and variation in color. Excised nevi should be examined histologically.

Keloids. Keloids are benign overgrowths of fibrous tissue at the site of a scar or trauma. They appear to be more prevalent among the black race. Keloids are asymptomatic but may cause disfigurement and cosmetic concern. The treatment, which is not always satisfactory, consists of surgical excision, intralesional corticosteroid therapy, and radiation.

Dermatofibroma. A dermatofibroma is a common benign tumor of connective tissue that occurs predominantly on the extremities. It is a firm dome-shaped papule or nodule that may be skin-colored or a pinkish-brown hue. Excisional biopsy is the recommended method of treatment.

Multiple Neurofibromata. These lesions occur in von Recklinghausen's disease. Any area of the body may be involved, and the number and size of the lesions is extremely variable. Small freckle-like spots and larger, lightly pigmented patches are common additional findings.

CANCER OF THE SKIN

The incidence of cancer of the skin appears to be increasing, but there is a 95 percent cure rate. The high curability is due to early diagnosis (the skin is accessible to direct visualization), the slow progression of most skin cancers, and the effective methods of treatment available.

Causes and Prevention

The sun is the leading cause of skin cancer; incidence is related to the total amount of exposure to the sun. Sun damage is cumulative, and harmful effects may be severe by the age of 20. The increase in skin cancer is probably due to changing life-styles and emphasis on sunbathing, etc. Therefore, protective measures should be started in childhood and carried on throughout life. Persons who do not produce sufficient melanin pigment in the skin to give protection to underlying tissue are very susceptible to sun damage: those at greatest risk are fair, blue-eyed, red-haired persons of Celtic ancestry or those with ruddy or light complexions, as well as those who suffer prolonged sunburn and do not tan. Others at risk are outdoor workers, such as farmers, sailors, fishermen, and people who are exposed to the sun over a period of time. Elderly persons with sun-damaged skin are also at risk, as are persons who have had a history of x-ray treatment (in years past) for acne or benign skin lesions. Workers exposed to certain chemical agents (*arsenic,* nitrates, tar and pitch, oils and paraffins) are also included in the risk group. People who have scars due to severe burns may develop skin cancer 20 to 40 years later. In fact, any condition causing scarring or chronic irritation may lead to cancer. Genetic factors are also involved.

Types of Skin Cancer

Skin cancer is diagnosed by biopsy and histologic evaluation. The most common types of skin cancer are *basal cell carcinoma, squamous cell (epidermoid) carcinoma,* and *malignant melanoma*.

Squamous cell carcinoma of the skin is a malignant proliferation arising from the epidermis, usually on sun damaged skin. It is of greater concern than basal cell carcinoma because it is a truly invasive carcinoma. The

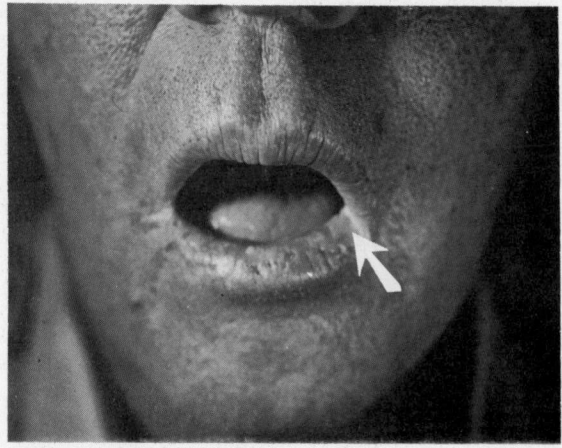

Figure 48-6. Leukoplakia on the lower lip. Progression to squamous cell carcinoma occurs in 20 to 30 percent of persons with chronic lesions. (Courtesy, Armed Forces Institute of Pathology, Negative No. 53-19363)

lesions may be primary, arising both on the skin and mucous membranes, or may develop from a precancerous condition such as actinic keratosis (lesions occurring in sun-exposed areas), leukoplakia (premalignant lesion of the mucous membrane) (Fig. 48-6), or scarred or ulcerated lesions. It appears as a rough, thickened scaly tumor that may be asymptomatic or may involve bleeding (Fig. 48-7). The border of the lesion may be wider, more infiltrated, and more inflammatory than that of basal cell carcinoma. Secondary infection can occur. Exposed areas, especially of the upper extremities and of the face, lower lip, ears, nose, and forehead, are common sites.

The incidence of metastases is related to the histological type and the level or depth of invasion. Usually tumors arising in sun damaged areas are less invasive and rarely cause death, whereas squamous cell carcinoma arising without a history of sun or arsenic exposure or scar formation appears to have a greater chance of meta-

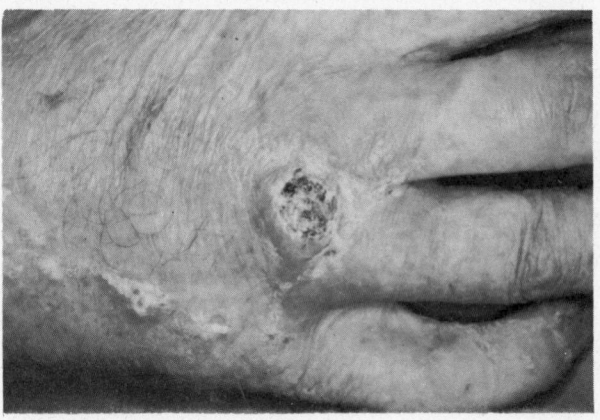

Figure 48-7. Squamous cell carcinoma. (Courtesy, Mervyn L. Elgart, M.D.)

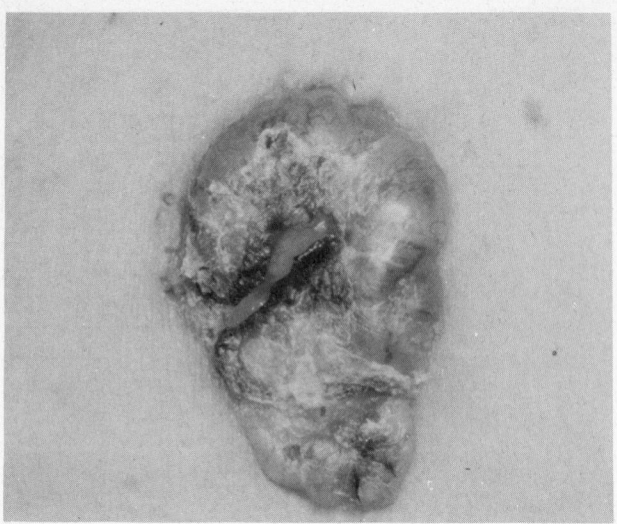

Figure 48-8. Basal cell carcinoma. (Courtesy, Mervyn L. Elgart, M.D.)

static spread. A careful evaluation of regional nodes must be made for evidences of metastases.

Basal Cell carcinoma (Epithelioma). Basal cell carcinoma is the most common type of skin cancer. It generally appears on the sun-exposed areas of the body and is more prevalent in regions where the population is subjected to intense and extensive exposure to the sun. The incidence is proportional to the age of the patient (average age of 60) and the total amount of sun exposure and inversely proportional to the amount of melanin pigment in the skin.

It usually presents as a small, waxy nodule with rolled, translucent, pearly borders with telangiectatic (dilation of end-blood vessels) vessels on the surface. As it grows, it undergoes central ulceration and sometimes crusting (Fig. 48-8). The tumors appear most frequently on the face between the hairline and the upper lip. Basal cell carcinoma is characterized by invasion and erosion of contiguous (adjoining) tissues but it rarely metastasizes. However, a neglected basal cell carcinoma can account for the loss of a nose, an ear, or a lip. Other lesions of this disease may appear as shiny, flat, gray, or yellowish plaques.

Management

The method of treatment depends on the tumor location, cell type (location and depth), cosmetic desires of the patient, history of previous treatment, whether or not the tumor is invasive, and if metastatic nodes are present.

The usual method of treatment of both basal cell carcinoma and squamous cell carcinoma is curettage followed by electrodesiccation and surgical excision. Unusual and extensive tumors are treated by chemotherapy.

Curettage followed by Electrodesiccation. Curettage is car-
ried out by excising the skin tumor by scraping it with a curette; electrodesiccation is then applied to achieve hemostasis and to destroy any viable malignant cells at the base of the wound or along its edges. It is useful for small lesions (less than 1 to 2 cm. [0.4 to 0.8 inch] in diameter). This method takes advantage of the fact that the tumor in each instance is softer than surrounding skin and therefore can be outlined by a curette, which "feels" the extent of the tumor. The tumor is removed and the base cauterized. The process is repeated three times. Usually healing occurs within a month.

Surgical Excision. Wide surgical excision may be necessary. The adequacy of excision is verified by microscopic study of sections of the specimen. Such a histologic study of excised tissue shows whether or not the margins are free of tumor. Skin grafting may be necessary if primary closure is not possible.

Irradiation (X-ray) Therapy. Irradiation therapy is frequently done for cancer of the eyelid, the tip of the nose, and areas in or near vital structures (facial nerve). It is reserved for older patients because x-ray changes may be seen after 5 to 10 years and malignant changes in scars may be induced by x-rays 15 to 30 years later.

The patient should be informed that the skin may become red and blistered. A bland skin ointment (prescribed by the physician) may be applied to relieve discomfort. The patient should also be cautioned against exposure to the sun.

Cryosurgery. Cryosurgery employs deep freezing to selectively destroy the tumor tissue. A thermocouple apparatus for deep freezing is inserted into the base of the tumor. Liquid nitrogen is sprayed onto the tumor until a temperature of −20° C. (4.0° F.) is reached at the tumor base. The tumor tissue is frozen at this temperature, allowed to thaw, and then refrozen. The site thaws naturally and then becomes gelatinous and heals spontaneously.

Chemosurgery. Chemosurgery combines the use of topically applied chemicals and serial surgical excisions of tumors layer by layer. Immediate microscopic examination is made of frozen sections for evidence of cancer cells. This procedure may be repeated daily until the specimens are cancer free and all peripheral extensions of the tumor are eradicated. Chemosurgery is useful for recurrent tumors or for infiltrating tumors whose margins cannot be determined.

Topical chemotherapy is the application of a topical antitumor agent (fluorouracil) to destroy cancer cells. The tumors are treated for a period of 3 to 4 weeks.

Patient Education

The follow-up treatment should be regular, including palpation of the adjacent nodes.

The following points of emphasis should be made by way of patient education.

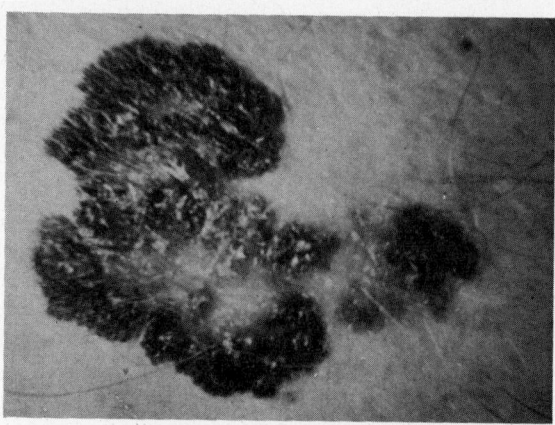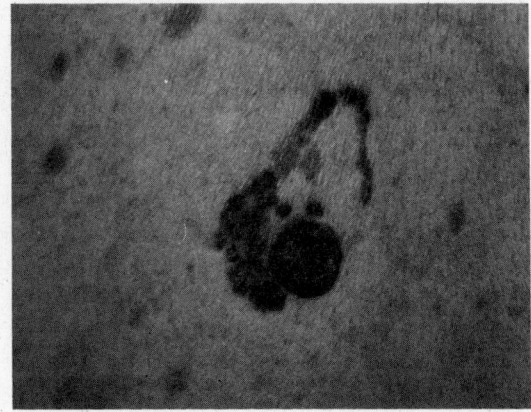

Figure 48-9. Malignant melanoma: (*Left*) Superficial melanoma. (*Right*) Nodular melanoma. (Courtesy, Mervyn L. Elgart, M.D.)

1. Avoid unnecessary exposure to the sun, especially during times when ultraviolet radiation light is most intense (10 A.M. to 2 P.M.).
2. Apply a protective sunscreen cream or lotion if an activity requires a long period of exposure.
3. Wear appropriate protective clothing (e.g., broad-brimmed hat, long-sleeved clothing, etc.). (These do not provide complete protection from ultraviolet rays.)
4. Have moles treated that are accessible to repeated friction and irritation.
5. Watch for indications of potential malignancy in moles (e.g., increase in size, ulceration, bleeding, or serous exudation).
6. Have follow-up evaluation throughout lifetime. Watch for development of new lesions. (There is also an incidence of internal malignancy associated with squamous cell cancer.)
7. Caution your children and grandchildren, especially those with fair skin, to avoid excessive exposure to the sun so as to prevent later skin cancers.

Malignant Melanoma

A malignant melanoma is a tumor of melanocytes (pigment cells) which can occur in one of three main forms: superficial spreading melanoma, lentigo-maligna melanoma, and nodular melanoma. Melanoma has a higher mortality rate than any other form of skin cancer. Melanomas frequently appear simultaneously with cancer of other organs.

The *superficial spreading melanoma* occurs anywhere on the body and is the most common form of melanoma. It usually affects persons of middle age and occurs most frequently on the trunk and lower extremities. The lesion tends to be circular with irregular outer portions. The margins of the lesion may be elevated and palpable (Fig. 48-9). This type of melanoma may appear in a combination of colors, with hues of tan, brown and black mixed with gray, bluish-black, or white. Sometimes there is a dull pink-rose color in a small area within the lesion.

The *lentigo-maligna melanomas* are slowly evolving pigmented lesions which occur on exposed skin areas, especially of the head and neck, in elderly people. They first appear as tan, flat lesions which in time undergo changes in size and color.

The *nodular melanoma* is a spherical blueberrylike nodule with a relatively smooth surface and relatively uniform blue-black color (Fig. 48-9). It may be dome-shaped with a smooth surface or rose-gray or black in color and is present as an elevated irregular plaque. A nodular melanoma invades directly into subjacent dermis (vertical growth) and hence has a poorer prognosis.

Prognosis. The prognosis is related to the depth of dermal invasion. The deeper and thicker the melanoma the greater the likelihood of metastases. If the melanoma is growing radially (horizontally), and is characterized by peripheral growth with minimal or absent dermal invasion, the prognosis is favorable. As the melanoma progresses to the vertical growth phase (dermal invasion), the prognosis is poor. The presence of ulceration correlates with a poor prognosis. Malignant melanoma can spread both through the bloodstream and the lymphatic routes and can metastasize to every organ of the body.

Malignant melanomas most frequently occur on the upper back (men), legs (women), head, neck, and trunk. About one tenth of melanomas occur in the eye. Melanomas of the trunk appear to have a poorer prognosis than those of other sites, perhaps because of the network of lymphatics in the trunk permitting metastasis to regional nodes. In the black race, melanomas are most apt to occur in the less pigmented sites: palms, soles, subungual areas, and mucous membranes.

Causes and Persons at Risk. The etiology is unknown, but ultraviolet rays are strongly suspected. Epidemiologic evidence indicates that the incidence and mortality rate of malignant melanoma has been increasing. In general, at greatest risk are patients with fair complexions, blue eyes, red or blonde hair, and freckles. These persons synthesize melanin more slowly. Persons of Celtic or Scandinavian origin are at greater risk. Persons who burn and do not tan are also at risk. In areas where sunlight is intense there is a disproportionate increase in incidence. There also appears to be a genetic component.

Assessment. A new or preexisting mole should be checked for irregular color, irregular border, irregular topography, and satellite lesions (lesions situated near the mole). Signs of *variegated* color should also be checked. Colors that may indicate malignancy in a brown or black lesion are shades of red, white, and blue. Shades of blue are considered ominous. White areas in a pigmented lesion are suspicious. Some malignant melanomas are not variegated but are uniformly colored; either bluish-black, bluish-gray or bluish-red.

If the mole has an *irregular border,* it should be checked for any angular indentation or a notch in the border. However some melanomas have a smooth surface.

Management. An excision biopsy specimen is taken to gain histological information. The therapeutic approach depends on the depth of the lesion.

Surgery. A wide excision of the primary site, usually followed by skin grafting, is accepted as proper management of the primary lesion. A regional lymph node dissection may be done depending on the level and depth of the tumor. The width of the excision and the need for node dissection are concepts which are undergoing revision at this time.

Chemotherapy. Chemotherapy is generally used when there is recurrence of metastatic disease. New drugs appear frequently and treatment is usually under the direction of a chemotherapist. Drugs in use include dacarbazine (DTIC), mercaptopurine, methotrexate, prednisone, adriamycin, bleomycin, vincristine, etc. The management of the patient undergoing chemotherapy is found in Chapter 16.

Regional Perfusion. If the lesion is anatomically accessible (e.g. on an extremity) regional perfusion chemotherapy is promising. A specific area is isolated by mechanically controlling its arterial inflow and venous outflow. This allows a high concentration of cytotoxic drugs to be delivered with less systemic toxicity.

Chemosurgery. In chemosurgery the tumor is removed layer by layer after it has been fixed in situ. The undersurface of each layer is examined microscopically by means of a frozen section. This technique is useful in the treatment of certain melanomas since the chance of dislodging melanoma cells is minimized and an extra margin of surface skin can be removed.

Immunotherapy. Immunotherapy involves the use of immune adjuvants to stimulate the patient's immunity. (See Chapter 50.) Bacillus Calmette-Guérin (BCG) administered intralesionally, intradermally, orally, or by scarification may limit the growth of the tumor as well as recurrence and may prolong the patient's life. At this time the role of immunotherapy in the treatment of malignant melanoma has not been firmly established.

Patient Education. The best hope of controlling the disease lies in the education of patients regarding the *early* signs of melanoma. The importance of examining and checking moles or new lesions should be emphasized repeatedly. The patient should report to the physician immediately moles that change color, enlarge, become raised or thicker, or itch. Treatment must be started immediately.

Metastatic Skin Tumors

The skin is an important although not common site of metastatic cancer. All types of cancer may metastasize to the skin, but carcinoma of the breast is the most frequent source. Next to carcinoma of the breast, cancers of the stomach, the uterus, and the lungs give rise to the majority of metastatic skin tumors. The clinical appearance of metastatic skin lesions is not distinctive except, perhaps, in some cases of breast cancer where diffuse brawny hardening of the skin of the involved breast is seen ("cancer en cuirasse"). In most instances, metastatic lesions occur as single or multiple cutaneous or subcutaneous papules or nodules of varying size that may be skin-colored or show different shades of red.

DERMATOLOGIC AND PLASTIC RECONSTRUCTIVE SURGERY

Reconstructive surgery is performed to repair extravisceral defects and malformations, both congenital and acquired, to restore function, and to prevent further loss of function. Frequently, plastic surgery is done primarily for aesthetic and cosmetic improvement; it is applicable to many parts of the body and to numerous structures such as bone, cartilage, fat, fascia, mucous membrane, muscle, nerve, and cutaneous structures. Bone inlays and transplants for deformities and nonunion can be done; muscle can be transferred; nerves can be reconstructed and spliced; and cartilage can be replaced. Lastly, but as important as any of these measures, is the reconstruction of the cutaneous tissues around the neck and the face; this is usually referred to as *cosmetic surgery*.

Living tissue may be transferred from one part of the body to another or it may be obtained from one person for use in another. A *graft* is a piece of tissue separated completely from its normal and original position and transferred by one or more stages to correct a distant defect. Transfers or transplants from the same person are termed *autografts;* those from a different person are called *allografts.* The autograft, after a "take," is permanent. The allograft, except in the case of identical twins, is temporary and lasts only a few days or weeks. Some transplant tissues may have been stored in "banks," including corneas of the eye, bone, fascia and collagen. At times tissue may be used from animal sources (*xenograft*).

Over the last several decades, kidney, lung, liver, and

heart transplants have been performed with varying degrees of success. With all transplants, the recipient reacts to the new tissue as to a foreign invader; the graft acts as an antigen causing the host to produce antibodies. The autoimmune reaction of the body is not fully understood, but attempts are made to avert such a reaction by immunosuppressive drugs.

Inert substances have long been used in plastic surgery. Such materials must not irritate the tissues of the recipient, nor must they alter in shape or consistency. On the other hand, the substance ought to match the quality of the part being replaced and provide proper function and cosmetic appeal. In the fascinating history of plastic surgery, a variety of substances have been used, such as metal, ivory, boiled inert bone, rubber, and wax. More recently, silicone and inert plastic materials such as Teflon and Dacron have been used with increasingly successful results.

The field of reconstructive and plastic surgery has been expanded to such an extent that often the problem requires the team work of several specialists, such as an orthopedist, a neurosurgeon, and a plastic surgeon to replace an extremity that had been accidentally severed. Maxillofacial reconstruction requires the work of an oral surgeon, a reconstructive surgeon, and an ear, nose and throat specialist. In addition to the nurse, the services of a sociologist, a psychologist, a psychiatrist, and chaplain may be required.

Availability of Facilities. The patient who is in need of plastic or reconstructive surgery may not know that such help is available. In this situation, the nurse, particularly the community health nurse, may be in a position to disseminate information. Parents who have a congenitally deformed child often delay in seeking assistance either because of guilt feelings, conviction that they must bear their own burden, false beliefs that perhaps the child will outgrow his handicap, or ignorance about what can be done.

Children and individuals (up to the age of 21) with congenital defects are eligible for financial support to meet the costs of plastic or reconstructive surgery. Plans for medical care of crippled children are available in each state; these, in turn, are partially supported by the Children's Bureau of the United States.

Initial Patient Assessment and Management

As in any other form of treatment, it is necessary to assess the status of the patient as a whole person and to view his problem in its entirety. Aside from the basic task of identifying the patient's problem, other aspects of the situation should be assessed—Is his defect a threat to his position or security among his daily contacts? Does the defect affect his interpersonal relations? Are personality changes out of proportion to the size or the nature of his physical problem?

The emotional reaction of the patient to his disfigurement or abnormality is most significant and must be understood if the repair process is to be progressive. The status of an adolescent girl may be threatened if she does not "look like" most of the other girls. The young man's scars may lead him to feel "inferior" to the other members of his class. Such feelings affect the personality, which in turn may affect the individual's level of performance and adjustment to the meaningful experiences of life. Feeling withdrawn and threatened, this person may lash out against his family, friends, and society. Some individuals have long blamed a history of disappointments, limited achievement and unhappiness on a deformity or disfigurement, and believe surgical repair will rechannel the future into a more wonderful course. The personality of the patient and his expectations must be clearly understood and guided, sometimes with professional assistance. The best possible results are obtained when the patient, nurse, and surgeon all follow the same plan of therapy in a cooperative effort.

Presurgical Preparation and Patient Instruction

Before the operation, the patient's physical state is assessed. Nutritional status is evaluated to see if increased vitamin and protein intake is needed to facilitate tissue healing. Hemoglobin and clotting time are also noted because their levels can affect the healing process. It is important that the tissues concerned be free of infection, and that other conditions, such as diabetes mellitus, be under control. The general condition of the patient with regard to nutrition, age, and morale should be at optimal levels.

Donor and recipient sites are prepared as for any surgical incision. The patient needs to know those aspects of postoperative care that can contribute significantly to a smooth recovery. The fact that the wound may appear unattractive, red, distorted, and puffy at first does not mean that the incision will not change. The fact that the size of the bandages (such as used with pressure dressings) may be voluminous does not mean that the surgery was correspondingly serious. Whether mirrors in the room should be removed would depend upon the circumstances. Of course, the family should be prepared for the postoperative appearance of the patient so that their surprised or disturbed expressions will not be conveyed to him on the first postoperative visit. Their genuine encouragement and support can mean a great deal to the apprehensive patient.

Wound Closure

Primary approximation of the skin and subcutaneous tissues is the ideal type of wound closure. Fine "hairline" scars can be achieved if the incision lines are parallel to skin lines of minimal tension, such as the "wrinkle lines" or lines of facial expression. If these cannot be followed, incision lines are placed at the junction of dissimilar tissues such as the hairline of the scalp and face, or the areolar and skin margins of the breast. If a lesion is to be excised, an elliptical incision parallel to skin lines where tension is minimal will give the best result. If sufficient tissue is not available, the next best cosmetic results can be achieved by using skin grafts or pedicle flaps.

SKIN GRAFTS

Prior to the removal of a graft of skin, the donor area is prepared by shaving it free of hairs and cleansing it thoroughly with a detergent-germicide. If the graft is to be successful, the area to be covered must be free of infection and sloughs because grafts "take" or grow only on a clean "granulating" surface.

Kinds of Grafts (Table 48-2)

Grafts are usually classified as *free* or *pedicle grafts*. Free grafts are completely separated from their donor sites, which means that their blood supply is completely inter-

rupted. Thus the survival of this graft depends upon the vascularization of the bed from the recipient site. Pedicle grafts are attached to the donor site or to an intermediate transfer site; they carry their own blood supply and therefore do not depend upon recipient sites for survival. Free grafts are usually split-thickness or full-thickness whereas pedicle grafts are usually full-thickness. Split-thickness grafts may be thin, intermediate, or thick (Fig. 48-10). Using standard donor areas such as the back or buttocks, these grafts will measure approximately as follows:

thin	0.010–0.012 inch
intermediate	0.016–0.018 inch
thick	0.022–0.024 inch

Because of the advent of microsurgery, a free flap may be used; this is a composite flap which can be taken, completely free of its donor site, and attached to the recipient site by the anastomosis of arteries and veins. This type of graft is gaining in popularity.

A graft is obtained by using a variety of instruments:

TABLE 48-2. KINDS OF GRAFTS

TYPE OF GRAFT	USES	RATIONALE	ADVANTAGES	DISADVANTAGES
Thin split-thickness	Infected wounds and those with poor vascularization	Thicker grafts do not take as well	Donor site heals readily	Contracture is great Little resistance to trauma Cosmetically poor
Thick split-thickness	Large superficial face wounds Noninfected wound on a flexor area	Thickest graft available	Less contracture than thin split-thickness and more resistant to trauma	Survives transplanting less well than thin split-thickness Donor site heals slowly
Full-thickness	Small superficial facial wound	Best cosmetic effect	Most similar to normal skin Minimal contracture Sensation good and cosmetically very good	Donor sites are less available Survives transplantation least well
Pedicle	Nasal tip Avulsed wounds with exposed nerves and tendons Good on avascular sites such as exposed cortical bone or cartilage, or a wound from a deep x-ray "burn"	Repair requires more skin than split- or full-thickness plus an additional blood supply Free grafts will not survive on avascular surfaces	Very little contraction Good sensation Good resistance to trauma Often helpful cosmetically if surgeon is adept	Requires a high degree of technical skill Usually requires several operative procedures
Free flap	Resurfaces a variety of wounds Covers exposed tendons, bones, or major blood vessels Closes wounds with deficient blood supply, i.e., irradiation ulcers	They can bring a large supply of tissue to a deficient area	A large area can be covered completely, more rapidly than with other types of grafts	This requires skill in technique of anastomosing arteries and veins (microsurgery) Long periods of immobilization of recipient site may be required

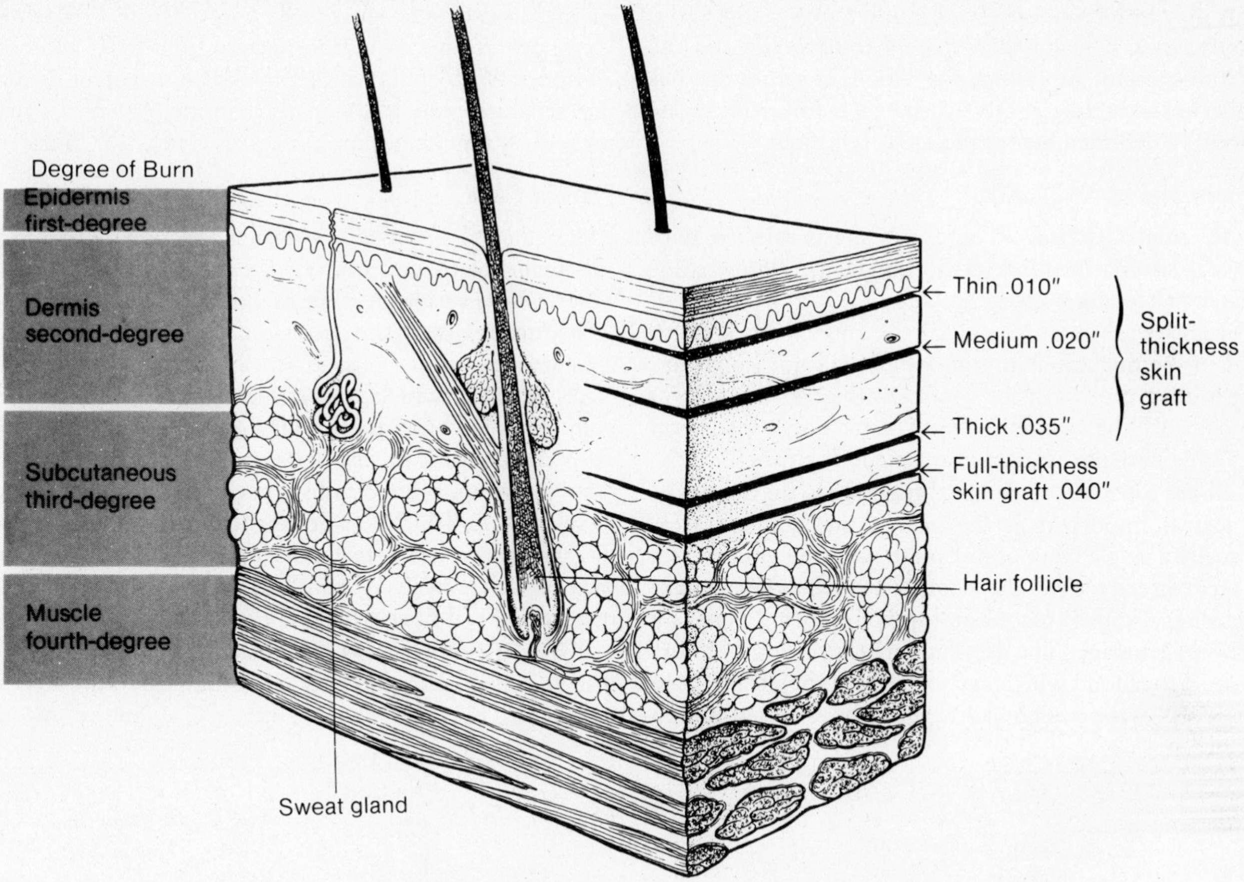

Degree of Burn

Epidermis
first-degree

Dermis
second-degree

Subcutaneous
third-degree

Muscle
fourth-degree

← Thin .010″
← Medium .020″ } Split-thickness skin graft
← Thick .035″
← Full-thickness skin graft .040″

── Hair follicle

Sweat gland

Figure 48-10.   Layers of skin showing split-thickness graft.

razor blade, skin-graft knives, or dermatomes of the manually operated or power-driven variety. Skin is obtained by suction or by adhering it to a drum. The skill of the operator, the nature of the donor site, the fine adjustment of the instrument, are all factors in obtaining the desired graft for the particular need.

Application of the Graft

The graft, when applied to the recipient site may or may not be sutured in place and may or may not be covered with dressings. It may be slit and spread apart for greater area coverage (Fig. 48-11). The exact size of the graft, correct thickness, proper condition or recipient site, all affect how well a graft "takes." When dressings are used, the initial covering often is a single layer of fine mesh gauze impregnated with an ointment to make it nonadherent. This is covered with several thicknesses of gauze cut to the exact size of the area; fluffy dressings are placed on top of this, and secured with a wraparound dressing for pressure.

Conditions Required for a Satisfactory "Take"

For a graft to survive and be effective, certain conditions must be met: (1) the recipient bed must be adequately vascularized, (2) the graft must be in complete contact with the bed, (3) immobilization must be as-

sured, and (4) the area must be free from infection. If infection is present in a wound before it is grafted, local saline compresses, local and systemic antibiotics, and careful debridement may provide an adequate recipient area of clean granulating tissue.

If the above conditions are obtained, skin graft dress-

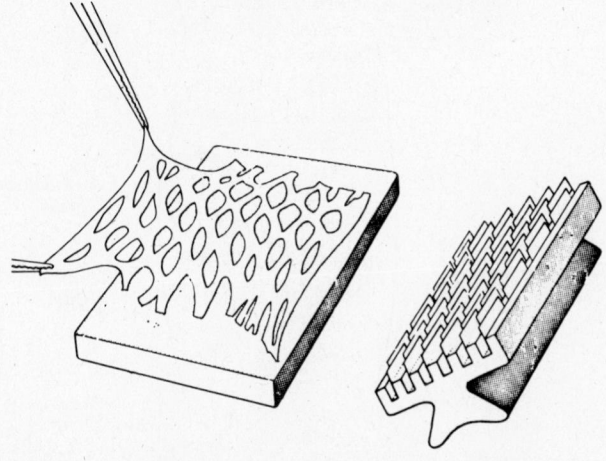

Figure 48-11.   Expansile graft. (Adapted from Feller, I., and Archambeault, C.: Nursing the Burned Patient. Ann Arbor, Michigan, The Institute of Burn Medicine)

ings may be left undisturbed for 5 to 7 days. Otherwise, the dressing is changed within 24 to 48 hours and the graft inspected. Any fluid, pus, blood, or serum that has collected should be gently evacuated and necrotic tissue carefully debrided before the site is redressed.

Donor Site

Selection Criteria. The donor site is selected with several criteria in mind: (1) to obtain the closest color match in keeping with the amount of skin graft required, (2) to match the texture and hair-bearing qualities, (3) to obtain the thickest skin graft which will not jeopardize the healing process of the donor site (Fig. 48-12), and (4) to consider the cosmetic effects of the donor site upon healing, so that it is in an inconspicuous location.

Donor Site Care. Detailed attention to the donor site is just as important as the care of the recipient area. Usually a single layer of fine mesh nonadherent gauze is placed directly over the donor site. Absorbent gauze dressings are then placed on top before being taped by pressure bandage. The dressings are checked in 24 hours to see if the blood which has oozed from the site has been absorbed. If the oozing has stopped, the dressings on top

of the nonadherent single layer are left off. If oozing continues, fresh sterile dressings are applied for another 24 hours. With epithelialization, the nonadherent dressing separates and is gradually trimmed away by the surgeon when the healing process is checked each day.

Pedicle Flaps

A pedicle flap is made by raising a section of skin and subcutaneous tissue from one site and moving it to another. However, a segment of skin always remains attached to its donor site. Pedicle flaps include a layer of subcutaneous adipose tissue beneath the skin along with nutrient vessels which must remain attached through the pedicle base in order to provide nourishment. The pedicle is far too thick to absorb its nourishment by osmosis from the wound surface; this is in contrast to this process in split- or full-thickness grafts. Newer work in microvascular anastomosis techniques (mainly experimental) may furnish a means of transferring thick pedicles without an attached base.

Types of Pedicle Flaps. Pedicle flaps may be local or distant depending upon how close they are to the recipient site. They also may be attached at one or more

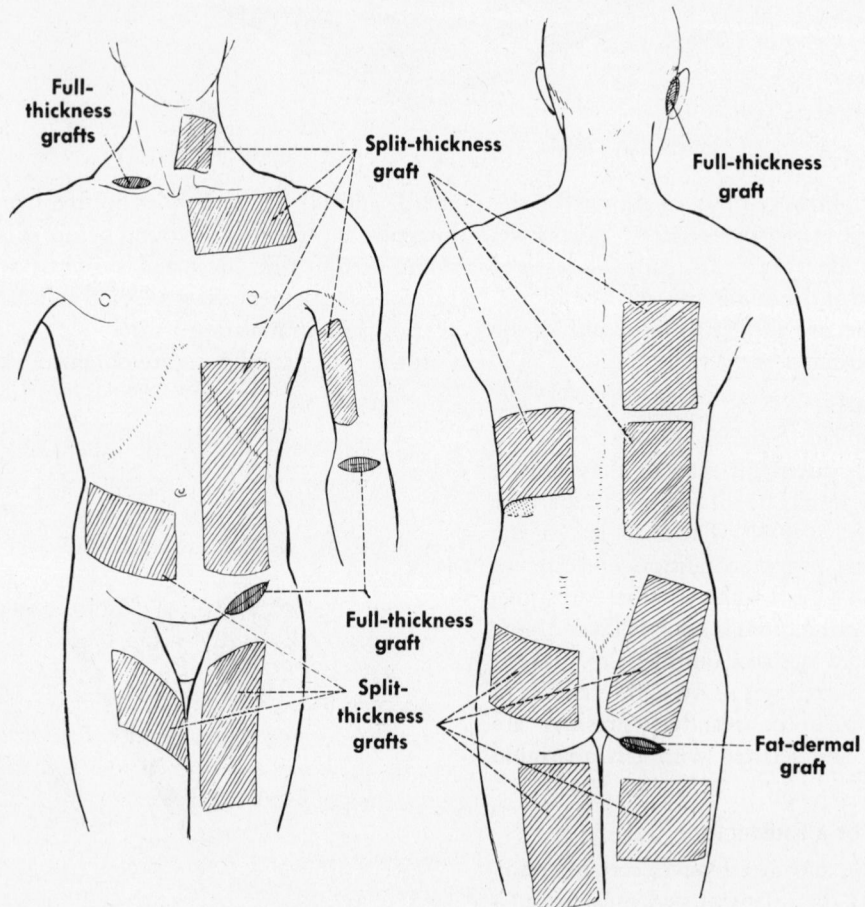

Figure 48-12. Commonly employed sites for donor areas of skin grafts. (From Converse, J. M., and Brauer, R. A.: Reconstructive Plastic Surgery. Philadelphia, W. B. Saunders)

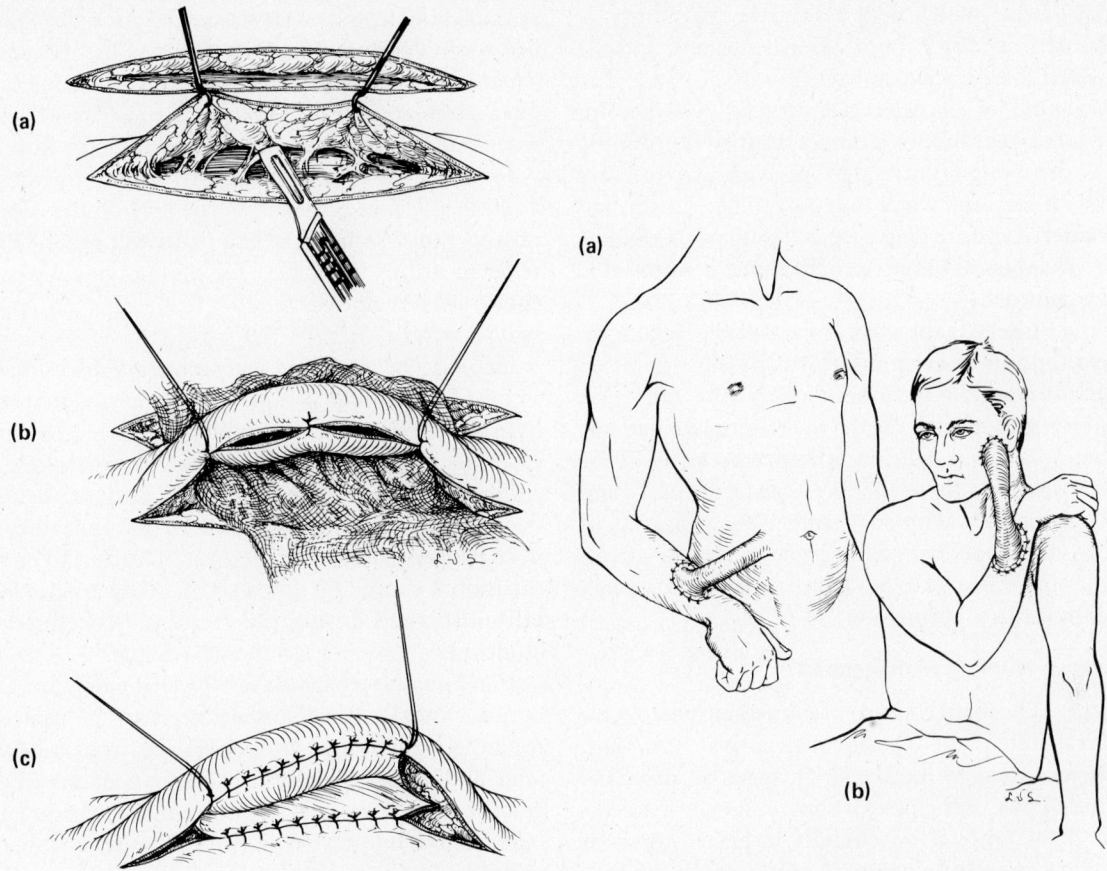

Figure 48-13. Tube pedicle. The skin and adjacent adipose layer between two parallel incisions are rolled and sutured together (*Left, a, b*). The closed flaps are suitable for transfer to a distant recipient site (*Left, c*). *Right a, b,* shows the transfer of pedicle graft via wrist carriers. (Reproduced, with permission, from Dunphy, J. E., and Way, L. W.: Current Surgical Diagnosis and Treatment, 3rd ed., 1977. Copyright 1977 by Lange Medical Publications, Los Altos, Calif.)

points, depending upon the number of attaching points. Pedicle grafts may be classified according to the manner in which skin is moved. This varies with the nature of the tissue and amount of skin desired. The various types of pedicle flaps include advancement flaps, transposed flaps, rotation flaps, tube pedicles (Fig. 48-13), island pedicles, and Z-plasty grafts.

FASCIAL TRANSPLANTS

Fascial transplants have numerous uses. They are obtained generally from the fascia lata of the thigh and are adaptable for use as suture material, for repair of hernia defects, and for replacement of tendon loss. Cartilage transplantation may be immediate and direct, taken from the costal cartilages and transferred to the nose. Bone grafts demand careful aseptic technique and rigid fixation in their new site. They may be taken from the crest of the tibia, the upper border of the iliac bone, or a rib. All donor areas should receive the same careful treatment given any other surgical wound.

MANAGEMENT OF THE PATIENT WITH MAXILLOFACIAL PROBLEMS

The face is a part of the body that every person desires to keep at its best. Many individuals try to improve on nature by using cosmetics or adopting their very own hair style. When the face becomes disfigured, an emotional reaction occurs. Consequently, an accident victim whose face is injured presents a problem that demands the utmost in understanding and care by the nurse.

The manner in which the person reacts to the medical and nursing personnel are all indices of his inner feelings and are most significant if appropriate measures are to be taken to help him.

Proper management of maxillofacial injuries or fractures depends on knowing how the injury occurred and carefully assessing how extensive the injury is. Initial care includes maintenance of an airway and treatment for shock.

Presurgical Nursing Management

The nurse is in a better position to prepare the patient before the operation when the physician has fully informed the patient about the surgical procedure, the functional defects which may result, the possibility of prosthesis, the necessity for additional surgery, and the possible need for a tracheostomy.

For any kind of maxillofacial surgery, whether for injury or cancer, the involved tissues must be thoroughly cleansed if the wound is to heal properly. All wounds are cleansed with soap and water to remove clots, crusts, and foreign material and are then irrigated with normal saline solution. Damaged tissue which appears nonviable should be debrided.

Since the surgery is directed at the maxillofacial area, the patient's mouth is made as clean as possible to lessen the danger of wound infection. Preoperative medication is prescribed with specific regard to relaxing the patient, diminishing pain, and reducing mouth secretions. If the person is male, the skin of the face is shaved closely and cleansed thoroughly with soap and water. Shaving of face, scalp, etc. should be done as requested by the physician. If the entire head is to be shaved, it is best to obtain the patient's written permission.

Postoperative Nursing Management

Airway. The main concern of immediate postoperative care is maintenance of an adequate airway. One sign of insufficient oxygen intake, air hunger, or anoxia is restlessness. Thus, if the patient shows signs of restlessness, the airway should be carefully inspected to see if there is laryngeal edema or accumulation of tracheobronchial mucus. Since signs of restlessness can alert the nursing staff to problems of anoxia, sedatives or narcotics should not be administered to the patient without the physician's permission.

Positioning. The position of the patient is determined by the nature of the surgery. If venous return is desired, the patient's head may be elevated. However, if hypotensive medications have been given, the patient should remain recumbent in the immediate postoperative period.

Suctioning. To avoid frequent change of dressings, portable wound suction may be used. Such suction is maintained at 40 to 60 mm. Hg and must be checked frequently to assure proper functioning.

Complications. Vital signs must be monitored regularly to maintain a check on possible complications.

Early hemorrhage may result from inadequate hemostasis, requiring simple aspiration or the removal of a hematoma. Bleeding may be controlled by inserting a gauze pad in the mouth and pressing it against the bleeding part of the jaw. The mouth can then be closed so that the lower teeth exert pressure against the gauze pad. If the patient is conscious, he can cooperate by biting on the pad. Should hemorrhage occur after the first week, it usually indicates infection and must be controlled immediately via direct digital pressure until suturing can be done in the operating room.

Venous congestion may give the face a purplish appearance and may be relieved by elevating the head of the bed to 30 degrees. Note the color of the extremities in order to be certain that discoloration is not due to inadequate circulation. Edema of the face also may be noted in some patients but usually subsides after the fifth day.

Pain. Pain is more likely to follow operations involving the jaw bones than the soft tissues alone. For postoperative pain, an icebag may offer relief. Whatever relief measures work best for the individual patient are employed. Analgesics ranging from aspirin to morphine may be required.

Pain may be more severe if secondary infection occurs, a complication which can be minimized if frequent oral hygiene is practiced. To avoid infection, the mouth is cleansed after each feeding. Mouthwash alone is not sufficient. A more effective method is to frequently swab the gums and the teeth with cotton on applicators soaked in hydrogen peroxide. The exact location of sutures in the mouth should be noted so that they are not accidentally disturbed during the cleaning procedures. Cold compresses may help to reduce edema.

Fluid and Nutritional Needs. Patients who have undergone maxillofacial surgery need not be denied fluids for any length of time after operation, as may be the case after abdominal operations. The patient may be given cracked ice or water as soon as postanesthetic nausea is over, and a liquid diet may be started as soon as the individual has a desire for food. Very often, soft diet is offered the day after surgery, if tolerated.

In many patients, particularly those with fractures of the jaws, the upper and lower teeth must be fastened together for weeks; hence only liquid food can be taken. Others are able to take soft food, but are unable to masticate. To meet optimum nutritional requirements, it often is necessary to utilize a nasogastric tube, cervical pharyngostomy, or gastrostomy. Blenderized foods are given for caloric needs and water for optimum hydration. The patient and perhaps the family may have to be taught to use these special techniques in feeding, particularly if the patient is discharged while still using a feeding tube.

Communication. Communication problems can present a major difficulty. The patient will find it easier to communicate if he can use gestures or respond to questions with a simple "yes" or "no" answer. The magic slate or pad and pencil can also be useful. Whatever the method of communication, patience and an empathetic understanding of this patient's problems are most helpful.

Psychological Support. The nurse is in a unique position to help these patients accept their many experiences more easily. Rehabilitation is often a combination of both physical and psychological considerations; it depends not only on eradication of a physical scar but also on the relief of psychic trauma that can be markedly influenced by the patient's social and emotional background.

If prosthetic devices are to be used, the patient must be taught how to use and care for them so as to gain a greater sense of independence. He needs to be able to accept his new self and adjust to his family and community. Later follow-up visits at a heath center are urged.

Many times, the ultimate objective requires a number of operations separated by long intervals of time. Patience is a real factor. Recreational, occupational, and spiritual therapies need to be explored fully, always keeping the interests of the individual patient intact.

Often, the kinds of dressings that have to be worn, the unusual positions that have to be maintained, and the temporary incapacities that must be experienced can be very upsetting to the most stable person. The nurse must be able to offer hope and encouragement and to combine this with a wholesome sense of humor. Tact, patience, and attention to small details will make the nurse an invaluable colleague as the patient regains self-assurance and more normal usefulness and appearance.

CHEMICAL FACE PEELING

Chemical face peeling is the application of an oil–water emulsion of a phenol-based chemical for the purpose of treating fine wrinkles, abnormal pigmentation, freckles, and acne scarring on the face. Prior to the treatment, the skin is cleansed thoroughly with soap and water followed by di-ethyl ether to remove oily residue. Pretreatment medication is designed to control apprehension.

Chemical Application. The chemical is carefully applied to the entire face with cotton-tipped applicators. Following this, a mask of waterproof adhesive tape is applied directly to the skin. This is molded closely but not too tightly. In 30 to 45 minutes following application of this medication, a burning sensation is experienced. It varies in intensity from person to person; some require additional pain medication.

Postchemical Application. After 6 or 8 hours, the face becomes edematous. No movement or facial activity is permitted for 48 hours except for bathroom privileges. Liquids are administered by straw to maintain nutrition and hydration. By the second day, the patient may feel moisture under the dressings as the chemically treated skin begins to weep.

Second Day. The dressings are removed after 48 hours, exposing skin similar to a second-degree burn. As the dressing is pulled away, the skin is pushed from the dressing with a sterile cotton applicator. Meperidine hydrochloride is administered to relieve pain. Thymol iodide powder, a bacteriostatic medication, is then ap-

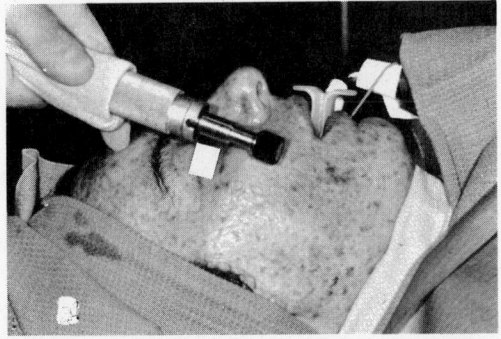

(A) The patient with acne before the dermabrasion procedure.

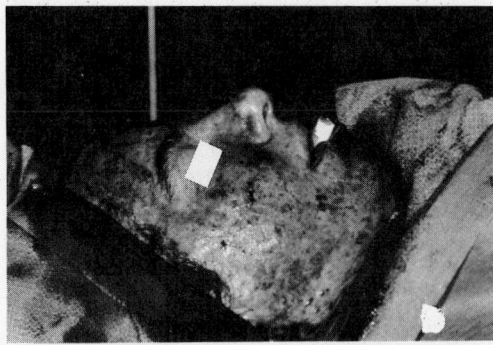

(C) A layer of petrolatum dressing is applied.

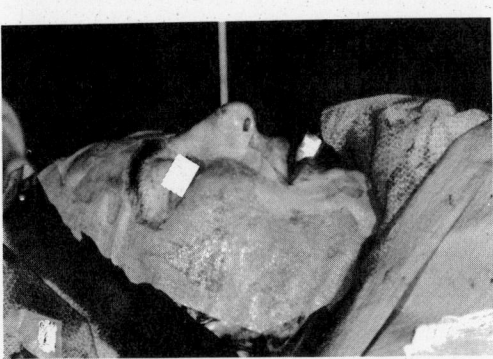

(B) The appearance of the skin after bleeding is controlled by pressure. Upper lip, eyelids, and nostril rims have not yet been abraded.

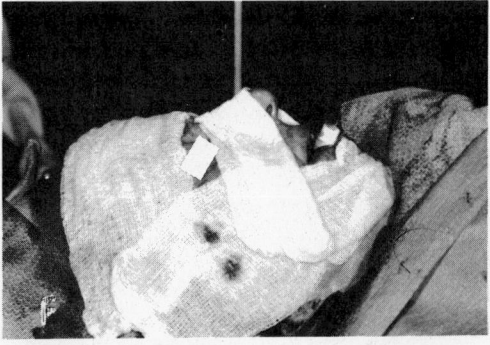

(D) Saline compresses are applied over the petrolatum dressing. This is done to absorb oozing and clotting, which are subject to infection.

Figure 48-14. Dermabrasion procedures. The saline compresses are discontinued after 12 to 24 hours and the petrolatum dressing is allowed to air dry in place. It is removed in 3 to 5 days. The skin will remain red for 6 to 8 weeks.

plied with a cotton applicator to the entire surface three or four times during the next 24 hours.

Twenty-four hours after the mask is removed, an ointment such as vitamin A and D ointment is applied to hasten the separation of the crust. In another 24 hours, the face may be washed with plain water. Crusting separates gradually.

Discharge Planning. By the fourth day, the patient is ready for discharge. For the next 2 to 3 weeks, the skin has a granular appearance. Treatment is limited to washing with clear water and applying an ointment. At the end of 3 weeks, cosmetics may be applied. Exposure to the sun is not permitted for 3 to 6 months because melanin (natural protective mechanism against the sun) in the basal layer of the epidermis is diminished.

Patients are carefully selected for chemical peeling and should realize that 3 to 4 weeks of social isolation is required and that they may have prolonged facial redness for several weeks.

SURGICAL PLANING (DERMABRASION)

Dermabrasion (scraping, sandpapering, brushing of the skin) is done in selected patients with facial disfigurements from scars resulting from acne, trauma, tattoo, nevi, freckles, and chickenpox or smallpox. The procedure involves the removal of the epidermis and some superficial dermis while preserving enough of the dermis to allow reepithelialization of the dermabraded areas (Fig. 48-14). Results are best in the face, because it is rich in intradermal epithelial elements. Planing is performed either manually with coarse abrasive paper, or mechanically with an abrader or a rapidly rotating wire brush.

Patient Instruction and Preparation. The primary reason for undergoing dermabrasion is to improve appearance. The surgeon explains to the patient what can be expected from dermabrasion. The patient should also be informed about the nature of the postoperative dressing, what discomfort may be experienced, and how long it will take before the tissues look normal. The extent of the surface to be planed will determine whether the procedure takes place in the surgeon's office, the clinic, or the hospital. Most often a general anesthetic is used, and the patient is hospitalized.

The skin is thoroughly cleansed with pHisoHex for several days before surgery. Shaving is not necessary in the female; however, the male shaves the morning of surgery.

In addition to general anesthesia, the use of a topical spray anesthetic (such as Frigiderm) for stabilizing and stiffening the skin may be desirable. The depth of planing can be readily gauged and the anesthetized area is momentarily bloodless.

During and after planing, copious saline irrigations remove debris and allow for inspection.

Postoperative and Convalescent Management. Usually, petrolatum gauze or perforated plastic-faced (Telfa) bandages are applied. Pressure dressings may or may not be used depending upon physician preference.

Edema occurs during the first postoperative day, and may cause the eyes to close. The patient should be informed that edema will subside within a day. After about 48 hours, dressings are removed and the sensation is that of a recent sunburn. When the crust forms, lanolin, cocoa butter, or hypoallergic cream relieves the sensation of tightness. When no dressings are used, oozing may be

TABLE 48-3. COMMON COSMETIC PLASTIC OPERATIONS

OPERATION	PURPOSE	SURGERY	POSTOPERATIVE EXPECTATIONS
Rhinoplasty (Nose)	To improve the shape of the nose in relation to the rest of the face	1 to 1½ hours. Excess bone or cartilage is removed; nose is reshaped	Nasal splint; soft intranasal packing; foam rubber dressings
Mentoplasty (Chin)	To improve the profile, such as is necessary with a receding chin	Incision approach is within the mouth. Silicone or plastic implant is positioned	Healing complete in a week
Rhytidoplasty (Face lift)	To remove wrinkles caused by loose skin and to tighten fatty tissues	Incision line is anterior to ear; facial skin is undermined and drawn taut	Improvement lasts from 5 to 10 years
Glabellar rhytidoplasty	To remove 2 vertical furrows between eyebrows	Dermabrasion and excision; skin graft may be required	
Otoplasty (Ear)	To correct deformed, flattened, or protruding ears	1 to 1½ hours. Silicone or plastic implant may be used	Ear bandaged for a week; protection during sleep required for 3 weeks
Blepharoplasty (Eyelid)	To remove wrinkles and bulges caused by aging or inheritance	1 to 1½ hours. Two incisions; one on upper lid and one on lower lid	Swelling and discoloration subsides in about 10 days

noticed. In some clinics, the drying process is facilitated by using a hair dryer turned to the warm setting and allowing the air to flow gently over the area. Within 14 days the crusts have separated, and although the skin is still red, most of the scars are gone. The patient is advised to avoid direct sunlight for 3 to 4 months and to use a sunscreen. Repeat treatments are usually advocated. The patient's chief complaint is that the procedure is more annoying than discomforting. The effects produced are well worth the inconvenience in those who are carefully selected for the procedure.

COSMETIC SURGERY

Cosmetic surgery is performed to improve the self-image; it affects mental health, which is as important as physical health. Cosmetic surgery may be done to correct deformities or visible scars, or to compensate for the aging process. Table 48-3 lists the common cosmetic operations.

Rhytidoplasty (Face Lift)

A rhytidoplasty is an operation on the face in which excess skin resulting from elastosis is removed and remaining skin is tightened; it is done for cosmetic purposes.

Preoperative Management. The face is cleansed thoroughly with a detergent germicide for 3 days prior to surgery, and the hair is shampooed the night before surgery. Once the patient reaches the operating room, the hair along the incision line is clipped slightly. After anesthesia has been induced, part of the skin is undermined and then stretched to give tension. Excess skin is excised.

Psychological preparation requires that the person recognize the limitations of surgery and understand that it will not necessarily solve all emotional problems. The patient also needs to know that when the dressings are removed after the operation, tissues will still be edematous and will give the face an unpleasant appearance. Several days are required for the edema to subside. Final results depend upon the condition of the patient's skin and the skill of the surgeon.

Postoperative Management. The patient is kept in bed for the first 2 days until dressings are removed. Relative quiet is recommended since hematomas are most likely to form during this time if there is too much movement. Thus excessive talking should be discouraged. The head and upper body may be elevated at least 30 degrees to lower venous pressure. A liquid diet may be given by means of straws; some surgeons will permit a soft diet.

If suction drains are used, it is important to maintain their patency. Although drugs may have to be prescribed for pain, the pain itself is not significant. Antibiotic therapy is usually prescribed to combat infection. A tran-

quilizer may be given to allay apprehension and maintain a relative degree of quietness.

Pressure dressings are left in place up to 48 hours. No dressings are reapplied; however, the matted hair may be gently combed out with a large-tooth comb dipped in soapy water. At this time the skin may be gently cleansed of caked blood and other debris.

Since there is edema, ecchymosis, and distortion of the tissues for the first few days, it is preferable that the patient not look into a mirror during this time.

The patient may be discharged in 2 or 3 days and treated in the physician's office thereafter. Activities are gradually increased. Sutures are removed on the fifth postoperative day in preauricular incisions and several days later for postauricular or temporal sutures. When all sutures are removed, the hair may be shampooed. Hair may be set and dried with warm, not hot, air.

A face lift will last for several years if the person has good skin tone and is between 45 and 55 years of age. It will not last as long for those in the older age group. Rhytidoplasty has been performed two or three times in some patients.

Rhinoplasty

Rhinoplasty is an operation to improve the shape of the nose. A deformed nose resulting from a fracture or a congenital malformation (a large hump, a bulbous nose, or a drooping tip) may be a source of sensitivity to a young man or woman. Cosmetic nasal reconstruction is suggested when the patient's nose is mature — at about 16 or 17 years of age. The operation is done through intranasal incisions, usually under local anesthesia. Hospitalization is brief, but postoperative edema and periorbital ecchymosis may be in evidence for several postoperative days.

Rhinoplasty is the most widely performed cosmetic surgical operation. If a nose problem is also associated with a receding chin, a mentoplasty may be done.

BIBLIOGRAPHY

BOOKS

Arndt, K. A.: Manual of Dermatologic Therapeutics. Boston, Little, Brown, 1978.

Behrman, H. T., Labow, T. A., and Rozen, J. H.: Common Skin Diseases. New York, Grune and Stratton, 1978.

Burks, J. W.: Dermabrasion and Chemical Peeling. Springfield, Charles C Thomas, 1979.

Burnett, J. W., and Robinson, H. M.: Clinical Dermatology, 2nd ed. New York, Yorke Medical Books, 1978.

Epstein, E., and Epstein, E., Jr.: Skin Surgery. Springfield, Charles C Thomas, 1976.

Fry, L.: Dermatology, 2nd ed. Fort Lee, Update Publishing International, 1978.

Goldschmidt, H.: Physical Modalities in Dermatologic Therapy. New York, Springer-Verlag, 1978.

Helm, F.: Cancer Dermatology. Philadelphia, Lea and Febiger, 1979.

Korting, G. W., and Denk, R.: Differential Diagnosis in Dermatology. Philadelphia, W. B. Saunders, 1976.

Mohs, F. E.: Chemosurgery. Springfield, Charles C Thomas, 1978.

Parrish, J. A., et al.: UV-A. New York, Plenum Press, 1978.

Stewart, W. D., Danto, J. L., and Maddin, S.: Dermatology: Diagnosis and Treatment of Cutaneous Disorders, 4th ed. St. Louis, C. V. Mosby, 1978.

Whitlock, F. A.: Psychophysiological Aspects of Skin Disease. Philadelphia, W. B. Saunders, 1976.

Williams, R. A.: Textbook of Black-Related Diseases. New York, McGraw-Hill, 1975.

ARTICLES

Acne

Caro, I.: Acne vulgaris: Recent advances in pathogenesis and treatment. J. Fam. Pract., 5:747-750, Nov. 1977.

Franz, E., Rohde, B., and Weidner-Strahl, S.: The effectiveness of topical antibacterials in acne: A double blind clinical study. J. Int. Med. Res., 6:72-77, 1978.

Heel, R. C., et al.: Vitamin A acid: A review of its pharmacological properties and therapeutic use in the topical treatment of acne vulgaris. Drugs, 14:401-419, Dec. 1977.

Kaminester, L. H.: Acne. JAMA, 235:2171-2172, May 19, 1978.

Spira, M.: Treatment of acne pitting and scarring. Plast. Reconstr. Surg., 60:38-44, July 1977.

Topicycline—a topical tetracycline for acne. Med. Lett. Drugs Ther., 20:35-36, Apr. 7, 1978.

Turner, T.: Acne vulgaris: yesterday, today and tomorrow. Int. J. Dermatol., 16:569-573, Sept. 1977.

Assessment and Therapy

Beare, J. M., Burrows, D., and Merrett, J. D.: The effects of mental and physical stress on the incidence of skin disorders. Brit. J. Dermatol., 98:553-558, May 1978.

Derbes, V. J.: Rashes: Recognition and management. Nursing '78, 8:54-59, Mar. 1978.

Galles, M. L.: Identifying dermatological conditions in blacks. J.E.N., 4:56-62, Nov.-Dec. 1978.

Hannigan, L.: Nursing assessment of the integument system. Occup. Health Nurs., 26:19-22, Jan. 1978.

Harlin, V. K.: Black skin. J. Sch. Health, 47:365-367, June 1977.

Hawkins, K.: Wet dressings. Putting the damper on dermatitis. Nursing '78, 8:64-67, Feb. 1978.

Matus, N. R.: Topical therapy: Choosing and using the proper vehicle. Nursing '77, 7:8-10, Nov. 1977.

Nadelson, T.: A person's boundaries: A meaning of skin disease. Cutis, 21:90-93, Jan. 1978.

Roach, L. B.: Color changes in dark skin. Nursing '77, 7:48-51, Jan. 1977.

Rubin, B. A.: Black Skin. R. N., 42:31-35, Mar. 1979.

Sykes, J., Kelly, A. P., and Kennedy, J. A.: Black skin problems. AJN, 79:1092-1094, June 1979.

Thorne, E. G.: Coping with pruritus—a common geriatric complaint. Geriatrics, 33:47-49, July 1978.

Other Skin Diseases

Brown, H.: Hand infections. Am. Fam. Phys., 18:79-85, Sept. 1978.

Dolin, R., et al.: Herpes zoster-varicella infections in immunosuppressed patients. Ann. Intern. Med., 89:375-388, Sept. 1978.

Lynch, P. J., Gallego, R. E., and Saied, N. K.: Pemphigus—a review. Arizona Med., 33:1030-1037, Dec. 1976.

McRae, M. E.: Scabies. Cutis, 20:90-92, July 1977.

Meislin, H. W., et al.: Anaerobic and aerobic bacteriology and outpatient management. Ann. Int. Med., 87:145-149, Aug. 1977.

Pankey, G. A., and Cortez, L. M.: Treatments of choice for bacterial infections of the skin. Med. Times, 105:92-99, Sept. 1977.

Rosen, T., and Rudolph, A. H.: Identifying and treating bacterial and fungal infections. Geriatrics, 33:71-82, Oct. 1978.

Zarratt, M.: Viral infections of the skin. Pediat. Clin. N. Am., 25:339-355, May 1978.

Psoriasis

Arnold, V., and Rose, S.: Photochemotherapy for psoriasis. AJN, 79:466-468, Mar. 1979.

Guilhou, J. J., Meynadier, J., and Clot, J.: New concepts in the pathogenesis of psoriasis. Brit. J. Dermatol., 98:585-592, May 1978.

Hashimoto, K., et al.: Psoralen-UVA-treated psoriatic lesions. Arch. Dermatol., 114:711-722, May 1978.

Loeffel, E. D.: The true heartbreaks of psoriasis. Med. Times, 105:49-56, June 1977.

Lynch, W. S., and Roenigk, H. H., Jr.: Essentials of PUVA therapy. Guidelines for photochemotherapy. Cutis, 20:494-501, Oct. 1977.

Nietsche, U. B.: Photochemotherapy for psoriasis. Int. J. Dermatol., 17:149-157, Mar. 1978.

Parrish, J. A., et al.: Photochemotherapy of psoriasis using methoxsalen and sunlight. Arch. Dermatol., 113:1529-1532, Nov. 1977.

Petrozzi, J. W., et al.: Updating the Goeckerman regimen for psoriasis. Brit. J. Dermatol., 98:437-444, Apr. 1978.

Roenigk, H. H., and Martin, J. S.: Photochemotherapy for psoriasis. Arch. Dermatol., 113:1667-1670, Dec. 1977.

Systemic Lupus Erythematosus

Blumenfield, M., ed.: Systemic lupus erythematosus: A symposium. Primary Care, 5:121-171, Mar. 1978.

Feely, R. H.: Systemic lupus erythematosus: a review. Rheumatol. Rehabil., 17:79-82, May 1978.

Fessel, W. J.: Systemic lupus erythematosus as seen in primary care. Postgrad. Med., 65:113-116, passim Mar. 1979.

Fialkow, R. Z., and Lee, S. M.: Lupus glomerulonephritis. Short review and guide to therapy. Arizona Med., 35:338-341, May 1978.

From the NIH: Awareness, better diagnosis and drug therapy increase outlook for systemic lupus erythematosus. JAMA, 241:23-24, Jan. 5, 1979.

Grigor, R., et al.: Systemic lupus erythematosus. A prospective analysis. Ann. Rheum. Dis., 37:121-128, Apr. 1978.

Hartley, B.: Systemic lupus: A patient perspective. Can. Nurse, *74*:16-20, Feb. 1979.

Kaplan, D., and Sadovsky, R.: Diagnosis and management of systemic lupus erythematosus. Am. Fam. Phys., *17*:133-138, Jan. 1978.

Quimby, F. W., and Schwartz, R. S.: The etiopathogenesis of systemic lupus erythematosus. Pathobiol. Ann., *8*:35-39, 1978.

Tumors/Melanoma

Callen, J. P., Chanda, J. J., and Stawiski, M. A.: Malignant melanoma. Arch. Dermatol., *114*:369-370, Mar. 1978.

Holmes, E. C., et al.: A rational approach to the surgical management of melanoma. Ann. Surg., *186*:481-490, Oct. 1977.

Kopf, A. W., and Bart, R. S.: Malignant melanoma: A review. J. Dermatol. Surg. Oncol., *3*:41-125, Jan.-Feb., 1977.

Lynch, H. T., and Frichot, B. C.: Skin, heredity and cancer. Semin. Oncol., *5*:67-84, Mar. 1978.

Nordlund, J. J., and Lerner, A. B.: On the causes of melanomas. Am. J. Pathol., *89*:443-448, Nov. 1977.

Teppo, L., Pakkanen, M., and Hakulinen, T.: Sunlight as a risk factor of malignant melanoma of the skin. Cancer, *41*:2018-2027, May 1978.

Wright, E. T.: Identifying and treating common benign skin tumors. Geriatrics, *33*:37-44, June 1978.

Plastic and Reconstructive Surgery

Care of cosmetic surgery patients. AORN J., *26*:926-927, Nov. 1977.

Chouinard, F., et al.: Vigilant nursing care after reconstructive microsurgery. Nursing '79, *9*:18-25, June 1979.

Finn, K. L.: Rebuilding skin, Part 1: A successful graft may be up to you. RN, *40*:41-45, Oct. 1977.

Johnson, C. M., and Anderson, J. R.: When the patient wants facial cosmetic surgery. Am. Fam. Phys., *16*:170-176, Sept. 1977.

Jones, C. A., and Feller, I.: Burns (or skin grafts). Nursing '77, *7*:72-81, Nov. 1977.

Magil, B.: Exciting changes in grafting techniques. Contemp. Surg., *10*:11-17, Mar. 1977.

Stark, R. B.: The growth of aesthetic surgery. Contemp. Surg., *11*:25-27, July 1977.

Stuart, M. S.: Skin flaps and grafts after head and neck surgery. AJN, *78*:1368-1374, Aug. 1978.

Vasconez, L. O., et al.: Musculocutaneous flaps in reconstructive surgery. Contemp. Surg., *14*:15-26, Jan. 1979.

AGENCIES

American Academy of Dermatology, 820 Davis St., Suite 380, Evanston, Ill. 60201.

American Academy of Facial Plastic and Reconstructive Surgery, 70 West Hubbard St., Suite 202, Chicago, Ill. 60610.

American Cancer Society, 777 Third Ave., New York, N.Y. 10017.

Lupus Foundation of America, Inc., 1167 Holly Springs Drive, St. Louis, Mo. 63141.

National Lupus Erythematosus Foundation, 5430 Van Nuys Blvd., Van Nuys, Calif. 91401.

National Psoriasis Foundation, Suite 250, 6415 S.W. Canyon Court, Portland, Ore. 97221.

49
MANAGEMENT OF THE BURN PATIENT

Approximately 12,000 persons die of burns each year in the United States. An additional 2 million experience pain, disability, and disfigurement as a result of burns. Some authorities estimate that reasonable caution and adherence to well-known safety measures could prevent 75 percent of all burn injuries. By taking advantage of opportunities to teach and to promote legislation for safety practices, the nurse can play an active part in preventing fires and burns.

Four major objectives relating to human burns are:
1. Prevention
2. Institution of life-saving measures for the severely burned person
3. Prevention of disability and disfigurement through early specialized, individual treatment
4. Rehabilitation of the individual through reconstructive surgery and rehabilitative programs

Emergency First Aid

- Once a burn has been sustained, the application of cold is the best first-aid measure. Soaking the burn area intermittently in ice water or applying cold towels give immediate and striking relief from pain and restricts local tissue edema and damage. However, one should avoid applying ice directly to the burn; such a procedure may worsen the lesion.
- The burn should also be covered as quickly as possible to minimize bacterial contamination and decrease pain by preventing air from coming into contact with the injured surface. Sterile dressings are best, but any clean, dry cloth can be used as an emergency dressing.
- Ointments and salves are not used. In fact, other than the dressing, no medication or material should be applied to the lesion.
- *Chemical burns*, which result from contact with a corrosive material, are irrigated immediately. Most chemical laboratories have a high-pressure shower for such emergencies; if such

an injury occurs at home, all areas that have come in contact with the chemical should be rinsed for several minutes in a shower or other source of continuously running water.
- If a chemical gets in or near the eyes, then the eyes should be flushed with cool, clean water. Following this, two or three drops of a mild oil (mineral or olive) are instilled, and a physician is promptly consulted.
- *When clothes catch on fire,* the flames can be extinguished if the victim falls to the floor or ground and rolls ("drop and roll"); anything available to smother the flames such as a blanket, rug, or coat may be used. Standing still would force the victim to breathe flames and smoke, and running would fan the flames.
- After the flames are extinguished, the hot clothing is soaked with cold water and the physician is notified. The physician, in turn, alerts the proper hospital personnel. Thus, life-saving measures can be initiated immediately by a trained team, with no time lost.

Prehospital Management. A burn victim awaiting transportation to the hospital should remain lying down; no attempt should be made to remove clothing. Exposed burned surfaces can be covered with the cleanest material available to prevent exposure to air and contamination; covering the person with a blanket will prevent loss of body heat. The victim should be kept warm during transportation to the treatment center.

Prevention of Shock. Prevention of shock in a person with a major burn is imperative. If the hospital cannot be reached within an hour, the physician may initiate fluid therapy intravenously.

- In rare instances in which definitive care is markedly delayed, an effective first-aid measure would be to give the conscious patient fluids to drink, if he can tolerate them. To a quart of water (1 L.), add one teaspoon (3 gm.) of salt and a half teaspoon (1.5 gm.) of soda bicarbonate. (Salt provides sodium and soda bicarbonate helps to combat acidosis.)

- Under ordinary circumstances, *nothing* should be given by mouth, and the patient should be placed in a position that will prevent aspiration of vomitus, since nausea and vomiting often occur as a result of paralytic ileus resulting from the stress of injury.

Usually an emergency medical technician (EMT) or ambulance or fire personnel will take steps to cool the wound, establish an airway, supply oxygen, and perhaps start an intravenous line. The victim is sent directly to the hospital; usually no pain medication is given before the victim reaches the hospital, where his condition can be assessed.

PATHOPHYSIOLOGY OF BURNS

Burns are wounds produced by various kinds of thermal, electrical, radioactive, or chemical agents, which kill cells by changing the protein substance of the cell. Because these agents attack the organism within its environment, the tissues in direct contact with that environment (e.g., the skin and mucosa of the respiratory tract and the upper alimentary tract) are the first to be damaged.

The pathophysiology of a burn may be divided into three stages. Although these stages overlap one another, in general they may be identified as: (1) the stage of fluid-loss shock, (2) the stage of infection and slough of burned tissue, and (3) the stage of repair or rehabilitation.

Stage of Fluid-Loss Shock

Although the local effects of a burn are most evident, the systemic effects pose a greater threat to life. These may be more easily understood if they are discussed in the order of their occurrence. The first effect a burn has is to produce a dilatation of the capillaries and small vessels in the area of the burn, thus increasing capillary permeability. Plasma seeps out into the surrounding tissues, producing blisters and edema. The type, the duration, and the intensity of the burn affect the amount and duration of the fluid loss.

- One of the first steps in the management of burns is to provide fluid replacement therapy.

Fluid loss reduces the blood volume, so that the blood becomes thicker, i.e., the volume of the cellular elements of the blood increases in relation to the volume of fluid (plasma) of the blood. This change reduces the efficiency of the circulation.

The loss of fluid volume is reflected in the fall of the blood pressure, causing shock. The relative increase in cell volume is reflected in the increasing hematocrit, which is a fairly accurate and reliable measure of the systemic effect of the burn.

- The hematocrit reading is used as a guide in estimating the fluid requirements of the patient; the aim is to provide enough fluids to bring the hematocrit back to normal.
- The amount of urinary output also indicates the extent of fluid loss from the blood. When the blood is concentrated by fluid loss and the hematocrit is elevated, the urinary output is reduced. Fluid administration during this period is adjusted so that a urinary flow of at least 30 to 70 ml. per hour is obtained.

The Stage of Infection and Sloughing

This stage of a burn is the period when the tissue killed by the burn (eschar) separates from the underlying viable tissue by a process of liquefaction called *slough formation*. The result is a large open wound that is usually infected, first by gram-positive organisms, then by gram-negative organisms, and finally by fungi.

The infection reveals itself by a gradually increasing fever and local tenderness, by tachycardia, and often by lymphangitis.

- Because infection is almost always a factor in burn treatment, the burn wound is closed as soon as possible and antibiotics are usually added to the intravenous solutions from the beginning.

Cultures are made, sensitivity tests are carried out, and the appropriate antibiotic is selected. The closure of a burn may be divided into two phases: (1) repair of the burned area and (2) systemic repair. The repair of a large wound left by a burn cannot begin until the area is free of sloughing tissue. In some cases the death of skin tissue may not have included deeper epithelial elements, so that some degree of epithelialization may occur from these remaining skin cells. When the entire thickness of the skin has been destroyed by the burn, repair must begin at the edges of the wound. This takes a long time in large burns, and permits an overgrowth of granulation tissue to occur.

To minimize this excessive overgrowth of granulation, the burn wound is covered with skin grafts, which also allows earlier healing. Sometimes the burn wound may be covered with cadaver skin (also called *homografts* or *allografts*) preserved in graft banks; this provides an excellent temporary covering but must be replaced by grafts of the patient's own skin. *Xenografts,* also called *heterografts* (pig skin), provide another method of temporary coverage. This biologic dressing is changed every 1 to 3 days, and is used to cover the wound temporarily and prepare it for autografting.

Systemic repair includes such measures as blood transfusions to overcome the anemia that always develops in the later stages of large burns, and a high calorie, high protein diet. The purpose of this diet is to aid in replacing the nutritional elements lost from the draining wound and to make up for the decreased food intake during the early phases of burn treatment. Extra calories are also needed because of the hypermetabolism experienced by the victim due to stress, an endogenous inability to metabolize carbohydrate, and the work required to evaporate large quantities of surface water. At times, particularly in large burns, the technique of intravenous hyperalimentation is needed in order to supply enough calories (page 728).

ASSESSMENT OF BURN INJURY (BURN APPRAISAL)

Initial assessment of a person with a burn is necessary in order to select the best method of treatment, to develop a guide for fluid management, and to determine the resources (personnel and equipment) available for patient care, since assessment influences outcome of care.

A burn is evaluated by determining the cause of the burn, the condition of the patient, the extent of surface area involved, and the depth of the burn. This initial evaluation is conducted in a clean environment by personnel who are conscious of the need to prevent pathogenic and resistant hospital bacteria from being introduced into an open burn wound. It is also necessary to ascertain if the patient was in an open, closed, or semi-closed area at the time of the injury in order to determine whether actual or potential endotracheal or pulmonary damage exists.

The Cause of Burn Injury

The cause of a burn may be:

1. *Thermal* — moist, as from steam or boiling water; dry, as from a flame, a hot-water bottle, hot metals, hot grease.
2. *Chemical* — strong acids, such as sulfuric or nitric acid; strong alkalies, such as caustic soda (lye). Other strong chemicals include phosphorus, mustard gas, etc.
3. *Electrical* — the effects vary widely, depending on the type, voltage, and amperage of the current. Burns usually are noted both where the current enters and where it leaves the body. In addition to these local effects, systemic changes that produce respiratory, circulatory, and central nervous system disturbances may be noted.
4. *Irradiation* — may be caused by ultraviolet rays, x-rays, and radium. Sunburn and burns from ultraviolet lamps usually are superficial and produce short-lived effects. Burns from x-rays and radium are slow to appear, so that the most marked effects, such as ulceration, may not occur for years.

Patient Assessment

The general condition and state of health of a burn victim, his approximate age, and when and how he was burned are important factors that may modify treatment. The elderly and very young are more likely to die than the young adult with the same percentage burn. The case of a debilitated 60-year-old man who fell asleep with a lighted cigarette that ignited the sofa would present a pathophysiologic and survival problem different from that of a 38-year-old man whose clothing caught fire while he was burning leaves. Associated trauma or pre-existing endocrine or pulmonary diseases, allergy, metabolic disease, a drug history, or joint limitations compound the problem and must be considered in planning care. The nurse has the responsibility to learn as much as possible about the patient, including his preburn weight and state of health, from his relatives and friends.

Additional information includes the place where the accident happened and the type of first-aid measures taken.

Extent of Surface Area Burned (Rule of Nine)

An estimation of the total body surface area (BSA) involved as a result of a burn is simplified by dividing the body into multiples of 9 (Rule of Nine — Figs. 49-1 and 49-2). The initial evaluation should be revised on the second and third postburn days, since the demarcation usually is not clear until then.

Depth of Burn

It is often difficult to immediately determine the depth of a burn. In such instances assessment remains a clinical judgment, so that often the depth is assessed after the

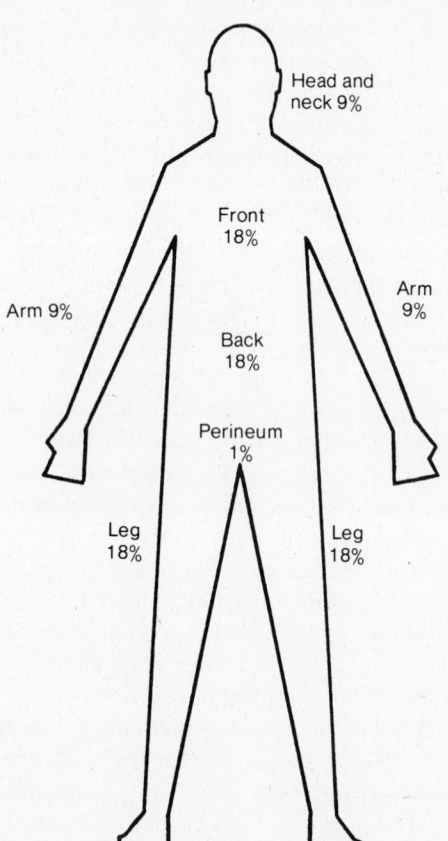

Figure 49-1. "Rule of Nine" chart for calculating percent of body burns in the adult. (Actual values have been modified for practical purposes.)

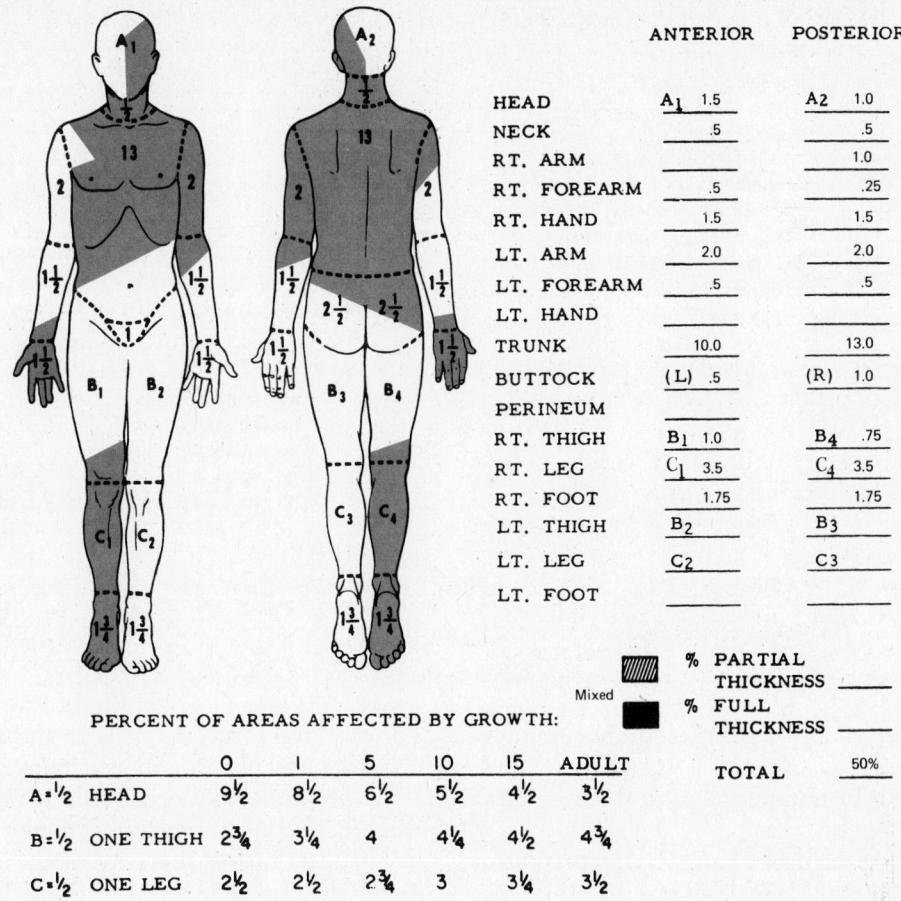

The chart portion with labels:

ANTERIOR   POSTERIOR

	ANTERIOR	POSTERIOR
HEAD	A₁ 1.5	A₂ 1.0
NECK	.5	.5
RT. ARM		1.0
RT. FOREARM	.5	.25
RT. HAND	1.5	1.5
LT. ARM	2.0	2.0
LT. FOREARM	.5	.5
LT. HAND		
TRUNK	10.0	13.0
BUTTOCK	(L) .5	(R) 1.0
PERINEUM		
RT. THIGH	B₁ 1.0	B₄ .75
RT. LEG	C₁ 3.5	C₄ 3.5
RT. FOOT	1.75	1.75
LT. THIGH	B₂	B₃
LT. LEG	C₂	C₃
LT. FOOT		

Mixed ▨ % PARTIAL THICKNESS ____
■ % FULL THICKNESS ____

PERCENT OF AREAS AFFECTED BY GROWTH: TOTAL   50%

	0	1	5	10	15	ADULT
A = ½ HEAD	9½	8½	6½	5½	4½	3½
B = ½ ONE THIGH	2¾	3¼	4	4¼	4½	4¾
C = ½ ONE LEG	2½	2½	2¾	3	3¼	3½

Figure 49-2.   Burn Evaluation Chart—estimation percent body burns. (Crozer-Chester Medical Center.)

fact—i.e., if it healed, it was partial thickness. However, classification of burns by degrees is helpful for description and identification (Table 49-1).

First-degree burns are not serious unless large areas of the body are involved. They produce pain and redness in the burned area.

Second-degree burns are those associated with blister formation (vesicles) in which the superficial layers of skin are destroyed, but the deeper layers escape injury. Patients with large areas of second-degree burns require hospitalization. Skin healing can take place from the deeper skin cells that have remained viable.

TABLE 49-1.   EVALUATION OF DEPTH OF A BURN

DEGREE	CAUSE OF BURN	SKIN INVOLVEMENT	SYMPTOMS	APPEARANCE	COURSE
Superficial (First)	Sunburn Low-intensity flash	Epidermis	Tingling Hyperesthesia Painful Soothed by cooling	Reddened; blanches with pressure Minimal or no edema	Complete recovery within a week Peeling
Partial thickness (Second)	Scalds Flash flame	Epidermis and part of dermis	Painful Hyperesthesia Sensitive to cold air	Blistered, mottled red base, broken epidermis, weeping surface Edema	Recovery in 2 to 3 weeks Some scarring and depigmentation Infection may convert to third-degree
Full thickness (Third)	Fire Prolonged exposure to hot liquids	Epidermis, entire dermis, and sometimes subcutaneous tissue	Painless Symptoms of shock Hematuria and hemolysis of blood likely	Dry; pale white or charred Broken skin with fat exposed Edema	Eschar sloughs Grafting necessary Scarring and loss of contour and function

TABLE 49-2. TYPES OF BURN INJURY AND RECOMMENDED TREATMENT SITES

TYPE OF INJURY	MAJOR BURN INJURY	MODERATE UNCOMPLICATED BURN INJURY	MINOR BURN INJURY
Definition	2nd degree burns > 25% 3rd degree burns > 10% smaller burns at extremes of age (< 2 or > 60) burns involving face, hands, feet, perineum burns with inhalation injury electrical burns burns with other trauma or illness	2nd degree burns 15-25% adults 10-20% children or elderly 3rd degree burns < 10% - • no complications • no extremes of age • no inhalation injury • no critical body areas • no other accompanying trauma or illness	2nd degree < 15% adults < 10% children 3rd degree < 2%
Recommended treatment site	Burn Unit/Center A (Advanced Level)	Burn Program or Burn Unit/Center I (Intermediate Level)	Hospital Emergency Dept. B (Basic Level)

Source: Specific Optimal Criteria for Hospital Resources for Care of Patients With Burn Injury. American Burn Association, Apr. 1976.

Third-degree burns imply destruction of the full thickness of the skin and often of the underlying fat, muscles, and even bone. Rapid transportation to the hospital is important.

In determining the depth of a burn, it is important that the following be known: (1) the causative agent, such as flame, a scalding liquid, etc., (2) the duration of exposure, and (3) the thickness of the skin. Hematuria and high plasma hemoglobin suggest deep burns. (See Table 49-2. Types of Burn Injury and Recommended Treatment Sites.)

Survival Prediction

The best survival expectancy is obtained in children and young adults, ages 5 to 40 years. In this group, burns of about 60 percent of the body are associated with a 50 percent mortality. A burn of over 20 percent of the body endangers life. Table 49-3 gives a clear picture of the effect of age and the percent of the body burned on survival rate.

Prognosis depends on the depth and extent of the burn as well as on the condition and age of the patient. Problems encountered are shock, infection, respiratory distress, cardiovascular and renal disturbances, fluid and electrolyte imbalance, and psychiatric derangements. Such difficulties may occur simultaneously or in sequence. Consequently, instead of thinking of patient care in terms of a "one-system" approach, it is necessary to consider this patient in terms of a "one-body" approach, which includes all systems.

LOCAL CARE OF THE BURN

Conscientious management of the burned area is of vital importance. When nonviable loose skin is removed, aseptic conditions must be established. Borderline normal skin near the burn wound is shaved to prevent possible contamination from hair follicles. A photograph is taken of all burned areas prior to initiation of treatment; this is filed on the patient's chart.

Infection is the major cause of death in patients who have survived the first few days following extensive burns. The infection begins within the burn site and then is carried into the bloodstream. Because of the danger of infection, cultures are taken of the burn wound on admission and twice weekly to monitor colonization of the wound by microbial organisms. Plastic liners are used in hydrotherapy equipment to prevent cross-infection.

A few of the bacteria ever present in our environment contaminate the wound. Bacteria such as staphylococci, *Proteus, Pseudomonas, E. coli,* and *Klebsiella* enterobacteria find optimal conditions for growth within the burn. The burn eschar is a nonviable crust with no blood supply, so that polymorphonuclear leukocytes and antibodies, even systemic antibiotics cannot reach the area. Phenomenal

TABLE 49-3. SURVIVAL RATE IN RELATION TO AGE AND PERCENTAGE OF BURN

AGE	PERCENT OF BODY BURNED	SURVIVAL	MORTALITY
5 and under	50%	66%	34%
5-40	50%	80%	20%
40-60	50%	51%	49%
Over 60	50%	9%	91%

numbers of bacteria — over one billion per gram of tissue — may appear and subsequently spread to the bloodstream or release their toxins, which reach distant sites.

Throughout the years, various approaches have been devised to combat these problems — exposure, occlusive dressings, open method with topical chemotherapy, and excision. All have advantages and disadvantages.

Exposure Method

The objective of this method is to control bacterial colonization by exposing the wound to light and maintaining a cool environment. This method is most frequently used to treat burns of the face, neck, perineum, and extensive areas of the trunk. Exposing a burn to the drying effect of air allows the exudate to dry and form a hard crust in about 3 days; this protects the wound. In a second-degree burn, regeneration of skin beneath the crust takes 2 to 3 weeks, at which time the eschar falls off. In a third-degree burn, no epithelialization occurs beneath the eschar. In the untreated burn, the eschar usually separates in 2 to 3 weeks. When full thickness burns occur circumferentially on the extremities or trunk, the eschar causes a tourniquet effect compromising distal circulation and chest expansion.

The success of the exposed method depends upon keeping the immediate environment free of organisms. Some practitioners maintain that everything coming in contact with the patient must be sterile. Linens are sterile; those who come in direct contact with the patient wear masks, sterile gowns, and gloves; visitors are instructed to wear gowns and masks and not to touch the bed or hand the patient anything. Some practitioners maintain a clean environment and rely on the amazing efficiency of the topical antibacterial agents to limit burn wound infection.

A cradle may be placed over the patient to prevent sheets from coming in contact with the burn area, to minimize the effects of air currents to which a burn patient is unusually sensitive, and to provide some form of covering. (Some persons are sensitive to being unduly exposed.) Heat shields or lamps may be required to maintain the patient's body temperature, since a loss of the microcirculation in the burned areas decreases the patient's ability to maintain body heat.

The use of a sterile "burn pack" facilitates the care of this patient; it may contain sheets, pillowcases, washcloth, bath blanket, loin cloth, halter, and perhaps a gown and mask for the attendant.

The room should be kept scrupulously clean; windows should have screens to keep out flies and other insects. Damp dusting and mopping are preferable to dry dusting and sweeping. Regulation of the room temperature and humidity is necessary for the patient's comfort and for optimal crust development. The patient is acutely aware of temperature changes and is most comfortable when the room is kept within the range of 34° C. ±2° (93° F. ± 4°). The most important characteristic of environmental conditions is that the ambient air temperature should be warmer than that of the burned skin.

The room temperature can be adjusted according to the patient's needs. A temperature that is too warm may cause fluid loss through perspiration and, in addition, may promote bacterial growth. If the temperature is too cool, a blanket may be spread over the cradle, or small light bulbs may be placed in the tent. When these lights are used, the patient may want to wear sunglasses or an eyeshade.

The preferred range of humidity in the room is between 40 and 50 percent. A room that is drier will cause burn eschar to crack and cause pain, whereas a room that is too moist will encourage softening and premature separation of eschar. Portable electric humidifiers or dehumidifiers are effective in controlling humidity.

A light sprinkling of sterile cornstarch on the lower sheet helps to prevent a burn area from sticking to the sheet. Alternatively, one may use Microdon sheeting (3M Co.) or aluminum foil such as Reynolds Wrap.

When linens are changed, care must be taken not to pull on those parts of the sheet that are adhering to the burn area. Sterile saline may be used to wet the area so that the sheet may be freed gently. Turning is encouraged to prevent pneumonia and contractures and to promote circulation. The patient may prefer to do this without assistance; if help is required, the nurse should don sterile gloves to handle nonburn areas. Even more importantly, the patient should be ambulated as soon as possible — even on the first day — and should be encouraged to use his arms, hands, fingers, and legs.

The advantages of the exposure method are: (1) there are no painful dressing changes; (2) less equipment is used; (3) infection can be detected early; and (4) large numbers of patients can be treated, making this method particularly suitable for disaster situations.

Disadvantages of this method are: (1) it is often not suitable for burns of the hands and feet because proper alignment and elevation are difficult to maintain; (2) it is unsuitable when the patient must be transported any distance, as from a battlefront to a base hospital; (3) it is less effective when other injuries exist that require the patient to be turned frequently; and (4) it may cause additional metabolic stress unless the patient's body temperature can be adequately maintained by controlling the immediate environment. Bandaging would be preferable in these instances.

Occlusive (Pressure) Dressings

Occlusive dressings are used primarily for burns of the feet and hands. Fine mesh gauze impregnated with a topical antimicrobial agent is applied lightly to the cleansed burn area and an appropriate dressing is applied. The dressing may consist of sterile absorptive fluffed or washed gauze placed in such a way that the material does not clump together.

Precautions are taken to prevent two body surfaces from touching, such as fingers or toes, ear and scalp, the areas under the breast, any point of flexion, or between the genital folds. Functional body alignment positions are maintained; thus, the fingers and thumb curve over fluffed gauze or a bandage roll, the foot is positioned to avoid pronation and dropfoot, and support is placed under the knees.

Some physicians fix the loose gauze in place with elastic bandage or stockinette; others apply abdominal pads before applying the conforming bandage. Another fixation bandage is Surgifix (Burn Treatment Skin Bank) which is a light, expansile, netlike, conforming overdressing available in many sizes (Fig. 49-3). Evenly distributed pressure is desired with no constriction to hinder circulation. Circulation may be checked every 3 or 4 hours by noting pulse, color, warmth, and symptoms of paresthesia. Having the tips of fingers or toes exposed provides areas where circulation can be easily checked.

Removal of Soiled Dressings. Dressings are changed in the patient's unit following the administration of an analgesic (20 minutes previously) or in the operating room with the patient anesthetized. If possible, dressings should be changed following or during hydrotherapy which facilitates the procedure and keeps the patient more comfortable. Otherwise, wetting the dressings

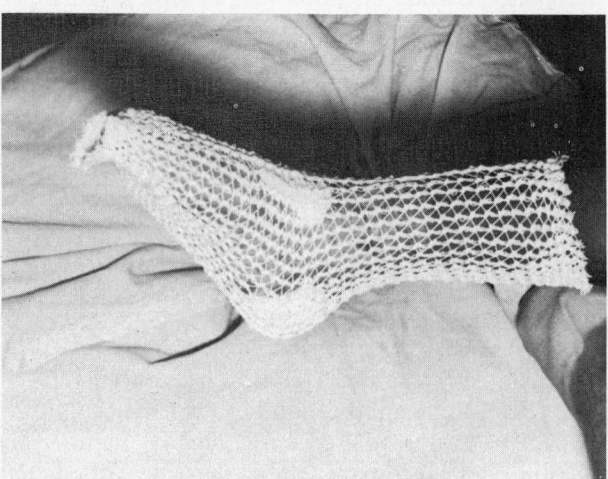

Figure 49-3. Use of tubular mesh overdressing (Surgifix) to hold gauze covering in place. Once a wound has been cleansed and debrided, a fine gauze impregnated with a topical antibacterial cream (silver sulfadiazine or mafedine) is applied in one layer. The gauze is cut to fit the wounds only and does not overlap onto unburned skin. The Surgifix overdressing, holding the gauze in place, is available in several sizes and is elasticized in order to facilitate application to all parts of the body. (Courtesy, Shriners Hospitals for Crippled Children, Burns Institute, Galveston, Texas)

(with warm saline, 2 parts to 1 part of 2 percent hydrogen peroxide) facilitates their removal by softening the exudate and eschar. If exudate stain is noted, indicating moisture, the wet dressings are replaced to encourage drying and to prevent the growth of microorganisms.

- Signs of infection are increased pulse, elevated temperature, and possibly odor, or greenish or yellowish coloring on the dressings.

Occasionally, with bacteremia from proteus or pseudomonas, the urine will become brownish to green in color.

To change the dressing, the nurse dons a mask and gloves, slits the outer dressings with blunt scissors and spreads the dressing open. The extremity is carefully lifted to withdraw the soiled dressings and the part is lowered onto a sterile towel. The remaining dressings are carefully removed with forceps and the gloved hand. Loose eschar is then debrided.

Debridement. Since the eschar is dead tissue, it can be cut safely up to the point of bleeding or pain. Using sterile gloves, a smooth forceps, and surgical scissors, the physician or specially trained nurse may debride the eschar. If there is bleeding from a torn small blood vessel, oxidized cellulose (Oxycel) and/or pressure may be applied for hemostasis. Medication and dressings are reapplied gently and smoothly. The area should be watched for further bleeding which may require ligation.

Redressing of the Burn. The prescribed topical antibacterial agent is applied according to the preference of the surgeon.

Burns of the extremities are elevated, usually on pillows, to prevent edema. In the case of a hand burn, a bucket-handle suspension device may be improvised.

Open Method and Topical Chemotherapy

The open method, the most popular method of treating burns, consists of a combination of the exposure method and the application of a topical agent. With this method, wound assessment is simpler, physical therapy occurs at an earlier point, and temperature is easier to control. However, there is a delay in eschar separation, as well as a risk of sepsis and patient discomfort due to body chilling.

Bacteriological cultures are required to monitor the effect of topical medications. Swab cultures or surface cultures (gauze capillarity) may be used. The procedures are noninvasive, simple, and painless but are limited to the area sampled. Wound biopsy cultures (invasive) may be required for quantitative sampling. Systemic antibiotics are used sparingly but are essential for pulmonary or other concomitant infections.

Criteria for topical agents include the following: (1) the agent is effective against gram-negative organisms, *Pseudomonas aeruginosa, Staphylococcus aureus,* and even fungi; (2) it is clinically effective; (3) it penetrates the eschar but is not systemically toxic; (4) it does not lose its effectiveness, thereby permitting another infection to develop; (5) it is cost-effective, available, and acceptable to the patient; and (6) it is inexpensive and easy to apply, minimizing nursing care time.

Silver Sulfadiazine (Silvadene)

Silver sulfadiazine, a popular topical medication used in this method of burn treatment, is synthesized by reacting silver nitrate with sodium sulfadiazine. It is available as a water-soluble cream in concentrations of 1 percent and is highly effective against gram-negative bacteria. It is more effective when the total burn area involves less than 60 percent of the body surface area.

Evidence indicates that the pseudomonas cells may split the agent so that silver is bound but sulfadiazine is released. This binding action may account for the potent inhibition of bacterial growth.

Compared with mafenide acetate and other antibacterial agents, silver sulfadiazine is more effective in controlling infection, causes no pain on application, does not disturb acid-base balance, electrolytes, or renal function, allows regeneration of epithelium to progress unhindered, and does not stain. Liberal amounts are applied topically with a gloved hand or on impregnated gauze rolls.

The medicated burn area can be left open or covered with a dressing. When silver sulfadiazine is applied to dermal burns, a proteinaceous gel (several millimeters thick) forms on the wound surface; after 72 hours, this pseudoeschar can be removed easily.

Recently it has been reported (Bridges and Lowbury) that a significant number of gram-negative bacilli can become highly resistant to sulfadiazine as a result of protracted use of this agent.

Silver Sulfadiazine – Cerium Nitrate. Cerium (a lanthanide element) has recently been incorporated into silver sulfadiazine to enhance its clinical effectiveness. A combination of just under 1 percent of silver sulfadiazine and 2.2 percent of cerium nitrate provides a thin cream which can be applied topically. It appears to be most effective against gram-negative bacteria and has been credited with lowering mortality rates. Occasionally a case of methemoglobinemia has been noted; however, on the whole it seems most effective and safe.

Cerium Nitrate Solution. Cerium nitrate solution (1.74%) can be used alone or in conjunction with the combination silver sulfadiazine-cerium nitrate cream as a wet soak to enhance the effectiveness of the antibacterial action of these agents. It must be rewet every 4 hours and applied with a bulky dressing for maximal effectiveness and to assist in maintaining the patient's body temperature at optimal levels. A dry top covering such as a bandaging layer of stockinette helps to reduce heat evaporation.

Silver Nitrate Solution
(0.5 percent aqueous solution)

Silver nitrate is an effective agent in preventing eschar contamination, particularly in burn injuries involving up to 40 or 50 percent of the body surface area. However, since the drug is unable to penetrate the eschar, infection can occur in the subeschar region. Because of this possibility, it is necessary to inspect the wound frequently and debride as necessary.

Disagreement still exists about whether the high mortality rate from extensive burns results from toxins produced by the burn or from inanition and overwhelming infection of the burn surface as well as evaporation of body heat from the burn surface. Those who support the latter theory note that covering the burn with continuous wet dressings of 0.5 percent silver nitrate solution effectively controls the infection. According to this thinking, the bactericidal action of the silver nitrate solution on burn wounds is so effective that cross-infection does not occur; therefore, isolation technique is not necessary. Caps, masks and gowns are not worn routinely, and relatives are permitted to visit freely and even feed the patient. However, cleanliness and hand washing are stressed. Clean (not sterile) strips of gauze are cut from large rolls and used as dressings. Further, masks and sterile gloves are used by personnel when they directly handle the patient.

The treatment begins soon after the patient reaches the hospital. The patient is placed in a sterile bath of warmed Locke's solution*, and all greases and ointments are carefully removed from the burn area; this facet of the treatment may take up to an hour. The burns are then covered with gauze dressings thoroughly soaked with 0.5 percent silver nitrate solution. Concentrations above 1 percent produce tissue necrosis, whereas those below 0.5 percent are ineffective antiseptically.

These dressings are kept wet with the silver nitrate solution, which is applied by means of bulb syringes. The best dressings are composed of six to eight layers of four-ply gauze applied wet and held in place with bandages of bias-cut wide stockinette. The gauze of the dressing *should not contain cotton between the layers* because this interferes with the efficient action of the silver nitrate solution and causes the dressing to stick to the wound. Catheters may be incorporated into the thick dressings to

---

*Modified Locke's solution for the sterile bath for the burned patient is a combination of various salts. It is best prepared from 2 stock solutions which are mixed at the time that the bath is prepared.

Solution A —gm./L.		Solution B —gm./L.	
NaCl	175.5	NaHCO$_3$	73.3
KCl	9.0	NaH$_2$PO$_4$ · H$_2$O	3.8
CaCl$_2$ · 2 H$_2$O	11.1		
MgCl$_2$ · 6 H$_2$O	9.13		

Add 1 volume of Solution A, followed by 1 volume of B, to 23 volumes of water.

permit saturation every 2 to 4 hours. The dressings are changed two or three times daily. The patient is covered with one or two dry sheets and a dry cotton blanket. These dry layers prevent or reduce the heat loss produced by vaporization from the wet dressings and from the burned surface. When the coverings become moist, they are changed. The patient is turned frequently to provide pressure and wetness to all areas. For the severely burned patient, the Stryker frame or circular bed may be used.

The use of 0.5 percent silver nitrate solution dressings is not without danger, because electrolytes, especially sodium and potassium, are withdrawn from the body fluids and pass into the dressings impregnated with silver nitrate solution. The withdrawal of sodium may occur very rapidly, especially in patients with extensive burns and in children, producing an acute electrolyte imbalance.

• In the early phases of the burn treatment, blood must be drawn at frequent intervals—every 2 to 4 hours—to determine sodium, chloride, potassium, and calcium levels. These electrolytes must be replaced, usually by the intravenous administration of Ringer's lactate solution.

Once the patient can take a normal diet, salt is added to the diet. Calcium depression is treated by the addition of calcium lactate or gluconate to the diet (usually within a few days postburn) and potassium depression by the administration of potassium gluconate elixir. Deficits in these constituents of the blood electrolytes naturally are more marked in more extensive burns (comprising 50 to 80 percent of the body surface).

The silver nitrate solution has the disadvantage of turning black in the sunlight. This means that everything touched by the solution is stained black, including clothes, hands, floors, and other objects. The nurse attending a patient being treated with silver nitrate solution must wear rubber gloves, as a protection against the silver nitrate stains. (Such stains may be prevented by applying an organic iodine preparation, such as Wescodyne or Betadine solutions, to objects which have come in contact with the silver solution and then rinsing them in water.) Stain-resistant floor and wall coverings are available, but such materials increase the cost of care.

Mafenide Acetate (Sulfamylon Acetate)

Mafenide acetate (10 percent) in cream form with a hydrophilic base diffuses rapidly through the burned skin and eschar and is effective against a broad range of gram-positive and gram-negative organisms in the subeschar area. It is limited in use to the treatment of localized invasive burn wound sepsis caused by organisms sensitive to this agent.

The cream is applied in a thick layer, 3 to 4 mm. (Fig. 49-4), once or twice daily; a fine mesh gauze may be applied in strips directly to the burn and changed daily or washed off in a whirlpool bath.

Although it is relatively nontoxic, mafenide acetate is a strong carbonic anhydrase inhibitor and may adversely affect the blood pH level, causing a reduction of the renal tubular buffering mechanism. With continued use, severe metabolic acidosis may occur, making it necessary to discontinue mafenide and monitor the respiratory rate, blood gases, and pH. Chest x-rays also may be justified because of possible pulmonary failure.

Another disadvantage of this form of treatment is the

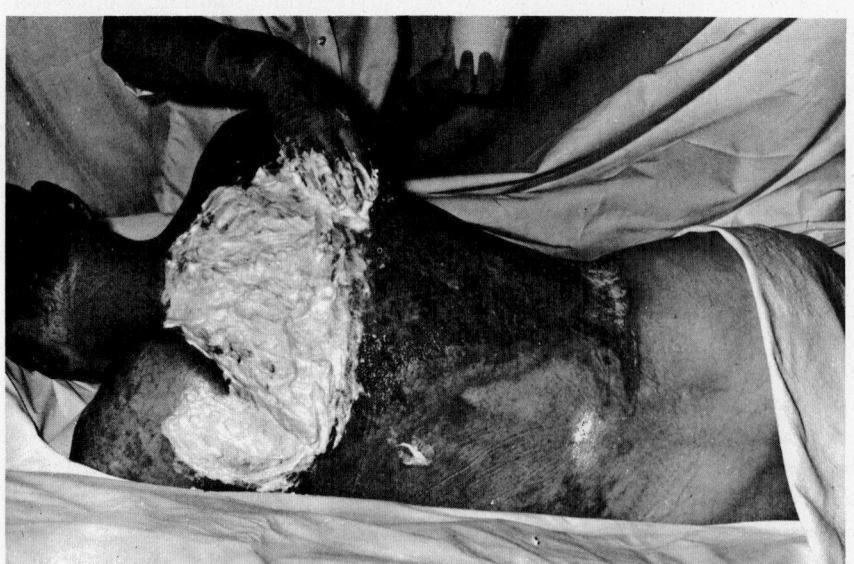

Figure 49-4. Photograph of back of patient with deep second-degree burn being treated with Sulfamylon. The Sulfamylon cream is put on in a thick layer with the gloved hand. (From Artz, C. P., and Mancrief, V. A.: The Treatment of Burns, Philadelphia, W. B. Saunders)

burning pain experienced by the patient for a few minutes following application of the cream. Thus, analgesics may be required before the ointment is applied. Another problem is that eschar separates very slowly, thereby delaying skin grafting unless the eschar is aggressively debrided.

Other Topical Agents

Povidone-iodine is commercially available as a brown water-miscible cream for topical use in which the iodine content is 1 percent. More information is needed in order to recommend its use.

Gentamicin sulfate is a bactericidal aminoglycoside available in a 0.1 percent cream for topical use. It is useful for short periods of time in small areas of invasive infection. Superinfection with resistant bacterial strains have been reported, indicating the need for very careful monitoring when it is used.

Excisional Therapy

When excisional therapy is the treatment of choice, all nonviable tissue is removed down to a viable base. This relatively new method of treating burns carries less danger of sepsis, creates less metabolic stress, and allows for earlier as well as quicker rehabilitation. When the excisional procedures are carried out, the patient's blood volume must be supported and adequate nutrition must be supplied. Expansion grafting techniques are used, and specific topical antimicrobial agents are selected.

A cold knife or laser scalpel is used to excise tissue. The laser is favored since is involves a minimal amount of blood loss. Usually the excision is done between the second and fifth postburn day, but it can be done in selected patients after that time. After the nonviable tissue is removed (not more than 25 percent of total body surface is excised at one time), the excised wounds are closed with expanded autografts or skin substitutes.

Temporary Wound Closure. As soon as nonviable tissue is removed, it is essential that the fresh wound be closed immediately. Sheet autografts are preferred. If the wound is large, involving over 50 percent of the total body surface, biological dressings (allografts) are the preferred temporary skin substitutes until sufficient autografts are available. The same donor site can be used every 2 to 3 weeks if healing is optimal and autograft skin can be meshed to increase the area that it will cover. (See page 1072 for skin grafting.)

Broad adherent and barrier dressings are being tried experimentally and appear to hold promise as the preferred method for providing temporary wound closure. Hydron (polyhydroxymethylmethacrylate) is an example of a barrier dressing that is sprayed on a fresh burn or excised burn wound. When incorporated with polyethylene glycol, this compound is converted into an adherent pliable membrane which discourages bacterial penetration. Hydron forms a bond to the underlying wound, is flexible, and permits the patient to engage in physical therapy.

Another excellent source is a skin bank in which skin is stored in liquid nitrogen. Such skin is typed and when needed can be thawed, washed in saline, and made ready for use in less than an hour.

Permanent Wound Closure. Skin grafts are acquired in a variety of sizes and thicknesses by means of a dermatome designed for this purpose. Meshing devices are available to provide for even expansion of sheet grafts. Skin expanded to the usual ratio of 3:1 makes it possible to cover greater surface areas; such grafts become adherent in approximately 3 to 4 days. Other types of grafts may be required, including rotation flaps, pedicle flaps, or free grafts. (See page 1072.)

Postgrafting Wound Care. The success of a graft depends upon applying the graft at the optimum time in the optimum way (following original skin lines) and with maximum control over infection. Thereafter, a multidisciplinary effort, including the surgeon, nurse, psychiatrist, physical and occupational therapists, social worker, and family, is required in order to carry out a planned rehabilitative program. Splints and braces may have to be worn to prevent contractures of burned joints. Elastic garments may be used to maintain the position of the tissue on the graft site and to reduce hypertrophic scarring. These devices may be worn for the first year. Massaging the scar area with topical steroids (or injections of steroid locally) may be required to reduce hypertrophic scar formation. Clear plastic splints are effective in maintaining positions and permitting visualization of pressure points.

An aggressive exercise program, with physical and occupational therapy conducted on an outpatient basis, plus conscientious lubrication of the skin and protection from trauma are examples of the kinds of continuing care required for successful rehabilitation.

MANAGEMENT OF THE BURN PATIENT

One of the greatest advances made in the care of the critically burned patient has been the development of burn teams. Initiated in the 1950s at the Brooke Army Hospital in San Antonio, Texas, the burn team consists not only of specially trained physicians, nurses, anesthesiologists, nutritionists, chaplains, respiratory and physical therapists, psychiatrists, and social workers but also of personnel trained in the areas of hyperalimentation, physiology, clinical engineering, microbiology, and immunology. Weekly interdisciplinary burn team conferences are effective in coordinating the roles of team members and in promoting mutual understanding. Ultimately and ideally, major burns will be cared for only in specialized centers. The number of such burn care services in the United States is increasing each year.

A well organized professional team simultaneously carries out many facets of burn management during the first hour of intensive care. These activities are directed toward lifesaving and comfort measures. One member may intubate the airway while another initiates fluid therapy and a third cares for the burned area.

Immediate management of the burn patient includes the following:
- An intravenous route via an indwelling catheter is established, preferably through an unburned area.
- Blood specimens are drawn for hematocrit, electrolyte, and blood gas determinations, and for typing and cross matching. These parameters must be followed closely in the resuscitation period.
- An indwelling urinary catheter is inserted so that urine volume and specific gravity can be monitored hourly. The amount of urine first obtained is recorded since it may assist in determining the extent of renal function. It should also be tested for hemoglobin. Urine volumes of less than 30 ml. per hour (10 ml. in children) are reported.
- The patient's vital signs are monitored at frequent intervals: temperatures over 38.3° C. (101° F.) or below 36.1° C. (97° F.) are reported.

Room Prepared to Receive the Burn Patient

When a bed is prepared for a burn patient, the mattress is completely covered with a plastic sheet, which is covered in turn with a sterile bottom sheet. Sterile Microdon sheeting (3M Co.) atop this bedding prevents the patient from sticking to the sheets as a result of the exudate's oozing from the burn. Caps, masks, and sterile gowns and gloves are available for those attending the patient. The equipment most likely to be required should be in the room, including intravenous therapy equipment, with polyethylene central venous catheters and fluids (i.e., plasmanate and Ringer's lactate solution); blood withdrawal syringes, needles, and tubes; catheterization tray and drainage equipment; urine testing devices; tracheostomy set; intubation equipment; venesection set; suction and oxygen therapy equipment; fresh, pathogen-free linens; overbed cradle; and side rails. The particular procedure to be followed in wound care determines additional needs.

In some clinics, patients with severe burns of the trunk are placed in circular beds and rotated from prone to supine position every 3 hours. The Stryker frame also may be used if it meets the individual patient's needs. An air fluidized bed or an "egg crate" pad or mattress may also be helpful.

POSTBURN PATIENT, FIRST TWO DAYS

Immediate Patient Care

When the patient is admitted to the hospital, his clothes are carefully removed, his weight and height are recorded, and he is placed on or between sterile sheets. Since this patient is usually frightened and may be in emotional shock, those in attendance should demonstrate concern for his care. Encouragement is offered and explanations are given when necessary. Should the patient express the desire to see a spiritual advisor, one should be notified.

Careful attention must be given to aseptic technique. Attending personnel must wear masks, caps, and gowns; sterile gloves are worn when the burn area is handled. The physician evaluates the patient's general condition, assesses the burn, determines the priorities, and directs the individualized plan of treatment, which is divided into systemic management and local care of the burned area.

Photographs should be taken of the burn areas at this time and periodically throughout the treatment. In this way, the progress of healing may be determined quickly. Such evidence is invaluable in insurance claims and courts of law.

Pulmonary Injuries in Burns

Pulmonary injury due to smoke inhalation and carbon dioxide intoxication is considered to be the leading cause of death in fire victims. It is estimated that *at least 50 percent of these deaths could have been prevented by such devices as smoke detectors.*

Pathophysiology. Extrinsic airway obstruction may be caused by circumferential burns of the neck, chest, or upper abdomen, or from foreign material in the nose, mouth, or throat. *Intrinsic airway obstruction* results from inhalation of smoke, steam, gases, or fire in an enclosed or semi-enclosed space, causing pulmonary injury.

Carbon monoxide is a prominent cause of inhalation injury. The pathophysiologic effects are due to tissue hypoxia. Carbon monoxide combines with hemoglobin to form carboxyhemoglobin, which competes with oxygen for available hemoglobin-binding sites. The affinity of hemoglobin for carbon monoxide is 200 times greater than for oxygen. Potentiating factors that enhance carbon monoxide poisoning are decreased oxygen in the burning area and added effects of smoke poisoning.

Smoke poisoning results from noxious chemicals formed in the burning process (particularly organic compounds such as plastics); these chemicals include hydrogen cyanide, hydrochloric acid, sulfuric acid, halogens, and benzene.

Smoke inhalation causes loss of ciliary action and severe mucosal edema. Congestion results in atelectasis. Expectoration of carbonaceous sputum may occur. In a few hours, sloughing of the tracheobronchial mucosa occurs, and the patient coughs up mucopurulent material.

Clinical Manifestations and Assessment Criteria. Criteria which suggest postburn pulmonary damage include the following: (1) a history indicating that the burn occurred in an enclosed area; (2) burns of the face, neck, or circumoral area; (3) singed nasal hair; (4) hoarseness, voice change, dry cough, sooty sputum; (5) bloody sputum, labored respiration, frank burns of the tongue or of the oral or pharyngeal mucosa.

Arterial blood gas values are obtained to serve as a baseline against which comparisons are later made in order to determine if there has been a lowering of oxygen tension, indicating possible pulmonary injury.

Management

- Immediate therapy is directed toward establishing an airway, possibly through oropharyngeal suctioning followed by the administration of 100 percent oxygen. Such a high concentration of oxygen may not be available under emergency conditions; however, oxygen by mask or nasal prongs is given initially.

In mild cases, inspired air is humidified and the patient is encouraged to cough so that secretions can be suctioned. For more severe situations, it is necessary to remove secretions by bronchial suctioning and administer bronchial dilators and mucolytic agents.

- When oropharyngeal edema is present, it may be necessary to intubate the patient. Hyperinflation hourly with an Ambu-bag helps to prevent atelectasis. Continuous positive airway pressure and mechanical ventilation may also be required.
- Arterial blood gases are evaluated (Swan-Ganz catheter may be required to monitor pulmonary artery wedge pressure) and urine output is checked.

Authorities differ on the administration of antibiotics. Gram stains of the sputum will help in determining antibiotic use: if gram-positive organisms and large numbers of neutrophils are present, penicillin or penicillinase-resistant antibiotics are given. Usually steroids are not given, because disadvantages outweigh advantages. Meticulous aseptic technique in all aspects of tracheal care is required in this infection-prone patient.

Management of Fluid Derangement (Plasma-to-Interstitial Fluid Shift) and Shock

Next to handling respiratory difficulties, the most urgent need is to replace lost fluid and to prevent irreversible shock. In extensive burns (more than 20 percent of the body surface) a dangerous systemic derangement of fluid balance occurs. This begins with the loss of fluid into the tissues surrounding the burn area and loss of fluid by exudation and evaporation from the surface of the burn. The result is a decrease in the circulating fluid of the entire body. Extravasation of fluid into the tissue begins within an hour and reaches its peak in 4 to 6 hours; fluid loss continues into the tissues up to 48 hours postburn (Table 49-4). The result is hemoconcentration—a relative increase in the ratio of blood cells to plasma. An increase in the hematocrit, a less efficient circulation, and a fall in the blood pressure result from the cumulative effects of

TABLE 49-4. WATER AND ELECTROLYTE CHANGES IN THE FIRST 48 HOURS OF MAJOR BURNS

FLUID ACCUMULATION PHASE (SHOCK PHASE) PLASMA → INTERSTITIAL FLUID (EDEMA AT BURN SITE)

OBSERVATION	EXPLANATION
1. Generalized dehydration	Plasma leaks through damaged capillaries
2. Reduction of blood volume	Brought about by plasma loss, fall of blood pressure, and diminished cardiac output
3. Decreased urinary output	Secondary to: Fluid loss Decreased renal blood flow Sodium and water retention caused by increased adreno-cortical activity (Hemolysis of red blood cells, causing hemoglobinuria and myonecrosis or myoglobinuria)
4. Potassium excess	Massive cellular trauma causes release of K^+ into extracellular fluid (ordinarily, most K^+ is intracellular)
5. Sodium deficit	Large amount of Na^+ is lost in trapped edema fluid and exudate and by shift into cells (ordinarily most Na^+ is extracellular)
6. Metabolic acidosis (base bicarbonate deficit)	Loss of bicarbonate ions accompanies sodium loss
7. Hemoconcentration (elevated hematocrit)	Liquid blood component lost into extravascular space

Adapted from Metheny, N. M., and Snively, W. D.: Nurses' Handbook of Fluid Balance. Philadelphia, J. B. Lippincott.

these processes. In addition to signs of restlessness and disorientation, determination of vital signs may reveal an accelerated heartbeat (tachycardia).

- A pulse rate in excess of 110 beats/minute should be reported immediately because it means that the heart is attempting to compensate for decreased blood volume.

Because of generalized cellular dehydration, the patient often exhibits extreme thirst. Shock is likely to occur, and the patient is seriously ill.

Fluid Replacement. There is no known way to stop the outpouring of fluids, but replacement of fluids is possible. The physician calculates the projected fluid requirements for the first 24 hours by evaluating the patient's burn injury (page 1084). Some combination of fluid categories may be appropriate: (1) colloids: whole blood, plasma, and plasma expanders; and (2) electrolytes: physiologic sodium chloride, Ringer's solution, Hartmann's solution.

Formulas have been evolved for estimating fluid loss based on the estimated percentage of body surface area burned and the weight of the patient. These are modified by physicians and individualized to meet the requirements of each patient.

The Evans Formula:

1. Colloids (blood, plasma, dextran): 1 ml. × percent burn × kg. body weight
2. Electrolytes (saline): 1 ml. × percent burn × kg. body weight
3. Glucose (5 percent) in water, 2,000 ml. (for insensible losses)

Second- and third-degree burns totaling over 50 percent are calculated on the basis of 50 percent. In any event, 10,000 ml. of total fluids is the maximal amount to be given in a 24-hour period. One half of the calculated fluid is given in the first 8 hours postburn; the remainder is spread evenly over the next 16 hours.

On the second postburn day, the patient receives one half of the colloid, one half of electrolyte, and all the insensible replacement (see chart, page 1096).

The Brooke Army Hospital Formula:

This formula differs from the Evans formula only in that the colloid fraction is reduced from 1.0 ml. to 0.5 ml. and the electrolyte fraction increased from 1.0 ml. to 1.5 ml. Instead of saline, the electrolyte preferred is lactated Ringer's solution because of its lower chloride content.

On the second postburn day, the patient receives one half of the colloid, one half of the electrolyte, and all the insensible replacement (see chart, page 1096).

The Parkland or Baxter Formula:

The patient is given 4.0 ml. of Ringer's lactate solution per percent burn, per kilogram body weight. One third is given in the first 8 hours and the rest over the next 16 hours. No fluids are calculated for the second postburn day (see chart, page 1096).

Nursing Management in Fluid Therapy

• The amount and speed of fluid given through an indwelling plastic vein cannula is gauged by the urinary output and the pulse rate. Urine flow from an indwelling catheter should be maintained at 30 to 70 ml. per hour. This means that the flow from the indwelling catheter must be collected, measured, and recorded every hour. Pulse should be less than 110 per minute. *These parameters are far more important in resuscitation than any formula.* Indeed the patient's individual response *is* the "formula."

• The following observations must be reported:

1. the presence of hematuria,
2. urine output below 30 ml. per hour—this suggests an inadequate rate of fluid resuscitation,
3. urine output above 100 ml. per hour, which may presage pulmonary edema or imminent water intoxication (suggested by the following signs: tremor, twitching, nausea, diarrhea, salivation, and disorientation).

Additional gauges of the fluid requirements include hematocrit and hemoglobin determinations. Blood samples for these examinations and for the determination of electrolytes are withdrawn at frequent intervals. If the hematocrit and hemoglobin determinations decrease, or if the urinary output is more than 50 ml. of urine per hour, the speed of flow of the intravenous solution may be decreased as shown in the 24-hour flow chart in Figure 49-5.

Antibiotics may be given by "piggy-back" if required. If nausea or vomiting occurs, a nasogastric tube is introduced into the stomach and attached to a suction apparatus.

The nurse needs to know the maximal amount of fluid the patient is allowed to have—usually fluids are given intravenously. Other feedings are started within a day or two, as soon as bowel sounds resume. High calorie and high protein or tube feedings (milk and egg) are initiated if the patient is intubated or unable to swallow or requires large amounts of calories.

Continued Assessment. Significant changes in the patient's condition must be reported promptly. The recording of patient problems and suggested means of solution are modified as the patient's condition changes. A progressive assessment is required of the patient's appearance and reactions, significant signs and symptoms, intake and output, and all therapies and treatments. Thus constant surveillance is required.

Preventing Infection

Aside from monitoring fluid requirements and providing constant care, the nurse is responsible for providing a clean and safe environment and for closely scrutinizing the wound in order to detect early manifestations of infection. Wound care includes cleansing and debridement, as well as application of topical or subeschar antimicrobial agents and perhaps physiologic dressings (page 1086).

Recent evidence suggests that the primary source of bacterial infection appears to be the patient's own intestinal tract. A major secondary source is the environment. Antibiotics seldom are given prophylactically today because of the tendency to promote resistant strains—except in patients with suspected respiratory injury. Sensitivity to antibiotics should be determined prior to administration. The choice of antibiotics for sepsis is based on the strains present in the patient's unit. The antibiotics chosen should be effective against *Staphylococcus aureus* and *Pseudomonas*. Serum antibiotic levels are monitored for maximal effectiveness and minimal toxicity.

Localized infection must be identified and eliminated. A prime nuring objective is to guard against resistance to antibiotics by maintaining strict isolation precautions. Combination drug regimens may be helpful.

• Ordinarily, a mask and sterile gloves are worn while caring for the patient with extensive burns, in order to prevent infection. Aseptic technique, with cap and gown, may be used when caring directly for burn wounds.

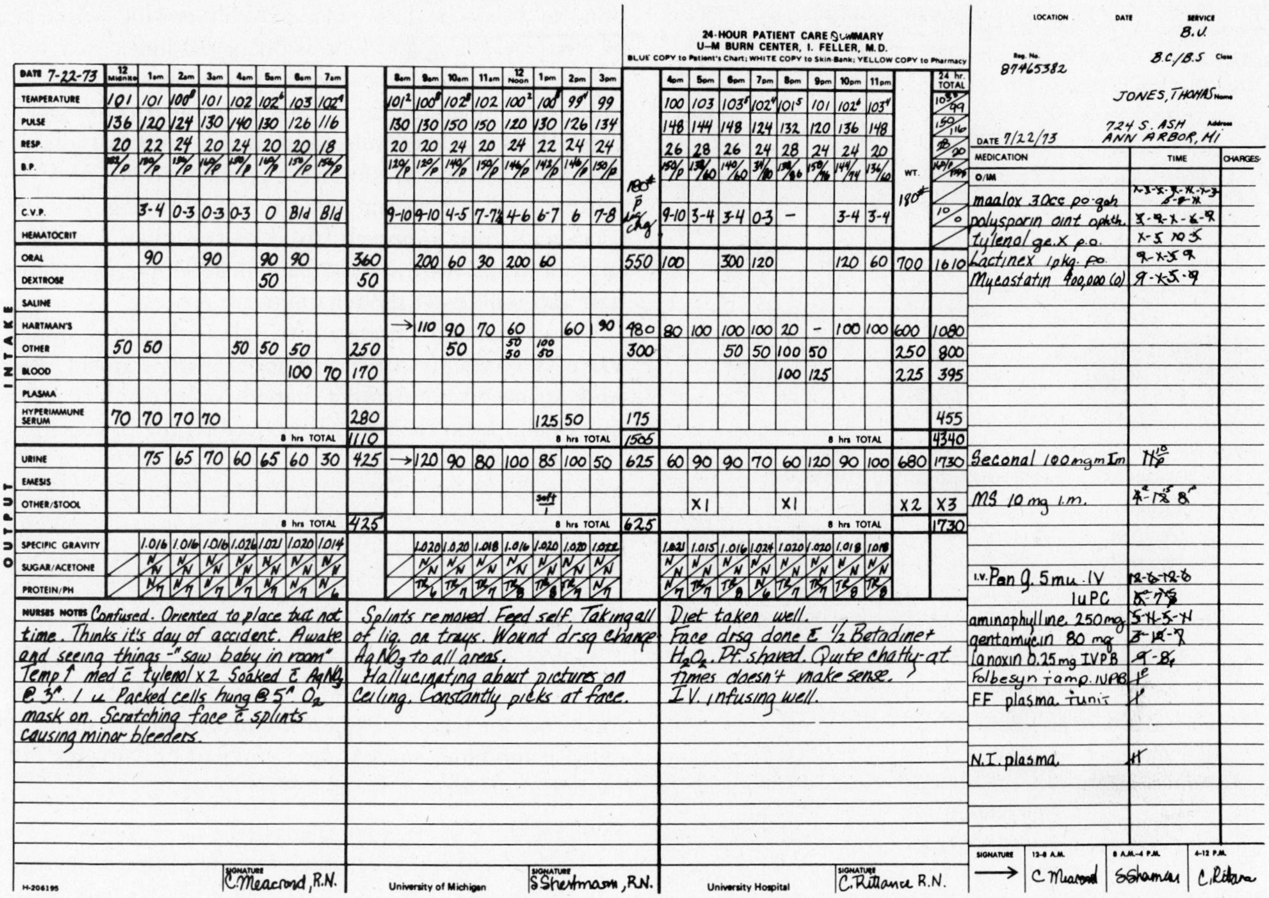

Figure 49-5. A 24-hour flow chart including vital signs, medications, CVP, intake, output, and nurse's notations. Note vital sign fluctuations, reported mental confusion, and attempt to stabilize fluid balance. The hourly recordings give a vivid picture of an unstable condition kept under control. (From Feller, I., and Archambeault, C.: Nursing the Burned Patient. Ann Arbor, Michigan, The Institute for Burn Medicine, 1973)

Wound cleansing and debridement are performed by the physician or a specially trained nurse. Warm bland soap solution or a detergent may be used for cleansing, at which time debridement may also be done. Hexachlorophene soaps are usually avoided because of limited evidence of neurotoxicity associated with absorption of the hexachlorophene.

Because burns are contaminated wounds, adequate tetanus prophylaxis is given. If the patient has been immunized or has had no booster dose in the preceding 4 years, a booster dose of adsorbed tetanus toxoid is administered. If the patient has never had immunizing toxoid, then hyperimmune human antitetanus globulin should be given. The amount given should depend on the extent of the burn and the environment in which the injury occurred. If the patient was rolled on the earth or has been lying on the earth, the danger of tetanus is increased, hence larger doses of antiserum are used.

Pain Relief

Intravenous morphine is usually prescribed to relieve pain in the burn patient. Subcutaneous or intramuscular routes are dangerous because of impaired circulation. For individuals with burns of the head and neck, morphine, which can depress respiration, is given in smaller dosages, intravenously.

• It should be emphasized that, in the presence of anemia, shock, and hypovolemia, especially in children, narcotics may cause cardiac arrest! For this reason, it is wise to give very small doses at short intervals (e.g., every 30–60 minutes) in the early, acute phase.

Pain is more severe in second-degree burns than in third-degree burns, because the nerve endings are destroyed in a third-degree burn. Exposed nerve endings are sensitive to cool, moving air; therefore, a sterile covering can help to reduce pain. Fright, hysteria, and severe pain can later cause neurogenic shock.

• Symptoms of restlessness and anxiety, often attributed to pain, may actually be due to hypoxia. Therefore, careful respiratory assessment is essential before giving analgesics in the early postburn period. Intravenous morphine or other narcotics are prescribed as needed, but large doses are avoided because of the danger of respiratory depression and the possibility of masking other symptoms.

FLUID REPLACEMENT

EXAMPLE: 70 kg. Patient with 70% B.S.A. (Burned Surface Area) Burn.

DAY 1

Evans:
1. Consider burn size as 50% B.S.A.
2. Calculate:
a. Colloid:	$1 \times 50 \times 70 =$	3,500 ml.
b. Electrolyte:	$1 \times 50 \times 70 =$	3,500 ml.
c. Insensible loss:		2,000 ml.
3. Total resuscitation: 9,000 ml.
   First 8 hours: 4,500 ml.
   Next 16 hours: 280 ml./hour

Brooke:
1. Consider burn size as 50% B.S.A.
2. Calculate:
a. Colloid:	$0.5 \times 50 \times 70 =$	1,750 ml.
b. Electrolyte:	$1.5 \times 50 \times 70 =$	5,250 ml.
c. Insensible loss:		2,000 ml.
3. Total Resuscitation: 9,000 ml
   Same as for Evans (above)

Parkland:
1. Consider burn size 70%
2. Calculate: $4 \times 70 \times 50 =$ 14,000 ml.
3. Administer:
First 8 hours:	4,700 ml.
Next 16 hours:	583 ml./hour

DAY 2

Evans:
1. Colloids: 1,750 ml.
2. Electrolyte: 1,750 ml.
3. Insensible loss: 2,000 ml.
                   5,500 ml.
4. Administer: 230 ml./hour

Brooke:
1. Colloids: 875 ml.
2. Electrolyte: 2,625 ml.
3. Insensible loss: 2,000 ml.
                   5,500 ml.
4. Administer: 230 ml./hour

Parkland:
Fluids by mouth. No formula.

NOTE: Total fluid over 2 days using the Brooke or Evans formula equals 14,500 ml. The salt content and water content of the Parkland formula are the same—only the formula is all given on Day 1.

Psychosocial Components of Care

Assessment of the emotional status of the patient often reveals an initial state of emotional stress manifested by confusion, fear for survival, uncontrolled emotions, and sleeplessness. This stage can be alleviated somewhat by the nurse's assuring the patient that these reactions are normal and temporary. By being attentive to the patient's needs, the nurse can relieve him of any fear of abandonment. Should he show signs of delirium or disorientation, he should be gently helped to understand where he is, what time it is, and who is caring for him.

The patient may have sustained many losses as a result of the fire, including family members or friends, and a home and/or possessions, as well as a potential loss of function. He must be allowed to go through the grieving process with caring support from the nursing staff. A consistent, firm approach based on truthful answers to any questions will help the patient develop trust in the staff and will foster the rehabilitative process.

Burn patients are often sensitive about their appearance and may be deeply concerned about disfigurement. Attendants need to remember that any indication of revulsion or shock on their part is noticed by the patient.

POSTBURN PATIENT FROM TWO TO FIVE DAYS

Pathophysiology

Following the shock period, the patient moves into the fluid mobilization phase (48 to 72 hours) (Table 49-5). At this time, the patient's response shifts from a position of defense and emergency to one of repair of damages and mobilization for recovery.

- During this period (2nd to 5th day), fluid is reabsorbed from the interstitial tissue and moves into the bloodstream, increasing the blood volume. An extra strain is placed on the heart, urinary output is greatly increased, and circulatory fluid overload may cause pulmonary edema. Any such changes should be reported immediately because it is imperative that fluid intake be restricted (particularly intravenous fluid intake).
- Of particular significance are signs of respiratory distress — moist rales, coughing of frothy liquid, and cyanosis — they may herald a fatal pulmonary edema.

Fluid, Electrolyte, and Blood Needs

The loss of fluids through the burned area may reach 3 to 5 liters. Water replacement can be measured by monitoring serum sodium and potassium; a sodium reading higher than 140 to 144 mEq./L. (normal) would suggest the need for water. More frequently, serum hyponatremia (sodium below 132 mEq./L.) occurs between the third and the tenth day with rapid fluid mobilization from the burned area.

Hypokalemia may occur at this time unless adequate oral intake of food and fluids is possible; the patient may need as much as 80 to 100 mEq. per day of potassium.

Other indications helpful in determining water replacement are urinary output and weight loss, which should not exceed 1 kg. per day. If the patient is not able to stand on a scale at the bedside, a bed scale might be used.

On the second or third postburn day, blood transfusions may be necessary to combat anemia. At this time, the patient should be observed for a possible transfusion reaction (page 677).

TABLE 49-5. WATER AND ELECTROLYTE CHANGES BEGINNING 48 HOURS AFTER MAJOR BURNS

FLUID REMOBILIZATION PHASE (STATE OF DIURESIS) INTERSTITIAL FLUID → PLASMA

OBSERVATION	EXPLANATION
1. Hemodilution (decreased hematocrit)	Blood cell concentration is diluted as fluid enters the vascular compartment; loss of red blood cells destroyed at burn site
2. Increased urinary output	Fluid shift into intravascular compartment increases renal blood flow and causes increased urine formation
3. Sodium deficit	With diuresis, sodium is lost with water; existing serum sodium is diluted by water influx
4. Potassium deficit (occurs occasionally in this phase)	Beginning on the 4th or 5th postburn day, K^+ shifts from extracellular fluid into cells
5. Metabolic acidosis	Loss of sodium depletes fixed base; relative carbon dioxide content increases

Adapted from Metheny, N. M., and Snively, W. D.: Nurses' Handbook of Fluid Balance. Philadelphia, J. B. Lippincott.

Nutrition Management and Gastrointestinal Disturbances

Gastric dilatation and paralytic ileus occur frequently and are indicated by vomiting and distention; therefore a nasogastric tube is passed early in the treatment. When oral alimentation is initiated, oral fluids should be administered *slowly*. The patient's tolerance is noted, and if vomiting, distention, or diarrhea do not occur, fluids may be slowly increased.

Fruit juices containing potassium are given after the serum potassium levels decrease. High-protein drinks are offered and provide an excellent means of supplementing the diet. A diet containing more solid food is usually begun toward the end of the first week, when the patient's tolerance for food improves. The catabolic response of the body is great, as is reflected in calorie expenditures of 5,000 to 6,000 calories a day. This means that, to meet nutritional demands, the patient must build up nutritional intake to a similar number of calories; he needs approximately 3 gm. of protein per kg. of body weight, 20 percent of the needed calories in the form of fats and the remainder in carbohydrates.

The incidence of *gastrointestinal tract ulcer* (Curling's ulcer) is in proportion to the extent of the burn area. This condition may first be manifested by hemorrhage, detected in bloody contents from nasogastric suction or in the stool. A sudden drop in hemoglobin concentration may be diagnostic even before the hemorrhage is evident. Gastric surgery may be indicated. This is not an uncommon complication. For this reason, frequent small feedings (e.g., six or more daily meals) and/or incorporation of milk and antacid in the diet is a part of proper management.

Proper Positioning and Mobilization

The prevention of pneumonia, the control of edema, and the prevention of pressure sores and contractures are guiding objectives in this facet of management. Deep breathing, turning, and proper repositioning are essential nursing practices modified to meet individual needs. Early ambulation may be encouraged according to the capability of the patient.

Whenever the lower extremities are involved in the burn, Ace bandages should be applied before the patient is placed in an upright position. Both passive and active range of motion exercises are initiated from day of admission and are continued after grafting within certain limitations.

Bathing

Wound care in many clinics includes immersing the patient in an electrolyte, soapy, or germicidal bath. A walk-in type bath, a tub, or a whirlpool may be used. The agitation in the whirlpool aids in cleansing and gently massaging the tissues. The temperature of the bath is maintained at 37.8° C. (100° F.), and the temperature of the room should be between 26.6° to 29.4° C. (80° to 85° F.).

During the bath, the patient should be encouraged to carry out as much activity as possible. Hydrotherapy provides an excellent medium for exercising the extremities and cleaning the entire body. When the patient is removed from the tub following the bath, any residue adhering to the body can be washed away with a spray or shower of clear water.

Psychosocial Response

Throughout the course of treatment the patient is subjected to a painful and distressing experience. Following the traumatic events related to the fire, the patient's life style has been dramatically changed from one of independence to one of dependence—within a strange and frightening environment where physical activity is limited, pain is prevalent, and life seems to hang in the balance, while the patient lies helpless, totally dependent on the care of strange people and equipment.

In such a situation, communication is of the utmost importance. Explanations must be given clearly and often repeatedly, so that the patient becomes involved and understands what is being done to, for, and with him. A major responsibility of the nurse is to constantly assess the patient's psychosocial reactions. Why is he fearful? Is he afraid of losing control of his bodily care, of his very sanity? Is he fearful of rejection by his family and loved ones? Is he fearful of being unable to cope with pain, the appearance of his body? Is he concerned about sexual function? Being aware of the patient's anxieties and understanding the basis of his fears will enable the nurse to provide support and to cooperate with other members of the health team in developing a plan of intervention to help the patient handle these feelings.

Such measures may include providing medication for adequate sleep, rest, and relief from pain and anxiety; including the patient in planning day-to-day care; soliciting the support of family members and collaborating with other personnel involved in providing burn care.

Aside from showing signs of fear, the patient frequently gives vent to angry feelings. At times the anger may be directed inward because of a sense of guilt—perhaps for causing the fire or even for surviving when loved ones perished; or the anger may reach outward toward those who escaped unharmed or even to those who are now providing care. One way to help the patient handle these emotions is to find someone to whom the patient can vent his feelings without fear of retaliation. A nurse, social worker, clergyman, or family member may fill this role successfully.

When feelings of guilt and depression are pronounced, the patient may need to be helped through the grieving process (page 172), since he may frequently be faced with a sense of loss resulting from disfigurement and the possible death of loved ones. In some instances it may help to provide diversion and physical activity, so that he is involved in more than just his own care.

If the patient becomes delirious, possibly because of psychosis or infection, efforts should be made to orient him to reality. People entering the unit should identify themselves; a clock, calendar, and radio can be used as points of reference for time and events; efforts can be made to give a sense of the hour of the day by placing the patient near a window. During this period of mental disequilibrium, no new personnel should attend to the patient. Familiar faces and voices will give the patient a sense of security and orientation.

Before the patient improves, there may be a period of regression during which he may become very dependent and even pessimistic about his recovery. He needs nursing support, honesty, candor, understanding, and firmness in setting reasonable goals of expectation. The family, too, will need guidance at this time so that they will understand the patient's emotional status. Of course the family will have been prepared to accept infection-control precautions and the appearance of the patient—the burn itself and its concomitant edema can cause disfiguring distortions, bandaging can appear voluminous, and certain treatments, such as silver nitrate, are most unattractive. Visitors must be instructed to conceal their own shocked reactions from the patient.

As the burn victim progresses, he becomes aware of daily improvement and begins to exhibit basic concerns: Will I be disfigured? How long will I have to be in the hospital? What about my job and family? Will I ever be independent again? How can I pay for my care? Was this the result of my carelessness? As he expresses his concerns, the nurse should take time to listen and to encourage him.

Wound Care and Skin Grafting

As the crusts of second-degree burns give way to tender, new pink skin, an active physical therapy program is instituted to recondition muscles and stimulate circulation.

After a week or two, the burned tissue tends to separate from the remaining normal tissue. The eschar can be separated from the underlying viable tissue (debridement), leaving a granulating, painful, bleeding wound. Physiologic dressings are used until the site is ready for autografting. Many of these wounds, which appear to be very deep, will be found to have some epithelium still remaining in them, and healing can take place from these islands of skin. In other areas where the skin is completely destroyed, nature must have some help to heal the tremendous wounds left by the burn. It is in these patients that skin grafts are most effective.

The burned area is frequently prepared for skin grafts with warm saline baths. The patient may be immersed in such a bath for an hour at a time, while the burned areas are washed gently to remove the debris that is usually attached to them. As soon as the burn wound becomes a red, granulating area without slough, skin grafts may be used. While giving care to the patient in the bath, the nurse should wear a gown, cap, mask, and sterile gloves in order not to infect the burned area.

The split-thickness type of skin graft is most often used to cover the area left after the eschar is removed. (See page 1073 for skin grafting management.) The hands, face, feet, and joints are high priority areas for grafting.

Nursing care is most important in adjusting the part to its most comfortable position and preventing the skin graft from being dislodged. Skin loss in areas such as the neck, the elbow, etc. produces scars that contract and cause marked deformities. It is in these areas especially that early skin grafting is most efficacious.

Large areas of burn often require hospitalization for a considerable time to permit healing. This is a trying period for the patient, and diversional therapy is most helpful. Occupational therapy and other types of diversion that take the patient's mind away from his troubles are very helpful. Television and/or radio at eye level and within the patient's control are most useful.

RECOVERY, CONVALESCENCE AND REHABILITATION

Nutritional Aspects

Patients lose a great deal of weight in the process of recovering from severe burns. Reserve fat deposits are tapped during the recovery, fluids have been lost, and calorie intake may have been limited. Because of low resistance to infection and disease, the patient's nutritional state must be improved even though he has a poor appetite and is still weak. Semisolid and then a regular diet are offered on the 3rd or 4th day postburn as tolerated. Encouraging him, catering to his preferences, and offering protein and vitamin supplement snacks are ways of tempting the patient to gradually increase his intake from 3,000 to as many as 6,000 calories a day. As a general rule, he should be permitted to eat what he likes — as much as he likes, as often as he likes — and then encouraged to eat more. A 70-kg. patient with a 50 percent burn must take in at least 4,200 calories per day to maintain weight.

Rehabilitation

The objective of rehabilitation is to return the patient to a productive place in society with the best possible emotional, cosmetic, and functional results. Emotional support is given throughout the postburn period. When passive exercises followed by active exercises are initiated, a team approach ensures that the nurse and the physical and occupational therapists are working toward the same goals.

Rehabilitative efforts may be concentrated in a particular division of the hospital. The patient is transferred to this unit when he is able to assume more and more responsibility for his own care. This is done gradually with continual daily assessment of his progress.

Dressings continue to need changing and special attention is given to healed areas, since tissue is tender at this stage. Padding is applied to areas that may be injured easily. Lubricating cream or lotion is applied to soften crusts.

Splints or functional devices may be applied to extremities for contracture control. The principles of care described on page 182 are applicable to prevent damage to nerves and blood vessels.

TABLE 49-6.   WATER AND ELECTROLYTE CHANGES AFTER 5 DAYS CONVALESCENT PHASE

OBSERVATION	EXPLANATION
1. Calcium deficit	Since calcium may be immobilized at the burn site in the slough and early granulation phase of burns, symptoms of calcium deficit may occur rarely.
2. Potassium deficit	Extracellular K^+ moves into the cells, leaving a deficit of K^+ in the extracellular fluid.
3. Negative nitrogen balance (present for several weeks following burns)	Secondary to: Stress reaction Immobilization Inadequate protein intake Protein losses in exudate Direct destruction of protein at burn site
4. Sodium deficit	

Adapted from Metheny, N. M., and Snively, W. D.: Nurses' Handbook of Fluid Balance. Philadelphia, J. B. Lippincott.

At this stage of recovery, attempts are made to establish positive nitrogen balance or anabolism, to promote healing (Table 49-6). Such a balance is achieved with a high-calorie, high-protein diet. Activities of daily living and principles of rehabilitation outlined in Chapter 12 are pursued. If reconstructive surgery is required, principles presented on pages 1070–1077 are applicable.

During the rehabilitation phase, the patient may be aware of unusual sensations, numbness, tingling, tightness, itching, heat sensitivity, and fatigue. Though such sensations are to be expected, they may be annoying. It helps to assure the patient that these feelings are not disabling and will subside with time. Before the patient is discharged, he and his family must be instructed in the care of small unhealed wounds, the general care of healed areas, and the method of carrying out the exercise and splinting program. The patient is encouraged to think about returning to work, school, and normal activities.

Psychosocial rehabilitation is addressed as a continuing process. Adjustments have to be made and bouts of depression and hostility need to be expressed by the patient, but patience, firmness and goal-setting must be continually practiced by the nursing staff and those on the rehabilitation team. Well planned family conferences are most effective in addressing problems of the patient prior to discharge from the hospital.

A possible complication which may occur a few weeks after a burn is the formation of heterotopic bone (a development of calcium deposits near tendons around joints). An early manifestation of beginning ossification is loss of joint function. Laboratory tests which may indicate such calcification are elevated alkaline phosphatase and decreased serum calcium. When x-ray confirms the presence of bone formation, and new formation appears to be halted, surgery may be performed. This is usually not sooner than 6 months after the initial burn injury. Afterwards, splinting, hydrotherapy, and exercises may be required to regain functional activity of the part.

BIBLIOGRAPHY

BOOKS

Aguilera, D. C., and Messic., J. M.: Crisis Intervention, 2nd ed. St. Louis, C. V. Mosby, 1974.

Artz, C., Miller, P., and Bayley, E.: Burns. Chap. 11 in Kintzel, K. C., ed.: Advanced Concepts in Clinical Nursing. Philadelphia, J. B. Lippincott, 1977.

Artz, C. P., and Weeter, J.: Thermal, Chemical, and Electrical Injuries. Chap. 25 in Artz, C. P., et al.: Brief Textbook of Surgery. Philadelphia, W. B. Saunders, 1976.

Artz, C. P., Moncrief, J. A., and Pruitt, B. A.: Burns: A Team Approach. Philadelphia, W. B. Saunders, 1979.

Bernstein, N.: Emotional Care of the Facially Burned and Disfigured. Boston, Little, Brown, 1976.

Feller, I., and Archambeault-Jones, C.: Nursing the Burned Patient. Ann Arbor, Mich. Nat'l. Institute for Burn Medicine, 1973.

Hall, J. E., and Weaver, B. R.: Nursing of Families in Crisis. Philadelphia, J. B. Lippincott, 1974.

Jacoby, F. G.: Nursing Care of the Patient with Burns, 2nd ed. St. Louis, C. V. Mosby, 1976.

Polk, H. C., and Stone, H. H.: Contemporary Burn Management. Boston, Little, Brown, 1971.

Practical Approaches to Burn Management, Flint Laboratories, Div. Travenol Laboratories, Inc., Deerfield, Ill. 1977.

Salisbury, R. E., and Pruitt, B. A.: Burns of the Upper Extremity, Philadelphia, W. B. Saunders, 1976.

ARTICLES

Burns

Allyn, P.: Inhalation Injuries. Crit. Care Quart., 1(3):37-42, Nov. 1978.

Andreasen, N. J. C., et al.: Management of emotional reactions in seriously burned adults. New Eng. J. Med., 286:65-69, Jan. 1, 1972.

Archambeault-Jones, C., and Feller, I.: Burn nursing is nursing. Crit. Care Quart. 1(3):77-92, Nov. 1978.

Artz, C. P., et al.: The burned patient: Current concepts of medical and nursing management. Chapt. 11 in Kintzel, K. C.: Advanced Concepts in Clinical Nursing, 2nd ed. Philadelphia, J. B. Lippincott, 1977, pages 252-271.

Bartlett, R. H., et al.: Rehabilitation following burn injury. Surg. Clin. N. Am., 58:1249-1262, Dec. 1978.

Baxter, C. R.: Problems and complications of burn shock resuscitation. Surg. Clin. N. Am., 58:1313-1322, Dec. 1978.

Baxter, C. R., et al.: The control of burn wound sepsis by the use of quantitative bacteriologic studies in subeschar clysis with antibiotics. Surg. Clin. N. Am., 53:1509-1518, Dec. 1973.

Bowden, M. L., and Feller, I.: Family reaction to a severe burn. AJN, 73:317-319, Feb. 1973.

Burke, J. F.: Use of antibiotics in management of the burn patient. J. Surg. Pract., 7:12-19, May-June 1978.

Burke, J. F., et al.: The contribution of a bacterially isolated environment to the prevention of infection in seriously burned patients. Ann. Surg., 186:377-387, Sept. 1977.

Curreri, P. W., and Luterman, A.: Nutritional support of the burned patient. Surg. Clin. N. Am., 58:1151-1156, Dec. 1978.

Davidson, S. P., and Noyes, R., Jr.: Psychiatric nursing consultation on a burn unit. AJN, 73:1715-1718, Oct. 1973.

Donovan, L.: Polyvinyl chloride: Fighting the secret killer in fires. RN, 41:59-63, Feb. 1978.

Doswell, W. M.: Karen A.: A patient with burns. RN, 40:59-68, May 1977.

Fitzgerald, R. T.: Prehospital care of burned patients. Crit. Care Quart., 1(3):13-24, Nov. 1978.

Fox, C. L., et al.: Topical chemotherapy for burns using cerium salts and silver sulfadiazine. Surg. Gyn. & Obstet., 144:668-672, May 1977.

Furste, W., and Aguirre, A.: Preventing tetanus. AJN, 78:834-837, May 1978.

Haburchak, D. R., et al.: Use of systemic antibiotics in the burned patient. Surg. Clin. N. Am., 53:1119-1132, Dec. 1978.

Harvey, S.: Drugs in burns. Nurse's Drug Alert, 2:154-158, Dec. 1978.

Hersperger, J. E., and Dahl, M. M.: Electrical and chemical injuries. Crit. Care Quart., 1(3):43-49, Nov. 1978.

Imbus, S. H., and Zawacki, B. E.: Autonomy for burned patients when survival is unprecedented. New Eng. J. Med., 297:308-311, Aug. 11, 1977.

Jacoby, F. G.: Individualized burn wound dressings. Nursing '77, 7:62-63, June 1977.

Jones, C. A., and Feller, I.: Burns: What to do during the first crucial hours. Nursing '77, 7:22-31, Mar. 1977.

————: Burns: Avoiding and coping with complications before and after grafting. Nursing '77, 7:72-81, Nov. 1977.

MacMillan, B. G.: Closing the burn wound. Surg. Clin. N. Am., 58:1205-1231, Dec. 1978.

Marvin, J.: Acute care of the burn patient. Crit. Care Quart., 1(3):25-35, Nov. 1978.

McGuire, A.: Prevention of burns. Crit. Care Quart., 1(3):1-11, Nov. 1978.

Mieszala, P.: Postburn psychological adaptation: An overview. Crit. Care Quart., 1(3):93-111, Nov. 1978.

Monafo, W. W., and Ayvazian, V. H.: Topical therapy. Surg. Clin. N. Am., 58:1157-1171, Dec. 1978.

Nathan, P., et al.: A new bromaterial (Hydron) for the control of infection in the burn wound. Trans. Am. Soc. Artif. Intern. Organs, 22:30, 1976.

New dressing aids burn healing. (editoral). JAMA, 236:335-336, July 26, 1976.

Parks, D. H., et al.: Prevention and correction of deformity after severe burns. Surg. Clin. N. Am., 58:1279-1289, Dec. 1978.

Pruitt, B. A., Jr.: Fluid and electrolyte replacement in the burned patient. Surg. Clin. N. Am., 58:1291-1312, Dec. 1978.

Rivers, E. A., et al.: The superiority of the transparent face mask in the prevention of hypertrophic scarring. Abstract 9th Ann. Mtg., Am. Burn Assoc. page 70, 1977.

Rosenthal, A.: Pulmonary problems associated with burn injury. Hosp. Med., 13:108-119, Feb. 1977.

Sato, R. M., et al.: Early excision and closure of the burn wound. Crit. Care Quart., 1(3):51-62, Nov. 1978.

Schumann, L., and Gaston, S.: Commonsense guide to topical burn therapy. Nursing '79, 9:34-39, Mar. 1979.

Shuck, J. M.: Outpatient management of the burned patient. Surg. Clin. N. Am., 58:1107-1117, Dec. 1978.

Stein, J. M., and Stein, E. D.: Safe transfer of civilian burn casualties. JAMA, 238:489-492, Aug. 8, 1977.

Steiner, H., and Clark, W. R.: Psychiatric complication of burned adults. A classification. J. Trauma, 17:134-143, Feb. 1977.

Stoddard, J. E.: Rehabilitation of the burn-injured patient. Crit. Care Quart., 1(3):63-76, Nov. 1978.

Tavis, M. J., et al.: Current status of skin substitutes. Surg. Clin. N. Am., 58:1233-1248, Dec. 1978.

Yarborough, M. F., et al.: 1. Thermal injury: Nutritional management of the severely injured patient. Contemp. Surg., 13:15-20, Aug. 1978.

West, D. A., and Shuck, J. M.: Emotional problems of the severely burned patient. Surg. Clin. N. Am., *58*:1189-1204, Dec. 1978.

Wilmore, D. W., and Aulick, L. H.: Metabolic changes in burned patients. Surg. Clin. N. Am., *58*:1173-1187, Dec. 1978.

Zawacki, B. E.: Reversal of capillary stasis and prevention of necrosis in burns. Ann. Surg., *180*:98-102, July 1974.

AGENCIES

American Burn Association, P. Wm. Curreri, M.D., Sec'y, Dept. of Surgery, Cornell Med. Ctr. — New York Hospital, 525 E. 68th St., New York, N.Y. 10021

International Society for Burn Injuries, c/o John A. Boswick, Jr., M.D., Dept. of Surgery, U. of Colorado Med. Center, 4200 East Ninth Ave., Denver, Col. 80220

National Institute for Burn Medicine, 909 East Ann St., Ann Arbor, Mich. 48104

50

ASSESSMENT AND MANAGEMENT OF PATIENTS WITH ALLERGIC DISORDERS

The human body is menaced by a host of potential invaders—for the most part, microbial organisms—which are constantly threatening its surface defenses. Having penetrated those defenses, these agents compete with the body for its nutrients and, if allowed to flourish unimpeded, disrupt its enzyme systems and destroy its vital tissues. Against these agents, the body is equipped with an elaborate blockade system. The first line of defense consists of the epithelial cells that coat the skin and compose the lining of the respiratory, gastrointestinal, and genitourinary tracts. The structure and continuity of these surfaces and the resistance to penetration are initial deterrents to invaders.

One of the most effective of the body's defense mechanisms is its capacity to equip itself rapidly with weapons (antibodies) individually designed to meet each new invader, namely, specific protein *antigens*. Antibodies react with antigens in a variety of ways: (1) by coating their surface, if they are particulate substances; (2) by neutralizing them, if they are toxic, or (3) by precipitating them out of solution, if they are dissolved. In any event, the antibodies prepare the antigen for handling by the phagocytic cells of the blood and the tissues.

1102

ALLERGIC REACTION: PHYSIOLOGIC OVERVIEW

Immunity

Some people are born with the ability to resist invasion by certain types of foreign agents. Most persons, however, acquire resistance by actually fighting off the invader.

It is also possible to acquire resistance by two other methods:
1. by *actively acquired immunization,* whereby an antigenic substance (one which has lost its ability to produce illness, but is able to stimulate antibody formation) is injected into the body (example: virus vaccine and tetanus toxoid), and
2. by *passively acquired immunization,* whereby resistance is brought about by the transfer of antibody-containing serum from a sensitized donor to a normal recipient (example: human gamma globulin and tetanus antitoxin).

Allergic Reaction

The term *allergy* has historically been defined as "altered reactivity"—that is, the body's response to a substance is different from its original response when initially exposed to that substance. Although such a defi-

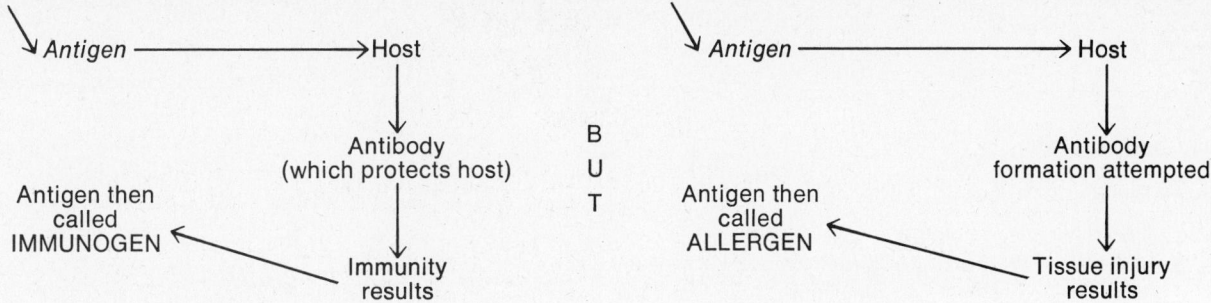

Figure 50-1. Diagram on the left describes the effect of an immunogen; that on the right describes the effect of an allergen.

nition proved to be fairly workable during the first half of this century, concepts and definitions have changed somewhat, as a result of a better understanding of the events which take place when the body recognizes "foreignness." Thus the definition of allergy has changed.

We have come to think of an *allergic reaction* as a manifestation of tissue injury resulting from an immunologic process (an interaction between an antigen and an antibody). When the host is invaded by the antigen, usually a protein which is recognized as foreign, a series of events takes place designed to render the invader harmless and to expel it. If white blood corpuscles of the lymphocyte series respond to such an invasion, antibodies may be produced by these cells.

An *antigen,* then, is any substance which, in the course of repeated contacts with the body, stimulates the body to produce another substance called an *antibody,* capable of combining with it in a very specific manner. This antibody may circulate freely in the blood as globulins or may be "fixed" in the tissues. Ordinarily, the net effect is one of protection of the host, in which case immunity results, and the stimulus is then defined as an *immunogen* (Fig. 50-1A). If, on the other hand, tissue injury results from the body's immune attempt, the stimulus is then defined as an *allergen* (Fig. 50-1B).

Exposure to the specific allergen causes the release of *mediators* (active chemical substances) (Fig. 50-2). These act directly or indirectly on the muscles and glands of the tracheobronchial tree to produce bronchial constriction, excess mucus, and edema. Such chemical mediators include histamine, kinins (polypeptides): serotonin, bradykinin, SRS-a (slow-reacting subsance of anaphylaxis), and acetylcholine.

Immunogens and allergens are usually protein in nature, but occasionally large-molecular-weight carbohydrates may also stimulate the initiation of an immune

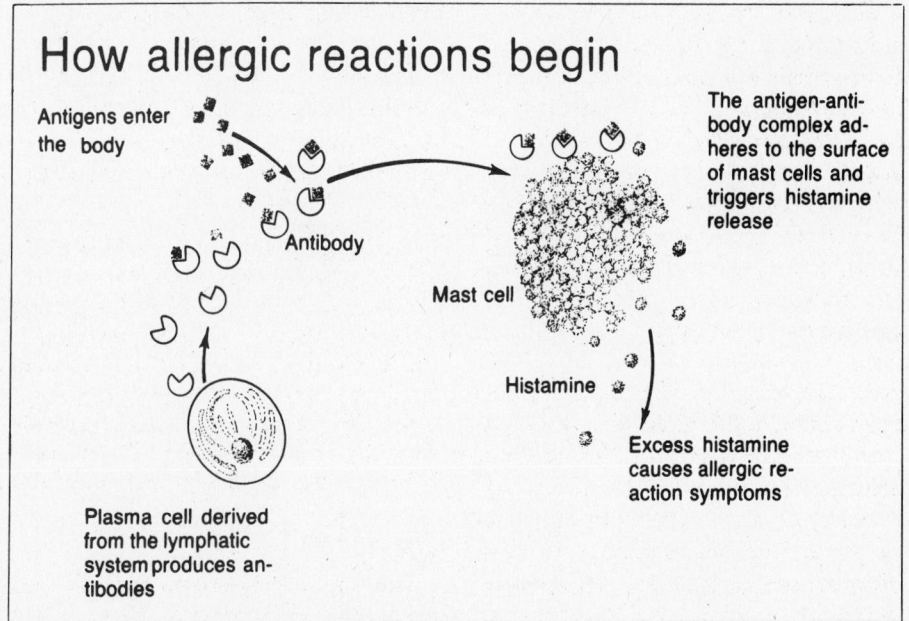

Figure 50-2. How allergic reactions begin. (Patient Care, Sept. 15, 1973, Copyright © 1973, Miller and Fink Corp., Darien, Conn. All rights reserved)

ALLERGY ASSESSMENT SHEET*

Name _____   Age_____ Sex_____ Date_____

I. Chief complaint:

II. Present illness:

III. Collateral allergic symptoms:

Eyes: Pruritus_____ Burning_____ Lacrimation_____
            Swelling_____ Injection_____ Discharge_____
Ears: Pruritus_____ Fullness_____ Popping_____
            Frequent infections_____
Nose: Sneezing_____ Rhinorrhea_____ Obstruction_____
            Pruritus_____ Mouth-breathing_____
            Purulent discharge_____
Throat: Soreness_____ Postnasal discharge_____
            Palatal pruritus_____ Mucus in the morning_____
Chest: Cough _____   Pain _____   Wheezing_____
            Sputum _____   Dyspnea _____
            Color _____   Rest _____
            Amount _____   Exertion _____
Skin: Dermatitis _____   Eczema _____   Urticaria_____

IV. Family allergies:

V. Previous allergic treatment or testing:
Prior skin testing:

Drugs: Antihistamines   Improved _____   Unimproved _____
            Bronchodilators   Improved _____   Unimproved _____
            Nose drops   Improved _____   Unimproved _____
            Hyposensitization Improved _____   Unimproved _____
                Duration _____
                Antigens _____
                Reactions _____
            Antibiotics   Improved _____   Unimproved _____
            Steroids   Improved _____   Unimproved _____

VI. Physical agents and habits:

Bothered by:

Tobacco for _____years   Alcohol _____   Air cond. _____
Cigarettes _____packs/day   Heat _____   Muggy weath. ____
Cigars _____per day   Cold _____   Weath. chngs. ____
Pipe _____per day   Perfumes _____   Chemicals _____
Never smoked _____   Paints _____   Hair spray _____
Bothered by smoke _____   Insecticides _____   Newspapers _____
                                      Cosmetics _____

VII. When symptoms occur:
Time and circumstances of 1st episode:
Prior health:
Course of illness over decades: progressing_____ regressing_____
Time of year: Exact dates
    Perennial_____
    Seasonal_____
    Seasonally exacerbated_____
Monthly variations (menses, occupation):
Time of week (weekends vs. weekdays):
Time of day or night:
After insect stings:

(Continued)

*From Patterson, R.: Allergic Diseases, Philadelphia, J. B. Lippincott.

ALLERGY ASSESSMENT SHEET (CONTINUED)

VIII. Where symptoms occur:
Living where at onset:
Living where since onset:
Effect of vacation or major geographic change:
Symptoms better indoors or outdoors:
Effect of school or work:
Effect of staying elsewhere nearby:
Effect of hospitalization:
Effect of specific environments:
Do symptoms occur around:
old leaves_____ hay_____ lakeside_____ barns_____
summer homes_____ damp basement_____ dry attic_____
lawn mowing_____ animals_____ other_____
Do symptoms occur after eating:
cheese_____ mushrooms_____ beer_____ melons_____
bananas_____ fish_____ nuts_____ citrus fruits_____
other foods (list) _____
Home: city_____ rural_____
house_____ age_____
apartment_____ basement_____ damp_____ dry_____
heating system_____
pets (how long)_____ dog_____ cat_____ other_____

Bedroom:	Type	Age	*Living room:*	Type	Age
Pillow	___	___	Rug	___	___
Mattress	___	___	Matting	___	___
Blankets	___	___	Furniture	___	___
Quilts	___	___			
Furniture	___	___			

Anywhere in home symptoms are worse: _____

IX. What does patient think makes him worse: _____

X. Under what circumstances is he free of symptoms: _____

XI. Summary and additional comments: _____

response. Many small-molecular-weight molecules may unite firmly with a tissue protein, the resultant combination then being recognized as foreign. These small molecules which form a union with proteins are called *haptens*. The metal nickel and many drugs such as penicillin are examples of haptens.

Immunoglobulins

Antibodies which are formed by lymphocytes and plasma cells in response to an immunogenic stimulus comprise a group of serum proteins called *immunoglobulins*. These can be found in lymph nodes, tonsils, the appendix, and Peyer's patches of the intestinal tract, or they may be found circulating in the blood and lymph. These antibodies combine with antigens in very special ways which have been likened to keys fitting into a lock. Antigens (keys) only fit certain antibodies (locks), hence the term *specificity* has been coined in relation to the specific reaction of an antibody to an antigen. There are many variations and complexities in these patterns.

Antibody molecules are bivalent, which means that they have two combining sites. Because of this, the antibody easily becomes a crosslink between two antigen groups, causing them to clump together (agglutination). By this action, invaders in the bloodstream are cleared. Agglutination is the means of determining blood group in laboratory tests.

There are five classes of immunoglobulins, designated as follows: IgG, IgA, IgM, IgD, and IgE. Antibodies of the IgM, IgG, and IgA classes have definite and well-established protective functions. These include neutralization of toxins and viruses and precipitation, agglutination, or lysis of bacteria and other foreign cellular material.

IgM ("gamma-M") is the largest molecule, which tends to stay in the bloodstream and is thus primarily engaged in defense in the intravascular compartment, such as in bloodstream infections. If it occurs in a pregnant woman, it will not cross the placenta from the mother to the fetus. Thus the finding of a high concentration of IgM in the newborn circulation is suggestive of an intrauterine infection.

IgG ("gamma-G"), the most abundant of the immunoglobulins, is one of the smallest immunoglobulins and thus can diffuse readily into the tissue spaces to assist in combating tissue toxins or infections. IgG has the property of crossing the placenta, so that antibodies of this family provide the baby with temporary immunity to many common diseases.

IgA ("gamma-A") circulates in the blood, but its role in that compartment of the body is uncertain. It is distinct in that it is produced in the external secretion, where it provides a primary defense mechanism. IgA is found in saliva, tears, and the respiratory, genitourinary, and gastrointestinal tracts.

The function of *IgD* ("gamma-D") has not yet been determined. It is small, like IgG, and has a molecular pattern distinct from the other known immunoglobulins.

IgE ("gamma-E"), the most recently described immunoglobulin, is responsible for most of the immediate types of allergic reactions which will be discussed later. It is present only in minute amounts in the blood serum. (In the normal person, one of 5,000 immunoglobulin molecules are of this class.) The unique feature of IgE is its great affinity for attaching to human epithelium.

A protective role for immunoglobulin-E has not yet been established, but it has been postulated that antibodies in this class may play a role in ridding the host of certain parasites. Deficiency of IgE has been associated with increased susceptibility to infection. The most important aspect regarding IgE is its association with immediate allergic reactions of the anaphylactic type. These reactions appear within minutes of an injection of antigen into a person having anaphylactic antibodies (or after two hours, if precipitin antibodies are present).

Delayed Hypersensitivity

The above reaction is in contrast to delayed hypersensitivity, which occurs when an antigen is brought into contact with the skin surface of a sensitized individual, with the inflammatory reaction reaching its peak within 24 to 48 hours. The reaction consists of erythema and induration.

Delayed hypersensitivity is mediated not by circulating immunoglobulins (described above) but rather by sensitized "T" (thymus-dependent) lymphocytes. Such lymphocytes, when stimulated on a second or subsequent occasion, elaborate a variety of factors which enhance the host's defense mechanism. The tuberculin skin test is an example of a delayed hypersensitivity reaction,

and advantage is taken of this action for diagnostic purposes. Also contact dermatitis (dermatitis venenata), such as poison ivy, detergent allergy, and skin reactions to a variety of chemicals, including medications, is an example of tissue injury resulting from re-exposure of a sensitized individual.

ATOPIC DISORDERS

Atopic disorders (allergic rhinitis, bronchial asthma, allergic dermatoses) are allergic manifestations which occur in persons who are genetically predisposed to forming *reagin,* a special antibody of the IgE class, when exposed to a variety of environmental allergens. Such allergens include various plant pollens, mole spores, domestic animal danders, and some foods. An estimated 7 to 10 percent of the population are subject to atopic disorders. The family history of related allergies can usually be elicited, but this is not always the case. There is recent evidence to show that the immune response gene resides near the HLA (tissue-type) locus on the chromosome. (HLA stands for Histocompatibility Locus Antigen and pertains to compatibility of tissue; that is, whether the recipient can tolerate a particular graft.)

If a sensitized individual is re-exposed to an allergen to which he has become sensitive, there is a release of histamine and other mediators which have a prompt and profound effect upon the tissues of the affected organ. These include dilatation of the walls of small blood vessels with loss of fluid from the blood into the tissue, causing swelling. There is also constriction of the smooth muscles surrounding the bronchi and the gastrointestinal tract. While clinical manifestations of atopy are most frequently caused by antigen-antibody interactions, some are initiated by other mechanisms. Nonspecific factors such as autonomic nervous system imbalance, hormonal disturbances, psychic factors, exertion, and changes in barometric pressure may result in tissue changes which mimic allergic reactions.

Nursing Management. The chief problems for the nurse are to get the patient to avoid medications or attitudes that can aggravate his condition. The nurse must understand the patient with an allergy, offering necessary services and lending an interested, friendly ear, as well as showing empathy for his problems. In the many contacts with the patient, the nurse gathers enough data and impressions to characterize the patient fairly accurately from the psychological standpoint, to discern with clarity the environment in which he habitually dwells, and to discover what factors are most important from the standpoint of "triggering" attacks. An assessment sheet such as is presented on pages 1104–1105 is effective in providing this information.

The nurse must be prepared to meet the dangerous

emergency that allergy creates on occasion in the form of anaphylactic shock or fulminating asthma, when swift and effective countermeasures may spell the difference between life and death.

ALLERGIC RHINITIS ("HAY FEVER," CHRONIC ALLERGIC RHINITIS, POLLINOSIS)

Allergic rhinitis is the most common form of respiratory allergy. It affects approximately 8 to 10 percent of the U.S. population. When untreated, many complications may result such as allergic asthma, chronic nasal obstruction, chronic otitis media with hearing loss, anosmia (absence of the sense of smell), and, in children, orofacial dental deformities. Consequently, early diagnosis and adequate treatment is strongly recommended.

Since allergic rhinitis is induced by airborne pollens, it is characterized by seasonal occurrences (see also Table 50-1):

TIME	SOURCE	EXAMPLE
Early spring	tree pollen	oak, elm, poplar
Early summer "rose-fever"	grass pollen	timothy, red top
Early fall	weed pollen	ragweed

Each year the attacks begin and end approximately on the same dates. (For pathophysiology, see page 113.)

Clinical Manifestations. Usually the rhinitis starts in the mucous membrane of the nose, which may become so edematous and swollen that the nostrils are closed completely. The nasal mucous membrane itches, burns, and secretes a thin irritating discharge. Violent paroxysms of sneezing are the rule. The eyes are usually involved, becoming red, and burning and lacrimating. During the "off season" a nasal examination reveals normal findings.

Management

The most effective treatment of allergic rhinitis, if the nasal passages and the paranasal sinuses are otherwise normal, and especially if the attacks began in childhood, is a seasonal change of climate. When and where, however, depends on the experience of the individual.

Nasal sprays containing ephedrine help some persons. Sinusitis or other nasal lesions that may be present should be treated thoroughly during the free seasons. Various eyewashes relieve the conjunctivitis.

The patient's hypersensitivity to the pollens that induce the attacks can usually be confirmed by proper skin, conjunctival, or intradermal tests. These reactions are not necessarily specific. A positive skin test does not necessarily mean that symptoms are due to that antigen. When properly performed and interpreted, these tests are quite specific in demonstrating reagin to the antigen in question. Accurate identification of the offending antigen, of course, depends upon close correlation with the patient's history.

Pharmacotherapy

Underlying Principle. Histamine is found in all body tissue and fluid and is concentrated in skin, lung, and gastrointestinal tissue. An enzyme, histidine decarboxylase, catalyzes histamine biosynthesis from histidine (a precursor amino acid). Histamine is concentrated in mast cells and basophils. When these are degranulated (histamine has been discharged) by certain agents, an anaphylacticlike reaction occurs. Hence the mast cell is considered the major target cell in acute allergic reactions.

Antihistamines. The basic structure of antihistamines is a substituted ethylamine.

Examples:
    Ethanolamine (Benadryl, Decapryn)
    Ethylenediamine (Pyribenzamine, Histadyl)
    Alkalamine (Chlor-Trimeton, Dimetane)

Antihistamines given orally are readily absorbed. They are most effective when given at the first signs of symptoms, since they prevent the development of new symptoms by preventing further histamine release. In actual practice, the effectiveness of these drugs is limited to certain patients with hay fever, vasomotor rhinitis, urticaria, and mild asthma; they are rarely effective in other conditions or in severe conditions of any sort. Side effects vary with the individual; therefore, individualization of dosage is required. Of the side effects, the most common are dryness of the mouth, dizziness, irritability, drowsiness, and gastrointestinal upset. These are often mild and temporary. Steroid hormones frequently are very helpful in ameliorating manifestations of allergy.

Azatadine maleate (Optimine) is a new potent antihistamine drug that is purported to offer longer-lasting relief than other antihistamines. The medication acts like other antihistamines and also dries secretions. The drug's antiserotonin activity helps relieve severe itching and reduces blocked nasal passages. The chief side effects are drowsiness and possibly dizziness, fatigue, and disturbed coordination. Since it may cause thickening of bronchial secretions, it is not recommended for patients with asthma and other chronic obstructive pulmonary conditions.

Sympathomimetic Drugs. The sympathomimetic drugs simulate the effects of the sympathetic nervous system.

The major agents are norepinephrine (noradrenaline) and epinephrine (Adrenalin). There are synthetic sympathomimetic drugs which have more specific actions, act longer, and may be taken orally—examples: isoproterenol (Isuprel) and phenylephrine (Neo-Synephrine). The major agents mentioned cannot be taken

TABLE 50-1. APPROXIMATE TIME OF APPEARANCE OF MAJOR POLLENS AND MOLDS IN VARIOUS REGIONS OF THE U.S.*

REGION	JAN.	FEB.	MAR.	APR.	MAY	JUNE	JULY	AUG.	SEPT.	OCT.	NOV.	DEC.
Northeast				Elm Maple	Oak	Grass	Alternaria †Hormod.	Ragweed Alternaria Hormod.	Ragweed Alternaria Hormod.	Alternaria Hormod.		
Southeast		Elm	Ash Maple	Oak Sycamore	Pecan Oak Bermuda grass	Bermuda grass Hormod.	Alternaria Hormod.	Ragweed Alternaria Hormod.	Ragweed Alternaria Hormod.	Ragweed Alternaria Hormod.	Hormod.	
North Central				Elm Maple	Oak	Grass Hormod.	Alternaria Hormod.	Ragweed Alternaria Hormod.	Ragweed Alternaria Hormod.	Alternaria Hormod.		
South Central		Elm	Oak Maple Sycamore	Pecan Alternaria	Bermuda grass Alternaria Hormod.	Bermuda grass Alternaria Hormod.	Alternaria Hormod.	Alternaria Hormod.	Ragweed Alternaria Hormod.	Ragweed Alternaria		
Plains			Maple	Cottonwood		Grass Hormod.	Russian thistle Kochia Hormod.	Ragweed Russian thistle Kochia Hormod. Alternaria	Ragweed Sagebrush			
Southwest	Alternaria	Alternaria Cottonwood	Alternaria Ash Mountain cedar	Alternaria Bermuda grass False ragweed	Bermuda grass	Bermuda grass Hormod.		Alternaria Russian thistle Kochia	Alternaria Russian thistle Kochia	Alternaria		
Intermountain Basin			Elm	Cottonwood	Sycamore	Grass		Russian thistle Kochia	Sagebrush			
Pacific Coast North			Alder	Maple Oak	Grass	Grass Plantain	Grass					
Pacific Coast South	Alternaria		Oak Walnut	Oak Walnut Olive	Bermuda grass	Bermuda grass	Bermuda grass	Various ‡Compos.	Elm Compos.	Elm Compos. Alternaria	Alternaria	Alternaria

*There is some variation from year to year. Locations in the northern part of the region usually lag behind locations in the southern parts. Small amounts of the various pollens and molds often are present before and after the season indicated in the table. Bermuda grass, which flourishes in the South, contains different antigens from the northern grasses, but the two regions overlap somewhat. There are many aero-allergens which are not listed which occur in small amounts or in restricted locations.

†Hormod.: Hormodendrum
‡Compos.: Compositae
(From Asthma, A Practical Guide for Physicians. American Lung Association in cooperation with the Allergy Foundation of America, 1973)

orally, since they are destroyed in the gastrointestinal tract.

Sympathomimetic drugs cause constriction of smooth muscle in skin, viscera, and mucous membranes and induce dilatation of muscular vasculature, bronchodilatation, and cardiac stimulation. Consequently, they reduce edema of the nasal mucous membrane, but they may induce nervousness and insomnia when given in large doses. Therefore, their use is recommended with caution in patients who have hypertension, heart disease, and hyperthyroidism.

The nurse must be aware of the effects caused by overuse of sympathomimetic agents in nose drops or sprays. A condition referred to as "rhinitis medicamentosa" may result. After topical application of the drug, a rebound period may occur in which the nasal mucous membranes become more edematous and congested than they were before the medication was used. Such a reaction encourages the use of more drug. A circular pattern of activity results much like a "cat chasing its tail." The topical agent must be discontinued immediately in order to correct this problem.

Rhinitis Medicamentosa

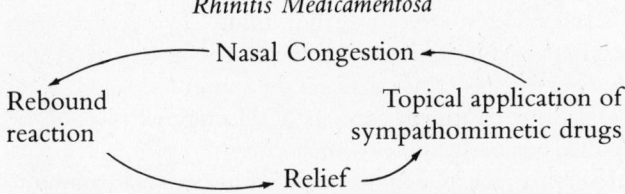

Systemic sympathomimetic drugs may be substituted. These agents must be used with caution in patients with hypertension, cardiovascular disease, diabetes, and thyroid disease.

Immunologic Management

Allergic reactions are triggered by the release of chemical mediators following the reaction of a specific antigen (example: ragweed, house dust) with its specific antibody (Fig. 50-2). To prevent this reaction, two methods of approach are possible: (1) avoidance of any exposure to the antigen (avoidance therapy), and (2) immunotherapy, or hyposensitization, which is an attempt to elevate the threshold level of the appearance of symptoms.

Avoidance Therapy

In avoidance therapy every attempt is made to remove those allergens which act as precipitating factors. For example, allergy due to animal dander would require that the pet be removed from the home environment and that feather pillows be replaced with a hypoallergenic Dacron pillow.

Aeroallergens are most difficult to avoid, since they are so widely distributed; however, the immediate surroundings may be altered. For example, irritating pol-

lens, dusts, and molds can be avoided by remaining in a building that has central air conditioning with an electrostatic precipitating filter. The limitation here is that one cannot remain indoors all the time. Without such a controlled environment, the rooms where the person spends most of his time can be modified. Mattress and box springs should be encased in elastic fabric casings; upholstered furniture, stuffed toys, chenille bedspreads, etc. should be removed from the bedroom. Another method is to travel to areas where the offending allergen is absent during certain times of the year. This method is becoming less effective (as well as expensive), since the atmosphere is becoming increasingly filled with allergens.

Sensitivity Tests and Immunotherapy (Hyposensitization)

A knowledge of the general concepts regarding therapy in allergic diseases is important, since the nurse is very apt to be an active participant in the treatment of these disorders and will almost certainly be in the position to advise patients who are potential candidates for one or another of these procedures.

Skin Tests. The most common method of treatment is the serial injection of one or more antigens which are selected in each particular case on the basis of *skin tests*. Skin testing (Fig. 50-3) entails the simultaneous intradermal inoculation (or superficial application), at separate sites, of several solutions containing individual antigens which comprise an assortment of those allergens deemed most likely to be implicated in the patient's disease. A positive reaction, evidenced by the appearance of an urticarial wheal (Fig. 50-4) or by localized erythema in the area of inoculation or contact, is regarded as evidence of sensitivity to the corresponding antigen.

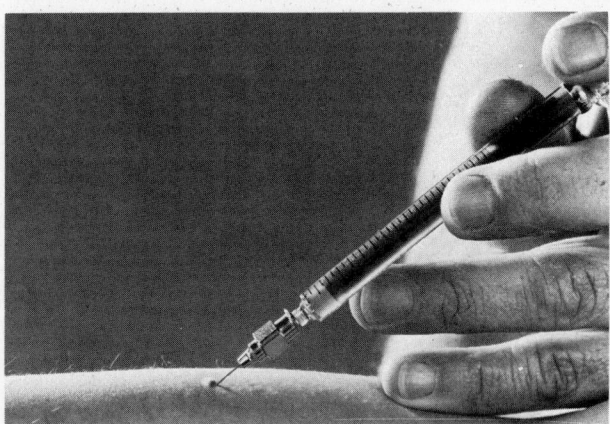

Figure 50-3. Intradermal testing. Cleanse the testing site with alcohol or ether. Tests are made on the volar surface of the lower arm and the outer surface of upper arm, omitting the antecubital space. Intradermal tests are limited to 10 or 20 at most. (Courtesy, Hollister-Stier Laboratories)

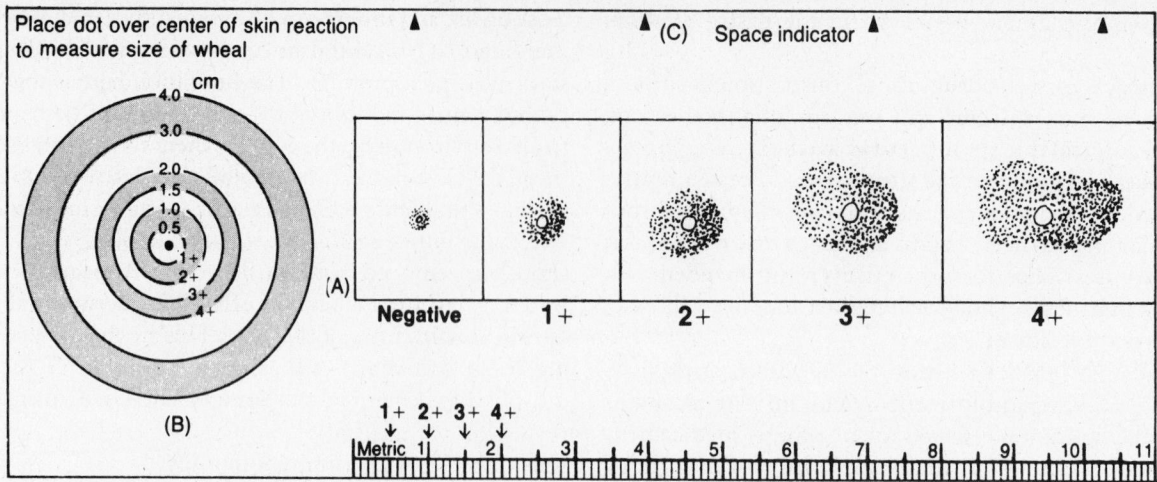

Figure 50-4. (A) These series of reactions indicate the sizes of wheals when the allergist refers to them as 1+, 2+, etc. A negative reaction is shown at the left. (B) The target wheal guide can be traced on a transparent sheet (acetate or x-ray film) and then placed over the wheal to measure the size in centimeters or according to plus-size. The relationship between the two is indicated on the lower metric scale. (C) Showing placement of test sites spaced uniformly. (Patient Care: Sept. 15, 1973, Copyright © 1973, Miller and Fink Corp., Darien, Conn. All rights reserved)

Skin tests lend important weight to other evidence obtained from the patient's history, indicating which of several antigens are most likely to provoke symptoms and providing some clue to the intensity of the patient's sensitization.

The dosage of the pollen injected is important also; the majority of patients are hypersensitive not to one but several pollens, and under testing conditions, they may not react to the specific pollens that induce their attacks, but they usually do. Ragweed seems to be the most potent of all. If there is any doubt regarding the validity of the skin test, a RAST (page 1111) may be done, or a provocative challenge of the suspected antigen to the shock organ tissue can be carried out. An example is applying the antigen to an affected organ such as the conjunctiva, nasal or bronchial mucosa, or gastrointestinal tract, and observing the response which follows.

Immunotherapy. Correlation of a positive skin test with a positive history is an indication for immunotherapy *if* the allergen cannot be avoided. The value of such injections has been fairly well established in those instances of allergic rhinitis and bronchial asthma that are clearly due to sensitivity to one of the common pollens or molds or to house dust. Although referred to as a "hyposensitization" procedure, the effects are very probably attributable to the opposite process, i.e., immunization, for it appears to stimulate the production of a new antibody with the capacity of neutralizing the allergy-provoking properties of the responsible allergen.

Immunotherapy, while helpful in a majority of patients, does not cure the condition. Before such a program is launched, the physician discusses with the patient what may be expected from immunotherapy and why it is important to continue the therapy for several years. When skin tests are done, they are to be correlated with clinical manifestations; the treatment is based on the patient's needs rather than on the skin tests.

Specific treatment consists of injecting extracts of the pollens or mold spores which cause symptoms in a particular patient. Injections begin with very small amounts and are gradually increased, usually at weekly intervals, until a maximum tolerated dose is attained. Maintenance "booster" injections are then given at 2- to 4-week intervals, frequently for a period of several years, before maximum benefit is achieved.

There are three methods of injection therapy: coseasonal, preseasonal, and perennial. When treatment is given on a *coseasonal basis,* it is initiated during the season when the patient experiences symptoms. This method has been used less widely in recent years; it is not an effective form of therapy, and there is increased risk of systemic reactions. *Preseasonal therapy* injections are given 2 to 3 months before symptoms appear, allowing time for hyposensitization to take place. This treatment is discontinued after the season. *Perennial therapy* is administered all year round, usually on a monthly basis, and is the preferred method because of more effective, longer-lasting results.

Precautions. Since there is a possibility that an injection of allergen may induce systemic reactions, it is only given in a physician's office where epinephrine is immediately available. Because of the dangers involved, injections ought not to be given by a lay person or by the patient himself. The patient is to remain in the physician's office for a minimum of 20 to 30 minutes and is observed for the possible development of systemic symptoms. If a large local swelling develops, the next dose should not be increased, since this may be a warning of a possible systemic reaction.

Complications. A systemic reaction is a serious complication which ranges from mild hives to an acute asthmatic attack, hypotension, or even anaphylactic shock. Emergency treatment is presented on page 1118.

RAST. The radioallergosorbent test (RAST) is a recently described technique for the laboratory determination of the presence of IgE antibodies in serum. The sensitivity of this procedure correlates very well with carefully conducted skin tests in the detection of immediate-type hypersensitivity. The RAST test is probably no more specific than direct skin testing but may be used to corroborate skin-test findings, especially in questionable cases. The RAST test may also substitute for skin testing when the latter may be considered hazardous or when a generalized dermatitis may preclude direct skin testing.

ALLERGIC DERMATOSES

Contact Dermatitis

Contact dermatitis (dermatitis venenata) is an inflammatory, often eczematous condition caused by a skin reaction to a variety of irritating or allergenic materials. Almost any substance can produce contact dermatitis. Poison ivy is probably the most common and best example; cosmetics, soaps, detergents and industrial chemicals are frequent offenders. The skin sensitivity may develop after brief or prolonged periods of exposure, and a clinical picture may appear hours or weeks after the sensitized skin has been exposed.

The symptoms include itching, burning, erythema, vesiculation, and edema, followed by weeping, crusting, and finally a drying up and peeling of the skin. In very severe responses, hemorrhagic bullae may develop. Repeated reactions may be accompanied by the development of thickening of the skin and pigmentary changes.

Secondary invasion by bacteria may develop in skin abraded by rubbing or scratching. Usually there are no systemic symptoms unless the eruption is widespread.

Diagnosis may sometimes be made easily on the basis of the location of the eruption and history of exposure. But in cases of obscure irritants or an unobservant patient, diagnosis may be extremely difficult, and many trial-and-error procedures may be involved before the etiology is correctly determined. Patch tests on the skin with suspected offending agents may clarify the picture.

The most important aspect of treatment is to remove the patient from further contact with the irritant or allergen. Burow's solution soaks (aluminum acetate) soothe the blistered erythematous skin and may be followed by corticosteroid ointments or creams. Antimicrobials are given if secondary invasion is present.

Atopic Dermatitis. Atopic dermatitis is chronic, pruritic, and familial in nature. It principally involves the skin of the neck, the face, and the flexural creases (Fig. 50-5) and will wax and wane in activity. It has a more prolonged course than simple contact dermatitis. It is frequently associated with allergic respiratory disorders, but the true cause remains unknown. Family history is usually positive for allergies such as allergic rhinitis, asthma, or eczema. Drying of the skin is an aggravating factor; wool and lanolin commonly compound the skin irritation of these patients. Allergy to foods has probably been overstressed but is, nonetheless, a factor. Emotional stress and nervousness aggravate the condition. The principles of treatment are the same as for contact dermatitis.

Drug Reactions (Dermatitis Medicamentosa)

Dermatitis medicamentosa is the term applied to skin rashes induced by the internal administration of certain drugs. While, as a rule, certain drugs tend to induce eruptions of similar types, individuals react differently to each of them.

In general, it may be said that drug rashes appear suddenly, have a particularly vivid color, present characteristics that are more spectacular than the somewhat similar eruptions of infectious origin, and, with the ex-

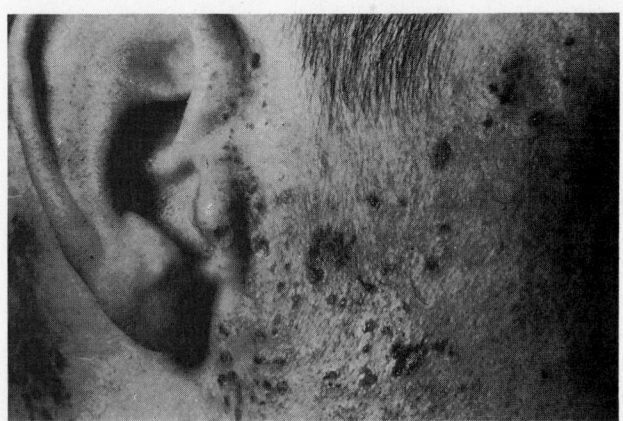

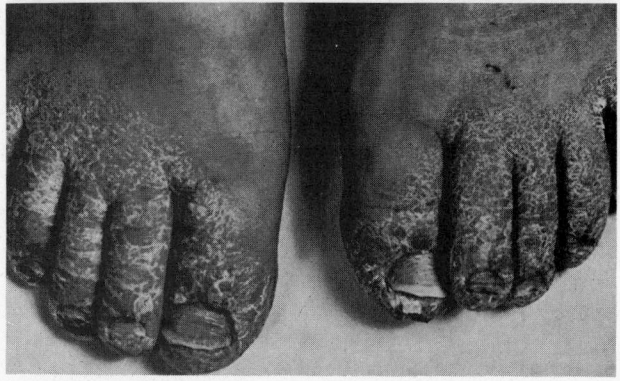

Figure 50-5. Atopic eczema. (From Sauer, G. C.: Manual of Skin Diseases. Philadelphia, J. B. Lippincott)

ception of the bromide and the iodide rashes, disappear rapidly after the drug is withdrawn. Some drug rashes are accompanied by constitutional symptoms. Upon discovery of a drug allergy, the patient is warned that he reacts peculiarly to a particular drug and is advised not to take it again. The nurse has an important responsibility in relation to drug eruptions, for these lesions offer a clue to more serious idiosyncrasies. By being in a primary position of initial contact with the patient, the nurse is able to report the appearance of the eruption so that early treatment is initiated.

Urticaria and Angioneurotic Edema

Urticaria (hives) is an allergic affection of the skin characterized by the sudden appearance of pinkish edematous elevations, which vary in size and shape, and itch and smart. They may involve any part of the body, including the mucous membranes, especially those of the mouth, the larynx (occasionally with serious respiratory complications), and the gastrointestinal tract. Each hive remains for a period varying from a few minutes to several hours, then disappears. For hours or days, crops of these lesions may come, go, and return, in a most capricious manner. If this sequence continues indefinitely, the condition is called *chronic urticaria*.

The swellings of angioneurotic edema involve the deeper layers of the skin, resulting in more diffuse swelling, rather than the discrete lesions characteristic of hives. On occasion, one may be seen that covers the entire back. The skin over it may appear normal, but often it has a reddish hue. It does not pit on pressure, as ordinary edema does. The regions most often involved are lips, eyelids, cheeks, hands, feet, genitalia, and tongue; also, the mucous membranes of the larynx, the bronchi, and the gastrointestinal canal may be affected, particularly in cases of the hereditary type. An eye may be completely closed; one lip may become so large that eating is impossible; one hand may become so huge that the fingers cannot be flexed. These swellings may appear suddenly, in a few seconds or minutes, or slowly, in 1 or 2 hours. In the latter case, their appearance often is preceded by itching or burning sensations. Seldom does more than a single swelling appear at one time, although one may develop while another is disappearing. Only infrequently do they recur in the same region. The individual lesions usually last from 24 to 36 hours. On rare occasions they recur with a remarkable periodicity at intervals of 3 or 4 weeks.

The swellings of angioneurotic edema along the gastrointestinal canal may cause acute crises of pain with vomiting, which suggest acute appendicitis, acute cholecystitis, renal colic, or intussusception; those in the throat (edema of the glottis) are especially critical because they may result in sudden suffocation.

Management. Many patients are relieved by anti-histamine drugs; others require injections of epinephrine. Corticosteroids usually give rapid resolution. Tracheostomy becomes necessary if laryngeal edema threatens to obstruct the glottis.

Hereditary Angioedema

Hereditary angioedema, although not an immunologic disorder in the usual sense, is included in this section because of its resemblance to allergic angioedema and because of the seriousness of this condition. Symptoms are due to edema of the skin, the respiratory tract, or the digestive tract. Attacks may be precipitated by trauma or may seem to occur spontaneously.

When the skin is involved, the swelling is usually rather diffuse, does not itch, and usually is not accompanied by urticaria. Gastrointestinal edema may cause abdominal pain severe enough to suggest the need for surgery. Edema of the upper respiratory tract may cause marked swelling of the uvula and of the larynx, resulting in suffocation. Acute laryngeal edema is the most serious manifestation of this disorder and has resulted in death due to asphyxiation in nearly 20 percent of these patients. Attacks usually subside within 3 to 4 days, but during this time the patient should be observed carefully for signs of laryngeal obstruction, which may necessitate tracheostomy as a life-saving measure. Epinephrine, antihistamines, and corticosteroids are usually employed in treatment, but the success of these agents is limited.

GASTROINTESTINAL ALLERGY

To a few persons, certain common foods are veritable poisons. There are those who cannot eat strawberries or shellfish without an attack of urticaria. Some people cannot eat pork or cheese, no matter how well disguised these foods may be. They vomit immediately or have diarrhea, often accompanied by considerable pain (owing, it is surmised, to urticarial lesions along the gastrointestinal mucosa). Often asthma and urticaria result as well.

BRONCHIAL ASTHMA

Asthma is a reversible form of bronchial obstruction characterized by paroxysmal wheezing, dyspnea, (predominantly expiratory in type), coughing, and sputum production. A hereditary tendency seems to be present in two-thirds of all patients. Attacks of allergic rhinitis in about 50 percent of all patients end as asthma. In adults, asthma is frequently preceded by upper respiratory infection, usually viral.

The stimuli of asthma are of four different kinds: extrinsic, intrinsic, mixed (extrinsic and intrinsic), and aspirin-sensitive (Table 50-2). Other causes are listed in Table 50-3.

TABLE 50-2. TYPES OF ASTHMA STIMULI

TYPES	CAUSATIVE AGENTS	CLINICAL FEATURES
1. Extrinsic (atopic)	Inhalant allergen causes an immediate allergic reaction Infection of the respiratory tract	Age: 5-40 High family incidence Skin-testing produces wheal-and-flare reaction Often seasonal Prognosis—good
2. Intrinsic (nonatopic)	Usually unknown (idiopathic), aggravated by respiratory-tract infection, irritating fumes, weather changes, emotions	Age: children below 3; adults over 40 No familial inheritance Skin-testing—negative Often associated with infections, emotional upsets, exertion, cold air Prognosis: less favorable; condition becomes chronic
3. Mixed (extrinsic and intrinsic)	Extrinsic and infectious factors coexist	Variable, depending upon which factor is predominant
4. Aspirin-sensitive	Aspirin intolerance	Resembles intrinsic type Age: 3rd decade—rhinitis and polyposis occur followed by asthma in 4th or 5th decade Aspirin causes urticaria and may continue to anaphylaxislike reactions Nonatopic

Clinical Manifestations

The asthmatic attack starts suddenly with coughing and a sensation of tightness in the chest. Then slow, laborious, wheezy breathing begins. Expiration is always much more strenuous and prolonged than inspiration, which forces the patient to sit upright and use every accessory muscle of respiration. He becomes blue from hypoxia and breaks out into a profuse sweat; the pulse is weak; the extremities are cold; there may be fever, and, occasionally, pain, nausea, vomiting, and diarrhea. The cough at first is tight and dry, but it soon becomes more violent; a distinctive sputum of thin mucus containing small round gelatinous masses is coughed up with much difficulty. The gelatinous masses are the "pearls of Laennec," which are molds of the smaller bronchi and contain Curschmann's spirals. The attack may last from one-half to several hours. Under certain circumstances, the attack may subside spontaneously, but this should not be counted upon. Such attacks are rarely fatal. However, occasionally "status asthmaticus" occurs, in which therapeutic measures fail and the patient has repeated attacks or continuous asthma. This condition is life-threatening (see page 1117).

Related Reactions. Allergic reactions related to asthma include: eczema (present at some time during life in 75 percent of asthma patients), urticaria, and angioneurotic edema (present in 50 percent of patients). Emotional stress may bring on an attack in those who are susceptible, just as any other organ system in the body may be stimulated by psychic factors.

Assessment

A clear history of hypersensitivity (at home or at work) to some known substance that may be inhaled or ingested, such as a pollen, a particular type of food, feathers, animal hair, face powder, etc., or a history suggesting the probability of such a sensitivity is very important in determining the type and cause of asthma presented in any given patient. The close association of the attacks with allergic rhinitis, together with the discovery, during the attack, of marked pallor and swelling of the nasal mucous membrane, aids in establishing the case as one of extrinsic allergic asthma. The finding of an abnormally high count of eosinophilic cells in the blood or the sputum tends to confirm this diagnostic impression. Blood gas evaluation and simple spirometry are useful in evaluating gas exchange and providing baseline data.

In an acute asthmatic attack, initial assessment is directed toward answering the following questions: How long has acute wheezing taken place? (If several days, the treatment will probably require hospitalization.) Can the patient use long sentences in responding to a question, or does he reply in short phrases, as he tries to get his breath? Can he speak at all?

However, "all that wheezes is not asthma," and it is important to be able to rule out congestive cardiac failure or bronchial obstruction due to a foreign body or a tumor as the underlying cause or precipitating factor that may explain the attack. Hence the necessity for careful radiologic and, often, bronchoscopic examination in every case of doubtful origin.

TABLE 50-3. INITIATING, AGGRAVATING, AND PERPETUATING FACTORS IN BRONCHIAL ASTHMA

MECHANISM-ASSOCIATION	SETTING	DIAGNOSTIC STUDY	TREATMENT
Immunologic			
Immediate hypersensitivity (reagin-mediated)	Exposure to inhalant, ingestant, or injected allergens precipitates asthmatic episode. Frequently associated rhinoconjunctivitis, urticaria, or anaphylaxis	Wheal-flare skin tests Inhalation/ingestion challenge	Avoidance of allergen Hyposensitization Symptomatic
Humoral antibody mediated	Microbial colonization or organic dust contamination of the bronchial tree	Sputum smear/culture Serum precipitins Inhalation challenge	Antimicrobial Corticosteroid Avoidance of allergen
Infection			
Sinusitis	Obstruction of sinus drainage by inflammatory, allergic, or vasomotor reaction, or a combination of these	Transillumination Sinus x-rays Culture of aspirate	Drainage Antimicrobial
Upper-respiratory tract infection	Relapse of asthma coincides/follows "head cold"	Nose-pharynx examination Viral culture Viral serology	Symptomatic
Purulent sputum	Relapse of asthma coincides/follows change of sputum production/color	Sputum/transtracheal Smears, cultures	Antimicrobial Symptomatic
Postviral onset	"Flulike" syndrome evolves into persistent cough, then asthma	Viral serology	Symptomatic
Aspirin Intolerance	Severe asthmatic episode follows ingestion of aspirin. Frequently associated nasal polyps and sinusitis	If history negative, cautious aspirin challenge	Avoidance of aspirin Corticosteroids
Isoproterenol abuse syndrome	Increased use (frequency and dose) of nebulizer with decreased symptom relief	Isoproterenol inhalation challenge	Discontinue isoproterenol
Irritant inhalation	Smoke or other irritant exposure	History	Avoidance Symptomatic
Exercise	Increased physical activity	Treadmill exercise provocation	Exercise modification Symptomatic
Atmospheric change	Temperature, humidity, or barometric pressure change	History	Symptomatic
Emotional	Emotional upset precedes relapse of asthma (not vice versa)	History	Symptomatic Psychotherapy
Associated disease			
Chronic bronchitis and emphysema	Acute bronchitis Precipitation of respiratory failure	Pulmonary function (irreversible airways obstruction, loss of elastic recoil)	As indicated
Cardiac disease ("cardiac asthma")	Cardiac failure	As indicated	As indicated
Esophageal disorder	Motility disturbance, acid reflux	As indicated	As indicated
Carcinoid tumor	Bronchial or systemic release of serotonin	Urinary 5-hydroxy indoleacetic acid	Surgery Symptomatic
Bronchial obstruction	Localized bronchial obstruction (foreign body, neoplasm)	Bronchoscopy	Surgery
Pulmonary embolus	Venous stasis/thrombosis	As indicated	As indicated
Unknown	Not recognized	Any of above if indicated	Symptomatic

(Source: Mathison, D. A., et al.: Clinical profiles of bronchial asthma. JAMA, *224*:1135, May 21, 1973)

Management

It should be remembered that asthma is a syndrome which may be produced by many widely different factors. However, the emotional response is more generalized. The hypoxic patient is understandably very anxious, and it is necessary that those who are in attendance relieve the patient's anxiety by acting calmly and confidently and, most importantly, by correcting the hypoxic state. It is thus necessary to relieve the obstruction and to supply sufficient supplementary oxygen to relieve the oxygen deficit.

Respiratory efficiency may be improved and comfort increased during an acute asthmatic attack by elevating the head of the bed and by strapping the pillows in a supporting position. The patient is likely to be most comfortable leaning forward, with arms supported on a pillow-upholstered over-bed table. Every opportunity for sleep and rest should be fostered after an acute asthmatic attack.

These patients are inclined to perspire excessively; thus they must be protected against chilling. Covers made of cotton are preferred, and frequent changes of bedclothes are carried out as needed.

Insofar as is possible, exposure to offending antigens should be reduced. Bronchial asthma is a chronic disease with exacerbations that produce symptoms at times, but with persistent subclinical obstruction. Because of this chronic nature, intermittent bronchodilator therapy is not as effective as continuous bronchodilator therapy.

Epinephrine (Adrenalin) is the drug of choice because of its potent bronchodilating effect and rapid action. It is injected subcutaneously in 1:1,000 solution (0.30-0.50 ml.). It may be repeated in 15 to 30 minutes if required. Side effects to be noted include headache, vomiting, agitation, hypertension, tachycardia, and arrhythmias.

Theophylline-aminophylline preparations are potent bronchodilators which have been found to be safe and effective. They come in various forms and are available either in tablet, liquid, or timed-release capsules. Blood levels (serum theophylline) need to be determined to prevent toxicity, and pulmonary-function tests are done to determine drug effectiveness. Nausea and vomiting may indicate toxicity.

Terbutaline sulfate (Brethine, Bricanyl) is a highly selective beta$_2$ stimulant. It has a longer duration of action than epinephrine and cannot be given as frequently. It is effective in dilating smooth muscles in the bronchial tree without stimulating the cardiac or central nervous systems. It does not cause hypertension. In some patients, it stimulates somatic muscles, which causes a tremor.

Synthetic products (beta agonists) such as metaproterenol (Alupent) and protokylol (Ventaire) are similar medications to terbutaline.

Corticosteroids are very effective in controlling asthma; however, because of serious side effects, they should be prescribed only when other, more conservative medications have failed. Hydrocortisone 100-200 mg. intravenously every 3 hours may be required to gain control of the attack. Thereafter, oral prednisone 10-30 mg. per day may be needed for several days to weeks, gradually tapering to the smallest dose necessary.

Cromolyn sodium (Aarane, Intal) is a therapeutic drug prescribed exclusively for prophylaxis of severe bronchial asthma; it is of no value in the treatment of an acute attack. It is an insoluble powder which is inhaled into the tracheal-bronchial tree. Its mechanism is to prevent the release of histamine and other mediators (after an antigen-antibody reaction) which are responsible for bronchial constriction. It seems to be most effective in allergic asthma, particularly for the patient who knows which extrinsic allergen is causing the problem. This means that the patient can inhale the medication one minute before entering an area where a known allergen exists (a house with a cat, or a field of ragweed) and be protected for some time. Cromolyn may be effective for asthma induced by exercise. Usually 2 to 4 weeks are required for maximum benefit. The patient needs to carry an inhaler with him; the cost is a factor to consider.

Mild throat irritation, cough, or hoarseness may occur and can be relieved by a bronchodilating aerosol. Hypersensitivity is noted in very few patients. If cromolyn provides no significant help after being used for a month, it should be discontinued slowly. To discontinue its use suddenly might trigger a severe asthma attack.

Antibiotics, sedatives, and tranquilizers are also part of the pharmacotherapeutic program. Antibiotics are given when infection is present; mild sedatives and tranquilizers are occasionally judiciously prescribed.

Use of Expectorants and Mucolytic Agents. *Acetylcysteine* (Mucomyst) is effective in liquefying sputum and is given with an intermittent positive pressure apparatus. Since it may initiate bronchospasm, Mucomyst is usually given with isoproterenol.

A person recovering from an asthma attack should be encouraged to increase fluid intake in order to maintain liquefied intrabronchial secretions. Otherwise, thickened retained secretions cause bronchial obstruction and atelectasis.

Management Beyond the Acute Phase: Health Teaching

Extrinsic and Mixed Asthma. Detailed and accurate instructions are to be provided the patient with regard to: (1) injections or aerosol inhalations to be administered at

MEDICATIONS TO BE AVOIDED BY PATIENTS WITH ASTHMA

TYPE OF ASTHMA	DRUG	RATIONALE
Acute or chronic	Antihistamines	They dry pulmonary secretions.
	Anticholinergics	They dry pulmonary secretions.
	Propranolol	May cause bronchospasm.
	Monoamine oxidase inhibitors	Initiates hypertensive crises when they combine with adrenergic drugs.
Status asthmaticus	Morphine Demerol Sedatives Tranquilizers	May suppress respiration.

home, (2) the types of contact that are considered potentially provocative of asthmatic attacks and are therefore to be avoided, (3) scheduling of return visits for observations during and following convalescence (the social worker may assist in securing new employment if a change of occupation is desirable), and (4) permissible activities and contraindicated activities, as follows:

Recommended Activities (Permissible).
Air conditioning may be helpful, although occasionally it aggravates symptoms in individual patients. Humidity kept at 30 to 50 percent is comfortable.

Instruct the patient as follows:
- Remain indoors during high-pollution days.
- Maintain adequate hydration and rest.
- Use an oral bronchodilator 15 to 30 minutes before exercise.
- Practice breathing exercises if they help expiratory function. However, explain to the patient that it is not known how effective such a practice really is.

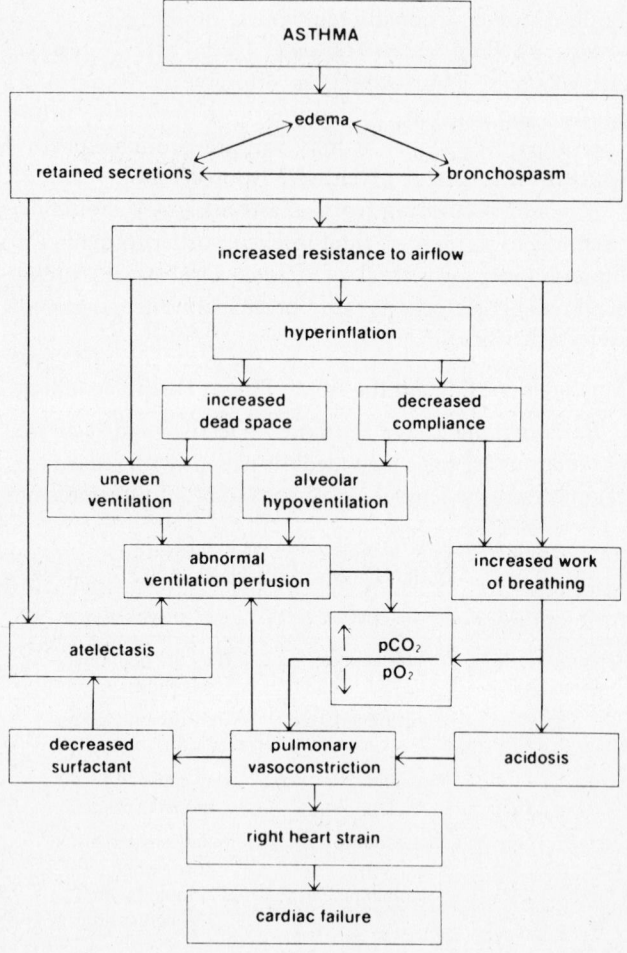

Figure 50-6. Diagrammatic representation of what can happen when asthma gets out of hand. (From Richards, W., and Siegel, S. C.: Emergency Medicine, 6:299, Feb. 1974)

- Promote practices recommended for allergy management, such as environmental controls, particularly in relation to dust, dander, and mold. Radiant heating systems are preferred to those which circulate air.

Contraindicated Activities

- Warn the patient that cigarette smoking enhances the development of bacterial bronchial infection by impairing ciliary movement.
- Instruct the patient *not* to use the hand nebulizer for more than four to six inhalation treatments per day. Overuse has deleterious effects and should be discouraged.

Intrinsic Asthma and Aspirin-sensitive Asthma.
Management is provided primarily through drug therapy. In the latter situation, it is important to avoid aspirin and aspirin-containing drugs to which the patient is sensitive.

Prevention

In every patient with recurrent asthma, evidence should be sought that might implicate a foreign protein to which the patient is hypersensitive and which might precipitate the attacks. If attacks chiefly occur at night when the patient is in bed, skin tests should be conducted with material from the mattress and pillows. If the test results are positive, then a mattress and pillow made from other materials should be substituted. If attacks appear to be associated with the presence of a particular species of animal, such as a horse or a cat, similar skin tests should be made with an antigen composed of hair or skin scrapings from the animal concerned. The physician should search for foci of bacterial infection, e.g., of chronically infected sinuses or teeth, because their eradication may be strikingly beneficial in certain patients. A seasonal incidence of attacks in a patient suggests an air-borne allergen as the chief etiologic agent. In such cases, therapy may be attempted with pollen extracts. Air conditioning offers possibilities in the prevention of attacks, depending on the extent to which the patient can restrict his life to air-conditioned rooms during the asthma season. A complete change of climatic environment to a locality with different flora during that period is the most satisfactory solution, when feasible.

Associated Psychotherapeutic Modalities

It is important to remember that asthmatic attacks, once started, may indicate that the patient will be susceptible to repeated attacks. In some patients, attacks may be induced by suggestion alone. Good general physical and mental health is most important.

Complications of Asthma

The acute asthmatic attack per se is seldom serious, although occasionally it does prove to be fatal through respiratory exhaustion, which is particularly possible if sedatives are administered too freely.

THE PATIENT WITH BRONCHIAL ASTHMA
Objectives and Principles of Management

The Problem: During an acute asthmatic episode, the ventilatory processes are altered due to airway obstruction. The ensuing hypoxia can be life-threatening to the patient.

I. TO TREAT THE PATIENT DURING THE ACUTE ASTHMATIC EPISODE:

A. Relieve the airway obstruction.
 1. Give medications as requested.
  a. Isoproterenol administered by nebulizer to oropharynx.
  b. Intravenous aminophylline administered slowly.
  c. Epinephrine administered subcutaneously.
  d. Corticosteroids given if needed, to treat inflammation and edema of the tracheobronchial tree.
 2. Evaluate patient's reaction to medication.
 3. Observe for symptoms of congestive failure.
 4. Prepare for bronchoscopic aspiration, to eliminate bronchial obstruction, if needed.

B. Relieve the hypoxia.
 1. Use intermittent positive pressure breathing (page 417) to assist respirations (if tolerated).
 2. Use nasal oxygen with caution.
 3. Observe for symptoms of carbon dioxide narcosis.

C. Liquefy the bronchial and the respiratory secretions.
 1. Replace fluid and electrolyte losses.
 2. Humidify the room.
 3. Add potassium iodide to intravenous solutions as requested.
 4. Encourage oral intake of fluids as soon as possible.

D. Alleviate the patient's anxiety and exhaustion.
 1. Use mild sedatives cautiously.
 2. Promote the comfort of the patient.
  a. Use supportive devices for orthopneic position.
  b. Keep the environment cool and quiet.
  c. Restrict visitors.
  d. Have a positive and calm approach to the patient.
  e. Ensure that patient sleeps undisturbed following attack.

II. TO INDIVIDUALIZE THE PATIENT'S THERAPY TO PREVENT FUTURE ATTACKS:

A. Avoid precipitating factors that will trigger an asthmatic attack.
B. Remove the patient from allergenic material.
C. Carry out a program of immunotherapy.
D. Conduct the program of maintenance therapy.
 1. Bronchodilators
 2. Sedatives
 3. Corticosteroids
 4. Inhalation treatments
E. Control secondary infections.
 1. Teach patient to call physician at first symptoms of respiratory infection.
 2. Observe the color of respiratory secretions.
 3. Treat "minor" respiratory infections vigorously.
 4. Avoid persons with colds and infections.
F. Promote the rehabilitation of the patient.
 1. Teach patient to call physician at first symptoms.
 2. Teach patient to avoid irritants.
 3. Keep environmental air humidified and filtered when possible.
 4. Institute balanced program of nutrition, rest, and exercise.
 5. Encourage the patient to express his anxieties.
 6. Assist the patient to have insight into his situational problems.

Complications of asthma include a ruptured bleb causing pneumothorax, mediastinal or subcutaneous emphysema, chronic and recurrent acute bronchitis, bronchiectasis, pulmonary hypertension, and hypertrophy of the right side of the heart with right-heart failure (pulmonary heart disease) (Fig. 50-6). Chronic hypoxia due to these complications leads to symptoms and personality changes.

STATUS ASTHMATICUS

Status asthmaticus is severe asthma that is unresponsive to conventional therapy with epinephrine and aminophylline and lasts longer than 24 hours. A vicious self-perpetuating cycle may occur as a result of infection, anxiety, overuse of tranquilizers, nebulizer abuse, dehydration, increased beta-adrenergic block, and non-specific irritants. An acute episode sometimes may be precipitated by hypersensitivity to acetylsalicylic acid.

Pathophysiology. A combination of factors, including constriction of the bronchiolar smooth muscle, swelling of bronchial mucosa, and/or thickened (inspissated) secretions all contribute to one pathologic problem—a decrease in the diameter of the bronchi. Another problem is the ventilation-perfusion abnormality that results from hypoxemia and respiratory acidosis or alkalosis. Therefore, blood gas determinations are an important guide to the severity of the condition and offer a reliable method of checking the patient's response to therapy.

There is a reduced arterial PO_2 and an initial respiratory alkalosis with a decreased PCO_2 and an increased pH. As the severity of status asthmaticus increases, the PCO_2 increases and the pH falls—reflecting respiratory acidosis. The rising PCO_2 suggests progressive pulmonary failure and requires aggressive drug intervention and other therapeutic measures to prevent death from respiratory failure.

Clinical Manifestations. Breathing is labored, with a greater effort made on exhalation. The neck and even face veins become engorged. Expelled air escapes with a wheeze; however, the amount of wheezing does not correlate with the severity of the attack. With greater obstruction, the wheeze may disappear.

Treatment is best given in a pulmonary intensive care unit where clinical management is in the hands of the allergist, pulmonary disease specialist, and anesthesiologist, as well as a nurse clinician.

Signs of dehydration are assessed by checking skin turgor and the tongue. Dehydration is one of the primary problems to be corrected, usually through the administration of intravenous fluids up to 3,000 to 4,000 ml./day. Fluid intake is essential to combat dehydration and to facilitate expectoration. Some physicians anticipate metabolic acidosis and add an ampule of sodium bicarbonate to intravenous fluids.

To treat dyspnea, cyanosis, and hypoxemia, oxygen therapy is intiated on low-flow humidified oxygen, either by Ventimask or nasal catheter. The amount is determined following blood gas determinations. Arterial PO_2 is kept between 65 and 85 mm. Hg.

Drug treatment is begun with agents that raise the concentration of cyclic $3',5'$ adenosine monophosphate (cyclic AMP); epinephrine hydrochloride is the drug of choice. Other beta-adrenergic drugs may be given such as ephedrine (isoproterenol usually is limited to children; in adults fibrillation may occur). Other, more specific $beta_2$ stimulators are useful, such as terbutaline sulfate (Brethine, Bricanyl). The methyl xanthines (theophylline) increase the concentration of cyclic AMP. Since, by definition, status asthmaticus is resistent to epinephrine and aminophylline, the blood levels are carefully monitored when these drugs are given.

Corticosteroids are also prescribed to restore bronchial reactivity. Mucolytic agents such as acetylcysteine (Mucomyst) are effective after bronchodilation. Cough suppressants and sedatives are avoided. If symptoms suggest the presence of an infection, antibiotics are given. The drugs of choice (if the patient is not sensitive to them) are tetracycline, erythromycin, and ampicillin. Appropriate agents are determined following gram-stain sputum studies.

Constant monitoring of the patient by the nurse is important for the first 12 to 24 hours, or until status asthmaticus is broken. The room should be quiet and free of respiratory irritants, including flowers and cigarette smoke. The patient should have a nonallergenic pillow.

Mechanical assistance may be required when maximum medical therapy fails. Volume respirators are preferable to pressure ventilators because large tidal volumes are necessary, to overcome airway resistance. During mechanical ventilation, the patient's cardiac function and blood gas volumes must be carefully monitored to avoid such complications as heart failure and pneumothorax.

Patient Education. This is an important part of posthospital care if recurrences are to be kept to a minimum. Bronchodilators may be required on an "around-the-clock" basis. Certain medications can be increased when asthmatic attacks occur. Adequate hydration must be maintained at home to keep secretions from thickening. The patient needs to recognize that infection is to be avoided, since it can trigger an attack.

SERUM SICKNESS

The illness known as serum sickness traditionally has resulted from the administration of therapeutic antisera of animal sources for the treatment or prevention of infectious diseases such as tetanus, pneumonia, rabies, diphtheria, and botulism and for bites of venomous snakes and black-widow spiders. However, with the advent of human antitetanus serum and antibiotics, true serum sickness is much less common now than in previous years. However, a variety of drugs, chief of which is penicillin, is now the main cause of a syndrome identical to that caused by foreign sera.

The symptoms are due to a reaction and immunologic attack upon the serum or the drug. Antibodies appear chiefly to be of the IgE and IgM classes. Early manifestations, beginning 6 to 10 days after the administration of the drug, include an inflammatory reaction at the site of injection of the drug, followed by regional and generalized lymphadenopathy. There is nearly always a skin rash, which may be urticarial or purpuric, and joints are frequently tender and swollen. Vasculitis may occur in any organ, but is most commonly observed in the kidney, resulting in proteinuria and, occasionally, casts. Cardiac involvement, mild to severe in nature, may occur. Peripheral neuritis may cause temporary paralysis of the upper extremities or may be widespread, causing the Guillain-Barré syndrome.

The usual untreated course lasts for several days to a few weeks but ordinarily responds promptly and completely if treated with antihistamines and corticosteroids.

ANAPHYLACTIC SHOCK

Anaphylactic shock is an immediate, shocklike (life-threatening) allergic reaction following exposure to a substance to which the person is exquisitely sensitive. Drugs, such as foreign sera, penicillin, nitrofurantoin (Furadantin), enzymes such as trypsin and chymotrypsin, allergenic extracts used in immunotherapy for extrinsic allergic conditions, and bee venoms, are the most common causes of anaphylaxis.

Initial symptoms may include a generalized feeling of warmth, itching of the palms and soles, itching around the eyes, itching in the ears, hoarseness, dysphagia, a sense of constriction in the throat, and a feeling of impending doom. The patient may experience tightness in the chest, with an audible expiratory wheeze. Fright may be evident, and pruritus severe. Hives may be localized and progress to massive facial angioedema, suggestive of upper-respiratory edema. Death may occur within minutes to several hours, due to respiratory failure brought on by laryngeal edema and/or bronchospasm, but if recovery occurs, it is usually complete and without sequelae.

Prevention. A careful history should be taken before the administration of any drug, to be certain that there is no known hypersensitivity to it. Any person who is known to be susceptible to anaphylaxis should carry an identification tag.*

Anyone who is endangered by the sting of hymenoptera (bees, wasps, hornets, yellow jackets) should carry an emergency kit (during spring and summer) containing parenteral epinephrine. An ANA-Kit (Hollister-Stier), which is available commercially, contains a prefilled syringe with epinephrine and the equipment required for self-administration.

If animal serum is to be given, it is mandatory that careful skin testing be carried out prior to injection of therapeutic doses.

The injection of any drug should, whenever possible, be given sufficiently distal on an extremity so that a tourniquet may be applied proximally in order to retard the absorption of the drug into the circulation.

In the presence of a positive skin test for a drug that must be given, a procedure of "desensitization" may be carried out. This is done by giving a minute amount of diluted drug or serum, followed by gradually increasing doses every 10 to 15 minutes, until a full therapeutic dose has been achieved. When carefully done, this is a fairly safe procedure but does not obviate the later development of a serum-sickness-like reaction (described above).

Management. Help should be summoned immediately, but the person suffering the attack should not be left unattended. Immediate assessment of vital functions is done to determine whether respiration or heartbeat has stopped. If so, closed-chest massage and/or mouth-to-mouth resuscitation is initiated.

Epinephrine (Adrenalin) is the most effective treatment of an acute allergic reaction. An intramuscular injection of 0.5 ml. of epinephrine 1:1,000 is given immediately into the opposite extremity. A tourniquet is then applied, if possible, proximal to the site of injection of the allergen. An additional 0.2 ml. of epinephrine is injected into the site of the allergen injection if tourniquet application is not feasible. Antihistamines and corticosteroids are also given as adjunctive agents, although it is important to emphasize that their effect cannot be relied upon, and they are given after the administration of epinephrine only to prevent relapse. Routine measures for shock including assuring an adequate airway, establishing the shock position, providing supplementary oxygen, and giving intravenous fluids are also indicated. Specific treatment for hypotension or for a known asthmatic condition would also be initiated.

BIBLIOGRAPHY

BOOKS

Frazier, C. A.: Psychosomatic Aspects of Allergy. New York, Van Nostrand Reinhold, 1977.

Lichtenstein, L. M., and Austen, K. F.: Asthma. Physiology, Immunopharmacology and Treatment, Second International Symposium. New York, Academic Press, 1977.

Middleton, E., Jr., et al.: Allergy, Principles and Practice. St. Louis, C. V. Mosby, 1978.

Patterson, R. (ed.): Allergic Diseases, Diagnosis and Management. Philadelphia, J. B. Lippincott, 1972.

Saunder, N. A., and McFadden, E. R., Jr.: Asthma—an update. Disease-a-Month. Chicago, Yearbook Med. Publ., Inc., Aug. 1978.

Simplified Techniques for Allergy Testing and Treatment, Atlanta, Ga., Hollister-Stier.

ARTICLES

General

Barclay, W. R.: Emergency treatment of insect-sting allergy (commentary). JAMA, *240*:2735, Dec. 15, 1978.

Burke, G. W., et al.: Allergic alveolites caused by home humidifiers. JAMA, *238*:2705-2708, Dec. 19, 1977.

Grazier, C. A.: The allergic surgical patient. AORN J., *26*:790-798, Oct. 1977.

Huntley, C. C.: Atopic dermatitis and contact dermatitis in children. Am. Fam. Phys., *16*:111-118, Aug. 1977.

Kintzel, K. C.: Nursing intervention for patients with allergic disorders. In Kintzel, K. C. (ed.): Advanced Concepts in Clinical Nursing, 2nd ed. Philadelphia, J. B. Lippincott, 1977.

Marks, M. B.: Recognizing the allergic person. Am. Fam. Phys., *16*:72-79, July 1977.

Oslick, T.: Aerosol sympathomimetic amines Am. Fam. Phys., *15*:146-148, June 1977.

Pap, L. F.: Anaphylaxis—the ever-present threat. Mod. Med., *45*:38-43, Aug. 15, 1977.

Speer, F.: Food allergy: the 10 common offenders. Am. Fam. Phys., *13*:106-112, Feb. 1976.

---

*Medic Alert Foundation, 1000 North Palm, Turlock, California 05380.

Bronchial Asthma

Ahmed, M., and Lindquist, C.: Bronchial asthma. Postgrad. Med., *62*:111-118, July 1977.

Ballin, J. C.: Evaluation of a new aerosolized steroid for asthma therapy. JAMA, *236*:2891-2893, Dec. 20, 1976.

Bardana, E. J.: Modern aspects in diagnosis and treatment of the asthmatic patient. Clin. Notes on Resp. Dis., Amer. Thoracic Society, *15*:3-13, Fall 1976.

Bergner, K., and Bergner, A.: Rational asthma therapy for the outpatient. JAMA, *235*:266-293, Jan. 19, 1976.

Cromoglycate and theophylline for asthma. Am. Fam. Phys., *16*:60-63, Aug. 1977.

DiPalma, J. R.: Helping your patient control his bronchial asthma. RN, *40*:78-81, Oct. 1977.

Farr, R. S.: Asthma in adults: the ambulatory patient. Hosp. Pract., *13*:113-123, Apr. 1978.

Greene, J. M.: Bronchial asthma: a chronic disease. Today's Clinician, *2*:33-35, Oct. 1978.

Imbeau, S. A., and Geller, M. L.: Aerosol beclomethasone treatment of chronic severe asthma. JAMA, *240*:1261-1262, Sept. 15, 1978.

Lovell, R. G., and Preuss, L.: Bronchial asthma: which drugs to use and why. *45*:34-36, Dec. 15, 1977.

Settipane, G. A., et al.: Adverse reactions to cromolyn. JAMA, *241*:811-813, Feb. 23, 1979.

Slater, E.: Cardiac tamponade and peripheral eosinophilia in a patient receiving cromolyn sodium. Chest, *73*:878-879, June 1978.

Slavin, R. G.: Asthma in adults: occupational asthma. Hosp. Pract., *13*:133-146, June 1978.

Wanna, A.: Management of ambulatory patients with asthma. Today's Clinician, *2*:57-62, Apr. 1978.

Wilson, A. F.: Drug treatment of acute asthma. JAMA, *237*:1141-1143, March 14, 1977.

Valentine, M. D.: A new era in asthma therapy. Mod. Med., *46*:44-48, Mar. 15, 1978.

Status Asthmaticus

Arkins, J. A.: Status asthmaticus — current therapy. Drug Ther. 7:39-42, Apr. 1977.

Harvey, S.: Drugs in pulmonary and neurologic emergencies: status asthmaticus. Nurses' Drug Alert, *2*:105-107, Sept. 1978.

Richerson, H. B.: Asthma in adults, II: the patient in status asthmaticus. Hosp. Pract., *13*:109-115, May 1978.

Scoggin, C. H., et al.: Status asthmaticus. JAMA, *238*: 1158-1162, Sept. 12, 1977.

AGENCIES

Allergy Foundation of America, 801 Second Avenue, New York, N.Y. 10017

Allergy Information Association, 3 Powburn Place, Western Ontario M9R 2C5, Canada

American Academy of Allergy, 225 East Michigan Street, Milwaukee, Wis. 53202

The American Lung Association, 1740 Broadway, New York, N.Y. 10019

Hay Fever Prevention Society, Inc., 2300 Sedwick (Rosewall Gardens, Suite 2-G), Bronx, N.Y. 10468

National Institute of Allergy and Infectious Disease, National Institutes of Health, Bethesda, Md. 20205

Sensorineural Problems

51

ASSESSMENT AND MANAGEMENT OF PATIENTS WITH VISION AND EYE DISORDERS

PHYSIOLOGIC OVERVIEW

The eyeball is a spherical organ situated in a bony cavity called the *orbit*. It is rotated easily in all the necessary directions by six muscles attached to its outer surface (Fig. 51-1); these muscles act in a manner similar to the reins on a team of horses. Four of the muscles are located on each side of the eye, and on the top and the bottom of the eye. Each of these four muscles, the *rectus* muscles, leads back to the apex of the orbit and turns the eye in or out, up or down. The other two muscles of the eye, the *oblique* muscles, run from the globe toward the medial wall of the orbit.

For the purpose of study, the eyeball may be divided into three coats or tunics. The dense white fibrous outer coat is called the *sclera*. Anteriorly, the sclera becomes continuous with the *cornea,* the translucent structure that bulges forward slightly from the general contour of the eye. Posteriorly, the sclera has an opening through which the optic nerve passes into the eyeball. The nerve spreads out over the posterior two-thirds of the inner surface of globe in a thin layer called the *retina*. In it are situated the tiny nerve endings, which, when properly stimulated, transmit visual impulses to the brain that are interpreted as sight.

Between the sclera and the retina is the pigmented middle coat known as the *uveal tract*. This tract is composed of three parts. The posterior part, the *choroid,* contains most of the blood vessels that nourish the eye. The anterior part is a pigmented muscular structure, the *iris,* which gives the characteristic color to the eye (blue, brown, and so forth). The circular opening at its center, the *pupil,* dilates or contracts according to the intensity of the light, by two sets of muscle fibers. Contraction of the circular fibers constricts the pupil; the radial fibers enlarge it. Between the iris and the choroid is the third portion of the uveal tract, a muscular body known as the *ciliary body*. It is composed of radial processes arising from a triangular-shaped muscle (ciliary muscle). Between these processes, and to them, are attached delicate ligaments that pass centrally and become inserted in the capsule of the crystalline lens.

The *lens* is a semisolid body enclosed in a transparent elastic capsule. It is capable of being modified to varying degrees of convexity by the contraction and the relaxation of the ciliary muscle, thus changing the focus of the eye as it looks from one object to another.

The cavity within the eye is divided by the lens into two parts. The posterior part contains a jellylike translucent substance called the *vitreous humor,* which is the chief factor in maintaining the form of the eyeball. The anterior part contains a clear, watery fluid, the *aqueous humor,* which is secreted by the ciliary processes. It bathes the anterior surface of the lens, escapes at the pupil, and enters the space between the iris and the cornea known as the *anterior chamber*. Finally it is drained from the eye

1123

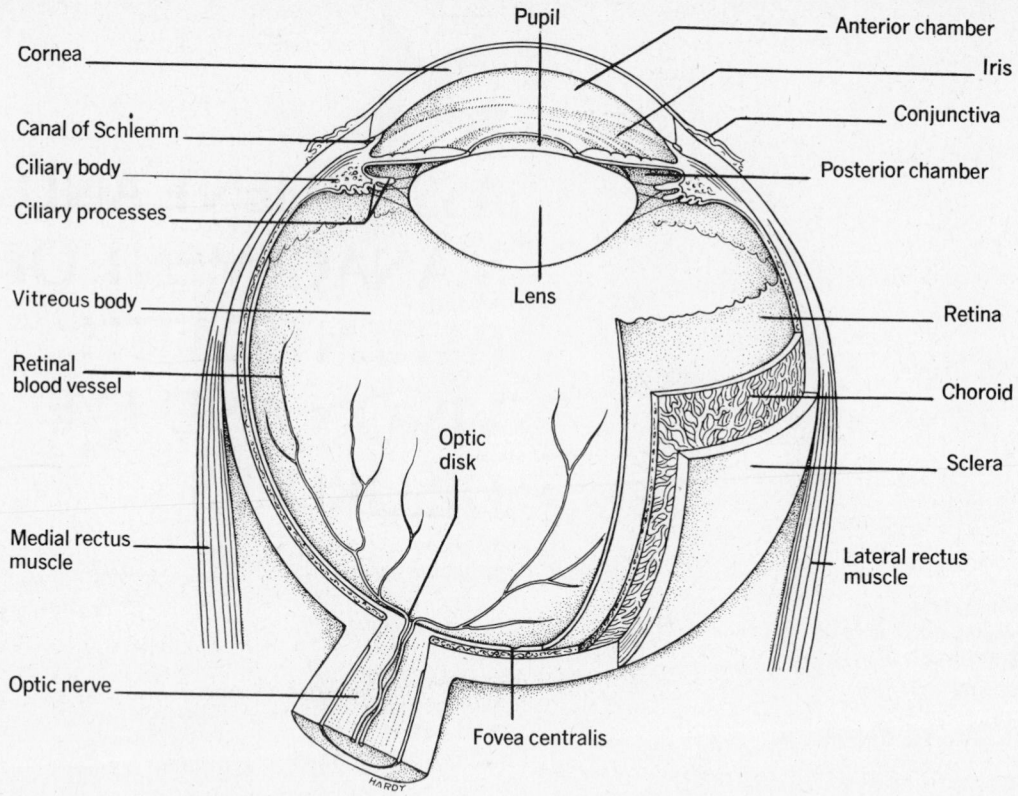

Figure 51-1. Transverse section of eye. (From Chaffee, E. E., and Greisheimer, E. M.: Basic Physiology and Anatomy. Philadelphia, J. B. Lippincott)

through lymph channels (the canal of Schlemm) located at the junction of the iris and the sclera.

APPENDAGES. The *eyelids* are the protective coverings of the eye. Lining the lids and entirely covering the anterior part of the eye is a highly sensitive membrane, the *conjunctiva,* the surface of which is kept moist by a constant flow of lacrimal fluid (tears). This fluid is excreted from the *lacrimal gland,* which is located in the upper and outer part of the orbit. It flows downward and inward across the eye and drains into tiny channels (lacrimal punctae). These channels conduct the fluid to the lacrimal sac and duct, which pass downward, backward, and outward and open into the nasal cavity beneath the inferior turbinate bone.

ASSESSMENT OF VISION

Eye-Care Specialists

The importance of adequate eye examination cannot be emphasized too strongly. Too often we find patients using a pair of glasses that belonged to a relative or was purchased at the local variety store.

The care of the eye is undertaken by four groups of specialists:

1. The *oculist,* the *ophthalmologist,* or the *ophthalmic physician* is a medical doctor who is skilled in the treatment of all conditions and diseases of the eye. Training and experience enable this physician to make a more thorough and complete examination of the eye for refractive errors and other changes.
2. The *optician* is not a physician, but is concerned with grinding, mounting, and dispensing lenses.
3. The *optometrist* is licensed to examine the eyes and related structures to determine the presence of vision problems, eye diseases, or other abnormalities, and to prescribe and adapt lenses or other optical aids.
4. The *ocularist* is a technician who makes artificial eyes and other prostheses used in ophthalmology.

Refractive Errors

Vision is made possible by the passage of rays of light from an object through the cornea, the aqueous humor, the lens, and the vitreous humor to the retina. In the normal eye, rays coming from an object at a distance of 6 meters or more are brought to a focus on the retina by the lens while perfectly at rest. Due to abnormalities in the eye structure or in the lens structure, defective vision may occur because objects are not focused correctly on the retina. If the rays of light are brought to a focus in front of the retina, the condition is spoken of as *myopia,* or nearsightedness, and if the rays are focused behind the retina, the condition is called *hyperopia* (farsightedness). In such conditions, glass lenses are prescribed. These, in association with the lenses of the eye, will correct the fault and restore a normal focus at the retina.

Rays from objects situated at shorter distances (less than 6 meters) require a "stronger" lens to focus them on the retina. This is brought about by a contraction of the ciliary muscle that relaxes the lens capsule and causes the lens to become more convex. This function is called *accommodation*. By means of accommodation, objects at different distances from the eye may be seen distinctly. With increasing age, the elasticity of the lens decreases, so that accommodation for near vision is not complete, a condition called *presbyopia*. This explains why it is so common to see older people reading a paper while holding it at arm's length. "Reading-glasses" may be prescribed for these patients to enable them to focus rays from near objects to the retina.

In the case of presbyopia, two different types of lenses may be used — bifocals — one for far distance and one for near vision and reading. Trifocal lenses are also available; these add a third dimension that gives sharp focus in the 68 to 127 cm. (27-50 inch) range. Most lenses are prescribed for use in "glasses," but in some cases the lens may be applied directly to the surface of the eye (contact lens).

Astigmatism results from uneven curvature of the cornea — instead of curving equally in all directions, the cornea is shaped somewhat like the bowl of a spoon. Two foci thus occur instead of one, and, as a consequence, the patient is unable to focus horizontal and vertical rays on the retina at the same time. These defects may be corrected with lenses called cylinder lenses. A patient may be myopic or hyperopic and also have astigmatism. In such a situation, a compound spherocylinder lens is ordered from the optician.

The strength and type of lens that will overcome refractive errors are determined by means of a retinoscope, which measures the refractive error. On the basis of this examination, an appropriate corrective lens is selected and then further refined by having the patient read letters on the Snellen chart through several different lenses.

Automated refractors, which rely on photoelectric devices sensitive to light, may also be used. The patient sits in front of the instrument and is instructed to look steadily at a target. A print-out on a card or graph indicates the refractive error to be corrected. Other types of automated refractors require the patient to make focusing adjustments by turning a knob. Such equipment is expensive, and although many can be operated by technicians, they need further evaluation to justify their replacing conventional refraction methods.

Contact Lenses

More and more people are wearing contact lenses as a means of correcting refractive errors, because of better techniques for measuring the eye and improved methods

---

ABBREVIATIONS AND TERMS USED IN OPHTHALMOLOGY

O.D. or R.E. (*oculus dexter*)—right eye
O.S. or L.E. (*oculus sinister*)—left eye
O.U. or O_2 (*oculi uterque*)—both eyes together
D. (diopter)—unit of measurement of strength or refractive power of lenses. (A 1-diopter lens brings parallel light rays to a focus at 1 meter from the lens.)
E.O.M.—extraocular muscles
H (hyperopia, hypermetropia)—farsightedness
HT (hypertropia)—upward deviation of one eye
ST (esotropia)—inward deviation of one eye
XT (exotropia)—outward deviation of one eye
+—plus or convex
−—minus or concave
Diplopia—seeing one object as two ("double vision")
Ectropion—turning out (eversion) of eyelid
Entropion—turning in of eyelid
Ptosis—drooping of upper lid
Epiphora—excessive production of tears
Hemianopia—blindness of one-half the field of vision
Photophobia—abnormal sensitivity to light
Presbyopia—lessening of power of accommodation owing to aging process

---

of supervising and instructing those who wish to wear the lenses. They are particularly effective in certain occupations and are desirable for cosmetic reasons. However, not everyone can wear contact lenses; therefore, all potential candidates should be thoroughly screened by an ophthalmologist.

Medical conditions in which corneal lenses are recommended include absence of lens (aphakia), absence of iris (aniridia), congenital absence of pigment, myopia and hyperopia, some types of astigmatism, cone-shaped deformity of the cornea (keratoconus), and turned-in eyelashes. Contraindications include allergic and inflammatory conditions (such as chronic blepharoconjunctivitis, corneal infection, iritis, uveitis), epiphora (abnormal overflow of tears), severe exophthalmus, pterygium, or local neoplasm.

Contact lenses are usually not recommended for people who do not require full-time visual correction or lack sufficient manual dexterity to insert and remove lenses.

Contact lenses are available in either hard or soft form. The hard lens was introduced in the early 1960s, the soft lens in the late 1960s. The most recent innovation has been a lens made of silicone rubber.

HARD CONTACT LENSES. The corneal lens is made of light-weight, paper-thin polymethylmethacrylate about 10 mm. or less in diameter. When properly fitted, contact lenses "float" on the fluid layer of the eyeball and are held loosely in place by the capillary attraction of the tears and the upper lid. The lens moves with the eye and is centered over the cornea.

Hard contact lenses have many advantages over framed lenses: they do not steam up when the wearer goes from the cold outside to a warm room; they are automatically cleaned with each blink of the eyelid; they can be worn safely during sports; they eliminate the need for less attractive lenses; they provide increased peripheral vision; and they do not break easily.

However, there are certain disadvantages and dangers in wearing contact lenses: contact lenses are more expensive than framed lenses; solutions used to clean the lenses are costly; the adjustment period in learning to use them properly is longer; contact lenses can be lost easily, such as down the sink drain or in a swimming pool; in the event of a chemical splash to the eye, the chemical agent may seep beneath the lens to cause extensive damage before the contact lens can be removed.

SOFT CONTACT LENSES. Soft lenses, a Czechoslovakian innovation, have been available in the United States since 1971 and are made of polymer gel, although new formulations are being tested as soft lenses grow in popularity. They are brittle when dehydrated but when immersed in saline or impregnated with tears, they absorb water and become flexible.

When fitting hard lenses, the ophthalmologist usually instills fluorescein into the eye in order to identify changes that occur in the formation of tear film as the lid blinks. However, fluorescein cannot be used with soft lenses because the dye stains the lenses permanently. To offset microbial contamination, special procedures are used to disinfect soft lenses while they are stored during the night.

Soft lenses have certain advantages over hard lenses. They are comfortable from the start and can be worn up to 18 hours a day. They are less easily displaced during wearing than hard lenses and therefore are less likely to drop from the eye. They appear to be superior to hard lenses for those who participate in sports, except for swimming. Since these lenses absorb pool chemicals and ocean salt, they should not be worn while swimming unless goggles and a mask are used. If they are worn only occasionally, rather than daily, the wearer will not lose his tolerance to them, as is the case with hard lenses. Finally, it is easier to switch from soft lenses to eyeglasses than from hard lenses to eyeglasses.

Soft lenses are inserted by placing the lens on the inferior conjunctiva while drawing the lower lid downward. With the release of the lid, the wearer then rolls his eye around or massages the eye through the closed lid to position the lens on the cornea. To remove, the lens is grasped between the clean thumb and forefinger.

EXTENDED-WEAR CONTACT LENSES. These highly permeable plastic lenses are thinner and more pliable than ordinary soft or hard contacts and can be worn continuously for weeks or months. These lenses are being tested and shortly may receive approval from the FDA (Food and Drug Administration). They are more expensive than soft contact lenses and are not completely trouble-free.

COMPLICATIONS. The improper use of contact lenses (both hard and soft) can cause corneal abrasions and ulcerations, which result from poorly fitted lenses, improper technique in applying or removing the lenses, and insufficient tear circulation under the lenses.

Patient Education

Although the advantages outweigh the disadvantages, precautions and safeguards must be understood by the nurse, the wearer, and his employer. The contact lens

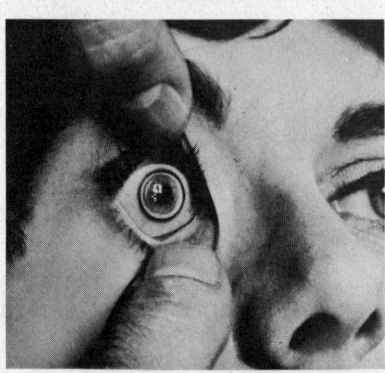 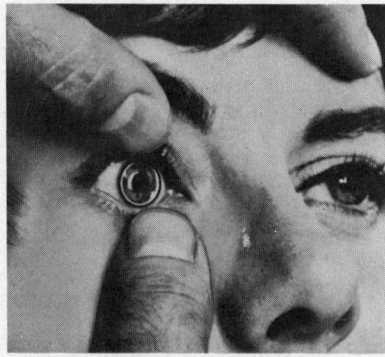 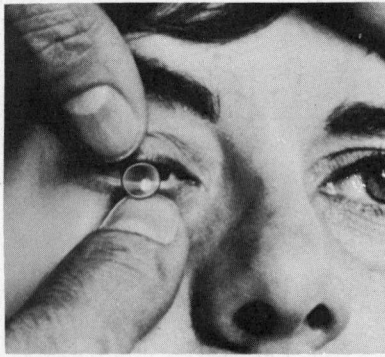

(A) After the eyelids have been separated and the corneal contact lens has been correctly positioned over the cornea, you widen the eyelid margins beyond the top and bottom edges of lens (as shown).

(B) After the lower eyelid margin has been moved near the edge of the bottom of the lens and then the upper eyelid margin has been moved near the edge of the top of the lens, you are ready to move under the bottom edge of the lens by pressing slightly harder on the lower eyelid while moving it upward.

(C) After the lens has tipped slightly, you move the eyelids toward one another and thereby cause the lens to slide out between the eyelids (as shown).

Figure 51-2. Emergency removal of hard contact lenses. (Reprinted with permission of the American Optometric Association)

must be regarded as a medical prosthesis, not a cosmetic device.

Care and precaution given to any medical prosthesis must be used with contact lenses.

1. Wash hands thoroughly before touching the lenses, whether applying them or removing them.
2. Cleanse lenses only with the recommended sterile solution (noncaustic).
3. Keep the storage kit clean.
4. Do not wear lenses beyond the prescribed time (maximal average is 10 to 16 hours).
5. Do not sleep with contact lenses in place; to do so may cause abrasion and erosion of the corneal epithelium.
6. Do not wet lenses with saliva before insertion; this can cause infection.
7. Restrict the wearing of contact lenses, in order to avoid potential corneal abrasions, if the following signs are present: photophobia, dryness, excessive burning, tearing.
8. Follow the physician's recommendations concerning eye makeup. Some ophthalmologists discourage patients from wearing eye makeup. Some advise applying mascara after lenses are in position.
9. Keep chemicals such as soaps, lotions, and creams away from lenses, since they may adversely affect the lens; instruct the wearer to keep his eyes tightly closed when applying hair, perfume, and deodorant sprays. Stay away from areas where household sprays are used.
10. Have an ophthalmologic examination every six months to ensure proper fit and to check corneal integrity.

Emergency Removal of Contact Lenses

Contact lenses are designed to be worn only while the person is awake and fully conscious. They should be removed as a safety measure if the wearer is incapacitated due to accident, sickness, or other cause. In emergency situations, the following directives should be followed:

1. Determine whether or not the patient is wearing contact lenses. If he is conscious or semiconscious, ask him directly, since he may be able to indicate that he is wearing contact lenses. He may even be able to remove the lenses by himself or with assistance, depending, of course, on his condition. If the patient is unconscious, check "Medic-Alert" tags (bracelets, necklaces, keychains, etc.), driver's licenses, and other identification cards which may reveal that the patient wears contact lenses. Look for observable indications that contact lenses are being worn by gently separating the patient's eyelids. Shining a light—preferably a small penlight—on the eye from the side will help.

2. Remove the patient's contact lenses if he cannot do so himself. With clean hands, position one thumb on the upper eyelid and one thumb on the lower eyelid, with thumbs near the margin of each eyelid. Separate the eyelids. A visible lens should slide easily with a gentle movement of the eyelids (Fig. 51-2). If the lens does not drop out easily, observe for possible lens position and follow instructions given in Figure 51-3 for removal of

A. When lens is directly over the cornea: This normal wearing position of a corneal contact lens is also the correct position for removing it. If the lens cannot be removed, however, slide it onto the sclera.

B. When the lens is on the sclera only: Here the lens can remain with relative safety until experienced help is available; other white areas of the eye to the side or above the cornea might also be used. If the lens is to be removed, however, slide it to a position directly over the cornea.

C. When the lens is on both the cornea and sclera: A lens in this position—or a similar one anywhere around the periphery of the cornea—should be moved as soon as possible. If the lens is to be removed, slide it to a position directly over the cornea; if the lens cannot be removed immediately, slide it onto the sclera.

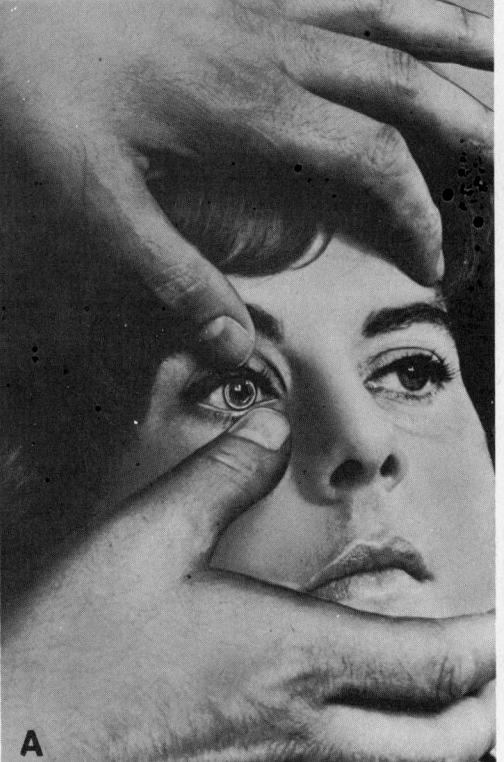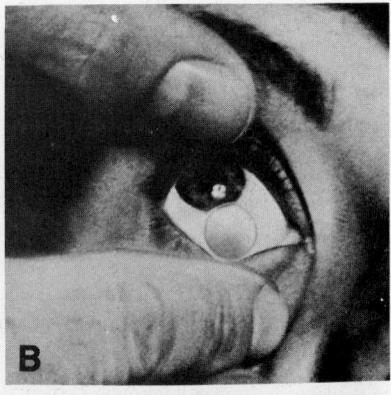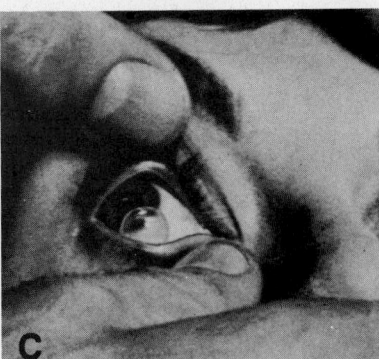

Figure 51-3. Emergency removal of hard lens which is (A) in normal position, (B) on the sclera, or (C) on both the cornea and the sclera. (Reprinted with permission of the American Optometric Association)

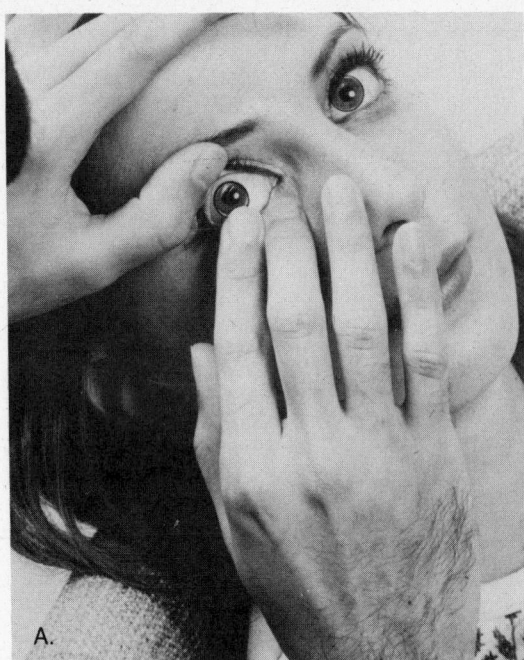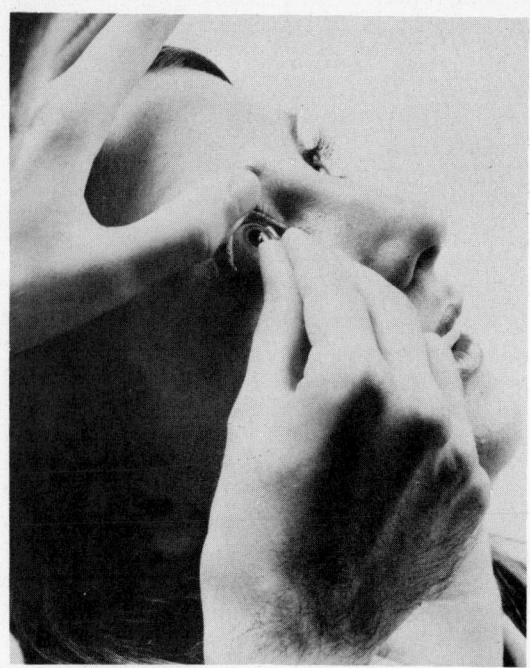

Figure 51-4.   Removal of soft contact lens. 1. With clean hands, pull down the lower lid with the middle finger and place the index fingertip on the lower edge of the lens (*A*). 2. Slide the lens down to the white part of the eye. 3. Compress the lens lightly between the thumb and index finger. 4. Bring thumb and index finger together in a "pinching" motion, causing the lens to double up between fingers, allowing air underneath (*B*). 5. Remove the lens from the eye. CAUTION: Inadequate tearing caused by severe injury or shock may cause the lens to adhere to the eye. If the lens resists removal, flush the eye with normal saline solution, wait several minutes, then follow the above five steps for removal. (Reprinted with permission of the American Optometric Association)

the lens. Remember that force should not be used. If the lens is seen but cannot be removed, gently slide it onto the sclera, where it can remain with relative safety until experienced help is available.

If the patient is wearing soft contact lenses, it is best to wait until someone experienced in removing these types of lenses is available to lend assistance. If flexible lenses are left in place for many hours, they will do little harm. However, if the emergency is such that they must be removed, then the steps described in Figure 51-4 should be followed.

GENERAL MANAGEMENT OF PATIENTS WITH EYE DISORDERS

It is well to remember that a patient with an eye problem may have other problems as well. Often other physical conditions are primary and affect the eye as a consequence. The appearance of the eye can alert the patient and the physician to difficulties or some disturbances in other parts of the body even before other symptoms present themselves. The mental anxiety frequently experienced by the ophthalmic patient requires as much consideration as does his physical condition.

Psychosocial Considerations

One's dependence on sight is emphasized when one faces a temporary or possible permanent loss of this vital sense. Worry, fear, and depression are common reactions in addition to tension, resentment, anger, and rejection. By encouraging the patient to express his feelings, the nurse may discover the basic problems involved and can then take steps to alleviate them.

SENSORY DEPRIVATION.   Many patients with eye disorders face unusual problems resulting from loss of sight. Such is the case of the postoperative patient whose eyes are bandaged and who suffers distortions in perception such as "eye-patch delirium," inappropriate behavior, loss of position sense in bed, and a sensation of floating. Often these problems are magnified and become frightening and upsetting. One way to assist the patient in overcoming these unsettling feelings is to constantly reorient him to reality and offer reassurance, explanations, and understanding.

Other helpful approaches may be followed: Anyone entering the patient's room should speak and identify himself so as not to startle the patient. If the patient is bothered by the restraint on his movements more than by an eye patch, a soothing back rub may offer relaxation.

When permissible, the radio and occupational therapy may be used to keep the patient's mind occupied. While it is important not to be oversolicitous, nonetheless, showing interest, empathy, and understanding enhances the patient's sense of well-being. Because of differences of personality, the approaches in overcoming the mental anxiety of individual patients vary. When permanent blindness is apparent, re-education may be done by specially trained personnel or similarly afflicted persons.

Daily Care

The daily care of ophthalmic patients should be the same as for other patients. The patient should be encouraged to carry out as much self-care as possible in order to promote a feeling of self-sufficiency. Nursing assistance is given as needed. A patient who cannot see is fed, but if he is accustomed to feeding himself, he is encouraged to do so. Proper elimination is promoted by proper diet, stool softeners, or enemas, as prescribed. Ambulatory patients are to have a daily rest period in the afternoon.

Ophthalmic patients are not to read, smoke, or shave unless given permission by the physician. They must be cautioned against rubbing their eyes or wiping them with a soiled handkerchief. All patients receiving atropine should wear dark glasses.

REDUCTION OF LIGHT. Because light causes pain in many conditions of the eye, and because the eyes should be rested as much as possible before and after undergoing operation, it is well to maintain subdued lighting in the room. If those assisting the patient need light to carry out their duties, then dimmed artificial lights may be used.

Eyedrops

Various drug solutions are inserted into the eyes in the treatment of nearly every kind of eye disorder (Table 51-1).

Before drops are instilled, it is important to see that the correct drug is being given. Some drugs (for example, miotics and mydriatics) act in exactly opposite ways. (Fig. 51-5). Therefore, if one of these drugs is indicated in the treatment of a certain eye disease, the other is contraindicated. It may seem needless to emphasize this warning, but experience has taught how easy it is to pick up the wrong bottle from a tray containing similar vials when the room is dimly lighted.

In addition, the solution should be checked for color changes or sedimentation, which indicates that the solution is decomposing. If this is so, the solution should be discarded and a fresh one ordered and sterilized for use. Patients especially should be warned to avoid using medication of any kind if it has been in the medicine cabinet at home for months or years. Of course the use of small sterile disposable containers has helped reduce this problem and has also eliminated the need for a separate dropper.

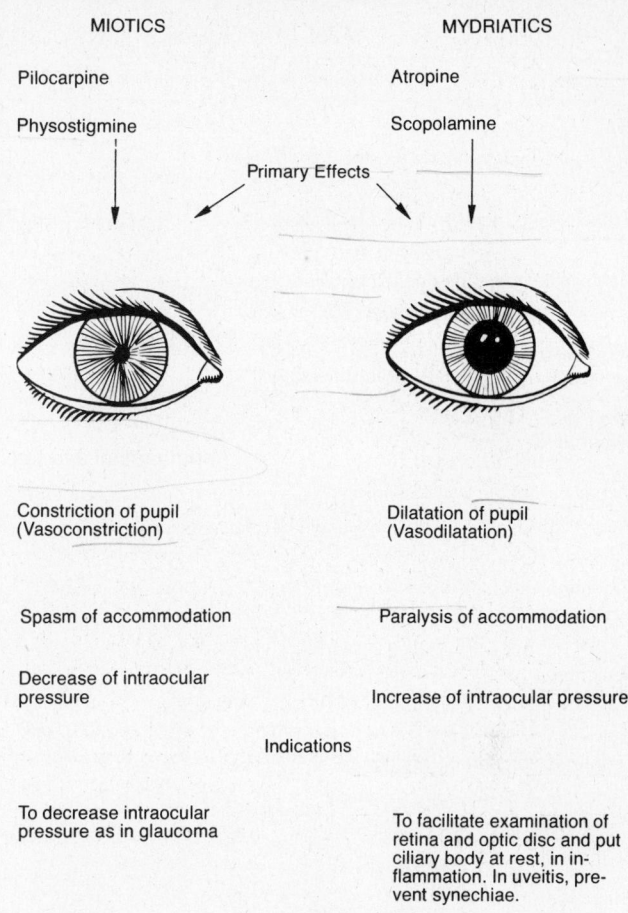

Figure 51-5. Effects and indications of miotics and mydriatics.

INSTILLATION. Before the medication is instilled into the eyes, the lids and the lashes are cleansed. Then the head of the patient is tilted backward (Fig. 51-6A) and inclined slightly to the side, so that the solution will run away from the tear duct. This latter precaution is especially necessary when toxic solutions, such as atropine, are employed, because absorption of the excess drug by way of the nose and the pharynx may lead to toxic symptoms. In most patients it is well to press the inner angle of the eye after instilling the drops to prevent the excess solution from entering the nose.

* The lower lid is depressed with the fingers of the left hand, the patient is told to look upward, and the solution is dropped on the everted lower lid.
* *Care must be taken that the pipette does not touch any part of the eye or the lids, to guard against contamination of the dropper and injury to the eye.*
* After the drops (1 or 2 at most) are placed in the eye, the lid is released, and any excess fluid is sponged gently from the lids and the cheeks with sterile cotton.
* After the medication is instilled, the patient is instructed to

TABLE 51-1. MEDICATIONS USED FREQUENTLY IN EYE CONDITIONS

MEDICATION	ACTION
Local Anesthetics	
Tetracaine hydrochloride (Pontocaine), 0.5%	Commonly used topical anesthetic Anesthesia produced in 1 to 2 minutes
Proparacaine hydrochloride (Ophthaine), 0.5%	More rapid in action Less discomfort during instillation
Benoxinate hydrochloride (Dorsacaine), 0.4%	Fewer allergic reactions than tetracaine
Procaine hydrochloride, 1 and 2%	Commonly used for injection in eye surgery Lasts about 45 minutes
Lidocaine hydrochloride (Xylocaine), 2%	Some favor this over procaine because its action is more rapid and it lasts longer
Antimicrobial and Chemotherapeutic Agents	
Neomycin sulfate (Mycifradin)	Topical application for external infections
Neomycin sulfate with polymyxin and bacitracin (Neosporin)	Broad-spectrum, ointment or solution Only disadvantage is its allergenic nature (allergy is to neomycin)
Chloramphenicol (Chloromycetin), 10 to 15% sol.; topically used in ¼% and ½%	Good penetrating power Very effective May sensitize a patient for future systemic use
Penicillin	Primarily used in newborns in ointment form Occasionally used for intraocular infection Primarily reserved for systemic use
Sodium methicillin (Staphcillin)	Used for penicillinase-producing organisms
Bacitracin, 500 units/gm. ointment	Good as a penicillin substitute for local eye uses against gram-positive organisms
Erythromycin	Effective as a penicillin substitute against resistant staphylococcal organisms

Sulfonamides:
    Sulfisoxazole (Gantrisin), 4% sol. or ointment
    Sulfacetamide sodium (Sulamyd Sod.)
	Used in treatment of conjunctivitis; sometimes effective against larger viruses

Dyes (For corneal staining to detect superficial abrasions)	
Fluorescein sodium	NOTE: Because *Pseudomonas aeruginosa,* highly pathogenic for corneal tissues, grows well in fluorescein solutions, the sterile single-dose containers or sterile Kimura fluorescein papers are recommended.
Rose Bengal, 2%	Selective dye to stain conjunctiva
Carbonic Anhydrase Inhibitor (Carbonic anhydrase is an enzyme present in body tissues. In the ciliary body, it is directly involved in the production of aqueous humor.)	
Acetazolamide (Diamox)	A sulfonamide used as a diuretic and also effective in decreasing production of aqueous humor by ciliary body in glaucoma. Because of side effects (gastric distress, shortness of breath, acidosis, tingling of extremities, dermatitis, ureteral stones), it is prescribed cautiously for selected patients.
Sympathomimetic Drugs (Used primarily for mydriasis and occasionally as vasoconstrictors)	
Phenylephrine hydrochloride (Neo-Synephrine), 2.5 to 10%	Action lasts 3 hours
Hydroxyamphetamine hydrobromide ophthalmic solution (Paredrine), 1%	Action lasts 3 hours
Epinephrine hydrochloride (Adrenalin), 1:1,000; (Glaucon), 2%	Lowers intraocular pressure in open-angle glaucoma (inhibits aqueous production)

TABLE 51-1. MEDICATIONS USED FREQUENTLY IN EYE CONDITIONS (CONTINUED)

MEDICATION	ACTION

Parasympathomimetic Drugs
(Used as miotics for controlling intraocular pressure in glaucoma)

Group I–Act directly on myoneural junction:

Pilocarpine hydrochloride, 0.5, 1, 2, 3, 4, and 6%	Drug of choice in glaucoma Action lasts 6 to 8 hours
Carbachol (Carcholin) 1.5 to 3%	Used if pilocarpine is ineffective

Group II–Cholinesterase inhibitors:

Physostigmine salicylate (Eserine), 0.25 and 0.5%	Action lasts 6 to 8 hours Because it is allergenic, unstable, and short in its action, it is gradually being replaced by Phospholine.
Echothiophate iodide (Phospholine Iodide), 0.06, 0.125, 0.25%	Water-soluble Causes less local irritation Action lasts 24 hours
Isoflurophate (diisopropyl fluorophosphate) (DFP) (Floropryl), 0.0025% ophthalmic ointment; 0.1%—ophthalmic solution	Oil-soluble miotic May produce side effects; watch for vomiting, diarrhea, tenesmus

Parasympatholytic Medications
(Used as mydriatics to facilitate ophthalmoscopic examination and for mydriasis and cycloplegia in refraction and in treatment of uveitis)

Mydriatics:

Epinephrine (Epitrate), 1 to 2%	Action lasts 12 hours
Eucatropine hydrochloride (Euphthalmine), 5.0%	Short-lived action Can dilate pupil without affecting accommodation

Cycloplegics:

Homatropine hydrobromide, 2 and 5%	A popular drug for cycloplegic refraction Action lasts 24 to 36 hours Allergic reactions rare
Scopolamine hydrobromide (hyoscine), 0.2% to 0.5%	Used in children's refraction Used in treating uveitis Because of low allergic reaction, it is preferred to atropine May cause dizziness and disorientation in older persons
Atropine sulfate, 0.5, 1, and 2%	Most powerful of this group Action lasts 10 to 14 days, during which eyes must be protected from bright light Used in treating uveitis Used in refraction of children Contraindicated in narrow-angle glaucoma 5% of persons are sensitive to it (symptoms: difficulty in swallowing, dizziness, flushed skin with circumoral pallor, rapid full pulse, delirium)
Cyclopentolate hydrochloride, (Cyclogyl), 0.5 and 1%	Action is less than 24 hours Very popular drug for cycloplegic refraction
Tropicamide (Mydriacyl), 0.5 and 1%	Newer, shorter acting—lasts 6 hours

Adrenal Corticosteroids
(Effective in treating inflammatory conditions of the eye: uveitis, episcleritis, chemical burns. Decreases vascularization and scarring following burns, trauma and severe inflammation.)

Cortisone acetate, 0.5 to 2.5%—suspension; 1.5%—ointment	Least expensive
Hydrocortisone, 0.5 to 2.5%—suspension; 1.5%—ointment	Greater potency than cortisone, so it can be used in lower concentrations
Prednisone, prednisolone, dexamethasone, and betamethasone	These are thought to be more potent than hydrocortisone
Fludrocortisone acetate (Florinef, Alflorone), 0.1%	

NOTE: These are highly dangerous when used in the presence of herpes simplex keratitis. The patient should definitely be under the care of an ophthalmologist with these medications. All steroids are now known to produce glaucoma in certain predisposed patients. Use of steroids locally or systemically must be carefully supervised.

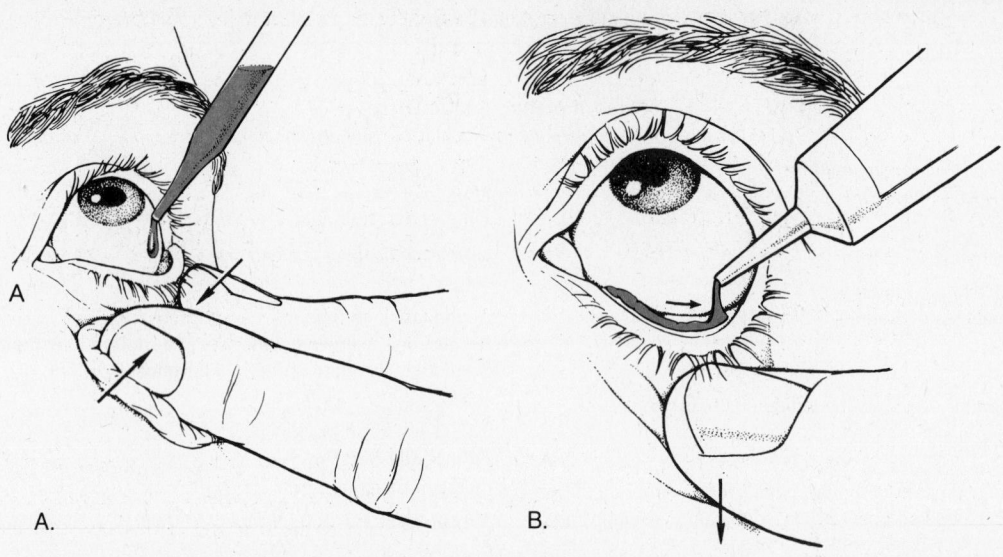

Figure 51-6. *A.* When instilling eye drops, instruct the patient to look upward, then lightly pinch the lower lid to form a receptacle for the dropped medication. *B.* In applying ointment, instruct the patient to look upward, then depress the lower lid and gently squeeze ointment along the everted lid beginning at the inner canthus (close to the nose) and then moving outward.

close his eyes gently; patients often have a tendency to "squeeze" their eyes closed, thereby expelling the medication.

- If the dropper has not been contaminated it may be replaced in the bottle, but is to be used only for this patient.

Ointments

Ointments of various kinds are used frequently in the treatment of inflammatory diseases of the lids, the conjunctiva, and the cornea. Those ordered most commonly are sulfonamides, bacitracin, neomycin, chloramphenicol, Terramycin, steroids, and various combinations.

Ointments are applied best by gently pulling down the lower lid and expressing a small amount of the ointment from the tube onto the conjunctiva of the lower lid. Care is taken not to touch the eye or the eyelid with the tube. The lid then may be massaged gently in such a way as to distribute the drug over the eyeball (Fig. 51-6B).

Ocular Irrigations

Ocular irrigations are indicated in treating various inflammations of the conjunctiva, in preparing the patient for eye surgery, and in removing inflammatory secretions. They are also used for their antiseptic effect. The fluid to be employed depends on the condition present and should be warmed before being used.

The irrigating apparatus is simple, consisting of a commercially prepared plastic irrigating bottle containing sterile ophthalmic solution (Blinx, Dacriose) and a small curved basin and cotton for catching the fluid and the secretions. Each patient should have his own solution in a plastic dispenser with cap.

- The patient lies flat on his back or sits with the head tilted backward and inclined slightly toward the side to be treated. The basin may be held by the patient, if he is sitting, or so placed that when he is lying down it will catch the fluid as it runs from the eye. The nurse stands in front of the patient.
- After the lids are carefully cleansed to remove dust, secretions, and crusts, the lids are held open with the thumb and the fingers of one hand and the eye flushed gently, directing the stream away from the nose. The fluid is never directed toward the nose, because of the danger that it may spill over into the other eye. The procedure is continued until the eye is entirely free of secretions.
- It must be remembered that very little force is to be used, because of the danger of injury. For the same reason, and to prevent contamination, no part of the irrigator should touch the eye, the lid, or the lashes.
- When the irrigation has been completed, the eye and the cheek are dried gently with cotton.

CONTINUOUS IRRIGATION OF THE EYE. Continuous irrigation is indicated in chemical burns, resistant corneal ulcers, enophthalmitis, uveitis, socket infections after enucleation, or conditions in which constant medication or debridement is indicated. Prior to irrigation, Ophthaine is instilled as a local anesthetic.

Hot Compresses

Heat relieves pain and increases the circulation, thereby promoting absorption and reducing tension in the eye. It is especially valuable for conjunctivitis accompanied by excessive secretions. Heat is best applied in the form of compresses composed of seven or eight layers of gauze or cotton just large enough to cover the eye.

- The patient is moved to the side of the bed, and a towel is used to cover the chest. The skin of the lids and the adjacent cheek may be anointed with cold cream or petrolatum.
- The compresses then are moistened in a basin of water or any other prescribed solution that has been heated.
- The fluid, which should be kept at a temperature between 46 to 49° C. (115-120° F.), should be expressed or squeezed from the pad, and the compress, after being tested for temperature on the back of the hand, should be placed gently over the closed lids.
- The pads should be changed every 30 to 60 seconds for 10 or 15 minutes, and the application should be repeated every 2 or 3 hours.
- At the completion of the period of application, the lids should be dried gently with cotton.
- New pads should be used for each application and, if the eyes have a purulent secretion, the compresses should be applied to one eye at a time, the solution and the basin being changed between applications in order not to carry infection from one eye to the other.

Cold Compresses

Cold causes a capillary constriction that tends to reduce the amount of secretion and relieve pain during the early stages of acute inflammatory conditions of the conjunctiva. Cold compresses are useful in relieving itching due to allergic conjunctivitis.

The patient is prepared in the same manner as for the application of hot compresses. The pads are moistened in boric-acid solution and placed in rows on a block of ice suspended by a gauze sling over a basin. They are applied to the closed lids and are changed every 15 to 30 seconds, for a period of 5 to 15 minutes each hour.

- Cold compresses are never used in the treatment of inflammations of the eye (iritis, keratitis), because cold, by constricting the capillaries, interferes with the nutrition of the cornea.

TRAUMA TO THE EYE

The prevention of eye injuries is a phase of child and adult education that cannot be emphasized too strongly. Children need to be reminded frequently of the dangers of sticks, arrows, and darts, BB guns, "sparklers," sling shots, rubber bands, and even harmless-looking toys. Precautions that should be taken when power tools are used need to be explained, along with the reasons protection is necessary from very bright lights, the sun shining on the snow, chemical fumes, sprays, and flying chips of wood. The use of goggles gives protection against most foreign bodies, but specially designed safety goggles or glasses with impact-resistant lenses are preferable if there is danger of flying metal or wood objects that may break the glass. Elderly persons or those unsure of their footing need safeguards where there is a possibility of injury.

General measures in caring for patients with eye injuries may include the following:

- Obtain a history of the injury first, then consult with an ophthalmologist immediately.
- Irrigate the eye with saline solution; however, note that irrigations may be dangerous in the instance of a penetrating eye injury.
- Stain the front surface of the eye with sterile fluorescein paper (Fluor-I-Strip) — the yellowish-green dye used to detect abrasions and ulcers.
- Irrigate the eye again.
- Evaluate the injury and manage as prescribed.
- Employ follow-up care.

Foreign Bodies

Foreign bodies (dust, cinders, and so forth) frequently cause considerable discomfort by irritating the sensitive conjunctiva. If the foreign body has been in the eye only a short time, it may be removed by a nurse. One way to detect foreign particles in the eye is to have the patient close his eyes, then darken the room and gently place a penlight on the lid. The foreign particle will show up as a black shadow.

The lower lid should be everted, the patient instructed to look up, and the lower half of the conjunctival sac examined.

If the particle is not found, the upper eye is examined by everting the upper lid. The examiner stands in front of the patient and instructs him to look down at his feet. The lashes are grasped between the thumb and fingers of one hand, and a matchstick, an applicator, or a toothpick is placed across the upper part of the lid. The lashes are pulled downward and forward, away from the eye, as the applicator is pressed downward, gently. The foreign body may be removed by touching it gently with a small applicator tipped with cotton and moistened in saline solution.

If this method is unsuccessful, or if the offending particle has been in the eye for a considerable time, no attempt should be made to remove it. It may have become embedded in cornea, and there is considerable danger of serious injury if removal is attempted by unskilled hands. The ophthalmologist usually requires local anesthesia, a hand lens, fluorescein, an eye spud, normal saline for irrigating the eye and, as a prophylaxis against infection, an antibiotic solution to instill after the offending particle is removed. If the particle is known to be a metal, the physician may use a magnet to remove it.

Acid and Alkali Burns

Careless use of hair sprays and other spray-on products has increased the incidence of chemical burns of the eye.

- Whenever acid or alkali gets on the lids or in the eye, an emergency exists, requiring that immediate action be taken. In such an instance, *the lids, the conjunctiva, and the cornea must be flushed copiously!*

The easiest and quickest way to flush the eye is to have the patient hold his head under a faucet and allow the water to run over the eye and wash it out. However, it is more satisfactory to flush the eye with a syringe, if available, taking care not to contaminate the other eye if it has not already been contaminated. Continuous flushing for at least 15 minutes is desirable. Plain tap water is adequate under such circumstances.

Actinic Trauma

Ultraviolet rays may damage the cornea as a result of excessive sunlight, snow blindness, and the use of a welder's arc ("welder's flash") or a sun lamp. Treatment consists of instilling anesthetic drops and patching both eyes.

Contusions and Hematoma ("Black Eye")

Trauma to the eye frequently results in hemorrhage. The bleeding that enters the loose tissues of the orbit spreads rapidly, discoloring the lids and surrounding skin. In itself the injury is not too serious, but frequently it is frightening to patients because the discoloration and swelling is so prominent. The bleeding usually stops spontaneously, but it may be reduced and the swelling lessened by the application of cold compresses. Absorption of the blood may be hastened after the first 24 hours by the use of hot compresses applied 15 minutes at a time, at intervals throughout the day. Drugs are now available to help hasten absorption of hematomas.

Corneal Abrasions

Lacerations of the cornea can be detected after being stained with sodium fluorescein (Fluor-I-Strip). A blue penlight more clearly identifies the abrasion than a white light.

Usually a local anesthetic and antibacterial drops are administered, and an eye patch is applied for 24 to 36 hours. The patient is instructed to keep the eyes at rest to promote comfort and facilitate the healing process. The danger to be guarded against with an abrasion is the development of a corneal ulcer. Therefore, if there is no improvement after 24 hours, an ophthalmic consultation is desirable.

Lacerations

Lacerations of the eyelids are serious because the lids become scarred and are unable to close. Injuries to the lids are treated in the same way as any other wound, but an ophthalmologist usually is requested to care for them.

Lacerations of the eyeball are more serious because visual defects may result. Since more extensive injuries may endanger the entire eye, such injuries are referred invariably to the ophthalmologist for appropriate care. Injuries of this type may entail transplantation of conjunctival flaps to prevent leakage of ocular fluids, excision of the prolapsed iris and, in severe injuries, even removal of the eye.

CONDITIONS OF THE EYELIDS (Table 51-2)

BLEPHARITIS. This common disorder of the lids can be controlled through cleanliness and the prevention of excessive dryness. Since blepharitis is frequently associated with seborrhea, attempts are made to keep the scalp clean. Daily cleaning of the eyelids by rubbing them gently with a clean wet washcloth helps to remove scales. Usually, an anti-infective ointment is prescribed, such as steroid-sulfa drops, to be applied to the lid margin twice a day. For pure staphylococcal blepharitis, local antibiotic solutions and application of moist heat are helpful.

STY (EXTERNAL HORDEOLUM). A *sty* is an infection of the Zeis's or Moll's glands that empty at the free edge of the eyelid. When a sty develops, this area becomes swollen,

TABLE 51-2. ASSESSMENT OF ACUTE EYE CONDITIONS

	ACUTE CONJUNCTIVITIS	ACUTE IRITIS	ACUTE GLAUCOMA	CORNEAL ULCER OR TRAUMA
Incidence	Very common	Common	Not common	Common
Vision	Normal	Some blurring	Marked blurring	Blurred (usually)
Pain	None	Moderate	Severe	May have pain
Intraocular pressure	Normal	Normal or low	Elevated	Normal
Cornea	Clear	Clear	Steamy	May have abrasion, foreign body, or ulcer
Ocular discharge	Moderate to copious	None	None	Watery and perhaps purulent
Pupillary response to light	Normal	Weak	Weak	Normal
Pupil size	Normal	Small	Dilated	Normal or small
Conjunctival vessels dilated	Yes	Mostly circumcorneal	Yes	Yes
Prognosis	Self-limited; 3 to 5 days	Good with treatment	Without proper treatment: Poor	Poor

red, tender, and painful. Frequently, a eyelash will be found in the center of the yellow point that appears. Hot compresses, applied in the early stage, hasten the pointing of the abscess. Removal of the central lash often is followed by drainage of pus, but incision sometimes is necessary. Antibiotic therapy hastens control of the infection.

CHALAZIA. A *chalazion* is a cyst of the meibomian glands. It appears as a small hard, painless lump in the lid and usually occurs secondary to infection of the gland which results when the opening on the lid margin becomes plugged. Occasionally, such a cyst may become infected. When this occurs, hot compresses are used; an incision and drainage also may be necessary. Incision and drainage are indicated if the mass distorts vision, causes astigmatism, or becomes a cosmetic blemish.

TRACHOMA. This chronic, highly communicable disease of the eyelids is one of the most common diseases of man and affects about 15 percent of the world's population (5 million). It is the greatest single cause for progressive loss of sight in the world. Trachoma is common in Asian countries, and countries around the Mediterranean Sea, particularly Egypt. In the United States, it is rare except among American Indians and Mexicans in the southwest.

The principal symptoms are mild itching and irritation. After an acute inflammatory process, follicles appear on the conjunctiva. Blurring of vision and increasing discomfort occur. The upper palpebral conjunctiva is affected.

The progress of the disease has been classified into four stages. In Stage I (incipient trachoma), immature follicles are present, especially in the upper tarsal conjunctiva. At the top of the cornea there is incipient pannus (abnormal vascularization). Stage II (established trachoma) consists of two types — type (a) and type (b). In type (a), follicular hypertrophy is predominant, while in type (b), papillary hypertrophy is predominant ("acute trachoma"). In Stage III, early conjunctival scarring is observed as fine white lines; corneal pannus also increases. In Stage IV, smooth scarring of the tarsal conjunctiva occurs, and vascular pannus becomes inactive. Secondary bacterial conjunctivitis increases the hazard of corneal ulceration, and this in turn leads to blindness.

Trachoma is spread by direct contact; therefore, personal cleanliness is a key factor in prevention. Isolating known cases and initiating antibiotic therapy early may help control the disease. If untreated, it will last for months or years. Medical treatment consists of a 3-week course of oral sulfonamide (trisulfapyrimidines) during which time the patient is closely observed for signs of toxicity. Should this occur, tetracycline is substituted for the sulfa drugs. The World Health Organization is making great strides in eliminating this curable disease, especially in Japan and the Philippines.

INFLAMMATIONS OF THE EYE

CONJUNCTIVITIS. Conjunctivitis may result from bacterial, viral, and rickettsial infections, or allergy, trauma, or chemical injury. However, no matter what the cause, the symptoms are similar: redness, pain, swelling, and lacrimation. The amount and the nature of discharge depend on the offending organisms; for instance, the pneumonococcus and the gonococcus cause an abundant purulent discharge. Frequent saline irrigations are required to remove the discharge. Warm compresses are recommended, to be applied for 15 minutes 3 or 4 times a day. Ointments such as sulfacetamide, Gentamicin, or chloromycetin drops or ointment may be instilled to clear the infection in 1 to 3 days. Untreated, the infection usually subsides in a week to 10 days. Precautions must be taken to prevent dissemination of infection to the other eye, as well as to other persons. Hands should be kept clean when treating the eye; individual clean washcloths and towels should be used.

UVEITIS. Uveitis is a general term for inflammatory conditions of the uveal tract (iris, ciliary body, choroid) which may be due to a number of causative agents. *Anterior uvetis* refers to *iritis* and *iridocyclitis,* whereas *posterior uveitis* refers to *choroiditis* and *chorioretinitis; panuveitis* involves the entire uveal tract. Uveitis (iritis) is usually unilateral and is characterized by pain, photophobia, blurring of vision, redness (circumcorneal flush), and a constricted pupil.

Some authorities prefer to classify the various forms of uveitis as granulomatous and nongranulomatous. In some aspects, the two forms are similar, but in others, there occurs a significant difference (see Table 51-3).

Complications and sequelae may result, should uveitis go untreated. Adhesions may result, impeding aqueous outflow at the anterior chamber angle, and causing glaucoma. If adhesions hinder the flow of aqueous humor from the posterior to the anterior chamber, then cataracts may develop. Even retinal detachment may

TABLE 51-3. COMPARISON BETWEEN GRANULOMATOUS AND NONGRANULOMATOUS UVEITIS

	GRANULOMATOUS	NONGRANULOMATOUS
Location	Any portion of uveal tract, but predilection for posterior part	Anterior portion; iris, ciliary body
Onset	Insidious	Acute
Pain	None or minimal	Marked
Circumcorneal flush	Slight	Present
Photophobia	Slight	Marked
Course	Chronic	Acute
Prognosis	Fair to poor	Good
Recurrence	Sometimes	Common

occur as a result of traction exerted on the retina by vitreous strands.

Management. Because the ophthalmologist can differentiate among the various forms of uveitis, treatment is directed to the specific type of involvement. For granulomatous uveitis, atropine is used, to reduce the likelihood of adhesions. Anti-infective chemotherapy may be initiated, and if the response is not favorable, it is followed with corticosteroids. Medications for comfort and relief of pain are also prescribed.

Nongranulomatous uveitis is also treated with atropine to keep the pupil dilated. Local, and possibly systemic steroids may be required.

Nongranulomatous uveitis subsides with treatment in a few weeks. Granulomatous uveitis may last months and even years in spite of treatment.

SYMPATHETIC OPHTHALMIA. Fortunately, this is a rare condition, but it may be suspected when there is a history of a penetrating eye injury in one eye (exciting eye) and the patient complains of photophobia, blurring vision, and injection in the other eye (sympathizing eye). Sympathetic ophthalmia is a severe granulomatous bilateral uveitis that may occur from 2 weeks to several years after an eye injury.

Medical management is directed in one of two directions: corticosteroids are administered both locally and systemically, while atropine is given locally. This treatment has proved effective. The other, more radical procedure is to suggest preventive enucleation of the severely injured eye before sympathetic ophthalmia develops. This decision is a difficult one; often, a patient can think more clearly and reach a satisfactory decision if he has the time and opportunity to express his thoughts and feelings about the operation. In such a case, it helps to understand the nature of the problem, the patient's ability and condition, and the desired goals of the ophthalmologist. Untreated, the disease progresses to bilateral blindness.

PTERYGIUM. Pterygium is an abnormal triangular fold of membrane that extends onto the cornea from the white of the eye; it always occurs toward the nose. It is thought to be caused by chronic irritation, as from dust or wind. Surgical intervention prevents its growth and protects against loss of vision. In some eye clinics, surgery is followed by beta-radiation therapy, which helps prevent recurrence of pterygium. Patients often erroneously refer to pterygium as a cataract.

THE PATIENT UNDERGOING EYE SURGERY

Preoperative Nursing Management

The preparation of the patient for an ophthalmic operation must be carried out with the most scrupulous care. The lower bowel is evacuated in the morning of the day of operation, and only liquid diet is given after that. The hair of female patients should be so arranged that it will remain in place for several days with bandages applied over it. Before the eyes are prepared for operation, the patient's head should be covered with a stockinet cap. This is followed by a normal cleansing of the face. Chloromycetin or gentamicin (Garamycin ophthalmic solution) are usually instilled as prescribed, prior to surgery, while the patient is awake.

Postoperative Nursing Considerations

Following surgery, the patient is placed in bed in a supine position with a small pillow under the head. Pillows are placed on each side of the head to keep the head still, and side rails are set in place to give the patient a sense of security. The patient is provided with a nurse-call system and instructed to ask for help rather than move or strain in an attempt to be self-sufficient. If a local anesthesia is used during the operation, the patient is usually ambulatory in a few hours after surgery.

The ophthalmologist is notified immediately if the patient has excessive pain or if the dressings are disturbed.

- Morphine is never given to ophthalmic patients unless it is certain that vomiting will not injure the eye.

Diversional or recreational therapy is important, but should be of such a nature that the eyes are not fatigued in any way. Even the environment of this patient is an important consideration. The walls and the ceiling should be painted in soft pastel shades. Light should be regulated so that it is not bright and does not produce a glare.

Prior to discharge, the patient is informed thoroughly regarding medications, eye aids (glasses), the type of work allowed, and follow-up visits.

STRABISMUS (SQUINT)

Strabismus, or *squint,* is a condition in which one eye deviates from the object at which the person is looking (lay term, "cross-eyed"). The deviating eye may turn in (*esotropia* — *ST*), or out (*exotropia* — *XT*), or up (*hypertropia* — *HT*). It may result from paralysis of the nerves supplying the extraocular muscles, due to injury or disease. Double vision or diplopia results.

A condition frequently associated with strabismus is amblyopia, a deficient acuity of central vision without apparent cause. (*Amblyopia ex anopsia* is amblyopia resulting from disuse.)

The following test may be used to determine whether strabismus is present. The patient fixes his vision on a light about 32.5 cm. (13 inches) from him. The reflex light is then observed to see if it falls in the center of each pupil.

In children, a strabismus due to ocular defects often develops. It is characterized by single vision, usually because the image seen by the nonfixing eye is suppressed involuntarily. The strabismus in children often may be corrected by properly fitted glasses.

Orthoptic training for muscle disturbances is successful in some instances, without operation. It consists of a series of muscle exercises carried out by means of various instruments, cards, and test objects. Patients with a marked degree of squint usually undergo operation after having had some training; after the eyes are straightened, the exercises are employed again. Early detection and immediate medical consultation are to be encouraged if the defect is to be corrected satisfactorily.

CORNEAL DISORDERS

Corneal Ulcers

Inflammation of the cornea (*keratitis*) with loss of substance, results in corneal ulcer. The inflammatory reaction often spreads deeper to the iris (iritis), resulting in the formation of pus which collects as a white or yellow deposit behind the cornea (hypopyon). If the ulceration perforates, the iris may prolapse through the cornea, or other serious complications may follow.

Because the cornea is so important to vision, any ulceration must be considered as a most serious condition. Scarring or perforation due to corneal ulceration is a major cause of blindness; 10 percent of all blindness is caused by corneal ulcers (6 percent in U.S.A.). The healing of all but the most superficial ulcers is attended with some degree of opacity of the cornea and, therefore, with some diminution of vision.

The symptoms of corneal ulceration are pain, marked photophobia, and increased lacrimation. The eye usually appears somewhat injected or "bloodshot."

Management. Prevention is much simpler and easier than cure. Therefore, prompt removal of foreign bodies and early treatment of infections may prevent the occurrence of a corneal ulcer.

Dark glasses are provided to relieve the photophobia. Mydriatics are given at frequent intervals. Optical anesthetics may be used to relieve pain. Fluorescein generally is used to outline the ulcers before the healing solutions are applied. Antibiotic solutions and chemotherapeutic agents are prescribed for the specific type of infection, since the microorganism may be bacterial, viral, or fungal.

Corneal Transplantation (Keratoplasty)

A keratoplasty may be done to repair a corneal opacity (scar), keratoconus, or chemical burn of the eye. The circular segment of cornea removed from the patient must be exactly matched and replaced by a similar segment of cornea from a donor eye. For best results, the graft should be removed within 5 or 6 hours following the death of the donor (to prevent softening of the cornea) and transplanted within 2 days.* Recent advances utilizing very fine monofilament nylon sutures, fine needles, operating microscopes, and soft contact lens have expanded the effective use of keratoplasty.

* The national eye bank (Eye-Bank for Sight Restoration, Inc., 210 E. 64th St., New York, N.Y. 10021) was founded in 1945. Eyes have been donated from persons all over the country and distributed to qualified ophthalmologists throughout the United States.

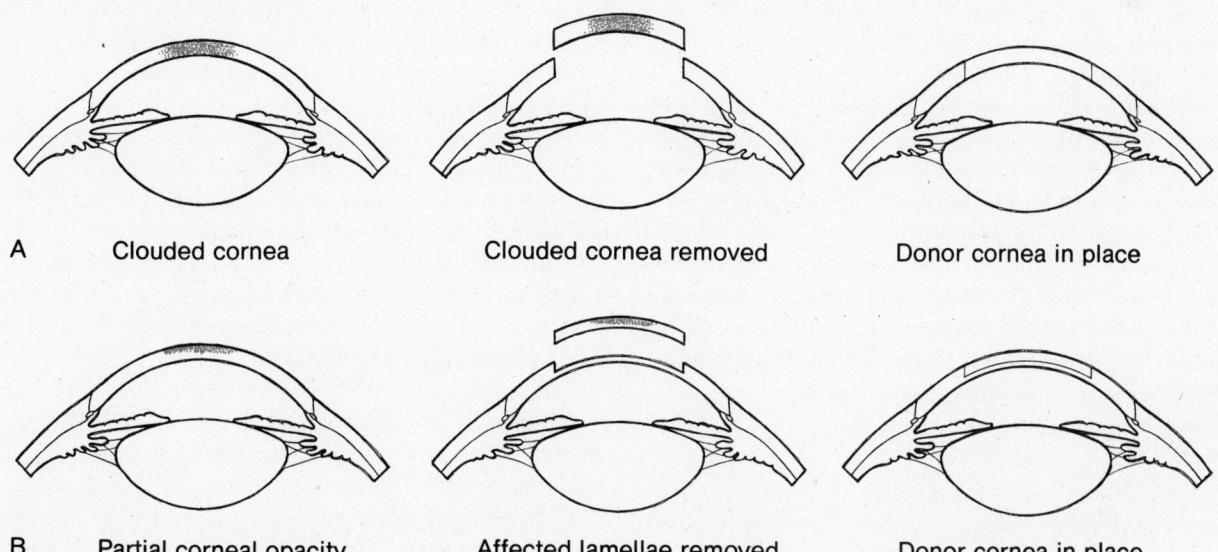

| A | Clouded cornea | Clouded cornea removed | Donor cornea in place |

| B | Partial corneal opacity | Affected lamellae removed | Donor cornea in place |

Figure 51-7. *A.* Penetrating keratoplasty: a full-thickness (7-8 mm.) disc is removed from the host and replaced with a matching full-thickness button from the donor. *B.* Lamellar keratoplasty: a thin layer of corneal tissue is excised from the host eye. Stroma and entire endothelium are spared.

The graft may be penetrating (including all layers of the cornea) or lamellar (involving only the outer layers of the cornea) (Fig. 51-7). The lamellar graft, popular in the past, is gradually being replaced by the penetrating graft.

Preoperative and Intraoperative Management. Since keratoplasty is elective surgery, the patient is probably aware of the nature of the operation and is no doubt optimistic about the likelihood of improved vision. The nurse, nevertheless, must allow time for the expression of concerns or questions that the patient may still have. Psychological and cultural concerns regarding the disability may have to be explored before the patient is in optimal condition for surgery. Physically, the patient should be free from respiratory or eye infections in order to promote postoperative healing.

Usually a transplant is done under local anesthesia and takes about an hour. A trephining instrument, having an end similar to that of a cookie cutter but the size of the cornea, is placed over the opacity, and the cornea is removed. The same instrument is used to remove the donor cornea so that the graft is a perfect fit. Ultrafine sutures are placed evenly to create a tight seal; this is done via an operating microscope.

Postoperative Management. Objectives of postoperative patient care are: (1) to avoid elevated intraocular pressure, as well as pressure upon the operated eye; (2) to provide rest for the eye so that healing progresses smoothly; and (3) to employ measures that will prevent infection of the eye.

Elevated intraocular pressure constricts the vascular supply and can cause retinal atrophy or damage to the graft. To prevent pressure from increasing within the eye, the nurse must be cognizant of those activities that can elevate pressure (see page 1143). Loss of aqueous humor through the suture line by increased pressure could cause dislocation of the newly transplanted cornea, prolapse of the iris, adhesions of the iris to the cornea, or malformation of the anterior chamber. To avoid these problems, when the patient is transferred from the operating table to the bed or stretcher, adequate personnel are required to move him horizontally in one smooth shift, giving adequate support to his head.

Intraocular pressure can be measured by sensitive electronic applanation tonometers. If the pressure is elevated, pharmacologic control can be achieved with such drugs as acetazolamide, which inhibits aqueous production.

Both eyes may be covered, to provide rest and to enhance healing. If one eye is uncovered, its movement will affect the operated eye because the two eyes move in unison. Healing is slow because the cornea is avascular, which also increases the possibility of infection. Thus, meticulous sterile technique is followed in dressing changes to protect the susceptible corneal epithelium from infection. Another means of reducing the chance for infection is to provide the patient with soft contact lenses, which protect the suture line. This is particularly effective in patients who have chemical burns. To prevent herpes simplex infection, the administration of antiviral agents may be indicated.

Graft rejection is controlled by topically applied corticosteroids; however, these are to be given only for short periods of time, since they retard healing. Even with the use of corticosteroids, graft rejection still occurs in about 20 percent of patients.

With this regimen of medical care, it is possible for the patient with a penetrating type of corneal transplant to have bathroom privileges the day of surgery and to be ambulatory the next day. The eye is unpatched on the third day, and the patient may be discharged in a week. Within a short time, normal activities may be resumed. The very fine sutures are well tolerated and need not be removed until 7 or 8 months after operation, when maximal healing has taken place. Periodic visits to the ophthalmologist will ensure that the patient is progressing as expected.

DETACHED RETINA

A *retinal detachment* occurs when the sensory retina separates from the pigment epithelium of the retina. The retina is that layer of the eye which perceives light and transmits impulses from its nerve cells to the optic nerve. When a tear occurs in the retina, vitreous humor and transudate seep out between the retinal layers, causing detachment. Tears or holes in the retina may occur suddenly or slowly, as a result of trauma or degeneration. It may also result from hemorrhage, exudation, or tumor in front of or behind the retina. Studies have shown that approximately 6 percent of the population have small holes or tears in the retina. Aging weakens these spots.

Assessment and Clinical Manifestations. The usual symptoms include flashes of light and blurred or "sooty" vision, sudden in onset; the patient may have the sensation of particles moving in his line of vision. These floating particles consist of retinal cells and blood that are released at the time of the tear and cast shadows on the retina as they drift by. Definite areas of vision may be blank, and in a few days the patient may have the sensation of a veil coming up or down in front of the eye, finally resulting in loss of vision.

The suddenness of the incapacity creates confusion and apprehension in most patients, as well as a fear of blindness. Usually, it means that the person must abandon his business or activity, with little or no time to make plans.

Conservative Management. The patient is treated with bed rest immediately. Both eyes are bandaged, in the hope that the retina will fall back into place as much as possible before surgery.

The patient should lie so that the area of detachment

will be in the dependent position. For example, a patient with a superior temporal detachment (the most common form) in the right eye should be supine, with the head turned to the right. For a left inferior nasal detachment of the retina, the patient should sit up, with the head turned to the right. Sedation and the tranquilizing drugs keep the patient comfortable and quiet.

Surgical Intervention

The objective in surgical treatment is to create a scar that seals the retina in place as it heals. Such treatment may be accomplished in one of several ways: electrodiathermy, cryosurgery, photocoagulation, or scleral buckling.

1. In *electrodiathermy,* an electrode needle is passed through the sclera, allowing the subretinal collection of fluid to escape. Because an exudate forms from the choroid, the torn retina adheres to the choroid, which in turn adheres to the sclera.

2. In *cryosurgery,* a supercooled probe is applied to the sclera, causing minimal damage; the choroid and retina adhere as a result of the scarring. The advantage of this method over the use of diathermy is the reduced damage to the sclera.

3. *Photocoagulation* makes use of a strong beam of light (from a carbon-arc source) that is directed through the dilated pupil to form a small burn, causing a choroid retinal inflammatory exudate. The *laser beam* (light amplification by stimulated emission of radiation) can be used in *photocoagulation.* This method of treatment is used for limited retinal detachments and also may be used after operation to reattach small areas.

4. In *scleral buckling,* the idea is to shorten the sclera to enhance contact between the choroid and retina. After the subretinal fluid is withdrawn, the detachment is treated by. one of the methods described above. The treated area is then indented, to "buckle" inward toward the vitreous humor (Fig. 51-8).

Postoperative Management

Both eyes are bandaged, and the patient is kept in bed for several days. This routine varies with the surgical procedure; patients with scleral buckling operations are permitted out of bed much sooner than those who have undergone diathermy. Precautions are taken to prevent the patient from bumping his head. After a gradual resumption of function, the patient may resume usual activities in 3 to 5 weeks.

The psychological nursing care of this patient is of major importance. Diversion that is relaxing is desirable, such as conversation, listening to music, having someone read a favorite book, and so forth.* These patients be-

---

* Recordings of books may be obtained from the public library or local association for the blind.

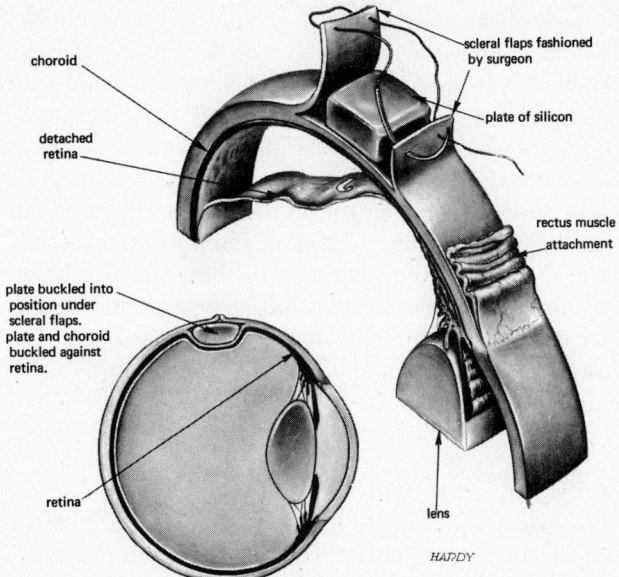

Figure 51-8. Scleral buckling for detached retina. (Ethicon, Inc.)

come depressed easily; therefore, every attempt should be made to prevent this reaction.

At the time of discharge the nurse should be sure that the patient understands all instructions for posthospital care and follow-up visits.

Prognosis. The prognosis for untreated retinal detachment is increasing detachment and eventual blindness. About 90 percent of patients can be cured with treatment. Some patients may require a second operation, which may be performed about 10 to 14 days after the first one. Ten percent of all detachments are or will become bilateral.

CATARACTS

A *cataract* is an opacity of the crystalline lens or its capsule. Occasionally it occurs at birth (congenital cataract) or in younger people, as a result of trauma or disease, but most commonly it occurs in adults past middle age (senile cataract).

Pathophysiology. The normal lens is a clear, transparent, buttonlike structure lying back of the iris; it possesses strong refractive powers. Physical and chemical changes may produce a loss of transparency of the lens. Swelling fibers, for example, cause a distortion of the image. Chemical change in lens protein may cause coagulation, thereby producing a cloudy appearance. Metabolic changes that result in a reduction of vitamins C and B_{12} in the lens also contribute to the formation of opacities. Although cataracts can be produced in the laboratory in many ways, the real cause of senile cataracts is still unknown.

Assessment.   Because the rays of light entering the eye must pass through the pupil and the lens to reach the retina, any opacity in the lens behind the pupil will produce alterations in vision. Objects may seem distorted, blurred, or hazy. In bright light, a cataract tends to scatter the light, causing an unpleasant glare. The patient experiences no pain, and visual loss is gradual. In time, the degenerative processes cause more opacification of the lens until the opacity becomes complete. Ordinarily, the lens is not visible; however, when a cataract develops, the pupil, which is normally black, becomes gray, and later milky-white. The cataract can be cured only by operation.

Management

In patients with uncomplicated senile cataracts, about 95 percent will regain satisfactory vision with surgery. Surgery for cataract is done at the convenience of the patient and is usually requested when the sight in the better eye causes problems. Because this particular surgery can be performed safely on elderly patients, even those in their nineties, the nurse is in a position to dispel family belief that the patient may be "too old" for the procedure. Improvement of a visual defect may make a person more independent and happier.

The patient is oriented to his room so that he will be familiar with his environment when his eyes are bandaged after the operation. The room is also arranged in such a way that the patient's personal needs are considered. For example, the nurse could place the bedside table on the side where the eye with better vision is. The patient can then see his belongings with a minimum of head movement. Preoperative teaching stresses those activities and restrictions he will experience after the operation, as well as what position he will be expected to maintain if he is kept in bed.

Preoperative Preparation.   Some clinics recommend a facial scrub the evening before and the morning of surgery in order to reduce pathogens and postoperative infection. Prophylactic antimicrobial eye drops may also be administered.

The patient is informed that a local anesthetic will be given in the operating room, that the injection may be uncomfortable at first, but that this discomfort will abate quickly. The surgeon may converse with him during the procedure.

Usually a sedative is prescribed the night before surgery, and a clear liquid breakfast given the morning of the operation, depending upon the time of day that the operation is scheduled. Preoperative medications in step-up fashion may be given in the morning, including a sedative, narcotic, and tranquilizer. Eye medications may include a topical mydriatic (which facilitates removal of the cataract when the pupil is dilated), and cycloplegics (to paralyze muscles of accommodation).

Surgical Intervention

Two general types of lens extraction may be performed: extracapsular and intracapsular. *Extracapsular extraction* is more often performed for congenital and traumatic cataracts than for senile cataracts. An incision is made through the sclera, barely outside of the cornea; the lens capsule is excised, and the lens is expressed by pressure exerted on the eye from below with a metal spoon. It is more conservative and simple to perform than the intracapsular extraction; however, in about 30 percent of patients, a secondary membrane forms that requires *discission* (a needling, or dividing, of the membrane).

The *intracapsular extraction* consists of removing the lens and the capsule which encases it.

Intraoperative Management.   The eyelids are held apart with a speculum (self-retaining retractor) placed inside the lids. Guideline and traction sutures are placed before the conjunctival incision is made at the 12 o'clock position; this incision is then extended to the 3 and 9 o'clock positions. The lens capsule is grasped, the cataract is delivered, and final suturing is done. If necessary, the surgeon reforms the anterior chamber with an injection of a balanced salt solution. Usually an iridectomy is performed at the time of cataract extraction.

When difficulty is expected in freeing the capsule of its zonules, a fibrinolytic and proteolytic enzyme, α-chymotrypsin, is injected into the anterior chamber under the iris. The lytic action is completed in 2 or 3 minutes and allows the lens to be extracted more easily.

Cryosurgery, a surgical technique in which freezing temperatures are used, is another method for extracting cataracts. All cryosurgical instruments operate on the principle that a cold metal adheres to a moist object. A thin pencil-like instrument with a metal-probe tip (straight or curved) is activated so that the temperature of the tip ranges from $-30°$ C. to $-40°$ C. The conjunctival flap is prepared and dissected as for a regular intracapsular extraction, after which the cryosurgical instrument is placed directly on the lens capsule. An ice ball forms in seconds, causing the capsule to adhere to the probe. A gentle upward and then sideward force frees and delivers the lens. The corneal flap is sutured back in place.

Cryoextraction is indicated for hypermature cataracts, which have a high incidence of capsular rupture, and in patients in whom a capsular rupture may exacerbate a glaucoma or uveitis.

Nursing implications both before and after operation are the same as for the conventional intracapsular extraction.

Phacoemulsification is an extracapsular removal of a lens by a mechanized instrument which is composed of three systems: irrigation, ultrasonic vibration, and aspiration. As the titanium tip of the instrument vibrates 40,000 times per second, the lens is broken up into minute particles, which are then aspirated. The procedure is generally done under local anesthesia, with the use of a microscope. Following surgery, glycerine drops, an eye pad, and an eye shield are applied; the next morning the dressing is removed, and the patient is discharged. Home care consists of instillation of cycloplegic and corticosteroid medications and a protective eye shield to be worn at night. The patient is permitted full activity with no restrictions.

An advantage of phacoemulsification over planned extracapsular or intracapsular extraction is that the cataract can be removed through a 2½ to 3 mm. corneoscleral incision. The small incision requires closure with only one or two sutures and thus allows the patient a much more rapid return to usual activities.

Intraocular Implant (IOL) is a prosthetic lens made of inert polymethylmethacrylate (Perspex, Plexiglas) with "wings" attached to the outer edges that permit the device to be attached to the iris in an anatomically correct position in the eye. This implant can be inserted following any type of cataract extraction.

The chief advantage in this procedure is the minimal distortion in the size or shape of the image. The ideal patient is one who is over 65 and possibly handicapped with arthritis, tremors, etc. (and who is therefore unable to manage spectacles or contact lenses).

Intraocular implants are not recommended for persons under 60 years of age, for a patient who already has an IOL and has developed a reaction, or for a patient who has cataracts in both eyes and is able to use spectacles or contact lenses.

The risk of infection is slightly higher than in simple cataract extraction. When there is extreme pupillary dilatation following lens implant, the implant may slip out of position.

Because existing safety data on the use of IOL is not currently available, the FDA published a regulation specifying the following clinical investigational procedures (applicable to physicians and manufacturers of intraocular lenses): (1) the sponsor of an IOL clinical investigation must receive prior approval from FDA (receiving an IDE — Investigational Device Exemption); (2) written informed-consent agreements must be signed by all prospective patients; and (3) all investigations are to be reviewed by Institutional Review Boards of each medical facility involved. These regulations are not designed to disrupt research or present difficulties which might impede the availability and benefits of intraocular implants.

Postoperative care for the patient with intracapsular lens implant is similar to the care for the cataract patient, described below. Constricting eyedrops are given to the patient having an iris-plane implant, to prevent it from dislodging. Steroid and antimicrobial eyedrops may be required. When the patient goes home, an eye patch or dark glasses must be worn for about a month if the eyes are sensitive to light and are watering.

Length of stay in the hospital following cataract sur-

gery may range from 24 hours to 10 days, depending upon the type of surgery performed; e.g., phacoemulsification, intraocular implant, or extra- or intracapsular extraction.

For an overall view of the care of the patient undergoing cataract surgery, see outline, page 1143.

Postoperative Management. Major objectives of postoperative care of the cataract patient (excluding phacoemulsification) are to prevent hemorrhage and stress on the sutures. The eye is kept bandaged for one day and an eye shield is worn over the dressing to protect the eye from injury. Only the operated eye is covered.

The patient is permitted a low, firm pillow immediately after operation and may have the head of the bed raised 30 to 45 degrees. Any strain felt by the patient may be relieved somewhat by placing pillows under the knees for short intervals and a small pillow under the small of the back. Later in the day he may be allowed out of bed, depending on his condition and the physician's preference. However, he is advised to move cautiously and slowly and to avoid straining for at least 3 weeks. For example, he ought not to stoop, pick up objects from the floor, or lift anything. Slip-in slippers will avoid the necessity to bend to tie laces. Even if the patient has vision in one eye, he should not walk through corridors alone; this will prevent his being bumped because of an inability to see objects or persons on the operated side.

Pain usually is slight after cataract extraction, but should it become severe the surgeon is to be notified at once, since it may be the symptom of a serious complication such as hemorrhage.

Liquid diet is supplemented with custards, junkets, and gelatin. Soft or regular diet is resumed when desired.

Atropine may be instilled 1 hour after operation by the surgeon to relieve pain. Dressings are changed twice daily by the physician for 3 to 5 days.

Patient instruction includes instillation of eye drops as prescribed, application of moist compresses, and use of a metal shield at night to protect the operated eye. The eyelids are not to be squeezed together, since this may injure the suture line or cause hemorrhage.

The effects of sensory deprivation can be minimized if the patient is kept interested in diversional activities such as the radio, "talking books," or visitors. He is discharged the day after surgery if no complications arise.

About 3 weeks after the operation, the aphakic (without lens) patient receives a temporary pair of thick biconvex glasses. Adjustment to these is gradual. The sides curve inward, the bottom curves upward, and the top curves down. Only through the center of the glass will the patient have clear vision. He must learn to turn his head to bring an object into central vision. The patient needs practice in judging distances, such as when climbing stairs or pouring liquids. Objects appear one-third larger than they really are. Contact lenses reduce this size discrepancy and allow adjustment to binocular vision

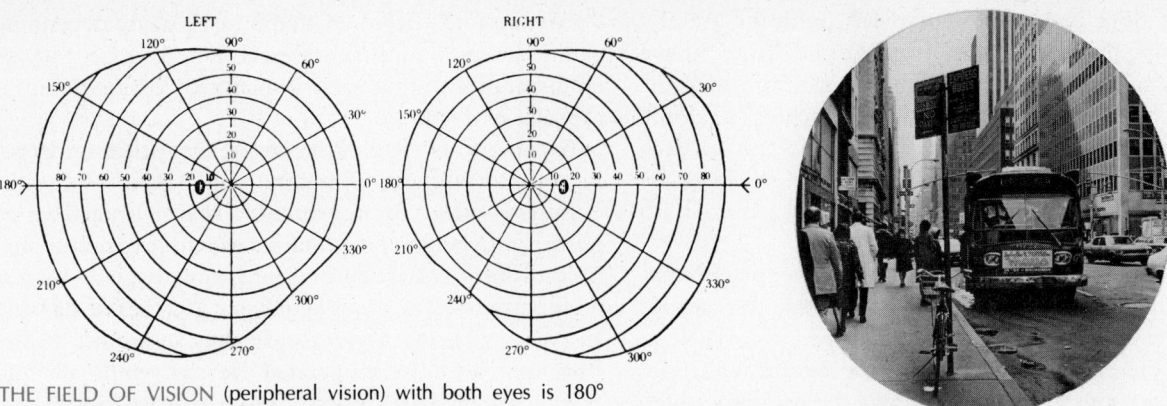

LEFT   RIGHT

THE FIELD OF VISION (peripheral vision) with both eyes is 180° recorded on these charts.

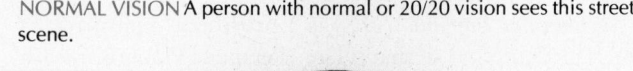

NORMAL VISION A person with normal or 20/20 vision sees this street scene.

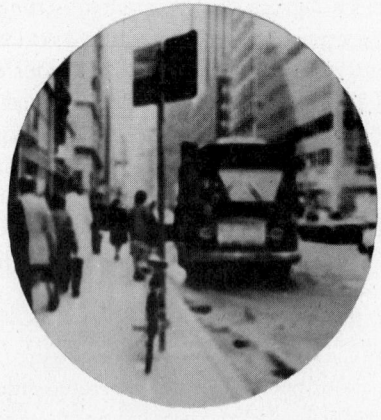

CATARACT diminished acuity from an opacity of the lens. The field of vision is unaffected. There is no scotoma, but the person has an overall haziness of the view, particularly in glaring light conditions.

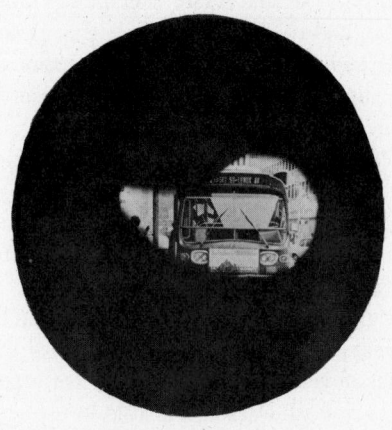

GLAUCOMA Advanced glaucoma involves loss of peripheral vision but the individual still retains most of his central vision.

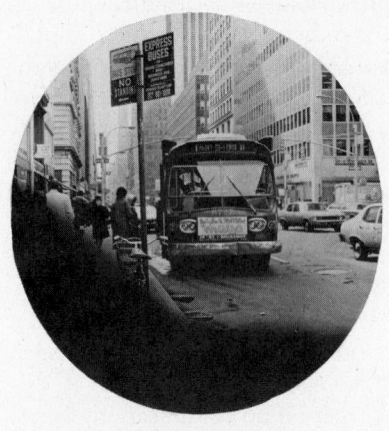

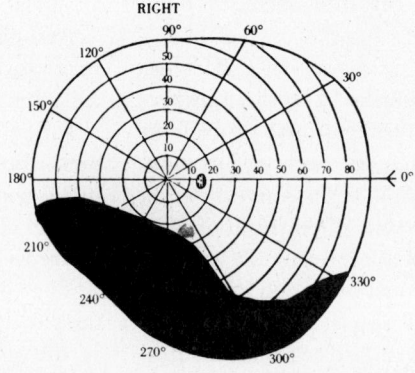

RIGHT

RETINAL DETACHMENT shown here in the active stage. There are many causes for detachment, but the hole or tear allows fluid to lift the retina from its normal position. This elevated retina causes a field or vision defect, seen as a dark shadow in the peripheral field. It may be above, or below as illustrated.

Figure 51-9. Photographs representing the eye diseases are done as if the camera were the right eye. The accompanying visual-field chart showing the area of visual loss also represents the right eye. (Photo courtesy The Lighthouse, The New York Association for the Blind)

more readily. However, not all individuals can adjust to contact lenses. In about 8 weeks, permanent lenses are ordered. By this time, the patient should be making a satisfactory psychological, physical, and visual adjustment.

GLAUCOMA

Glaucoma is a disease characterized by increased tension or pressure within the eye and progressive loss of visual field (Fig. 51-9). It ordinarily occurs in individuals past 40 and may be classified as primary or secondary:

1. *Primary:*
   a. Chronic simple glaucoma (open-angle)
   b. Congestive glaucoma (closed-angle)
      (1) Acute
      (2) Chronic
2. *Secondary:*
   Many types secondary to such conditions as trauma, aphakia, iritis, tumor, hemorrhage, etc.

The cause of primary glaucoma is unknown. Some evidence indicates that chronic simple glaucoma, the most common form, is inherited.

This disorder is the second most common cause of blindness in the United States. In view of the fact that about 1 million Americans have undiagnosed glaucoma, the health professions have a responsibility to encourage annual eye checkups, because *early detection could substantially reduce the incidence of blindness from glaucoma.*

Pathophysiology and Diagnostic Assessment. Intraocular pressure increases when the patient exerts energy, as in running, climbing the stairs, bending over to pick up an object, sneezing, or turning the head suddenly.

It also occurs in relation to emotional upsets (e.g., apprehension about the nature and prognosis of surgery may cause an increase in pressure). Apparently, both physical and emotional factors are involved in increasing pressure within the eye. The underlying mechanism is episcleral venous pressure engorgement transmitted by the Valsalva phenomenon.

The total volume and pressure of intraocular fluid is regulated by the balance between formation and reabsorption of aqueous humor. Ordinarily, the pressure-regulating mechanism maintains an almost constant balance throughout life. The exact operation of this mechanism is not known; however, pathologic changes at the iridocorneal angle usually increase intraocular pressure. Early detection of increased ocular pressure (22–30 mm. Hg) does not necessarily mean the patient will develop frank glaucoma.

Measurement of Intraocular Pressure. An increase in

THE PATIENT UNDERGOING CATARACT SURGERY

OBJECTIVES AND PRINCIPLES OF NURSING MANAGEMENT

I. **To prepare the patient for cataract surgery:**
   A. Orient the patient to his new environment.
      1. Walk with the patient around the unit.
      2. Explain the plan of care.
      3. Provide side rails on bed if patient is elderly.
   B. Begin rehabilitation measures as soon after admission as possible.
      1. Teach patient to turn to side of the unaffected eye only.
      2. Instruct the patient how to close his eyes slowly without squeezing the lids.
   C. Reduce the conjunctival bacterial count.
      1. Obtain a conjunctival culture, if prescribed.
      2. Use local broad-spectrum antibiotics as prescribed.
      3. Use aseptic technique when doing eye treatments and procedures.
   D. Prepare the affected eye for surgery.
      1. Identify beyond a doubt the proper eye to be operated upon.
      2. Instill local mydriatic if prescribed.
      3. Determine whether the pupil is dilated after the instillation of a mydriatic is completed.

II. **To give optimal nursing care after the operation:**
   A. Reorient the patient to his surroundings.
   B. Prevent increased intraocular pressure and stress on the suture line.
      1. Instruct the patient not to cough, sneeze, or move too rapidly.
      2. Position the patient on his back and unoperated side.
      3. Elevate the head of the bed 30 to 45 degrees for comfort.
      4. Keep the eye shield on the operated eye to protect it from injury.
   C. Promote the comfort of the patient.
      1. Position him to relieve back pain.
      2. Give mild analgesics to control pain.
      3. Maintain a quiet and relaxed environment.
      4. Inform the patient when you enter the room.
   D. Observe and treat for complications of hemorrhage or pain.
      1. Notify physician immediately if patient complains of sudden pain in eye.
      2. Observe for, and try to allay restlessness.

III. **To promote the rehabilitation of the patient:**
   A. Encourage the patient to become independent.
      1. Teach him to increase his activities gradually.
      2. Walk with him when he gets out of bed.
   B. Instruct the patient and his family about the use of eyedrops.
   C. Refer the patient to proper agencies if home assistance is needed.
   D. Assist the patient to participate in a program of diversional activities during the convalescent period.
   E. Inform the patient that:
      1. Dark glasses may be used after the eye dressing is removed.
      2. Temporary corrective lenses may be prescribed during the convalescent period.
      3. Permanent lenses will be prescribed 6 to 8 weeks after surgery, unless the patient has intraocular implant(s).

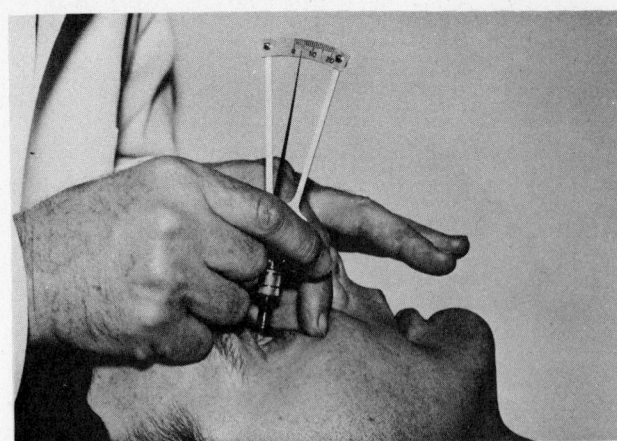

Figure 51-10. After a local anesthetic is instilled into the eye, the Schiotz tonometer is gently rested on the eyeball; the indicator measures in mm. Hg the ocular tension. (Courtesy, F. H. Roy, M.D.)

intraocular pressure or hardening of the eyeball may be noted with the fingers, but more accurately it is measured by means of a *tonometer* (Fig. 51-10). This is a simple and painless test in which the patient tilts his head back and looks to the ceiling. The cornea of the eye is anesthetized with a drop of 0.5 percent Ophthaine. The sterile footplate of the tonometer is placed on the cornea; a small pressure is applied to the central plunger, causing the central cornea to be displaced inward. Pressure within the eye exerts a force that moves an indicator. A normal reading is 11 to 22 mm. Hg.

Electronic tonometry can be done, but it involves expensive equipment. Tonography units provide a graphic presentation of intraocular pressure for a 4-minute test period. This is a valuable index that assists the physician in determining movement of the aqueous humor.

Primary (Open-Angle) Glaucoma

Primary open-angle glaucoma is the most common form of glaucoma, occurring in about 2 percent of the population over the age of 40; it occurs in about 10 percent of those whose blood relatives have had glaucoma. Symptoms are insidious and develop slowly. The patient may have mild discomfort, such as a tired feeling in the eye. Impairment of peripheral vision occurs long before any effects are noted on central vision. The patient may become aware of peripheral visual impairment by bumping into things that he did not see at his side; driving a car may be a hazard to others because he may not be able to see pedestrians or approaching vehicles laterally. The patient may also note halos around lights.

PHARMACOTHERAPY AND SURGICAL MANAGEMENT. Primary (open-angle) glaucoma often is treated by one or a combination of the following medications: (1) miotics, such as pilocarpine or carbachol, to increase outflow of aqueous humor, (2) carbonic anhydrase inhibitors, such as acetazolamide (Diamox) or dichlorphenamide (Daranide), to decrease the production of aqueous humor, (3) anticholinesterase, such as echothiophate iodide (Phospholine Iodide), or demecarium bromide (Humorsol), to facilitate the outflow of aqueous humor, (4) epinephrine drops, to decrease production of aqueous humor and promote its outflow from the eye.

Timolol maleate (Timoptic), a beta-adrenergic receptor blocking agent has recently been approved for the treatment of primary open-angle glaucoma, aphakic glaucoma, and selected patients with secondary glaucoma. It appears to be better tolerated than previously used drugs. When applied topically, timolol decreases production of aqueous humor and reduces intraocular pressure for as long as 24 hours. Pupillary size is not changed nor is the tone of the ciliary body altered; hence this medication does not interfere with vision.

Drug dosage is usually one drop twice a day. Occasionally mild eye irritation or brief blurred vision occurs with timolol. This medication is prescribed with caution for patients who may have adverse effects from systemic use of beta-adrenergic receptor blocking agents (such as patients with asthma, heart block, or heart failure).

Remissions may occur, but, if there is no improvement, surgery may be done. In the preoperative treatment of these patients, irrigations of both eyes are often prescribed, and weaker solutions of pilocarpine are instilled in the unaffected eye.

The surgeon makes a small opening with a circular knife at the junction of the cornea and the sclera. This operation, called *corneoscleral trephining,* leaves a permanent opening through which aqueous humor may drain. Usually it is covered by a flap of conjunctiva.

After the operation, the patient is kept flat and relatively quiet for 24 hours in order to prevent prolapse of the iris through the incision. He may turn to the unoperated side. Straining, coughing, squeezing the eyelid, and any other activity which can raise intraocular pressure is to be avoided. A liquid diet is permitted. Narcotics or sedatives may be given if necessary. After the first dressing is changed, the patient is allowed more freedom. The hospital stay usually lasts three days. Regular visits to the ophthalmologist are required, since glaucoma is a condition that must be followed periodically.

Acute (Closed-Angle) Glaucoma

When pressure increases rapidly, severe pain occurs in and around the eye. Artificial lights appear to have a rainbow around them, and vision becomes cloudy or blurred. Nausea and vomiting, as well as pupil dilatation, also may be noted. This is an emergency situation, which, if left untreated, may lead to blindness.

PHARMACOTHERAPY. Miotic drugs will cause the pupil

to contract and the iris to draw away from the cornea, thus allowing the aqueous humor to drain through the lymph spaces into the canal of Schlemm. Pilocarpine, eserine, or DFP (diisopropyl fluorophosphate) are the drugs employed. Dosage and frequency of drops are regulated to meet the individual requirements.

Another kind of medication (carbonic anhydrase inhibitor) restricts the action of the enzyme that is necessary to produce aqueous humor. Diamox is an example of such an agent. This aids in getting some patients in better condition for surgery and may control tension in other patients to such an extent that surgery is not necessary.

Ordinary U.S.P. glycerin (oral) reduces intraocular pressure through the mechanism of osmotic balance exchange. Glycerin has a high osmotic pressure; it withdraws fluid from the eye through the membrane, and lowers pressure. Mannitol (20%) intravenously may also be used.

SURGICAL INTERVENTION. In acute closed-angle glaucoma, an incision is made through the cornea so that a portion of the iris may be drawn out and excised (*iridectomy*). This may be peripheral or sector (keyhole) iridectomy. An iridectomy prevents the iris from bulging forward to crowd the chamber angle and permits drainage of aqueous humor from the anterior chamber, thereby reducing intraocular tension. Other operations on the iris (*iridencleisis*) are modifications having the same objective, that is, the escape of fluid.

Patient Education

Although glaucoma cannot be cured, it can be controlled, to a great extent. Whether the patient has had surgery or not, certain limitations must be set.

Activities that may increase intraocular pressure and should be avoided are:
1. Excessive fluid intake.
2. Use of antihistamines or sympathomimetic medications without proper medical management.

A recommended activity is carrying a card or "dog tag" indicating that the individual has glaucoma.

ENUCLEATION

Removal of the eyeball, *enucleation,* is necessitated by a variety of factors, including trauma that forces the contents of the globe to escape, infections, and other injuries which threaten to lead to sympathetic ophthalmia (see page 1136). During the removal of the eye, muscles are cut as close to the globe as possible. These muscles are approximated with sutures over a plastic prosthesis, thereby providing the means for coordinated motion of the prosthesis with the patient's real eye. A plastic, gold,

or teflon ball is placed in the area of the removed eyeball to form a stump on which the ocularist fixes the prosthesis (artificial eye). This prosthesis is colored to match the patient's eye. In successful cases, it is difficult to distinguish the prosthesis from the normal eye.

In certain cases, the sclera can be retained and the rest of the contents of the eye "scooped" out; this procedure is known as *evisceration.* The main advantage of evisceration is that it provides better motion to the artificial eye. The disadvantage is that sympathetic ophthalmia may occur.

Exenteration is usually performed in advanced malignancy or severe war injuries. In this procedure, the eyelids, the eyeball, and all contents of the orbit are removed, down to the bone. This operation is *very* disfiguring, and although the ocularist may attempt to build a prosthesis, it very often appears rather poor and unlifelike. These patients usually wear a black patch.

THE NEWLY BLIND

The number of blind people in the world is estimated at 40 million, or approximately 1 percent of the population; in some areas this figure approaches 4 percent. Between 15 and 25 million of these people have preventable, or easily curable blindness.

There are about 1,000,000 blind persons in America, and each year nearly 50,000 more go blind. Of these newly blind cases, approximately half could have been prevented with our present knowledge.

When an individual has marked visual impairment or is newly blind, he needs a great deal of help in making a healthy adjustment. For the most part, this help is entrusted to those skilled in such rehabilitation. However, a nurse can follow certain practices when caring for such a person.

A blind person always should be treated with the dignity accorded any other human being. Avoid expressions of pity. Keep the patient from becoming discouraged by seeing to it that he has someone with whom he can talk or some other form of diversion, such as a radio. Help him to overcome his feeling of awkwardness as he performs simple activities.

If he is allowed out of bed, the blind person should survey his room by walking around and touching the furniture. Thereafter, the nurse should be sure that the furniture remains in the same position. Never leave a door half-open; it should be either open or shut. When walking with a blind person, allow him to follow you by lightly touching your elbow; do not push him ahead of you. When he walks alone, he should learn to use a lightweight walking stick to warn him of obstacles.

Personal appearance is a significant part of the patient's care. He should be allowed to dress by himself; a woman even can learn to fix her hair and use cosmetics. Table etiquette, writing, etc., are activities that can be acquired with practice. The nurse should be familiar with the programs offered by such groups as The Seeing Eye, Inc., Morristown, N.J., where blind persons learn to work with a dog guide.

BIBLIOGRAPHY

BOOKS

Brady, F. B.: A Singular View (The Art of Seeing with One Eye). Oradell, N.J., Medical Economics Co., 1972.

Hales, R.: Contact Lenses: Clinical Approaches to Fitting. Baltimore, Williams & Wilkins, 1978.

Heilmann, K. (ed.): Glaucoma: Conceptions of a Disease. Philadelphia, W. B. Saunders, 1978.

Hill, E., and Ponder, P.: Orientation and Mobility Techniques: A Guide for the Practitioner. New York, American Foundation for the Blind, 1976.

International Guide to Aids and Appliances for Blind and Visually Impaired Persons. New York, American Foundation for the Blind, Inc., 1977.

Jaffe, N. S.: Cataract Surgery and its Complications, 2nd ed. St. Louis, C. V. Mosby, 1976.

Kintzel, K. C. (ed).: Advanced Concepts in Clinical Nursing, 2nd ed. Chap. 19: Nursing implications in the care of the patient experiencing sensory deprivation. Philadelphia, J. B. Lippincott, 1977.

Lowenfeld, B.: The Changing Status of the Blind. Springfield, Charles C Thomas, 1975.

New Orleans Academy of Ophthalmology: Symposium on Strabismus. St. Louis, C. V. Mosby, 1978.

Rose, F. C. (ed.): Medical Ophthalmology. St. Louis, C. V. Mosby, 1976.

Scheie, H. G., and Albert, D. A.: Textbook of Ophthalmology, 9th ed. Philadelphia, W. B. Saunders, 1977.

Vaughan, D., et al.: General Ophthalmology. Los Altos, California, Lange Medical Publications, 1977.

Wilson, F. M.: So You Have a Retinal Detachment: A Guide for Patients. Springfield, Charles C Thomas, 1977.

ARTICLES

General

Automated eye refraction. Med. Letter, 20:91-92, Oct. 6, 1978.

Baum, J. L.: Current concepts in ophthalmology: ocular infections. New Eng. J. Med., 299:28-31, July 6, 1978.

Cohen, K. L., and Hyndrick: Ocular emergencies. Am. Fam. Phys., 18:178-184, Oct. 1978.

Fenwick, A., et al.: Traumatic blindness. Nursing '79, 9:37-41, Jan. 1979.

Leone, C. R., Jr.: Eye disorders, treatment of baggy eyelids. Postgrad. Med., 61:205-210, Mar. 1977.

Ostler, H. B., et al.: Opportunistic ocular infections. Am. Fam. Phys., 17:134-140, Apr. 1978.

Records, R. E.: Primary care of ocular emergencies: 1. Traumatic injuries. Postgrad. Med., 65:143-152, May 1979; 2. Thermal, chemical, and nontraumatic eye injuries. 65:157-163, June 1979.

Smith, J. P.: Ophthalmic care of comatose patients and those under general anesthesia. Res. & Staff Phys. 25:104-105, Mar. 1979.

Waddleton, C. A.: Eye openers: uses and precautions. Nurses' Drug Alert, 2:132-134, Nov. 1978.

———: Drugs in eye infections. Nurses' Drug Alert, 2:100-103, Sept. 1978.

Contact Lenses

Boyd-Monk, H.: Taking a closer look at contact lenses. Nursing '78, 8:38-43, Oct. 1978.

Dixon, W. S.: Contact lenses: do they belong in the workplace? Occup. Health Saf., 47:36, May-June, 1978.

Garcia, G. E.: Extended wear of CAB (cellulose acetate butyrate) contact lenses in aphakic patients. Ophthal., 86:332-339, Feb. 1979.

Cornea

Boyd-Monk, H.: Helping the corneal transplant patient to see again. Nursing '78, 8:47-50, Feb. 1978.

Cataract

Bettman, J. W., et al.: Symposium: modern aspects of cataract operations. Ophthal., 85:39-81, Jan. 1978.

Boyd-Monk, H.: Cataract surgery. Nursing '77, 7:56-61, June 1977.

Drews, R. D.: The management of patients with intraocular lenses. Ophthal. Surg., 10:56-64, Feb. 1979.

New standards and procedures for intraocular lenses. FDA Drug Bull., 8:4, Jan.-Feb. 1978.

Taylor, D. M., et al.: Intraocular lenses: 500 consecutive intracapsular cataract extractions with lens implantation compared with 500 intracapsular extractions—observations and comments. Ophthal. Surg., 9:29-55, Feb. 1978.

Smith, J.: Focusing your care for the patient with an intraocular lens implant. RN, 41:46-50, Mar. 1978.

Symposium on intraocular lenses. Ophthal., 86:197-255, Feb. 1979.

Wilkinson, C. P.: Retinal detachment after phacoemulsification. Am. J. Ophthal., 87:628-631, May 1979.

Glaucoma

The noncontact tonometer. Med. Letter, 19:91, Nov. 4, 1977.

Techo, U., et al.: A clinical trial with Piloplex—a new long-acting pilocarpine compound: preliminary report. Annals Ophthal., 11:555-561, Apr. 1979.

Timolol maleate—a new drug for glaucoma. Med. Letter, 20:109-110, Dec. 15, 1978.

Understanding glaucoma: preventing silent blindness. Harvard Med. School Health Letter, 4:1-2, Apr. 1979.

Zimmerman, T. J.: Glaucoma editorial, pilocarpine update. Annals Ophthal., 11:631-632, Apr. 1979.

AGENCIES

American Association of Ophthalmology, 1100 17th St., N.W., Washington, D.C. 20036.

American Council of the Blind, 501 N. Douglas Ave., Oklahoma City, Okla. 73106.

American Foundation for the Blind, 15 West 16th St., New York, N.Y. 10011.

American Optometric Association, 7000 Chippewa St., St. Louis, Miss. 63119.

Better Vision Institute, Inc., 230 Park Ave., New York, N.Y. 10017.

Contact Lens Society of America, Inc., 301 First National Building, Lexington, Ky. 40507.

Eye-Bank Association of America, Inc., 3195 Maplewood Ave., Winston-Salem, N.C. 27103.

Eye-Bank for Sight Restoration, Inc., 210 E. 64th St., New York, N.Y. 10021.

John Milton Society for the Blind, 366 Fifth Ave., Room 503, New York, N.Y. 10001.

Leader Dogs for the Blind, 1039 Rochester Rd., Rochester, Mich. 48063.

National Braille Press, Inc., 88 St. Stephen St., Boston, Mass. 02115.

National Federation of the Blind, 218 Randolph Hotel Building, Des Moines, Iowa 50309.

National Society for the Prevention of Blindness, Inc., 79 Madison Ave., New York, N.Y. 10016.

Recording for the Blind, Inc., 215 East 58th St., New York, N.Y. 10022.

The Seeing Eye, Inc., Morristown, N.J. 07960.

52

ASSESSMENT AND MANAGEMENT OF PATIENTS WITH HEARING AND EAR DISORDERS

The ear is a very complex sense organ with a dual function—hearing and the maintenance of equilibrium (Fig. 52-1). The early detection and the accurate diagnosis of ear and hearing disorders are important in both children and adults. Among those who take an important part in the diagnosis of auditory disorders are pediatricians, otolaryngologists, psychiatrists, neurologists, psychologists, speech pathologists, educators, and audiologists. Before a child can speak, he must first be able to hear, then to interpret what he hears, and, lastly, to express himself in speech. Disorders due to birth injury, bacterial and viral infections in childhood, toxic drug effects, damage to the ear by noise, and changes in the ear as the result of aging are only a few of the problems that require assessment, treatment, and rehabilitation.

NOISE AND ITS EFFECT ON HEARING

One of the waste products of the twentieth century is noise (unwanted and unavoidable sound). The sheer volume of noise that surrounds us daily has grown from a simple annoyance into a potentially dangerous source of physical and psychological damage.

In terms of physical impact, loud persistent noise can cause constriction of peripheral blood vessels, alterations in blood pressure and heart rate (because of increased output of adrenalin), disturbances in equilibrium, and increased gastrointestinal activity. Additional research is required to answer many questions regarding the overall effects of noise on the human body. However, one thing seems beyond dispute—a quiet environment is more conducive to peace of mind; in the hospital, patients are happier and less upset when noise is kept to a minimum.

SOUND INTENSITY AND FREQUENCY. Scientists measure sound *intensity* (pressure exerted by sound) in decibels. For example, the shuffling of papers in quiet surroundings represents about 15 decibels; a low conversation, 40 decibels; and a jet plane 100 feet away about 140 decibels. Sound above 80 decibels begins to grate harshly upon the human ear.

Over the last several decades the loudest sounds to which humans are exposed have grown from 120 decibels (the roar of a small two-engine prop plane) to 150 decibels (the blast of a giant four-engine jet). Experiments have shown that 160 decibels are lethal for small fur-bearing animals. Research at many universities shows that exposure to noise of 90 decibels or more can cause the skin to flush, the stomach muscles to constrict, and tempers to be short.

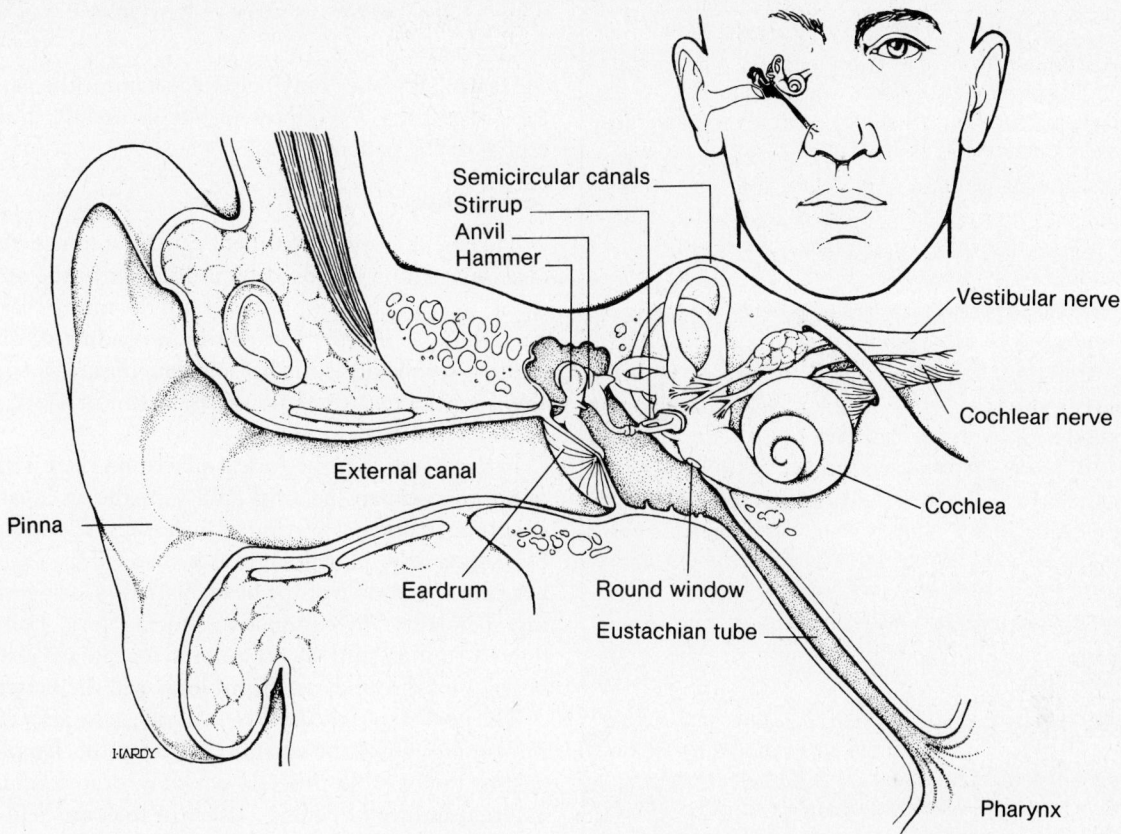

Figure 52-1. Anatomy of the ear.

Frequency refers to the number of sound waves emanating from a source per second — cycles per second (cps or Hz). *Pitch* is the term used to describe frequency; a tone with 100 cps or Hz is considered low pitch; a tone of 10,000 cps or Hz is considered high pitch. Generally, a young adult can distinguish frequencies from 16 cps to 20,000 cps.

HEARING LOSS

Psychosocial Considerations

Impairment of hearing may cause changes in personality and attitude, in ability to communicate, in awareness of surroundings, and even in the ability to protect onself. In a classroom, a student with impaired hearing may show disinterest, inattention, and failing grades. A woman at home may think the "world is dead" because she no longer can hear the clock chime, the refrigerator hum, the birds sing, or the traffic pass. A pedestrian may attempt to cross the street at the wrong time because of failure to hear an approaching car. The person with a hearing loss may miss parts of a conversation and may feel that people are talking about him. Many individuals are not even aware that their hearing is gradually becoming impaired.

More than 20 million persons in the United States suffer from some form of hearing loss. Approximately 90 percent of these people can be helped through medical or surgical measures or with a hearing aid. The nurse and the family physician play a major role in diagnosing hearing loss and guiding patients toward some type of assistance. Although some hearing difficulty may be due to impacted cerumen (wax), which is readily treated, proper assessment is best done by an otologist.*

Not infrequently, a person with a hearing loss refuses to seek medical attention, because of fear that hearing loss is a sign of advancing age; many people refuse to wear a hearing aid for this reason. Others feel self-conscious when they do wear an aid. These attitudes and behaviors should be taken into account when counseling patients who need hearing assistance.

Manifestations of Hearing Loss

The symptoms of hearing loss are varied, complex, and often subtle, as is indicated in the danger signals listed in the chart on page 1150.

*The *otologist* is a physician who specializes in the diagnosis and treatment of problems of the ear.
An *otolaryngologist* is a physician who specializes in problems relating to the ear, nose, and throat.
An *audiologist* is a person who specializes in nonmedical evaluation and rehabilitation of hearing disorders; educational preparation usually includes an M.A. or Ph.D. degree.

SYMPTOMS OF HEARING LOSS

SPEECH DETERIORATION—If a person slurs his words or drops word endings, or if speech is "flat" sounding, he may not be hearing correctly! The ears guide the voice, both in loudness and pronunciation.

FATIGUE—If a person tires easily when listening to conversation or to a speech, fatigue may be the result of straining to hear. Under these circumstances, he may become irritable or "touchy" very easily.

INDIFFERENCE—It is easy for a person to become depressed and disinterested in life in general when he can't hear what others are saying.

SOCIAL WITHDRAWAL—Not being able to hear what is going on around him causes the hard of hearing person to withdraw from situations which might prove embarrassing.

INSECURITY—Lack of self-confidence and fear of mistakes create a feeling of insecurity in many hard of hearing persons. No one likes to "say the wrong thing" or do something that might tend to make him look foolish.

INDECISION—PROCRASTINATION—Loss of self-confidence makes it increasingly difficult for hard of hearing persons to make decisions.

SUSPICIOUSNESS—Because he often hears only part of what is being said, the hard of hearing person may suspect that others are talking about him or that portions of the conversation relating to him are deliberately spoken softly so that he will not hear them!

FALSE PRIDE—The hard of hearing individual wants to conceal his hearing loss. Consequently, he often pretends he is hearing when he actually isn't.

LONELINESS AND UNHAPPINESS—Though everyone wishes for quiet now and then, *enforced* silence can be boring and even somewhat frightening. Persons with a hearing loss often feel "left out of things."

TENDENCY TO "HOG" THE CONVERSATION—Many hard of hearing people tend to dominate the conversation, knowing that so long as it is centered on them and they can control it they are not so likely to be embarrassed by some mistake.

(Courtesy, Maico Hearing Instruments)

The signs of significant ear disease which require referral to an otolaryngologist have been identified by the National Hearing Aid Society (NHAS).*

1. Visible congenital or traumatic deformity of the ear.
2. Active drainage from the ear within the previous 90 days.
3. Sudden or rapidly progressive hearing loss.
4. Acute or chronic dizziness or tinnitus.
5. Unilateral hearing loss of sudden or recent onset.
6. Significant air-bone gap (which can be recognized only from hearing tests).
7. Visible evidence of cerumen accumulation or a foreign body in the ear canal.
8. Pain or discomfort in the ear.

*National Hearing Aid Society, 20361 Middlebelt, Livonia, Mich. 48152

ASSESSMENT OF HEARING ABILITY

Hearing tests not only help to determine the particular type of hearing defect present but also establish the potential of the patient's hearing.

Tuning Fork

This inexpensive instrument can differentiate between *conductive deafness* (caused by a disorder in the auditory canal, the eardrum, the ossicles and the middle ear itself, e.g., fluid, as in the most common conductive disorder today—serous otitis media) and *sensorineural (perceptive) deafness* (due to a disorder of the organ of Corti or the auditory nerve).

In the *Weber test,* the fork is placed on the forehead in order to compare hearing ability in the two ears. For example, in normal hearing or in deafness that is equal on both sides, the patient indicates that vibrations can be heard in the middle of the head. Variations suggest hearing inequality. In conductive hearing loss, bone-conducted sounds shift to the poorer ear. In sensorineural hearing loss, sounds are heard louder in the better ear.

The next step is the *Rinne test.* In this test, after striking the tuning fork, the examiner places the handle first against the mastoid process, which is located behind the external auditory opening. Then the tines are held beside the ear and the patient is asked to tell where he heard the sound better or longer. A "Rinne positive" result means that the tone was heard longer by air conduction—this indicates perceptive loss. A "Rinne negative" result occurs when the tone is heard longer by bone conduction—this indicates conductive loss. "Rinne equal" means that the tone is heard the same by air and bone conduction.

These two tests do not give quantitative information, which can be obtained by audiologic study (audiogram).

Audiogram

In the detection of deafness, the audiometer is the single most important diagnostic instrument. Audiometric testing is of two kinds: (1) *pure-tone audiometry,* in which the sound stimulus consists of a pure or musical tone (the louder the tone before the patient perceives it, the greater the hearing loss; the unit of measure of loudness or intensity of sound is the *decibel*); (2) *speech audiometry,* in which the spoken word is used to determine the ability to understand and discriminate sounds.

For accuracy, audiometric tests should be done in a soundproof room. The patient wears earphones and is instructed to signal when he hears the tone and again when he no longer hears it. When the tone is applied directly over the external auditory opening, air conduction is measured. When the stimulus is applied to the mastoid bone, thereby bypassing the conductive mechanism, nerve conduction is tested.

The normal human ear perceives sounds ranging from

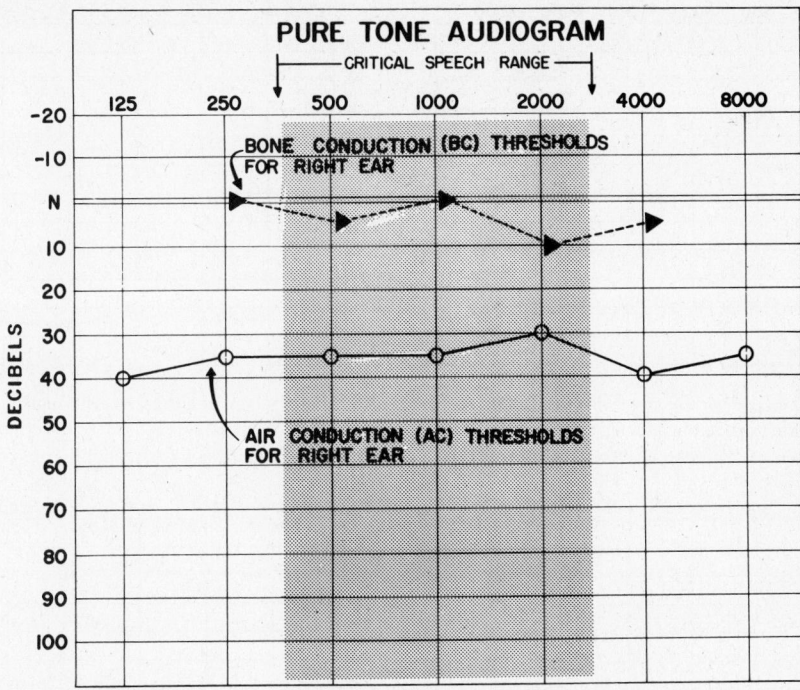

Figure 52-2. An audiogram presents a graphic outline of the individual's hearing as measured by tones of different pitches ranging from 125 through 8,000 cycles per second (cps or Hz). Thresholds for these different tones as heard by air and bone conduction are plotted on this graph. The information is important for determining the type of hearing loss. Also, by testing through the critical speech range (approximately 300 to 3,000 cps), one can predict how much difficulty there may be in hearing and understanding speech. (From Nilo, E.R.: Hearing Impairment. *In* Saunders, W. H., et al.: Nursing Care in Eye, Ear, Nose, and Throat Disorders. St. Louis, C. V. Mosby)

about 20 cycles per second (cps or Hz) to 20,000 cycles per second; however, only the frequencies from 500 to 2,000 are important in understanding everyday speech. Clinically, this range is referred to as *speech range*. The critical level of loudness is around 30 decibels. In treating patients surgically to improve hearing loss, the aim is to improve the hearing level to 30 decibels or better within the speech frequencies (Figs. 52-2 and 52-3).

CLASSIFICATION OF HEARING LOSS

Conductive Loss. Conductive loss results from an impairment of the outer ear, middle ear, or both. The inner ear is not involved in this type of loss; it can analyze clearly the sounds that come to it. Correction of the problem (see pages 1153–1161) may be all that is necessary to treat and correct this type of impairment. If the problem cannot be corrected, these individuals benefit greatly from hearing aids because in most instances they require only amplification of sounds.

Sensorineural (Perceptive) Loss. A disease of the inner ear or nerve pathways produces a type of hearing loss in which sensitivity to and discrimination of sounds are impaired. Sounds may be conducted properly through the external and middle ear but are not analyzed correctly in the inner ear. Because of poor sensitivity to sound, hearing aids are not as helpful as they are to those with conductive loss. However, a hearing aid should not be ruled out until the patient's hearing is evaluated in relation to hearing aids, that is, until a variety of aids are tested against the patient's hearing loss.

Combined Hearing Loss. A combined hearing loss indicates that the patient has both a conductive and a sensorineural loss.

Psychogenic Hearing Loss (Nonorganic, Functional). Hearing loss of this type is unrelated to detectable structural changes in the hearing mechanism. Usually it is a manifestation of an emotional disturbance, and the loss is frequently total. *Malingering* is similar to psychogenic hearing loss except that in this instance the patient really does hear.

REHABILITATION

It is important to classify the kinds of hearing impairment so that rehabilitative efforts can be directed at meeting a particular need. The Conference of Executives of

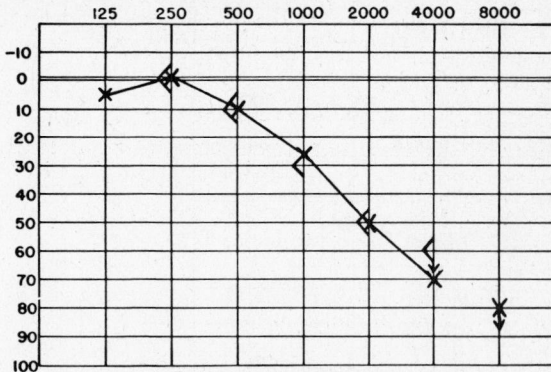

(A) Audiogram typical of presbycusis (hearing loss due to age). Air and bone conduction are equally affected, and loss is mainly in higher tones. No improvement can be expected from surgery.

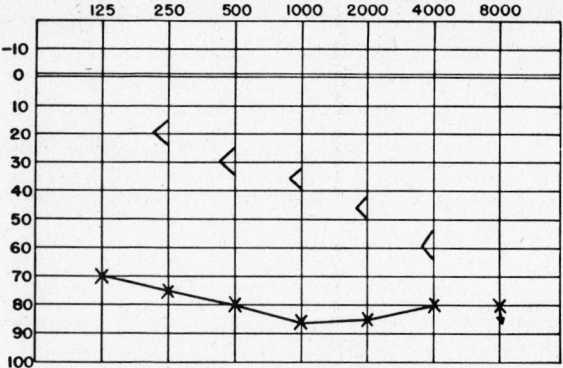

(B) Severe mixed hearing loss. Although a great differential exists between air conduction and bone conduction, considerable high-tone deafness is inescapable, regardless of the results of surgery.

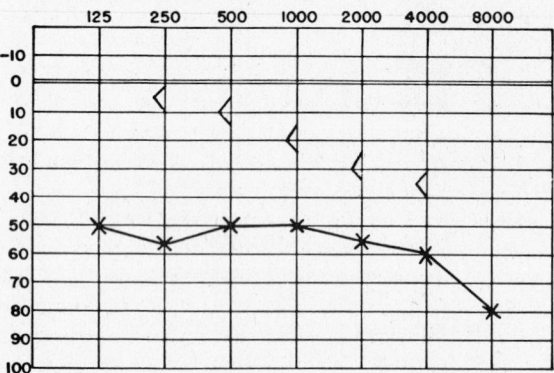

(C) Moderately severe mixed hearing loss. Hearing may be considerably improved by surgery, but perception of the higher frequencies may be inadequate.

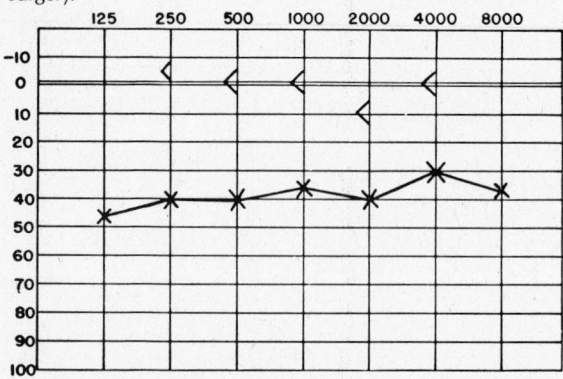

(D) This audiogram illustrates a pure conduction loss because of uncomplicated otosclerosis. In such a case, surgery should give excellent results.

Figure 52-3. Conventional audiograms. (From Ciba, Clinical Symposia, Vol. 14, No. 2)

American Schools for the Deaf* proposed the following classification based on (1) time of onset of hearing loss and (2) functional status of hearing:

1. The deaf—those in whom the sense of hearing is nonfunctional for ordinary purposes of life. This general group is made up of two distinct classes:
   (a) The congenitally deaf—those who lose hearing before speech is developed.
   (b) The adventitiously deaf—those who are born with normal hearing but then suffer some illness or accident that causes their hearing to become nonfunctional.

2. The hard of hearing—those in whom hearing, although defective, is serviceable with or without a hearing aid.

Hearing Aids

A *hearing aid* is an instrument through which sounds, both speech and environmental, are received by a microphone, converted into electrical signals, amplified, and

*Saunders, W. H., *et al.*: Nursing Care in Eye, Ear, Nose, and Throat Disorders. St. Louis, C. V. Mosby.

reconverted to acoustical signals. A hearing aid is not a new ear. It is as its name implies, only an aid to hearing. Many aids available for nerve deafness depress the low tones and give better hearing for the high tones.

Whether an individual would benefit by a hearing aid can best be determined by an otologist in conjunction with an audiologist. When the hearing loss is more than 30 decibels in the range of 500 to 2,000 cycles per second in the better ear, a patient may benefit (but not with certainty) from a hearing aid used with this ear. A variety of aids are available; the problem is to select the best aid for the individual patient. The decision should be made with the advice of an otologist and audiologist. Even this does not ensure optimal benefit from such an instrument. Psychological factors such as vanity may be involved, as well as other types of sensitivity.

The patient needs to know that the aid will not restore hearing to the level of the person with normal hearing but will improve it in the range of 300 to 3500 cycles per second (range of primary speech). (See Fig. 52-2.)

A hearing aid makes speech louder but it does not always make it clear enough for the deaf person to understand what is said. The wearer must experiment and adjust the controls for optimal results. He needs to recognize that he will never hear what others cannot hear, nor will he hear as well as one who has no hearing impairment. It may be necessary to receive auditory training and lessons in speech reading (lip reading) in order to make the new hearing aid effective. With such assistance, this person can learn to interpret sounds and use advantageously whatever hearing remains. Speech reading can help fill in the gaps of those words that might be missed. In auditory training, speech discrimination and listening skills are emphasized. The otologist, nurse clinician, or the hearing center can direct the patient to such classes.

A problem with most hearing aids is that background noise is also amplified, which may be distressing to the wearer. Binaural aids, that is one for each ear, may be indicated. Such aids can be concealed in the arms of specially made eyeglasses as may a single aid.

FDA Regulations. In August, 1977, the Food and Drug Administration (FDA) established a new regulation on hearing aids to protect the health and safety of individuals with hearing impairments.

1. A medical evaluation of the impairment by a licensed physician (preferably one specializing in diseases of the ear) must be obtained within 6 months prior to the purchase of a hearing aid.
   a) Such a written statement from a physician, however, may be waived by the client (a fully informed adult 18 years of age or older) upon signing a document.
   b) Children must be evaluated by a physician.
2. Hearing aid dispensers are required to refer prospective users to physicians if any of the eight specified otologic conditions is evident. (See list, page 1150).
3. A *User Instructional Brochure* is to accompany every hearing aid device. In this brochure, the following information is presented:
   a) Proper use and maintenance of the device.
   b) Good health practice requires a medical evaluation before purchasing a hearing aid.
   c) Any of the designated otologic conditions should be investigated by a physician before client purchases an aid.
4. Medical evaluation is required to insure appropriate medical diagnosis and care.

Care of a Hearing Aid. A hearing aid must be cared for carefully. The ear mold, which is the only part of the instrument that may be washed, should be washed in soap and water every day and the cannula should be cleansed with a small applicator or pipe cleaner. The mold must be dry before it is snapped into the receiver. The transmitter usually is worn off the body—behind the ear or in the frame of eyeglasses. A spare battery and cord should be carried by the wearer at all times. (This is suggested, but most patients do not do it.)

When a hearing aid is not functioning properly, the following steps should be taken: (1) note whether the on-off switch is on; (2) check the positioning of the batteries; (3) try a new battery; (4) examine the cord for breaks and whether it is plugged in correctly; (5) examine the ear mold for cleanliness. If the aid still will not work, notify the local service agency. Meanwhile, if the unit requires days to repair, the agency from whom it was purchased may lend an aid, or one may be borrowed from the local Chapter of the American Hearing Society.

Communicating With a Person Who Has a Hearing Impairment

Terry and co-workers* offer the following suggestions for better communication with deaf persons whose speech is difficult to understand:

1. Devote full attention to what the person is saying. Look and listen—do not try to give attention to another task while listening.
2. Engage him in conversation when it is possible for you to anticipate his replies. This will enable you to become accustomed to any peculiarities in speech patterns.
3. Try to catch the essential context of what is being said; you can often fill in the details from context.
4. Do not try to appear as if you understand when you do not.
5. If you cannot understand at all or have serious doubt about your ability to understand what is being said, have the person write his message rather than risk misunderstanding. Having him repeat the message in speech, after you know its content, will also aid you in becoming accustomed to his pattern of speech.

Suggestions for better communication with deaf persons who lip-read:

1. When speaking, always face the person as directly as possible.
2. Make sure your face is as clearly visible as possible; locate yourself so that your face is well-lighted; avoid being silhouetted against strong light; do not obscure that person's view of your mouth in any way; avoid talking with any object held in your mouth.
3. Be sure the patient knows the topic or subject of your verbal expression before going ahead with what you plan to say—this will enable him to use contextual clues in his lip-reading.
4. Speak slowly and distinctly, pausing more frequently than you would normally.
5. If you question whether the patient has understood some important direction or instruction, check to be certain that he has the full meaning of your message.
6. If for any reason your mouth must be covered (as with a mask) and you must direct or instruct the patient, there is no alternative but to write the message for him.

PROBLEMS OF THE EXTERNAL EAR

The auricle or external ear, which varies in size, shape, and position on the head, aids in the collection of sound waves and their passage into the external auditory canal.

*Terry, F. J., *et al.*: Rehabilitation Nursing. St. Louis, C. V. Mosby.

The external auditory canal is a skin-lined tube that ends at a disk-like structure, which is also lined with skin, the eardrum. The skin of the canal contains highly specialized glands that secrete a brown wax-like substance, *cerumen* (earwax). This material serves as a protection for the skin. Hair follicles and sweat glands are also present.

Infections (External Otitis)

Bacterial or fungal infections may result from an abrasion of the ear canal or from swimming in contaminated water; they appear more commonly during the summer. Since such infections are painful, management is directed toward relieving the discomfort. Even touching or moving the auricle increases pain. (In a middle ear infection, movement of the auricle does not increase pain.) Aspirin, codeine, and applications of heat provide comfort. If the tissues are edematous, it may be necessary to insert a wick of cotton gently through the canal to the eardrum so that liquid medications (such as Burow's solution [5% aluminum acetate] or antibiotics) may be introduced. Later, these medications may be given by dropper at room temperature. Such medications usually are combinations of antibiotics and agents to soothe the inflamed membranes. Systemic antibiotic therapy may also be required. The patient is cautioned to avoid swimming or allowing water to enter the ear when shampooing or showering.

Patients prone to "swimmer's ear" (otitis externa) should wear specially fitted ear plugs, which are made from instant plastic material molded to exact measure. The patients should also be reminded to avoid self-cleansing of the ear — Q-tips are not to be used.

The chronic form of external otitis is often due to a dermatosis such as psoriasis or seborrheic dermatitis. Even allergic reactions to hair spray, hair dye, and permanent wave lotions can cause dermatitis which clears when the offending agent is removed.

Furuncle of the External Canal

Infection of the skin and the subcutaneous tissue of the external canal usually results in a great deal of pain in the affected ear. There may be fever, severe headache and enlargement of the local lymph nodes. This disorder may be mistaken for mastoid infection. The early administration of antibiotics and application of hot packs usually results in resolution of the furuncle. Incision and drainage is rarely done since such measures may result in perichondritis or chondritis. It is better for the furuncle to localize (point) and open spontaneously or resolve by itself.

Cerumen in the Ear Canal

Earwax normally accumulates in the ear in varying degrees and color. While it does not ordinarily need to be removed, on occasion it may become impacted, causing otalgia (earache) and hearing difficulties. Attempts to clear the external auditory canal with matches, hair pins, and other implements is dangerous, since trauma to the skin may result in infection or damage to the eardrum.

Wax deposits may be softened by instilling a few drops of warmed glycerine, mineral oil or acetic acid (0.5%) solution. Other ceruminolytic agents such as peroxide in glyceryl (Debrox) are available. However, these compounds may cause an allergic reaction in the form of a dermatitis. If the wax deposits cannot be dislodged by this method, the cerumen may be removed with a curet or another suitable instrument used under magnification. As a last resort, the ear canal may be irrigated, although this mode of treatment is the least preferred because (1) it may cause discomfort, (2) it is messy, (3) it may cause vertigo if the temperature of the solution is higher or lower than room temperature, (4) it tends to macerate the skin, increasing the possibility of an external otitis, and (5) it could permit fluid to enter and contaminate the middle ear if the tympanic membrane is perforated.

Foreign Bodies in the External Canal

Small objects are at times inserted into the ear, usually by young children. Such objects may be nonirritating and remain for years without symptoms. An insect in the ear may be disturbing, but can be easily managed by instilling oil drops that smother the insect and allow it to be floated or flushed out.

However, vegetable foreign bodies have a tendency to swell, so irrigation is contraindicated. Attempts at removal may be dangerous in unskilled hands, because the object may be pushed completely into the bony portion of the canal, lacerating the skin of the canal and perforating the drum. Serious infections of the middle ear and the mastoid, with ensuing deafness, may result. When such an object is trapped in the ear of a very young child, it should be removed with a special instrument under general anesthesia; when this procedure is skillfully performed, there are no sequelae.

Earlobe Piercing

Women and particularly young girls often have their earlobes pierced so that they can wear earrings without fear of losing them. However, piercing of the ears is contraindicated in persons having diabetes, skin disease, or keloids. When ear piercing is permissible, it is suggested that a physician perform the procedure. A large (18-gauge) straight needle with a sterilized and flexible gold wire is inserted into the bevel and then inside the needle. After a little local anesthesia is applied, the needle is inserted through the back of the earlobe, then withdrawn, leaving the wire in the ear. The wire is tied loosely in place — serving as a type of primitive earring — and is removed 10 days to 2 weeks later. During this time, the area is cleansed daily with soap and water or alcohol, followed by a mild antiseptic ointment, and the wire is removed from time to time to ensure patency of the opening in the earlobe. Hair should be kept away from the lobes; hair and perfume spray, bleach, or dye should be avoided for 3 weeks. Swimming also should be avoided until the ears have healed.

Some difficulties have been experienced with all types of ear-piercing procedures, among them, premature closure of the puncture, hemorrhage into the earlobe, secondary infection, and keloid formation. Many individuals develop contact dermatitis and are sensitive to alloy metals. For this reason, it is recommended that only 14 K gold posts be worn. Any early sign of pain, redness, swelling or tightness should be reported to the physician.

Irrigation of the External Auditory Canal

Irrigation of the ear canal is used less frequently today than in the past. When it is used, the purposes are (1) to carry out the caloric test for labyrinthine function, (2) to facilitate surgery on the external ear and (3) to remove impacted cerumen (done by the physician).

The solutions for irrigating the ear should be at a temperature of about 40.6–43.3° C. (105–110° F.). Solutions that are too hot or too cold or are used with too much force may cause pain or dizziness. The patient may sit or lie with head tilted toward the side of the affected ear. The curved basin can be supported under the ear to catch the solution. To be effective the fluids must reach the eardrum. To achieve this end, the auricle is pulled upward and backward in order to straighten the external auditory canal. (In children this canal may be straightened by pulling the auricle down and back.) Extreme gentleness should be used, and care must be taken that the fluid has free exit so that it is not driven into the middle ear. After the irrigation, the external opening should be plugged lightly with sterile cotton, which is changed when necessary. After the procedure, the patient is instructed to lie on the affected ear so that gravity facilitates drainage.

- *Note:* If injury to the tympanic membrane is suspected, irrigation should not be performed.

PROBLEMS OF THE MIDDLE EAR

The middle ear, with its ossicles and ligaments and their connection to the eardrum, is vitally concerned with the function of hearing. The middle ear connects with the posterior portion of the nose by means of the eustachian tube; thus equal air pressure is maintained on both sides of the eardrum. The tube, which is normally closed, opens by action of the muscles of the palate on yawning or swallowing. The tube serves as a drainage channel for normal and abnormal secretions of the mid-

dle ear and equalizes pressures in the middle ear to that of the atmosphere. When the membrane of this tube is inflamed, it offers an easy passage for infection into the middle ear.

Sound waves transmitted by the drum to the ossicles of the middle ear are transferred to the *cochlea,* the organ of hearing, lodged in the labyrinth or inner ear. An important ossicle is the stapes, which rocks on its posterior portion, not unlike a piston, and sets up vibrations in fluids contained in the labyrinth. The fluid waves cause the basilar membrane in which the hair cells of the organ of Corti rest to move in a wave-like manner. The waves set up electrical currents which stimulate the various areas of the cochlea. The hair cell sets up a neural impulse which is encoded and then transferred through the auditory nerve to the auditory cortex in the brain where it is decoded into a sound message.

Middle Ear Effusion (Serous Otitis Media)

Secretory Otitis Media. Exudates in the middle ear may be retained as a result of allergy or after an acute inflammation that has been treated with antibiotics or after a bout with the common cold. It may also occur with nasopharyngeal tumors and in a rapidly descending plane or in deep diving without equalizing.

This condition, known as secretory otitis media, is commonly seen today in patients treated with wide-spectrum antibiotics. When unrecognized, it can be a common cause of persistent deafness in children and in adults. Symptoms such as ear pain and fever may subside, but, although the exudates in the middle ear have been rendered sterile they are not evacuated, thereby leading to tubal inflammation and abnormal ventilatory function. Deafness and a sense of fullness in the ear caused by the exudates persist. If long-term decongestants or antihistamines and antibiotics fail to resolve the problem, surgical intervention may be required.

Simple *myringotomy,* or incision of the drum (see page 1156), and aspiration by suctioning will evacuate the contents of the middle ear; healing takes place within a few days. Frequently a plastic tube is inserted into the tympanic membrane to act as a secondary eustachian tube and provide a means of ventilation to the middle ear.

When such a ventilatory tube is in place, certain precautions must be observed: (1) Water must not get into the external ear canal (when taking a shower or bathing, the patient is to place a cotton ball coated with petrolatum in the intubated ear); (2) Swimming may be permitted if well-fitted ear plugs are used; (3) Diving is contraindicated because of increased pressure on the tympanic membrane and even on the round and oval windows of the inner ear.

Aerotitis Media. Aerotitis media is a form of serous otitis media in which fluid and/or air is trapped in the middle ear due to sudden descent in an airplane (barotrauma). The condition usually lasts a short time, but it may continue for days. For this reason many people avoid flying when they have an upper respiratory infection. Preventive measures to be taken by flight passengers are to chew gum, suck on hard candy, yawn, or swallow several times during the descent of the plane. Those flying should be taught to inflate their ears by the so-called Valsalva method. In this technique the nostrils are held tightly, and the ears are inflated by vigorous blowing; thus pressure in the middle ear is equalized to relieve annoying symptoms.

Acute Otitis Media
(Infection of the Middle Ear)

Acute otitis media is an acute infection (or abscess) of the middle ear. The essential cause of acute otitis media is the entrance of pathogenic bacteria into the normally sterile middle ear when the resistance is lowered or the virulence of the organism is great enough to produce inflammation. Bacteria commonly found, in the order of importance, are: the hemolytic streptococcus, the pneumococcus, the staphylococcus, and the influenza bacillus. The mode of entry of the bacteria in most patients is spread by way of the auditory canal or the eustachian tube during the indiscriminate use of nose drops or nasal douching, forcible blowing of the nose, or sneezing; in rare cases, infection may enter after fracture of the skull.

Nursing Assessment. The symptoms may vary with the severity of the infection and may be either very mild and transient or very severe and fraught with serious complications. Pain in and about the ear is the first symptom. It may be intense and is relieved after spontaneous perforation of the drum or after myringotomy (see below). Fever varies and in severe cases may range between 40.0-40.6° C. (104-105° F.). Deafness, ear noises, headache, loss of appetite, nausea and vomiting are other symptoms.

Management. The end results of otitis media depend on the virulence of the bacteria, the efficiency of the therapy, and the resistance of the patient. With early and appropriate wide-spectrum antibiotic therapy, otitis media may clear with healing, with no serious sequelae.

It is important to note that symptoms may be masked by the antibiotic therapy and that during the course of treatment of an acute middle ear infection, symptoms such as headache, slow pulse, vomiting, and vertigo are all significant and should be recorded carefully for evaluation by the otologist. The appropriate antibiotic, often determined by culture and sensitivity tests, is important to the prognosis for eventual cure.

The condition may become subacute, with long-persistent purulent discharge from the ear. Healing may take place with permanent deafness. Perforation as the result of rupture of the eardrum may persist and develop into a chronic form of otitis media. Secondary complications, with involvement of the mastoid, and other serious intracranial complications such as meningitis or brain abscess may result.

Myringotomy. In mild cases treated early, myringotomy may not be necessary. However, if pain persists, this procedure is important for promoting surgical drainage. It also offers a ready means of identifying the type of organism present to test its sensitivity to chemotherapeutic agents.

An incision is made in the posterior inferior aspect of the tympanic membrane. Even though a sweeping incision is made to relieve pressure and pus from a middle ear infection, the incision heals rapidly and hearing is not impaired. This procedure is now performed much less frequently than it was before the advent of antibiotic therapy. Usually when myringotomy is done, a plastic tube is inserted through the eardrum.

Chronic Otitis Media

Chronic otitis media results from repeated attacks of otitis media causing persistent perforation of the drum. It is due to particular virulence of the infecting organism or to bacterial resistance to antibiotic therapy. The chronically infected ear is characterized by persistent or recurrent purulent discharge, with or without pain, and varying degrees of deafness, usually conductive or mixed. Most chronic otitis media begins in childhood and may persist to adult life.

Classification. Chronic suppurative middle ear infection has been classified into five groupings as indicated in Table 52-1.

Clinical Manifestations and Diagnosis. The symptoms of chronic otitis media may be minimal, with varying degrees of deafness and the presence of a persistent or intermittent foul-smelling discharge of variable quantity. Pain may or may not be present. Symptoms such as sudden facial paralysis, unusually profound deafness or dizziness, onset of headache with dizziness, and stiff neck may herald a beginning meningitis or brain abscess or erosion into the semicircular canals. The diagnosis is corroborated by the physical findings, but, in addition, roentgenograms of the mastoids usually show pathologic changes.

Management. Local treatment consists of (1) careful cleansing of the ear, (2) instillation of antibiotic drops, (3) application of antibiotic powders, and (4) x-ray and study. Tympanoplastic procedures may be required early to prevent further damage to hearing and more serious complications.

Mastoiditis and Mastoidectomy

Mastoiditis is an inflammation of the mastoid, resulting from an infection of the middle ear; if untreated, osteomyelitis may occur. Symptoms are pain and tender-

TABLE 52-1. CLASSIFICATION OF CHRONIC OTITIS MEDIA*

TYPE	SPECIFIC CONDITION	INVOLVEMENT	MANIFESTATION
I	Chronic otitis media simplex	Central perforation of the tympanic membrane	Mucoid serous discharge
II	Chronic otitis media with cholesteatoma†	Usually attic perforation (posterior superior part of eardrum) With or without perforation	Usually odorous discharge
III	Chronic adhesive otitis media	Marked retraction of tympanic membrane	No discharge Marked hearing loss
IV	Chronic otitis media with tympanosclerosis	Tympanosclerosis, a degenerative process in eardrum and middle ear Plaque of amorphous connective tissue	Severe hearing loss No discharge
V	Chronic serous otitis media	If untreated or neglected may result in severe deafness, chronic adhesive otitis media, cholesteatoma† or tympanosclerosis	Repeated bout of serous or fluid ear

*By Woodrow D. Schlesser, M.D.: Personnel communication.
†*Cholesteatoma* is due to the ingrowth of the skin of the external ear canal (squamous epithelium) into the middle ear. The skin from the external canal forms the outer sac which fills with degenerated skin and sebaceous material. The sac is attached to the structures of the middle ear and mastoid and produces changes by pressure necrosis.

ness behind the ear, discharge from the middle ear, and swelling of the mastoid. Usually this is successfully treated with antibiotics and occasionally myringotomy.

When there is recurrent or persistent tenderness, fever, headache, and discharge from the ear, it may be necessary to remove the mastoid process (mastoidectomy).

Preoperative Management. Aside from general preoperative preparation of the patient, the postauricular area is cleansed thoroughly. To keep hair out of the operative field, a water-soluble jelly (KY jelly) may be applied to the hairline in the operating room or a commercially available plastic drape with a small central hole to expose the operative site may be used. (The edge of the hole adheres to the skin with adhesive.)

During the operation, the infection is removed completely from the mastoid process, and the middle ear is drained, thus preventing spread of the infection to surrounding structures. The middle ear can be saved from further damage, and possible permanent hearing loss prevented.

Postoperative Management. Sedatives usually are indicated after the operation and during the first postoperative days to control pain and restlessness. Fluids are given freely when the anesthetic reaction clears. The mastoid is drained by means of a small Teflon drain. The small patch dressing is changed in about 4 or 5 days.

A complication after mastoidectomy is facial paralysis. The nurse may be the first to note this serious indication of facial nerve inflammation or injury. The patient shows immobility of the side affected, so that the eye cannot be closed and the mouth droops. He is unable to drink without water dripping from the mouth, and he is unable to whistle. When the patient attempts to speak or grimace, the facial paralysis is more pronounced, due to the immobility of the paralyzed side. Any evidence of facial paralysis should be reported immediately to the otologist. The patient may be taken back to the operating room, the wound opened, and repair of the facial nerve done at once.

Trauma to the Tympanic Membrane (Perforation)

Permanent perforation of the tympanic membrane occurs most frequently as a result of auto accidents with skull fracture. The next most frequent cause is infection—perforations of the drum membrane that fail to heal are often the end result of acute or chronic suppurative otitis media. Traumatic damage may also result from the blast effects of high explosives or from intense compression caused by a severe blow on the ear that can rupture the drum. The drum may also be burned by a spark from a welder's equipment.

Less frequently, perforation is caused by foreign objects, water, burns of the face that include the external ear and the drum membrane, postmyringotomy defects, scuba diving, accidental or deliberate blows to the face. Perforations may also occur when people use cotton-tip applicators to clean their ears. A person may insert one into the external ear and inadvertently turn around, jamming the applicator deeper into the ear. Or the tip may be bumped and pushed into the canal. Either occurrence may result in severe destruction of the drum, ossicles, and even the inner ear. Thus all attempts to clean the ear with applicator sticks must be discouraged.

Management. Most accidental perforations of the drum membrane heal spontaneously. Some persist because of the growth of scar tissue over the edges of the perforation, thus preventing extension of the epithelial areas across the margins and final healing.

• In suspected traumatic perforations, warn the patient against irrigating the ear. Cleanse the outer ear carefully with sterile cotton but leave the ear canal alone until an otologist can aspirate blood and inspect the drum for evidence of perforation.

TABLE 52-2. TYMPANOPLASTIC PROCEDURES

TYPE	DAMAGE OF MIDDLE EAR	METHODS OF REPAIR
I	Perforated tympanic membrane with normal ossicular chain	Closure of perforation; same as myringoplasty
II	Perforation of tympanic membrane with erosion of malleus	Closure with graft against incus or remains of malleus
III	Destruction of tympanic membrane and ossicular chain *but with* intact and mobile stapes	Graft contacts normal stapes; also gives sound protection for round window
IV	Similar to type III, but head, neck, and crura of stapes missing; foot-plate mobile	Mobile foot-plate left exposed; air pocket between round window and graft provides sound protection for round window
V	Similar to type IV plus *fixed* foot-plate	Fenestra in horizontal semicircular canal; graft seals off middle ear to give sound protection for round window

(From DeWeese, D. D., and Saunders, W. H.: Textbook of Otolaryngology, ed. 5. St. Louis, C. V. Mosby, 1977)

If the patient has sustained a head injury, he is kept under observation to detect any evidence of cerebrospinal otorrhea, such as clear watery drainage. Such fluid can be checked in the laboratory to determine whether its source is the cerebrospinal canal.

Tympanoplasty

Tympanoplasty denotes a number of reconstructive operations on middle ear structures that have become diseased or are congenitally deformed (see Table 52-2). Utilizing an illuminated binocular microscope, the otologist is able to visualize and reconstruct defective conductive mechanisms to maintain or improve hearing. Chemotherapy and/or antibiotics maintain an infection-free area so that healing is promoted.

Physiologic Principles Underlying Sound Conduction. The conductive function of the eardrum and the ossicles transforms sound waves from airborne vibrations to mechanical stimulation of the endolymphatic fluids. The prevailing physiologic concept holds that the ratio of the large tympanic membrane to the smaller oval window, combined with the lever action of the ossicles, transforms stimuli from the air to the inner ear fluids with great increase in force.* Obviously, defects in the tympanic membrane or interruption of the ossicular chain will disturb that mass relationship to the oval window and will cause a loss of the sound-pressure ratio, resulting in hearing loss.

*Wever and Lawrence (*Physiological Acoustics*. Princeton University Press) indicate that an actual ratio is 21:1, but an effective ratio is 14:1 (23 decibels). Since ordinarily sound-transfer from air to liquid sustains a loss of 30 decibels, this is compensated for by the action of the tympanic membrane and the ossicles (up to 23-25 decibels).

The functional physiology of the round and oval windows plays an important role as well. The oval window is bordered by the annular ligament, and the unimpeded motility of the stapes foot-plate receives impulses transmitted by the incus and the malleus from the drum membrane. The round window, opening on the opposite side of the cochlear duct, permits motion of the endolymphatic fluids with sound-wave stimulation. With the normally intact drum membrane, sound waves stimulate the oval window first, and a lag occurs before the terminal effect of the stimulus reaches the round window. This phase lag, normally present with an intact drum, is changed by a perforation of the drum that is large enough to allow sound waves to impinge on both the round and oval windows simultaneously. This effect cancels the lag and prevents the maximal effect of labyrinth fluid motility and its subsequent effect in stimulating the hair cells in the organ of Corti. The result is a reduction in hearing ability.

Pathophysiology. Pathologic sequelae vary after otitis media, with minimal or large defects remaining in the tympanic membrane. In protracted or virulent infections, necrotic involvement of the ossicles may occur. Involvement of motility may result with fibrosis or necrosis of all or part of the ossicular chain. The malleus commonly is involved, the handle lost by osteonecrosis as the perforation in the drum enlarges. The lenticular process of the incus often is involved because of its tenuous blood supply. Osteonecrosis may involve the entire ossicular chain, so that the stapedial foot-plate is the only portion remaining. The oval and round windows may be impeded functionally by granuloma, polyps, fibrous, or bony plaques. Otosclerosis may exist along with the pathologic sequelae of otitis media. Obstruction of the tympanic orifice of the eustachian tube by pathologic tissue deposits or fibrotic stenosis may result in dysfunction of this structure.

Procedures. Tympanoplasty is performed to reestablish two functions of the middle ear, (1) the transformer action and (2) sound protection for the round window.

Originally five types of tympanoplastic procedures were described (Table 52-2). Since then, modifications and innovations have been devised. In the original procedures of Types I, II, and III, both of the above objectives were achieved; however, with Types IV and V, only sound protection was provided for the round window. Variations of these operations are being done with the following innovations: incus interposition and prosthetic replacement.

Incus interposition is a procedure in which the incus is detached from the malleus, diseased segments of the incus are removed, and the remains of the incus are balanced on the head of the stapes; the contact is maintained with pieces of Gelfoam.

Homologous tympanic membrane, including annulus and malleus, may be taken from a cadaver and used in place of a fascial graft. Other prostheses may include tragal cartilage or a piece of shaped cortical bone from the patient's own mastoid.

Tympanoplasty, Type I (Myringoplasty)

Indications and Management. *Myringoplasty* is a plastic surgical procedure designed to close perforations of the tympanic membrane. The operation has a dual purpose: (1) to create a closed middle ear cavity by graft over the perforation and (2) to improve hearing.

The most important advantage of the closed tympanic membrane is the avoidance of the risk of contamination of the middle ear during bathing, swimming, or diving. The reactivation of a chronic otitis media and/or mastoiditis thus may be prevented. Dramatic improvement in hearing may result from closure of a perforation if there is no involvement of the ossicles. The probability of improved hearing after closure of the drum membrane can be prognosticated to some degree by an audiometric study with evaluation of the air–bone conduction levels. Preoperative testing, with and without a patch prosthesis over the perforation, usually provides a fairly accurate estimate of the degree of hearing levels. Temporary patching of the defect with glazed paper, latex, or a cotton collodium disk should be a routine maneuver during the preliminary examination of the patient. When the patching of a perforation of the drum is not followed by audiometric improvement, one must consider involvement of the ossicular chain. During the surgical repair of a perforation, a careful inspection of the middle ear contents, with particular attention to the continuity of the ossicles, is important.

Contraindications. Medical or surgical closure of perforations of the drum in the presence of an active infection usually is contraindicated. In chronic disease of the middle ear with malfunction of the eustachian tube, and therefore inadequate drainage from the middle ear (the only avenue for egress of discharges), surgery is contraindicated. Involvement of the nasopharynx because of chronic infectious discharge from sinusitis or allergy, plus a history of acute exacerbations of otitis media, is an obvious contraindication.

Postoperative Management. An antibiotic is administered routinely for at least 5 days after surgery. The patient remains in the hospital for 1 or 2 days at most, and the dressing is left undisturbed except for the external bandage, which may be changed if it becomes soiled from bleeding. The gauze strip is removed from the canal on the seventh day; the Gelfoam is left undisturbed. No suction or probing is carried out at this time.

On the twentieth day, capillary suction can be used carefully to remove the Gelfoam or crusted debris. Gen-

tle inflation may be carried out to test the efficiency of the closure of the perforation by the graft.

The patient is seen at 5-day intervals and is instructed to avoid contaminating the ear by shampooing or showering. Antibiotics are given for 1 week, but may be continued if there is evidence of complicating respiratory infection. An antihistaminic with an ephedrine derivative is used routinely for 1 month postoperatively. In those patients with known seasonal or perennial rhinologic allergy, an antihistaminic is continued.

Tympanoplasty, Types II-V and Modified Versions

Tympanoplasty may be done by various techniques. Either the postauricular or endaural approach is used. Skin grafts have been replaced by fascial grafts. The operation may be done in one or two stages. When done in two stages, the first is performed to clear the infection and/or remove cholesteatoma, whereas the second stage is directed to mechanical correction of the deficient sound-transmission system.

Preoperative Care. The bacterial flora in all patients should be studied by culture and sensitivity tests. In those whose treatment is accompanied by the parenteral administration of an appropriate antibiotic, the postoperative morbidity is reduced. Topical and systemic antibiotic treatment should precede surgery when the patient's ear is continuously or frequently discharging.

Operative Procedure. Part of the tympanoplastic procedure includes restoring the continuity of the sound mechanism, when it is involved. Ossicular interruption is most frequent in otitis media, but problems of reconstruction occur with malformations of the middle ear and ossicular dislocations due to head injuries.

Polyethylene tubing, stainless steel wire, bone and cartilage have been used as replacements, either to utilize the remaining parts of the ossicles or to create a columella (little column) effect for the transmission of impulses from the tympanic graft to the oval window.

A two-stage procedure may be necessary — the first for the surgical eradication of all pathology and the establishment of a healed, dry middle ear, and the second for the reconstructive process. The ear should remain dry for 2 or 3 months before the second stage for the exploration of the window niches and the restoration of a conductive mechanism. Remaining parts of the ossicular chain may be repositioned to establish impulse transmission to the oval window.

Postoperative Care. Outer dressings may be reinforced if soiled with blood or drainage, but the inner dressing is undisturbed. The patient is hospitalized for 3 or 4 days.

The patient must be assisted the first time out of bed since dizziness and nystagmus are typical reactions. Medications to combat vertigo and nausea may be prescribed. The patient is cautioned to avoid blowing his nose or wetting the dressings during bathing. Eventually he will be permitted to resume showering and swimming.

Clinical Results. Patients with a lengthy history of disease may regain as much hearing as those with less protracted infections. In patients whose otitis media has been healed and whose ear has remained dry for a lengthy period, hearing improvement may be marked after tympanoplasty. Younger patients achieve better results than older patients. The simpler the surgery, the better the chance for hearing gain; this, of course, relates directly to the functional integrity of the ossicular chain and the efficiency of the newly-created tympanic covering.

Continued research is being done to improve tympanoplasty procedures. In some instances, clinical failures have been due to infection, poor technique, and tissue rejection of graft or prosthesis.

Otosclerosis

Otosclerosis or otospongiosis is the term applied to a form of progressive deafness caused by the formation of new spongy bone in the labyrinth which locks the shape in a fixed position (clinical otosclerosis) and prevents sound transmission by the vibrating ossicles to the inner ear fluids.

The cause of this condition is unknown, but it occurs most commonly in women, beginning after puberty, and it has a hereditary basis. The condition, which usually involves both ears about equally, begins with insidious loss of hearing and a ringing or buzzing in the ears. The patient gives a history of slowly progressive hearing loss without middle ear infection.

Assessment. The diagnosis is evident from the findings of the audiometer test. Sound transmission by air as tested with a tuning fork is markedly reduced, while intensification of sound is noted by placing the tuning-fork handle over the mastoid and recording the marked difference in hearing between air and bone. The bone conduction is far better than air conduction, which is the reverse of normal. There is no known medical treatment for this form of deafness other than the help offered by amplification with an electric hearing aid or preferably, a stapedectomy.

Stapedectomy

A stapedectomy involves removing the otosclerotic lesion at the footplate of the stapes and creating a suitable tissue implant with a prosthesis to replace this portion of the conductive mechanism.

Indications. As a consequence of the increasing numbers of regressions that occurred after stapes mobilization, stapedectomy was employed as a secondary operative technique to salvage the failures of initial mobilization attempts. With the initial success of this operation, the indications have extended to all classes of otosclerosis; and in some clinics where this technique is carried out, virtually all patients with otosclerosis are treated by a routine stapedectomy. Others use the procedure only after failure of a stapes mobilization (seldom done today since stapedectomy is the operation of choice).

Microsurgery. The otologic binocular microscope is of distinct value in this operation. To bridge the gap between the incus and the inner ear, Schuknecht uses steel wire and fat implant, whereas House's technique employs Gelfoam and prefabricated stainless steel wire (two popular procedures). Kos uses wire and a segment of a vein as a plug in the oval window, and Shea advocates a vein graft with polyethylene tubing (Fig. 52-4). In any case, the prosthetic device should be fashioned and ready preliminary to the removal of the stapedial footplate.*

Postoperative Management. The position that the patient assumes in bed in the immediate 24-hour postoperative period varies with the preference of the physician. Some prefer the patient to lie on the operated ear to facilitate drainage; others desire the operated ear to be uppermost in order to prevent graft displacement. Still others allow the patient to chose the most comfortable position and one which does not cause vertigo. If dizziness is noted, the patient should be instructed to change from one position to another slowly; Benadryl and/or Valium may also be prescribed. The patient can be prevented from falling by keeping side rails up when he is in bed and assisting him when he gets out of bed. This precaution is mandatory if the patient is dizzy.

Unusual symptoms such as fever, headache, vertigo or ear pain are to be noted and the patient instructed to avoid blowing his nose or sneezing. If he must do so, he should take care to avoid violent head movements. In addition, smoking should be forbidden.

Any subjective symptoms such as pain, taste changes, a "sloshy" feeling in the ear or unusual sensations should be noted and reported.

Patient Education. The patient is discharged in 3 to 4 days and may be depressed because his hearing has not improved appreciably. Since initial hearing gain at the time of operation is masked by ear packing and subsequent edema of the tissues, the patient should be reassured that hearing gain may be noted from one to several weeks after surgery. Packing is removed about the fifth or sixth day in the physician's office.

Before leaving the hospital the patient is instructed as follows:
• Avoid sudden head movements and risks of infections.
• Do not wet head (in showers or swimming) for about 6 weeks.
• Postpone washing hair for 2 weeks; after this time, when washing hair be careful to avoid getting water into the ear for an additional 4 weeks.
• Avoid flying for several months and stay away from people who have upper respiratory infections.

*Most surgeons use a tissue graft and wire prosthesis. Most commonly used are vein grafts or fat grafts.

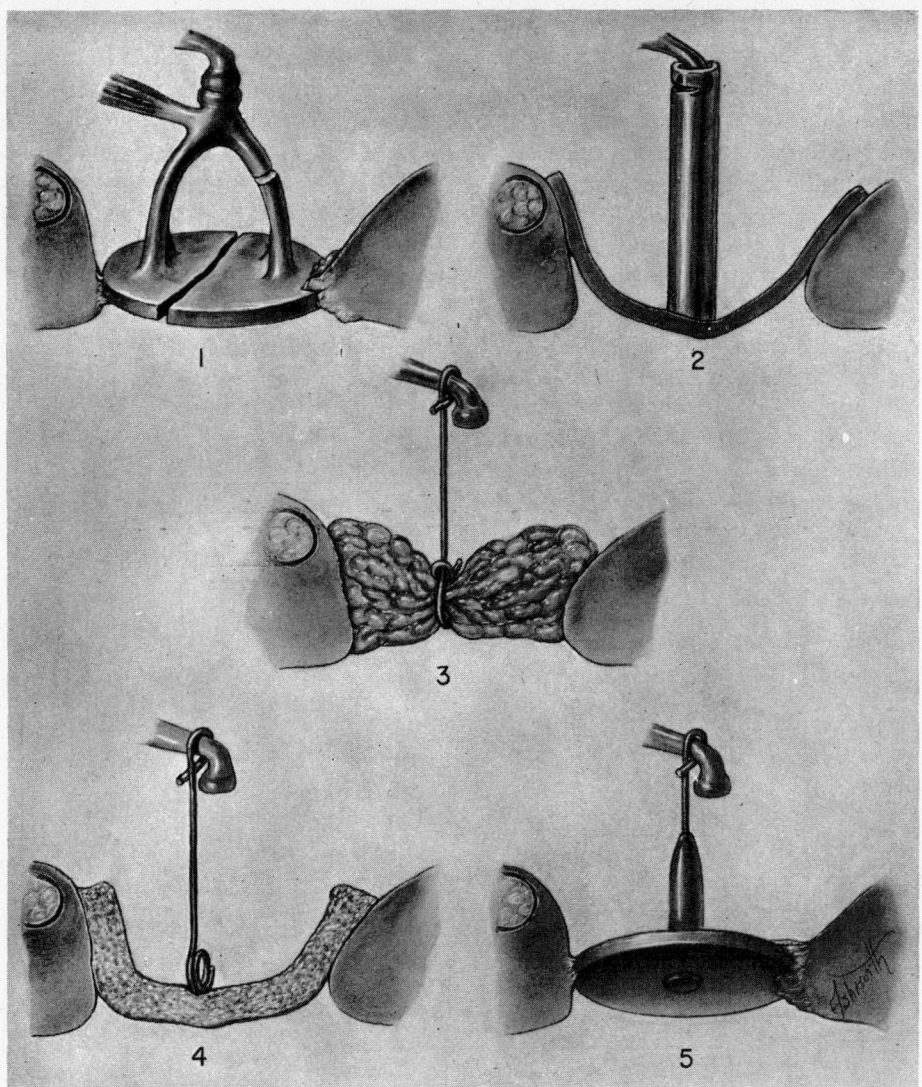

Figure 52-4.   Techniques of stapedectomy. (*1*) Partial stapedectomy by cutting anterior crus and bisecting footplate. The posterior crus and remaining footplate are mobile (Hough). (*2*) Stapes removed and replaced with a vein graft. Polyethylene strut provides continuity (Shea). (*3*) Wire-fat prostheses replacing the stapes (Schuknecht). (*4*) Oval window covered with Gelfoam (House). Preformed wire placed on Gelfoam. (*5*) Footplate not removed. Footplate drilled and preformed wire-Teflon piston placed through hole in footplate (Shea; Guilford). Note otosclerotic fixation of the anterior footplate margin shown in (*1*) and (*5*). (DeWeese and Saunders: Textbook of Otolaryngology. St. Louis, C. V. Mosby)

PROBLEMS OF THE INNER EAR

Body balance is maintained by the cooperation of muscle, joint, tendon, visceral senses, the eyes, and the inner ear or vestibular apparatus. The last is the most important in this function. The inner apparatus of the ear provides feedback regarding the movements and the position of the head in space, coordinates all body muscles, and positions the eyes during rapid motion or head movement.

The vestibular apparatus consists of the utricle, the saccule, and the semicircular canals, of which there are three in each ear. Each canal lies in a plane at right angles to the others, with the entire apparatus grouped in working pairs for this complex function. The mechanism of action of the semicircular canals may be likened to the cochlea or organ of hearing. Here, also, fluids are set in motion by head or body movement which, in turn, stimulate extremely delicate nerve fibers which transmit messages as electric impulses along the nerve to centers in the brain where they are interpreted.

Hydrops of the Labyrinth (Meniere's Syndrome)

Meniere's disease or *syndrome* is an inner ear problem stemming from a labyrinthine dysfunction, the cause of which has not been definitely established. Many theories have been advanced, such as an increase in pressure in the endolymph, sodium retention, vasomotor changes causing a spasm of the internal auditory artery, emotional or endocrine disturbance, or an allergic reaction.

Clinical Manifestations. Meniere's syndrome is characterized by the presence of a triad of symptoms: paroxysmal whirling vertigo, tinnitus, and sensorineural hearing loss. At the onset of the condition perhaps only one or two of these symptoms are manifested; however, the disease is not diagnosed as Meniere's syndrome until all three signs are present (Fig. 52-5).

Vertigo, the outstanding symptoms of Meniere's disease, occurs as a sudden attack, appearing at irregular intervals of hours, days, or months. Some patients have an aura or some warning sign such as a sense of pressure or fullness in the ear that tells them an attack is coming on. This gives them time to lie down, stop the car, etc. Each attack lasts from a few minutes to several hours or all day and the patient complains of the room appearing to spin around him. Any sudden motion of the head may induce vomiting. This symptom complex often occurs in persons who have had previous ear trouble and allergic symptoms, especially vasomotor rhinitis. When vasospasm of the blood vessels occurs, the mucous membrane of the cochlea becomes swollen and congested, the fluid increases in quantity, and the resultant pressure on the labyrinth produces the symptoms of Meniere's syn-

drome. This patient may also complain of headache, nausea, vomiting and incoordination; however, there is no pain or loss of consciousness. The patient generally prefers to lie quietly with eyes shut.

Between attacks, the patient works or proceeds normally and complains only of tinnitus or hearing impairment. Tinnitus is characteristically a low fluctuating buzzing sound in the ears. It is often louder preceding and during an attack. Sensorineural loss applies to low tones and usually occurs in only one ear. It gets progressively worse and may cause severe cochlear damage if untreated.

Diagnostic Evaluation. The caloric test is not done during an acute attack but when the patient is in remission and free of vertigo. It is important to check to make sure the patient is not taking an antihistamine or tranquilizer since this modifies the test. Electronystagmography (ENG) is the preferred test, since it is more accurate in stimulus, is not influenced by the subjective interpretation of the examiner, and provides a permanent record on cardiogram paper.

The patient with Meniere's disease has a normal or hyperactive response early in the disease. As the disease becomes chronic and the hearing decreases, the responses become hypoactive or absent. In acoustic neuroma, the labyrinthine response is hypoactive or absent. If the nystagmus is not present with water at 30° C. (86° F.), ice

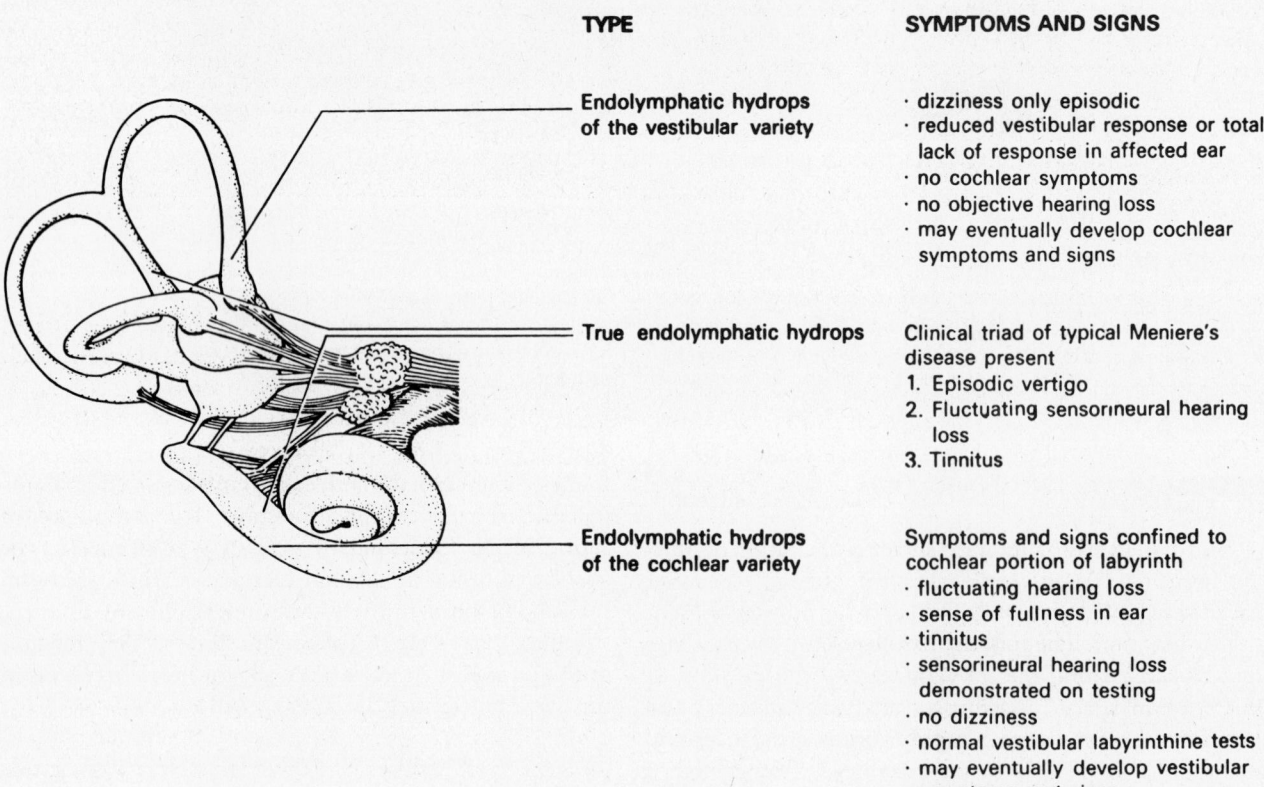

TYPE	SYMPTOMS AND SIGNS
Endolymphatic hydrops of the vestibular variety	· dizziness only episodic · reduced vestibular response or total lack of response in affected ear · no cochlear symptoms · no objective hearing loss · may eventually develop cochlear symptoms and signs
True endolymphatic hydrops	Clinical triad of typical Meniere's disease present 1. Episodic vertigo 2. Fluctuating sensorineural hearing loss 3. Tinnitus
Endolymphatic hydrops of the cochlear variety	Symptoms and signs confined to cochlear portion of labyrinth · fluctuating hearing loss · sense of fullness in ear · tinnitus · sensorineural hearing loss demonstrated on testing · no dizziness · normal vestibular labyrinthine tests · may eventually develop vestibular symptoms and signs

Figure 52-5. A practical classification of Meniere's disease.

water is used. If there is no response to 15 ml. of ice water, the labyrinth is considered nonresponsive. Recent study of the balance function relies on ENG (electronystagmography). This measures the electropotential of the eye movements, when nystagmus is produced, and provides a graphic record of labyrinthine function.

In suspected acoustic tumors of intracranial lesions, the Hollpike bithermal (hot and cold water) test is used to study the directional preponderance and localize a lesion. In Meniere's disease with a nonfunctioning labyrinth and severe hearing loss, compensation is already occurring and the opposite ear is taking over. In situations of this type, these patients are candidates for total labyrinthectomy.

Management. The main objective of treatment is to eliminate vertigo and improve or stabilize the patient's hearing. This is accomplished by a combination of methods done early in the disease in order to avoid severe hearing loss. For an acute attack, the patient is permitted to assume whatever position is most comfortable. Usually an intravenous line is started to permit the administration of medications such as diazepam (Valium) which is given slowly to control vertigo. Vital signs and the patient's condition are monitored. On occasion a rectal suppository of dimenhydrinate (Dramamine) may be prescribed.

Three-quarters of the patients respond to the treatment of a salt-free diet (see box, this page) and ammonium chloride. If there is an immediate favorable reaction to this regime, it is continued for 2 or 3 months before the amount of ammonium chloride is gradually decreased. The patient, however, never returns to a full use of salt. Food allergy is investigated and may require that certain elements be eliminated from the diet.

Vasodilating drugs, such as nicotinic acid, tolazoline hydrochloride (Priscoline), and methantheline bromide (Banthine), improve tinnitus.

For patients with a history of allergy (about 5 percent of these patients), relief may be obtained from dimenhydrinate (Benadryl and Dramamine). Phenobarbital may be prescribed to relieve the tension factor. Antivertiginous (against dizziness) drugs are effective for prolonged control. Alcohol is contraindicated and smoking is discouraged because of the vasospastic action of nicotine.

The nursing approach to the individual who has vertigo attacks is two-pronged. First, the patient needs understanding and encouragement, because many find it difficult to define a problem that has subjective symptoms. The patient looks well enough to work, but he does not feel well. Secondly, he needs assistance in slowing down his movements so that he does not precipitate an attack. This need for self-protection is extended when an attack takes place; his best place is lying in a bed equipped with side rails, but, if he is standing, he needs

---

DIET FOR MENIERE'S DISEASE (FURSTENBERG DIET)*

1. Fluids not restricted; however, excessive quantities of water discouraged.

2. Proteins unrestricted or forced; calories permitted as indicated; sodium allowance low.

3. All foods to be prepared and served without salt.

4. The following foods to be eaten daily:
   Eggs, meat, fish, and fowl as desired.
   Bread as desired.
   Cereal, one of the following: farina, oatmeal, rice, puffed rice, or puffed wheat.
   Potato and at least one of the following: macaroni, spaghetti, rice, corn, plums, prunes, or cranberries.
   Any fruit and any vegetable not listed below.
   Milk as desired.
   Butter, cream, honey, jellies, jam, sugar, and candy (except chocolate) as desired.

5. The following foods are to be avoided at all times:
   Salted meats and fish
   Bread, crackers, and butter prepared with salt

Carrots	Clams	Olives
Spinach	Oysters	Raisins
Endive	Cheese	Caviar
Cow peas	Condensed milk	

6. The following foods may be taken no more than twice weekly:

Chard	Radishes	Muskmelon
Kohlrabi	Celery	Dried currants
Pumpkin	Cantaloupe	Dried coconut
Watercress	Strawberries	Buttermilk
Beets	Limes	Peanuts
Cauliflower	Peaches	Horseradish
Turnips	Figs	Mustard
Rutabagas	Dates	

*(From DeWeese, D. D., and Saunders, W. H.: Textbook of Otolaryngology, 5th ed. St. Louis, C. V. Mosby, 1977)

---

help to avoid injury from a possible fall. The patient should be taught to lie down, avoid sudden motion, and, if driving, pull off the road and stop the car. The lifestyle of the individual with excessive work habits needs to be investigated and perhaps adjusted.

Surgical Management. A variety of medical and surgical treatments exist for Meniere's disease, one of which may give a particular patient the relief he needs. Research continues in an effort to find the cause of this syndrome, which will more clearly suggest definitive therapy.

Cryosurgery is one surgical approach in which a postauricular incision is made and the horizontal semicircular canal is approached through a simple mastoidectomy. The cryogenic probe ($-160°$ C.) is applied for a total of 6 minutes. Fascia and skin are then closed. Postoperatively, the patient is moderately dizzy for about 2 days; unsteadiness may persist for 2 or 3 weeks. The patient is hospitalized for 6 or 7 days. Within a month of discharge he may resume work.

An *endolymphatic shunt* is another procedure; it involves decompressing the endolymphatic sac and sectioning the vestibular nerve.

Ultrasonic surgery is one technique that has been tried but is seldom used now. A mastoidectomy incision is made to gain access to the horizontal semicircular canal. Ultrasonic energy is then applied directly to the bone in the canal by means of a probe. Proponents claim that hearing is preserved while vertigo is eliminated.

Total labyrinthectomy. When medical management fails (in about 10 to 20 percent of cases) and the patient has had progressive hearing loss and experiences severe vertigo attacks (loss of hearing, 60 decibels, loss of nerve response, and poor discrimination), the destruction of the membranous labyrinth (inner ear) is probably the most helpful technique (total labyrinthectomy). This is done through the ear canal in the same manner as a stapedectomy. The stapes is removed and the endolabyrinth is aspirated with suction. The inner ear is packed with streptomycin.

Postoperatively, the patient who has had a surgical destruction of the labyrinth may experience vertigo for up to 48 hours, after which it gradually subsides and permits him to get out of bed. Some unsteadiness and vertigo may persist as long as 3 to 6 weeks, but this may be controlled if the patient moves easily.

As for ultrasonic surgery the destructive effects of ultrasonic vibrations last for 3 to 5 days. Usually the patient is able to be up and about in 2 to 3 days, leaves the hospital in a week, and returns to work in 3 weeks.

Bell's palsy (a peripheral facial weakness attended by aching pain near the angle of the jaw or behind the ear) may be a postoperative complication, but this clears between 2 weeks and 3 months. The patient should be forewarned about the possibility of this sequelae.

BIBLIOGRAPHY

BOOKS

Ballantyne, J.: Synopsis of Otolaryngology, 3rd ed. Chicago, Yearbook Medical Pub., 1978.

Ballinger, J. J.: Diseases of the Nose, Throat and Ear, 12th ed. Philadelphia, Lea and Febiger, 1977.

DeWeese, D. D., and Saunders, W. H.: Textbook of Otolaryngology. St. Louis, C. V. Mosby, 1977.

Goodhill, V.: Ear Diseases, Deafness, and Dizziness. New York, Harper and Row, 1979.

Hartbauer, R. E.: Aural Rehabilitation. Springfield, Ill., Charles C Thomas, 1975.

Katz, J., ed.: Handbook of Clinical Audiology, 2nd ed. Baltimore, Williams and Wilkins, 1978.

Noble, W.: Assessment of Impaired Hearing: Critique and a New Methodology. New York, Academic Press, 1978.

ARTICLES

Hearing

Carney, A. E.: Management of sensorineural hearing loss: Educational, social, and psychologic aspects. Postgrad. Med., *62*:135-138, Oct. 1977.

Farrell, D. E.: Hearing loss in the geriatric patient. Nurse Pract., *3*:30-32, Nov.-Dec. 1978.

Holm, C. S.: Deafness: Common misunderstandings. A.J.N., *78*:1910-1912, Nov. 1978.

Linthicum, F. H.: Viral causes of sensorineural hearing loss. Otolaryng. Clin. N. Am., *11*:29-33, Feb. 1978.

Lipscomb, D. M.: Noise induced sensorineural hearing loss: Implications for the practicing clinician. Otolaryng. Clin. N. Am., *11*:49-53, Feb. 1978.

McNamee, C.: Communicating with the hard-of-hearing. Canad. Nurse, *74*:27-29, Mar. 1978.

Paparella, M. M.: Hearing loss. The physicians responsibility. Postgrad. Med., *62*:94-98, Oct. 1977.

Prado, S., and Paparella, M. M.: Sensorineural hearing loss secondary to bacterial infections. Otolaryng. Clin. N. Am. *11*:35-41, Feb. 1978.

Pulec, J. L.: Surgically treatable sensorineural hearing loss. Postgrad. Med., *62*:121-131, Oct. 1977.

Shambaugh, G. E., Jr.: Sensorineural deafness due to cochlear otospongiosis: Pathogenesis, clinical diagnosis, and therapy. Otolaryng. Clin. N. Am. *11*:135-154, Feb. 1978.

Smyth, G. D. L.: Immediate and delayed alterations in cochlear function following stapedectomy. Otolaryng. Clin. N. Am., *11*:105-112, Feb. 1978.

Wolf, E. M.: Communicating with deaf surgical patients. AORN J. *26*:39-47, July 1977.

Hearing Devices

Bussic, S. N., et al.: Pointers for detecting hearing loss. Pat. Care, *11*:174-202, Aug. 15, 1977.

Cochlear implant hearing devices provide interpretable sound. JAMA, *237*:621-622, Feb. 14, 1977.

Gardner, G.: Hearing aids. Am. Fam. Phys., *15*:94-96, June 1977.

Goode, R. L.: Implantable hearing aids. Otolaryng. Clin. N. Am., *11*:155-161, Feb. 1978.

Hearing aid devices: professional and patient labeling and conditions for sale. Fed. Reg., *42*:9286-9296, Feb. 15, 1977.

Sanders, J. W.: The successful hearing-aid user. Otolaryng. Clin. N. Am., *11*:187-193, Feb. 1978.

Ventura, F. D.: Counselling the hearing-impaired geriatric patient. Pat. Counselling & Health Educ., *1*:22-25, 1st Quart. 1978.

Vernon, J. A.: Some questions about an implantable hearing instrument. Otolaryng. Clin. N. Am., *11*:163-171, Feb. 1978.

Weber, H. J., and Pirkey, W. P.: Selection of hearing aids. Otolaryng. Clin. N. Am., *11*:173-186, Feb. 1978.

Ear Problems

Fairbanks, D. N. F.: How to remove middle ear fluid without surgery. Consult., *18*:112-118, Sept. 1978.

Fee, W.: Earlobe to cochlea. Emerg. Med., *10*:43-52, Feb. 1978.

Fletcher, M. M.: The painful ear. Med. Times, *106*:23-29, Sept. 1978.

Huber, H. L.: Draining the "fluid ear" with myringotomy and tube insertion. Nursing '78, 8:28-30, July 1978.

McCurdy, J. A., Jr.: Middle ear effusion: Current concepts. Am. Fam. Phys., 17:107-111, Apr. 1978.

Meyers, A. D.: Managing cerumen impaction. Postgrad. Med., 62:207-209, July 1977.

Ruben, R. J.: Otolaryngologic problems of the old. Hosp. Pract., 12:73-87, Aug. 1977.

AGENCIES

American Academy of Ophthalmology and Otolaryngology of the American Medical Association, 15 Second Street, S.W., Rochester, Minn. 55901

American Organization for the Education of the Hearing Impaired, c/o Alexander Graham Bell Association for the Deaf, 3417 Volta Place, N.W., Washington, D.C. 20007

American Speech and Hearing Association, 1081 Rockville Pike, Rockville, Md. 20852

Deafness Research Foundation, 366 Madison Avenue, New York, N.Y. 10017

National Association for Hearing and Speech Action, 814 Thayer Avenue, Silver Spring, Md. 20910

National Association for the Deaf, 814 Thayer Avenue, Silver Spring, Md. 20910

National Hearing Aid Society, 20361 Middlebelt, Livonia, Mich. 48152

53

ASSESSMENT OF NEUROLOGIC FUNCTION

PHYSIOLOGIC OVERVIEW

The nervous system is comprised of the brain and the spinal cord, together with all extensions therefrom and neural connections thereto. Its function is to control and to coordinate cellular activities throughout the body. The signaling device that it employs involves the transmission of electrical impulses, a system which permits each stimulus to be placed accurately in the area that is intended to receive it. These impulses are routed by way of nerve fibers, pathways that are direct and continuous, and the responses that these elicit are practically instantaneous, because changes in electrical potential transmit the signals.

The Brain

The brain is divided into the cerebrum, brain stem, and cerebellum. It is enclosed in a rigid, bony box — the skull or cranium. At the base of this box is the *foramen magnum,* an opening through which the spinal cord forms a continuous connection with the brain (Fig. 53-1). The brain has three coverings: (1) the *dura,* the outer covering of dense fibrous tissue that closely hugs the inner wall of the skull, (2) the *arachnoid,* and (3) the *pia mater,* which adheres closely to the brain and the spinal cord.

The *brain stem* consists, from top down, of midbrain, pons, and medulla oblongata.

The *cerebrum* is divided into two hemispheres and consists of four lobes: frontal, parietal, temporal, and occipital (Fig. 53-2). The cerebrum is the largest part of the brain, and on its surface or cortex are located the "centers" from which motor impulses are carried to the muscles, and to which sensory impulses come from the various sensory nerves.

The *midbrain* connects the pons and the cerebellum with the cerebral hemispheres. The *cerebellum* is located below and behind the cerebrum. Its function is the control or the coordination of muscles and equilibration.

The *pons* is situated in front of the cerebellum between the midbrain and the medulla and is a bridge between the two halves of the cerebellum as well as between the medulla and the cerebrum.

The *medulla oblongata* transmits motor fibers from the brain to the spinal cord and sensory fibers from the spinal cord to the brain. The majority of these fibers decussate at this level. The pons also contains important centers controlling heart, respiration, and blood pressure and gives origin to the fifth, sixth, seventh, and eighth cranial nerves.

There are two glands present in the brain: the pituitary and the pineal. The pituitary gland is frequently approached surgically. It lies at the base of the brain in a bony fossa termed the sella turcica, just posterior to the optic chiasm, upon which it may press when the gland is enlarged.

CEREBRAL CORTEX. While the cells in the cerebral cortex are quite similar in appearance, their functions vary widely, depending on their geographic location. Figure 53-2 depicts the topography of the cortex in relation to certain of its specific functions. The posterior portion of each hemisphere, i.e., the occipital lobe, is devoted to all aspects of visual perception; the lateral region, or temporal lobe, incorporates the hearing center. The mid-central zone, or parietal zone, posterior to the fissure of Rolandi, is concerned with sensation; the anterior portion is concerned with voluntary muscle movements. The large uncharted area beneath the forehead, i.e., the frontal lobes, contains the association pathways that determine emotional attitudes and responses and contributes to the formation of thought processes. Damage to the frontal lobes as a result of trauma or disease is by no

1166

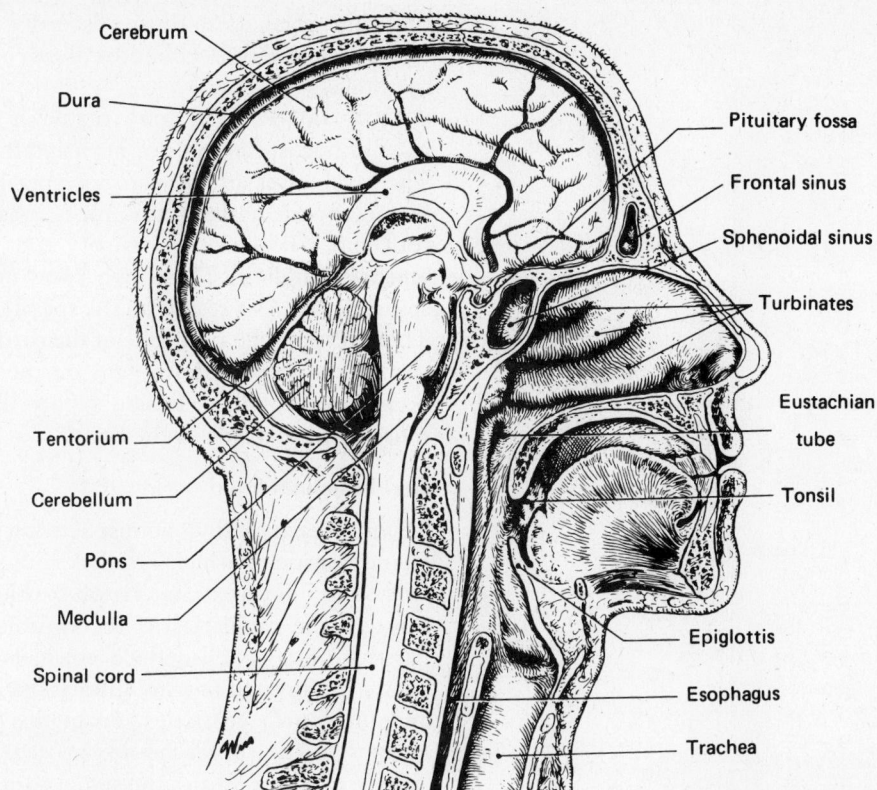

Figure 53-1. Cross-sectional view, showing the anatomic position and the relation of structures of the head and the neck.

means incapacitating from the standpoint of muscular control or coordination, but has decided effect on the personality of the individual, as reflected by basic attitudes, sense of humor and propriety, self-restraint, and motivations.

INTERNAL CAPSULE, PONS, AND MEDULLA. Nerve fibers from all portions of the cortex converge in each hemisphere and make their exit in the form of tight bundles known as the "internal capsule." Having entered the pons and the medulla, each bundle crosses the corresponding bundle from the opposite side. Some of these axons make connections with axons from the cerebellum, basal ganglia, thalamus, and hypothalamus; some connect with the cranial nerve cells. Other fibers from the cortex and the subcortical centers are channeled through the pons and the medulla into the spinal cord.

The Spinal Cord and Its Connections

The spinal cord, a direct continuation of the medulla oblongata, is that part of the nervous system contained within the vertebral column (Fig. 53-3). It is a cord about 45 cm. (18 inches) long and approximately the thickness of a finger, extending from the foramen magnum of the skull, where it is continuous with the medulla oblongata, to the first lumbar vertebra, where it tapers off into a fine thread of tissue. The spinal cord is an important center of reflex action for the body and contains the conducting pathways to and from the higher centers in the cord and

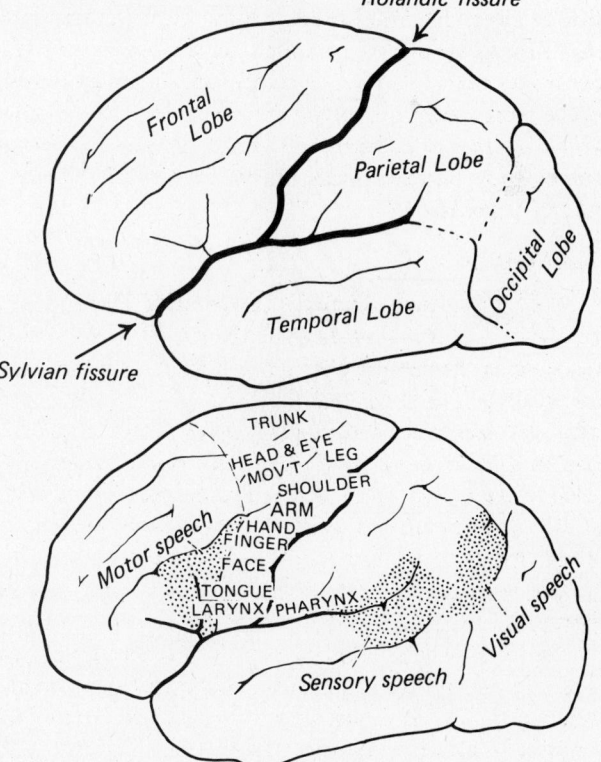

Figure 53-2. (*Top*) Diagrammatic representation of the cerebrum, showing relative locations of various lobes of the brain and the principal fissures. (*Bottom*) Diagrammatic representation of cerebral localization for motor movements of various portions of the body.

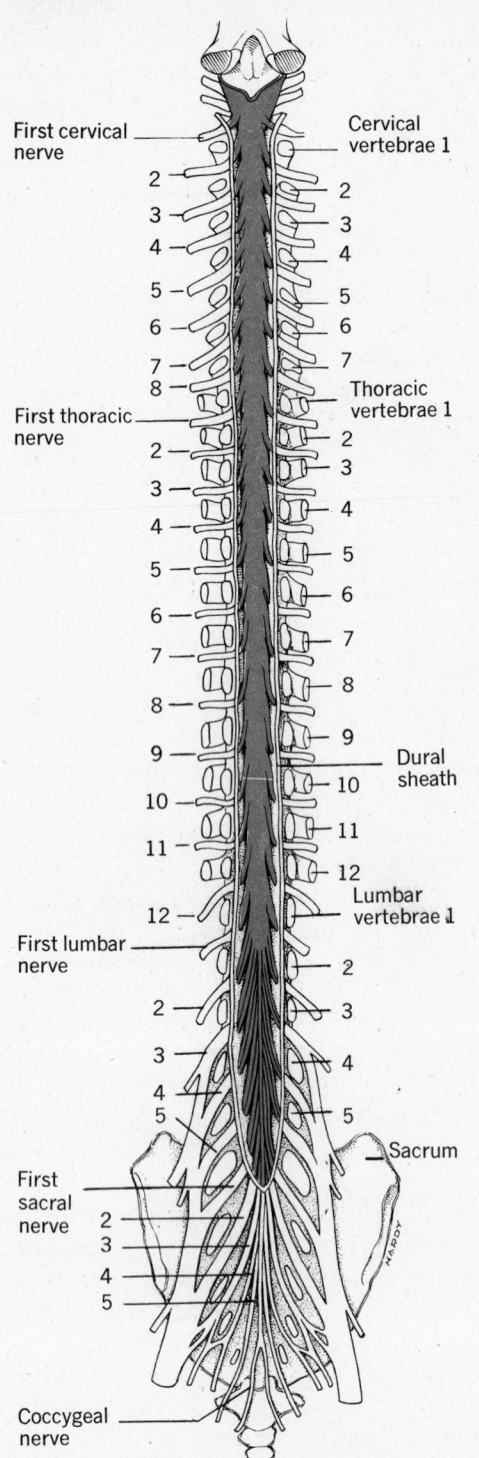

First cervical nerve

Cervical vertebrae 1

First thoracic nerve

Thoracic vertebrae 1

Dural sheath

Lumbar vertebrae 1

First lumbar nerve

Sacrum

First sacral nerve

Coccygeal nerve

Figure 53-3. Spinal cord lying within the vertebral canal; spinous processes and laminae have been removed; dura and arachnoid have been opened. Spinal nerves are numbered on the left side; vertebrae are numbered on the right side. (From Chaffee, E. E., and Greisheimer, E. M.: Basic Physiology and Anatomy, 4th ed. J. B. Lippincott, 1979)

the white fibers, both those of sensory tracts running up to the brain and those of motor fibers coming down from the brain.

GRAY MATTER. The gray matter is shaped like two pairs of horns, the anterior horn and the posterior horn. The cord gives off 31 pairs of spinal nerves. Each is formed by the union of two roots, an anterior or motor root and a posterior or sensory root on which is the sensory ganglion. These two roots unite to form one spinal nerve. As a result, all the spinal nerves are mixed. Those leaving the right side of the cord supply the muscles, the skin, and the organs on the right side of the body; those of the left side supply the corresponding muscles on that side of the body.

Cerebrospinal Fluid

Within each cerebral hemisphere is a central cavity, the lateral ventricle, which is filled with clear *cerebrospinal fluid*. This fluid is extracted from the blood as it circulates through the capillaries of the choroid plexus. It then passes through well-defined channels from the lateral ventricles through narrow tubular openings to the third and the fourth ventricles. From this narrow cavity it escapes to the subarachnoid space to bathe the entire surface of the brain and the spinal cord. The cerebrospinal fluid normally is absorbed by the large venous channels of the skull and along the spinal and the cranial nerves.

The spinal fluid is clear and colorless, having a specific gravity of 1.007. The average patient's ventricular and subarachnoid systems contain about 150 ml. of this fluid. The organic and inorganic contents of the cerebrospinal fluid is very similar to that of the plasma; however, their concentration is somewhat different.

Disease produces changes in the composition of the cerebrospinal fluid. Determinations of the protein content and the quantity of glucose and chloride present constitute the chief chemical examinations. In a state of health there are a minimal number of white cells and no red cells in the spinal fluid.

By replacing cerebrospinal fluid with air, the radiologist is able to visualize with x-rays the size, shape, and position of the ventricles. Any interference or distortion may be suggestive of a space–occupying lesion.

PATHOPHYSIOLOGY

Vision and Cortical Blindness

There is a definite area in the rear of each hemisphere where the fibers of the corresponding optic nerve end. It is by means of these receiving cells that vision is possible. The eyes may be normal and the optic nerve perfect, but if these cells in one hemisphere are diseased, the person is half-blind and has *cortical blindness*. He cannot see to one side of the midline. He sees only half of any object. This is known as *hemianopsia* (half-blindness).

the brain. Like the brain, it consists of gray and white matter, but, although in the brain the gray matter is external and the white internal, in the cord the gray matter is in the center and is surrounded on all sides by

Cortical blindness of one optic area (that is, of the posterior tip of one cerebral hemisphere) always affects both eyes equally. Total blindness in one eye may be due to disease of that eye itself or to disease of its optic nerve. Just behind the two eyes, however, the two optic nerves become confluent (the chiasm), then again become separate and continue to the brain as two optic tracts.

In each of these tracts is just half of each optic nerve, so that if one tract is injured, there is complete blindness of exactly one-half of each retina. For example, if the right tract is injured, the patient is blind on the right half of each retina, so that with either eye he can see nothing to his left but will see perfectly to his right. If the cortical optical area of the hemisphere to which that tract runs is destroyed, this same form of hemianopsia occurs.

The pituitary gland is located just beneath the chiasm; a tumor of this gland often disturbs the chiasm and produces blindness of both inner halves of the retinas, since it is only the fibers in the nasal halves of the optic nerves that cross. In many cases of blindness it is thus possible to locate the disorder.

Motor Controls: Paralysis and Dyskinesia

A vertical band of cortex on each cerebral hemisphere governs the voluntary movements of the body. This region, known as the "motor cortex," can be located accurately.

We know the exact location of the cells in which originate the voluntary movements of the muscles of the face, the thumb, the hands, the arm, the trunk, or the leg. Before a person can move a muscle, these particular cells must send the stimulus down along their fibers. If these cells are stimulated with an electric current, the muscles they control will contract.

En route to the pons, as described previously, the motor fibers converge into a tight bundle known as the *capsule*. A comparatively small injury to the capsule causes paralysis in more muscles than does a much larger injury to the cortex itself.

The brain is like a telephone station, in which one blow of an axe can sever all the wires at the point where they leave the building, but a similar blow on the switchboard would sever only a few.

The ordinary cause of a stroke, followed by paralysis of one half of the body (hemiplegia), is usually a small hemorrhage from a blood vessel in the capsule. A much larger hemorrhage nearer to or in the cortex might paralyze one limb, but hardly half of the body. Hemiplegia may be due to the rupture of a miliary aneurysm of a tiny artery running to the internal capsule or to the plugging of this artery by a thrombus or an embolus, and the subsequent death of the fibers which it supplies with blood.

Immediately after a stroke, one half of the body, as a rule, is paralyzed. Then, gradually, the person recovers the use of certain muscles, usually those of the leg, often those of the upper arm, least often those of the hand. Although the hemorrhage actually destroys the fibers of only a few nerves, it temporarily injures all those in its neighborhood, perhaps by the pressure of the escaped blood or by the edema that surrounds it. As the swelling from the hemorrhage diminishes, these latter fibers resume their function, but those actually destroyed never do.

Within the medulla the motor axons from the cortex form two well-defined bands known as the *corticospinal* or *pyramidal tracts.* Here the majority of these fibers cross (or decussate) to the opposite side, continuing thereafter as the "crossed pyramidal tract." The remaining fibers then enter the spinal cord on the original side as the "direct pyramidal tract," each fiber in this tract finally crossing to the opposite side of the cord near the point of termination and coming to an end within the gray matter comprising the anterior horn on that side, in close proximity to a motor nerve cell. Fibers of the crossed pyramidal tract terminate within the anterior horn and make connections with anterior horn cells on the same side. All of the motor fibers of the spinal nerves represent extensions of these anterior horn cells, with each of these fibers communicating with only one particular muscle fiber.

Thus each muscle fiber is under voluntary control through a combination of two nerve cells. One is located in the motor cortex, its fiber in the direct or crossed pyramidal tract, and the other is located in the anterior horn of the spinal cord, its fiber running to the muscle. The former is referred to as the upper motor neuron; the latter, as the lower motor neuron. Every motor nerve serving a muscle is a bundle comprised of several thousand lower motor neurons.

Several motor nerve tracts, other than the corticospinal, are contained in the spinal cord. Some represent the pathways of the so-called "extrapyramidal system," establishing connections between the anterior horn cells and the automatic control centers located in the basal ganglia and the cerebellum. Others are components of reflex arcs, forming synaptic connections between anterior horn cells and sensory fibers that have entered adjacent or neighboring segments of the cord.

Motor Paralysis. Paralysis of a muscle may be due to pathologic changes in either the upper or the lower motor neuron. If a motor nerve is cut somewhere between the muscle and the spinal cord, the muscle becomes paralyzed, and the individual is not able to move it. Furthermore, it takes no part in reflex movements. Moreover, this muscle becomes limp and wastes away; that is, it atrophies owing to disuse. The injury to the spinal nerve trunk may heal, and the patient may regain the use of the muscles that it supplies. But if the anterior horn motor nerve cells are destroyed, the nerve cannot regenerate, and that muscle never will be useful again. This is exactly what occurs in anterior poliomyelitis.

If the upper motor neuron is destroyed, a different

condition exists in the muscle. It is paralyzed as far as voluntary movement is concerned, but not necessarily for reflex (involuntary) movements, because these originate in the nerve cells in the cord or the medulla. The muscle does not atrophy, and it will not become limp; on the contrary, it remains permanently more tense than normal. This paralysis seldom affects a part of one muscle, one single muscle or only a few muscles; it usually affects a whole limb, both limbs or an entire half of the body (hemiplegia).

A good illustration of this form of paralysis is the spastic (stiff) paralysis of those infants who during birth receive some mechanical injury that may have caused the rupture of a blood vessel in the meninges of the brain. The long-continued pressure of the escaped blood may injure large areas of cortex; hence these children are frequently mentally defective. Many have convulsions. When such a child begins to walk, the legs and the arms are stiff. During life, movements are awkward, stiff, and weak. Since those muscles that draw the feet and the knees toward each other (the adductor muscles) are naturally stronger than those that spread those limbs apart (the abductor muscles), these persons walk by a cross-legged progression, called also the *scissors gait;* that is, in each step the leg is moved not only forward but is swung round across the front of the other. When both legs are paralyzed, the condition is called *paraplegia;* and when the arm and the leg on the same side are paralyzed, the term *hemiplegia* is used. Paralysis of all four extremities is *quadriplegia.*

A common illustration of upper motor neuron paralysis is hemiplegia. If a hemorrhage, an embolus, or a thrombus destroys the fibers from the motor area in the internal capsule, the arm and the leg of the opposite side promptly become stiff and more or less paralyzed, and the reflexes are exaggerated. Another illustration of upper neuron disease is seen in adults with spastic paraplegia, a chronic stiffness of both legs due to a gradual degeneration of the fibers in the pyramidal tract. The person so afflicted walks stiffly, as though wading through water, the knees always touching each other and the feet scarcely raised from the ground (the spastic gait).

Both an upper and a lower motor neuron paralysis may result from an injury that crushes the spinal cord, a type of injury that is all too common. A boy diving into too-shallow water, for example, strikes his head and "breaks" his neck. That is, at one point the vertebrae are no longer in line, and the cord is badly crushed at the point of the dislocation. Knuckling of the backbone due to tuberculosis may accomplish the same thing, only more slowly. The result of such crushing of the cord leads to a rigid paralysis on both sides of all muscles whose nerves leave the cord below the crushed spot. Limp paralysis also occurs in those muscles whose motor nerve fibers come from cells in the crushed area. There also will be insensibility of the skin below the crush, since the sensory fibers from below the injury no longer reach the brain. Tumors of the cord ultimately cause this same picture. At first, only that part of the cord directly involved is disturbed, but as the tumor grows, it may completely crush the cord.

EXTRAPYRAMIDAL MOTOR CONTROLS. The smoothness, the accuracy and the strength that characterize the muscular movements of a normal individual are attributable to the influence of the cerebellum and the basal ganglia.

The cerebellum (Fig. 53-1), nestled beneath the posterior lobe of the cerebrum, chief assistant to the higher motor centers in the cerebral cortex, is responsible for coordinating, balancing, timing, and synergizing with precision all muscular movements that originate in those centers. Through the agency of the cerebellum, the contractions of opposing muscle groups are adjusted in relation to each other to maximal mechanical advantage; muscular contractions can be sustained evenly at the desired tension and without significant fluctuation, and reciprocal movements can be reproduced at high and constant speed, in stereotyped fashion and with relatively little effort.

The basal ganglia are masses of gray matter in the midbrain beneath the cerebral hemispheres. These border or project into the lateral ventricles and lie in close apposition to the internal capsule. It is their function to control habitual or automatic acts and to maintain a "postural background" against which voluntary movements are performed. These ganglia, aided by their connections with the organs of special sense, keep the contractile tone of every muscle in the trunk and the extremities in a constant state of adjustment, so that an individual is able to keep his balance regardless of the posture of his body, in darkness as well as in light and irrespective of the status underfoot. Moreover, thanks to this control station, the individual is equipped to react swiftly, appropriately and automatically to any smell, sight or sound that demands an immediate response.

Dyskinesias. Loss of cerebellar function, which may occur as a result of intracranial injury, hemorrhage, abscess or tumor, results in muscular flabbiness, weakness, and fatigue. The patient exhibits a coarse involuntary tremor that increases in intensity in association with voluntary movements. He is unable to control his movements accurately or to coordinate his muscles efficiently or smoothly, every act being performed in disjointed fashion, according to stages, or "by the numbers." He is incapable of performing alternating movements with speed or uniformity, a characteristic of cerebellar disease called "adiadochokinesis." When he walks, he staggers, lurching from side to side as though intoxicated, feet wide apart but steps short and not stamping, i.e., with the vertiginous, reeling gait of cerebellar ataxia.

Destruction or dysfunction of the basal ganglia does

not lead to paralysis but to muscular rigidity, with consequent disturbances of posture and movement. Such patients are afflicted by a tendency to display involuntary movements. These may take the form of coarse tremors, characterized by approximately six oscillations per second; *athetosis,* namely, movements of a slow, squirming, writhing, twisting type; or *chorea,* marked by spasmodic, purposeless and grotesque motions of the trunk and the extremities, and facial grimacing. Clinical syndromes based on lesions involving the basal ganglia include parkinsonism (page 1232), Huntington's disease (page 1235), Wilson's disease, or "hepatolenticular degeneration," and spasmodic torticollis.

Sensory Pathways and Disturbances

THE THALAMUS. The thalamus, major receiving and communication center for the afferent sensory nerves, is a large and complicated structure located in the midbrain. It lies in close relation to the third ventricle, forming its lateral wall, and to the lateral ventricle, forming its floor, and is in close proximity to the basal ganglia and adjacent to the internal capsule. To the thalamus may be attributed the vague awareness of sensations described as "feelings" of pleasure, discomfort or pain. Moreover, it is responsible for the routing of all sensory stimuli to their many destinations, including the cerebral cortex, which receives them and translates them automatically into appropriate responses.

SENSORY PATHWAYS. The transmission of sensory impulses from their points of origin to their cerebral destinations involves three neuron relays; moreover, there are three major pathways by which they may be routed, depending on the type of sensation that is registered. Specific knowledge regarding these paths is of great importance from the standpoint of neurologic diagnoses, being indispensable for the accurate localization of brain and cord lesions in many patients.

The axon of the nerve in which the sensory impulse originates enters the spinal cord by way of the posterior root. Axons conveying sensations of heat, cold, and pain immediately enter the posterior gray column of the cord, where they make connections with the cells of secondary neurons. Pain and temperature fibers cross immediately to the opposite side of the cord and course upward to the thalamus. Fibers carrying sensations of touch, light pressure, and localization do not connect immediately with the second neuron but ascend the cord for a variable distance before entering the gray matter and completing this connection. The axon of the secondary neuron crosses the cord and proceeds upward to the thalamus.

The third category of sensation, produced by stimuli arising from muscles, joints and bones, includes position sense and vibratory sense. These stimuli are conveyed, uncrossed, all the way to the brain stem by the axon of the primary neuron. In the medulla, synaptic connections are made with cells of the secondary neurons, whose axons then cross to the opposite side and proceed to the thalamus.

Sensory Losses. Severance of a sensory nerve results in total loss of sensation in its area of distribution. Transection of the spinal cord yields complete anesthesia below the level of injury. Selective destruction or degeneration of the posterior columns of the spinal cord, a characteristic of combined system disease, is responsible for a loss of position sense in segments distal to the lesion, unaccompanied by loss of touch, pain or temperature perception. Such individuals, unless they look, cannot tell where their feet are, or in what direction they are pointing. Moreover, they cannot perceive vibrations in the affected area. A lesion such as a cyst in the center of the cord causes dissociation of sensation, that is, loss of pain at the level of the lesion. This is explainable on the basis of the fact that the fibers carrying pain and temperature cross the cord immediately upon entering; thus, any lesion that divides the cord longitudinally divides these fibers likewise. Other sensory fibers ascend the cord for variable distances, some even to the medulla itself, before crossing, thereby bypassing the lesion and avoiding destruction.

Dysesthesias. Irritative lesions affecting the posterior spinal nerve roots may cause intermittent severe pains that are referred to their areas of distribution. This phenomenon explains the pains of tabes dorsalis. The sensation of tingling of the fingers and the toes constitutes a prominent symptom of combined systems disease, presumably due to degenerative changes in the sensory fibers that extend to the thalamus, i.e., belonging to the spinothalamic tract.

AUTONOMIC NERVOUS SYSTEM

The contractions of muscles that are not under voluntary control, including the heart muscle, the secretions of all digestive and sweat glands and the activity of certain endocrine organs as well, are controlled by a major component of the nervous system known as the *autonomic nervous system.* The term "autonomic" refers to the fact that the operations of this system are independent of the desires and the intentions of the individual. It is not subject to his will; i.e., it is in a sense autonomous.

To the extent that it is not subject to regulation by the cerebral cortex, the autonomic nervous system resembles the extrapyramidal systems that are centered in the cerebellum and the basal ganglia. However, in other respects it is unique. First, its regulatory effects are exerted not on individual cells but on large expanses of tissue and on entire organs. Second, the responses that it elicits do not appear instantaneously, but only after a lag period, and they are sustained far longer than other neurogenic responses, a type of response that is calculated to ensure maximal functional efficiency on the part of receptor organs, such as the blood vessels and the hollow viscera.

The quality of these responses is explained by the fact that the autonomic nervous system transmits its impulses only partly by way of nerve pathways, the remainder of

TABLE 53-1. COMPARISON OF PARASYMPATHETIC AND SYMPATHETIC EFFECTS ON SPECIFIC ORGANS AND TISSUES*

ORGAN OR TISSUE	PARASYMPATHETIC EFFECTS	SYMPATHETIC EFFECTS
Vessels:		
Cutaneous	—	Constriction
Muscular	—	Variable
Coronary	Constriction	Dilatation
Salivary gland	Dilatation	Constriction
Buccal mucosa	—	Dilatation
Pulmonary	Variable	Variable
Cerebral	Dilatation	Constriction
Of abdominal and pelvic viscera	—	Constriction
Of external genitalia	Dilatation	Constriction
Heart	Inhibition	Acceleration
Eye:		
Iris	Constriction	Dilatation
Ciliary muscle	Contraction	Relaxation
Smooth muscle of orbit and upper lid	—	Contraction
Bronchi	Constriction	Dilatation
Glands:		
Sweat	—	Secretion
Salivary	Secretion	Secretion
Gastric	Secretion	Inhibition? Secretion of mucus
Pancreatic		
Acini	Secretion	—
Islets	Secretion	—
Liver	—	Glycogenolysis
Adrenal medulla	—	Secretion
Smooth muscle:		
Of skin	—	Contraction
Of stomach wall	Contraction (predominantly)	Inhibition (predominantly)
Of small intestine	Increased tone and motility	Inhibition
Of large intestine	Increased tone and motility	Inhibition
Of bladder wall (detrusor muscle)	Contraction	Inhibition
Of trigone and sphincter	Inhibition	Contraction
Of uterus, pregnant	None	Contraction
Of uterus, nonpregnant	None	Inhibition

*Best, C. H., and Taylor, N. B.: Physiological Basis of Medical Practice, 6th ed. Baltimore, Williams and Wilkins.

the route being serviced by chemical mediators, resembling in this respect the endocrine system. Electrical impulses, conducted through nerve fibers, stimulate the formation of specific chemical agents at strategic locations within the muscle mass, the diffusion of these chemicals being responsible for the contraction.

THE HYPOTHALAMUS. Overall supervision of the autonomic nervous system is considered a function of the hypothalamus. The *hypothalamus* is a portion of the diencephalon (interbrain) located immediately beneath and lateral to the lower portion of the wall of the third ventricle. It includes among its components the optic chiasm, the tuber cinereum, the pituitary stalk, which originates from the latter, and the pituitary gland itself. Large cell groups in adjacent portions of the hypothalamus have been assigned the role of the probable centers of autonomic regulation. These centers are richly endowed with connections linking the autonomic systems with the thalamus, the cortex, the olfactory apparatus and the pituitary gland. Here reside the mechanisms for the control of visceral and somatic reactions that were designed originally for defense or attack, but in man these are associated with his emotional states, i.e., his fears, anger, anxiety; for the control of metabolic processes, including fat, carbohydrate and water metabolism; for the regulation of body temperature, arterial pressure and all muscular and glandular activities of the gastrointestinal tract; the genital functions; and the sleep rhythm. The close proximity, histologic similarity and multiple connections between the pituitary gland, master gland of the endocrines, and this portion of the brain suggest that here may be located the supreme headquarters of the endocrine and autonomic nervous systems, commanding all vital processes.

Sympathetic and Parasympathetic Nervous Systems

The *autonomic nervous system* comprises two divisions that are anatomically and functionally distinct, referred to as the sympathetic and the parasympathetic nervous systems. The majority of the tissues and the organs under autonomic control are innervated by both systems. Sympathetic stimuli are mediated by norepinephrine; parasympathetic impulses, by acetylcholine. These chemicals produce opposing and mutually antagonistic effects, as indicated in Table 53-1.

SYMPATHETIC NERVOUS SYSTEM. Sympathetic neurons are located in the thoracic and the lumbar segments of the spinal cord; their axons, called *preganglionic fibers*, emerge by way of all anterior nerve roots from the eighth cervical or first thoracic segment to the second or third lumbar segment, inclusive. A short distance from the cord these fibers diverge to join a chain composed of 22 linked ganglia that extends the entire length of the spinal column, flanking the vertebral bodies on both sides. Some form multiple synapses with nerve cells within the chain. Others traverse the chain without making connections or losing continuity to join large "prevertebral" ganglia in the thorax, the abdomen or the pelvis, or one of the "terminal" ganglia in the vicinity of an organ, such as the bladder or the rectum. Postganglionic nerve fibers originating in the sympathetic chain rejoin the spinal nerves that supply the extremities and are distributed to blood vessels, sweat glands and smooth muscle tissue in the skin. Postganglionic fibers from the prevertebral plexuses, i.e., the cardiac, the pulmonary, splanchnic and the pelvic plexuses, supply structures in the head and the neck, the thorax, the abdomen and the pelvis, respectively, having been joined in these plexuses by fibers from the parasympathetic division.

The adrenals, the kidneys, the liver, the spleen, the stomach and the duodenum are under the control of the giant celiac plexus, familiarly known as the "solar plexus." This receives its sympathetic nerve components by way of the three splanchnic nerves, composed of preganglionic fibers from nine segments of the spinal cord (i.e., T4 to L1), and is joined by the vagus nerve, representing the parasympathetic division. From the celiac plexus, fibers of both divisions travel along the course of blood vessels to their target organs.

PARASYMPATHETIC SYSTEM. The preganglionic nerve cells of the sympathetic division, as described above, are consolidated in consecutive segments of the cord, from C7 to L1 or L2. Those of the parasympathetic system, on the other hand, are located in two sections, one in the brain stem and the other from spinal segments below L2. On this account the parasympathetic system is referred to as the "craniosacral" division, as distinct from the "thoracolumbar" division of the autonomic nervous system.

The cranial parasympathetics arise from the midbrain and the medulla oblongata. Fibers from cells in the midbrain travel with the third oculomotor nerve to the ciliary ganglia, whence postganglionic fibers of this division are joined by those of the sympathetic system. Forming the ciliary nerve, these channel to the ciliary muscles of the eye to control the caliber of the pupil. Parasympathetic fibers from the medulla travel with the seventh (facial), ninth (glossopharyngeal), and tenth (vagus) cranial nerves. Those from the facial nerve end in the spleno-palatine ganglion, whence emanate the fibers that innervate the lacrimal glands, the ciliary muscle, and the sphincter of the pupil. Those from the glossopharyngeal nerve innervate the parotid gland. The vagus nerve carries preganglionic parasympathetic fibers without interruption to the organs that it innervates, joining ganglion cells within the myocardium and within the walls of the esophagus, the stomach and the intestine.

Preganglionic parasympathetic fibers from the anterior roots of the sacral nerves coalesce to become the pelvic nerves, consolidate and regroup in the pelvic plexus, and terminate around ganglion cells in the musculature of the pelvic organs. These innervate the colon, the rectum and the bladder, inhibiting the muscular tone of the anal and the bladder sphincters and dilating the blood vessels of the bladder, the rectum and the genitalia.

The vagus, the splanchnic, pelvic and the other autonomic nerves carry impulses generated in the viscera to the dorsal nucleus of the vagus, where connections are made with efferent parasympathetic neurons, forming a series of reflex arcs. These provide the basis for self-regulation, a cardinal feature of the autonomic nervous system, and one reason for "autonomy."

Autonomic Functions and Dysfunctions. A detailed listing of the effects produced by the two divisions of the autonomic nervous system is supplied in Table 53-1. This listing provides impressive evidence of the scope and the importance of autonomic activity in relation to all bodily functions and from the standpoint of survival itself. Both sympathetic and parasympathetic divisions are in a constant state of activity, the activity of each relative to the other being one of controlled opposition, with a delicate balance maintained between the two at all times.

Sympathetic Syndromes. Certain syndromes are distinctive of diseases of the sympathetic nerve trunks. Among these are dilatation of the pupil of the eye on the same side as a penetrating wound of the neck (evidence of disturbance of the cervical sympathetic cord); temporary paralysis of the bowel (indicated by the absence of peristaltic waves and the distention of the intestine by gas) following fracture of any one of the lower dorsal or upper lumbar vertebrae with hemorrhage into the base of the mesentery; and the marked variations in pulse rate and rhythm that often follow compression fractures of the upper six thoracic vertebrae.

GENERAL ASSESSMENT

The nurse's observations relative to all systems of the body may be of great assistance in establishing the diagnosis of many neurologic disorders.

- Of utmost importance are changes in muscle strength and disturbances of sensation.
- The appearance of pain, its type and location, should be noted with care.
- Oliguria and incontinence should be reported as well as any episode of vomiting with a full description of when and how it occurred (whether or not it was accompanied by nausea, what its relationship to the preceding meal was, and the nature of the vomitus).
- Mental and nervous symptoms should be observed and studied analytically, because their complete description is likely to be of value in the diagnosis and the therapeutic management of the patient. The general attitude of the patient may reveal depression or euphoria; the mood swings may run the gamut of irritability, apprehension, anger, and elation.

• Disturbances of vision, hearing, speech, smell, taste, touch, pressure or pain may be elicited in the course of patient management, possibly indicating a new development in the patient's neurologic status.

The diagnostic value of the nurse's findings, when described completely and accurately, are very significant.

For an overview of general neurological assessment pertaining to levels of consciousness, cranial nerve function, reflex actions, muscle strength, sensory perception, mental status, etc. see pages 83–88 of Chapter 5, Physical Assessment.

DIAGNOSTIC ASSESSMENT

Cranial Nerve Tests

In addition to the usual complete physical examination, every patient suspected of having a neurologic disorder and every neurosurgical patient is subjected to a systematic and detailed neurologic examination. This involves the testing of each cranial nerve in the manner specified in Table 53-2. Maximal cooperation of the patient is essential for the proper conduct of this diagnostic routine and can be elicited only if he understands what he is expected to do. All equipment for these tests should be available in one place.

Examination of the peripheral motor and the sensory systems also is done. Motor tests include observation of posture and gait, reflex tests, coordination observations, etc. Sensory tests determine skin sensation and deeper tissue sensation, as well as the ability to recognize objects by the sense of touch.

The nurse should know the results of the findings of the neurologic and the physical examination, because only then is one able to observe intelligently the symptoms and aberrant reactions of the patient. These deviations must be recorded accurately if they are to be meaningful.

Computerized Tomography (Computed Axial Tomography; CAT Scanning)

Computed tomography makes use of a narrow beam of x-ray to scan the head in successive layers (Fig. 53-4). The images that are produced provide cross-sectional views of the brain, with distinguishing differences in tissue densities of the skull, cortex, subcortical structures and ventricles. A computer printout is obtained of the absorption values of the tissues in the plane that is being scanned. The data is transformed into an image through a series of complex equations. Therefore, the brightness of each portion or "slice" of brain in the final image is

TABLE 53-2.   NEUROLOGIC EXAMINATION FOR TESTING CRANIAL NERVES*

NERVE	EQUIPMENT	CLINICAL EXAMINATION
1. Olfactory	Four small bottles of volatile oils, such as (1) turpentine, (2) oil of cloves, (3) oil of wintergreen, (4) vanilla	Instruct the patient to sniff and to identify the odors. Each nostril is tested separately. The patient is asked if he perceives the smell and if he can identify it.
2. Optic	Ophthalmoscope	In darkened room the patient is asked to look straight ahead at a distant object while the examiner looks for choked disc, optic atrophy, and retinal and vascular lesions. Special equipment is used for examination of visual fields. Eye chart is used to check visual acuity.
3. Oculomotor 4. Trochlear 6. Abducens	Flashlight	Because of close association, these nerves are examined collectively. They innervate pupil and upper eyelid and are responsible for extraocular muscle movements.
5. Trigeminal	Test tube of hot water Test tube of ice water Cotton wisp from cotton applicator stick Pin	*Sensory* branch—Vertex to chin tested for sensations of pain, touch and temperature. This includes reflex reaction of cornea to wisp of cotton. *Motor* branch—Ability to bite is tested.
7. Facial	Four small bottles with solutions which are salty, sweet, sour, and bitter (Four wet cotton applicators)	Observe symmetry of face and ability to contract facial muscles. Instruct patient to taste and to identify substance used. He should rinse his mouth well between each drop of solution. This is a test for the anterior ⅔ of tongue.
8. Acoustic	Tuning fork	Tests for hearing, air and bone conduction.
9. Glossopharyngeal	Cotton applicator stick	Test posterior ⅓ of tongue for taste, and check gag reflex.
10. Vagus	Tongue depressor	Checking voice sounds, observing symmetry of soft palate will give suggestion of function of vagus.
11. Spinal Accessory		Since this innervates the sternocleidomastoid and the trapezius muscles, the patient will be instructed to turn and to move his head and to elevate shoulders with and without resistance.
12. Hypoglossal		Observe tongue movements.

*See also Neurological Examination, pages 83-88.

proportional to the degree to which it absorbs x-ray. The image is displayed on an oscilloscope or TV monitor and photographed (Fig. 53-5).

Lesions within the brain are seen as variations in tissue density differing from the surrounding normal brain tissue. Abnormalities of tissue density indicate possible tumor masses, brain infarction, displacement of the ventricles, cortical atrophy, etc.

Computed tomography is usually done first without contrast material and then with intravenous contrast enhancement. The patient lies on an adjustable table, with his head held in a fixed position, while the scanning system rotates around the head. (The patient is used as the axis and the machine is rotated around this axis, resulting in a cross-cut image). The patient must lie with the head held perfectly still, and with a careful effort not to talk or move the face as head motion causes considerable artifact.

Computed tomography is the most revolutionary development in neurological diagnosis in this century. It is non-invasive, painless and has a high degree of sensitivity for detecting lesions.

Air Studies

The cerebrospinal fluid spaces in and around the brain may be seen in x-ray examination when the fluid is replaced with a gas. This is based on the principle that gas, replacing the fluid within the ventricular and subarachnoid systems, serves as a contrast medium, because air is less dense than fluid to roentgen rays. The cerebrospinal fluid may be partially replaced with air through *pneumoencephalography* and *ventriculography*.

Pneumoencephalography is a diagnostic procedure in which air or gas is instilled through a lumbar puncture as a means of demonstrating the ventricular system and subarachnoid space overlying the hemispheres and basal cisterns. A small amount of cerebrospinal fluid is removed and an equivalent amount of air injected. A special chair allows the patient to be rotated in all directions so that air may be placed selectively in the desired cavities. Films are then taken and studied.

This procedure is usually done under local or neuroleptic anesthesia and may be accompanied and followed by unpleasant side effects including severe headache associated with nausea, vomiting, photophobia, diaphoresis, pallor, restlessness and syncope. Adequate personnel should be available to treat the complications. The patient may be informed that the air inserted into the spine can be felt rising up to the ventricles and that a "sloshing sound" may be heard as a result of the air in the ventricles as the head is repositioned.

Although used less frequently since the advent of computed tomography, pneumoencephalography is useful in demonstrating lesions in the parasellar region and in assessing intraventricular and brainstem lesions.

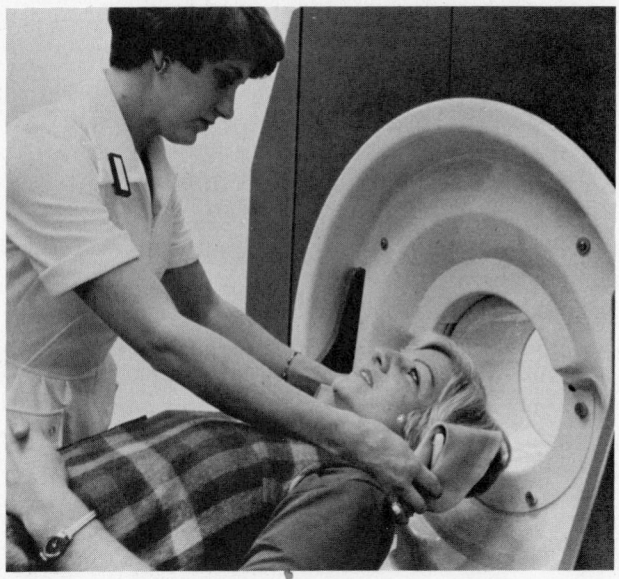

Figure 53-4. Computerized tomography. Scan of the brain. Courtesy EMI Medical, Inc.

A *ventriculogram* is an x-ray taken of the lateral ventricles following withdrawal of cerebrospinal fluid and injection of air or gas into the lateral ventricles through openings in the skull. This procedure is usually done under local anesthesia with the patient sitting in a special chair. The posterior half of the head is prepared and draped. Trephines (burr holes) are made through scalp incisions, and the ventricles are punctured by a special needle. (In infants this study may be done through fontanelle puncture without burr holes.) The fluid is replaced with air, the cannulae are withdrawn, and the scalp wounds are closed. If a lesion is present, there is a

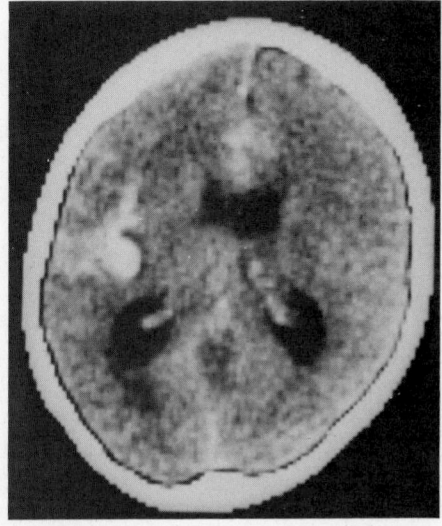

Figure 53-5. CT scan of the brain. A dense clot can be seen in the left sylvian and interhemispheric fissures. Note the peripheral zone of edema around the left sylvian clot. (Scan courtesy of Toronto General Hospital) (See also Figure 16-8, page 289.)

change in size, shape or position of the ventricular, subarachnoid, or cisternal spaces.

During this procedure, the patient develops a mild headache, may become nauseated, may retch and very rarely may have a convulsive seizure. The reaction to this procedure is usually milder than that attending pneumoencephalography.

Preparation of the Patient. The night before encephalography or ventriculography, the patient should have a good rest. On the morning of the test, breakfast is withheld since nausea and vomiting are side effects of these procedures.

Appropriate sedatives and analgesics are administered before the patient is taken to the operating room or x-ray department. The back of the head should be shaved before ventriculography. The entire head is shaved if craniotomy is to follow. All hairpins should be removed; however, long hair should *not* be braided before pneumoencephalography, since braids cast shadows on the x-ray films. As with other surgical procedures, dentures are removed.

Postprocedure Assessment. The patient is observed for signs of increased or decreased intracranial pressure (page 1184) or shock. Disturbances of intracranial pressure may cause downward herniation of the supratentorial and posterior fossa contents. If this occurs, preparations should be made for a ventricular tap and prompt decompression. Special care must be taken to see that the patient does not aspirate any vomitus. Vital signs are taken frequently until they are stabilized, and neurological checks, especially level of responsiveness, are made. Parenteral fluids may be necessary for the first 24 hours.

Since a pounding headache is the major complaint following these procedures, an ice cap may be placed on the head and adequate analgesics given while the headache lasts. The duration of the headache depends on how quickly the intracranial air is absorbed.

Since the discomforts are related to the amount of air used, the instillation of smaller amounts of air has reduced the frequency, severity, and duration of the symptoms.

Cerebral Angiography

Cerebral angiography is an x-ray study of the cerebral circulation following injection of contrast material into a selected artery. The contrast material may be injected into the common carotid, vertebral or subclavian artery or the arch of the aorta. Selective catheterization may also be done via a femoral or brachial artery. After injection of the selected arteries, x-rays are made of the arterial and venous phases of circulation through the brain. As the dye is injected, serial films are taken by means of an automatic, computer-programmed rapid film changer. The procedure may be done under local or general anesthesia.

Cerebral angiography is the primary investigative tool for intracranial aneurysm, arteriovenous malformation and cerebral vascular occlusive disease. It also has value in localizing mass lesions and may aid in preoperative diagnosis. It is frequently done prior to craniotomy.

Preprocedure Management. The meal preceding the test is withheld. A sedative may be given before the patient is taken to the x-ray department. He is informed that he should try to lie quietly while the dye is injected and that a burning sensation, lasting a few seconds, may be felt behind the eyes, or in the jaw, teeth, tongue or lips as the dye is injected. In a small percentage of patients, an allergic reaction to the contrast media may occur, requiring that prompt resuscitation procedures be carried out.

Postprocedure Management. In some instances patients may experience major or minor arterial block due to embolism, thrombosis or hemorrhage. Signs of such an occurrence include alterations in the level of responsiveness and consciousness, weakness on one side of the body, motor or sensory deficits or speech disturbances. It is necessary to observe the patient repeatedly for these signs and to report them immediately if they occur.

The injection site is observed for hematoma formation, and an ice cap is applied intermittently to the puncture site to relieve swelling and discomfort. Since a hematoma at the puncture site or embolization to a distant artery will affect the peripheral pulses, these signs are monitored frequently. The color and temperature of the involved extremity are also noted as a means of detecting possible embolism.

Myelography

A *myelogram* is an x-ray of the spinal subarachnoid space taken after an opaque medium or air is injected into the spinal subarachnoid space through a spinal puncture. It outlines the spinal subarachnoid space and shows any distortion of the spinal cord or spinal dural sac caused by tumors, cysts, herniated intervertebral discs or other lesions.

After the contrast medium is injected, the head of the table is tilted down and the course of the contrast medium is observed radioscopically. After the examination is completed, the contrast material (Pantopaque) may be removed by syringe and needle aspiration. The patient may complain of sharp pain down the leg during aspiration if a nerve root is affected. Should this occur, the needle point is rotated or the depth of the needle adjusted. Newer water-soluble contrast media (metrizamide [Amipaque]) may be injected through a smaller needle and need not be removed by aspiration from the thecal sac because it is highly soluble and clears relatively quickly from the cerebrospinal fluid.

Nursing Management. Since most patients have some misconceptions about this procedure, the nurse can answer questions and clarify the explanation offered by the physician. The patient should be aware that the x-ray table will be tilted in varying positions during the study. The meal that would normally be eaten prior to the procedure is omitted. The patient may be given a light sedative to help cope with a rather lengthy test.

Following a procedure in which Pantopaque is used, the patient should lie in a recumbent position for the amount of time specified by the physician. Usually he is permitted to turn from side to side. When a water-soluble medium has been used, the patient lies in bed with the head of the bed elevated 15 to 30 degrees to reduce the rate of upward dispersion of the medium. The patient may be kept in a horizontal position for an additional number of hours at the discretion of the physician.

The patient is encouraged to drink liberal amounts of fluid for rehydration and replacement of cerebrospinal fluid and to decrease the incidence of postlumbar puncture headache. The blood pressure, pulse, respiratory rate and temperature are monitored, as well as the patient's ability to void. Other untoward signs to watch for include: fever, stiff neck, photophobia or signs of chemical or bacterial meningitis.

Other X-ray Procedures

Lumbar Epidural Venography. In this procedure a catheter is inserted percutaneously into the femoral vein and guided into the ascending lumbar vein and/or internal iliac veins. The contrast medium is injected to fill the epidural veins overlying the disc spaces and to opacify the epidural venous plexus. The procedure may be useful in the diagnosis of herniated lumbar discs that are not demonstrated by myelography. It reveals deviation or compression of the epidural veins due to a herniated disc or tumor. The procedure is relatively easy to perform, well tolerated, fairly painless and not associated with arachnoiditis. Lumbar epidural venography and myelography may be done as complimentary diagnostic studies.

Following the test, the site is observed for evidence of hematoma formation.

Discography. Discography is the injection of a radiopaque substance directly into the intervertebral disc, followed by x-ray studies. While this procedure may be done in suspected instances of herniated discs, it is infrequently used.

Lumbar Puncture

A lumbar puncture is carried out by inserting a needle into the lumbar subarachnoid space in order to withdraw cerebrospinal fluid for diagnostic and therapeutic purposes. The purposes are to obtain spinal fluid for examination, to measure and relieve spinal fluid pressure, to determine the presence or absence of blood in the spinal fluid, to detect spinal subarachnoid block and to administer antibiotics intrathecally in certain cases of infection.

The needle is usually inserted into the subarachnoid space between the third and fourth lumbar spinous interspace. Since the spinal cord divides into a sheaf of nerves

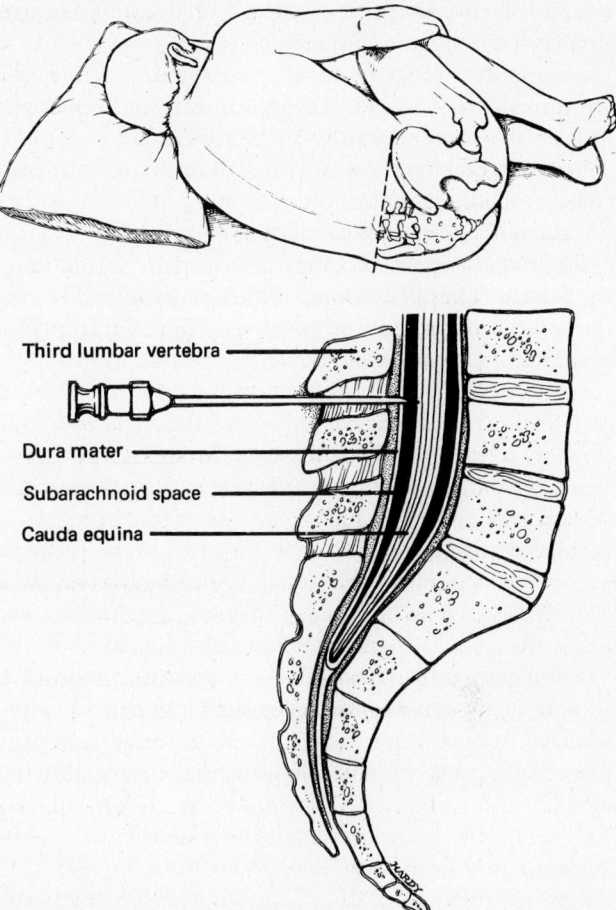

Figure 53-6. Technique of lumbar puncture. The interspaces between the spines of L3 and L5 are just below the line joining the anterosuperior iliac spines.

at the first lumbar vertebra, the needle is inserted below the level of the third lumbar vertebra (Fig. 53-6) to prevent the spinal cord from being punctured.

A successful lumbar puncture requires that the patient be relaxed, since an anxious patient may become tense, thereby causing an increase in the pressure reading. The normal range of spinal fluid pressure with the patient in a lateral position is 70 to 180 mm. of water. Pressures over 200 mm. of water are considered abnormal. A lumbar puncture may be quite dangerous in the presence of an intracranial mass lesion because when pressure is released, the intracranial contents may herniate.

Lumbar Manometric Test (Queckenstedt Test). This test is done when a spinal subarachnoid block (by tumor, vertebral fracture or dislocation) is suspected. Pressure may be applied manually by pressing firmly and simultaneously upon the jugular veins on each side of the neck for a period of 10 seconds. Or a blood pressure cuff may be placed around the patient's neck and inflated to a pressure of 20 mm. Hg. The increase in the pressure caused by the compression is noted. Then the pressure is released and pressure readings are made at 10 second intervals. In normal persons, the cerebrospinal fluid pressure rises rapidly in response to compression of the jugular veins and returns quickly to normal when the compression is released. A slow rise and fall in pressure indicates a partial block due to a lesion compressing the spinal subarachnoid pathways. If there is no pressure change, then a complete block is indicated. This test is not done if an intracranial lesion is suspected.

Nursing Support. During the initial explanations, the patient should be assured that inserting a needle into the spine will not result in paralysis. Prior to the lumbar puncture, the bladder and bowel should be emptied. The patient is placed on his side with his back toward the physician. The thighs and head are flexed as much as possible to increase the space between the spinous processes of the vertebrae and afford easier entry into the subarachnoid space. A pillow fixed between the legs will prevent the upper leg from rolling forward. A small pillow is placed under the patient's head so that the spine is maintained in a horizontal position. The nurse may assist the patient to maintain the position in order to avoid sudden movement which can produce a traumatic (bloody) tap. During the procedure, the patient is instructed to breathe normally since hyperventilation may lower an elevated pressure. Following the procedure the

patient is encouraged to lie quietly for 6 to 12 hours. A liberal fluid intake is encouraged.

Examination of the Cerebrospinal Fluid. Spinal fluid should be clear and colorless. Bloody spinal fluid may indicate cerebral contusion, laceration, or subarachnoid hemorrhage. Usually specimens are sent to the laboratory for cell count, culture, and chemical analysis. The specimens should be sent immediately, since changes will take place and alter the result if the specimens are allowed to stand. (See Appendix for the normal values of cerebrospinal fluid.)

Post-Lumbar Puncture Headache. A post-lumbar puncture headache, ranging from mild to severe, may appear in a few hours to several days following the procedure. It is a throbbing bifrontal and/or occipital headache, dull and deep in character, that is particularly severe when the patient sits or stands upright, but lessens or disappears when he lies down in a horizontal positon.

The cause of this unpleasant complication is the leakage of spinal fluid at the puncture site. The fluid continues to escape into the tissues by way of the needle tract from the spinal canal. It is then absorbed promptly by the lymphatics, never having accumulated in sufficient volume to be detected. As a result of this leak, the supply of cerebrospinal fluid in the cranium is depleted to a point at which it is insufficient to maintain proper mechanical stabilization of the brain. The brain becomes displaced caudally, exerting traction on the dural attachments to the venous sinuses, thereby causing headache. Traction on these pain-sensitive structures is maximal, and the pain is most severe when the patient is in a vertical position; both traction and pain are lessened and the leakage reduced when the patient lies down.

The lumbar puncture headache may be avoided if a needle with a small bore is used and if the patient is encouraged to remain recumbent for 6 to 12 hours following the procedure. Other complications of a spinal puncture include herniation of the intracranial contents, spinal epidural abscess, spinal epidural hematoma and meningitis.

Electroencephalography (EEG)

An *electroencephalogram* represents a record of the electrical activity generated in the brain and obtained through electrodes applied on the scalp surface or through microelectrodes placed within the brain tissue. It provides physiologic assessment of cerebral activity. EEG is a useful test for diagnosing seizure disorders such as the epilepsies, and is a screening procedure for coma or organic brain syndrome. It also serves as an indicator of brain death. Tumors, abscesses, brain scars, blood clots and infection may cause electric changes to differ from normal patterns of rhythm and rate.

Electrodes are arranged on the scalp to record the electrical activity in various regions of the head (Fig.

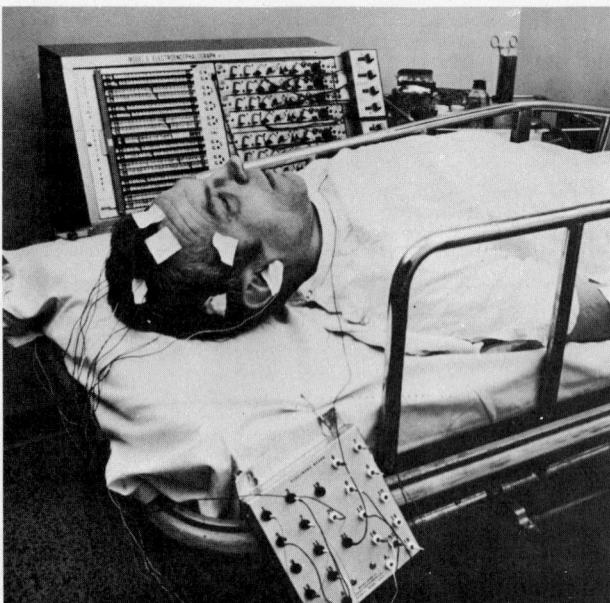

Figure 53-7. The electroencephalograph (EEG) is the most useful diagnostic and research tool yet developed to study the epilepsies. The nurse's function in this diagnostic examination is to reinforce the patient's understanding of the procedure and to listen to his concerns. Reassure the patient that he will not receive an electrical shock and that the EEG is not a form of treatment. The recording procedure takes approximately 45 minutes. While the examination is in progress, the patient need only relax and rest. Towards the end of the procedure he may be requested to breathe deeply or perform some simple type of mental activity. (Courtesy of Roche Laboratories)

53-7). The amplified activity of the neurons is recorded on a continuously moving paper sheet. For a baseline recording, the patient lies quietly with his eyes closed. Then he may be asked to hyperventilate for 3 to 4 minutes and then to look at a bright flashing light for photic stimulation. These are activation procedures done to evoke abnormal electrical discharges, especially seizure potentials. A sleep EEG may be recorded following sedation because some abnormal brain waves are seen only when the patient is asleep. If the epileptogenic area is inaccessible to the conventional scalp electrodes, nasopharyngeal electrodes may be used.

Patient Preparation. Tranquilizers and stimulants may be withheld 24 to 48 hours before an EEG since these medications can alter the EEG wave patterns or mask the abnormal wave patterns of seizure disorders. Coffee, tea or cola drinks are omitted in the meal before the test because of their stimulating effect. However, the meal is not omitted because an altered blood sugar level can also cause changes in the brain wave patterns.

The patient is informed that the EEG will take approximately 45 to 60 minutes, or longer if a sleep EEG is performed. At the same time, the patient is assured that the procedure will not cause an electric shock and that the EEG is a test, not a form of treatment.

Electromyography (EMG)

An *electromyogram* is obtained by introducing needle electrodes into the skeletal muscles in order to study changes in the electrical potential of the muscles and the nerves leading to them. The electrical potentials are shown on an oscilloscope and amplified by a loudspeaker so that both the sound and the appearance of the waves can be analyzed and compared simultaneously. EMG is useful in determining the presence of a neuromuscular disorder. It helps distinguish weakness due to neuropathy (functional and/or pathologic changes in the peripheral nervous system) from weakness due to other causes. EMG is also useful in the evaluation and follow-up of patients with peripheral nerve injuries.

No special patient preparation is required. The patient is told that he will experience a sensation similar to that of an intramuscular injection as the needle is inserted into the muscle.

Radioisotope Brain Scanning

In this procedure the patient is given an intravenous injection of a radiopharmaceutical. The radioactivity subsequently transmitted through the skull is traced by a scanner which prints out a picture based on the number of counts received from the brain as it is scanned. A more recent imaging device, a gamma camera, prints out an image without any actual scanning taking place.

This test is based on the principle that a radiopharmaceutical may diffuse through a disrupted blood-brain barrier into abnormal cerebral tissue or in areas where there is new vascularization. (Normal brain tissue is relatively impermeable.) There is an increased uptake of radioactive material at the site of pathology.

Brain scanning is particularly useful in evaluating vascular lesions of the brain and meninges and in locating vascular neoplasms. It is useful in the early detection and evaluation of stroke, abscess, and follow-up of surgical or radiation therapy of the brain. Newer techniques permit the evaluation of cerebral circulation during the brain scan.

The patient may be pretreated with Lugol's solution or potassium perchlorate to block the radiopharmaceutical uptake in the thyroid, salivary glands, choroid plexus and gastrointestinal mucosa. The patient is asked to lie quietly during the scan.

Echoencephalography

Echoencephalography is the recording of echos from the deep structures within the skull by means of ultrasound (high frequency sound waves). Ultrasonic transducers are positioned over specified areas of the head, while echoes are transcribed into images that are stored on the oscilloscope. Echoencephalography is a rapid and useful technique to determine the position of midline structures of the brain and the distance from the midline to the lateral ventricular wall or the third ventricular wall. Therefore it is done to detect a shift of the cerebral midline structures caused by subdural hematoma, intracerebral hemorrhage, massive cerebral infarction and neoplasms. It is useful in the evaluation of hydrocephalus since it can detect dilation of the ventricles.

The nurse may explain that this is a noninvasive test, and that some type of liquid (mineral oil) may be used to eliminate the air gap between the hand-held transducer and the patient's head.

Other Methods for Studying Cerebral Circulation

In addition to angiography and isotope angiography other methods have been developed for studying cerebral circulation.

Thermography is used to measure the heat radiating from the face (a function of blood circulation). Decreased circulation to the face is detected by "cold spots."

Circulatory changes in retinal vessels may be observed directly, providing information on intracranial circulation.

An *indicator dilution test* may also be used. The amount of an indicator substance removed from the arterial blood during passage through the brain is measured in the expired air or venous blood.

In *acoustical detection of blood flow* an ultrasonic beam can be directed toward an artery and the echoes corresponding to the artery monitored as they move synchronously with the arterial pulse. The varying diameters of the artery as well as small changes in the position of the artery (represented by displacement of the echoes) may be noted.

BIBLIOGRAPHY

BOOKS

Adams, R. D., and Victor, M.: Principles of Neurology. New York, McGraw-Hill, 1977.

Conway, B. L.: Carini and Owens' Neurological and Neurosurgical Nursing, 7th ed. St. Louis, C. V. Mosby, 1978.

Ganong, W. F.: The Nervous System. Los Altos, Calif., Lange Med. Pub., 1977.

Goldensohn, E. S., and Appel, S. H., eds.: Scientific Approaches to Clinical Neurology. Vols. 1 & 2. Philadelphia, Lea and Febiger, 1977.

Heilmann, K. M., Watson, R. T., and Greer, M.: Handbook for Differential Diagnosis of Neurologic Signs and Symptoms. New York, Appleton-Century-Crofts, 1977.

Lewis, A. J.: Mechanisms of Neurological Disease. Boston, Little, Brown, 1976.

Mayo Clinic and Mayo Foundation. Clinical Examinations in Neurology. Philadelphia, W. B. Saunders, 1976.

Merritt, H. H.: A Textbook of Neurology, 6th ed. Philadelphia, Lea and Febiger, 1979.

Patten, J.: Neurological Differential Diagnosis. New York, Springer-Verlag, 1977.

Patton, H. D., et al.: Introduction to Basic Neurology. Philadelphia, W. B. Saunders, 1976.

Ross, R. T.: How to Examine the Nervous System. Springfield, Ill., Charles C Thomas, 1978.

Swift, N., and Mabel, R. M.: Manual of Neurological Nursing. Boston, Little, Brown, 1978.

Treip, C. S.: Color Atlas of Neuropathology. Chicago, Year Book Medical Pub., 1978.

Vick, N. A.: Grinker's Neurology, 7th ed. Springfield, Ill., Charles C Thomas, 1976.

Walton, J. N.: Essentials of Neurology, 4th ed. Philadelphia, J. B. Lippincott, 1976.

ARTICLES

Diagnosis

Andriola, M. R.: Role of EEG in evaluating central nervous system dysfunction. Geriatrics, *33*:59-65, Feb. 1978.

Baker, M., et al.: Developing strategies for biofeedback. Applications in neurologically handicapped patients. Phys. Therapy, *57*:402-408, Apr. 1977.

Baker, R. A., et al.: Sequelae of metrizamide myelography in 200 examinations. Am. J. Roentgenol., *130*:499-502, Mar. 1978.

Kieffer, S. A., et al.: Contrast agents for myelography: Clinical and radiological evaluation of Amipaque and Pantopaque. Radiology, *129*:695-705, Dec. 1978.

Ramirez, B.: When you're faced with a neuro patient. RN, *42*:67-76, Jan. 1979.

O'Dell, C. W., Coel, M. N., and Ignelzi, R. J.: Ascending lumbar venography in lumbar-disc disease. J. Bone Joint Surg. (Am.), *59*:159-163, Mar. 1977.

Quisling, R.: Using computerized tomography to identify neurological problems. Geriatrics, *33*:37-45, Mar. 1978.

54

MANAGEMENT OF PATIENTS WITH NEUROLOGIC DYSFUNCTION

SCOPE OF NEUROLOGIC NURSING

Recovery from organic disease of the nervous system is not always followed by complete restoration of function. The rehabilitation needs of these patients are usually complex, their solution requiring physical therapy, guidance, recreational opportunities, and reeducation of the most difficult sort.

Through optimism, nursing ability, and concern for the patient as a person, the nurse can help to ease many of the difficulties experienced by the patient and family. Upon realizing that the behavior and the personality of a person can be affected markedly by organic lesions of the brain, one is less inclined to think of a patient as being uncooperative or having a foul disposition; instead he becomes a person who needs help and understanding. His reactions may be beyond his control; anyone caring for these patients must realize this.

The many interesting diagnostic tests in which the nurse participates are much like solving a puzzle. But the diagnosis is not the end; it is merely a steppingstone to the removal of the cause. Surgery must be done accurately, otherwise the penalty may be the death of the patient or the reduction of his mental or physical abilities to the level of mere existence. Although surgery has many successful outcomes, there are cases in which an injury is too great to repair, or a tumor too extensive to remove, and the patient's prognosis is hopeless. It is important that even in these instances the nurse exercise as much concern for the comfort and the feelings of the patient as in situations in which the prognosis is more encouraging.

This kind of care is significant, not only from the point of view of the individual patient but also from that of the family.

The nurse has an opportunity to carry out sound, conscientious patient management. It is important to apply the principles of good body mechanics, since the position of the patient must be changed frequently. From the moment the patient shows response, the nurse is on the alert to assist in rehabilitation. Often every activity may have to be relearned, such as using the fingers to hold a spoon, learning to say words and sentences, and acquiring the ability to write. In struggling with these problems, the patient needs psychological assistance in the form of encouragement. The nurse, as the key person who is with the patient day and night, is responsible for much of the progress made.

SPECIAL PROBLEMS OF NEUROLOGIC PATIENTS

SKIN CARE. Special nursing problems arise from paralyses, sensory disturbances, psychosis, and coma. If hyperesthesia is present, superficial pain may be aroused through slight stimulation of the terminals of the affected nerve branches. Even air drafts or gentle friction can cause marked discomfort.

Disturbances in the skin innervation may cause anesthesia, thereby favoring the development of pressure sores. In order to relieve the pressure, the patient's position should be changed frequently. Small foam rubber pads placed under pressure areas are beneficial. The skin must be kept scrupulously clean and dry. Provision should be made for frequent nursing inspection of areas susceptible to pressure sores. Special skin care (bathing and massage in a circular motion) should be done at specified intervals.

NUTRITIONAL NEEDS. Nutritional problems arise if there is any disturbance connected with the swallowing reflex. Such problems may be overcome by homogenizing the patient's meals in a food blender and feeding him through a tube. Vitamin preparations usually are added to the feeding. The blenderized meal is tolerated well, since the patient's gastrointestinal tract is accustomed to this type of diet, and there is less incidence of diarrhea. Plastic drinking tubes should be used by patients who are subject to convulsions, and dentures, of course, are removed from the mouths of such patients, as well as from those in coma.

ORAL HYGIENE. The condition of the patient's mouth should be checked often, because the buccal structures tend to become exceedingly dry after a short period of mouth breathing. The lips, the tongue, and the gums should be lubricated systematically, and the hydration of the patient should be maintained at an adequate level.

EYE CARE. When facial palsy, from any cause makes it impossible to shut the eyes, special eye care must be given, such as irrigating the eyes with sterile saline and lubricating the outer lids with trace amounts of mineral oil to prevent drying and ulceration of the cornea. These procedures should be carried out several times each day, and the eyes should be inspected regularly for signs of inflammation. An eye shield should be worn at night. Patients who are conscious and cooperative can administer their own eye care with proper instruction and supervision.

THE INCONTINENT PATIENT. Many patients with diseases of the central nervous system initially or eventually, temporarily or permanently, exhibit urinary and fecal incontinence. The hygienic care of patients with incontinence is an important nursing priority, because it is essential that the patient be kept clean and dry.

The management of bladder disturbances due to a lesion of the nervous system is discussed on page 914. The management of urinary incontinence from other causes is discussed on page 202. Promotion of a bowel training program is described on page 202.

PREVENTION OF DEFORMITIES. Any paralyzed extremity deserves careful attention. Care must be taken lest a patient lie on it, or circulation to the part become impeded in any way. Footboards or cradles prevent pressure from weighty bed linens.

To prevent contractures, the nurse must see that the patient is positioned correctly, and that the joints are moved, either actively or passively, through their range of motion several times daily. When the condition of the patient permits, active exercises (bathing, walking, therapeutic exercises) are desirable. Massage may be instituted and perhaps later supplemented by electrical stimulation. Passive exercises and, as soon as possible, active motions are prescribed for the purpose of developing strength.

PSYCHOLOGICAL CONSIDERATIONS. Various emotional disturbances appear in neurologic patients and complicate their care in hospital and home. However, it is important that the patient's feeling and behavior be accepted in a nonjudgmental way. The consulting psychiatrist will guide the medical therapy and give suggestions regarding the proper approach for meeting the personality requirements of the individual. If the family attitude becomes unsympathetic and a feeling of reserve and tension and a general lack of understanding develops, the health care team must offer the family a helping relationship, recognizing their feelings and problems.

Occasionally patients are admitted to the nursing units with a manic psychosis. They obviously require treatment in the psychiatric division of the hospital where the environment is better suited to their care. Meanwhile, good nursing practice requires that adequate protection, understanding, and care be given.

HEADACHE

Possibly the most common of all human afflictions is headache or *cephalgia* ("condition of head pain"). Headache may arise from a variety of sources due to a variety of mechanisms such as vascular spasms caused by muscle contraction or inflammation of pain-sensitive structures inside or outside the skull. Most headaches are not caused by structural diseases but are a symptom of the patient's problems in coping or adapting to a life situation.

Assessment

When data are obtained for the nursing history, the patient should be given a chance to describe his headache *in his own words* as related to the following questions:

- What is the location? Is it unilateral or bilateral?
- What is the quality—dull, aching, steady, boring, burning, intermittent, continuous, paroxysmal?
- Are there any precipitating factors (foods, exertion, etc.)?
- What makes the headache worse (coughing, straining)?
- What time (day/night) does it occur?
- Are there any associated symptoms (facial pain, lacrimation, scotomas (blind spots in field of vision)?
- What usually relieves the headache (aspirin, ergot preparation, food, heat, rest, neck massage)?
- Is there nausea, vomiting, weakness, numbness in the extremities?
- Does the patient have insomnia, poor appetite, loss of energy?
- Is there a family history of headache?
- What is the relationship of the headache to the life style: physical/emotional stress?

The physical examination includes clinical assessment of the head and neck, a neurological examination of the cranial nerves, evaluation of the size and reactions of the pupils, a funduscopic examination of the eyes and a test of motor and sensory systems.

Other diagnostic tests that may be carried out are skull x-rays, electroencephalography, and thermography (assessment of blood flow by determining body temperature). As indicated by the findings of these procedures, more specialized studies such as computed tomography, cerebral angiography and myelography are reserved for those patients requiring additional tests when a structural lesion is suspected.

Types of Headaches

TENSION HEADACHE (SCALP MUSCLE CONTRACTION HEADACHE). Emotional or physical stress may cause contraction of the muscles in the neck and scalp, resulting in tension headache. The headache may be characterized by a steady, pressing ache, which usually begins in the forehead, the temple, or the nape of the neck. It is often band-like and is located at the base of the skull. Tension headaches tend to be more chronic than severe and are probably the most common type of headaches.

Various pharmacologic agents are useful in the treatment of severe tension headache, including analgesics, such as aspirin, phenacetin, and codeine; muscle relaxants; and tranquilizing agents. To obtain long-term relief, however, the person needs to understand the source of any emotional conflicts and attempt to reduce stressful and anxiety-producing situations.

TEMPORAL ARTERITIS (VASCULITIS). Inflammation of the temporal artery is characterized by a unilateral or bilateral temporal and frontal headache lasting for weeks or months. Sometimes a thickened artery is visible and palpable, and loss of vision may occur due to thrombosis of the central retinal artery.

Treatment consists of early administration of a corticosteroid drug to prevent the possibility of loss of vision. Analgesic agents are given for comfort. The temporal artery is sometimes excised to relieve the pain.

HEADACHE IN BRAIN TUMOR. Headache is a common sign of brain tumor, particularly a rapidly expanding tumor that produces traction on pain-sensitive structures of the head. If the tumor is slow growing, the headache may be mild or transitory. In about one third of the patients, the headache occurs in the area overlying the tumor. If the patient has not had a previous history of headaches, a headache of recent onset is significant. The headache is usually accompanied or overshadowed by other complaints: weakness, visual loss or seizures.

HEADACHE IN MENINGITIS. Inflammation and stretching of the meninges and blood vessels are the cause of headache in meningitis. The headache is rapid in onset, usually generalized and accompanied by a stiff neck. A slight movement of the head may markedly aggravate the headache. Photophobia and fever are common.

HEADACHE IN SUBARACHNOID HEMORRHAGE. This headache is severe, sudden in onset and has been described as a "violent bursting sensation in my head." It is commonly located in the occipital region but becomes generalized rather quickly. If the hemorrhage is severe, there is almost immediate loss of consciousness followed rapidly by death. More often, consciousness is lost for a short interval. Vomiting frequently accompanies the early stage and within an hour or so there is neck stiffness and a positive Kernig's sign indicating meningeal irritation. The severe, constant and generalized headache gradually subsides and is usually amenable to analgesics such as codeine. (Subarachnoid hemorrhage is discussed on page 1224.)

HYPERTENSIVE HEADACHE. This type of headache may take any form, but it is typically a dull, pounding, occipital headache, which is present upon awakening in the morning and tends to wear off during the day. The precise mechanism of the headache is not certain, but it is thought to emanate from overly-stretched extra- and intracranial arteries. The headache is relieved by antihypertensive therapy.

FEBRILE HEADACHE. The pain in a febrile headache may be throbbing or steady, and may be frontal, occipital, or generalized. It is thought to be caused by stretched extra- and intracranial arteries. Relief is usually achieved with aspirin and similar analgesic medication.

Vascular Headaches: Migraine

Migraine is a symptom-complex characterized by unilateral (or generalized) periodic attacks of severe headache. The cause of migraine has not been clearly demonstrated but it is primarily a vascular disturbance that occurs more commonly in women. A positive family history is present in 65 percent of patients with migraine.

A "preheadache" phase or an "aura" (warning sign) may occur, forewarning the patient of an impending attack and providing enough time to take the prescribed medication in order to avert a full blown attack. The aura may be in the form of visual, sensory or motor symptoms. These sensations preceding the headache are described at times as "scintillating scotomata" or "visual field defects" and are attributed to intracranial vasoconstriction. Other neurological phenomena preceding the attacks include paresis of an extremity, aphasia or confusion.

Pathophysiology and Clinical Manifestations. The cerebral symptoms and signs of migraine are the results of cortical ischemia of varying degree. The typical attack begins with vasoconstriction affecting the arteries of the scalp and certain cerebral or retinal vessels. The patient appears pale and may experience sensory, motor, and mood disturbances. Extracranial and intracranial blood vessels dilate causing pain and discomfort. Studies suggest that the dilated artery becomes hyperpermeable and that sterile local inflammatory reactions occur in the vicinity of the painful dilated arteries. It is proposed that vasoactive substances (histamine, serotonin, plasmokinins) participate in this sterile inflammatory reaction.

The pain begins in the supraorbital, retro-orbital or temporal areas on one side and increases in such intensity that the patient is prostrated, frequently with nausea and vomiting. The attack may last 2 hours to several days. Sleep tends to relieve the symptoms.

Prevention. The first step in assessing the problem is to obtain a careful medical and neurologic evaluation as well as a survey of social, environmental, and personality factors. Although there is a wide variation in the personality types who are subject to migraine, there is evidence that the hard driving, somewhat compulsive perfectionist is most vulnerable to this condition.

The patient can be helped to develop insight into his feelings, behavior, and conflicts and to make the necessary modifications in life style on the basis of these analyses. Regular periods of exercise and relaxation are suggested and any offending or provoking factors (allergens, fatigue, foods, environmental stresses) are removed or reduced in order to obtain relief. A record may be kept of the circumstances surrounding the attacks (activities, food, feelings) to determine if there is a pattern to the migraine episodes. If so, a change in the pattern may help avoid the attacks.

Management of Acute Attack. The objective of management during an acute attack is to prevent the painful dilation of cranial vessels. Ergotamine preparations (taken orally, sublingually, intramuscularly, by rectum or inhaled) may be effective in aborting the headache if taken early in the migraine process. Ergotamine tartrate acts on smooth muscle, causing prolonged constriction of the cranial blood vessels. Each patient's dosage is titrated according to individual needs. Side effects include aching muscles, paresthesias, nausea and vomiting. During the acute attack the patient may find relief by lying quietly in a darkened room with the head slightly elevated. Drinking black coffee may also be helpful in counteracting the attack. Symptomatic therapy for migraine includes analgesics, sedatives and antianxiety agents.

Management Between Attacks. Methysergide maleate (Sansert) is an effective prophylactic agent in preventing frequent and severe migraine attacks. Troublesome side effects include abdominal discomfort, muscle cramps, edema, numbness, tingling of extremities, and depression. The drug should not be given longer than 6 months because of the potential complication of retroperitoneal fibrosis and pleuropulmonary and cardiac fibrosis.

It has been found that migraine headaches may disappear in patients who are taking propranol hydrochloride (Inderal) for coexisting heart problems. In selected patients this drug is being used with varying success for the treatment of migraine. Cyproheptadine hydrochloride (Periactin), which is an antagonist to serotonin and histamine, reduces the severity of pain in some patients.

Antidepressants, barbiturates and tranquilizers may help the patient to cope with stress. Because of the diversity of treatment for migraine, the patient must be treated on an individual basis and followed closely.

Cluster Headache. Cluster headache is another form of vascular headache and is considered by some to be a variant of migraine. It is seen most frequently in men. The attacks come in "clusters," or groups, with severe and excruciating pain that is localized on one side of the forehead. It is accompanied by watering of the eye and nasal congestion. The duration of the pain is quite short, lasting less than an hour. Cluster headaches may be precipitated by alcohol, nitrates, vasodilators, and histamines. Eliminating these factors helps in preventing the headaches. Cluster headache responds to vasoconstrictors and amine antagonists.

INCREASING INTRACRANIAL PRESSURE

The usual causes of increased intracranial pressure are head injury, cerebral edema, cerebrovascular accidents, inflammatory lesions, or brain tumor. In the majority of patients undergoing cranial surgery, varying degrees of cerebral edema or bleeding (rare) occur, causing increased intracranial pressure. Therefore, it is important to know the following signs:

1. CHANGES IN THE LEVELS OF RESPONSIVENESS. The level of responsiveness/consciousness is the most important measure of the patient's condition.

• The earliest sign of increasing intracranial pressure is *lethargy*. Watch for slowing of speech and a delay in response to verbal suggestions.

Any sudden change in condition, such as shifting from quietness to restlessness (without apparent cause), from orientation to confusion, or increasing drowsiness, has neurologic significance. These signs may result from compression of the brain due to either swelling from hemorrhage or edema or an expanding intracranial lesion (hematoma or tumor) or a combination of both.

As pressure increases, the patient may react only to loud auditory or painful stimuli. At this stage, serious impairment of brain circulation is probably taking place and immediate surgical intervention may be required. If the stupor deepens, the patient responds to painful stimuli by moaning but may not attempt to withdraw. As the condition worsens, the extremities become flaccid and reflexes are absent. The jaw sags and the tongue becomes flaccid, producing inadequate respiratory exchange. When the coma is profound, with the pupils dilated and fixed and the respirations impaired, a fatal outcome is usually inevitable.

Nursing Assessment. The nursing assessment for determining the patient's level of responsiveness can be organized on three levels:
1. response to commands,
2. assessment of spinal motor reflexes, and
3. observation of spontaneous activities.

The first two levels involve purposeful nursing intervention. In order to provide all nursing personnel with information on the baseline condition and the patient's present status, a neurological observation record is kept of the following points of assessment:

I. Response to commands:
   1. Answers questions readily and correctly.
   2. Can perform a complex maneuver.
   3. Responds to simple command.
   4. Shows delayed or unequal response.
   5. Reacts only to loud voice.
   6. Does not respond.

II. Assessment of spinal motor reflexes (pinch Achilles tendon, arm or other body site):
   1. Prompt purposeful withdrawal
   2. Sluggish or nonpurposeful movement of extremities
   3. Facial expression—grimace
   4. Involuntary voiding
   5. No response

III. Observation of patient's spontaneous activity:
   1. Verbal or other communication
   2. Changes in posture (frequency)
   3. Breathing pattern
   4. Retching, vomiting
   5. Restlessness, twitching, tremors, convulsions.

2. SUBTLE CHANGES. Restlessness, headache, forced breathing, purposeless movements and mental cloudiness may be early clinical indications of rising intracranial pressure.

3. CHANGES IN VITAL SIGNS. Alterations in vital signs may be a late sign of increased intracranial pressure.

- As the pressure increases, the pulse rate and respiratory rate are slowed and the blood pressure and temperature rise. Special signs to look for are arterial hypertension, bradycardia, respiratory irregularity; the development of any of these signs warrants further investigation. (Cheyne-Stokes or Kussmaul breathing are the respiratory irregularities frequently seen.)

The body signs compensate as long as the major circulation of the brain is preserved. If, as a result of brain compression, the major circulation begins to fail, the pulse and respirations become rapid and the temperature usually rises but does not follow a consistent pattern. The pulse pressure (the difference between the systolic and diastolic pressure) widens; this is considered a serious development. Immediately preceding this reversal of clinical responses, there is usually a period of rapid fluctuations in pulse, varying from a slow rate to a rapid one. Surgical intervention is indicated or death will ensue.

- The vital signs may not always be altered, even in the event of increased intracranial pressure. They are assessed for changes in the level of responsiveness and for the presence of shock (Table 54-1), to aid in evaluation.

4. HEADACHE. The headache is constant, increasing in intensity, and aggravated by movement or straining.

5. VOMITING. Vomiting is recurrent and may be projectile.

6. PUPILLARY CHANGES. Increasing pressure or an expanding clot can displace the brain against the oculomotor or optic nerves producing pupillary changes.

- The pupils are periodically inspected with a flashlight to evaluate size, configuration and reaction to light. Both eyes are compared for similarities or differences.
- Gaze is evaluated as to whether it is conjugate (paired; working together) or dysconjugate.
- The ability of the eyes to abduct (cranial nerve function) and adduct (cranial nerve function) is assessed.
- The retina and optic nerve are inspected for hemorrhage and papilledema.

7. TENSENESS OR BULGING OF WOUND AREA. In patients who have undergone a craniotomy, part or all of the temporal bone may be removed for the purpose of relieving postoperative brain edema. This area is located in front of the ear on the side of operation, and its tension is an indication of the degree of intracranial pressure. The area should be palpated periodically and the degree of tension noted, with care being taken not to contaminate the wound.

Management

- Increased intracranial pressure constitutes a true emergency and must be treated promptly. As pressure rises, the brain substance is compressed. Secondary phenomena caused by circulatory impairment and edema may lead to death.

Osmotic diuretics (mannitol, urea, glycerol solution) may be given to dehydrate the brain and reduce cerebral edema. (Since hyperosmolar solutions produce diuresis when administered parenterally, an indwelling urethral catheter should be inserted.) The value of steroids (dexamethasone) is uncertain in the treatment of intracranial pressure due to head injury. Since the removal of even 1 or 2 ml. of cerebrospinal fluid may dramatically reduce intracranial pressure, such steps may be taken if the patient is being monitored (see page 1186). An elevation of temperature is to be avoided since fever increases

TABLE 54-1. COMPARISON OF MANIFESTATIONS OF INCREASED INTRACRANIAL PRESSURE AND SHOCK

	THE PATIENT WITH INCREASING INTRACRANIAL PRESSURE	THE PATIENT WITH SHOCK
Levels of Responsiveness	Variable: Alert and active Lethargic → drowsy Stuporous → comatose	Alert → coma
Pulse	Slowing rate to 60 or below, Increasing rate to 100 or above	Rapid
Respiration	Slowing of rate with lengthening periods of apnea Irregular respirations may occur, with Cheyne-Stokes or Kussmaul breathing	Rapid and shallow
Blood Pressure	Falling diastolic pressure Widening pulse pressure	Falling
Temperature	Moderately elevated Does not usually rise until brain compression is quite extensive	Subnormal
Skin Temperature (by palpation)	Normal until hyperthermia develops	Cold, moist and clammy, unless hyperthermia develops

cerebral metabolism and increases the rate at which cerebral edema forms. Conversely, hypothermia will decrease intraventricular pressure.

- If measures are taken to reduce the patient's temperature, cardiac output is monitored with a Swan-Ganz catheter.
- Hypercapnea and hypoxia must be prevented through proper ventilatory management (see Chapter 23). Therefore, the patient may be hyperventilated with a volume ventilator to reduce the blood volume in the brain and promote constriction of the cerebral vasculature, which in turn decreases intracranial pressure.

Certain positions and activities are to be avoided in instances of increased intracranial pressure.

- The prone position, flexion of the neck, and extreme hip flexion should be avoided.
- The Valsalva maneuver which can be produced by straining at the stool or even moving in bed is to be avoided. In this last instance, the patient can be instructed to exhale while moving or turning in bed.
- Isometric muscle contractions are also contraindicated since they raise the systemic blood pressure and hence the intracranial pressure.
- Nursing care must be planned so that activities that initiate increased intracranial pressure are properly paced.

A neurological observation sheet (page 1250) is kept and all observations are made from the baseline condition of the patient. Repeated assessments of the patient are made (sometimes minute by minute) so that improvement or deterioration may be noted immediately. If the patient's condition deteriorates, preparations are made for surgical intervention (page 1206).

Intracranial Pressure Monitoring

Intracranial pressure monitoring is the recording of the pressure exerted within the skull by the brain, cerebral blood and cerebral spinal fluid. The volume of any of these elements can expand as a result of tumor, trauma, edema, bleeding, cerebral vessel dilatation, etc.

The purposes of intracranial pressure monitoring are (1) to provide a warning before cerebral damage occurs, (2) to reduce elevated pressures by withdrawing cerebrospinal fluid and (3) to evaluate the effectiveness of treatment.

Intracranial pressure is not in a steady state but fluctuates as indicated by waves of high pressure and troughs of relatively normal pressure. These waves have been classified as A waves (plateau waves), B waves and C waves. The plateau waves (A waves) are transient, paroxysmal, recurring elevations of intracranial pressure that may last from 5 to 20 minutes and range in amplitude between 50 to 100 mm. Hg. Plateau waves have clinical significance and are usually related to cerebral dysfunction caused by brain shift or distortion. They may increase in amplitude and frequency, causing cerebral ischemia and brain damage that can occur before overt signs and symptoms of raised intracranial pressure are seen clinically. This is especially true in the unconscious patient. Rapid variations of pressure waves may also indicate a potentially serious intracranial situation. Therefore intracranial pressure monitoring provides a more objective evaluation of early or changing trends of intracranial pressure than other forms of observation.

There are a large number of devices available that monitor ICP by means of sensors or transducers that are either connected to an intraventricular catheter or implanted in the skull (Fig. 54-1).

Ventricular Catheter Monitoring. Ventricular catheter monitoring consists of placing a fine catheter into the frontal horn of a lateral ventricle via a burr hole or twist drill hole and holding it in place with a rubber plug. The intraventricular catheter is connected to an external pressure monitor by means of tubing filled with normal saline. The transducer transmits the impulses, and the pressures are recorded. The device can be mounted on a stand located beside the bed at the level of the patient's foramen of Monro (the reference point). Or a smaller transducer can be fixed on the patient's head. The output from the pressure transducer is amplified and displayed on a chart recorder. In addition to obtaining continuous

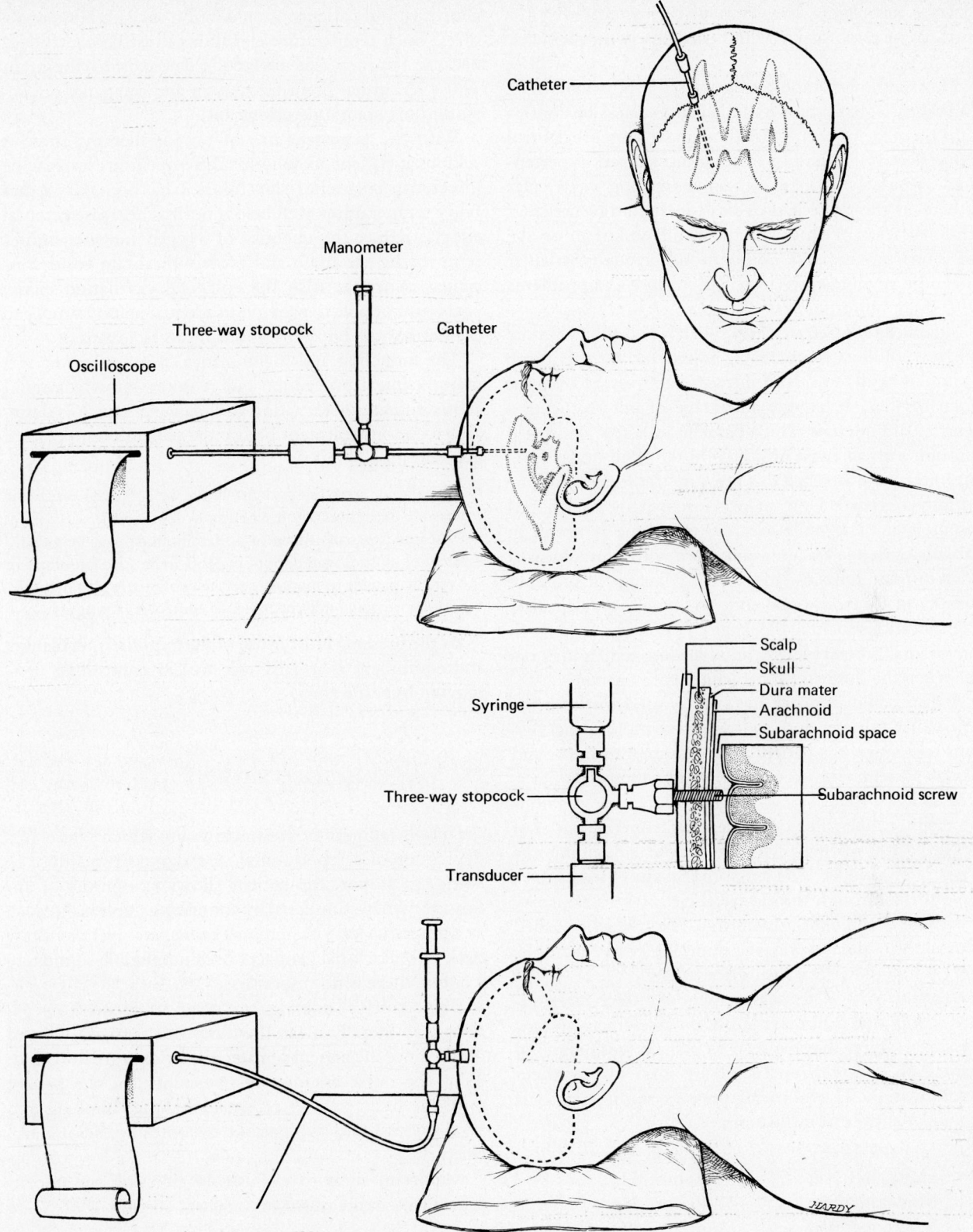

Figure 54-1. Intracranial pressure monitoring. (*top*) Ventricular catheter. (*center*) Subarachnoid or hollow screw. (*bottom*) Monitoring system connected to pressure transducer and display system.

Catheter

Manometer

Three-way stopcock

Catheter

Oscilloscope

Syringe

Scalp
Skull
Dura mater
Arachnoid
Subarachnoid space

Three-way stopcock

Subarachnoid screw

Transducer

pressure recordings, the ventricular catheter allows for drainage of cerebrospinal fluid particularly during acute rises in pressure.

This method of monitoring is useful in patients with infratentorial brain tumors and aneurysms. Also continuous drainage of ventricular fluid under pressure control is an effective method of treating intracranial hypertension. Another advantage of an indwelling ventricular catheter is the route it provides for the intraventricular administration of drugs and the instillation of air or dye for ventriculography. Complications include ventricular infection, meningitis, ventricular collapse and problems with the monitoring system.

Subarachnoid Screw. (Fig. 54-1) The subarachnoid screw is a hollow screw that is bolted into the calvarium (dome of skull) to record intracranial pressure over the brain cavities. It has the advantage of not requiring a ventricular puncture. The subarachnoid screw is inserted through a small twist drill hole in the skull under local anesthesia; it is attached to a pressure transducer, and the output is recorded on an oscilloscope for continuous monitoring. The hollow screw technique is useful in patients with head trauma and those with supratentorial brain tumors. It has the additional advantage of avoiding complications from brain shift and small ventricle size. Complications include blockage of the screw from high intracranial pressure levels, and bleeding which may occur when the dura and subarachnoid are opened.

A disposable stopcock network is used for both the ventricular catheter and hollow screw monitoring systems to connect the patient to a pressure transducer and display system. The network contains a three-way stopcock attached to the screw or ventricular catheter, a nondistensible saline-filled tubing leading from one outlet of the three-way stopcock to a manifold containing the pressure transducer. The pressure transducer transmits a wave form through the electrical circuitry to a display system for continuous monitoring. The system is flushed with sterile saline at varying time intervals (example: every 6 hours) to keep the device patent.

Implications. The measurement of intracranial pressure is only one parameter in patient assessment. A low pressure reading may be seen in patients with signs of brain stem compression caused by mass displacement and herniation. The following pressure readings are part of the patient's total evaluation:

Normal level:	1-10 mm. Hg
Slight increase:	11-20 mm. Hg
Moderate increase:	21-40 mm. Hg
Severe increase:	More than 40 mm. Hg

HYPERTHERMIA

Because of severe intracranial infection or damage to the heat-regulating center in the brain, neurologic and neurosurgical patients often develop very high temperatures. Such temperature elevations must be controlled, because the increased metabolic demands by the brain will overburden brain circulation and oxygenation, resulting in cerebral deterioration.

With the persistent use of proper therapy, there is seldom a patient in whom the temperature cannot be lowered in a matter of a few hours. It has been shown that body temperatures well below normal decrease cerebral edema, reduce the quantity of oxygen and metabolites required by the brain and protect the brain from continued ischemia. Also the collateral circulation in the brain may be able to provide an adequate blood supply to the brain if the body metabolism can be lowered.

The induction and maintenance of hypothermia is a major clinical procedure and requires knowledge and skilled nursing observation and management. It is desirable to begin treatment before the patient's temperature gets too high.

- All bedding over the patient should be removed (with the possible exception of a light sheet or loin cloth).
- Repeated doses of aspirin or acetaminophen may be given.
- Alcohol or cool water sponging and an electric fan blowing over the patient to increase surface cooling are also helpful.
- Chlorpromazine may be given to control shivering.

At the present time the use of the hypothermia blanket and equipment is usually effective in controlling neurogenic hyperthermia.

THE UNCONSCIOUS PATIENT

Unconsciousness is a condition in which there is a depression of cerebral function, ranging from stupor to coma. In stupor, the patient shows symptoms of annoyance when stimulated by something unpleasant, such as a pinprick, loud clapping of hands, etc. He may draw back or make facial grimaces or unintelligible sounds. In a coma, there is no response.

The quality of nursing care given an unconscious patient may literally mean the difference between life and death, since the patient's protective reflexes are impaired. Thus the nurse assumes responsibility for the patient until the basic reflexes return (coughing, blinking and swallowing) and the patient becomes conscious and oriented.

Important signs to evaluate in assessing the unconscious patient are noted in the chart on page 1190.

- The most important consideration in the management of the unconscious patient is to establish and maintain the airway.

SECRETIONS. The accumulation of secretions in the pharynx presents a serious problem that demands intelligent and conscientious management. Since the patient is unable to swallow and lacks pharyngeal reflexes, these secretions must be removed to eliminate the danger of aspiration.

- The patient is positioned in a lateral or semiprone position to facilitate drainage of respiratory secretions. (*Never allow an unconscious patient to remain on his back.*)
- Suction is employed to remove secretions from the posterior pharynx and upper treachea.

With the suction turned *off*, a whistle-tip catheter is lubricated with a water-soluble lubricant and maneuvered to the desired level. Then the suction is turned on (negative pressure) while the aspirating catheter is withdrawn with a twisting motion of the thumb and forefinger. This twisting maneuver prevents the suctioning end of the catheter from irritating the tracheal or pharyngeal mucosa, since irritation merely increases secretions and produces mucosal bleeding. The suction catheter should be kept meticulously clean. (If the patient has a tracheostomy, it should be kept sterile.) The frequency of suctioning is determined by the amount of secretions present.

MOUTH CARE. The mouth of the unconscious patient is an area that also needs conscientious care. The mouth should be swabbed carefully and rinsed thoroughly. The tongue as well as the space underneath must be included. A soothing lubricant within the mouth and on the lips prevents drying and the formation of encrustations.

NUTRITION. The nutritional needs of this patient are met by giving the required fluids intravenously.

- Intravenous solutions and blood transfusions for patients with intracranial conditions must run in slowly. If given too rapidly, they may increase the intracranial pressure.

A nasogastric tube may be passed, and the patient can be given liquid and blenderized feedings (see page 726).

One way of testing to see whether the patient is able to swallow without choking is to give him a wet swab to suck.

- Never give fluids by mouth to the patient who cannot swallow.

ELIMINATION CONCERNS. Urinary incontinence may be managed by inserting a 3-way catheter attached to continuous drainage or by instituting tidal drainage. This is important if diuretics are used. Clamping the catheter at intervals helps to prevent contracture of the bladder, as this procedure more closely approximates normal functioning. A full bladder, on the other hand, may be the overlooked cause of incontinence. Colonic irrigations administered every second or third day eliminate fecal incontinence or reduce the frequency of involuntary stools. Frequent loose stools are an indication of fecal impaction.

POSITIONING. Special attention is given to uncon-scious patients because they are insensitive to external stimuli. They must be turned frequently and positioned properly. To effectively prevent pressure sores, attention should be given to those areas where pressure is greatest. Sheets must be free of wrinkles, crumbs, and moisture. A lotion with lanolin may be used to keep the skin lubricated.

Maintaining correct body position is important; equally important is passive exercise of the extremities, so that contractures are prevented. The use of a footboard aids in the prevention of footdrop and eliminates the pressure of bedding on the toes. Trochanter rolls supporting the hip joints keep the legs in good position (page 184). The arm should be in abduction, the fingers lightly flexed, and the hand in a position of slight supination.

TEMPERATURE. The temperature of the environment is determined by the patient's condition. An elevated temperature would call for a minimum amount of bed clothing—a sheet or perhaps only a loin cloth.

The room may be cooled to 18.3° C. (65° F.). However, if the patient is older and does not have an elevation of temperature, a warmer atmosphere is needed. Regardless of the temperature, the air should be fresh and free from odors.

- The body temperature of an unconscious patient never is taken by mouth. Rectal temperature is preferred to the less accurate axillary temperature.

EYE CARE. Because there are occasions when the corneal reflex is absent, the cornea is likely to become irritated or scratched. It may be necessary to irrigate the eyes with normal saline solution and to lubricate them with sterile mineral oil. Often, periocular edema occurs following head surgery. Cold compresses may be used, and care must be exerted to avoid contact with the cornea.

FLUID SEEPAGE. If there is ear or nasal bleeding, or oozing of cerebrospinal fluid, the physician should be notified immediately. A small sterile cotton pledget may be placed loosely in the nostril or ears, but no attempt to clean them should be made until the patient is further evaluated.

SAFETY. For the protection of the patient, side-rails should be provided. If there is any chance that the patient may sustain injury against the side attachments, they should be padded satisfactorily. Every measure that is available and appropriate for calming and quieting the disturbed patient should be carried out. Any form of restraint is likely to be countered by rebellion, whether the patient is fully conscious or not, and fury so incited may lead to self-injury or to a dangerous increase in intracranial pressure.

A summary of the nursing management of the unconscious patient is found on pages 1192 to 1195.

EXAMINATION	CLINICAL ASSESSMENT	CLINICAL SIGNIFICANCE
Level of responsiveness or consciousness	See page 1184	
Respirations	Cheyne-Stokes	Lesions deep in both hemispheres, area of basal ganglia and upper brain stem
	Hyperventilation	Systemic acidosis
	Ataxic respiration with irregularity in depth and rate	Grave sign of imminent failure of medullary centers
Eyes: Pupils	Progressive dilatation	Indicates increased cranial pressure
	Equal or unequal diameter	Localizing sign
Size		
Equality		
Reaction to light	Pupils react or do not react to light	Localizing sign
Eye movements	Eyes move from side to side	Absent in lesions of brain stem or pons
Corneal reflex	When cornea is touched with a wisp of clean cotton, blink response is normal	Absent in deep coma Tests cranial nerves V and VII Localizing sign if unilateral
Facial symmetry	Asymmetry (sagging; decrease in wrinkles)	Sign of paralysis
Swallowing reflex	Drooling versus spontaneous swallowing	Absent in coma Paralysis of cranial nerves X and XII
Neck	Stiff neck	Subarachnoid hemorrhage; meningitis
	Absence of spontaneous neck movement	Fracture or dislocation of cervical spine
Response of extremity to pain	Firm pressure on a joint of the upper and lower extremity	Asymmetrical response in paralysis Absent in deep coma
Deep tendon reflexes	Tap patellar and biceps tendons	Brisk response may have localizing value Asymmetrical response in paralysis Absent in deep coma

NURSING ASSESSMENT OF THE UNCONSCIOUS PATIENT (CONTINUED)

EXAMINATION	CLINICAL ASSESSMENT	CLINICAL SIGNIFICANCE
Pathologic reflexes	Firm pressure with blunt object on sole of foot moving along lateral margin and crossing to the ball of foot	Flexion of the toes, especially the great toe is normal except in newborn Dorsiflexion of toes (especially great toe) indicates contralateral pathology of corticospinal tract (Babinski reflex) Localizing signs
Pathologic posturing	Decerebrate rigidity (*left, below*) Decorticate rigidity (*right, below*)	Implies brain stem pathology; poor prognostic sign Seen with cerebral hemisphere pathology

Decerebrate rigidity   **Decorticate rigidity**

Muscle tone	Flexor or extensor rigidity or limb flaccidity	Indicates paralysis

APHASIA

Aphasia is a disturbance of language function resulting from injury or disease of the brain centers. It may involve impairment of the ability to read and write as well as to speak, listen and comprehend. (See Glossary, page 1196.) Nearly 1,000,000 to 1,500,000 adults in this country have a chronic disabling aphasia.

The cortical area that is responsible for integrating the myriad association pathways required for the comprehension and formulation of language measures little more than a square inch in extent (marked Motor speech in Fig. 53-2). The principal speech center, called *Broca's area,* is located in a convolution adjoining the middle cerebral artery. Here are stored the combinations of muscular movements necessary to speak each word. They are not the cells that govern the muscles of speech; these cells are in the motor area itself. Each word requires for its utterance a combination or sequence of combinations of muscular contractions. Not only must the muscles of the vocal cords contract, but also those of the throat, the tongue, the soft palate, the lips and the chest wall. These combinations are stored in the cells of Broca's convolution. They direct the cells of the motor area, which make the muscles contract at the proper time and with the proper force.

Broca's area is so near the left motor area that a disturbance in the motor area often affects speech area. This is the reason that so many persons paralyzed on the right side (due to a lesion of the left hemisphere) are unable to speak, whereas in those paralyzed on the left side, speech disturbances are less common. Some patients are affected, but these usually are left-handed persons whose speech area is located on the right hemisphere.

PREDOMINANTLY EXPRESSIVE APHASIA. The destruction of Broca's convolution by stroke, hemorrhage, thrombosis, or tumor results in motor aphasia. The patient understands most of what is said to him; he knows the words he wants to say; he may be able to write them and read them; but he cannot produce the sequence of movements necessary to utter them, and, if he tries, he makes an unintelligible noise. He is conscious of this defect (verbal apraxia), and it distresses him greatly. To cause a permanent motor aphasia, however, the lesion must (and usually does) affect the white matter beneath this convolution where the fibers are going to and coming from other parts of the brain. When only the gray matter of Broca's convolution is destroyed, the aphasia may be transitory.

PREDOMINANTLY RECEPTIVE APHASIA. There are many varieties of aphasia affecting the ability to speak, gesture, comprehend the spoken word, read, write, or calculate.

(Text continues on page 1195)

The basic nursing principles underlying the care of an unconscious patient are applicable to any unconscious patient regardless of the clinical cause. There are two major threats to the patient: (1) the disease or trauma that produced unconsciousness and (2) the threat of the unconscious state. The primary problem is that the patient's normal protective reflexes are impaired. The nursing goal is to assume these protective mechanisms for the patient until he is aware of himself and can function in his environment.

Nursing Action	Rationale/Amplification
I. To establish and maintain an adequate airway	Inadequate respiratory exchange promotes CO_2 retention, which can produce diffuse cerebral edema. Airway obstruction will aggravate cerebral swelling and may be a cause of continuing or deepening unconsciousness.
1. Place the patient in a three-quarters prone position or a lateral recumbent position with his face dependent.	1. A dependent position prevents the tongue from obstructing the airway, encourages drainage of respiratory secretions, and promotes oxygen and carbon dioxide exchange.
2. Insert oral airway if tongue is paralyzed or is obstructing airway.	2. *A noisy airway is an obstructed airway.* (An obstructed airway increases intracranial pressure.) The use of an oropharyngeal airway is considered a short-term measure.
3. Prepare for insertion of cuffed endotracheal tube if patient's condition requires.	3. Endotracheal intubation is more effective in permitting positive-pressure ventilation. The cuffed tube seals off the digestive tract, thus preventing aspiration, and allows efficient removal of tracheobronchial secretions.
4. Utilize humidified oxygen therapy, positive pressure assisted breathing techniques or mechanical ventilation with a ventilator when there is indication of impending respiratory failure.	4. When arterial blood gas measurements reveal the patient has insufficient ventilation and gas exchange, respiratory failure may ensue.
5. Keep the airway free of secretions with efficient suctioning.	5. With the absence of the cough and swallowing reflexes, secretions rapidly accumulate in the posterior pharynx and upper trachea and can pave the way to fatal respiratory complications.

a. Attach open-end catheter to Y-tube.
    b. Keep one end of Y-tube open while inserting the catheter.
    c. When catheter is at desired level, close the open-end of Y with finger.
    d. Turn the suction *on* and slowly withdraw catheter with a twisting motion of the thumb and forefinger.
	d. Negative pressure (suction on) is applied only as the catheter is withdrawn. The twisting motion of the suction catheter reduces prolonged contact with the pharyngeal mucosa. Forceful suction irritates the mucosa, increases the amount of secretions, produces mucosal bleeding, and can precipitate infection.

e. Gently turn the head from side to side while suctioning.
      (1) Limit tracheal aspiration to intervals of a few seconds.
      (2) Allow patient to rest between aspirations.
      (3) Oxygenate the patient between aspirations as required.	

6. Carry out periodic determinations of arterial pO_2 and pCO_2.	6. These evaluations determine adequacy of treatment.

Nursing Action	**Rationale/Amplification**
7. Prepare for tracheostomy if coma is deepening and there are evidences of inadequate respiratory exchange.	
a. Keep trachestomy tube meticulously clean.	
(1) Carefully inject 3 to 5 ml. saline solution through trachea stoma and then suction.	(1) The dryness of the respiratory tract produces rapid formation of mucous plugs, which are difficult to remove. The careful washing (3 to 5 ml. of saline) of the trachea also stimulates the cough reflex, which helps clear the tracheobronchial tree.
b. Wear sterile gloves and use a sterile catheter each time the tracheostomy is aspirated.	
c. Suction trachea around cannula and through tube.	c. Keeping the upper respiratory tract clean and free of mucous plugs and dried secretions lessens subsequent pulmonary complications.
d. Have adequate humidification.	
8. Assess cardiac function.	
9. Give antibiotics as per schedule.	9. A screen of broad spectrum antibiotics may be given to the unconscious patient to prevent infectious and pulmonary complications.
10. Assist with diagnostic tests.	
II. To assess the level of responsiveness	
1. Maintain a constant assessment of the patient's level of consciousness and changes in responsiveness.	1. The level of consciousness is the most important measure of the patient's condition. Unconscious patients may deteriorate rapidly from numerous clinical causes.
2. Record the patient's *exact reactions,* movements, and quality of speech.	
a. Request the patient to speak.	
b. Ask the patient to perform some activity (raise arm, protrude tongue, etc.)	
c. Apply painful stimuli if there is no response (pinching skin of arms, thighs, etc.) and assess patient's perception of pain.	c. No response or a delayed or unequal response is an unfavorable clinical sign.
III. To evaluate the progression of vital signs	
1. Know the patient's base-line (initial) vital signs and alert the physician if there are significant fluctuations of blood pressure and instability of the pulse and respiratory cycles.	1. Fluctuations of vital signs indicate a change in intracranial homeostasis. Monitoring of vital signs is also essential to alert personnel for hidden bleeding.
2. Take blood pressure readings, pulse and respiratory rate, and temperature at frequently specified intervals until there is clinical evidence of stabilization.	2. Taking and recording of temperature is mandatory since temperature-regulating mechanisms may be disturbed. Hyperthermia is an unfavorable prognostic sign.
IV. To maintain fluid and electrolyte balance	
1. Give intravenous fluids as indicated (use vein in hand).	1. Serial laboratory electrolyte evaluations are made when the patient is maintained on intravenous fluids to ensure proper balance.

(Continued)

Nursing Action	**Rationale/Amplification**
2. Initiate nasogastric feedings.	2. Feeding through a gastric tube ensures better nutrition than does intravenous feeding. Electrolyte and protein balance is maintained by selective absorption. Also, paralytic ileus is fairly frequent in the unconscious patient, and a nasogastric tube assists in gastric decompression.
a. Insert small gastric tube through nose into stomach.	
b. Aspirate stomach before each feeding.	b. If aspirated residual exceeds 50 ml., the patient may be developing an ileus. Gastric distention and vomiting may result.
c. Elevate patient's head and thorax and give 100 to 150 ml. blenderized formula slowly. Give small amount at first and gradually increase until 400 to 500 ml. are given at each feeding.	c. Elevation of the patient's head before, during, and after feeding reduces likelihood of esophageal reflux regurgitation and aspiration.
d. Give 2000 to 2500 ml. of fluid through tube daily.	d. An unconscious patient requires adequate fluids daily. High protein feedings can produce a solute diuresis which will produce dehydration and hyperosmolar coma unless an adequate fluid intake is ensured. Fever, excessive sweating or fluid loss elsewhere in the body increase the fluid requirements.
e. Rinse the tube with water or cranberry juice after each feeding.	
f. Keep tube feeding refrigerated.	
g. Prepare for gastrostomy if patient's condition indicates.	g. Prolonged nasogastric intubation can cause esophagitis (from gastric reflux) and erosion of the nasal septum.
V. To give nursing support as the patient's changing condition indicates	
1. Be aware of the varying phases of restlessness.	1. A certain degree of restlessness may be favorable, as it may indicate the patient is regaining consciousness. However, restlessness is quite common in cerebral anoxia or when there is a partially obstructed airway, distended bladder, overlooked bleeding, or fracture; it may be a manifestation of brain injury.
a. Avoid restraints if at all possible.	
b. Have adequate lighting in the room to prevent hallucinations in the patient who is regaining consciousness.	
c. Pad side rails, apply mitts or boxing gloves on hands, or use other devices to protect patient.	
d. Avoid oversedating the patient.	d. Sedatives and narcotics depress the level of responsiveness which is a guide to clinical assessment. Certain drugs affect pupillary size and reaction which is an important sign.
e. Speak softly to the patient calling him by name.	
f. Touch him as gently as possible.	
2. Keep the skin clean, dry, and free of pressure.	2. Comatose patients are susceptible to the formation of pressure sores. All these activities are to prevent the formation of pressure sores on pressure-sensitive areas.
a. Lubricate skin with emollient lotions to prevent sheet irritation, dryness, chafing, and cracking.	
b. Inspect pressure areas for evidences of skin redness and breakdown.	
c. Clip patient's nails to prevent skin excoriation.	

NURSING MANAGEMENT OF THE UNCONSCIOUS PATIENT (CONTINUED)
Objectives, Principles, and Rationale of Care

Nursing Action	**Rationale/Amplification**
3. Put all extremities through range of motion exercises 4 times daily.	3. Contracture deformities develop early in unconscious patients.
4. Turn the patient from side to side at regular intervals.	4. Turning relieves pressure areas and helps keep lungs clear by mobilizing secretions. Prolonged pressure on extremities produces nerve palsies and pressure sores.
5. Observe the patient for indications of an overdistended bladder. a. Utilize external sheath catheter (condom catheter) for male patient. b. If patient is unable to void, insert 3-way indwelling catheter with continuous drainage. c. Tape the catheter to the lower abdomen or the penis horizontally to the side of the male patient and the inner thigh of the female to prevent traction on the urethra.	a. Involuntary voiding indicates an impaired state of consciousness. b. Infection invariably follows prolonged use of an indwelling catheter that is attached to straight drainage.
6. Protect the eyes from corneal irritation. a. Routinely inspect size of pupils and condition of eyes using a flashlight. b. Remove contact lenses if worn. c. Irrigate eyes with sterile prescribed solution and instill ophthalmic ointment in each eye. d. Prepare for temporary tarsorrhaphy (suturing of eyelids in closed position) if unconscious state is prolonged.	a. The cornea functions as a shield. If the eyes remain open for long periods, corneal drying, irritation, and ulceration are apt to result.
7. Protect the patient during convulsive seizures (see page 1244). a. Protect the patient from self-injury. b. Observe the patient during the seizure and record observations. c. Give prescribed anticonvulsant medications via the nasogastric tube.	7. A patient with head trauma is a potential candidate for convulsive seizures.
8. Be alert for complications. a. Respiratory complications (infection, aspiration, obstruction, atelectasis). b. Fluid and electrolyte imbalance. c. Infection (urinary, pressure sores, central nervous system). d. Bladder and gastrointestinal distention. e. Convulsive disorders.	
9. Give the patient an explanation of what has happened during period of unconsciousness. Permit him to question and talk about the experience of unconsciousness.	9. This will help the patient cope with anxieties, mobilize psychological defenses and promote psychological recovery.

Auditory aphasia is the inability of a person to understand and to repeat words spoken to him. Often he talks jargon, but he is unaware that he is not talking correctly. This defect is the result of lesions in the posterior part of the left superior temporal convolution, where the memory of sounds is stored. The patient has difficulty in naming objects set before him, and yet he understands their use. The disturbance in silent reading comprehension (alexia) is due to lesions in the angular gyrus.

The most common type of aphasia is the result of cerebral hemorrhage that injures the left internal capsule and the surrounding fibers and also produces marked hemiplegia without loss of sensation and often a homonymous hemianopsia (see page 1197) which is loss of vision in corresponding halves of the visual field in both eyes. This is the mixed type of aphasia with loss of voluntary speech, impaired ability to read, and difficulty in the comprehension of spoken words.

In some cases it would seem as though another part of the cortex can take over the work of the destroyed area, for through careful retraining a person with motor aphasia may learn to talk again.

Nursing Management

There are a variety of symptoms and disorders underlying aphasia. The treatment is individualized and is based on the patient's background and interest. Recovery depends on the extent of brain damage, the patient's personality and the support system available (family and friends). The potential for recovery is assessed by the speech pathologist or therapist in cooperation with the neurologist. Some patients with extensive brain damage never regain speech.

GLOSSARY OF SELECTED TERMS RELATING TO APHASIA*

Acalculia; dyscalculia—difficulty in dealing with mathematical processes or numerical symbols in general

Agnosia—failure to recognize familiar objects perceived by the senses

Auditory agnosia—inability to recognize significance of sounds

Color agnosia—inability to recognize differences in color

Tactile agnosia—inability to recognize familiar objects by touch or feel

Visual object agnosia—inability to recognize objects; visual acuity may or may not be intact

Agraphia; dysgraphia—disturbances in writing intelligible words

Alexia; dyslexia—difficulty in reading

Anomia; dysnomia—difficulty in selecting appropriate words, particularly nouns

Apraxia—inability to perform certain purposeful movements without the loss of motor power, sensation or coordination

Verbal apraxia—difficulty in forming and organizing intelligible words although the musculature is intact

Dysarthria—defects of articulation due to neurological causes

Hemianopia—blindness for one-half of the field of vision in one or both eyes

Paraphasia—a frequently observed characteristic in many asphasic patients; uses wrong words, word substitutions, grammatical errors, faults in word usage; may be observed in both oral and written language.

Perseveration—continued and automatic repeating of an activity or word or phrase that is no longer appropriate

*The prefix a means "without" or "absence." The prefix dys refers to "difficulty" or "disordered." These prefixes are frequently used interchangeably in these conditions.

A patient with aphasia should be given as much psychological security as possible. The same manner is used with this patient as with a young child learning to speak. At the same time the patient is treated as an adult. A kind, unhurried manner combined with encouragement, patience and a willingness to invest time are required. Relearning speech and language skills may take several years. The goal is to help the patient communicate.

First the patient is encouraged to *listen.* Speaking is thinking out loud, and the emphasis is on *thinking*. The patient must think and sort out incoming messages and formulate a response. Listening requires mental effort, yet the patient must struggle against mental inertia and needs time to organize an answer.

In working with the aphasic patient, the nurse must remember to *talk* to the patient while caring for him. This provides social contact for the patient.

It is best to face the patient and establish eye contact, at the same time speaking in a normal manner but in short phrases, pausing between phrases. The emphasis here is on ensuring that the patient understands what is being said. Conversation should be confined to practical and concrete matters, and supplemented with gestures. As the patient handles and uses the object, the word should be stated; it helps when words are matched with actions. Consistency is important and the same wording and gestures are used each time instructions are given and questions are asked. Since the patient is easily fatigued and distracted, extraneous noises and sounds must be kept at a minimum since the patient cannot sort out messages when there is too much noise and confusion in the environment.

When the patient attempts to communicate, the nurse should make a real effort to understand him and to treat him as an intelligent adult. It is important to behave in a way that shows acceptance of the patient as a worthwhile human being. The patient should never be forced to correct his mistakes since this merely adds to his tension. During periods of emotional lability, the patient should be approached in a calm, accepting, and deliberate manner since frustration and depression are frequent reactions to the inability to communicate. Since speech that is motivated by emotions usually comes first (i.e., swearing), the content of this speech should be ignored by the nursing personnel. Patients with aphasia must be stimulated both internally and externally to action. Therapy is based on a recognition of the patient's needs, *previous* interests, drives, and motivation. If the patient's speech is unintelligible or filled with jargon, his gestures may offer a clue to his intent. Continue to listen to him. Nod and make neutral statements occasionally. When appropriate, shift the topic to gain another point of interest and frame of reference.

The environment should provide sensory input, with auditory stimulation supplemented with visual stimulation. Reading is encouraged for a few minutes at a time, and the patient can look at pictures while another person talks about them. Games stimulate the mind and help organize the thoughts. For more relaxed forms of communication, the television, radio and tape recorder can be used.

Accept the patient's behavior, relieve his embarrassment, and give support by assuring him that there is nothing wrong with his intelligence and that you realize he knows what he wants to say. The environment should be relaxed and permissive, and the patient should be encouraged to socialize with family and friends. The typical aphasic individual has almost an obsession with orderliness. Thus nurses and family members should return items in the room to their proper place.

FAMILY SUPPORT. The attitude of the family is an important factor in helping the patient adjust to this deficit. They are encouraged to act naturally and treat the patient in the same manner as before his illness. They should be aware that the patient's ability to speak may vary from day to day and that fatigue will have an adverse effect on speech. They should also be aware that the patient may strike out verbally when his emotional controls are lowered. The strain of the constant adjustment to the patient's illness, demands, and needs, as well as the financial drain and the change in life style can produce explosive pressures on the family. In addition to the family learning as much as possible about the support of the patient with aphasia, they should also be counseled to continue a life of their own and to seek the aid of a social worker, pastor or psychologist if they need additional help in dealing with their frustrations and pressures.

NEUROLOGIC DEFICITS DUE TO STROKE

A stroke or cerebral vascular accident can produce an array of neurological deficits that require extensive and careful nursing management from onset through rehabilitation. See page 1222 for a complete discussion of stroke and cerebrovascular disease.

EFFECTS OF A STROKE

MOTOR LOSS. Stroke is a disease of the upper motor neurons and results in loss of voluntary control over motor movements. Since the upper motor neurons decussate, a disturbance of voluntary motor control on one side of the body may reflect damage to the upper motor neurons on the opposite side of the brain. The most common residual effect is *hemiplegia* (paralysis on one side of the body).

In the early stage of stroke, the initial clinical feature may be flaccid paralysis and loss or decrease in the deep tendon reflexes. When these deep reflexes reappear (usu-

ally by 48 hours), increased tone is observed along with spasticity (resistance to motion) of the extremities on the affected side. In the hemiplegic patient, the greatest amount of neurologic recovery occurs in the first 4 to 6 weeks.

COMMUNICATION LOSS. Other brain functions affected by stroke are language and communication. Dysfunction in these areas may be manifested by *dysarthria* (difficulty in speaking) as demonstrated by poorly intelligible speech caused by paralysis of the muscles responsible for producing speech; *dysphasia* or *aphasia* (defective speech or loss of speech) which is mainly expressive or receptive in nature (page 1191); or *apraxia* (inability to perform a previously learned action) as may be seen when a patient picks up a fork and attemps to comb his hair with it. (The nursing management of aphasia is discussed on page 1196.)

VISUAL LOSS. *Homonymous hemianopia* (loss of half of the visual field) may occur from stroke and may be temporary or permanent. In such instances, the patient will not be able to see food on half of the tray; only half of the room will be visible. This decreased field of vision must be kept in mind during all rehabilitation procedures. Personnel should approach the patient on the side where visual perception is intact. All visual stimuli (clock, calendar, television) should be placed on this side. The patient can be taught to turn his head in the direction of the defective visual field in order to compensate for this loss.

If there is a disturbance in *visual perception* (seen more frequently in left hemiplegia), the patient will have problems in performing those tasks involving spatial analysis and perceptual organization.

SENSORY LOSS. Minor sensory loss from stroke may take the form of slight impairment of touch or it might be more severe with loss of position sense or hemianesthesia, loss of awareness of half of the body.

BLADDER IMPAIRMENT. Following a stroke the bladder becomes atonic with impaired sensation in response to bladder filling. Sometimes control of the external urinary sphincter is lost or diminished. During this period, an indwelling catheter with a closed drainage system is used. When muscle tone increases and deep tendon reflexes return, bladder tone increases and spasticity of the bladder may develop. Because the patient's sense of awareness is clouded, persistent urinary incontinence may be symptomatic of bilateral brain damage. Continuing bladder and bowel incontinence may reflect extensive neurologic damage.

IMPAIRMENT OF MENTAL ACTIVITY AND PSYCHOLOGICAL EFFECTS. If damage has occurred to the frontal lobe, then learning capacity, memory or other higher cortical intellectual functions may be impaired. Such dysfunction may be reflected in a limited attention span, forgetfulness and a lack of motivation, which causes these patients to encounter frustrating problems in their rehabilitation programs. Depression is a natural response to such a catastrophic illness. Other psychological problems are myriad and are manifested by emotional lability, hostility, frustration, resentment and noncooperation.

NURSING MANAGEMENT OF THE PATIENT WITH A STROKE

A patient who is in a deep coma on admission to the hospital is considered to have a poor prognosis. Conversely, a fully conscious patient faces a more favorable outcome.

The Acute Phase

The immediate goal in the acute phase of management is to keep the patient alive. Skilled nursing is required while the patient is unconscious. (The principles underlying the management of the unconscious patient are summarized on pages 1192 to 1195.)

One of the primary nursing objectives is to maintain a patent airway.
- The patient is placed in a lateral or semiprone position with the head of the bed slightly elevated to lower cerebral venous pressure.
- Endotracheal intubation and mechanical ventilation are necessary for patients with massive stroke since respiratory arrest is usually the life-threatening factor in this situation.
- If stertorous respirations are present, an artificial airway should be inserted. The negative pressure produced by the stertorous respirations causes an increase in the amount of secretions.
- If oropharyngeal suctioning is indicated, the catheter should be lubricated with water, "pinched off" and inserted through

the nose to the epiglottis. This initiates the cough reflex and serves to make the suctioning procedure more efficient. Repeated irritation to the mucous membrane by suctioning produces an increase of secretions, which is the direct opposite of its purpose. Suctioning may also cause an increase in intracranial pressure and therefore could be dangerous in the presence of brain hemorrhage.
- Adequate oxygenation of blood to the brain is necessary to minimize cerebral damage. During the acute stage the cerebral vessels involved are maximally dilated due to tissue acidosis and ischemia. The blood pressure and cardiac output must be maintained to sustain cerebral blood flow, and hydration (intravenous fluids) must be ensured to reduce blood viscosity and improve cerebral blood flow. Oxygen should be given at adequate perfusion pressure.

A neurological flow sheet is maintained to reflect the following significant observations:
1. A change in the level of responsiveness as evidenced by movement, resistance to changes of position, and response to stimulation; orientation to time, place, and person
2. Presence or absence of voluntary or involuntary movements of the extremities; the tone of the muscles; the body posture and the position of the head
3. Stiffness or flaccidity of the neck
4. The comparative size of the pupils and pupillary reactions to light
5. The color of the face and the extremities; the temperature and the moisture of the skin
6. The quality and the rates of pulse and respiration; the body temperature and the arterial pressure
7. The volume of fluids ingested or administered, and the volume of urine excreted each 24 hours
8. The ability to speak
9. Arterial blood gas measurements.

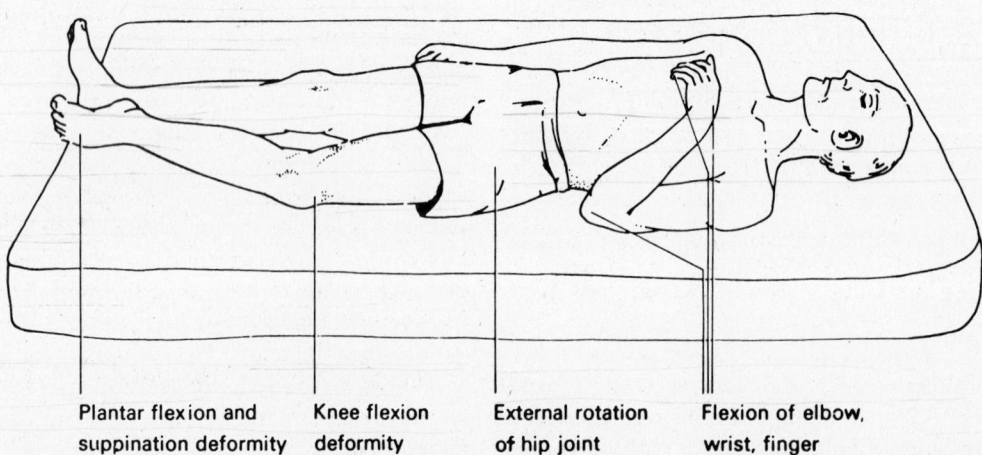

| Plantar flexion and suppination deformity | Knee flexion deformity | External rotation of hip joint | Flexion of elbow, wrist, finger |

Figure 54-2. Hemiplegic deformities. The involved leg immediately falls into external rotation. The knee almost invariably flexes. As soon as knee flexion occurs, abduction of the upper leg follows. The foot falls into plantar flexion, so that there is always a footdrop and a shortening of the Achilles tendon. This position of the leg is assumed whether the leg is flaccid or spastic.

The arm on the affected side is held against the body. Often, a flail arm is placed across the body for convenience in handling the patient, but if spastic, the elbow flexes to about 90 degrees. With the arm across the body, the wrist is dropped. If the arm is spastic, the fingers curl into a fist, with the thumb adducted and flexed under the fingers. (After Covalt, N.K.: Preventive technics of rehabilitation for hemiplegic patients, G.P. *17*:131)

When the patient begins to regain consciousness, signs of extreme fatigue and confusion will be apparent as a result of the cerebral edema that follows a stroke. To offset any anxiety, efforts should be made at frequent intervals to orient the patient to time and place and to reassure him that he has not lost his mind. Some aphasia can be expected to accompany right-sided hemiplegia. (See nursing support of the patient with aphasia, page 1196.) As soon as the patient has passed the acute stage, rehabilitation measures are started.

REHABILITATION PHASE

Rehabilitation begins on the day the patient has the stroke. A hemiplegic patient has a unilateral paralysis and requires intensive rehabilitation nursing.

The *immediate nursing goals* are (1) to prevent deformities, (2) to retrain the affected arm and leg, and (3) to help the patient gain independence in personal hygiene and dressing activities.

When control of the voluntary muscles is lost, the strong flexor muscles exert control over the extensors. The arm tends to adduct (adductor muscles are stronger than abductors) and to rotate internally. The elbow and the wrist tend to flex, the affected leg tends to rotate externally at the hip joint and flex at the knee, while the foot at the ankle joint supinates and tends toward plantar flexion (Fig. 54-2).

Positioning

Correct positioning in bed is of prime importance (Fig. 54-3) in order to prevent contractures, relieve pressure and assist in maintaining good body alignment. A bed board under the mattress provides firm support for the body. The patient should remain flat in bed except when engaged in activities of daily living. Maintaining the upright position in bed for extended periods of time is one of the greatest contributors to hip flexion deformity. A footboard may be used at intervals to keep the feet at right angles to the legs when the patient is in a supine (dorsal) position. This prevents footdrop and the heel cord from shortening as a result of contracture of the gastrocnemius muscle. However, many therapists feel that the continuous use of the footboard will stimulate the plantar surfaces of the feet producing plantar flexion. If the affected extremity is spastic, a bed cradle is used to keep the bedding off the extremity.

Figure 54-3A. Positioning for a patient following a stroke. (Dark side of pajamas represents affected or hemiplegic side.) (*right*) A pillow is placed in the axilla to prevent adduction of the affected shoulder. Pillows are placed under the arm, which is in a slightly flexed position with each joint positioned higher than the preceding one.

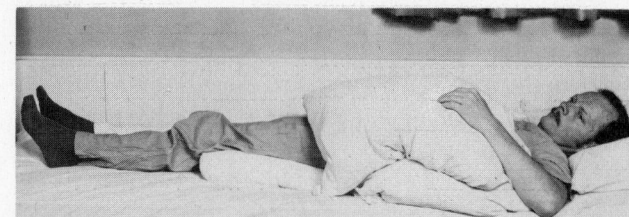

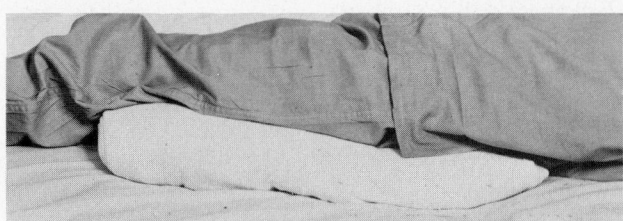

B.   The trochanter roll should extend from the crest of the ilium to the midthigh, since the hip joint lies between these 2 points. The trochanter roll acts as a mechanical wedge under the projection of the greater trochanter and prevents the femur from rolling.

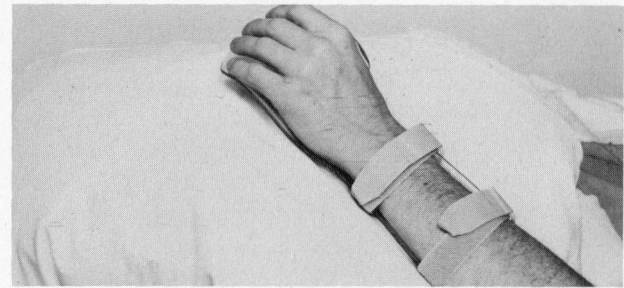

C.   A volar resting splint may be used to support the wrist and hand if the upper extremity is flaccid.

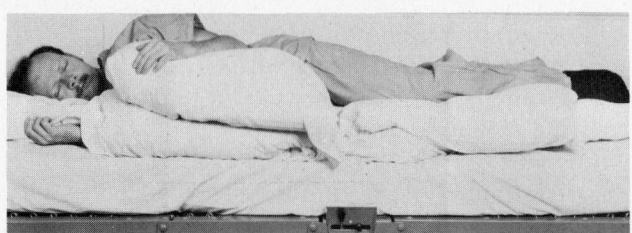

D.   Lateral or side-lying position. The patient should be turned on his unaffected side. The upper thigh should not be acutely flexed.

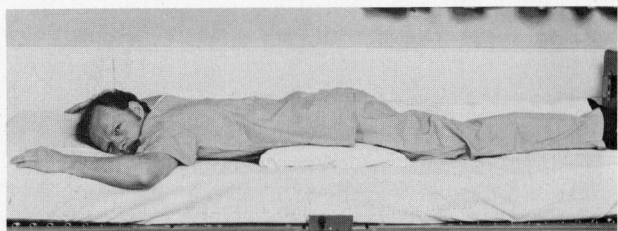

E.   Prone position. A pillow is placed under the pelvis to help promote hyperextension of the hip joints, which is essential for normal gait. Note position of arms.

Because flexor muscles are stronger than extensor muscles, it may be necessary to apply a posterior splint at night to prevent flexion of the affected extremity. If such a splint is not available, it may be improvised by applying a cast to the affected extremity, bivalving it and padding the posterior portion. The heel portion should be well padded with foam rubber or lamb's wool. The leg is positioned in the cast and wrapped with an elastic bandage to keep it in an extended position. The posterior splint is used only at night to maintain correct positioning while the patient is sleeping.

To prevent external rotation at the hip joint, a trochanter roll is used, extending from the crest of the ilium to the midthigh, since the hip joint lies between these two points (Fig. 54-3B). Sandbags applied laterally to the leg will not prevent external rotation inasmuch as this motion originates in the ball and socket joint of the hip. The knee has no such rotating function. The trochanter roll acts as a mechanical wedge under the projection of the greater trochanter and prevents the femur from rolling.

To prevent adduction of the affected shoulder, a pillow is placed in the axilla (Fig. 54-3A). This keeps the arm away from the chest. A pillow is placed under the arm, and the arm is placed in a neutral (slightly flexed) position, with each joint positioned higher than the preceding one. Thus the elbow is higher than the shoulder, and the wrist is higher than the elbow. The elevation of the arm helps to prevent edema and the resultant fibrosis that will prevent normal range of motion if the patient regains control of the arm.

The fingers are positioned so that they are barely flexed. The hand is placed in slight supination, which is its most functional (i.e., useful) position. If the upper extremity is flaccid a volar resting splint can be used to support the wrist and hand in a functional position (Fig. 54-3C). If the upper extremity is spastic, a hand roll is *not* desirable as it stimulates the grasp reflex. In this instance, a dorsal splint is useful in allowing the palm to be free of pressure.

CHANGING POSITIONS. The patient's position should be changed every 2 hours. To place a patient in a lateral (side-lying) position, a pillow is placed between the legs before the patient is turned. The patient may be turned from side to side, but the amount of time spent on the affected side should be limited because of impaired sensation. The upper thigh should not be acutely flexed (Fig. 54-3D).

The patient should be placed in a prone position for 15 minutes to a half hour several times a day. A small pillow or a support is placed under the pelvis extending from the level of the umbilicus to the upper third of the thigh (Fig. 54-3E). This helps to promote hyperextension of the hip joints, which is essential for normal gait. The prone position also helps to drain bronchial secretions and prevents contractural deformities of the shoulders and knees.

Exercise

The affected extremities are exercised passively and put through a full range of motion 4 to 5 times a day to prevent contractures.

Repetition of an activity forms new pathways in the central nervous system and therefore encourages new patterns of motion. At first the extremities are usually flaccid. If tightness occurs in any area, the range of motion exercises should be done more frequently. (See pages 188 to 190 for techniques of range of motion exercises.) Signs to watch for include: shortness of breath, chest pain, cyanosis, and increasing pulse rate during the exercise period.

Frequent short periods of exercise always are preferred to longer periods at infrequent intervals. *Regularity* in exercise is most important. Improvement in muscle strength and maintenance of range of motion can be achieved only through daily exercise.

The patient is encouraged and reminded to exercise the unaffected side at intervals throughout the day. It is well to work out a written time schedule that can be used to remind the patient of the exercise activities. The nurse has the responsibility of supervising and supporting the patient during these activities. The patient can be taught to put the unaffected leg under the affected one to move it when turning and exercising. Bed exercises prepare the patient for ambulation and give the patient a goal. Quadriceps muscle setting and gluteal setting exercises are started early to improve the muscle strength needed for walking. These are done at least 5 times daily for 10 minutes at a time.

QUADRICEPS SETTING

Instruct the patient to contract the quadriceps muscle (on the anterior portion of the thigh) while raising the heel and pushing the popliteal space against the mattress. The muscle contracture is held until the count of 5, then relaxed until the count of 5. Repeat. This exercise is performed by each extremity.

GLUTEAL SETTING

Contract or "pinch" the buttocks together until the count of 5. Then relax until the count of 5. Repeat.

CARE OF AFFECTED UPPER EXTREMITY. If the patient's arm is paralyzed completely, subluxation (incomplete dislocation) at the shoulder can occur from the weight of the paralyzed arm. A sling will prevent this complication and will help the patient maintain balance when ambulating. Subluxation can be avoided when the patient is seated by placing a pillow under the arm for support or resting the arm on the arm of the chair. The sling is discarded when spasticity develops, because spasticity of the shoulder muscles will help prevent subluxation.

Another painful and difficult condition to reverse is frozen shoulder, which comes as a result of lack of motion. The patient may exercise the affected arm by raising and lowering it with the unaffected one. A clothesline may be strung through a pulley attached to a door jamb (or over a shower rod) and tied on the affected hand. The patient pulls the rope up and down with the unaffected hand and so exercises the affected arm and shoulder. The combination of sling support and range of motion exercises will prevent painful frozen shoulder and subluxation. If the position of the chair is changed, other shoulder motions may be carried out. The patient is instructed to flex the affected wrist at frequent intervals and to move all the joints of the affected fingers.

Mobilizing the Patient

As soon as possible the patient is assisted out of bed. Usually when hemiplegia has resulted from a thrombosis, an active rehabilitation program is started as soon as the patient regains consciousness, whereas a patient who has had a cerebral hemorrhage cannot participate actively until all evidence of bleeding is gone.

SITTING BALANCE

A hemiplegic patient tends to lose his sense of balance and needs to learn to maintain balance in a sitting position before learning to balance himself in the standing position.
- Before the patient attempts to rise from a recumbent position, blood pressure should be checked since orthostatic hypotension may occur. A fall in blood pressure may further damage the ischemic area.

The patient may be helped to a sitting position in bed as follows:

1. The patient grasps the involved arm at the wrist and places his forearm over his waist.
2. The strong elbow that is flexed at a 90-degree angle should then be pressed into the mattress.
3. The patient comes to a sitting position by transferring the weight to the forearm and then to the hand while contracting the abdomen.
4. Extend the patient's arm with his hand flat on the bed.

The patient is then helped to come to a sitting position on the edge of the bed. This may be achieved in the following manner:

1. Adjust the bed to the low position.
2. Instruct the patient to place the strong leg beneath the weak leg and lift it toward the side of the bed.
3. Instruct the patient to press the strong elbow that is flexed to a 90-degree angle into the mattress and come to a sitting position by transferring weight to the forearm and then to the hand, while lifting the uninvolved leg with the strong leg over the edge of the bed. The force of gravity, set in motion by pushing against the hand and moving the legs, is sufficient to pivot the patient's torso on the buttocks.
4. Extend the patient's strong arm with his hand flat on the bed behind him to assist in balancing.
5. Stand in front of the patient to observe and, if necessary, help him to maintain this posture.
- A change in color, shortness of breath, increasing pulse rate or profuse perspiration is an indication that the patient should be placed in bed again. The sitting time is increased as rapidly as the patient's condition permits.

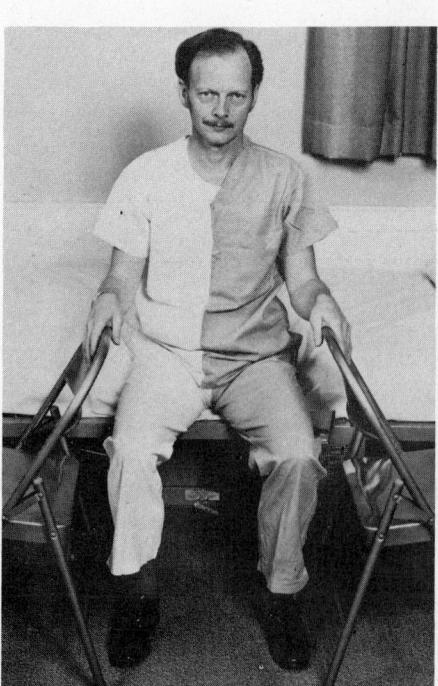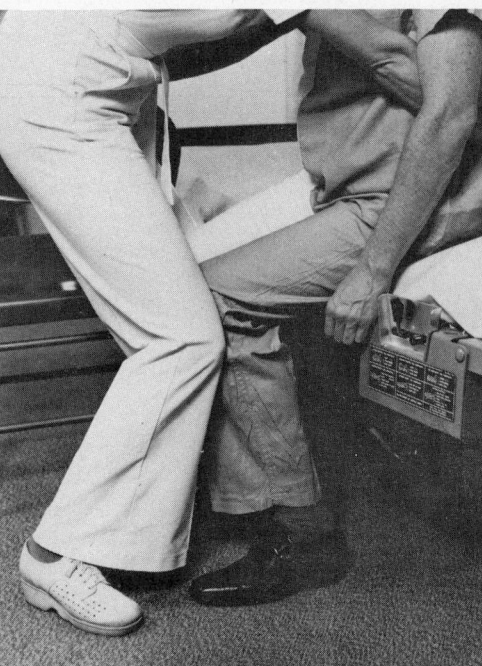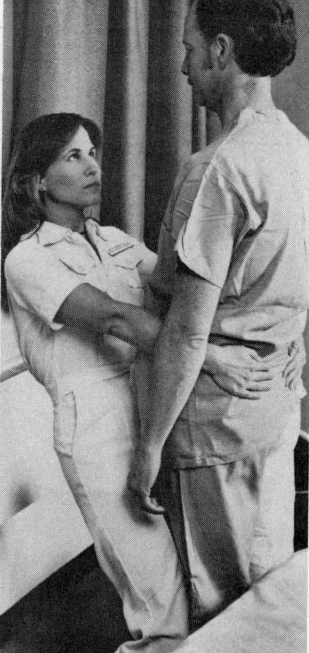

Figure 54-4. Getting the patient out of bed following a stroke. *(left)* Place the bed in the low position so that the feet are resting on the floor. Observe the patient's reaction and increase the sitting time as rapidly as the patient's condition permits. *(center)* Getting ready to arise to a standing position. Positioning the nurse's knees on the outside of the patient's knees will prevent the patient's knees from buckling. *(right)* Stabilizing the patient as he assumes a standing position. Note that the nurse is (1) stabilizing the patient's lower back and knees and (2) assessing his reaction to standing. (Courtesy Washington Adventist Hospital, Glenn Dalby, photographer)

STANDING BALANCE

As soon as the patient is able to balance while sitting, he is taught standing balance. He should wear walking shoes with a strong shank for all ambulation activities.

- Seat the patient on the edge of the bed, and place a straight-back chair on each side of him (Fig. 54-4). If the patient lacks strength to grasp and to push the chair with his affected hand, the hand can be tied to the top of the chair. This stabilization gives the patient greater support.
- Help the patient to come to a standing position by supporting his lower back with your hands and positioning your knees on the outside of the patient's knees. This will give the patient maximum support in the standing position and will prevent his knees from buckling. The patient should be reminded to lean forward when he comes from a sitting to a standing position. The patient's arms must be left free for balance and support.
- Stand behind the patient and stabilize him at his waist. Place a waistband or a belt (a scultetus binder can serve as a waistband) around the patient's waist and grasp it for patient support.
- Dizziness, pallor, and an increasing pulse rate indicate that the patient should be permitted to rest in a sitting position. If the symptoms continue, the patient should be put back in bed. With repeated effort the patient will tolerate this activity for longer periods.

If the patient has difficulty in achieving standing balance, a tilt table will help him assume an upright position. There should be frequent periods of standing before walking is started.

WALKING

Parallel bars are useful when the patient first starts to walk. A chair or wheelchair should be readily available in the event of sudden fatigue or vertigo.

The following method is one way to ambulate the patient:
1. Instruct the patient to stand between the parallel bars or beside one rail with his weight evenly distributed on both feet and his strong arm on the rail 10 cm. (about 4 inches) in front of his body.
2. Have the patient shift the weight to the strong leg and advance the involved leg while pushing *down* on the rail.
3. The patient then shifts the weight to the weak leg. (If the patient has poor muscle tone and cannot advance his involved leg, functional electrical stimulation may be used. Stimulating muscles electrically may increase strength, reverse atrophy and enhance voluntary control.)

The training periods for ambulation should be short and frequent. As the patient gains in strength and confidence he can begin to walk with an adjustable aluminum cane. Generally a three- or four-prong cane provide a more stable support in the early phases of this training program.

BRACING

If the patient has a weakened or absent quadriceps muscle, the knee joint may be supported with a splint applied to the back of the knee. Reflex contractures of those muscles used in standing are brought into play by putting on a posterior knee brace and having the patient stand. Temporary splints can be constructed from light-weight thermoplastic material and Velcro straps.

Splinting the extremity and helping the patient to a standing position early in the rehabilitation program offers the following advantages: (1) the muscle tone is maintained through reflex action, (2) the patient develops a better command of balance, and (3) position sense is retained. After a period of time has elapsed, the physician determines whether the patient needs to be fitted with a short- or a long-leg brace.

WHEELCHAIR

If the patient needs a wheelchair, the folding type with hand brakes is the most practical since it allows the patient to manipulate the chair. The chair should be low enough so that the patient can propel it with the uninvolved foot and narrow enough to permit it to be used in the home. To propel the wheelchair, the patient places the strong hand on the hand rim and the stronger foot on the floor to guide and direct the chair.

When the patient is transferred from the wheelchair, the brakes are applied on both sides of the chair. The technique for transferring from a wheelchair is as follows:

- The patient lifts the foot pedals out of the way and moves forward in the chair.
- He pushes down on the arm rest with the uninvolved arm while leaning forward and then comes to a standing position.
- The knee of the uninvolved leg is kept as straight as possible so the patient can pivot on this extremity and then transfer to another seat (toilet; bed).

Wheelchair mobility provides greater independence in self-care activities. When a permanent wheelchair is needed, it is ordered with specific instructions for the individual patient.

Activities of Daily Living

As soon as the patient is able to sit up, he is encouraged to assist in his personal hygiene. The first step is to have the patient carry out all self-care activities on the unaffected side. Such activities as combing the hair, brushing the teeth, shaving with an electric razor, bathing, and eating can be carried out with one hand and are suitable for self-care. While the patient may feel awkward at first, the various motor skills can be learned by repetition, and the unaffected side will become stronger with use. Assistive devices will help make up for some of the patient's deficits.

DRESSING ACTIVITIES. The patient's morale will improve if ambulatory activities are carried out while he is fully dressed. The family is instructed to bring in clothing that is preferably a size larger than that normally worn. Clothing, fitted with front or side fasteners, is the most suitable. The patient has better balance if most of the dressing activities are done in a seated position.

In the early stages, when the patient needs to be helped or supported by the nurse, he should not be permitted to become overfatigued and discouraged.

The following procedure for dressing has been found to be workable for many patients. However, the nurse must use judgment in assisting the patient to work out individual modifications.

Underclothing

Use a flare leg or boxer-type shorts with an elastic waistband.

With the unaffected hand, place the affected ankle in a resting position on top of the unaffected knee.

Place the unaffected hand through the outside opening of the shorts. Thrust the hand through the shorts, grasp the affected foot firmly and shake the garment off the unaffected hand and well over the affected foot.

While holding the garment, allow the affected foot to rest on the floor. Draw the shorts up the affected leg.

Then put the unaffected leg into the shorts, and pull them up as far as possible.

To complete the procedure of bringing the shorts up over the buttocks, roll to each side and pull up the shorts on the opposite side.

Undershirt

Place the undershirt in the lap, with the back of the shirt facing upward.

Thread the paralyzed arm through the appropriate armhole to above the elbow.

Introduce the normal arm through its armhole.

With the good arm, pull the garment on the affected side up to the shoulder and over the head, and adjust the garment with the normal hand.

Brassiere

Stabilize one end of the garment with the affected arm while fastening it in the front with the unaffected hand.

Slide the garment around the body, so that the fastener is in the back.

Use the unaffected hand to pull the affected arm through the strap and place the strap over the shoulder. Then place the unaffected arm through the other strap.

Shirt, Blouse, or Front-fastening Dress

Button the cuff on the normal side.

Thread the sleeve over the paralyzed arm to the shoulder.

Place the hand and the arm through the other sleeve.

Button the sleeve on the affected side.

It is wise to wear collars a size larger than normal, because buttoning a tight neckband is difficult. Snap-on ties may be worn, or four-in-hand ties may be loosened and slipped over the head without being untied.

Trousers

The use of suspenders makes it easier to pull up the trousers. Trousers are put on in the same manner as shorts. If the patient prefers, he can pull the shorts and the trousers up over the buttocks at the same time. When more balance has been achieved, an over-the-head garment (dress, slip, sweater) is put on in the same manner as is the undershirt. It is suggested that stretchable clothing be used.

Patient and Family Education

The family plays an important role in the patient's recovery. However, they may have difficulty in accepting the patient's disability and be unrealistic in their expectations. The family must be counseled to avoid doing for the patient those things which he can do for himself. Assure them that their loving and warm interest is part of the patient's therapy. The family needs to be informed that the rehabilitation of the hemiplegic patient requires many months and that progress may be slow. All should approach the patient with a supportive and optimistic attitude.

If the patient has some brain damage, he may be emotionally labile. The family should be prepared to expect occasional episodes of emotional instability. The patient may laugh or cry easily and is likely to become depressed. Explain to the family that his laughing does not necessarily mean the patient is glad nor does crying mean that he is sad. Advise the family that the patient will tire easily, will become irritable and upset by small events and is apt to show less interest in things. As progress is made in the rehabilitation program, these problems will diminish. The family can help by supporting the patient and giving honest praise for the progress that is being made.

Usually the home environment has to be rearranged for the patient's activities and safety. A shower is more convenient than a tub for the hemiplegic patient as most patients do not gain sufficient strength to get up and down from a tub. Sitting on a stool of medium height with rubber suction tips will permit him to wash with greater ease. A long-handled bath brush with a soap container is helpful to the patient who has only one functional hand. If a shower is not available, a stool may be placed in the tub and a portable shower hose attached to the faucet. Handrails may be attached by the bathtub and the toilet. There are numerous self-help devices on the market that can assist the patient in the activities of daily living.

When feasible, it is best if the patient can return to work or some modification of his former job. The local or the regional branch of the State Office of Vocational Rehabilitation provides individual evaluation and retraining services, depending on the needs of the patient.

All nurses coming in contact with the patient, whether as members of the hospital health team, community health nurses, or office or industrial nurses, should encourage the patient *to keep active,* faithfully adhere to the exercise program, accept the limitations, and yet, confidently continue to remain as self-sufficient as possible.

NEUROSURGICAL TREATMENT OF PAIN

The management of long-term pain requires a multidisciplinary approach. (The reader is referred to Chapter 14 for a discussion of the basic theories of the psychophysiology of pain and its management.)

Intractable pain refers to pain that cannot be relieved satisfactorily by drugs, without causing drug addiction or incapacitating sedation. Such pain usually is the result of malignancy (especially of the cervix, bladder, prostate and lower bowel), but it does occur in many other conditions, such as postherpetic neuralgia, tic douloureux, spinal cord arachnoiditis and uncontrollable ischemia and other forms of tissue destruction. Surgical intervention should be considered before narcotic addiction and debilitation become problems.

The objective of neurosurgical procedures for the management of intractable pain is to interrupt the pathways by which painful sensations are perceived. Pain-conducting fibers can be interrupted at any point from their origin to the cerebral cortex. The challenge is to select the appropriate level. The range of diverse surgical techniques points to the fact that the ultimate treatment of pain has not yet been found. With surgery there is destruction of some part of the nervous system which can result in varying amounts of neurologic deficit and incapacity. In time, pain usually returns as a result of either regeneration of axonal fibers or the development of alternate pain pathways.

Rhizotomy

A posterior or spinal *rhizotomy* is the surgical interruption of selected posterior spinal nerve roots between the ganglion and the cord. This results in permanent loss of sensation and may be done at any spinal level. In the head or torso the resultant numbness is not troublesome. In the extremities, however, the extremity is useless (even though muscle strength is intact) as there is loss of positional feedback to the spinal cord and cerebellum.

Rhizotomy is used in controlling the severe chest pain that may be experienced in lung cancer and is used to give pain relief in head and neck malignancies.

The length of the incision for rhizotomy varies directly with the number of nerves that are to be cut. This requires a fairly extensive laminectomy and the patient should be in condition to tolerate a major operative procedure.

Since many patients with metastatic malignancies may not be able to tolerate an open rhizotomy, a *percutaneous rhizotomy* may be done, whereby a radiofrequency current is used to selectively coagulate the pain fibers, while the fibers concerned with touch and proprioception are preserved.

A *chemical rhizotomy* is one in which alcohol, phenol or a mixture of drugs is injected into the subarachnoid space. The medication is maneuvered over the affected nerve roots by tilting the patient to the desired level. This renders the sensory nerve roots functionless. The patient's perception of pain is absent but the motor nerve roots are usually not affected.

Cordotomy and Sympathectomy

CORDOTOMY. An *open cordotomy* is the surgical division of the anterolateral columns of the spinal pain fibers high in the thoracic or cervical region. This procedure interrupts or destroys conduction of pain and temperature sense, while touch and position sense are preserved. The cord is exposed by laminectomy. Cordotomy is used most frequently in controlling the severe pain of terminal cancer. Since a significant percentage of cordotomies lose their effectiveness in 1 to 5 years, the procedure is used for pain associated with conditions in which survival time is limited.

Postoperative Nursing Management. The principles of nursing management following a laminectomy are applicable in the postoperative and rehabilitation requirements of this patient. (See page 1260.) Following a cordotomy the patient may be kept flat for the prescribed time period, because there is less tension on the incision when this position is assumed. A patient with a thoracic cordotomy may be turned to the prone position. In instances of a cervical incision, pillows should not be used when the patient is in a supine position. Trauma to the surgical site is eliminated when the neck is kept in a neutral position. The patient is turned as a unit ("log" fashion) by two persons using a turning sheet to avoid twisting the body and putting pressure on the incision.

Assessment for Complications. The patient is watched for respiratory complications, as well as for signs of fatigue and weakening of the voice. The patient may ventilate adequately while awake but may experience progressive hypercarbia and hypoxia while asleep. Therefore, arterial blood gases are monitored, and assisted mechanical ventilation initiated when required.

Since hemorrhage may result in motor and sensory loss, the motion, strength and sensation of each extremity must be tested every few hours (or more frequently if necessary) during the first 48 hours postoperatively. If hemorrhage is indicated, immediate surgical intervention is imperative. Because the patient has no sense of temperature, the skin should be felt at intervals to ascertain any changes in temperature. Since pressure sores may develop without the patient realizing it, the patient should be taught to inspect his skin using a hand mirror to view the hard-to-see places.

Urinary retention is usually transient. If there is permanent loss of motor control from a high cervical procedure, a bladder training program is carried out (page 914).

Percutaneous Cordotomy. The percutaneous approach (which is a simplified form of surgical cordotomy) uses radiofrequency currents to produce lesions in the anterolateral spinal cord. Under local anesthesia, a needle is inserted into the neck below and behind the mastoid process. It is guided into the spinal cord under x-ray control and then an electrode is inserted through it. By means of radiofrequency currents, a lesion is made at the desired spinal cord level.

Verification of electrode placement is determined by the patient's response to stimulation. The procedure is tolerated by wasted and debilitated patients and gives complete relief of pain in approximately 80 percent of patients. Percutaneous cordotomy is replacing open cordotomy as the procedure of choice.

Patient and Family Education. Since temperature sense is permanently lost, the patient is instructed concerning external temperature changes. Bath water should be tested by a family member before the patient gets into the tub. Because frostbite and sunburn can occur without any sense of discomfort, protection must be taken against inclement weather. Warn the patient of the danger of impaired circulation and the need to avoid constricting clothing, such as tightly tied shoes. Sexual function is usually impaired in males.

SYMPATHECTOMY. *Sympathectomy* is the interruption of afferent pathways in the sympathetic division of the autonomic nervous system. It is used to control the pain in patients with vascular insufficiency, particularly Raynaud's disease. The operation eliminates vasospasm and improves peripheral blood supply. A sympathectomy may be done to relieve visceral pain as this procedure destroys the visceral afferents that accompany the sympathetic fibers to the viscera. (See also page 620.)

Psychosurgical Approaches

The purpose of these procedures is to alter the patient's response to pain. A *thalamotomy* is the destruction (either unilateral or bilateral) of the target centers within the thalamus. Burr holes are made in the skull, electrodes are placed in the target area by stereotaxic techniques, and a radiofrequency current is then directed through the electrodes to create the lesion. This procedure represents the highest level in the central nervous system in which pain pathways can be interrupted and is usually done for malignancy of the head and neck.

Cingulumotomy is a unilateral or bilateral interruption of the anterior cingulate bundle in the frontal lobe of the brain. It is accomplished either by an open or stereotaxic approach. It tends to modify the patient's affective reaction to pain.

Electrical Stimulation for the Control of Pain (Neuromodulation)

Electrical stimulation or neuromodulation is a method of suppressing pain by applying an electronic device that stimulates the different parts of the nervous system for pain relief. This therapy is based on the gate control theory (page 241) that explains how nondestructive stimuli can interfere with the transmission of pain within the central nervous system. The neural mechanism in the

dorsal horns of the spinal cord acts like a gate which can increase or decrease the flow to the central nervous system. Electrical stimulation is thought to relieve pain by preventing messages from reaching the brain. It is accomplished through electrodes applied to the skin, by stimulation of the peripheral nerves or peripheral nerve plexuses, by stimulation of the anterior and posterior surfaces of the spinal cord or by implants into selected areas within the brain. Currently, flexible electrodes are being implanted into the spinal epidural space percutaneously to stimulate the spinal cord. This newer procedure eliminates a major operation. At the present time, transcutaneous electrical stimulation and dorsal column stimulation are the procedures most frequently done. Electrical stimulation techniques may be the wave of the future in the management of severe pain.

Transcutaneous Nerve Stimulation

Transcutaneous nerve stimulation (TNS) is the passage of small electrical currents through the skin for the purpose of controlling pain. The stimulating electrodes are placed over the site of pain or along the course of the major peripheral nerves innervating the area or over the peripheral plexus. The patient operates the amplitude control until stimulation, detected by a buzzing or tingling sensation, is felt. The amplitude is increased until the sensation is strong but not uncomfortable. The patient controls the amplitude, frequency and duration of stimulation.

Patient Education. The skin is cleansed and electrode gel is applied to the electrodes which are then placed over the nerves that serve the painful area. The electrodes are secured with nonallergenic tape. The patient is given the instruction booklet provided by the manufacturing company that explains care of the skin, the electrodes and generator. The major problems of transcutaneous nerve stimulation are skin reactions to electricity and the inability of some patients to learn to use the device.

Dorsal Column Stimulation (DCS)

Dorsal column stimulation (DCS) is a technique used for the relief of chronic intractable pain in which a surgically implanted device allows the patient to apply pulsed electrical stimulation to the dorsal aspect of the spinal cord to block pain impulses. It is hypothesized that electrical stimulation of larger peripheral nerve fibers causes a negative feedback to "close the gate" in the spinal cord, preventing the transmission of pain sensation to the brain. Some researchers feel that the mechanism of peripheral nerve stimulation is actually a blockade of the nerve. The explanation for pain relief from electrical stimulation is not yet available.

The dorsal column stimulation unit consists of a radiofrequency stimulation transmitter, a transmitter antenna, a radiofrequency receiver and a stimulation electrode. The battery-powered transmitter and antenna are worn externally while the receiver and electrode are implanted. A laminectomy is performed above the highest level of pain input and the electrode is placed in the epidural space over the posterior column of the spinal cord. (The placement of the stimulating systems is varied.) The subcutaneous pocket is constructed over the clavicular area or some other site for placement of the receiver. The two are connected by a subcutaneous tunnel.

Postoperative Nursing Management. The postoperative nursing management is similar to that following a laminectomy. The patient is assessed for evidences of paraplegia, quadriplegia and urinary incontinence. The extremities are evaluated for movement. Leakage of cerebrospinal fluid at the laminectomy site is also checked since the dura is opened during surgery. The implant sight is checked for signs of infection. As soon as the patient is fully alert the dorsal column stimulation system may be tested, although initial testing may not be accurate because a bandage may cover the receiver site.

Patient Education. The patient is given the manufacturer's booklet to become acquainted with the system. Proper skin care is taught as well as the method for attaching the antenna to the skin, connecting the transmitter, and adjusting the settings. Different stimulation

frequencies should be tried to determine which one gives the best pain relief. A record is to be kept of the stimulation used. The patient is also instructed to keep several batteries in reserve. (Battery life depends on the extent of use.) The transmitter and antenna are cleaned according to the manufacturer's directions.

THE PATIENT UNDERGOING INTRACRANIAL SURGERY

In recent years, certain technological advances have helped to refine existing neurological procedures and develop newer ones. Superior neuroradiologic techniques have made it possible to localize intracranial lesions, while microsurgical instruments with improved illumination and magnification have made it possible to obtain a three-dimensional view of the field of operation (Fig. 54-5).

It is now possible to coagulate vessels adjacent to structures without causing injury to the structures themselves. Microsurgical instruments (miniaturized probes, hooks, clamps, needle holders) allow delicate tissue to be separated without trauma. Suture material smaller than a strand of human hair permits very small nerves and vessels to be sutured and anastomosed.

Surgical Approaches

A *craniotomy* is the surgical opening of the skull to gain access to intracranial structures. This procedure is done to remove a tumor, relieve intracranial pressure, evacuate a blood clot and control hemorrhage. In general, two approaches are used: (1) above the tentorium (supratentorial craniotomy) into the supratentorial compartment and (2) below the tentorium into the infratentorial (posterior fossa) compartment.

The intracranial structures may be approached through burr holes (Fig. 54-6) which are circular openings made in the skull by either a hand drill or an automatic craniotome (which has a self-controlled system to stop the drill when the bone is penetrated). Burr holes may be used to determine the level of brain tension and the size and position of the ventricles. They are also a means of evacuating an intracranial hematoma or abscess, making a bone flap in the skull and allowing access to the ventricles for decompression purposes, ventriculography or shunting procedures.

Other cranial procedures include *craniectomy* (an excision of a portion of the skull and *cranioplasty* (repair of a cranial defect by means of a plastic or metal plate).

Preoperative Assessment and Management

Proper assessment of the postoperative status of the patient requires an awareness of the patient's symptoms so that a comparison may be made between the preopera-

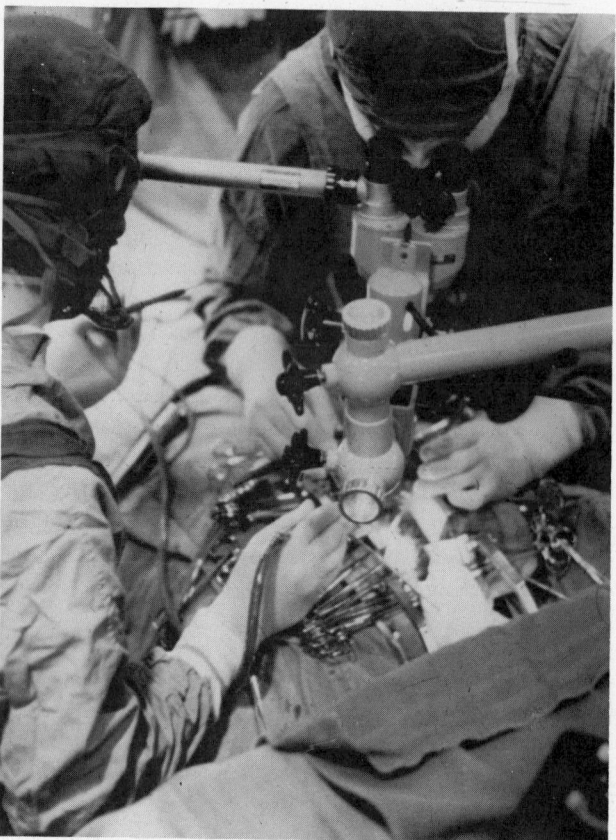

Figure 54-5. Intracranial surgery.

tive and postoperative conditions. Included in this assessment are observations of paralysis, vision, personality, speech, and incontinence. Motor function of the hands can be tested by the hand grip. Observations of leg movement should be especially noted if the patient is not ambulatory.

If there is paralysis of the extremities, trochanter rolls should be applied to both extremities and the feet positioned against a footboard. Patients who have speech difficulties, failing vision, and hearing loss are a challenge to the nurse's ingenuity. If the patient is aphasic, writing materials or picture and word cards showing the bedpan, glass of water, blanket, etc., may be supplied to help improve communication. If the patient is able to ambulate, he should be encouraged to do so in a quiet, unhurried way.

The emotional preparation of the patient is also important. The patient may not realize that he is about to undergo surgery. Even so, encouragement and attention to his needs usually will reinforce his confidence. Whatever the state of awareness of the patient, the family needs reassurance and consideration, since they recognize the seriousness of a brain operation.

Preparation for Operation. The scalp is shaved just prior to surgery so that any resultant superficial abrasions will not have time to become infected. A preoperative enema is not given to a patient who has increased intracranial pressure since straining to expel the enema may increase the pressure and contribute to brain herniation.

Morphine sulfate usually is not given to neurosurgical patients because it acts as a respiratory depressant and also masks pupillary signs. Other preoperative *anticipatory* measures include giving preoperative steroids to decrease brain volume and inserting an indwelling urethral catheter to assess urinary volume during the dehydrating operative period.

Phenytoin (Dilantin) may be given prophylactically prior to surgery.

Postoperative Nursing Management

Following an intracranial operation, nursing assessment and management will affect the patient's clinical course. Since the patient will be unconscious during the initial postoperative care, the reader is referred to the nursing management of the unconscious patient outlined on pages 1192–1195. The nursing management of a patient undergoing an intracranial operation is summarized on page 1209.

Postoperative Positioning. Following a supratentorial operation the patient is placed on his side (unoperated side if a large lesion was removed) with one pillow under his head. The head of the bed may be elevated 15 to 45 degrees according to the level of the intracranial pressure and the neurosurgeon's directives. (Usually the patient is kept in relatively the same position as during the

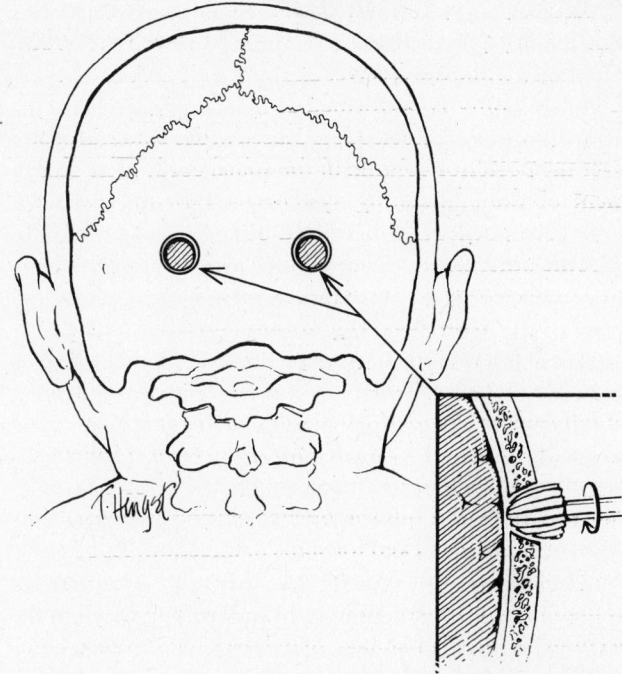

Figure 54-6. (*posterior view*) Burr holes in intracranial surgery.

operation.) Following a posterior fossa operation (infratentorial), the patient is kept flat on his side (off his back) with his head on a small firm pillow. He may be turned on either side, but his head should not be flexed on his chest. When the patient is being turned, his body should be turned as a unit to prevent strain on the wound and possible tearing of the sutures.

The patient's position is changed every two hours and skin care is given frequently. If the position is changed too frequently, the intracranial monitoring equipment will be disrupted. A turning sheet from the head to the mid-thigh level will make it easier to move the patient. Whatever the patient's position, the bed should be so arranged as to permit easy access to his head.

Dressings. The dressing is often stained with blood in the immediate postoperative period. It is important to reinforce the dressing with sterile pads so that contamination and infection may be avoided. (Blood is an excellent culture medium for bacteria.) If the dressing is heavily stained or displaced, it should be reported immediately. A rubber drain is sometimes placed in the craniotomy wound to facilitate drainage. This is usually removed by the surgical staff within 24 hours. The wound is usually dressed on the third to the fifth postoperative day and sutures are removed.

Following suboccipital operations, cerebrospinal fluid may leak through the wound. This complication is dangerous because of the possibility of meningitis. Any sudden discharge of fluid from a cranial or spinal wound should be reported at once.

Patients with suboccipital surgery are sometimes dressed with firm adhesive strappings to prevent movement of the head and the neck.

Drainage. Ventricular catheters are frequently inserted in patients undergoing surgery for tumors of the posterior fossa. These catheters are connected to an external drainage bottle. The patency of the catheter can be noted by the pulsations of the fluid in the tubing. In addition, the degree of intracranial pressure can be determined by the height of the fluid level in the tube above the level of the ventricle. The catheter is removed when the ventricular pressure is normal and no further fluid is draining (usually within 2 or 3 days). The neurosurgeon should be notified if at any time the catheter appears to be obstructed. A more recent innovation is the use of ventriculoatrial shunts to lower intracranial pressure before certain operations, particularly in patients with posterior fossa tumors.

When drainage catheters are not used, a hematoma frequently forms under the scalp and spreads down to the orbit, producing an area of ecchymosis (black eye). Sometimes the eyes cannot be opened for a few days due to edema of the eyelids.

Drug Therapy. Some degree of local swelling of the brain usually occurs following brain surgery. Usually cerebral edema reaches its peak 72 hours after operation and may be treated with the intravenous administration of dehydrating agents (mannitol; dexamethasone; oral glycerol). Antacids are given with steroids to protect the gastric mucosa.

Sometimes external decompression is achieved by removing the bone flap. Fluids may need to be restricted and electrolyte surveys carried out. (See page 1185 for treatment of increased intracranial pressure.)

There will be a certain amount of headache following craniotomy which is mostly attributed to stretching or irritation of the nerves of the scalp that occurs during operation. Codeine, given parenterally, is usually sufficient to relieve headache. Anticonvulsant medication (diazepam; phenytoin) is given to patients who have undergone supratentorial craniotomy because of the high risk of epilepsy following this procedure.

Fluid and Electrolyte Balance. Electrolyte imbalance, particularly sodium imbalance, may contribute to the development of postoperative brain edema. Sodium retention is observed in the immediate postoperative period. Serum and urine electrolytes, BUN, blood glucose, weight and clinical status are evaluated. The input and output are measured in view of the losses incurred from fever, respiration, and ventricular/spinal drainage. The postoperative fluid regimen is calculated on an individual basis. Fluid overload is scrupulously avoided.

Postoperative Complications. Complications that may develop within hours following surgery include intracranial bleeding, cerebral edema, and water intoxication.

- A drop in blood pressure, a fast pulse and respiration, and a pale and cold body are usually manifestations of a hypovolemic shock following long operations. This type of shock is best treated by blood transfusion.
- Conversely, an increase in blood pressure and decrease in pulse with respiratory failure may indicate increased intracranial pressure.

Aside from the immediate postoperative complications, other complications may occur during the first 2 weeks or later and may endanger the patient's recovery. The most important of these are pulmonary infection, pressure sores, urinary infection, and thrombophlebitis. The majority of these complications may be avoided by frequent change of position, nasopharyngeal suctioning, observation and auscultation for pulmonary complications, and urinary bladder and skin care as is described in the care of patients with cerebrovascular disease.

Status epilepticus (occurrence of prolonged seizures without recovery of consciousness in the intervals between seizures) may occur after craniotomy as a result of the intracranial lesion. Intravenous phenobarbital, phenytoin (Dilantin) or diazepam (Valium) may relieve the seizures. Sometimes general anesthesia is necessary to halt the seizures. Other complications are summarized on page 1211.

Rehabilitation and Patient Education

The convalescence of a neurosurgical patient depends on the extent of trauma and the success with which treatment was carried out. When a benign tumor is removed successfully, it is most gratifying to help the patient toward recovery. Good nursing management eliminates untoward complications and permits the major emphasis to be placed on regaining function. Helping the patient to gradually exercise his arms and legs, get out of bed, and feed himself are methods by which the nurse can encourage self care. Doing everything for the patient hinders successful rehabilitation. However, he should be accompanied when he is walking, because sudden attacks of dizziness or unconsciousness may occur.

Close cooperation between the nurse and the physical therapist helps the patient to achieve good muscle function. If the patient is aphasic, speech therapy may be necessary. This is likely to become a long-term and time-consuming project—one demanding great patience and continual encouragement on the part of the nurse (see page 1196.)

The family must be aware of the limitations of the patient, but should be informed of his progress and how they can help to promote his recovery.

When tumor, injury, or disease is of such a nature that the prognosis is poor, care is directed toward making the patient as comfortable as possible.

With return of the tumor or cerebral compression the patient becomes less alert and aware. Other possible sequelae include: paralysis, blindness or seizures. When the family is kept informed of the progress of the patient by the surgeon, many times the real expression of their emotions takes place after the physician leaves. It is then that the nurse must help them to work out their feelings.

Often the care of this patient is transferred to some member of the family. Whoever is responsible must have proper instruction regarding the physical and emotional care of the patient. If a family member is not able to give this care, perhaps some arrangements can be made for a community health nurse to assume part care as needed. The medical social worker may be consulted in making financial arrangements or in helping to place the patient in an extended care facility.

Pituitary Surgery

Pituitary tumors (which comprise 10 percent of all intracranial tumors) may be treated by surgery or radiation. Surgical removal may be carried out through an open craniotomy (usually transfrontal) or through the transsphenoidal approach. The choice is determined by anatomical considerations and the extent and nature of the pathologic process.

TRANSSPHENOIDAL PITUITARY SURGERY. Tumor located within the sella turcica (intrasellar) and small adenomas of the pituitary can be removed by way of the nasal sphenoid sinus (transsphenoidal approach). This approach, which is being used with greater frequency, offers direct access to the sella with minimal risk of trauma and hemorrhage. It avoids many of the risks of craniotomy and the postoperative discomfort is similar to that of other transnasal operations.

The preoperative work-up includes a series of endo-crine tests, rhinologic evaluation and neuroradiologic studies. Funduscopic examination and visual field determinations are done, as the most serious effect of pituitary tumor is localized pressure on the optic nerve or chiasm. In addition, the nasopharyngeal secretions are cultured. Cortisone is usually given, and antibiotics are administered prophylactically on the morning of surgery and continued until the nasal packing is removed postoperatively.

While the initial surgical opening may be made by a rhinologic surgeon, the neurosurgen completes the opening into the sphenoid sinus and exposes the floor of the sella. Microsurgical techniques provide improved illumination, magnification and visualization so that nearby vital structures can be avoided.

Postoperative Management. The vital signs are monitored and the intake and output are measured as a guide to fluid and electrolyte replacement. Fluids are given when nausea ceases, and the patient progresses to a regular diet in 24 to 48 hours. Medications include antimicrobials which are continued until the nasal packing is removed, cortisone, analgesics and agents for the control of diabetes insipidus (pitressin).

The nasal packing is withdrawn slowly and is generally allowed to fall out from the 4th to 7th day. However, the patient must be cautioned against blowing his nose or engaging in any activity that raises intracranial pressure. The patient may be given an external metal nasal mold and tape and instructed to apply this mold at bedtime for a prescribed time period.

Excessive manipulation of the posterior pituitary gland during operation may produce transient diabetes insipidus of several days duration which is treated with pitressin. Occasionally there is permanent diabetes insipidus. Another complication may be postoperative meningitis.

SUMMARY: NURSING MANAGEMENT OF THE PATIENT HAVING INTRACRANIAL SURGERY
Objectives, Principles, and Rationale of Care

PREOPERATIVE CARE:
Objective: To determine the precise location of the lesion (clot, tumor, aneurysm).
1. Assist the patient undergoing diagnostic tests and frequent neurologic examinations.
2. Evaluate and record patient's symptoms and signs before the operation in order to make postoperative comparisons.
3. Support the patient with motor and sensory defects.
    a. Position paralyzed extremities correctly to prevent contracture deformities.
    b. Familiarize the blind patient with his environment.
       (1) Personnel entering the room should announce themselves—helps the patient understand incoming stimuli.

  (2) Help the patient to assume an active role in his care.
    c. Assist the aphasic patient to communicate by means of picture cards, writing materials, gestures, etc.
    d. Protect the confused patient.
       (1) Remove disturbing environmental stimuli.
       (2) Keep the patient oriented to time and place; place wall calendar and clock where he can see them.
    e. Instruct and encourage the patient and his family about the impending surgery.
4. Prepare the patient physically for surgery.
    a. Shave entire scalp immediately before surgery as directed; save the hair.
    b. Shampoo the scalp and report evidences of scalp infection.

(Continued)

PREOPERATIVE CARE (CONTINUED):

  c. Give enemas only as directed—straining upon defecation raises intracranial pressure.

  d. Give medications and treatments as indicated.

    (1) Steroids—to decrease brain edema

    (2) Indwelling spinal catheter connected to a stopcock—to decrease brain edema. Lumbar drainage can be stopped and started as required during procedure

    (3) Indwelling urethral catheter—to assess urinary volume during dehydrating operative period

POSTOPERATIVE MANAGEMENT:

Objectives: 1. To watch for life-threatening complications, namely increasing intracranial pressure from edema and bleeding.

          2. To improve the functional status of the patient.

1. Establish proper respiratory exchange—to eliminate systemic hypercarbia and hypoxia which increase cerebral edema.

  a. Keep the patient in a lateral or a semiprone position—to facilitate respiratory exchange.

  b. Employ tracheopharyngeal aspiration—to remove secretions.

  c. Carry out arterial blood gas studies—to determine respiratory adequacy.

  d. Elevate the head of the bed 30.5 cm. (12 inches) after patient is conscious—to aid venous drainage of the brain.

  e. See that the patient has nothing by mouth until an active coughing and swallowing reflex is demonstrated.

2. Assess patient's level of responsiveness:

  a. Response to commands

    (1) Answers questions readily and correctly.

    (2) Can perform a complex maneuver.

    (3) Responds to simple command.

    (4) Shows delayed or unequal response.

    (5) Reacts only to loud voice.

    (6) Does not respond.

  b. Assessment of spinal motor reflexes: (pinch Achilles tendon, arm, or other body site.)

    (1) Prompt, purposeful withdrawal

    (2) Sluggish or nonpurposeful movement of extremities

    (3) Facial grimace

    (4) Involuntary voiding

    (5) No response

  c. Observation of patient's spontaneous activity:

    (1) Verbal or other communication

    (2) Changes in posture (frequency)

    (3) Breathing pattern

    (4) Retching, vomiting

    (5) Restlessness, twitching, tremors, convulsions

3. Keep the patient normothermic during the postoperative period, since temperature control may be lost in certain neurologic states and a higher temperature increases the metabolic demands of the brain.

  a. Take rectal temperature at specified intervals.

    (1) Extremities may be cold and dry due to paralysis of heat-losing mechanisms (vasodilation and sweating).

  b. Employ measures to reduce excessive fever when present.

    (1) Remove blankets; place loincloth over patient.

    (2) Give aspirin if indicated. (High fever of central origin is less responsive to salicylates.)

    (3) Apply ice bags to axillae and groin—application of cold over large superficial vessels helps lower body temperature.

    (4) Give tepid water or alcohol sponge.

    (5) Place a fan so that it will blow on patient and increase surface cooling.

    (6) Use hypothermia blanket.

    (7 Give chlorpromazine (IM)—to prevent shivering.

    (8) Utilize ECG monitoring to detect arrhythmias during hypothermia procedures.

4. Evaluate for signs and symptoms of increasing intracranial pressure.

  a. Assess patient (minute by minute, hour by hour) for:

    (1) Diminished response to stimuli

    (2) Fluctuations of vital signs

    (3) Restlessness

    (4) Weakness and paralysis of extremities

    (5) Increasing headache

    (6) Changes or disturbances of vision; dilated pupils

  b. Control postoperative cerebral edema.

    (1) Keep patient *slightly* underhydrated—to combat cerebral edema.

    (2) Record urinary specific gravity at intervals—especially indicated for surgery of the pituitary and hypothalamus.

    (3) Evaluate electrolyte status:

      (a) Early postoperative gain indicates fluid retention; a greater than estimated weight loss indicates negative water balance.

      (b) Loss of sodium and chlorides will produce weakness, lethargy, and coma.

      (c) Low potassium will cause confusion and decreased level of responsiveness.

    (4) Give steroids, osmotic dehydrating agents, and glycerol in selected patients in the postoperative period.

    (5) Institute hypothermia procedures (see above) to decrease brain metabolism.

    (6) Elevate head of bed 20 to 30 degrees to reduce intracranial pressure and to facilitate respirations.

5. Perform supportive measures until the patient is able to care for himself.

  a. Change the position frequently, since pain and pressure responses are variable.

  b. Give analgesics that do not mask the level of responsiveness (codeine, aspirin).

SUMMARY: NURSING MANAGEMENT OF THE PATIENT HAVING INTRACRANIAL SURGERY (CONTINUED)
Objectives, Principles, and Rationale of Care

POSTOPERATIVE MANAGEMENT (CONTINUED):

   c. Support the patient if convulsive seizures occur (page 1244).

   d. Relieve signs of periocular edema.

     (1) Lubricate eyelids and around eyes with petrolatum.

     (2) Apply light cold compresses in pliofilm (taped over eye) at specified intervals.

     (3) Watch for signs of keratitis if cornea has no sensation.

   e. Put extremities through range of motion exercises.

   f. Use aseptic measures in management of indwelling 3-way urethral catheter (see page 911).

   g. Evaluate and support patient during episodes of restlessness.

     (1) Evaluate for airway obstruction, distended bladder, meningeal irritation from bloody cerebrospinal fluid.

     (2) Pad patient's hands and bed rails—to protect from injury.

   h. Watch for leakage of cerebrospinal fluid, since there is an ever present danger of meningitis.

     (1) Differentiate between cerebrospinal fluid (CSF) and mucus.

       (a) Collect fluid on Dextrostix; if CSF is present the indicator will have a positive reaction since cerebrospinal fluid contains sugar.

       (b) Assess for moderate elevation of temperature and mild neck rigidity.

     (2) Keep cerebrospinal pressure low.

       (a) Periodic lumbar punctures—to reduce cerebrospinal fluid pressure and decrease its force against the wound.

       (b) Ventricular catheters may be inserted in patient undergoing surgery of posterior fossa; catheter(s) connected to an external drainage bottle.

       (c) Elevate head of bed as prescribed.

       (d) Give antibiotics as indicated.

   i. Reinforce bloodstained dressings with sterile dressing; blood-soaked dressings act as a culture medium for bacteria.

   j. Evaluate patient with hypophysectomy (surgery upon pituitary) for diabetes insipidus.

     (1) Weigh daily.

     (2) Keep input and output record.

6. Assess for complications.

   a. Intracranial hemorrhage. (Postoperative bleeding may be intraventricular, intracerebral, intracerebellar, subdural or extradural.)

     (1) Watch for progressive impairment of state of responsiveness, signs of increasing intracranial pressure.

     (2) Prepare patient for cerebral angiography.

     (3) Prepare patient for re-operation and evacuation of hematoma.

   b. Brain edema.

   c. Postoperative meningitis.

   d. Wound infections (scalp, bone flap)—wound may have to be reopened.

   e. Pulmonary complications.

   f. Epilepsy. (There is a greater risk of epilepsy with supratentorial operations.)

     (1) Give anticonvulsants on a long-term basis.

     (2) Watch for status epilepticus which may occur after any intracranial operation.

   g. Gastrointestinal ulceration (signs and symptoms of hemorrhage and perforation or both).

BIBLIOGRAPHY

BOOKS

Adams, R. D., and Victor, M.: Principles of Neurology. New York, McGraw-Hill, 1977.

Allen, M. B., Jr., et al.: A Manual of Neurosurgery. Baltimore, University Park Press, 1978.

American Nurses Association, Division Medical-Surgical Nursing Practice and the American Association of Neurosurgical Nurses: Standards of Neurological and Neurosurgical Nursing Practice. Kansas City, American Nurses Association, 1977.

Appenzeller, O.: Pathogenesis and Treatment of Headache. New York, Spectrum Pub., 1976.

Brown, A.: Physiological and Psychological Considerations in the Management of Stroke. St. Louis, Warren H. Green, 1976.

Buerger, A. A., and Tobis, J. S., eds.: Neurophysiologic Aspects of Rehabilitation Medicine. Springfield, Ill., Charles C Thomas, 1974.

Cohen, L. K.: Communication Aids for the Brain Damaged Adult. Minneapolis, Sister Kenny Institute, 1976.

Conway, B. L.: Carini and Owens' Neurological and Neurosurgical Nursing, 7th ed. St. Louis, C. V. Mosby, 1978.

Crickmay, M. C.: Helping the Stroke Patient To Talk. Springfield, Ill., Charles C Thomas, 1977.

Darmody, W. R.: Management of the Unconscious Patient. St. Louis, C. V. Mosby, 1976.

Eliasson, S. G., Prensky, A. L., and Hardin, W. B.: Neurological Pathophysiology, 2nd ed. New York, Oxford University Press, 1978.

Goldensohn, E. S., and Appel, S. H., eds.: Scientific Approaches to Clinical Neurology. Vols. 1 & 2. Philadelphia, Lea and Febiger, 1977.

Haynes, W. O., and Greenberg, B. R.: Understanding Aphasia: A Guide for Medical and Paramedical Personnel. Danville, Ill., Interstate Prints and Publishers, 1976.

Howe, J. J. R.: Patient Care in Neurosurgery. Boston, Little, Brown, 1977.

Jacox, A. K., ed.: Pain: A Source Book for Nurses and Other Health Professionals. Boston, Little, Brown, 1977.

Johnston, M.: The Stroke Patient: Principles of Rehabilitation. New York, Churchill Livingston, 1976.

Lee, J. F., ed.: Pain Management. Symposium on the Neurosurgical Treatment of Pain. Baltimore, Williams and Wilkins, 1977.

LeRoy, P. L., Boulos, M. I., and Goloskov, J.: Current Concepts in the Management of Chronic Pain. New York, Stratton Intercontinental Medical Book Corp., 1976.

Leutenegger, R. R.: Patient Care and Rehabilitation of Communication-Impaired Adults. Springfield, Ill., Charles C Thomas, 1975.

Licht, S.: Stroke and its Rehabilitation. Baltimore, Waverly Press, 1975.

Lipton, S.: Persistent Pain: Modern Methods of Treatment. Vol. 1. New York, Grune and Stratton, 1977.

Lewis, A. J.: Mechanisms of Neurological Disease. Boston, Little, Brown, 1976.

Marshall, J.: The Management of Cerebrovascular Disease, 3rd ed. Oxford, Blackwell Scientific Publications, 1976.

Merritt, H. H.: A Textbook of Neurology, 6th ed. Philadelphia, Lea and Febiger, 1979.

Mossman, P. L.: Problem Oriented Approach to Stroke. Springfield, Ill., Charles C Thomas, 1976.

O'Brien, M. T., and Pallet, P. J.: Total Care of the Stroke Patient. Boston, Little, Brown, 1978.

O'Connor, A. B., ed.: Nursing in Neurological Disorders. New York, American Journal of Nursing Co., 1976.

Patton, H. D., et al.: Introduction to Basic Neurology. Philadelphia, W. B. Saunders, 1976.

Robinson, J., and Gyetan, M.: Coping with Neurological Problems Proficiently. Horsham, Pa., Intermed Communications, 1979.

Siev, E., and Freishat, B.: Perceptual Dysfunction in the Adult Stroke Patient. Thorofare, N. J., Charles B. Slack, 1976.

Samuels, M. A., ed.: Manual of Neurologic Therapeutics. Boston, Little, Brown, 1978.

Swift, N., and Mabel, R. M.: Manual of Neurological Nursing. Boston, Little, Brown, 1978.

Treip, C. S.: Color Atlas of Neuropathology. Chicago, Year Book Medical Pub., 1978.

Vick, N. A.: Grinker's Neurology, 7th ed. Springfield, Ill., Charles C Thomas, 1976.

Walton, J. N.: Essentials of Neurology, 4th ed. Philadelphia, J. B. Lippincott, 1976.

ARTICLES

Surgery

Calcaterra, T. C., and Rand, R. W.: Current adjuncts for surgery of the sphenoid sinus and pituitary gland. Laryngoscope, *86*:1692-1698, Nov. 1976.

Cannon, M.: To Sharon, with love. AJN., *79*:642-645, Apr. 1979.

Kern, E. B., et al.: A transseptal, transsphenoidal approach to the pituitary. Postgrad. Med., *63*:97-108, June 1978.

May, P. B.: Initial evaluation and management of patients with suspected pituitary tumors. Prim. Care, *4*:89-125, Mar. 1977.

Ontjes, D. A., and Ney, R. L.: Pituitary tumors. CA, *26*:330-350, Nov.-Dec., 1976.

Rhoton, A. L.: Neurologic surgery. Surg. Gyn. Obstet., *142*:205-208, Feb., 1976.

Headache

Friedman, A. P., ed.: Headache and related pain syndromes. Med. Clin. N. Am., *62*:427-620 (entire vol.), May, 1978.

Freemon, F. R.: Evaluation and treatment of headache. Geriatrics, *33*:82-85, May 1978.

Medina, J. L., and Diamond, S.: The clinical link between migraine and cluster headaches. Arch. Neurol., *34*:470-472, Aug. 1977.

Saper, J. R.: Migraine. JAMA, *239*:2380-2383, June 2, 1978.

Intracranial Pressure Monitoring

Barker, J.: Postoperative care of the neurosurgical patient. Br. J. Anaesth., *48*:797-804, Aug. 1976.

Fleischer, A. S., Patton, J. M., and Tindall, G. T.: Monitoring intraventricular pressure using an implanted reservoir in head injured patients. Surg. Neurol., *3*:309-311, June 1975.

Goloskov, J. W., and LeRoy, P. L.: The role of the nurse in quantitative intracranial pressure determinations. J. Neurosurg. Nurs., *10*:17-19, Mar. 1978.

Johnson, M., and Quinn, J.: The subarachnoid screw. AJN, *77*:448-450, Mar. 1977.

Miller, J. D.: Intracranial pressure monitoring. Br. J. Hosp. Med., *19*:497-503, May 1978.

Mitchell, P. H., and Mauss, N. K.: Intracranial pressure: Fact and fancy. Nursing '76, *6*:53-57, June 1976.

———: Relationship of patient-nurse activity to intracranial pressure variations: A pilot study. Nurs. Res., *27*:4-10, Jan.-Feb. 1978.

Rosner, M. J., and Becker, D. P.: ICP monitoring: Complications and associated factors. Clin. Neurosurg., *23*:494-519, 1976.

Taylor, F. A., and Schutz, H.: Symptoms caused by intracranial pressure waves. J. Neurosurg. Nurs., *9*:144-146, Dec. 1977.

White, R. J.: Chronic monitoring of head injury with an implantable ventricular module. J. Trauma, *17*:521-525, July 1977.

Winn, H. R., Dacey, R. G., and Jane, J. A.: Intracranial subarachnoid pressure recording: Experience with 650 patients. Surg. Neurol., *8*:41-47, July 1977.

Pain

Davis, A. J.: Teaching your patients to use electricity to ward off pain. RN, *41*:43-45, Feb. 1978.

Gramse, C. A.: For control of severe pain: Dorsal column stimulation. AJN, *78*:1022-1025, June 1978.

Loeser, J. D.: Neurosurgical control of chronic pain. Arch. Surg., *112*:880-883, July 1977.

Ostrowski, M. D., and Dodd, V. A.: Transcutaneous nerve stimulation for relief of pain in advanced malignant disease. Nurs. Times, *73*:1233-1238, Aug. 11, 1977.

Perret, G., and McDonnell, D.: Neurosurgical control of pain in the patient with cancer. Curr. Probl. Cancer, *1*:1-27, Mar. 1977.

Pineda, A.: Complications of dorsal column stimulation. J. Neurosurg., *48*:64-68, Jan. 1978.

Stroke Rehabilitation

Anderson, T. P., and Kottke, F. J.: Stroke rehabilitation: A reconsideration of some common attitudes. Arch. Phys. Med. Rehabil., *59*:175-181, Apr. 1978.

Bellows, J. G.: Stroke prevention. Compr. Ther., *4*:3-4, Feb. 1978.

Coleman, L.: The objectives and final goals of physical therapy. Geriatrics, *31*:91-95, May 1976.

Fox, M. J.: Patients with receptive aphasia: They really don't understand. AJN, *76*:1596-1598, Oct. 1976.

Guentz, S., and Navales, R. D.: New approaches to the nursing care of the stroke patient. Clin. Orthopaed. & Related Res., *131*:90-96, Mar.-Apr. 1978.

Heaney, L. M.: Cardiac and respiratory monitoring of acute stroke patients. Heart Lung, *6*:469-474, May-June 1977.

Isaacs, B.: Problems and solutions in rehabilitation of stroke patients. Geriatrics, *33*:87-91, July 1978.

Thompson, R. A., and Green, J. R., eds.: Stroke. Adv. in Neurol., *16*:1-225 (entire vol.), 1977.

Waters, R. L., ed.: Symposium on stroke rehabilitation. Clin. Orthopaed. and Related Res., *131*:2-122, Mar.-Apr. 1978.

AGENCIES

Governmental

Division for the Blind and Physically Handicapped, Library of Congress, Washington, D.C. 20542

National Institute of Neurological and Communicative Disorders and Stroke, National Institutes of Health, Bethesda, Md. 20205

Voluntary

American Speech and Hearing Association, 10801 Rockville Pike, Rockville, Md. 20852

National Easter Seal Society for Crippled Children and Adults, 2023 W. Ogden Ave., Chicago, Ill. 60612

55

MANAGEMENT OF PATIENTS WITH NEUROLOGIC DISORDERS

CRANIAL, SPINAL AND PERIPHERAL NEUROPATHIES

1st Cranial (Olfactory) Nerve

Disturbances of the olfactory bulbs due to intracranial diseases reveal themselves when the sense of smell is lost (anosmia) or altered (perversions).

ANOSMIA. Loss of smell follows fractures of the base of the skull which cause lacerations of the olfactory nerves (fine filaments that pass from the bulb to the olfactory mucous membrane through small holes in the cribriform plate of the ethmoid bone). Falls or blows on the back of the head that merely jar the skull but cause contusion of these filaments may also produce temporary anosmia.

2nd Cranial (Optic) Nerve

Diseases of and injuries to the optic nerves, whatever their nature, cause reduction in the acuity of vision and contraction of the visual fields-symptoms that may progress to complete blindness.

PAPILLEDEMA OR CHOKED DISK. Edematous swelling of the head of the optic nerve appears in all conditions that increase the intracranial pressure, such as brain tumors, abscess, and acute hemorrhage into the brain.

SECONDARY OPTIC ATROPHY. Optic atrophy is the out-come of prolonged severe choking of the optic disk, neuritis of the optic nerve, closure of its central artery, pressure against it by brain tumors, and fractures of the base of the skull that involve the optic foramen (through which the optic nerve leaves the skull). Optic atrophy is also an important early sign of multiple sclerosis. It is one of the manifestations of central nervous system syphilis and an effect of methanol poisoning.

3rd, 4th and 6th Cranial Nerves (Oculomotor, Trochlear, and Abducens)

The oculomotor nerve supplies all but two of the muscles that move the eyeball. One of these two, the superior oblique, is innervated by the 4th cranial (trochlear) nerve; the other, the external rectus muscle, which rotates the eyeball outward, is innervated by the 6th cranial (abducens) nerve. Paralysis of any one of these three nerves produces a particular type of strabismus (squint) (depending on the muscle paralyzed). Paralysis of the 3rd nerve produces ptosis and dilation of the pupils as well. Such paralysis follows poisoning by alcohol, lead, or carbon monoxide and infections, such as botulism, measles, and encephalitis. Much more often, the cause is related to syphilis, multiple sclerosis, fractures of the base of the skull, and middle ear infections.

1214

5th Cranial (Trigeminal) Nerve

The trigeminal nerve supplies all the sensory fibers to the skin of the face (except the angle of the jaw and the anterior half of the scalp), the teeth, the conjunctivae, the mucous membrane covering the inside of the mouth, the nose, the paranasal sinuses, and the greater part of the tongue. The lowest branch of this nerve also contains the motor fibers that control the muscles of mastication (see Fig. 55-1).

One, two, or all three branches of this nerve (ophthalmic, maxillary, and mandibular) may be affected by disease and by trauma, and the disturbances that follow always correspond exactly to the areas of distribution of the branch affected. Severe injury to one of these nerves, such as contusions over the supraorbital notch or the intraorbital foramen, may be followed by anesthesia of the area it supplies. If the trauma merely irritates or compresses the nerve, then pain follows. If, however, the trauma causes bleeding into the tissue in the area of the nerve, the scar tissue that forms afterward may so compress its fibers that months later localized pain appears in the forehead or the cheek. This pain may continue indefinitely.

HERPES ZOSTER. The ophthalmic branch of the trigeminal nerve may be affected by herpes zoster. Herpes zoster (shingles) is caused by a virus which produces a painful vesicular eruption in the cutaneous areas supplied by peripheral sensory nerves arising in the affected root ganglia. It most commonly attacks the chest wall, but when it involves the ophthalmic branch of the trigeminal nerve, it produces painful lesions on the eyelid, conjunctiva, and cornea. The patient experiences severe pain over the affected nerve followed by an eruption of vesicles that may rupture to form a crust. The healing of pustules on the cornea may cause scarring and impaired vision. Therefore, patients with ophthalmic herpes zoster should be examined by an ophthalmologist.

Frequently, *postherpetic neuralgia* occurs long after the lesions have healed. The pain is particularly severe in the elderly. Pain is controlled with analgesics, and topical steroids are given to promote healing. Systemic corticosteroids are sometimes indicated. Herpes zoster may indicate the presence of serious internal disease (Hodgkin's disease, leukemia, malignancy) in persons past middle age.

OTHER CAUSES OF FACIAL PAIN. Facial pain related to the trigeminal nerve may result from lesions that directly irritate the trigeminal nerve or its ganglion or from diseases of other organs that refer their pains to the area distributed by the trigeminal nerve. Among such lesions are inflammatory processes and neoplasms in the soft tissues and the bones of the face; paranasal sinus infections; infected teeth; unerupted third molar teeth; tumors

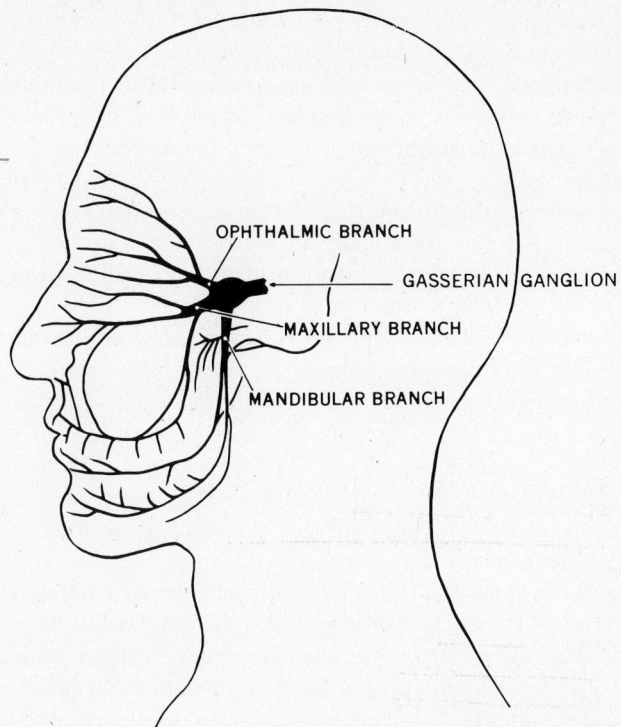

Figure 55-1. The main divisions of the trigeminal nerve are the ophthalmic, maxillary, and mandibular. Sensory root fibers arise in the Gasserian ganglion.

and aneurysms about the base of the skull; venous sinus thrombosis; basilar meningitis; tumors of the Gasserian ganglion; diseases of the sphenopalatine ganglion, the middle ear, and the orbit of the eye; such conditions as eyestrain, migraine, and multiple sclerosis; and occasionally syphilis, diabetes, nephritis, and malaria. Facial pain for which no cause can be demonstrated is referred to as atypical facial pain. A very specific type of facial pain is trigeminal neuralgia or tic douloureux (see below).

Trigeminal Neuralgia (Tic Douloureux)

Trigeminal neuralgia is a condition of the 5th cranial nerve characterized by an explosive onset of pain similar to an electric shock or a lancinating burning sensation in the area distributed by one or more branches of the trigeminal nerve. The pain ends as abruptly as it starts. Each pain episode can be described as stabbing and explosive and produces contraction of some of the facial muscles, such as a sudden closing of the eye or a twitch of the mouth; hence the name, tic douloureux (painful twitch). The etiology is not known, but some investigators believe that it may be due to vascular pressure from structural abnormalities (loop of an artery) encroaching upon the trigeminal nerve, Gasserian ganglion, or root entry zone. Early attacks, appearing most often in the fifth decade of life, are usually mild and brief. Pain-free intervals may be measured in terms of minutes, hours, days, or longer. With advancing years, the painful episodes tend to become more and more frequent and agonizing.

The pain of this neuralgia is felt in the skin, not in the deeper structures, but it is more severe at the peripheral areas of distribution of the affected nerve, notably over the lip, the chin, the ala nasi, and in the teeth. Paroxysms are aroused by any stimulation of the terminals of the affected branches, such as washing the face, shaving, brushing the teeth, eating, and drinking. A draft of cold air and direct pressure against the nerve trunk may also cause pain. Certain areas are called *trigger points,* since the slightest touch immediately starts a paroxysm. To avoid stimulating these areas, patients with trigeminal neuralgia try not to touch or wash their faces, shave, chew, or do anything else that might cause an attack. Behavior of this type is a clue to diagnosis.

Management. The antiepileptic drugs carbamazepine (Tegretol) and phenytoin (Dilantin) will relieve pain in most patients. Carbamazepine is taken with meals, in gradually increased dosages until relief is obtained. Side effects include nausea, dizziness, hematosuppression, and hepatic dysfunction. The patient's blood is monitored for bone marrow depression. Phenytoin also produces such side effects as nausea, dizziness, somnolence, ataxia, and skin allergies.

Alcohol injection of the Gasserian ganglion and peripheral branches of the trigeminal nerve will relieve pain for several months. However, the pain returns after the nerve regenerates.

Percutaneous Radiofrequency Trigeminal Gangliolysis. Surgical interruption of the trigeminal system is considered when drugs do not relieve pain without causing considerable side effects. Percutaneous radiofrequency interruption of the Gasserian ganglion, whereby the small unmyelinated and thinly myelinated fibers which conduct the pain are thermally destroyed, is becoming the procedure of choice.

Under local anesthesia, the needle is introduced through the cheek on the affected side. Under fluoroscopic control, the needle electrode is guided through the foramen ovale into the Gasserian ganglion. The divisions of the Gasserian ganglion (mandibular, maxillary, and ophthalmic) are encountered sequentially. The nerve is stimulated with a small current, while the patient is awake. The patient then reports when a tingling sensation is felt. When the electrode needle is in the desired position, the patient is anesthetized briefly and a radiofrequency current (heating current to destroy the nerve) is passed in a controlled manner to thermally injure the trigeminal ganglion and rootlets (Fig. 55-2). The patient is then awakened from the anesthetic and examined for sensory deficits. Repeat lesions may be produced until the desired effect is achieved. The operative procedure takes less than one hour and gives permanent pain relief in most patients. Touch and proprioceptive functions are left intact.

Microvascular Decompression of the Trigeminal Nerve. An intracranial approach (retromastoid craniectomy) can be used to decompress the trigeminal nerve since tic douloureux may be caused by vascular compression of the entry zone of the trigeminal root by an arterial loop and occasionally by a vein. With the aid of an operating microscope, the artery loop is lifted from the nerve in order to relieve the pressure, and a small prosthetic device is inserted to prevent recurrence of impingement on the nerve. The postoperative management is the same as for any intracranial operation.

Preoperative Management. Preoperative management of a patient with trigeminal neuralgia includes recognizing that certain factors may aggravate excruciating facial pain, such as food that is too hot or too cold or jarring the bed. Even washing the face, combing the hair, or brushing the teeth may produce acute bouts of pain. The nurse can lessen these discomforts in a variety of ways—by using cotton pads to wash the patient's face, substituting a blunt-tooth comb to comb the hair, etc.

7th Cranial (Facial) Nerve

The facial nerve is the chief motor nerve of the muscles of the face. Its few sensory fibers are disregarded in this discussion.

FACIAL PARALYSIS. There are three types of facial paralysis: peripheral, nuclear, and upper motor neuron. The peripheral type is produced by interruption or dysfunction of the facial nerve when the trunk of the nerve is involved distal to its exit from the skull or within the

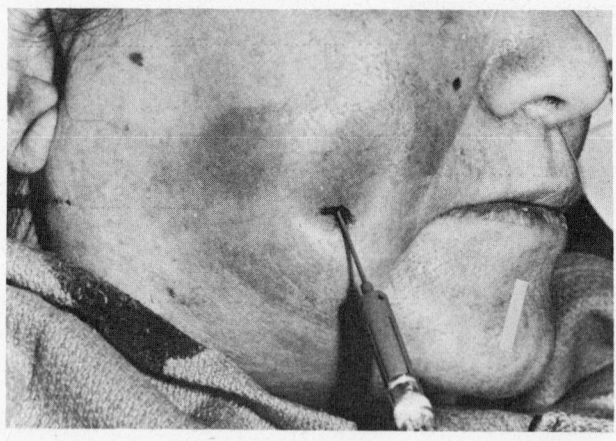

Figure 55-2. Percutaneous radio-frequency rhizotomy for relief of pain from trigeminal neuralgia. The needle electrode has been inserted so that it may be advanced under x-ray control to the area where the heat lesion will be made. This procedure requires only a brief hospital stay without the time, expense, and hazards of an open cranial procedure. (From Silverberg, G. D.: Percutaneous radio-frequency rhizotomy in the treatment of trigeminal neuralgia. Western J. Med., Aug. 1978, p. 98)

temporal bone through which it courses. External lesions are usually the result of direct trauma or a suppurative infection of the parotid gland, whereas those occurring within the skull are encountered as complications of mastoiditis, mastoid surgery, or fractures of the skull that involve the temporal bone.

Peripheral facial neuritis is manifested by complete paralysis of the face on the same side as the lesion. As a result, the mouth is drawn toward the normal side, the wrinkles of the forehead and the nasolabial fold are obliterated on the paralyzed side, and the eye remains open, its upper lid drooping and its lower lid slightly everted, allowing the tears to escape over the cheek. The patient cannot puff out the cheek, close the mouth, or show the teeth on the paralyzed side. One form of peripheral paralysis is Bell's palsy.

Bell's Palsy

Bell's palsy (facial paralysis) is due to peripheral involvement of the 7th cranial nerve on one side which results in weakness or paralysis of the facial muscles. The etiology is unknown, although possible causes may include vascular ischemia, viral disease (herpes simplex; herpes zoster), autoimmune disease, or a combination of all of these factors.

Pathophysiology. Bell's palsy is considered by some to represent a type of pressure paralysis. The inflamed, edematous nerve becomes compressed to the point of damage, or its nutrient vessel is occluded to the point of producing ischemia necrosis of the nerve within its long canal—a channel in which the fit at best is very snug. There is distortion of the face from paralysis of the facial muscles, increased lacrimation (tearing), and painful sensations in the face, behind the ear, and in the eye. The patient may experience speech difficulties and may be unable to eat on the affected side because of relaxation of the facial muscle.

Management. The objectives of treatment are to maintain the muscle tone of the face and to prevent or minimize denervation. The patient should be reassured that he has not had a stroke and that spontaneous recovery occurs within 3 to 5 weeks in the majority of cases.

Steroid therapy (prednisone) may be given to reduce inflammation and edema, which in turn reduces vascular compression and permits restoration of blood circulation to the nerve. Early administration of the drug appears to diminish the severity of the disease, relieves the pain, and helps prevent or minimize denervation.

While the paralysis lasts, the involved eye must be protected. Frequently the patient's eye does not close completely and the blink reflex is diminished so that the eye is vulnerable to dust and foreign particles. Corneal irritation and ulceration are a major threat to this patient. Sometimes there is an overflow of tears down the cheek (epiphora) from keratitis caused by drying of the cornea and lack of the blink reflex. The laxity of the lower lid

alters the proper drainage of tears. To counter these problems, the eye should be covered with a protective shield at night. However, the eye patch may abrade the cornea, since there is some difficulty in keeping the partially paralyzed eyelids closed. The application of eye ointment at bedtime will cause the eyelids to adhere to one another and remain closed during sleep. If this approach does not work, the eyelids may have to be temporarily sutured together. Wraparound sunglasses or goggles are worn to decrease normal evaporation from the eye.

Face pain is controlled with salicylates or codeine. Heat may be applied to the involved side of the face to promote comfort and the flow of blood through the muscles. If the nerve is not too sensitive, the face may be massaged several times daily to maintain muscle tone. The technique is to massage the face with a gentle upward motion. Facial exercises, such as wrinkling the forehead, blowing out the cheeks, and whistling, may be performed with the aid of a mirror and are intended to prevent muscle atrophy. The face should be kept warm.

Electrical stimulation may be applied to the face to prevent atrophy of the muscle until reinnervation occurs.

In selected cases, surgical decompression of the facial nerve has been recommended to allow the edematous facial nerve to expand into the stylomastoid foramen. The decision as to which patient should be treated surgically is a difficult one and is made on the basis of the patient's clinical status, electrical testing of the facial muscles, and the physician's clinical experience. Although most patients recover with conservative treatment (80–90 percent) surgical intervention is necessary in some patients to help regain maximum function of the facial nerve and to avoid and minimize the complications of degeneration and regeneration.

Other forms of facial paralysis include nuclear facial paralysis and upper motor neuron facial paralysis:

NUCLEAR FACIAL PARALYSIS. The nuclear type of facial palsy is caused by destruction of the nuclei from which the fibers of the 7th nerve originate. Neoplastic vascular or degenerative lesions in the pons are usually responsible for this form of facial palsy.

UPPER MOTOR NEURON FACIAL PARALYSIS. If this type of paralysis is due to lesions (such as tumors, abscesses, depressed skull fractures, etc.) which injure the motor cortical area governing the face, only the muscles of the lower half of the face become paralyzed. The muscles around the eyes and the forehead escape because they are bilaterally innervated from the cortex. The paralysis occurs on the side opposite that of the lesion. Patients with facial palsy of the upper motor neuron type cannot force a smile no matter how hard they try, but they do smile involuntarily when amused. Their 7th nerve connections to the cortex are severed, but the nerve itself is intact, and the subcortical centers are in sole control.

8th Cranial (Auditory-Vestibular) Nerve

Each 8th cranial nerve has two divisions: the auditory (cochlear) and the vestibular portions (the nerve to the semicircular canal system). Disturbances of the auditory nerve impair hearing; disturbances of the vestibular nerve produce vertigo (sensations of turning or falling) and nystagmus. Meniere's disease, a disease of the 8th cranial nerve, is discussed in Chapter 52.

9th Cranial (Glossopharyngeal) Nerve

GLOSSOPHARYNGEAL PARALYSIS. This paralysis (usually in association with disturbances of the vagus nerve) results in difficulty in swallowing, anesthesia of the upper portion of the pharynx, and loss of taste over the posterior third of the tongue on the same side as the lesion. It most often is due to brain diseases—such as tumors.

GLOSSOPHARYNGEAL NEURALGIA. Neuritis of the 9th nerve causes glossopharyngeal neuralgia which is characterized by severe pain radiating from the base of the tongue to deep in the ear. There is also an increase in salivation. Resection of this nerve may cure the problem.

10th Cranial (Vagus) Nerve

The vagus nerve is the motor nerve of the voluntary muscles of the throat and the larynx, and is the nerve that slows the rate of heartbeat and supplies the parasympathetic nerves to the lungs, the stomach, the esophagus, and other abdominal organs.

NEURITIS. Neuritis of this nerve occasionally occurs in such acute infections as pneumonia and influenza and results from the action of such poisons as alcohol, lead, and arsenic. The vagus nerve (usually in association with the glossopharyngeal) frequently is injured by lesions of the pons and the base of the skull.

PARALYSIS. Paralysis of one vagus nerve causes unilateral paralysis of the larynx, with resultant impairment of speech, difficulty in swallowing, temporary changes in the heart rate and rhythm and, occasionally, vomiting, abdominal pain, and anorexia. Complete paralysis of both vagi is followed by permanent tachycardia, since the accelerator nerves of the heart (sympathetic fibers) then lack the normal inhibition of the vagi.

The recurrent laryngeal branch of this nerve, because of its position, is injured easily. The result is paralysis of the larynx and, therefore, hoarseness. This may be caused by the pressure of mediastinal tumors, masses of enlarged lymph nodes in the mediastinum or the neck, aneurysms of the aorta or the subclavian artery, and malignant growths of the thyroid gland or adjacent structures. This nerve is occasionally severed by wounds and operations on the neck, such as thyroidectomy.

11th Cranial (Spinal Accessory) Nerve

The spinal accessory nerve, entirely motor in nature, supplies the sternomastoid muscle and the upper portion of the trapezius muscles. Injuries to and diseases of this nerve, therefore, weaken the power to rotate the head to the side opposite the lesion and cause a slight drooping of the shoulder on the side of the lesion. Such paralysis may result from penetrating wounds and operations on the neck, fractures of the skull, injuries to and diseases of the cervical vertebrae, rickets, unilateral poliomyelitis, and all diseases that involve the upper portion of the cervical cord.

12th Cranial (Hypoglossal) Nerve

The hypoglossal nerves, entirely motor in character, innervate the muscles of the tongue only. Injury to one of these nerves, with resultant paralysis of that side of the tongue, is rare but can occur from deep penetrating wounds, abscesses and tumors of the neck, and trauma to and tuberculosis of the first cervical vertebra; much more frequently, this paralysis is evidence of brain disease.

The tongue, when paralyzed on one side, will deviate toward the weak side when it protrudes from the mouth. When both hypoglossal nerves are paralyzed, the tongue cannot be moved; hence, speech, mastication, and swallowing cannot be performed properly.

The Brachial Plexus

Paralysis of the brachial plexus and the nerves arising from it occasionally follows violent movements of the shoulder, the head, and the arm, which overstretch or even tear the root of this plexus. (Erb's palsy of the infant results from dislocation during birth of the humerus, which forcibly pushes the head of the bone against this plexus.) The brachial plexus (and also its roots) occasionally suffers from the pressure of local tumors, aneurysms, and masses of enlarged lymph nodes in the neck or the axilla.

CERVICAL RIBS. A cervical rib is one or a pair of extra ribs attached usually to the 7th cervical vertebra. If a pair is present, one only may produce symptoms. They are found more frequently in women than in men, occasionally in several members of the same family, and usually in association with other anatomic anomalies.

A cervical rib is a lifelong hazard to the brachial plexus. Because of its presence, the plexus may be crushed by accidents that suddenly force or pull the shoulder down; this trauma is followed by pain and numbness, felt first in the fingers and gradually extending up the forearm, and later by weakness, followed by atrophy of the muscles of that hand and arm. The continuous pressure of a cervical rib on the brachial plexus (the symptoms of which seldom appear before middle life) affects first its sympathetic nerve fibers, as shown by such vasomotor signs as cyanosis, coldness, paleness, and edema (a syndrome that at first may suggest Raynaud's disease). Later this pressure causes disturbances of sensation and finally atrophy of the muscles of the arm and the hand.

Since the presence of a cervical rib frequently produces developmental abnormalities in the pattern of the brachial plexus, the findings on physical examination often are puzzling. Thus, various muscles and skin areas of the arm and the hand seem to be supplied by the wrong nerves; the arteries of the shoulder region may lie in an unusual position or be abnormal in their relative size; and often the pulse volume of the radial artery of that arm is unusually small and the blood pressure low. Cervical ribs are not always visible on x-ray films, since some constitute merely fibrous bands. However, they exert pressures just as serious as those produced by bone.

The Nerves of the Arms

FLEETING NEURALGIC PAINS. Pains referred to the shoulder and the upper arm are common following exposure to cold and occur frequently in chronic and often latent general infections and in cases of spondylitis and chronic subdeltoid bursitis. To this region, particularly on the left side, are referred the pains of aortitis and coronary artery disease (for example, angina pectoris), and to both sides, those of acute pleuritis. More constant pain, with or without accompanying muscular weakness, results from pressure against the roots of the brachial plexus by spinal tumors, by a herniated cervical disk, and occasionally by the scalenus anticus neck muscles between which these nerves course. A true toxic neuritis, which affects the radial nerve in particular, is one of the features of lead poisoning.

RADIAL NERVE PARALYSIS. This paralysis, causing *wrist-drop,* may be the result of pressure against the trunk of the radial nerve as it lies in the axilla. Such pressure may be caused by a crutch or the back of a bench over which the arm is thrown. It also follows blows against the outer aspect of the upper arm, where this nerve lies in an unprotected position. The same type of paralysis also may be caused by a tourniquet that is applied to the arm too tightly or allowed to remain on for too long a time. Late radial paralysis, appearing 3 to 4 weeks following fracture of the humerus, results from the gradual compression of this nerve by either excessive callus formation or—more often—by contracting scar tissue formed in tissues infiltrated by blood.

ULNAR NERVE. The ulnar nerve is often traumatized at the elbow, where it lies in an exposed position. To hit the "crazy bone" really is to strike the ulnar nerve. Even the simple act of reclining on the elbow may cause a pressure paralysis of several weeks' duration in the muscles that this nerve supplies. Dislocation of the elbow and fracture of the bones near this joint may stretch or compress this nerve, causing immediate paralysis of the same muscles or weakness due to delayed neuritis.

The Intercostal Nerves

The intercostal nerves may be injured by trauma to the chest wall and fracture of the ribs, causing pain in their areas of distribution. Anesthesia never results if only a single nerve is injured, because of the overlapping of the areas supplied by the two adjacent nerves.

NEURITIS. Intercostal neuritis is usually due to disease of the nerve proper (as in herpes zoster) or of the nerve roots in the spinal canal (as in exostoses of the vertebrae in hypertrophic osteoarthritis or in metastatic malignancy of the vertebrae). The sensation is generally described as a sore, burning or shooting "electric" pain.

The Lumbar and Sacral Plexuses

THE LUMBAR PLEXUS. Tumors of the vertebrae, retroperitoneal neoplasms, enlarged inflamed pelvic lymph nodes, and psoas abscesses occasionally cause enough pressure on the lumbar plexus to cause weakness or paralysis of the anterior thigh muscles that are supplied by the femoral nerve.

THE SACRAL PLEXUS. The sacral plexus may be torn by fractures of the lower lumbar vertebrae and the sacrum or it may be subjected to pressure from large fibroid tumors of the uterus and malignant growths within the pelvis. It may also be traumatized during difficult labor. The chief symptom produced is spasmodic or continuous pain, often called *sciatica.*

SCIATICA. The term *sciatica* refers to any condition in which the most prominent symptom is pain along the course of the sciatic nerve. Its etiology in many instances is uncertain. Some patients give a past history of sprain of the lumbosacral or the sacroiliac joints. In other instances, spondylitis, spondylolisthesis, or a ruptured intervertebral disc pressing on the cauda equina may be responsible. In some instances, primary neuritis is assumed to be responsible.

Peripheral Neuropathies (Polyneuritis)

NEURITIS. Neuritis is the term applied to both demonstrable inflammatory or degenerative changes in peripheral nerves and (less scientifically) to symptoms that suggest these changes. The patient has resultant motor weakness, sensory loss, and varying degrees of pain.

Neuritis may involve one nerve only (*mononeuritis*), or several nerves (*polyneuritis* or *multiple neuritis*). In all cases of the latter, the same nerves on the two sides of the body are involved similarly. The symptoms of all types of neuritis, according to the character of the nerves involved, are sensory, motor, and vasomotor, these signs always being limited to the structures that the affected nerves supply. Mononeuritis and polyneuritis, however, differ much in their etiology, course, and treatment.

Neuritis of a sensory nerve causes pain and disturbances of sensation, provided that the nerve is able to function in some degree. Anesthesia occurs if the process is severe. In the case of nerves that are partly or wholly motor, the result of neuritis is either weakness or complete paralysis of the muscles that they control, depending on the degree of severity.

MONONEURITIS. Mononeuritis is limited to a single

peripheral nerve and its branches. It arises when the trunk of the nerve is *traumatized,* as when bruised by a blow; *overstretched,* as in cases of dislocation of a joint; *pressed upon,* as by a tumor, a cervical rib, a crutch, or bony exostoses (e.g., in that type of arthritis that narrows the apertures between adjacent vertebrae through which the spinal nerves pass); *punctured* by a needle used to inject a drug or poisoned by the drugs thus injected; or *inflamed* because of the extension to its trunk of an adjacent infectious process. Mononeuritis is frequently seen in the diabetic patient.

One type of mononeuritis appears many months after an injury that caused considerable bleeding into the tissues surrounding a nerve. In tissues thus infiltrated with blood, considerable scar tissue forms, which contracts and slowly compresses the nerve. Similarly, delayed nerve paralysis follows the healing of an abscess, the encapsulation of a foreign body or sequestra of bone, and the healing of fractured bone. In this last case, however, the nerve trunk is caught in the callus.

Pain is seldom a conspicuous symptom of mononeuritis due to trauma, but in patients with complicating inflammatory conditions, such as arthritis, this feature is prominent. Such pain is increased by all body movements that tend to stretch, strain, or cause pressure on the injured nerve, and by all sudden jars of the body, such as those incident to coughing and sneezing. The skin in the areas supplied by nerves that are injured or diseased may become reddened and glossy; its subcutaneous tissue may become edematous, and the nutrition of the nails and the hair in this area, defective. Chemical injuries to a nerve trunk, such as those caused by drugs injected into or near it, often are permanent.

Management. The objective of treatment of mononeuritis is to remove the cause if possible, such as by freeing the enmeshed nerve. The pain may be relieved by aspirin or codeine, and the function of the muscles may be maintained by weak galvanic currents.

CAUSALGIA. Causalgia (Greek words for heat and pain) refers to the group of symptoms and signs that follow peripheral nerve injuries. The nerves most often affected, in order of frequency, are the median, the ulnar, the radial, and the internal and external popliteals.

The chief symptom of causalgia is severe burning pain along the course of the injured nerve. The pain may be described as "hot," "burning," "stabbing," or "crushing." This is more or less persistent, but becomes severe following such physical stimuli as the contact of clothes. The skin over the affected limb becomes hot, shiny, and, at times, swollen; it shows abnormalities in sweating and eventually undergoes atrophic changes involving also the nails. The patient holds the extremity quiet, since each movement tends to increase the pain. Sympathetic nerve blocks, repair of local nerve lesions, and aggressive physical therapy are part of the treatment program. Experi-

ence in the Vietnam conflict revealed that active and passive exercises with very early mobilization appeared to reduce the incidence of causalgia following wounds of the extremities.

POLYNEURITIS. Polyneuritis is a disease that involves many nerves, particularly those of the legs and arms; the same nerves on both sides of the body are affected. Although the symptoms of this disease suggest that the terminal branches of the affected nerves alone are involved, multiple peripheral neuritis involves entire nervous pathways—that is, terminal branches, trunks and related fibers in the spinal cord and possibly in the brain.

Causes. The most common cause of polyneuritis in the United States is heavy alcohol intake, since nutritional deficiency results when alcohol becomes the main source of calories. Peripheral neuritis may occur in the course of various infectious diseases and may result from poisons and toxins circulating in the bloodstream. Among exogenous poisons important in the causation of this disease are methyl alcohol, lead, bismuth, mercury, arsenic, sulfonamides, carbon disulfide, aniline and other coal-tar products, emetine and several less common drugs and poisons.

Although in cases of multiple neuritis all the peripheral nerves have an equal opportunity to become affected, each poison or toxin attacks certain nerves in particular. Thus, botulinus toxin injures the nerves to the muscles of the eyes and the throat, and lead poisoning, those to the muscles of the hands and the feet.

Other causes include dietary deficiency involving the B complex vitamins, notably thiamine. A deficiency of thiamine causes disturbances in the metabolism of nerve tissue, and as a result, this tissue is unable to utilize carbohydrates normally. This inability gives rise to symptoms of muscle pains, tenderness, and weakness.

Anatomical polyneuritis is much slower to heal and involves reflex changes, skin hyperesthesias or hypoesthesias, motor weakness, or diminution or loss of the deep-tendon reflexes. It is probably due to deficiencies involving other components of the water-soluble vitamin group. The deficient diet of habitual drinkers now is considered to be altogether responsible. Similar are the polyneuritides of beriberi, diabetes, pregnancy, and malnutrition (particularly if there is a preponderance of carbohydrate in the diet).

Symptoms. Polyneuritis, whatever its cause, when well-developed presents a fairly uniform clinical picture. The symptoms may be sensory only, but they are never exclusively motor; sensory changes always accompany any muscular weakness or paralysis that appears. The hands and the feet are affected most often. Sensations of numbness, hyperesthesia, and diminution of heat perception and cold perception appear early and may last for weeks. Sometimes there is a slight fever.

The initial symptoms are followed by anesthesia of the

fingers and toes, which gradually extends toward the trunk. Associated with this is marked tenderness of the affected nerve trunks and of the skin overlying their branches. Pain is a marked early feature in some patients. There is more or less loss of the deep sensations, hence the pseudotabetic (ataxic) gait occasionally present, observed particularly in the cases of complicating diabetes mellitus and chronic alcoholism.

Muscular weakness then follows, either suddenly or over a period of days. Since the fibers to the extensor muscles of the feet and hands are more suceptible to the effects of toxins than are those to the flexor muscles, the first motor symptom to appear is an ankledrop or a wristdrop; but after a week or two, paralysis of the entire limb may become complete. Convulsions may occur, frequently in children, because (as was stated above) the pathology is not limited solely to the peripheral nerves.

In the majority of patients, the symptoms of polyneuritis are superimposed on those of the primary disease, but in a few patients they so overshadow all others that it is difficult to determine the cause.

Management. The treatment of polyneuritis is first aimed at the cause—for example, to eliminate all exposure to lead, to supply the needed B vitamins via the diet and by parenteral injection, and to treat any infection present.

Since the nerves require months to recover, during which time the muscles they control may become so weak and atrophied as to become permanently useless, the muscles should be kept in good condition by daily massage, passive movements, or galvanic stimulation. Often splints are indicated to prevent footdrop and wristdrop. Analgesic drugs may be necessary.

POLYRADICULITIS. Polyradiculitis (*Landry-Guillain-Barré syndrome*; infectious polyneuritis) is a clinical syndrome of unknown cause involving the nervous system and characterized by varying degrees of motor and sensory disturbances. In the majority of patients the syndrome is preceded by an infection (respiratory or gastrointestinal), but in some instances it has occurred following vaccination and surgery. It may be due to a primary viral infection, an immune reaction, some other process, or a combination of processes. One hypothesis is that a viral infection induces an autoimmune reaction which attacks the myelin of the peripheral nerves.

Proximal portions of the nerves tend to be affected most often, and the nerve roots within the subarachnoid space are commonly involved. Autopsy findings have revealed inflammatory edema and demyelination with some lymphocytic infiltration that is especially prominent in the spinal nerve roots.

Clinical Manifestations. There is variation in the mode of onset. The initial neurological symptoms are paresthesia (tingling and numbness) and muscle weakness of the legs which may progress to the upper extremities, trunk, and facial muscles. Muscle weakness may be followed quickly by complete paralysis. The cranial nerves are frequently involved, resulting in marked difficulty in swallowing, talking, and chewing. Sensory disturbances include loss of sensation and sphincter disturbances of the bladder and rectum. There may be back pain, muscle soreness, and loss of position sense, as well as diminished or absent tendon reflexes. Spinal fluid shows elevation in total protein with no increase in cell count.

Management. Since the cause of the disease is unknown, there is no specific therapy. The treatment is supportive. A course of corticosteroid therapy may be beneficial in the early phase of the disease.

• *Careful and continued assessment of respiratory function is necessary since respiratory insufficiency and failure may develop quickly.* Since respiratory failure is the main cause of death, vital capacity should be monitored. Signs to watch for are breathlessness while talking, shallow and irregular breathing, increasing pulse rate, use of accessory muscles while breathing, and any *change* in the respiratory pattern. If difficulties develop, the patient may require tracheostomy and mechanical ventilation.

When bulbar nerves are involved, the airway must be protected against the hazards of regurgitation and vomiting. If the patient is unable to swallow, nasogastric tube feedings are instituted.

• The heart is monitored for arrhythmias since cardiac arrest may occur if the vagus nerve becomes affected.

Urinary retention may be encountered during the acute phase of the disease. The paralyzed extremities are supported in functional positions and given passive range of motion exercises at least twice daily. The prevention of contracture deformities (page 182) and pressure sores (page 187) is a major nursing challenge. For severely paralyzed patients, the principles of nursing management of the unconscious patient (page 1192) may be applied, although these patients are in full possession of their mental faculties.

Because of paralysis, tracheostomy, and intubation, the patient is unable to talk, laugh, or cry and thus has no outlet for emotional expression. These problems are compounded by boredom, dependency, isolation, and frustration. To establish some form of communication, lip reading and the use of picture cards, combined with a system of blinking the eyes to indicate "yes" or "no," may be tried. Diversional therapy (television, radio, visits from the family) can alleviate some of the frustrations encountered by these patients.

Patients with polyradiculitis are dependent on quality medical and nursing management for recovery. Unless there is fatal respiratory failure, the rate of recovery is usually related to the degree of involvement and may take many months for some patients.

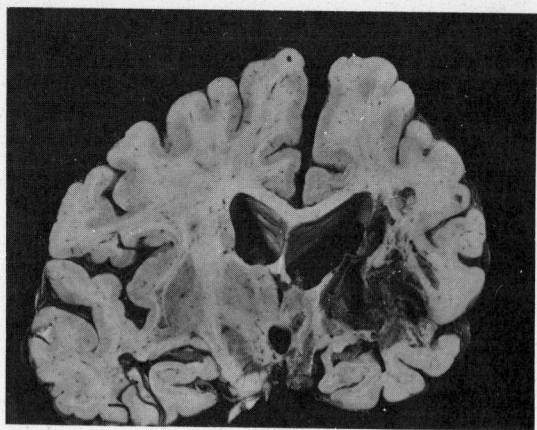

Figure 55-3. Impairment of cerebral circulation leading to a stroke. Note the area of cerebral infarction. (Armed Forces Institute of Pathology: Neg. No. 55-13956)

CEREBROVASCULAR DISEASE

Cerebrovascular disease is the third ranking cause of death in the United States and strikes over 500,000 persons in this country every year. Of the 2,500,000 who have survived these attacks over the years, 30 percent return to work or their usual activities, 55 percent are disabled but can carry on their activities of daily living, sometimes with assistance, while 15 percent are incapacitated and require lifelong total care.

Pathophysiology. Cerebrovascular disease refers to any functional abnormality of the central nervous system caused by interference with the normal blood supply to the brain. The pathology may involve an artery, a vein, or both, when the cerebral circulation becomes impaired as a result of partial or complete occlusion of a blood vessel or hemorrhage resulting from a tear in the vessel wall.

Vascular disease of the central nervous system may be caused by arteriosclerosis (most common), hypertensive changes, arteriovenous malformations, vasospasm, inflammation, arteritis, or embolism. As a result of vascular disease, blood vessels lose their elasticity, become hardened, and develop atheromatous deposits, or plaques, which may be the source of an embolus. The lumen of the vessel may gradually close, causing impairment of cerebral circulation and ischemia of the brain. If cerebral ischemia is transient, there is usually no neurologic deficit. However, occlusion of a large vessel produces cerebral infarction (Fig. 55-3). The vessel may rupture and produce hemorrhage. (See page 1224.)

STROKE (CEREBROVASCULAR ACCIDENT)

Cerebrovascular accident (commonly referred to as *stroke*) is a sudden loss of brain function resulting from a disruption of the blood supply to a part of the brain.

Frequently it is the culmination of cerebrovascular disease of many years standing.

A stroke is usually brought on by one of four events: (1) thrombosis (a blood clot within a blood vessel of the brain or neck); (2) cerebral embolism (a blood clot or other material carried to the brain from another part of the body); (3) stenosis of an artery supplying the brain; and (4) cerebral hemorrhage (rupture of a cerebral blood vessel with bleeding or pressure into the brain substance). The result is an interruption in the blood supply to the brain, causing temporary or permanent loss of movement, thought, memory, speech, or sensation.

Risk Factors and Prevention of Stroke

Prevention of stroke is the best possible approach; steps are taken to alter those factors which predispose certain people to stroke or increase their risk of having a stroke.

- The persons at risk must be identified and assisted in managing the underlying condition which predisposes them to stroke. This is especially true of patients with hypertension, since this disease is highly correlated with stroke.
- The prevalence of transient ischemic attacks among the elderly seems to be related to the occurrence of cerebral vascular accident in this patient population. Signs of transient ischemic attacks (TIA) include weakness or transient paralysis of an extremity, loss of or change in speech, visual problems, light-headedness, dizziness, or blackouts. (See below.) Stroke in people with these manifestations may be prevented with surgery or drugs.
- Persons receiving oral anticoagulants should be monitored to assure that their prothrombin times are kept within the range necessary to prevent intracerebral bleeding.
- Patients with abnormalities of heart rhythm and heart sounds or those with electrocardiogram abnormalities should be under medical treatment, since cerebral embolism of cardiac origin is a cause of stroke.
- Oral contraceptives are still considered to be a risk factor by some researchers in light of the number of strokes that have been documented in young women who were taking these drugs, yet had no evidence of other risk factors.
- An excessive or prolonged fall of blood pressure following shock, hemorrhage, surgery, diagnostic procedures, and ingestion of certain drugs may cause general cerebral ischemia. In these instances the patient requires careful monitoring.
- In younger persons, attention should be directed at controlling blood lipids (particularly cholesterol), blood pressure, cigarette smoking, and obesity.

Transient Ischemic Attacks (Little Strokes)

A *transient ischemic attack* (TIA) is a transient or temporary episode of neurological dysfunction commonly manifested by a sudden loss of motor, sensory, or visual function, lasting a few seconds or minutes but no longer than 24 hours. Complete recovery usually occurs between attacks. As was indicated above, a TIA may serve as a warning of impending stroke. The cause of this clinical entity is a temporary impairment of blood flow to a specific region of the brain due to a variety of reasons, including atherosclerosis of the vessels supplying the brain, a fall in cerebral perfusion pressure, cardiac arrhythmias, etc.

The most common sites of atherosclerosis in the extracranial arteries are located at the bifurcation of the common carotid and at the origin of the vertebral arteries (Fig. 31-5). Among the intracranial arteries, the middle cerebral artery is the most common location of atherosclerosis. If the ischemia arises in the carotid system, the patient may experience hemiparesis, blindness in one eye, aphasia, or confusion. If the ischemia occurs in the vertebral basilar system, vertigo, blindness, disturbances of consciousness, and various signs of motor and sensory impairments may occur.

Management of TIA. Following various diagnostic procedures—including angiographic evaluation of the diseased vessels, cerebral blood flow, and computerized tomography of the head and neck (if available)—some patients are treated by reconstructive vascular procedures such as carotid endarterectomy or extracranial/intracranial bypass graft.

CAROTID ENDARTERECTOMY. A carotid endarterectomy of the internal carotid artery at the bifurcation in the neck may be done to prevent the onset of stroke in persons with extracranial occlusive disease. A temporary bypass shunt is made to give the brain maximum protection during the surgical procedure. The artery is occluded below and above the lesion. The atheromatous lesion or thrombus and a portion of the artery are then removed.

- Following endarterectomy, a neurologic flow sheet is kept to maintain close assessment of the neurologic status. The neurosurgeon must be notified immediately if the patient develops any motor or sensory deficits. The primary complications of carotid endarterectomy are myocardial infarction and mild to severe neurologic deficits.

EXTRACRANIAL/INTRACRANIAL BYPASS GRAFTING. In patients with extracranial and intracranial lesions, a relatively new procedure may be done to prevent stroke. Microvascular techniques are used to help establish an anastomosis of the superficial temporal artery to the middle cerebral artery or one of its branches in order to augment the collateral blood supply to the ischemic areas of the brain.

Postoperative assessment includes monitoring the blood pressure and measuring the central venous pressure. Blood pressure and blood volume are maintained with infusions of colloid, pressors, or nitroprusside. When the patient becomes ambulatory, the blood pressure is controlled with oral agents. To keep the graft patent, aspirin and dipyridamole are given twice daily for six months.

DRUG THERAPY. Patients who are not candidates for surgical intervention may be placed on anticoagulant therapy (Coumadin) in order to prevent future attacks and a possible massive cerebral infarction. Antiplatelet aggregation drugs (particularly aspirin) are very useful in decreasing the occurrence of cerebral infarction in patients who have experienced multiple TIAs.

Other Cerebral Circulation Problems Causing Stroke

CEREBRAL THROMBOSIS. Cerebral arteriosclerosis and slowing of the cerebral circulation are major causes of cerebral thrombosis.

Headache is rather uncommon at the onset of cerebral thrombosis. Some patients may experience dizziness, mental disturbances, or convulsions, and some may have an onset indistinguishable from that of intracerebral hemorrhage or cerebral embolism. In general, cerebral thrombosis does not develop abruptly, and a transient loss of speech, hemiplegia, or paresthesias in one half of the body may precede the onset of a severe paralysis by a few hours or days.

CEREBRAL EMBOLISM. Pathologic abnormalities of the left heart, such as infective endocarditis, rheumatic heart disease, and myocardial infarction, as well as pulmonary infections, are the sites where emboli originate. It is possible that the insertion of a prosthetic heart valve may precipitate a stroke since there seems to be an increased incidence of embolism following this procedure. The incidence of stroke following this procedure can probably be reduced with postoperative anticoagulant therapy. Atrial fibrillation and cardioversion for atrial fibrillation are other possible causes of cerebral emboli and stroke.

The embolus usually lodges in the middle cerebral artery or its branches, where it disrupts the cerebral circulation.

- Sudden onset of hemiparesis or hemiplegia with or without aphasia or loss of consciousness in a patient with cardiac or pulmonary disease is characteristic of cerebral embolism.

Although endarterectomies of the intracranial arteries are being performed, the treatment of cerebral thrombosis and embolism consists chiefly of medical and nursing management similar to that given patients with intracerebral hemorrhage.

CAVERNOUS SINUS THROMBOSIS. Infections of the upper half of the face, orbit, and nasal sinuses may extend into the cavernous sinus and, by causing thrombosis, interrupt the venous drainage of the eye and other veins that drain the brain. Initially, edema, congestion, proptosis (bulging of the eyeball), and pain occur in the homolateral eye, and later in the contralateral eye as well because of extension of the infection to the other cavernous sinus. These patients are treated by antibiotic and anticoagulant medications and occasionally by surgical intervention.

SAGITTAL SINUS THROMBOSIS.   Infective processes involving the frontal or nasal sinuses and osteomyelitis of the skull may extend into the sagittal sinus and disturb the cerebral venous drainage, producing cerebral congestion and edema. Usually, there are no localizing signs, but symptoms and signs of increased intracranial pressure may develop.

CEREBRAL ARTERIOVENOUS MALFORMATION.   There are two types of congenital cerebral arteriovenous (A-V) malformation: (1) the cryptic type, which usually occurs mainly in the brain stem, and (2) the large type, which is usually located on or near the surface of the cerebral hemisphere, particularly in the parietal region. They commonly produce either spontaneous subarachnoid hemorrhage or focal seizures. The treatment consists of anticonvulsive medications or surgical removal of the A-V malformation.

CAROTID CAVERNOUS FISTULA.   This condition is usually post-traumatic, occurring either from a small tear in the intracavernous portion of the internal carotid artery, or from disruption of one of its branches in this location. Through this abnormal communication, the high pressure carotid flow enters the cavernous sinus and disturbs the sinus drainage.

The clinical manifestations consist of headaches, noise in the head, congestion of the eye (chemosis), proptosis, papilledema, and bruit in the homolateral eye. Carotid angiography demonstrates the arterial flow into the cavernous sinus.

Management consists of one of the several surgical procedures designed to obliterate the fistula.

Hemorrhage as a Cause of Stroke

In the Framingham Study on Heart Disease and Stroke which covered 24 years of study, hemorrhage was found to be the mechanism of stroke in 15 percent of the patients. Hemorrhage may occur outside the dura mater (extradural hemorrhage), beneath the dura mater (subdural hemorrhage), in the subarachnoid space (subarachnoid hemorrhage), or within the brain substance (intracerebral hemorrhage).

EXTRADURAL HEMORRHAGE.   Extradural hemorrhage (epidural hemorrhage) is a neurosurgical emergency that requires urgent care. If the patient is not treated within hours following the accident, he has very little chance of survival. (This is discussed under head injuries on page 1248.)

SUBDURAL HEMORRHAGE.   This type of hemorrhage (excluding the acute subdural) is basically the same as an epidural hemorrhage, except that in subdural hematoma usually a bridging vein is torn. Thus, a longer period of time (longer lucid interval) is required for the hematoma to form and cause pressure on the brain. (This is discussed under head injuries on page 1248.)

SUBARACHNOID HEMORRHAGE.   Subarachnoid hemorrhage (hemorrhage occurring in the subarachnoid space) may occur as a result of trauma or hypertension, but the most common cause is a leaking aneurysm in the area of the circle of Willis and congenital arteriovenous malformations of the brain. Any artery within the brain can be the site of an aneurysm. The treatment of intracranial aneurysms is discussed on page 1228.

INTRACEREBRAL HEMORRHAGE.   Hemorrhage or bleeding into the brain substance is most common in patients with hypertension and cerebral atherosclerosis, since degenerative changes due to these diseases usually cause rupture of the vessel. The bleeding is usually arterial and occurs particularly around the basal ganglia. Intracerebral hemorrhage is occasionally due to hemorrhagic disorders, such as leukemia or thrombocytopenia, or may be a complication of anticoagulant therapy. The clinical picture and the prognosis depend mainly on the degree of hemorrhage and brain damage. Occasionally the bleeding ruptures the wall of the lateral ventricle and causes intraventricular hemorrhage, which is frequently fatal.

Usually the onset is abrupt, with severe headache. Nuchal rigidity is generally noted. As the hematoma enlarges, a more pronounced neurologic deficit occurs in the form of decreased alertness and abnormalities in the vital signs. If the bleeding is limited or develops gradually, there may be no significant pressure effects. On the other hand, the full deficit may evolve in a matter of hours. A marked reduction in consciousness (stupor/coma) in the early phase of the bleeding episode usually has an ominous prognosis.

The treatment of intracerebral hemorrhage is controversial. If the hemorrhage is small, the patient is treated conservatively and symptomatically.

• The blood pressure is carefully lowered with nitroprusside sodium (Nipride), if there is a crisis situation, or by other antihypertensive drugs. The patient's neurologic deficit may worsen if the blood pressure is dropped too low or lowered too rapidly. The most effective form of treatment is the prevention of hypertensive vascular disease.

Management

The management of stroke patients is discussed in detail in Chapter 54. See page 1197 for the effects of a stroke, page 1198 for nursing management, and pages 1199-1203 for the rehabilitation phase.

BRAIN TUMORS

A brain tumor is a localized intracranial lesion which occupies space within the skull and tends to cause a rise in intracranial pressure.

In 95 percent of patients with tumors of the brain, the tumor originates in the brain (including the roots of the cranial nerves and the meninges). The remaining 5 percent are either metastases from primary growths elsewhere in the body or malignancies of the skull that have ulcerated through into the cranial cavity. The highest incidence of intracranial tumors occurs between the ages of 50 and 70 years. Brain tumors rarely metastasize outside the central nervous system but cause death by impairing vital functions either by direct involvement or by increasing intracranial pressure.

Classification

Brain tumors may be classified into several groups: (1) those arising from the coverings of the brain, such as the dural meningioma; (2) those developing in or on the cranial nerves, best exemplified by the acoustic neuroma and the optic nerve spongioblastoma polare, (3) those originating in the brain tissue, such as the various gliomas, and (4) metastatic lesions originating elsewhere in the body. (See also Table 55-1.) Tumors may be benign or malignant. However, because a benign tumor may occur in a vital area, it may have effects as serious as those of a malignant tumor.

Specific Tumors

GLIOMAS. The malignant glioma is the most frequently seen brain neoplasm. Usually these tumors cannot be totally removed, because they spread by infiltrating into the surrounding neural tissue.

POSTERIOR FOSSA TUMORS. These are the most common brain tumors found in children and are manifested by staggering gait, headaches (gradually become very severe) and vomiting. Since tumors in the cerebellum lie very near the medulla oblongata, death may occur very suddenly.

PITUITARY GLAND TUMORS. The pituitary gland is a small, olive-shaped body located in a small pocket just below the optic nerves. The activity of this gland may be increased or decreased by the presence of a tumor. Increased function (hyperpituitarism) accelerates growth, which in children results in gigantism. In adults, the face becomes coarse and the hands large, a condition called *acromegaly*. Hyperfunction of the gland may cause other conditions such as Cushing's disease, lactation, etc.

A decrease in function leads to hypopituitarism, characterized by changes in skin pigmentation, anemia, and loss of sexual characteristics. In addition to these disturbances of function, the tumor, by exerting pressure on the optic nerves, causes a progressive loss of vision that results in blindness.

Computerized tomography and roentgenograms are important aids in diagnosis since they can reveal an enlargement or deformity of the bony shell surrounding the pituitary gland. Visual field examinations are also part of the diagnostic workup.

ANGIOMAS. Brain angiomas (masses composed largely of abnormal blood vessels) are found either in or on the surface of the brain. Some persist throughout life

TABLE 55-1. CLASSIFICATION OF BRAIN TUMORS

Tumors Originating in the Brain Tissue

Gliomas; infiltrating tumors that may invade any portion of the brain; most common type of brain tumor

- Glioblastoma multiforme
- Astrocytoma
- Ependymoma — Subclassified according to cell type
- Medulloblastoma
- Oligodendroglioma
- Mixed

Tumors Arising from Covering of Brain

Meningioma; encapsulated, well-defined, growing outside the brain tissue; compresses rather than invades brain

Tumors Developing in or on the Cranial Nerves

Acoustic neuroma; derived from sheath of acoustic nerve
Optic nerve spongioblastoma polare

Metastatic Lesions (most commonly from lung and breast)

Tumors of the Ductless Glands

Pituitary
Pineal

Blood Vessel Tumors

Hemangioblastoma
Angioma

Congenital Tumors

without causing symptoms, others give rise to symptoms of brain tumor. Occasionally, the diagnosis is suggested by the presence of another angioma somewhere in the head or by a bruit audible over the skull. Since the walls of the blood vessels in angiomas are thin, a cerebral vascular accident frequently occurs. In fact, cerebral hemorrhage in persons under 40 years of age always should suggest the possibility of an angioma.

ACOUSTIC NEUROMA. An acoustic neuroma is a tumor of the 8th cranial nerve, the nerve of hearing and balance. It usually arises just within the internal auditory meatus where it frequently expands before filling the cerebellopontine recess.

An acoustic neuroma may grow slowly and attain a considerable size before it is correctly diagnosed. The patient usually experiences progressive unilateral nerve deafness, tinnitus, and episodes of vertigo and staggering. As the tumor becomes larger, painful sensations of the face may occur on the same side, as a result of the tumor's compressing the 5th cranial nerve.

With improved radiological techniques and the use of the operating microscope and microsurgical instrumentation, even large tumors can be removed through a relatively small craniotomy.

Clinical Manifestations

The manifestations of brain and meningeal tumors may be divided into general and local symptoms.

General Symptoms. These symptoms are caused by

a gradual compression of the brain due to the growth of the tumor. The effect is to disrupt the equilibrium that exists between the brain, the cerebrospinal fluid and the cerebral blood—all located within the skull. As the tumor grows, compensation may occur through compression of intracranial veins, reduction of cerebrospinal fluid volume (by increased absorption or decreased production) and reduction of intra- and extracellular brain tissue mass. When these compensatory mechanisms fail, the patient develops signs and symptoms.

The most common symptoms produced by increased intracranial pressure are headache, vomiting, papilledema (choked disk) with associated blurring of vision and diplopia, and stupor. Headache, though not always present, is most common in the early morning and is made worse by coughing, straining, or sudden movement.

Headaches are usually described as deep or expanding or as dull but unrelenting. Frontal tumors usually produce a bilateral frontal headache; pituitary gland tumors produce pain radiating between the two temples (bitemporal), whereas in cerebellar tumors the headache may be located in the suboccipital region.

Vomiting, usually unrelated to food intake, is usually due to irritation of the vagal centers in the medulla. If the vomiting is of the forceful type it is described as "projectile" vomiting.

Papilledema (edema of the optic nerve) is present in a large percentage of patients.

Localizing Symptoms. Localizing symptoms occur when specific regions of the brain are disrupted, resulting in locally referable signs, such as sensory and motor abnormalities, visual alterations, and convulsive seizures.

The *progression* of the signs and symptoms is important, because it indicates tumor growth and expansion.

Because the functions of the different parts of the brain are known, the location of the tumor can be determined, in part, by identifying those functions which are affected by the presence of the tumor. For example, a tumor of the motor cortex manifests itself by causing convulsive movements localized to one side of the body, spoken of as "Jacksonian seizures." Tumors of the occipital lobe cause blindness in half of each eye (hemianopsia) by involving the centers of the tracts for vision of one side of the brain. Tumors of the cerebellum cause dizziness and a staggering gait, with a tendency to fall toward the side of the lesion, and marked muscle incoordination and nystagmus (rhythmical vibration of the eyeballs). Tumors of the frontal lobe frequently produce personality disorders and a disinterested mental attitude. The patient often becomes extremely untidy and careless and may use obscene speech.

Tumors of the cerebellopontine angle usually originate in the sheath of the acoustic nerve and give rise to a sequence of symptoms that is the most characteristic of all brain tumors. First, tinnitus and vertigo appear, soon followed by progressive nerve deafness (8th nerve dysfunctions); next, numbness and tingling of the face and the tongue (due to involvement of the 5th nerve); still later, weakness or paralysis of the face (7th nerve involvement); and finally, since the enlarging tumor presses on the cerebellum, abnormalities in motor control may be present.

Many tumors are not so easily localized, because they lie in the so-called silent areas of the brain (i.e., areas where functions are not definitely determined).

Diagnostic Evaluation

The history of the illness and the manner in which the symptoms evolved is important. A neurological examination indicates the areas of the central nervous system involved. To assist in the precise localization of the lesion a battery of tests is performed. A skull x-ray will reveal intracranial calcification, displacement of intracranial structures, and signs of increased intracranial pressure and bone destruction. Computerized tomography will give specific information concerning the number, size, and density of the lesion(s) and the extent of secondary cerebral edema. It also provides information about the ventricular system. Cytologic studies of the cerebrospinal fluid may be done to detect malignant cells. An electroencephalogram can detect abnormal brain waves in regions occupied by the tumor and can evaluate temporal lobe seizures. Echoencephalography can show whether certain structures have been displaced from the midline by a lesion in one hemisphere. Cerebral angiography provides visualization of cerebral blood vessels and can localize most cerebral tumors. These procedures have largely supplanted air studies in the diagnosis of brain tumor.

A brain scan may be valuable since an abnormal amount of radioactive material will accumulate in the area of the tumor and can be localized with a scintillation counter.

Management

An untreated brain tumor ultimately leads to death, either from progressively increasing intracranial pressure or from primary brain damage. Patients with possible brain tumor should be investigated and treated as soon as possible before irreversible damage occurs.

The objective of management is to remove as much or all of the tumor as possible without increasing the neurological deficit (paralysis, blindness). The treatment of brain tumor is surgical extirpation (page 1206), when possible, followed by radiation therapy or chemotherapy when indicated. In general, patients with meningiomas, acoustic neuromas, cystic astrocytomas of the cerebellum, colloid cyst of the third ventricle, congenital tumors such as dermoid cyst, and some of the granulomas can be cured by surgical removal of the tumor. A complete extirpation of the infiltrating gliomas is not possible. In these patients the treatment consists of: biopsy to establish the diagnosis, partial removal, decompression if necessary, and radiation therapy. Certain chemotherapeutic agents combined with radiation therapy are also being used. Newer drugs are continually being evaluated, and there is hope that these will be more successful in the future. Sometimes a by-pass operation is performed to relieve obstructive hydrocephalus.

Cerebral Metastases

A significant number of patients (15 to 20 percent in one cancer institute) suffer central nervous system complications as a result of systemic cancer and neurologic symptoms caused by cerebral metastases. Cancer of the lung commonly metastasizes to the brain, as do tumors of the breast, thyroid and kidney and melanoma. Neurologic symptoms include headache, personality changes, mental changes, focal weakness, paralysis, and seizures. These problems may be devastating to the patient and the family.

The treatment is palliative and involves eliminating or reducing serious symptomatology. Bear in mind that even when palliation is the goal, distressing signs and symptoms can be resolved, thereby improving the quality of life that remains. Patients with intracerebral metastases who are not treated have a steady downhill course with a very limited survival time.

Treatment may include adrenocorticosteroid hormones which are helpful in relieving headache and alterations of consciousness. It is thought that adrenocorticosteroids (dexamethasone; prednisone) reduce inflammatory reaction around the metastatic deposits and decrease the edema surrounding them. Other drugs include osmotic agents (mannitol; glycerol), which are useful because of their ability to reduce intracranial pressure, and anticonvulsant drugs (phenytoin), which are used for patients with focal or generalized seizures.

Radiation to the whole brain is the foundation of treatment of intracerebral metastases, although surgical removal may be appropriate for a single metastatic brain tumor. At this time there is no significant statistical difference between the survival rates produced by radiation therapy and by surgery. With the advent of nitrosourea derivatives that cross the blood-brain barrier, there have been encouraging results with the use of chemotherapy. (See also the care of the patient with advanced cancer, page 275.)

INTRACRANIAL ANEURYSMS

An intracranial (cerebral) aneurysm is a dilation of the walls of a cerebral artery, resulting in a saclike formation (Fig. 55-4). An aneurysm may be due to a congenital defect in the media of the artery, but most often it results from acquired factors such as atherosclerosis, hypertensive vascular disease, and advancing age. The aneurysm

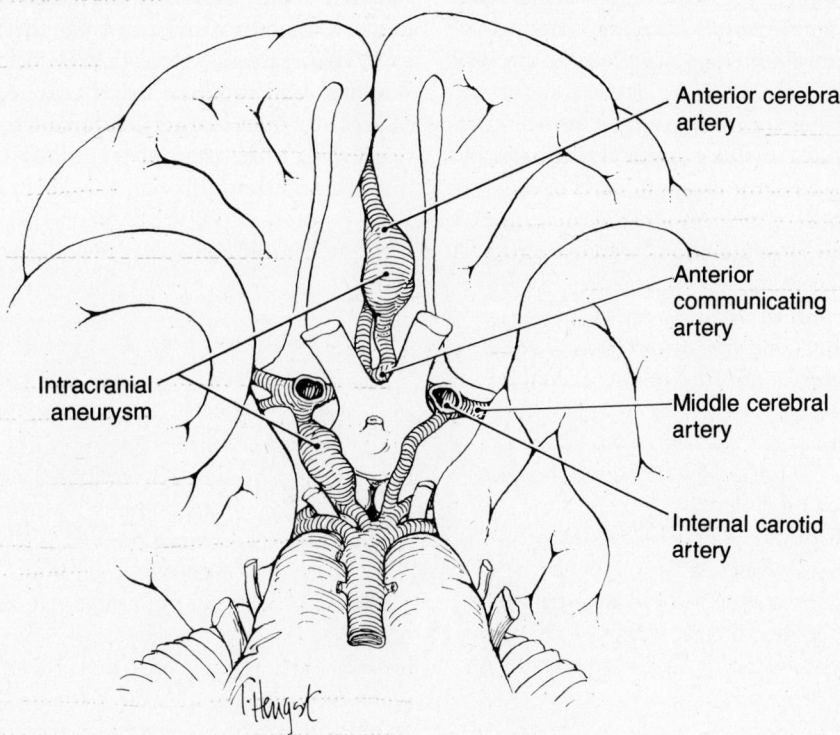

Figure 55-4. Intracranial aneurysm.

is most commonly located on the internal carotid, anterior cerebral, anterior communicating, and middle cerebral arteries. A small percentage develop in the vertebrobasilar territory. Multiple cerebral aneurysms are not uncommon.

Symptoms are produced when the aneurysm enlarges and presses on nearby cranial nerves or brain substance or, more drastically, when the aneurysm ruptures, causing subarachnoid hemorrhage. Rupture of the aneurysm usually produces a *sudden* severe localized headache with stiff neck and often loss of consciousness for a variable period of time. There may be pain and rigidity in the back of the neck and spine due to meningeal irritation. Visual disturbances (visual loss, diplopia, ptosis), tinnitus, dizziness, and hemiparesis may also occur. The diagnosis is confirmed by the presence of blood in the cerebrospinal fluid and by cerebral angiography. Subarachnoid hemorrhage has a high early mortality rate.

At times an aneurysm will "leak" blood, leading to the formation of a clot that seals the site of rupture. In this instance, the patient may show little neurological deficit. Or there may be severe bleeding, resulting in coma followed rapidly by death. Aneurysms that produce subarachnoid hemorrhage occur most frequently in middle life.

Management

The objective of management is to stop or diminish the flow of blood in the aneurysmal sac. The patient is placed on immediate and strict bed rest since activity and stress may elevate the blood pressure and potentiate bleeding. Any activity requiring exertion is forbidden. Because of this consideration, stool softeners are given to prevent straining. The head of the bed may be elevated slightly to promote venous drainage although some neurologists prefer that it remain flat to increase cerebral perfusion and thus reduce hypoxia.

One method of management is to establish a hypotensive state. The blood pressure is kept low to reduce the systolic arterial thrust on the weakened arterial wall as well as to reduce the chance of bleeding by diminishing the blood pressure in the region of the circulatory break. Hypotensive agents may be used to keep the blood pressure just above the range of cerebrovascular insufficiency. Barbiturates may be administered for their sedative and/or anticonvulsive effects. Antifibrinolytic medication (aminocaproic acid [Amicar]) is given to decrease fibrinolysis in the hope of retarding dissolution of the clot that forms at the site of hemorrhage. Mannitol and other osmotic diuretics are used to reduce intracranial pressure. Oxygen is frequently necessary to reduce hypoxia.

• Periodic observations are made to assess for signs of a decrease in mental alertness, an increase in headache, and alteration in the size of the pupils. Any of these changes are reported immediately, since they usually signify additional bleeding. Quick action is necessary if a fatal hemorrhage is to be prevented.

Cerebral vasospasm (constriction of intracranial blood vessels as a result of smooth muscle contraction) is a serious complication of subarachnoid hemorrhage and often is correlated with a poor clinical condition. The mechanism responsible for vasospasm is not clear. The spasm initially occurs immediately after the bleed, which probably exerts a protective effect for the affected artery. Spasm frequently recurs during the second week. It is also during this time that the clot undergoes the lytic process (dissolves) and increases the chances of rebleeding. The major vessels at the base of the brain may be affected, thereby compromising the blood flow in the area. Hemiparesis, visual field defects, seizures, mental clouding, and paralysis may occur. An Aminophylline-Isuprel regimen is one method of treatment currently being used in an attempt to modify vasospasm and increase blood flow through the cerebral vessels.

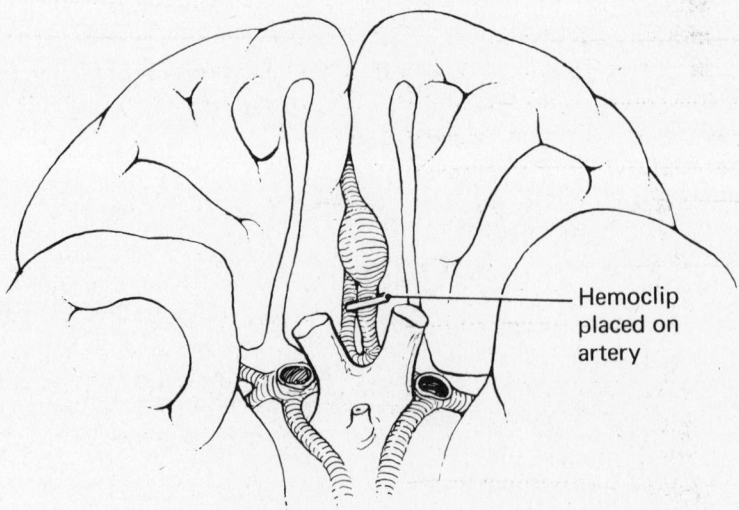

Hemoclip placed on artery

Figure 55-5.   Cerebral aneurysm isolated by means of a hemoclip.

Other complications following subarachnoid hemorrhage from a ruptured aneurysm include epilepsy, hydrocephalus, and psychiatric and psychological difficulties due to brain damage. Anxiety and depressive states may be complicating factors.

After the acute phase of bleeding is over, the patient is maintained on bed rest for a number of weeks.

Surgical Approach

There is considerable controversy concerning the timing of surgery for the low-risk patient. A patient severely affected by massive hemorrhage is usually not a candidate for surgery. Since the advent of the operative microscope and microsurgical techniques there has been a decreased morbidity and mortality in low-risk patients. Magnified vision and improved lighting allow the neurosurgeon to see the details of the vascular relationships and identify aneurysms deep in the brain.

The objective of surgery is to protect the patient from further hemorrhage. This is done by isolating the aneurysm from its circulation or by strengthening its wall. An aneurysm may be treated by excluding it from the circulation by means of a ligature or a clip across its neck (Fig. 55-5). If this is not anatomically possible, the aneurysm can be reinforced by wrapping it with plastic, muscle, or some other substance. Or, an extracranial method may be used, whereby the carotid artery is occluded in the neck in order to reduce pressure within the blood vessel. Following ligation of the carotid artery, there is some risk of cerebral ischemia and sudden hemiplegia. In anticipation of these complications, measurements of cerebral blood flow and internal carotid pressure may be taken in order to identify those patients who are at risk for postoperative ischemic episodes.

(The management of the patient following intracranial surgery is discussed on pages 1207 to 1209.)

CEREBRAL INFECTION—BRAIN ABSCESS

True brain abscesses are collections of pus within the substance of the brain itself. They may occur by *direct invasion of the brain* from intracranial trauma or surgery; by *spread of infection from nearby sites* (otitis media, sinusitis, or mastoiditis); or by *spread of infection from other organs* (lung infections, infective endocarditis). As a preventive measure, otitis media, mastoiditis, sinusitis, and systemic infections should be promptly treated to prevent brain abscesses.

Clinical Manifestations. The clinical manifestations result from alterations in intracranial mass dynamics (edema, brain shift), infection, or the location of the abscess. Headache, usually worse in the morning, is the patient's most constant symptom. Vomiting is also common. Focal neurologic signs (weakness of an extremity,

decreasing vision, seizures) may occur depending on the site of the abscess.

Any localizing symptoms that occur are not as typical as those seen in patients with brain tumor. When they do occur, they usually indicate pathology in either the temporal lobe or the cerebellum, since so many abscesses are aural in origin. There may be a change in the patient's mental alertness as reflected in lethargic, confused, or disoriented behavior. A thick-walled abscess may cause a subnormal temperature.

Repeated neurological examinations and continuing nursing assessment of the patient are necessary to determine accurately the location of the abscess. Computerized tomography is invaluable in showing the site of the abscess and following the course of treatment.

Management

- A neurological flow chart is maintained and the patient is monitored frequently for signs and symptoms of increased intracranial pressure (page 1184), which may result suddenly from cerebral edema caused by a rapidly growing abscess. Secondary compression of the midbrain and brain stem can quickly lead to coma and death.

Cerebral edema may be treated with dexamethasone, although use of this drug is controversial since steroids reduce resistance to infection. Antimicrobial therapy is given to eliminate the causative organism or reduce its virulence. Large doses are necessary to penetrate the abscess cavity until it becomes encapsulated and ready for surgical intervention. Anticonvulsant medications (phenytoin, phenobarbital) may be given as a prophylaxis against seizures. Multiple abscesses may be treated with appropriate antimicrobial therapy alone, with the patient closely followed by computer-assisted tomography.

The definitive treatment of a brain abscess is surgical intervention, either aspiration or excision. Pus may be evacuated by a needle or catheter that is placed through burr holes into the abscess cavity. The catheter may be left in place for intermittent aspiration and irrigation for several days, or the abscess may be excised via a craniotomy.

Postoperative Management

- Following surgery, drainage may be copious. Dressings are reinforced as soon as they become moist, and strict aseptic technique is maintained. The patient should lie on the operative side to promote drainage.
- The antimicrobial agents are administered on an exact time schedule because *meningitis is an ever present danger*. These patients must be watched carefully for retraction of the head, stiffness of the neck, headache, chill, sweats, etc.—symptoms suggestive of a postoperative meningitis.
- It is important that the patient be maintained on a high-calorie diet.

Serial computerized tomographic examinations are carried out to see if the infection has been eradicated. The mortality rate is fairly high and relapse is common. Neurological deficits following treatment of brain abscess include hemiparesis, seizures, and visual defects.

Patient Education. Antimicrobial agents may be continued for 3 to 4 weeks or longer after the brain abscess is excised or drained. It is important that the patient remember to take the prescribed anticonvulsant medication daily for an indefinite period of time.

MULTIPLE SCLEROSIS

Multiple sclerosis is a chronic, frequently progressive disease of the central nervous system, characterized by the occurrence of small patches of demyelination in the brain and spinal cord. (Demyelination refers to the destruction of myelin, the fatty and protein material that ensheathes certain nerve fibers in the brain and spinal cord.) In this disease, the demyelination is scattered irregularly throughout the central nervous system with relative sparing of the axon (Fig. 55-6). In time, myelin peels off the axis cylinders and the axons themselves degenerate. The plaques or patches in the involved areas become sclerosed, interrupting the flow of nerve impulses and resulting in a variety of manifestations, depending on which nerves are affected. The areas most frequently affected are the optic nerve and chiasm, the margins of the lateral, third, and fourth ventricles, the pons, medulla and cerebellar peduncles, and the spinal cord.

This is one of the most disabling neurologic diseases of the young adults (20 to 40 years of age) in this country. Its occurrence among the young maximizes the medical, psychological, social and economic problems encountered by the patient and the family.

Clinical Manifestations. The signs and symptoms of multiple sclerosis are varied and multiple, reflecting the location of the demyelination within the central nervous system.

Early symptoms of multiple sclerosis can be easily mistaken for neurosis, peripheral neuritis, or spinal lesions, since many systems or parts of the body are involved.

Symptoms include visual disturbances due to lesions in the optic nerves or their connections; nystagmus; "scanning" speech (slow, monotonous, and slurred); and intention tremor and loss of tonicity due to cerebellar lesions. Spastic weakness of the extremities and loss of

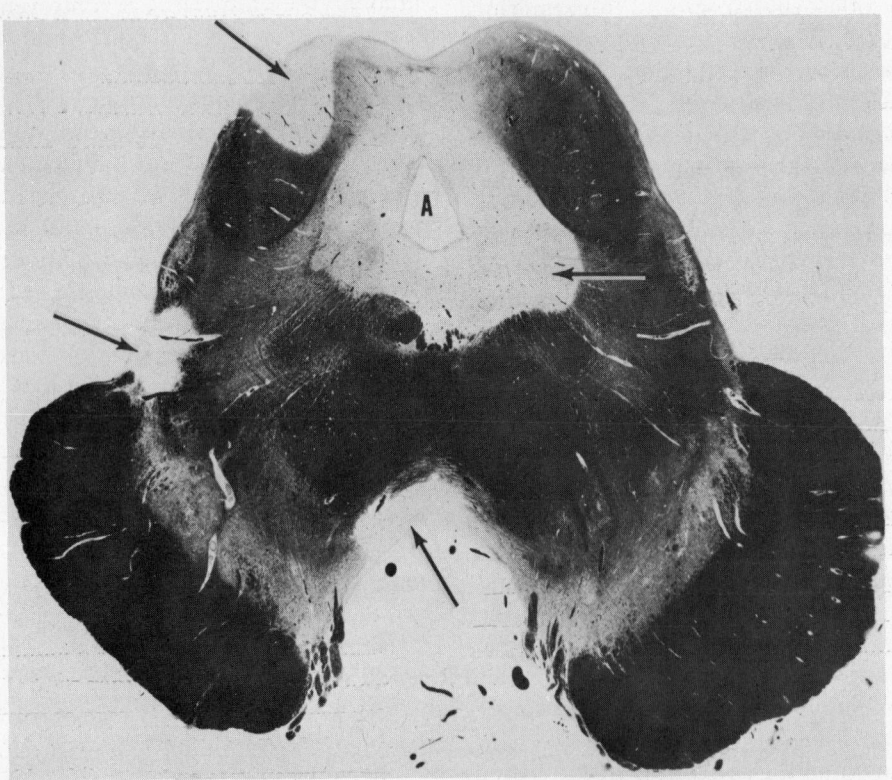

Figure 55-6. Cross section from the midbrain (enlarged approximately 3 times) of a patient with chronic MS. Specimen stained to show myelin (black). The four white areas indicated by the arrows are typical plaques in which the myelin has been destroyed. The plaque to the right of the aqueduct (*A*) impinges upon periaqueductal gray matter. The nerve fibers in these plaques have lost their myelin sheaths and as a consequence, conduction of stimuli in these areas would be impeded or lost. (Courtesy of Cedric S. Raine, M.D., Professor of Pathology [Neuropathology] and Neuroscience. Albert Einstein College of Medicine of Yeshiva University)

the abdominal reflexes are due to involvement of the main motor pathways (pyramidal tracts) of the spinal cord. Euphoria and emotional hyperexcitability result from loss of the control connections between the cortex and the basal ganglia. Vertigo, with nausea and vomiting, may occur if the vestibular nuclei or their connections are diseased; bladder, rectal, and genital disturbances also occur if the process involves the cord pathways connected with the sacral plexus. The most common group of symptoms includes spastic paraplegia with slight speech disturbance and nystagmus.

The disease is characterized by long remissions and exacerbations, with symptoms abating and recurring with increased frequency and severity for many years. The prognosis for a fairly prolonged life is good.

Causes and Epidemiology. The cause of multiple sclerosis is not known. Research evidence suggests that the plaques and subsequent scars which damage the brain and spinal cord are precipitated by an autoimmune response. It may be that this defective immune response developed in relation to some illness or injury in childhood. Certain individuals with a particular genetic makeup (having certain tissue antigen types) may be more susceptible to the disease. There has been a great deal of interest in the role of a slow virus in causing the disease. Although the initiating mechanism may stem from some form of viral infection, a defective immune response probably plays a major role in the pathogenesis of multiple sclerosis.

Epidemiological factors have been the subject of much research. Findings indicate that this disease is rare in tropical countries. It is aggravated by exposure to cold, damp weather and improves when and where the climate is mild and dry. Relapses are often associated with periods of emotional and physical stress (illness, injuries, inoculations).

Management. At this time there is no cure for multiple sclerosis; therefore there is no specific treatment. Many drugs have been used to treat the disease, but it is difficult to evaluate their effectiveness since a high percentage of patients will show spontaneous improvement. During acute exacerbations, high dosages of ACTH may be beneficial, possibly by reducing the area of edema surrounding the plaques. (However, controversy surrounds this theory.) The patient is informed that this drug suppresses the symptoms but does not cure the disease.

Nursing Management and Rehabilitation

The objectives of management are *to keep the patient active* and in as good physical condition as possible and to prevent the complications of urinary infections, pressure sores, and contracture deformities. The patient is treated symptomatically, and an individualized program of physical therapy, rehabilitation, and education is combined with emotional support.

Although rehabilitation measures will not alter the disease process, it is the aim of the rehabilitation program to bring about functional improvement, so that the patient can perform activities of daily living whether he is ambulatory, in a wheelchair, or confined to bed. If the patient's disease is not progressing too rapidly, the goal is to return the patient to satisfying employment or to keep him happily engaged in his present employment. An individualized therapeutic program is established after an appraisal has been made of the extent of disability and muscle strength.

Sometimes the patient presents the clinical picture of hemiplegia, although more commonly he may have the same disabilities as the patient with paraplegia. Any one extremity or combination of extremities may be involved. Therefore, the principles of rehabilitation of these conditions can be used for the patient who has similar problems due to multiple sclerosis (see page 1199).

COMBATING MUSCLE DYSFUNCTION. Daily exercises for muscle stretching are prescribed to minimize joint contractures. Special attention is given to hamstrings, gastrocnemius muscles, hip adductors, biceps, wrist, and finger flexors. A stretch-hold-relax routine is helpful for relaxing and treating muscle spasticity, which is common in MS patients. Splinting, muscle relaxant drugs, and surgery to relieve contractures have all been used to treat spasticity.

Relaxation and coordination exercises promote muscle efficiency. Progressive resistive exercises are used to strengthen weak muscles since diminishing muscle power is a significant problem. The patient is encouraged to work up to the point just short of fatigue. However, prolonged exercise that fatigues an extremity may cause paresis, numbness, or incoordination. The patient is advised to take frequent short rest periods, preferably lying down. Extreme fatigue may be a contributing factor in exacerbation.

Walking exercises improve the gait, particularly when there is a loss of position sense of the legs. If certain muscle groups are irreversibly affected, other muscles can be trained to take over their action. Warm baths, packs, and muscle relaxants may be beneficial if painful muscle spasm is present.

If motor dysfunction causes problems of incoordination, clumsiness or ataxia may be apparent. To overcome this disability, the patient can be taught to walk with his feet wide apart in order to widen the base of support and increase walking stability. A cane or walker affords additional support. If incoordination and intention tremor of the upper extremities occur, weighted bracelets or wrist cuffs are helpful. The patient is trained in transfer activities and activities of daily living to promote as much independence as possible.

BLADDER AND BOWEL TRAINING. Management of bladder and bowel control are among the patient's most difficult problems if sphincter control is impaired. Bladder dysfunction may lead to progressive renal failure. However, an indwelling catheter should be inserted only if absolutely necessary. A high level of fluid input helps to reduce the urinary bacterial count, minimizes urinary crystals and subsequent stone formation, and reduces encrustation of the indwelling catheter.

The patient with urinary frequency, urgency, or incontinence requires special support. The sensation of the need to void must be heeded immediately, hence the bedpan or urinal should be readily available. A voiding time schedule should be set up (every 1½ to 2 hours initially, with gradually lengthening time intervals). The patient is instructed to drink a measured amount of fluid every 2 hours and then attempts to void 30 minutes after drinking. An alarm clock may be set for the patient with diminished warning sensation.

If the female patient has permanent urinary incontinence, a urinary diversion procedure (ileal conduit) may have to be performed. The male patient may wear a condom appliance for urine collection. A bowel-training program is effective if there is loss of bowel control (page 202).

PROGRESSIVE DYSFUNCTION. During periods of exacerbation of the disease, the patient is encouraged to remain on bed rest for a few days, since continued activity appears to worsen the attack. Any aspects of the patient's life style which might cause exacerbation — cold, infection, emotional upset, etc. — should be avoided.

As the patient's disease progresses, self-help devices that include feeding devices, handrails, canes, braces, wheelchairs, and ramps are utilized to maintain independency for as long as possible. Corrective action is taken as each new problem arises. Creative nursing calls for inventiveness, adaptation, and modification of equipment that can be used for self-help devices so that the patient will not lose ground.

SENSORY IMPAIRMENT. Measures may be taken if optic and speech defects occur (the cranial nerves relating to sight and speech are affected by multiple sclerosis). An eye patch or frosted lens may be used to block visual impulses of one eye when the patient has diplopia (double vision). When the vision begins to fail, painting the cane tip and shoe tips with fluorescent paint helps. Persons with any physical limitations preventing them from reading regular print materials are eligible for the free talking book services of the Library of Congress (address at end of chapter).

When the cranial nerves controlling the mechanisms of speech are involved, dysarthrias (defects of articulation) marked by slurring, low volume of speech, and difficulties in phonation are seen. There are problems with shallow breathing and low breath pressure. A speech pathologist may recommend therapy to alleviate these problems.

Since sensory loss may occur in addition to motor loss, pressure sores are a continuing threat to skin integrity. Confinement to a wheelchair compounds the threat. (See page 187 for a discussion of the prevention and treatment of pressure sores.)

Psychological Support and Patient Education

Multiple sclerosis imposes numerous stresses on the patient and the family. Embarrassing and humiliating symptoms may result in "inappropriate" responses by the patient. As there may be organic changes in the brain, MS patients may be forgetful and easily distracted and may show emotional instability. Patients adapt to illness in a variety of ways — denial (with euphoria), depression, withdrawal, and hostility. Compassion and significant emotional support are required to help the patient adapt to a new identity as a handicapped person (a new self-image) and cope with the disruption in his life. The patient should be encouraged to remain in the mainstream of life as much as possible and to keep up social interests and activities. Hobbies help the patient's morale and provide satisfying interests when the disease has progressed to the stage in which normal activities cannot be pursued.

The nurse has the responsibility of emphasizing to the patient and the family the importance of a regular program of exercise, work, and recreation. Once certain abilities are lost, they are almost impossible to regain. Physical abilities may vary from day to day. Physical and emotional stresses should be avoided as much as possible, since these worsen symptoms and impair performance. The patient must remain under continuing medical supervision.

Encourage the patient to contact the local chapter of the National Multiple Sclerosis Society for services, publications and contact with other MS patients. Local chapters give direct services to patients. Through group participation, the patient has an opportunity to learn self-help methods in a social environment.

PARKINSON'S DISEASE

Parkinson's disease is a progressive neurologic disorder affecting the brain centers that are responsible for control and regulation of movement. It is characterized by bradykinesia (slowness of movement), tremor, and muscle stiffness or rigidity.

Pathophysiology. The major lesion appears to result in a loss of pigmented neurons, particularly those in the substantia nigra of the brain. (The substantia nigra is a collection of midbrain nuclei which project fibers to the corpus striatum). One of the major neurotransmitters in this area of the brain, and in other parts of the central nervous system, is dopamine, which has an important inhibiting function in the central control of movement. Although dopamine normally exists in high concentration in certain parts of the brain, in Parkinson's disease it is depleted in the substantia nigra and the corpus striatum. Depletion of dopamine levels in the basal ganglia is associated with bradykinesia, rigidity, and tremors.

In the majority of patients the cause of the disease is unknown. Arteriosclerotic parkinsonism is seen more frequently in older age groups. It may follow encephalitis, poisoning or toxicity (manganese; carbon monoxide) or hypoxia.

More than 500,000 persons in the United States are affected by this crippling disease; estimates range from one case per 1000 to one case per 200 population. The disease most frequently attacks persons in their 50s and 60s.

Clinical Manifestations. The chief manifestations of Parkinson's disease are impaired movement, muscular rigidity, tremor, and weakness. Early signs include a stiffening of the limbs and a waxlike rigidity in the performance of all movements. The patient has difficulty in initiating, maintaining, and performing motor activities, and experiences some delay in carrying out normal activity. As the disease progresses, the tremor begins, frequently in one hand and arm, then the other, and later in the head, although the tremor may remain unilateral (Fig. 55-7).

The tremor is characteristic; it is a slow, turning motion (pronation-supination) of the forearm and the hand, and a motion of the thumb against the fingers, as if rolling a pill between the fingers. If the patient gets excited, the tremor becomes worse; when he makes a voluntary motion, it ceases, allowing him to perform the most delicate acts, such as picking up a pin.

Other characteristics of the disease affect the face, stature, and gait. Eventually the rigid limbs become definitely weaker. Since there is limited movement in the muscles, the face has so little expression that it is said to be masklike, a feature that can be recognized at a glance. The patient stands with head bent a little forward and walks as if in danger of falling on his face. Frequently, these patients show signs of depression.

Mental manifestations may appear in the form of cognitive, perceptual, and memory deficits. Mental confusion may be a feature of the disease as well as a side effect of drug treatment.

Management

The aim of treatment is to *keep the patient functionally useful and productive for as long as possible.* This is done with appropriate drug therapy, physical therapy, rehabilitation techniques, and patient and family education.

LEVODOPA THERAPY. Levodopa (L-dopa, Larodopa,

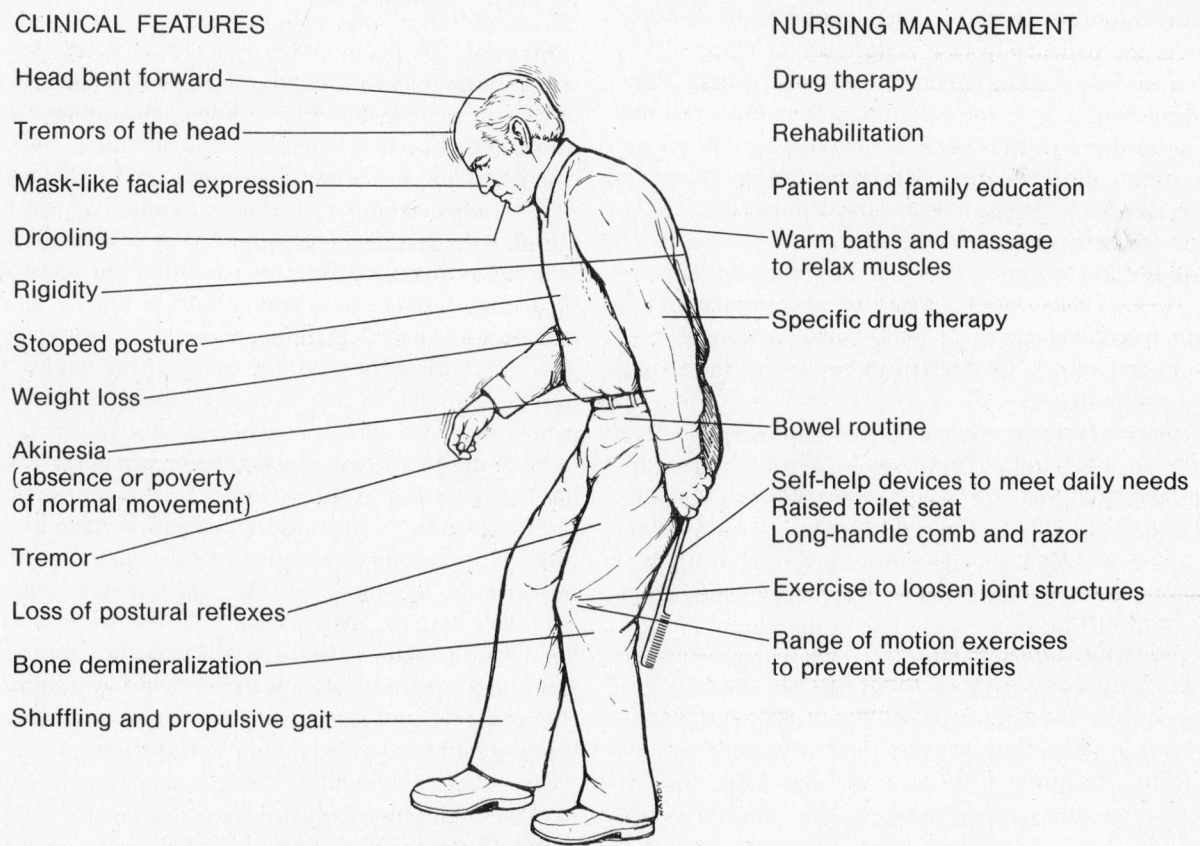

CLINICAL FEATURES

Head bent forward
Tremors of the head
Mask-like facial expression
Drooling
Rigidity
Stooped posture
Weight loss
Akinesia
(absence or poverty
of normal movement)
Tremor
Loss of postural reflexes
Bone demineralization
Shuffling and propulsive gait

NURSING MANAGEMENT

Drug therapy

Rehabilitation

Patient and family education

Warm baths and massage
to relax muscles

Specific drug therapy

Bowel routine

Self-help devices to meet daily needs
Raised toilet seat
Long-handle comb and razor

Exercise to loosen joint structures

Range of motion exercises
to prevent deformities

Figure 55-7. Clinical manifestations and nursing management of the patient with parkinsonism.

Benodopa, Dopar) constitutes an important facet of treatment. Early efforts to replace dopamine were unsuccessful since dopamine would not cross the blood-brain barrier (a protective biochemical mechanism which screens substances passing from the blood into the cells of the central nervous system). However, levodopa (a precursor of dopamine) was found to be effective because it traverses the blood-brain barrier. Levodopa is not a cure for parkinsonism but is effective in controlling symptoms, particularly bradykinesia and rigidity, for a period of time. However, levodopa must be given in large enough doses and for a long enough period of time to build up an effective and stable blood level. The dosage is increased gradually until side effects begin to appear, including nausea, vomiting, anorexia, postural hypotension, mental changes (confusion, agitation, mood alterations), cardiac arrhythmias, and twitching.

The beneficial effects of levodopa are most pronounced in the first few years of treatment. Benefits to the patient begin to wane and adverse side effects become more severe with the passage of time. Confusion, hallucinations, depression, and sleep alterations are associated with prolonged use of the drug. The patient may experience an "on-off" reaction in which he has sudden periods of near immobility (freezing).

LEVODOPA IN COMBINATION WITH CARBIDOPA. Carbidopa is a selective decarboxylase inhibitor, a substance which slows down the peripheral metabolism of dopa. The administration of carbidopa with levodopa makes more levodopa available for transport to the brain. Sinemet (a combination of carbidopa and levodopa) potentiates the therapeutic effects of levodopa by blocking extracerebral metabolism of levodopa thus permitting a reduction in the dosage level and incidence of side effects.

DOPAMINE AGONISTS. These drugs mimic the action of dopamine by directly affecting the postsynaptic receptors in the striatum. They bypass the enzymatic conversion of levodopa to dopamine. Bromocriptine and lergotrile are ergot alkaloids that have been shown to give improvement.

ANTICHOLINERGIC THERAPY. Anticholinergic drugs, such as trihexyphenidyl (Artane) and benztropine (Cogentin) continue to be useful for patients who have a mild disability or those who respond poorly to levodopa or are sensitive to it. These anticholinergic drugs may also be used in combination with levodopa. They counteract the action of acetylcholine in the central nervous system. (Relative cholinergic dominance appears to play a role in symptomatology.) With the administration of anticholinergics there is some degree of impairment of mental acuity ranging from mild difficulty in concentration and recall to confusion and hallucinations. Other side effects include dry mouth, blurred vision, constipation, and urinary hesitancy. Patients with prostatic hyperplasia as well as Parkinson's disease must be monitored for urinary retention, which may result from a combined effect of the enlarged prostate and the drug treatment for parkinsonism.

Antihistaminic drugs (diphenhydramine [Benadryl]) may be effective for tremor, possibly as a result of their anticholinergic properties.

Amantadine hydrochloride (Symmetrel) has been shown to reduce rigidity, tremor, and bradykinesia with a low risk of adverse reactions. Antidepressant drugs (imipramine [Tofranil]) are given to reduce depression.

SURGICAL INTERVENTION. In some selected patients, surgery may be effective in providing some relief of tremor and rigidity that encompasses one side of the body. The purpose of the surgery is to destroy a part of the thalamus (stereotaxic thalamotomy) in order to relieve certain types of excessive muscle contraction.

The stereotaxic technique allows the neurosurgeon to precisely position and localize a small target deep within the brain. Special guiding instruments and rapid x-rays are used to place an electrode or freezing probe with pinpoint precision in the target area of the brain. A lesion is then created at that point.

Although this procedure provides a certain amount of relief, it does not alter the course of Parkinson's disease, nor does it assure permanent improvement.

Supportive Management

EXERCISE. A progressive program of daily exercise will increase muscle strength, improve coordination and dexterity, reduce muscular rigidity, and prevent contractures that occur when muscles are not used. Walking, riding a stationary bicycle, swimming, and gardening are all exercises that help maintain joint mobility. Stretching exercises (stretch-hold-relax) will help loosen the joint structures. Postural exercises are important to counter the tendency of the head and neck to be drawn forward and down. Special walking techniques must also be learned to offset the shuffling gait and the tendency to lean forward. There are defective balancing reflexes. The patient may also walk off balance because of the rigidity of his arms. (Arm swinging is necessary in normal walking.) The patient is taught early in the course of the disease to concentrate on walking erect, to keep his eyes on the horizon and to use a broad-based gait, i.e., walking with the feet separated. A conscious effort must be made to swing the arms and raise the feet while walking and to use a heel-toe, heel-toe gait in fairly long strides. Breathing exercises while walking help to mobilize the rib cage. Frequent rest periods are important during the training period to avoid fatigue and frustration.

Every effort should be made to encourage the patient to carry out his own daily needs and to retain his independence. "Doing things" for the patient merely to save time runs contrary to this basic goal of management.

There should be a planned program of activity throughout the day to prevent too much daytime sleeping as well as disinterest and apathy. These patients have difficulty turning in bed and getting in and out of bed. Bedrails on the bed at home will provide assistance. A bedside commode is important.

SPEECH. The low-pitched monotonous speech of the patient with parkinsonism requires that he make a real effort to speak slowly. A small electronic amplifier (such as that used by the laryngectomee) is useful if the patient has a weak voice.

BOWEL ROUTINE. A patient with parkinsonism has severe problems with constipation. Among the factors causing this condition are weakness of the muscles used in defecation, lack of exercise, and an inadequate fluid intake. The drugs used for the treatment of the disease also inhibit normal intestinal secretions. A regular bowel routine may be established by seeing that the patient follows a regular habit time, consciously increases fluid intake, and eats high-residue foods. A raised toilet seat is a useful device to facilitate toilet activities, since the patient has difficulty in changing from a standing to a sitting position.

NUTRITIONAL CONSIDERATIONS. The patient also has a problem in keeping his weight up. He becomes embarrassed by his slowness and untidiness in eating. His mouth is dry from the medications, and he experiences difficulty in chewing and swallowing. (This last factor can result in aspiration pneumonia, which occurs fairly commonly in this disease.) Because of problems in eating, the patient in time suffers a sizable weight loss. Demineralization starts in the bones as a result of malnutrition. Thus there is the added threat of fractures occurring should the patient fall. Supplementary feedings will keep calorie intake up, and an electrical warming tray will keep food hot and permit the patient to rest during the prolonged time that it takes to eat.

PATIENT EDUCATION. It is important that the patient understand this ailment and that every effort be made to explain the nature of the disease in order to offset anxieties and fears that may be as disabling as the disease. The disease may be described as one that affects a small motor control station at the base of the brain. Although it progresses in severity, it does so very slowly, with lengthy periods of 5 to 15 years occurring between stages in the progression of symptoms.

Faithful adherence to an exercise and walking program helps to delay the progress of the disease. Encouragement and reassurance can be given by praising the patient for his perserverance and pointing out that his activities are being maintained through active participation. A combination of physiotherapy, psychotherapy, drug therapy, and sociotherapy may be necessary to help combat the depression that so often accompanies this condition.

HUNTINGTON'S DISEASE

Huntington's disease is a chronic progressive neurological disease of hereditary origin which affects men and women of all races. Because it is transmitted as an autosomal dominant genetic disorder, each child of a parent with Huntington's disease has a 50 percent risk of inheriting the illness.

The basic pathology involves an unexplained loss of cells in the basal ganglia and portions of the cerebral cortex. Recent research suggests that the disease may be related to a lack of important brain chemicals (gamma-aminobutyric acid [GABA] and acetylcholine [ACh]) which inhibit nerve action. Onset usually occurs between the ages of 35 to 45; the patient slowly progresses toward death in 10 to 20 years. Approximately 10 percent of victims are children. There is at present no means of detecting the HD gene before symptoms appear.

Clinical Manifestations

The most prominent clinical features of the disease are abnormal involuntary movements (chorea), intellectual decline, and, often, emotional disturbance. As the disease progresses, a constant writhing, twisting, uncontrollable movement may involve the entire body. These motions are devoid of purpose or rhythm, although patients may try to turn them into purposeful movement. All of the body musculature is involved. Facial movements produce tics and grimaces. Speech is affected, becoming slurred, hesitant, often explosive, and eventually unintelligible. Chewing and swallowing are difficult and there is a constant danger of choking and aspiration. Like speech, the gait becomes disorganized to the point that ambulation eventually is impossible. Although independent ambulation should be encouraged for as long as possible, a wheelchair is usually necessary at some point; eventually the patient is confined to bed. Bladder and bowel control is lost. The sensorium likewise is usually involved. There is progressive intellectual impairment, although the patient is generally aware that the disease is responsible for the myriad dysfunctions he experiences.

The mental and emotional changes may be more devastating to the patient and family than the abnormal movements. Patients may be nervous, clumsy, irritable, or impatient. Particularly in the early stages of the illness, patients are subject to uncontrollable fits of anger; profound, often suicidal depression; apathy; or euphoria. Judgment and memory are impaired. Hallucinations, delusions, and paranoid thinking may even precede the appearance of disjointed movements. Emotional symptoms often become less acute as the disease progresses, although dementia eventually ensues. Despite a ravenous appetite, often for sweets, patients usually become emaciated and exhausted. Eventually patients succumb from heart failure, pneumonia, or infection, or die as a result of a fall or choking.

THE CHALLENGES OF A PATIENT WITH HUNTINGTON'S DISEASE

Nursing Objective: To develop creative approaches until the complex needs of the patient are met.

Problem	Nursing Approach	Problem	Nursing Approach
CONSTANT MOVEMENT	Pad the sides and head of the bed. Use lamb's wool padding for heel and elbow protection.	**FEEDING (CONTINUED)**	Use *blenderized meals* if patient cannot chew; do not give the same strained baby foods.
Skin excoriation Abrasions or pressure sores	Keep the skin meticulously clean. Apply emollient skin lotion frequently. Use *soft* sheets and bedding.		For swallowing difficulties: Rub fingers in circles on patient's cheeks. Rub fingers simultaneously down each side of patient's throat.
Falls	Tie the patient (only if absolutely necessary) in bed or chair with padded protective devices, making sure that they are loosened frequently. Encourage ambulation with assistance to maintain muscle tone.		Know the Heimlich maneuver (to be used in the event of choking).
		PSYCHOLOGICAL SUPPORT AND COMMUNICATION	Respect the patient as a fellow human being with rights and needs.
FEEDING*		Grimacing Unintelligible speech	Use eye contact. Touch the patient. *Talk,* even though the patient may not be able to answer.
Constant movement Difficulty in chewing or swallowing Choking Emaciation	Talk to the patient before mealtime to help him relax; use mealtime for social interaction. Give your undivided attention.		Try to devise a communication system, perhaps using cards with words or pictures of familiar objects, before verbal communication becomes too difficult.
	Learn the position that is best for *this* patient. Keep patient as close to upright as possible while feeding. Stabilize patient's head gently with one hand while feeding.		Patients can indicate correct card by hitting it with hand, grunting, or blinking the eyes.
	Encircle patient with one arm and get as close as possible to provide stability and support. Use pillows and wedges for additional support.		Learn how this particular patient expresses needs and wants; particularly nonverbal messages (widening of eyes, responses).
	Do not interpret stiffness, turning away, or sudden turning of head as rejection; these are uncontrollable choreiform movements.		Patient can understand even if he cannot speak. Do not isolate patient by ceasing to communicate with him.
	Use a long-handled spoon (iced-tea spoon). Place spoon in middle of tongue and exert slight pressure.	**PROGRESSIVE INTELLECTUAL IMPAIRMENT AND EMOTIONAL DISTURBANCE**	Have a clock, calendar, and wall posters in view.
	Place bite-size food between teeth.		Interact with the patient in a *creative* manner.
	Wait for patient to chew and swallow before introducing another spoonful. Make sure that bites are tiny.		Use every opportunity for one-to-one contact.
	Give between-meal feedings. Constant movement burns more calories. Patients are often voracious, particularly for sweets.		Use music for relaxation. Keep patient in the social mainstream. Recruit and train volunteers for social interaction. Set a good example.
	Avoid too many milk drinks (produces mucus).		Do not abandon a patient because the disease is eventually terminal. Patients are *living* until the end.

*Adapted from Perske, R., et al.: Mealtimes for Severely and Profoundly Handicapped Persons. Baltimore. University Park Press, 1977.

Management

Although no treatment halts or reverses the underlying process, several methods of management have fairly good palliative action. The phenothiazine or butyro-phenone antipsychotic drugs improve the chorea in many cases. Haloperidol (Haldol), fluphenazine (Prolixin), mesoridazine (Serentil), trifluoperazine (Stelazine), chlorpromazine (Thorazine), and perphenazine (Triavil; Trilafon) are being used in this country. The patient's motor signs must be assessed and evaluated on a continuing basis so that optimal therapeutic drug levels may be reached. Akathisia (motor restlessness) in the overmedicated patient is a danger since it may be mistaken for the restless fidgetiness of the illness and consequently overlooked.

In certain types of the disease in which hypokinetic motor impairment resembles parkinsonism, some benefit may be obtained from antiparkinsonism therapy (page 1233). Patients who have emotional disturbances, particularly depression, may be helped by antidepressant medications. Psychotic symptoms usually respond to antipsychotic drugs. It is imperative that nurses look beyond the disease to focus on the patient's needs and capabilities. (See Chart, page 1236.)

A program combining medical, psychological, social, occupational, speech, and physical rehabilitation services is needed to help the patient and family cope with this severely disabling illness. More than most disorders, Huntington's disease exacts enormous emotional, physical, social and financial tolls of every member of the patient's family. Since there is no test to determine the carriers of the disease, entire families often live under a heavy burden of uncertainty, anxiety, and guilt. Not only is genetic counseling crucial, but patients and their families also require access to long-term psychological counseling, marriage counseling, and emotional, financial, and legal support. Some form of home care assistance, work and recreation day centers, respite care, and eventually skilled long-term care is necessary to help the patient and family cope with the constant strain of the illness. Although nothing can stop the relentless progress of the disease, families who have had good care have benefited tremendously.

VOLUNTARY HEALTH ORGANIZATIONS. Voluntary health organizations are major aids to families and have been largely responsible for bringing the illness to national attention. The Hereditary Disease Foundation, The Committee to Combat Huntington's Disease, and the National Huntington's Disease Association are oriented toward helping patients and their families by providing information, referrals, family and public education, and support for research.

NEUROMUSCULAR DISEASES
MYASTHENIA GRAVIS

Myasthenia gravis is a disorder affecting the neuromuscular transmission of the voluntary muscles of the body; the etiology is unknown. It affects young adults most commonly but may occur in the elderly. The disease is characterized by *extreme muscular weakness* and easy fatigability which generally is worse after effort and is relieved by rest.

Patients with this disease tire on such slight exertion as combing the hair, chewing, and talking, and must stop for rest. Symptoms vary according to the muscles af-

fected. Symmetrical muscles are involved, first and foremost those innervated by cranial nerves. Because of the involvement of the ocular muscles, diplopia (double vision) and ptosis (drooping) of the eyelids are early symptoms. The patient has a sleepy, masklike expression because the facial muscles are affected. Weakness of the laryngeal and pharyngeal muscles causes the voice to be weak and presents a danger of choking and aspiration of food. *Progressive weakness of the diaphragm and intercostal muscles may produce respiratory distress or myasthenic crisis, which is an acute emergency.*

Pathophysiology. The basic abnormality in myasthenia gravis is a defect in the transmission of impulses from nerve to muscle cells. Conduction of these impulses is presumably mediated by acetylcholine (ACh). In view of the observation that the injection of acetylcholine corrects the defect, briefly at least, it is quite possible that the principal difficulty resides in the inadequate synthesis or release of acetylcholine at the neuromuscular junction. Support for this view is provided by the fact that chemicals that delay the enzymatic destruction of acetylcholine in the body (i.e., compounds with anticholinesterase activity) such as neostigmine, produce temporary remissions of the disease, as evidenced by transient gains in muscle strength.

Other evidence indicates that myasthenia gravis may be an autoimmune disturbance in which circulating antibodies attack and damage the patient's own tissues. It has been found that one third of these patients have circulating antibodies against skeletal muscle and the thymus. These antibodies are found in almost all patients with myasthenia gravis who have tumors of the thymus. Researchers hypothesize that the defect in nerve transmission located at the neuromuscular junction is possibly secondary to and caused by an aberration in the metabolism of the nerve cell body. The circulating factor from the thymus and related tissue may be exerting the detrimental influence.

Diagnostic Assessment. The signs and symptoms of myasthenia gravis are sometimes so striking that a presumptive diagnosis can be made on the basis of the patient's history and physical examination. An injection of edrophonium (Tensilon), a drug that facilitates the transmission of nerve-muscle messages, is used to confirm the diagnosis. Within 30 seconds of an intravenous injection of edrophonium, most patients will improve substantially, but only temporarily. Improvement in muscle strength following administration of this agent usually confirms the diagnosis of myasthenia. Electromyography (EMG) is used to measure the electrical potential of muscle cells.

Management

Anticholinesterase drugs are given to increase the response of the muscles to nerve impulses and to improve strength. Drugs in current use include pryridostigmine bromide (Mestinon), ambenonium chloride (Mytelase) and neostigmine bromide (Prostigmin). Most patients prefer pyridostigmine because it produces less marked side effects. The dosage is increased gradually until maximal benefits are obtained, although normal muscle strength may not be achieved, and the patient may have to adapt to some disability. Anticholinesterase medications are given with milk, crackers, or other buffering substances. Their side effects include abdominal cramps, nausea, and vomiting. Small doses of atropine, given once or twice daily, may ameliorate or prevent these side effects. Other side effects of anticholinesterase therapy include adverse effects on skeletal muscles such as fasciculations (fine twitching), spasm, and weakness. The effects on the central nervous system include irritability, anxiety, insomnia, headache, dysarthria, syncope, coma, and convulsions. Increased salivation and lacrimation, increased bronchial secretions, and moist skin may also be noted.

- The nursing (and patient) priority is to give the drug prescribed according to an exact time schedule in order to control the patient's symptoms. *Any delay in drug administration may result in the patient's losing his ability to swallow.* Watch for an increase in muscle weakness within one hour after the patient takes the anticholinesterase drug, and be particularly alert for signs of respiratory distress.

After the initial medication doses have been adjusted, the patient learns to take the medication according to his needs and time plan. Further adjustments may be necessary in the presence of physical or emotional stress and intercurrent infection. Timespan Mestinon is sometimes taken at bedtime for its prolonged effect.

IMMUNOSUPPRESSIVE THERAPY. Corticosteroid therapy may benefit the patient with severe generalized myasthenia. Steroids exert their effect by suppressing the patient's immune response, thus decreasing the amount of blocking antibody. The anticholinesterase dosage is lowered while the patient's ability to maintain effective respirations and to swallow is monitored. The steroid dosage is gradually increased and the anticholinesterase medication is slowly withdrawn. Prednisone, taken on alternate days because of lower incidence of side effects, appears to be successful in suppressing the disease. Sometimes the patient will show a marked decrease in muscle strength right after steroid therapy is started but this is usually only temporary. He is given a tap bell to use in emergency situations.

PLASMAPHERESIS. Removal of the plasma containing the IgG antibodies (plasmapheresis) to lower antibody levels may improve muscle strength in patients who do not respond to anticholinesterase therapy, corticosteroids, and thymectomy (see this page). This process is combined with prednisone and azathioprine therapy and has caused remarkable improvement in some patients. (Plasmapheresis is discussed on page 676.)

THYMECTOMY. In some patients, histologic abnormalities have been identified in the thymus gland. Thymectomy (surgical removal of the thymus) causes substantial remission of the disease, especially in patients with tumor or hyperplasia of the thymus gland. Thymectomy is carried out through the transcervical or sternal-splitting (median sternotomy) approach. Following surgery, the patient is monitored in an intensive care unit; special attention is given to ventilatory function.

Myasthenic Crisis

Myasthenic crisis is the sudden onset of muscular weakness in patients with myasthenia. It may be manifested by sudden respiratory distress and an inability to swallow or speak. Weakness of respiratory, laryngeal, pharyngeal, and bulbar musculature causes respiratory depression and airway obstruction as well as cerebral hypoxia with its attendant sequelae of central nervous system injury and death.

Myasthenic crisis may result from progression of the disease, emotional upset, upper respiratory infection, surgery, or trauma, or it may be brought about by ACTH therapy.

Cholinergic crisis occurs from overmedication with anticholinesterase drugs which release too much acetylcholine at the neuromuscular junction. *Brittle crisis* occurs when the receptors at the neuromuscular junction become insensitive to anticholinesterase medication. It is not controlled by increasing or decreasing anticholinesterase therapy.

Recognition and Intervention for Myasthenic Crisis. Respiratory distress combined with varying signs of dysphagia (difficulty in swallowing), dysarthria (difficulty in speaking), eyelid ptosis, and diplopia are symptoms of impending crisis.

- Providing adequate ventilatory assistance takes precedence in the immediate management of the patient with myasthenic crisis.
- The patient is suctioned, since aspiration is a common problem. Arterial blood is drawn for arterial blood gas analysis. Endotracheal intubation and mechanical ventilation may be needed (see Chapter 24). The patient is placed in an intensive care unit for constant monitoring, since this condition is marked by intense and sudden fluctuations.

Intravenous edrophonium (Tensilon) is given to differentiate the type of crisis. It improves the condition of the patient in myasthenic crisis, temporarily worsens that of the patient in cholinergic crisis, and is unpredictable in brittle crisis. If the patient is in true myasthenic crisis, neostigmine methylsulfate (Prostigmin) is administered intramuscularly or intravenously.

If the edrophonium (Tensilon) test is uncertain or there is increasing respiratory weakness, all anticholinesterase drugs are withdrawn and atropine sulfate is given to reduce excessive secretions.

Other supportive measures include:

- Monitoring arterial blood gases, serum electrolytes, input and output, and daily weight.
- Establishing postural drainage by elevating the foot of the bed for 20 minutes each hour, followed by turning and suctioning the patient.
- Feeding the patient via nasogastric tube (200 ml. at a time) if he is unable to swallow. (Postural drainage should not be done for one half hour after feeding.)
- Avoiding use of sedatives and tranquilizing drugs, since these agents aggravate hypoxia and hypercapnia and can cause respiratory and cardiac depression.
- Establishing a method of maintaining communication: hand bell, picture cards, hand signals, etc.
- Reassuring patient that the crisis should pass and that he will not be left alone.

Patient Education. To be a participant in his treatment the patient should learn the basic facts about anticholinergic drugs: their action, timing, dosage adjustment, symptoms of overdose, and toxic effects. Stress the importance of taking the medication on time. Anticholinesterase drugs are not to be taken with morphine, ether, quinine (commercial cold products), procainamide, and certain antibiotics. Novocain is usually not well tolerated.

Mealtimes should coincide with the peak effects of anticholinesterase, if the patient has difficulty in swallowing. If choking occurs frequently, blenderized food may be easier to swallow. Standby suction should be available at home.

Certain factors may increase weakness and precipitate a myasthenic crisis: emotional upset, infections (particularly respiratory infections), vigorous physical activity, and exposure to heat and cold. These situations should be avoided. To avoid the risk of fatigue, it is best to rest *before* becoming too tired. Adaptive or self-help devices are available and are useful in helping the patient handle the disease more effectively, enabling him to live as full a life as possible.

AMYOTROPHIC LATERAL SCLEROSIS

Amyotrophic lateral sclerosis (ALS, Lou Gehrig's disease) is a disease of unknown cause in which there is a loss of motor neurons (nerve cells controlling muscles) in the anterior horns of the spinal cord and the motor nuclei of the lower brain stem. As these cells die, the muscle fibers which they supply undergo atrophic changes. The degeneration of the neurons may occur in both the upper and lower motor neuron systems.

ALS affects more men than women, with onset occurring usually in the fifth or sixth decade. In this country it is often referred to as "Lou Gehrig's disease" after the famous ballplayer who died from it.

The chief symptoms are fatigue, weakness, and muscle atrophy and fasciculations (twitching). The clinical picture depends on the location of the affected motor neurons, since specific neurons activate specific muscle fibers. Loss of motor neurons in the anterior horns of the spinal cord will result in progressive weakness and atrophy of the muscles of the arms, trunk, or legs. Spasticity is usually present and the stretch reflexes become brisk and overactive. When bulbar muscles are affected there is progressive difficulty in speaking and swallowing. The voice assumes a nasal sound and speech articulations become so disrupted that the patient is unintelligible. Some emotional lability may be present, but intellectual function usually is not impaired. The prognosis generally is based on the speed with which the disease progresses.

ALS is a progressively incapacitating and fatal disease. The patient and family facing this cruel affliction need compassionate and caring support. It is often agonizing to discuss this disease with the patient and his family. When all voluntary movement becomes impossible, the patient is helpless—unable to feed himself or even turn or move in bed. Yet he is alert and aware of his plight. Weakness of the posterior tongue and palate impairs the ability to laugh, cough, or even blow the nose. Sometimes the patient cannot swallow. Eventually respiratory function is compromised. Understandably the patient is depressed and frustrated by the relentlessly progressive course of the disease.

Management

No specific treatment is available. Symptomatic treatment and rehabilitative measures are employed to support the patient and improve the quality of life. The patient should remain active as long as possible without tiring the involved muscles. Active exercises and range of motion exercises help to strengthen uninvolved muscles and maintain muscle power at maximum levels. Stretching exercises (stretch, hold, relax) are beneficial. Such devices as ankle-foot orthoses for patients with weak dorsiflexors, which impair dorsiflexion of the ankle, help keep the patient mobile. Hand splints can provide a stronger grip and more effective use of the hand. The use of Velcro to fasten clothing aids the patient in dressing.

As the muscles grow weaker, the patient may use a wheelchair for activities outside of the house. Assistive devices are used to help the patient function independently for as long as possible. When the illness has progressed to the point where the patient is confined to a wheelchair, an electrically powered model can be used. At this stage, the prevention of contractures is important. When the patient becomes dependent, transfer devices (Hoyer lift) will be needed and special instructions will have to be given to the family concerning the best way to position the patient for the greatest comfort.

The most serious complication in the later stages of the disease is respiratory difficulty, since all muscles involved in breathing may be affected. Respiratory aids (tracheostomy, ventilator) may be necessary when this occurs. (The use of respiratory aids is discussed in Chapter 24.)

THE MUSCULAR DYSTROPHIES

The muscular dystrophies are a group of chronic muscle disorders characterized by progressive weakening and wasting of the skeletal or voluntary muscles. Most of these diseases are inherited.

The pathological features include muscle fiber necrosis, variation in muscle fiber size, cellular reaction, increased internal nuclei, and replacement of muscle tissue by connective tissue.

The common characteristics of these diseases include: varying degrees of muscle wasting and weakness; abnormal elevation in serum creatine phosphokinase, indicating a leakage of muscle enzymes; a myopathic electromyographic pattern and myopathic findings on muscle biopsy. The differences center around the pattern of inheritance, the muscles involved, the age of onset and the rate of progression.

Management

There is no specific treatment at this time for the muscular dystrophies. The objectives of supportive management are to keep the patient as active and normal as possible and to minimize functional deterioration. A therapeutic exercise program is prescribed for the individual patient to prevent muscle tightness, contractures, and disuse atrophy. Night splints and stretching exercises are used to delay contractures of the joints, especially the ankles, knees, and hips. Braces may compensate for muscle weakness. If the patient becomes confined to a wheelchair, he is fitted with a Silastic jacket, or a spinal fusion is done to prevent collapse of the trunk. Other surgical procedures may be carried out to correct deformities. Self-help devices can assist in achieving a greater degree of independence. Additional self-help devices become necessary as more muscle groups become affected.

Intercurrent illnesses, upper respiratory infections, and fractures from falls must be vigorously treated in such a way as to minimize immobilization, since joint contractures will become worse if the patient's activities are restricted more than usual. Aside from muscle weakness and contractures, a variety of other difficulties may be manifested in relation to the underlying disease. Dental and speech problems may result from weakness of the facial muscles, which makes it difficult to attend to dental hygiene and to speak coherently. Additional problems affect the gastrointestinal tract, resulting in gastric dilatation, rectal prolapse, and fecal impaction. Finally, cardiomyopathy appears to be a common complication in all forms of muscular dystrophy.

Because of the genetic nature of this disease, parents and siblings of the patient are advised to seek genetic counseling. The Muscular Dystrophy Association works to combat neuromuscular disease through scientific research, programs of patient services and clinical care, and professional and public education.

CONVULSIVE DISORDERS

Seizures

Seizures (convulsions) are symptomatic of focal or diffuse pathology of the brain. They are sudden and transient and can be described as motor, sensory, autonomic, or pyschic episodes that have associated electroencephalographic change. The causes are varied and are classified as idiopathic (genetic, developmental defects) and acquired. Among the causes of acquired seizures are hypoxemia of any cause, including vascular insufficiency, fever (childhood), head injury, hypertension, central nervous system infections, metabolic and toxic conditions (renal failure, hyponatremia, hypocalcemia, hypoglycemia, pesticides, etc.), brain tumor, drug withdrawal, and allergies. Often there is memory loss for the convulsive episode and for a short time thereafter.

The immediate therapeutic objective is to control the seizure and the long-term goal is to seek out and control the cause. See below for a discussion of epilepsy (the most common clinical syndrome of recurrent seizures) and the nursing management of the patient with seizures.

THE EPILEPSIES

The epilepsies are a symptom-complex of several disorders of brain function characterized by brief episodes of unconsciousness that may or may not be associated with convulsions, sensory phenomena, erratic behavior, or a combination of all three. Thus, epilepsy is not a disease but a symptom. An epileptic seizure is a manifestation of an abnormal and excessive discharge of neurons in the brain.

The basic problem is thought to be an electrical disturbance (dysrhythmia) in the nerve cells in one section of the brain that give off abnormal, recurring, uncontrolled electrical discharges. The characteristic epileptic seizure is a manifestation of this excessive neuronal discharge.

Incidence. An estimated 1 percent of the population (more than 2 million) in the United States have epilepsy at an annual cost of 3 billion dollars. There has been an increasing incidence of this condition, probably due to a number of factors. Improved obstetrical and pediatric care salvages babies who previously would have succumbed from cerebral birth defects; these persons are predisposed to intermittent seizures. The improved medical, surgical, and nursing managment of patients with head injuries, brain tumors, meningitis, and encephalitis saves those whose conditions may produce cerebral changes with resultant seizures. Also, advances in electroencephalography have aided in the identification of patients with epilepsy. Education has served to enlighten the general public and has lessened the stigmata associated with the condition, so that more persons are more willing to admit that they have epilepsy.

Altered Physiology. Messages from the body are carried by the neurons (nerve cells) of the brain by means of discharges of electrochemical energy that sweep along them. These impulses occur in bursts whenever a nerve cell has a task to perform. Sometimes certain of these cells or groups of cells continue firing after a task is finished. It is as if a switch sticks in the "on" position until the power source runs down, then closes to allow recharge. During the period of unwanted discharges, parts of the body controlled by the errant cells may perform erratically. Resultant discomfort and dysfunction range from mild to incapacitating and usually cause unconsciousness. When these uncontrolled, abnormal discharges happen repeatedly, a person is said to have epilepsy. The erratic physical movements are called "seizures."*

Causes. No one knows what makes brain cells in some people cause epilepsy. Scientists have produced seizures in experimental animals through surgical injury or chemical or electrical stimulation. Epilepsies often follow birth trauma, head injuries, some infectious diseases, and drug or alcohol intoxication. They are also associated with brain tumors, abscesses, and congenital malformations. In many instances the epilepsies are termed "idiopathic" (cause unknown). There is evidence that susceptibility to some types may be inherited, but it is not conclusive. Epilepsy strikes before the age of 18 in more than 75 percent of patients.

The epilepsies have little to do with intelligence in most cases. If the person with epilepsy does not have other brain or nervous system disabilities he will fall within the same intelligence ranges as the overall population. Epilepsy is not synonymous with mental retardation or illness. However, many who are retarded because they have serious neurological damage often have epilepsy too, thus pulling the mean IQ for all epilepsy victims below that of the so-called normal range.

Diagnostic Assessment

The diagnostic assessment is aimed at determining the *type* of seizures, their frequency and severity, and the factors that precipitate them. A developmental history is taken, including events of pregnancy and childbirth, to seek evidence of preexisting injury. A search is made for illnesses or head injuries that may have affected the brain. In addition to a physical and neurologic examination,

*Adapted from report of the National Institure of Neurological Disease and Stroke.

diagnostic examinations include biochemical, hematologic, and serologic studies. Computerized tomography may be used to determine whether a tumor or other abnormality is present in the brain.

Of all the tests now available, the most illuminating is the *electroencephalogram* (EEG), which furnishes positive diagnostic evidence in a substantial proportion of epileptic patients, aids in classifying the type of seizure, and serves as a guide in establishing a prognosis (Fig. 55-7). Abnormalities in the electroencephalogram usually continue to be apparent between attacks, or, if concealed, may be brought out by hyperventilation or during sleep. In addition, microelectrodes can be inserted deep in the brain to probe the action of single brain cells. It should be noted, however, that some persons with seizures may have normal EEGs whereas persons who have never had seizures may have abnormal EEGs. Telemetering and computer equipment developed by space technology are being used to take and store electroencephalographic readings on computer tapes while patients pursue their normal activities. Videorecording of seizures taken simultaneously with EEG telemetry is useful in determining the type of seizure as well as its duration and magnitude. These tools help to identify seizure patterns before and after they occur.

Classification of Seizures

Epileptic seizures may vary from a twitch of the eyelid or a pain in the stomach to violent tremors of all parts of the body. The variations in seizures have been classified internationally as partial (simple and complex), generalized, unilateral, and unclassified (Table 55-2). The accompanying glossary provides a further breakdown in definition.

In *simple partial* seizures, only a finger or hand may shake or the mouth may jerk uncontrollably. The person may speak nonsense, may be dizzy, and may experience unusual or unpleasant sights, sounds, odors, or tastes, but without loss of consciousness.

In *complex partial* seizures, the person either remains motionless or moves automatically but inappropriately for time and place. Or he may experience excessive emotions of fear, anger, elation, or irritability. Whatever the manifestations, the person does not remember the episode when it is over.

Generalized seizures, more commonly referred to as *grand mal,* involve both hemispheres of the brain, causing both sides of the body to react. There may be intense rigidity of the entire body followed by jerky alternations of muscle relaxation and contraction (generalized tonic-clonic). Often the tongue is chewed, and stools and urine may be passed involuntarily. After 1 or 2 minutes the convulsive movements begin to subside; the patient relaxes and lies in deep coma, breathing noisily. The respirations at this point are chiefly abdominal. In the

---

Glossary

Generalized seizure (formerly termed *grand mal*)—a seizure characterized by loss of consciousness, tonic spasms of the trunk and extremities rapidly followed by repetitive generalized clonic jerking.

Partial seizures (formerly termed *petit mal*)—attacks of brief impairment of consciousness often associated with flickering of eyelids and slight twitching of the mouth.

Psychomotor seizures—attacks characterized clinically by impairment of consciousness and amnesia for the episode; may be accompanied by motor and psychic activity which is irrelevant for time and place.

Focal seizures—seizures beginning with a focal disturbance of cerebral function.

Jacksonian seizures—focal motor or sensory convulsions.

---

postseizure state the patient may be confused and suffer from headache, malaise, and nausea.

Included under general seizures are those which affect only infants (infantile spasms) and those which cause muscle flabbiness (atonic), muscle rigidity (tonic), muscle spasms (clonic), rapid rhythmic muscle jerks (myoclonic), and complete muscle collapse (akinetic).

TABLE 55-2.   INTERNATIONAL CLASSIFICATION OF EPILEPTIC SEIZURES

I.   PARTIAL SEIZURES (seizures beginning locally)

   A. Partial seizures with elementary symptomatology (generally without impairment of consciousness)
      1. With motor symptoms (*includes Jacksonian seizures*)
      2. With special sensory or somatosensory symptoms
      3. With autonomic symptoms
      4. Compound forms

   B. Partial seizures with complex symptomatology (generally with impairment of consciousness)
      (*temporal lobe or psychomotor seizures*)
      1. With impairment of consciousness only
      2. With cognitive symptomatology
      3. With affective symptomatology
      4. With "psychosensory" symptomatology
      5. With "psychomotor" symptomatology (automatisms)
      6. Compound forms
   C. Partial seizures secondarily generalized

II.   GENERALIZED SEIZURES (bilaterally symmetrical and without local onset)

      1. Absences (*petit mal*)
      2. Bilateral massive epileptic myoclonus
      3. Infantile spasms
      4. Clonic seizures
      5. Tonic seizures
      6. Tonic-clonic seizures (*grand mal*)
      7. Atomic seizures
      8. Akinetic seizures

III.   UNILATERAL SEIZURES (or predominantly)

IV.   UNCLASSIFIED EPILEPTIC SEIZURES (due to incomplete data)

Abstracted from: Gastaut, H.: Clinical and electroencephalographical classification of epileptic seizures. Epilepsia, *11*:102-113, 1970.

Prevention of Epilepsy.   A full scale attack incorporating a wide range of measures must be mounted for the prevention of epilepsy. Since the infants of epileptic mothers who take certain antiepileptic medications are at risk, these women need to be monitored carefully, including blood studies to detect the level of antiepileptic drugs taken throughout pregnancy. High-risk mothers (teenagers, women with histories of difficult deliveries, drug addicts, those with diabetes and hypertension) should be identified and supervised closely during pregnancy since brain lesions or injury that ultimately causes epilepsy may occur to the fetus during pregnancy and delivery.

Childhood infections (measles, mumps, bacterial meningitis) should be controlled with appropriate vaccination. Lead poisoning is another preventable cause of epilepsy.

Head injury is one of the main causes that can be prevented. Through highway safety programs and occupational safety precautions, not only can lives be saved, but the possible development of epilepsy from head injury can be prevented.

Screening programs to detect children with seizure disorders at an early age and seizure prevention programs with the judicious use of antiepileptic medications and modification of life style are part of this prevention plan.

Management

The management of epilepsy is planned according to a long-range program, one that is tailored to meet the special needs of each patient and not just to manage and prevent seizures. There is no simple solution, since some forms of epilepsy arise from brain damage and others depend upon alterations of brain chemistry.

The aims of medical and nursing management are to determine and treat (if possible) the primary underlying cause of seizures, to prevent recurrence of seizures, and to gain an understanding of the patient and his relationship to his environment.

The patient must learn to adapt to his disease and control its manifestations. The patient's life style and environment should be examined to determine whether certain factors precipitate the seizures: emotional disturbances, fever, new environmental stresses, onset of mestruation. The patient is encouraged to follow a regular and moderate routine in life style, diet, exercise, and rest. Moderate activity is good therapy, but excessive expenditure of energy is to be avoided, as is emotional overstimulation such as watching late night television. Since seizures are known to follow alcoholic intake, alcoholic beverages are restricted. All in all, the best therapy is to follow the therapeutic program.

DRUG THERAPY.   Many antiepileptic drugs are available to control seizures, although the mechanisms of their actions are still unknown. The objective of drug therapy is to control the number and/or severity of seizures. Drug therapy is a form of control, not cure. The drug is selected according to the type of seizure being treated and the effectiveness and safety of the drug. If properly prescribed and taken, these drugs will result in control of more than 50 percent of patients with recurring seizures and will partially control another 30 percent. The condition of approximately 20 percent of patients will not be improved by any currently available drugs.

Usually treatment is started with a single drug, and the dose is increased slowly until seizures are controlled or toxic symptoms develop. If there is no improvement, another drug is tried. A second drug is added in the same manner, if there is partial improvement. Initially the drug levels are monitored in the blood, since the rate of drug absorption varies among people. The drug may have to be adjusted because of intercurrent illness, weight gain, or increases in stress. Sudden withdrawal of antiepileptic medication can cause seizures to occur with greater frequency or can precipitate the development of status epilepticus.

The side effects of these medications may be divided into three groups: (1) idiosyncratic or allergic disorders which present primarily as skin reactions; (2) acute toxicity which may be manifested when the drug is initially prescribed or (3) chronic toxicity which occurs late in the course of drug therapy. The manifestations of drug toxicity are variable and any organ system may be involved. Periodic physical examinations and laboratory tests are done on patients receiving drugs known to have toxic effects on the hematopoietic, genitourinary, or hepatic systems. Table 55-3 summarizes the antiepileptic drugs in current use.

One of the most significant advancements in the treatment of epilepsy has been the development of an accurate method for measuring levels of antiepileptic drugs in the blood. Patients metabolize these drugs at different rates, and the usual drug dose may be either insufficient or too much for a given individual. Through the use of gas tomography, radioimmune assay, and immunoassay techniques, the drug dosage can be adjusted more precisely and drug levels can be monitored to determine if the patient is taking the medication. It is of special value to researchers studying the effectiveness of old or new drugs.

SURGERY FOR EPILEPSY. Surgery is indicated for patients whose epilepsy results from intracranial tumors, abscess, cysts, or vascular anomalies.

Some patients have intractable seizure disorders and do not respond to drug therapy. There may be a focal atrophic process secondary to trauma, inflammation, stroke, or anoxemia. If the seizures originate in a reasonably well circumscribed area of the brain which can be excised without producing significant neurologic deficits, the removal of the epileptogenic focus generating the sei-

TABLE 55-3. ANTIEPILEPTIC DRUGS*†

GENERIC NAME	TRADE NAME	SIDE EFFECTS
carbamazepine	Tegretol	Dizziness, drowsiness, eye muscle imbalance causing blurred vision and nystagmus, nausea, vomiting, headache, skin rashes, blood dyscrasias
clonazepam	Clonopin	Drowsiness, ataxia, neurologic symptoms, behavior changes, palpitations, hair loss, anorexia
diazepam	Valium	Drowsiness, fatigue, ataxia, depression, headache, tremor
ethosuximide	Zarontin	Nausea, drowsiness, lethargy, headache, euphoria, anorexia
ethotoin	Peganone	Dizziness, fatigue, skin rash, insomnia, diplopia
mephenytoin	Mesantoin	Nervousness, ataxia, nystagmus, pancytopenia, exfoliative dermatitis, drowsiness
mephobarbital	Mebaral	Dizziness, headache, nausea, facial edema, skin rash
metharbital	Gemonil	Drowsiness, dizziness, gastric distress, irritability, skin rash
methsuximide	Celontin	Nausea, vomiting, anorexia, ataxia, rash, drowsiness, dizziness, blood dyscrasias
paramethadione	Paradione	Nausea, anorexia, insomnia, diplopia, skin rash, bleeding gums, blood dyscrasias
phenacemide	Phenurone	Gastrointestinal disturbances, anorexia, drowsiness, insomnia, paresthesias, psychic changes, hepatitis, blood dyscrasias, skin rash, nephritis
phenobarbital	Luminal	drowsiness, dermatitis
phensuximide	Milontin	Nausea, ataxia, dizziness, drowsiness, skin eruptions, blood dyscrasias, hematuria
phenytoin	Dilantin	Ataxia, slurred speech, nystagmus, mental confusion, motor twitching, nausea, rash, gingival hyperplasia, hirsutism
primidone	Mysoline	Ataxia, vertigo, anorexia, fatigue, hyperirritability
trimethadione	Tridione	Bone marrow depression, pancytopenia, exfoliative dermatitis, photophobia, nephrosis, hepatitis
valproate sodium	Depakene	Gastrointestinal disturbance, altered bleeding time, liver toxicity

*Side effects and sensitivity to antiepileptic drugs vary among patients and at different times in the same patient. The dose for each patient is based on the patient's clinical response (free of seizures and side effects).
†Adapted from Official Names of Antiepileptic Drugs. Epilepsia, 18:123, 1977.

zures seems to give long-term control and improvement. This type of neurosurgery has been aided by several modern advances, including microsurgical techniques, improved illumination and hemostasis, and the introduction of neuroleptanesthetic drugs (droperidol and fentanyl). These techniques, combined with local infiltration of scalp incisions, enable the neurosurgeon to perform surgery on an alert and cooperative patient. With special testing devices, electrocortical mapping and the patient's response to stimulation, the boundaries of the epileptogenic focus are determined. Any abnormal epileptogenic cortex (i.e., abnormal area of the brain) is then removed.

Other neurosurgical techniques which are considered promising but still experimental are stereotaxic surgery, disconnection surgery, cerebellar stimulation, and cerebral cooling.

Nursing Management During a Seizure

During a convulsive seizure the nursing objective is to prevent injury to the patient. This includes not only physical support but psychological support as well.

- Provide privacy and protect the patient from curious onlookers. (The patient who has an *aura* [warning of an impending seizure] may have time to seek a safe place.)
- Ease the patient to the floor, if there is enough time.
- Protect the head with a pad to prevent injury (from striking a hard surface).
- Loosen constrictive clothing.
- Push aside any furniture that may be struck by the patient during the attack.
- If the patient is in bed, remove the pillows.
- If an aura precedes the seizure, insert a handkerchief between the teeth to reduce the possibility of the tongue or cheek being bitten. *Do not attempt to pry open jaws that are clenched in a spasm to insert a mouth gag.* Broken teeth and injury to the lips and tongue may result from such an action.
- No attempt should be made to restrain the patient during the seizure, since muscular contractions are strong and restraint can produce a fracture.
- If possible, place the patient on his side, because he is unable to swallow during a convulsive episode and a lateral position facilitates drainage of mucus and saliva.
- After the seizure, keep the patient turned on his side to prevent aspiration. Make sure he has an adequate airway.
- When the patient awakens, reorient him to his environment. If the patient experiences severe excitement following a seizure (postictal), try to handle him with calm persuasion and gentle restraint.

Nursing Assessment During a Seizure.
A major responsibility of the nurse is to observe and to record the sequence of symptoms. The nature of the seizure usually indicates the type of treatment that is employed.

During an attack, the following should be noted:
1. The first thing the patient does in an attack—where the movements or the stiffness starts; position of the eyeballs and the head at the beginning of the attack. This information gives clues as to the location of the epileptogenic focus in the brain. (In recording, always state whether or not the beginning of the attack was observed.)
2. The type of movements of the part involved.
3. The parts involved. (Turn back bed covers and expose patient.)
4. The size of both pupils.
5. Incontinence of urine or feces.
6. Duration of each phase of the attack.
7. Unconsciousness, if present, and its duration.
8. Any obvious paralysis or weakness of arms or legs after the attack.
9. Inability to speak after the attack.
10. Movements at the end of the seizure.
11. Whether or not the patient sleeps afterward.

Psychosocial Considerations*

It has been noted that the social, psychological, and behavioral problems frequently accompanying epilepsy can be more of a "handicap" than the actual seizures. Epilepsy imposes feelings of fear, alienation, depression, and uncertainty. The patient must cope with the ever present fear of a seizure and its embarrassing consequences. Children with epilepsy may be ostricized and excluded from school and peer activities. These problems are compounded in the teen years and add to the challenges of dating, not being able to drive, and "being different." Adults face all of these problems plus the burden of finding employment and decisions concerning marriage and childbearing, noninsurability, stigma of all kinds, and legal barriers. Alcohol may complicate matters. The burden on the family is great, and family problems run the gamut of outright rejection to overprotection. As a result of all these factors, many persons with epilepsy have psychological and behavioral problems.

Counseling is a must for helping the individual and the family to understand the condition and the limitations imposed by it. Social and recreational opportunities are necessary for good mental health. Some persons are not able to cope with epilepsy; others have psychological problems resulting from brain damage. Those with seizures originating in the temporal lobes of the brain (areas controlling thought and emotions) have particular mental problems. Symptoms of schizophrenia, hyposexuality, and impulsive or irritable behavior may be due to brain damage associated with temporal lobe seizures. These patients require comprehensive mental health services.

Patient and Family Education

The complete cooperation of the patient and family is of the utmost importance. They must have confidence in the value of the regimen that is prescribed. It must be

*Commission for the Control of Epilepsy and Its Consequences: Plan for Nationwide Action on Epilepsy. Vol. 1, DHEW Pub. No. (NIH) 78-276.

emphasized that the prescribed antiepileptic drug must be taken on a continuing basis and that the medicine is not a habit-forming "dope." It may be taken without fear, for many years if necessary, if the patient is under medical supervision and following instructions faithfully.

Of all the services that are contributed by the nurse in the care of the person with epilepsy, perhaps the most valuable are efforts to reorient the attitude of the patient and family to the disease itself. Concepts that reflect all of the ignorance and brutality that might be associated with the Middle Ages still prevail regarding epilepsy. For other patients, public sympathy and support abound; for the epileptic, common responses are abhorrence, rejection, unemployment, and legal shackles.

For the average person an epileptic seizure is a terrifying or a repulsive spectacle; thus, for the individual who experiences them, every seizure is inevitably a source of humiliation and shame, which in turn breeds anxiety, depression, hostility, secrecy, and deceit, to which the public reacts with abhorrence, etc., and the vicious cycle is complete. The reaction of shame and the recourse to deceit are not confined merely to persons with epilepsy but extends to their families as well.

In order to escape from this vicious cycle, patients who have epilepsy, their families, and the public at large need facts. These are the facts: Epilepsy is not a mysterious disease; it does not reflect the supernatural. It is not a stigma. Epilepsy is no more disgraceful than diabetes, pernicious anemia, or hyperthyroidism. It is not a form of insanity. It does not tend to get worse with time. It can be controlled effectively. It should not prevent the child from completing his schooling or keep the adult from work. *Activity tends to inhibit, not stimulate, epileptic seizures.* Some 50 percent of patients with epilepsy now may have their symptoms controlled.

Enlightenment of the public will give new hope to those facing centuries-old prejudices. Continuing encouragement should be given patients to mobilize their inner resources to overcome feelings of inferiority and self-consciousness resulting from seizures.

The hereditary transmission of epilepsy has not been proved. The matter of marriage and children must be decided on an individual basis, but this right should not be denied to the person with epilepsy merely because he has the disease. However, genetic counseling is advised.

SERVICES TO PATIENTS. Since epilepsy is a long-term disorder, the continuous use of expensive medications may present a sizable burden to the patient and his family. The Epilepsy Foundation of America offers a low-cost pharmacy service. A prescription, authorized and signed by the patient's physician, is filled by registered pharmacists and sent by mail to the patient. Life insurance protection is also available through this organization. The patients with epilepsy should carry an Emergency Medi-cal Identification card in his wallet or have an identification bracelet around the wrist.

For many, employment problems still remain the greatest handicap of epilepsy. Studies have demonstrated that the epileptic who is properly placed in his work has a satisfactory job performance. The director of each State Vocational Rehabilitation agency can provide information about vocational rehabilitation. If the individual's seizures are not well controlled, information about workshop opportunities may be obtained. Counseling and job training are provided for qualified persons through the Veterans' Administration. The U.S. Civil Service Commission now grants government jobs to individuals if seizures are controlled and the person is otherwise qualified. The Rehabilitation Act of 1972 specifies that employers having government contracts of $2,500 or more must employ qualified handicapped individuals. Private firms are becoming enlightened, and the number of employers who knowingly hire persons with epilepsy is increasing.

Status Epilepticus

Status epilepticus (acute prolonged seizure activity) is a series of generalized convulsions which occur without recovery of consciousness between attacks. The series of convulsions may last for hours or days and is considered a major medical emergency. Status epilepticus produces cumulative effects. There is some respiratory arrest at the height of each seizure which produces venous congestion and hypoxia of the brain. Repeated episodes of cerebral anoxia and swelling may lead to irreversible and fatal brain damage.

The objective of treatment is to stop the seizures as quickly as possible, to ensure adequate cerebral oxygenation, and to maintain the patient in a seizure-free state. Intravenous diazepam (Valium) has been found effective in the control of status epilepticus. Good results have been obtained by anesthetizing the patient with one of the volatile anesthetic agents.

Other antiepileptic drugs (phenytoin, phenobarbital) are given after diazepam is administered to maintain a seizure-free state. An intravenous line is established and kept open to monitor electrolytes, blood urea, and glucose. EEG monitoring may be useful in determining the nature of epileptogenic activity. Of course, vital and neurologic signs are monitored on a continuing basis. As soon as control of seizures is achieved, serum concentration of the antiepileptic drug is measured, since a low level will suggest that the patient was not taking the medication or that the dosage was too low. Patients recovering from status epilepticus may die within a few days from cardiac involvement or respiratory depression.

HEAD INJURIES

Injuries to the head are among the most frequent and serious neurologic disorders and have reached epidemic proportions as a result of traffic accidents. Studies and estimates reveal that head injury occurs in 71 percent of persons injured in automobile accidents and in 50 percent of persons injured in motorcycle accidents. Injuries in the home and at work are also frequent, as is indicated by the fact that head injuries occur in 70 percent of persons injured in accidental falls in the home and in 70 percent of compensable work-related injuries.

The most important consideration in any head injury is whether or not the brain has been injured. The brain dies when its blood supply is interrupted for only a few minutes; there is no regeneration of damaged neurons. *Injuries to the cervical spine frequently coexist with head injuries.* The patient may also be in shock from other body injuries.

If a person has suffered a head injury and is to be transported from the scene of the accident, he should be placed on a board or stretcher with his head and neck maintained in alignment with the axis of the body. Slight traction should be maintained on the head.

SCALP INJURY

Because of the many blood vessels, the scalp can bleed profusely when injured. Trauma may result in an abrasion ("brush wound"), contusion, laceration, or avulsion. Before such a wound can be cared for properly, an area about 5 cm. (2 inches) should be shaved around the wound. The injection of procaine makes it easier for the wound to be cleaned and treated. If the patient is unconscious and showing evidence of shock, this type of wound is the last to receive attention except to stop the bleeding and apply a sterile dressing.

SKULL INJURY—FRACTURE OF THE SKULL

Fracture of the skull is treated as a neurosurgical condition, because the fracture in itself is of less importance than the possibility of a brain injury (Fig. 55-8). For this reason, every patient with head injury, even though it appears to be slight, should be under constant observation for several days. If a depressed fracture has occurred, then increased intracranial pressure may be likely and should be watched for.

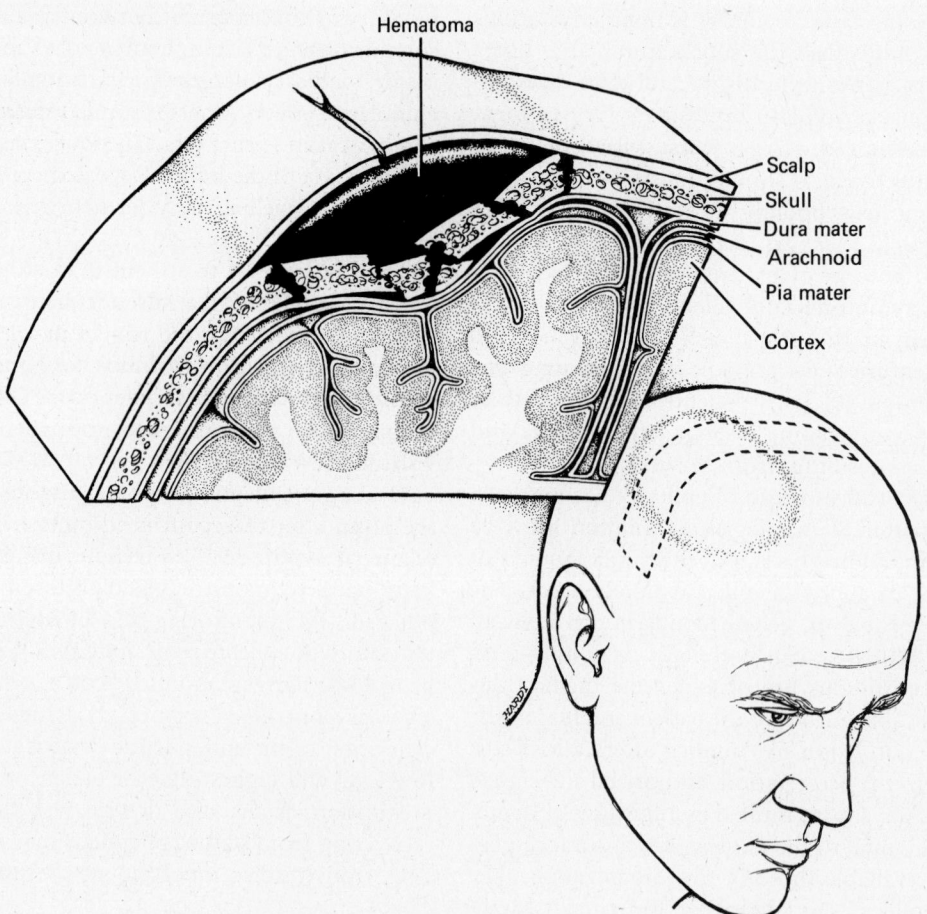

Hematoma

Scalp
Skull
Dura mater
Arachnoid
Pia mater
Cortex

Figure 55-8.   Depressed fracture of the skull.

- All patients with fractures of the skull should be suspected of having brain injury until proved otherwise. It is possible that the patient may have other injuries that are masked by the head injury.

Clinical Manifestations. The symptoms, besides those of the local injury, depend on the amount and the distribution of brain injury. Pain, persistent or localized, suggests that a fracture is usually present. Fractures of the vault produce swelling in the region of the fracture, and for this reason an accurate diagnosis cannot be made without a roentgenogram. Fractures of the base of the skull frequently produce hemorrhage from the nose, the pharynx, or the ears, and blood may appear under the conjunctivae. An area of ecchymosis may be seen over the mastoid. The escape of cerebrospinal fluid from the ears (otorrhea) and the nose (rhinorrhea) suggests skull fracture. Bloody spinal fluid, if present, suggests brain laceration or contusion.

Diagnostic Evaluation. Although a rapid physical examination and evaluation of the neurologic status will reveal the more obvious brain injuries, the less apparent abnormalities found in head injuries may be detected by cranial computerized tomography, which can differentiate subtle changes in the degree to which the soft tissue absorbs x-ray. It is accurate and safe in determining the presence, nature, location, and extent of the lesion as well as detecting cerebral edema, contusion, intracerebral or extracerebral hematoma, subarachnoid and intraventricular hemorrhage, and late traumatic changes (infarct; hydrocephalus).

If computerized tomography is not available, cerebral angiography will demonstrate the presence of supratentorial, extracerebral and intracerebral hematomas and cerebral contusion.

Management. In general, nondepressed skull fractures usually do not require surgical treatment. However for depressed skull fractures, surgery is indicated. The scalp is shaved and cleansed and the fracture exposed. The skull fragments are elevated and the area is debrided. Closure of the dura is carried out if possible, and the wound is closed. Large defects in the skull can later be repaired with metallic or plastic plates if necessary. In instances of a clean wound and an intact dura, the elevated fragments can be replaced, making a later cranioplasty unnecessary. Penetrating wounds require surgical debridement to remove foreign bodies and devitalized brain tissue and to control hemorrhage. Antibiotic treatment is immediately instituted and blood transfusions are made available.

Fractures of the base of the skull are serious because of the danger of grave cranial complications and meningitis. The nasopharynx and the external ear should be kept clean, and usually a plug of sterile cotton is placed in the ear to absorb discharges.

BRAIN INJURY

Serious brain injury may occur following blows or injuries to the head, with or without fracture of the skull.

A cerebral *concussion* may occur following a head injury in which there is neither structural damage nor persistent neurologic deficit. The jarring of the brain may be so slight as to cause only dizziness and spots before the eyes (spoken of as "seeing stars"), or there may be complete loss of consciousness for a time. If the brain tissue in the frontal lobe is affected, the patient may exhibit bizarre irrational behavior, whereas disruption of brain tissue in the temporal lobe can produce temporary amnesia or disorientation. The treatment of concussion is to observe the patient for headache, dizziness, and nervous instability (postconcussional syndrome) which may follow this type of injury.

A *cerebral contusion* is a more marked cerebral injury in which the brain is bruised, with possible surface hemorrhage. The victim will be unconscious for a considerable period. The symptoms as would be expected, are more marked. The patient may lie motionless; the pulse will be feeble, the respiration shallow, and the skin cold and pale. Often there is involuntary evacuation of the bowels and the bladder. The patient may be aroused with effort but soon slips back into unconsciousness. The blood pressure and the temperature are subnormal, and the picture is somewhat similar to that of shock.

In general, persons with diffuse injury who have abnormal motor function, abnormal eye movements, and raised intracranial pressure have a poor outcome. On the other hand, the patient may recover consciousness completely and perhaps pass into a stage of cerebral irritability.

In the stage of cerebral irritability the patient is no longer unconscious. On the contrary, he is easily disturbed by any form of stimulation, noises, light, and voices, and may become hyperactive at times. Gradually, the pulse, the respiration, the temperature, and the other body functions return to normal. However, recovery is not complete at once. Residual headache and vertigo are common, and often impaired mentality or epilepsy occurs as a result of irreparable cerebral damage.

Epidural, Subdural, and Intracerebral Hemorrhage

The most serious injuries are caused by hematomas that develop within the cranial vault (Fig. 55-9). The hematoma may be epidural, subdural, or intracerebral depending upon the location. *The signs and symptoms of brain ischemia resulting from clot compression are variable and depend upon the speed with which vital areas are encroached upon.* In general, a small hematoma that develops rapidly may be fatal, whereas the patient may adapt to a more massive hematoma if it develops slowly.

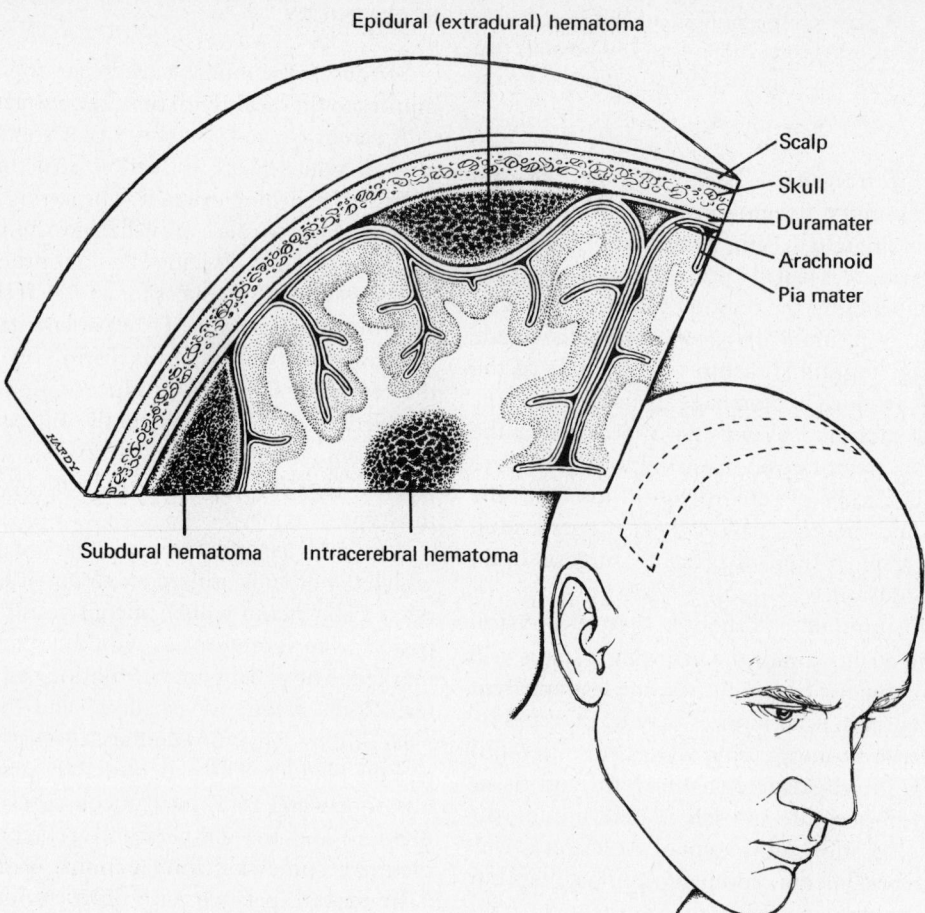

Figure 55-9. Diagrammatic views showing epidural, subdural, and intracerebral hematomas.

Epidural Hematoma
(Extradural Hematoma or Hemorrhage)

Following a head injury, bleeding may occur in the epidural (extradural) space between the skull and the dura. This often results from fracture of the skull that causes rupture or laceration of the middle meningeal artery, which runs between the dura and the skull; hemorrhage from this artery causes pressure on the brain.

More frequently, bleeding sites along the fracture line produce acute hematomas. Epidural hematomas most frequently occur in the temporal area.

The symptoms are caused by the expanding hematoma. There is usually a momentary loss of consciousness at the time of injury followed by an interval of apparent recovery (lucid interval). However, a lucid interval is not always present with an epidural hematoma although it may occur with a subdural hematoma. Then, often suddenly, signs of compression appear, usually with muscular twitchings or convulsions, because the clot presses on the region of the cortex that sends impulses to the muscles (the motor cortex). There may be headache, focal neurologic signs such as dilatation and fixation of a pupil, and weakness and paralysis of an extremity.

Management. An epidural hematoma is considered an extreme emergency, since marked neurologic deficit or even cessation of breathing may occur within minutes. The treatment consists of making openings through the skull (burr holes), removing the clot, and controlling the bleeding point.

Subdural Hematoma

Not infrequently, either with or without injury, hemorrhage may take place over the surface of the brain underneath the dura. A subdural hemorrhage is more frequently venous in origin, and the blood spreads over the brain surface. A subdural hematoma may be either acute, subacute, or chronic, depending on the size of the involved vessel and the amount of bleeding present. Usually the patient is comatose and the clinical signs are similar to those of epidural hematoma. A rising blood pressure with slowing of pulse and respirations indicates a rapidly increasing hematoma.

The mortality rate for patients with acute subdural hematomas is high, although the condition is amenable to early surgical intervention. The clot may be evacuated and the hemorrhage controlled. Postoperative cerebral edema is treated by such drugs as mannitol and steroids.

Chronic subdural hematoma imitates other conditions and may be mistaken for a stroke. In fact, it has been termed "the great imitator." The bleeding is less profuse and there is compression of the intracranial contents. The blood within the brain changes in character in 2 to 4 days, becoming thicker and darker. In a few weeks the clot breaks down and has the color and consistency of motor oil. Eventually calcification or ossification of the clot takes place. The brain adapts to this foreign body invasion and the patient's clinical signs and symptoms fluctuate. There may be severe headache which tends to come and go, alternating focal neurologic signs, personality changes, mental deterioration, and focal convulsions. Unfortunately, the patient may be labeled "neurotic" or "psychotic" if the cause of the symptoms is overlooked.

The treatment of chronic subdural hematoma consists of surgically evacuating the clot by suctioning or irrigating the blood. The procedure may be carried out through multiple burr holes, or a craniotomy may be performed in which the dura is opened and the blood evacuated, along with the membranes, if necessary.

Intracerebral Hematoma

Intracerebral hemorrhages are more frequently seen in the elderly and occur after a fall. In severe injuries to the brain, scattered petechial hemorrhages or a large parenchymal hematoma may occur. The neurologic signs and symptoms may be masked by coma and confusion. The clot may be evacuated by means of a craniotomy, but the associated mortality rate is high.

Assessment

When the patient is admitted to the emergency department, a complete history is obtained, if possible. Any observers of the accident should be interviewed. A head injury may be obscured if the patient is under the influence of alcohol or drugs, or attention may be diverted from a head injury because of serious trauma elsewhere in the body.

The following questions are significant in assessing head injuries:
- What caused the injury? a high velocity missile? an object striking the head? a fall? What was the direction and force of the blow?
- Was there a loss of consciousness? What was the duration of the unconscious period? Could the patient be aroused? (A history of amnesia and unconsciousness after a head injury indicates a significant degree of cerebral dysfunction.)
- Was there bleeding from the orifices? eyes? ears? nose? mouth?
- Was there paralysis or flaccidity of the extremities?

Management

As soon as the initial assessment is made, a neurological observation record is started and maintained (see page 1250).

Airway. One of the most important nursing objectives in the management of the patient with a head injury is to establish and maintain an adequate airway. Death may occur following head injury as a result of cerebral anoxia from an inadequate airway or from injury to the brain caused by contusion, laceration, or compression. The patient must be adequately ventilated to preserve cerebral function. Hypercarbia causes cerebral engorgement and increases intracranial pressure.

Therapeutic and nursing activities to ensure an adequate exchange of air are summarized on pages 1192-1193 and include the following:
- Keeping the unconscious patient in a semiprone or prone position with the head of the bed elevated about 30 degrees to decrease intracranial venous pressure.
- Monitoring arterial blood gases.
- Providing for endotracheal intubation with mechanical ventilation.
- Establishing effective suctioning procedures.
- Guarding against aspiration and respiratory insufficiency.

An equally important nursing objective is constant assessment of the level of responsiveness, since irreversible changes occur rapidly. This nursing priority, discussed in detail on pages 1184-1185, includes:
- Determine the orientation of the patient, his reaction to auditory and painful stimuli, response to command.
- Determine the presence or absence of paralysis as well as observations of spontaneous activity.
- Note any change or variation, no matter how subtle, in the patient's level of responsiveness. Deterioration of the patient's condition may be due to an expanding intracranial hematoma and progressive brain engorgement or edema.

Shock. Although the presence of shock is rarely the result of a head injury, it is apt to occur in the patient who has associated injuries. Fracture of the extremities, fractured vertebrae, chest wounds, ruptured internal organs, etc. may be extracranial causes of shock in the patient with multiple injuries. Since the presence of shock is life-threatening, its immediate treatment has first priority. Table 54-1 gives comparative data to assist in the clinical assessment of the patient.

- *A brain-injured patient who is in shock is not placed in a head-low position, because this would increase the likelihood of cerebral edema and hemorrhage.* The extremities may be elevated to increase return of blood to the heart.
- Shock is treated with intravenous fluids, plasma, or dextran until blood transfusions can be started.
- An indwelling catheter is inserted to measure hourly urinary volume, which indicates adequacy of perfusion.
- An intake and output record is maintained. Monitoring of central venous pressure is useful in determining adequate

NEUROLOGICAL OBSERVATION RECORD*

	Time 7/14 9³⁰ AM	10⁰⁰ AM	
Spontaneous behavior	Quiet; lies in bed; little activity; complains of headache	No spontaneous activity	
Level of responsiveness to stimulation	Drowsy; can be aroused — Responds to voice	Less response; more difficult to arouse but does respond to deep pain (supra-orbital pressure)	
Orientation (time/place)	Oriented to place; knows year but not day or month	—	
Movements: Rt. and left arm Rt. and left leg	Moves all 4 extremities but left less than right.	Moves right side in response to pain; left side gives decerebrate response	
Pupil size (draw) Rt. Left reaction	Rt. ◯ Left ○ Rt. reacts sluggishly to light	Rt. ◯ Left ○ Fixed Slight reaction	
Speech Clear Rambling Incoherent Aphasic	Slightly slurred	No speech	
Vital Signs Blood pressure	150/60	200/60	
Pulse	60	48	
Respirations	18	12	
Temperature	37°C (98.6°)	37°C	
Seizures	None	None	
Position of Patient	Supine	Supine	
Input Output			
Other observations			

*Based on following patient study:

Mr. Elliott Smith, a 36-year-old computer-programmer, sought the services of an ophthalmologist because he had been having generalized headaches for a period of "several months." Moderate papilledema and a left hemianopia field defect (loss of vision in one-half of the visual field of one or both eyes) was noted upon examination. He was admitted immediately to the hospital with a possible brain tumor and increasing intracranial pressure. These nursing observations were part of a continuing assessment record and were made 36 hours after admission.

amounts of fluid intake. The patient may be kept slightly dehydrated to reduce extracellular fluid volume.

- Serial studies of blood and urine electrolyte and osmolality are carried out, since head injuries may be accompanied by disorders of sodium regulation. Sodium retention may last several days followed by sodium diuresis. Watch for lethargy, confusion, and convulsions due to electrolyte imbalance.
- A record of daily weight is kept, especially if the patient has hypothalamic involvement and must be watched for the development of diabetes insipidus.

After 3 to 4 days of parenteral fluids, nasogastric feedings may be started. Small frequent feedings lessen the possibility of diarrhea and vomiting. Elevating the head of the bed and aspirating the tube before feeding (for evidences of residual feeding in the stomach) are measures used to prevent distention, regurgitation, and aspiration pneumonia. (The principles and technique of nasogastric feeding are discussed on page 726.)

Vital Signs. Although deterioration of the patient's

The Patient With a Head Injury

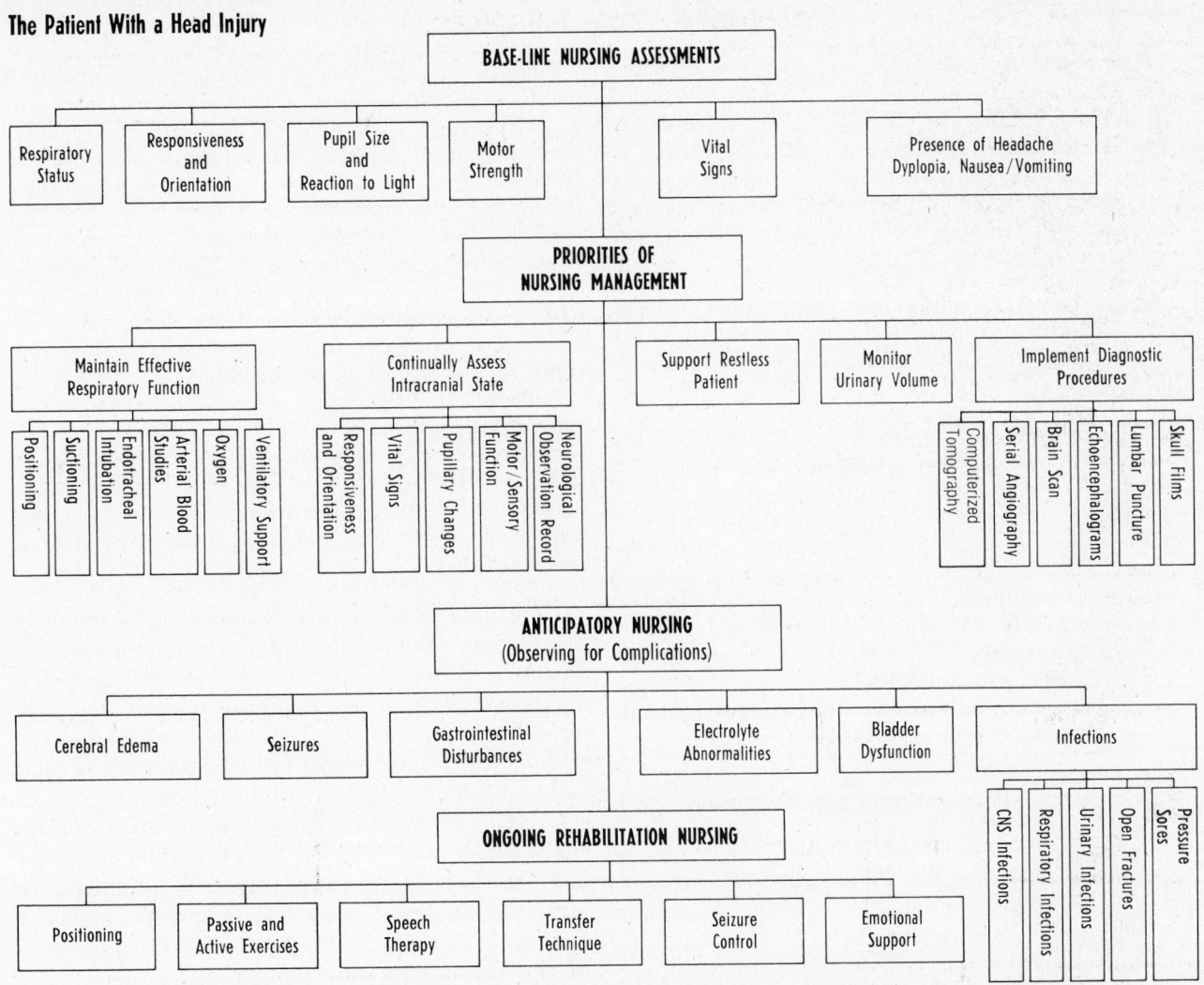

level of consciousness is the most sensitive neurologic indication of impending danger, vital signs are monitored at frequent intervals to assess the intracranial state.

- Signs of rapidly increasing intracranial pressure include slowing of the pulse and respirations and a rapid increase in blood pressure and temperature.
- If brain compression encroaches upon cerebral circulation, the vital signs tend to be reversed — the pulse and respiration become rapid, and the blood pressure may fall. This is an ominous development, as is a rapid fluctuation of vital signs.
- A rapid rise in body temperature is regarded unfavorably because hyperthermia increases the metabolic demands of the brain. (The nursing management of the patient with hyperthermia is discussed on page 1188.)
- The size of the pupils and their reaction to light are evaluated. A unilaterally dilated and poorly responding pupil may indicate a developing hematoma with subsequent pressure on the 3rd cranial nerve due to shifting of the brain. If both pupils become fixed and dilated, overwhelming injury and intrinsic damage to the upper brain stem usually are indicated.

Motor Function. Motor function is checked frequently by observing the patient's spontaneous movements, requesting him to raise and lower the extremities, and comparing the power of his hand grip. Notice whether he moves one extremity less frequently than the other. Also determine the patient's ability to speak and note the quality of the speech.

Cerebrospinal Fluid (CSF) Discharge. The orifices (eyes, ears, nose, mouth) require careful scrutiny.

- To determine whether a fluid discharge is spinal fluid otorrhea or rhinorrhea, blot the area with sterile gauze. If the discharge is bloody (which is readily observed), a red spot forms on the gauze, but if the discharge also contains cerebrospinal fluid, a clear wet halo encircles the bloody spot.
- Cerebrospinal fluid may also be differentiated from mucus by means of a Dextrostix (used to measure blood sugar). If the indicator turns blue, sugar is present — cerebrospinal fluid contains sugar; mucus does not.
- Drainage of cerebrospinal fluid from the nose or ears indicates a basal skull fracture. If the patient is conscious, caution him against sneezing or blowing his nose.

- A sterile cotton pad may be taped loosely against the ear or under the nose to collect the draining fluid.
- The head sometimes is elevated approximately 30 degrees to reduce intracranial pressure and promote spontaneous closure of the leak. However, some neurosurgeons prefer that the bed be kept flat. Persistence of spinal fluid otorrhea or rhinorrhea usually requires surgical intervention. Also, cerebrospinal fluid leakage may mask the usual clinical signs of an expanding intracranial hematoma by preventing brain compression.

Restlessness. Restlessness may indicate injury to the brain, but it is also a sign that the unconscious patient is regaining consciousness. (Some restlessness may be beneficial.)

- Make sure that the patient's airway is adequate and the bladder is not distended. Likewise, bandages and casts should be checked for constriction.
- It is not wise to treat restlessness with opiates and narcotics, because these substances depress respiration, constrict the pupils, and alter the level of the patient's responsiveness. However, small doses of chloral hydrate, paraldehyde, or tranquilizing drugs may be given for restlessness.
- To keep the patient from hurting himself and dislodging body tubes, siderails are padded and the patient's hands are wrapped in mitts. Restraints should be avoided because straining against them can increase intracranial pressure.

MANAGEMENT OF SEVERE HEAD INJURIES

1. Establish the airway. Ensure adequate respiratory exchange and ventilation. Monitor blood gases.
2. Place the patient in a semiprone or prone position, with the head turned to one side.
3. Monitor temperature (rectally), blood pressure, pulse, and respirations every 15 minutes to ½ hour until vital signs become stabilized. Monitor central venous pressure.
4. Make frequent neurological assessments and maintain neurological flow sheet.
5. Give oxygen therapy.
6. Give intravenous infusion of osmotic diuretic; osmotic dehydrating agent transiently reduces intracranial pressure and thus allows time for more definitive treatment.
   a. In the more seriously injured patient, glucosteroids (dexamethasone) may be given to reduce cerebral edema.
   b. Give antacids via nasogastric tube to reduce likelihood of gastric bleeding from steroids.
7. Insert indwelling urinary catheter for assessment of urinary volume.
8. Obtain ECG: cardiac arrhythmias frequently accompany head injury.
9. Give nasogastric tube feedings and maintain positive nitrogen balance.
10. Do not give sedation or morphine derivatives.
11. Administer prophylactic anticonvulsant medication (phenytoin) as directed.

- Lubricate the skin with oil or emollient lotion to prevent irritation from sheets.

Catheterization. If incontinence is a problem, an external sheath catheter may be used on the male patient. Since prolonged use of an indwelling catheter inevitably produces infection, a catheter employing a continuous antibacterial drip and attached to a closed drainage system is used, or the patient is catheterized on an intermittent schedule.

Seizures. Seizures following head injury may occur from bruising of the cortex or may be associated with intracranial hemorrhage. Intravenous diazepam (Valium) is used to control seizures, and phenytoin (Dilantin) is given after control is obtained. (The Nursing management of the patient during convulsive seizures is discussed on page 1244.)

Rehabilitation. Rehabilitative techniques are employed, including range of motion exercises, correct positioning to prevent contractures, proper skin management to prevent pressure sores, and a graded program of exercises. The patient is kept oriented to time, place, and person, especially if he is emerging from an unconscious state. Adequate lighting may prevent visual hallucinations.

Complications. Complications following a traumatic head injury include pneumonia, epilepsy, cerebral edema, infection, and vascular complications. Aftereffects of head injury, usually directly related to the severity of the trauma, include headache, dizziness and vertigo, emotional instability or irritability, brain damage, and post-traumatic neuroses and psychoses.

General Management. Management of these patients encompasses every phase and facet of nursing. No group of patients presents greater opportunities for the exercise of clinical judgment and nursing competency, and in no category of disease does therapeutic success depend more on excellent nursing care.

Patient Education

The patient is encouraged to continue on his rehabilitation program following discharge, since improvement in status may continue up to three or more years following injury. Headache may be the most reliable guide to recovery. A second pillow or backrest at night may be helpful to alleviate some head discomfort.

The patient is encouraged to return gradually to his usual activities. Since there may be brain damage, the family needs to understand and set limits in coping with outbursts of anger, crying, etc., and in realistically evaluating the patient's capabilities. It is difficult to understand and accept alterations in a loved one's behavior.

If the patient is discharged from the hospital in a relatively short time after a head injury, the family is instructed to look for the following signs and to notify the physician or clinic or bring the patient back to the Emergency Department if they occur: difficulty in awakening, difficulty in speaking, confusion, severe headache, vomiting, pulse change, development of unequal pupils, or weakness of one side of the body.

SPINAL CORD INJURY

Spinal cord injury is a major health problem affecting about 100,000 persons in this country, with an estimated 7,500 to 10,000 new injuries occurring each year. Half of these injuries result from motor vehicle accidents, whereas most of the others occur from falls, sporting and industrial accidents, and gunshot wounds. Over two thirds of the accident victims are males under 36 years of age. The vertebrae most frequently involved in spinal cord injuries are the fifth, sixth and seventh cervical (neck), the twelfth thoracic, and the first lumbar vertebrae. These vertebrae are the most susceptible because there is a greater range of mobility in the vertebral column in these areas.

Prevention. To prevent this devastating and catastrophic injury, the following steps should be taken: (1) reduction in driving speed; (2) use of seat belts; (3) educational programs directed against driving while intoxicated; (4) continuing education concerning the dangers of diving in shallow water; (5) prevention of falls; and (6) the use of protective devices in sports. Paramedical personnel are taught the importance of properly removing a car-crash victim from a motor vehicle and of following proper methods in transporting the victim to the Emergency Department in order to avoid further and possibly permanent damage to the spinal cord.

Pathogenesis of Spinal Cord Injury. Damage to the spinal cord ranges from transient concussion (from which the patient fully recovers) to contusion, laceration, and compression (either alone or in combination), to complete transection of the cord (which renders the patient paralyzed below the level of the injury). When hemorrhage occurs in the area of the spinal cord, the blood may seep into the extradural, subdural, or subarachnoid spaces of the spinal canal. Immediately after injury (contusion or tear) the nerve fibers begin to swell and disintegrate. Not only is there injury to the spinal cord vasculature, but there also appears to be a pathogenic process responsible for the progressive damage of acute spinal cord injury. A secondary chain of events produces ischemia, hypoxia, edema, and hemorrhagic lesions, which in turn result in destruction of myelin and axons.

If the cord has not suffered irreparable damage, some method of early treatment is needed to prevent partial damage from developing into total and permanent damage. The effectiveness of using cooling techniques or hypothermia perfusion on the injured area of the spinal cord to counteract the autodestructive forces that follow this type of injury is being studied. The use of high dosage steroids to maintain the vascular integrity of the cord following acute injury is viewed as promising by researchers.

Immediate Management

The immediate management of the patient at the scene of the accident is critical, because improper handling can cause further damage and loss of neurological function. Any victim of a motor vehicle or diving accident, a contact sport injury, falls, or any direct trauma to the head and neck should be suspected of having a spinal cord injury until such an injury is ruled out.

- At the scene of the accident, the victim should be placed in a neutral position (head, back, legs, knees, and arms straight). If he is lying in a twisted position, his extremities should be straightened with extreme caution.

A cervical collar reinforced with steel stays is applied without moving the patient's head. If this device is not available, the head is immobilized with sandbags. At least four persons should slide the victim carefully onto a board for transfer to the hospital. Any twisting movement may irreversibly damage the spinal cord by causing a bony fragment of the vertebra to cut into, crush, or sever the cord completely.

Assessment

If the patient is conscious, he will probably complain of acute local pain, which may radiate peripherally along the involved nerve. Often he will say that he is afraid he has broken his neck or back.

Breathing Pattern

- The breathing pattern must be noted, since respiratory problems are frequently seen in patients with cervical spine injuries because of possible paralysis of the intercostal and abdominal muscles. (The C-4 segment provides the major innervation to the diaphragm by the phrenic nerve.) If endotracheal intubation is necessary every attempt is made to accomplish this without moving the head backward.

Motor and Sensory Function

- As soon as possible, the patient is evaluated for motor and sensory changes. It is necessary to record these findings so that changes or progression from the baseline neurological status can be evaluated accurately.
- Motor ability is tested by requesting the patient to spread his fingers, squeeze the examiner's hand, and move his toes or turn his feet.
- Sensation is evaluated by pinching the skin or pricking it with a pin, starting at the shoulder level and working down both sides of the extremities. The patient is asked where he feels the sensation. The presence or absence of sweating is also noted, since perspiration does not occur on paralyzed areas.
- Edema of the spinal cord may occur with any severe cord injury and may further compromise spinal function. Therefore, the patient is watched constantly for any changes in motor or sensory loss and symptoms of progressive neurologic damage (Fig. 55-10). These, of course, are reported immediately. It may be impossible in the early stages of injury

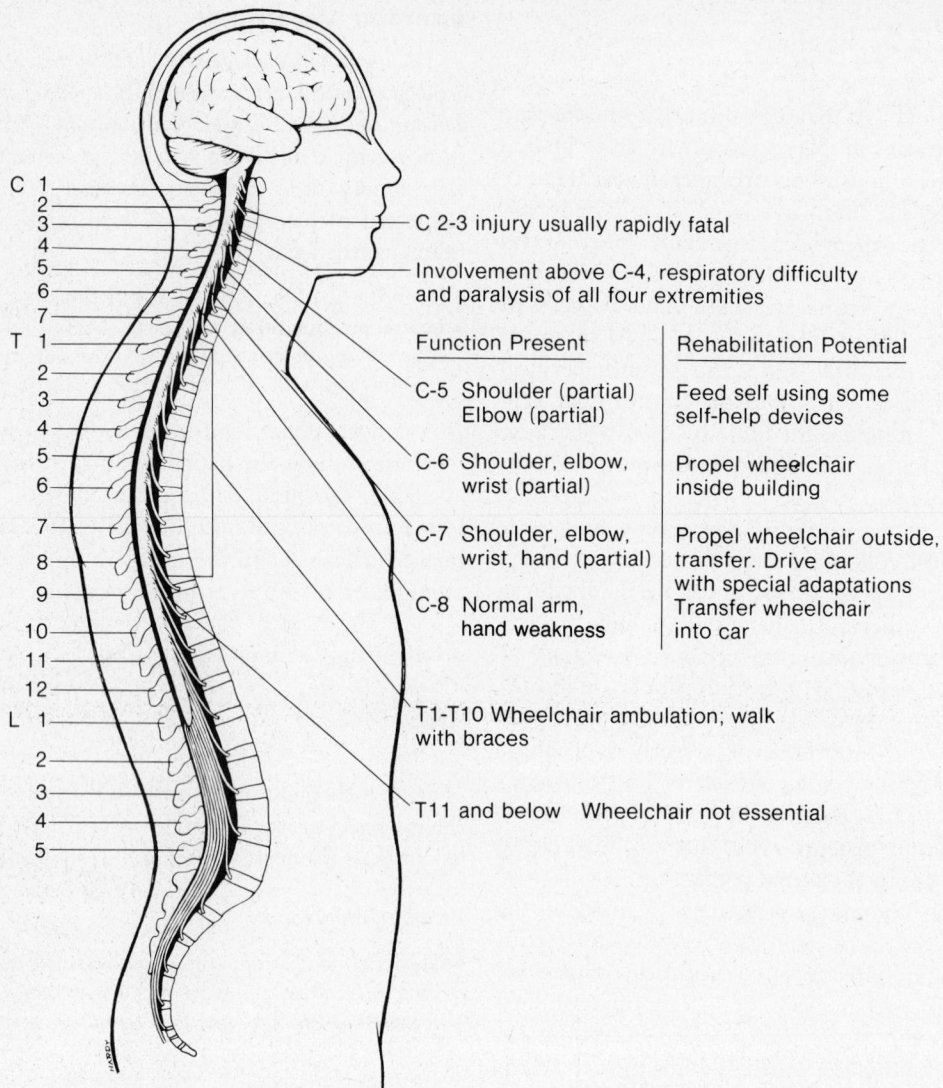

C 2-3 injury usually rapidly fatal

Involvement above C-4, respiratory difficulty and paralysis of all four extremities

Function Present	Rehabilitation Potential
C-5 Shoulder (partial) Elbow (partial)	Feed self using some self-help devices
C-6 Shoulder, elbow, wrist (partial)	Propel wheelchair inside building
C-7 Shoulder, elbow, wrist, hand (partial)	Propel wheelchair outside, transfer. Drive car with special adaptations
C-8 Normal arm, hand weakness	Transfer wheelchair into car

T1-T10 Wheelchair ambulation; walk with braces

T11 and below   Wheelchair not essential

Figure 55-10.   Sequelae of spinal cord injury and rehabilitation challenges. (The vertebrae are numbered on the left side of the drawing and the spinal nerves are numbered on the right.)

to determine whether the cord has been transected, since signs and symptoms of cord transection are indistinguishable from those of cord edema.

Bladder Function

- Immediately after a spinal cord injury the urinary bladder becomes atonic and cannot contract by reflex activity. Since the patient has no sensation of bladder distention, damage to the urinary tract may occur from overstretching of the bladder. If the hospital has an intermittent catheterization team, the patient is placed on this regimen. If not, an indwelling catheter is inserted. Gastric intubation and suction are initiated to reduce gastric distention and prevent vomiting and aspiration.

Definitive Management

Management of a cervical spinal injury requires *immobilization, early reduction, and stabilization.*

SKELETAL TRACTION.   To reduce the fracture dislocation

and maintain alignment of the cervical spine fracture some form of skeletal traction with skull calipers or tongs is applied, or the halo-cast or halo-vest technique is used.

A variety of skeletal tongs are available, including the Crutchfield (Fig. 55-11), Barton and Vinke tongs all of which need to be inserted into the skull. These are usually placed in the outer table of the skull through holes made with a special drill under local anesthesia. The Gardner-Wells tongs require no predrilled holes and the pins are tightened by hand to the proper depth. These procedures are usually done in the Emergency Department under local anesthesia.

Traction is applied to the tongs by weights (4.5 to 9 kg., 10 to 20 pounds or more), depending on the patient's size and the degree of displacement. The traction force is exerted along the longitudinal axis of the vertebral bodies with the neck in a neutral position. Then the traction is

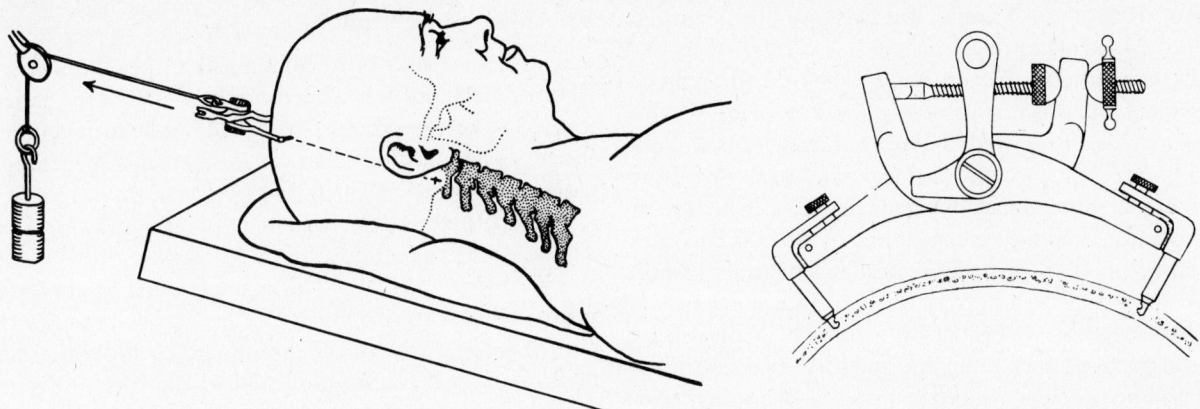

Figure 55-11. Diagrammatic drawing shows the method of application of skull traction. Note that the pegs extend through the outer layer of the skull and thus produce direct skeletal traction. (Courtesy University of Virginia)

gradually increased by the addition of more weight until reduction is obtained. Once reduction is achieved, as verified by cervical spine films and neurological examination, the weights are gradually removed until the amount of weight needed to maintain the alignment is obtained (usually 10 to 30 pounds). The weights should hang free so as not to interfere with the traction. The patient is placed on a turning frame if one is available. (See page 1256 for a method of transfer to the turning frame.) Some neurosurgeons do not advocate the use of the circOlectric bed for spinal injuries because excessive pressure is placed on the fracture when the patient is turned in a vertical fashion.

• The patient's skull is assessed for signs of infection, including drainage around the tongs. The back of the head is checked periodically for signs of pressure and is massaged at intervals, care being taken not to move the neck.

Halo Traction. Halo skeletal traction for cervical spine injuries offers some advantages over skull-tong traction. Not only is it relatively simple to apply and comfortable to the patient but hospitalization time is markedly reduced. Halo traction devices consist of a stainless steel "halo ring" which fits around the head and is attached to the skull by four skull pins inserted through threaded holes in the ring. It can be connected to a plaster body cast or to a plastic halo vest or girdle which suspends the weight of the unit circumferentially around the chest (Fig. 55-12).

The patient may experience a slight headache or discomfort around the skull pins for several days after the pins are inserted. Initially the patient may not appreciate the rather startling appearance of this apparatus, but he can readily adapt to it because of the comfort the device provides to the unstable neck. He may complain of being "caged in" and of noise created by any object coming in

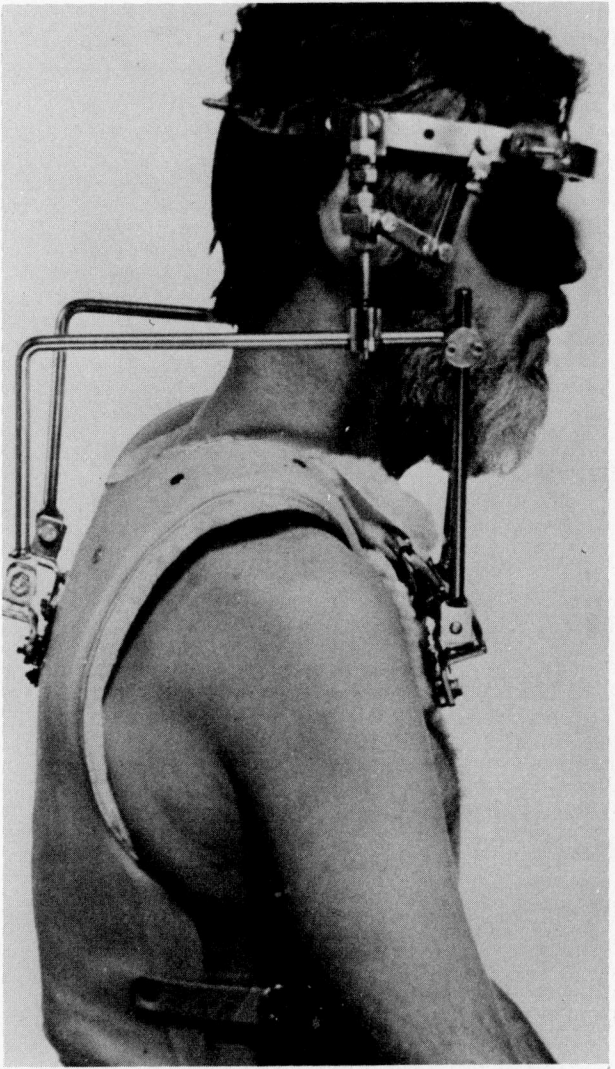

Figure 55-12. Halo plastic vest for immobilization of the cervical spine. (Courtesy of Richard Young, C.O.)

contact with the steel frame, but he should be reassured that he will adapt to this.

The hair around the pin tracts is shaved to facilitate assessment and prevent infection. Some drainage around the pin site is anticipated. These areas are cleansed daily and observed for redness, drainage, and pain. A torque screwdriver should be readily available in case the screws on the frame need tightening. If one of the pins becomes detached, stabilize the patient's head in a neutral position while another person notifies the neurosurgeon.

LAMINECTOMY. If reduction cannot be achieved by skeletal traction, open reduction and surgical decompression will be necessary in order to reduce the spinal fracture or dislocation. The cord may undergo extrinsic damage from a variety of sources, including displaced bone fragment, compression from vascular insufficiency that affects a portion of the spinal cord, intrinsic damage to the spinal cord, or a combination of any of these factors.

A laminectomy may be indicated in the instance of an ascending neurological lesion, suspicion of epidural hematoma, and penetrating wounds that require surgical debridement. Or, surgery may be done to permit direct visualization and exploration of the cord. (The care of the patient following a laminectomy is discussed on page 1260.)

TRANSFERRING THE PATIENT. During treatment in the emergency and x-ray departments, the patient is kept on the transfer board.

The transfer of the patient to a bed presents a definite nursing problem.

- The patient always must be maintained in an extended position. No part of the body should be twisted or turned, nor should the patient be allowed to assume a sitting position.

The patient should be placed on a Stryker frame when he is to be transferred to bed. Later, if it is proved that there is no cord injury, the patient always can be moved to a conventional bed without harm; the reverse, however, is not true. If a Stryker frame is not available, the patient should be placed on a firm mattress with a bedboard under it.

The patient may be transferred from the board to the Stryker frame in the following manner:

- The board on which the patient is strapped is placed directly on the posterior frame.
- Unstrap the patient from the board, but do not remove the head strappings.
- Place a blanket roll between the legs.
- Place the anterior frame in position, and secure the frame straps.
- Turn the frame so that the patient is in the prone position.
- Remove the frame straps and the posterior frame. Remove the head strapping with care. Then remove the transfer board.

Prevention of Deformities

The patient must be maintained in proper alignment at all times. Usually he is turned every 2 hours. If the patient is not on a turning frame, he should not be turned unless the physician has indicated so. (Directives for turning a patient not on a Stryker frame are found on page 1259.)

POSITIONING. The patient is placed in a dorsal or supine position as follows:

The feet are positioned against a padded footboard to prevent footdrop. There should be a space between the end of the mattress and the footboard to allow free suspension of the heels. A wooden block on either end of the mattress prevents the mattress from pushing against the footboard. Trochanter rolls are applied from the crest of the ilium to the midthigh of both extremities to prevent external rotation of the hip joints.

EXERCISING. Atrophy of the extremities will result from disuse. To avoid this complication, the physician may direct that passive range of motion exercises be started on the affected extremities within 48 to 72 hours after injury. These exercises preserve joint motion and stimulate circulation. A joint that is immobilized too long becomes fixed as a result of tendon and capsule contracture. Toes, metatarsals, ankles, knees, and hips should be put through a full range of motion at least 4 and ideally 5 times daily. Range of motion exercises can prevent many complications.

Complications

SPINAL SHOCK. Spinal shock represents a sudden loss of reflex activity in the spinal cord (arreflexia) below the level of injury. In this condition, the muscles innervated by the part of the cord segment situated below the level of the lesion become completely paralyzed and flaccid, and the reflexes are absent. The blood pressure falls, and the parts of the body below the level of the cord lesion are paralyzed and without sensation. The reflexes that initiate bladder and bowel function likewise are affected. (The management of the patient with a neurogenic bladder—i.e., a bladder disturbance due to a lesion of the central nervous system—is discussed on page 914.) Bowel distention and paralytic ileus caused by depression of the reflexes may be treated with intestinal decompression. The patient does not perspire on the paralyzed portions of his body, since sympathetic activity is blocked. Therefore he must be watched carefully for an abrupt onset of fever. (Hyperthermia is treated as outlined on page 1188.)

- The patient's body defenses are supported and maintained until spinal shock abates and the system has recovered from the traumatic insult. Special attention must also be directed to the respiratory system. There may not be enough intrathoracic pressure for the patient to cough effectively. Chest physical therapy is used to help clear pulmonary secretions.

- Symptoms of cord compression depend on the level at which the compression occurs. A neurological flow sheet is kept so that signs of cord compression and their progression may be quickly noted. The patient is repeatedly evaluated for loss of sensation and inability to move the extremities.
- During spinal shock and subsequent periods of immobilization, the patient is assessed for signs of venous thrombosis since pulmonary embolism is a major cause of death in the first few weeks after injury. Subcutaneous low-dose heparin may be started.

Usually the acute period of spinal shock is transient, but residual results may linger for a much longer time. If the injury is incomplete the prognosis is uncertain.

PRESSURE SORES.   Because a patient with a spinal cord injury is immobilized for a period of time, there is an ever present, life endangering threat of pressure sores. In areas of local tissue ischemia where there is continuous pressure and where the peripheral circulation is inadequate as a result of the spinal shock and recumbency, pressure sores have been known to develop within 6 hours.

Turning not only aids in the prevention of pressure sores but also prevents the pooling of blood and tissue fluid in the dependent areas.

- Every few hours the patient's skin should be washed with a mild soap, rinsed well, and *blotted* dry. Sacrum, trochanters, ischia, iliac spines, knees, and heels are especially susceptible to pressure. These areas should be kept soft and well lubricated with an emollient lotion. Massage should be done gently with a circular motion. The linen under the patient is kept dry.

OTHER COMPLICATIONS.   Kidney and bladder complications and autonomic hyperreflexia may also occur. These problems are discussed elsewhere in the text: for kidney and bladder complications, see page 914; for autonomic hyperreflexia, see page 1263.

Ambulation

After a period of absolute immobilization (either by skeletal tongs or halo traction), the duration of which depends on the severity and mechanism of injury, the patient may be allowed to gradually assume an erect position. The patient will require bracing to reduce movement of the cervical spine and to allow bone healing. The commonly used orthoses are either a two-poster firm brace placed under the chin and the subocciput with a chest extension, or a four-poster cervical brace with chest extension. For the patient with a cervical fracture without neurological deficit, reduction in traction followed by rigid immobilization for 16 weeks will restore skeletal function in most cases. (The rehabilitation of the patient with a permanent spinal cord injury, i.e., the paraplegic patient, is discussed on page 1261.)

HERNIATION OR RUPTURE OF AN INTERVERTEBRAL DISC

The intervertebral disc is a cartilaginous plate that forms a cushion between the vertebral bodies. This tough gristle-like material is incorporated in a capsule. A ball-like condensation in the disc is called the *nucleus pulposus*. In herniation of the intervertebral disc (ruptured disc), the nucleus of the disc protrudes into the annulus (the fibrous ring around the disc) with subsequent nerve compression. Following trauma (falls, accidents, and repeated minor stresses such as lifting) the cartilage may be injured.

In most patients the immediate symptoms of trauma are short-lived, and those resulting from injury to the disc do not appear for months or years. Then with degeneration in the disc, the capsule pushes back into the spinal canal, or it may rupture and allow the nucleus pulposus to be pushed back against the dural sac or against a spinal nerve as it emerges from the spinal column (Fig. 55-13). This sequence produces pain due to pressure in the area of distribution of the involved nerve.

Continued pressure may produce degenerative changes in the involved nerve, such as changes in sensation and reflex action. A myelogram usually demonstrates the area of pressure and localizes the herniation of the disc. A lumbar venogram may also be useful.

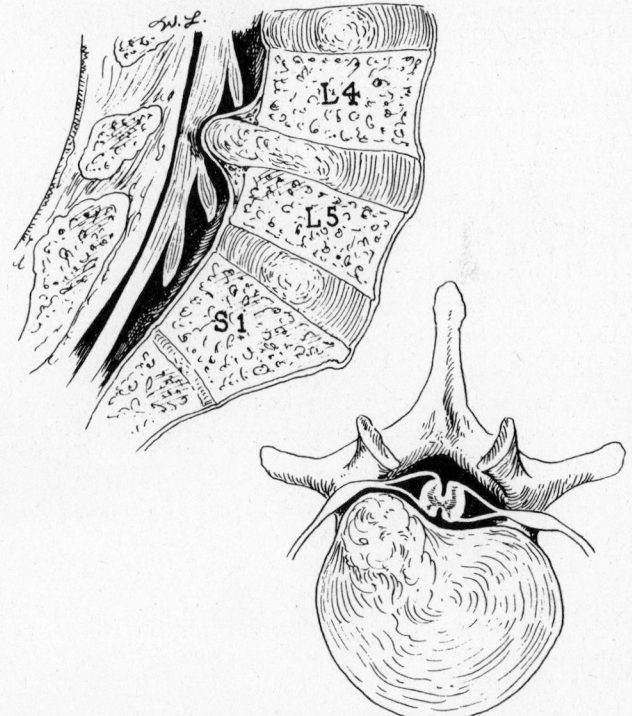

Figure 55-13.   Diagram shows herniation of the nucleus pulposus. The upper drawing shows how such herniation presses upon the structures of the spinal cord. The lower drawing shows how such herniation may press upon the exit of the spinal nerve and produce pain and other symptoms.

Clinical Manifestations

A herniated disc with accompanying pain may occur in any portion of the spine: cervical, thoracic (rare), or lumbar. The clinical manifestations depend on the location, the rate of development (acute or chronic), and the effect on the surrounding structures.

A *cervical disc herniation* usually occurs at the C5–C6 and C6–C7 interspaces. Pain and stiffness may occur in the neck, the top of the shoulders and the region of the scapulae. At times, the patient may interpret these signs as symptoms of heart trouble or bursitis. Pain may also occur in the upper extremities and head, accompanied by paresthesia and numbness of the upper extremities.

The majority of *lumbar disc herniations* occur at the L4–L5 or the L5–S1 interspaces. A lumbar disc produces low back pain accompanied by varying degrees of sensory and motor impairment. The patient may complain of pain in the buttock and thigh radiating to the calf and ankle. Pain is aggravated by actions that increase intraspinal pressure (sneezing, straining, lifting). There is usually some type of postural deformity, since pain causes an alteration of the normal spinal mechanics. If the patient lies on his back and attempts to raise his leg in a straight position, pain will radiate into the leg because this maneuver (straight-leg raising) stretches the sciatic nerve. Additional signs include muscle weakness, alterations in tendon reflexes, and sensory loss.

Management: Cervical Disc Herniation

The goals of treatment are (1) to rest and immobilize the cervical spine to give the soft tissues time to heal and (2) to reduce inflammation in the supporting tissues and the affected nerve roots in the cervical spine. Bed rest (usually 2 weeks) is important since it eliminates the stress of gravity and frees the cervical spine from having to support the weight of the head. It also relieves pressure on the nerve roots. Proper positioning on a firm mattress with a bedboard between the mattress and springs may bring dramatic relief from pain.

The cervical spine may be rested and immobilized by a cervical collar, cervical traction or a brace. A collar allows maximal opening of the intervertebral foramina and holds the head in a neutral or slightly flexed position. The patient may have to wear the collar 24 hours a day during the acute phase. The skin site under the collar is inspected for irritation. When the patient is free of pain, cervical isometric exercises are started to strengthen the muscles in the neck.

Cervical traction is accomplished by means of a head halter attached to a pulley and weight (Fig. 55-14). It increases vertebral separation and thus relieves pressure on the nerve roots. The head of the bed is elevated to provide countertraction. If the skin becomes irritated, the halter can be padded. Experience has shown that a male patient may suffer more skin irritation if he shaves; the beard offers a natural form of padding.

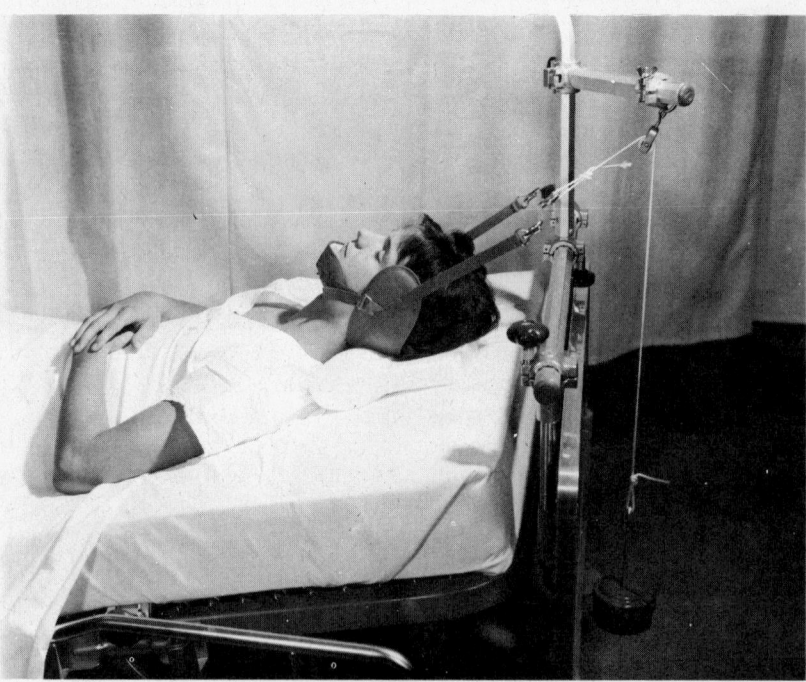

Figure 55-14. Cervical traction. The patient should be assessed for pressure sores developing under chin or occiput.

Hot moist compresses (10 to 20 minutes) applied to the back of the neck several times daily will increase blood flow to the muscles and help to relax the spastic muscles as well as the patient. Analgesics are given during the acute phase to relieve pain, and sedatives may be administered to control the anxiety often associated with cervical disc disease. Muscle relaxants are administered to interrupt the cycle of muscle spasm and allow for patient comfort. Anti-inflammatory drugs (aspirin, phenylbutazone [Butazolidin], oxyphenbutazone [Tandearil]) or steroids are given to treat the inflammatory response which usually occurs in the supporting tissues and affected nerve roots. Occasionally an injection of a corticosteroid drug into the epidural space may be tried as a means of relieving radicular pain. Food and antacids are given with anti-inflammatory agents to prevent gastrointestinal irritation. Periodic blood evaluations should be carried out to detect the development of blood dyscrasias.

Surgical excision of the herniated disc may be necessary when there is a significant neurological deficit, progression of a neurological deficit, signs of cord compression, or no improvement or worsening of pain. In the lumbar area, a hemilaminectomy and discectomy may be the procedures of choice, whereas in the cervical area an anterior or posterior discectomy may be done.

Patient Education. The patient must be cautioned against flexing, extending, or rotating the neck in any extreme manner while working. When sleeping, the patient should avoid the prone position and should keep his head in a neutral position, using a feather or down-filled pillow. The patient should be cautioned not to prop himself up in bed with several pillows since this produces neck flexion.

Long automobile rides during the acute phase should be avoided because vibration associated with such trips has an adverse effect on the spine. It may take up to 6 weeks to recuperate from a significant disc herniation.

Management: Herniated Lumbar Disc

The objectives of treatment are to relieve the pain and slow the progress of the disease and to increase the functional ability of the patient. Bed rest is encouraged to free the disc from stress. The patient is allowed to assume a comfortable position; usually a semi-Fowler's position with moderate hip and knee flexion is most satisfactory. A hinged bedboard is placed under the mattress to limit spinal flexion.

Since muscle spasm is prominent during the acute phase, muscle relaxants (methocarbamol [Robaxin]; carisoprodol [Soma]) are used. Anti-inflammatory drugs and systemic steroids may be administered to counter the inflammation that usually occurs in the supporting tissues and the affected nerve roots. Moist heat and mas-

TURNING THE PATIENT WITH CRUTCHFIELD TONGS
(Not on Stryker Frame)

If Crutchfield tongs are used and the patient is not on a Stryker frame, an order from the physician must be obtained before the patient is turned. The patient's head *never should be flexed,* neither forward nor laterally, and at all times should be kept in a direct line with the axis of the cervical spine.

TO TURN THE PATIENT:

The nurse supporting the head gives the commands for turning. Place a pillow between the legs of the patient to prevent the upper leg from slipping forward and jarring the patient's head.

Place a pillow longitudinally on the chest, with the patient's upper arm resting on it. The pillow prevents the shoulder from sagging and pulling on the neck as the patient is turned.

Three persons should turn the patient in a logrolling fashion, making sure that the shoulder turns with the head and the neck. One nurse should support the head; the second nurse or attendant, the shoulders; and the third person, the hips and the legs.

As the patient is turned, the traction should be moved carefully to keep it in direct line with the cervical spine. The patient's position should be adjusted so that the traction, the patient's head and the cervical spine are in correct alignment.

While the nurse still supports the head in the lateral position, a small pillow is placed under the head to maintain cervical alignment.

sage help to relax spastic muscles and produce a sedating effect on the patient.

Chemonucleolysis. Chemonucleolysis is an investigational method of treating a slipped lumbar disc accompanied by root irritation. The procedure consists of injecting chymopapain (Discase) into the diseased disc. Chymopapain is an enzyme derived from the papaya plant; it has a proteolytic action which dissolves the nucleus pulposus, reducing the pressure on the adjacent nerve roots and thus removing low back pain.

This technique is regarded as the last step in the conservative treatment of lumbar disc herniation and not as an alternative to laminectomy. An anaphylactoid reaction is possible with this drug.

Surgical Intervention. Muscle weakness and atrophy, loss of sensory and motor function, and unrelieved acute pain are indications of a significant neurological deficit. When these manifestations occur, surgical intervention (hemilaminectomy with removal of the ruptured disc) is undertaken. If more than one disc is involved, pain and disability tend to recur, requiring another operation. In this event, a spinal fusion may be done.

Patient Education and Rehabilitation. The patient with a lumbar disc can begin to ambulate gradually when the inflammatory reaction and edema from the disc herniation have subsided. For patients with weak abdominal muscles, a corset or brace may be necessary to help pull the abdomen in and alter the lumbar sacral curve, so as to relieve the strain on the ligaments.

To correct underlying mechanical problems which commonly contribute to painful derangements of the low back, an exercise program is designed to strengthen the abdominal and paraspinous musculature without stressing the back or legs.

The patient is instructed as follows:
1. Lie on the floor, knees bent, with feet flat on the floor and arms folded across the chest.
2. Slowly elevate the head and shoulders; relax. Continue several times and increase daily.
3. Slowly flex the trunk; relax.
4. Continue the exercises daily for an indefinite period of time.

The patient is taught to sleep on his side with the knees and hips in a position of flexion (pillow between the legs). Caution him not to sleep in a prone position since this hyperextends the spine. He should be taught to lift correctly by bending the knees and keeping the back straight and to avoid lifting anything above the elbows.

Disc Surgery

Surgical excision of a herniated disc is done when there is evidence of a progressing neurological deficit (muscle weakness and atrophy, loss of sensory and motor function, loss of sphincter control) and continuing pain and sciatica. The objective of surgical treatment is to relieve pressure on the nerve root in order to relieve pain. In the cervical area, an anterior approach may be used through a transverse incision in the neck to remove disc material that has herniated into the spinal canal and foramina. Or a posterior approach may be used at the desired level of the cervical spine. In the lumbar region, the surgical treatment is excision through a posterolateral laminotomy (division of the lamina of a vertebra). A *laminectomy* involves removing the lamina in order to expose the neural elements in the spinal canal, so that the spinal canal can be inspected. The herniated disc is identified and removed, relieving the pressure on the cord and roots. Microsurgical techniques allow for improved illumination and magnification during disc operations. During these procedures, spinal cord function can be monitored electrophysiologically.

Sometimes, an additional stabilizing procedure is added (spinal fusion), in which a bone graft from the iliac crest is used to fuse the spinous processes. The spinal fusion has the purpose of bridging over the defective disc to stabilize the spine.

Preoperative Management. Most patients fear surgery on any part of the spine and therefore need assurance and explanations all along the way. When data is being collected for the nursing history, any complaints of pain, paresthesia, and muscle spasm are recorded in order to have a baseline for comparison after surgery. Preoperative assessment should also include an evaluation of movement in the extremities as well as bladder and bowel function. To facilitate the postoperative turning procedure, the patient is taught to turn himself as a unit (logrolling) as part of the preoperative preparation. Other facets of the postoperative regimen which should be practiced before the operation are deep breathing, coughing, and muscle setting exercises which will help maintain muscle tone.

Cervical Disc: Postoperative Management. Throughout the postoperative period, vital signs are monitored frequently to detect any signs of respiratory difficulty. Occasionally during surgery the recurrent laryngeal nerve may be injured by retractors, resulting in hoarseness and inability to cough effectively. The elimination of pulmonary secretions then becomes a problem requiring chest physical therapy. Usually the major complaint of the patient is a sore throat, which can be relieved by throat sprays (Chloraseptic spray). Throat sprays or lozenges that numb the throat are avoided since the numbness may result in choking. The patient may complain of dysphagia, which is probably due to edema of the esophagus. In this event, a blenderized soft diet may be given. One sign to watch for following an anterior cervical discectomy is a sudden return of radicular pain, which may indicate that the spine has become unstable.

Lumbar Disc Excision: Postoperative Management. Following surgery, the vital signs are checked frequently and the wound is inspected for evidence of hemorrhage. Since postoperative neurological deficits may occur from nerve root injury, the sensation and motor power of the lower extremities are evaluated at specified intervals, along with the color and temperature of the legs and sensation of the toes. Another important sign to check is possible urinary retention, which may indicate that a hematoma has developed at the operative site.

To position the patient, a pillow is placed under his head, and the knee rest is elevated slightly since slight knee flexion relaxes the muscles of the back. However, when the patient is lying on his side, extreme knee flexion must be avoided. The patient is encouraged to move from side to side to relieve pressure. But first he is reassured that no injury will result from moving. When the patient is about to be turned, the bed is placed in a flat position and a pillow is placed between his legs. He is then turned as a unit (logrolling) without twisting the back.

Following surgery, the patient may experience varying degrees of pain and sensory manifestations in the legs and may worry about these sensations. Usually they represent a temporary manifestation due to inflammatory changes, edema, and swelling of the compressed nerve. Occasionally they may be caused by the presence of disc material adjacent to a nerve root. Narcotics and sedatives are given during the early postoperative period to relieve pain and anxiety.

Spinal fusion involves the added danger of a longer procedure carrying a greater potential of shock. The patient has an additional wound since bone fragments are usually taken from the iliac crest to serve as wedges in the spine. Therefore, the leg wound must be attended to after surgery and attention must be given to moving the leg that was operated on. Pillows must be adjusted for support and comfort, and care must be taken to avoid sudden flexion and extension at the knee, which will cause pain. The recovery period is somewhat slower than in those patients who have undergone removal of the ruptured portion of the disc without a spinal fusion, because bony union must take place.

Early ambulation is encouraged. To assist the patient out of bed, the head of the bed is raised while the patient lies on his side. The patient's head and shoulders are supported while he pushes himself up to a sitting position. At the same time, another person eases the patient's legs over the side of the bed. Coming to a sitting or standing posture should be accomplished by one long smooth motion.

Complications. Unfortunately a person requiring a disc procedure at one level usually has degenerative processes at all levels of the vertebral column. A herniation relapse may occur at the same level or elsewhere, so that the patient is apt to become a candidate for another disc procedure. Arachnoiditis may occur after operation (and after myelography) in which there is an insidious onset of diffuse, frequently burning pain in the lower back, radiating into the buttocks. Disc excision can leave adhesions and scarring around the spinal nerves and dura, which then produce inflammatory changes that can create chronic neuritis and neurofibrosis. Disc surgery may relieve pressure on the spinal nerves, but it does not reverse the effects of neural injury and scarring and the pain which ensues.

Patient Education. The patient is advised that since it takes up to 6 weeks for the ligaments of the muscles to heal, activity is to be gradually increased up to the point of tolerance. Activities that produce flexion strain on the spine (automobile riding) should be avoided until healing has taken place. Heat may be applied to the back to soothe and relax muscle spasm and help absorb exudates in the tissues. Scheduled rest periods are important. Usually the patient is advised to avoid heavy work for 2 to 3 months after surgery. Exercises are prescribed to strengthen the abdominal and erector spinae muscles. A back brace or corset may be necessary if back pain persists.

SPINAL CORD TUMORS

Tumors that occur within the spinal cord or exert pressure on it cause symptoms that are in effect the same as those caused by fractures of the spine, except that they develop more slowly. Usually sharp pain occurs in the area that is innervated by the spinal roots which arise from the cord in the region of the tumor. In addition, increasing paralysis develops below the level of the lesion. The level of the tumor usually may be determined by a neurologic examination; however, myelography is necessary for exact localization.

Surgical Management. The surgical management consists of a laminectomy to remove the tumor. The patient is placed in a prone position while the spinal cord is exposed. A median incision is made over the spinous processes, and the soft tissues are separated on each side. These bony projections are removed with large bone-cutting forceps, and the posterior part of the vertebral arch is removed to expose the dura. After a bloodless field is obtained, the dura is incised and the tumor or clot is removed. The dura is then closed, the soft tissues are sutured over it, and an adhesive dressing is applied.

THE PARAPLEGIC PATIENT*

Paraplegia (loss of motion and sensation in lower extremities) most frequently follows trauma due to accidents and gunshot wounds, but may be the result of spinal cord lesions (intervertebral disc, tumor, vascular lesions), multiple sclerosis, infections and abscesses of the spinal cord, and congenital defects. The patient requires extensive rehabilitation which will be less difficult if appropriate nursing management has been carried out during the acute phase of the injury or illness. (See the management of spinal cord injuries, page 1253.) The nursing care is one of the determining factors in the success of the rehabilitation program.

Psychological Support

It is usually some time before the patient comprehends the magnitude of the disability. He may go through stages of adjustment including shock and disbelief, denial, depression, grief, and acceptance. During the acute phase of the injury, denial can be a protective mechanism to shield the patient from the overwhelming reality of what has happened. As he realizes the finality of para-

---

*Quadriplegia (tetraplegia) is loss of motion and sensation involving both upper and lower extremities. These patients require the same meticulous nursing management to prevent complications that are given patients with paraplegia. Their rehabilitation problems and procedures are more complex. Therefore patients with quadriplegia are treated in rehabilitation centers with personnel and facilities that can meet their special needs.

plegia (or quadriplegia), the grieving process may be prolonged by the awareness of "what will never be." A period of depression follows as the patient experiences a loss of self-esteem in areas of self-identity, sexual functioning, and social and emotional roles. Self-esteem is related to being strong, loved, and lovable—all of which are threatened by the injury. To be able to work through this depression, the patient must be able to see some hope for relief in the future. Thus he is guided toward a sense of confidence in his ability to achieve self-care and relative independence. The role of the nurse ranges from caretaker during the acute phase to teacher, counselor, and facilitator as the patient gains mobility and independence.

Acceptance of the disability leads to the development of realistic goals for the future, making the best of those abilities that are left intact. Rejection of the disability will cause self-destructive neglect and noncompliance with the therapeutic program. This leads to more frustration and depression. The family usually requires counseling social services and other support systems to help them cope with the changes that will be made in their life style and socioeconomic status. (The psychological implications of a disability are discussed also on page 181.)

Weight-bearing Activities

A patient with complete severance of the cord can begin weight-bearing early, because no further damage can be incurred. The sooner muscles are strengthened, the less chance they will atrophy (disuse atrophy). The earlier the patient is brought to a standing position, the less opportunity there will be for osteoporotic changes to take place in the long bones. Weight-bearing also diminishes urinary infections and the formation of renal calculi and enhances many other metabolic processes.

Postural Hypotension. Because vasomotor tone is lacking in the lower extremities, the patient may become hypotensive when placed in an upright position. Postural hypotension results because the reflex arcs that normally produce vasoconstriction in the upright position have been interrupted.

To counteract this problem, a tilt table may be used to help the patient overcome vasomotor instability and tolerate the upright posture. Other possible measures include wearing elastic stockings to facilitate venous return in the legs and applying an abdominal binder to alleviate the pooling of blood in the abdominal area.

When a tilt table is used, the patient is gradually elevated to an upright position. At first he may be able to tolerate only an elevation of 45 degrees (or less), but gradually the angle of elevation is increased. The patient should be observed closely for signs of intolerance, including nausea, perspiration, pallor, dizziness, and syncope. The patient's blood pressure is taken before he is allowed up and as soon as he is positioned on the tilt table,

since periods of recumbency also favor the development of orthostatic hypotension.

If no tilt table is available, a high-back reclining wheelchair with extension leg rests may be used. To overcome the effects of hypotension, the backrest is raised slowly and the leg rests are lowered gradually over a period of 7 to 10 days. While in the wheelchair, the patient may experience dizziness, tachycardia, hypotension, and blackouts. If he becomes dizzy, the brakes should be placed in the "on" position and the wheelchair tilted back for several minutes. If hypotension is prolonged, cerebral anoxia is a distinct threat and must be avoided.

Bowel Training Program

The objective of a bowel training program is to establish bowel evacuation through reflex conditioning. This technique is described on page 202. If a cord injury occurs above the sacral segments or nerve roots and there is reflex activity, the anal sphincter may be massaged to stimulate defecation. (If the cord lesion involves the sacral segment or nerve roots, anal massage is not done because the anus may be relaxed and lack tone. Massage is also contraindicated if there is spasticity of the anal sphincter.) The anal sphincter is massaged by inserting a gloved finger (which has been adequately lubricated) 2.5 to 3.7 cm. (1 to 1½ inches) into the rectum and moving it in a circular motion or from side to side. It will soon become apparent which area triggers the defecation response. This procedure should be done at the same time (usually every 48 hours) after a meal and at a time that will be convenient for the patient when he returns home. The patient is also taught the symptoms of impaction (frequent loose stools; constipation) and cautioned to watch for the development of hemorrhoids. A diet with sufficient bulk is essential to a bowel training program.

Muscle Exercises

The diet for a paraplegic usually is high in protein, vitamins, and calories. The unaffected parts of the body are built up to optimal strength to enable the patient to ambulate with braces and crutches. The muscles of the hands, arms, shoulders, chest, spine, abdomen, and neck must be strengthened, since the patient must bear full weight on these muscles. The triceps and the latissimus dorsi are important muscles used in crutch-walking. The muscles of the abdomen and the back also are necessary for balance and the maintenance of the upright position.

To strengthen these muscles, the patient can do "push-ups" when he is in a prone position and "sit-ups" while he is in a sitting position. Extending the arms while he holds weights (traction weights can be used) also develops muscle strength. Squeezing rubber balls or crumpling newspaper promotes hand strength.

Through the encouragement of all of the members of

the rehabilitation team, the patient develops the increased exercise tolerance needed for gait training and ambulation activities.

Mobilization

When the spine is stable enough to allow the patient to assume an upright posture, mobilization activities are initiated. A brace or vest may be used, depending on the level of the lesion. Braces and crutches enable some patients to ambulate for short distances and even to drive manually operated automobiles. Modern technological developments, such as motorized wheelchairs and specially equipped vans, are contributing to the greater independence and mobility of patients with high level spinal cord injuries.

A major goal of nursing management is to help the patient overcome his sense of futility and to encourage him in the emotional adjustment that must be made before he is willing to venture into the "outside world." To achieve this goal it is important to realize that an excessively sympathetic attitude may cause the patient to develop an overdependence that defeats the purpose of the entire rehabilitation program.

Teach and help when necessary, but do not take over activities that the patient can do for himself with a little effort. This type of nursing care more than repays itself in the satisfaction of seeing a completely demoralized and helpless patient begin to find meaning in his newly emerging life style.

Complications

Autonomic dysreflexia (autonomic hyperreflexia) is an acute emergency that occurs as a result of exaggerated autonomic responses to stimuli. This syndrome is characterized by a severe, pounding headache with paroxysmal hypertension, profuse sweating (most often of the forehead), nasal obstruction, and bradycardia. It occurs among patients with cord lesions above the T4 to T6 segments (the sympathetic splanchnic visceral outflow). The sudden rise in blood pressure may cause a rupture of one or more cerebral blood vessels or lead to an increase in intracranial pressure. A number of stimuli may trigger this reflex: distended bladder (the most common cause), distended bowel, stimulation of the skin (tactile, pain, thermal stimuli) or distention or contraction of the visceral organs.

Since this is an emergency situation, the objective is to remove the triggering stimulus and to avoid the possible serious complications.
- Place the patient in a sitting position to lower the blood pressure.
- Drain the bladder via the catheter. If the catheter is not patent, irrigate it with a small amount of irrigating solution or insert another catheter.

- After the symptoms subside, the rectum is examined for a fecal mass. If one is present, Dibucaine ointment is applied 10 to 15 minutes before the mass is removed, since visceral distention or contraction can cause autonomic dysreflexia.
- Any other stimuli that can be the triggering event, such as an object on the skin or a draft of cold air, must be removed.
- If these measures do not relieve the patient's hypertension and excruciating headache, a ganglionic blocking agent (hydralazine hydrochloride [Apresoline]) is given slowly by vein.
- The patient's chart should be tagged with an allergic marker.

Any patient with a lesion above the T6 segment should be informed that such an episode is possible and may even occur many years after the initial injury.

OTHER COMPLICATIONS. Other complications of paraplegia include bladder and kidney infections, which are discussed under neurogenic bladder (page 914), pressure sores (page 187), and depression (pages 181 and 1261).

Sexuality of the Paraplegic Patient. Most patients with cord injury can have some form of meaningful sexual relationship, although some modifications will have to be made to cope with anxiety. The patient and his partner will benefit from counseling on special techniques, positions, etc. Sexual education and counseling services are being included in the rehabilitation services at Spinal Centers. Small group meetings in which the patients can share their feelings, receive information, and discuss sexual concerns and practical aspects are helpful in producing effective attitudes and adjustments. The reader is referred to the bibliography at the end of the chapter for readings on this topic.

Home Care: Continuing Medical and Rehabilitation Care

The patient with a spinal injury is at risk the first few weeks after his return home. Urinary infections, pressure sores, and deconditioning resulting in contractures may appear and may require rehospitalization. To avoid these complications, a family member is taught skin care, catheter care, range-of-motion exercises, etc., while the patient is still in the hospital. The community health nurse provides follow-up evaluation to reinforce previous teaching and to answer questions. The local counselor for the Division of Vocational Rehabilitation works with the patient with respect to job placement or additional educational or vocational training.

The patient requires continuing lifelong follow-up by the physician, physical therapist, and other rehabilitation team members because the neurological deficit is permanent and new problems can erupt that require prompt attention before they take their toll in physical impairment, time, morale, and money.

BIBLIOGRAPHY

BOOKS

Adams, R. D., and Victor, M.: Principles of Neurology. New York, McGraw-Hill, 1977.

Allen, M. B., Jr., et al.: A Manual of Neurosurgery. Baltimore, University Park Press, 1978.

American Nurses Association, Division Medical-Surgical Nursing Practice and the American Association of Neurosurgical Nurses: Standards of Neurological and Neurosurgical Nursing Practice. Kansas City, American Nurses Association, 1977.

Andrew, J. M., and Johnson, R. T.: Amyotrophic Lateral Sclerosis. New York, Academic Press, 1976.

Brooke, M. H.: A Clinician's View of Neuromuscular Disease. Baltimore, Williams and Wilkins, 1977.

Conway, B. L.: Carini and Owens' Neurological and Neurosurgical Nursing, 7th ed. St. Louis, C. V. Mosby, 1978.

Eliasson, S. G., Prensky, A. L., and Hardin, W. B.: Neurological Pathophysiology, 2nd ed. New York, Oxford University Press, 1978.

Forster, F. M.: Reflex Epilepsy, Behavioral Therapy and Conditional Reflexes. Springfield, Ill., Charles C Thomas, 1977.

Ganong, W. F.: The Nervous System. Los Altos, Calif. Lange Med. Pub., 1977.

Goldensohn, E. S., and Appel, S. H., eds.: Scientific Approaches to Clinical Neurology. Vols. 1 & 2. Philadelphia, Lea and Febiger, 1977.

Gregory, M. F.: Sexual Adjustment. A Guide for the Spinal Cord Injured. Bloomingdale, Ill., Accent Special Publications, 1974.

Guttmann, L.: Spinal Cord Injuries. Oxford, Blackwell Scientific Publications, 1976.

Hoppenfeld, S.: Orthopaedic Neurology. Philadelphia, J. B. Lippincott, 1977.

Howe, J. J. R.: Patient Care in Neurosurgery. Boston, Little, Brown, 1977.

Hughes, J. T.: Pathology of the Spinal Cord. London, Lloyd-Luke Medical Books, 1978.

Lewis, A. J.: Mechanisms of Neurological Disease. Boston, Little, Brown, 1976.

McLaurin, R. L., ed.: Head Injuries. New York, Grune and Stratton, 1975.

Marshall, J.: The Management of Cerebrovascular Disease, 3rd ed. Oxford, Blackwell Scientific Publications, 1976.

Matthews, B.: Multiple Sclerosis. The Facts. New York, Oxford University Press, 1978.

Merritt, H. H.: A Textbook of Neurology, 6th ed. Philadelphia, Lea and Febiger, 1979.

O'Brien, M. T., and Pallet, P. J.: Total Care of the Stroke Patient. Boston, Little, Brown, 1978.

O'Connor, A. B., ed.: Nursing in Neurological Disorders. New York, American Journal of Nursing Co., 1976.

O'Doherty, D. S.: Handbook of Neurologic Emergencies. Garden City, N.Y., Medical Examination Pub. Co., 1977.

Patton, H. D., et al.: Introduction to Basic Neurology. Philadelphia, W. B. Saunders, 1976.

Pierce, D. S., and Nickel, V. H.: The Total Care of Spinal Cord Injuries. Boston, Little, Brown, 1977.

Perske, R., et al.: Mealtimes for Severely and Profoundly Handicapped Persons. Baltimore, University Park Press, 1977.

Pippenger, C. E., Penry, J. K., and Kutt, H.: Antiepileptic Drugs: Quantitative Analysis and Interpretation. New York, Raven Press, 1978.

Richens, A.: Drug Treatment of Epilepsy. London, Henry Kimpton Publishers, 1976.

Roaf, R.: Spinal Deformities. Philadelphia, J. B. Lippincott, 1977.

Robinson, J., and Gyetan, M.: Coping with Neurological Problems Proficiently. Horsham, Pa., Intermed Communications, 1979.

Rubin, L. R.: Reanimation of the Paralyzed Face. St. Louis, C. V. Mosby, 1977.

Russell, W. R.: Multiple Sclerosis: Control of the Disease. New York, Pergamon Press, 1976.

Siegel, I. M.: The Clinical Management of Muscle Disease. Philadelphia, J. B. Lippincott, 1977.

Samuels, M. A., ed.: Manual of Neurologic Therapeutics. Boston, Little, Brown, 1978.

Solomon, G. E., and Plum, F.: Clinical Management of Seizures. Philadelphia, W. B. Saunders, 1976.

Swift, N., and Mabel, R. M.: Manual of Neurological Nursing. Boston, Little, Brown, 1978.

Treip, C. S.: Color Atlas of Neuropathology. Chicago, Year Book Medical Pub., 1978.

Vick, N. A.: Grinker's Neurology, 7th ed. Springfield, Ill., Charles C Thomas, 1976.

Vinken, P. J., Bruyn, G. W., and Braakman, R., eds.: Handbook of Clinical Neurology. Injuries of Spine and Spinal Cord. Part 1. New York, American Elsevier, 1976.

Vinken, P. J., and Bruyn, G. W.: Handbook of Clinical Neurology. Tumours of the Spine and Spinal Cord. Parts I and II. New York, American Elsevier, 1976.

Walton, J. N.: Essentials of Neurology, 4th ed. Philadelphia, J. B. Lippincott, 1976.

Yashon, D.: Spinal Injury. New York, Appleton-Century-Crofts, 1978.

ARTICLES

Brain Tumor, Abscess

Calcaterra, T. C., and Rand, R. W.: Current adjuncts for surgery of the sphenoid sinus and pituitary gland. Laryngoscope, *86*:1692-1698, Nov. 1976.

Cannon, M.: To Sharon, with love. AJN., *79*:642-645, Apr. 1979.

Hirsh, L. F.: Metastatic brain tumors. Postgrad. Med., *65*:145-154, Feb. 1979.

Joubert, M. J., and Stephanov, S.: Computerized tomography and surgical treatment in intracranial suppuration. J. Neurosurg., *47*:73-78, July 1977.

May, P. B.: Initial evaluation and management of patients with suspected pituitary tumors. Prim. Care, *4*:89-125, Mar. 1977.

Ontjes, D. A., and Ney, R. L.: Pituitary tumors. CA, *26*:330-350, Nov.-Dec., 1976.

Persaud, D. H.: Nursing implications. Cerebral vasospasms — Rx: Aminophylline-Isuprel regime. J. Neurosurg. Nurs., *10*:63-65, June 1978.

Posner, J. B.: Management of central nervous system metastases. Semin. Oncol., *4*:81-91, Mar. 1977.

Vick, N. A., Khandekar, J., and Bigner, D. D.: Chemotherapy of brain tumors. Arch. Neurol., *34*:523-526, Sept. 1977.

Walker, M. D.: Treatment of brain tumors. Med. Clin. N. Am., *61*:1045-1051, Sept. 1977.

Wheeler, P.: Care of the patient with a cerebellar tumor. AJN, 77:263-266, Feb. 1977.

Yorke, C. H., and Levin, V. A.: Intracranial malignant growth, primary and metastatic. Curr. Probl. Cancer, *1*:1-46, Feb. 1977.

Wilson, C. B., et al.: Single agent chemotherapy of brain tumors. Arch. Neurol., *33*:739-744, Nov. 1976.

Zulch, K. J., and Mennel, H. D.: New aspects of brain tumor research. J. Neurol., *214*:241-250, 21 Mar. 1977.

Epilepsy

Conomy, J. P.: Long-term use of the major anticonvulsant drugs. Am. Fam. Phys., *18*:107-116, Oct. 1978.

Livingston, S.: Medical treatment of epilepsy. South. Med. J., *71*:Part 1: 298-310, Mar. 1978; Part 2: 432-447, Apr. 1978.

Rapport, R. L.: Surgical management of epilepsy. West. J. Med., *127*:185-189, Sept. 1977.

Swift, N.: Helping patients live with seizures. Nursing '78, *8*:24-31, June 1978.

Sypert, G. W.: New concepts in the management of epilepsy: Medical and surgical. Clin. Neurosurg., *24*:600-641, 1976.

Valproic acid and sodium valproate approved for use in epilepsy. FDA Drug Bulletin, *8*:14-15, Mar.-Apr. 1978.

Head Injury

Adams, N. R.: Prolonged coma. Your care makes all the difference. Nursing '77, 7:20-27, Aug. 1977.

Koo, A. H., and LaRoque, R. L.: Evaluation of head trauma by computed tomography. Radiology, *123*:345-350, May 1977.

Kunkel, J., and Wiley, J. K.: Acute head injury: What to do, when—and why. Nursing '79, *9*:22-33, Mar. 1979.

Lewin, W.: Changing attitudes to the management of severe head injuries. Br. Med. J., *2*:No. 6046: 1234-1239, 20 Nov. 1976.

Meyd, C. J.: Acute brain trauma. AJN, 78:40-44, Jan. 1978.

Schnaper, N.: The psychological implications of severe trauma: Emotional sequelae to unconsciousness. J. Trauma, *15*:94-98, Feb. 1975.

Wahl, S.: Only a concussion. Nursing '76, *6*:44-45, Aug. 1976.

Intervertebral Disc

Bullard, J. R., and Houghton, F. M.: Epidural steroid treatment of acute herniated nucleus pulposus. Anesth. Anal., *56*:862-863, Nov.-Dec. 1977.

Farrell, J.: Caring for the laminectomy patient: How to strengthen your support. Nursing '78, *8*:65-69, May 1978.

Macnab, I.: The surgery of lumbar disc degeneration. Surg. Annu., *8*:447-480, 1976.

Sampson, P.: Chymopapain: A case study in federal drug regulation. JAMA, *240*:195-219, July 21, 1978.

Neuromuscular Conditions: Amyotrophic Lateral Sclerosis; Guillain-Barré Syndrome; Myasthenia Gravis

Boyle, M. A., and Cicua, R. L.: Amyotrophic lateral sclerosis. AJN, 76:66-68, Jan. 1976.

Dau, P. C., et al.: Plasmapheresis and immunosuppressive drug therapy in myasthenia gravis. New Eng. J. Med., *297*: 1134-1140, Nov. 24, 1977.

Free, J. W., and McPhillips, C.: Huntington's disease. RN., *40*:44-46, Aug. 1977.

Furukawa, T., and Peter, J. B.: The muscular dystrophies and related disorders. JAMA, *239*:1537-1542, Apr. 14, 1978.

Galdi, A. P.: Essentials in the management of myasthenia gravis. Am. Fam. Phys., *17*:95-102, June 1978.

Goldblatt, D.: Treatment of amyotrophic lateral sclerosis. Adv. in Neurol., *17*:265-283, 1977.

Griggs, R. C., and Moxley, R. T., eds.: Treatment of neuromuscular diseases. Adv. in Neurol., *17*:1-364, 1977.

Havard, C. W.: Progress in myasthenia gravis. Br. Med. J., *2*, No. 6093:1008-1011, Oct. 15, 1977.

Jaretzki, A., et al.: A rational approach to total thymectomy in the treatment of myasthenia gravis. Ann. Thorac. Surg., *24*:120-130, Aug. 1977.

Kealy, S. L.: Respiratory care in Guillain-Barré syndrome. AJN, 77:58-60, Jan. 1977.

Kennedy, R. H., et al.: Guillain-Barré syndrome: A 42-year epidemiologic and clinical study. Mayo Clin. Proc., *53*:93-99, Feb. 1978.

Ketenjian, A. Y.: Muscular dystrophy: Diagnosis and treatment. Orthoped. Clin. N. Am., *9*:25-42, Jan. 1978.

McCleave, D. T., Fletcher, J., and Cruden, L. C.: The Guillain Barré syndrome in intensive care. Anaesth. Intensive Care, *4*:46-52, Feb. 1976.

Merritt, H. H.: Diagnosis and treatment of muscle disease. Med. Times, *105*:35-44, Aug. 1977.

Mulder, D. W., and Howard, F. M., Jr.: Patient resistance and prognosis in amyotrophic lateral sclerosis. Mayo Clin. Proc., *51*:537-541, Sept. 1976.

Sinkai, M. S., and Mulder, D. W.: Rehabilitation techniques for patients with amyotrophic lateral sclerosis. Mayo Clin. Proc., *53*:173-178, Mar. 1978.

Raine, C. S.: The etiology and pathogenesis of multiple sclerosis: Recent developments. Pathobiol. Annu., 7:347-384, 1977.

Schneitzer, L.: Rehabilitation of patients with multiple sclerosis. Arch. Phys. Med. Rehabil., *59*:430-437, Sept. 1978.

Parkinson's Disease

Calne, D. B.: Developments in the treatment of parkinsonism (editorial). N. Eng. J. Med., *295*:1433-1434, Dec. 16, 1976.

———: Parkinsonism. Clinical and neuropharmacologic aspects. Postgrad. Med., *64*:82-88, Aug. 1978.

Cohen, M. M., and Scheife, R. T.: Pharmacotherapy of Parkinson's disease. Am. J. Hosp. Pharm., *34*:531-538, May 1977.

Davis, J. C.: Team management of Parkinson's disease. Am. J. Occup. Ther., *31*:300-308, May-June 1977.

Fahn, S., and Calne, D. B.: Considerations in the management of Parkinsonism. Neurology, *28*:5-7, Jan. 1978.

Fischbach, F. T.: Easing adjustment to Parkinson's disease. AJN, 78:66-69, Jan. 1978.

Godwin-Austen, R. B.: The treatment of Parkinson's disease. Postgrad. Med. J., 53:729-731, Dec. 1977.

Lieberman, A., et al.: Treatment of Parkinson's disease with lergotrile mesylate. JAMA, 238:2380-2382, Nov. 28, 1977.

Synder, B. D.: Selected aspects of Parkinsonism: Therapeutics. Minn. Med., 60:284-286, Apr. 1977.

Stern, G. M., and Lees, A. J.: Choice of treatment in Parkinson's disease. Practitioner, 219:537-541, Oct. 1977.

Tyler, H. D.: Update on Parkinson's disease. Med. Times, 106:10d-17d, Apr. 1978.

Winkelman, A. C.: Update on drug treatment of Parkinsonism. Am. Fam. Phys., 16:118-120, July 1977.

Yahr, M. D.: Parkinson's disease—overview of its current status. Mt. Sinai J. Med. (N.Y.), 44:183-191, Mar.-Apr. 1977.

Spinal Cord Injury

Abramson, A. S.: Management of the neurogenic bladder in perspective. Arch. Phys. Med. Rehabil., 57:197-201, May 1976.

Bricolo, A., et al.: Local cooling in spinal cord injury. Surg. Neurol., 6:101-106, Aug. 1976.

Clark, J. A., and Roemer, R. B.: Voice controlled wheelchair. Arch. Phys. Med. Rehabil., 58:169-175, Apr. 1977.

Donovan, W. H., Kiviat, M. D., and Clowers, D. E.: Intermittent bladder emptying via urethral catheterization of suprapubic cystocath: A comparison study. Arch. Phys. Med. Rehabil., 58:291-296, July 1977.

Doss, G. H., Miller, J. M., and Rhodes, M.: The home health team: Continuing care for spinal cord patients. Rehab. Counsel. Bull., 18:272-278, June 1975.

Eisenberg, M. G., et al.: Sex education and counseling program on a spinal cord injury service. Arch. Phys. Med. Rehabil., 57:135-140, Mar. 1976.

Fast, A.: Reflex sweating in patients with spinal cord injury: A review. Arch. Phys. Med. Rehabil., 58:435-437, Oct. 1977.

Feuer, H.: Management of acute spine and spinal cord injuries. Arch. Surg., 111:638-645, June 1976.

Hamric, A., et al.: Caring for the totally dependent patient. Nursing '76, 6:38-43, July 1976.

Hansen, A. M.: Towards independence for paraplegics. Can. Nurse, 72:24-31, Dec. 1976.

Kursh, E. C., Freehafer, A., and Persky, L.: Complications of autonomic dysreflexia. J. Urol., 118:70-72, July 1977.

Opitz, J. L.: Bladder retraining: An organized program. Mayo Clin. Proc., 51:367-372, June 1976.

Stewart, T. D.: Coping behaviour and the moratorium following spinal cord injury. Paraplegia., 15:338-342, Feb. 1978.

Stewart, T. D., and Rossier, A. B.: Psychological considerations in the adjustment to spinal cord injury. Rehabil. Lit., 39:75-80, Mar. 1978.

Wagner, F. C.: Management of acute spinal cord injury. Surg. Neurol., 7:346-350, June 1977.

Stroke, Cerebrovascular Disease

Bellows, J. G.: Stroke prevention. Compr. Ther., 4:3-4, Feb. 1978.

Breunig, K. A.: After the blow up—how to care for the patient with a ruptured cerebral aneurysm. Nursing '76, 6:37-45, Dec. 1976.

Caplan, L. R., and Mohr, J. P.: Intracerebral hemorrhage: An update. Geriatrics, 33:42-52, May 1978.

Eastman, D. G., et al.: Identifying and reducing stroke risks. Patient Care, 10:71-88, Apr. 15, 1976.

Gotshall, R. A., and Harker, L. A.: Using antithrombotic therapy in ischemic cerebrovascular disease. Geriatrics, 32:101-104, Nov. 1977.

Kester, R. C.: Surgery for strokes resulting from extracranial arterial occlusion. Nurs. Times, 74:59-62, Jan. 12, 1978.

Langfitt, T. W.: Conservative care of intracranial hemorrhage. Adv. Neurol., 16:169-180, 1977.

McDowell, F. H.: The extracranial/intracranial bypass study. Stroke, 8:545, Sept.-Oct. 1977.

Moran, J. M., Reichman, H., and Baker, W. H.: Staged intracranial and extracranial revascularization. Arch. Surg., 112:1424-1428, Dec. 1977.

Rodvien, R., and Mielke, C. H.: Platelet and antiplatelet agents in strokes. Curr. Concepts of Cerebrovascular Dis., 13:5-8, Mar.-Apr. 1978.

Stanford, J. R., Lubow, M., and Vasko, J. S.: Prevention of stroke by carotid endarterectomy. Surg., 83:259-263, Mar. 1978.

Thompson, R. A., and Green, J. R., eds.: Stroke. Adv. in Neurol., 16:1-225 (entire vol.), 1977.

Troupp, H.: The management of intracranial arterial aneurysms in the acute stage. Adv. in Tech. Standards in Neurosurg., 3:35-46, 1976.

Webb, P. H.: Neurological deficit after carotid endarterectomy. AJN, 79:654-658, Apr. 1979.

Trigeminal Neuralgia

Dalessio, D. J.: Evaluation of the patient with chronic facial pain. Am. Fam. Phys., 16:84-92, Sept. 1977.

Loeser, J. D.: What to do about tic douloureux. JAMA, 239:1153-1155, Mar. 20, 1978.

Loeser, J. D., Cavin, W. H., and Howe, J. F.: Pathophysiology of trigeminal neuralgia. Clin. Neurosurg., 24:527-549, 1976.

Ostrow, L. S.: New hope for patients with trigeminal neuralgia. AJN, 76:1301-1303, Aug. 1976.

Silverberg, G. D., and Britt, R. H.: Percutaneous radiofrequency rhizotomy in the treatment of trigeminal neuralgia. West. J. Med., 129:97-100, Aug. 1978.

AGENCIES

Governmental

Commission for the Control of Huntington's Disease and Its Consequences, Room 8A11, Building 31, National Institutes of Health, Bethesda, Md. 20205

Division for the Blind and Physically Handicapped, Library of Congress, Washington, D.C. 20542

National Institute of Neurological and Communicative Disorders and Stroke, National Institute of Health, Bethesda, Md. 20205

Voluntary

ALS Society of America, 12011 San Vicente Blvd., Suite 350, Box 49001, Los Angeles, Calif. 90049

American Parkinson's Disease, Assoc., Inc., 147 E. 50th Street, Suite 103, New York, N.Y. 10022

American Speech and Hearing Association, 10801 Rockville Pike, Rockville, Md. 20852

Committee to Combat Huntington's Disease, 250 W. 57th St., Suite 2016, New York, N.Y. 10019

Epilepsy Foundation of America, 1828 L. Street, N.W., Suite 406, Washington, D.C. 20036

Muscular Dystrophy Association, Inc., 810 Seventh Ave., New York, N.Y. 10019

Myasthenia Gravis Foundation, 230 Park Ave., New York, N.Y. 10017

National ALS Foundation, Inc., 185 Madison Ave., New York, N.Y. 10016

National Easter Seal Society for Crippled Children and Adults, 2023 W. Ogden Ave., Chicago, Ill. 60612

National Epilepsy League, Six N. Michigan Ave., Chicago, Ill. 60602

National Huntington's Disease Association, Suite 501, 1441 Broadway, New York, N.Y. 10018

National Multiple Sclerosis Society, 205 E. 42nd St., New York, N.Y. 10017

National Paraplegia Foundation, 333 N. Michigan Ave., Chicago, Ill., 60601

National Parkinson Foundation, 1501 N.W. Ninth Ave., Miami, Fla. 31316

Paralyzed Veterans of America, 7315 Wisconsin Ave., Suite 300 W, Washington, D.C. 20014

Parkinson's Disease Foundation, Inc., William Black Medical Research Building, Columbia Presbyterian Medical Center, 640 W. 168th St., New York, N.Y. 10032

United Parkinson Foundation, 220 S. State St., Chicago, Ill., 60604

Musculoskeletal and Locomotion Problems

UNIT FOURTEEN

56

ASSESSMENT OF MUSCULOSKELETAL FUNCTION

PHYSIOLOGIC OVERVIEW

The musculoskeletal system is composed of bones, muscle, cartilage, ligaments, tendons, and fascia, organized into a complex system that protects the body, gives it a structural framework, and provides it with its means of locomotion. The muscle mass accounts for approximately half of normal body weight, while the bony structures and connective tissue add an additional 25 percent. Therefore, the musculoskeletal system collectively constitutes the largest organ system in the body.

The Skeletal System

ANATOMY OF THE SKELETAL SYSTEM. There are 206 bones in the human body—divided into four categories: long bones (i.e., the femur), short bones (i.e., the tarsals), flat bones (i.e., the sternum), and irregular bones (i.e., the vertebrae).

The center of a typical long bone is called the *shaft* or *diaphysis*. The ends of the long bones, called the *epiphyses,* are separated in childhood from the shaft of the bone by a plate of actively proliferating cartilage called the *epiphyseal plate*. In the adult, this plate is calcified. The ends of the long bones, at which point they articulate with other bones, are covered with cartilage (articular cartilage). Running through the shaft of long bones (and in flat bones as well) is a vascular tissue in which the cellular elements of blood are manufactured. This tissue, called *bone marrow,* is the principal tissue engaged in hematopoiesis. Bone marrow is found particularly in the skull, vertebrae, ribs, sternum and ileum. Surrounding the bone and containing most of its blood vessels is a thin fibrous tissue called the *periostium*. Bone tissue is well vascularized. It is estimated that the blood flow to bone in man is about 8 percent of the total cardiac output.

BONE FORMATION. Bone is composed of cells, a protein matrix, and minerals, primarily calcium and phosphorous. Sodium, magnesium, and carbonate are also present but in small amounts. The protein matrix is predominantly collagen, that is, produced by the cellular elements of the bone. The collagen molecule is somewhat unique in that it contains practically all of the hydroxyproline (an amino acid) that is present in the body. Collagen is secreted into the extracellular space in a soluble form and then undergoes a maturation process which consists of cross-linking between adjacent strands to form a tough, fibrous insoluble material. Calcium and phosphorous are then deposited in the collagen matrix to give bone its characteristic hardness. This process, called *ossification,* depends on formation of an insoluble calcium and phosphate complex called hydroxyapatite, which has the chemical composition $Ca_{10}(PO_4)_6(OH)_2$. The maintenance of bone structure is dependent on normal cellular production of collagen and on the availability in the body of adequate amounts of calcium and phosphorous. The enzyme, alkaline phosphatase, may accelerate bone formation by releasing phosphates from organic material thereby raising the local phosphate concentration. Elevated alkaline phosphatase activity in the blood is commonly found during periods of rapid bone formation.

The mineral in the skeleton is constantly being laid down and reabsorbed. Calcium in bone in an adult human is replaced at the rate of about 18 percent a year. This indicates that bone is a dynamic tissue in a constant state of turnover. The important regulating factors that determine the balance between bone formation and bone resorption include local stress, vitamin D, and parathyroid hormone. Local stresses act to stimulate local bone resorption and formation and can result in extensive remodeling. In this way, deformed bones may tend to straighten out. This phenomenon also explains why important weight bearing bones are thick and strong. Vitamin D functions to increase the amount of calcium in the blood by promoting absorption of calcium from the gastrointestinal tract and accelerating deposition of calcium in the collagen matrix. In the absence of vitamin D, insufficient calcification occurs resulting in the clinical conditions known as rickets and osteomalacia. Parathyroid hormone regulates the concentration of calcium ions in the blood, in part by promoting mobilization of calcium from the bones. Excessive mobilization of calcium due to excess parathyroid hormone results in demineralization of the skeleton and formation of bone cysts.

Bone tissue contains three different types of cells: osteoblasts, osteocytes, and osteoclasts. Osteoblasts are the bone-forming cells that secrete the collagen which forms the bone matrix. Osteocytes and osteoclasts are the cells that are responsible for reabsorption of the calcified matrix. The bone structure represents the balance between the formative and reabsorptive activities of the bone cells.

FUNCTIONS OF THE SKELETON. The human body as we know it owes its shape to the skeletal system. The skeleton is also the structure which allows the body to move, lift, and fight. The bony skeleton provides the support in which all other organs are placed and suspended and also provides protection for them. Since more than 99 percent of the total body calcium is present in the bones, they serve as the main storage depot for this mineral, and to a certain extent for phosphorous also. Bone is also a good chemical buffer and so helps to prevent rapid changes in hydrogen ion concentration of the body fluid.

JOINTS. The junction of two or more bones is called a *joint* or an *articulation.* In freely moving joints, the bones that comprise the joint are separated by fluid. In immovable joints, there is close contact between two adjacent bones which are fused. A partially movable joint is one in which limited motion is possible. The bones in this type of joint are separated by fibrous cartilage as in the union between the two pubis bones.

Movable joints are of several different types. The *ball and socket* type, best exemplified by the hip or the shoulder, permits full freedom of movement. *Hinge* joints permit bending in one direction only and are best exemplified by the elbows and knees. A *biaxial* joint, for example, the wrist, is one in which movement can occur in two planes. The *pivot* joint is characterized by the articulation between the radius and the ulna in the forearm; it permits only rotation.

At a typical movable joint, the ends of the articulating bones are covered with a smooth hyaline cartilage. The space between the bones is surrounded by a sheath of tough fibrous tissue called a *joint capsule*. The joint capsule is strengthened by bands of connective tissue, called *ligaments,* which help to maintain the bones in proper relationship to each other. Ligaments occur both along the outside of the joint capsule and also within the joint capsule where they bridge the gap between the bones. The joint capsule is lined with a membrane which secretes fluid into the synovial cavity between the bones. The synovial fluid functions as a shock absorber as well as a lubricant to allow the joint to move freely in the appropriate directions.

Skeletal Muscles

ANATOMY OF THE SKELETAL MUSCLES. The skeletal muscles, through contraction and relaxation, move the bones around the joints to provide locomotion and other body movements. The ends of skeletal muscles are connected to the bones by tough, fibrous tissue called *tendons.* Skeletal muscles vary greatly in size or weight in different parts of the body. However, all skeletal muscles are composed of many muscle cells in parallel.

Muscles also vary in their pigmentation. The two basic categories are red muscle and white muscle. Red muscle is given its color by the presence in its cells of myoglobin, a hemoglobin-like protein. Myoglobin is thought to function both as a store of oxygen and as a facilitator of the movement of oxygen from capillary blood into the muscle cell. White muscle contains little myoglobin. Most skeletal muscles are combinations of fibers of more than one type providing broad functional capacity. The speed of contraction of various muscles varies greatly but the slower ones are predominantly red muscles.

Each muscle cell (also referred to as a muscle fiber) contains myofibrils which in turn are composed of a series of sarcomeres, the actual contractile units of skeletal muscle. The components of the sarcomeres are known as thick and thin filaments. The thin filaments are composed mainly of a protein known as actin. The thick filaments are composed mainly of myosin, another protein material.

TYPES OF MUSCULOSKELETAL MOTION. Contraction of most skeletal muscles causes two bones to move relative to each other around the joint between. Usually one of the bones tends to remain stationary while the other bone moves. By convention, the end of the muscle attached to the stationary bone is called its *origin* and the end that is attached to the movable bone is called its *insertion.* For most movements around a joint, there are muscles that have opposing actions. Such muscles are referred to as *agonists* and *antagonists.* For example, contraction of the biceps causes flexion while contraction of the triceps causes extension of the elbow joint. Normally when an individual voluntarily flexes the elbow, the biceps muscle (the agonist) contracts while the triceps (the antagonist) relaxes.

Besides flexor and extensor muscles, examples of which are given above, contraction of other skeletal muscles results in a variety of body movements. *Adductor* muscles tend to bring a portion of the body toward the midline; *abductor* muscles do the opposite. *Pronation* (for example, turning palms down) and *supination* (turning palms up) are movements involved in rotation. Circumduction, inversion, and eversion are additional descriptions of body movements.

MUSCLE CONTRACTION. The contraction of muscle fibers can result in either isotonic or isometric contraction of the muscle. In *isometric contraction* the length of the muscles remains constant but the force generated by the muscles is increased. An example of this is when one pushes against an immovable wall. *Isotonic contraction,* on the other hand, is characterized by shortening of the muscle with no increase in tension within the muscle. An example of this is flexion of the forearm. In normal activities, many muscle movements are a combination of isometric and isotonic contraction. For example, during walking, isotonic contraction results in shortening of the leg, while during isometric contraction, the stiff leg pushes against the floor.

Contraction of a muscle is due to the contraction of each of its component sarcomeres. The muscle shortens because each sarcomere shortens. The contraction of a sarcomere is due to interactions between the thick filaments and the thin filaments brought about by a local increase in the calcium ion concentration. The interaction between the actin and the myosin causes the thick and thin filaments to slide across one another. When calcium concentration in the sarcomere subsequently falls, the myosin and actin filaments cease to interact and the sarcomere returns to its original resting length (relaxation). Intracellular metabolic energy stored in the form of adenosine triphosphate (ATP) is required to break the actin and myosin bonds and allow relaxation. Interaction between actin and myosin does not occur in the absence of calcium because of the presence on the thin filaments of the proteins tropomyosin and troponin. In the presence of calcium, the configuration of these inhibitory proteins is altered and the cross bridges between the myosin and actin filaments can occur.

EXCITATION-CONTRACTION COUPLING. Muscle fibers contract in response to electrical stimulation. Muscle cells when stimulated generate an action potential in a manner similar to that described for nerve cells. These action potentials propagate along the muscle cell membrane and lead to the release in the muscle cell of calcium ions that are stored in specialized organelles called the *sarcoplasmic reticulum.* The release of calcium allows the interaction of actin and myosin in the sarcomere. Very shortly after the muscle cell membrane is depolarized, it recovers its resting membrane voltage. Calcium is rapidly removed from the sarcomeres by active reaccumulation in the sarcoplasmic reticulum, and the muscle relaxes.

Depolarization of the muscle cells normally occurs in response to a stimulus delivered by a nerve cell. The communication between the nerve cell and the muscle cell takes place at the motor end plate. The neurons that control the activity of skeletal muscle cells are called *lower motor neurons* which originate in the anterior horn of the spinal cord.

ENERGY SOURCE FOR MUSCLE CONTRACTION. Energy is consumed during muscle contraction and relaxation. The rate of energy utilization by skeletal muscle is variable; it increases markedly during exercise. The source of energy for the muscle cells is ATP that is generated through cellular oxidative metabolism. Creatine phosphate, also present in muscle cells, functions as a second reservoir of metabolic energy: it can be converted to ATP when necessary. At low levels of activity, the skeletal muscle synthesizes ATP from the oxidation of glucose to water and carbon dioxide. During periods of high activity when sufficient oxygen may not be available, glucose is metabolized primarily to lactic acid. Although ATP is generated during production of lactic acid, the process is inefficient compared with oxidative pathways. Therefore, increased amounts of glucose are required and are supplied by muscle glycogen. Glycogen is a starch that is produced from glucose, stored in the cells during periods of rest, and utilized during periods of activity. Muscle fatigue is thought to be caused by a rapid rate of work of the muscle resulting in depletion of glycogen and energy stores and accumulation of lactic acid. As a result, the cycle of muscle contraction and relaxation cannot continue.

HEAT PRODUCTION. During muscle contraction, the energy released from ATP is not completely utilized by the contractile apparatus. This excess energy is dissipated in the form of heat. During isometric contraction, almost all the energy is released in the form of heat, while during isotonic contraction some of the energy is expended in mechanical work. In some situations such as shivering, the need for generation of heat is the primary stimulus for muscle contraction.

MUSCLE SIZE. When a muscle is repeatedly caused to develop maximum or close to maximum tension over a long period of time, as in regular exercise with weights, the cross-sectional area of the muscle increases. This is due to an increase in the cross-sectional area of each muscle fiber without increase in the number of muscle fibers. This increase in the size of the individual muscle fibers is called *hypertrophy.* Hypertrophy will persist only if the exercise is continued. The opposite phenomenon occurs with disuse of muscle over a long period of time. This decrease in the size of a muscle is called *atrophy.*

GENERAL ASSESSMENT

Management of orthopedic problems starts with accurate assessment of the patient's problems. Important information can be obtained from the patient history and the physical assessment. Principles of clinical interviewing are found in Chapter 4 and the technique of physical assessment in Chapter 5.

The patient is assessed for muscle atrophy or swelling in addition to any problems in posture and gait. The joints are examined for shape, alignment, circumference, range of motion, stability, instability and the presence of abnormal joint fluid. The bone(s) are evaluated for integrity, size and any signs of swelling and tenderness. The skin overlying bone is palpated for local swelling, tenderness and skin temperature. Muscle strength is measured as well as the length and circumference of the extremities. Usually a neurological assessment is carried out at the same time.

DIAGNOSTIC ASSESSMENT

Radiological Procedures

X-rays are important in evaluating patients with musculoskeletal disorders. Bone films determine bone density, texture, erosion and changes in bone relationships. X-ray of the cortex of the bone detects widening, narrowing and any signs of irregularity. Joint x-rays will reveal the presence of fluid, irregularity, spur formation, narrowing and changes in the joint structure.

Laminography or tomography shows in detail a specific plane of involved bone.

Myelography, the injection of radiopaque dye into the subarachnoid space of the lumbar spine, is carried out to determine disc herniation or the site of a tumor. This technique is discussed on page 1176.

Arthrography is the injection of a radiopaque substance and/or air into the joint cavity in order to outline soft tissue structures and the contour of the joint. The joint is put through its range of motion while a series of radiographs are taken. Arthrography is useful in identifying acute or chronic tears of the joint capsule or supporting ligaments of the knee, shoulder, ankle, hips or wrist. (If a tear is present, the dye will leak out of the joint and show on x-ray.)

Computed tomography can be useful in orthopedic diagnosis by identifying tumors of the soft tissue or injuries to the ligaments or tendons. It is helpful in identifying the location and extent of fractures in difficult to define areas (i.e., the acetabulum). The technique of computed tomography is discussed on page 289.

Other Studies

An *arthrocentesis* is carried out to obtain synovial fluid for purposes of examination. A needle is inserted into the joint, and fluid is then aspirated. Since this procedure has the potential for introducing bacteria into the joint, aseptic techniques must be followed. Following aspiration no special precautions are necessary.

Normally synovial fluid is clear, pale, straw-colored and scanty in volume. The fluid is examined grossly for volume, color, clarity, and viscosity and formation of mucin clot. It is examined microscopically for cell count, cell identification, Gram stain, and formed elements. Examination of synovial fluid is helpful in the diagnosis of rheumatoid arthritis and other inflammatory arthropathies, and will reveal the presence of hemarthrosis (bleeding into joint cavity) which suggests trauma or a tendency to bleed.

Electromyography provides information on the electric potential of the muscles and nerves leading to them. The purpose of this procedure is to determine any abnormal physiology involving the motor unit.

A *bone scan* reflects the degree to which the crystal lattice of bone "takes up" a bone-seeking radioactive isotope that is injected into the system. The degree of nuclide uptake is related to blood flow to the bone. An increased uptake of isotope is seen in primary skeletal disease (osteosarcoma), metastatic bone disease, inflammatory skeletal disease (osteomyelitis) and certain types of fractures.

Thermography measures the degree of heat radiating from the skin surface. It is used to investigate the pathophysiology of inflamed joints (rheumatoid arthritis) and to assess the patient's response to anti-inflammatory drug therapy.

Arthroscopy is an endoscopic procedure which allows direct visualization of a joint, especially the knee. The procedure is carried out in the operating room, under sterile conditions and following infiltration of a local anesthetic agent or a general anesthesia. A large bore needle is inserted into the suprapatellar pouch and the joint is distended with saline. The arthroscope is introduced and the knee joint visualized, including the synovium, articular surfaces and menisci. If an arthrotomy is not indicated, the puncture wound is covered with a sterile Band-Aid and the limb is wrapped from the midthigh to the midcalf with a compressive wrap that is worn for 24 hours for support. The patient may be advised to limit his activities for three days. When arthroscopy is combined with arthrography a high degree of accuracy is achieved in diagnosing lesions and internal derangement of the knee.

ASSESSMENT OF MUSCULOSKELETAL DISCOMFORT

Pain

Most patients with diseases and traumatic conditions of muscles, bones, and joints experience pain. *Bone pain* is characteristically described as a dull, deep ache that is boring in nature, whereas *muscular pain* is considered sore and aching and is frequently referred to as muscle cramps. *Fracture pain* is sharp and piercing and is relieved by immobilization. Sharp pain may also result from *bone infection* with muscle spasm or pressure on a sensory nerve.

Most musculoskeletal pain is relieved by rest. Pain that increases with activity may indicate joint sprain or muscle strain, while steadily increasing pain points to a progression of an infectious process (osteomyelitis), a malignant tumor or vascular complications. Radiating pain is seen in conditions in which pressure is exerted on a nerve root. Pain is variable and its assessment and nursing management must be individualized.

Assessment of Pain

- What was the patient doing before he complained of pain?
- Is his body in proper alignment?
- Is there pressure from traction, bed linen, a cast, or other appliances?
- Is he overly tired from lack of sleep, exciting stimuli, or too much activity?
- Can he localize the pain?
- How does he describe it?
- What was the manner of onset?
- Is there radiation of pain? If so, in what direction does it occur?
- Is there pain in any other part of the body?
- What is the character of the pain (sharp, dull, boring, shooting, throbbing, cramping)?
- Is it constant?
- What relieves it?
- What makes it worse?

Management. Because orthopedic conditions require long periods of treatment, the management of the patient with pain is important. Regardless of the cause, the presence of pain is exhausting. If the pain is prolonged, the patient may become self-centered and dependent. Whatever the cause and however intense the pain, successful management depends on obtaining the patient's cooperation and involving him in his rehabilitation program.

The nurse should observe the patient carefully to evaluate the effect of any physical, emotional, and social factors that may be present. Since sharp or sudden movements are painful, painful parts of the body should be supported and moved slowly and with a steady motion. When possible a turning sheet should be used. Care should be exercised not to bump the bed, as this greatly increases discomfort. Provision is to be made to allow the patient regular periods of rest.

Heat or cold may be beneficial in relieving muscle spasm and joint and bone pain. Cold applications, especially in inflammatory conditions, may give comfort. Analgesics are given when necessary, but symptoms of physical or psychological tolerance should be watched for and evaluated. Muscle relaxant drugs may or may not be effective.

Since pain always is worse at night, sedatives, soporifics, and ataractic drugs may prove helpful. Of course, the administration of backrubs and warm drinks, and the presence of a sympathetic, understanding nurse are all adjunctive measures in the management of pain. (See Chapter 14 for the nursing management of the patient with pain.)

Contracture Deformities

Contracture deformities are caused by limitation of motion and disuse. Pain and muscle spasm produce limitation of motion. Inflammation also limits the motion of a joint and causes the formation of fibrous tissue that in turn may produce fibrous or bony ankylosis (abnormal joint rigidity).

Any weight-bearing joint that has its normal motion restricted for a prolonged period loses motion.

Prolonged immobility in other than a neutral position affects the resting length of a muscle. A patient may easily develop a flexion deformity if his extremities are placed in nonfunctional positions. The patient is unable to extend his extremities, and thus crippling flexion deformities result.

Nursing Assessment. It is the aim of orthopedic nursing to prevent contracture deformities and to maintain as much function as possible. The following are part of the nursing assessment:

- When was the deformity noted?
- Was the onset accompanied by injury?
- Is the deformity increasing? Decreasing?
- Is there neurological loss (sensory or motor deficit)?
- Is there hypoesthesia, paresthesia, hyperesthesia?
- Is there weakness, stiffness, difficulty in walking?
- Is there paralysis? Time and mode of onset?
- Are there any disturbances in control of bladder and bowel?

Positioning. To prevent muscle contractures and loss of joint function, the patient must be positioned in accordance with correct principles of body alignment. The mattress should be firm or placed on a bedboard. The bed should be flat, unless otherwise ordered. To keep the patient in a semi-upright position for prolonged periods of time is highly undesirable; this position promotes flexion deformities of the hip. If possible, the patient should be placed in a prone position several times daily. The nurse should exercise ingenuity in the use of supportive devices, such as pillows and sandbags.

Muscle Exercises. If a patient becomes inactive as a result of trauma, infection, paralysis, or any other cause, the musculature loses strength, joint mobility becomes restricted, and deformities are likely to ensue. To avoid these complications the physician prescribes therapeutic exercises that may be performed under the guidance and with the assistance of the physical therapist or the nurse. The nature and the objectives of the exercise program are dictated by the patient's disease and his general condition. In general, if a joint is injured, it should be rested and the musculature moved; an injured muscle should be rested, but the accompanying joint should be moved.

Exercises, properly performed, help (1) to maintain or to improve muscle strength, (2) to maintain or to restore optimal joint function, (3) to prevent deformities, (4) to stimulate circulation, and (5) to build endurance. (See pages 182-184.)

BIBLIOGRAPHY

BOOKS

Aegerter, E. E., and Kirkpatrick, J. A., Jr.: Orthopedic Diseases. Philadelphia, W. B. Saunders, 1975.

Farrell, J.: Illustrated Guide to Orthopedic Nursing. Philadelphia, J. B. Lippincott, 1977.

Larson, C. B., and Gould, M.: Orthopedic Nursing. 9th ed. St. Louis, C. V. Mosby, 1978.

Turek, S. L.: Orthopaedics. Principles and Their Application, 3rd ed. Philadelphia, J. B. Lippincott, 1977.

ARTICLES

Buck, B. I. (ed.): Symposium on orthopedic nursing. Nurs. Clin. N. Am., *11*:639-730, Dec. 1976.

Greenfield, L. D., and Bennett, L. R.: Bone scanning. Am. Fam. Phys., *11*:84-89, Mar. 1975.

Janecki, C. J., Jr., Hill, D. H., and Eubanks, R. G.: Arthroscopy of the knee. Am. Fam. Phys., *17*:109-116, Mar. 1978.

AGENCIES

Governmental

National Institute of Arthritis, Metabolism and Digestive Diseases, National Institutes of Health, Bethesda, Md. 20205

Voluntary

American Physical Therapy Association, 1156 15th St., N.W., Washington, D.C. 20005

American Podiatry Association, 20 Chevy Chase Circle, N.W., Washington, D.C. 20015

National Easter Seal Society for Crippled Children and Adults, 2023 W. Ogden Ave., Chicago, Ill. 60612

(See also Rehabilitation Agencies, Chapter 12)

57

MANAGEMENT OF PATIENTS WITH MUSCULOSKELETAL DYSFUNCTION

SURGICAL MANAGEMENT

Preoperative Preparation

In general, the principles of preoperative care are the same as those that apply to the care of any surgical patient (see Chapter 17). Only the differences are stressed here.

PSYCHOLOGICAL SUPPORT. Most patients with acute musculoskeletal problems have pain and anxiety, experiencing a curious mixture of fear and anticipation before surgery. If an individual has been handicapped and dependent for most of his life, he faces reconstructive surgery with added concern. Some patients have faced repeated operations, so that patience and hope are almost gone. These are the people who need much help from an understanding nurse. One way to allay the patient's fear and to prepare him for the surgical experience is to inform him about the procedure and what to expect in the postoperative period. When possible he is instructed during the preoperative period about the postoperative exercises, the presence of traction or a cast and the use of crutches or ambulatory aids. If he is to be immobilized after surgery, he should practice using the bedpan and urinal in a recumbent position before surgery.

PHYSICAL CARE. Whatever the method used in preparing the patient's skin for surgery, the principles remain the same. The procedure usually is more painstaking because of the difficulty in controlling infection in the bone, should that occur. A meticulous nontraumatizing cleansing of the skin with germicidal soap and water is done the day before surgery and is repeated at the time of surgery.

It is known that the number of bacteria on the skin can be reduced by daily washing with a germicidal soap. If the operation is an elective one, the orthopedist may advise the patient to use a germicidal soap for skin cleansing for a period of time before hospital admission.

Permanent disability can result should infection occur within a bone or a joint. In no instance should one rely on the antibiotics to control infection and thereby justify slipshod preoperative preparation.

Adequate hydration is always an essential objective in orthopedic patients, particularly those immobilized for a long period of time. This prevents the occurrence of stones, infection, and kidney complications. Notice should be taken of urinary output.

It should be determined if the patient has had previous therapy with corticosteroids the year prior to surgery, especially the person with rheumatoid arthritis. Steroid therapy, whether current or past, may adversely affect his response to anesthesia. The prescribed dose of steroid should be given preoperatively to cover the anticipated stress of surgery.

Postoperative Care

Patients who have bone and joint surgery experience real *pain*. Many times, the person who has undergone surgery to correct a foot condition is much more uncomfortable than one who has had extensive abdominal surgery. Narcotics and other pain-relieving measures are given, taking into consideration the type of surgery and the size and age of the patient. However, in the long-term patient it is well to remember that habit-forming possibilities may pose a considerable problem. After surgery the extremity is elevated. Icecaps may be applied around the operative site intermittently. Even though a patient has had an orthopedic operation, pain may not result from the wound and the operative trauma. Swelling frequently follows, and when it occurs under tight bandages or casts, there may be interference with the blood supply, which also produces excruciating pain. This type of pain may be suspected when there is blueness and swelling beyond the limits of the cast, and it may be relieved by releasing the pressure (cutting the cast or bandages).

Another type of pain occurs in orthopedic patients when there is prolonged pressure over bony prominences such as areas of the heel, the head of the fibula on the lateral side of the leg just below the knee, and the tuberosity of the tibia. Even though they have been well padded before the cast has been applied, these areas eventually may become painful. The pain is characteristically of a burning type. It is wise not to treat this with narcotics but to call it to the attention of the surgeon, who may wish to cut away areas of the cast to relieve the pressure.

In major orthopedic surgery, *shock* may be a problem, especially since orthopedic wounds have a tendency to ooze and bleed more than other surgical wounds. As a result, the nurse must be on the alert for the symptoms of shock. A rising pulse rate or slowly falling blood pressure indicates persistent bleeding or the development of a state of shock. Changes in the respiratory rate or in the patient's color indicate obstruction of respiratory exchange, and pulmonary or cardiac complications. Fat embolus (page 1299) and thrombophlebitis (page 635) are other orthopedic complications.

Bone does not mend as rapidly as soft tissues. Therefore, even though the skin incision is well-healed, bony structures underneath still need time to repair. This is especially important to remember in surgery of the lower extremities, for in addition to normal movement, bone must be able to bear weight in ambulation.

Other complications that may occur are similar to those of general surgical patients. They are abdominal distention, wound infection, and pulmonary and circulatory problems. In addition, elderly men usually have some degree of prostatism and may have difficulty in voiding. Thus it is important to watch the urinary output.

The patient is placed on a normal diet as soon as possible. However, large amounts of milk should not be given to orthopedic patients who are on bed rest, since this only adds to the calcium pool in the body and requires that more calcium be excreted by the kidneys which favors formation of urinary calculi.

Orthopedic operations may require prolonged periods in bed. Hence the development of pressure sores are a constant threat. Turning, washing, drying, and massaging the skin frequently are necessary to avoid this complication. Plasma and vitamins are given as necessary to prevent hypoproteinemia and avitaminosis, conditions which make pressure sores resistant to treatment. Vitamin C is given to promote tissue integrity.

Rehabilitation

An important nursing principle in the management of orthopedic patients is to *mobilize the patient*. Prolonged immobility leads to loss of muscle bulk, decreased exercise tolerance, dimunition in blood flow, loss of calcium, changes in protein metabolism and osteoporosis of bone. Exercise is encouraged of all unaffected parts and the patient is instructed to move in bed. When encouraging the patient to help himself, be sure he is taught the proper way. The physical therapist working with the physician and the nurse can guide the patient in the proper use of his muscles and joints. Emphasis is placed on activities of daily living so that he will be able to perform those functions which allow him independence.

When he goes home, the patient should have explicit instructions that he understands, indicating those activities which he may and may not perform. It is not enough to bid him "good-bye, and take it easy." The patient must know any untoward signs and symptoms that should be reported to his physician. He must be aware of the importance of follow-up visits. If he has any difficulties, he ought to know where and how to get help. The nurse has a major part of the responsibility for educating the patient before he leaves the hospital. (See Chapter 12, Principles of Rehabilitation.)

MANAGEMENT OF THE PATIENT IN A CAST

Casts

A *cast* is an immobilizing device, made of layers of plaster bandages, fiberglass or a thermolabile plastic material. The purposes of a cast are to immobilize and hold bone fragments in reduction, to apply uniform compression of soft tissues, to permit early mobilization, to improve function by stabilizing a joint, and to correct and prevent deformities.

Types of Casts. The following casts are commonly used in fracture immobilization (Fig. 57-1):

Short-arm cast—extends from below the elbow to the proximal palmar crease

Gauntlet cast—extends from below the elbow to the proximal palmar crease, including the thumb (thumb spica)

Long-arm cast—extends from the upper level of the axillary fold to the proximal palmar crease; the elbow usually is immobilized at right angle

Short-leg cast—extends from below the knee to the base of the toes

Long-leg cast—extends from the junction of the upper and middle third of the thigh to the base of the toes; the foot is at a right angle in a neutral position

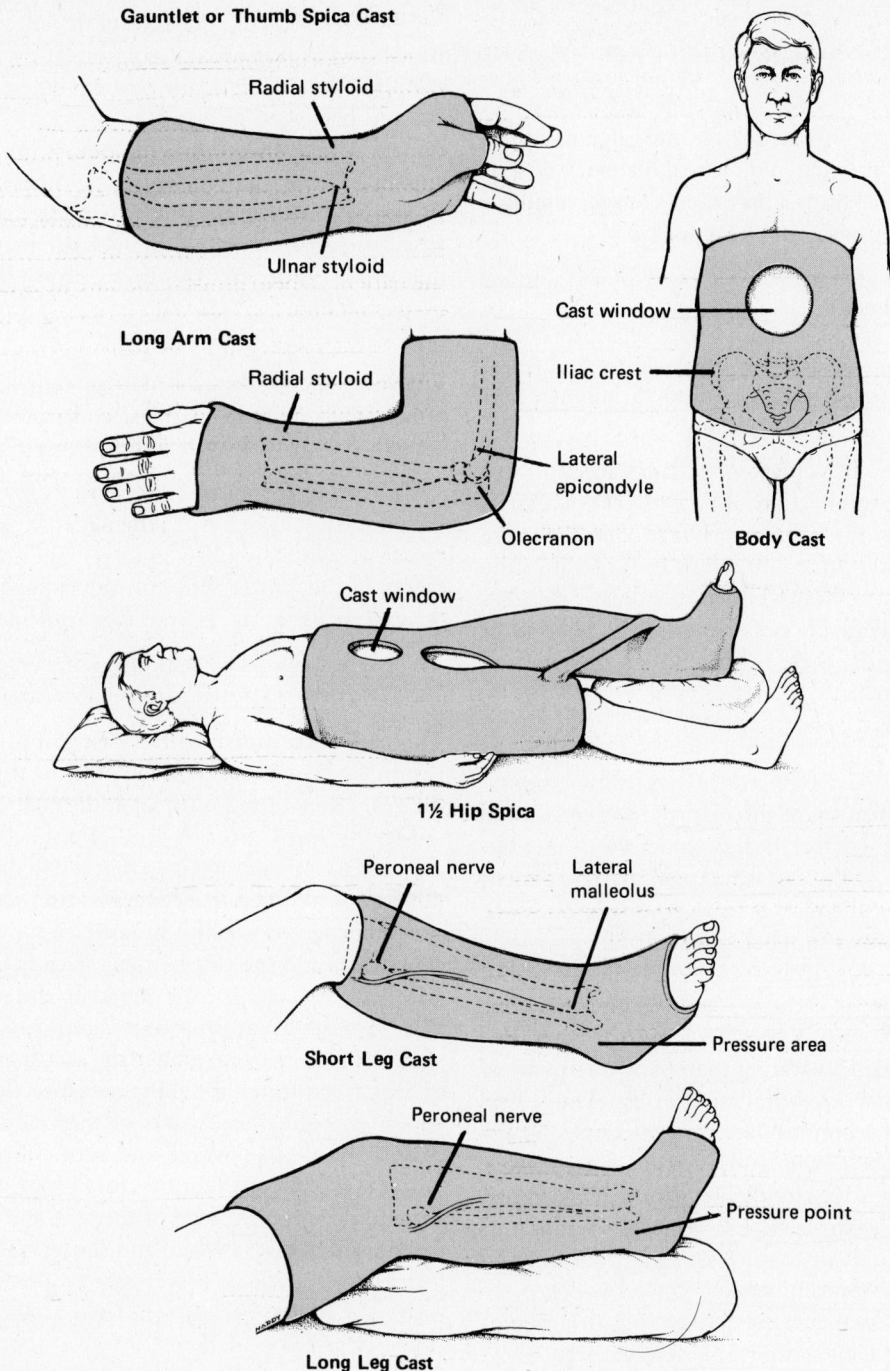

Gauntlet or Thumb Spica Cast

Radial styloid

Ulnar styloid

Long Arm Cast

Radial styloid

Lateral epicondyle

Olecranon

Cast window

Iliac crest

Body Cast

Cast window

1½ Hip Spica

Peroneal nerve

Lateral malleolus

Pressure area

Short Leg Cast

Peroneal nerve

Pressure point

Long Leg Cast

Figure 57-1. Pressure areas in different types of casts.

Walking cast —a short- or long-leg cast with a walking device

Spica or body cast —incorporates the trunk and an extremity

    a. *Shoulder spica cast* —a body jacket that encloses the trunk and the shoulder and elbow

    b. *Hip spica cast* —encloses the trunk and a lower extremity; may be a single or double hip spica cast

Cast Preparation

Plaster of paris is the most common form of fracture immobilization. Plaster of paris bandages consist of rolls of crinoline impregnated with a solid crystalline material known as gypsum or calcium sulfate dihydrate. Gypsum is reduced to a powder to break up the crystals and then subjected to intense heat to drive off the water in the crystal. The product of this action is plaster of paris.

$$\text{2CaSO}_4 \cdot \text{2H}_2\text{O} \xrightarrow{\Delta} \text{(CaSO}_4)_2 \cdot \text{H}_2\text{O} + \text{3H}_2\text{O}\uparrow$$
(gypsum)   (plaster of paris)

When water is added to the plaster, the calcium sulfate dihydrate absorbs the water and recrystallizes or "sets" as calcium sulfate or gypsum. This process of recrystallization gives off heat (exothermic reaction).

- Because a cast gives off heat in the process of drying, a freshly applied cast should not be placed on a pillow or mattress or covered with a blanket. Such action insulates the cast from air and causes a sharp temperature rise that could give the patient a burn. Most casts begin to cool 5 to 15 minutes after application.

Figure 57-2 shows how plaster bandages are saturated with water prior to application. A clean bucket is essential, since plaster residue (which may have collected at the bottom of the bucket during previous use) can alter the plaster's setting times. Plaster knives, benders and shears should be readily available because once the process of applying a cast begins, there is little time to lose before the critical setting period.

Cast Application

Prior to the application of the cast, the patient should be informed that he will feel the heat under the plaster but that the application of the cast is not painful. The patient is draped to prevent the plaster from smearing on those parts of the body that are not being casted. The part to be casted is cleansed with soap and water and dried. Alcohol may be applied for its drying action. Some surgeons spray the extremity with a nonallergenic adhesive. Before the cast is applied a padding material, usually made of cotton or cellulose (Webril, Sof-Rol, Stockinet) that can be stretched to accommodate various shapes, is applied to the area to be casted. Padding is used to prevent pressure areas, minimize circulatory problems, and pad the sharp margins of the cast. Extra pieces of padding, such as orthopedic felt or foam plastic padding may be placed over any bony prominences.

Plaster of paris is available in bandage rolls of different widths. Three speeds of setting time are available: extra fast setting (2 to 4 minutes), fast setting (5 to 6 minutes), and slow setting (10 to 18 minutes).

The plaster bandage is applied evenly on the extremity, turn upon turn, with each turn overlapping the preceding turn by one-half the width of the roll. The motion is continuous, without pause, while the bandage is maintained in constant contact with the surface of the extremity. The turns or layers of the bandage are smoothed and rubbed as the cast is applied to form a smooth, solid and well-contoured cast. Plaster splints may be used to reinforce places where strain will take place (i.e., back of the knee) to increase the strength of the cast.

Plaster Splints. Plaster splints may be used when rigid immobilization is not required or when a significant amount of swelling is anticipated. These splints are pre-cut and packaged in a variety of sizes. The extremity is wrapped with sheet wadding before the plaster splint is applied. The plaster reaches its maximal temperature 5 to 15 minutes after application; therefore, the splint is usually not overwrapped with an elastic bandage until after this time. Figure 57-3A shows how plaster splints are prepared. Figure 57-3D shows a posterior splint in place on an extremity.

- When the splint is handled, the fingers of the hand supporting the splint should be extended under the splint in order to avoid denting or distorting the cast while it is still "green."

Trimming the Cast. As soon as the cast is applied, the plaster is cleaned from the patient's skin with a damp towel. If plaster is allowed to remain on the skin, small pieces of the plaster will crumble and slide down under the cast, causing the patient a great deal of discomfort.

- Any complaints by the patient of painful areas under the plaster should be reported and investigated.

The cast is trimmed with a cast knife, after which the padding or stockinet is folded over the top and bottom of the cast and secured with an additional roll of plaster.

Drying the Cast. A freshly applied cast should be exposed to circulating air so that it will dry. A cast should not be covered because covers restrict the escape of heat and moisture, especially in large casts. As the moisture evaporates and the cast hardens, heat is generated. A fan will help circulate the air and keep the patient comfortable. If a cast dryer is used, it is important to realize that skin burns may occur under the cast from overexposure to heat even though the skin is not directly exposed. If the patient is cold, those parts of the body not encased in plaster should be covered and kept warm.

It takes up to 48 hours for a cast to become dry, depending upon the size of the cast and the moisture in the air; a dry cast is white and shiny, resonant and odorless as well as firm; a wet cast is gray and dull in appearance, dull to percussion, feels damp and has a musty odor.

- After a cast has cooled and starts to harden, the arm or leg in the cast is elevated above the level of the heart to reduce swelling. The cast should not be allowed to rest on hard surfaces or sharp edges that can cause a dent in the cast and subsequent pressure sores.

Other Casting Systems. A newer type of casting system (Lightcast II*) consists of an open weave, fiberglass tape impregnated with a photosensitive resin which becomes rigid when exposed to a special lamp. The casting tape is applied in the usual manner and then is

*Merck and Co., Inc.

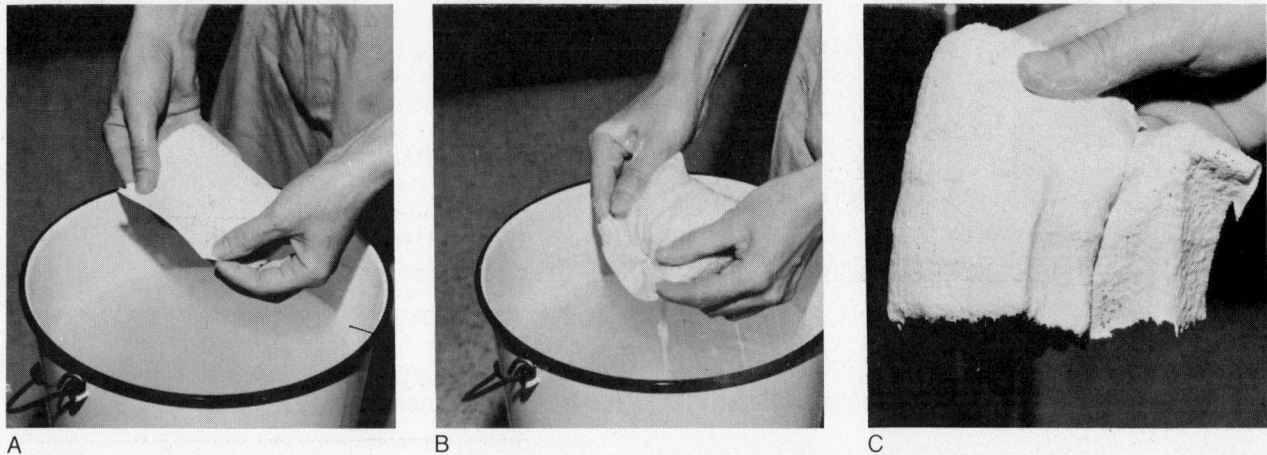

A   B   C

Figure 57-2.   Preparing plaster of paris bandages. Plaster may come in a plastic bag encasement. This can be used as the "bucket" for the plaster by filling the bag with water and standing it on end until the plaster is saturated. Other forms of plaster bandages are wrapped in individual rolls. (*A*) Unwind the end of the bandage for a few inches so it will be easily grasped when the bandage is wet. Some manufacturers indicate the end of the plaster with a colored paper tab. Submerge the plaster *vertically* in water at room temperature (70-75° F.) until it ceases to yield bubbles of air. Do not disturb the bandage while it is soaking in the water. (*B*) Expel the excess water by gently squeezing the ends with the palms of the hands. The end "pinch" prevents the center of the wet roll from falling out during application. (*C*) Pass the plaster bandage so that the starting end is easily grasped.

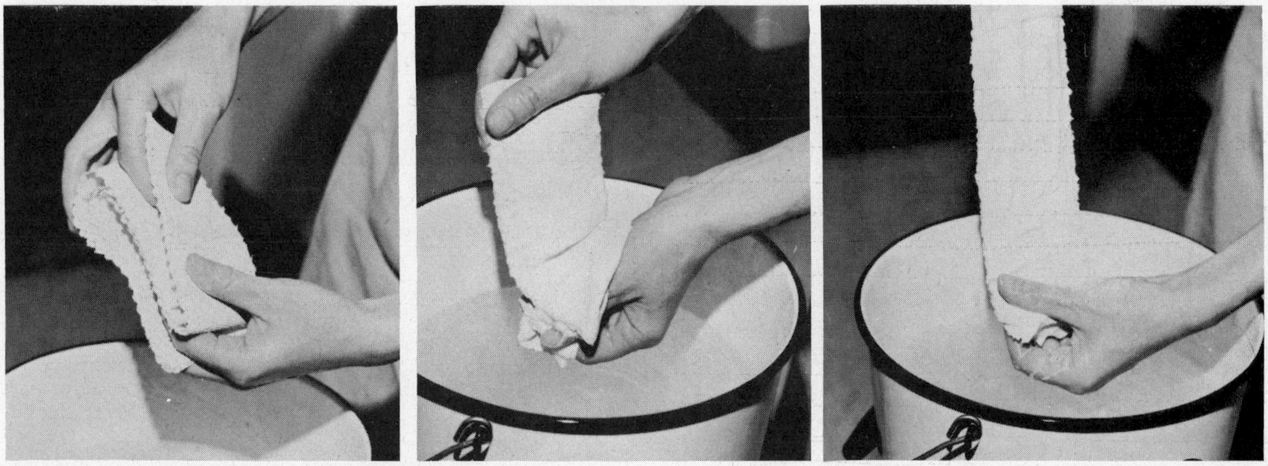

A   B   C

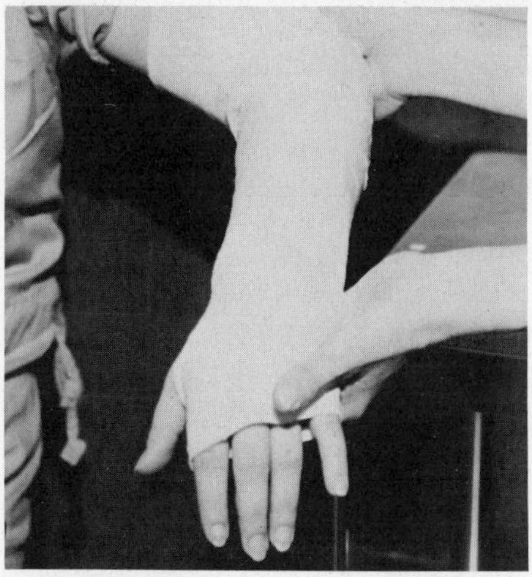

D

Figure 57-3.   Preparing plaster splints. *A.* Splints are prepared by loosely fanfolding the plaster bandage in the hand before they are dipped. *B.* Dip the splints in a vertical position in warm water. *C.* Excess water is removed by rubbing the splint carefully on the side of the bucket or by passing it between the index and the middle finger in a "squeeze" action to remove excess water. *D.* Posterior splint in place.

exposed to the special lamp for 3 minutes, after which the cast becomes functional. It takes 5 to 10 minutes for the cast to harden completely. The finished cast is approximately one-half to one-third the weight of a plaster cast. The use of this type of cast permits immediate weight bearing, facilitates ambulation and exercise and, with medical permission, allows the patient to return to near normal levels of functioning. The cast is porous and supposedly will not deteriorate if wet, thus allowing the patient to shower or bathe. However, if the cast is wet too frequently or for a prolonged period, skin maceration may occur.

Immediate Cast Care Following Application

The main concern following the application of a cast is to avoid complications. Experience has taught that any complaint of discomfort must not go unheeded. Two types of complications occur: *constriction of circulation* and/or *pressure on tissues and bony parts.*

Constriction of Circulation. Trauma or surgery affecting an extremity will produce swelling due to hemorrhage and edema. Unrelieved swelling may result in vascular insufficiency, thereby reducing or obliterating the blood supply to an extremity. If circulation is restricted for too long a period, gangrenous necrosis may occur. Signs of circulatory impairment are noted by assessing the toes and fingers of a leg or arm that has recently been placed in a cast. The toes and fingers should be pink in color, warm to the touch and easily moved (wiggled) if the patient is requested to do so. The blanch test may be carried out as another means of assessing circulatory sufficiency. The nail beds and pulp of fingers/toes are pressed lightly and then released to check how quickly color returns, thereby indicating return of capillary action. A blue tinge to the toes or fingers suggests venous obstruction, while white and cold fingers or toes suggest arterial obstruction. The temperature of the injured extremity is compared with the uninjured one as are the pulses. Inability to move the fingers or toes, pain on extension of the hand or foot, and coldness of an extremity are indicative of ischemia. If there is swelling, the cast will seem tight.

- Unrelieved pain, swelling, blanching or discoloration, tingling, numbness, inability to move fingers and toes, or any temperature change must be reported immediately to avoid possible paralysis and necrosis.

Nursing Intervention for Cast Constriction and Pressure. If the patient continues to have pain, the cast may be exerting pressure on a nerve, blood vessel, or bony prominence.

- If constriction of circulation is suspected, the cast may be bivalved to relieve pressure.

The procedure for bivalving a cast is as follows:
1. Cut the cast into two halves.

2. Cut the underlying padding since blood-soaked padding may shrink and constrict the circulation. (The anterior and posterior parts of the cast may be held together with an elastic compression bandage.)
3. Then spread the cast sufficiently to relieve constriction.
4. After the cast is bivalved elevate the extremity until the circulation is restored and swelling diminishes.

Bivalving a cast does not disturb the alignment of the fracture.

Another method of checking the cause for discomfort or viewing a surgical wound is to cut a *window* in the cast. After the window is opened, a soft plastic foam pad is inserted and the "window" is replaced with tape to prevent the skin from swelling through the window and forming pressure areas around the margins of the window.

Pressure on Tissues or Bony Parts. Any cast that presses on tissues may cause necrosis (tissue death) pressure sores and nerve palsies or paralysis, such as may occur when a leg cast damages the peroneal nerve. Severe initial pain over bony prominences is a warning symptom of an impending pressure sore. If the pain then disappears, it might very well mean that ulceration has occurred. Those sites most susceptible to pressure on the lower extremity are the heel, malleoli, dorsum of the foot, the head of the fibula, and the anterior surface of the patella. On the upper extremity, the main pressure sites are located at the medial epicondyl of the humerus and the ulnar styloid. (Fig. 57-1)

- If the patient complains of pain, analgesics should not be given until the cause of the pain is determined. The first step in determining the cause is to ask the patient to localize the exact site of the pain.

Body or Hip Spica Cast

When a large cast, such as a body or hip spica cast, is applied, the bed is prepared before the patient is received. A board under the mattress provides the necessary firmness to the bed. The curves of the cast can be supported with small plastic-covered flexible pillows to prevent the cast from cracking while it is drying. Three pillows placed crosswise on the bed will suffice for the body cast; for a hip spica, one pillow placed crosswise at the waist and two pillows placed lengthwise for the affected leg are necessary. If both legs are involved, two additional pillows are necessary. It is important that the pillows be next to each other, because any spaces in between will allow the damp cast to sag, become weak, and possibly break. It is also important to see that a pillow is not placed under the head and shoulders (of a patient in body cast) while the cast is drying since this causes pressure on the chest.

When a patient is moved from side to side in a large cast, at least three people are necessary. Only the palms of the hands are used to lift the cast; fingers make indentations in soft plaster. Support should be given to the entire cast and most particularly at such vulnerable points as the hip and the knee. When the head of the bed is elevated or when the patient is on the bedpan, the cast is to be kept level by elevating the lumbar sacral area with a small pillow.

Cast Syndrome. One important complication that can develop from a body cast is *cast syndrome* (acute obstruction of the duodenum).

- The primary symptom of cast syndrome is *nausea*. Respiration also may be compromised by pressure on the diaphragm.
- Should cast syndrome occur, the patient is placed in a prone position to relieve pressure symptoms. It may be necessary to remove the cast entirely.

Surgical intervention may be required when conservative measures (nasogastric suction, intravenous fluid replacement) fail to relieve duodenal obstruction. It is important to realize that the patient receives first consideration; the cast is secondary in importance.

Turning the Patient in a Spica Cast

The patient is moved to the side of the bed with a steady, even pulling motion. Pillows are placed along the other side of the bed; one for the chest and two (lengthwise) for the legs. Turning is done as follows:

1. Instruct the patient to place his arms at his sides or above his head, whichever is most comfortable.
2. One nurse stands at the other side of bed to reach out and support the patient's shoulders.
3. A second nurse supports the affected leg, while the third nurse supports the patient's back as he is turned.
4. The patient is turned *as a unit* toward the free leg or toward the unoperated side if both legs are in plaster.
5. The cross bar of the spica cast must not be grasped to move the patient. (The purpose of the bar is to strengthen the cast.)
6. The patient's body should not be twisted.

The patient is turned to a prone position twice daily in order to provide postural drainage of the bronchial tree and relieve pressure on the back. A small pillow under the abdomen will be an added comfort measure. Placing a pillow lengthwise under the dorsum of the feet will prevent the toes from being forced into the mattress. Allowing the toes to hang over the edge of the mattress is a welcome change.

Skin and Hygiene Care. The skin around the edges of the cast must be inspected frequently for signs of irritation. The area under the cast can be inspected by pulling the skin taut and using a flashlight. Accessible skin should be massaged with an emollient.

Pressure areas may develop over any bony prominence. A common site of pressure from a large cast is the buttocks. When the patient is turned on his abdomen, the exposed skin can be washed carefully and massaged. The rough edges of the cast can be padded by pulling the inside stockinette over the edge of the cast and fixing it with plaster to the outside. This will eliminate cast crumbs and make the edge smooth. Reaching up under the cast edges as far as possible with the fingers may help to remove plaster crumbs and to massage the skin area.

A patient in a body cast will appreciate a "back scratcher," consisting of a length of flannel that is 2.5 cm. (1 inch) wide and 10 cm. (4 inches) longer than the cast and is inserted inside the back of the cast by a long alligator forceps. (A thoughtful nurse might suggest that this type of flannel strip be put in place before the cast is applied.) By holding each end of the flannel, it is possible to give the patient a gentle back rub. At no time should the patient be allowed to insert coat hangers or other objects to "scratch" under the cast.

The area of the cast around the perineum needs to be protected from excretions. If the opening in the cast is inadequate for hygienic care, the nurse should report this. When the cast is dry, the perineum is covered with a towel and the perineal area of the cast sprayed with aerosol plastic spray. Strips of thin polyethylene sheeting 10 cm. (4 inches) long may be tucked under the cast and fastened to the exterior, allowing for adequate coverage of the outside of the cast. These may be replaced as necessary.

Shoulder Spica Cast. The shoulder spica cast is applied to the upper torso and envelops a part or all of an arm, holding it in a position of abduction. Such a cast is used for humeral neck fractures. The pressure areas of concern in this cast may involve the median epicondyl

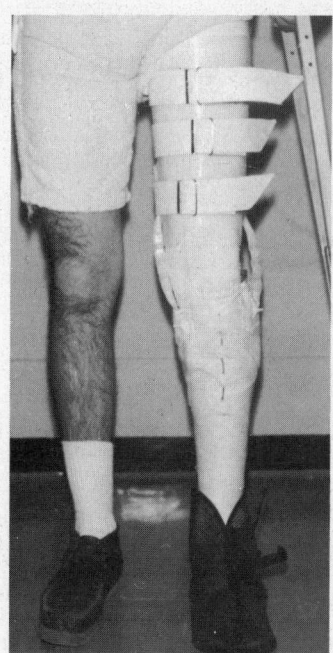

Figure 57-4. Cast-brace. A cast-brace provides circumferential support to a segment of a fractured extremity while allowing mobility of nearby joints.

and the adjacent ulnar nerve. To avoid this complication, the patient is encouraged to exercise his fingers and thumb frequently.

The Cast-Brace

A *cast-brace* (fracture orthosis) consists of two separate weight-bearing casts: a patellar weight-bearing cast on the lower leg and an ischial weight-bearing cast on the thigh. The two are joined at the knee by a pair of gliding-action hinges (Fig. 57-4). The foot and ankle may be included in the cast and a walking heel or boot applied. Or the foot and ankle joint may be freed by a removable shoe attached to the cast by a brace joint. Some cast braces are constructed with hinges at the hip, elbow, wrist and ankle.

Cast bracing is based on the concept that weight-bearing is always physiologic and will promote the formation of bone and contain fluid within a tight compartment. It is widely used in the treatment of fractures of the distal femur and upper tibia to maintain motion at the knee and to allow early ambulation with partial weight-bearing on the fracture. Early weight-bearing promotes healing by adding pressure to the fracture site, improving circulation by mobilizing muscles and lessening edema in the capsules and joint structures. Thus, the patient can be discharged from the hospital at an earlier date.

Nursing Assessment. Usually the patient is permitted to get up 24 to 48 hours after the cast-brace is applied. A 3-point crutch gait is used so that normal gait and rhythm are established. The patient is closely monitored to detect any signs of angular deformity which may occur during the first few weeks of ambulation. The skin is assessed for breakdown and circulatory problems, and the exposed area of the knee assessed for excessive swelling. Any complaints of numbness are duly noted. Since the cast may extend to the groin, measures should be taken to protect this area of the cast from becoming soiled with urine and feces. To promote venous return, the cast-brace is elevated when the patient is not walking. It is changed at intervals as required.

Management After the Cast Dries

Leg Cast. After the leg cast is applied, the therapeutic objective is to prevent or lessen swelling by elevating the extremity above the level of the heart and applying ice bags to each side of the cast. After the patient begins to ambulate, he should be encouraged to elevate the cast when he is seated. Several times during the day, he should lie down because a sitting position does not promote complete drainage. If the skin has become irritated at the cast edges, moleskin padding may be used.

Excessive pressure is checked by examining the toes and foot for blanching or cyanosis or swelling and by testing the patient's ability to move his toes. Numbness, tingling, burning, or a cold sensation may be due to

peroneal nerve injury from pressure at the head of the fibula.

- Injury to the peroneal nerve as a result of pressure is a common cause of footdrop.

Arm Cast. To diminish and control swelling when the patient is lying down, the arm is elevated, with each joint positioned higher than the preceding joint (e.g., elbow higher than the shoulder, hand higher than the elbow). When the patient becomes ambulatory, a sling may be used. However, a sling keeps the arm in a dependent position. For adequate drainage, the limb should be higher than the level of the heart. Thus the patient should be encouraged to remove the arm from the sling frequently and to extend it above his head.

Circulatory disturbances in the hand may become apparent with signs of cyanosis, swelling, and an inability to move the fingers.

- One serious effect of circulatory constriction in an arm cast is *Volkmann's contracture,* in which contracture of the fingers and wrist occurs as the result of ischemia due to the obstruction of arterial flow to the forearm and hand. This serious complication can be prevented by nursing surveillance and proper care.

Exercising the Patient in a Cast. While the patient is in a cast he should be taught to tense or to contract his muscles without moving the joints. The patient may actually forget how to "will" a motion through the central nervous system pathways to the immobilized muscle. Therefore isometric muscle contractions (contracting the muscle without moving the part) may be carried out to prevent atrophy and maintain muscle strength.

- If the patient is in a leg cast, place your hand under the knee and instruct the patient to "push down." If the patient has an arm cast, instruct him to "make a fist."

Isometric muscle contractions should be done at least hourly while the patient is awake. He is taught to exercise his fingers and his toes frequently and actively.

Patient Education

After the Application of a Cast
1. Although it takes minutes for a cast to harden, it will take up to 48 hours or longer for the cast to dry.
2. Avoid covering the cast with bedding until it is dry.
3. Avoid resting the cast on hard surfaces or sharp edges which will dent the cast and cause pressure areas.
4. Keep the affected limb elevated above the heart.
5. Watch for these danger signs (for arm or leg cast): blueness or paleness of toenails or fingernails accompanied by pain and tightness, numbness, cold or tingling sensation.
   Elevate the affected limb above the heart and wiggle the toes or fingers. Call the physician if the condition persists.

When the Cast is Dry
1. Move about as normally as possible.
2. Do the prescribed exercises faithfully.

3. Do not cover a leg cast with plastic or rubber boots as this causes condensation and wetting of the cast. Avoid walking on wet floors or sidewalks. Wetness destroys the hardness of the cast.
4. Report to the physican if the cast breaks; do not attempt to fix it yourself.
5. To clean a cast:
   a. Remove surface soil with a damp cloth.
   b. Touch up stained areas with white shoe polish.
6. Do not attempt to scratch the skin under the cast with any foreign object; this may cause a break in the skin and result in the formation of a cast sore.

After Removal of a Cast
1. Cleanse the skin gently with bland soap and water. *Blot* dry.
2. Apply baby powder, cornstarch, or baby oil; avoid scratching the skin.

Removing a Cast. A cast may be removed with a cast cutter—an electric saw with a circular blade that oscillates through the plaster. Before the procedure the patient should be assured that the cast cutter will cause vibration but will not be painful. The usual method of cutting the cast is to bivalve it—i.e., cutting the cast in a longitudinal manner. On a lower extremity cast, the cutting line should be in front of the lateral malleolus and behind the medial malleolus.

The cutter is grasped as illustrated in Figure 57-5. The thumb is allowed to touch the plaster in order to serve as a depth gauge and to act as a guard in front of the blade. The thumb comes in contact with the cast as the saw blade cuts. The saw is pushed firmly and gently through the cast. A firm resistance will be felt as the blade cuts through the plaster which will "give" suddenly when the cut is completed, at which point the blade is immediately lifted up a degree (but not out of the cutting groove) and advanced 1.2 cm. (½ inch) in the direction of the cut. The cast is then cut by a series of alternating pressures and linear movements along the line of the cut. If the saw blade is left against the padding too long, the patient will feel a burning sensation on the skin from the rapidly oscillating blade. As a last step, the padding is cut by scissors.

Care of the Patient After the Cast is Removed. One of the most important things to remember when a cast has been removed is that the part or parts involved have been immobilized for a considerable period of time. When the support and protection of the cast have been removed, stresses and strains are placed on parts that have been at rest. The patient complains of pain and stiffness, often much different from the original injury, and he is depressed and discouraged, because the anticipated release from the cast has only added to his problems.

The responsibility of the nurse is to help the patient adjust to this new discomfort. This can be accomplished by supporting the part so that it is maintained in the same position as when in the cast. A small pillow can be used to

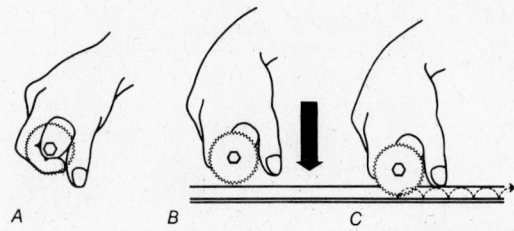

Figure 57-5. Operating a cast cutter. (Courtesy, Stryker Corporation)

support the knee, the lumbar spine, etc. The support is then gradually removed. When the extremity is moved, adequate support must be provided and the limb moved gently. After the cast has been removed, exercises are prescribed to redevelop and to increase strength. If the patient has been doing isometric muscle contractions, he will not have to relearn to contract his muscles and will progress more rapidly with his rehabilitation program.

Once the cast is removed, there will be a considerable amount of desquamated epithelium (dead skin) that may adhere to the underlying skin surface. The skin is washed carefully with detergent or germicidal soap, blotted dry, and some type of lanolin cream is applied. The patient should be cautioned against rubbing or scratching the skin, which could cause a break in the skin.

If a new cast is to be applied, the skin is washed and dried carefully. The skin and the underlying tissues must be handled carefully until normal function is gradually restored. Atrophy of the part may be noted but this disappears gradually with the return of muscle function. Should the patient go home with a cast, he must be instructed in methods of cast care (page 1284). Swelling after a cast is removed is common and is treated by elevating and supporting the tissues with elastic bandages or an elastic stocking.

MANAGEMENT OF THE PATIENT IN TRACTION

Traction is force applied in a longitudinal direction. It is used to reduce and immobilize a fracture, to treat muscle spasm, and to help regain normal length and alignment of an injured extremity. Traction may be applied directly to the skin (skin traction) or to the bone (skeletal traction).

Skin Traction

Skin traction is accomplished by a weight that pulls on tape, sponge rubber, or plastic materials that have been attached to the skin. Traction on the skin transmits traction to the musculoskeletal structures. However, only limited traction can be applied with skin traction. This type of traction is used as a temporary measure in adults—Buck's extension for hip fractures and Russell's

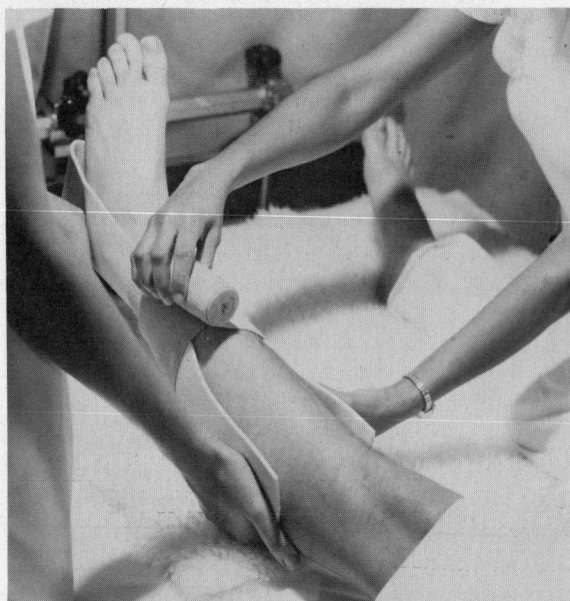

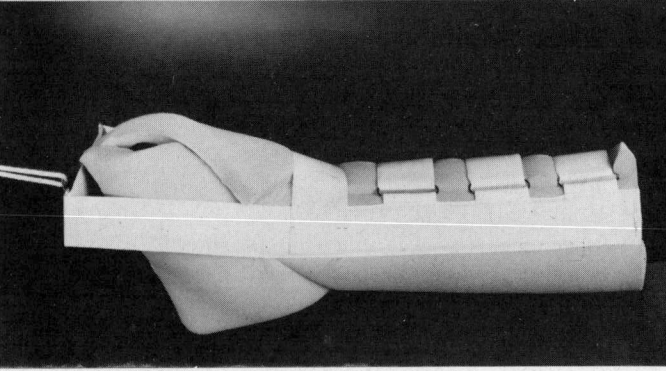

Figure 57-6. (*Left*) Applying elastic bandage for Buck's extension traction. (*Above*) Prepadded boot that may be used in Buck's extension. (Photo of boot courtesy of All Orthopedic Appliances)

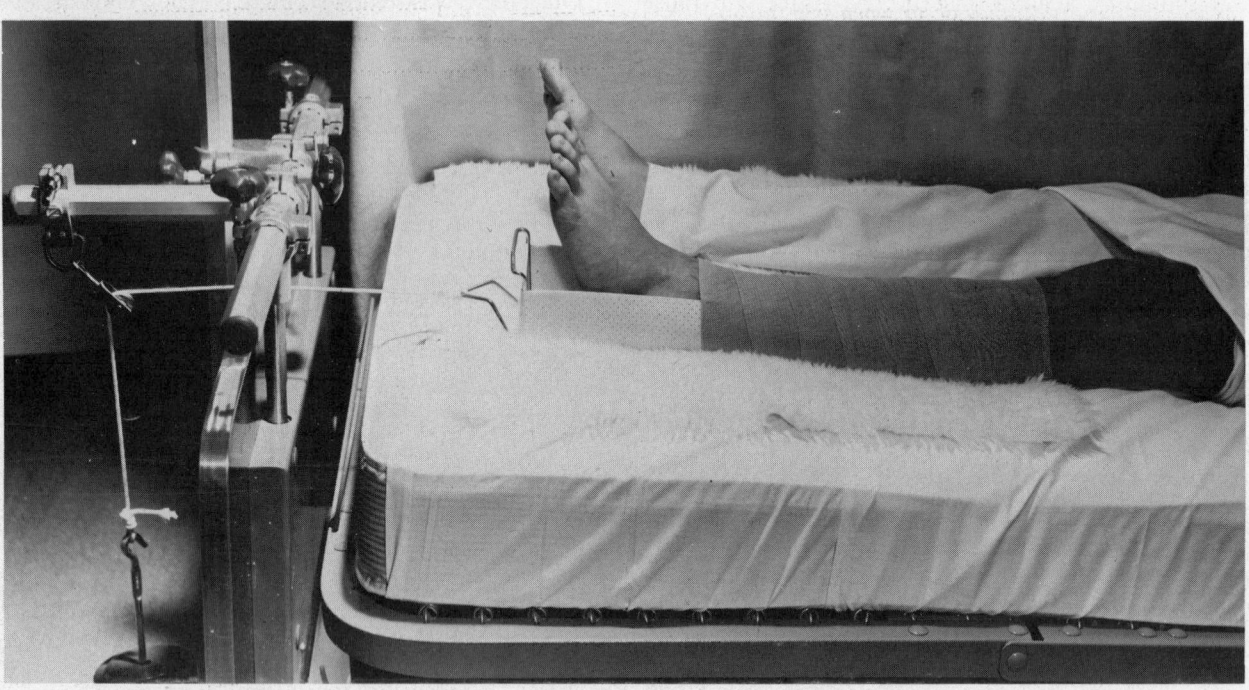

Figure 57-7. Lower extremity in Buck's extension traction.

traction for applying traction to the femoral shaft with the knee flexed.

Buck's extension (unilateral or bilateral) is a form of skin traction in which the pull is exerted in one plane when partial or temporary immobilization is desired (Figure 57-6). It is used following injuries to the hip while the patient is awaiting surgical fixation.

Before the traction is applied, the skin is inspected for abrasions and circulatory disturbances since the skin must be in healthy condition to tolerate the traction. The extremity should be clean and dry before the traction tape or bandage is applied so as to enable the tape to adhere to the skin. The malleoli and proximal fibula are padded with cast padding to prevent pressure sores and skin necrosis. Foam rubber padded straps are applied with the foam surface against the skin on each side of the affected leg. (Prepadded boots are frequently used, Figure 57-7.) When the leg is wrapped, a loop of tape about 10 to 15 cm. (4 to 6 inches) is extended beyond the sole of the foot. Then while one person elevates and supports the extremity under the patient's ankle and foot, another person wraps the elastic bandage circumferentially over the traction tape beginning at the ankle and wrapping up to the tibial tubercle. The elastic bandage helps the tape to adhere to the skin and prevents slipping. A spreader is applied to the distal end of the tape to prevent pressure along the side of the foot. A rope is attached to the spreader and passed over a pulley fastened to the end of the bed. Then a weight is attached to the rope. A sheepskin pad is placed under the leg to reduce the friction of the heel against the bed.

Nursing Assessment. Skin traction can irritate the skin and cause pressure on peripheral nerves. The circumferential wrappings around the skin tapes should not impair circulation, but must be firm enough to ensure that the tapes will remain in contact with the skin.

- To detect pressure points in skin traction, the area over the traction tapes should be palpated daily. The area over the Achilles tendon should be inspected several times daily since pressure in this region may occur when skin traction is applied to the leg. Care must be taken to avoid pressure on the peroneal nerve at the point at which it passes around the neck of the fibula just below the knee. Pressure at this point can cause footdrop.
- When skin traction is applied to the arm, the area around the elbow where the ulnar nerve is located should not be wrapped tightly.
- The wrappings applied around the leg should be removed daily and the skin inspected. During these checks, the foot is assessed for loss of sensation, weakness of the dorsiflexor muscles and inversion of the foot which may be caused by tight traction tape and pressure on the common peroneal nerve. Inspection should also be carried out if the patient complains of persistent itching or burning.

- Proper positioning must also be maintained to keep the leg in a neutral position. The patient should not turn from side to side to prevent bony fragments from moving against one another.

The chief limitation of skin traction is that no more than 2 to 3 kg. (4.5 to 7 pounds) of traction can be used on a part. Therefore, when prolonged or heavy traction weight is necessary, skeletal traction is used, not skin traction. See also page 1289 for additional nursing principles.

Skeletal Traction

Skeletal traction is traction applied directly to the bone. This method of traction is used most frequently in the treatment of fractures of the femur, the humerus, and the tibia. The traction is applied directly to the bones by the use of a metal pin or wire (Kirschner wire, Steinmann pin) inserted into or through a bone distal to the fracture. Usually the pin or wire is inserted through a small opening in the skin made under local anesthesia. The pin or wire is sterilized and inserted by a drill under aseptic conditions. Following insertion of the pins, the wound is covered with a small gauze square. A cork or adhesive is applied over the exposed sharp edges of the pin. Traction is applied by weights and pulleys as described for skin traction.

The Thomas splint with the Pearson attachment is usually used with skeletal traction in fractures of the femur (Figure 57-8). It may be used with skin traction and other balanced suspension apparatus. Because upward traction is required for these fractures, the patient is placed on a fracture bed. Figures 57-9 and 57-10 show various types of *suspension traction*.

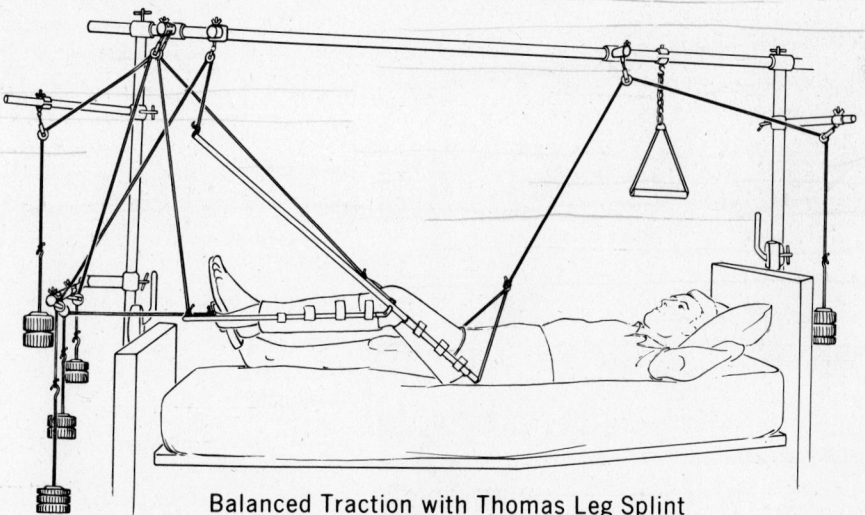

Balanced Traction with Thomas Leg Splint

Figure 57-8. Principles of balanced suspension traction. Vertical movement of the patient is permitted as long as longitudinal forces are maintained. Force means to push or pull. Force, as used in traction, means push or pull in a given direction. In the nursing management of the patient in traction one has to understand the direction in which the force is operating. Study the line drawing carefully. Notice that the force produced by the weights is changed in direction by the pulleys.

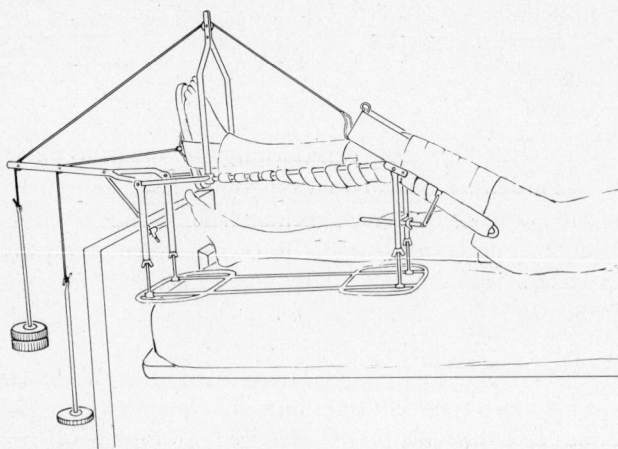

Figure 57-9. Unilateral leg traction using Bohler-Braun splint.

• One problem with skeletal traction is *infection*, which may develop in or around the pin tract. The site must be inspected daily for odor and signs of inflammation. Daily cleaning of the tract with sterile applicators and prescribed medication and ointment is necessary to clear the tract and pin of the slight drainage that always occurs. The drainage dries at the mouth of the tract and about the pin and forms a plug, setting up conditions for bacterial invasion of the tract and bone.

Inasmuch as fractures occur under varying circumstances and involve individuals of different ages, weights, and body builds, no two fractures are alike, and every fracture patient requires individualized treatment. By the same token, traction procedures may be modified in many ways to meet a variety of special requirements, as exemplified by the so-called balanced suspension traction, and running traction procedures. These pro-

cedures, and the special nursing implications involved with them, are outlined on page 1289. These basic nursing principles for traction procedures in general, apply equally to all other modified forms of traction.

Management

The importance of frequent inspection of the fracture dressing in the first 24 hours after application cannot be impressed too strongly. A bandage that appears sufficiently loose when applied may in a very few hours cause serious constriction which, if not relieved, may lead to gangrene of the extremity.

Dressings are applied in such a way as to leave the tips of the fingers and toes exposed. Any cyanosis, loss of temperature, tingling, or loss of sensation in these parts is a warning that the dressings are too tight. If the condition is caused by a single turn of the bandage, the turn may be divided with the scissors, but it is usually advisable to notify the surgeon. After the first 24 hours, the fracture dressing should be inspected at least 3 or 4 times daily. Evidences of constriction should be noted and pressure points checked. It is also important to ask the patient if there are any painful areas.

When traction is being used, the apparatus should be checked to see that the ropes are in the wheel groove of the pulleys, that the supporting apparatus is free of the pulleys, that the weights hang free, and that the patient

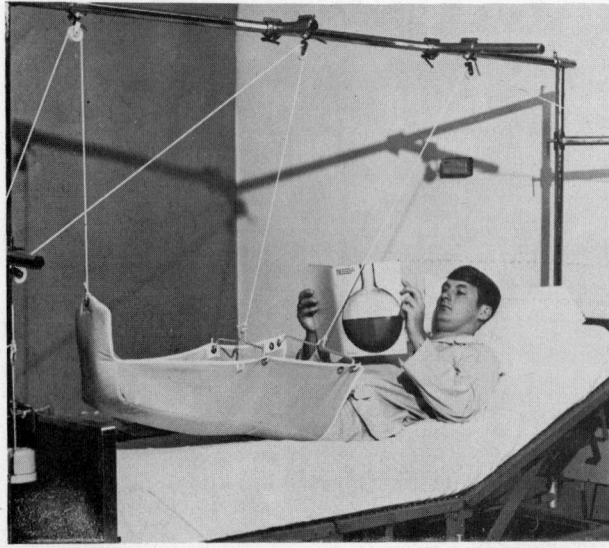

Figure 57-10. A type of balanced suspension for the lower extremity. Patient's leg supported by weights to balance the injured leg in the sling. (Photo courtesy of Richards Manufacturing Co.)

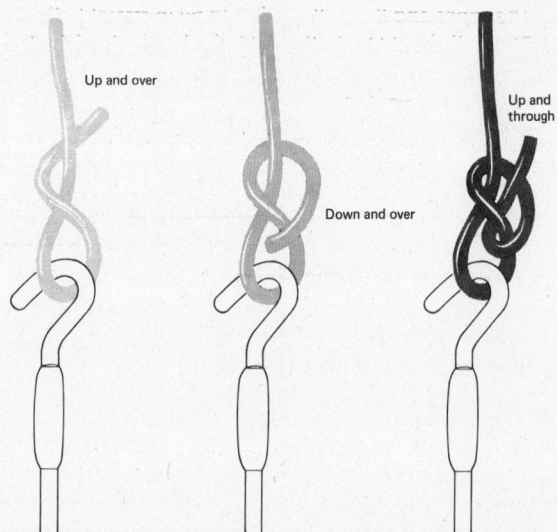

Figure 57-11. Guidelines for traction knot tying. Tying knots correctly is an orthopedic nursing activity essential for the safety of the patient in traction. To save time, follow this simple phrase:

Up and over
Down and over
Up and through.

Practice a few times with a traction cord. It is a good idea to secure all knots tightly with adhesive tape. (Courtesy Zimmer Manufacturing Company)

has not slipped down in bed. Since the rope sometimes frays, it too must be inspected at least daily. The foot must be in a natural position; rotation outward or inward should be reported. Footdrop is to be avoided, and the patient's foot must be maintained in a neutral position supported by appropriate orthopedic devices. The skin around the traction is inspected for evidence of circulatory impairment since weights are necessary to provide constant force.

It is especially important that the knots on the traction rope be tied securely (Fig. 57-11). Enough weight is applied at first to overcome the shortening tendency of the injured limb, but it is gradually lessened as the fracture becomes more fixed.

- *Weights should never be removed from a patient with a fracture unless a life-threatening situation occurs. Weight and pulley traction is applied to secure constant corrective extension. If the weights are removed to move the patient from one department to another, the whole purpose of their use has been defeated.*
- *When there is a pull in one direction, there must be an equal pull in the opposite direction. (For every action there is an equal and opposite reaction—this is Newton's third law of motion.)*

Countertraction is supplied by the patient's body weight and friction against the bed.

When traction frames are used, a trapeze may be suspended overhead within easy reach of the patient. This apparatus is of great help in assisting the patient to move about in bed and on and off bedpans. It is also a help to the nurse in caring for these patients. When a patient is not permitted to turn on one side or the other or on his abdomen, the nurse must make a special effort to provide good back care and to keep the bed dry and free of crumbs and wrinkles. This can be accomplished by having the patient raise his hips from the bed by holding onto the overhead trapeze. Often a patient uses the heel of his good leg to act as a brace when he raises himself. This digging of the heel into the mattress may cause injury to the tissues; hence, the heel must be massaged with lanolin and inspected for pressure areas. Some physicians wrap both legs in elastic bandage in an attempt to decrease the incidence of thrombophlebitis. If the patient is unable to raise himself, the nurse can push down on the mattress with one hand, leaving space for the other hand to massage the skin.

NURSING MANAGEMENT OF THE PATIENT IN TRACTION

NURSING PRINCIPLES AND IMPLICATIONS

The purposes of traction, regardless of how it is achieved, are (1) to reduce and to immobilize a fracture, (2) to lessen or to eliminate muscle spasm, and (3) to prevent fracture deformity. Nursing implications underlying all traction procedures include the following:

1. The patient is placed on a firm mattress often with a hinged bedboard beneath it.
2. The ropes and the pulleys should be in straight alignment.
3. The pull should be in line with the long axis of the bone.
4. Any factor that might reduce the pull or alter its direction must be eliminated.
   (a) Weights should hang free.
   (b) Ropes should be unobstructed.
   (c) Help the patient to pull himself up in bed at frequent intervals. Traction is *not* accomplished if the knot in the rope or footplate is touching the pulley or the foot of the bed, or if the weights are resting on the floor.
5. The amount of weight applied in skin traction must not exceed the tolerance of the skin. The condition of the latter must be inspected frequently.

6. A possibility always to be kept in mind in connection with skeletal traction is the risk of a complicating bone infection. The nurse is alert to detect odors, signs of local inflammation or other evidence of infection.
7. The patient's skin should be examined frequently for evidence of pressure or friction over bony prominences.
8. Provision should be made for supplying additional countertraction by increasing the pull in the opposite direction, i.e., by raising the bed in such a manner that the weight of the patient's body tends to oppose the pull of the traction.
9. Active motion of all unaffected joints are encouraged.
10. Every complaint of the patient in traction is to be investigated immediately.

PRINCIPLES OF BALANCED SUSPENSION TRACTION

Definition: Balanced suspension traction is produced by a counterforce other than the patient's body weight. The extremity balances or floats in the traction apparatus. The line of traction on the extremity remains fairly constant despite changes in position of the patient.

Example: Russell's leg traction for treating fractures of the femoral shaft.

Activities permitted patient:
The patient may sit, turn slightly and move as desired.

Nursing implications:

1. The angle of hip flexion is 20 degrees. (This is the angle between the thigh and the bed.)
2. The ropes and the pulleys are freely movable, and the traction is applied securely to the leg.
3. Observe for skin irritation around the traction bandage.
4. Check the patient for signs of odor and infection.
5. Observe for pressure under the sling at the popliteal space.
6. The patient should have foot supports to prevent footdrop.
7. The traction must be continuous to be effective.

(Continued)

NURSING MANAGEMENT OF THE PATIENT IN TRACTION (CONTINUED)

PRINCIPLES OF RUNNING TRACTION

Definition: Running traction is a form of traction in which the pull is exerted in one plane. It may utilize skin or skeletal traction, and it may be either unilateral or bilateral.

Example: Buck's extension.

Activities permitted patient:

1. The head of the bed may be elevated to the point of countertraction (e.g., if the countertraction is 20 cm. [8 inches], the head of the bed may be elevated 20 cm.).
2. The patient may not turn from side to side, because the position of the leg on the bed will cause the bony fragments to move against each other.

Nursing implications:

1. The foot is inspected for circulatory difficulties within a few minutes and then periodically after the elastic bandage has been applied.
2. Special care is given to the back at regular intervals, because the patient maintains a supine position.
3. Any complaint or burning sensation under the traction bandage is reported immediately.
4. Observe for wrinkling or slipping of the traction bandage.
5. The patient should have foot supports to prevent footdrop.
6. Check peripheral pulses and the color and temperature of the fingers and toes.
7. Check for calf tenderness and for possible Homan's sign for signs of thrombophlebitis.

BIBLIOGRAPHY

BOOKS

Adams, J. C.: Outline of Fractures, 7th ed. New York, Churchill Livingstone, 1978.

Brashear, H. R., Jr., and Raney, R. B.: Shands' Handbook of Orthopaedic Surgery, 9th ed. St. Louis, C. V. Mosby, 1978.

Devas, M.: Geriatric Orthopaedics. New York, Academic Press, 1977.

Epps, C. H. (ed.): Complications in Orthopaedic Surgery, vols. 1 and 2. Philadelphia, J. B. Lippincott, 1978.

Farrell, J.: Illustrated Guide to Orthopedic Nursing. Philadelphia, J. B. Lippincott, 1977.

Hartman, J. T.: Fracture Management: A Practical Approach. Philadelphia, Lea & Febiger, 1978.

Iverson, L. D., and Clawson, D. K.: Manual of Orthopaedic Therapeutics. Boston, Little, Brown, 1977.

Larson, C. B., and Gould, M.: Orthopedic Nursing, 9th ed. St. Louis, C. V. Mosby, 1978.

Lewis, R. C., Jr.: Handbook of Traction, Casting and Splinting Techniques. Philadelphia, J. B. Lippincott, 1977.

Rockwood, C. A., and Green, D. P.: Fractures, vols. 1 and 2. Philadelphia, J. B. Lippincott, 1975.

Ryan, J. R.: Orthopedic Surgery. Flushing, Medical Examination Pub. Co., 1977.

Stewart, J. D. M.: Traction and Orthopaedic Appliances. New York, Churchill Livingstone, 1975.

Turek, S. L.: Orthopaedics, Principles and Their Application, 3rd ed. Philadelphia, J. B. Lippincott, 1977.

AGENCIES

Governmental

National Institute of Arthritis, Metabolism and Digestive Diseases, National Institutes of Health, Bethesda, Md. 20205

Voluntary

American Physical Therapy Association, 1156 15th St., N.W., Washington, D.C. 20005

National Easter Seal Society for Crippled Children and Adults, 2023 W. Ogden Ave., Chicago, Ill. 60612

(See also Rehabilitation Agencies, Chapter 12)

58

MANAGEMENT OF PATIENTS WITH MUSCULOSKELETAL TRAUMA

MUSCULOSKELETAL TRAUMA

Injury to one part of the system usually produces injury to other parts and to the structures enclosed or supported by them. If the bones are broken, the muscles cannot function; if the nerves do not send impulses to the muscles, as in paralysis, the bones cannot move; if the joint surfaces do not articulate normally, neither the bones nor the muscles can function properly. Thus, although a fracture primarily affects the bone, it may also produce injury to the muscles surrounding the injured bone and to the blood vessels and the nerves in the vicinity of the fracture.

In the treatment of injury to the musculoskeletal system, support is provided for the injured part until nature has time to heal it. Support may be accomplished by bandages, adhesive strapping, splints, or plaster casts, applied externally. Support may be applied directly to the bone in the form of pins or plates. In other instances, it may be necessary to overcome overlapping and to correct deformity by applying weighted traction.

After the immediate and the painful effects of the injury have passed, consideration must be given to the prevention of fibrosis and the resulting stiffness in the injured muscles and the joint structures. Active function by the patient is the best form of treatment to guard against this disability. In some cases, the support applied may permit active function almost from the start. In other cases, the nature of the injury may not permit function, and even in those instances in which partial function is possible, na-

ture may be aided in the healing process and recovery of function may be hastened by various forms of physical therapy.

CONTUSIONS, SPRAINS, AND DISLOCATIONS

Contusions

A *contusion* is an injury to the soft tissues, produced by blunt force (a blow, kick, fall, etc.). There is always some hemorrhage into the injured part (ecchymosis), due to the rupture of many small vessels. This produces the well-known discoloration of the skin (black-and-blue spot), which gradually turns to brown and then to yellow, and finally disappears as absorption becomes complete. When the hemorrhage is sufficient to cause an appreciable collection of blood, it is called *hematoma*. The local symptoms (pain, swelling, and discoloration) are easily explained.

Management. Treatment consists of elevating the affected part and applying moist or dry cold for the first 8 or 10 hours to produce vasoconstriction which results in decreased hemorrhage and edema. Application of cold should be continued for 20 to 30 minutes. In the recovery phase, moist heat is applied for 20 minutes at a time to promote absorption and repair. Since heat causes swelling and increases tissue fluid which may impair function, hot compresses may be followed by cold applications to minimize the secondary effects of heat. Pressure in the form of an elastic adhesive bandage also is of distinct value in reducing contusion, hemorrhage, and swelling.

Sprains/Strains

A *sprain* is an injury to the ligamentous structures surrounding a joint, caused by a wrench or a twist. The function of a ligament is to maintain stability while permitting mobility. A torn ligament loses its stabilizing function. As is the case with contusions, blood vessels are ruptured, resulting in rapid swelling due to the extravasation of blood within the tissues. The movement of the joint becomes painful. To be certain that there is no bone injury, all these patients should have an x-ray examination.

A *strain* is an injury to the musculotendinous unit caused by excessive force or stretching. There is usually hemorrhage into the muscle.

Management. Sprains or strains are treated with intermittent cold compresses (15 to 20 minutes, 4 times daily). The vasoconstricting effect of cold retards the extravasation of blood and lymph and suppresses pain. The part should be elevated and rested. Sometimes additional support is provided with either temporary splinting or elastic bandages to reduce swelling and edema.

After 24 hours, mild heat may be applied (15 to 30 minutes, 4 times daily) to promote absorption. If the sprain is severe (torn muscle fibers and disrupted ligaments), surgical repair or cast immobilization is necessary so that the joint will not lose its stability.

Joint Dislocations

A *dislocation* of a joint is a condition in which the articular surfaces of the bones forming the joint are no longer in anatomical contact. The bones are literally "out of joint."

Dislocations may be (1) congenital (present at birth, due to some maldevelopment, most often noted at the hip); (2) spontaneous or pathologic, owing to disease of the articular or the periarticular structures, and (3) traumatic, owing to injury, such as the application of force in such a manner as to produce disruption of the joint.

The signs and symptoms of a traumatic dislocation are (1) pain, (2) change in contour of the joint, (3) change in the length of the extremity, (4) loss of normal mobility, and (5) change in the axis of the dislocated bones.

Roentgenograms confirm the diagnosis and should be made in every case, because frequently there is an associated fracture.

Management. The part is immobilized while the patient is transported to the emergency department, x-ray, or clinical unit. The dislocation is reduced (i.e., displaced parts brought into normal position), usually under anesthesia. The head of the dislocated bone is manipulated back into the joint cavity, and the joint is immobilized by

bandages and splints and kept immobile in a stable position until healing takes place.

The nursing management following reduction of a dislocation is essentially the same as that following the reduction of fractures. The part must be kept immobilized for a sufficient time to permit the ligamentous structures about the joint to heal. Therefore, splints and casts are the usual dressings. Complications that are common with such appliances must be watched for, including cyanosis, pain, and the disturbance or the loss of sensation which are familiar signs of circulatory impairment due to tight dressings. Attention must be paid to the slightest complaint by the patient. Signs of pressure both within and outside the immobilization dressing must be assessed regularly.

FRACTURES

A *fracture* is a break in the continuity of bone and is defined according to type and extent (Fig. 58–1). While the bone is the part most directly affected, other structures also may be involved, resulting in soft tissue edema, hemorrhage into the muscles and joints, joint dislocations, ruptured tendons, severed nerves, and damaged blood vessels. Body organs may be injured by the force that caused the fracture or by the fracture fragments.

Types of Fractures

A *complete* fracture involves a break across the entire cross-section of the bone and is frequently displaced (removed from normal position). In an *incomplete* fracture, the break occurs only through part of the cross-section of the bone and is usually undisplaced.

An *open* fracture is one that extends through the skin and mucous membrane. In a *closed* fracture, the fracture does not communicate with the outside area.

The following are specific types of fractures (Fig. 58–1):

Greenstick —a fracture in which one side of a bone is broken and the other side is bent

Transverse —the fracture is straight across the bone

Oblique —a fracture occurring at an angle across the bone (less stable than transverse)

Spiral —a fracture twisting around the shaft of the bone

Comminuted —a fracture in which bone has splintered into several fragments

Depressed —a fracture in which fragment(s) is (are) in-driven (seen frequently in fractures of skull and facial bones)

Compression —a fracture in which the fractured bone has been compressed by another bone(s) (seen in vertebral fractures)

Pathologic —a fracture that occurs through an area of diseased bone (bone cyst, Paget's disease, bony metastasis, tumor)

Avulsion —fragment of bone pulled off by ligament or tendon and its attachment

Epiphyseal —separation of the epiphysis from the rest of the bone

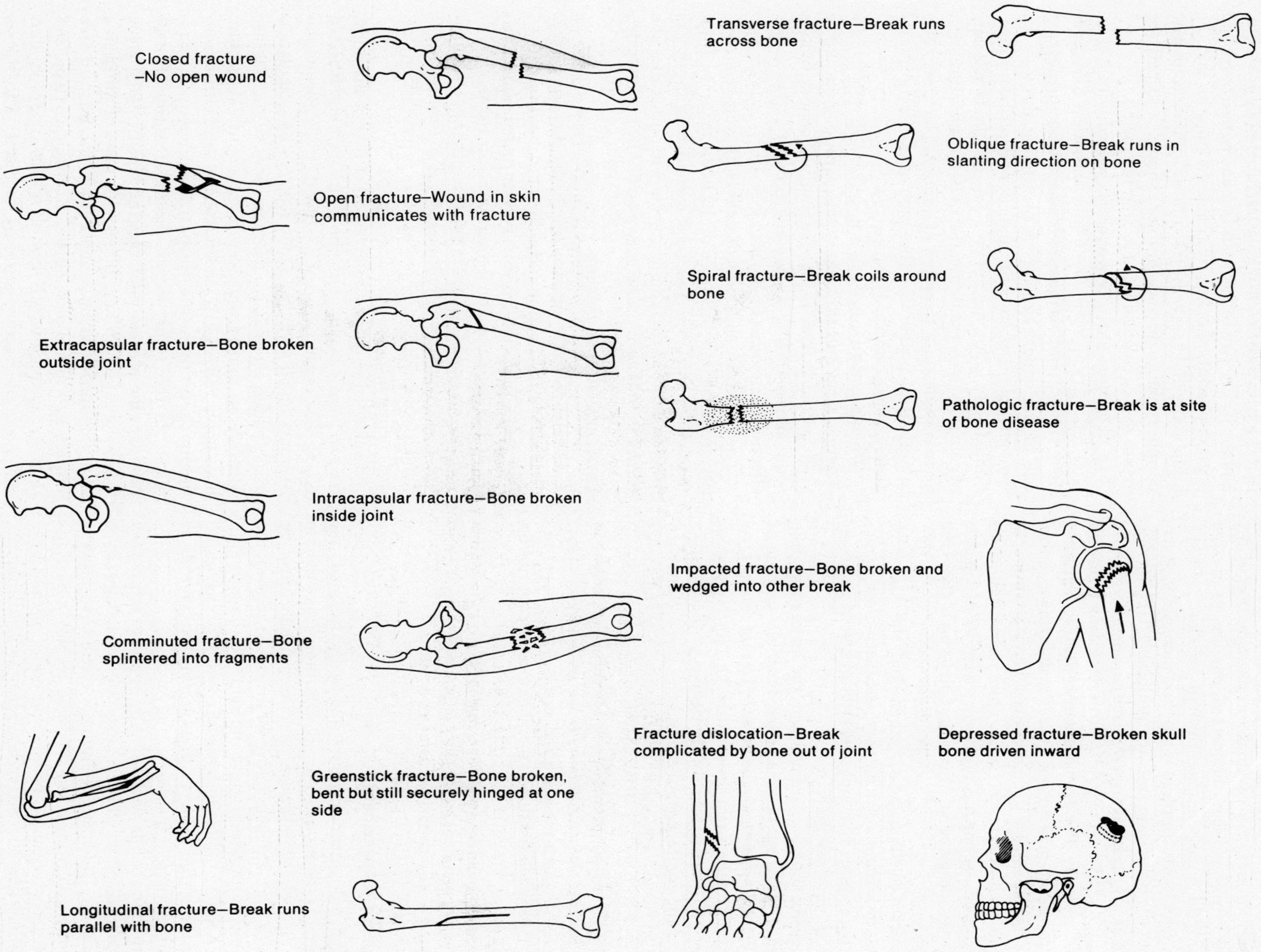

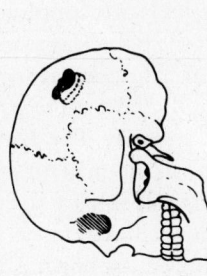

Transverse fracture—Break runs across bone

Oblique fracture—Break runs in slanting direction on bone

Spiral fracture—Break coils around bone

Pathologic fracture—Break is at site of bone disease

Impacted fracture—Bone broken and wedged into other break

Fracture dislocation—Break complicated by bone out of joint

Depressed fracture—Broken skull bone driven inward

Closed fracture —No open wound

Open fracture—Wound in skin communicates with fracture

Extracapsular fracture—Bone broken outside joint

Intracapsular fracture—Bone broken inside joint

Comminuted fracture—Bone splintered into fragments

Greenstick fracture—Bone broken, bent but still securely hinged at one side

Longitudinal fracture—Break runs parallel with bone

Figure 58-1. Types of fractures. (Courtesy Ethicon, Inc.)

1293

Clinical Manifestations

The clinical manifestations of a fracture are pain, loss of function, localized swelling and discoloration of the skin, deformity, false motion and crepitation. In an open fracture, the bone penetrates through the skin.

The *pain* is of a continuous type and increases in severity until the bone fragments are immobilized. Following the break, the part cannot be used and tends to move unnaturally (false motion) instead of remaining rigid as it normally would. The displacement of the fragments in a fracture of the arm or leg causes a deformity (either visible or palpable) of the extremity when it is compared to the normal extremity. The extremity cannot function properly because normal function of the muscles depends upon the integrity of the bones to which they are attached.

Localized swelling and discoloration of the skin occur as a result of trauma and hemorrhage that follow a fracture. These signs may not develop for several hours or days following the injury.

When the limb is examined with the hands, a grating sensation, called *crepitus,* can be felt due to the rubbing of the fragments one upon the other. (Testing for crepitation can produce further tissue damage.) In fractures of long bones there is actually shortening of the limb because of the contraction of the muscles that are attached above and below the site of the fracture. The fragments may often overlap as much as an inch or two.

All of these symptoms are not necessarily present in every fracture. When there is a linear or fissure fracture, or in cases where the fractured surfaces are driven together (impacted fractures), many of these symptoms do not occur.

The diagnosis of a fracture is dependent on the symptoms of the patient, the physical signs, and x-ray examination. Usually there is a history of injury.

Emergency Management

When the patient is transported to the hospital, the fractured extremity is rendered as immobile as possible *before the patient is moved.* If an injured patient must be removed from a vehicle before splints can be applied, the extremity is supported above and below the fracture site, and traction is applied in accordance with the line of the long axis of the bone to prevent rotation as well as angular motion.

Immobilization is established by applying temporary well-padded splints which are then firmly bandaged over the clothing. Adequate splinting is essential to prevent the soft tissue from being damaged by the bony fragments. Immobilization of the long bones of the lower extremities may also be accomplished by bandaging the extremities together, with the sound extremity serving as a splint for the injured one. In an upper extremity injury, the arm may be bandaged to the chest, or an injured forearm may be placed in a sling. It must be remembered that the pain associated with a fractured bone is severe, and the surest way to decrease pain and hemorrhage and prevent possible shock is by fixing the bone so that the joints above and below the fracture are immobilized. The peripheral pulses distal to the injury should be palpated to assure that circulation has not been hampered.

In an *open fracture,* the wound is covered with a clean (sterile) dressing to prevent contamination of deeper tissues. No attempt is made to reduce the fracture, even if one of the bone fragments is protruding through the wound. Splints should be applied as described above. Immediately following injury, a patient who is in a state of confusion may not be aware that he has a fracture, i.e., he may walk on a fractured extremity. Therefore, it is important to immobilize that part of the body immediately when a fracture is suspected.

When a patient comes to a hospital suffering from a fracture, a narcotic sufficient to relieve the pain should be given provided there is no head injury. The intravenous route allows smaller dosage and prompt action and is effective in a patient in shock.

Then with care and gentleness the clothes are removed, first from the uninjured side of the body, and then from the injured side. The fractured extremity is moved as little as possible to avoid disturbing it; sometimes the patient's clothing must be cut away on the injured side.

Physiology of Bone Healing

A bone fracture, initiates all of the physiologic responses of inflammation and wound healing. In addition, new bone formation must be reconstructed rather than the area being patched together with scar tissue.

There are several stages in fracture healing: (1) hematoma, (2) cellular proliferation, (3) callus formation, (4) callus ossification or union, and (5) consolidation and remodeling into mature bone (Fig. 58-2).

As in wound healing in every other part of the body, fracture repair begins with the clotting of extravasated blood. The organization of the blood clot begins within 24 hours on all surfaces, and is replaced by granulation tissue within a few days. The torn ends of the fracture (periosteum, endosteum, bone fragments) at the fracture line supply cells. These proliferate and differentiate into fibrous connective tissue, fibrocartilage, and hyaline cartilage. At this stage, except for the predominance of cartilage, the process resembles the repair of any tissue following injury. In long bones, this mass of differentiated preliminary tissue bridges across the fracture area and acts as a model or template of connective tissue and cartilage, through which new bone cells are drawn into and across the fracture gap from each side. The fibrous connective tissue and cartilage form a complex structure termed *callus.*

SEQUENCE OF FRACTURE HEALING AND POSSIBLE COMPLICATIONS

1. HEMATOMA STAGE

The local clot serves as a fibrin network for subsequent cellular invasion

POSSIBLE COMPLICATIONS:

Prevention of coagulation
Loss of hematoma
—through open fracture
—through debridement
—through action of fibrinolytic synovial fluid

2. CELLULAR PROLIFERATION STAGE

Fibroblastic and endothelial cells invade and colonize the fibrin scaffolding of the clot

POSSIBLE COMPLICATIONS:

Devitalization of periosteal, intramedullary or extraosseous mesenchymal tissues from which red cells arise
—by original trauma
—by surgery

Unbridgeable gaps between bone ends
—due to loss of bone substance
—due to interposed soft tissue

Hostile environment due to inadequate blood supply

Interruption of vascular network
—by motion
—by infection

3. CALLUS FORMATION STAGE

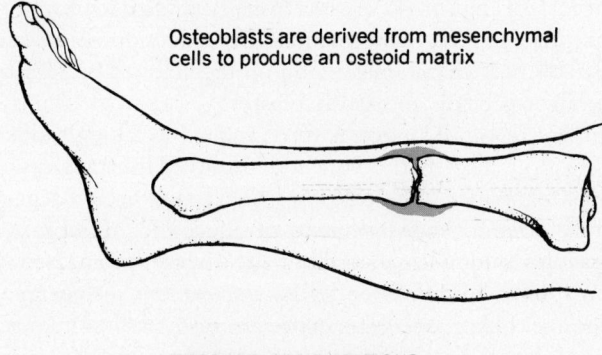

Osteoblasts are derived from mesenchymal cells to produce an osteoid matrix

POSSIBLE COMPLICATIONS

The collagen matrix may be rendered nonossifiable
—by hypercortisonism
—by scurvy

4 CALLUS OSSIFICATION OR UNION STAGE

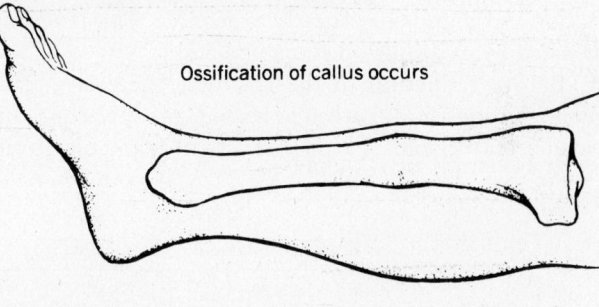

Ossification of callus occurs

5. CONSOLIDATION AND REMODELING

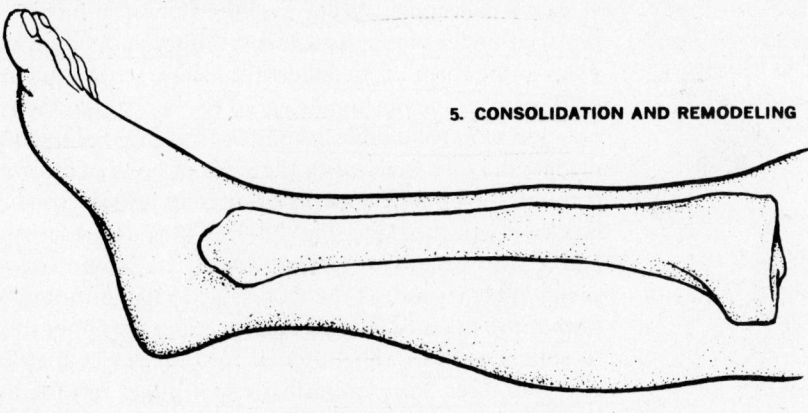

Stages of callus ossification and remodeling do not seem to be related to delayed union and nonunion, so that those influences which lead to delayed union must be in action during the early stages of repair

Figure 58-2.   Sequence of fracture healing and possible complications. (From Moe, J. H.: Delayed union and nonunion of long-bone fractures. Hosp. Med., 9:35, Feb. 1970)

The external callus of the healing fracture develops in great part from the periosteum. The contribution of the periosteum to the repair of bone is of major importance. The vascular network of the callus is a new growth of small arteries, capillaries, and veins arising from the vascular supply of surrounding muscle, periosteum, and bone marrow.

The shape of the callus and the volume of tissue required to bridge the defect is directly proportional to the amount of bone damage and displacement and the manner in which the bones are fixed. The healing time depends on the total volume of damaged tissue, the area of the fracture as well as the regional condition of blood supply and the age of the patient.

Collagen and ground substance are produced by the bone-forming cells called *osteoblasts.* The collagen and ground substance are called *osteoid.* It is this osteoid that is "calcified" and appears on the x-ray, providing evidence of progressive healing at the fracture site.

Principles of Fracture Management

The principles of fracture treatment include reduction, immobilization, and regaining of normal function and strength (rehabilitation). (See Table 58-1.)

FRACTURE REDUCTION

Reduction of a fracture ("setting" the bone) refers to restoration of the fracture fragments into anatomical rotation and alignment as nearly as possible. This is accomplished by closed or open manipulation.

Before reduction of the fracture, there is usually enough time for the patient to be undressed, washed, and made comfortable. A limb that is to be manipulated and dressed in a splint or a cast should be cleaned and elevated.

In treating a fracture, the most important objectives are: (1) to regain the function of the involved part, (2) to regain and maintain the correct position and alignment and (3) to return the patient to his usual activities in the shortest time.

Methods Employed to Obtain Fracture Reduction

Several methods may be used to obtain reduction of a fracture; the method selected depends on the nature of the fracture. Variations of these methods are carried out, but the underlying principles are the same. Usually fractures are reduced as soon as possible inasmuch as tissues may lose their elasticity if infiltrated by edema or hemorrhage. In most cases, fracture reduction becomes more difficult as the hemorrhage at the fracture site becomes organized.

CLOSED REDUCTION. In most instances, closed reduction is accomplished by bringing the bone fragments into apposition (ends in contact) by *manipulation* and *manual traction.* Anesthesia is given to relieve the patient's pain and relax the muscles. Following the manipulation, x-ray films are taken to determine that the bone fragments are in correct alignment. A cast is usually applied to immobilize the extremity and maintain the reduction. A second person may maintain traction on the affected extremity while it is being encased in plaster.

TRACTION. Traction is force applied in a longitudinal direction. This method may be employed for fractures of all long bones. The purposes of traction are to regain normal length and alignment, to reduce and immobilize a fracture, and to lessen or eliminate muscle spasm. It may be applied to an extremity by *skin traction,* using tape, sponge rubber, or plastic materials, or by *skeletal traction,* using wires, pins, or tongs placed through bone. To apply the needed force a system of ropes, pulleys and weights is used. The nursing management of a patient in traction is discussed more fully on page 1289.

OPEN REDUCTION OR OPEN OPERATION. Some fractures require an operation or open reduction. This necessitates a formal incision in order that the bone fragments be replaced under direct visualization. Internal fixation devices in the form of metallic pins, wires, screws, plates, nails, or rods may be used to hold the bone fragments in position until solid bone healing occurs. Internal fixation devices may be attached to the sides of bone or inserted through the bony fragments or directly into the medullary cavity of the bone (Fig. 58-3). These devices assure better maintenance of alignment of the fracture fragment. After closure of the wound, external immobilization of the fracture is often employed by the application of splints or casts. The internal fixation device may be removed after bony union has taken place, but for the majority of patients it is not removed unless it produces symptoms.

TABLE 58-1.   THE TREATMENT OF FRACTURES

Principles of Care in Treating Fractures
1. Restore fracture fragments to their normal anatomic position (reduction)
2. Maintain reduction in place until healing occurs (immobilization)
3. Regain normal function and strength of the affected part (rehabilitation)

Methods Used to Obtain Fracture Reduction
1. Closed reduction
2. Traction
3. Open reduction

Methods Used to Maintain Fracture Reduction (Fixation)
1. Plaster cast or cast-brace
2. Splints
3. Continuous traction
4. Pin and plaster technique
5. Internal fixation devices
    a. Nails   c. Screws   e. Rods
    b. Plates   d. Wires

Nursing Management Following Open Reduction

During the immediate postoperative period following open reduction, the nursing management is the same as for any other major surgical procedure (Chapter 20). Before the patient leaves the recovery room, the bed on the unit should be made ready with traction apparatus appropriate to his needs. The affected part is elevated, and the circulation of the part evaluated at frequent intervals, by comparing the affected extremity with the unaffected one for color and skin temperature.

- Symptoms of pain, pallor, pulselessness, paralysis (the four P's), or coolness indicate abnormal circulatory changes and consequent neurovascular disturbances.
- The orthopedist should be notified immediately so that the dressings may be loosened or the cast bivalved in order to relieve pressure. Dressings should be inspected at regular intervals.

The assessment and management of postoperative pain is an individualized problem. Remember that upon awakening, the patient is susceptible to suggestion. Reassure him that the operative procedure is over and that someone is with him. During the immediate postoperative period narcotics may be necessary. In general, an elderly patient requires less narcotic than a younger patient. As soon as possible, oral non-narcotic analgesics should be given, since patients who have undergone orthopedic operations may have prolonged musculoskeletal complaints. Restlessness, anxiety, and general discomfort may be relieved by appropriate nursing measures, reassurance, physical therapy, tranquilizers, and other forms of treatment.

Orthopedic wounds have a tendency to ooze more than other surgical wounds. External muscle dissection frequently produces wounds in which hemostasis is poor. Wounds that are closed while under tourniquet control may bleed when the tourniquet is released in the postoperative period.

Redressings are required for many fractures dressed with splints, especially those that involve or are near the joints. Fractures complicated by joint involvement, or those treated by the application of a cast often benefit from a regimen of physical therapy after union is firm enough for external support to be discontinued. Under ordinary conditions, with proper treatment, the fragments of the broken bone unite by the formation of a soft callus in which are deposited calcium salts, so that in time a patch of bone results that is as strong as the original part.

FRACTURE IMMOBILIZATION

After the fracture has been reduced, bone fragments must be immobilized or held in position until union has had time to take place. Immobilization may be accom-

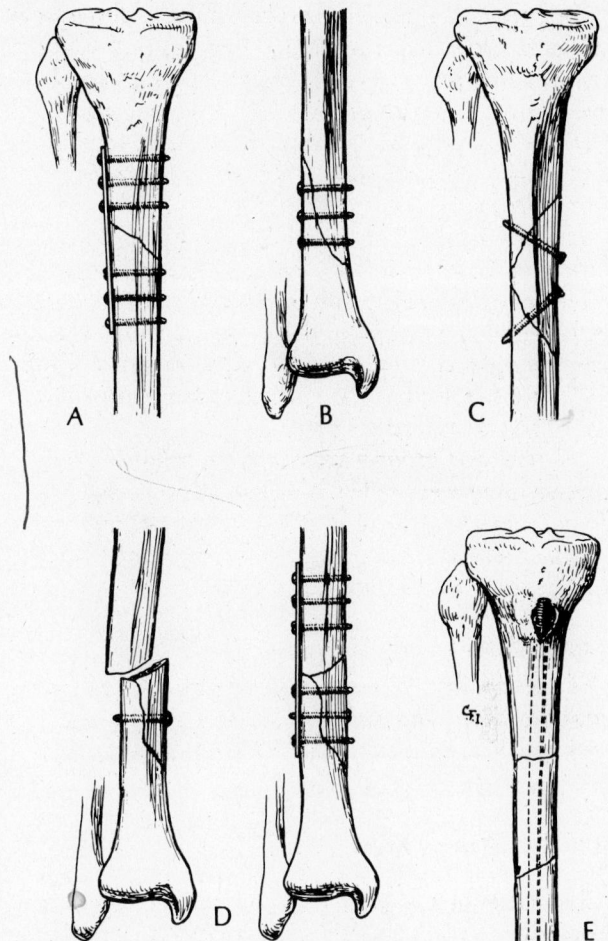

Figure 58-3. Techniques of internal fixation. (*A*) Plate and six screws for a transverse or short oblique fracture. (*B*) Screws for a long oblique or spiral fracture. (*C*) Screws for a long butterfly fragment. (*D*) Plate and six screws for a short butterfly fragment. (*E*) Medullary nail for a segmental fracture. (From Smith, H.: Fractures. *In* Crenshaw, A. H. (ed.): Campbell's Operative Orthopaedics, vol. 1. St. Louis, C. V. Mosby, 1971)

plished by external or internal fixation. Methods of external fixation include bandages, plaster casts, splints, continuous traction or pin and plaster technique. Internal fixation devices (metal implants) include nails, plates, screws, wires and rods. These serve as internal splints to hold the fractured bones in alignment while healing takes place.

Bandages of muslin or elastic are used commonly to immobilize certain fractures. The *Velpeau* bandage is used for fractures of the scapula, clavicle and humerus (Fig. 58-4). Certain fractures are treated with elastic compression bandages. Splints (wooden, plastic or plaster) may be used for temporary or permanent immobilization, especially for fractures of the upper extremity. Air splints are quite commonly used by emergency paramedical personnel. Any splint that does not fit the curve of the extremity should be well-padded to prevent pressure.

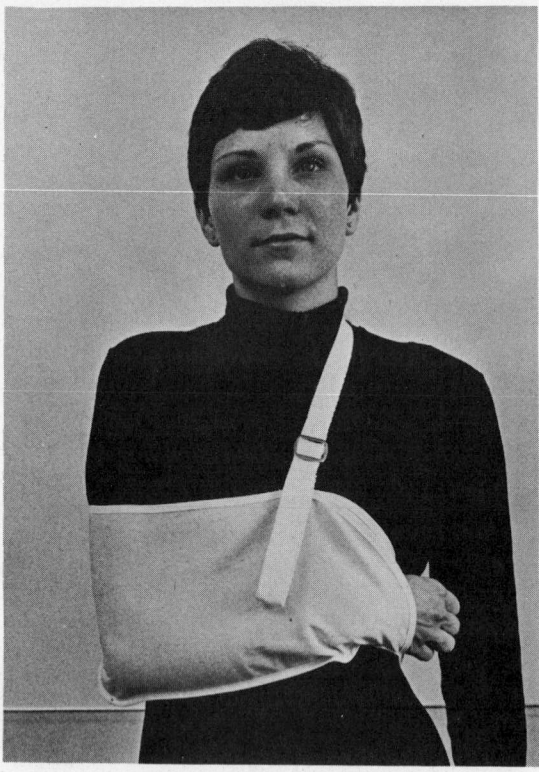

Figure 58-4.   The Velpeau sling splints the arm to the chest to immobilize the shoulder girdle. It is used to treat fractures of the scapula, clavicle, and humerus.

TABLE 58-2.   APPROXIMATE IMMOBILIZATION TIME NECESSARY FOR UNION

FRACTURE SITE	NUMBER OF WEEKS
Phalanx	3-5
Metacarpal	6
Carpal	6
Scaphoid	10
	(or until x-ray shows union)
Radius and ulna	10-12
Humerus:	
Supracondylar	8
Midshaft	8-12
Proximal (impacted)	3
Proximal (displaced)	6-8
Clavicle	6-10
Vertebra	16
Pelvis	6
Femur:	
Intracapsular	24
Intratrochanteric	10-12
Shaft	18
Supracondylar	12-15
Tibia:	
Proximal	8-10
Shaft	14-20
Malleolus	6
Calcaneus	12-16
Metatarsal	6
Toes	3

(From Compere, E. L. *et al.*: Pictorial Handbook of Fracture Treatment. ed. 5. Chicago, Yearbook Medical Publishers)

MANAGEMENT OF OPEN FRACTURES

In an *open* fracture (one associated with an open wound extending throughout the skin surface and down to the area of bone injury) there is risk of *infection* — osteomyelitis, gas gangrene and tetanus. The objectives of management are to minimize the chance of infection of the wound, soft tissue and bone and to promote healing of soft tissue and bone.

The patient is taken to the operating room where the wound is cleansed, debrided (foreign matter and devitalized tissue removed) and irrigated. Swabs are taken for culture and sensitivity studies. Devitalized bone fragments are usually removed. The fracture is carefully reduced and stabilized by external fixation. Repair of damage to blood vessels, soft tissue, muscles, nerves and tendons is usually carried out. A heavily contaminated wound may be left open, dressed with sterile gauze and not closed until it is clear that infection has been aborted or overcome. Later the wounds may be closed by suture or by autogenous skin or flap grafts. Tetanus prophylaxis is given. Usually intravenous antibiotics are started to prevent or treat serious infection.

When the patient returns from the operating room he is observed for signs of shock since considerable loss of blood usually occurs during surgery. The distal pulses are palpated and the extremity observed for evidences of ischemia. The temperature is taken at regular intervals and the patient is observed for signs that indicate infection.

HEALING TIME OF FRACTURES

Many factors influence the speed with which healing occurs. The reduction of the displaced fracture fragments must be accurate and successfully maintained to assure healing. The affected bone must have an adequate blood supply. In addition the age of the patient and the type of fracture affect healing time. In general, fractures of flat bones (pelvis, scapula) heal quite rapidly. Fractures at the ends of long bones where the bone is more vascular and cancellous heal more quickly than do fractures in areas where the bone is dense and less vascular (midshaft). Electrical stimulation is being investigated as a means of promoting fracture healing. Table 58-2 shows the approximate immobilization times necessary for union of the most common types of fractures.

COMPLICATIONS OF FRACTURES

The immediate complications following a fracture are *shock*, which may be fatal within a few hours after injury; *fat embolism,* which may occur within 48 hours or longer; *infection; thromboembolism* (pulmonary embolism), which may cause death several weeks after injury; and *disseminated intravascular coagulation*.

SHOCK. Hypovolemic or traumatic shock, resulting from hemorrhage (both external and nonvisible blood loss) and loss of extracellular fluid into damaged tissues, may occur in fractures of the extremities, thorax, pelvis, and spine. Because the bone is very vascular, large quantities of blood may be lost as a result of trauma, especially in femoral and pelvic fractures.

Treatment consists of replacing the depleted blood volume, relieving the patient's pain, providing adequate splinting, and protecting the patient from further injury.

FAT EMBOLISM SYNDROME. Following a fracture, fat embolism syndrome may occur from innumerable fat globules being released into the bloodstream and occluding small blood vessels that supply the brain, lungs, kidneys and other organs. The onset may occur within 48 hours after injury and is more apt to develop in patients with multiple fractures, particularly of the long bones (femur and tibia) and pelvis.

The presenting feature is usually cerebral disturbance manifested by bizarre mental symptoms varying from mild agitation and confusion to delirium and coma which occur in response to hypoxia which results from fat emboli lodging in the brain.

- Personality changes, restlessness, irritability or confusion in a patient who has sustained a fracture is an indication that immediate blood gas studies should be done. Occlusion of a large number of small vessels causes the pulmonary pressure to rise, possibly resulting in acute right heart failure. Edema and hemorrhages in the alveoli impair oxygen transport leading to hypoxia. There is an increase in respiratory rate, precordial chest pain, cough, dyspnea, and acute pulmonary edema.

With systemic embolization, petechiae are noted in the buccal membranes and conjunctival sacs, on the hard palate, on the fundus of the eye, and over the chest and anterior axillary folds. Free fat may be found in the urine when emboli reach the kidneys.

Management. The objectives of management are to support the respiratory system and to correct homeostatic disturbances. Arterial blood gas analysis is done to determine the degree of respiratory impairment, as respiratory failure is the most common cause of death. Respiratory support is provided with oxygen given in high concentrations. Controlled volume ventilation with positive end-expiratory pressure (PEEP) may be employed to decrease and inhibit the formation of pulmonary edema. Steroids to treat the inflammatory lung reaction and to control cerebral edema may be given. Low molecular weight dextran may improve pulmonary and capillary flow because of its desludging effect.

OTHER COMPLICATIONS. *Thromboembolism* (discussed on page 635), *infection* (all open fractures are considered to be contaminated — page 1298), and *disseminated intravascular coagulation (DIC)* are other possible complications of fractures. DIC includes a group of bleeding disorders with diverse causes, including massive tissue trauma. Manifestations include ecchymoses, unexpected bleeding after surgery, and bleeding from the mucous membranes, venipuncture sites and gastrointestinal and urinary tract. The treatment of DIC is discussed on page 674.

Delayed Complications of Fractures

DELAYED UNION AND NONUNION. Delayed union occurs when healing does not advance at a normal rate for the location and type of fracture. *Nonunion* results from failure of the ends of a fractured bone to unite. Delayed union and nonunion are caused by infection at the fracture site, tissue becoming interposed between the bone ends, motion that converts healing callus to fibrous tissue and a combination of limited bone contact and restricted blood supply. If union does not result by adequate immobilization, the fracture is said to be *ununited*.

In nonunion, only fibrous tissue exists between the bone fragments; no bone salts have been deposited. In such instances, a false joint (pseudoarthrosis) often develops at the site of the fracture. When such an unfortunate result occurs, braces may be used to make the limb useful. An operation may be performed by which the ends of the bone are freshened, and an attempt is made to unite them by means of a graft removed from another bone, which is placed in position to span the fragments. Fractures of the middle third of the humerus, of the neck of the femur in elderly people, and of the lower third of the tibia most frequently result in nonunion.

AVASCULAR NECROSIS OF BONE. Avascular necrosis may occur when the bone loses its blood supply or when infection occurs. It may be idiopathic or follow a fracture or dislocation. The blood supply to the head and neck of the femur may be disrupted due to injury of the blood vessels which can cause severe damage to the bone. The dead bone may be reabsorbed and replaced by new bone. If revascularization takes place, the structure may collapse. Healing can occur in the presence of avascular necrosis, but the patient may develop a painful arthritis. Usually the interruption of the blood supply is an unpreventable complication that occurs at the time of injury.

FRACTURES OF SPECIFIC SITES

Management of a patient with a fracture requires an understanding of the extent of the fracture, the therapeutic aim, the management to accomplish this aim as well as

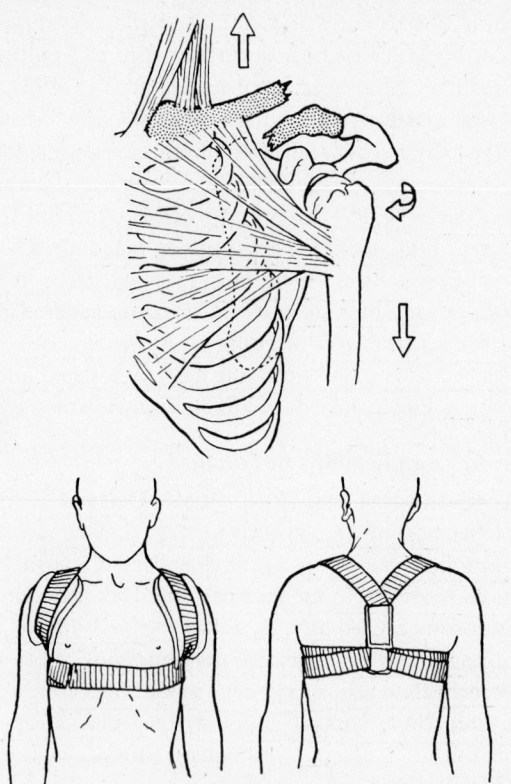

Figure 58-5. Fracture of the clavicle. (*Top*) Anteroposterior view, showing typical displacement of midclavicle fracture. (*Bottom*) Method of immobilization with a clavicular strap. (From Hardy, J. D.: Rhoads Textbook of Surgery. Philadelphia, J. B. Lippincott, 1977)

the care required through convalescence. The overall objective is to restore the function of the affected part to as near normal as possible.

An injury to the skeletal structure may vary from a simple linear fracture to a severe crushing injury. The therapeutic program is determined by the type and location of the fracture and the degree of involvement of surrounding structures.

Fractures of the skull and cervical spine have been considered in Chapter 55 on the management of patients with neurological disorders. Fracture of the mandible is discussed in Chapter 23.

CLAVICLE (COLLAR BONE) FRACTURES

Fracture of the collar bone is one of the most common fractures encountered and is usually the result of a fall on the shoulder or an outstretched hand or a direct blow. The clavicle helps to hold the shoulder upward, outward, and backward from the thorax. Therefore, when the clavicle is fractured, the objective of management is to hold the shoulder in its normal position by means of closed reduction and immobilization with external splinting in the form of a clavicular strap, sling, figure-8 bandage or T-splint.

If the fracture is medial to the coracoclavicular ligament, a figure-8 bandage or a commercially available clavicular strap (Fig. 58-5) may be used to pull the shoulders back and hold them in that position. When a clavicular strap is used, the axillae are well padded to prevent a compression injury to the brachial plexus and axillary artery. There should be no restriction of circulatory or nerve function in either arm.

When more secure shoulder immobilization is desired, a plaster shoulder spica cast may be used. When an undisplaced fracture occurs lateral to the coracoclavicular ligament, the shoulder may be held in place with a sling. If proper reduction and immobilization cannot be maintained, open reduction with internal fixation may be required. Complications of clavicular fractures include trauma to the nerves of the brachial plexus or injury to the subclavian vein or artery from a bony fragment.

Patient Education. The patient is cautioned not to elevate his arm above shoulder level until the fracture has united. He is also encouraged to exercise the elbow, wrist and fingers as soon as possible. When the patient is able, shoulder exercises (Fig. 58-6) are prescribed to obtain full shoulder motion.

RIB FRACTURES

Uncomplicated fractures of the ribs occur frequently and usually unite with no resultant impairment of function. However, fractures of the ribs produce painful respirations. Thus the patient tends to decrease his respiratory excursions and refrains from coughing. As a result, tracheobronchial secretions are not coughed up, aeration of the lung is diminished, and a predisposition to pneumonia and atelectasis is created. Intercostal nerve blocks with procaine are done to relieve respiratory pain and permit productive coughing.

Other serious problems may result from rib fractures. Multiple rib fractures may lead to a flail chest (page 498), while severe rib fractures may result in puncture of the lung with the escape of air into the pleural space (pneumothorax) or of blood into the pleural space (hemothorax). The management of these patients is discussed on page 499.

UPPER EXTREMITY FRACTURES

Fractures of the Humeral Neck

Fractures of the neck of the humerus may occur through either the surgical or the anatomical neck. The most common fracture in the upper arm and the shoulder is that of the surgical neck of the humerus. Such a fracture occurs most often from a person falling and striking the ground with his outstretched arm (impacted fracture). The patient comes for aid with the affected arm hanging limp at the side and supported by the uninjured hand.

Many of the impacted fractures of the surgical neck of

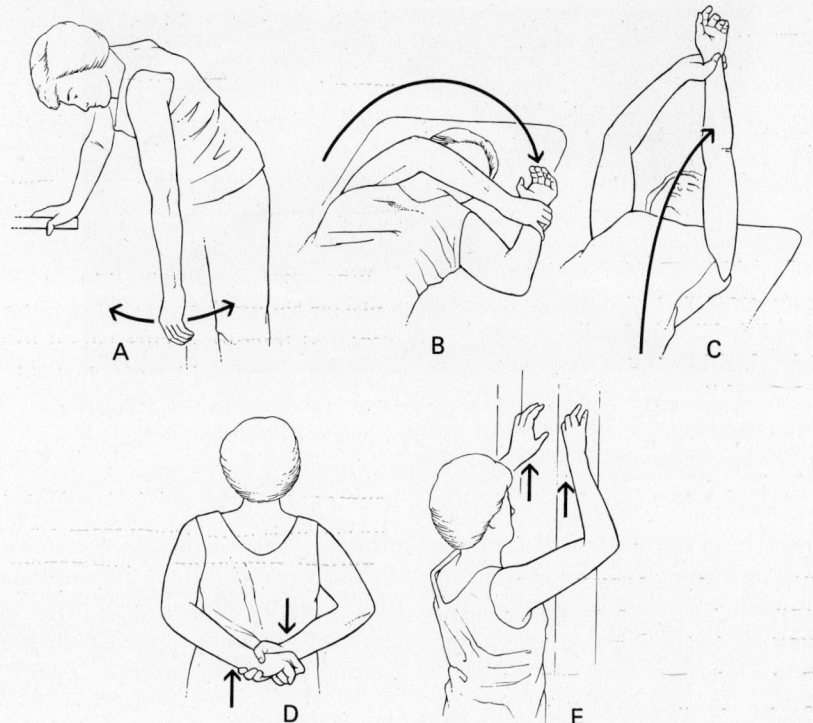

Figure 58-6. Exercises to develop range of motion of shoulder. *A.* Pendulum exercise. *B.* External rotation. *C.* Elevation. *D.* Internal rotation. In all of these, the unaffected arm is used for power. *E.* Wall climbing.

the humerus do not require reduction. The arm is supported by a sling supplemented by a modified Velpeau bandage (Fig. 58-4). When this type of "sling" is used, a soft pad is placed in the axilla to prevent skin maceration.

In any fracture of the arm, limitation of motion and stiffness of the shoulder occur from disuse. Therefore, pendulum exercises are begun as soon as tolerated by the patient. (In pendulum or circumduction exercises, the patient is instructed to lean forward and to allow the affected arm to abduct and rotate [Fig. 58-6]). Early motion of the joint does not displace the fragments if motion is carried out within the limits imposed by pain.

When a surgical neck fracture is displaced, treatment consists of closed reduction under x-ray control, open reduction or replacement of the humeral head with a prosthesis. In this type of fracture there must be a specified period of immobilization before exercises are started.

Patient Education.   If the fracture is not displaced, active motion of the shoulder joint is started *early* to prevent limitation of motion and stiffness of the shoulder.

Fractures of the Shaft of the Humerus

Fractures of the shaft of the humerus are most frequently caused by (1) direct violence which results in a transverse, oblique or comminuted fracture or (2) an indirect twisting force that results in a spiral fracture. The radial nerve may be injured in this fracture because it lies immediately adjacent to the midportion of the humerus in the musculospiral groove.

Frequently, the weight of the arm helps to correct any displacement so that surgery is not required. A hanging cast may be applied to an oblique, spiral, or displaced fracture which has resulted in shortening of the humeral shaft. A hanging cast must be dependent (allowed to hang free without support) since the weight of the cast is the means by which continuous traction is applied to the long axis of the arm. The patient is advised to sleep in a fairly upright position so that traction is maintained constantly. Finger exercises are started as soon as the cast is applied, while pendulum exercises are done as directed to provide active movement of the shoulder, thereby preventing adhesions of the shoulder joint capsule. After the cast is removed, a sling is applied and exercises of the shoulder, elbow and wrist are begun.

Supracondylar Fractures of the Humerus (Above the Elbow)

This fracture occurs close to the median nerve and brachial artery. Therefore, the most serious complication of a supracondylar fracture of the humerus is Volkmann's ischemic contracture which results from compression or damage to the brachial artery (Fig. 58-7).

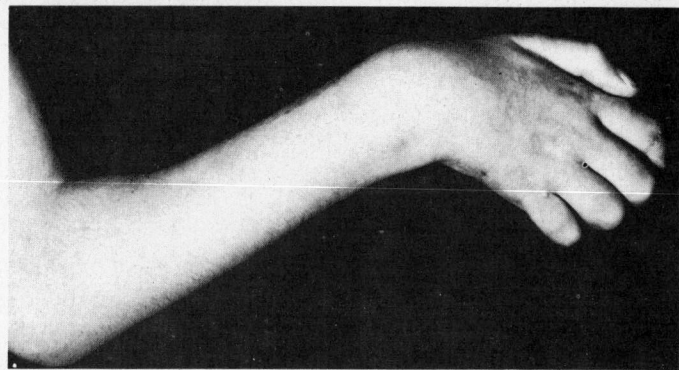

Figure 58-7. Photograph of the forearm and hand of a patient with late Volkmann's ischemic contracture. (From Rockwood, C. A., and Green, D. P. (eds.): Fractures, vol. 1. J. B. Lippincott, 1975)

The treatment for this type of fracture varies. If possible, the bones are aligned by manipulation under general anesthesia. After reduction, the bone fragments are maintained in alignment by keeping the elbow in an acutely flexed position in a long-arm cast.

For more severe injuries, skeletal traction is applied with the arm suspended over the face (Fig. 58-8) or in a sidearm position (Fig. 58-9). The traction is established from a Kirschner wire placed through the olecranon process. These methods serve to maintain traction, keep the fracture reduced, decrease edema and aid the circulation, thereby reducing the risk of Volkmann's contracture. Sometimes open reduction and pin-or-screw fixation may be necessary.

An important nursing function when managing the patient with a supracondylar fracture of the humerus is to assess for signs of impaired circulation in the forearm and hand.

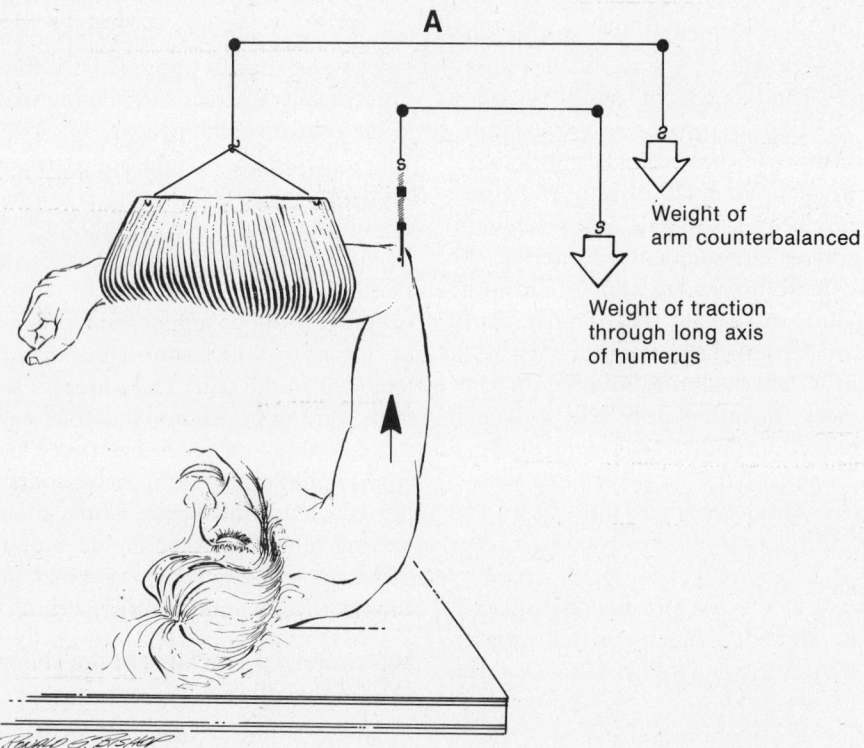

Figure 58-8. Treatment of supracondylar fracture: over-the-face traction is useful when swelling is great enough to compromise circulation. This type of traction reduces swelling by creating a very effective elevation of the extremity. (From Lewis, R. C.: Handbook of Traction, Casting and Splinting Techniques. Philadelphia, J. B. Lippincott, 1977)

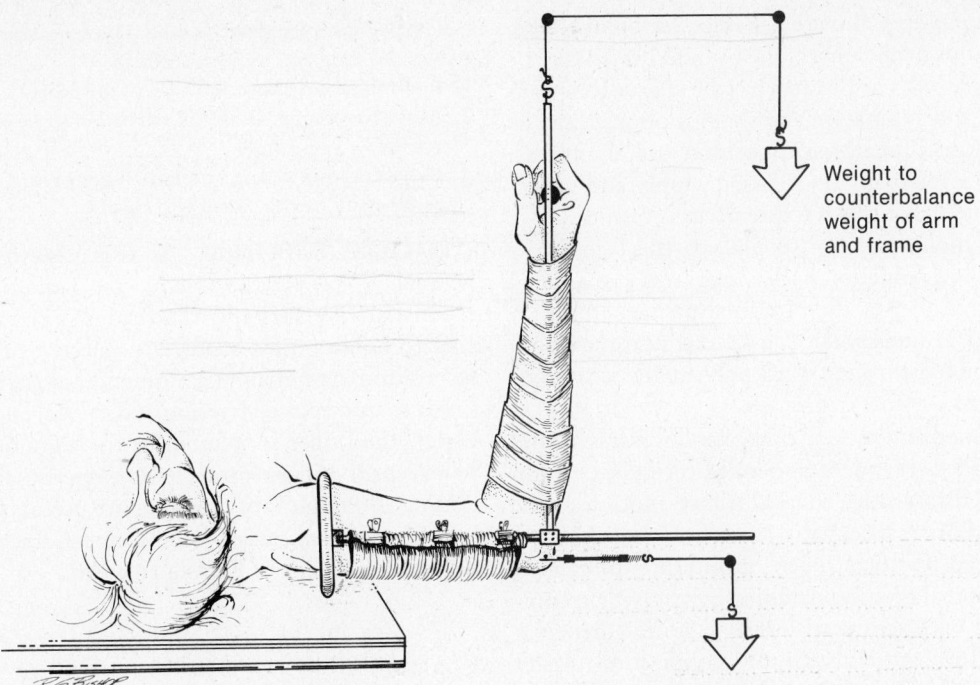

Figure 58-9. Balanced side-arm traction. The arm is passed through the ring, which is then passed up so that it encompasses the shoulder. The upright attachment for the forearm may be moved in either direction to accommodate the length of the humerus. A cloth sling is placed on the horizontal segment to provide a surface on which the arm may rest. The olecranon extends just past the vertical limb, so that the pin drilled through the olecranon will be clear and allow unimpeded traction. The forearm is placed between the two upright supports, and usually held there with a circumferentially applied elastic bandage. A rope is attached to the vertical section and is passed through pulleys. A weight is attached to exactly counterbalance the weight of the arm and the frame. Skeletal traction is then applied in the desired amount through the pin in the olecranon. The entire extremity is counterbalanced so that a balanced traction system is created. (From Lewis, R. C.: Handbook of Traction, Casting and Splinting Techniques. Philadelphia, J. B. Lippincott, 1977)

- Observe the hand for swelling, skin color (blueness and blanching of the nailbeds) and temperature, comparing it with the unaffected hand.
- Evaluate the amplitude of the radial pulse. If it weakens or disappears, the orthopedic surgeon must be informed *immediately* since irreversible ischemia may result. Fasciotomy may become necessary.
- Assess for paresthesias (prickling and burning sensations) in the hand since such signs may indicate nerve injury or impending ischemia. Early treatment is indicated to restore circulation before irreparable damage occurs.
- Encourage the patient to move his fingers frequently.

Fractures and Dislocations Above the Elbow

Fractures above the elbow usually occur from a fall on the elbow or an outstretched hand or by a direct blow such as may occur in a side-swipe injury. If the fracture is not displaced, the arm is immobilized in a cast with the elbow at 45 to 90 degrees of flexion; or the elbow may be supported with a pressure dressing and a sling.

A displaced fracture is usually treated by open reduction and internal fixation. Sometimes the bone fragments are excised. Additional external support with a plaster splint is then applied.

This type of fracture may result in nerve damage from injury to the median, radial or ulnar nerves. The patient is evaluated for paresthesias and also for signs of compromised circulation in the forearm and hand. Active exercise of the elbow is carried out when prescribed as limitation of motion is common unless an intensive rehabilitation program is done.

Radius and Ulna

HEAD AND NECK OF THE RADIUS. These fractures are usually produced by a fall on the outstretched hand with the elbow in extension. If blood has collected in the elbow joint (hemarthrosis) it is aspirated to relieve pain and allow early range of motion. Immobilization is accomplished by a plaster slab or sling.

If the fracture is displaced, an open operation is required, with excision of the radial head when necessary. Postoperatively the arm is immobilized in a posterior plaster splint and sling. The patient is encouraged to carry out a program of active motion of the elbow and forearm when prescribed.

FRACTURES OF THE SHAFTS OF THE RADIUS AND ULNA. Fractures of the shaft of the bones of the forearm occur frequently in children and are not uncommon in adults. Either the radius or the ulna alone or both bones may be broken at any level. The forearm has the unique functions of pronation and supination and those motions must be preserved by good anatomical position and alignment. The ulna has a relatively poor blood supply and unfortunately nonunion of this fracture occurs at times.

If the fragments are not displaced, the fracture is treated by closed reduction with a long-arm cast applied from the upper arm to the proximal palmar crease. A wire loop may be incorporated in the cast near the elbow and a sling pulled through it to prevent the cast from sagging against the forearm.

The circulation and motion of the hand is assessed after the cast is applied. Frequent finger flexion and extension are encouraged to reduce edema. Active motion of the involved shoulder is essential.

For displaced fractures, open operation is frequently done with internal fixation obtained by applying a compression plate with screws or inserting some other fixation device. The arm is usually immobilized in plaster splints or a cast until there is evidence of healing.

Fractures of the Wrist and Hand

FRACTURES OF THE WRIST. A fracture of the distal radius (Colles' fracture) is a common fracture and is usually the result of a fall on an open hand. It is frequently seen in an elderly person whose bones are osteoporotic.

Treatment usually consists of closed reduction and immobilization with a cast or plaster-and-pin fixation to control pronation and supination so that reduction will not be lost. (A sugar-tong splint is sometimes used.) For more severe fractures, traction may be used to maintain length or a Kirschner wire inserted through the distal fragments to maintain reduction.

The wrist and forearm are elevated for 48 hours after reduction. Swelling of the fingers (from decreased venous and lymph return) is watched for and actively treated. Observe for constricting bandages or cast.

The patient is taught to do the following finger exercises to reduce swelling and prevent stiffness:
1. Hold the hand above the level of the heart.
2. Move the fingers from full extension to flexion. Hold and release.
3. Repeat at least 10 times every half hour when awake as long as the hand has a tendency to swell.

FRACTURES OF THE HAND. Since trauma to the hand can be such a complex problem, one requiring extensive reconstructive surgery, the reader is referred to specialized books on the hand. The objective of treatment is always to regain maximum function of the hand.

For an undisplaced fracture of the distal phalanx (finger bone), the finger is splinted to the adjoining finger to relieve pain and to protect the fingertip from further trauma. Boxing glove dressings are useful in those hand injuries that may cause swelling. Open fractures may be reduced by means of Kirschner wires.

LOWER EXTREMITY FRACTURES

The objectives of management of a fracture of the lower extremity are (1) to obtain adequate bony union with full length and normal alignment and without rotational or angular deformity, (2) to restore muscle power and joint motion, and (3) to allow weight bearing.

Special Rehabilitation Nursing Measures

- A fractured lower extremity is not to be placed in a dependent position for prolonged periods since *edema is a common problem* following all injuries of the lower extremities.
- The patient is encouraged to exercise regularly all joints which do not move the bone fragments.
- The extremity is elevated intermittently when the patient becomes ambulatory to minimize recurrence of edema. It is best for the patient to lie down when elevating the cast.
- After the cast is removed, elastic stockings can be worn to support venous circulation, thus reducing the problem of edema.

Since practically all fractures of the lower extremity require the use of crutches during convalescence, adjustable crutches should be secured for the patient. They should be about 2.5 cm. (1 inch) longer than the distance from the axilla to the heel and should be fitted with rubber suction tips as well as axillary and hand cushions. (The various gaits used in crutch walking are discussed in Chapter 12.)

Femur

Fractures of the femur can occur at several sites (Fig. 58-10). When the head, neck, or trochanteric region of the femur is involved, a hip fracture results. The management of this type of fracture will be covered after fractures of the shaft of the femur are discussed.

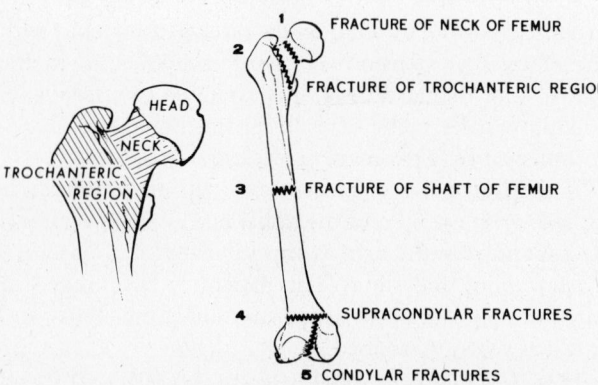

Figure 58-10. Sites of fracture of the femur.

SHAFT OF THE FEMUR. In adults considerable violence is required to break the shaft of the femur. Therefore, extensive damage to soft tissue and muscle, severe displacement of bone fragments and blood loss usually accompany this injury. These fractures occur most commonly in youth and middle age.

Fixation with an intramedullary (within the bone) nail or a compression plate can constitute the treatment of uncomplicated fractures of the femoral shaft. When there is evidence of early union across the fracture site, the patient may be started on weight-bearing activities. Once stability is achieved, a cast-brace may be used in conjunction with internal fixation.

If the fracture is comminuted, reduction may be accomplished by traction in which a Thomas splint is used to support the limb. A Pearson attachment applied to the splint allows knee flexion and supports the leg below the knee. Skeletal traction in the long axis of the thigh is applied by means of a Kirschner wire (or a Steinmann pin). Some orthopedic surgeons apply upward as well as horizontal traction on the lower fragment (Fig. 58-11). This treatment requires a traction frame to which pulleys may be attached for traction.

The fracture may be immobilized for 10 to 12 weeks, at the end of which time the patient may be permitted to walk with the aid of crutches. Full weight-bearing is not usually allowed for at least 6 months. To preserve the muscle strength, the patient should exercise the lower leg, foot, and toes on a regular regimen. A more recent variation in this treatment consists of applying a cast-brace (page 1284) after 2 to 4 weeks of traction, at which time the patient begins partial weight-bearing.

A common complication following fracture of the femoral shaft is restriction of knee motion. Thus quadriceps setting exercises and foot and ankle exercise should be started early. Active and passive knee exercises are done when enough healing has occurred.

Hip Fractures

There is a high incidence of hip fractures among elderly people because their bones are brittle from osteoporosis and they fall readily from weakness of the quadriceps as well as from general fraility due to age and a sedentary existence. Falls in the elderly also occur because of conditions which produce a decrease in cerebral arterial perfusion (transient ischemic attacks, anemia, emboli, cardiovascular disease, drug effects). Their therapeutic and nursing management is further complicated by associated medical diseases (cardiovascular, pulmonary, renal and endocrine disorders). Hip fractures are the most frequent cause of traumatic death after the age of 75, occurring more frequently in women, often after insignificant injuries. A hip fracture is viewed by the patient and the family as a catastrophic event that will make a negative impact on the patient's life style.

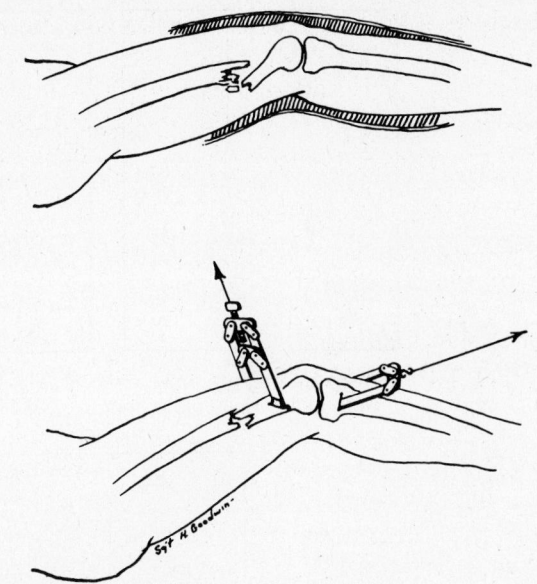

Figure 58-11. Diagrammatic representation of 2-wire skeletal traction for fracture of femur in distal third. (*Top*) Deformity on admission to hospital. (*Bottom*) Adequate reduction when additional wire is inserted in lower femoral fragment and vertical lift is secured. (From Hampton, O. P., Jr.: Wounds of the Extremities in Military Surgery. St. Louis, C. V. Mosby, p. 273)

Classification. Several types of hip fractures may occur: fractures of the neck of the femur (intracapsular), fractures of the trochanteric region of the femur (includes fractures between the base of the neck and the lesser trochanter of the femur) and subtrochanteric fractures.

Fractures of the neck of the femur have more difficulty in healing than those of the trochanteric region, because the vascular system supplying blood to the head and neck of the femur may be easily damaged with the fracture. The nutrient vessels within the bone may be interrupted and the bone cells may die. For this reason, nonunion or aseptic necrosis is common in patients with these types of fractures.

Clinical Manifestations. Because of the fracture, the leg is shortened and externally rotated. The patient complains of severe pain and is usually not able to move the extremity. If the fracture is impacted, shortening and external rotation may not be evident, and the patient may complain of slight pain in the groin or in the medial side of the knee. The diagnosis is confirmed by roentgenograms.

Preoperative Management. Surgical intervention is carried out as soon as possible after the injury. The preoperative objective is to ensure that the patient is in as favorable condition as possible. Temporary skin traction in the form of Buck's extension (page 1286) can be applied to relieve pain and allow for some mobility. Thromboembolism is the most common complication following hip fracture and occurs frequently without clinical signs. To prevent thromboembolism, anticoagulation therapy

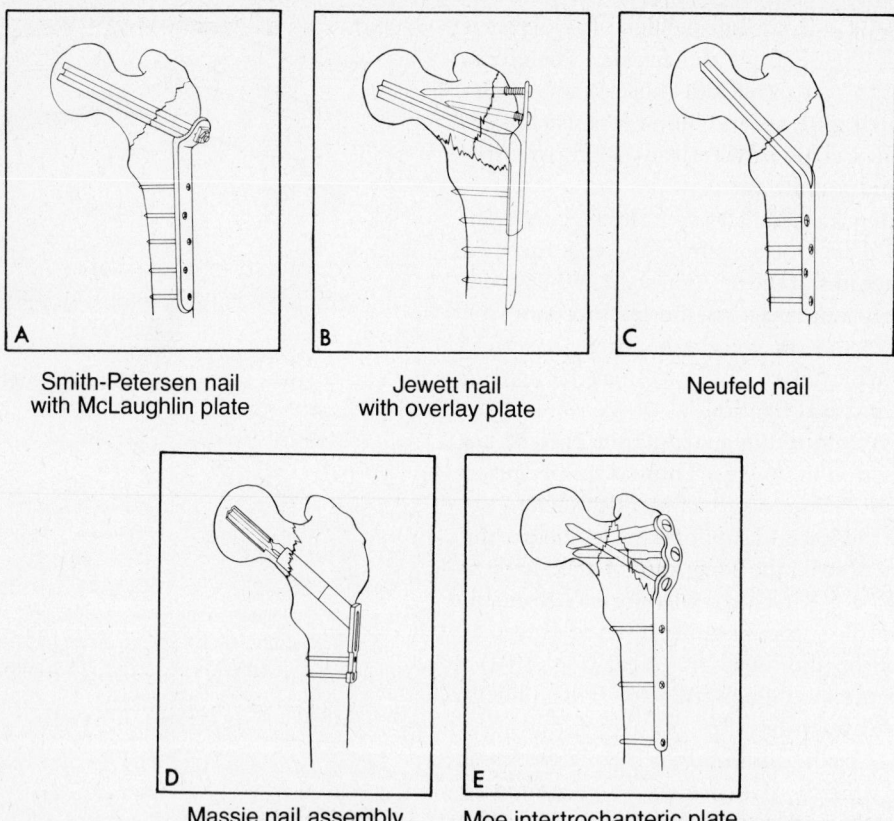

A Smith-Petersen nail with McLaughlin plate

B Jewett nail with overlay plate

C Neufeld nail

D Massie nail assembly

E Moe intertrochanteric plate

Figure 58-12.   Examples of internal fixation for trochanteric fractures. In fractures of the femoral neck and trochanteric region, internal fixation is achieved through the use of nails which are flanged in various configurations for stability inside the bone, and with plates which provide additional stability and fixation. *A.* Smith-Petersen nail with McLaughlin plate. *B.* Jewett nail with overlay plate. *C.* Neufeld nail. *D.* Massie nail assembly. *E.* Moe intertrochanteric plate. (Courtesy Zimmer-USA, Warsaw, Ind.)

such as subcutaneous low dose heparin, warfarin, low-molecular weight dextran or aspirin may be given from the time the patient is admitted to the hospital until he or she is fully mobilized.

During the preoperative period, the patient should be assessed as to orientation to time, place and person. Many of these elderly persons are confused, not only as a result of stress of the trauma but also because of underlying systemic illness. Mental alertness, bright facial expression and good skin turgor are considered signs of a favorable prognosis. Additional nursing management is directed toward assessing for possible dehydration, which is frequently seen in elderly patients, and encouraging movement of all but the involved hip and knee, along with deep breathing and coughing exercises to ensure adequate pulmonary ventilation.

Operative Treatment.   Operative treatment consists of (1) reduction of the fracture and internal fixation or (2) replacement of the femoral head with a prosthesis.

After general or spinal anesthesia, the fracture is reduced under radiographic control using an image-intensifier. A stable fracture is usually fixed with nails, a nail-and-plate combination, multiple pins, screws, etc. (See Fig. 58-12). The choice of fixation device is determined by the fracture site and the preference of the orthopedic surgeon.

When the nails are placed through the trochanter along the neck of the femur and into the head, the patient may be up and in a chair within a few days or less. It is desirable that these patients be taught to use a walker as soon as possible and that no weight or only partial weight be placed on the affected extremity, depending on the fracture and the type of fixation used.

In a trochanteric fracture of the femur, the operative method is carried out with a nail-plate type of fixation. This patient may also be out of bed using a nonweight-bearing technique (see page 1308). Although the blood supply in a trochanteric fracture is maintained fairly well so that fractures at this site almost always unite, there is a fairly high mortality rate, mainly because the patients are generally older (70 to 85) and are poorer operative risks. Their conditions are further compromised by the degree of soft tissue damage that occurs at the time of injury. Added difficulties can be anticipated when the fracture is comminuted and unstable, as is frequently the case.

Replacement of the head of the femur with a prosthesis

Primary objectives: 1. To prevent physical, psychological and social dependence
2. To restore the ambulatory function of the hip joint (if the patient was ambulatory before the fracture)

Nursing Action	Rationale

PREOPERATIVE MANAGEMENT

I. To attain mobilization of the patient:

Elderly patients tolerate inactivity poorly. Inactivity predisposes to pressure sores, thromboembolism, pneumonia and senile dementia.

A. Prepare the bed with a trapeze and flotation mattress.
B. Alleviate the pain.
   1. Handle the affected extremity gently.
   2. Give analgesics as patient's condition indicates.
   3. Utilize proper positioning techniques.
   4. Keep the skin dry and relieve pressure areas.

Pressure sores develop rapidly in the preoperative period from immobilization.

   5. Assist with the application of Buck's extension as indicated.

Buck's extension is used in intertrochanteric fractures to afford patient mobilization and relieve pain until the operative procedure is performed.
A patient with an intracapsular fracture will assume a flexed position. The extremity may be supported in this position with pillows until surgery is performed.

     a. Inspect the heel daily. Massage area around the heel at intervals.

A patient with a painful hip tends to let the weight of the leg press the heel against the bed. The heel loses sensation when the blood supply diminishes resulting in necrosis of nerve endings.

     b. Place a sheepskin pad under the leg.
     c. Check compression wrap and traction frequently.
C. Ensure that the patient is in as favorable condition as possible preoperatively.
   1. Coordinate ECG, blood chemistry studies, arterial blood gas analysis, and x-ray evaluation procedures.

Elderly patients in poor condition with prefracture disabilities and associated diseases are considered poor risks.

   2. Give intravenous infusions *slowly.*

Patients with limited cardiac reserve cannot stand additional circulatory loading.

   3. Carry out ongoing nursing assessment.

Mental alertness, bright facial expression and good skin turgor are considered favorable prognostic indications.

     a. Determine if patient is oriented to time, place and person.

Mental confusion may be due to underlying systemic illness, particularly cardiopulmonary disease with inadequate cerebral oxygen transport.

     b. Use anticipatory nursing assessment and techniques to avoid complications.

Thromboembolism is the most common complication following hip fracture, and it frequently occurs without clinical signs.

       (1) Give prescribed anticoagulant (warfarin, aspirin, etc.)
       (2) Elevate foot of bed 25 degrees to promote venous drainage.

POSTOPERATIVE NURSING MANAGEMENT

II. To maintain physical and mental capabilities:
A. Encourage the patient to move independently as much as possible.

Active motion decreases the likelihood of complications (thromboembolism, diminished cerebral perfusion, aspiration of secretions and pneumonia, gastrointestinal stasis, urinary problems, increase in bone mineral loss and pressure sores).

   1. Teach the patient to assist with turning by grasping the bedrails for support.
   2. Support the affected extremity in a position of abduction when the patient turns on his side.

(Continued)

Objectives, Principles and Rationale of Nursing Management

Nursing Action	Rationale

POSTOPERATIVE NURSING MANAGEMENT (CONTINUED)

II. To maintain physical and mental capabilities (continued):

    3. Place pillow between legs while patient is in side-lying position.

    4. Start the prescribed exercise program.

  B. Get the patient out of bed as soon as possible.

    1. Wrap the lower extremities with elastic compression bandages or elastic hose.

> Wrapping the extremities supports venous circulation and helps minimize dependent edema. Active motion is an effective method of relieving edema.

    2. Use the tilt table as soon as patient's condition permits.

> With the use of the tilt table the patient becomes accustomed to the upright position. Circulatory and respiratory functioning improve.

    3. Assist the patient into a wheelchair several times daily as prescribed.

      a. With the aid of the overhead trapeze, encourage the patient to move into the dangle position (use a Hi-lo bed).

      b. Assist the patient to stand on the *unaffected extremity* and to transfer to a chair.

> Getting out of bed is valuable exercise; it helps the patient avoid hypotension, helps maintain strength, aids pulmonary function and is beneficial psychologically. However, certain types of fractures must be supported until bone union is secure and displacement of fracture unlikely. Sometimes the patient may have to be lifted in the chair or transferred to the chair using a non-weight-bearing technique.

      c. If weight-bearing is permitted, the patient may be encouraged to ambulate with a walker, applying as much weight to the extremity as is comfortable.

      d. For patient with replacement prosthesis—the hip should be kept in abduction, extension and slight external rotation.

    4. Encourage the patient to participate in activities of daily living (eating, bathing, hair care, dressing).

> Participation in A.D.L. helps condition the patient for future ambulation activities and establishes a degree of independence. Getting dressed is an outward symbol of independence and a release of the sick role. It is also excellent exercise.

    5. Start active exercises as soon as pain and soreness subside to prepare the patient to walk.

      a. Encourage quadriceps setting exercises hourly.

> The quadriceps femoris muscle extends the leg and is one of the major muscles necessary for ambulation.

      b. Do heel cord stretching of both legs.

      c. Use isometric muscle contractions of the abdominal and gluteal muscles.

> Isometric muscle contractions strengthen the muscles.

      d. Assist the patient to perform arm strengthening exercises (flexion and extension of the arms).

> The muscles in the shoulder girdle and upper extremities must be strong enough to bear the patient's weight when a walker is used.

      e. Assist the patient to learn to use the walker ambulating with a nonweight-bearing or partial weight-bearing technique *depending on the type of fracture and its fixation.*

> Remind the patient *not* to bear weight on the affected extremity until the orthopedist gives permission and the x-rays reveal sufficient healing. Early weight-bearing before bony union exerts too much stress and may bend or break the pin, crush the bone, or cause loss of fixation due to the device cutting through the bone.

III. To be alert for and prevent complications:

> Complications have a serious prognostic significance leading to death in the elderly. Anticipation of complications help in their prevention.

  A. Watch for signs and symptoms of:

    1. Thromboembolism: Examine for evidence of thrombophlebitis.

> Prophylactic anticoagulation may be given preoperatively and postoperatively.

Nursing Action	Rationale

POSTOPERATIVE NURSING MANAGEMENT (CONTINUED)

III. To be alert for and prevent complications (continued):

2. Pneumonia	Pneumonia is a common terminal event in the elderly.
a. Have the patient breathe deeply and cough at intervals.	
b. Use incentive spirometer to maximize voluntary lung inflation as prescribed.	
3. Fat embolism (characterized by fever, tachycardia, dyspnea, cough) (See page 1299.)	Fat embolism sometimes occurs after fractures of the long bones, particularly in elderly patients.
4. Heart failure	
5. Knee contractures	There is a functional inter-relationship of the knee joint with the hip joint that is essential for ambulation. There is a tendency to flex the knee when hip joint pain is present.
a. *Maintain the knee in a position of extension while in bed.*	Do not place a pillow under the knee, because this encourages flexion contraction.
b. *Flex the knee in a 90-degree angle while the patient is in the chair.*	Avoid extending the knee when the patient is in a sitting position, because extension produces undue strain on the fractured hip.
c. Move the knee through assisted range of motion exercises.	
6. Urinary tract infection	
a. Avoid the routine use of an indwelling catheter.	Infection almost always follows the presence of an indwelling catheter. A urinary tract infection can cause a prolonged period of morbidity and incontinence in the elderly.
b. Watch the color, odor and volume of urinary output.	
c. Maintain a liberal fluid intake (within limits of cardiorenal function).	
7. Pressure sores	Peripheral arterial insufficiency, poor nutrition and lack of movement from pain contribute to skin breakdown.
a. Encourage the patient to move about freely using the overhead trapeze as an assistive device.	
b. Inspect the heels daily.	
(1) Use protective heel padding.	
(2) Massage reddened areas.	
8. Infection	Infection is usually related to intercurrent medical problems, debility and infection elsewhere in the body.
9. Nonunion and avascular necrosis	
10. Dislocation of the prosthesis	
11. Internal fixation device cutting through bone	

is usually reserved for a fracture that cannot be satisfactorily reduced or securely nailed. Some orthopedists prefer this method because nonunion and avascular necrosis of the head are common complications of internal fixation techniques. However, it appears that after prosthetic replacement, the morbidity rate (infection and dislocation of the prosthesis) and mortality rates are higher than with reduction by internal fixation. Total hip replacement (page 1336) may be used in selected patients who cannot be treated satisfactorily.

Postoperative Nursing Care

Turning

The patient may be turned on the unaffected extremity by means of the following method:

• A pillow is placed between the legs to keep the affected leg in an abducted position. Then the patient is pulled over gently on his or her side. After initial soreness has gone and the incision is healed, the patient usually may be turned in the same manner on the affected hip.

Exercise

It is also important that the patient exercise as much as possible by means of the trapeze suspended from the fracture bed. However, despite the use of the trapeze, triceps and shoulder exercises should be continued preparatory to ambulatory activities.

(The nursing management of the patient with a hip fracture is summarized on pages 1307–1309.)

Complications. Elderly persons who suffer hip fractures are particularly prone to develop complications that may require more vigorous treatment than the fracture itself. In some instances, the shock of the injury may prove fatal. In less drastic responses, shock following this traumatic experience may cause bladder incontinence, although urinary control is usually gradually regained. In general, the routine use of an indwelling catheter is to be avoided. Yet urinary problems may occur. Therefore, the color, odor, and the volume of urine are monitored to detect problems such as urinary retention, which is common following orthopedic operations, especially in the elderly. To assure proper kidney function, a liberal fluid intake is important.

As in many postoperative situations, thromboembolism is the most common complication. To prevent thromboembolism, preoperative and postoperative prophylactic anticoagulation therapy is frequently used. To detect its occurrence, the patient's legs are checked daily for evidence of thrombophlebitis.

Pulmonary complications are also a threat in elderly patients undergoing hip surgery. Deep breathing exercises, a change of position at least every 2 hours and possible use of an incentive spirometer help to prevent the development of respiratory complications.

Because patients with hip fractures generally have poor circulation and tend to remain in one position, pressure sores frequently develop. Giving proper skin care, especially to the back and heels and under the hips and shoulders, helps relieve the constant pressure. An air or flotation mattress may provide adequate protection by relieving pressure.

Fracture of the Tibia and Fibula

The most common fracture below the knee is a fracture of the lower portion of the fibula which results from "twisting the ankle." Frequently associated with such a fracture is fracture of the internal malleolus and the posterior portion of the articular surface of the tibia. Swelling and discoloration about the ankle are marked. Fractures of the shafts of the tibia and fibula may occur in association with each other. Considerable swelling also accompanies such fractures. These fractures may require prolonged immobilization because union is slow due to the poor blood supply to the distal part of the tibia.

The treatment of tibial fractures is somewhat challenging because an open fracture may be involved due to the fact that the tibia lies superficially beneath the skin throughout its entire length. With open fractures, there is a high incidence of infection. Opinion varies on the treatment of these fractures. The fracture(s) may be managed by manipulation and the reduction maintained by the application of a long-leg plaster cast. In time the long-leg cast may be replaced with a below-the-knee functional cast which permits motion at the knee joint and weight-bearing. Or a cast-brace may be used (Fig. 57-4).

A more complicated fracture (oblique or spiral fracture) usually requires open reduction and fixation (intermedullary nail or plate) as determined by the etiology, type of trauma and type of fracture.

Internal Derangement of the Knee

Injury to most joints consists of a tear of the supporting ligaments. In the knee joint, however, there may also be a displacement or tear of the semilunar cartilages, which are two crescent-shaped cartilages attached to the edge of the shallow articulating surface of the head of the tibia. They normally move slightly backward and forward to accommodate the change in the shape of the condyles of the femur when the leg is in flexion or extension. In sports and in certain accidents, the body is often twisted with the foot fixed. Since little torsion movement is normally permitted in the knee joint, either the cartilage is torn from its attachment to the head of the tibia or an actual tear or fracture of the cartilage itself occurs.

These injuries leave a loose cartilage in the knee joint that may slip between the femur and the tibia, preventing full extension of the leg. If this happens when the patient is walking or running, he often describes his disability as his "leg giving way" under him. The patient may hear or feel a click in his knee when he walks, especially when he extends the leg bearing his weight, as in going upstairs. When the cartilage is attached front and back, but torn loose laterally (bucket-handle tear), it may slide between the bones to lie between the condyles and prevent full flexion or extension. As a result, the knee "locks."

These various types of injury are spoken of as internal derangements of the knee joint, and they produce a disturbing disability because the patient never knows when the knee will give him trouble. The treatment of this disability is removal of the injured cartilage. This can be done through an incision into the knee joint. The joint function can return to normal, and no apparent disability will result from the loss of the cartilage.

Postoperative Nursing Care. After suture of the wound, a pressure dressing is applied, and at times a posterior splint. The leg should be elevated on pillows with a slight bend at the knee. The most common complication is an effusion into the knee joint which produces marked pain. If this occurs, the physician should be called. Relief can be obtained by cutting the pressure dressing and reapplying it more losely. The joint may be aspirated under local anesthesia and pressure relieved by withdrawing the fluid in the joint.

To prevent atrophy of the thigh muscles, these patients are instructed to contract their quadriceps muscles while in bed. After 1 or 2 days the patient may be up using crutches to bear his weight. In a short time (1 to 2 weeks), full unsupported weight-bearing is possible. The knee usually is supported for another few weeks by an elastic bandage. Additional exercises are given to continue the quadriceps building program. Full and normal function may be expected in 6 to 8 weeks from the time of operation.

FRACTURES OF THE LUMBAR AND DORSAL SPINE

The Vertebral Body

Injuries to the vertebrae of the dorsal and lumbar spine may involve (1) the vertebral body, (2) the lamina and articulating processes and (3) the spinous processess or transverse processes. Fractures of the vertebral body are compression fractures. They are often multiple and comprise the most common type of fractures of the spine. The majority of vertebral fractures seem to be related to osteoporosis.

A person with a fracture of a vertebral body complains of severe pain in the back, which may radiate down the legs or to the abdomen and chest. *The most important considerations are to determine if there is injury to the spinal cord and if the fracture is stable or unstable.* Spinal cord injury may occur if any of the vertebra has been dislocated. Assessment and treatment of patients with spinal cord injury is discussed on pages 1253-1257.

• Frequently, after a compression fracture of the lower dorsal or lumbar spine, the patient experiences paralytic ileus and difficulty in voiding the first few days. Undoubtedly, this is the major nursing problem at this time. The treatment and nursing aspects of the patient with paralytic ileus are found on page 789.

If the fracture of the lower dorsal or lumbar spine is without complication, the patient is placed on a firm mattress and kept at bed rest until the pain subsides (days to weeks). When ready for ambulation he may be fitted with a back support or a full-length back brace to support the region of the fracture. Exercises are prescribed to increase and maintain the strength of the back muscles. Patients with stable injuries to the vertebrae are treated symptomatically for pain and encouraged to ambulate immediately.

If the fracture is displaced or unstable, it may be reduced by postural positioning, protracted periods of immobilization or open operation with internal fixation. The patient may then be placed in a body case for immobilization. The nursing care of a patient in a cast is discussed on pages 1282-1285.

Fractures of the Transverse Process

For fractures of the transverse process, the patient is permitted to ambulate if the fracture is not severe. If there is displacement and soft tissue injury the patient is placed on bed rest followed by support in a corset or brace.

Following a fracture of the lumbar and dorsal spine, the patient is mobilized when physical examination and x-ray examination determine that there is no displacement or neurological deficit.

Pelvic Fractures

Pelvic fractures commonly occur as a result of automobile accidents, crush injuries and falls from buildings and scaffolds. General symptoms include local swelling, tenderness over the symphysis pubis, anterior spines, iliac crest, sacrum or coccyx, and inability to bear weight without discomfort. In addition, shock and hemorrhage may occur. Pelvic fractures are serious because at least two-thirds of these patients have significant and multiple injuries. (The care of the patient with multiple injuries is discussed on page 1424.) Therefore a high mortality rate accompanies these fractures. Death may ensue from local hemorrhage in view of the rich blood supply to the pelvis and the possibility of massive and hidden bleeding in the retroperitoneal region. Bleeding also arises from the cancellous surfaces of the fracture fragments and the laceration of veins and arteries by bone spicules. There is also the added danger of intra-abdominal hemorrhage from a torn iliac artery. In addition to hemorrhage, the bladder, the urethra or the intestines may be ruptured, a condition that can prove to be more serious than the fracture itself.

Management. The objective of management is to carry out ongoing and continuing nursing assessment for injuries to the bladder, rectum, intestines and intra-abdominal organs. To check for possible damage to the urinary tract, the patient is requested to void so that the urine can be examined for blood. All subsequent urine and stools are saved for a period of time and examined for blood. A cystourethrogram and intravenous urogram are often done if injury to the urinary tract is suspected. Since hemorrhage is possible in these injuries, the abdomen is examined for evidence of intra-abdominal hemorrhage. The peripheral pulses of both lower extremities are palpated since absence of peripheral pulses may indicate the possibility of a torn iliac artery or one of its branches. The patient is carefully and gently handled to minimize further bleeding and shock.

If there is evidence of bleeding, the immediate objective is to restore the circulating volume and initiate emergency treatment of intrathoracic, intra-abdominal and intracranial injuries. An external compression suit (Medical Anti-Shock Trousers [MAST]) may be applied to the body below the diaphragm to control the hemorrhage and combat shock. The suit is deflated at intervals to evaluate whether or not hemorrhaging has recurred and to inspect the skin. Pulmonary support (humidified oxygen, arterial gas measurement, endotracheal intubation, and mechanical ventilation, PEEP) may be required. Operative treatment is usually required for ruptured abdominal or pelvic viscera and occasionally for hemorrhage. Bleeding from the bones and the veins may stop spontaneously unless the fractures are not prevented from moving.

Most fractures of the pelvis heal rapidly since the in-

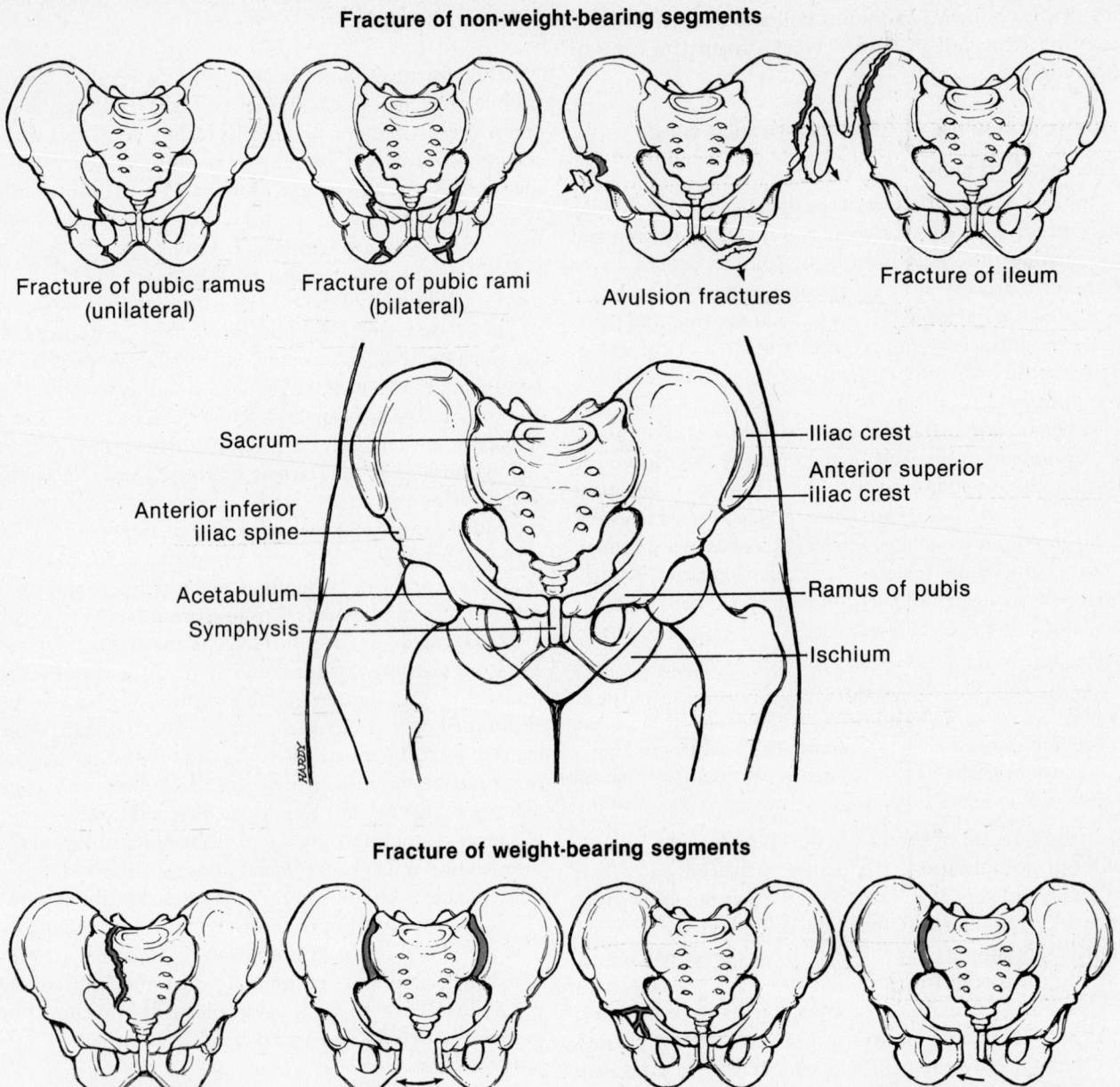

Fracture of non-weight-bearing segments

Fracture of pubic ramus
(unilateral)

Fracture of pubic rami
(bilateral)

Avulsion fractures

Fracture of ileum

Sacrum

Anterior inferior
iliac spine

Acetabulum

Symphysis

Iliac crest

Anterior superior
iliac crest

Ramus of pubis

Ischium

Fracture of weight-bearing segments

Fracture of sacrum

Separation of symphysis

Fracture of acetabulum

Fracture of hemipelvis

Figure 58-13.   Fractures of the pelvis.

nominate bones are made up mostly of cancellous bone which has a rich blood supply. Nonoperative treatment consists of bed rest, skeletal traction with a pelvic sling or the application of a double hip spica cast to immobilize the fracture. The type of immobilization depends on the location of the fracture.

For many patients with fractures of the sacrum and pelvis without disruption of the pelvic ring (Fig. 58-13), rest in bed is all that is required. A bedboard is desirable under the mattress to give more stability. The patient is turned as a unit. For fractures that disrupt the pelvic ring or involve weight-bearing areas (Fig. 58-13), skeletal traction is used.

When both sides of the pelvis are fractured, a pelvic sling is used to immobilize the pelvis into a single unit so that the patient can move the rest of his body with less pain. The pelvic sling lifts the weight of the pelvis very slightly from the mattress (Fig. 58-14A). The sling may be folded back over the buttocks in order to permit the patient to use the bedpan. (Some orthopedists permit the sling to be loosened for certain nursing care activities if the patient's condition permits.) Since skin care is a problem, sheep skin may be used to line the sling to prevent excoriation. It is necessary to reach under the sling to give skin care.

If separation of the symphysis pubis has occurred, a compression force must be applied. This is obtained by crossing the ropes from the sling to the weights on the opposite side (Fig. 58-14B). The pelvic sling is adjusted to exert a compression effect from side to side to correct the separation of bones. Since the sling exerts pressure over the trochanteric region, the patient may become quite uncomfortable from soreness over the area. When acetabular fractures occur, open reduction is usually necessary.

When bony healing has taken place in a pelvic fracture, the patient is mobilized with a method of progressive weight-bearing, usually with crutches.

AMPUTATION

Amputation of an extremity is frequently necessary as a result of peripheral vascular disease, trauma (destruction by crushing injuries, burns, frostbite, electrical burns), congenital deformities and malignant tumor. Of all these reasons, vascular disease accounts for the majority of amputations of the lower extremities.

Psychological Considerations. Amputation forces anyone to make a major adjustment. Even those patients who have suffered with debilitating and painful diseases due to circulatory problems of the legs must adjust to the loss of an extremity. The way a patient adapts to an amputation depends not only on his physical condition and the ability to use a prosthetic device, but also on his perception of the disability. An amputation produces a permanent physical handicap that certainly thwarts some physiological, psychological, and social needs. The patient must accept these limitations realistically. Physicians, nurses, prosthetists, and physical therapists share the task of helping the amputee make the necessary changes in the pattern of living, with minimal interference in life activities.

LOWER EXTREMITY AMPUTATIONS

Preoperative Care. Before surgery, the circulatory status of the limb must be assessed in relation to surface temperature, color changes when the limb is elevated or placed in a dependent position, oscillometric readings and arteriography. The circulatory status of the sound limb is also evaluated. Effort is made to control infection or gangrene. If the limb is gangrenous, it may be packed in ice to reduce absorption of toxic products and improve the condition of the patient. The patient's nutritional status is determined and improved if necessary. Dehydration, anemia, cardiac insufficiency and diabetes mellitus are treated so that the patient is in the best possible condition to withstand the trauma of surgery.

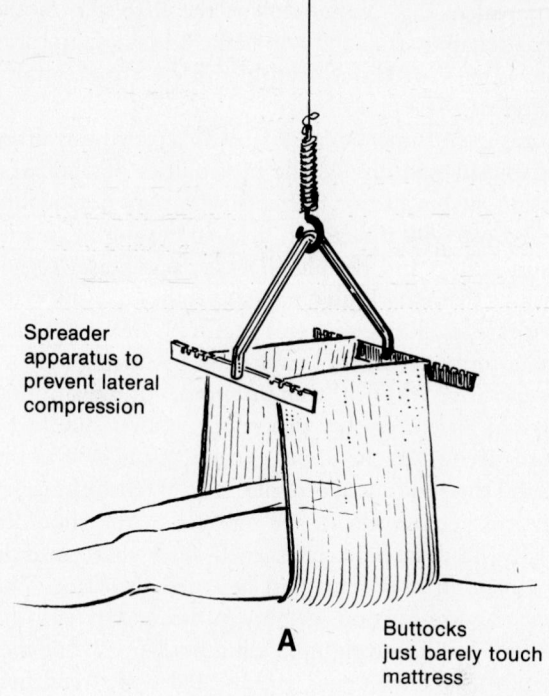

Spreader apparatus to prevent lateral compression

A

Buttocks just barely touch mattress

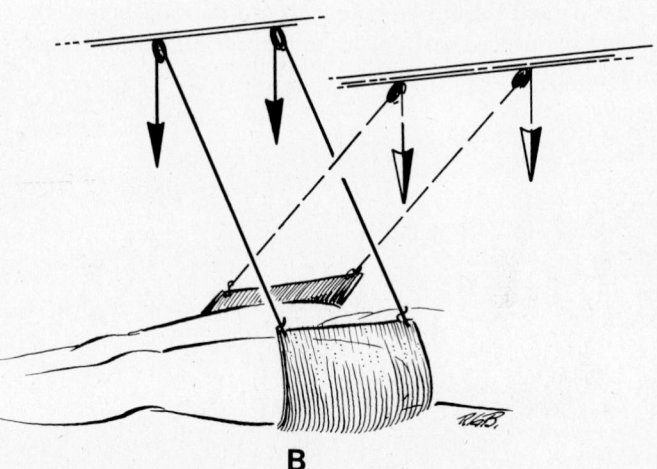

B

Figure 58-14. Pelvic sling suspension for fractures of the pelvis. (A) A suspension of the pelvis without an attempt at compression. The sling is suspended by means of a large metal frame, and weight is applied so that the pelvis is largely counterbalanced and becomes, to a certain extent, "weightless." Movement can then occur without moving the pelvic fragments. (B) The method for applying compression when there has been separation of the anterior pelvic ring, particularly at the symphysis pubis. The suspension in this type of traction is not as great, but is effective to a certain extent. This suspension compresses the pelvis from side to side to correct any diastasis that may have occurred. Pain developing at pressure points over the trochanters is unavoidable; it will often limit the duration of time that compression traction is useful. (From Lewis, R. C.: Handbook of Traction, Casting and Splinting Techniques. Philadelphia, J. B. Lippincott, 1977)

Psychological preparation should not be neglected. Knowing what to expect helps reduce anxiety. Optimism and motivation can be fostered by helping the patient realize that amputation is the first step in the patient's rehabilitation and will make it possible to carry out activities of daily living and be functionally independent.

Some patients may be candidates for a prosthesis. If so, the physician will discuss the possibilities of obtaining and using such a device. Patients who may not qualify include those with infections, delayed healing of an amputation stump and peripheral vascular disease. Other conditions that may limit a patient's ability to walk with a prosthesis include: diabetes mellitus, heart disease, stroke, arteriosclerosis obliterans and advancing age.

Preoperative Physical Conditioning. If the amputation is not an emergency procedure, efforts should be made to strengthen the upper extremities as well as the trunk and the abdominal muscles. The extensor muscles in the arm and the depressor muscles in the shoulder especially need to be strengthened since these muscle groups play an important part in crutch walking. The patient may use traction weights to flex and extend the arms while holding weights. Doing push-ups while in a prone position and sit-ups while seated will strengthen the triceps muscles.

In addition to strengthening the muscles in the arms, the patient should be taught to crutch-walk before the surgical procedure in order to prepare for postoperative mobility (see page 198).

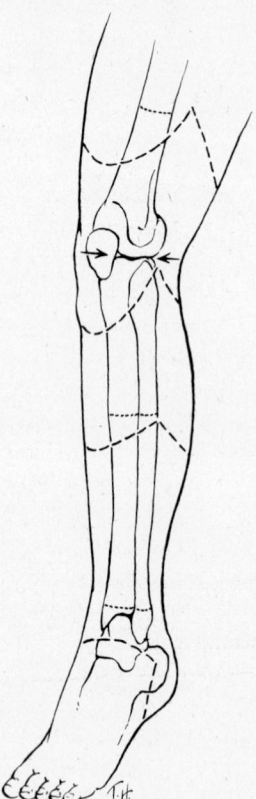

Figure 58-15. Levels of amputation are determined by circulatory adequacy, type of prosthesis, function of the part, and muscle balance.

Surgical Approach

Levels of Amputation. Amputations are usually performed by making soft-tissue flaps, which are used to cover the bone end. The site of the amputation is determined by two factors: circulation in the part and the requirements of the prosthesis. For the most part every attempt is made to preserve as much length as possible and to keep the knee and elbow joints intact. (Figure 58-15 shows the different levels at which a limb may be amputated.) Almost any level of amputation can be fitted with a prosthesis.

Often when amputations of the lower extremity are performed for gangrene of the foot due to vascular impairment, the stump is left open to allow for drainage. This is referred to as an open amputation. Frequently, following the amputation of one leg, the remaining leg may deteriorate from disuse and poor blood supply. If circulation is a problem in both legs, as may be the case with obliterative arteriosclerotic vascular disease, both limbs may need to be amputated in what is known as a bilateral lower extremity amputation.

Postoperative Management

Following the surgical procedure, a soft compression dressing or a rigid dressing may be applied. Each type of dressing requires a different type of management. The following discussion applies to the soft compression dressing. Management for the rigid dressing is discussed on page 1317.

The postoperative objectives are to rehabilitate the patient by promoting healing, preventing prolonged disability and attaining the best possible function of the residual portion of the extremity.

- Since hemorrhage is a possible postoperative complication, the patient should be watched carefully for any signs or symptoms of bleeding, including any evidence noted in the suction drainage. Immediate postoperative bleeding may develop slowly or take the form of a massive hemorrhage resulting from a loosened ligature.
- As a precaution against sudden hemorrhage, a tourniquet should be in plain sight so that if severe bleeding occurs, it can be applied to the stump and pulled sufficiently tight until the surgeon can be notified. The dressing is reinforced as required using aseptic techniques.

According to the surgeon's preference, the stump may be placed in an extended position or elevated for a brief period following surgery.

If the stump is to be elevated, the foot of the bed should be raised.

- The stump should not be placed on a pillow because a flexion contraction of the hip may result. A contracture of the next joint above the amputation is a frequent complication.

On occasion, especially when the amputation has been done for infection, a guillotine-type operation may be performed without any attempt to suture the skin. In such patients, to prevent the retraction of the skin, traction may be applied and eventual healing brought about. The principles given under Nursing Care of the Patient in Traction (page 1289) apply here.

During the first 24 hours, especially in older patients, a shock-like state frequently occurs so that the patient does not fully realize that the leg has been amputated. Often the realization may come as a shock, even though the patient knew before the operation that an amputation was to be performed. Because of the psychological trauma involved, it is important to accept the frustrations and behavior of the patient and to help him modify his self-image after the amputation; it will take time for the patient to make this adjustment.

Rehabilitation

Effective preprosthetic care is important to assure proper fitting of the prosthesis. The major problems that can delay the prosthetic fitting during this period are (1) flexion deformities, (2) nonshrinkage of the stump, and (3) abduction deformities of the hip. These deformities can be avoided.

In a lower extremity amputation after the first 24 to 48 hours, depending on the physician's preference, the patient should be encouraged to turn from side to side and to assume a prone position to stretch the flexor muscles and to prevent flexion contracture of the hip. A pillow can be placed under the abdomen and the stump with the forefoot resting over the edge of the mattress. The legs should remain close together while the patient is in the prone position to prevent an abduction deformity. It is important that the patient recognize the value of moving the stump.

The remaining leg and foot are examined daily and protected from injury. The pressure of the bedding should be kept off the foot.

Range of motion exercises (pages 183–190) are started early because contracture deformities develop rapidly. Range of motion is carried out to the hip and knee for below-the-knee amputations and to the hip for above-the-knee amputations.

If possible, an overhead trapeze can be used by the patient to change position and strengthen the biceps. However, this set of muscles is not as necessary in crutch-walking as are the triceps. The triceps can be strengthened by pressing the palms against the bed while pushing the body upward (push-up exercises). Exercises, such as hyperextension of the stump, conducted under the supervision of the physical therapist, also aid in strengthening muscles as well as increasing circulation, reducing edema, and preventing atrophy. When the patient gets out of bed, good posture must be maintained.

The patient should be fairly adept at balancing himself on one leg and walking with crutches before he leaves the hospital. Several weeks or many months may elapse before the patient is fitted with a prosthesis.

Exercises that assist in developing balance are:
1. Arising from a chair and standing
2. Standing on toes while holding on to a chair
3. Bending the knees while holding on to a chair
4. Balancing on one leg without support
5. Hopping on one foot while holding on to a chair

The nurse may stand behind the patient and stabilize him by his waist while he is learning to perform these exercises. While crutch-walking, the patient should learn to use a normal gait. The stump should move back and forth while the patient is walking with his crutches. The stump should not be held up in a flexed position to prevent a permanent flexion deformity from occurring.

Stump Conditioning. After the wound has healed, the stump should be bandaged as indicated by the surgeon. The patient or some member of the family can be taught the correct method of bandaging.

The stump has to be conditioned if a prosthesis is to be fitted properly. (However, not every patient can be fitted for a prosthetic device.) The stump must be shrunk and shaped into a conical form to permit accurate measurement and maximum comfort and fit of the prosthetic device. This is done by applying bandages, an elastic stump shrinker or an air splint. In some instances, a cast (rigid dressing) is applied soon after surgery.

Bandaging supports the soft tissue and minimizes the formation of edematous fluid while the stump is in a dependent position. The bandage is applied in such a manner that the remaining muscles required to operate the prosthesis are as firm as possible, while those muscles that are no longer useful will atrophy (Fig. 58-16). An improperly applied elastic bandage contributes to circulatory problems and a poorly-shaped stump. A guide to bandaging an amputation stump is found on page 1316.

In order to "toughen" the stump in preparation for a prosthesis, stump-conditioning activities are usually prescribed. The patient begins by pushing the stump into a soft pillow, then into a firmer pillow and finally against a hard surface. The patient is taught to massage the stump to mobilize the scar, decrease tenderness, and improve vascularity. Massage is usually started when healing takes place and is first done by the physical therapist.

When amputations of the leg have been performed on elderly, debilitated patients, especially those with diabetes and arteriosclerosis, particular care is taken to protect the stump against external infection. Such patients frequently become incontinent of urine and feces, and not infrequently the dressing and the wound of the stump may become soiled. In this event the stump is washed with soap and water. Plastic material secured by a wide

BANDAGING AN ABOVE-THE-KNEE AMPUTATION STUMP*

PURPOSE: The purpose for bandaging a stump is to shrink and to shape the stump for the application of an artificial leg.

PROBLEMS: Improper bandaging will produce:
a. Constriction of the stump
b. Delayed healing
c. Skin abrasions
d. Formation of creases or adipose tissue at distal end

BASIC PRINCIPLES: The bandage is applied before the patient gets out of bed after periods of recumbency. The bandage should be maintained continuously and reapplied when tension is lost. Pressure should be applied under moderate tension to the entire stump, guarding against any tourniquet-like action at the proximal portion of the stump. The stump is kept in *hyperextension* while the bandage is applied.

TECHNIQUE OF APPLYING BANDAGE

1. Begin the recurrent vertical turns on the anterior surface of the stump just inferior to the level of the inguinal ligament (Fig. 58-16A).

   Pass the bandage over the distal end of the stump posteriorly to the gluteal fold. The patient assists by holding the recurrents in pace.

   Make two additional recurrents over the medial and the lateral aspects of the end of the stump.

2. Anchor the recurrents by several horizontal circular turns of the bandage (Fig. 58-16B).

   When anchoring the recurrents, the circular turns begin at the lateral side and run posteriorly to the medial side.

   When the recurrents are firmly secured, bring the bandage down and around the stump and up again using oblique turns or a modified figure-8.

   Keep the pressure away, up, and out from the distal portion of the stump to eliminate creases. Do not use circular turns which are not oblique, since they tend to constrict circulation.

3. Start the hip spica from the anterior medial aspect of the stump and bring it laterally across the anterior surface of the stump in the inguinal region (Fig. 58-16C). (The hip spica anchors the bandage and covers the tissue high in the groin and the lateral surfaces of the hip, thus eliminating the formation of bulges in this area.)

   Bring the bandage around the body on a level with the iliac crest.

4. Return around the stump, making a figure-8, and bring the bandage around the pelvis again. Finish the bandaging by making oblique turns on the stump.

   Anchor the bandage with safety pins at the lateral or the anterior surface of the stump. Fasten where bandage ends and at crossing of spica at the hip (Fig. 58-16D).

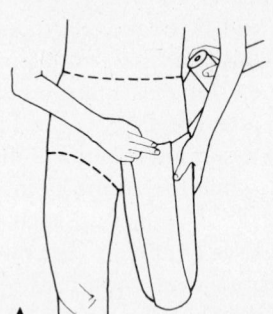 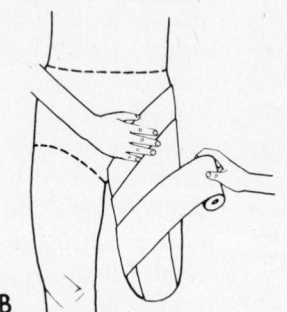 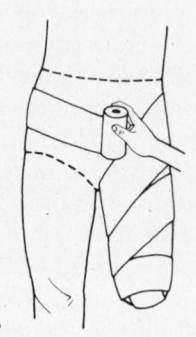 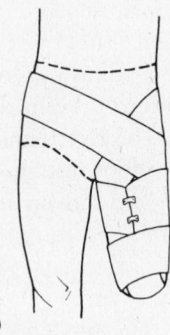

A   B   C   D

Figure 58-16. Bandaging an above-the-knee amputation stump. In applying the elastic bandage, take care to apply it smoothly, with no folds that can produce circulatory problems and skin abrasions.

*(Text from Nattress, L. W., Jr.: Orthopedic and Prosthetic Appliance Journal)

adhesive strip about the leg above the dressing has proved to be a good method of protecting the stump from becoming soiled.

Often during convalescence, while the stump muscles are adjusting themselves, twitching and spasms may occur. This discomfort may be alleviated by applying heat, changing the patient's position or placing a light sandbag on the thigh stump to counteract the psoas action. After the bandage is removed, the stump is exposed to the air and sun.

During the early postoperative stage, the patient may complain of phantom limb sensation (sensation that the amputated extremity is still there). This feeling will eventually disappear, but while it lasts it can have a disquieting effect on the patient. The pathogenesis of phantom limb phenomena is unknown. However, *keeping the patient active* helps decrease the occurrence of phantom limb pain. Phantom limb pain may occur 2 to 3 months after amputation and is seen more frequently in above-knee amputations.

The complete rehabilitation of an amputee requires the concerted efforts of the entire rehabilitation team. The orthopedic surgeon, the physiatrist, the prosthetist (limb maker), the physical therapist, and the occupational therapist all unite their efforts to condition and train the patient to make a satisfactory adjustment to the prosthesis. The establishment of prosthetic clinics has improved the outlook of amputees. With vocational

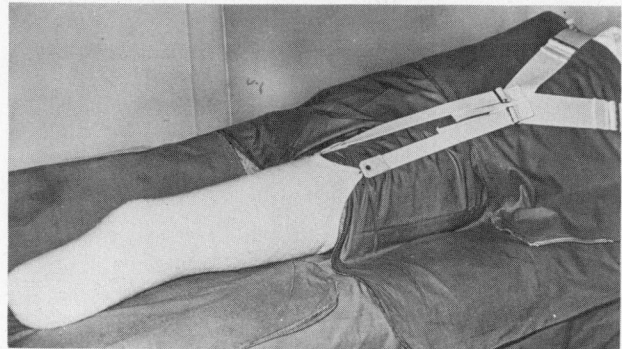

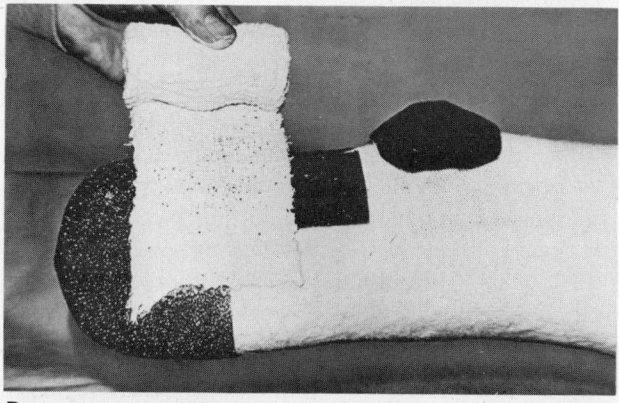

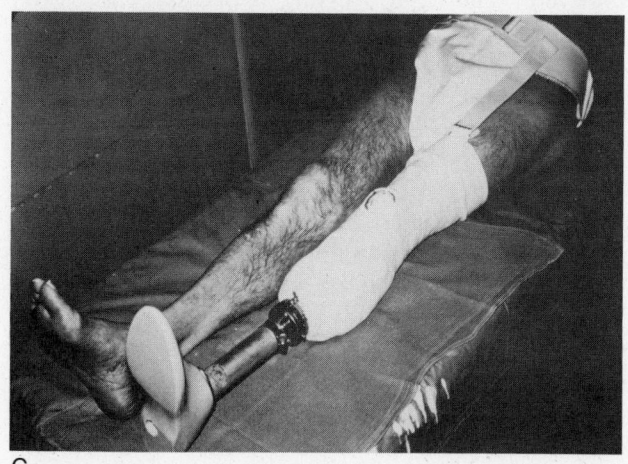

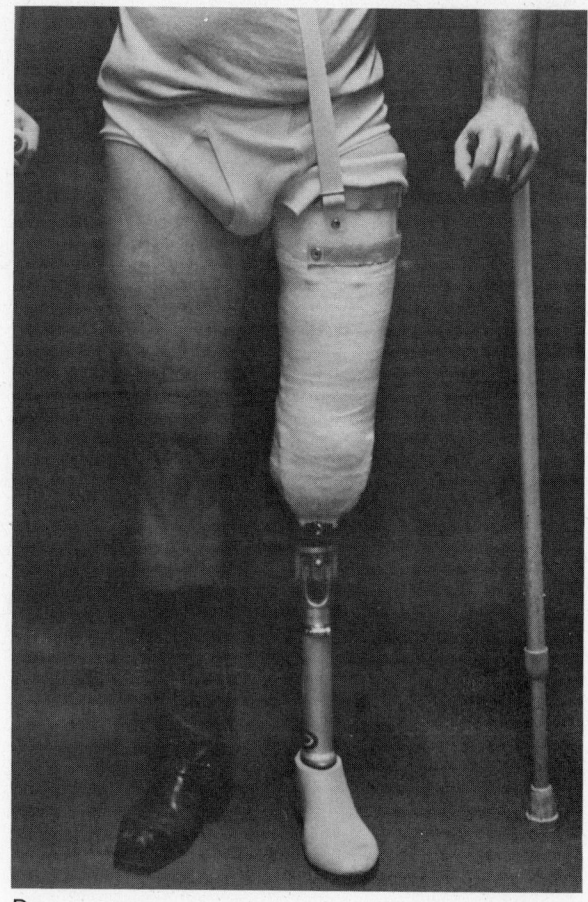

Figure 58-17. Immediate prosthetic fitting after amputation. *A.* Sterile stocking held under firm tension as the rigid dressing is applied. *B.* Pressure relief pads and distal polyurethane pad in place prior to application of the plaster of paris rigid dressing. *C.* Complete assembly of components for the immediate postsurgical prosthetic fitting of the below-knee amputee. *D.* Immediate postsurgical prosthetic fitting of the above-knee amputee. (Courtesy of the Prosthetics Research Study, Veterans Administration Contract V663P-784)

counseling and job-retraining where necessary, many of these patients can return to work.

Problems most frequently encountered in rehabilitation are obesity, circulatory insufficiency, and hypertension which increases with effort. If it is not possible for the patient to use a prosthesis, he can be taught to participate in self-care activities in a wheelchair.

A special wheelchair designed for amputees is advocated for persons who have lost one or both legs. Because of the decreased weight in the front, a regular wheelchair is in danger of tipping backwards when an amputee sits in it. In an amputee wheelchair the rear axle is set back about 5 cm. (2 inches) to compensate for this danger.

Rigid Dressing Approach

Immediately following surgery, a rigid plaster dressing may be applied, consisting of a prosthetic extension (pylon) and an artificial foot. Following the amputation, a sterilized stump sock is applied to the stump. Felt pads are placed over pressure-sensitive areas. Starting from the

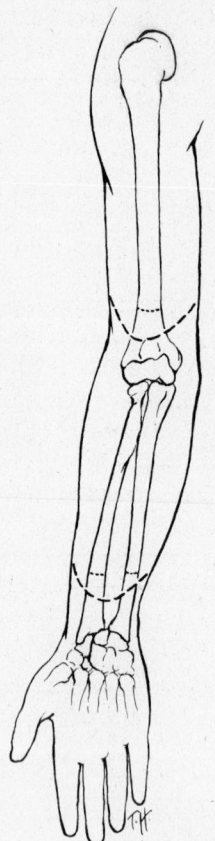

Figure 58-18. Levels of amputation of upper extremity.

distal end, the stump is wrapped with elastic plaster of paris bandages while firm, even pressure is maintained (Fig. 58-17). Care is taken not to constrict circulation. This rigid dressing technique is used as a means for creating a socket for immediate postoperative prosthetic fitting. It controls edema, minimizes pain on movement, and results in improved wound healing and maturation of the stump. It seems to be the major advance in early rehabilitation of patients. As soon as the rigid dressing has dried, the prosthetic unit, consisting of a prosthetic extension and foot, can be applied. The length of the prosthesis is tailored to the individual patient in the operating room after the amputation is performed.

The patient is brought to an upright position as soon as possible after surgery and allowed to extend the artificial foot to the floor. This promotes continuity of proprioception and helps to prevent the sensation of one-leggedness. It also allows for early ambulation. Earlier fitting of the prosthesis shortens the interval between amputation and walking and is of tremendous psychological value to the patient. It is more economical and helps avoid complications that can result from inactivity.

Nursing Management. The patient returns from the recovery room with the special plaster cast on the stump and the prosthetic extension and foot attached or nearby.

• *A most important consideration is that the amputation stump remain in the plaster cast socket during the patient's entire hospitalization.* If the cast inadvertently comes off, the stump must be immediately wrapped tightly with an elastic compression bandage and the surgeon notified so that another cast can be applied. Excessive edema will develop in a very short time and will result in a delay in rehabilitation.

Any signs of complications are assessed including: increasing stump pain, hematoma, odor emanating from the cast, infection and stump necrosis. If at any time the patient complains of severe pain, the cause is probably undue pressure on the bony prominence. This is relieved by splitting the cast or replacing it. Of course the surgeon is notified.

Explain to the patient that he may "feel" the amputated foot for a time and that this sensation will help him direct the movement of the artificial foot while he is learning to use the prosthesis. As soon as he is ready, the patient may stand between parallel bars or be raised to an upright position on a tilt table to allow him to extend the foot to the floor with *minimal* weight-bearing. Excessive pressure is to be avoided since it may compromise wound healing. At this time the prosthetist aligns the adjustable prosthetic unit. How soon after surgery the patient is allowed to "touch down" his artificial foot depends on his age and physical status and the condition of the other foot, etc. The rigid dressing is necessary but early weight-bearing is not always feasible. Patients who are debilitated or have severe diabetes or peripheral vascular disease may not be able to tolerate the degree of pressure required to "touch down" the foot and thus must wait a longer period before starting this activity.

Early minimal weight-bearing produces surprisingly little pain. In fact these patients do not complain of the severe pain and phantom limb discomfort that is experienced by patients who are treated by the more conventional method. Usually only mild opiates are needed to relieve pain during the immediate postoperative period.

The patient usually stands between parallel bars twice daily. As his endurance increases, ambulation is started within the parallel bars, but full weight-bearing is not permitted on the amputated side. The original cast may be left on for 10 to 14 days unless contraindicated by elevated body temperature, severe pain, loose fitting cast, etc. A second cast is then applied and changed usually 10 to 14 days after the initial cast change. At this time the patient may be measured for the definitive prosthesis. Crutch-walking is started when balance is achieved, but full weight-bearing is not permitted until the permanent prosthesis is fitted. A light plaster cast or a tensor bandage is provided to limit edema during the times the patient is not wearing his permanent prosthesis. Gait training is continued under the supervision of a physical therapist until optimal gait is achieved. Adjustments of the prosthetic socket are made by the prosthetist to accommodate the stump changes that take place during the first 6 months to a year after surgery.

UPPER EXTREMITY AMPUTATIONS

The loss of an upper extremity can be a greater catastrophe than the loss of a lower extremity, because the upper limb has such a highly specialized function. The major reasons for upper extremity amputation are severe trauma (acute injury, electrical burns, frostbite), malignant tumors, infection (fulminating gas gangrene, chronic osteomyelitis) and congenital malformations.

If time permits (and it usually does *not* with acute trauma), the patient is able to find out about the available prosthetic replacement and one-handed devices that aid independence. Regardless of what assistive devices are available, psychological support is essential to help the patient adapt to changes that will be made in lifestyle.

The objective of surgery is to conserve as much limb length as possible, consistent with eradicating the disease process (Fig. 58-18). Following surgery, a rigid plaster dressing with provision for the application of a temporary prosthesis or a compression bandage will be applied. Usually suction drainage is used to eliminate hematoma and achieve better approximation of tissues. At first the stump may be elevated to prevent edema.

Stump exercises (muscle-setting and joint-mobilizing exercises) are started as soon as tolerated to strengthen the muscles and mobilize the joints. These exercises are usually done under the supervision of the physical therapist. The muscles of both shoulders are exercised since an upper-extremity amputee uses both shoulders to operate the prosthesis. The patient is instructed how to carry out the activities of daily living with one arm. An over-the-bed trapeze helps in transferring out of bed. A patient with an above-the-elbow amputation or shoulder disarticulation is likely to develop a postural abnormality that is caused by loss of weight of the amputated extremity. Thus, postural exercises are helpful.

Usually the wound is inspected and sutures removed 7 to 10 days after surgery. If the patient is being treated with the rigid dressing, a new plaster socket with a temporary prosthetic device is applied. This type of management enables the patient to practice with the prosthesis and be fitted for a permanent device.

If a compression dressing is used, the stump is rewrapped 3 to 4 times daily to maintain proper tension in the bandage in order to reduce the edema and shape the stump so that a prosthesis may be eventually fitted. The stump is kept securely wrapped throughout the 24-hour period except for periods of bathing and exercise.

The patient is started on one-handed self-care activities as soon as possible. The occupational therapist teaches self-feeding, bathing, grooming, etc. The fitting of the prosthesis depends on the level of the amputation, the patient's age, and whether or not the joints proximal to the amputation site are weak or have limited range of motion.

Complications of an upper extremity amputation include the formation of a neuroma (a sensitive tumor of nerve cells growing at the end of severed nerves) and skin problems. Skin problems occur from contact dermatitis that results from irritants in the prosthetic components and from lack of ventilation and poor skin hygiene. Stump contracture or stump contour problems may develop. Infection, necrosis of the skin edges and phantom sensations (feeling that the arm is still present) are other complications. Psychological problems (denial, withdrawal) may be influenced by the type of support the patient receives from the rehabilitation team and by how quickly one-handed activities are taught and learned. Knowing the full options and capabilities available in the various prosthetic devices can give the patient a sense of control over the disability. The patient is not fully rehabilitated until he has been fitted with a prosthesis and has learned how to use it. Training of this nature is best accomplished in a specialized rehabilitation unit or center.

Patient Education. Careful skin hygiene is essential to prevent skin irritation, infection and breakdown. The stump should be washed and dried (gently) at least twice daily. Usually a stump sock is worn to absorb perspiration and avoid direct contact between the skin and the prosthetic socket. The stump sock is changed daily and must fit smoothly to avoid the irritation caused by wrinkles. The socket of the prosthesis should be washed with a mild detergent, rinsed and dried thoroughly with a clean cloth. The patient is advised that the socket must be thoroughly dry before the prosthesis is applied. An upper extremity amputee may wear a cotton tee shirt to prevent contact between the skin and shoulder harness and to promote absorption of perspiration. The prosthetist will advise about cleaning the washable portions of the harness.

BIBLIOGRAPHY

BOOKS

Adams, J. C.: Outline of Fractures, 7th ed. New York, Churchill Livingstone, 1978.

Bender, L. F.: Prosthesis and Rehabilitation After Arm Amputation, Springfield, Charles C. Thomas, 1974.

Brashear, H. R., Jr., and Raney, R. B.: Shands' Handbook of Orthopaedic Surgery, 9th ed. St. Louis, C. V. Mosby, 1978.

Devas, M.: Geriatric Orthopaedics. New York, Academic Press, 1977.

Epps, C. H. (ed.): Complications in Orthopaedic Surgery, vols. 1 and 2, Philadelphia, J. B. Lippincott, 1978.

Farrell, J.: Illustrated Guide to Orthopedic Nursing. Philadelphia, J. B. Lippincott, 1977.

Friedmann, L. W.: The Psychological Rehabilitation of the Amputee. Springfield, Charles C. Thomas, 1978.

Haimovici, H.: Vascular Surgery: Principles and Techniques. N.Y. McGraw-Hill, 1976.

Hartman, J. T.: Fracture Management: A Practical Approach. Philadelphia, Lea & Febiger, 1978.

Iverson, L. D., and Clawson, D. K.: Manual of Orthopaedic Therapeutics. Boston, Little, Brown, 1977.

Larson, C. B., and Gould, M.: Orthopedic Nursing. 9th ed. St. Louis, C. V. Mosby, 1978.

Lewis, R. C., Jr.: Handbook of Traction, Casting and Splinting Techniques. Philadelphia, J. B. Lippincott, 1977.

Muckle, D. S.: Femoral Neck Fractures. New York, John Wiley, 1977.

Rockwood, C. A., and Green, D. P.: Fractures, vols. 1 and 2. Philadelphia, J. B. Lippincott, 1975.

Ryan, J. R.: Orthopedic Surgery. Flushing, Medical Examination Pub. Co., 1977.

Stewart, J.D. M.: Traction and Orthopaedic Appliances. New York, Churchill Livingstone, 1975.

Turek, S. L.: Orthopaedics. Principles and Their Application, 3rd ed. Philadelphia, J. B. Lippincott, 1977.

Washam, V.: The One-Hander's Book. New York, Day, 1973.

ARTICLES

Amputation

Carlen, P. L., et al.: Phantom limbs and related phenomena in recent traumatic amputations. Neurology, *28*:211-217, Mar. 1978.

DesGroseilliers, J. P., et al.: Dermatologic problems in amputees. Can. Med. Assoc. J., *118*:535-537, March 4, 1978.

Quinn, L.: It's worth the effort . . . I know. RN, *39*: 57-68, Oct. 1976.

————: What to tell your below-knee amputees. RN, *39*:60-61, Oct. 1976.

Fractures

DeSouza, L. J.: Changing management of hip fractures. Minn. Med., *60*:339-343, May 1977.

Hunter, G.: Treatment of fractures of the head of the femur. Can. Med. Assoc. J., *117*:60-61, July 9, 1977.

Jackson, R. P., Jacobs, R. R., and Neff, J. R.: External skeletal fixation in severe limb trauma. J. Trauma, *18*:201-205, Mar. 1978.

McFarland, M. B.: Fat embolism syndrome. AJN, *76*:1942-44, Dec. 1976.

Seinsheimer, F.: Subtrochanteric fractures of the femur, J. Bone Joint Surg., *60*:300-306, Apr. 1978.

AGENCIES

Governmental

National Institute of Arthritis, Metabolism and Digestive Diseases, National Institutes of Health, Bethesda, Md. 20205

Voluntary

American Orthotic and Prosthetic Association, 1440 N St., N.W., Washington, D.C. 20005

American Physical Therapy Association, 1156 15th St., N.W., Washington, D.C. 20005

National Amputation Foundation, 12-45 150th St., Whitestone, N.Y. 11357

National Easter Seal Society for Crippled Children and Adults, 2023 W. Ogden Ave., Chicago, Ill. 60612

(See also Rehabilitation Agencies, Chapter 12)

59

MANAGEMENT OF PATIENTS WITH MUSCULOSKELETAL DISORDERS

BONE AND JOINT INFECTIONS

OSTEOMYELITIS

Osteomyelitis is an infection involving all or parts of a bone. It is essentially a disease of childhood and adolescence, caused most frequently by *Staphylococcus aureus*, although other pathogenic bacteria may be involved, including streptococcal organisms, *Salmonella*, *Proteus* and *Pseudomonas*. The infection is usually blood-borne from other foci of infection, but it may follow trauma or surgery or occur from direct infection of the bone resulting from open fractures.

Clinical Manifestations and Pathophysiology

When the infection is carried by the blood, the onset is usually sudden, occurring often with a chill, high fever, rapid pulse and general malaise. In children, in whom the disease usually begins as an acute epiphysitis, these constitutional symptoms at first may overshadow the local signs completely. As the infection extends from the marrow cavity through the cortex of the bone, it involves the periosteum and the soft tissues, with the limb becoming painful, swollen and extremely tender. Thus an abscess of bone is formed.

In the natural course of events, the abscess may point and drain but, more often, incision and drainage are done by the surgeon. The resulting abscess cavity has in its walls areas of dead tissue, as in any abscess cavity; however, in this case the dead tissue is bone, which cannot liquefy easily and be discharged as pus. This dead bone is called a *sequestrum*. Healing in a bone abscess is more difficult than in an abscess in soft tissue, because the cavity cannot collapse and heal. New bone, the *involucrum*, forms as the body attempts to repair. Often it grows so as to surround a sequestrum. Thus, even though healing appears to take place, a chronically infected sequestrum remains that is prone to produce recurring abscesses throughout the life of the individual. This is the so-called chronic type of osteomyelitis.

In *chronic osteomyelitis*, all dead, infected bone and cartilage must be removed before permanent healing takes place. This operation, which is called a *sequestrectomy*, consists of the removal of enough involucrum with mallet and chisel to enable the surgeon to remove the sequestrum. Often sufficient bone is removed to convert a deep cavity into a shallow saucer (saucerization). Muscle sometimes is used to help in obliterating the resulting wound. These operations are becoming increasingly rare since the advent of effective antimicrobial chemotherapy. Primary healing may be obtained frequently by the use of an appropriate antibiotic if the cavity can be closed and the skin approximated. Sometimes the granulating wound may be covered by a split-thickness skin graft.

When osteomyelitis occurs in an open fracture by direct implantation of the offending organism, there is no preceding septicemia, but the treatment generally follows that outlined above, except that the fracture must be treated in addition.

1321

Management

The antibiotic to which the causative organism has demonstrated sensitivity is the drug treatment of choice. Usually the antibiotic is given intravenously or intramuscularly in large doses to maintain a sustained therapeutic level.

Osteomyelitis is a disease that demands careful nursing management. The wounds themselves frequently are very painful and must be handled with great care and gentleness. The joints above and below the affected part should be supported and the extremity moved in a smooth manner. The affected part may be immobilized with a splint until the wound has healed. Immobilization decreases pain and muscle spasm. Careful handling is also essential because of the possibility of cross infection. Hot packs may be prescribed for indurated areas. These patients should be watched carefully for any development of painful areas or sudden rises in temperature as these symptoms usually indicate the formation of a secondary abscess. If there is a draining wound the patient is isolated and secretion precautions or wound and skin precautions followed depending on the extent of infection.

Suspected regions of pus may be evacuated by needle aspiration. If the patient does not respond to treatment, surgery is carried out whereby the involved bone is exposed, the purulent and necrotic material removed, and the area irrigated directly with a suitable antibacterial agent.

BONE AND JOINT TUBERCULOSIS

Tuberculosis is an infectious disease caused by the tubercle bacillus, *Mycobacterium tuberculosis*. While the lungs are the organs usually invaded directly, involvement of bones and joints is secondary to tuberculosis elsewhere in the body. Therefore when the bones are affected, a search is made for other active foci of disease.

Tuberculosis of a bone or joint is usually a low grade and slowly progressive infection. Characteristically one joint (mono-articular) or one bone (mono-osseous) is affected. The spine is involved most commonly, while the hip, the knee and the ankle may also be affected in some patients. Local symptoms and signs include swelling (caused by synovial inflammation), pain and tenderness, muscle spasm, early stiffness progressing to limitation of active and passive motion (from fibrous ankylosis), slight warmth about the involved site, increased amounts of joint fluid and muscle atrophy. Constitutional manifestations include fatigue, anorexia, weight loss and low-grade fever.

Management. A combination of antituberculosis drugs is given to eradicate the microbial organisms as rapidly as possible and to minimize the opportunity for the persistence of drug-resistant organisms. (Drug therapy is discussed on page 1379.) Usually a period of 18 to 24 months of drug therapy is recommended. Secondary infection of the bone is treated with the appropriate antimicrobial agent. Orthopedic surgery is indicated when drainage of abscesses, excision of bone and fixation of a joint are necessary. Other facets of care and patient education are discussed under the management of the patient with tuberculosis, page 1379.

Tuberculous Tenosynovitis and Bursitis. *Tuberculous tenosynovitis* most often develops in association with tuberculosis of nearby bones and joints. The tendons most frequently affected are those about the wrists—either the flexor or the extensor group, seldom both.

Tuberculous bursitis may be the only demonstrable focus of this infection in the body. This type of bursitis develops very slowly, distending the sac with a serous fluid, in which, later, great numbers of rice bodies (cartilaginous particles) appear. Such swelling generally is painless, but it may interfere with the motions of the part which the bursa is intended to aid.

Management. These periarticular infections, as in the case of other tuberculous lesions, respond quite readily to vigorous chemotherapy and surgery.

ARTHRITIS

No other disease causes more prolonged misery to a greater number of persons in this country than does arthritic and rheumatic disease. Over 24 million people in the U.S. have arthritis severe enough to seek medical help. It ranks second only to heart disease as the most widespread chronic disease in the U.S. Authorities estimate that it costs the nation billions of dollars per year, with a staggering loss of human productivity.

Definition and Classification. The term "arthritis" implies inflammation and destruction of joints, specifically the joint lining. "Rheumatism" is a more general term and refers to symptoms from pain, stiffness, or deformity of joints, muscles, and related structures. The term "rheumatic diseases" refers to musculoskeletal disorders in which the changes take place in the tissues comprising or surrounding the joints. (One can readily understand how these terms have come to be used interchangeably.)

The two main types of arthritis are rheumatoid arthritis and degenerative joint disease (osteoarthritis). The American Rheumatism Association and the Arthritis Foundation list about a hundred disorders under the combined heading of arthritis and rheumatism and group them into 13 different categories (Table 59-1).

TABLE 59-1.   CLASSIFICATION OF THE RHEUMATIC DISEASES*

I. **Polyarthritis of unknown etiology**
   A. Rheumatoid arthritis
   B. Juvenile rheumatoid arthritis (including Still's disease)
   C. Ankylosing spondylitis
   D. Psoriatic arthritis
   E. Reiter's syndrome
   F. Others

II. **"Connective tissue" disorders (acquired)**
   A. Systemic lupus erythematosus
   B. Progressive systemic sclerosis (scleroderma)
   C. Polymyositis and dermatomyositis
   D. *Necrotizing arteritis and other forms of vasculitis*
      1. *Polyarteritis nodosa*
      2. *Hypersensitivity angiitis*
      3. *Wegener's granulomatosis*
      4. *Takayasu's (pulseless) disease*
      5. *Cogan's syndrome*
      6. *Giant cell arteritis (including polymyalgia rheumatica)*
   E. Amyloidosis
   F. Others
      (See also Rheumatoid arthritis, I, A; Sjögren's syndrome, VI, G)

III. **Rheumatic fever**

IV. **Degenerative joint disease (osteoarthritis, osteoarthrosis)**
   A. Primary
   B. Secondary

V. **Nonarticular rheumatism**
   A. Fibrositis
   B. Intervertebral disc and low back syndromes
   C. Myositis and myalgia
   D. Tendinitis and peritendinitis (bursitis)
   E. Tenosynovitis
   F. Fasciitis
   G. Carpal tunnel syndrome
   H. Others
      (See also Shoulder-hand syndrome, VIII, C)

VI. **Diseases with which arthritis is frequently associated**
   A. Sarcoidosis
   B. Relapsing polychondritis
   C. Schönlein-Henoch purpura
   D. Ulcerative colitis
   E. Regional enteritis
   F. Whipple's disease
   G. Sjögren's syndrome
   H. Familial Mediterranean fever
   I. Others
      (See also Psoriatic arthritis, I, D)

VII. **Associated with known infectious agents**
   A. Bacterial
      1. Gonococcus
      2. *Meningococcus*
      3. Pneumococcus
      4. *Streptococcus*
      5. Staphylococcus
      6. Salmonella
      7. Brucella
      8. Streptobacillus moniliformis (Haverhill fever)

      9. Mycobacterium tuberculosis
      10. Treponema pallidum (syphilis)
      11. Treponema pertenue (yaws)
      12. Others
         (See also Rheumatic fever, III)
   B. Rickettsial
   C. Viral
      1. *Rubella*
      2. *Mumps*
      3. *Viral hepatitis*
      4. *Others*
   D. Fungal
   E. Parasitic

VIII. **Traumatic and/or neurogenic disorders**
   A. Traumatic arthritis (the result of direct trauma)
   B. Neuropathic arthropathy (Charcot joints)
      1. Syphilis (tabes dorsalis)
      2. Diabetes mellitus (diabetic neuropathy)
      3. Syringomyelia
      4. *Myelomeningocele*
      5. *Congenital insensitivity to pain (including familial dysautonomia)*
      6. Others
   C. Shoulder-hand syndrome
   D. Mechanical derangement of joints
   E. Others
      (See also Degenerative joint disease, IV; Carpal tunnel syndrome, V, G)

IX. **Associated with known or strongly suspected biochemical or endocrine abnormalities**
   A. Gout
   B. *Chondrocalcinosis articularis ("pseudogout")*
   C. Alkaptonuria (ochronosis)
   D. Hemophilia
   E. Sickle cell disease and other hemoglobinopathies
   F. Agammaglobulinemia (hypogammaglobulinemia)
   G. Gaucher's disease
   H. Hyperparathyroidism
   I. Acromegaly
   J. *Thyroid acropachy*
   K. Hypothyroidism
   L. Scurvy (hypovitaminosis C)
   M. Hyperlipoproteinemia type II (xanthoma tuberosum and tendinosum)
   N. *Fabry's disease (angiokeratoma corporis diffusum or glycolipid lipidosis)*
   O. *Hemochromatosis*
   P. Others
      (See also Inherited and congenital disorders, XII)

X. **Neoplasms**
   A. Synovioma
   B. Primary juxta-articular bone tumors
   C. Metastatic malignant tumors
   D. Leukemia
   E. Multiple myeloma
   F. Benign tumors of articular tissue
   G. Others
      (See also Hypertrophic osteoarthropathy, XIII, I)

(Continued)

---

*Adapted from the 1963 ARA Nomenclature and Classification of Arthritis and Rheumatism (tentative). Additions and modifications are italicized.
Reproduced from the 7th edition Primer on the Rheumatic Diseases prepared by the American Rheumatism section of the Arthritis Foundation.

TABLE 59-1. (Continued)

XI. Allergy and drug reactions
  A. Arthritis due to specific allergens (eg, serum sickness)
  B. Arthritis due to drugs
  C. Others
     (See also Systemic lupus erythematosus, II, A, for Drug-induced lupus-like syndromes, e.g., hydralazine and procainamide syndromes; Hypersensitivity angiitis, II, D, 2)

XII. Inherited and congenital disorders
  A. Marfan syndrome
  B. *Homocystinuria*
  C. Ehlers-Danlos syndrome
  D. *Osteogenesis imperfecta*
  E. *Pseudoxanthoma elasticum*
  F. *Cutis laxa*
  G. *Mucopolysaccharidoses (including Hurler's syndrome)*
  H. *Arthrogryposis multiplex congenita*
  I. *Hypermobility syndromes*
  J. *Myositis (or fibrodysplasia) ossificans progressiva*
  K. *Tumoral calcinosis*

  L. *Werner's syndrome*
  M. Congenital dysplasia of the hip
  N. Others
     (See also Arthropathy associated with known biochemical or endocrine abnormalities, IX)

XIII. Miscellaneous disorders
  A. Pigmented villonodular synovitis and tenosynovitis
  B. Behçet's syndrome
  C. Erythema nodosum
  D. *Relapsing panniculitis (Weber-Christian disease)*
  E. Avascular necrosis of bone
  F. Juvenile osteochondritis
  G. Osteochondritis dissecans
  H. Erythema multiforme (Stevens-Johnson syndrome)
  I. Hypertrophic osteoarthropathy
  J. Multicentric reticulohistiocytosis
  K. *Disseminated lipogranulomatosis (Farber's disease)*
  L. *Familial lipochrome pigmentary arthritis*
  M. Tietze's syndrome
  N. *Thrombotic thrombocytopenic purpura*
  O. Others

RHEUMATOID ARTHRITIS

Rheumatoid arthritis is a chronic systemic disease of unknown cause, characterized most prominently by recurrent inflammation involving the synovium or lining of the joints, leading to destructive changes in the joints. It occurs more frequently in women (4:1), although in the severe progressive forms of the disease, the ratio drops to 3:1 or 2:1.

Clinical Manifestations

The disease usually begins with unusual fatigue, morning stiffness (lasting 30 minutes or more), loss of appetite and painful swelling in one or more joints, often in the fingers (second and third metacarpophalangeal joints). The swelling is due in part to the accumulation of fluid in the joints or to hypertrophy of the joint lining.

Following one or several attacks, some of the joints involved never quite return to normal, but remain stiff and sore. During subsequent acute exacerbations, other joints likewise become chronically injured, and each attack leaves the involved joints more damaged than before.

The disease affects primarily the joint cartilages and the articular surfaces of the bones, destroying the joint cavity, which becomes filled with adhesions. Subsequent difficulties include crepitation, dislocations, ankyloses, and muscular contractures. Atrophic changes appear early, involving the soft tissues about the affected joints.

The clinical course is variable, ranging from a mild episode to an unremitting disorder causing severe disease in 20 to 30 percent of patients affected. Usually mild deformities develop slowly and the patient at first experiences only mild discomfort.

The clinical picture presented in a well-marked case of this condition is typical. The patient appears chronically ill; the muscles of the extremities, especially of their distal segments, are apt to be wasted; the subcutaneous fat often is greatly decreased. The joints become deformed—some of them dislocated. If the condition is extreme, the patient can scarcely move a single joint in the body. The early immobility of the joints, however, does not result from bony ankylosis but from tense muscular spasm.

The appearance of the hands reflects the deformity of the joints as well as soft-tissue damage. The distal phalanges are hyperextended, the proximal flexed, and there is ulnar deviation of the fingers. The skin covering the fingertips is thin, pale, smooth, and shiny, the nails are rough and brittle, and the intrinsic muscles of the hand are wasted. A large number of patients show clinical or radiographic evidence of disease of the cervical spine. In more advanced stages of rheumatoid arthritis the spine may be stiff and the jaw partly fixed. The severity of the disease may vary from this marked degree of involvement to a mild stiffening and swelling of the finger joints.

Although joint pain and destruction are the most apparent problems, rheumatoid arthritis is a systemic disease. There may be associated inflammation of connective tissue. The skin, eyes and nervous system may be affected by vasculitis, which may produce thrombosis and ischemia. The rheumatoid process may affect changes on the serosal surfaces of the heart and lungs. Any or every organ or system may be involved by the rheumatic disease.

Other abnormal clinical findings observed in addition to the joint involvement include subcutaneous nodules which in many respects are indistinguishable from those of rheumatic fever; frequent generalized lymphadenopathy and splenomegaly; fever, which may be high and prolonged; anemia, leukocytosis, and elevation of the sedimentation rate.

Etiology

The etiology of rheumatoid arthritis is unknown and its relation to rheumatic fever is not clear. As indicated below, many regard it as a disorder of autoimmunity because the body, for unknown reasons, produces high levels of certain types of gamma globulins (rheumatoid factors) that are directed against its own tissues.

Some researchers believe that rheumatoid arthritis may be due to infection from bacteria, viruses, or Mycoplasma. Some feel that rheumatoid arthritis is a reaction to an infectious agent that evolves in certain susceptible people. There is evidence for support of both infection and autoimmunity as causes of rheumatoid arthritis. In fact the concept of a single cause for rheumatoid arthritis may be restrictive.

Pathophysiology (Fig. 59-1)

The disease is thought to be due to an immunological response that is centered upon the synovial joints. The pathological changes are seen first as inflammation occurring in the synovial tissue.

Each of the synovial joints may be the site of inflammation, with swelling and pain, edema and infiltration with lymphocytes and plasma cells. The lymphocytes and plasma cells begin to make IgG, IgA and IgM antiglobulin antibodies (rheumatoid factors) which react with antigen (IgG) to form immune complex. These generate inflammatory reactions characterized by release of lysomal enzymes and lymphokines. There is an increase of phagocyte cells to remove the debris. Phagocyte cells produce enzymes which create more destruction—hyperemia, edema, swelling and thickening of the synovial lining continue. Clear or slightly turbid fluid collects in the joint. Granulation tissue covers the articular cartilage (pannus), gradually replacing it with fibrous connective tissue. As the process spreads, the joint is destroyed as the articular cartilage becomes eroded, exposing the bone in the joint. Destruction of the joint produces ankylosis and deformity. The muscles are affected as the muscle fibers undergo degenerative changes with loss of muscle elasticity and contractile power.

In approximately 25 percent of patients, subcutaneous rheumatoid nodules are present. These occur particularly in the subcutaneous tissue adjacent to the joints but they may appear in the myocardium, aorta and lung. Cardiac, pleural, and ocular involvement results. What actually starts this whole process is unknown, but the cause is the object of intensive research.

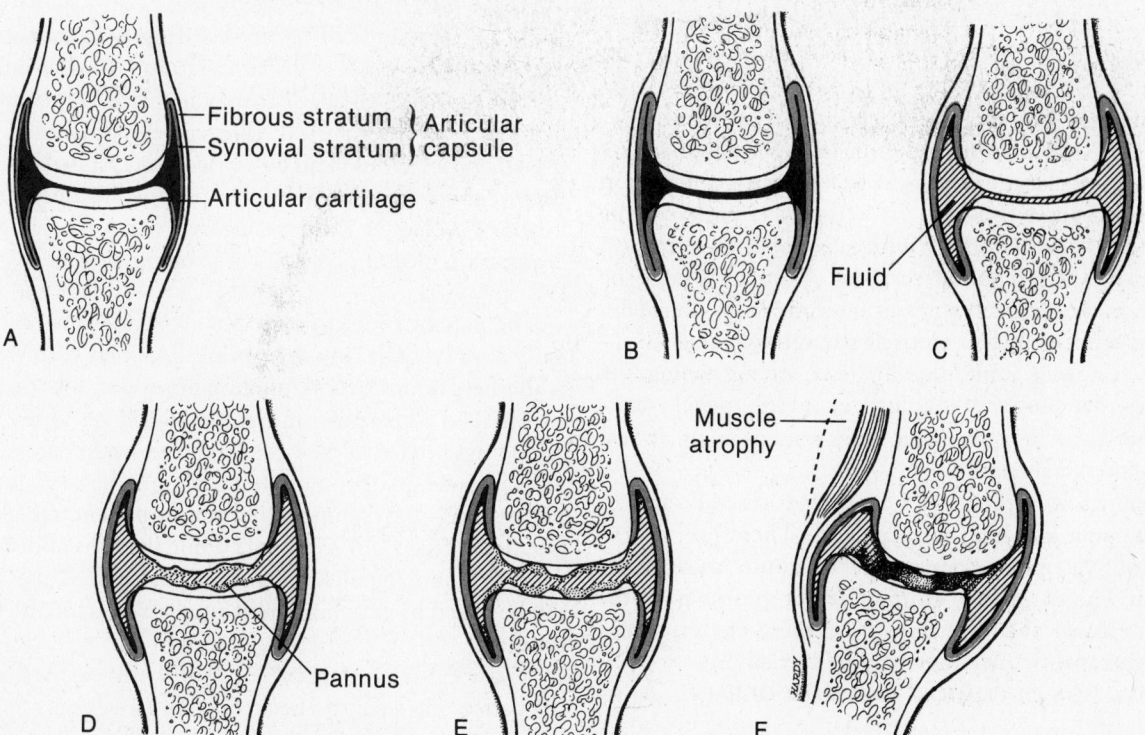

Figure 59-1.   Pathophysiology of rheumatoid arthritis. (A) Normal (B) Synovial swelling (C) Fluid collects in joint (D) Pannus (E) Eroded articular cartilage (F) Ankylosis and muscle atrophy.

Management

The primary objectives of treatment in the acute stage of rheumatoid arthritis are to keep the patient at a satisfactory level of function and to prevent crippling deformities. Other therapeutic goals include (1) to maintain joint mobility and muscle strength; (2) to promote comfort; (3) to halt the activity of the disease; (4) to help the patient and his family to adjust to his chronic disability; and (5) to assist the patient to become functionally independent as soon and as completely as possible.

The patient is instructed about the disease and placed on a program of rest (systemic, emotional, and articular), physical therapy, and an extended course of treatment with salicylates supplemented by other anti-inflammatory agents as necessary.

MAINTENANCE OF JOINT MOBILITY AND MUSCLE STRENGTH. Inflammation, scarring, or other structural damage to joint structures results in pain and disability. The patient, in an effort to avoid pain, tends to immobilize the affected joints, and muscular spasm further limits their motion. If acutely inflamed, these joints should be rested by applying splints, bivalved casts, or any other mechanical device that will maintain them in functional positions. Simple splints provide rest, support the joint in optimal position to relieve pain and spasm, and help prevent deformity. Above all, the joints should not be permitted to "freeze" in positions of flexion, which is their natural tendency because of the predominant strength of the flexor muscles. The knee is splinted at full extension and the wrist at slight dorsiflexion. Splints may need to be modified when changes occur in joint structure.

Joints may lose their normal range of motion due to deformity and atrophy of the muscles. This loss can be prevented to a large extent by systematic range of motion exercises (page 183–190). If activity is painful, the nurse may help the patient (with active-assisted exercises) to perform the required motions. Emphasis must be placed on the need to carry out these exercises on a daily basis in order to increase muscle strength which is essential in restoring joint mobility and strengthening the muscles that support the joints. Isometric muscle exercises are especially valuable. The joint is kept at rest during these exercises.

Rheumatoid arthritis is a long-term disease, and its management is a long-term project. Therefore, a program of systematic exercises in the home must be included. The pamphlet, Home Care Programs in Arthritis* explains and illustrates how these exercises and other therapeutic measures may be carried out.

PROMOTION OF COMFORT AND RELIEF OF PAIN. Anti-

inflammatory drugs (nonsteroidal or steroidal) are given to relieve inflammatory changes that are responsible for the symptoms of pain, swelling, stiffness and impaired function. At first salicylates are given in large doses in accordance with the patient's response. Table 59-2 outlines the drugs in use for rheumatoid arthritis.

Heat applications are also helpful to relieve pain, stiffness, inflammation, and muscle spasm. Superficial heat may be supplied in the form of warm tub baths and warm moist compresses. Paraffin baths (dips) offer concentrated heat and are helpful to patients with wrist and small joint involvement (page 1331). Therapeutic exercises can be carried out more comfortably and effectively after heat has been applied. However, in some patients, heat may actually increase pain, muscle spasm and synovial fluid volume. If the inflammatory process is acute, cold applications may be tried in the form of moist packs or an ice bag. Cold at first produces a superficial vasoconstriction, which causes pallor, and then superficial vasodilation which results in rubor. Both heat and cold are analgesic to nerve pain receptors and relax muscle spasm.

Rest also helps to allay pain. Since arthritis is a systemic disease, the whole patient—not merely the joints—must be treated. The amount of rest required is indicated by the amount of inflammatory involvement and the feelings of the patient. When in bed, the patient should lie flat on a firm mattress with only one pillow under the head because of the risk of dorsal kyphosis. (At no time should a pillow be placed under the knees, as this promotes flexion contractures of those joints.)

Frequent periods of bed rest during the day take the weight off the joints and relieve fatigue. If joint inflammation is severe, the patient may be placed on complete bed rest for a brief period. (Nevertheless, range of motion exercises should still be carried out.) At bed rest, the patient should lie flat, with feet propped against a footboard. Trochanter rolls are utilized when the patient is lying in the dorsal position for prolonged periods (page 191).

The patient should lie on the abdomen several times daily to prevent flexion deformities. As joint stiffness and tenderness diminish and function improves, the patient is encouraged to perform more out-of-bed activities. Pain can be anticipated in the knees and hips when rising from a chair. The nurse should select a straight-back chair with a seat that is high enough to permit the patient to keep the feet flat on the floor (or stool) while the hips and shoulders are resting against the back of the chair. Toilet seats can be raised by attaching built-up seats to standard toilet fixtures.

A cervical collar to prevent cervical motion may help if the patient has a painful neck. Stretch gloves may control hand and finger pain by providing a mild splinting action and presumably by reducing joint swelling and stasis of blood.

*Arthritis Foundation, 3400 Peachtree Road, N.E., Atlanta, Georgia 30326

When the foot is involved, pain is due to synovial proliferation, distention of the joint capsule and lax supporting ligaments which contribute to mechanical deformities. Pain about the metatarsal area of the forefoot may be relieved by placing a metatarsal bar proximal to the point of impact on the metatarsal heads in order to relieve weight bearing. Pads may be placed in strategic places to relieve stress and irritation. These may be fitted to standard shoes by an expert shoemaker. When there are significant deformities of the feet (bunion, subluxation [partial dislocation] of the metatarsophalangeal [MTP] joints, hammer toes), custom-made shoes molded to the contours of the feet will permit more comfortable walking. The patient is advised that the foot may continue to change shape and that modifications will need to be made on the shoes. In many instances, corrective surgery can restore function and relieve pain.

Drug Therapy (Table 59-2)

Drug therapy is used to relieve inflammation and pain and arrest the progress of the disease. The salicylates (aspirin), when used in full dosage, have an anti-inflammatory as well as analgesic action in the treatment of rheumatoid arthritis. They provide an effective and inexpensive relief of pain and stiffness. Salicylates reach their peak level in the blood approximately 2 hours after oral ingestion and then gradually decline. To be most effective the patient should take aspirin every 3 hours, beginning from the moment he awakes in the morning and regularly throughout the day. The serum salicylate level is usually kept at 20 to 30 mg./100 ml. which usually requires 12 to 20 aspirin tablets daily. There are sustained-released salicylate preparations for bedtime usage to maintain a therapeutic blood level at night. Because heavy and continual use of aspirin can produce side effects, the patient is advised to have periodic hematocrit determinations for the presence of occult gastrointestinal bleeding. However, he should be assured that chronic use of aspirin does *not* lead to tolerance or addiction.

Other anti-inflammatory drugs used are ibuprofen (Motrin), naproxen (Naprosyn), tolmetin (Tolectin) and fenopren (Nalfon) and indomethacin (Indocin). Phenyl-butazone and oxyphenbutazone are useful for acute flareups. However, these drugs are capable of producing severe toxic side effects.

Systemic hormonal therapy (taken orally) with one of the corticosteroids (such as prednisone) does not alter the course of rheumatoid arthritis but reduces inflammation and pain and increases the sense of well-being. Corticosteroids are used when the patient has a rapid downhill course or when extraarticular manifestations occur. Corticosteroid therapy has undesirable side effects including sodium and water retention, potassium depletion, hypertension, glucosuria, menstrual irregularities,

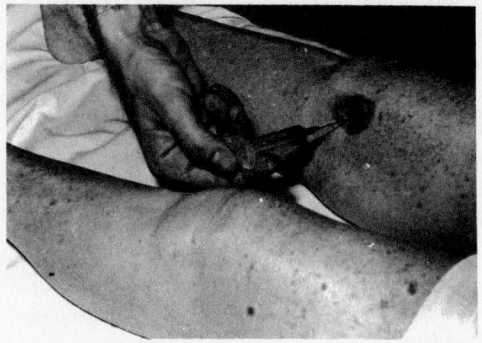

Figure 59-2. Intra-articular injection of the knee joint with a steroid preparation. Note that the knee is in full extension and the needle is inserted laterally and parallel to the plane of the patella. (From Ehrlich, G. E., ed.: Total Management of the Arthritic Patient. Philadelphia, J. B. Lippincott, 1973)

and other features of the Cushing syndrome as well as osteoporosis, psychosis and psychologic dependency.

To halt the disease process, joints that are severely inflamed and fail to respond promptly to the measures outlined above may be treated by the local injection of a corticosteroid (Fig. 59-2). This maneuver suppresses local inflammation and provides temporary relief from pain and disability.

If significant inflammation persists, gold therapy may be tried, in which weekly intramuscular injections of gold compounds are given. The patient should be advised of possible dermatologic, hematologic and renal complications resulting from this therapy.

Immunosuppressive drugs that are thought to affect the production of antibodies at the cellular level are under investigation for the treatment of rheumatoid arthritis. These include methotrexate, penicillamine, cyclophosphamide (Cytoxan), and azathioprine (Imuran). However, these drugs are highly toxic and can produce bone marrow depression, anemia, gastrointestinal disturbances and skin rashes.

Table 59-2 summarizes the drugs used in the treatment of rheumatoid arthritis. The nurse, especially the community health nurse and the nurse in the outpatient clinic, should be familiar with the side effects and potential toxicity of all these drugs.

Psychological Support

In addition to the physical limitations imposed by rheumatoid arthritis, this disease can affect the personality and limit the person socially. The psychosocial factors of motivation, intelligence, and personal and social adjustment influence the patient's response to therapy as well as his ability to maintain psychological equilibrium in the presence of a chronic disability. Patients with arthritis show the same fundamental psychological responses to their disease as persons with other chronic diseases—fear or anxiety, dependency, anger, and loss of

TABLE 59-2. DRUGS USED IN RHEUMATOID ARTHRITIS

DRUG	ACTION	NURSING IMPLICATION AND ASSESSMENT FOR DRUG INTOLERANCE
Anti-inflammatory Agents **Salicylates**		
Acetylsalicylic acid (aspirin) (may be buffered or enteric coated)	Acetylsalicylic acid is the cornerstone of treatment, especially in early phase of disease. Has anti-inflammatory, antipyretic and analgesic effects. Optimum dosage will produce blood salicylate levels of 20-30 mg./100 ml. Can be used in combination with other analgesics and anti-inflammatory agents.	Take salicylates with antacid or milk to protect against gastric irritation. Watch for complaints of tinnitus, gastric intolerance, or GI bleeding and purpuric tendencies.
Newer Nonsteroidal **Anti-inflammatory Agents**		
Ibuprofen (Motrin)	Anti-inflammatory action.	Gastrointestinal irritation and hemorrhagic erosions but less frequently than aspirin. Used in patients who cannot tolerate or who do not respond to aspirin.
Fenoprofen (Nalfon)	Mechanism of action may be related to inhibition of prostaglandin synthetase (prostaglandins have a role in inflammatory process, pain and fever).	Variation among patients in response to these drugs.
Naproxen (Naprosyn)	Longer half-life, thus permits less frequent administration.	Dosage individualized for each patient.
Tolmetin (Tolectin)		
Sulindac (Clinoril)	Anti-inflammatory, analgesic antipyretic properties.	Peptic ulceration and gastrointestinal bleeding have been reported.
Other Anti-Inflammatory Agents		
Indomethacin (Indocin)	Used for short-term treatment of active synovitis.	Can produce significant side effects: Gastrointestinal effects; CNS effects.
Phenylbutazone (Butazolidin) Oxyphenbutazone (Tandearil)	Nonsteroidal antirheumatic agents for adjunctive treatment of rheumatoid arthritis. Exerts analgesic, antipyretic, anti-inflammatory action. Sometimes remarkably effective in control of articular symptoms. Patient should be under close medical supervision. Can cause salt and water retention. Usually used only for short periods.	Observe for untoward effects: Gastrointestinal effects: Nausea, vomiting, epigastric distress, precipitation and reactivation of peptic ulcer. Hematologic: Bone marrow depression, anemia, leukopenia, agranulocytosis, thrombocytopenia purpura. *Irreversible blood element depression may occur rapidly despite careful supervision and frequent testing.*
Antimalarial Compounds Hydroxychloroquine sulfate (Plaquenil)	Appears to be no rational basis for the comparative success of these drugs at this time.	Useful for severe and destructive forms of arthritis. Stress that patient should have regular ophthalmologic examination every 4-6 months; *drug has potential retinal effects.* Toxic effects: Headache, dizziness, GI complaints, ocular toxicity and retinopathy.
Gold Therapy (Chrysotherapy)		
Gold sodium thiomalate (Myochrysine)	Gold salts are useful when rheumatoid activity is uncontrolled by nonsteroidal therapy.	Toxic effects: Dermatitis, stomatitis, nephropathy, blood dyscrasias. Blood count performed before each injection.

TABLE 59-2. (Continued)

DRUG	ACTION	NURSING IMPLICATION AND ASSESSMENT FOR DRUG INTOLERANCE
Gold Therapy (Chrysotherapy) *(Continued)* Aurothioglucose (Solganal)	Gold therapy is cumulative with slow onset of beneficial effects. Mechanism of action unknown; exerts an inflammatory-suppressive effect. Can produce a long-sustained remission when treatment continued indefinitely. Induces remission; 8-14 weeks may pass before benefit is noted.	Question patient at each visit concerning pruritus, rash, sores in mouth, metallic taste. Read package insert before drug administration. Administer deep I.M. into the ventrogluteal area to avoid local irritation or necrosis of nerves, a potential lethal complication of injection.

Corticosteroids
Corticotropin
Adrenocorticotropic hormone (ACTH)
	Corticosteroids used in treatment of incapacitating active rheumatoid arthritis when other conservative measures fail to control the disease.
	Use of corticosteroids for long periods has wide range of adverse effects.
	Steroids should be used with caution in small doses and for limited periods.
		Toxic effects:
		  Osteoporosis and fractures.
		  Gastric ulcers, psychiatric problems, infection.
		  Hirsutism, acne, moon facies, abnormal fat deposition, edema, emotional disorders, menstrual disorders.

Intra-articular Corticosteroid Injections	Given when rheumatoid arthritic reaction has been suppressed and 1 or 2 joints are not responding to treatment. Given when only 1-2 joints affected. Given to patient with extremely painful joints so he can undergo physical therapy. Relieves pain; benefit may last from weeks to months.	An inflamed joint may respond to local injection when it has failed to come under control with other general systemic measures. Joints most amenable to corticosteroid injections are ankles, knees, hips, shoulders and hands.

Immunosuppressive Drugs
Cyclophosphamide (Cytoxan)
Azathioprine (Imuran)
	Mechanisms underlying action of these drugs not known; thought to affect the production of antibodies at the cellular level.
	Suppress auto-immune mechanism.
	Used only in advanced rheumatoid arthritis that is unresponsive to conventional therapy.
	These drugs have teratogenic potential.
		Highly toxic:
		  Bone marrow depression, GI ulcerations.
		  Skin rashes, alopecia. Bladder toxicity.
		  Reduces patient's resistance to infections.
		Patient must be monitored with weekly blood evaluation and urinalysis.
		Advise patient of contraceptive measures.

gratification. An understanding of these factors is important in the patient's comprehensive management.

Rheumatoid arthritis alters all aspects of the person's life, including work, family and leisure. The nurse and family should try to understand the patient's personality and his emotional reactions to the disease. Presenting a realistic but optimistic view by pointing out that only a small percentage of patients become disabled can help reassure the patient. At the same time the prospects of a favorable outcome must be linked to a faithful adherence to the rehabilitation program that is designed to improve functioning. The patient can be reassured that something can be done to relieve his pain and mobilize his joints.

Patients with rheumatoid arthritis require long-term support and *continuing explanations* of the treatment program in order to cope with the anxiety related to the fear of becoming crippled and disabled. Patients with chronically painful joints may be hostile, angry, and bitter.

Such behavior should not be reciprocated with an equally negative response. It is better for the patient to express hostility than to suppress it and to ultimately stop trying to communicate with the health care team. Failure of communication also leads to deterioration of inter-family relationships.

Ideally the community health nurse appraises the home environment, monitors and encourages the patient to carry out the prescribed program, interprets the disease process to the patient and the family, and supplies the feedback data to the physician.

Patient Education and Rehabilitation

In order for the patient to become functionally independent, he must be instructed and trained by the nurse and others of the rehabilitation team in activities of daily living. It is important that the nurse work with the patient to achieve the goals of self-care and independence.

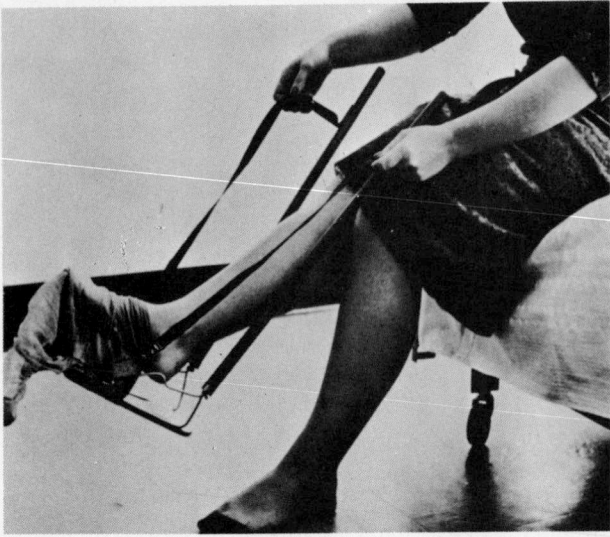

Figure 59-3. The purpose of self-help devices is to conserve energy and help the patient maintain his independence. There are many such devices available. Ingenious nurses working with patients can invent "gadgets" to solve individual problems. Simple things are not easy if you are crippled with arthritis. (The Arthritis Foundation)

There are many self-help devices available to assist with dressing, bathing, and eating (Fig. 59-3). Corrective shoes are helpful in treating and preventing foot deformities and will make walking easier. Canes or crutches may be prescribed as assistive devices to reduce the amount of weight-bearing on the joints of the lower extremities.

As the patient gains more independence, vocational counseling and job placement services may be used to help secure employment.

To correct pre-existing deformities, progressive resistive exercises that have been individually prescribed for the patient are carried out by the physical therapist. (See principles of rehabilitation nursing, Chapter 12.) Reconstructive surgery of the hips, knees, hands, feet and other joints may restore some function and reduce pain (page 1335).

Although there is no specific "cure" for rheumatoid arthritis, much can be done to alleviate suffering and prevent crippling by applying specific therapeutic measures. For the program to be effective the patient must be wholeheartedly involved in the therapeutic program. The federal government has established arthritis centers across the U.S. to carry out research and apprise patients and medical personnel of the newest advances in arthritis therapy. The summary outline on pages 1331-1332 includes the major aspects of patient education and rehabilitation.

DEGENERATIVE JOINT DISEASE (OSTEOARTHRITIS)

Osteoarthritis is a degeneration of the articular cartilage in the joints. It is the most common of all joint diseases. By the age of 50, about 50 percent of the population show the characteristic pathologic changes both clinically and on x-ray.

Pathophysiology. As a person ages, the elasticity of the joint capsules, articular cartilages and ligaments is reduced. The articular plate is thinned and its function as a shock absorber is decreased. There is narrowing of the joint space and loss of stability. When the articular plate disappears, spurs form at the edges of the joint surfaces and the capsule and synovial membranes thicken. The joint cartilages degenerate and atrophy, the bones harden at their articular surfaces, and the ligaments calcify. Nevertheless, the joint spaces themselves remain preserved; no adhesions form in them. Sterile joint effusions not infrequently develop, particularly in the knees.

Causes. Osteoarthritis is to be regarded essentially as a senescent process—the result of prolonged wear and tear of the joint surfaces which has produced changes, not only in the bony structures but also in the cartilaginous and soft tissue components of the joints. Other precipitating factors include repeated trauma, faulty body posture and mechanics, excessive joint use, strenuous physical labor and obesity, which subject the weight-bearing joints to unusual strain and diminish vascular supply due to developing vascular sclerosis.

Clinical Manifestations. The common symptoms are pain and stiffness. The pain is usually worse after inactivity but also increases with continued use and is improved by rest. There usually is some restriction of movement. Among the joints most frequently involved are those of the fingers, which may give rise to *Heberden's nodes,* bony nodules that appear on the distal joints of some or all of the fingers. These nodes, which appear most often among middle-aged women, may develop abruptly with pain and inflammation but when fully developed cause no pain. No known treatment modifies their development.

Osteoarthritis of the first metatarsophalangeal (MTP) joint of the foot is common. Since weight-bearing joints are particularly involved, the hips and knees may be the site of severe disability. The spine is a common site of degenerative joint disease especially in the midcervical, midthoracic and the L3-L4 areas, which are the regions of greatest movement in the spine. Films of the spine demonstrate spur formation and gross irregularities involving the margins and the articular surfaces of the vertebral bodies, which causes localized pain and stiffness.

Management. The objectives of management are to relieve discomfort, preserve joint function, and protect the joints from undue stress and trauma. Treatment is largely symptomatic and is generally the same as that used in rheumatoid arthritis: rest with alternating periods of activity, analgesics, regulated exercise, and later, corrective surgery.

A summary of nursing objectives, guidelines, and teaching points for the management of persons with osteoarthritis is found on page 1333.

Goal: To maintain function of all joints

A. To understand the disease in order to learn to live with it
1. Learn the nature of the disease and its treatment.
2. Have confidence in your physician and individualized treatment program.
3. Avoid "miracle cures"—drugs not prescribed by your physician and other forms of "quackery."
4. Report to the physician or clinic *regularly* for evaluation.
   a. Joints must be examined at regular intervals to measure range of motion.
   b. X-ray evaluations of hands, wrists and feet can detect disease activity (erosion, cartilage destruction).
5. Have regular medical and functional reevaluation to determine whether there is any loss of joint function.
6. Accept the *realities* of the disease and live within the limits imposed by it.
7. Maintain your independence.
   a. Rely on your own capabilities.
   b. Participate in as many activities as possible without producing fatigue.
   c. Use self-help devices and "gadgets" to conserve energy and expand efficiency.
   d. Study and use methods of work simplification.
   e. Build up muscle strength and endurance by participating in an exercise program.
   f. *Pace yourself.* Avoid overdoing on "good" days.
   g. Alternate sitting and standing tasks.
8. Try to avoid anxiety, worry, and emotional crises.

B. To relieve pain and reduce inflammation
1. Achieve a balance between rest and activity.
2. Have scheduled rest periods in bed to reduce joint stresses and control fatigue.
   a. Use a bedboard under the mattress to prevent sagging.
   b. Use a bed cradle when the joints of ankles and feet are involved.
   c. Rest in positions of extension maintaining good posture.
   d. Place only one pillow under the head.
   e. Avoid putting pillows under painful joints to prevent flexion deformities.
   f. Turn in prone position twice daily to prevent hip flexion and knee contractures.
   g. Modify rest time gradually as improvement is seen.
   h. Secure a long period of sleep at night (at least 10 hours).
3. Rest and support inflamed joints.
   a. Use prescribed splints and supports to relieve pain and muscle spasm.
   b. Support inflamed joints in their most functional position.
   c. Wear splints during sleeping hours.
   d. Keep in mind that the splint may need to be altered every week or two.

e. Avoid stroking and rubbing joints that are swollen and painful.
f. Avoid overactivity that produces fatigue.
g. Take salicylates 1½ hours before arising in the morning to relieve stiffness.
4. Use heat treatments for muscle relaxation and relief of pain and postrest stiffness.
   a. Take a warm shower or tub bath upon arising to relieve morning stiffness.
      (1) Rest in bed 20 to 30 minutes if possible after warm bath
   b. Apply warm moist compresses to especially painful joints *as directed* several times daily.
      (1) Leave hot application on only for prescribed length of time
      (2) Cover moist compresses with hot water bottle, plastic wrap, and a heavy towel to prevent rapid loss of heat
   c. Use paraffin dips as prescribed for the hands (Fig. 59-4).
      (1) Melt paraffin in a double boiler (4 lbs. paraffin to 1 pint of light mineral oil), or use a slow cooker.
      (2) Use a candy thermometer to determine exact temperature (52-54° C. or 126-130° F.).
      (3) Allow mixture to cool until a film forms on top.
      (4) Immerse part in warm paraffin quickly, allow wax to harden, withdraw and immerse again (Fig. 59-4).
         (a) Repeat procedure 8 to 10 times until paraffin glove is formed.
         (b) Cover with a towel to retain heat.
         (c) Leave in place for 15 to 20 min. or until cool.
         (d) Peel off paraffin and re-use at next treatment time.
         (e) Do finger and hand exercises immediately after treatment.
   d. Use contrast baths (hot and cold) as prescribed.
   e. If heat intensifies pain, discontinue heat treatments and notify physician.
   f. Try cold packs or ice applied to acutely inflamed painful joints.
   g. Try an electric blanket to ascertain its usefulness in relieving morning stiffness.
5. Take prescribed drugs for pain relief on a regular schedule, and exactly as prescribed.
   a. Aspirin must be taken in divided doses throughout the day. Take with food (a buffering agent).
   b. Develop an awareness of the *amount* of aspirin or sodium salicylates necessary to provide individual relief of pain and stiffness.
   c. Report symptoms of ringing in the ears or decreased hearing as this is a guide in controlling dosage.
   d. Watch for symptoms of gastric irritation and diminished hearing.

(Continued)

---

e. Do not substitute Empirin or Tylenol for aspirin: these possess no anti-inflammatory properties but are pain relievers.

C. To preserve joint function and prevent deformities

1. Do the prescribed exercises to preserve joint motion and to gain muscular strength and endurance.
   a. Know the purpose of each exercise.
   b. Perform the exercise slowly.
   c. Perform one set of exercises after using systemic heat (shower/bath).
2. Carry out range of motion exercises several times daily.
   a. Do muscle setting (isometric) and deep breathing exercises at 1- or 2-hour intervals.
   b. Start active exercises and progress to resistive exercises when condition permits.
3. Increase gradually the frequency and duration of the exercise period.
   a. Do the exercises 2 to 4 times daily.
   b. Decrease the time if pain persists more than 2 hours following exercise.

4. Use swimming pool for exercise periods when available; muscles are exercised and water supports the joints.
5. Avoid prolonged sitting, which produces stiffness and flexion adduction deformities.
6. Wear proper shoes (not slippers) and tarsal and metatarsal supports when necessary.
7. Use supports (crutches, braces) during periods of exacerbation of disease of the weight-bearing joints.
8. Wear stretch gloves at night to relieve numbness and tingling of fingers.
9. Protect the joints from further injury.
   a. Sit in chairs with higher seats to avoid "collapsing" into chair with resultant knee and hip joint trauma.
   b. Avoid continued standing and walking when fatigued.
   c. Refrain from sudden, jerky movements.
   d. Avoid obesity which places greater strain on weight-bearing joints.

TRAUMATIC ARTHRITIS

Of all joints, those most susceptible to injury resulting in arthritis are the knee and the lumbosacral and sacroiliac joints. The joint may be involved directly by injury (fracture of articular surface) or indirectly by a twisting or wrenching motion that causes rupture of the tendons, tears of the semilunar cartilage, and disruption of the joint capsule with dislocation or subluxation.

If dislocated pieces of cartilage (for example, the semilunar cartilage of the knee) have been chipped off into the joint cavity as the result of injury and are not removed by operation, the joint remains painful and its movements limited. Joint movements may be limited permanently by scar tissue formed in the capsules.

Following a sprain, inflammation of the interior joint lining (the synovial membrane) may develop, and, later, in the course of a few weeks, degenerative changes may occur in the cartilaginous articular surfaces and in underlying bones. When structures in the joint are injured hemorrhage may occur into the joint (hemarthrosis). The blood can incite an inflammatory reaction in the synovium which again is capable of producing scar tissue leading to erosion of articular surfaces.

ANKYLOSING SPONDYLITIS (MARIE-STRUMPELL DISEASE)

Ankylosing spondylitis is a systemic inflammatory disease of the joints of the spine — the cartilaginous joints between the vertebral bodies and the gliding joint between the vertebral arches of the spine. The disease may range from minimal involvement to severe disability.

If the disease progresses, there is ossification and ankylosis (fixation) of the joints, and the entire spine and the thorax become extensively ankylosed. Peripheral joints may be involved and extra-articular manifestations

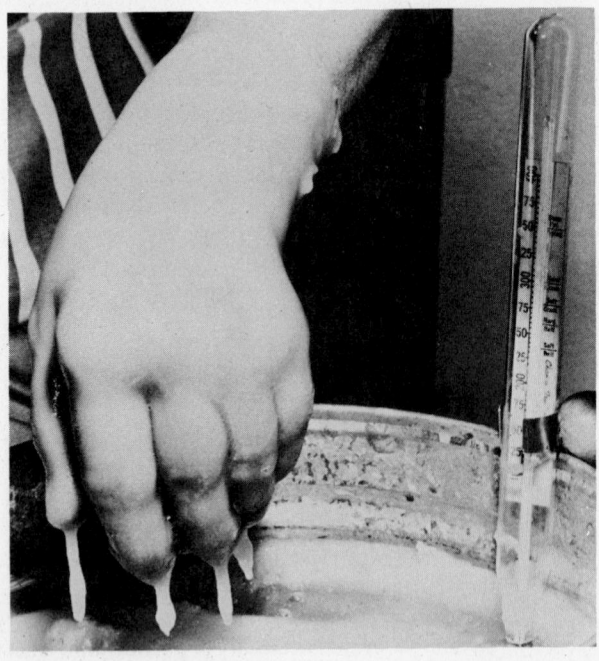

Figure 59-4. Hot paraffin applications are useful for the patient with arthritis because they provide uniform heat. Paraffin dips are particularly effective for painful hands and wrists. See page 1331 for instructions to the patient for the use of paraffin applications. (The Arthritis Foundation)

MANAGEMENT OF THE PATIENT WITH DEGENERATIVE JOINT DISEASE (OSTEOARTHRITIS)
Summary of Objectives and Guidelines of Nursing Management and Patient Education

A. To relieve strain on the affected joints advise the patient to:
1. Rest in a recumbent position twice daily; symptoms worsen when joints are overused.
2. Rest the involved joints with splints, braces, cervical collars, etc.
3. Use correct posture and body mechanics.
4. Use cane, crutches, braces, or walker when indicated to reduce weight-bearing stress of hips and knees.
5. Wear stretch gloves at night to relieve pain and stiffness of fingers.
6. Sleep with a rolled terrycloth towel under the neck for relief of cervical osteoarthritis.
7. Do not engage in excessive activity and unusual exercise or effort.

B. To control the pain:
1. Relieve pain, stiffness, and muscle spasm with prescribed forms of heat and physical therapy.
   a. Use hot packs, warm soaks, tub baths, paraffin dips.
   b. Try cold applications if heat is not effective.
   c. Do isometric exercises to maintain muscle tone.
2. Give anti-inflammatory agents when synovial inflammation is present.
3. Give analgesics for pain control.
4. Use muscle relaxants when muscle spasm is present.
5. Support the patient undergoing intra-articular (into the joint) injections of long-acting steroids.

6. Advise the patient to use positive coping mechanisms to deal with emotional strain which increases muscle tension and joint strain.

C. To avoid trauma and further wearing of the weight-bearing joints the patient should be instructed as follows:
1. Do postural exercises to correct poor posture.
2. Wear corrective shoes for foot disorders.
3. Carry out weight reduction under medical and nursing supervision to decrease stress on weight-bearing joints.
4. Stop excessive weight-bearing activities, such as lifting, carrying heavy loads, excessive vigorous overhead reaching.
5. Avoid continuous standing.

D. To restore function to the maximal extent:
1. Use range of motion exercises to prevent capsular and tendon tightening.
2. Avoid flexion deformities by splinting and proper positioning.
3. Use corrective and graded exercises to improve muscle strength around the involved joint.
4. Support the patient undergoing orthopedic surgery for severely disabling joint involvement.
   a. Surgery for joint malalignment to alleviate abnormal joint stiffness.
   b. Debridement of loose bodies (cartilage, bone, large spurs).
   c. Osteotomy to redistribute joint forces.

---

may be apparent. The disease predominates in men, typically occurring between the ages of 15 and 30 years, and it appears to have a genetic predisposing factor.

The initial symptoms are usually in the lower back with aching pain, morning stiffness, and sacroiliac tenderness. In a significant number of patients, the peripheral joints are involved, usually the knee or hip. To ease the backache, the patient bends over, so that a thoracic curvature (kyphosis) develops which in time can lead to impaired pulmonary function.

Associated Conditions. At some point in the disease, as many as 25 percent of the patients have acute anterior uveitis. Cardiovascular abnormalities (aortic insufficiency, cardiomegaly, pericarditis), pulmonary fibrosis, and amyloidosis are associated conditions.

Management. The immediate objective is to relieve pain, while the long-range goals are to retard the disease process (if possible) and prevent spinal deformity.

Drugs are given to relieve inflammation, pain, stiffness and spasm so that the patient can follow a program of exercise. Aspirin is effective, as is indomethacin which has an analgesic and anti-inflammatory action. The butazones (phenylbutazone and oxyphenbutazone) are effective but have toxic reactions and must be administered with caution.

Patient Education. Particular attention is paid to posture. The patient is advised to sit on straight-back chairs and stand erect, avoiding the temptation to slouch.

An extra-firm mattress should be used or a bed board placed under the mattress. A small cervical neck roll can be used instead of a pillow. Regular intervals of rest are beneficial along with periods of lying prone which help prevent a hip flexion abnormality.

Exercise is essential to prevent postural deformities and limitation of movement in the spine, chest and peripheral joints. Specific exercises to build up muscles and to strengthen the extensor muscle groups are usually taught by the physical therapist. Swimming is an excellent general exercise for all muscle groups, although special breathing exercises are important to maintain maximum chest expansion.

Reconstructive surgery is performed when indicated. If a significant flexion deformity develops, removal of a portion of the vertebra (wedge osteotomy) to allow straightening of the spine may be indicated. Total hip replacement may be required in order to restore hip movement.

Since this disease is manifest in the prime of adult life, pain, disability and deformity have an impact which requires psychological adaptation. Sexual counseling is

TABLE 59-3. SURGICAL INTERVENTION FOR ARTHRITIS

Underlying Considerations:
1. Surgical intervention is advocated before joints are destroyed and surrounding musculature becomes contracted and atrophied.
2. Surgery is done to prevent further joint destruction. Priority is given to weight-bearing joints.

Objectives:
1. To keep the patient functional by restoring motion and stability.
2. To relieve pain.

TYPE OF SURGERY	DESCRIPTION	INDICATIONS	NURSING IMPLICATIONS
Articular Surgery			
Arthroplasty (Total joint replacement) (Fig. 59-5)	Reconstruction of a joint	Relief of pain Restore movement and stability Correct deformity	Surveillance for postoperative infection Special emphasis placed on positioning Support patient with exercise program.
Synovectomy	Excision of hypertrophied, inflamed synovial membrane within a joint	Prevents erosive bone changes that cause joint destruction Usually considered a palliative measure; performed on knee, finger, wrist and elbow joints	Suction drainage in immediate postoperative period. Knee exercises and gentle motion started after suction tube is removed.
Arthrodesis	Fusion of a bone to eliminate a joint; results in loss of joint motion	Performed to obtain a stable, painless joint Especially effective in the wrist	
Para-articular Surgery			
Osteotomy	Surgical cutting of bone that changes the alignment, with or without bone removal	Osteotomy of tibia or femur corrects valgus or varus deformities of the knee joint	
Tendon Surgery			
Tenorrhaphy	Repair of ruptured tendon; diseased synovium invades tendon and interferes with its nutrition leading to necrosis and rupture	Restore function Rupture of extensor tendons fairly common in arthritis causing difficulty in extending part	Repair of tendons does not usually give full extension postoperatively
Tenosynovectomy	Excision of thickened tendon sheath and other tissue surrounding tendon		Institute early joint motion to prevent stiffness and adhesions of flexor tendons
Tendon transfer	Redirecting an intact tendon from one position to another	Done to replace or help muscle function lost from nerve damage, rupture of tendon	
Neurolysis Surgical procedure in which entrapped nerve is relieved from pressure by diseased synovium	Surgical decompression for carpal tunnel syndrome (compression of median nerve within the carpal tunnel)	Nerve entrapment can produce loss of motor and nerve function	Encourage patient to exercise hand postoperatively to prevent adhesions and loss of function
	Surgical decompression of ulnar nerve entrapment (excision and release of synovial tissue)	Entrapment of deep peroneal nerve, posterior tibial nerve (tarsal tunnel syndrome) also occurs	Nerve entrapment syndromes characterized by disturbances of sensation, painful tingling and weakness

advocated if the patient has hip flexion contractures (see bibliography on the sexuality of the disabled, Chapter 12). With treatment and continuing follow-up, the majority of patients will lead nearly normal lives.

The role of the nurse is one of supporting and reinforcing health teaching, encouraging the patient to carry out the remedial exercises and emphasizing good posture.

SURGERY FOR ARTHRITIS AND OTHER JOINT PROBLEMS

In spite of good therapeutic management, the arthritic process may progress to a point at which the patient's condition deteriorates. In such instances a variety of corrective procedures can be performed for joint deformity secondary to arthritic damage in both rheumatoid arthritis and osteoarthritis. The aims of surgical treatment are to improve function and relieve pain. In order for the surgeon to select the best procedure available and to achieve the best result, surgery should be performed before the surrounding musculature becomes contracted and atrophied and serious structural abnormalities occur. In general, surgery is indicated for progressive synovitis, severe joint deformity, loss of function, constant severe pain, faulty alignment, tendon ruptures, nerve compression and ankylosis. Surgical therapies in current use for joint disease include: excision of diseased tissues (example, synovectomy), repair of damaged structures such as a ruptured tendon, immobilization or fusion of a joint (arthrodesis) and replacement of all or parts of a joint (joint arthroplasty). Partial or total prosthetic replacements are being done with increasing frequency. Table 59-3 summarizes some of these procedures.

Complications of surgery for arthritis are similar to other operative procedures. In addition these patients are frequently anemic and bones may be softened due to disuse and corticosteroid therapy. The skin in these patients also tends to heal slowly because it has become thin, fragile and friable from long-term steroid therapy. Finally, dislocation of the prosthesis, fracturing of osteoporotic bones and hypotension secondary to steroid-induced adrenal suppression may occur.

Total Hip Replacement

Total hip replacement is the replacement of a severely damaged hip with an artificial joint. Although a large number of implants are available, most consist of a metal femoral component topped by a spherical ball fitted into a plastic acetabular socket and held in the bone with methyl methacrylate (bone cement) (Fig. 59-5). Following a successful operation, the hip is free or nearly free of pain, has good motion, is more stable, and usually permits normal or near normal ambulation.

The operation is usually reserved for patients over 45 or 50 with unremitting pain and/or irreversibly damaged hip joints. The following conditions are amenable to this type of surgery: arthritis (degenerative joint disease; rheumatoid arthritis), complications of femoral neck fractures, failure of previous reconstructive surgery (osteotomy, cup arthroplasty, femoral head replacement) and problems resulting from congenital hip disease. More recently, selected patients with pathologic fractures from metastatic cancer have benefitted from total hip-joint replacement.

Preoperative Nursing Management. Total joint replacement is an exacting and meticulous procedure. A complete preoperative evaluation is carried out with emphasis on cardiovascular, respiratory, renal and hepatic function since this surgery is done on the older age group. Every effort is made to prevent pulmonary embolism as this is the most common cause of postoperative mortality. Obesity, preoperative leg edema, history of deep vein thrombosis, varicose veins and osteoarthritis

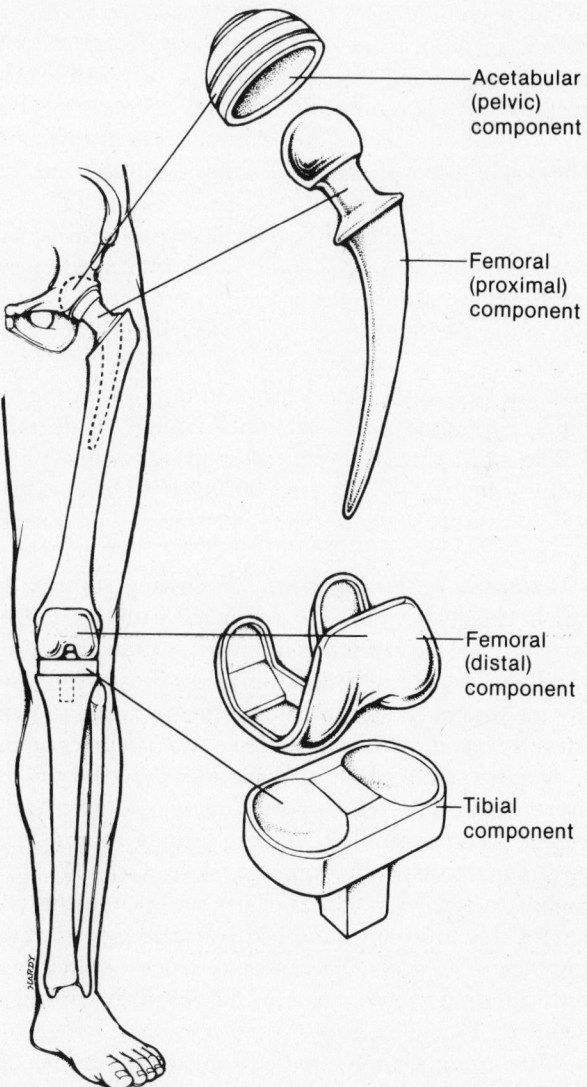

Acetabular (pelvic) component

Femoral (proximal) component

Femoral (distal) component

Tibial component

Figure 59-5. Hip and knee replacement.

increase the risk of postoperative pulmonary embolism. Prophylactic anticoagulation is used with aspirin, dextran or warfarin. The patient is typed and cross-matched in the event transfusions are required.

Infection is the most feared complication, because it generally means that the implant unit must be removed. A search is made before the operation for any possible source of infection, since an untreated infection anywhere in the body precludes surgery. Preoperative urine cultures are taken since urinary tract infection is a likely portal of entry for bacteria. The use of preoperative antibiotics is controversial but many surgeons use bactericidal antibiotics that are effective against Gram positive and Gram negative organisms during the preoperative, intraoperative, and postoperative period. Research suggests that the majority of deep infections are caused by bacteria that are implanted into the wound at the time of surgery, mostly from airborne sources. During operation there is strict adherence to aseptic principles including double gloves, double masks, special gowns with waterproof fronts and sleeves and devices used to make the operating area as bacteria-free as possible. The operative area is scrubbed twice daily preoperatively as microorganisms on the skin can cause latent infection. The on-call preoperative medication is injected into the uninvolved extremity.

The patient is taught isometric exercises of the quadriceps and gluteal muscles and is fitted with crutches and instructed in a nonweight-bearing gait (no weight-bearing on the affected extremity) to facilitate postoperative ambulation. The patient is also taught how to transfer from the bed to the wheelchair without flexing the hip joints beyond the prescribed limits—usually 45 degrees. At the same time, the patient is shown some of the equipment that will be used during the postoperative period: overbed traction frame, the trapeze, and the abduction splint.

Postoperative Management. Following surgery the patient usually is positioned flat in bed with the affected extremity held in abduction by either an abduction splint or pillows to prevent dislocation of the prosthesis. Usually the patient is not turned until the physician so indicates. At first the patient is turned only 45 degrees on the unoperated side with the hip kept fully abducted and the entire length of the leg supported by two pillows. As the patient becomes familiar with the turning routine he is encouraged to assist by using the overbed trapeze. He is also instructed not to adduct or flex the operated hip. As part of this procedure, the bed is usually not elevated more than 45 degrees. There are numerous modifications with differing requirements in the postoperative management of these patients.

When using the fracture bed pan, the patient should flex the unoperated hip and knee and use the trapeze to lift the pelvis onto the pan. He is instructed not to bear down on the operated hip in flexion when getting on the bed pan.

An ice cap may be prescribed intermittently to the operative site to reduce edema. Portable suction of the wound is used to decrease the incidence of wound hematoma which is a possible focus of infection. If an indwelling urethral catheter is used, it must be meticulously cared for and removed as early as possible to prevent sepsis.

The circulation in the operated extremity is assessed by checking the sensation, pulses, color and temperature of the leg. These signs are compared with the unoperated extremity. A sudden onset of pain in the extremity may be due to hematoma, especially if the patient is on anticoagulation therapy.

On the day following surgery, active foot and ankle motion may be started to prevent circulatory stasis and decrease the chance of postoperative thrombosis. Specific exercises are supervised by the physical therapist. Pain medication is given one half hour before the exercise session as required by the patient. A knee sling may be placed on the extremity to begin active flexion and extension of the knee, hip, and foot (Fig. 59-6). By using the sling, the patient may start gentle abduction when permitted. The exercises are carried out to increase range of motion and muscle strength in the operative hip and to work toward the goal of independence in ambulation.

When the patient is helped out of bed, an abduction splint or pillows are kept between the legs. Once the patient is out of bed, the hip is kept at maximum extension. The procedure for assisting the patient out of bed consists of instructing the patient to pivot on the unaffected extremity while the nurse supports the extremity that has the implant. An aged or weakened patient may need to be lifted into a chair by several persons.

At first the patient may merely be able to stand because of weakness or light-headedness from orthostatic hypotension. When he is ready to ambulate he is taught to use a walker by first advancing the walker and then advancing the involved extremity to the walker, bearing most of his weight on his hands. After he has mastered ambulating with the walker he progresses to crutch walking at which time he is taught the 3-point gait which requires that he lead with the uninvolved extremity while simultaneously moving the involved extremity and the crutches together.

Complications. Patients who have undergone surgery for total hip replacement have a higher incidence of thromboembolic disease than patients who have undergone other surgical procedures. Fatal pulmonary emboli occurs in approximately 2 percent of patients over 40 who have not received prophylaxis (heparin, warfarin, dextran, aspirin). Other measures which help reduce the incidence of thrombosis include exercising the ankles and legs (to accelerate blood flow and prevent venous stasis) and applying elastic stockings. The extremities are checked daily for calf edema and tenderness.

Deep infection is the most serious complication following total hip replacement. Deep infection may occur as late as 8 years after operation and almost always requires removal of the implant. It may result from bacteria introduced at the time of operation or from a transient septicemia. Other complications include dislocation of the hip, loosening of the prosthesis, heterotropic ossification (formation of bone in the periprosthetic space), avascular necrosis or dead bone caused by loss of blood supply.

Patient Education Following Total Hip Replacement. A program of patient education involves teaching the patient how important it is that the hip be maintained in abduction at all times and that stooping be avoided. The patient should also be reminded that until otherwise instructed he should use a pillow between his knees when lying in a supine or side-lying position and when turning. This prevents possible dislocation of the affected hip before the soft tissue has had a chance to heal and adequate muscle control has been restored. He is not to sleep on the operated side until directed to do so by the surgeon, and he should keep the operated leg elevated when he is seated. At no time should he cross his legs. Positions of flexion during sexual activity are to be avoided to prevent adduction and subluxation of the prosthesis.

Over exertion is to be avoided to prevent pain. However taking frequent walks is excellent exercise. Low back chairs should be avoided as well as sitting for more than 30 minutes at a time to minimize hip flexion and the risk of prosthetic dislocation and to prevent hip stiffness and flexion contracture. Traveling long distances is also to be avoided unless frequent changes in position are possible.

Crutches are used for the length of time prescribed for the individual patient, usually 6 weeks. After the patient is able to walk well with crutches, a cane may be used. The cane is usually discarded when sufficient muscle tone has returned to permit normal gait.

The patient is advised to be faithful in the daily exercise program in order to maintain the functional motion of the hip joint and strengthen the abductor muscles of the hip. It will take time to strengthen and reeducate the muscles. Swimming is beneficial. In general, by three months the patient is able to resume all routine daily living activities with the exception of strenuous sports such as tennis and skiing. Heavy loads, excessive bending and twisting (lifting, shoveling snow, forceful turning) are to be avoided.

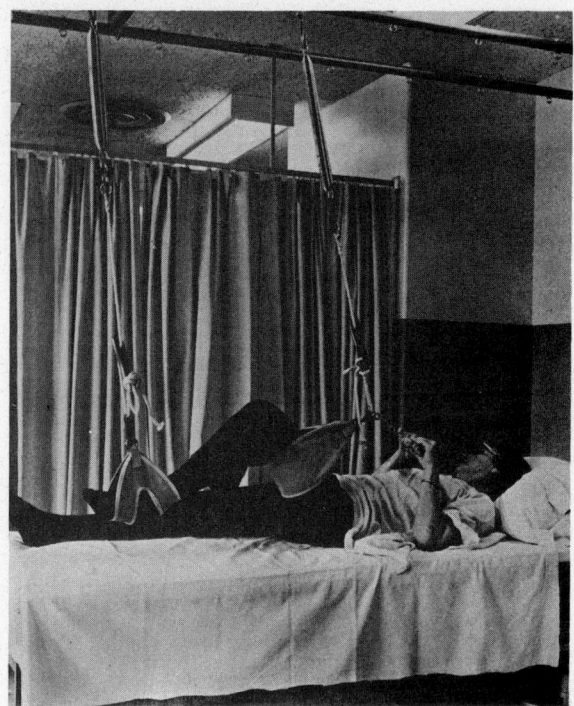

Figure 59-6.   A proximal knee sling is used in this patient with a total hip replacement. Hip and knee flexion is assisted by a handle fastened to the proximal knee sling. (Reprinted with permission of Physical Therapy, 52:826, 1972)

Total Knee Replacement

Total knee replacement is an implant procedure in which both the tibial and femoral joints are replaced because of destroyed knee joint(s). There are over 300 different knee prostheses in use but most fall into two classifications: the hinge variety (Young or Walldius prosthesis) or the unattached variety in which the tibial and femoral components are cemented in place and articulate with one another, but are unattached; instead they are held together by muscle action (geometric or polycentric knee).

The indication for total replacement of the knee is advanced destruction of the joint with marked instability or restriction of motion. The patient may need replacement therapy for both knees.

Preoperative Management. Since thromboembolism is a complication following surgery for total knee replacement, the patient may be given low weight dextran or warfarin to prevent thromboembolism and pulmonary embolism. Before surgery every effort is made to eradicate any foci of infection, with prophylactic antibiotic therapy given before and after the operation. The same principles for the prevention of infection are observed as those carried out for total hip replacement (page 1335).

Postoperative Management. Following surgery, the knee is bandaged with a firm compression bandage.

Some surgeons use a long-leg plaster cast or an extension splint for immobilization to overcome the tendency of some patients to develop flexion contractures in the immediate postoperative period. The leg may be elevated on pillows above the level of the heart, and the foot of the bed may be elevated to decrease the possibility of postoperative thrombophlebitis. The head of the bed is not elevated except while meals are eaten. Ice packs may be applied to the operative area to minimize swelling.

The operative area is checked for excessive drainage. A suction catheter is in place to provide constant drainage of the knee to remove excessive accumulation of blood. Suction drainage should not exceed 300 ml. in 6 to 8 hours.

Quadriceps setting exercises are generally started on the first postoperative day and flexion and extension of the feet and hips are encouraged. An inability to flex the foot could indicate peroneal nerve palsy due to pressure exerted by the dressing or cast on the Achilles tendon or at the head of the fibula.

When prescribed, the physical therapist starts gentle knee flexion exercises which may then be actively carried out with the aid of a pulley and sling exerciser. Ambulation with crutches or a walker is allowed when the patient can perform straight leg raising and flex and extend the knee adequately. Full weight-bearing is usually not tolerated for 6 weeks to allow time for repair of those tissues damaged at the site of the bone-cement interface. If the patient is not able to flex the knee satisfactorily (60 degrees of flexion by the 14th postoperative day), gentle manipulation is carried out under general anesthesia.

Early complications of total knee replacement are infection, thromboembolism, and peroneal nerve palsy. Deep infection, loosening of the prosthetic components, dislocation and wearing of the implant, as well as fatigue fracture of the tibial plateau are late complications.

Patient Education. A resting splint may be prescribed for nighttime use for several weeks to maintain the knee at extension. The patient is instructed to continue the exercise program until at least one year after surgery. A stationary bicycle is helpful in improving range of motion and strengthening the muscles. The patient is instructed to lift weights with the affected leg, starting with one-half pound and increasing the weight per physician's directions. Because there is a large implant present and the development of deep infection can be catastrophic, some orthopedists advocate preventive antibiotic therapy if the patient needs any type of subsequent surgical instrumentation such as tooth extraction or cystoscopy.

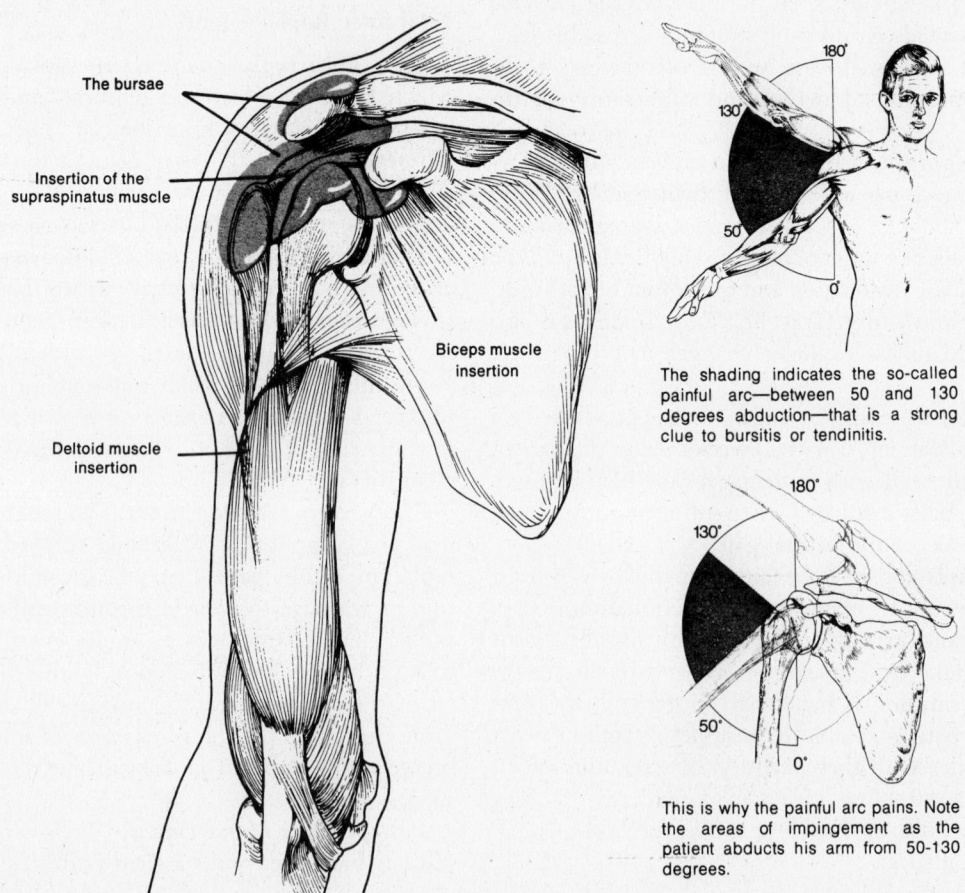

The shading indicates the so-called painful arc—between 50 and 130 degrees abduction—that is a strong clue to bursitis or tendinitis.

This is why the painful arc pains. Note the areas of impingement as the patient abducts his arm from 50-130 degrees.

Figure 59-7. Principal sites of pain in bursitis and calcific tendonitis. (From Nursing Update, Oct. 1973. Copyright © 1973, Miller and Fink Corporation, Darien, Conn. All rights reserved)

TABLE 59-4.   PAINFUL SHOULDER SYNDROMES*

SYNDROMES	CLINICAL FEATURES	CLINICAL MANIFESTATIONS	MANAGEMENT
Supraspinatus tendonitis Tenosynovitis	Reaction to mechanical stress and strain plus a degenerative process with traumatic inflammation	Pain in shoulder; "catching" sensation Patient grabs affected shoulder with opposite hand Night pain; inability to lie on affected side Painful arc beyond 60° abduction (as tendons and cuff impinge under coracoacromonial arch (Fig. 59-7)	Intermittent heat/cold applications Pendulum exercises Anti-inflammatory medications—salicylates (aspirin) to tolerance Local injection of steroid and/or anesthetic agent into shoulder joint
Calcific tendonitis	Calcific deposits develop in tendons; causes reaction in overlying bursa Calcific tendonitis and bursitis often coexist	Occurs in younger and more active persons Abrupt onset of severe aching pain, 1-4 days All shoulder and arm movement is painful Acute phase followed by pain relief	Infiltration of subacromial area and aspiration of deposit Analgesics for pain Anti-inflammatory agents (aspirin, phenylbutazone, indomethacin) Applications of heat/cold Injection with local anesthetic agent and steroid Operative treatment may be necessary for excision of calcified deposits
Tears and rupture of rotator cuff	Tears occur at the insertion of rotator cuff into the bone, probably from degenerative changes	Occur most commonly after 50 Abrupt shoulder pain in deltoid area Weakness/inability to abduct shoulder "Clicking" sensation felt in shoulder on abduction/rotation	Partial rupture usually responds to conservative management Infiltration with local anesthetic to relieve pain Confirmation of defect by arthrogram Surgical repair for complete rupture

Bicipital syndromes (lesions on the long head of biceps muscle)
  Tendonitis
  Tenosynovitis
	Long head of biceps affected by arm and shoulder movement	Chronic pain in anterolateral area of shoulder associated with muscle spasm and pain in trapezius, scalenus, deltoid	Rest of the limb
			Gentle exercises within tolerance
			Salicylates
			Heat applications to reduce inflammation
			Avoid movements that put biceps tendon on stretch

Bursitis	Almost all cases of subacromial bursitis have preceding tendonitis and tenosynovitis in the rotator cuff, biceps tendon and sheath or an inflammatory process in bone or joint; the spread of inflammation to bursa is a secondary event	Deep-seated ache in shoulder Pain upon rotation of the arm	Treatment consists of locating and treating the primary process causing the bursitis

*Adapted from: Bateman, J. E.: The Shoulder and Neck. Philadelphia, W. B. Saunders, 1978.

PAINFUL SHOULDER SYNDROME

The structures in and about the shoulder are frequently the site of painful syndromes. With aging, degenerative alterations occur in all joints, including the articulations comprising the shoulder joint (glenohumeral, sternoclavicular and acromioclavicular). Pain may arise from supraspinatus tendonitis or bicipital tendonitis with the inflammation spreading to the tendon sheaths, other tendons and their sheaths (tenosynovitis), the bursa, capsule, synovium, cartilage, bone and surrounding muscles. Frequently encountered syndromes are listed in Table 59-4.

Patient Education

The following are teaching points to protect the shoulder from further injury:
1. Support the affected arm on pillows while sleeping to keep from rolling over on the shoulder.
2. Avoid working and lifting above the shoulder level or pushing an object against a "locked" shoulder.
3. Do prescribe daily range of motion exercises to strengthen the shoulder girdle and glenohumeral muscle.

Other Hand and Finger Deformities

DUPUYTREN'S CONTRACTURE. Dupuytren's deformity is a slowly progressive contracture of the palmar fascia causing flexion of the little finger, the ring finger, and frequently the middle fingers, which renders them more or less useless. It is a fairly common abnormality, but its cause is unknown. It starts as a thickening of the palmar fascia. The fibrous thickening extends to involve the skin in the distal palm and produces a contracture of the fingers to which the palmar fascia is inserted. This condition always starts in one hand, but eventually both become symmetrically deformed. Plastic surgery, consisting of total excision of the involved palmar fascia, offers excellent relief.

GANGLION. A ganglion is a round, firm projection, usually near the wrist. It is a collection of gelatinous-like material near the tendon sheaths and joints. It is caused by strains, contusions, or a series of repeated minor strains, as a result of which the tissues of the sheath or sac involved have gradually become weakened and distended. As a rule, the ganglion is painless, but the affected joint often is weak and moderately painful. A ganglion has a tendency to rupture and disappear; it can also be dispersed by firm local pressure, but it will slowly reappear. The ganglion is surgically excised if it is painful or disfiguring.

LOW BACK PAIN

Low back pain is characterized by an uncomfortable or acute pain in the lumbosacral area associated with severe spasm of the paraspinal muscles. It is one of the most ubiquitous complaints of man. In fact backache is becoming the most common leveler of Americans, resulting in great discomfort, loss of time from work, and disability.

The causes of the condition are multiple. In the young and active person, it frequently represents acute and chronic muscle strains, ligament sprains and possibly pericapsular sprains of the joints of the vertebrae. Lack of physical activity and exercise, structural abnormalities, postural problems, obesity and systemic diseases are all possible causes. The pathological basis of backache may originate outside the spine. Pain, referred to the back, may result from other problems: gastrointestinal (penetrating ulcer, pancreatic tumor), genitourinary (renal calculi), gynecologic (tumor), peripheral vascular (aneurysm) or central nervous (spinal cord tumor). This type of pain is usually not aggravated by activity nor relieved by rest.

Back pain may also be due to herniation of a vertebral disc, which acts as a joint between the vertebral bodies and is subject to injury (usually flexion-rotation) and degeneration. The central nucleus pulposus of the disc may herniate causing symptoms of nerve root compression. Disc pain is usually worse upon sitting or bending and is improved by lying down. (Intervertebral disc disease is discussed on page 1257.)

Management

The objectives of management are (1) to relieve muscle spasm (painful contraction of muscles), (2) to gain normal elasticity of affected muscles, (3) to return the joint to normal function, and (4) to correct any underlying condition. The initial treatment for low back pain is conservative. Treatment is symptomatic and is directed at rest, heat, and appropriate medication. No specific treatment will alter degenerative changes in the discs.

The patient is advised to rest in bed in a Fowler's position with hips and knees flexed to remove stress from the lumbosacral area, to relax the muscles, relieve tension on sciatic nerves and open the posterior aspect of the intervertebral spaces. When the patient lies on his side, a pillow is placed between the flexed knees. If there is no nerve involvement or other serious underlying disease, acute spasm should subside in 3 to 7 days. Warm moist heat followed by massage relaxes muscle spasm and relieves discomfort. Sometimes cold applications may be equally as effective for secondary muscle spasm. Pain medications, muscle relaxants, and tranquilizers are also used. Injecting the trigger points with hydrocortisone and/or xylocaine may give dramatic pain relief. Pelvic traction and manipulation may also be utilized. The patient with a neurologic deficit should be evaluated more aggressively since the problem could stem from a disc herniation.

Usually low back pain is accompanied by weak abdominal muscles, which are the anterior supporting muscles of the spine. After acute symptoms subside the patient is started on exercises to strengthen these abdominal muscles. Exercises are prescribed to lessen lordosis while strengthening the abdominal and gluteal muscles. One simple exercise (gluteal tensing) is to contract the abdominal muscles (pull umbilicus toward spine) while exhaling forcibly. This exercise increases the tone of the gluteus maximus muscles of the buttocks. Other exercises are prescribed to strengthen the back muscles, increase mobility of the spine, stretch contracted structures and improve posture (Fig. 59-8). Pelvic tilt (pressing the small of the back against a flat surface) decreases lordosis.

Some patients, especially those who are obese, benefit by a light corset or back brace. Heel lifts may be necessary to level the pelvis, but high heels are to be avoided as they throw the body forward and increase lumbar lordosis.

Most patients get over the acute attack in 2 to 3 weeks. During this time, the patient can be reassured that normally the chances of recovery are good. If the patient shows no improvement after 10 to 14 days of conservative treatment, further diagnostic studies are indicated. If the

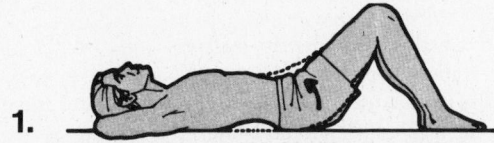

1.

Lie on your back with knees bent and hands clasped behind neck. Feet flat on the floor. Take a deep breath and relax. Press the small of your back against the floor and tighten your stomach and buttock muscles. This should cause the lower end of the pelvis to rotate forward and flatten your back against the floor. Hold for five seconds. Relax.

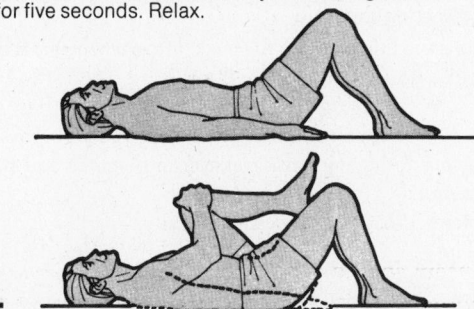

2.

Lie on your back with knees bent. Feet flat on the floor. Take a deep breath and relax. Grasp one knee with both hands and pull as close to your chest as possible. Return to starting position. Straighten leg. Return to starting position. Repeat with alternate leg.

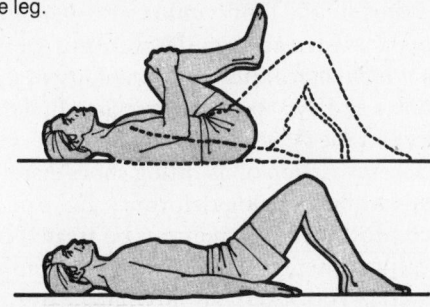

3.

Lie on your back with knees bent. Feet on the floor. Take a deep breath and relax. Grasp *both* knees and pull them as close to your chest as possible. Hold for three seconds, then return to starting position. Straighten legs and relax.

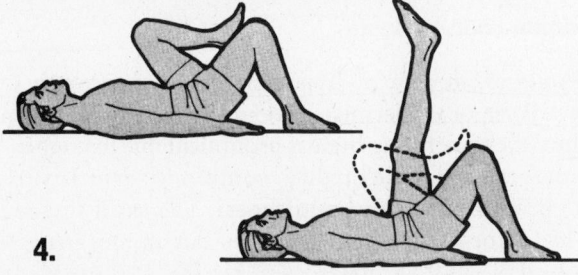

4.

Lie on your back with knees bent. Feet flat on the floor. Take a deep breath and relax. Draw one knee to chest. Then point leg upward as far as possible. Return to starting position. Relax. Repeat with alternate leg.

NOTE: This exercise is useful in stretching tight hamstring muscles, but is not recommended for patients with sciatic pain associated with a herniated disc.

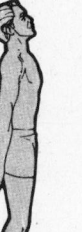 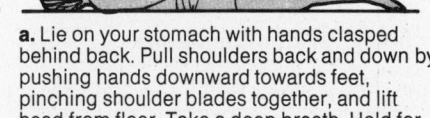

5.

a. Lie on your stomach with hands clasped behind back. Pull shoulders back and down by pushing hands downward towards feet, pinching shoulder blades together, and lift head from floor. Take a deep breath. Hold for two seconds. Relax.

b. Stand erect. With one hand grasp the thumb of other hand behind the back, then pull downwards toward the floor; stand on toes and look at the ceiling while exerting the downward pull. Hold momentarily, then relax. Repeat 10 times at intervals of two hours during the working day. Take an exercise break instead of a coffee break!

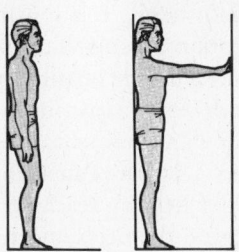

6. Stand with your back against doorway. Place heels four inches away from frame. Take a deep breath and relax. Press the small of your back against doorway. Tighten your stomach and buttock muscles, allowing your knees to bend slightly. This should cause the lower end of the pelvis to rotate forward (as in Exercise 1). Press your neck up against doorway. Press both hands against opposite side of doorway and straighten both knees. Hold for two seconds. Relax.

The following exercises (7, 8, 9) should not be started until you are free of pain and the other exercises have been done for several weeks.

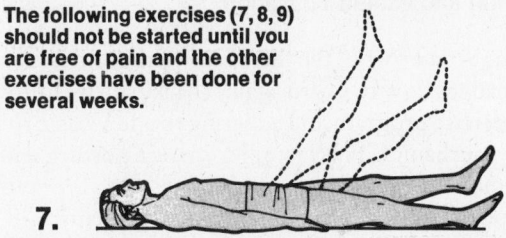

7.

Lie on your back with your legs straight out, knees unbent and arms at your sides. Take a deep breath and relax. Raise legs one at a time as high as is comfortable and lower to floor as slowly as possible. Repeat five times for each leg.

8.

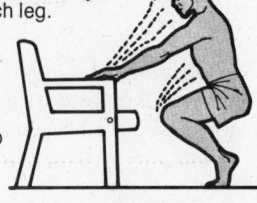

May be done holding onto a chair or table. After squatting, flex head forward, bounce up and down two or three times, then assume erect position.

9.

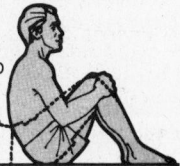

Lie on your back with knees bent. Feet flat on floor. Take a deep breath and relax. Pull up to a sitting position keeping knees bent. Return to starting position. Relax. Having someone hold your feet down facilitates this exercise.

A SERVICE OF RIKER LABORATORIES, INC.   91578 PRINTED IN U.S.A. DECEMBER 1973

Figure 59-8.   Back exercises: These exercises have been provided courtesy of Riker Laboratories, Inc. and Everett J. Gordon, M.D., Clinical Associate Professor, Orthopedic Surgery, Georgetown University.

pain is related to a ruptured disc, operative intervention consisting of a laminectomy with disc excision may be necessary (page 1260).

Psychological Considerations

Sometimes low back pain can be a psychosomatic illness or a reaction to environmental and life stresses. Emotional problems resulting from anxiety and stress can evoke muscle spasm which produces a cycle of anxiety, tension, more spasm and pain. In some persons, mental conflicts are manifested in physical symptoms. There are psychologic components in all illness and chronic pain has an emotional impact. In trying to help the patient, one needs insight into family relationships, environmental variables, and work problems. If the back problem stems from a recent accident, the possibility of pending litigation may be a factor. Psychiatric intervention may be necessary for the patient with chronic depression and low back syndrome. There are Pain Centers throughout the country that offer help by teaching the patient the significance of pain and the skills and techniques of coping with it (see page 248).

Prevention and Patient Education

An important part of the therapeutic program is teaching the patient how to guard against back pain by following an exercise program and adhering to a few basic rules of body mechanics. For example, correct posture and a correct method for lifting objects are essential to avoid strain upon muscles, joints, bones and ligaments.

Standing, sitting, lying and lifting properly are necessary for a healthy back:

STANDING
- Avoid prolonged standing and walking.
- When standing for any length of time, rest one foot on a small stool or box to relieve lumbar lordosis.

SITTING
Stress on the back may be greater in the sitting position than in the standing.
- Avoid sitting for prolonged periods.
- Sit in a straight back fairly high-seated chair. Sit with the knees higher than the hips. Use a foot stool.
- Eradicate the hollow of the back by sitting with the buttocks "tucked under."
- Avoid knee and hip extension. When driving a car, have the seat pushed forward as far as possible for comfort. Place a cushion in the small of the back for support.
- Guard against extensional strains—reaching, pushing, sitting with legs straight out.
- Alternate periods of sitting with walking.

LYING
- Rest at intervals as fatigue contributes to spasm of the back muscle.
- Place a firm bedboard under the mattress.
- Avoid sleeping in a prone position.
- When lying on the side, place a pillow under the head and one between the legs which should be flexed at the knees.

LIFTING
- When lifting, keep the back straight and hold the load as close to the body as possible. Lift with the legs, not the back.
- Avoid trunk twisting, lifting above waist level and reaching up for any length of time.
- Squat down while keeping the back straight when it is necessary to pick something off the floor.

EXERCISE
- *Daily exercise is important in the prevention of back problems.*
- Walking outdoors with progression in distance and pace is recommended.
- Do prescribed back exercises twice daily.

COMMON FOOT PROBLEMS

Disabilities of the human foot not only develop from poorly fitting shoes but may be the result of hereditary influence. Probably the foot would cause man little pain or disability on its own account if it were not for modern civilization which disregards the physiology of the foot. Fashion, vanity and eye appeal, rather than function, are for the most part the determining factors in the design of footwear. The restriction of ill-fitting shoes distorts normal anatomy while inducing deformity and pain.

The discomfort of foot strain can be treated by rest, elevation, physiotherapy, supportive strappings, and orthotic devices. Foot exercises in which active motion occurs will benefit the circulation and help strengthen the feet. Walking is considered the best form of exercise.

Common Foot Ailments

A *corn* is an area of hyperkeratosis (overgrowth of horny layer of epidermis), produced by pressure from within (the underlying bone is prominent due to congenital or acquired abnormality, commonly arthritis) or from pressure from without (shoes). The usual sites are the lesser toes, mainly the fifth toe, but all toes may be involved.

Corns are treated by soaking and scraping off the horny layer with an instrument, by applying protective shield or pads, or by surgical removal of the underlying offending osseous structure.

Soft corns are located between the toes and are kept soft by moisture and maceration. Treatment consists of drying the affected web spaces and separating the affected toes. Usually a podiatrist will be needed to treat the underlying cause.

A *callus* is a discretely thickened area of the skin that has been exposed to persistent pressure or friction. Faulty foot mechanics usually precede the formation of a callus. Treatment consists in eliminating the underlying causes and having the callus pared by a podiatrist if it is painful. A keratolytic ointment may be applied and a thin plastic cup worn over the heel if the callus is on this area. Felt padding with adhesive backing is also used to prevent and relieve pressure. Orthotic devices can be made to remove the pressure from the bony protuberance. The protuberance may be excised.

An *ingrown toenail* (onychocryptosis) is a condition in which the free edge of a nail plate has penetrated the surrounding skin, either laterally or anteriorly. It may be accompanied by secondary infection and/or granulation tissue. This painful condition is caused by improper self treatment, external pressure (tight shoes or stockings), internal pressure (deformed toes; growth under the nail), trauma and infection. Trimming the nails properly can prevent this problem. Active treatment consists of relieving the pain by decreasing the pressure on the surrounding soft tissue by the nail plate. A toenail may have to be excised if there is severe infection. If a neoplasm or gangrene is associated with an ingrown toenail, the patient is immediately hospitalized for appropriate care.

Common Deformities of the Foot (Fig. 59-9)

FLATFOOT.   Flatfoot (pes planus) is a common disorder and occurs in various forms. It is most often inherited. Exercises to strenghten the muscles and to improve posture and walking habits are helpful. A number of foot devices are available to give the foot additional support. Severe flatfoot problems are usually treated by an orthopedic surgeon or a podiatrist.

HAMMER TOE.   Hammer toe is a flexion deformity of the interphalangeal joint and may involve several toes (Fig. 59-9). The condition is usually an acquired deformity. Tight socks or shoes may push an overlying toe

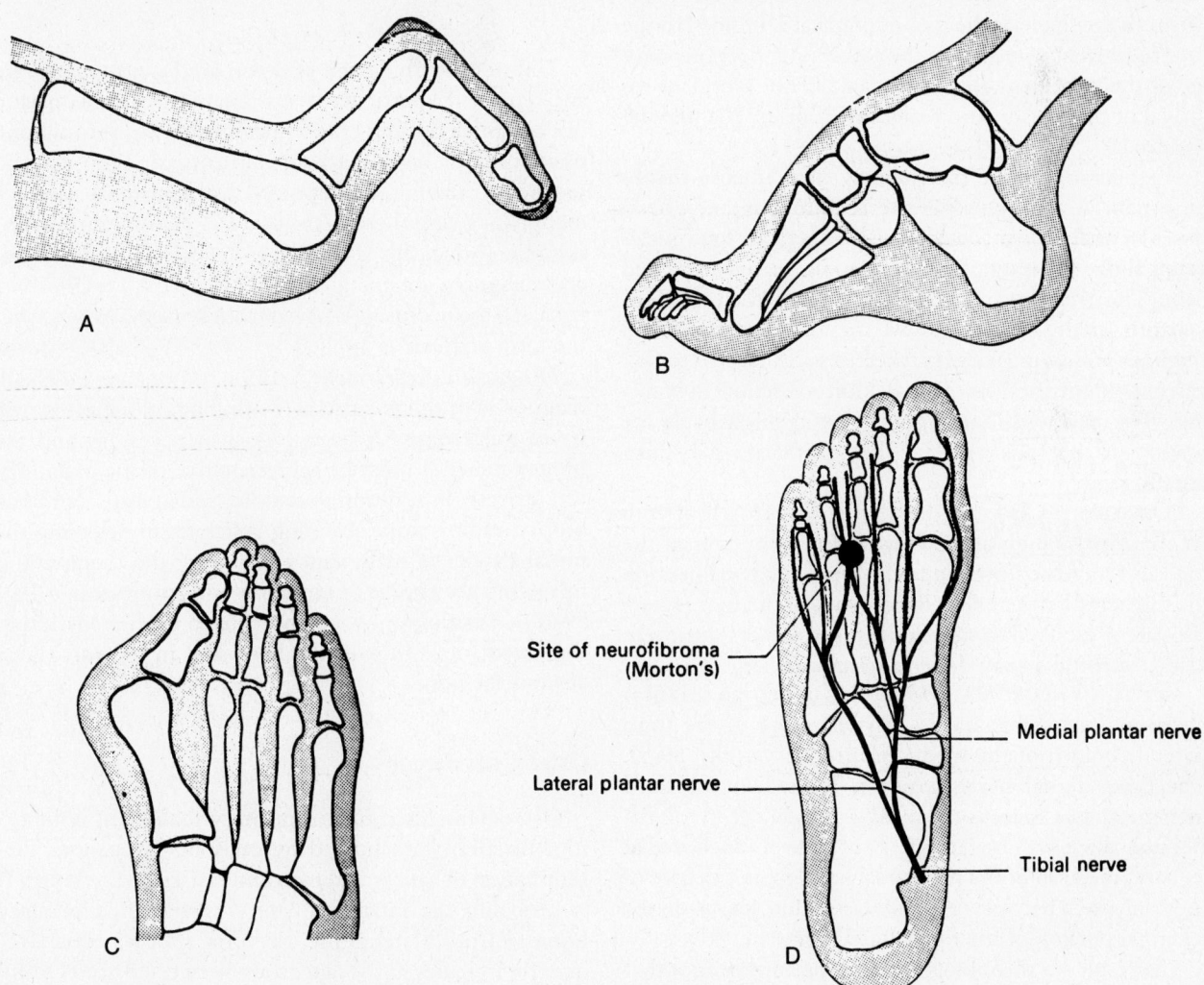

Figure 59-9.   Common foot deformities: (*A*) Hammer toe; (*B*) Clawfoot (pes cavus); (*C*) Hallux valgus; (*D*) Sites for Morton's neuroma.

back into the line of the other toes. The toes usually are pulled upward forcing the metatarsal points (ball of foot) downward. Corns develop on top of the toes and tender calluses under the metatarsal area. The treatment consists of conservative measures: carrying out manipulative exercises, wearing open-toed sandals or shoes that conform to the shape of the foot; protecting the protruding joints with pads. Surgical correction is necessary for an established deformity.

HALLUX VALGUS.   Hallux valgus is a progressive deformity in which the great toe deviates laterally (Fig. 59-9). Associated with this is a marked prominence of the medial aspect of the first metatarsal—phalangeal joint, with osseous enlargement of the medial side of the first metatarsal head, over which a bursa may form (secondary to pressure and inflammation). This bursa is commonly known as a *bunion*.

Treatment depends on the patient's age, the degree of deformity, and the severity of symptoms. If a bunion deformity is uncomplicated, wearing a shoe that conforms to the shape of the foot or one that is molded to the foot to prevent pressure on the protruding portions may be all the treatment that is needed. If not, surgical removal of the bunion and realignment of the toe may be required.

Postoperatively the patient may have intense throbbing pain at the operative site requiring rather liberal doses of analgesic medication. The operated foot is elevated above the level of the heart to decrease edema and pain. The great toe is watched for impaired circulation, warmth, color, ability to move the toes, numbness and tingling. Following surgery, exercises are initiated to flex and extend the toes, since toe flexion is essential in walking. The patient should avoid wearing high heels for prolonged periods because they push the toes into dorsiflexion.

CLAWFOOT.   Clawfoot (pes cavus) refers to a foot with an abnormally high arch. This causes shortening of the foot and increased pressure which produces calluses on the metatarsal area and on the dorsum of the foot. Exercises are prescribed to stretch the toe extensors. In severe cases, osteotomies are done to reshape the feet.

MORTON'S NEUROMA.   Morton's neuroma (plantar neuroma; neurofibroma) is a hypertrophy of the third (lateral) branch of the medial plantar nerve (Fig. 59-9). The third digital nerve which is located in the third intermetatarsal space is the most common site involved. Because the fourth metatarsal is not securely anchored at its base, the head of the metatarsal has a greater degree of motion which becomes a chronic irritating source on the terminal portion of the third digital nerve.

The result is a throbbing, burning pain in the foot that is usually relieved when the patient rests. Pain sometimes radiates up the leg. Conservative treatment consists of inserting innersoles, metatarsal bars and pads designed to spread the metatarsal heads and balance the foot posture. Local injections of hydrocortisone and a local anesthetic may give relief. If these fail, surgical intervention is necessary.

OTHER FOOT PROBLEMS.   Several systemic diseases affect the feet. In the case of rheumatoid arthritis, deformities result. Diabetics are prone to develop corns and peripheral neuropathies with diminishing sensation leading to ulcers over pressure points of the foot. Persons with peripheral vascular disease and arteriosclerosis complain of burning and itching feet with attendant scratching and excoriations. Dermatologic problems commonly affect the feet in the form of fungal infections and plantar warts. The specifics of these problems and others can be found in the discussions of the various dysfunctions covered throughout the text.

MALIGNANT BONE TUMOR

Tumors involving the skeleton are by no means rare and represent a particularly malignant form of neoplastic disease. Such tumors may be primary, arising from bone tissue cells or bone marrow elements, or they may be secondary, having metastasized from primary sites of malignancy elsewhere in the body. A benign tumor arising from bone cells is known as an *osteoma;* tumors that are malignant are grouped under the term *osteogenic sarcoma*. To the neoplasm derived from bone marrow tissue, the term *myeloma* is applied.

Diagnostic Assessment.   Bone tumors are a difficult diagnostic problem since x-ray findings alone are sometimes misleading. A bone biopsy is necessary and the biopsy material must be representative of the pathological process. In addition to radiologic diagnosis and bone biopsy, radioisotope scanning is helpful in detecting the initial extent of malignancy, planning the therapy and following the course of radiation or chemotherapy (Fig. 59-10). Arteriography has been used in demonstrating the extent of lesions in the bone and in the soft tissue around the bone.

Osteogenic Sarcoma

Osteogenic sarcoma is a primary malignant bone tumor usually characterized by early hematogenous dissemination of cancer and micrometastasis in the lungs. It is probably the most frequently encountered primary bone tumor. Osteogenic sarcoma appears most frequently in males in the age group between 10 and 25 and in older persons with Paget's disease. It is manifested by pain, swelling, limitation of motion and weight loss; the latter is considered an ominous finding. The bony mass

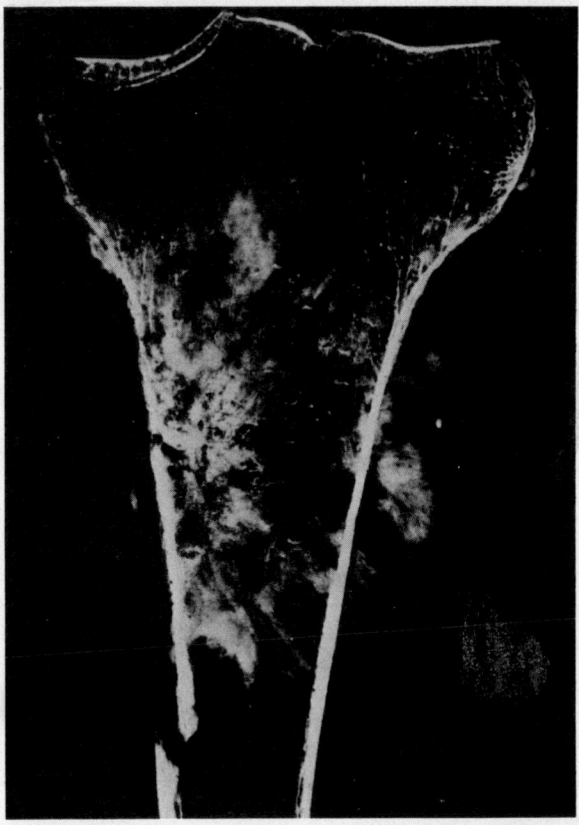
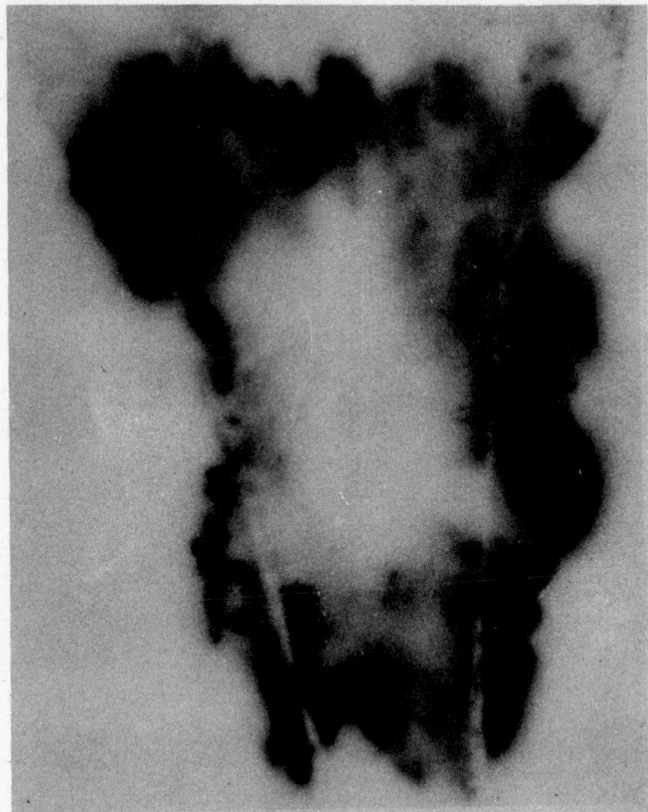

Figure 59-10. (*Left*) X-ray showing osteosarcoma at the proximal end of the tibia. Note the destruction of the normal anatomy of the bone. (*Right*) Contact autoradiograph of the same patient. The patient has received ^{85}Sr. intravenously for bone scanning. Note the high uptake (black areas) in the peripheral growing margin and the relative lack of uptake centrally. (Armed Forces Institute of Pathology. Negative numbers 67-4-8, 67-4-9)

may be palpable, tender and fixed with an increase in skin temperature over the mass and venous distention. The primary lesion may involve any bone; the most common sites are the lower end of the femur, the upper end of the tibia and the upper end of the humerus. The tumor carries a high mortality rate since the cancer frequently has spread to the lungs by the time the patient seeks treatment.

Management.   The goal of management is to destroy or remove malignant tissue by the most effective method possible. This requires a multidisciplinary approach, possibly in a cancer treatment center.

Surgical removal of the tumor usually requires that the affected extremity be amputated, with the line of amputation extending through the bone or joint above the tumor in order to achieve local control of the primary lesion. (See nursing management of the patient following an amputation, page 1314.) Some centers are now performing local bone resection without amputation using metallic prosthetics or allografts for bone replacement. These procedures are still considered investigational.

Because of the real danger of metastasis with these tumors, combined chemotherapy is started before and after surgery in an effort to eradicate micrometastatic lesions. The hope is that combined chemotherapy will achieve a greater response at a lower toxicity rate with a minimum amount of resistance to the drugs. Vincristine, high dose methotrexate with citrovorum factor, doxorubicin, and cyclophosphamide are used in various combinations. Large doses of methotrexate inhibit DNA synthesis and are made more acceptable by the concomitant administration of citrovorum factor which "rescues" the patient from the excess toxicity of methotrexate. Chemotherapy is also used in combination with radiation therapy. Exciting gains in survival times are being achieved in osteogenic sarcoma with surgery, radiation, chemotherapy and immunotherapy. The nursing management of the patient undergoing chemotherapy can be found on page 270. A patient with a bone tumor requires understanding and support to cope with the disagreeable side effects of treatment and the uncertain outcome of the disease.

Giant Cell Tumor

A giant cell tumor (osteoclastoma) is a neoplasm that develops within the bone and apparently arises from the mesenchymal cells of the connective tissue framework. It is rare before the age of 20 or after 55. These tumors almost always arise from the end of a long bone with a later secondary involvement of the shaft of the bone. (The majority of these tumors develop in the lower end of the femur, upper end of the tibia, and the lower end of the radius.) Usually the tumor grows insidiously and has attained an appreciable size before the patient is aware of its existence. He may complain of pain, swelling, limitation of motion, and tenderness.

Management. Surgery and radiation are the most important methods of treating primary bone tumors. The surgical approach varies from wide excision of bone to hemipelvectomies and interscapulothoracic amputations. Now emphasis is placed on thorough local resection of tumors of low grade malignancy and on procedures to restore bone continuity with various types of bone grafts. Whether or not chemotherapeutic agents are effective (systemically or by infusion or perfusion) depends on whether or not the tumor is sensitive to the agent being administered.

Multiple Myeloma

Multiple myeloma (plasma cell myeloma, plasmacytoma) is a malignant disease of plasma cells that infiltrates bone and soft tissues and occurs characteristically in middle-aged females. This tumor has its origin and principal location in the bone marrow, although the cause is unknown. In later stages the lymph nodes, liver, spleen, and kidneys may become involved. There is a widespread proliferation of immature plasma cells in the marrow cavity throughout the skeleton. The bones most commonly affected are those which are the site of active hemopoietic marrow—the spine, skull, ribs, sternum, pelvis, and the upper ends of the humerus. There is a constant threat of hypercalcemia, hypercalciuria, and hyperuricemia due to skeletal destruction. The malignant plasma cells may produce abnormal amounts of an immunoglobulin or parts of immunoglobulin protein (Bence Jones protein) that usually can be detected in the serum or urine by immunoelectrophoresis.

Clinical Manifestations. The patient has constant severe bone pain especially on movement due to the bone marrow being infiltrated with plasma cells and the presence of destructive bone lesions. Skeletal lesions produce swelling, tenderness, pain, and pathological bone fractures. Low back pain is the most characteristic symptom.

Anemia occurs as a result of the marrow being replaced with neoplastic cells. Symptoms of renal failure occur due to the precipitation of the immunoglobulin in the tubules, or to pyelonephritis, hypercalcemia, increased uric acid, infiltration of the kidney with plasma cells (myeloma kidney) and renal vein thrombosis.

A pathologic tendency to bleed is characteristic of myeloma for two major reasons: (1) a numerical deficiency of platelets (thrombocytopenia), due to destruction of the megakaryocytes, their parent cells, in the marrow; and (2) platelet dysfunction, the macroglobulin tending to coat these elements and to interfere with their hemostatic functions.

Management. The major objectives of therapy are to suppress the plasma cell growth and to control the pain. Alkylating agent chemotherapy to reduce the tumor mass is the foundation of treatment. Combination drug therapy appears more effective than single dose therapy in most patients. Malphalen (Alkeran) and cyclophosphamide (Cytoxan) with or without prednisone are commonly used. Other chemotherapeutic agents are tried when the patient fails to respond to the prescribed regimen. (The care of the patient undergoing chemotherapy is discussed on page 270.)

A major problem of the patient is bone pain. To relieve this discomfort, the above mentioned chemotherapy and steroids are helpful. Radiotherapy is given to relieve bone pain from large lesions (especially from nerve compression and fractures) and to reduce the size of extraskeletal plasma cell tumors. When pain is severe, analgesics and narcotics may be necessary.

It is important that the patient be kept ambulatory as long as possible unless lesions in the spine (extradural plasmacytomas) produce danger of cord compression. If this occurs the patient may be given radiation therapy to prevent paraplegia, or a laminectomy is done for cord compression or vertebral fractures, since the patient is susceptible to pathologic fractures.

The patient is kept well hydrated (2500–3000 ml. urine output daily) to control serum calcium levels and prevent hypercalcemia and hyperuricemia. Dehydration which can precipitate acute renal failure must be avoided.

- Thus patients with multiple myeloma should *not* have their fluids severely restricted prior to x-ray or laboratory tests.

Allopurinol may be given to control hyperuricemia.

Complications. Because of impaired antibody production the health care team is on the alert for recurring infection. Infection also occurs because of extensive bone marrow involvement and the effects of chemotherapy, radiotherapy, and steroids, which contribute to leukopenia. The temperature is closely monitored, and signs of respiratory and urinary tract infection are checked. Patients on steroids may not have overt symptoms of infection. Therefore more subtle signs of apathy and lethargy are to be noted.

In addition to infection, neurologic complications (paraplegia from collapse of supporting structures, infiltration of nerve roots, or cord compression from plasma cell tumors), pathologic fractures, renal and hematologic complications are ever-present threats to the patient's life. A disordered immune system makes the patient susceptible to multiple tumor involvement.

Compassionate management and supportive care are essential nursing tools as the disease is ultimately fatal.

A discussion of this disease as it relates to the blood-forming organs is found on page 670.

Metastatic Bone Cancer

Tumors arising from tissues other than the bone may invade the bone, producing localized bone destruction with results that are clinically quite analogous to those occurring in primary bone tumors. Those most frequently metastasizing to bone include carcinomas of the kidney, the prostate, the lung, the breast, the ovary, and the thyroid. A sign of diagnostic importance in patients with metastatic carcinoma of the prostate is an elevation of the serum acid phosphatase. The first indication of disease in such cases may be a pathologic bone fracture; in later stages, the peripheral blood may show evidences of bone marrow interference. If the bone marrow becomes seriously crowded by the invading malignancy, a myelophthisic anemia is produced.

The treatment of metastatic bone cancer is palliative and the therapeutic goal is to relieve the patient's discomfort as much as possible. Surgery may be indicated in long bone fractures.

OTHER DISORDERS OF BONE

OSTEOMALACIA

Osteomalacia is a metabolic bone disease characterized by failure of normal mineralization of bone. (A similar condition in children is called rickets). As a result of this faulty mineralization there is softening and weakening of the skeleton, causing pain, tenderness to the touch and bowing of the bones. In these patients a large amount of osteoid or remolded bone does not calcify. It is thought that the primary defect is a defective supply of calcium and phosphate from the extracellular fluid to the calcification sites in the bones.

Vitamin D aids in the maintenance of calcium homeostasis. It increases absorption of calcium and, secondarily, phosphate from the small intestine. Its primary effect is the transfer of calcium from the lumen of the intestine to the blood. The defect of demineralization occurring in osteomalacia may be the result of a combined deficiency or resistance to vitamin D or phosphate or a defect in production of alkaline phosphatase or bone matrix. Thus ingested vitamin D undergoes synthesis in the body that is regulated in response to homeostatic demands and can be regarded as a hormone as well as a vitamin.

Etiology

There are a variety of causes of osteomalacia resulting from a generalized disturbance in mineral metabolism. Risk factors for the development of osteomalacia are dietary deficiencies, malabsorption problems, gastrectomy, chronic renal failure and prolonged drug absorption (phenytoin; phenobarbital).

Osteomalacia may occur as a result of inadequate dietary intake of calcium or phosphate ions, failure of these ions to be absorbed or excessive loss of these materials from the body.

The malnutrition type (deficiency of vitamin D often associated with poor intake of calcium) is mainly due to poverty, but food faddism and lack of knowledge of nutrition may be factors. It occurs in parts of the world where vitamin D is not added to food and where dietary deficiencies exist and sunlight is scarce.

Gastrointestinal disorders in which fats are inadequately absorbed are prone to produce osteomalacia through loss of vitamin D (among other fat-soluble vitamins) and calcium, the latter being excreted in the feces in combination with fatty acids. Such disorders include sprue, celiac disease, chronic biliary tract obstruction, chronic pancreatitis and small bowel resections or operative shunts (gastrectomy) that involve the small intestine.

Diseases of the kidney lead to a reduced serum phosphate concentration which leads to impaired mineralization of bone. Also liver and kidney diseases can produce a lack of vitamin D as these are the organs which convert vitamin D to its active form. Finally, hyperparathyroidism leads to skeletal decalcification, and thus to osteomalacia, through the promotion of phosphate excretion in the urine.

Clinical Manifestations

The most common and distressing symptom of osteomalacia is bone pain and tenderness. As a result of calcium deficiency there is usually muscle weakness. The patient develops a waddling or limping gait. In the more advanced disease, the legs become bowed (due to body weight and muscle pull). The softened vertebrae become compressed, thus shortening the patient's trunk and deforming the thorax. The sacrum is forced down and forward and the pelvis is compressed laterally. These two deformities explain the characteristic shape of the pelvis that often necessitates cesarean section in pregnant women who are affected with this disease. Weakness and unsteadiness present a danger of falls and fractures.

Management

Osteomalacia can be treated with gratifying results on an individualized basis. The underlying cause is corrected as far as possible. Vitamin D is given in the treatment of many forms of osteomalacia. Its various therapeutic actions combine to raise the concentrations of calcium and phosphorus in the extracellular fluid and thus make these ions available for mineralization. If osteomalacia is dietary in origin, a normal diet plus vitamin D is given. If vitamin D deficiency is due to malabsorption, larger doses of vitamin D are required in addition to supplementary doses of calcium. High doses of vitamin D are toxic and enhance the risk of hypercalcemia. Therefore the patient's serum calcium is monitored. With malabsorption the patient may also be treated with ultraviolet irradiation. The patient is encouraged to expose his skin to sunlight as the ultraviolet portion of sunlight is necessary to transform a cholesterol substance (7-dehydro-) present in the skin into vitamin D. Newer compounds or metabolites of vitamin D (Rocaltrol) are currently being investigated.

Prevention. In the elderly, who are economically and socially deprived, special attention to a nutritious diet is important. Since sunlight is necessary, older people should be encouraged to spend some time in the sun.

OSTEOPOROSIS

Osteoporosis is a disorder in which there is a reduction in the amount of total bone mass without a change in chemical composition. There is an imbalance between bone formation and bone resorption (loss). It is characterized by generalized loss of bone density and tensile strength. The bones become progressively more porous and fragile, eventually leading to fractures (from minimal stress), collapse of vertebral bodies and skeletal deformity (Fig. 59-11). An estimated 6 million persons in this country suffer annually from spontaneous fractures due to osteoporosis; of these, 5 million are sustained by postmenopausal women. Thus osteoporosis has serious sequelae.

Causes and Pathogenesis

Normally the skeleton rebuilds itself in a constant and systematic way. Old bone is continually reabsorbed by the body and new bone is produced. However, bone loss occurs with aging, especially in women, as a result of changes in hormonal balance. With the decline and disappearance of estrogen production, postmenopausal osteoporosis occurs. Men are less likely to develop osteoporosis apparently due to the fact that the male gonads continue to produce androgens for most of their lives and there is not a sudden diminution of their production as occurs in women at menopause.

A low calcium intake is responsible also for osteoporosis. If the body does not receive or absorb enough calcium or if excessive amounts are lost from the body, the calcium is taken from bone in order to maintain the serum calcium at a normal level. (The parathyroid hormone keeps the amount of calcium in the blood at normal levels). Persons who do not drink milk usually have a daily calcium intake between 200 and 300 mg. which is well below the 1 gm. necessary to maintain adequate calcium balance. Vitamin D is necessary for calcium absorption and deficiencies of this vitamin also occur in people who do not get adequate sunshine or do not ingest food supplemented with vitamin D. Probably an inadequate supply of protein, minerals and vitamins over a period of years contributes to its development as well as poor use of nutrients and an imbalance of hormones.

Other factors producing bone loss are malabsorption syndrome from gastrointestinal disease, disuse atrophy from immobilization or physical inactivity, hyperthyroidism, hyperparathyroidism, Cushing's syndrome and the prolonged use of cortisone or related drugs.

Clinical Manifestations

The patient may be asymptomatic for a long time or complain of generalized backache as the spine begins to collapse and the spinal curvature increases, forcing the ligaments to bear more weight. A sudden severe pain in the low back is the result of a compression fracture of the vertebrae. Some postmenopausal women may lose 2 to 15 cm. (1 to 6 inches) in height from vertebral collapse. Roentgenograms show decreased skeletal density, changes in the lower thoracic and lumbar vertebrae and possible multiple compression fractures which produce the gradual loss of height with an associated kyphosis (dowager's hump) (Fig. 59-12).

Other fracture sites commonly seen are those of the femoral neck, and distal radius and ulna (Colles' fracture). The pain may subside from one fracture and appear suddenly when another fracture occurs.

Bone biopsy may be necessary to rule out malignant disease. Bone mass is measured using densitometric or radiologic methods.

Management and Patient Education

The objectives of management are to keep the patient active, to provide optimal nutrition and to prevent fractures.

The treatment of osteoporosis varies with the individual cause. In general, a diet high in calcium, protein and vitamin D is prescribed to slow the rate of bone loss. This would include two or more servings of meat, chicken or fish or protein equivalent and three glasses of skim or whole milk daily. A calcium preparation (calcium carbonate) is given to add sufficient calcium to the diet as many older persons frequently suffer from a deficiency in dietary calcium. Vitamin D, necessary for calcium absorption, is frequently added in the form of vitamin D-fortified milk or calcium supplements containing vitamin D.

Estrogen replacement therapy (Premarin) may be given to retard bone loss, relieve low back pain and promote a sense of well-being. However it may be of little value in long-term care. During estrogen therapy, the patient must examine her breasts monthly and report for a pelvic examination including a Pap smear and aspiration of endometrial secretions for histologic examination since estrogens may produce breast and endometrial hyperplasia and cancer.

Physical activity is most essential to strengthen muscles, prevent disuse atrophy and further bone demineralization. Daily activity, preferably outdoors in the sunshine, is necessary. Sometimes a back brace is prescribed to encourage the patient to return to normal activities of daily living. The most rational measure to prevent bone demineralization is an adequate calcium intake throughout life combined with physical activity and regular exercise. A woman who has had her ovaries removed or has undergone a premature menopause may develop osteoporosis at a fairly young age. Estrogen replacement is considered in this patient.

The patient is instructed to avoid sudden jarring, heavy lifting and bending. Lifting should be done correctly to avoid compression fractures of the vertebral bodies. Potential sources of falls should be removed. Sleeping with a bedboard under the mattress may help relieve the back pain.

PAGET'S DISEASE

Paget's disease (of the bone) is a bone disease of unknown cause marked by excessive bone resorption (bone loss) and disordered formation of bone. There is thought to be a primary proliferation of osteoclasts which produce bone resorption followed by a compensatory increase in osteoblastic activity which repairs the bone resorbed. This bone destruction and formation (turnover) causes distortion of normal bone anatomy, e.g., enlarged and deformed bones with increasing vascularity. The increase in the number, size and activity of the bone cells is responsible for the biochemical abnormalities of Paget's disease. The serum alkaline phosphatase and the level of urinary hydroxyproline excretion are usually increased. In general, the level of alkaline phosphatase correlates with the extent and activity of the disease. Bone scans may detect the disease quite early, while roentgenograms also may show striking changes. The disease occurs more often in men after the age of 40.

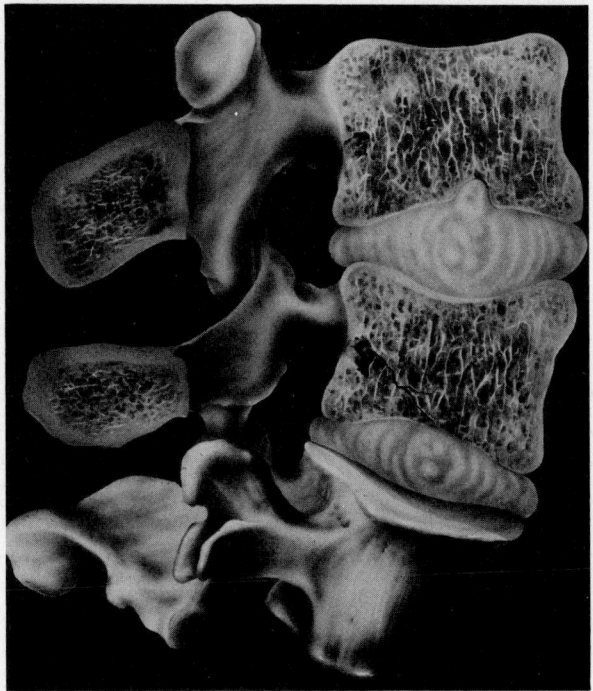

Figure 59-11. Artist's conception of progressive osteoporotic bone loss and compression fractures. (Printed with permission of Ayerst® Laboratories, New York, New York)

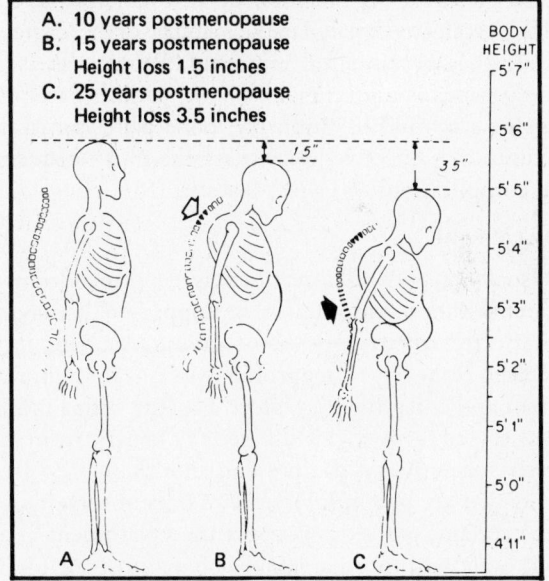

A. 10 years postmenopause
B. 15 years postmenopause
Height loss 1.5 inches
C. 25 years postmenopause
Height loss 3.5 inches

BODY HEIGHT
5'7"
5'6"
5'5"
5'4"
5'3"
5'2"
5'1"
5'0"
4'11"

Figure 59-12. Typical loss of height associated with osteoporosis and aging. (Courtesy, Wilson Research Foundation)

Clinical Manifestations

The disease usually begins insidiously. Although it may start in any part of the skeleton, it ususally begins in the skull, vertebral column, pelvis or long bones. Pain and tenderness on pressure may be noted in the bones. Such pain, which is wrongly attributed to old age or arthritis by the patient, may precede the skeletal changes by years. There is an increase in skin temperature overlying the bone from increased vascularity of the bone. In the majority of patients there is deformity involving the skull or long bones. The skull may be thickened and the patient may complain that his hat no longer fits. In well-marked cases of Paget's disease, the cranium is much enlarged, but not the face, which therefore appears small and triangular in shape. Most patients with skull involvement have impaired hearing.

The spine is bent forward and is rigid; the chin rests on the chest. The thorax is compressed and immobile on respiration. The trunk is flexed on the legs to maintain equilibrium; the arms, which are bent outward and forward and appear long in relation to the shortened trunk, give to the patient an ape-like appearance; and the legs are greatly bowed, hence the gait is labored and waddling. As a result of the kyphosis and the bowing of the legs, the patient's height may be reduced as much as 30 cm. (12 inches). The bones involved are brittle and fractures occur frequently.

Complications. Associated problems include high output cardiac failure from the increased blood flow to the affected bone, neurologic sequelae secondary to pressure on the brain, cranial nerves and spinal nerve roots by pathologic bone degeneration or vascular insufficiency and hypercalcemia related to the inability of the kidney to excrete the increased calcium load. Paget's disease in some patients is a precursor of bone tumor, mainly osteogenic sarcoma. In summary, bone pain, deformity, fractures and defective hearing are the most frequently seen complications of Paget's disease.

Management

Usually no particular treatment is recommended in the patient without symptoms. The supportive and symptomatic treatment consists of giving Aspirin, indomethacin (Indocin) or ibuprofen (Motrin) for pain relief and/or anti-inflammatory effect. Patients with a moderate to severe form of the disease may benefit from suppressive therapy. At the present time there are several agents that are potent inhibitors of bone resorption and under certain conditions may permit replacement of diseased bone with normal lamellar bone: the calcitonins, sodium etidronate (EHDP) and mithramycin. These agents all suppress bone resorption but are mediated by different mechanisms.

Calcitonin, a polypeptide hormone, retards bone resorption by decreasing the number and availability of osteoclasts. It is used to relieve bone pain and helps alleviate neurologic and biochemical complications. Three species of calcitonin are available: salmon, porcine and human. Calcitonin is given by injection, with the subcutaneous route used for self-administration. Flushing of the face and nausea are side effects.

Sodium etidronate (EHDP), a diphosphonate compound, produces rapid reduction of bone turnover and relief of pain. It also reduces elevated serum alkaline phosphatase and urinary hydroxyproline levels. It is easy to administer since it can be taken by mouth. Diarrhea may be a side effect; it is alleviated by spacing the dose.

Mithramycin (Mithracin), a cytotoxic antibiotic, is used to control the disease, since Paget's disease is similar in some ways to a low-grade neoplastic process. It has dramatic effects on the serum calcium, alkaline phosphatase and urinary hydroxyproline levels, possibly due to the fact that mithramycin is toxic to osteoclasts. It is given by intravenous infusion and requires that hepatic, renal and bone marrow function be monitored during therapy.

BIBLIOGRAPHY

BOOKS

Aegerter, E. E., and Kirkpatrick, J. A., Jr.: Orthopedic Diseases. Philadelphia, W. B. Saunders, 1975.

American Academy Orthopaedic Surgeons: Symposium on Reconstructive Surgery of the Knee. St. Louis, C. V. Mosby, 1978.

Bateman, J. E., and Fornasier, V. L.: The Shoulder and Neck. Philadelphia, W. B. Saunders, 1978.

Brashear, H. R., Jr., and Raney, R. B.: Shands' Handbook of Orthopaedic Surgery, 9th ed. St. Louis, C. V. Mosby, 1978.

Dahlin, D. C.: Bone Tumors, 3rd ed. Springfield, Charles C Thomas, 1978.

Devas, M.: Geriatric Orthopaedics. New York, Academic Press, 1977.

Epps, C. H. (ed.): Complications in Orthopaedic Surgery, vols. 1 and 2. Philadelphia, J. B. Lippincott, 1978.

Farrell, J.: Illustrated Guide to Orthopedic Nursing. Philadelphia, J. B. Lippincott, 1977.

Fisk, J. W.: A Practical Guide to Management of the Painful Neck and Back. Springfield, Charles C Thomas, 1977.

Gschwend, N., and Debrunner, H. V.: Total Hip Prosthesis. Baltimore, Williams & Wilkins, 1976.

Helfet, A. J., and Lee, D. M. G.: Disorders of the Lumbar Spine. Philadelphia, J. B. Lippincott, 1978.

Hollingsworth, J. W.: Management of Rheumatoid Arthritis and Its Complications. Chicago, Year Book Med. Publ., 1978.

Hughes, G. R. V.: Modern Topics in Rheumatology. London, Wm. Heinemann Medical Books Ltd., 1976.

Iverson, L. D., and Clawson, D. K.: Manual of Orthopaedic Therapeutics. Boston, Little, Brown, 1977.

Jowsey, J.: Metabolic Diseases of Bone. Philadelphia, W. B. Saunders, 1977.

Katz, W. A.: Rheumatic Diseases. Philadelphia, J. B. Lippincott, 1977.

Larson, C. B., and Gould, M.: Orthopedic Nursing. 9th ed. St. Louis, C. V. Mosby, 1978.

Lichtenstein, L.: Bone Tumors, 5th ed. St. Louis, C. V. Mosby, 1977.

Macnab, I.: Backache. Baltimore, Williams & Wilkins, 1977.

Marmor, L.: Arthritis Surgery. Philadelphia, Lea & Febiger, 1976.

Melvin, J. L.: Rheumatic Disease: Occupational Therapy and Rehabilitation. Philadelphia, F. A. Davis, 1977.

Ruge, D., and Wiltse, L. L.: Spinal Disorders. Philadelphia, Lea & Febiger, 1977.

Ryan, J. R.: Orthopedic Surgery. Flushing, Medical Examination Pub. Co., 1977.

Scott, J. T. (ed.): Copeman's Textbook of the Rheumatic Diseases, 5th ed. New York, Churchill Livingstone, 1978.

Swezey, R. L.: Arthritis: Rational Therapy and Rehabilitation. Philadelphia, W. B. Saunders, 1978.

Turek, S. L.: Orthopaedics. Principles and Their Application, 3rd ed. Philadelphia, J. B. Lippincott, 1977.

Walker, P. S.: Human Joints and Their Artificial Replacements. Springfield, Charles C Thomas, 1977.

Weinstein, P. R., Ehni, G., and Wilson, C. B.: Lumbar Spondylosis: Diagnosis, Management and Surgical Treatment. Chicago, Year Book Med. Pub., 1977.

ARTICLES

Arthritis

Calin, A.: Rheumatoid arthritis. Am. Fam. Phys., *18*:89-94, July 1978.

Bland, J. H., Merrit, J. A., and Boushey, D. R.: The painful shoulder. Semin. Arthritis Rheum., 7:21-47, Aug. 1977.

Feibel, A., and Fast, A.: Deep heating of joints: a reconsideration. Arch. Phys. Med. Rehabil., *57*:513-514, Nov. 1977.

Healy, L. A.: More on the new arthritis drugs. Res. and Staff Phys., *23*:109-110, Feb. 1977.

Lewis, J. R.: New antirheumatic agents. JAMA, *237*:1260-1261, Mar. 21, 1977.

Person, D. A., and Sharp, J. T.: The etiology of rheumatoid arthritis. Bull. Rheum. Dis., *27*:888-893, 1976-1977.

Philips, V. K.: Intramuscular gold for rheumatoid arthritis. Compr. Ther., *3*:26-31, June 1977.

Scherbel, A.: Nonsteroidal antiinflammatory drugs: new alternatives for rheumatic disease. Postgrad. Med., *63*:69-74, Mar. 1978.

Zeitlin, D. J.: Psychological issues in the management of rheumatoid arthritis. Psychosomatics, *18*:7-14, Aug. 1977.

Low Back Pain

Crown, S.: Psychological aspects of low back pain. Rheumatol. Rehabil., *17*:114-124, May 1978.

Hastings, D. E.: Back pain: a multifaceted syndrome. Postgrad. Med., *62*:159-165, July 1977.

Pheasant, H. C.: The problem back. Current practice in Orthopaed. Surg., 7:89-115, 1977.

Mooney, V., and Cairns, D.: Management in the patient with chronic low back pain. Orthop. Clin. N. Am., *9*:543-557, Apr. 1978.

Osteoporosis/Osteomalacia

Albanese, A. A. (ed.): Bone Loss: Causes, detection and therapy. Current Topics in Nutrition and Disease, *1*:1-178, 1977.

Albanese, A. A., Lorenze, E. J., and Wein, E. H.: Osteoporosis: effects of calcium. Am. Fam. Phys., *18*:160-167, Oct. 1978.

Chalmers, G. L.: Disorders of bone. Practitioner, *220*:711-721, May 1978.

Frame, B., and Parfitt, M.: Osteomalacia: current concepts. Ann. Intern. Med., *89*:966-982, Dec. 1978.

Habener, J. F., and Mahaffey, J. E.: Osteomalacia and disorders of vitamin D metabolism. Annu. Rev. Med., *29*:327-342, 1978.

Jowsey, J. J.: Osteoporosis. Postgrad. Med., *60*:75-79, Aug. 1976.

———: Osteoporosis: dealing with a crippling bone disease of the elderly. Geriatrics, *32*:41-50, July 1977.

———: Why is mineral metabolism important in osteoporosis? Geriatrics, *33*:39-42, Aug. 1978.

Sissons, H. A.: Osteoporosis and osteomalacia. Bones and Joints, *17*:25-38, 1976.

Smith, D. M., and Edmondson, J. W.: Common adult osteopenic states: osteoporosis and osteomalacia. Am. Fam. Phys., *14*:160-166, Nov. 1976.

Surgery for Arthritis

Bowden, S. A.: New surgery for arthritic hands. Nursing '76, *6*:46-48, Aug. 1976.

Feinstein, P. A., and Habermann, E. T.: Selecting and preparing patients for total hip replacement. Geriatrics, *32*:91-96, July 1977.

Jennings, K. R.: The cheerful operation: total hip replacement. Nursing '76, *6*:32-37, July 1976.

Harris, W. H.: Total joint replacement. New Engl. J. Med., *297*:650-651, Sept. 22, 1977.

Miller, G. D.: Orthopedic case study: adult orthopedics. Bilateral total hip arthroplasty. ONA J., *4*:281-289, Nov. 1977.

Murray, W. R.: The hip. Proceedings of the 4th Open Scientific Meeting of the Hip Society. 1-285 (entire volume), 1977.

Sculo, C. D., and Sculo, T. P.: Management of the patient with an infected total hip arthroplasty. AJN, *76*:584-587, Apr. 1976.

Other Orthopedic Conditions

Banks, H. H. (ed.): Symposium on care of the critically ill orthopedic patient. Orthoped. Clin. N. Am., *9*:587-864, July 1978.

Berger, M. R.: Dupuytren's contracture. AJN, *78*:244-245, Feb. 1978.

Berger, M. R., and Froimson, A. I.: Hands that hurt: carpal tunnel syndrome. AJN, *79*:264-266, Feb. 1979.

Buck, B. I. (ed.): Symposium on orthopedic nursing. Nurs. Clin. N. Am., *11*:639-730, Dec. 1976.

Carron, H.: Relieving pain with nerve blocks. Geriatrics, *33*:49-57, Apr. 1978.

Douglass, H. O.: Osteosarcoma: survival gains resulting from multidisciplinary therapy. Progress in Clin. Cancer, 7:83-96, 1978.

Greenfield, L. D., and Bennett, L. R.: Bone scanning. Am. Fam. Phys., *11*:84-89, Mar. 1975.

Janecki, C. J., Jr., Hill, D. H., and Eubanks, R. G.: Arthroscopy of the knee. Am. Fam. Phys., *17*:109-116, Mar. 1978.

Mass, R. E.: Diagnosing and managing plasma cell (multiple) myeloma. Geriatrics, *33*:53-61, July 1978.

Wallach, S. (ed.): Paget's disease. Clinical orthopaedics and related research, *127*:2-110, Sept. 1977.

AGENCIES

Governmental

National Institute of Arthritis, Metabolism and Digestive Diseases, National Institutes of Health, Bethesda, Md. 20205

Voluntary

American Physical Therapy Association, 1156 15th St., N.W., Washington, D.C. 20005

American Podiatry Association, 20 Chevy Chase Circle, N.W., Washington, D.C. 20015

Arthritis Foundation, 3400 Peachtree Rd., N.E., Suite 1101, Atlanta, Ga. 30326

National Easter Seal Society for Crippled Children and Adults, 2023 W. Ogden Ave., Chicago, Ill. 60612

(See also Rehabilitation Agencies, Chapter 12)

Other Acute Problems

UNIT FIFTEEN

60

MANAGEMENT OF PATIENTS WITH INFECTIOUS DISEASES

THE CHALLENGE OF INFECTIOUS DISEASES

Infectious diseases are still the major health problem of the vast majority of people inhabiting the earth. In the developing countries, the principal causes of death are infectious and parasitic diseases which drain the capabilities of humans to work and to learn. Thus the conquering of these diseases is necessary for economic self-sufficiency and national development. In the industrialized countries, the mortality from infectious diseases has declined dramatically, but these diseases represent the most frequent problems requiring professional attention, accounting for a large portion of the cost of health care.

Although many infectious diseases have been conquered, new and emerging problems have been created. There is an increase in the number of organisms that have developed resistance to a variety of available antimicrobials. Then, too, there is a rapidly growing number of people whose normal host defenses have been compromised by immunosuppressive therapy related to other disorders. As a result, they are susceptible to organisms that are not usually considered pathogenic.

On the other hand, the advances in modern medicine have led to the development of more antimicrobial drugs and the ability to cultivate viruses in tissue cultures, as well as an increased knowledge about immunity.

THE INFECTIOUS PROCESS

Epidemiology is the science concerned with the study of the history and occurrence of a disease, along with those factors that may directly or indirectly favor the development of a disease. (See Table 60-1, page 1360.)

A chain of events is necessary for the continual spread of an infectious disease, beginning with a *causative agent* or invading organism, which may be bacterial, viral, rickettsial, protozoal, fungal, or helminthic. Infection by each type of organism gives rise to specific reactions in the infected organism.

GLOSSARY OF INFECTIOUS DISEASE TERMS

Antigen—agent that when introduced into body of susceptible person is capable of producing antibodies

Antiserum—a serum containing antibodies given to provide immunity against a specific disease. Usually regarded as temporary protection

Attenuation—the weakening of the toxicity or virulence of an infectious agent

Bacteremia—presence of bacteria in the circulating blood

Bactericidal—lethal or killing to bacteria

Carrier—one who harbors and eliminates organisms causing a specific disease, although he gives no evidence of having the disease

Case—a particular instance of disease

Communicable—transmissible from person to person, directly or indirectly

Contact—a person known or believed to have been exposed to an infectious disease

Contaminated—persons or objects that have come in contact with infectious agents or materials

Disinfection—destruction of pathogenic organisms by chemical or physical means

Endemic—a disease occurring habitually within a given geographic area

Epidemic—a disease attacking many people in a community simultaneously

Exanthem—an eruption on the skin

Fomites—inanimate vehicles other than food, milk, water, and air that may harbor, or be the means of transmission of organisms

Immune—protected against disease

Incubation period—the development of an infection from the time it gains entry into the body until the appearance of the first signs and symptoms

Infectious—capable of causing infection or disease

Infestation—invasion of body by arthropods; including insects, mites, mosquitoes, and ticks, and by helminths

In vitro—within the test tube

In vivo—within a living body

Isolation—procedures directed toward separating one patient from others

Morbidity rate—the number of illnesses compared to the population. The rate may be measured in *incidence* or *prevalence*: *incidence*—the number of cases occurring in the population in a year; *prevalence*—the average number of cases existing in the population

Mortality rate—the number of deaths compared to the population

Nosocomial infection—infection acquired during hospitalization; not present or incubating at the time of admission to hospital

Pandemic—disease affecting a large portion of the population; extensive epidemic

Pathogenic—disease-producing

Prodromal—symptoms occurring at the beginning stage of the disease

Prophylaxis—measures taken to prevent disease

Surveillance—dynamic system of collecting, tabulating, analyzing, and reporting data on the occurrence and distribution of disease.

Toxin—a poison elaborated by a microorganism

Toxoid—a modified toxin capable of stimulating the production of antibodies

Vaccine—a suspension of attenuated or killed microorganisms given to build up an active immunity against an infectious disease

---

The second link in the chain is a *reservoir*—a place for the invading organisms to live and multiply. The reservoir is the environment in which the agent is found, whether it be human, animal, or nonanimal; e.g., humans are the reservoir for syphilis; soil is the reservoir for tetanus; and animals are the reservoir for brucellosis. In humans, infectious diseases most often arise from contact with infected persons.

The next link is the *mode of escape* from the reservoir, including various body systems, such as the respiratory tract (most common when the reservoir is a human), intestinal tract, and genitourinary tract; open lesions; or mechanical escape, including the bite of insects.

After the infectious organism has escaped from its reservoir, it is dangerous only if it finds a way of reaching a host. This *mode of transmission* (the next link) may be direct (direct contact) or indirect (transfer without close contact). An example of an organism spread by indirect transmission would be the typhoid bacillus, which is able to survive for a long period of time outside the body. Disease may also be transmitted by the vehicle route (contaminated food, water, drugs, blood), by air (droplets), or by vector (arthropod).

The fifth link in the chain is the *mode of entry* of organisms into the human body. These correspond somewhat to the mode of escape and include the respiratory tract, gastrointestinal tract, direct infection of mucous membranes, or infection through a break in the skin.

The sixth link in the chain is a *susceptible host*. The presence of an infectious agent does not inevitably produce disease. Whether or not the person becomes ill following the entrance of infectious organisms into the body depends on numerous factors, including the number of organisms, the duration of the exposure, the person's age, general physical, mental, and emotional health and nutritional state, as well as the status of the hematopoietic system, the absence of immunoglobulins (or the presence of abnormal immunoglobulins), the number of T-lymphocytes, and their ability to function.

Removing one link in the chain of the infectious process controls infections, which is the purpose of all public health measures.

REPORTING OF DISEASE

When a communicable disease occurs in the community, the practicing physician has the legal responsibility of reporting its occurrence to the local health department. The method of reporting may be by telephone, telegraph, or a special written form provided for the purpose. The local health department forwards this information to the state health department, which sends weekly reports to the Center for Disease Control in Atlanta, Georgia, where data about communicable and chronic disease are compiled and published in the *Morbidity and Mortality Weekly Report.* This publication is fed back to all local health departments and practicing physicians. Thus, the occurrence of any local communicable disease becomes part of a huge network of health surveillance.

Among the most frequently reported cases of specified notifiable diseases in the United States are gonorrhea, chickenpox, syphilis, measles, tuberculosis, hepatitis A, salmonellosis, mumps, rubella, hepatitis B, and shigellosis.

The World Health Organization receives data about communicable diseases from all countries. Regional epidemiologists keep a careful watch on regional disease trends and disseminate this information to the appropriate individuals and services within the various countries. Computers are used to help in this rapid dissemination of information.

Diseases subject to international health regulation are cholera, yellow fever, plague, and smallpox. Other diseases receiving emphasis in global surveillance include influenza, poliomyelitis, measles, German measles, venereal diseases, malaria, relapsing fever, and typhus. Health problems vary from country to country, as do the available medical personnel and financial resources necessary to carry out effective surveillance programs. Only through unrelenting vigilance will it be possible to predict outbreaks of disease and take countermeasures for their control.

ASSESSMENT

Many early symptoms of infectious diseases are nonspecific. The illness may begin with malaise and all its attendant sequelae—listlessness, light-headedness, headache, anorexia, arthralgia, and weight loss. As the disease progresses, there is usually fever, although elderly people, in general, do not have as vigorous a febrile response as younger people. Nor will patients who have previously received antibiotics or are taking immunosuppressive agents exhibit fever. Fever may be preceded by a chill in certain infections such as pneumococcal pneumonia, streptococcal infection, influenza, etc. Repeated chills may be seen in the course of fevers caused by

bacteremias and in certain other infections, such as malaria.

The first step in identifying an infectious disease is to try to find out the *order and progression* of symptoms.
- Has the patient had a local or systemic infection?
- History of travel?
- Any contact with animals or animal products—raw wool, animal hides, blood?
- Has he had an animal or insect bite, cat scratch, exposure to birds?
- In addition, it is important to determine if the patient has a systemic disease that compromises host defenses, such as chronic renal disease, malignant disease (especially the leukemias and lymphomas), or if immunosuppressive agents or steroids are being taken which increase susceptibility to infection.

The physical examination helps in identifying infectious diseases, since many physical findings are diagnostic. An inflamed throat and enlarged lymph glands are compatible with a number of infectious diseases. Characteristic skin rashes and lesions may be present and may be pointed out by the patient who complains "Look at this rash!" Table 60-2, p. 1364, lists the diseases that produce exanthems (rashes) and describes the nature of the eruption as well as the other clinical features of the disease.

Laboratory examination of exudates (pus, sputum, wound swabbings), body fluids (urine, cerebrospinal fluid, synovial fluid), and tissues (blood, bone marrow) is often essential in the diagnosis of infections.

PRINCIPLES OF MANAGEMENT IN INFECTIOUS DISEASES

The management of a patient with any of the infectious diseases requires an understanding of the following information:
1. What is the nature of the infecting organism?
2. Where is this organism harbored in the host (i.e., the carrier or patient)?
3. How is the pathogen disseminated by the host?
4. What is the principal portal of entry for this organism?
5. How does the infective agent survive outside the host (i.e., under what circumstances, and how long is it likely to survive)?
6. How is immunity to this agent acquired or conferred, and how long is it effective?
7. What precautions or isolation techniques are indicated while caring for a patient with this infection?

Isolation Procedures

The purposes of isolation techniques in health care facilities are to prevent the spread of the infectious agent and to protect the patients, personnel, and visitors from infection. A committee of experts of the Center for Disease Control reviewed the isolation techniques for hospitalized persons with infectious diseases and established recommended procedures for isolating the disease—not the patient. (See Table 60-3, pages 1365-1367.)

All isolation techniques fall into one of the following categories:

Strict isolation
Respiratory isolation
Protective isolation
Enteric precautions
Wound and skin precautions
Discharge precautions
Blood precautions

The principles of isolation can be applied in almost any health care facility, including hospitals, extended care facilities, and mental institutions, although the specific techniques may need to be modified.

Protective (or reverse) isolation is carried out to protect patients with decreased resistance to disease.

• Patients requiring protective isolation include those with agranulocytosis, those receiving immunosuppressive drugs and large doses of radiation, and certain patients with lymphomas and leukemias.

The objective is to maintain a level of asepsis similar to that of the operating room. The patient is placed in a clean single room with bath. All personnel and visitors wear clean caps and sterile masks and gowns in the room. Gloves are worn by all persons having direct contact with the patient. Everything touching the patient should be either clean or sterile.

The following considerations are applicable in the care of all patients with communicable infections.

Handwashing

Handwashing is the foundation of controlling infectious disease. Ideal facilities for handwashing include a sink with foot or knee controls, hot and cold water, liquid, bar or powdered soaps or detergents, and paper towels. Effective handwashing consists of wetting, soaping, and lathering, applying friction to all surfaces of the hands, rinsing, and then repeating the process a second time. Uncontaminated lotion is used, since a break in the skin is a portal of entry for infection.

Personnel must wash their hands in the following instances: when coming on duty, when their hands are soiled, when they are between patients, before and after they wipe or blow their nose, after they use the toilet, when they leave an isolation unit, after they handle dressings, urinals, bedpans, needles, syringes, and catheters, and when they complete duty.

Gowns

Gowns are worn by *all* personnel when they enter the room of a patient with a disease that requires strict isolation and protective isolation, and are to be worn by those coming in direct contact with patients who require enteric, wound, and skin precautions. Gowns are to be used once (individual gown technique) and then discarded in an appropriate container before the user leaves the contaminated area. Clean, freshly laundered or disposable gowns should be available outside the isolation area. Sterile gowns are used for patients in protective isolation or for patients with extensive burns or wound infections.

Masks

Masks, when worn, should cover the nose and mouth and are to be used only once. A mask is to be discarded when moist, and not worn longer than an hour. Neither should the mask be lowered and then reused. The mask is discarded in a receptacle before anyone leaves the patient's room. The high-efficiency disposable masks are considered more effective than the cotton gauze masks. Supplies of clean masks are kept outside of the isolation unit.

Gloves

Disposable (single-use) gloves are worn when the patient requires strict isolation, protective isolation, and enteric, wound, and skin precautions. In some instances, sterile gloves will be necessary. The gloves are changed after direct contact with the patient's excretions or secretions even if the care of the patient has not been completed.

Dressings, Tissues, and Disposable Items

For the safe disposal of oral and nasal discharges, the patient is supplied with paper tissues and a disposable paper bag at his bedside. Disposable sputum cups with tops are to be provided, and the patient instructed in their proper use. All disposable supplies, including tissues, sputum cups, and contaminated dressings, as well as disposable drinking cups, dishes, and utensils, and table wastes wrapped in paper, are to be collected at frequent intervals and placed in a large plastic bag (securely sealed) for burning. Burning is the most effective method of destroying organisms.

Urine and Feces

Each patient should have his own bedpan and urinal; disposable ones, which can be placed in a bag and incinerated upon the patient's discharge, are preferable. If the bedpan is not disposable, it is cleaned and *autoclaved* when the patient is discharged. In most institutions the sanitary facilities permit disposal of all excreta through the public sewage system that serves the hospital. However, if such facilities are not available, then all stools, urine, vomitus, and liquid food waste should be pooled in a covered can containing a disinfectant solution, such as 5 percent chlorinated lime or 5 percent creosol, and allowed to stand for an hour before they are emptied into the sewage system. Feces should be broken up into fine particles, so that the lime comes in contact with all parts.

Linen

Contaminated bed linen should be collected and enclosed securely in a color-coded bag which is removed from the room and enclosed in a second clean bag marked "Contaminated." All contaminated clothing and linen should be sterilized by autoclaving before they are laundered with noninfectious goods. In the home, linens may be thoroughly washed with soap or detergent and *hot* water.

Instruments and Equipment

All instruments and items used on the patient are to be cleaned, rinsed, dried, double-bagged, and sent to Central Supply for decontamination and disinfection or sterilization. Gas sterilization (ethylene oxide) is used in the sterilization of many items that cannot be autoclaved. Disposable syringes, needles, and other equipment are available commercially and are recommended for use whenever possible.

Environmental Control

Microorganisms on the floor or other surfaces become airborne during sweeping, dry mopping, and dusting, and when mechanical buffers and unfiltered vacuum cleaners are used. Such practices should be avoided, and housekeeping personnel should be instructed in the proper methods of maintaining a clean environment. Since bedmaking contributes to the bacteriological pollution of hospital air, it is best to avoid shaking bed linens. Proper ventilation also is essential. The patient's door is to be kept closed, and an effective artificial ventilating system used, i.e., one that takes the room air to the outside. Currently, research is being directed at assessing the practical value of laminar airflow units in such areas as surgery, intensive care, and isolation units.

The most effective way to remove dust is to use a damp cloth and a wet vacuum pick-up with a filtered exhaust system for the floor. If mops are used, disposable or freshly laundered and machine-dried mops and cleaning cloths are necessary. The mop head is to be changed at least every 4 hours. A dirty, wet mop merely serves as a brush to paint the floor with live bacteria. When disinfectant is used in the mop bucket, the soil and bacterial load can reach a heavy enough level to inactivate the disinfectant. The water in the mop bucket must be changed frequently, and the bucket disinfected before being refilled. The buckets are not used outside the isolation area. Painted walls and flat surfaces (other than floors) rarely present a contamination problem. A spray bottle of disinfectant should be used instead of a bucket.

Terminal cleaning of the room upon discharge of the patient includes incinerating disposable items, cleaning and bagging equipment for disinfection or sterilization in Central Supply, washing furniture and mattress covers, washing grossly soiled areas on walls, and wet vacuuming or mopping the floors by means of the double-bucket technique.

IMMUNITY

Immunity is the resistance that a person has against disease. Specific immunity to a particular organism implies that an individual either has generated the appropriate antibody in his own body or has received ready-made antibodies from another source. Immunity may be natural (not acquired through previous contact with the infectious agent) or acquired. Not much is known about the processes responsible for natural immunity or resistance. More is known about acquired immunity, which has been identified as being either active or passive.

Active Immunization. Active immunization is produced by natural or acquired stimulation, so that the body produces its own antibodies. It may result from clinical or subclinical infection (e.g., the person "gets the disease"). Or it may be produced by administering live or killed microorganisms or their antigens or inactivated vaccines and toxoids.

Active immunization is the most important and effective tool in preventive medicine. It has been most effective with bacterial exotoxins (diphtherial and tetanus toxoids) and with viruses. Most live-virus vaccines produce antibody responses that consist of prompt (but transient) production of specific immunoglobulins: (IgM followed by a sustained production of specific IgG). Live-virus vaccines may produce mild clinical illness, with fever and rash appearing in some patients.

Inactivated vaccines and toxoids give a less complete response after a single injection and may have to be administered in repeated doses according to a prescribed schedule for long-lasting IgG response and sustained protection against infection. Following injection with inactivated vaccines and toxoids, there may be a mild local reaction at the site of injection and occasional systemic symptoms of fever, malaise, and headache.

Active immunization agents that are available for adults include tetanus and diphtheria toxoid, adult-type tetanus toxoid, influenza virus vaccines, mumps virus vaccine, poliomyelitis vaccine, measles vaccine, and rubella virus vaccine. Vaccines are also available for plague, rabies, typhoid, typhus, yellow fever, Rocky Mountain spotted fever, and smallpox.

Current recommendations for the use of vaccines and other biologics used in the prevention of disease are available from the Public Health Service Advisory Committee on Immunization Practices, Center for Disease Control, Atlanta, Georgia 30333. The recommendations are based on an analysis of the scientific evidence, weighing the benefits and the risks of protection against the effects of infectious or communicable diseases.

Passive Immunity. Passive immunity provides temporary protection to a disease and is produced by the injection of serum that contains antibodies which have been formed in another host. It is given for temporary protection against a disease when active immunizing agents are not available (example: immune serum globulin for hepatitis A), or when there is insufficient time to acquire active immunization following exposure to disease. (Passive immunity is not totally satisfactory because of the risk inherent in providing antibodies of one animal to another.)

There are several types of preparations in use for passive immunity: standard immune serum globulin (for general use), human immune serum globulin with a known antibody content for specific illnesses, and animal antiserum or antitoxins. Products made with animal serum may cause an anaphylaxislike reaction or serum sickness. Therefore products made with human serum are given whenever possible.

Immunization Programs. A national immunization program has been supported by federal legislation (Vaccination Assistance Act) to assist states and communities in carrying out intensive vaccination programs against poliomyelitis, diphtheria, pertussis, tetanus, measles, rubella, and other infectious diseases for which a preventive agent is available. Studies show that socially deprived and low-income groups do not receive the protection of immunization programs; this is a challenge to all medical personnel. A person's acceptance of this type of preventive care may help him to accept other medical services. Nurses, using gentle persuasion, can reach out and listen to the fears of the people and teach them the benefits of immunization.

TABLE 60-1. EPIDEMIOLOGY, THERAPY, AND CONTROL OF COMMUNICABLE INFECTIONS

DISEASE	INFECTIVE ORGANISM	INFECTIOUS SOURCES	ENTRY SITE	METHOD OF SPREAD	INCUBATION PERIOD	CHEMOTHERAPY*	PROPHYLAXIS
Amebiasis	*Entamoeba histolytica*	Contaminated water and food	Gastrointestinal tract	Patients and carriers; fecal-oral route	Variable	Metronidazole; emetine; chloroquine; diiodohydroxyquin; chlortetracycline	Detection of carriers and their removal from food handling; plumbing safeguards
Bacillary Dysentery	*Shigella* group	Contaminated water and food	Gastrointestinal tract	Patients and carriers; fecal-oral route	24-48 hours	Ampicillin; chloramphenicol; tetracycline; Sulfa-trimethoprim	Detection and control of carriers; inspection of food handlers; decontamination of water supplies
Brucellosis	*Brucella melitensis* and related organisms	Milk, meat, tissues, blood, absorbed fetuses and placentas from infected cattle, goats, horses, pigs	Gastrointestinal tract	Ingestion of or contact with infective material	6-14 days	Tetracycline and streptomycin or chloramphenicol	Milk pasteurization; control of infection in animals
Chancroid	Ducrey bacillus	Human cases and carriers	Genitalia	Direct sexual contact	2-5 days	Sulfonamides; streptomycin; tetracycline	Effective case-finding and treatment of infection
Chickenpox (Varicella)	Virus	Human cases	Probably nasopharynx	Probably respiratory droplets	14-16 days	None	Zoster immune globulin (ZIG) (an investigational drug) provided by Center for Disease Control to high-risk susceptible children exposed to varicella zoster within 72 hours
Diphtheria	*Corynebacterium diphtheriae*	Human cases and carriers; fomites; raw milk	Nasopharynx	Nasal and oral secretions; respiratory droplets	2-5 days	Diphtheria antitoxin; penicillin; erythromycin	Active immunization with diphtheria toxoid
Encephalitis, epidemic (eastern and western equine)	Viruses	Chicken and wild-bird mites; horses; hibernating garter snakes	Skin	Mosquitoes	Variable	None	Eastern equine encephalitis vaccine, dried (available from Center for Disease Control)
Gonorrhea	*Neisseria gonorrhoeae*	Urethral and vaginal secretions	Urethral or vaginal mucosa; pharynx; rectum	Sexual activity	2-9 days	Aqueous Procaine Penicillin G, preceded by probenecid or alternative regimen outlined by U.S.P.H.S.	Examination culture, and treatment of sexual partners
Granuloma Inguinale	Donovan body (bacillus)	Infectious exudate	External genitalia; cervix	Sexual intercourse	Unknown, presumably 8-80 days	Tetracyclines; erythromycin	Chemotherapy of carriers and contacts; case-finding and treatment of patients

*Research developments produce changes in drug therapy. The reader is referred to drug brochures and digests to keep abreast of changing dosages and uses.

TABLE 60-1. (Continued)

DISEASE	INFECTIVE ORGANISM	INFECTIOUS SOURCES	ENTRY SITE	METHOD OF SPREAD	INCUBATION PERIOD	CHEMOTHERAPY*	PROPHYLAXIS
Type A Hepatitis (HAV)	Hepatitis A virus	Person-to-person contact; contaminated food or water; feces; blood; urine	Gastrointestinal tract; skin	Fecal-oral route; ingestion of or parenteral inoculation with infected blood or blood products	15–45 days	None	Enteric and blood precautions for infected cases. Immune serum globulin (ISG) offers protection against clinical manifestations if given early in incubation period
Type B Hepatitis (HAB)	Hepatitis B virus	Infected blood donor; contaminated injection equipment	Skin	Parenteral injection of human blood, plasma, thrombin, fibrinogen, packed cells, and other blood products from an infected person; contaminated needles and syringes; venereal contact	60–180 days	None	Screening of blood donors; avoidance of unnecessary use of blood and blood derivatives Hepatitis B immume globulin (HBIG) given under certain conditions
Infectious Mononucleosis	E-B virus	Human cases and carriers	Mouth	Probably oral-pharyngeal route; via blood transfusion in susceptible recipients	2–6 weeks	None	None
Influenza	Virus (types A and B)	Human cases; animal reservoir	Respiratory tract	Respiratory	24–72 hours	Amantadine(?)	Specific virus vaccine
Lympho-granuloma Venereum	Chlamydia trachomatis	Human cases	External genitalia; urethral or vaginal mucosa	Sexual intercourse; indirect contact with contaminated articles/clothing	5–21 days	Tetracyclines	Case-finding and treatment of infection

(Continued)

TABLE 60-1. (Continued)

DISEASE	INFECTIVE ORGANISM	INFECTIOUS SOURCES	ENTRY SITE	METHOD OF SPREAD	INCUBATION PERIOD	CHEMOTHERAPY*	PROPHYLAXIS
Malaria	*Plasmodium vivax, falciparum, malariae,* and *ovale*	Human cases	Skin	Mosquitoes (Anopheles)	Variable, depending on strain	Chloroquine; primaquine; amodiaquine; quinine; proguanil	Coordinated measures for wide-scale mosquito control; prompt detection and effective treatment of cases; suppressive drugs in malarious areas
Measles	Virus	Human cases	Respiratory mucosa	Nasopharyngeal secretions	8-13 days	None	Measles vaccine
Meningococcal Meningitis	*Neisseria meningitidis*	Human cases and carriers	Nasopharynx; tonsils	Respiratory droplets	2-10 days	Penicillin; chloramphenicol	Meningococcal polysaccharide vaccine to persons at risk; rifampin for carriers or contacts
Mumps	Virus	Human cases (early)	Upper respiratory tract	Respiratory droplets	12-26 days (avg. 18 days)	None	Live mumps vaccine
Paratyphoid Fever	*Salmonella paratyphi A and B* and related organisms	Contaminated food, milk, water; rectal tubes; barium enemas	Gastrointestinal tract	Infected urine and feces	7-24 days	Chloramphenicol; ampicillin; sulfa-trimethoprim	Control of public water sources, food vendors, food handlers; treatment of carriers
Pneumococcal Pneumonia	*Streptococcus pneumoniae*	Human carriers; patient's own pharynx	Respiratory mucosa	Respiratory droplets	Variable	Penicillin	Polyvalent pneumococcal vaccine; control of upper respiratory infections; avoidance of alcoholic intoxication
Poliomyelitis	Polioviruses (Types I, II, III)	Human cases and carriers	Gastrointestinal tract	Infected feces; pharyngeal secretions	7-12 days	None	Wide-scale application of parenteral (Salk) and oral (Sabin) poliovirus vaccines; case isolation
Rocky Mountain Spotted Fever	*Rickettsia rickettsii*	Infected wild rodents, dogs, wood ticks, dog ticks	Skin	Tick bites	3-10 days	Tetracyclines; chloramphenicol	Avoidance of tick-infected areas, or wearing of protective clothing in such areas; frequent search for, and prompt removal of ticks from body; specific vaccination of exposed persons
Rubella (German Measles)	Virus	Human cases	Respiratory mucosa	Nasopharyngeal secretions	14-21 days	None	Rubella virus vaccine; immune serum globulin (human) given to contacts of rubella; rubella in early stages of pregnancy legally recognized as indication for abortion
Scarlet Fever	Group A streptococcus	Human cases; infected food	Pharynx	Nasal and oral secretions	3-5 days	Penicillin	Case isolation; prophylactic chemotherapy with penicillin; asepsis during obstetrical procedures; specific chemoprophylaxis for persons with rheumatic fever

TABLE 60-1. (Continued)

DISEASE	INFECTIVE ORGANISM	INFECTIOUS SOURCES	ENTRY SITE	METHOD OF SPREAD	INCUBATION PERIOD	CHEMOTHERAPY*	PROPHYLAXIS
Syphillis	Treponema pallidum	Infected exudate or blood	External genitalia; cervix; mucosal surfaces; placenta	Sexual activity; contact with open lesions; blood transfusion; transplacental inoculation	10–70 days	Penicillin; erythromycin; tetracycline	Case-finding by means of routine serologic testing and other methods; adequate treatment of infected individuals
Tetanus	Clostridium tetani	Contaminated soil	Penetrating and crush wounds	Horse and cattle feces	4–21 days (avg. 10 days)	Tetanus immune globulin (human) [TIG] and penicillin	Wound debridement; toxoid booster injections for patients previously immunized; tetanus toxoid and tetanus immune globulin (separate sites and separate syringes) for nonimmune persons
Trichinosis	Trichinella spiralis	Infected pigs	Gastrointestinal tract	Ingestion of infected pork, undercooked	2–28 days	Steroids; thiabendazole	Regulation of hog breeders; adequate meat inspection; thorough cooking of pork
Tuberculosis	Mycobacterium tuberculosis	Sputum from human cases; milk from infected cows (rare in U.S.)	Respiratory mucosa	Sputum; respiratory droplets	Variable	Isoniazid; ethambutol; rifampin; streptomycin	Early discovery and adequate treatment of active cases; milk pasteurization
Tularemia	Pasteurella tularensis	Wild rodents and rabbits	Eyes; skin; gastrointestinal tract	Handling infected animals; ingestion of undercooked infected meat; drinking contaminated water; bites from infected flies, ticks	1–10 days	Streptomycin; tetracyclines; chloramphenicol	Use of rubber gloves when skinning/handling potentially infectious wild animals; avoidance of contact with potentially infected rodents; adequate cooking of wild rabbit dishes; vaccination of hunters, butchers, laboratory workers risking heavy exposure
Typhoid Fever	Salmonella typhi	Contaminated food and water	Gastrointestinal tract	Infected urine and feces	1–3 weeks	Chloramphenicol; ampicillin; sulfa-trimethoprim	Decontamination of water sources; milk pasteurization; individual vaccination of high risk persons; control of carriers
Typhus, endemic	Rickettsia typhi (mooseri)	Infected rodents	Skin	Flea bites	1–2 weeks	Tetracyclines; chloramphenicol	Delousing procedures; case quarantine
Whooping Cough (Pertussis)	Bordatella pertussis	Human cases	Respiratory tract	Infected bronchial secretions	Commonly 7 days	Erythromycin; ampicillin	Active immunization with vaccine; case isolation

1363

TABLE 60-2. DIAGNOSTIC FEATURES OF SOME ACUTE EXANTHEMS

DISEASE	PRODROMAL SIGNS AND SYMPTOMS	NATURE OF ERUPTION	OTHER DIAGNOSTIC FEATURES	LABORATORY TESTS
Measles (rubeola)	3-4 days of fever, coryza, conjunctivitis, and cough.	Maculopapular, brick-red; begins on head and neck; spreads downward. In 5-6 days rash brownish, desquamating.	Koplik's spots on buccal mucosa.	White blood count low. Virus isolation in cell culture. Antibody tests by hemagglutination inhibition and complement fixation or neutralization.
Rubella (German measles)	Little or no prodrome.	Maculopapular, pink; begins on head and neck, spreads downward, fades in 3 days. No desquamation.	Lymphadenopathy, postauricular or occipital.	White blood count normal or low. Serologic tests for immunity and definitive diagnosis (hemagglutination inhibition, complement fixation).
Chickenpox (varicella)	0-1 day of fever, anorexia, headache.	Rapid evolution of macules to papules, vesicles, crusts; all stages simultaneously present; lesions superficial, distribution centripetal.	Lesions on scalp and mucous membranes.	Specialized complement fixation and virus neutralization in tissue culture. Fluorescent antibody test of smear of lesions.
Smallpox (variola)	3 days of fever, severe headache, malaise, chills.	Slow evolution of macules to papules, vesicles, pustules, crusts; all lesions in any area in same stage; lesions deep-seated, distribution centrifugal.		Virus isolation. Serologic tests for immunity. Fluorescent antibody test of smear of lesions.
Scarlet fever	½-2 days of malaise, sore throat, fever, vomiting.	Generalized, punctate, red; prominent on neck, in axilla, groin, skinfolds; circumoral pallor; fine desquamation involves hands and feet.	Strawberry tongue, exudative tonsilitis.	Group A hemolytic streptococci cultures from throat, antistreptolysin O titer rise.
Exanthem subitum	3-4 days of high fever.	As fever falls by crisis, pink maculopapules appear on chest and trunk; fade in 1-3 days.		White blood count low.
Erythema infectiosum	None. Usually in epidemics.	Red, flushed cheeks; circumoral pallor; maculopapules on extremities.	"Slapped-face" appearance.	White blood count normal.
Meningo-coccemia	Hours of fever, vomiting.	Maculopapules, petechiae, purpura.	Meningeal signs, toxicity, shock.	Cultures of blood. Cerebrospinal fluid. High white blood count.
Rocky Mt. spotted fever	3-4 days of fever, chills, severe headaches.	Maculopapules, petechiae, distribution centrifugal.	History of tick bite.	Agglutination (0 × 19, 0 × 2), complement fixation.
Typhus fevers	3-4 days of fever, chills, severe headaches.	Maculopapules, petechiae, distribution centripetal.	Endemic area, lice.	Agglutination (0 × 19), complement fixation.
Infectious mononucleosis	Fever, adenopathy, sore throat.	Maculopapular rash resembling rubella, rarely papulovesicular.	Splenomegaly, tonsillar exudate.	Atypical lymphocytes in blood smears; heterophil agglutination. Monospot test.
Enterovirus infections	1-2 days of fever, malaise.	Maculopapular rash resembling rubella, rarely papulovesicular or petechial.	Aseptic meningitis.	Virus isolation from stool or cerebrospinal fluid; complement fixation titer rise.
Drug eruptions	Occasionally fever.	Maculopapular rash resembling rubella, rarely papulovesicular.		Eosinophilia.
Eczema herpeticum	None.	Vesiculopustular lesions in area of eczema.		Herpes simplex virus isolated in tissue culture; complement fixation. Fluorescent antibody test of smear of lesions.

(From Krupp, M. A., and Chatton, M. J. (eds.): Current Medical Diagnosis and Treatment. Los Altos, Calif., Lange Medical Publications, 1979)

TABLE 60-3. CLASSIFICATION OF INFECTIOUS DISEASES REQUIRING ISOLATION OR PRECAUTIONS*

STRICT ISOLATION

Private room—*necessary*; door must be kept closed.
Gowns—must be worn by all persons entering room.
Masks—must be worn by all persons entering room.
Hands—must be washed on entering and leaving room.
Gloves—must be worn by all persons entering room.
Articles—must be discarded or wrapped before being sent to Central Supply for disinfection or sterilization.

Diseases Requiring Strict Isolation†
1. Anthrax, inhalation
2. Burn wounds (major) infected with *Staphylococcus aureus* or group A streptococcus
3. Congenital rubella syndrome
4. Diphtheria (pharyngeal or cutaneous)
5. Disseminated neonatal *Herpesvirus hominis* infection (herpes simplex)
6. Herpes zoster, disseminated
7. Lassa fever
8. Marburg virus disease
9. Plague, pneumonic
10. Pneumonia, *Staphylococcus aureus* or group A streptococcus
11. Rabies
12. Skin infection (major) infected with *Staphylococcus aureus* or group A streptococcus
13. Smallpox
14. Vaccinia (generalized and progressive, and eczema vaccinatum)
15. Varicella (chickenpox)

RESPIRATORY ISOLATION

Private Room—*necessary*; door must be kept closed.
Gowns—not necessary.
Masks—must be worn by any person entering room unless that person is not susceptible to the disease.
Hands—must be washed on entering and leaving room.
Gloves—not necessary.
Articles—those contaminated with secretions must be disinfected.

Diseases Requiring Respiratory Isolation†
1. Measles (rubeola)
2. Meningococcal meningitis
3. Meningococcemia
4. Mumps
5. Pertussis (whooping cough)
6. Rubella (German measles)
7. Tuberculosis, pulmonary—including tuberculosis of the respiratory tract, suspected or sputum-positive (smear)

PROTECTIVE ISOLATION

Private room—*necessary*; door must be kept closed.
Gowns—must be worn by all persons entering room.
Masks—must be worn by all persons entering room.
Hands—must be washed on entering and leaving room.
Gloves—must be worn by all persons having direct contact with patient.
Articles—See *Isolation Techniques for Use in Hospitals.*

Conditions That May Require Protective Isolation†
1. Agranulocytosis
2. Dermatitis; noninfected vesicular, bullous, or eczematous disease, when severe and extensive
3. Extensive, noninfected burns in certain patients
4. Lymphomas and leukemia in certain patients (especially in the late stages of Hodgkin's disease and acute leukemia)

ENTERIC PRECAUTIONS

Private room—*necessary for children only.*
Gowns—must be worn by all persons having direct contact with patient.
Masks—not necessary.
Hands—must be washed on entering and leaving room.
Gloves—must be worn by all persons having direct contact with patient or with articles contaminated with fecal material.
Articles—special precautions necessary for articles contaminated with urine and feces. Articles must be disinfected or discarded.

Diseases Requiring Enteric Precautions†
1. Cholera
2. Diarrhea, acute illness with suspected infectious etiology
3. Enterocolitis, staphylococcal
4. Gastroenteritis caused by:
   Enteropathogenic or enterotoxic *Escherichia coli*
   Salmonella species
   Shigella species
   Yersinia enterocolitica
5. Hepatitis, viral, type A, B, or unspecified
6. Typhoid fever (*Salmonella typhi*)

WOUND AND SKIN PRECAUTIONS

Private room—desirable.
Gowns—must be worn by all persons having direct contact with patient.
Masks—not necessary except during dressing changes.
Hands—must be washed on entering and leaving room.
Gloves—must be worn by all persons having direct contact with infected area.
Articles—special precautions necessary for instruments, dressings, and linen.

Diseases Requiring Wound and Skin Precautions†
1. Burns that are infected, except those infected with *Staphylococcus aureus* or group A streptococcus that are not covered or not adequately contained by dressings (see Strict Isolation)
2. Gas gangrene (due to *Clostridium perfringens*)
3. Herpes zoster, localized
4. Melioidosis, extrapulmonary with draining sinuses
5. Plague, bubonic
6. Puerperal sepsis—group A streptococcus, vaginal discharge
7. Wound and skin infections that are not covered by dressings or that have copious purulent drainage that is not contained by dressings, except those infected with *Staphylococcus aureus* or group A streptococcus, which require strict isolation

(Continued)

*From *Isolation Techniques for Use in Hospitals,* 2nd ed., U.S. Department of Health, Education and Welfare, Center for Disease Control, 1975.
†See *Isolation Techniques for Use in Hospitals* for details and recommended duration of isolation.

TABLE 60-3. (Continued)

WOUND AND SKIN PRECAUTIONS (CONTINUED)

8. Wound and skin infections that are covered by dressings so that the discharge is adequately contained, including those infected with *Staphylococcus aureus* or group A streptococcus; minor wound infections, such as stitch abscesses, need only secretion precautions

DISCHARGE PRECAUTIONS

A. *Secretion Precautions—Lesions*
   1. Use a "no-touch" dressing technique (do not touch the wound or dressings with the hands (when changing dressings on these lesions.
   2. Employ proper handwashing procedures.
   3. Wash hands before and after patient contact; use sterile equipment when changing dressings; double-bag soiled dressings and equipment.
   4. These precautions apply only with lesions from which there is a discharge.

Diseases; Duration of Precautions
   1. Actinomycosis, draining lesions—for duration of drainage
   2. Anthrax, cutaneous—until culture-negative
   3. Brucellosis, draining lesions—for duration of drainage
   4. Burn, skin, and wound infections, minor—for duration of drainage
   5. Candidiasis, mucocutaneous—for duration of illness
   6. Coccidioidomycosis, draining lesion—for duration of drainage
   7. Conjunctivitis, acute bacterial (including gonococcal)—until 24 hours after start of effective therapy
   8. Conjunctivitis, viral—for duration of illness
   9. Gonococcal ophthalmia neonatorum—until 24 hours after start of effective therapy
   10. Gonorrhea—until 24 hours after start of effective therapy
   11. Granuloma inguinale—for duration of illness
   12. *Herpesvirus hominis* (herpes simplex), except disseminated neonatal disease—for duration of illness. For disseminated neonatal disease, see Strict Isolation; for oral *H. hominis* disease, see Secretion Precautions, Oral.
   13. Keratoconjunctivitis, infectious—for duration of illness
   14. Listeriosis—for duration of illness
   15. Lymphogranuloma venereum—for duration of illness
   16. Nocardiosis, draining lesions—for duration of illness
   17. Orf—for duration of illness
   18. Syphilis, mucocutaneous—until 24 hours after start of effective therapy
   19. Trachoma, acute—for duration of illness
   20. Tuberculosis, extrapulmonary draining lesion—for duration of drainage
   21. Tularemia, draining lesion—for duration of drainage

B. *Secretion Precautions—Oral*
   1. The diseases listed in this section can be spread to susceptible persons by contact with oral secretions.
   2. Attention should be given to the proper disposal of oral secretions to prevent spread of infection.
   3. Instruct the patient to cough or spit into disposable tissues held close to the mouth; discard tissues in an impervious (impenetrable) bag at the bedside.
   4. If the patient has nasotracheal suction or tracheostomy, the suction catheter and gloves should be placed in an impervious bag for disposal.
   5. Seal the bag before discarding in the trash.

Diseases; Duration of Precautions
   1. Herpangina—for duration of hospitalization
   2. Herpes oralis—for duration of illness
   3. Infectious mononucleosis—for duration of illness
   4. Melioidosis, pulmonary—for duration of illness
   5. Mycoplasma pneumonia—for duration of illness
   6. Pneumonia, bacterial (if not covered elsewhere)—for duration of illness
   7. Psittacosis—for duration of illness. (It may be desirable to place patient with acute psittacosis who is coughing and raising sputum in respiratory isolation.)
   8. Q fever—for duration of illness
   9. Respiratory infectious disease, acute (if not covered elsewhere)—for duration of illness
   10. Scarlet fever—until 24 hours after start of effective therapy
   11. Streptococcal pharyngitis—until 24 hours after start of effective therapy

C. *Excretion Precautions*
   1. The diseases listed in this section can be spread to susceptible persons through the oral route by contact with fecal excretions from a person infected with the organism.
   2. Strict attention should be paid to careful handwashing following any patient contact and especially following contact with excretions.
   3. Instruct the patient on the necessity of careful handwashing after defecating.
   4. Make sure there is proper sanitary disposal of excretions; a standard sewage system is adequate.

Diseases; Duration of Precautions
   1. Amebiasis—for duration of illness
   2. *Clostridium perfringens (C. welchii)* food poisoning—for duration of illness
   3. Enterobiasis—for duration of illness
   4. Giardiasis—for duration of illness
   5. Hand, foot, and mouth disease—for duration of hospitalization
   6. Herpangina—for duration of hospitalization
   7. Infectious lymphocytosis—for duration of hospitalization
   8. Leptospirosis (urine only)—for duration of hospitalization
   9. Meningitis, aseptic—for duration of hospitalization
   10. Pleurodynia—for duration of hospitalization
   11. Poliomyelitis—for duration of hospitalization
   12. Staphylococcal food poisoning—for duration of symptoms
   13. Tapeworm disease (only with *Hymenolepsis nana* and *Taenia solium* [pork])—for duration of illness

TABLE 60-3. (Continued)

DISCHARGE PRECAUTIONS (CONTINUED)

14. Viral diseases, other (ECHO or Coxsackie gastroenteritis, pericarditis, myocarditis, meningitis)—for duration of hospitalization

D. *Blood Precautions*
1. The diseases in this category are associated with circulation of the etiologic agent in blood; be aware of the route of transmission.
2. Blood precautions should be taken for the duration of clinical disease or for as long as the etiologic agent can be demonstrated in the blood. Blood precautions should be taken with anyone who is HB_sAg-positive.
3. Disposable needles and syringe should be used for patients in isolation. They must not be reused.
4. Used needles need not be recapped; they should be placed in a prominently labeled, impervious, puncture-resistant container designated for this purpose. Needles should not be purposefully bent, because accidental needle puncture may occur.

5. Used syringes should be placed in an impervious bag. Both needle and syringe bags should be incinerated or autoclaved before discarding.
6. Rinse reusable needles and syringes thoroughly in cold water after use; place the needle in a puncture-resistant rigid container; wrap syringes and needles using double-bag technique and return to proper department for decontamination and sterilization.
7. These specifications pertain to needle and syringe precautions and to labeling of blood specimens. Label blood specimens with patient's diagnosis (so that necessary precautions will be taken).

Diseases; Duration of Precautions
1. Arthropod-borne viral fever (dengue, etc.)—for duration of hospitalization
2. Hepatitis, viral, type A, B, or unspecified (also listed under Enteric Precautions)—for duration of hospitalization
3. Malaria—for duration of hospitalization

NURSING SUMMARY: THE PATIENT WITH AN INFECTIOUS DISEASE

Objectives and Guidelines

A. **TO ASSIST IN IDENTIFYING THE ETIOLOGIC AGENT AND ESTABLISHING THE DIAGNOSIS:**
1. Obtain specimens of blood, urine, stools, sputum, throat swabbings, nasal secretions, and pyogenic exudates for bacteriologic study.
2. Assist in securing smears of blood and other materials for microscopic examination.
3. Assist with aspirations of spinal fluid, bone marrow, and other body fluids or tissues for cytologic, serologic, and bacteriologic tests.
4. Carry out appropriate skin tests for specific diagnostic reactions as directed.

B. **TO CONTROL THE INFECTION IN THE PATIENT:**
1. Administer the appropriate antimicrobial agents as requested.
2. Assist in administering specific immune therapy, if available, employing immune antiserum, gamma globulin, antitoxin, toxoid, vaccine, or an appropriate mixture of antigen and antibody, depending on the circumstances.
3. Observe patient carefully for evidences of drug or serum sensitivity.

C. **TO PREVENT SPREAD OF THE INFECTION TO OTHERS:**
1. Carry out isolation technique as required by the disease.
2. Observe asepsis as indicated.
3. Use mask technique effectively. (Masks are not used now as much as in the past.)
   a. Change mask frequently—moisture increases the mask's permeability, promoting bacterial growth.
   b. Refrain from handling the mask while in use.

4. Use gown as required by disease of patient.
   a. Use gown once and discard in proper receptacle.
   b. Collect linen in water-soluble bags; double-bag, and mark "ISOLATION."
5. Use gloves when indicated by the patient's condition.
   a. Disposable single-use gloves are preferable.
   b. Use once and discard in appropriate receptacle.
6. Handle needles and syringes with extreme care.
   a. Rinse nondisposable needles and syringes in cold water and wrap using the double-bag technique.
   b. Place in a clean bag in contaminated area and then in a second clean bag outside the patient's room.
7. Wash hands immediately after each patient contact and after every contact with material that may be contaminated and is potentially infectious.
   a. Use paper towel to turn off faucet if sink is not equipped with foot, knee, or elbow-operated faucets.
   b. Use individualized soap tissues.
8. Disinfect and handle wastes with all due precautions.
9. Handle bed linens and fomites with care.
10. Carry out concurrent disinfection of fomites.
11. Control dissemination of infectious droplets.
    a. Encourage patient to cover nose and mouth when coughing or sneezing.
    b. Wrap contaminated tissues and articles in paper before disposal.

(Continued)

---

12. Control dust.
   a. Avoid creating aerosols—example, shaking bed linens.
   b. Require damp dusting of furniture and wet vacuum cleaning of floors.
   c. Maintain cleanliness of surroundings; wash soil from walls as soon as it appears.
   d. Reduce to a minimum the activity of personnel in the patient's room.
13. Ventilate the patient's room properly with a system that directs room air to the outside.
   a. Keep the door to the room closed.
   b. Disinfect room air with a laminar airflow system, if available.

D. TO PROVIDE PHYSIOLOGIC SUPPORT OF THE PATIENT:
1. Ensure adequate hydration in the face of excessive fluid loss through vomiting, diarrhea, or excessive sweating.
   a. Encourage the ingestion of fluids.
   b. Prepare for the administration of intravenous fluids as required.
2. Reduce the fever when indicated.
   a. Administer antipyretic drugs, as prescribed.
   b. Employ cool sponges cautiously, as indicated.
3. Measure and record body temperature, pulse, and respiratory rates frequently.
4. Measure arterial blood pressure at regular intervals if patient exhibits a tendency to vascular collapse.
5. Weigh patient periodically, preferably at same hour of day on same scale.

E. TO PROVIDE SYMPTOMATIC RELIEF:
1. Combat generalized aching and malaise.
   a. Utilize warm applications and massage, as indicated.
   b. Apply cold compresses for headache.
   c. Administer analgesic medications as prescribed.
   d. Attend to oral hygiene.
   e. Limit physical activity.
2. Relieve cough.
   a. Humidify inspired air.
   b. Administer warm gargles and throat irrigations.
   c. Supply expectorants or cough depressants as indicated and prescribed.

3. Relieve anxiety and depression.
   a. Recognize loneliness of the isolated patient.
   b. Lend strong encouragement to patient faced with prospect of prolonged convalescence.

F. TO PROTECT EXPOSED INDIVIDUALS AND PUBLIC AT LARGE AGAINST INFECTIOUS ILLNESS:
1. Make available, facilitate or perform whatever vaccination procedures are known to be effective and are indicated for the stimulation of active immunity in exposed and susceptible individuals.
2. Furnish specific immune serum (heterologous or human convalescent) or human gamma globulin, if indicated, to provide passive immunity and temporary protection to contacts who are particularly vulnerable.
3. Isolate patients with communicable infections, as well as known carriers and contacts, when required.
4. Educate the public with respect to:
   a. Availability and importance of prophylactic immunizations.
   b. Manner in which infectious illnesses are spread and methods of avoiding spread.
   c. Importance of seeking medical advice in the event of a febrile illness or skin eruption.
   d. Importance of environmental cleanliness and personal hygiene.
   e. Importance of adequate housing and nutrition.
   f. Means of preventing the contamination of food and water supplies.
      (1) Discipline, cleanliness, and inspection of food handlers.
      (2) Dangers of "perishable" foods; the identity of foods that tend to promote bacterial growth; and methods of food preservation.
      (3) Significance of milk pasteurization.
      (4) Indications for, and methods of, sterilizing food by means of heat.
      (5) Importance of meat inspection.
   g. Knowledge of insect, rodent, and other animal vectors, and reservoirs of human infections, and importance of eliminating them.

SPECIFIC BACTERIAL INFECTIONS

NOSOCOMIAL (HOSPITAL-ACQUIRED) INFECTIONS

A nosocomial infection is an infection acquired during hospitalization; it is neither present nor incubating at the time of admission unless it is related to a previous hospitalization.

Approximately 5 percent of the 30 million persons admitted to hospitals in this country acquire an infection. It is estimated that a patient with such a problem spends an average of 10 extra days in the hospital, with an economic impact of more than 1 billion dollars.

Gram-Negative Bacterial Infections

The major cause of hospital-acquired infections in the United States is gram-negative bacteria, such as *Escherichia coli*, *Enterobacter* species, *Klebsiella pneumoniae*,

Pseudomonas aeruginosa, the *Proteus* species, and *Serratia marcescens.* In recent years, these organisms have invaded the bloodstreams (bacteremia) of more hospitalized patients than the staphylococcal organisms which were previously responsible for most cases of bacteremia. Such infections arise from the patient's own bacterial flora or may be acquired from other sources. Gram-negative bacilli frequently are responsible for infections of the bloodstream and of the urinary and respiratory tracts. Most gram-negative bacilli are not invasive in normal hosts but become invasive in hospitalized patients who have underlying disease and low resistance, have undergone immunosuppressive therapy, or have cardiac prostheses.

- These organisms can infect burns or wounds, can be introduced into the bladder by indwelling catheter, inhaled into the lung by contaminated ventilatory equipment (particularly reservoir nebulizers), or transported directly into the bloodstream by intravenous catheters. Gastrointestinal and biliary surgery, tracheostomies, and contaminated devices account for a significant number of infections.

The risk of developing nosocomial infection parallels the severity of the underlying disease. Gram-negative infections occur in the very young, the elderly, patients with impaired immune systems, blood dyscrasias, burns, trauma, or poorly controlled diabetes, those undergoing prolonged procedures that result in extensive tissue damage, or those in whom a foreign body has been implanted. Potent immunosuppressive and cytotoxic drugs, steroids, radiation, etc., further diminish the patient's defense mechanisms. Antibiotics add to the problem by altering the patient's normal flora and encouraging overgrowth of hospital pathogens that are resistant to antibiotics. Thus the susceptible patient who is exposed to invasive diagnostic and monitoring equipment is predisposed to develop a gram-negative infection.

Table 60-4 shows the site, the precipitating event, and the agents producing the most frequently seen gram-negative infections.

Prevention. Awareness of the possible risk of infection among hospitalized patients is the first step in preventing such infections.

- Fundamental to the control of infection is correct handwashing procedures, as well as strict aseptic technique applied to all diagnostic and therapeutic procedures involving the use of catheters, cardiac pacing, intravenous therapy, tracheostomies, tube drainage, and wound care.

As indicated so many times throughout this text, catheterization should be avoided if at all possible, since a patient can be infected with gastrointestinal flora present on the perineum. If an indwelling catheter is required, a closed urinary drainage system is essential. At the same time, the outside of the catheter and the urine in the catheter and the drainage bag must be regarded as highly contaminated. Routine periodic culture of urinary catheters is advocated. Ideally, patients who have indwelling

TABLE 60-4. ORIGIN, PRECIPITATING EVENTS, AND ETIOLOGIC AGENTS OF BACTEREMIA

SITE OF ORIGIN	PRECIPITATING EVENTS	MOST FREQUENT ETIOLOGIC AGENTS
Genitourinary tract	Indwelling catheters Instrumentation Obstruction	*E. coli* *Klebsiella-* *Enterobacter-* *Serratia* *Proteus sp.* *Ps. aeruginosa*
Gastrointestinal tract		
Bowel	Obstruction Perforation Abscesses Neoplasia Diverticuli	*Bacteroides sp.* *E. coli* *Klebsiella-* *Enterobacter-* *Serratia* *Salmonella*
Billiary tract	Cholangitis Obstruction (stones) Surgical procedures	*E. coli* *Klebsiella-* *Enterobacter-* *Serratia*
Reproductive system	Abortion Instrumentation Postpartum	*Bacteroides sp.* *E. coli*
Vascular system	Venous cutdowns Intravenous catheters Intracardiac pacemakers Surgical procedures	*Ps. aeruginosa* *Herellea sp.* *Serratia* *Erwinia* *E. cloacae*
Skin	Leukemia Agranulocytosis Immunosuppressive and cancer chemotherapeutic agents	*Ps. aeruginosa* *Herellea* *Serratia*
Respiratory tract	Tracheostomy Mechanical ventilatory assistance	*Ps. aeruginosa* *Klebsiella-* *Enterobacter-* *Serratia* *Herellea sp.* *E. coli*
	Aspiration	*E. coli* *Bacteroides sp.* *Klebsiella-* *Enterobacter-* *Serratia*

(From McCabe, W. R.: Gram-Negative Bacteremia. Disease-A-Month, Dec., 1973. Copyright © 1973 by Year Book Medical Publishers, Inc. Used by permission)

catheters should not occupy the same room, since infection may spread from patient to patient.

Prolonged intravenous therapy should be avoided, and when used, the intravenous catheter should be securely anchored to prevent it from moving in the vein. Scrupulous attention should be paid to inserting the needle properly, protecting the needle site, and observing and caring for the intravenous setup. Intravenous cannulae should be changed at least every 72 hours.

Great care must be exercised in using and disinfecting ventilatory equipment. IPPB therapy should be replaced, when possible, by equally effective and simpler forms of therapy, such as deep breathing or incentive spirometry. Respirator tubing should be changed at least every 24 hours. Every precaution should be taken to reduce the possibility of aspiration.

Ideally, every hospital should appoint special personnel to monitor infection-control procedures. However, every staff member should use all surveillance methods known to prevent these problems.

MANIFESTATIONS. Gram-negative bacteremia may be self-limited, transient, intermittent, or continuous. Onset is usually abrupt, with fever, often as high as 40° C. (105°-106° F.), possible chills, nausea, vomiting, and diarrhea. Vascular collapse and shock occur in about 25 percent of the patients.

As bacilli are destroyed by the host's defense mechanisms, endotoxins are liberated from the bacterial cells. Among the effects that ensue are inadequate perfusion, circulatory insufficiency, increased peripheral resistance, pooling of blood in the microcirculation, and diminished cardiac output and hypoxia. As cerebral blood-flow diminishes and shock occurs, the patient becomes confused and disoriented and shows signs of hypotension, tachycardia, weak, thready pulse, cool, clammy skin, peripheral cyanosis, oliguria, and respiratory alkalosis followed by metabolic acidosis. Death may occur as a result of vascular collapse.

Management. The objectives of management are to recognize and treat the bacteremia and to improve perfusion to the vital organs.

Treatment of gram-negative bacteremia includes:
1. a careful search for underlying infection,
2. administration of appropriate antimicrobial agents,
3. drainage of any localized infections,
4. removal of any foreign bodies, such as venous or bladder catheters, when possible, and
5. prevention and treatment of shock resulting from the bacteremia.

The patient is examined to identify the source of sepsis, and the etiologic agent is isolated and identified through blood cultures or cultures of any extravascular sites of infection. Usually the patient is too ill to await the result of culture and sensitivity tests. Therapy is usually started immediately, with agents effective against a broad-spectrum of bacteria, and with consideration given to the prevalence of resistant strains of bacteria in the hospital. Drugs in frequent use include the cephalosporins, aminoglycosides (gentamicin), chloramphenicol, and carbenicillin.

Any possible source of infection, such as an intravenous or urinary catheter, is removed. Surgical drainage of localized infection is carried out. The patient is monitored and treated for shock and other complications.

• The following variables must be monitored and recorded: state of responsiveness, skin temperature, moisture, color, turgor, appearance of mucous membranes and nails, respiratory rate, pulse, blood pressure, and intake and urinary output.

Two or three large intravenous catheters may have to be inserted to provide rapid replacement of fluid and blood, the amount and rate of which is determined by central venous pressure measurements. Blood, plasma, low-molecular-weight dextran or saline may be used to replace fluid volume and to combat vascular collapse. A Swan-Ganz catheter may be inserted to monitor pulmonary artery pressure, and blood gas and pH determinations are carried out to detect respiratory alkalosis early in the course of bacteremia. Inadequate respiratory exchange is a frequent cause of death in gram-negative shock. Metabolic acidosis, which appears later, is treated with sodium bicarbonate. Serum electrolytes are monitored. Vasoactive drugs, digitalis, diuretics, and other pharmacologic agents are given as required.

STAPHYLOCOCCUS (STAPH) INFECTIONS

Staphylococci are widely distributed in nature, with humans serving as the predominant reservoir. These bacteria constitute a good part of the common body flora and are found on the skin surface and in the mouth, nose, and throat. It is estimated that 30 to 50 percent of healthy, nonhospitalized adults carry *S. aureus* in their noses. Organisms carried in the nose can be spread to other people or inanimate objects, principally by hand contact. This is frequently how food becomes contaminated by a contaminated food handler who carries the bacteria in the nose, or in skin lesions. (The primary mode of transmission of staphylococci is by direct hand transfer.) Staphylococci are also transmitted through the air (thereby contaminating a wound during dressing changes), via contaminated needles, and through animal sources.

When the continuity of the skin has been disrupted or by-passed (abrasion, wounds, surgical incision, burns, cutaneous viral infection) the patient is a candidate for infection by staphylococci.

Staphylococci are responsible for most human skin infections. The furuncle, or common boil, is almost always a staphylococcal abscess, and the familiar carbuncle on the back of the neck represents a coalition of staphylococcal abscesses. Most staphylococcal abscesses are located in superficial subcutaneous tissues and do not extend beyond the original site. Eventually, their purulent contents, under mounting pressure, perforate the overlying skin and are evacuated externally, leaving the empty cavities to fill in with granulation tissue, close over, and heal.

This common, usually benign, sequence of events might be misconstrued as evidence that the staphylococcus is a relatively innocuous microbe. Far from it! From the standpoint of aggressiveness, destructiveness, tenacity, and talent for survival, this organism has few equals. Although staphylococci cause most superficial infections, they also produce serious infections of the lungs, pleural space, heart valves, bones, kidneys, and surgical wounds. Some strains produce an enterotoxin which is responsible for foodborne disease (staphylococcal food poisoning).

The tendency of the organism to localize in superficial areas of the body merely establishes its potency as an antigen that arouses the defense mechanisms to feverish activity; and the voluminous pus that typifies its lesions demonstrates the lethal effect that it has on tissue cells and defending leukocytes.

Systemic Staphylococcal Infections

If the peripheral defenses are unable to contain the staphylococcus, the infection may spread or invade the bloodstream, attended by profound toxemia. Invasion of the lymphatics may result in axillary, cervical, mediastinal, retroperitoneal, or subdiaphragmatic abscesses. Bloodstream invasion may produce acute bacterial endocarditis, staphylococcal pneumonia, empyema, perinephric abscess, hepatic abscess, staphylococcal enteritis, pyogenic arthritis, meningitis, osteomyelitis, or generalized sepsis. Constitutional symptoms are extremely severe.

Irrespective of location, staphylococcal lesions possess many characteristics in common, including varying degrees of necrosis, a tendency to localize, and a tendency to persist, despite intensive chemotherapy, until the exudate finds an escape route or is evacuated.

Its resistance to therapy is explained in part by the extraordinary ability of the staphylococcus to adapt itself to an unfavorable environment. Resistance to the commonly used antibiotics is frequently observed in strains of staphylococci. Thus, responsiveness to antibiotic chemotherapy, however gratifying at the onset, may diminish to the point of true refractoriness.

Hospital Staphylococcal Infections

Many hospitals throughout the world have experienced serious outbreaks of staphylococcus infections that have been responsible for a number of fatalities.

- Patients who are chronically ill or debilitated, those receiving systemic steroids or cancer chemotherapy, and those undergoing major or prolonged surgery, as well as infants in the nursery, are susceptible and at risk for staphylococcal infections.

Many factors have conspired to produce this situation, among them the capacity of the staphylococcus to develop resistance to most antibiotics, the ability of this organism to penetrate skin and destroy tissue, and the prevalence of the staphylococcus, especially in hospitals, where its presence is ubiquitous.

Control Measures and Prevention. The major means by which staphylococci are transmitted within the hospital is through person-to-person transmission. The prevention of hospital staphylococcosis requires the combined and coordinated efforts of many individuals, from all departments of the hospital.

The following measures are recommended as a means of controlling hospital "staph" infections:
1. All hospitals and extended care facilities should enforce aseptic techniques supervised by the infection control committee of the individual health agency.
2. Personnel with staphylococcal lesions should not work in the health agency until the lesion has healed or cultures have become negative after treatment.
3. Patients with staphylococcal infections should be placed under strict isolation precautions until antibiotic treatment has rendered cultures negative for staphylococci.
4. The cross-traffic between those areas of the hospital that house infected patients and those in which noninfected patients are quartered should be reduced.

Management. The drug selected for treatment is the one most apt to eradicate the infection rapidly. Penicillinase-resistant penicillins (oxacillin, methicillin, nafcillin) and the cephalosporins (cephalothin) are among the most effective antistaphylococcal drugs available. Intravenous administration is the route usually selected, because of the large doses required. Serious staphylococcal infections may have to be treated for 4 to 6 weeks to prevent infection of the heart valves.

Nursing Isolation Procedures Required for Staphylococcal Disease (*S. aureus*)

1. Burns—strict isolation, wound and skin precautions or secretion precautions, depending on extent of infection, for duration of illness; (wounds or lesions: until they stop draining).
2. Enterocolitis—enteric precautions until patient is off antibiotics and is culture-negative
3. Gastroenteritis—excretion precautions for duration of illness
4. Lung abscess, draining—strict isolation for duration of illness (until drainage stops)
5. Pneumonia—strict isolation for duration of illness

6. Skin infection—strict isolation, wound and skin precautions, or secretion precautions for duration of illness (depending on extent of infection)
7. Wound infection—strict isolation, wound and skin precautions, or secretion precautions (depending on extent of infection) for duration of illness.

STREPTOCOCCAL INFECTIONS

There are many strains of hemolytic streptococci, but Group A streptococci accounts for the majority of pathogenic infections in humans. Included in this group are the beta hemolytic streptococci, which gain entrance to the body primarily through the upper respiratory tract from persons with streptococcal infections or those who are asymptomatic carriers. Included in these infections are streptococcal pharyngitis, scarlet fever, sinusitis, otitis media, peritonsillar abscess, pericarditis, pneumonia and empyema, and various wound and skin infectious—impetigo, puerperal infections, erysipelas. Rheumatic fever and acute glomerulonephritis may occur as a sequel of Group A streptococci infection.

Streptococcal Pharyngitis

The most common type of streptococcal infection is streptococcal pharyngitis (strep throat) with Group A organism. The organism establishes itself in the lymphoid tissues and produces an abrupt onset of illness, with sore throat, fever (38.2° C [101° F.]), chills, and headache. The patient may complain bitterly of throat pain which is aggravated by swallowing or even turning the head. Nasal discharge, cough, and earache may also occur. Upon inspection, the pharynx shows varying degrees of redness and edema and may be covered with an exudate. (A throat culture should be done to confirm the presence of streptococci.) In some patients, a rash appears, starting over the neck and chest and spreading over the skin of the abdomen and extremities. If the rash becomes pronounced, the patient has scarlet fever. (The rash of scarlet fever often disappears in 12 to 18 hours.) Although these are the usual symptoms associated with streptococcal pharyngitis, most patients have some, but not all, of these symptoms.

Management. Penicillin, in a variety of forms, is the drug of choice in streptococcal infections (except for enterococcal Group D infections). If the patient is sensitive to penicillin, one of the cephalosporins, erythromycin, or clindamycin, may be used. Therapy is continued for at least 10 days to eliminate the organisms, reduce the frequency of suppurative complications, prevent the majority of cases of rheumatic fever (and to a lesser extent, acute glomerulonephritis), and help prevent further spread of streptococci.

The patient must understand the importance of *completing* the course of antibiotic treatment in order to prevent the development of complications of this infection, namely, acute rheumatic fever and acute glomerulonephritis.

In addition to penicillin therapy, the therapeutic regimen and nursing support are directed at relieving the patient's symptoms.

Nursing Isolation Procedures
Streptococcal disease (group A)
1. Burns—strict isolation, wound and skin precautions or secretion precautions (depending on extent of infection) until wounds or lesions stop draining
2. Endometritis (puerperal sepsis)—wound and skin precautions until 24 hours after initiation of effective therapy
3. Pharyngitis—secretion precautions until 24 hours after initiation of effective therapy
4. Pneumonia—strict isolation until 24 hours after initiation of effective therapy
5. Scarlet fever—secretion precautions until 24 hours after initiation of effective therapy
6. Skin infection—strict isolation, wound and skin precautions or secretion precautions (depending on extent of infection) until wounds or lesions stop draining
7. Wound infection—strict isolation, wound and skin precautions or secretion precautions (depending on the extent of infection) until wound stops draining
8. Streptococcal disease (not group A) unless covered elsewhere—none

Prevention and Patient Education. Ongoing health education programs are required to emphasize the relationship of streptococcal infections to heart disease and glomerulonephritis. People with these conditions, especially rheumatic heart disease, are at risk and may require long-term prophylaxis with penicillin. As part of prevention, in other situations, those hospitalized patients who are at risk—and this includes the obstetrical patient—must be protected from personnel or visitors with respiratory or skin infections. For the health of the public at large, food handlers should be instructed about hygienic procedures and closely monitored to assure compliance.

GONORRHEA

Gonorrhea is an infectious disease characterized by inflammation of the mucous membranes of the genitourinary tract. It is caused by the gonococcus *Neisseria gonorrhoeae,* and is transmitted sexually, except in the case of gonococcal ophthalmia of the newborn, or nonvenereal transmission from an infected member to a child below the age of 1 year.

There are an estimated 70 million cases of gonorrhea in the world. In the United States it is the most common reportable disease, with approximately 3 million persons acquiring the disease each year. In fact, it has reached epidemic proportions, due in part to liberalized attitudes, personal mobility, and changing sexual habits (premarital, extramarital, anogenital or agenital sexual practices, and homosexuality).

The highest rate of gonorrhea occurs among the 20-to-24 year age group, followed by the 15-to-19 year group, with a rapid rise occurring in teenagers less than 15 years of age. (One in four new cases is in the age range of 10 to 14.)

One factor that contributes to the rapid spread of gonorrhea is its short incubation period. The problem is further compounded by the fact that the disease is relatively asymptomatic in females (and increasingly so in males), in addition to which the organism is becoming increasingly resistant to penicillin.

Persons who are repeatedly reinfected tend to have problems with interpersonal relationships, low self-esteem, and a negative attitude toward society. They tend to be less well educated, come from broken homes, and have problems with alcohol, infections (hepatitis; tuberculosis), and injuries.

Pathophysiology. The gonococcus (*Neisseria gonorrhoeae*) causes a surface infection, ascending, in almost all cases, by way of the lower genital tract. The primary infection takes place in or near the urethra, in males, and in the epithelium of the endocervix in females. If drainage is good, it subsides spontaneously and clears in the course of a few days or weeks. However, infection of the prostatic urethra in the male and also of the female urethral and vaginal glands predisposes to chronic infection, with occasionally very serious sequelae. Females are apt to contract secondarily a mixed infection of the endometrium and, thereafter, of the tubes, constituting pelvic infection, with resultant pelvic peritonitis. The upward spread of the infection into the reproductive tract is precipitated by such factors as menstruation, douches, and the trauma associated with sexual intercourse or instrumentation.

Clinical Manifestations and Complications

In males the incubation period lasts for 3 to 4 days, after which an acute anterior urethritis occurs, along with painful urination accompanied by mucopurulent urethral discharge. The infection may extend to involve the posterior urethra and spread to the prostate, seminal vesicles, and epididymis, causing prostatitis, inguinal lymphadenitis, pelvic pain, and fever. A major complication in men is urethritis and urethral stricture, with all its attendant problems—difficulty in voiding, delay in emptying the bladder, with subsequent infection, etc. A particularly serious problem, recently discovered, is the possibility that the male may be an asymptomatic carrier of gonorrhea for considerable periods of time.

In females, the infection is very frequently silent, so that a large percentage of women are asymptomatic and unaware that they are infected. A small number have vaginal discharge, abnormal uterine bleeding, urinary frequency, and dysuria. The sites most frequently involved are the urethra and cervix. As the endocervical gonococcal infection spreads upward into the reproductive tract, it causes pelvic infection (pelvic inflammatory disease), with endometritis, salpingitis, or pelvic peritonitis. An estimated 15 to 17 percent of women infected with the gonococcus develop pelvic infection, as evidenced by abdominal pain, adnexal tenderness, fever, and vaginal discharge. Pelvic infection causes adhesions about the pelvic organs and rectum. Strictures of the cervix and uterine (fallopian) tubes are responsible for many cases of infertility.

Other Manifestations of Gonorrhea. *Anal manifestations* consist of anal itching and irritation (from erythema and edema of the anal crypts), a sensation of rectal fullness, anal discharge, and painful defecation.

Oral manifestations may be the result of the direct contact of the infecting organisms with the oral cavity, or of their transmission to the oral cavity from infection elsewhere in the body. Although the majority of pharyngeal infections are asymptomatic, the following oral manifestations are seen: sore throat, painful ulcerative inflammation of the lips, reddened, spongy, and tender gingivae, reddened, dry tongue, and redness and edema of the soft palate and uvula. The oropharynx may be covered with vesicles.

Systemic manifestations may become apparent, since secondary foci of infection may develop in any organ system, causing gonococcal bacteremia (disseminated gonococcal infection), gonococcal arthritis, endocarditis, peritonitis, and perihepatitis. Disseminated gonococcal infection (DGI) occurs in 1 to 3 percent of patients with gonorrhea. It has been suggested that some gonococci are more likely to cause DGI than others. Men and women alike may be the victims of these systemic complications.

Diagnostic Assessment

There are a variety of ways of identifying gonorrhea through laboratory diagnosis. The gram-negative intracellular diplococci may be found in smears or through direct fluorescent antibody tests, or may be cultured with selective media, such as modified Thayer-Martin media (TM). The pharyngeal and rectal sites should be cultured in persons who engage in oral and/or rectal sex.

In the male, a smear of urethral discharge is taken for microscopic examination. A culture may also be made, especially in the asymptomatic male, by passing a sterile swab or a bacteriologic loop 2 to 4 cm. into the urethra (Fig. 60-1A). If culture specimens are obtained from the pharynx and rectum, they are inoculated on separate modified Thayer-Martin culture plates.

In women, cultures are collected from the endocervix and rectum and inoculated on separate modified Thayer-

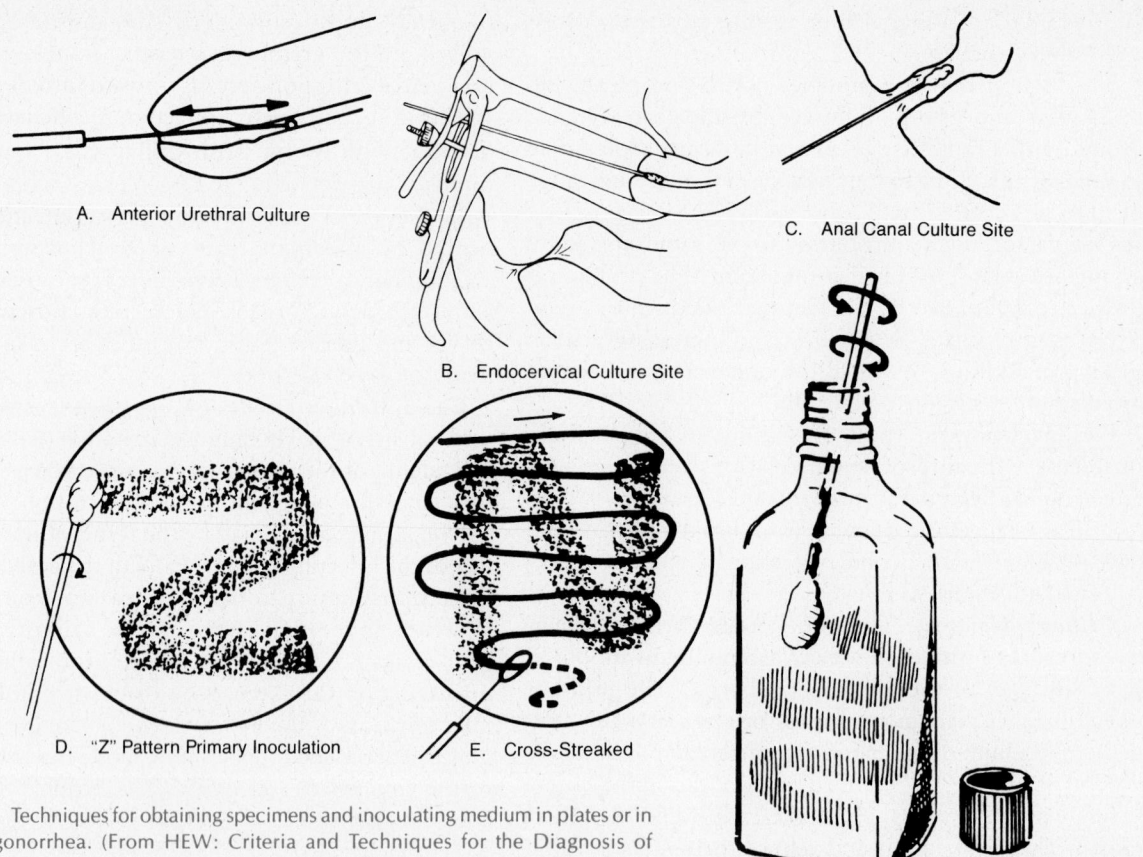

A. Anterior Urethral Culture

B. Endocervical Culture Site

C. Anal Canal Culture Site

D. "Z" Pattern Primary Inoculation

E. Cross-Streaked

F. MTM Medium in Bottle

Figure 60-1. Techniques for obtaining specimens and inoculating medium in plates or in bottles for gonorrhea. (From HEW: Criteria and Techniques for the Diagnosis of Gonorrhea)

Martin culture plates. Pharyngeal cultures may also be taken.

To collect an endocervical specimen:
1. Moisten the vaginal speculum with warm water; do not use any other lubricant.
2. Insert a cotton-tipped swab into the endocervical canal (Fig. 60-1B) and move it from side to side a few seconds allowing the organisms to be absorbed on the swab.
3. Transfer the swab to the culture plate.

To take an anal canal culture:
1. Insert a clean cotton-tipped swab 2.5 cm. (1 inch) into the anal canal (Fig. 60-1C).
2. Move the swab from side to side to obtain a sample from the anal crypts.
3. If the swab is inadvertently pushed into feces, use another swab to obtain the specimen.

To inoculate the modified Thayer-Martin medium in plates:
1. Roll the swab in a large Z pattern on MTM-medium in a round or rectangular plate (Fig. 60-1D).
2. Cross-streak immediately with a sterile wire loop or the tip of the swab (Fig. 60-1E). This preferably should be done in the clinical facility, but if inadvertently omitted, it should be done in the laboratory before incubation.
3. Place the culture in a CO_2 enriched atmosphere (e.g., candle jar) within 15 minutes, as successful recovery of *N. gonorrhoeae* requires an atmosphere enriched in carbon dioxide.

When the modified Thayer-Martin medium in bottles is used:
1. Inoculate the bottle in an upright position, to prevent CO_2 loss.
2. Remove the cap of the bottle only when ready to inoculate the medium.
3. Soak up all excess moisture in the bottle with the specimen swab, and then roll the swab from side to side across the medium, starting at the bottom of the bottle (Fig. 60-1F).
4. When possible, incubate the bottle in an upright position at 35°-36° C. for 16 to 18 hours before sending it to a central bacteriologic laboratory.

Management

The objective of treatment is to eradicate the organisms. Pencillin is the drug of choice, since it is effective, inexpensive, and will abort incubating syphilis. The patient should wait in the clinic 20 to 30 minutes after penicillin treatment in case of an anaphylactoid reaction. Each year a number of deaths occur from anaphylactic reactions to penicillin.

Unfortunately, certain gonococcus strains have become resistant to penicillin. In at least 16 countries (including the U.S.) pencillinase-producing *Neisseria gonorrhoeae* (PPNG) fail to respond to treatment with any penicillin or ampicillin regimen. This may result in major changes in future treatment practices.

Treatment schedules presently recommended by the United States Public Health Service are outlined in Table 60-5. There are now four drug regimens which can be used for the treatment of uncomplicated gonorrhea.

All patients with gonorrhea should undergo a serologic test for syphilis at the time of diagnosis. Patients with both gonorrhea and syphilis must be given additional treatment, depending on the stage of the disease. The patient is instructed to avoid reinfection with untreated sexual contacts until they have been treated. It is imperative that follow-up cultures be obtained from appropriate sites 3 to 7 days after completion of treatment, since no therapy is 100 percent effective. Cultures are also obtained 4 to 6 weeks after treatment to detect reinfection. A positive reculture is most often due to reinfection by infectious contacts. The treatment of complications (endocarditis, bacteremia, etc.) is individualized.

Each patient must be interviewed for the names of contacts. Then the contacts must be investigated and treated within 10 days. Public health programs are geared to trace contacts and prevent further spread through reporting, diagnosis, treatment, and follow-up.

Patient Education

The following are important points to stress:
1. Venereal disease (VD) is acquired by sexual contact (vaginal sexual intercourse, anal intercourse, oral intercourse) and by close and direct contact with an infected person.
2. A person who thinks that he or she may have VD or who has been exposed to someone who might have it should have a checkup. Immediate treatment should be sought if symptoms develop.
3. Anyone who is sexually active with a number of sexual partners should have regular checkups.
4. Washing the sex organs (before and after sexual contact) and the use of a condom may give limited protection against VD.
5. Birth control pills and IUDs give no protection against VD.
6. Gonorrhea and syphilis are different diseases, caused by different germs; they attack the body in different ways but are spread in the same manner. A person may have both gonorrhea and syphilis at the same time.
7. There appears to be no natural or acquired immunity to gonorrhea and syphilis. A person can get gonorrhea and syphilis again and again.
8. Pregnant women may pass infection of syphilis to unborn child. Pregnant women may pass gonorrhea to a baby during the birth process.
9. Bacteria from gonorrhea may enter the bloodstream and affect joints, joint linings, heart valves, etc.

PULMONARY TUBERCULOSIS

Tuberculosis is an infectious disease caused by *Mycobacterium tuberculosis, M. bovis,* or rarely *M. avium.* It usually involves the lungs, but it also involves and sometimes produces gross lesions in other organs and tissues.

TABLE 60-5. GONORRHEA: CDC RECOMMENDED TREATMENT SCHEDULES, 1979

Note: Physicians are cautioned to use no less than the recommended dosages of antibiotics. The major change from the 1974 published treatment schedule is that there are now 4 drug regimens which can be used for the treatment of uncomplicated gonorrhea.

Uncomplicated Gonococcal Infections in Men and Women

DRUG REGIMENS OF CHOICE

Aqueous procaine penicillin G (APPG): 4.8 million units injected intramuscularly at 2 sites, with 1.0 gm. of probenecid by mouth, **OR**

Tetracycline hydrochloride*: 0.5 gm. by mouth 4 times a day for 5 days (total dosage 10.0 gm.). Other tetracyclines are not more effective than tetracycline hydrochloride. All tetracyclines are ineffective as a single-dose therapy, **OR**

Ampicillin or amoxicillin: Ampicillin, 3.5 gm. or amoxicillin, 3.0 gm.—either with 1 gm. probenecid by mouth. Evidence shows that these regimens are slightly less effective than the other recommended regimens.

Patients who are allergic to the penicillins or probenecid should be treated with oral tetracycline, as above. Patients who cannot tolerate tetracycline may be treated with spectinomycin hydrochloride, 2.0 gm. in 1 intramuscular injection.

SPECIAL CONSIDERATIONS

Single-dose treatment is preferred in patients who are unlikely to complete the multiple-dose tetracycline regimen. The APPG regimen is preferred in men with anorectal infection.

Pharyngeal infection is difficult to treat. High failure rates have been reported with ampicillin and spectinomycin.

Tetracycline treatment results in fewer cases of postgonococcal urethritis in men. It may eliminate coexisting chlamydial infections in men and women.

Patients with incubating syphilis (seronegative, without clinical signs of syphilis) are likely to be cured by all of the above regimens except spectinomycin. All patients should have a serologic test for syphilis at the time of diagnosis.

Patients with gonorrhea who also have syphilis or are established contacts of syphilis patients should be given additional treatment appropriate to the stage of syphilis.

*Food, and some dairy products, interfere with absorption. Oral forms of tetracycline should be given 1 hour before or 2 hours after meals.
(From Center for Disease Control: Morbidity and Mortality Weekly Report, *28*, January 19, 1979)

The organisms multiply slowly and are characterized as acid-fast aerobic organisms which can be killed by heat, sunshine, drying, and ultraviolet light.

The strain, *M. tuberculosis* var. *hominis,* is responsible for almost all tuberculous infections in humans in the United States. Another strain, *M. tuberculosis* var. *bovis,* exhibits similar morphologic criteria and is responsible for producing tuberculous infections in cattle. The latter strains may produce human infections, especially of the tonsils, cervical lymph nodes, and gastrointestinal tract, after ingestion of infected milk. Infections with the bovine strain of tubercle bacillus still remain a significant problem in underdeveloped countries. Public-health control measures have almost completely eradicated bovine tuberculosis in cattle and dairy herds in the United States.

In contrast with the majority of infectious diseases, the bacillus of tuberculosis, once it has gained a foothold in the body, is likely to remain there, quiescent, for years after the forces of immunity have controlled the original infection. If, during this quiescent period, the resistance of the host is weakened, the germ at once begins to multiply, causing any one of many tuberculous diseases. If the patient's body proves able to recover from this illness, then the tubercle bacilli again become dormant.

Transmission; Risk Factors. Tuberculosis is an airborne disease transmitted by droplet nuclei, usually from the respiratory tract of an infected person who expels the organisms during talking, coughing, or sneezing. To acquire the infection, a person must be constantly exposed to the air exhaled by an infected person.

Persons at high risk for acquiring the disease are those in close contact with someone who has infectious tuberculosis; persons whose tuberculin skin tests have recently converted from negative to positive; those with lowered resistance because of alcoholism, general debilitation or the presence of other diseases (diabetes, silicosis); those with malignancies or immune-deficiency disease; those who have undergone recent gastrointestinal surgery or steroid therapy; and women who are pregnant.

Crowded living conditions, low incomes, substandard housing, and inadequate health care contribute to the spread of tuberculosis.

Types of Tuberculosis

Since tubercle bacilli can establish themselves in almost every type of human tissue, and since there is no organ system that they cannot colonize, the clinical manifestations of tuberculosis are extremely numerous and varied. Most common, by far, of all variants of this infection is pulmonary tuberculosis, in which there is involvement of some portion of the lung parenchyma, together with the bronchi and the bronchioles within it, the mediastinal nodes that drain it, and the pleura that covers it. In other patients the principal site of involvement is in the upper respiratory tract, as in patients with tuberculous tonsillitis and laryngitis. The most prominent lesion may be a tuberculous laryngitis. Lymph nodes that guard the lymphatic drainage may become infected, producing the picture of tuberculous adenitis. Organisms that are swallowed and later absorbed from the small bowel may localize in the mesenteric or retroperitoneal lymphatic system, giving rise to tuberculous mesenteric adenitis or

peritonitis, and later to tuberculous ileitis or splenitis, or renal tuberculosis. The infection may spread from retroperitoneal to mediastinal nodes, producing tuberculous mediastinitis, pleuritis, or pericarditis. From lymph nodes in the neck, the mediastinum, or the retroperitoneum, the infection may extend to the spine, causing tuberculous osteomyelitis, with resultant vertebral collapse and deforming kyphosis, or it may enter the spinal canal and infect the meninges, producing tuberculous meningitis. Transported by way of the bloodstream, which it has many opportunities to enter, the tubercle bacillus finds access to, and may localize within the brain, forming a "tuberculoma"; cause tuberculous uveitis; or, when in a joint, produce tuberculous arthritis. Or it may implant and grow simultaneously in hundreds of sites throughout the body, which is the situation in "miliary tuberculosis."

Pathophysiology

Tuberculosis is one of the so-called *granulomatous* diseases; that is, when the organism invades normal tissues, the response is the formation of new tissue masses which are called *infectious granulomas*. The tubercle (little tumor), the characteristic lesion of tuberculosis, is a tiny, spherical infectious granuloma just large enough to be seen with the naked eye. Another more diffuse, and equally characteristic tissue reaction also occurs in response to the tubercle bacillus.

Tubercle bacilli, swept along by the lymph and bloodstream, lodge in susceptible tissues in small clumps. The neighboring tissue cells quickly accumulate around each of these "clumps", forming a protective wall that checks their further spread, and may kill them. If immunity is successful, after a long time the germs die, and the tubercle becomes transformed into a tiny mass of fibrous tissue. At the same time, the tissue of the tubercle may become necrotic and transformed into a cheesy mass, a process known as *caseation*. If this occurs, the germs are liberated from the imprisonment and lymph sweeps them into the surrounding tissues, which respond by enclosing these freed germs in new tubercles. In this way, the original miliary (like millet seeds) tubercle grows into larger and larger irregular masses, some as large as a fist.

The fate of the patient depends on which of these two processes prevails. If the tissue barriers survive, then the imprisoned tubercle bacilli cease to multiply, and may die. Lime salts from the blood are deposited in the dead caseous material, and scar tissue forms around the infected area, which remains throughout life as a healed, calcified mass. However, if the germs survive and are freed from the tubercle, they multiple and are swept along by the lymph stream into the neighboring tissues, and by the bloodstream into other organs, where they lodge and repeat the same process.

Host Defense Mechanisms. Individuals who have experienced a primary tuberculous infection are sensitized or allergic to the chemical constituents of the organism. Henceforth, contact with the bacillus, whether it is alive or killed, produces an acute local tissue inflammation. This is the basis of the tuberculin test, in which a suspension of ground-up killed tubercle bacilli obtained from a culture is injected into the skin. If the patient is allergic—that is, has at one time had a tuberculous infection—a local skin reaction results, whereas if there is no allergy, no reaction is obtained. According to the Center for Disease Control, there are 15 million persons in the United States who are tuberculin-positive reactors.

A similar inflammatory reaction develops in the lung of a person who has been sensitized previously to the tubercle bacillus if this lung is invaded later by more organisms than the immune processes can handle at the time. In contrast with the relatively bland, silent, primary type of pulmonary tuberculosis, the course of the reinfection type is complicated by necrosis, with resulting ulceration of the infected lung tissue. Clusters of tubercles, as in the primary type of tuberculosis, form at once around the nest of organisms, but now, due to the tissue sensitivity, these become surrounded by zones of inflammatory reaction. The alveoli in the area become filled with exudate; in other words, a tuberculous bronchopneumonia develops. The tuberculous tissue in this area gradually becomes caseous and ulcerates into a bronchus, causing a cavity. At the same time, as the ulcerations heal, considerable scar tissue forms locally, especially around the cavities. The pleura over the infected lobe, more often an upper lobe, becomes inflamed, then thickened and retracted by scar tissue.

This cycle of inflammatory bronchopneumonia proceeds to ulceration with cavitation, followed by scarring. Unless the process can be arrested, it spreads slowly downward toward the hilum and later extends into adjacent lobes. The activity of the process may be very prolonged and characterized by long remissions, when the disease may appear to be arrested, only to be followed by periods of renewed activity.

Depending on whether the predominant pathologic feature of the infection is ulceration or fibrosis, an infection is designated as *chronic ulcerative pulmonary tuberculosis* or *chronic fibroid tuberculosis*. Fibroid tuberculosis is that form of the infection in which the healing process is sufficient to prevent gross caseation of the tuberculous areas, yet cannot halt the infection. The result is a gradual transformation of a lobe, or of the entire lung, into a mass of fibrous tissue. The pleurae become thick and adherent, and the bronchi dilated, their walls pulled apart by the contracting scar tissue in the lung, while the chest on the affected side becomes shrunken, the spine curved laterally.

Clinical Manifestations

Chronic pulmonary tuberculosis is insidious in its onset and course. A person with active tuberculosis may have no symptoms until there is extensive disease. The early symptoms seldom suggest the lungs as the seat of the disease. Often the patient notices first that he is losing weight; that, although he feels very well on rising in the morning, he becomes fatigued a little more easily than previously, especially in the afternoon. He becomes a trifle pale, his appetite gradually fails, and he may suffer from "indigestion." He gradually acquires a cough, or at any rate he "clears his throat" every morning. His temperature, although normal in the morning, may be elevated each afternoon. He may think he has a cold that is just "hanging on."

With the progress of the disease, the anorexia and the "indigestion," may be marked. Abdominal pain or even vomiting may occur after meals. The cough, for weeks passed off as bronchitis or a cigarette cough, gradually becomes more troublesome, and the sputum increases. There is no longer doubt as to the afternoon fever; the patient may have night sweats. Loss of weight and strength is rapid.

Hemoptysis (expectoration of blood or blood-streaked sputum) is common in pulmonary tuberculosis. It may be the first symptom noticed by the patient. These hemorrhages are usually only slight in quantity, but on rare occasions, when an artery ulcerates, the bleeding

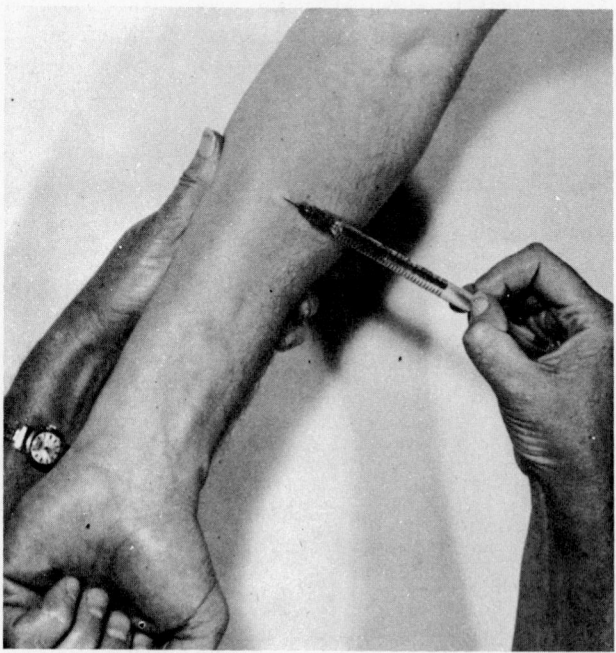

Figure 60-2. The Mantoux intracutaneous test. A tuberculin syringe and a subcutaneous needle, with the bevel up, are used to inject tubercle bacillus extract into the skin of the forearm to form a wheal. (American Lung Association)

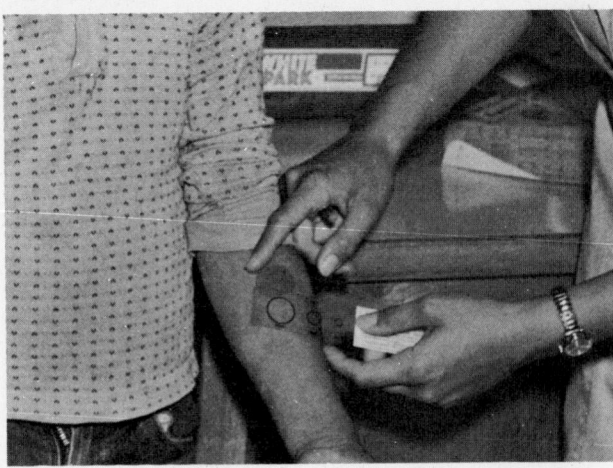

Figure 60-3. Interpretation of Mantoux test. The area of induration is measured most accurately with the aid of a plastic ruler containing concentric circles of specific diameters. (American Lung Association)

may be profuse or even fatal. The bleeding occurs unexpectedly, and quite independent of exertion or activity. In fact, it may occur during sleep. On the other hand, there may just be slightly blood-streaked sputum.

Diagnostic Assessment

The initial diagnostic evaluation includes a tuberculin skin test, examination of a sputum sample (smear and culture) and an x-ray evaluation of the chest.

TUBERCULIN SKIN TEST: MANTOUX TEST. The Mantoux intracutaneous test is the standard test used to identify the infected person. Tubercle bacillus extract (tuberculin) is inoculated into the intradermal layer of the inner aspect of the forearm. Intermediate strength of purified protein

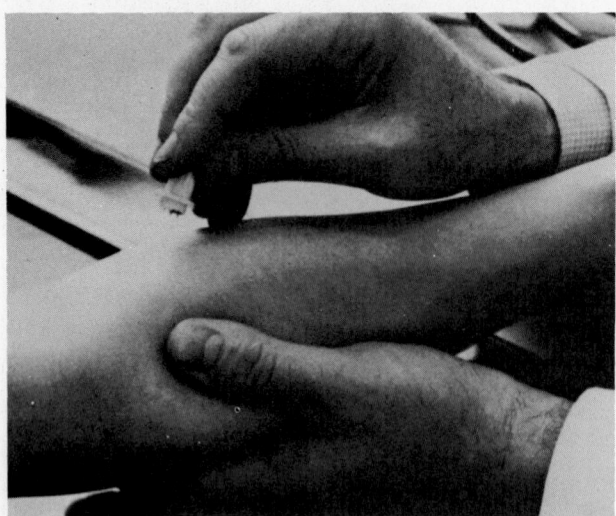

Figure 60-4. This test to detect tuberculosis in humans is easy to apply and is disposable and accurate. Called the Tuberculin Tine Test, it was developed by Lederle Laboratories, a Division of American Cyanamid Company.

derivative (PPD) is usually used. The tuberculin syringe should be held close to the skin, so that the hub of the needle (26 or 27 gauge) touches it as the needle is introduced, bevel up. This reduces the needle angle at the skin surface and facilitates the injection of tuberculin into the superficial layer of the skin, to form a wheal (Fig. 60-2). The test is read 48 to 72 hours after injection since tuberculin skin tests are tests of delayed hypersensitivity.

Test reactions should be read in a good light, with the forearm slightly flexed at the elbow. After the area is inspected for the presence of induration (hardening or thickening of tissues), it is lightly palpated across the injection site, from the area of normal skin to the margins of induration. A pencil mark is made where the area of induration is felt. Then the diameter of the induration (*not erythema*) is measured in millimeters, at its widest width (Fig. 60-3). Erythema or redness without induration is generally considered to be of no significance. The size of the induration is documented, as well as the antigen strength, the date the testing was conducted, the date when the reading was taken, and the lot number used, if available.

Interpretation of Skin Test. An area of *induration* measuring 10 mm. or more in diameter is interpreted as a positive reaction.

Doubtful reactions measure 5 through 9 mm. and require that the test be repeated at a different site. (Individuals who are close contacts of persons with active tuberculosis and who have reactions in the 5- through 9-mm. range should be considered positive reactors and should receive preventive treatment. A negative reaction is an induration of 0 to 4 mm. This shows either a lack of tuberculin sensitivity or low-grade sensitivity that probably is not caused by *M. tuberculosis.*

- *A positive reaction indicates that a patient has had contact with the tubercle bacillius. It does not necessarily mean that active disease is present in the body.* The vast majority (more than 90 percent) of people who are tuberculin-positive reactors will *not* develop clinical tuberculosis. (However, all positive reactors are candidates for active tuberculosis.)

In general, the more intense the reaction, the greater the likelihood of an active infection. A negative test is even more valuable diagnostically, for it practically rules out the presence of active tuberculosis, except in patients with miliary tuberculosis, who may lose their capacity to react to tuberculin, and those who are receiving one of the corticosteroid drugs and may react negatively in the face of an active infection.

A *tuberculin converter* is a person whose tuberculin reaction changes from less than 10 mm. in diameter to more than 10 mm. in diameter, with the increase measuring at least 6 mm. (This usually indicates recent infection.)

OTHER SKIN TESTS. Multiple-puncture skin tests, such as Tine, Mono-Vac, and Heaf, are utilized for surveying and screening large groups and are not intended to establish positive diagnosis, since there is no way to standardize the amount of tuberculin introduced. The tests are administered by instruments that pierce the skin at several points simultaneously (Fig. 60-4). The test is read on the third day after administration. If vesiculation is present, the test may be interpreted as positive. Since the dosage is not controlled, the size of reaction does not have much significance. All positive reactors should be retested with the Mantoux test, and should have a chest x-ray.

The majority of new cases of active tuberculosis arise from previously quiescent lesions that have become activated. Tuberculin testing serves to identify the group at greatest risk of developing active disease.

SPUTUM TESTING. Diagnosis is also made by finding the acid-fast bacilli in smears of sputum. Sputum can be coughed up directly or induced by inhaling aerosols which irritate the trachea and produce coughing. Bronchoscopic aspiration via fiberoptic bronchoscope or transtracheal aspiration are other possible means of obtaining a sputum specimen. An early-morning specimen is more apt to be productive and less contaminated. If the patient is unable to expectorate but has swallowed sputum, then a gastric specimen may be obtained via a nasogastric tube, provided that the patient has not eaten recently. Tubercle bacilli may also be obtained and cultured from ascitic fluid, pleural fluid, cerebrospinal fluid, urine, and pus that has been aspirated or drained from abscesses. Tissue such as liver, bone marrow, and lymph nodes may also be cultured.

CHEST X-RAY. Tuberculosis is a possibility in anyone with an abnormal chest x-ray. A chest x-ray is obtained to determine the presence and extent of the disease. Also, subsequent x-rays are made to determine how effective treatment has been.

Management

- Every active case of tuberculosis must be reported to the local health department so that close contacts may be examined and followed. Contacts are usually placed on preventive therapy (usually isoniazid) to prevent the development of active disease.

The objectives of management are (1) to relieve pulmonary and systemic symptoms by eliminating all viable tubercle bacilli, (2) to return the patient to health, work, and family life as quickly as possible and, (3) to prevent transmission of the infection. The patient may be hospitalized for a more careful and complete diagnostic workup if the infection is serious, if supportive care is required, and if respiratory isolation (page 1365) cannot be achieved at home.

CHEMOTHERAPY. Active tuberculosis is usually treated with simultaneous administration of two or more drugs

to which the organisms are suceptible. Such therapy is carried out until the disease is brought under control. Multiple drug regimens are used to destroy as many viable microbial organisms as quickly as possible, and to minimize the emergence of organisms resistant to the various antituberculosis drugs. Although the tubercle bacillus is susceptible to several drugs, there are no drugs to which it cannot develop resistance. Such resistance results from genetic mutations of the organism. Using a variety of drugs enables one agent to destroy those mutants that are resistant to the initial drug. Using a variety of drugs enables one agent to destroy those mutants that are resistant to the initial drug.

Treatment is continued until x-rays demonstrate improvement and negative sputum cultures are obtained. Then the patient is placed on continuing drug therapy for an additional period of time. The total treatment time varies and is approximately 18 to 24 months.

If effective medications are taken as prescribed, it is possible to treat and "cure" at least 95 percent of patients with newly detected, initially treated pulmonary tuberculosis.

The choice of drug regimens vary. The drugs most commonly used for initial treatment (so called first-line drugs) are isoniazid (INH), ethambutol (EMB), rifampin, and streptomycin (SM) (Table 60-6).

Isoniazid is the principal drug used, because it is highly effective and low in toxicity and cost. Serious side effects have infrequently occurred, but the patient should be monitored for *early* signs of hypersensitivity—fever and rash. The major side effect, hepatitis, is thought to be related to some of the metabolic products of isoniazid that are toxic to the liver. Other side effects of isoniazid are outlined in Table 60-6. For patients receiving more than the usual dosage of INH or those with a poor dietary history or alcoholism, the prophylactic use of pyridoxine may be given to combat peripheral neuritis.

Ethambutol (EMB), is used with isoniazid in initial treatment because it is effective, easy to administer, and has low toxicity. The drug can cause optic neuritis in persons receiving larger doses and prolonged treatment. Visual acuity and determination of red-green color discrimination should be tested before the drug is administered and at monthly intervals during treatment. However, this problem is usually not encountered when lower dosages are given.

Rifampin is a remarkably effective drug in treating both initial and recurrent infections. It is usually combined with isoniazid. Rifampin is slightly more toxic than isoniazid. Other disadvantages include its relatively high cost, plus the fact that organisms can develop resistance to it if it is used alone. Side effects include hepatitis, hypersensitivity reactions, thrombocytopenia, and leukopenia.

Streptomycin was the first clinically effective drug to

TABLE 60-6.   TREATMENT OF MYCOBACTERIAL DISEASE (TUBERCULOSIS)

DRUG	DOSAGE		SIDE EFFECTS	MONITORING	REMARKS
First-Line Drugs	*Daily*	*Twice Weekly*			
Isoniazid	5-10 mg./kg. up to 300 mg. PO or IM	15 mg./kg. PO or IM	Peripheral neuritis, hepatitis, hypersensitivity	SGOT/SGPT (not routine)	Bactericidal; for neuritis, pyridoxine. 10 mg. as prophylaxis; 50-100 mg. as treatment daily.
Ethambutol	15 mg./kg. PO	50 mg./kg. PO	Optic neuritis (reversible, with discontinuation of drug; very rare at 15 mg./kg.); skin rash	Red-green color discrimination and visual acuity	Use with caution in renal disease or when eye testing is not feasible.
Rifampin	10-20 mg./kg. PO up to 600 mg.		Hepatitis, febrile reaction, purpura (rare)	SGOT/SGPT (not routine)	Bactericidal; orange urine color, benign.
Streptomycin	15-20 mg./kg. up to 1 gm. IM	25-30 mg./kg.	8th nerve damage, nephrotoxicity	Vestibular function, audiograms, BUN, and creatinine	Use with caution in older patients or those with renal disease.
Second-Line Drugs	*Daily*				
Viomycin	15-30 mg./kg. up to 1 gm. IM		8th nerve damage, nephrotoxicity, vestibular toxicity (rare)	Vestibular function, audiograms, BUN, and creatinine	Use with caution in older patients, rarely use with renal disease.
Capreomycin	15-30 mg./kg. up to 1 gm. IM		8th nerve damage, nephrotoxicity	Vestibular function, audiograms, BUN, and creatinine	Use with caution in older patients, rarely use with renal disease.
Kanamycin	15-30 mg./kg. up to 1 gm. IM		8th nerve damage, nephrotoxicity, vestibular toxicity (rare)	Vestibular function, audiograms, BUN, and creatinine	Use with caution in older patients, rarely use with renal disease.
Ethionamide	15-30 mg./kg. up to 1 gm. PO		Gastrointestinal, hepatotoxicity, hypersensitivity	SGOT/SGPT	Divided dose may help GI side effects.
Pyrazinamide	15-30 mg./kg. up to 2 gm. PO		Hyperuricemia, hepatotoxicity	Uric acid, SGOT/SGPT	Combination of pyrazinamide and amino-glycoside is bactericidal.
Para-amino-salicylic acid	150 mg./kg. up to 12 gm. PO		Gastrointestinal, hypersensitivity, hepatotoxicity, sodium load	SGOT/SGPT	GI side effects very frequent, making cooperation difficult.
Cycloserine	10-20 mg./kg. up to 1 gm. PO		Psychosis, personality changes, convulsions, rash	Psychologic testing	Very difficult drug to use. Side effects may be blocked by pyridoxine, ataractic agents, or anticonvulsant drugs.

Check product labeling for detailed information on dose, contraindications, drug interaction, adverse reactions, and monitoring.
(American Thoracic Society: Treatment of Mycobacterial Disease. Based on a Statement by an Ad Hoc Committee, 1976)

be used in the treatment of tuberculosis. It is now used in combination with other antituberculous agents, particularly in patients with extensive or cavitary disease. It can only be given by injection. Streptomycin may cause damage to the 8th cranial nerve (vertigo and, rarely, deafness) and renal damage.

Second-line drugs (viomycin, capreomycin, kanamycin, ethionamide, pyrazinamide, para-aminosalicylic acid, cycloserine) are antituberculous drugs used for treatment of recurring tuberculosis or whenever the first-line drugs are not suitable. They have a high rate of toxicity and are less acceptable to the patient. In patients with severe constitutional symptoms or who have tuberculous meningitis, tuberculous pericarditis, or tuberculous peritonitis, corticosteroids may also be of value in quickly reducing inflammation and toxicity.

SURGICAL TREATMENT.   Since the advent of chemotherapy, surgical intervention is rarely necessary for tuberculosis. Pulmonary resection may be performed when the possibility of cancer coexists. It may also be carried out for the purpose of eliminating lesions that have ceased to decrease in size after several months of therapy. Such lesions are particularly apt to contain resistant bacilli or to reactivate at a future date. Other indications for surgery may be recurrent or massive hemoptysis and a bronchopleural fistula occurring from tuberculous empyema.

ISOLATION PROCEDURES. Although tuberculosis is a contagious disease, its infectiousness quickly subsides once chemotherapy is started. However, respiratory isolation (page 1365) is advocated until effective therapy puts a stop to infectiousness, as demonstrated by a decline in malaise, fever, cough, and the absence of bacilli in the sputum smear. Often these goals are achieved within 2 weeks after drug treatment is initiated. The duration of respiratory isolation is adjusted to each patient's situation.

Until the signs of recovery are definite, the patient is placed in a private room with the flow of air carried to the outside. One of the most important considerations in preventing the spread of tuberculosis is adequate ventilation to reduce the number of droplet nuclei in the air.

The patient should be instructed to cover his mouth and nose with double-ply tissue when he coughs or sneezes; these should be discarded in a bag, and burned. (Covering the mouth with the bare hand does not stop small droplets.) If the patient refuses to, or cannot cover his mouth, then he should wear a mask.

Fomites do not constitute a significant infection hazard. Therefore, no special dishwashing or laundering techniques are required. Proper hand-washing removes tubercle bacilli from the hands.

Patient Education and Prevention

Continuing medical and nursing support and supervision are essential. Aspects of the disease should be explained to the patient and any close contacts supervised. Frequent visits to the physician or clinic to determine if the patient is taking the drugs are also important follow-up measures. The booklet, "Understanding Tuberculosis Today: A Handbook for Patients,"* is available from the local Lung Association and will help improve insight and knowledge of the disease.

• *A major reason for treatment failure is that patients do not take their medications regularly and for the period of time prescribed.* One of the teaching functions of the community health nurse is to stress the importance of uninterrupted and long-term chemotherapy.

The side effects of drug therapy are reviewed with the patient, and he is told to report them immediately if they occur. The patient must understand the importance of periodic physical examinations, including roentgenograms of the chest, until drug treatment has been successfully completed.

The patient and family should be instructed carefully in regard to possible complications, including hemorrhage, pleurisy, and other untoward symptoms that are

*American Lung Association, 1740 Broadway, New York, N.Y. 10019.

indicative of a possible recurrence of tuberculous activity. Chronic alcoholism is a troublesome complication which makes ambulatory treatment difficult. This patient should be referred to an alcoholic clinic or appropriate health agency.

Usually the patient can return to his former employment. However, he should avoid exposure to excessive amounts of silicone (dusty jobs in foundry, rock quarry, sand blasting), since silicone dioxide dust may be harmful to the lungs.

Preventive Treatment. Eradicating tuberculosis depends on prevention, detection, health education, and improved standards of living. Most cases of tuberculosis occur in persons known to be positive tuberculin reactors. These patients are the reservoir from which more than 90 percent of active disease develops. Infected persons must be identified, and preventive therapy (isoniazid) given to those at risk of developing disease and becoming transmitters.

Another means of prevention is the vaccine BCG (bacille Calmette-Guérin) which is considered for persons who are not infected but are likely to become infected. Its use is restricted to persons who are tuberculin negative, because it does not benefit persons who have already been infected. However, BCG vaccination will convert a negative tuberculin reactor to a positive one (for a period of time) thus abolishing the diagnostic value of the tuberculin test. The vaccine is infrequently used in the United States, because the medical and socioeconomic conditions are more favorable here than in some other parts of the world, and there are better methods of control and treatment.

In the developing countries, where tuberculosis is a major health problem, it has been found that BCG gives substantial protection against tuberculosis. BCG vaccination has been a major tool of the World Health Organization's efforts to control tuberculosis in countries with high rates of transmission.

The American Lung Association is a voluntary, nonprofit health agency dedicated to the prevention and control of lung diseases. The association's official publication is the *Bulletin,* which disseminates information about tuberculosis and respiratory diseases to lay and professional groups. The American Thoracic Society is the medical arm of the American Lung Association, and has a monthly publication, *The American Review of Respiratory Diseases,* which is a journal for professional readers.

Miliary Tuberculosis

Miliary tuberculosis is the result of bloodstream invasion by the tubercle bacillus. It is the most serious form of tuberculosis. The origin of the bacilli that flood the bloodstream is either some chronic focus that has ulcerated into a blood vessel, or multitudes of miliary tubercles lining the inner surface of the thoracic duct. The germs, poured from these foci into the bloodstream, are carried throughout the body and locate throughout all tissues, everywhere inducing tubercle formation. Definite evidence of this tubercle formation almost always is found on x-ray examination of the lungs. Another location of diagnostic importance is the choroid of the eye, where these tubercles become visible on ophthalmic inspection.

The clinical course of miliary tuberculosis is varied, depending on which organs are involved earliest and most severely. The usual picture is one of prolonged high, irregular fever, without chills, and gradually progressive inanition, weight loss, and prostration. At first there may be no localizing signs except for splenomegaly, anemia, and leukopenia, or at least the absence of leukocytosis, which distinguishes it from most other bacteremias. Within a few weeks, however, a roentgenogram of the chest reveals small densities scattered diffusely throughout both lung fields; these are the miliary tubercles, which gradually increase in size. Very few physical signs may be elicited on physical examination of the chest, but at this stage the patient suffers from a severe harassing cough, dyspnea, and cyanosis. Treatment is the same as that described for pulmonary tuberculosis.

Atypical Mycobacteria

In recent years, it has been recognized that some bacteria which give a staining reaction similar to that of *Mycobacterium tuberculosis,* but which have distinctly different growth and cultural characteristics, may produce an infection that is clinically indistinguishable from tuberculosis. When tuberculosis was a much more common disease than at present, and when more sophisticated bacteriologic techniques were not used, these infections were overlooked, or the organisms discarded as contaminants. Today, these strains of mycobacteria, termed *atypical mycobacteria,* are classifed more precisely. In some localities, infections with these atypical mycobacteria comprise 10 percent of cases of suspected tuberculosis. These organisms not only produce infections indistinguishable from tuberculosis, but because of their chemical similarity to the tubercle bacillus, infected patients often have a positive tuberculin skin test.

These organisms have been divided into four groups. Group 1 organisms are often termed *photochromogens.* When grown in the dark, these bacteria produce nonpigmented colonies resembling tubercle bacilli. After exposure to light, the colonies develop a bright yellow pigmentation. Group 2 organisms show bright yellow-to-orange pigmentation when grown in the dark and are termed *scotochromogens* (from *skotos,* the Greek word for darkness). Group 3 organisms are referred to as *nonchromogens,* or *Battey bacilli* (after Battey State Hospital, in Georgia, where they were first identified). Group 4 bacilli are termed *rapid growers,* because they produce

visible colonies within a few days of culture, whereas 3 to 4 weeks are usually required for cultivation of *M. tuberculosis.* None of these bacilli are pathogenic for guinea pigs, and this characteristic is used to distinguish them from *M. tuberculosis.* In addition, other laboratory procedures are used to distinguish these strains from *M. tuberculosis,* and from one another.

Of these atypical mycobacteria, Group 1 and 3 bacilli are pathogenic for man and often produce pulmonary infections indistinguishable from pulmonary and, less often, other forms of tuberculosis. Organisms belonging to Group 2 scotochromogens rarely cause pulmonary disease, but often produce suppurative infections in the lymph nodes of the neck in young children. The Group 4 rapid growers rarely produce human infection. In addition, organisms of all four groups may be isolated from healthy people with no evidence of disease, and their isolation alone is not always indicative of disease.

Little is known about the epidemiology of infections with atypical mycobacteria. Available evidence suggests that there is little hazard of person-to-person transmission. Treatment of infections with these atypical mycobacteria is often quite difficult, since they are usually resistant to most, if not all, antituberculous drugs.

LEGIONNAIRES' DISEASE

Legionnaires' disease refers to an acute respiratory infection from a gram-negative bacterium with the proposed name *Legionella pneumophila.* It is named after an outbreak of the disease that occurred in Philadelphia, in 1976, among persons attending the state convention of the American Legion. While the organism was first isolated in 1977 from autopsy tissues of patients who died from the disease, it is now known that it caused disease as far back as 1965.

Epidemiological evidence indicates that Legionnaires' disease is acquired from environmental sources. It is proposed that one way in which the aerobic gram-negative bacillus finds its way from the soil into humans is through the evaporation pans and filters of large air conditioners, where the bacteria multiply and are discharged as an infectious aerosol through fans and exhaust vents. The disease is not considered highly infectious. Persons at risk are the middle-aged and older, especially those who smoke.

Clinical Manifestations. The target organ appears to be the lungs. The earliest symptoms are profound malaise, myalgias, mild headache, and a dry cough. Within a day, the patient experiences a rapidly rising fever, and chills. The fever remains high and unremitting (39-41° C. [102-105° F.]) until specific therapy is started. Occasionally, diarrhea precedes other symptoms. Associated manifestations include pleuritic pain, confusion, and impaired renal function. A chest x-ray will document evidence of pneumonia. Tachypnea and dyspnea may reflect the extent of the pneumonic process. The diagnosis is made on the basis of an increase in specific serum antibodies and by culture of the organisms on appropriate culture media.

Pathophysiology. Autopsy specimens from tissues of patients with Legionnaires' disease have shown different amounts of lung consolidation in varying distributions. The histologic pattern has been that of an acute fibrinopurulent pneumonia, which resembles a stage of lobar pneumonia. An exudate containing neutrophils, macrophages, and fibrin is found in the alveolar spaces.

Management. Erythromycin is the drug of choice in treatment. These patients may be seriously ill, and 15 percent of known cases have been fatal. The nursing management is that described for pneumonia (page 475).

Nursing Isolation Procedure: Respiratory isolation is recommended for persons whose illness is strongly suspicious of Legionnaires' disease.

SALMONELLA INFECTIONS (SALMONELLOSIS)

Salmonellosis is a form of food poisoning caused by certain species of the genus *Salmonella;* it produces acute gastroenteritis. There are 1,500 known serotypes of salmonella. The most common in the United States are *S. typhimurium, S. enteritidis, S. newport, S. heidelberg, S. infantis,* and *S. st. paul.*

The diseases resulting from these infections are quite similar, clinically, and the infecting organisms are spread in exactly the same manner as the typhoid bacillus. The patient is infected by ingesting the organism in food contaminated by infected feces of man or animal, in whole eggs and egg products, in meat and meat products, in poultry (especially turkey), and in pharmaceuticals of animal origin. There has been a steady increase in the incidence of salmonellosis due to the enormous reservoir of contaminated food products and a changing pattern of mass food processing and distribution. It has been proposed that large numbers of eggs and chickens on the market are contaminated by salmonella microorganisms. Common foods causing salmonella infections include commercially processed meat pies, poultry, sausages, foods containing eggs or egg products, and unpasteurized milk or dairy products.

Clinical Manifestations. Symptoms usually develop within 8 to 48 hours after ingestion of contaminated food. The patient experiences headache, abdominal discomfort, low-grade fever, and a watery diarrhea which may contain blood and mucus. Some patients only have a headache and occasional loose stools. The infectious agent may localize and cause necrosis in any body tissue,

producing abscesses, cholecystitis, arthritis, endocarditis, meningitis, pericarditis, pneumonia, and pyelonephritis. Petechiae, splenomegaly, and leukopenia may also be manifested.

Early in the disease, every attempt should be made to recover and identify the infecting organism from stools, blood, vomitus, and urine. Later, after acute infection subsides, serologic agglutination tests are useful in establishing the diagnosis.

Management. The treatment is supportive, and includes restriction of food until the abdominal pain subsides. Clear liquids are offered as tolerated. Fluid and electrolyte depletion may have to be corrected intravenously. Antimotility drugs (anticholinergics, paregoric) may be counterproductive, since a slowed peristaltic activity may extend the period of infection by interfering with an effective cleansing mechanism. Enteric precautions are used for the duration of the illness. If a patient has a focal infection (abscess) or systemic infection, treatment is similar to that of typhoid fever (page 1385).

Prevention and Patient Education. There is no active or passive immunization. Raw eggs or egg drinks should not be eaten, nor should dirty or cracked eggs be used, since salmonellae can penetrate cracked eggs. All foods from animal sources, especially fowl, egg products, and meat dishes, should be *thoroughly cooked.* Food service workers should be instructed about food-borne illnesses and given guidelines on avoiding food contamination, storing and preparing food, and maintaining service areas and good personal hygiene.

SHIGELLOSIS (BACILLARY DYSENTERY)

Shigellosis is an acute bacterial disease of the intestinal tract. There are approximately 40 serotypes of shigellae divided into 4 serogroups: *S. dysenteriae, S. flexneri, S. boydii,* and *S. Sonnei* (most common serotype isolated in industrialized countries). The source of infection is feces from an infected person, with the route of spread being fecal-oral. Shigellosis may be passed through toilet paper onto the fingers. The bacilli have also been recovered from milk, eggs, cheese, and shrimp.

While encountered in all countries, bacillary dysentery is endemic in the tropics, where serious epidemics are frequently found. It continues to pose a very substantial problem for the citizens of this country, especially those with a substandard environment and those living in a closed-group population—day care centers, military installations, institutions for mentally retarded children, etc.

Pathogenesis. The pathology of shigellosis, in severe cases, consists of organisms reaching the small intestine, where they multiply and release a toxin which initiates secretion of water and electrolytes from the jejunal area.

The shigellae are thought to invade the distal ileum and colon, where they establish themselves in epithelial cells, multiply, spread to adjacent cells, and destroy them. The invading pathogens are capable of initiating an intense inflammatory response in the mucosa, followed by small patches of ulceration, which may coalesce to form large ulcers.

Clinical Manifestations. Initially there is cramping abdominal pain. Diarrhea soon appears, followed by frank dysentery, with the passage of varying amounts of blood, mucus, and pus. There may be high fever. At the height of the active infection, the symptoms are severe and the prostration quite profound. The patient has a constant desire to defecate, and the straining is severe during the attempts. Patients with mild cases recover in 8 to 10 days. Some cases last 2 or 3 weeks, and chronic cases last several months, or even years, unless adequately treated. In severe cases, death may ensue in a few days.

Management. The organism may be recovered from the stool, and sensitivity tests done in order to determine the appropriate antibiotic, since the organism may be resistant to certain drugs. Antimotility drugs (Lomotil) are not given, since they may abolish antibiotic effectiveness in reducing diarrhea and positive cultures, thus impeding the body's normal defense mechanisms.

Antibiotics which are absorbed from the intestinal tract and to which the shigellae are sensitive (ampicillin, tetracyclines, sulfa-trimethoprim, chloramphenicol) shorten the clinical course and decrease the duration of excretion of the organisms.

The objectives of treatment are to maintain fluid and electrolyte balance and to eliminate the spread of shigellosis to the patient's contacts; e.g. eliminate the carrier state.

Intravenous fluids of physiologic saline are administered to maintain the electrolyte balance and prevent profound dehydration owing to an excessively large loss of water and salts in the diarrheic stools. The patient is assessed for weight loss, skin turgor, and dryness of mucous membranes, and his vital signs and urinary volume are monitored. The patient may require supplemental potassium. Clear fluids are offered by mouth during the acute stage.

Nursing Isolation Procedures: Enteric nursing precautions are carried out until three successive cultures of feces, taken 24 hours apart after cessation of antimicrobial therapy, are negative.

Prevention. Dysentery bacilli are spread by drinking water polluted by infected human excreta and by food handled carelessly by shigella carriers, some of whom have the active disease, others being entirely asymptomatic. Thus, the same precautions must be observed, and the same control of water sources and food handling enforced, in the prevention of dysentery as of typhoid

fever. This includes proper handwashing, effective sanitation, adequate sewage disposal, and detection of carriers.

TYPHOID FEVER

Typhoid fever is a bacterial infection transmitted by water, milk, shellfish, or foods contaminated by *Salmonella typhi,* which is harbored in human excreta. This bacillus produces no spores. However, under suitable conditions it can live for months outside the body, and, since it is eliminated in the stools and the urine of patients, it is very likely to find its way into food and water through sewage, flies, and dirty fingers. Today it is spread chiefly by carriers, patients who have recovered from this fever, but whose stools or urine may spread these bacilli for years. Another common source is the ingestion of oysters and shellfish infected from offshore sewage-disposal depots.

Pathophysiology. The organism enters the body by way of the mouth and invades the walls of the gastrointestinal tract. There, multiplying rapidly, it gives rise to a massive bacteremia which continues for about 10 days. The chief localization of the organism is in the mesenteric lymph nodes and the masses of lymphatic tissue in the mucous membrane of the intestinal wall, which are called *Peyer's patches,* and in small solitary lymph follicles, numerous in the ileum and the colon. The blood vessels of the Peyer's patches become thrombosed, and the swollen mass of lymphatic tissue dies and sloughs away, leaving clean ulcers in the mucous membrane, the floor of which may be the muscularis, or even the peritoneum. If the latter, they may perforate, causing peritonitis. The solitary follicles may or may not ulcerate, but they are so tiny that they do little harm.

Clinical Manifestations

The distinctive clinical features of typhoid fever consist of prolonged fever, rose-spot rash, enlarged spleen, slow pulse, and leukopenia. The incubation period of typhoid fever lasts from 3 to 20 days, with the disease beginning as a subacute illness. Without therapy, the temperature rises steadily, reaching its highest level—usually from 40.9° C. (105.6° F.)—in from 3 to 7 days. During this period of rising temperature, most patients suffer with a severe headache and a nonproductive cough. During the second week, if the patient is not treated, the temperature remains consistently high. During the third week, however, it becomes more and more remittent, a little lower each morning and not quite so elevated each afternoon.

The pulse, in typhoid fever at its height, is usually remarkably slow (between 80 and 90). Also, one often feels the dicrotic wave so distinctly that there is danger of mistaking it for a separate beat.

Other clinical manifestations are hepatomegaly,

splenomegaly, delirium, rose spots (rose-red papules appearing over the abdomen) and intestinal bleeding.

Diagnostic Assessment. The white blood cell count usually declines below 5,000, sometimes to a level as low as 1,500 cells per cu. mm. (leukopenia). The blood and stool cultures are positive for the organism after the first week. Urine cultures, however, may or may not show signs of the organism. The blood serum agglutination test usually becomes positive by the end of the second week.

Complications. Many structures may become infected in the course of typhoid fever, including the lungs, the pleura, the pericardium, the heart, the kidneys, and the bones. However, the most common of the dangerous complications are intestinal hemorrhage and perforation of the bowel with resultant peritonitis. Since the advent of effective chemotherapy, such incidences have decreased.

Intestinal hemorrhages, from erosion of blood vessels in the ulcerated small intestine, occur during the third week in about 10 percent of patients. Some patients have many such hemorrhages. Signs of hemorrhage include apprehension, sweating, pallor, weak, rapid pulse, hypotension, and bloody or tarry stools. During these episodes, food is withheld and blood transfusions given.

Intestinal perforation, the most serious complication, may happen at any time, but most often occurs during the third week. The perforation usually takes place in the lower ileum. It occurs when the ulcer causing the slough involves the entire thickness of the bowel wall. The intestinal contents pour into the abdominal cavity, at once causing peritonitis. The patient may experience a sudden drop in temperature or an increase in pulse rate, and complain of acute abdominal pain. There is associated abdominal tenderness and rigidity. However, the pain may only last a few seconds and then stop, with the patient falling sound asleep within a few minutes. If such signs occur, a nasogastric tube is passed and intravenous fluids started, to correct fluid and electrolyte balance. Surgical closure of perforation is usually carried out.

Other complications of typhoid fever include thrombophlebitis, urinary infections, cholecystitis, anemia, and typhoid hepatitis. Cholecystitis, marked by the development of crampy right upper quadrant pain, accompanied by tenderness, nausea, vomiting, and jaundice, may occur from direct infection of the gallbladder by the typhoid bacillus. This is treated conservatively with sedatives, antispasmodics, and parenteral fluids.

Management

Drug therapy. Chloramphenicol is the most commonly used drug for typhoid fever. When this drug is used, the blood count is monitored to detect chloramphenicol toxicity. Amoxicillin also appears to be effective, as does a combination of sulfamethoxazole and trimethoprim which is active against chloramphenicol-resistant *S. typhi* strains.

The fever usually subsides in 3 to 5 days following initiation of antibiotic therapy. However, bacteriologic cure is not achieved in all patients. Relapses have occurred and positive stool cultures have been obtained after one course, and even repeated courses of antibiotic therapy. Thus, while chloramphenicol has reduced the fatality rate of typhoid fever significantly and has curtailed the excretion of typhoid bacilli during convalescence, it has not reduced the frequency of complications or the incidence of the chronic carrier state following typhoid fever.

Nursing Management. The objectives of nursing management are to give supportive care and to observe for complications such as bacteremia which occurs frequently in patients with typhoid fever.

Delirium is common in the severe form of the disease, and the patient will require special support during this period. He may be drowsy, indifferent to his surroundings, and incontinent of urine and feces. Temperature should be taken by rectum, since the patient may not be able to keep his mouth closed while holding the thermometer. Fever sponges are given for temperatures of 40° C. (104° F.), and a high fluid intake is encouraged, to counteract loss by perspiration.

The patient should be awakened when it is time to turn him, take his temperature, and administer medications, fluid, and food.

Many patients are so toxic that they lose the urge to void, with the result that the bladder becomes distended. Input and output must be measured and recorded, in order to obtain quantitative data concerning the status of fluid balance.

Retention of feces, as well as urine, may pose a problem. Low saline enemas are given to relieve this problem. But they are to be given under low pressure, to diminish the chances of intestinal perforation caused by an increase in the pressure or the volume of the fluid within the colon. Distention may be reduced by inserting a rectal tube for short intervals (20 minutes). A high-calorie, low-residue diet is given during the febrile stage.

Nursing Isolation Procedure: Enteric precautions are used until three consecutive stool cultures (taken after cessation of antimicrobials) are negative for *S. typhi.*

Follow-up. Since typhoid fever is a very serious disease, the process of recovery may be a slow one. Once a patient has recovered, stools must be checked, to see if he has become a carrier, as will be the case in 2 to 5 percent of typhoid patients. Such carriers harbor the organism and excrete it in their urine and stools. A positive stool culture after 6 to 12 months indicates a carrier. Such people must not become food or milk handlers. Public health agencies maintain surveillance of carriers, because the occurrence of typhoid fever almost always is traceable to a known or undetected carrier.

Prevention and Patient Education

The prevention of typhoid fever depends on personal hygiene, cleanliness in food preparation and intake, and proper sewage disposal. Water supplies should be protected and purified. Milk and dairy products require pasteurization and refrigeration. All persons handling food should use proper handwashing techniques. There is no substitute for good sanitation.

Routine typhoid vaccination is no longer recommended for persons in the United States.

Selective immunization is, however, indicated for the following:*

1. Persons with intimate exposure to a documented typhoid carrier, such as would occur with continued household contact.
2. Travelers to areas where there is a recognized risk of exposure to typhoid because of poor food and water sanitation. It should be emphasized, however, that even after typhoid vaccination, there should be careful selection of foods and water in these areas.

There is no evidence that typhoid vaccine is of value in the United States in controlling common-source outbreaks. Furthermore, there is no reason to use typhoid vaccine for persons in areas of natural disaster, such as floods, or for persons attending rural summer camps.

PRIMARY IMMUNIZATION. On the basis of the above recommendations, adults (and children over 10 years old) may be given 0.5 ml. of typhoid vaccine subcutaneously on two occasions separated by 4 or more weeks. A booster dose is given at least every 3 years, under conditions of continued or repeated exposure.

MENINGOCOCCAL MENINGITIS

Meningitis is an inflammation of the meningeal tissues covering the brain, and is caused by bacterial, mycobacterial, or viral agents. The bacteria most frequently encountered in acute bacterial meningitis are *Neisseria meningitidis, Streptococcus pneumoniae* (in adults), and *Haemophilus influenzae* (in young children).

Meningitis is often asymptomatic, but may start as an infection of the nasopharynx or the tonsils, followed by meningococcal septicemia which extends to the meninges of the brain and the upper region of the spinal cord. It can be one of the most fulminating of infectious diseases.

Meningococcal disease is endemic in the United States and throughout the world, and occurs most frequently in the winter and spring months. Epidemics are most apt to occur when people live in crowded quarters, notably in cities, crowded institutions, military installations, or prisons, but the disease also occurs in rural regions.

*Recommendation of the Public Health Service Advisory Committee on Immunization Practices, July, 1978.

The germ is spread by the droplet method, the portals of entry being the mucous membrane of the nose and the tonsils. Of those exposed to it, the great majority do not develop the infection but become carriers, harboring this organism in the posterior nasopharynx for months.

Pathophysiology. Predisposing factors include upper respiratory tract infections, otitis media, mastoiditis, sickle cell anemia (or other hemoglobinopathies), recent neurosurgical procedures, head trauma, and immunologic defects. The venous channels serving the posterior nasopharynx, middle ear, and mastoid drain toward the brain and are near the veins draining the meninges. This favors bacterial proliferation.

The meningococci enter the bloodstream and cause an inflammatory reaction in the meninges and underlying cortex, which may result in vasculitis with thromboses and reduced cerebral blood flow. The cerebral tissue is metabolically impaired from the presence of meningeal exudate, vasculitis and underperfusion, and cerebral edema. A purulent exudate may spread over the base of the brain and spinal cord. The inflammation spreads also to the membrane lining the cerebral ventricles. In acute cases, however, the patient dies from the toxin of the bacteria before meningitis develops. In these patients meningococcemia is overwhelming, with adrenal damage, circulatory collapse, and associated widespread hemorrhages (Waterhouse-Friderichsen syndrome) occurring as a result of endothelial damage and vascular necrosis caused by the meningococci.

Clinical Manifestations

The onset may be abrupt or insidious. The symptoms result first from the infection, and then from increased intracranial pressure.

During each epidemic some patients are scarcely ill; others, at once overwhelmed by the toxemia, develop either a high or a subnormal temperature, with purpura on the skin, and die within a few hours of the onset (the fulminant type).

The disease may follow two patterns. Usually the patient presents with a sudden onset of severe headache, neck pain and stiffness (from spasm of the extensor muscles, due to meningeal irritation), and fever. In addition to neck stiffness, other signs of meningeal irritation are positive Kernig's sign (inability to extend the leg completely when the thigh is flexed); positive Brudzinski's sign (flexion of the opposite leg when one leg is flexed, and flexion of both legs when the neck is flexed by the examiner); hyperextension of the head, and hyperirritability. Convulsions and vomiting may occur, along with lethargy, mental confusion, and a hemorrhagic rash ranging from petechiae to a combination of petechiae and ecchymoses.

In approximately 10 percent of the patients, a fulminating infection occurs, with signs of overwhelming septicemia: an abrupt onset of high fever, extensive purpuric lesions (over face and extremities), shock and signs of intravascular coagulation. Death may occur within a few hours after onset.

Diagnostic Assessment. Cerebrospinal fluid, obtained from a lumbar puncture, will contain the organism, as might the blood. The cerebrospinal fluid, instead of being clear, contains so much pus that it looks like thin milk; it is under high pressure, and the gram stain of the fluid may reveal the organisms immediately. On occasion, the cerebrospinal fluid is clear, which may occur as a result of prior therapy with antimicrobial agents active against the particular microorganisms. When cerebrospinal cultures are sterile, counter immunoelectrophoresis is used to detect small amounts of bacterial antigen in the cerebrospinal fluid of patients with certain types of meningeal disease. Blood cultures are likewise often positive for the meningococcus.

Management

In general, the mortality of untreated meningococcal infection ranges from 25 to 90 percent, with an average of about 50 percent. The immediate objective of care is to observe and treat for vasomotor collapse and shock with appropriate fluid replacement and cardiorespiratory support.

The antimicrobial therapy depends upon the infecting organism, and the aim is to eradicate the organisms from the subarachnoid space. Penicillin or ampicillin in high, intravenous doses (to achieve high blood concentration of antibiotic) is the agent of choice for the most common varieties of bacterial meningitis. The patient is maintained on large doses of intravenous antibiotics, since most antimicrobials enter the cerebrospinal fluid and central nervous system inefficiently.

- The patient's outcome may depend on the supportive care given. In meningitis of all causes, the patient's clinical status and vital signs are constantly assessed, since altered consciousness may lead to airway obstruction. Arterial blood gas determinations, insertion of a cuffed endotracheal tube (or tracheostomy), and mechanical ventilation may be necessary. Oxygen may be given to maintain the arterial pO_2 at desired levels.
- The central venous pressure is monitored to assess for incipient shock, which precedes cardiac or respiratory failure. Generalized vasoconstriction, circumoral cyanosis, and cold extremities may be noted. The high fever must be reduced, to decrease the load on the heart and the brain's oxygen demand.
- Rapid intravenous fluid replacement may be necessary, but care is taken not to overhydrate the patient because of risk of cerebral edema.

The combination of fever, dehydration, decreased fluid intake, and subsequent alkalosis often predispose to convulsive seizures. Airway obstruction, respiratory arrest, or cardiac arrhythmias may follow. Acute cerebral edema may occur. Osmotic diuretics (IV mannitol, urea) are given to decrease cerebral edema. Diazepam (Valium) followed by phenytoin (Dilantin) may be administered to control convulsive seizures. (The care of the patient with seizures is discussed on page 1244 and the care of the unconscious patient on page 1188.

The continuing nursing management requires ongoing assessment of the patient's clinical status, attention to skin and oral hygiene, monitoring of input and output, promotion of comfort, and protection during seizures and while comatose.

Nursing Isolation Procedure: Use respiratory isolation precautions (page 1365) until 24 hours after initiation of effective therapy.

Prevention and Patient Education. Persons having close contact with the patient should be considered as candidates for antimicrobial prophylaxis, in which case rifampin is given for 2 to 5 days. Close contacts are observed, and immediately examined if fever or other signs and symptoms of meningitis develop.

Three meningococcal polysaccharide vaccines, monovalent A, monovalent C, and bivalent A-C vaccine, are licensed for selective use in the United States. The monovalent vaccines for the specific serogroup are recommended to control outbreaks of meningococcal disease caused by *N. meningitidis* serogroup A or C. Vaccine may be of benefit for some travelers visiting countries which are experiencing epidemic meningococcal disease. Vaccination should also be considered as an adjunct to antibiotic chemoprophylaxis for anyone living with a patient who has meningococcal disease caused by serogroups A or C. At present there is no effective vaccine for prevention of group B meningococcal disease.

TETANUS (LOCKJAW)

Tetanus is an acute disease caused by the tetanus bacillus, *Clostridium tetani,* whose spores are introduced into the body when an open wound is contaminated with soil, street dust, or animal and human feces. The bacillus is an anaerobe (cannot live in presence of oxygen). It is found most commonly in wounds with small external openings and is also seen in drug addicts. It may occur in any deep wound that is contaminated with soil or harbors foreign bodies. Frequently the presumed site of infection is a "minor wound." Not infrequently, the wound entrance is so insignificant that it cannot be found. Wounds may be minor injuries, scratches, bee stings, lacerations, frostbite, animal injuries, abortions, circumcision, surgery and dental and orofacial trauma. The incidence is greater among low-income groups (not receiving immunization) and among women, and the elderly, who never were immunized as children, or have lost their immunity.

Pathophysiology and Clinical Manifestations. *Clostridium tetani* is known to produce 3 exotoxins: tetanospasmin, which is a neurotoxin with a special affinity for nervous tissue, especially in the spinal cord and cranial nerves, and which produces intense and severe muscle spasms; nonconvulsive neurotoxin; and tetanolysin, which may have hemolytic and cardiotoxic effects. These neurotoxins are absorbed by the peripheral nerves and carried to the spinal cord, where they produce a reaction that amounts to a stimulation of the nervous tissue. The sensory nerves become sensitive to the slightest stimuli, and the hypersensitive motor nerves carry impulses that produce spasms of the muscles that they supply.

Early symptoms include irritability, restlessness, headache, low-grade fever, and muscle rigidity. The jaw muscles are the first group affected, making it difficult to open the mouth because of spasms of the masticatory muscles (trismus). This characteristic symptom has given the disease the common name of *lockjaw*. The spasms of the facial muscles produce a distorted smile (risus sardonicus) which is quite characteristic for the disease and persists even during convalescence.

The spasm rapidly involves other groups of muscles, until the whole body is affected. The spasm is continuous, but the least stimulus—a door banging, or a loud voice—may cause a generalized convulsion, with every muscle in violent contraction. In fact, fractures of the vertebral bodies can occur during severe spasms. Because the extensor muscles are stronger than the flexors, the head is retracted, the feet are extended fully, and the back is arched, so that during a convulsion the whole body may be supported on the back of the head and the feet. This condition is called *opisthotonos*. Death may occur from asphyxia, due to spasms of the respiratory muscles, and from pneumonia.

Management

If the disease has already developed, the patient is immediately given tetanus immune globulin (TIG) to neutralize the toxin and to ensure that circulating levels of the drug will be present when the wound is debrided. Since the half-life of immune globulin is 30 days, active immunization with tetanus toxoid is also started, to give more permanent protection. The wound is debrided and left open. Immune globulin may also be infiltrated into the wound site. Usually penicillin G (or an alternate antibiotic) is given intravenously or intramuscularly in high doses to eradicate persisting *C. tetani*, stop the production of any new toxin, and eradicate other pathogens from the wound.

- In severe tetanus infection, one of the most important nursing objectives and priorities is constant supportive care of the patient to assure respiratory function. Convulsive paroxysms, especially those involving the respiratory muscles, impair pulmonary gas exchange by preventing normal swallowing and by obstructing the airway.

- Tetanic spasms of the larynx, pharynx, and respiratory muscles usually occur during convulsions and can lead to asphyxiation and death. Rigidity and spasm of the trunk muscles also contribute to ventilatory failure. In fact, ventilation ceases during a tetanus convulsion.

- The patient requires expert respiratory management in an intensive care unit, with early endotracheal intubation and mechanical ventilation. Oral secretions are usually constant and heavy, requiring frequent suctioning.

Diazepam is used to sedate the patient, relax the muscles, and increase the threshold of tetanus spasm. It may be combined with chlorpromazine or meprobamate for added effectiveness. Curariform drugs are given, for severe convulsions. The nursing management of the patient with convulsions is discussed on page 1244.

Since the slightest stimulation may trigger paroxysmal spasm, sudden stimuli and light must be avoided. The patient is placed in a quiet room, to minimize spasms and seizures. Nursing activities are carried out during the periods when sedation has its maximum effect, so that the patient is disturbed as little as possible, since tactile stimulation often provokes spasms. Usually a vein is kept open for emergency situations such as cardiac or respiratory arrest, and for infusions to maintain careful fluid and electrolyte balance. Insensible water loss and caloric expenditure may be high due to the energy output caused by muscular contractions. To offset this loss, parenteral nutrition may be required, as opposed to direct food intake, since aspiration pneumonia is a hazard.

Constant attention is given to the eyes, mouth, skin, and bladder and bowels. The patient is monitored for signs of infection (skin, urinary tract, aspiration pneumonia). Overactivity of the sympathetic nervous system, as manifested by tachycardia, arrhythmias, labile blood pressure, hyperpyrexia, and excessive sweating and salivation, may eventually lead to circulatory failure and death. A significant increase in the heart rate and mean arterial blood pressure may indicate a need for an adrenergic blocking agent (propranolol), to lessen the possibility of catecholamine-induced myocardial damage. Therefore, cardiac monitoring is essential. Even with expert care, the mortality rate of tetanus ranges between 25 and 75 percent.

Prevention. Tetanus can be prevented through proper immunization programs. For primary immunization of adults, three doses of adult-type tetanus and diphtheria toxoids should be given, followed by a booster dose every 10 years.

Every break in the skin must be considered a potential portal of entry for *C. tetani*.

- The most important step in the prevention of tetanus is the thorough washing and cleaning of the wound, with removal of all foreign material and devitalized tissue. This helps eliminate tetanus bacilli from wounds and removes the material that forms a focus in which tetanus spores can develop.

Following injury, the immunization status of the patient will determine whether tetanus can be avoided. The nature and age of the wound, the conditions under which it was incurred, and the treatment must all be considered.

CLOSTRIDIAL MYONECROSIS (GAS GANGRENE)

Gas gangrene is a severe infection caused by several species of gram-positive clostridia which may complicate trauma, compound fractures, contusions, or lacerated wounds by producing exotoxins that destroy tissue. These organisms (*Clostridium perfringens, C. novyi, C. septicum,* and others) are anaerobes and spore-formers and are found normally in the intestinal tract of man and in soils. Their growth occurs primarily in deep wounds where the oxygen supply is reduced, a situation enhanced by the presence of foreign bodies or necrotic tissue, which leads to further reduction of oxygen tension in wounds.

In contaminated wounds in which the vascular supply may be impaired, the environment is suited for the growth of spores and the production of exotoxins which cause hemolysis, vessel thrombosis, and damage to the myocardium, liver, and kidneys.

Spores formed by anaerobic bacilli are highly resistant to heat, cold, sunlight, drying, and many chemical agents. Because the gas bacillus is an inhabitant of the human intestinal tract, it is likely to be the infecting organism in thigh wounds following amputations, especially if the patient is incontinent. Peripheral vascular disease, gangrene, incontinence, and debility often are combined in patients with diabetes, and it is in the amputation stump of diabetic patients that gas gangrene is most likely to occur.

Clinical Manifestations. The onset of gas gangrene is usually attended by sudden, severe pain at the site of injury, usually occurring 1 to 4 days following the injury. The wound is very tender. The surrounding skin initially appears normal, or white and tense, but later becomes bronzed, brown, or even black in color. Vesicles filled with red, watery fluid appear, and crepitus (crackling) produced by gas in the tissue may be felt. Frothy fluid with a foul, sweetish odor may escape from the wound. The gas and edema fluid increase local pressure and impair the blood supply and drainage. The involved muscles become black or reddish purple (necrosis). The infection may spread quickly, resulting in systemic toxicity.

The patient is pale, prostrated, and apprehensive, but usually quite alert. Pulse and respirations are rapid, but the temperature usually does not exceed 38.3° C. (101° F.). Anorexia, diarrhea, vomiting, and vascular collapse may occur. Death from toxemia is frequent.

Another, more benign form of clostridial infection (clostridial cellulitis) may involve the skin and sub-cutaneous tissue. It may be differentiated from gas gangrene by the absence of muscle involvement and relatively less severe systemic manifestations.

Management

Gas gangrene may be prevented if all devitalized and infected tissue is excised and debrided, with wide incisions made, to render the wound unsuitable for the growth of clostridium. Antibiotic therapy (penicillin) may be combined with prompt surgical debridement of the wound. In the patient with established infection, antibiotics may be of questionable value, since they cannot effectively penetrate the anoxic and ischemic areas in which anaerobic infections occur. However, since mixed infections frequently occur, antibiotic therapy may be of benefit. Amputation of an affected extremity often is necessary.

Hyperbaric oxygen (oxygen administered under pressure greater than atmospheric, in specially designed chambers) has proven extremely effective in treating gas gangrene. This increases the dissolved oxygen in the arterial system by increasing the partial pressure of oxygen breathed by the patient. Toxin formation and microbial replication (reproduction) may thereby be reduced. With hyperbaric oxygen therapy, it may not be necessary to amputate the extremity or debride as extensive an area. Since gas gangrene produces an intense toxemia, pulmonary capillary wedge pressure, central venous pressure, and urinary output are monitored. Intravenous fluids are given, to support the cardiovascular system and to maintain fluid and electrolyte balance.

Nursing Isolation Procedure: Wound and skin precautions (page 1365) are taken until the wound stops draining.

BOTULISM

Botulism is a type of poisoning which affects the central nervous system. It is caused by eating food in which *Clostridium botulinum* has grown and produced toxins. These toxins are extremely potent and are rapidly absorbed by the GI tract, becoming bound to neural tissue and producing a neuroparalytic syndrome. People usually become ill after eating contaminated foods preserved in jars and tins.

Of the eight toxigenic serotypes of *C. botulinum;* types A, B, E, and F have been shown to produce disease in humans.

Home-processed foods pose a serious danger of *C. botulinum,* because this germ is a spore-bearer and is not killed rapidly at boiling temperature. (Reliable commercial packing houses sterilize their products at 120° C. [248° F.], which kills all the spores.) Preserved foods in which this germ has been growing look soft, contain gas bubbles, and give off an odor of decay. Since the toxin is destroyed rapidly by heat (within a few seconds at temperatures over 82.2° C. [180° F.]), foods containing it are safe if heated to the boiling point before being eaten; but if allowed to cool and stand for a while, the organism will immediately proceed to form more toxin. Vegetables, including mushrooms, beans, tomatoes, beets, okra, peppers, corn, and asparagus have been implicated, while meats, fish and poultry have also accounted for some outbreaks.

Clinical Manifestations. The symptoms appear 12 to 48 hours after ingestion of the contaminated food. If the symptoms appear in less than 24 hours after ingestion, a more severe illness and a higher fatality rate are usually encountered.

Cranial nerve symptoms include diplopia, ptosis and blurred vision (extraocular muscle involvement), dysphagia and pharyngeal pain (involvement of pharynx), and dysphonia (involvement of larynx). Paralysis then occurs, slowly descending through the body and affecting all muscle groups, usually in a symmetrical fashion. Throughout the ordeal, the patient's mind remains clear. Almost three-fourths of the patients have respiratory problems. In addition, there may be nausea, vomiting, abdominal pain, early diarrhea, dizziness, and, occasionally, urinary retention.

The diagnosis is confirmed by finding the toxin in the serum, gastric contents, stools, and incriminated food. Local, state, and federal public health officials are notified when a case of botulism is diagnosed.

Management. The objectives of treatment are to prevent respiratory failure and to eliminate the toxin and *C. botulinum* from the gastrointestinal tract.

If the toxin type is unknown, the patient is given a botulinal antitoxin to counteract the effect of the toxin (usually for types A, B, and E). This is available from the Center for Disease Control. Ventilatory equipment and emergency drugs should be readily available, in the event of a life-threatening reaction.

Organisms are eliminated from the gastrointestinal tract by means of gastric lavage, cathartics, and enemas. In instances of respiratory paralysis or an ileus, these procedures may not be prescribed.

- Since the neurotoxins produced by *C. botulinum* may result in neuroparalytic syndromes, the patient is given respiratory care and support as the basic management, to prevent the pulmonary complications which are responsible for most fatalities due to botulism. The patient is prepared for endotracheal intubation and mechanical ventilation. (The respiratory care of the paralyzed patient is discussed in detail in Chapter 24.)

The patient's heart is monitored in order to detect immediately any signs of cardiac arrest. Skin care and positioning are also important facets of management, to prevent pressure sores and musculoskeletal complications.

Guanidine hydrochloride may be given, as it is purported to enhance the release of acetylcholine from the nerve terminals. Its use is controversial.

Nursing Isolation Procedure: No precautions are necessary, since botulism is an intoxication, not an infection.

LEPROSY (HANSEN'S DISEASE)

Leprosy is a chronic infectious disease caused by *Mycobacterium leprae,* a bacillus that produces lesions in the skin tissues and peripheral nerves. This organism resembles the tubercle bacillus in appearance and staining characteristics. However, it differs from the tubercle bacillus in that it does not infect animals and cannot be cultivated. It is not known exactly how leprosy bacilli enter the body, but they are probably transmitted to a susceptible individual by direct skin-to-skin contact. There is evidence that large numbers of bacilli can be discharged from the nose of an untreated patient with advanced leprosy.

As the bacilli multiply, they invade adjoining skin areas and find their way into the axis cylinders of nerves by way of the axon-plasma filaments, i.e., the ultimate terminals of the nerves supplying the skin. As the infection spreads, organisms break out of the nerves at various points in the skin to produce macules and papules. These are painless, since the bacilli that caused them to form had already destroyed the nerve supply.

Incidence. An estimated 11 to 12 million persons throughout the world suffer from this ancient, feared, and disfiguring disease. While it is most prevalent in Africa and some parts of Asia, sporadic outbreaks have occurred in the United States, in Florida, Louisiana, Texas, California, and Hawaii. It has been suggested that in the majority of cases in the United States, the disease was contracted outside the country.

Clinical Manifestations. The earliest manifestation is a single skin lesion, located anywhere on the body. The lesions are either tuberculoid or lepromatous in appearance. In the tuberculoid form, the tuberculoid patches are few in number, and either colorless or reddish-brown. The earliest sign is usually a loss of feeling in a small area of the skin, as a result of nerve involvement. Eventually, muscle damage occurs. In the lepromatous form, the bacillus grows unchecked, with skin lesions or nodules appearing over most of the body. These nodules, resembling skin tumors and sores, may appear anywhere on the body. When the face is involved, the nodules, together with the loss of the eyebrows and eyelashes, give the face a typical leonine appearance. Because the nodules are easily infected, giving rise to deep ulcers that heal slowly, scars deform the face. This process often dissects the nose, fingers, and toes, and destroys sight.

Diagnosis is made on the basis of the appearance of the lesions and the discovery of the leprosy bacilli, obtained by punch biopsies of the skin lesions.

Management. Leprosy is best treated with sulfone drugs (related chemically to the sulfonamides), especially DDS (4,4-diaminodiphenyl sulfone, dapsone) which inhibits the multiplication of *M. leprae*. Therapy is continued until all *M. leprae* have disappeared from the skin. Improvement often is evident within 3 to 6 months, and is described by the majority of patients after 3 to 5 years of treatment. Clofazimine, rifampicin, and thiacetazone are also active against leprosy, but are more expensive and toxic than dapsone. Dapsone-resistant leprosy, is now being seen with increasing frequency and is becoming a source of anxiety in leprosy control programs.

Mucosal lesions respond most readily, disappearing within a few months, resulting in relief of nasal obstruction and clearing of laryngeal lesions. The smaller nodular lesions in the skin shrink and are absorbed, leaving only pigment spots. Larger lesions disperse, with eventual scar formation. However, bacilli can persist following treatment, resulting in relapse at a later date.

Reconstructive surgery and rehabilitation to restore damaged hands, feet, face, etc. require the services of reconstructive and plastic surgeons, physical therapists, orthopedists and others. Because the disfigurement of leprosy is such a stigma, surgery is absolutely necessary if the patient is to return to society.

To counter the crippling effects of the disease, the patient must realize the importance of maintaining mobility of the affected extremities and preventing fixed deformities. The principles are similar to those stressed in patient education for rheumatoid arthritis (page 1331).

The United States Public Heath Service maintains a center for leprosy care in Carville, Louisiana, which serves as a treatment, research, and training facility. Other U.S.P.H.S. hospitals and clinics with a special interest in leprosy are located in New Orleans, San Francisco, and Staten Island, New York. Research is still being conducted in hopes of finding a specific skin test for leprosy, as well as a vaccine.

Nursing Isolation Procedures: No isolation precautions are required, since the infection declines rapidly under chemotherapy.

ORNITHOSIS (PSITTACOSIS)

Ornithosis is an infectious and atypical form of pneumonia transmitted to humans by certain birds. The agents responsible for ornithosis belong to the genus *Chlamydia,* (obligate intracellular organisms that were formerly considered viruses but are now classed as bacteria). The chlamydiae cause trachoma, lymphogranuloma venereum, and ornithosis; they may be found in nasal secretions and in the feathers, feces, and blood of sick birds. The organisms are transmitted to humans through person-to-person contact or inhalation of aerosolized particles—droplets, droplet nuclei, and dust. Birds of the parrot family (parakeets, parrots, cockatoos, budgerigars), as well as many other species of birds (canaries, sparrows, pigeons, turkeys) may be infected.

Clinical Manifestations. The illness may appear as a transient, influenzalike illness or a severe pneumonia, or it may be asymptomatic. After an incubation period lasting 7 to 14 days (it may be as long as 6 weeks in man, 6 months in a parrot), the disease begins abruptly, with malaise, headache, photophobia, and chills. Its course is characterized by high fever, great weakness, marked depression, and delirium, with surprisingly slow pulse and respiration. Cough is a prominent symptom. The lungs become involved, with edema, mononuclear cells and lymphocytes appearing in the alveoli and interstitial areas. Chest x-ray may reveal an interstitial pneumonitis. Convalescence is apt to be prolonged.

Management. Ornithosis responds to the tetracyclines. Active immunity is acquired as a result of the infection. Supportive therapy includes bed rest, oxygen (when necessary), and measures to reduce the fever.

Prevention. Persons at risk are those who work in pet shops or around poultry and pigeons, or workers who may handle infected birds in the food processing and marketing business. Care should be taken to avoid dust from feathers and bird-cage contents. No protective vaccination is available.

Nursing Isolation Procedures: Secretion precautions are necessary for the duration of the illness.

ACTINOMYCOSIS

Actinomycosis is a chronic suppurating granulomatous disease, usually caused by an anaerobic grampositive bacterium, *Actinomyces israelii*. This organism may be found in the tonsillar crypts of apparently healthy individuals, as well as in scrapings from teeth and gums and in the gastrointestinal tract. Minor trauma, aspiration, or surgical manipulation may initiate the infectious process. Actinomycosis has traditionally been classified as a mycotic or fungal disease because it characteristically resembles the deep mycoses, but the actinomycetes are now classified as bacteria.

Clinical Manifestations. The characteristic lesions appear as firm, indurated granulomas which spread slowly to adjacent tissues and break down to form multiple sinus tracts which penetrate to the surface. The exudate from the sinus tracts contains the characteristic sulfur granules which are visible masses of the organism.

Actinomycosis of the head and the neck, the most common locations, starts as a swelling in and around the teeth, and extends into the submaxillary region and the neck, producing a flat, hard, painless tumor mass, with a smooth, regular surface and uniform dense consistency, which is fixed firmly to the jawbone. From this mass a firm nodular induration extends into the neck, covered by skin that is wrinkled and dusky red in color. Later this granuloma breaks down, and becomes riddled with abscesses which perforate externally. The process may extend into the cheek, skull, and brain.

In the abdominal type, any viscera may be affected, including the pelvic organs, especially the ovaries and the tubes, but most commonly the appendix and the cecum. Here, in time, an uneven tumor mass develops, resembling carcinoma. The tumor may spread, involving the abdominal wall and discharging externally through open sinuses.

In the thoracic form, induced by inhaling actinomyces spores, the acute and chronic inflammatory reaction may involve the lungs, pleura, mediastinum, or chest wall, producing chest pain, fever, cough, and hemoptysis.

Management. Actinomycotic lesions respond to penicillin, which is the drug of choice. Large doses are given daily, without interruption for weeks to months. Alternate antibiotics are given if the patient is allergic to penicillin. Surgical drainage and resection of damaged tissues, and excision of sinuses and fistulous tracts may be required.

Nursing Isolation Procedures: For draining lesions, secretion precautions are necessary until the wound stops draining.

RAT-BITE FEVER

Rat-bite fever is caused by *Streptobacillus moniliformis* or *Spirillum minus,* bacteria which are found in the normal oropharyngeal flora of rodents. The patient will give a history of rodent contact followed by signs of intermittent fever, skin rash, and lymphadenitis. However, there are different manifestations between streptobacillary fever and spirillar fever.

Streptobacillary fever, caused by the gram-negative bacillus *Streptobacillus moniliformis,* is the major cause of rat-bite fever in the United States and may be acquired by the bite of a rat, mouse, weasel, cat, or squirrel.

Within a week to three weeks following the infecting bite, the patient develops fever, chills, malaise, and headache. A maculopapular or petechial rash may appear, along with polyarthritis.

Management. The wound is cleansed with a topical anesthetic agent, and some form of antimicrobial is prescribed. Penicillin is the drug of choice, while tetracycline or erythromycin are effective for persons who are allergic to penicillin. Usually the patient responds quickly to therapy.

SPIROCHETAL INFECTIONS

SYPHILIS (LUES)

Syphilis is an acute and chronic infectious disease caused by *Treponema pallidum* (a spirochete). It is acquired by sexual contact, or may be congenital in origin.

A single initial lesion appears at the point where the treponemata entered the body; widespread transistory cutaneous and visceral manifestations then appear, and, years later, scattered destructive granulomatous lesions develop.

Treponema pallidum is a threadlike, actively motile spirochete 6 to 20 micra long, which always produces its effects locally—never at a distance, as through toxins. It is killed quickly by a few minutes' exposure to cold or drying.

Open, untreated lesions contain spirochetes. These sores and any infected material are capable of transmitting the disease. In the pregnant woman, the fetus is infected from the mother by way of the placenta. The vast majority of cases are contracted through sexual intercourse; the danger of transmission by direct contact is greatest in the first 4 years of the disease.

Syphilitic infection arouses powerful forces of resistance in the recipient, and temporary immunity to further infection develops early in the course of the disease. Probably 10 to 15 percent of untreated cases of syphilis go on to develop manifestations many years later in the central nervous system, heart, bone, skin, and viscera.

Community and Epidemiologic Aspects

Following the development of penicillin therapy in the 1940s, the incidence of reported cases of syphilis fell dramatically. Relaxation of concern has led to a rising incidence again in recent years, leaving no doubt that the disease is far from being eradicated and that there is still a need for mass screening and strong epidemiologic measures. New cases today are seen particularly among teenage groups, young people, homosexuals, and the lower socioeconomic classes. It is more prevalent in males than females, and more cases are seen in the large urban centers. Each person with syphilis is a potential source for a small outbreak, since each infected individual has an average of 4.6 recent contacts, 2 of whom are infected.

Epidemiologic measures are geared to trace the source and spread of the disease by interviewing known patients for sexual contacts. Rapid investigation must be done to identify these contacts within a minimal time period, to prevent the further spread of the disease. Then all known contacts must receive preventive treatment.

Diagnostic Evaluation

Since syphilis is the great imitator of many diseases, the clinical history and laboratory evaluation are very important.

There are two types of serologic tests:

1. *Nontreponemal* or *reagin tests* are screening tests which detect antibodylike substances called reagin found in the serum of infected patients. The most widely used are the Venereal Disease Research Laboratory (VDRL) slide test and the rapid plasma reagin (RPR) card tests. Both tests are highly reliable and low in cost.

2. *Treponemal tests* are tests to measure specific antibodies to *Treponema pallidum*. These tests are recommended for patients who have reactive reagin tests and atypical signs of primary or secondary syphilis and for diagnosis of late syphilis. The treponemal tests are the fluorescent treponemal antibody absorption test (FTA-ABS) and the microhemagglutination test (MHA-TP).

Clinical Manifestations

Syphilis is capable of destroying tissue in almost any organ in the body, so that a wide variety of clinical manifestations are produced. Some of the manifestations of syphilis are designated as early and others as late. The time interval between early and late syphilis is about 4 years, during which period the patient has developed a partial immunity and an altered tissue response to the spirochete.

The incubation period is 10 to 90 days, with an average of 21 days. No symptoms or lesions are noted. However, the patient's blood contains the spirochetes and is infective.

Primary Stage. During the *primary (early) stage,* the most infectious stage, the chancre, or primary sore, appears at the site where the treponema enters the body — genitalia, rectum, oral cavity, breasts and fingers (Fig. 60-5) — generally related to the pattern of sexual behavior. The typical primary sore (chancre) is an indurated, painless papule which becomes eroded and heals after 4 to 6 weeks. In some patients no primary sore can be found. Invariably, the regional lymph nodes become enlarged. Serologic tests usually become positive shortly after the appearance of the chancre. In the untreated patient, the chancre heals within 3 to 6 weeks.

Even before the chancre appears, and while it is present, the treponema have begun to spread throughout the entire body by way of the lymph system and bloodstream. Some patients become listless, run a slight fever, and lose weight; others show no symptoms during this period of general dissemination.

Secondary Syphilis. In 6 to 8 weeks following the appearance of the chancre, the so-called secondary symptoms appear. These include cutaneous manifestations (see below), generalized enlarged lymph nodes and painful joints, as well as enlargement of the spleen and liver. Acute iritis in some patients may be the first and only symptom. Sometimes there is hoarseness and chronic sore throat.

The skin manifestations (which may fail to appear) vary to such a degree that they may simulate practically every known skin disease. However, certain features are more or less common to all variations: the lesions are bilaterally symmetrical in distribution, and the distribution is generalized; the eruptions are almost invariable polymorphous (that is, almost never are the skin lesions of any one type only, as macules alone, or papules alone); although they last for weeks, they cause no itching and no pain. If untreated, they gradually fade. If treated, they disappear quickly. Concomitantly, the hair often drops out, sometimes in patches, giving the scalp a motheaten appearance.

The macular eruption, which usually appears early, may cover the entire trunk, sparing the face. It may be merely a diffuse rosy blush, rose-colored spots, or an eruption of slightly elevated copper-colored macules. Papular luetic lesions, covered with scales, may appear on

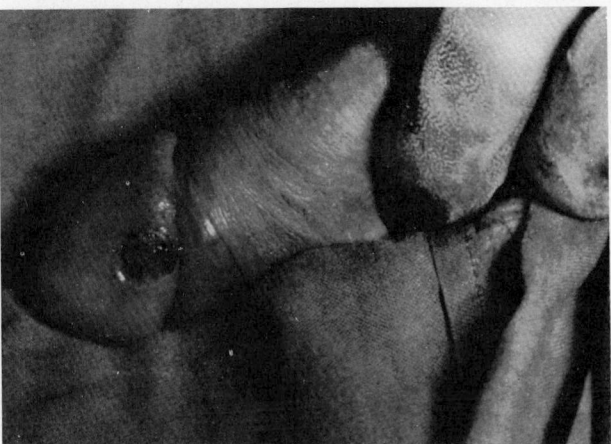

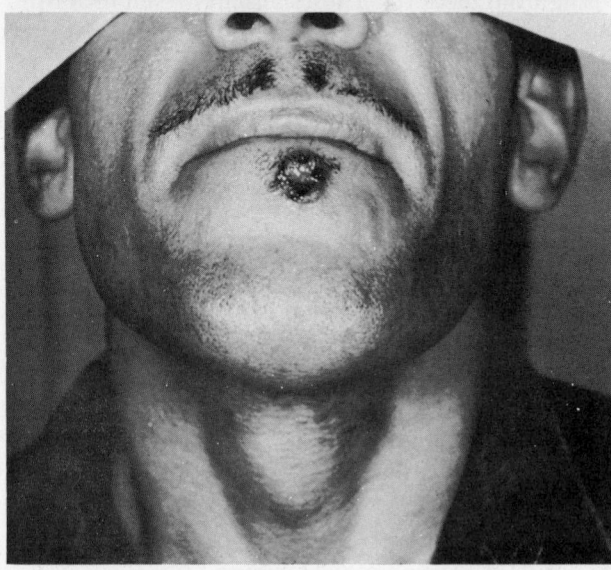

Figure 60-5. (*Top*) Syphilitic chancre on the external surface of the prepuce. (From Elliott, H., and Rhyz, K.: Venereal Diseases: Treatment and Nursing. London, Bailliere Tindall, 1972.) (*Bottom*) Primary syphilis. Typical Hunterian chancre on lower lip. (From Syphilis—A Synopsis. U.S. Department of Health, Education and Welfare, Public Health Service)

the body surface. These papules are prone to become secondarily infected, and the resultant pustular eruption may resemble acne vulgaris, impetigo, or even smallpox. Nodular skin lesions—small, bluish-red or brown in color—also may develop. These nodules may persist for years and, on disappearing, leave areas of pigmentation.

The lesions that develop on moist skin surfaces, for example, about the anus or genitalia, take the form of broad wartlike plaques (the so-called condylomata), which tend to crack and ulcerate. Those that appear on the mucous membranes of the mouth and the tongue are glistening, slightly elevated, flat circumscribed patches, usually covered with a white or yellowish exudate. These papules, the so-called mucous patches, are the most characteristic, persistent, and infectious of all luetic lesions. Other papules, dry and scaly in character, develop on the palms and the soles. Those on the fingertips occasionally destroy the bed of the nails, which become brittle and fissured.

Late Syphilis. After the early manifestations disappear (in untreated, or inadequately treated patients) there follows a period of apparent good health. Many patients have no further trouble, with or without treatment. But in some people, after 3 to 10 years or longer, signs of late (formerly called *tertiary*) syphilitic lesions appear. These granulomatous lesions are found mainly in the skin and bones, but may also involve the liver, cardiovascular system, and central nervous system. In fact, any organ of the body may be attacked. The inflammatory reaction may involve the heart and great vessels, with lesions occurring in the aorta, pulmonary artery, or great vessels arising from the aorta. The lesions may result in aortitis and aneurysm. Syphilis invades the central nervous system during the early stage of the infection, but in the absence of treatment some patients will develop symptomatic neurosyphilis, including meningovascular and/or parenchymatous syphilis. Meningovascular syphilis results in cerebrovascular occlusion, infarction, and encephalomalacia, while the parenchymatous form includes syphilitic paresis and tabes dorsalis, with personality changes and varing neurologic signs.

The skin lesions of late syphilis produce large, deep, punched-out ulcers on the lower legs; upon healing, these leave characteristic scars with sinuous borders, pigmented areolae, and atrophied bases. On the arm, the lesions seen around the elbow consist of peculiar many-layered crusts. The lesions in the mouth, the throat, and the nose ulcerate and perforate the soft palate or the septum and give rise to the "saddle-nose" appearance and the diffuse thickening of the tongue.

Management

The Public Health Service recommends the following treatment schedule, according to the stage of syphilis:*

*Center for Disease Control: Recommended Treatment Schedules for Syphilis, 1976.

Early Syphilis (primary, secondary, latent syphilis of less than one year's duration)
- Benzathine penicillin G—2.4 million units total by intramuscular injection at a single session. (This is the drug of choice because it provides effective treatment in a single visit.)

    OR
- Aqueous procaine penicillin G—4.8 million units total: 600,000 units by intramuscular injection daily for 8 days.

    OR
- Procaine penicillin G in oil with 2 percent aluminum monostearate (PAM)—4.8 million units total by intramuscular injection: 2.4 million units at first visit, and 1.2 million units at each of two subsequent visits 3 days apart.

Patients who are allergic to penicillin are given tetracycline or erythromycin according to a schedule advocated by the Public Health Service.

Treatment of syphilis of more than one year's duration:
In general, treatment schedules for syphilis of greater than one year's duration require higher-dose therapy. This includes:
- Benzathine penicillin G—7.2 million units total: 2.4 million units by intramuscular injection weekly for three successive weeks

    OR
- Aqueous procaine penicillin G—9.0 million units total: 600,000 units by intramuscular injection daily for 15 days.

Although therapy is recommended for established cardiovascular syphilis, there is little evidence that antibiotics reverse the pathology associated with this disease. Cerebrospinal fluid (CSF) examination is mandatory in patients with suspected symptomatic neurosyphilis and is also desirable in other patients with syphilis greater than one year's duration, to exclude asymptomatic neurosyphilis.

Prevention: Patient Education
1. Patients who have been exposed to infectious syphilis within the preceding 3 months should be treated as for early syphilis.
2. All patients with early syphilis should return for repeat nontreponemal tests 3, 6, and 12 months after treatment. Patients with syphilis of more than one year's duration should, in addition, have a serologic test 24 months after treatment.
3. The patient is to be instructed to refrain from sexual contact with previous partners not under treatment.
4. A program of sex education and epidemiologic screening should be ongoing. Mass screening of special groups with a known high incidence of venereal disease should be conducted.

Nursing Isolation Procedures: If the patient has skin and mucous membrane manifestations, secretion precautions (page 1366) are carried out until 24 hours after initiation of effective therapy.

VIRAL INFECTIONS

NATURE OF VIRUSES

Viruses are submicroscopic particles that pass through bacterial filters. They are known as filtrable particles or filtrable viruses and can be visualized only by electron microscopy. Viruses may be made of RNA or DNA. They cannot propagate outside living tissue, but require tissue cells of the host or tissue culture preparations (in contrast to bacteria, which will grow on artificial culture media). Viruses infect cells and cause disease by subverting the cellular metabolism to their own needs for growth. The infected cell is often killed in the process. Like bacteria, viruses are antigenic and stimulate the host to produce antibodies. This fact is useful both as an aid to diagnosis and in conferring immunity to the same disease. It is not known why one virus will infect the respiratory tract and another the central nervous system; they tend to be specific in the type of cells they invade.

Viruses may infect the human being from embryo stage throughout life, though particularly during childhood. The severity of the initial virus infection tends to increase with increasing age (except for the neonatal period). For example, poliomyelitis and viral hepatitis have more severe sequellae in adults than in children. Some viruses, like that of herpes simplex, maintain a persistent presence in the host and recur from time to time, especially in the presence of other illness (e.g., the fever blisters in pneumonia are reactivations of latent herpes simplex infection and are activated by the febrile illness of pneumonia). Currently, viruses are not susceptible to antibiotics or chemotherapy, but prophylactic vaccines are available for many of them.

INFLUENZA

Influenza is an acute infectious disease caused by an RNA-containing myxovirus. It is characterized by respiratory and constitutional symptoms. It has swept through the entire civilized world approximately every 20 years, attacking as many as 40 percent of the people in the affected areas. The striking features of these epidemics have been the speed with which they have spread and an extremely high attack rate.

Typical epidemics of influenza have been characterized by three successive waves, separated by brief intermissions. The first wave lasts from 3 to 6 weeks, is explosive in outbreak, widespread, and mild in form in the majority of cases, with few complications. The second wave also is widespread, but lasts longer; the cases are more severe, and the complications are serious. The third wave lasts still longer (from 8 to 10 weeks), involves fewer persons, but the complications are quite severe. During the years succeeding a major epidemic, there follow scattered local waves of decreasing severity, with sporadic cases of influenza occurring during the intervals.

Etiology

The primary factor in the etiology of influenza is a filtrable virus, of which three major strains have been isolated, designated Types A, B, and C. Type A is the major pathogen in humans. The numerous variants within a given type are called subtypes.

It is difficult to control influenza because the surface antigens of the virus have the capacity to undergo antigenic variation. Major antigenic shifts and new human pandemic influenza strains arise from time to time. Therefore, previously acquired antibodies against earlier influenza strains may not be effective against the new emerging strain, depending upon the extent of the surface change. Recent pandemic outbreaks have been caused by an antigenic variant of Type A (Victoria, Texas, Swine influenza, Russian "flu"). It has been observed that when a new influenza virus strain becomes prevalent throughout the country, the old virus strain disappears.

Transmission is by close contact or by droplets from the respiratory tract of an infected person. The virus is airborne and multiplies in the upper respiratory tract, invading the nasal, tracheal, and bronchial mucosal cells.

Clinical Manifestations

In the majority of patients, influenza begins as an acute coryza, after a short incubation period of approximately 2 days (range of 1 to 4 days). The patient has fever, either low-grade or as high as 41.1° C. (106° F.), headache, and profound malaise. Respiratory features include a dry cough, sore throat, nasal obstruction, and discharge. Aching occurs in the substernal area and the muscles, especially in the back and legs. Other patients start with acute sinusitis, bronchitis, pleurisy, or bronchopneumonia. These symptoms are always abrupt in onset, and prostrating. In still another group there are gastrointestinal symptoms of nausea, vomiting, abdominal pain, and diarrhea; and finally, in each epidemic, cases develop without local symptoms but with chills or a continuous fever. The patient usually recovers within a week if there are no complications.

Complications. Persons at risk of developing the complications of influenza are the elderly (over 65), persons with chronic pulmonary or cardiac disease (especially rheumatic valve disease), and those with diabetes or other chronic metabolic disorders or chronic renal disease. The influenza virus damages the ciliated epithelium of the tracheobronchial tree, rendering the patient vulnerable to the development of secondary invaders such as pneumococci or staphylococci, *Hemophilus influenzae,* various streptococci, and other organisms.

Dyspnea early in the course of the disease points to bronchopneumonia, which is potentially life-threatening. This pneumonia may be viral, mixed viral, or bacterial in origin. Other symptoms include coughing of viscid sputum, tachycardia, and cyanosis. Vigorous supportive care is indicated, including tracheal aspiration, oxygen, and possibly mechanical ventilation. Other complications include myocarditis, myositis, and meningoencephalitis.

Management

The objectives of treatment are to give symptomatic management and to prevent and treat complications. There is no specific treatment for influenza. Usually the patient will go to bed because of prostration. Antipyretics and analgesics, such as aspirin, will reduce fever and relieve headache and myalgia. Such drugs should be taken regularly to avoid marked swings of temperature with sweating and chills, leading to exhaustion and dehydration. When the patient resumes activities, he should be sure that any sense of well-being and reduction of temperature are not being caused by the aspirin.

Cough syrup may be soothing for a dry, hacking cough. A vaporizer is helpful in reducing irritation of the respiratory mucosa. A liberal fluid intake is advised because of fever.

Prevention and Patient Education. Active immunization consists of a single dose of influenza virus vaccine for either primary or annual booster vaccination. However, influenza vaccination has not been recommended as a routine primary procedure because uncomplicated influenza is a self-limited disease with a low mortality rate. The effectiveness of influenza vaccine has been variable, and protection has been relatively brief. Recent vaccine has more antigen than prior products and should give better results. However, annual vaccination is recommended for high-risk persons. Influenza vaccine should be given by mid-November.

The National Influenza Immunization Program of 1976 revealed an association of Guillain-Barré Syndrome with influenza vaccination; the syndrome appears 10 to 12 times more frequently in vaccinated persons than in unvaccinated individuals.

The risk of developing influenza is also related to crowding and close contact of groups of individuals. Therefore, visiting privileges within health care facilities should be restricted during epidemics to minimize any chance of introducing influenza.

Amantadine hydrochloride (Symmetrel), an antiviral drug, can prevent clinical infection with influenza A virus. (It blocks an early step in the replication of this virus.) It is given only to certain high-risk patients, since most patients exposed to influenza require no prophylaxis. Amantadine is also given for the treatment of symptomatic influenza A infection and may shorten the duration and diminish the severity of illness. Adverse effects, occurring mainly in the elderly, include central nervous system toxicity, confusion, dizziness, slurred speech, headache, sleep disturbances, and visual hallucinations. To be effective, amantadine should be given prior to, and for the duration of exposure to type A influenza virus.

Nursing Isolation Procedure: No isolation or precautions are necessary for the usual patient. There may be instances when respiratory isolation is indicated, especially if the diagnosis can be made on admission, or shortly thereafter.

INFECTIOUS MONONUCLEOSIS

Infectious mononucleosis ("mono," glandular fever) is an acute infectious disease of the lymphatic system caused by the Epstein-Barr virus (EBV), a DNA virus of the herpes virus group. Another virus, cytomegalovirus, can cause virtually identical symptoms. A third infecting organism, Toxoplasma (a protozoan) can also produce a similar clinical picture.

Epidemiology and Clinical Manifestations

Epidemiology. Infectious mononucleosis is encountered most frequently in the 15 to 25 age group. It has been shown that when natural primary infection with EBV develops in childhood, a mild and nonspecific or inapparent illness occurs, and the child has immunity for many years. Infectious mononucleosis only occurs in individuals without antibody to EBV. If natural primary infection does not take place in childhood and a susceptible person (adolescent/young adult) acquires the infection, this event will lead to clinical manifestations of infectious mononucleosis in about 50 percent of cases. Thus infectious mononucleosis is more frequently encountered in countries with a high standard of living, whereas in developing countries or among deprived socioeconomic groups, primary infection almost always occurs in early childhood, so that the disease is virtually unknown. In this country, in persons of college age, the rate of clinical attack is 3 to 5 times that of the population at large.

Transmission of infectious mononucleosis is by oral contact. The virus may persist in the pharynx for weeks or months. This suggests that a large number of young adults are probably convalescent carriers of this disease. The virus can also be spread by blood transfusion. The incubation period ranges from 30 to 50 days.

Clinical Manifestations. The early clinical manifestations are usually vague and masquerade as those of streptococcal sore throat, leukemia, and hepatitis. The triad of fever, sore throat, and cervical lymphadenopathy suggests infectious mononucleosis. A typical attack begins with fever and chills, anorexia, sore throat, and myalgia. Headache and diarrhea are often seen. On the second or third day, the lymph nodes begin to swell and become tender, usually the posterior cervical group first, and then the anterior groups. This causes pain in the neck. Generalized lymphadenopathy may occur. Early in the course of the disease, supraorbital edema occurs and the spleen enlarges in 50 to 75 percent of patients. Although hepatomegaly occurs in less than 25 percent of patients, the majority of patients have abnormal liver-function tests. A faint erythematous or maculopapular eruption may appear in the early stage of the disease.

Diagnostic Evaluation. The diagnosis is made on the basis of the typical picture of clinical illness, as well as such laboratory findings as lymphocytosis with many atypical lymphocytes, abnormal liver-function tests, a positive heterophil antibody test, and the persistence of antibody to Epstein-Barr virus. In the heterophil test (positive in 90 percent of cases), heterophil antibodies in a small amount of blood from the patient with infectious mononucleosis will clump red blood cells from sheep or horses. This test can now be done in less than 3 minutes in the physician's office, using a specially prepared slide on which there are sheep or horse red blood cells stabilized by formaldehyde. (Heterophil-negative disease has been reported.) Antibodies to Epstein-Barr virus also develop, and a blood test can identify EBV-specific IgM and IgG antibodies.

Management

The treatment is symptomatic and supportive. The patient is encouraged to remain on bed rest while fever lasts and to rest at intervals during recovery. Aspirin is given for headache and muscle pains. Steroids may be used when severe or life-threatening complications develop—marked hepatic dysfunction, neurological manifestations, thrombocytopenia, hemolytic anemia, and airway obstruction. Most patients recover in 1 to 3 weeks.

Patient Education. The enlarged spleen of the patient with infectious mononucleosis is vulnerable to injury and may rupture if subjected to relatively mild trauma. Thus strenuous physical activity and competitive sports should be avoided until recovery is complete. For the athlete, this may mean up to 6 months. However, the exact length of time is uncertain, since the spleen may rupture after clinical, hematologic, and serologic evidence reveals complete recovery.

The consequences of a ruptured spleen are potentially serious because of the substantial volume of blood that may be lost into the peritoneal cavity. Abdominal pain usually heralds the presence of splenic rupture. The presence of free intraperitoneal blood may irritate the diaphragm and may cause shoulder pain. The treatment is blood transfusions and immediate splenectomy.

RABIES (HYDROPHOBIA)

Rabies is a severe viral infection of the central nervous system communicated to humans from the saliva of infected animals and commonly transmitted by a bite or by contact of the animal's saliva with a mucous membrane or open wound. The disease occurs among wildlife, especially skunks, foxes, raccoons, and bats, and is becoming more prominent. The rabies virus is classified with the rhabdoviruses. The virus is spread from the wound to the central nervous system by way of the nerves.

Rabies in Animals. Early signs of rabies in animals include an altered disposition, fever, loss of appetite, and a change in the tone of bark (in dogs).

Dogs, fortunately, usually present evidence of the disease before becoming infective. The etiologic agent is an ultramicroscopic virus present in the saliva and the central nervous sytem. Negri bodies (round objects about one-quarter the size of red blood corpuscles) are found in the brain tissues so constantly in this disease that their presence is sufficient for diagnosis.

The course of rabies in dogs is characterized by an incubation period of 14 to 30 days. This is followed by a period of restlessness, agitation, and excitement, when the animal becomes vicious. The excitement stage may not be evident at all or may be entirely absent. Paralysis then develops, first involving the hind legs and thereafter becoming general. Death occurs within 10 days following the first symptom.

Diagnostic Evaluation. The diagnosis is made on the basis of the history of exposure (the patient was bitten by an animal), the development of characteristic symptoms, and the demonstration of rabies antibodies in the patient's blood, along with the characteristic Negri bodies in samples of brain tissue taken from the infected animal.

Prophylactic Management

Local Treatment of Wound. The bite wounds should be cleansed immediately and thoroughly with soap and water to remove the saliva from the area. Squeezing the wound to make it bleed helps cleanse it. The patient is then taken immediately for emergency treatment, at which time the wound is cleansed with aqueous benzalkonium chloride (Zephiran). The patient is given tetanus prophylaxis and antibacterial therapy to counter any other possible infection transmitted by the animal.

Postexposure Prophylaxis. The decision to give postexposure treatment is made on an individual basis and depends on the species of the animal, the circumstances surrounding the exposure incident, the vaccination status of the animal, and the presence of rabies in the region.

A combination of passive and active immunization (immune globulin and vaccine) is recommended for the treatment of patients bitten by animals suspected of having rabies and for nonbite exposure inflicted by animals suspected of being rabid.

Human Rabies Immune Globulin (RIG) is administered once at the beginning of antirabies therapy. Part of the RIG dose is infiltrated around the wound and the rest is administered intramuscularly in the patient's buttock. If RIG is not available, antirabies serum (equine) (ARS) is given, although adverse reactions are more frequently associated with ARS. Active immunization with duck embryo rabies vaccine (DEV) is given in conjunction with either RIG or ARS. A total of 23 doses is given, beginning on the day passive immunization is administered. It is given subcutaneously in the abdomen, lower back, or lateral aspects of the thighs. The schedule of administration may be 21 daily doses or 14 doses in the first 7 days (two injections per day) and then 7 daily doses. This is followed by 2 booster doses given according to the product insert directives.

Local reactions to DEV include immediate pain, stinging and/or burning at the injection site, and local erythema and tenderness. The vaccine schedule may be discontinued if fluorescent antibody (FA) tests of the animal killed at the time of the attack are negative.

A new rabies vaccine (human diploid cell strain rabies vaccine) has been developed by inactivating a strain of rabies grown in human cell tissue. It is claimed to give a higher level of protection against rabies and produces minimal adverse reaction, compared to existing duck embryo vaccine. It is currently being used in human field trials in the United States and Israel.

Management of the Biting Animal. The animal inflicting the bite is captured (if possible) and kept under surveillance. This may enable the bitten person to avoid undergoing unnecessary rabies vaccination. If the animal remains healthy for 7 to 10 days it is assumed that it was not infective.

However, if the animal becomes sick, the health department is notified. The animal is humanely killed, and its head shipped, under refrigeration, to a qualified laboratory where the brain is examined for the characteristic Negri bodies. A wild animal that bites a person without provocation is killed at once, and the brain sent for examination. If the brain of the animal is negative for rabies (by fluorescent antibody examination) it is assumed that the saliva contained no virus and that the bitten person need not be treated.

Clinical Course in Man. The incubation period in humans is extremely variable, depending on the location and severity of the wound and the length of the nerve over which the virus must travel before it reaches the brain. The incubation period may only be 10 days to several weeks for bites around the face, or from 60 to 90 days and up to a year for a bite in another part of the body.

There are several clinical phases of rabies in humans. During the prodromal phase of the illness there are abnormal sensations around the site of infection, and the individual experiences an uneasy feeling, accompanied by depression and irritability. The patient may have headache, nausea, sore throat, and loss of appetite, or may experience unusual sensitivity to sound, light, and changes in temperature.

Then follows the stage of excitement. There are episodes of irrational excitement alternating with periods of alert calm. During this stage, convulsions occur. Attempting to swallow or even looking at liquids induces such severe and painful spasms of the muscles of swallowing and respiration that the patient writhes and the ensuing choking may produce apnea. (Hence the older name for rabies is *hydrophobia,* or fear of water.)

If the patient survives this stage, the muscle spasms and agitation cease. The paralytic phase is one of usually progressive ascending paralysis terminating in coma and death.

Management

There is no specific treatment for rabies, and the care of the patient is supportive. Barbiturates, phenothiazines, and paraldehyde are used symptomatically. The patient is placed in the intensive care unit and receives continuing cardiac and pulmonary monitoring. The room should be quiet and darkened. The outcome is usually fatal.

- Bear in mind that the rabies virus is contained in the saliva of patients with this disease, constituting a distinct hazard to personnel caring for him. All personnel must be on guard against being bitten by such a patient or allowing saliva to contaminate a skin abrasion. If this occurs, personnel must receive the same treatment as the patient, including antirabic serum and rabies vaccine.

Nursing Isolation Procedure: Strict isolation precautions are carried out for the duration of the illness.

RICKETTSIAL INFECTIONS

RICKETTSIAE

The rickettsial diseases, of which the three most common on this continent are typhus fever, Rocky Mountain spotted fever, and trench fever, are named after Dr. H. T. Ricketts, in honor of his pioneering work in this field. They are vermin-spread infections caused by tiny organisms found in the patient's tissues and in the bodies of insect vectors, such as ticks, fleas, and lice. As in the case of viruses, these organisms make their habitat, thrive, and produce their effect within the tissue cells, as contrasted with the bacteria, whose activities are extracellular. Like viruses, the rickettsiae cannot live apart from animal cells, and their culture, to date, has proved impossible in artificial media other than that containing live tissue. It is obvious from this fact that the survival of these organisms in nature depends on the accessibility of suitable living hosts, or *reservoirs,* such as rodents, monkeys, dogs, dog ticks, and wood ticks. Individuals harboring rickettsiae are likely to exhibit fever and skin eruptions and to be afflicted with disorders of the central nervous system.

Typical of all rickettsial infections is the appearance in the blood serum of a bacterial agglutinin that has the property of agglutinating bacilli of the Proteus OX group. (The reason for this is obscure, for there is no other relationship known between Proteus OX and the rickettsiae.) The phenomenon is the basis for a diagnostic test known as the Weil-Felix test, useful in differentiating this group of diseases, as a whole, from other infectious diseases. A more specific serologic test, such as the complement fixation test, appears to be more accurate. Fur-

TABLE 60-7. SUMMARY OF SOME EPIDEMIOLOGIC FEATURES OF SELECTED RICKETTSIAL DISEASES OF MAN

DISEASE	ORGANISM	NATURAL CYCLE		USUAL MODE OF TRANSMISSION TO MAN	COMMON OCCUPATIONAL OR ENVIRONMENTAL ASSOCIATION	GEOGRAPHIC DISTRIBUTION
		Arthropod Vector	*Reservoir/* Mammalian Host			
Typhus group						
Murine typhus	*Rickettsia mooseri* (*R. typhi*)	Flea	Rodents	Infected flea feces into broken skin or aerosol to mucous membranes	Rat-infested premises (shops, warehouses, grain elevators)	Scattered foci, worldwide
Epidemic typhus	*R. prowazekii*	Body louse	Man*	Infected crushed louse or feces into broken skin or aerosol to mucous membranes	Lousy human population with louse transfer	Worldwide
Brill's disease	*R. prowazekii*	Recrudescence months to years after primary attack of louse-borne typhus			Unknown; ?stress	Worldwide
Spotted fever group (selected examples)						
Rocky Mountain spotted fever	*R. rickettsii*	Ixodid ticks	Ticks, small mammals	Tick bite, mechanical transfer to mucous membranes, ?airborne	Tick-infested terrain, houses, dogs	Western Hemisphere
Boutonneuse fever	*R. conorii*	Ixodid ticks	Ticks, rodents, dogs	Tick bite	Tick-infested terrain, houses, dogs	Mediterranean, littoral, Africa, ?Indian subcontinent
Rickettsialpox	*R. akari*	Mouse mite	Mite, mice	Mouse mite bite	Unique mouse- and mite-infested premises (incinerators)	United States, U.S.S.R., Korea, ?Central Africa
Scrub typhus						
Tsutsugamushi disease	*R. tsutsugamushi* (multiple serotypes)	Chigger	Chigger, ?rodents	Chigger bite	Chigger-infested terrain; secondary scrub, grass airfields, golf courses	Asia, Australia, New Guinea, Pacific islands
Q fever†	*Coxiella burnetii*	?Ticks	Ticks, mammals	Inhalation of dried airborne infective material; ?tick bite	Domestic animals or products, dairies, lambing pens, slaughterhouses	Worldwide
Trench fever†	*Rochalimaea quintana*	Body louse	Man	Infected crushed louse or feces into broken skin; ?aerosol to mucous membranes	Lousy human population with louse transfer	Africa, Mexico, ?South America, ?Eastern Europe

(From Beeson, P. B., McDermott, W., and Wyngaarden, J. W.: Cecil Textbook of Medicine, 15th ed., Philadelphia, W. B. Saunders, 1979)

*Recent isolations of putative *R. prowazekii* from flying squirrels in the eastern United States have not been evaluated as reservoirs for human infection. Previous claims of involvement of domestic animals are now largely discounted.

†Though *C. burnetii* and *R. quintana* are not strictly "rickettsiae" and Q fever and trench fever differ clinically from the others, they are conventionally considered with the rickettsiae.

ther differentiation of one rickettsial disease from another is made possible by the use of tissue cultures and protection tests (inoculating suspected material into susceptible animals previously vaccinated with rickettsiae of known identity).

A summary of certain important epidemiological and clinical characteristics of rickettsial diseases is found in Table 60-7.

ROCKY MOUNTAIN SPOTTED FEVER

Rocky Mountain spotted fever (tick-borne typhus fever) is characterized by a continuous fever. It is caused by the bite of an infected tick, by an infected tick being crushed on the skin, or by the conjunctiva becoming contaminated with infected tick juice. The organism responsible is the *Rickettsia rickettsii*.

Clinical Manifestations

During infection in humans, *R. rickettsii* localize and proliferate in the vascular endothelium of small vessels, where they produce widespread swelling and degeneration. This generalized vasculitis accounts for the manifestations of the disease, both the cutaneous lesions and visceral disturbances. It may involve virtually every organ.

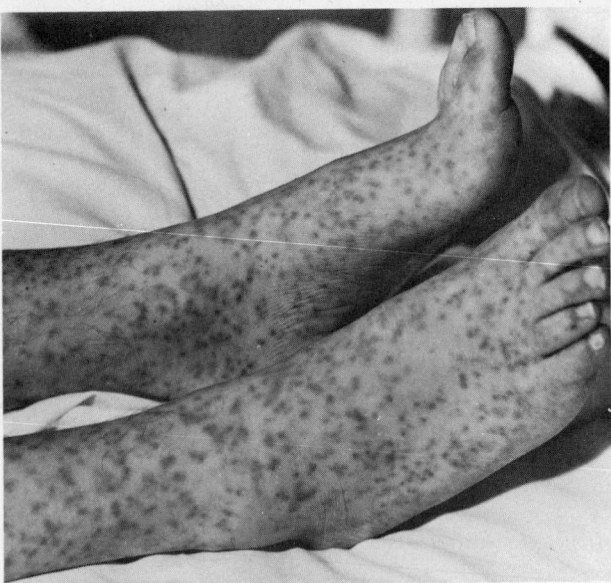

Figure 60-6. The rash of Rocky Mountain Spotted Fever. (Armed Forces Institute of Pathology photograph, Neg. No. N-67987-3)

Early symptoms, appearing several days after an infected tick bite, are severe headache, malaise, anorexia, photophobia, slight fever, and muscle and joint pain. Within a few days, the fever, rash, and edema are quite pronounced. The rash is the most specific manifestation of the infection and consists of rose-colored macules of variable size that appear on the wrists, ankles, soles, and palms, gradually spreading over the entire body. It becomes papular, darker red, and slightly dusky, and after a few days has a petechial or purpuric character (Fig. 60-6). Large subcutaneous hemorrhages may appear. In severe forms of the disease, areas of skin necrosis appear as a result of endarteritis (inflammatory blockage of arterioles). This necrosis may involve the ear lobes, fingers, toes, and scrotum — those areas at the extreme periphery of the vascular system. There may be marked thrombocytopenia due to inflammation of the vessels communicating with the bone marrow. As a result of generalized vascular involvement and resulting escape of serum, generalized edema occurs.

Restlessness, insomnia, and hyperesthesias are distressing symptoms of this disease. Delirium is common at the height of the fever, but convulsions rarely occur. The spleen is large and tender. There are a slight leukocytosis and a slight secondary anemia. Pneumonia may occur. Mental confusion, deafness, and visual disturbances are common and may last for weeks.

The early diagnosis is important and is almost always made on clinical grounds. The Weil-Felix agglutinins and complement fixing antibodies do not rise until 10 to 14 days after the onset of the disease.

Management

One of the tetracyclines or chloramphenicol is effective if administered in the *early* stages of the disease. (Usually one of the tetracyclines is given, since chloramphenicol can produce bone marrow depression.) Rocky Mountain spotted fever can run a rapid and fulminating course, and despite the effectiveness of tetracycline or chloramphenicol in treatment, the morbidity and mortality rates are still significant. Because Rocky Mountain spotted fever is an infectious vasculitis, the patient may display marked physiological disturbances, including circulatory collapse, hypotension, oliguria, azotemia, hypoproteinemia, and edema. Central venous pressure measurements are used to guide fluid and electrolyte replacement. The patient may be given transfusions of packed red blood cells and platelets. Severe coagulation disturbances may be treated with heparin. Supportive nursing measures are used to combat fever, restlessness, and pain, and to promote patient comfort. The majority of patients recover if treated early.

Prevention and Patient Education. Rocky Mountain spotted fever continues to increase in the United States, with 80 percent of the cases occurring in the South Atlantic and South Central States. (The disease has almost vanished from its original home in the Rockies.)

As increasing numbers of Americans participate in backpacking and other camping activities, more people will be exposed to this disease. Important aspects of prevention are wearing protective clothing and conscientiously searching for and removing ticks. Persons living in tick-infested areas, or visiting such places, should examine their scalp, skin, and clothing 2 to 3 times daily for ticks. This is important, as an infected tick must usually be attached and feeding several hours before it can transmit the disease. Tick repellent should be applied to the exposed parts of the body and clothing, especially socks and trouser cuffs and any openings in the clothing (neck, top of pants, button areas).

Ticks may be removed from the body by grasping the tick with tweezers (or if these are not available, a bent twig or the fingers, covered with paper) and pulling it gently and firmly outward from the body. Care should be taken not to crush the tick, thus avoiding contamination of the broken skin with infectious tick secretions. The tick bite should be disinfected immediately. The hands should be protected with gloves or paper while the tick is being removed. Other means of removing a tick are to touch it with gasoline or cover it with a thick ointment. Household pets should be examined for ticks on a regular basis.

The Advisory Committee on Immunization Practices recommends vaccine routinely only for those persons with laboratory exposure to *R. rickettsii* (rickettsiologists and their technicians) and those with regular occupational exposure.

A promising new tissue-culture grown vaccine appears to be more immunogenic than the previously available commercial preparations.

PROTOZOAN INFECTIONS

PROTOZOA

Protozoa are single-celled animals which, despite their unicellular structure, possess protoplasmic devices adapted for several different functions. They are considerably more complicated structurally than are the bacteria. Most of them possess, to varying degrees, the ability to move about under their own power and are equipped with differential tissue structures that enable them to feed, breathe, eject excreta, and attach themselves to other objects.

Varieties of protozoa include the *Sporozoa*, which are without organs of feeding or locomotion; the *Sarcodina*, which move about by means of pseudopodia (temporary projections of their bodies), and the *Mastigophora*, which are protozoa possessing flagella (whiplike appendages) for purposes of locomotion. The Sporozoa of greatest importance to man is the *Plasmodium*, the genus causing malaria. Of the Sarcodina, the most hazardous for humans is of the genus *Entamoeba*, responsible for amebic dysentery. In this country, the most common Mastigophora infestations producing symptoms is that of *Trichomonas vaginalis*, but in Africa and the Orient diseases are found of much more serious consequence, caused by protozoa of this group—for example, kala-azar, caused by the *Leishmania*, and African sleeping sickness, a *Trypanosoma* infection.

MALARIA

Malaria is an acute infectious disease caused by protozoa, which are transmitted by way of an intermediate host, the bite of an infective female *Anopheles* mosquito. This mosquito, resting on a wall, can be recognized at a distance, because instead of standing hunchbacked, as does the ordinary mosquito (*Culex*), it stands with body, thorax, and bill in a straight line, forming with the wall an angle of about 30 degrees. Malaria has also been transmitted via blood transfusions and from the needles and syringes shared by drug addicts.

Incidence. Malaria affects approximately 150 to 200 million people in the world. It is claimed that in Africa, one-fourth of all adults suffer from malarial fever at one time or other. It causes more disability and a heavier economic burden than any other parasitic disease. International travel has been responsible for a resurgence in many nontropical countries.

Types of Malaria. There are four species of malarial parasites, grouped under the generic name *Plasmodium*, each causing a different type of malaria. Each malarial parasite lives within a red blood corpuscle, utilizing the hemoglobin as food. When full grown, it divides (segments) into 10 to 20 small, young parasites, called *hyalines* (or segments), which burst the cell; this bursting of cells causes chills in the patient. The majority of these hyalines die, but a few find their way into new red cells, and the process described above is repeated.

Clinical Manifestations. The majority of patients present with fever, with or without other findings, including chills or sweats, splenomegaly, and anemia. Intense headache and muscle aches, especially in the back, may be present. Paroxysms of chills and fever may last about 12 hours, after which the cycle may be repeated daily, every other day, or every third day.

Patients with severe malaria of any form may become comatose and die (pernicious malaria); they may develop renal failure (due to the precipitation of free hemoglobin in the kidney tubule); a serious gastrointestinal disturbance; or cerebral symptoms (due to an accumulation of the parasites in the blood vessels of the affected organ).

Diagnostic Evaluation. The patient should be asked where he has been. Travel or residence in an endemic area where malaria is endemic is an important diagnostic clue. The diagnosis is confirmed by the finding of the plasmodium in the patient's blood. The blood should be examined as soon as the patient presents for treatment. More than one blood examination may be required, since the diagnosis can be missed on a routine smear.

Management

The objective of treatment is to destroy the blood trophozoites and schizonts of *Plasmodium* that cause the clinical manifestations and the pathologic effects that characterize the disease.

The use of antimalarial drugs depends on the stage of the life cycle of the parasite which is affected. The species of parasite infecting the patient is determined by way of a blood smear. The drugs used to cure the acute attack caused by *P. vivax, P. malariae, P. ovale,* or a chloroquine-sensitive strain of *P. falciparum* is a three-day course of chloroquine phosphate, hydroxychloroquine sulfate, or amodiaquine hydrochloride.

Other supportive measures include the administration of aspirin, to control fever, muscular aches, and headaches, and the lowering of fever by cool sponges. The fluid balance must be appraised on each patient. Complications are treated as they arise.

Unfortunately, *P. falciparum* (especially from Southeast Asia and Central and South America) is often drug-resistant, and the diagnosis is made when the patient is critically ill. Patients with this type of malaria should be hospitalized. In fact, this is considered a medical emergency. If the patient comes from an area known to harbor drug-resistant malaria, the treatment is quinine (orally if possible, or by slow infusion in severely ill patients), pyrimethamine, or one of the sulfonamides. A new synthetic quininelike drug, mefloquine, is being used in clinical trials and appears successful in treating strains of *Plasmodium* that are resistant to chloroquine.

Oxygen may be given, as tissue anoxia is thought to be common. Jaundice is evaluated and is related to the density of *P. falciparum* parasitemia (presence of malarial parasites in the blood). Abnormalities of hepatic function are common in this type of malaria. The degree of anemia is related to the severity of infection. Abnormal bleeding (nosebleeds, oozing of blood from venipuncture sites, passage of blood in the stool) may be due either to decreased production of clotting factors by a damaged liver or to disseminated intravascular coagulation.

Nursing Isolation Procedures: Blood precautions should be used for the duration of the patient's hospitalization. A screened room is required for the patient who is ill in a tropical climate.

Prevention and Patient Education. The essence of malaria control is the eradication of malaria as an endemic disease. In several areas of the world, this goal has been achieved. To escape malaria, one must avoid *Anopheles* mosquitos that have fed on the blood of patients with malaria about 3 weeks previously. To protect against these mosquitoes, houses should be well screened, pools of stagnant water (in which mosquitoes breed) must be eliminated, and walls of dwellings (where mosquitoes habitually rest) should be sprayed.

The Center for Disease Control (Atlanta, Georgia) publishes *Health Information for International Travel,* which lists the areas of the world where there is risk of infection with malaria, and also the areas with strains of *Plasmodium falciparum* that are resistant to chloroquine. The drugs of choice for prophylaxis for persons traveling to malarious areas are chloroquine phosphate, amodiaquine, or hydroxychloroquine. The drug is taken once a week, beginning two weeks before entering the malarious area and continued once a week for six weeks after leaving the area. Primaquine may be taken on return to prevent infection with *P. vivax* or *P. ovale.* There are alternative regimens.

AMEBIASIS (AMEBIC DYSENTERY)

Amebae are protozoa, larger than leukocytes, which move by ameboid action. Only a few amebae infect man. One of the most important of these is *Entamoeba histolytica,* the cause of amebic dysentery. These amebae survive outside the body in resistant encysted forms.

Amebiasis is a worldwide parasitic disease of the large intestine. It is acquired through the ingestion of the cyst stage of *Entamoeba histolytica* in food or water contaminated by infected human feces, flies, or the hands of infected food handlers.

In parts of the world where there is lack of hygiene and sanitation, infection rates of 50 percent or more occur. In the United States, the average rate of infection is 2 to 5 percent, and the mode of transmission is usually person-to-person. Persons at risk in this country are immigrants and visitors from developing countries, travelers returning from these areas, and people who are institutionalized.

Pathophysiology. The amebae burrow their way into the intestinal mucosa, where they feed mainly on bacteria. Pus pockets may form, with only a small orifice opening into the bowel from which numerous burrows extend for considerable distances in all directions under the mucous membrane. Here the amebae live. Abscesses form in the mucous membrane, and eventually slough off, exposing an underlying ulcer which may enlarge to sizes of 1 to 2 cm. in diameter. The large bowel may be so covered by such ulcers that very little normal mucous membrane is left. Usually the floor of these ulcers is the muscle wall of the bowel, but they may perforate its entire wall and cause fatal peritonitis.

In the small intestine, the organism may erode intestinal mucosa, invade the bloodstream, and gain access to the liver through the portal vein.

Clinical Manifestations and Course. The clinical manifestations depend on the site of involvement. In some instances, the patient may be asymptomatic. If the intestines have been affected, the chief symptoms are diarrhea, with abdominal cramping and pain. Diarrhea may be mild, with loose stools, or there may be severe dysentery with stools containing considerable amounts of blood, exudate, and mucus, the latter swarming with amebae. Persons with chronic disease usually have associated weight loss and anemia.

The two important features of this disease are its chronicity (one attack of acute dysentery following another, separated by periods of constipation which lasts for months) and the tendency of the infection to cause liver abscess, as a result of metastases to the liver by way of the portal vein. Complications include peritonitis, abscess formation, hemorrhage, and extraintestinal disease.

The diagnosis is made by finding trophozoites or cysts in fecal samples within an hour after passage. Rectal biopsy may reveal the organism. If the test is suspected as being falsely negative, there are serological techniques available to detect amebiasis.

Management

The objectives of treatment are to eradicate the organism, to give symptomatic relief, and to replace fluids and electrolytes.

There is uncertainty about what constitutes the best treatment. At the present time, the drug diloxanide furoate (Furamide) is being used when cysts are found in the fecal matter. This drug causes minimal toxicity, and excessive flatulence is the only reported side effect. It is considered an investigational drug in the United States.

In patients with trophozoites (the active, feeding stage of the organism) found on stool examination, metronidazole (Flagyl) may be effective, but some patients fail to respond to recommended dosages. Patients taking metronidazole should be cautioned against drinking alcohol during treatment, since the combination may cause a severe reaction. Emetine and dehydroemetine are drugs usually reserved for the patient who cannot take oral medications, or for those who are critically ill.

To support the patient's general condition, intravenous infusions are given as required to correct fluid and electrolyte imbalance resulting from severe diarrhea. If diarrhea is acute, the patient remains on bed rest and is offered low-residue, bland foods. Follow up study of the stools are necessary, since relapses are common.

Control; Patient Education. Methods of control include sanitary disposal of human feces, protection of the public water supply, and an ongoing program of health education in personal hygiene, including hand-washing after defecation and before preparing and eating food. Contacts of recently diagnosed patients should be examined.

Nursing Isolation Procedures: Excretion precautions should be observed for the duration of the illness.

AMEBIC LIVER ABSCESS

Amebic liver abscess represents the most common extraintestinal complication of amebiasis. It occurs when the amebae infiltrate the liver from the portal circulation. It is found in approximately 3 to 9 percent of patients with amebiasis.

In most patients, the right lobe of the liver is involved. The major complaint is pain in the right upper abdomen (caused by the liver's enlarging rapidly and stretching of its capsule); right upper chest pain (due to the liver's enlarging in an upward direction); fever, anorexia, and loss of weight. Physical examination reveals an enlarged, tender liver (due to hepatic abscess) and ausculatory abnormalities of the right lung field (from direct extension or rupture of a contiguous liver abscess). If the abscess is in the left lobe of the liver, a tender epigastric mass is noted. A liver scan suggests the diagnosis and is useful in following the resolution of the abscess. Immunological techniques, mainly serological methods, are also used in diagnosis. One point to be emphasized is that not infrequently the abscesses are found unexpectedly in patients who have had few or no symptoms suggesting amebiasis.

Usually the patient responds promptly to amebicidal therapy. Metronidazole (Flagyl) has generally been successful. If the patient does not respond to this drug, combinations of emetine, dehydroemetine, chloroquine, di-iodohydroxyquin, and tetracycline have been used. Needle drainage of the abscess may be necessary if there is concern that the abscess may rupture and cause peritonitis, or when clinical illness persists after adequate drug therapy. The supportive treatment is that outlined for amebiasis.

SYSTEMIC MYCOTIC INFECTIONS (FUNGAL INFECTIONS)

Fungi are primitive organisms that take their nourishment from living plants and animals and decaying organic material. Fungi have the ability to exist as yeasts or as molds and may alternate between the yeast and mold form. The fungi present difficult problems in control because they are so widespread in nature—in soil, decaying vegetation, and bird excreta. Although there are thousands of known species of fungi, only about 50 kinds of fungi cause disease in humans.

The three main types of mycoses (fungal infections), as determined by the tissue level at which the fungus settles, are:
1. Systemic or deep mycoses involving primarily the internal organs, usually centering in the lungs.
2. Subcutaneous mycoses which involve the skin, subcutaneous tissue, and sometimes the bone.
3. Superficial or cutaneous mycoses that grow in the outer layer of skin (epidermis), the hair, and the nails.

The systemic mycoses have occurred more frequently in recent years, since they are more common in patients with impaired immunological resistance and in patients receiving immunosuppressive agents (steroids, antilymphocyte serum, chemotherapy for cancer). Many patients who are receiving such treatment, or who are debilitated or severely ill and have reduced defenses, become prey to invasion by fungi which they could ordinarily withstand.

In addition to those receiving immunosuppressive agents, patients at risk for invasive fungal infections are those with certain immunological deficiencies; those with advanced malignancies; kidney or other organ-transplant patients; open heart surgery patients; the severely burned; patients receiving prolonged intravenous feedings; and those with renal failure and diabetes.

Systemic infections are usually acquired by accidental inhalation (spores carried on wind currents), occasionally by traumatic implantation (from contaminated soil or plant materials), or by the pathologic takeover of a normal inhabitant when the resistance of the host is lowered. It is not transmitted person-to-person.

HELMINTHIC INFESTATIONS

There are three major groups of helminths (worms) that are intestinal parasites in man: the nematodes (roundworms), the cestides (tapeworms), and the trematodes (flukes).

TRICHINOSIS (TRICHINELLOSIS)

Trichinosis is infestation by the parasite *Trichinella spiralis,* one of the roundworms. It is acquired by consuming infected meat, usually pork.

Clinical Manifestations and Course. This is a disease of pigs in the continental United States and of bears in Alaska. Tiny embryos of the parasite, *Trichinella spiralis* become encysted in the muscle fibers of an infected pig. These calcified cysts, barely visible to the naked eye, appear in the meat like tiny grains of sand. If such pork is insufficiently cooked and then eaten, the embryos are set free by the gastric juice and develop in the intestine during the following week into adult worms, about 3 to 4 mm. in length. These worms make their way into the mucous membrane and there produce myriad embryos. The intestinal phase starts about 24 hours after larval ingestion, causing symptoms of gastrointestinal disturbance: nausea, vomiting, diarrhea, and abdominal pain.

The embryos, carried by the bloodstream and by their own activity, migrate to all parts of the body. The patient's symptoms, arising from muscle invasion (due to an inflammatory process in the muscles), include edema of the eyelids, scleral hemorrhages, pain on eye motion, and generalized pain and soreness of muscles. Trichinosis causes high fever. Peripheral eosinophilia is a constant finding. Occasional heart irregularities (due to trichinae in the heart muscle) may be seen, and may be fatal. Difficulties in breathing, masticating, swallowing, or speaking may also occur.

Diagnostic Evaluation. A biopsy specimen taken from a painful muscle (deltoid, biceps, gastrocnemius) reveals the larvae. Serologic tests may be positive, with demonstrable titers 3 to 4 weeks after the infection. Usually the eosinophil count begins to rise in the second week. A skin test based on an extract of trichinae as the test antigen becomes positive after 16 to 20 days and may be positive for years afterward.

Management. The treatment of trichinosis is symptomatic. Thiabendazole (Mintezol) produces clinical improvement, but its effect on larvae that have migrated to muscles is not conclusive. Side effects of this drug include nausea, vertigo, headache, and weakness. The patient is kept on bed rest and given analgesics to relieve muscle pain. Corticosteroids may be given during the acute phase to minimize the allergic reaction and relieve the patient's symptoms. Electrocardiograms are taken to determine the evidence of myocarditis.

Prevention; Patient Education. The public should be educated regarding the importance of thoroughly cooking all pork and pork products, especially sausage. There should be no trace of pink in cooked pork. Smoking, pickling, seasoning, or spicing does not make pork safe unless it is cooked. Beef hamburger may be contaminated by a meat grinder that has been used for pork.

Garbage intended for hogs should be cooked. And finally, pork should be inspected by regular meat inspectors, to determine if the disease is present.

HOOKWORM DISEASE (Ancylostomiasis)

Hookworm disease is the result of infestation of the small intestine by one of two quite similar roundworms about 1.2 cm. (one-half inch) long. Two species are parasitic in the human intestinal tract: *Necator americanus* and *Ancylostoma duodenale.* The infection is usually acquired by walking barefoot, whereby infected larvae of the worms penetrate the skin.

Incidence. Approximately 25 percent of the world's population is infected with hookworm. It is found mainly in tropical and subtropical regions, notably Asia, the Mediterranean area, South America and Africa, and in most of the western hemisphere. In the United States hookworm infections are most prevalent in the southeastern states.

Pathology and Clinical Course. The embryos of this worm, hatched from eggs passed in the stools, live in dirt, sand, and clay, and easily infest man. They enter by mouth when food is eaten with dirty hands, or they bore through the skin of bare feet (ground itch). Having gained access to the blood or lymph vessels, they are carried by the bloodstream to the lungs, and migrate from the pulmonary capillaries into the alveolar sacs. The larvae migrate up the bronchi and trachea, pass over the epiglottis and down the esophagus, and into the bowel. The worms attach themselves to the intestinal mucosa and suck the blood of the host. The effect of the blood-sucking and hemorrhages at the attachment sites is iron-deficiency anemia. The resultant anemia makes the patient apathetic. A patient with a chronic infection develops malnutrition, hypoproteinemia, and profound anemia leading to cardiac symptoms. Maturation of the worms in the intestine may cause diarrhea and other gastrointestinal symptoms. A dry cough and dyspnea develop when the larvae rupture through the capillary bed and are spread throughout the bronchial tree.

Management. Mebendazole and pyrantel are both effective for hookworm disease. The patient should be placed on a nutritious diet, since hookworm disease occurs in persons suffering from malnutrition. Protein and iron supplementation is administered to aid in the correction of the anemia. Occasionally, blood transfusions are necessary.

Prevention. The prevention of hookworm disease depends on sanitary disposal of human excreta and the wearing of shoes. Night soil (human excrement used as fertilizer) and sewage affluents should not be used for fertilizer.

ASCARIASIS

Ascariasis is an infection by the nematode *Ascaris lumbricoides* (intestinal roundworm), that may live in the intestine of man. The infestation occurs throughout the world, with an estimated 644 million persons thought to harbor this parasite. Ascariasis occurs in approximately 1 million Americans and is more common in the southern states.

This disease is usually found in overcrowded areas with poor sanitation. Contamination of the soil by human feces is a factor in its spread. Indiscriminate defecation in the fields, streets, and doorways provides a major source of infective eggs. Man is infected by ingestion of the eggs in contaminated raw vegetables and drinking water. Children usually acquire the infection from fecal contamination of toys, soil, and fingers.

Life Cycle and Clinical Features. The eggs are swallowed and pass into the intestine, where they hatch as larvae. The larvae enter the bloodstream and pass through the pulmonary circulation, migrate through the lungs, and return to the gastrointestinal tract, where they grow, mature, and mate. Large numbers of worms may migrate into various organs of the body and cause obstruction—to the trachea, bronchi, bile duct, appendix, and pancreatic duct. Masses of worms in the intestine cause gastrointestinal discomfort, severe abdominal pain, and vomiting. Fever, chills, dyspnea, cough, and pneumonia may develop from invasion of the lungs by large numbers of larvae. Adult worms may migrate into the ampulla of Vater and then to the pancreatic or biliary ducts, causing acute and agonizing pain.

Ascariasis is diagnosed by detecting ova, larvae, or adult worms in the feces.

Management. Mebendazole (least toxic), pyrantel, and piperazine have been used successfully for treating intestinal ascariasis.

Nursing Isolation Procedures: No isolation or precautions are required.

Prevention. Preventive measures include providing adequate toilet facilities and teaching the importance of personal hygiene. All patients with the infestation should be treated.

ENTEROBIASIS (OXYURIASIS; PINWORM DISEASE)

Enterobiasis (oxyuriasis) is the most common helminthic infection in the United States. The pinworm (*Enterobius vermicularis*) is a small, white threadlike

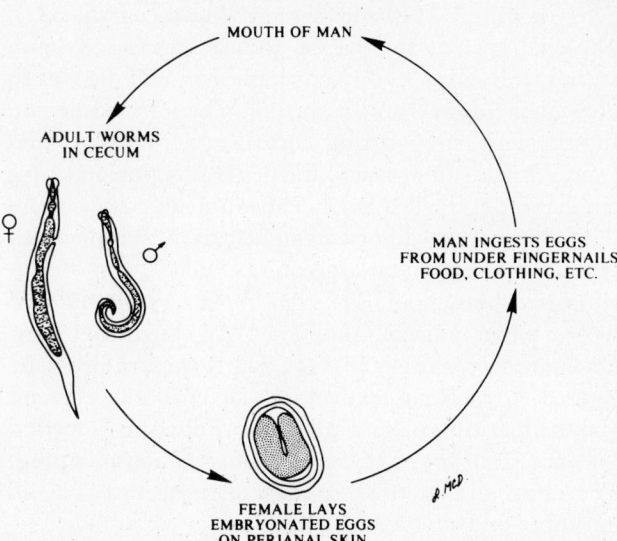

ENTEROBIASIS
ENTEROBIUS VERMICULARIS

MOUTH OF MAN

ADULT WORMS IN CECUM

MAN INGESTS EGGS FROM UNDER FINGERNAILS FOOD, CLOTHING, ETC.

FEMALE LAYS EMBRYONATED EGGS ON PERIANAL SKIN

Figure 60-7. Life cycle of *Enterobius vermicularis*. (Armed Forces Institute of Pathology photograph, Neg. No. 75-10881-13)

worm, about half a centimeter long, commonly found in the rectum of children. It is a worldwide infestation, and infections tend to affect groups (families; institutionalized populations).

The life cycle of the pinworm begins with the mating of the male and female worms in the human intestinal tract (Fig. 60-7). The gravid female migrates down the large intestine to the anus and deposits eggs on the perianal and perineal skin. These eggs are infectious. One pinworm may produce 5,000 to 15,000 eggs. Anal pruritus and scratching promote anal-to-oral transmission by contaminated fingers. Infection may also occur by ingesting eggs in food, dust, and fomites.

The chief symptoms are intense nocturnal itching around the anus, restlessness, and nervousness. Vaginitis may occur if the pinworms migrate into the vagina.

Worms may be seen on freshly passed stool or about the anus. Confirmation of the diagnosis can be obtained by securing anal impressions on transparent tape in the morning, before defecation and bathing, since the eggs remain adherent to the skin of that region. The tape is then applied to a slide, where microscopic examination will reveal numerous eggs.

Management. Pyrantel, mebendazole, or pyrvinium pamoate are usually effective when given in a single dose. Therapy may have to be repeated in two weeks. All members of the family should be treated on the same day, or reinfection is apt to occur.

Prevention of Reinfection; Patient Education. The fingernails should be cut short and nail biting discouraged, since eggs may be retained under the nails of infected persons. Children who bite their nails should be encouraged to wear gloves until the infection has been controlled. Fingernails should be scrubbed with a brush before bedtime. The hands should be washed frequently. The anal area of the patient should be washed upon arising, and salve or ointment applied around the area to prevent the eggs from dispersing. The infected person should wear snug-fitting cotton underpants to discourage hand contact with the perianal region and contamination of the bed linen. The infected person should sleep alone, and bedding and nightwear must be handled carefully. There are a large number of eggs in a contaminated household. The eggs remain viable for two weeks under normal conditions. All potentially contaminated clothing, sheets, and furniture must be cleaned, to prevent reinfection. The airborne element makes this a household infection. Pinworm infection does not mean poor hygiene or indifferent housekeeping. The nurse should reassure these patients that it is an infection, and anyone can get it.

Nursing Isolation Procedures: Excretion precautions for the duration of illness.

TAPEWORMS (INTESTINAL CESTODIASIS)

Beef Tapeworm. *Taenia saginata,* the beef tapeworm is the most prevalent endemic tapeworm in the United States, and is acquired by eating insufficiently cooked "measled" beef (that is, beef containing this worm in its larval form). In the bowel of man, this worm grows to a length of 4.5 to 6 m. (15 to 20 ft.). The head, about the size of a common black-headed pin, is provided with suckers only, and the largest links are about a half-centimeter broad and one centimeter or more long (quarter-inch broad to a half-inch or more long). Broken-off chains of links, full of eggs, often are passed in the stools.

Pork Tapeworm. *Taenia solium,* the pork tapeworm, rare in America, is acquired by eating insufficiently cooked infested pork. It is smaller than the beef tapeworm, being only from 1.8 to 3.6 m. long, and has somewhat smaller links. Its head, also smaller, is provided with suckers and hooks. This worm is much more difficult than the beef worm to expel.

Cysticercosis is infection by the larval stage of the tapeworm.

If a person swallows an egg instead of the larval form of the pork tapeworm, an embryo will be hatched in the bowel. This penetrates the intestinal mucous membrane and may be carried by the bloodstream to almost any organ of the body (heart, lungs, liver, kidneys, brain). Wherever it settles, it becomes encysted, and in this larval cyst, about a centimeter in diameter, only the head of the tapeworm develops.

The internal organs and the skin of an infested person may contain one or thousands of these cysts. If the cysts are located in the skin or subcutaneous tissues, there may be painless swelling of the area. However, in the eye, cysticeri (larval form of worm) may produce pain and visual symptoms, and in the brain may cause meningitis, epilepsy, and increased intracranial pressure.

The treatment of these cysts is surgical removal.

Fish Tapeworm. *Diphyllobothrium latum,* a tapeworm common in Europe and the Far East, but comparatively rare in America, is acquired by eating uncooked, infested fish. It may grow to a length of 7.6 to 9.1 meters (25 to 30 ft.).

Manifestations and Diagnosis

The beef and pork tapeworms cause few, if any, symptoms, except those suggested by the patient's knowledge that he has the worm. The fish tapeworm, however, occasionally precipitates an anemia which scarcely can be distinguished from pernicious anemia.

The diagnosis of all large tapeworms is easy, because their links appear in nearly every stool which the patient passes, and when seen, cannot be mistaken. Ova of the worms may be found on microscopic examination of the stool.

Management

Tapeworm infections may be treated by a single dose of the drug niclosamide (Yomesan), given on an empty stomach. (The drug is obtained from the Center for Disease Control.)

Nursing Isolation Procedures: Excretion precautions are required for patients with pork tapeworm for the duration of the illness. No isolation or precautions are required for persons with the beef tapeworm.

Prevention. There must be adequate inspection, refrigeration, and thorough cooking of fish, beef, and pork products. Other preventive measures include the treatment of human infections and carriers, the proper disposal of human excreta, and good personal hygiene.

BIBLIOGRAPHY

BOOKS

Barrett-Connor, E., et al.: Epidemiology for the Infection Control Nurse. St. Louis, C. V. Mosby, 1978.

Barua, D., and Burrows, W.: Cholera. Philadelphia, W. B. Saunders, 1974.

Binford, C. H., and Connor, D. H.: Pathology of Tropical and Extraordinary Diseases, vols. 1 and 2. Washington, D.C.: Armed Forces Institute of Pathology, 1976.

Cluff, L. E., and Johnson, J. E.: Clinical Concepts of Infectious Diseases, 2nd ed. Baltimore, Williams and Wilkins Co., 1978.

Cundy, K. R., and Ball, W.: Infection Control in Health Care Facilities: Microbiological Surveillance. Baltimore, University Park Press, 1976.

Dubay, E. C., and Grubb, R. D. (eds.): Infection: Prevention and Control, 2nd ed. St. Louis, C. V. Mosby, 1978.

Evans, A. S.: Viral Infections of Humans: Epidemiology and Control. New York, Plenum Medical Books Co., 1976.

Gardner, P., and Provine, H. T.: Manual of Acute Bacterial Infections. Boston, Little, Brown, 1975.

Hoeprich, P. D. (ed.): Infectious Diseases, 2nd ed. Hagerstown, Harper and Row, 1977.

Hook, E. W., et al.: Current Concepts of Infectious Diseases. New York, John Wiley and Sons, 1977.

Jones, G. L., and Hebert, G. A.: "Legionnaires' ". The disease, the bacterium and methodology, Washington, D.C., U.S. Dept. HEW, 1978.

King, A., and Nicol, C.: Venereal Diseases, 3rd ed. Baltimore, Williams and Wilkins Co., 1975.

Kurstak, E., and Kurstak, C.: Comparative Diagnosis of Viral Diseases, vols. 1 and 2. New York, Academic Press, 1977.

Maegraith, B.: Adams and Maegraith: Clinical Tropical Diseases, 6th ed. Oxford, Blackwell Scientific Publications, 1976.

Mims, C. A.: The Pathogenesis of Infectious Disease. New York, Grune and Stratton, 1976.

Minor, T. E., and Marth, E. H.: Staphylococci and Their Significance in Foods. New York, Elsevier Scientific Publishing Co., 1976.

Ramsay, A. M., and Emond, R. T. D.: Infectious Diseases, 2nd ed. London, William Heinemann Medical Books, Ltd., 1978.

Roberts, R. B. (ed.): The Gonococcus. New York, John Wiley & Sons, 1977.

Rothschild, H., Allison, F., Jr., and Howe, C.: Human Diseases Caused By Viruses. New York, Oxford University Press, 1976.

Rubin, R. H., and Weinstein, L.: Salmonellosis. New York, Stratton Intercontinental Medical Book Corp., 1977.

Schachter, J., and Dawson, C. R.: Human Chlamydial Infections. Littleton, Mass., PSG Publishing Co., Inc., 1978.

Schuhardt, V. T.: Pathogenic Microbiology. Philadelphia, J. B. Lippincott Co., 1978.

Spink, W. W.: Infectious Diseases. Minneapolis, Univ. Minnesota Press, 1978.

Top, F. H., et al. (eds.): Communicable and Infectious Diseases, 8th ed. St. Louis, C. V. Mosby, 1976.

U.S. Department of Health, Education and Welfare: Isolation Techniques for Use In Hospitals, 2nd ed. Washington, D.C., U.S. Govt. Printing Office, 1975.

Williams, J. D. (ed.): Modern Topics in Infection. London, William Heinemann Medical Books, Ltd., 1978.

Youmans, G. P.: Tuberculosis. Philadelphia, W. B. Saunders, 1979.

ARTICLES

Bacterial Infections

Clostridial Infections
(Botulism, Gas Gangrene, Tetanus)

Benedict, C. R., and Kerr, J. H.: Assessment of sympathetic overactivity in tetanus. Br. Med. J., 2:806, Sept. 24, 1977.

Darke, S. G., King, A. M., and Slack, W. K.: Gas gangrene and related infection: classification, clinical features and aetiol-ogy, management and mortality. A report of 88 cases. Br. J. Surg., 64:104-112, Feb. 1977.

El-Naggar, M.: Management of tetanus. Compr. Ther., 2:64-72, July 1977.

Furste, W., and Aguirre, A.: Preventing tetanus. AJN, 78:834-837, May 1978.

Henderson, D. K., et al.: Infectious disease emergencies: the clostridial syndromes. West. J. Med., 129:101-120, Aug. 1978.

Horwitz, M. A., et al.: Food-borne botulism in the United States, 1900-1975. J. Infect. Dis., 136:153-159, July 1977.

Kinahan, C. C., and Holden, F. A.: Tetanus in a 67-year-old man. Postgrad. Med., 62:233-237, Nov. 1977.

Mohr, J. A., et al.: Clostridial myonecrosis ("gas gangrene") during cephalosporin prophylaxis. JAMA, 239:847-849, Feb. 1978.

Morse, H. E., Kent, J. N., and Rothschild, H.: Tetanus — review of literature and report of case. J. Oral Surg., 36:462-466, July 1978.

Nursing Ground Rounds: Temple University: A little caution may be too much. Nursing '77, 7:52-56, Jan. 1977.

Rothstein, R. J., and Baker, F. J.: Tetanus, JAMA, 240:675-676, Aug. 18, 1978.

Skiles, M. S., Covert, G. K., and Fletcher, H. S.: Gas-producing clostridial and nonclostridial infections. Surg. Gynecol. Obstet., 147:65-67, July 1978.

Bacterial Enteric Diseases
(Salmonellosis, Shigellosis, Typhoid fever)

Butler, T., et al.: Typhoid fever. Arch. Intern. Med., 138: 407-410, Mar. 1978.

DuPont, H. L.: Salmonellosis and shigellosis. Hospital Med., 13:57-80, Oct. 1977.

Fontaine, R. E., et al.: Raw hamburger: an interstate common source of human salmonellosis. Am. J. Epidemiol., 107:36-45, Jan. 1978.

Geddes, A. M.: The antibiotic treatment of typhoid fever. J. Antimicrob. Chemother., 3:382-383, Sept. 1977.

Hornick, R. B., and Greisman, S.: On the pathogenesis of typhoid fever. Arch. Intern. Med., 13:357-359, Mar. 1978.

Jobson, K. F.: Typhoid perforations of the ileum. Trop. Doct., 8:76-77, Apr. 1978.

Nasrallah, S. M., and Nassar, V. H.: Enteric fever: a clinico-pathologic study of 104 cases. Am. J. Gastroenterology, 69:63-69, Jan. 1978.

Nolan, C. M., and White, P. C., Jr.: Treatment of typhoid carriers with amoxicillin. JAMA, 239:2352-2354, June 2, 1978.

Gonorrhea

Barlow, D., and Phillips, I.: Gonorrhoea in women. Diagnostic, clinical and laboratory aspects. Lancet, 1:vol. 8067, 761-764, Apr. 8, 1978.

Brooks, G. F., Darrow, W. W., and Day, J. A.: Repeated gonorrhea: an analysis of importance and risk factors. J. Infect. Dis., 137:161-169, Feb. 1978.

Chan, M. A., and Goldner, M.: A review of multiple drug resistance in Neisseria gonorrhoeae. J. Antimicrob. Chemother., 4:39-45, Jan. 1978.

DiCaprio, J. M., et al.: Ampicillin therapy for pharyngeal gonorrhea. JAMA, 239:1631-1633, Apr. 21, 1978.

Fiumara, N. J.: The treatment of gonococcal proctitis. JAMA, *239*:735-737, Feb. 20, 1978.

Handsfield, H. H.: Gonorrhea and nongonococcal urethritis: recent advances. Med. Clin. N. Am., *62*:925-943, Sept. 1978.

Huffman, J. W.: Gonorrhea: unmasking asymptomatic or atypical infection. Postgrad. Med., *63*:205-207, Jan. 1978.

McChesney, M. B., Chang, A., and Wallace, H. M.: Gonorrhea screening in teenage registrants of a children and youth project. Clin. Pediatrics, *17*:266-270, Mar. 1978.

Roberts, P. O.: Containing the gonorrhea epidemic (editorial). Am. J. Pub. Health, *68*:13-14, Jan. 1978.

Sattler, F. R., and Ruskin, J.: Therapy of gonorrhea. JAMA, *240*:2267-2270, Nov. 17, 1978.

Siegel, M. S., et al.: Penicillinase-producing *Neisseria gonorrhoeae:* results of surveillance in the United States. J. Infect. Dis., *137*:170-175, Feb. 1978.

Sparling, P. F., and Lee, T. J.: Gonorrhea: new insights and problems. Seminars in Infectious Disease, *1*:34-67, 1978.

Legionnaires' Disease

Callan, J.: "Creature comfort," culprit in Legionnaires' disease. JAMA, *241*:124, Jan. 12, 1979.

Friedman, H. M.: Legionnaires' disease in non-legionnaires. Ann. Intern. Med., *88*:294-302, Mar. 1978.

Kirby, B. D., et al.: Legionnaires' disease. Clinical features of 24 cases. Ann. Intern. Med., *89*:297-309, Sept. 1978.

Leprosy

Browne, S. G.: The treatment of leprosy today and tomorrow: the LEPRA consultation on chemotherapy. Lepr. Rev., *48*:283-286, Dec. 1977.

Leiker, D. C.: On the mode and transmission of *Mycobacterium leprae.* Lepr. Rev., *48*:9-16, Mar. 1977.

Meade, T. W.: How effective is the treatment of leprosy? Lepr. Rev., *48*:3-8, Mar. 1977.

Rea, T. H., and Levan, N. E.: Current concepts in the immunology of leprosy. Arch. Dermatol., *113*:345-352, Mar. 1977.

Williams, H. W.: Leprosy — a social disease. Can. Med. Assoc. J., *116*:834-835, Apr. 23, 1977.

Tuberculosis

Bailey, W. C., et al.: Tuberculosis and alcoholism. A partial solution through detection. Chest, *73*:183-185, Feb. 1978.

Barlow, P. B.: Treatment of tuberculosis. Basics of R.D., *5*:1-6, Sept. 1976.

Buckingham, W. B.: Modern medical management of pulmonary tuberculosis. Compr. Ther., *3*:28-32, Jan. 1977.

Comroe, J. H.: T.B. or not T.B. Part I. The cause of tuberculosis. Am. Rev. Respir. Dis., *117*:137-143, Jan. 1978; Part II. The treatment of tuberculosis. *117*:379-389, Feb. 1978.

Edwards, P. Q.: Tuberculosis, now and the future: short-term therapy, preventive therapy and bacillus Calmette-Guérin. Bull. N.Y. Acad. Med., *53*:526-531, July-Aug. 1977.

Eickhoff, T. C.: The current status of BCG immunization against tuberculosis. Ann. Rev. Med., *28*:411-433, 1977.

Farer, L. S.: Preventing tuberculosis. Compr. Ther., *3*:45-48, Dec. 1977.

Guernsey, B. G., and Alexander, M. R.: Tuberculosis: review of treatment failure, relapse and drug resistance. Am. J. Hosp. Pharm., *35*:690-698, June 1978.

Keim, L. W., Schuldt, S., and Bedell, G. N.: Tuberculosis in the intensive care unit. Heart Lung, *6*:624-634, July-Aug. 1977.

Middleton, J. R., et al.: Death-producing hemoptysis in tuberculosis. Chest, *72*:601-604, Nov. 1977.

Peterson, L. D., and Green, J. H.: Nurse-managed tuberculosis clinic. AJN, 77:433-435, Mar. 1977.

Reichman, L. B., and McDonald, R. J.: Practical management and control of tuberculosis. Med. Clin. N. Am., *61*: 1185-1204, Nov. 1977.

Reichman, L. B.: New challenges in ambulatory care of tuberculosis. Bull. N.Y. Acad. Med., *53*:516-525, July-Aug. 1977.

———: Diagnosis of tuberculosis today. Compr. Ther., *3*:25-31, Dec. 1977.

Meningitis

Fraser, D. W.: Vaccines against bacterial meningitis. Postgrad. Med., *62*:105-109, Aug. 1977.

Smith, A. L.: How to evaluate and treat meningitis. Med. Times, *105*:79-87, Sept. 1977.

Nosocomial Infection

Britt, M. R., Schleupner, C. J., and Matsumiya, S.: Severity of underlying disease as a predictor of nosocomial infection. JAMA, *239*:1047-1051, Mar. 13, 1978.

Pegram, S., Jr., and Philp, J. R.: Managing anaerobic infections. Am. Fam. Phys., *17*:186-195, Mar. 1978.

Spengler, R. F., and Greenough, W. B.: Hospital costs and mortality attributed to nosocomial bacteremias. JAMA, *24*:2455-2458, Nov. 24, 1978.

Protozoan Infections

Apte, V. V., and Packard, R. S.: Tinidazole in the treatment of trichomoniasis, Giardiasis, and amoebiasis. Drugs, *15*, suppl 1:43-48, 1978.

Archampong, E. Q.: Amoebic liver disease. Trop. Doct., 7:161-168, Oct. 1977.

Barrett-Connor, E.: Chemoprophylaxis of malaria. Ann. Intern. Med., *89*:417-418, Sept. 1978.

———: Latent and chronic infections imported from Southeast Asia. JAMA, *239*:1901-1906, May 5, 1978.

———: Where are you going? (editorial). Ann. Intern. Med., *86*:236-237, Feb. 1977.

Chin, W.: Recent developments in malaria. South. Med. J., *71*:97-99, Feb. 1978.

Gabaldon, A.: What can and cannot be achieved with conventional anti-malaria measures. Am. J. Trop. Med. Hyg., *27*:653-658, July 1978.

Krogstad, D. J., et al.: Amebiases: epidemiologic studies in the United States. Ann. Intern. Med., *88*:89-97, Jan. 1978.

Krogstad, D. J., Spencer, H. C., and Healy, G. R.: Current concepts: amebiasis. New Engl. J. Med., *298*:262-265, Feb. 2, 1978.

Lyster, A.: Nursing care study: malaria. Nurs. Times, *72*:1796-1799, Nov. 18, 1976.

O'Holohan, D. R.: Clinical and laboratory presentation of malaria. An analysis of one thousand subjects with malaria parasitaemia. J. Trop. Med. Hyg., *79*:191-196, Sept. 1976.

Peters, W.: Current concepts in parasitology. Malaria. New Engl. J. Med., *297*:1261-1264, Dec. 8, 1977.

Shabot, J. M., and Patterson, M.: Amebic liver abscess: 1966–1976. Am. J. Dig. Dis., *23*:110–118, Feb. 1978.

Trenholme, G. M., and Carson, P. E.: Therapy and prophylaxis of malaria. JAMA, *240*:2293–2295, Nov. 17, 1978.

Spirochetal Diseases

Anderson, D. C., et al.: Leptospirosis: a common-source outbreak due to Leptospires of the Grippotyphosa serogroup. Am. J. Epidemiol., *107*:538–544, June 1978.

Benedek, T. G.: The "Tuskegee study" of syphilis: analysis of moral versus methodologic aspects. J. Chronic Dis., *31*: 35–50, Jan. 1978.

Dans, P. E., and Judson, F. N.: How to use the newer serologic tests for syphilis. Illinois Med. J., *152*:499–503, Dec. 1977.

Drusin, L. M., et al.: Infectious syphilis mimicking neoplastic disease. Arch. Intern. Med., *137*:156–160, Feb. 1977.

The Jarisch-Herxheimer reaction (editorial). Lancet, 1, no. 8007, 340–341, Feb. 12, 1977.

McQuillan, W. J.: Leptospirosis. Nurs. Times, *73*:535–536, Apr. 14, 1977.

Meade, R. H.: A swollen labium. Hosp. Prac., *13*:33–34, Apr. 1978.

Mohr, J. A., et al.: Neurosyphilis and penicillin levels in cerebrospinal fluid. JAMA, *236*:2208–2209, Nov. 8, 1976.

Viral Diseases

Amantadine for high-risk influenza. Med. Lett. Drugs Ther., *20*:25–26, March 10, 1978.

Ellenbogen, C.: Postexposure antirabies therapy. Am. Fam. Phy., *15*:138–145, Mar. 1977.

Epstein, M. A., and Achong, B. G.: Recent progress in Epstein-Barr virus research. Annu. Rev. Microbiol., *31*: 421–445, 1977.

Epstein, M. A., and Achong, B. G.: Pathogenesis of infectious mononucleosis. Lancet, *2*:no. 8051, 1270–1272, Dec. 17, 1977.

Matzek, M. J., and Daniel, W. A., Jr.: Infectious mononucleosis — new perspectives. A current review. Ala. J. Med. Sci., *14*:26–30, Jan. 1977.

Pons, V. G., and Dolin, R.: Influenza. Hosp. Med., *14*:78–91, Oct. 1978.

Public Health Service Advisory Committee on Immunization Practices: Rabies. Morbidity and Mortality Weekly Report, *25*:403–406, Dec. 31, 1976.

Rutkow, I. M.: Rupture of the spleen in infectious mononucleosis. Arch. Surg., *113*:718–720, June 1978.

Schleupner, C. J., and Overall, J. C.: Infectious mononucleosis and Epstein-Barr virus. 1. Epidemiology, pathogenesis, immune response. Postgrad. Med., *65*:83–88; 2. Clinical picture, diagnosis, management. 95–105, Jan. 1979.

Seyal, M., Ziegler, D. K., and Couch, J. R.: Recurrent Guillain-Barré syndrome following influenza vaccine. Neurology, *28*:725–726, July 1978.

Other Infectious Diseases

Ascher, M. S., et al.: Initial clinical evaluation of a new Rocky Mountain Spotted Fever vaccine of tissue culture origin. J. Infect. Dis., *138*:217–220, Aug. 1978.

Riley, H. D., Jr.: "Rocky Mountain" Spotted fever. Hosp. Practice, *12*:51–57, Apr. 1977.

Weinstein, L.: Perspectives in infectious diseases. N.Y. State J. Med., *76*:1836–1841, Oct. 1976.

AGENCIES

Governmental

Center for Disease Control, Atlanta, Ga. 30333.

National Institute of Allergy and Infectious Diseases, National Institutes of Health, Bethesda, Md. 20205.

U.S. Department of Health, Education and Welfare, U.S. Public Health Service, Washington, D.C. 20201.

International

World Health Organization (Regional Office for the Americas), Pan American World Health Organization, 525 23rd St., N.W., Washington, D.C. 20037.

World Health Organization, Palais de la Sante, Geneva, Switzerland.

Voluntary

American Lung Association, 1740 Broadway, New York, N.Y. 10019.

American Public Health Association, 1015 18th St., N.W. Washington, D.C. 20036.

American Social Health Association, 260 Sheridan Ave., Palo Alto, Calif. 94306.

American Venereal Disease Association, 4716 Benton Smith Rd., Nashville, Tenn. 37215.

61
EMERGENCY MANAGEMENT

NURSING IN EMERGENCY CONDITIONS

Emergency management has traditionally referred to the care given to patients with urgent and critical needs. The philosophy of emergency care has broadened to include the concept that an emergency is whatever the patient or his family considers it to be. The staff have an obligation to treat the patient with understanding and to respect the anxiety which he undoubtedly feels. If they downgrade his complaint, the therapeutic process may very well be impaired.

A large number of people seek emergency help for serious life-threatening cardiac conditions such as myocardial infarction, acute congestive failure and pulmonary edema, and cardiac arrhythmias. The priorities of management of such cardiac conditions together with the ECG patterns evoked by the arrhythmias are discussed in Chapters 27 and 30. This chapter will deal mainly with the emergency management of trauma and other conditions not found elsewhere in this book. *It is assumed that treatment is given under the direction of a physician.*

PSYCHOLOGICAL MANAGEMENT OF PATIENTS AND FAMILIES IN EMERGENCIES AND CRISIS SITUATIONS

Approach to the Patient

Body trauma presents a threat to both physiological and psychological well-being. In an emergency situation, one of the objectives is to prevent the patient from becoming psychologically incapacitated.

If the patient is unconscious, he should be treated as if he were conscious—by touching him, calling him by name, and explaining every procedure that is being done. As soon as the patient regains consciousness, a primary concern is to orient him—by stating his name, the date, and the place. If necessary, this basic information should be repeated over and over. The patient is brought back into reality in a calm, reassuring way.

Patients experiencing sudden injury or illness are often overwhelmed by anxiety since they have not had time to mobilize their resources to adapt to the crisis. They experience real and terrifying fear—of death, mutilation, immobilization, and other assaults on their personal identity and body integrity. Those caring for the patient should act confidently and competently to help relieve his excessive anxiety. Personalizing the situation as much as possible and speaking, reacting, and responding to the patient in a warm manner contributes to a sense of security. In addition, explanations should be given on a level that the patient can grasp—an informed patient can cope with psychological and physical stress in a more positive manner. An ongoing human contact helps reduce the panic of the severely injured person, and reassuring words aid in dispelling fear of the unkown. It helps the emotionally distressed patient and family to mobilize their own psychological resources when the emergency department staff conveys optimism and concern for the welfare of the patient with a calm and reassuring manner.

Approach to the Family

In the admitting area the family is told where the patient is and that he is receiving expert care. When the crisis of trauma, severe disfigurement and sudden death are confronted, the family goes through several stages, beginning with "unbearable anxiety" and progressing through denial, remorse, grief, anger, and reconciliation. The family members are encouraged to recognize and talk about their feelings of anxiety. The approach here is to tune into the family's thinking and to deal with reality as gently and as quickly as possible. Although denial is an ego-defense mechanism that protects one from recognizing painful and disturbing aspects of reality, it cannot be encouraged or supported, since the family must be prepared for the reality of what has happened (and not for what they wish it could be) and for what may come.

Expressions of remorse and guilt are frequently heard, with members accusing themselves (or each other) of negligence or minor omissions. The nursing approach is to allow expressions of remorse, over and over, if need be until the family realize that there was probably little that they could have done to prevent the accident or illness.

Grief is a complex emotional response to anticipated or actual loss. In this stage the nursing intervention is to help family members work through their grief and to support their usual coping mechanisms, letting them know that it is normal and acceptable for them to cry and feel this way.

Expressions of anger are common in crisis situations. It is a way of handling anxiety. The anger is frequently directed at the patient, but it is also expressed toward someone else—the physician, the nurse, the admitting officer. Without condemnation or rejection, the therapeutic approach is to allow the anger to be ventilated in order to help the family identify their feelings of frustration.

The following are guidelines for helping a family deal with sudden death in the emergency department:
- Take the family to a private place.
- Talk to all of the family together.
- Assure the family that everything possible was done.
- Allow the family to talk about the deceased and what he meant to them.
- Encourage them to talk about events preceding admission to the emergency department.
- Encourage the family to support each other and express feelings of loss, anger, helplessness, etc.
- Avoid volunteering unnecessary information (the patient was drinking, etc.).
- Avoid giving sedation to family members, since this may mask or delay the grieving process which is necessary to achieve emotional equilibrium and prevent prolonged depression.
- Allow the family members to view the body if they wish to do so (unless there is severe mutilation). They may need to see that the deceased is "really dead."

PRIORITIES AND PRINCIPLES OF EMERGENCY MANAGEMENT

Priorities of Emergency Management

When care is being given to a patient in an emergency situation, many crucial decisions must be made. Such decisions require sound judgment based on an understanding of the condition that produced the emergency and its effect on the person.

The major objectives of emergency medical treatment are (1) to preserve life, (2) to prevent deterioration before more definitive treatment can be given, and (3) to restore the patient to useful living.

When the patient is first received into the emergency department the goal is to determine the extent of injury (illness) and to establish priorities for the initiation of treatment. These priorities are determined by the comparative threat to the person's life. Injuries or conditions interfering with vital physiologic function (obstructed airway, massive bleeding) take precedence. Usually injuries of the face, neck, and chest which impair respiration command the highest priorities. Every member of the emergency team must be alert to the total problem of the patient since the body cannot be isolated into parts.

Principles of Emergency Management

The following principles are applicable to the emergency management of any patient:
1. Maintain a patent airway, employing resuscitation measures when necessary. Assess for chest injuries with subsequent airway obstruction.
2. Control hemorrhage and its consequences.
3. Evaluate and restore cardiac output.
4. Prevent and treat shock; maintain or restore effective circulation.
5. Carry out a rapid and ongoing physical examination; the clinical course of the injured or seriously ill patient is not static.
6. Protect wounds with sterile dressings.
7. Splint suspected fractures, including fractures of the cervical spine in patients with head injuries.
8. Check to see if the patient has a Medic Alert or similar identification designating allergies.
9. Start a flow sheet of patient's vital signs, blood pressure, neurological status, etc.

Obtaining Data from the Patient

If possible a brief history of the accident or illness is taken from the patient or the person accompanying him to the emergency department.

As part of the history, the following questions should be answered:
1. What were the circumstances, forces, location, and time of the injury?
2. When did the symptoms appear?
3. How did the patient reach the hospital?
4. What was the health status of the patient before the accident or illness?

5. Is there a past history of illness? of past admissions?
6. Is the patient currently taking any medications: especially hormones, insulin, digitalis, anticoagulants?
7. Does the patient have any allergies?
8. Does the patient have any bleeding tendencies?
9. When was the last meal eaten? (Important if an anesthetic is to be given.)
10. Is the patient under a physician's care? name of physician?
11. What was the date of the patient's last tetanus immunization?

Recording of Data

Consent to examine and treat the patient is part of the Emergency Department record. More sophisticated procedures (angiography, lumbar puncture) should be specifically consented to by the patient. If the patient is unconscious and brought to the Emergency Department without family or friends, this fact should be documented. Following treatment, a notation is made on the record concerning the patient's condition on discharge or transfer and the instructions that are given for follow-up care.

EMERGENCY RESUSCITATION MEASURES

The first priority in the treatment of any emergency condition is the maintenance of an open airway. If the airway is obstructed, the ensuing hypoxia will produce

Mouth-to-mouth resuscitation

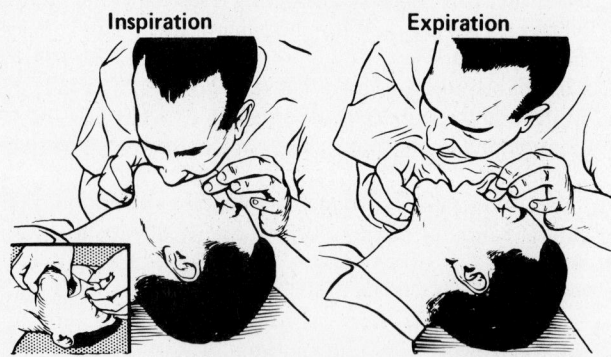

Inspiration   **Expiration**

Mouth-to-nose resuscitation

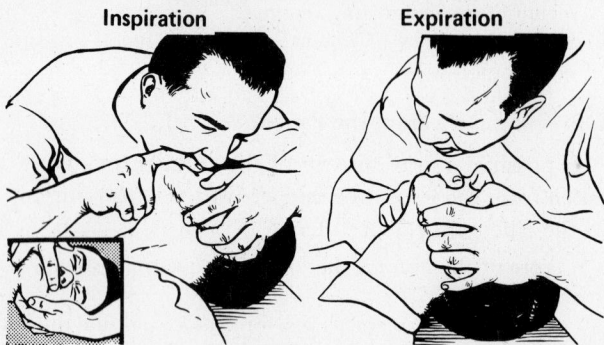

Inspiration   **Expiration**

Figure 61-1. Techniques for mouth-to-mouth and mouth-to-nose resuscitation. (From Gordon, Archer S., et al.: Mouth-to-mouth versus manual artificial respiration for children and adults. JAMA, 167:326)

permanent brain damage or death within 3 to 5 minutes, depending on the age of the patient.

Complete airway obstruction is readily recognized—the patient is not breathing and is unconscious and in complete collapse.

Partial airway obstruction which interferes with air flow will produce an apprehensive look, inspiratory and expiratory stridor, labored use of accessory muscles (suprasternal and intercostal retraction), flaring nostrils, and progressive anxiety, restlessness, and confusion. Cyanosis of the earlobes and nail beds may be a late sign. Partial obstruction of the airway can produce progressive hypoxia and hypercarbia and can lead to respiratory and cardiac arrest.

EMERGENCY MANAGEMENT

1. Turn patient on his side or turn his head to one side—to prevent the tongue from occluding the airway.
2. Place your fingers behind the angle of the mandible and pull forward while extending the patient's head at the atlanto-occipital joint.
3. If the patient is still having respiratory distress:
   a. Grip the tongue and pull forward.
   b. If the jaws are locked, insert the index finger behind the last molar and pry the jaw open; then grip the tongue and pull it forward.
   c. Clear any material from the mouth with a finger of the other hand or suction if equipment is available.
4. If these maneuvers do not clear the airway and if the patient is still not breathing:
   a. Apply the Heimlich maneuver (if patient is choking)—page 1414.
   b. Take one of the following steps: (1) insert an oropharyngeal airway (page 1414) and start bag-mask resuscitation, (2) insert esophageal obturator airway (page 1414), (3) insert endotracheal tube (page 1415), or (4) perform cricothyroidotomy.
5. Start artificial ventilation as soon as upper airway obstruction is cleared.

ARTIFICIAL VENTILATION

Artificial ventilation is instituted on a person who is not breathing. It is accomplished by means of mouth-to-mouth resuscitation and mouth-to-nose resuscitation (see below).

If the patient is unresponsive and there is no palpable carotid or femoral pulse, cardiopulmonary resuscitation (CPR) is initiated immediately. CPR consists of establishing an effective airway, and providing artificial ventilation and artificial circulation by external cardiac compression (see page 548). Advanced CPR involves electrical defibrillation (page 536), endotracheal intubation (page 450), and drug therapy (page 548).

Airway management and artificial ventilation are discussed in detail under "Respiratory Insufficiency and Failure," Chapter 23.

GUIDELINES: GIVING MOUTH-TO-MOUTH AND MOUTH-TO-NOSE RESUSCITATION*

Action	Rationale/Amplification

OPEN THE AIRWAY.

1. Place the patient on his back.
2. Tilt the patient's head backward as far as possible by placing one hand beneath the patient's neck and the other hand on his forehead.
3. Lift the neck gently with one hand and tilt the head backward by pressure with the other hand on the patient's forehead.

4. If the head cannot be tilted back successfully, place your fingers behind the angles of the patient's jaw and forcefully displace the mandible forward while tilting the head backward and using your thumbs to retract the lower lip—to allow patient to breathe through his mouth as well as his nose (jaw thrust technique).

VENTILATE THE PATIENT.

2. In an unconscious, supine patient, the base of the tongue falls against the posterior wall of the pharynx, obstructing airflow into the trachea.
3. This extends the neck and lifts the tongue away from the posterior pharynx; the mouth opens, and the obstruction of the airway is relieved, since the tongue no longer occludes the back of the throat.
4. This provides additional forward displacement of the lower jaw.

If the patient does not breathe spontaneously after this maneuver, search for presence of vomitus or of a foreign body in the mouth. Start artificial ventilation.

Absence of ventilation is determined by minimal or absent respiratory effort, failure of chest or upper abdomen to move, and inability to detect air movement through mouth or nose.

Mouth-to-Mouth Ventilation (Fig. 61-1)

1. Keep one hand behind the patient's neck.

2. Pinch the patient's nostrils together with the thumb and index finger of the other hand while also continuing to exert pressure on the forehead to maintain the backward tilt.
3. Open your mouth wide. Take a deep breath. Make a tight seal with your mouth around the patient's mouth and blow into his mouth.
4. For the *initial* ventilatory maneuver, give the patient 4 quick full breaths without allowing time for full lung deflation between breaths.
5. Remove your mouth from the patient's and allow him to exhale passively.
6. Repeat this cycle once every 5 seconds as long as respiratory inadequacy persists (12 ventilations per minute).

1. This maintains the head in a position of maximum backward tilt.
2. If the jaw thrust technique is used, keep the patient's mouth open with your thumbs and seal his nose by placing your cheek against it.

5. Watch the patient's chest fall.
6. Adequacy of ventilation is ensured by:
   a. Seeing the patient's chest rise and fall.
   b. Feeling in your own airway the resistance and compliance of the patient's lungs as they expand.
   c. Hearing and feeling the air escape during exhalation.

Mouth-to-Nose Ventilation

This is performed when it is impossible to open the patient's mouth, when it is impossible to ventilate through his mouth, when his mouth is seriously injured, or when it is difficult to achieve a tight seal around the mouth.

1. Tilt the patient's head with 1 hand on the forehead while using the other hand to lift the lower jaw.
2. Take a deep breath. Seal your lips around the patient's nose and blow in until you feel his lungs expand.
3. Remove your mouth from the patient's nose and allow him to exhale passively.

4. Repeat the cycle every 5 seconds (12 ventilations per minute).

1. This maneuver seals the lips.

3. Watch his chest fall when he exhales. It may be necessary to open the patient's lips to allow air to escape during exhalation since the soft palate may cause nasopharyngeal obstruction.

*From Standards for Cardiopulmonary Resuscitation (CPR) and Emergency Cardiac Care (ECC). JAMA, 227:837-851, February 18, 1974.

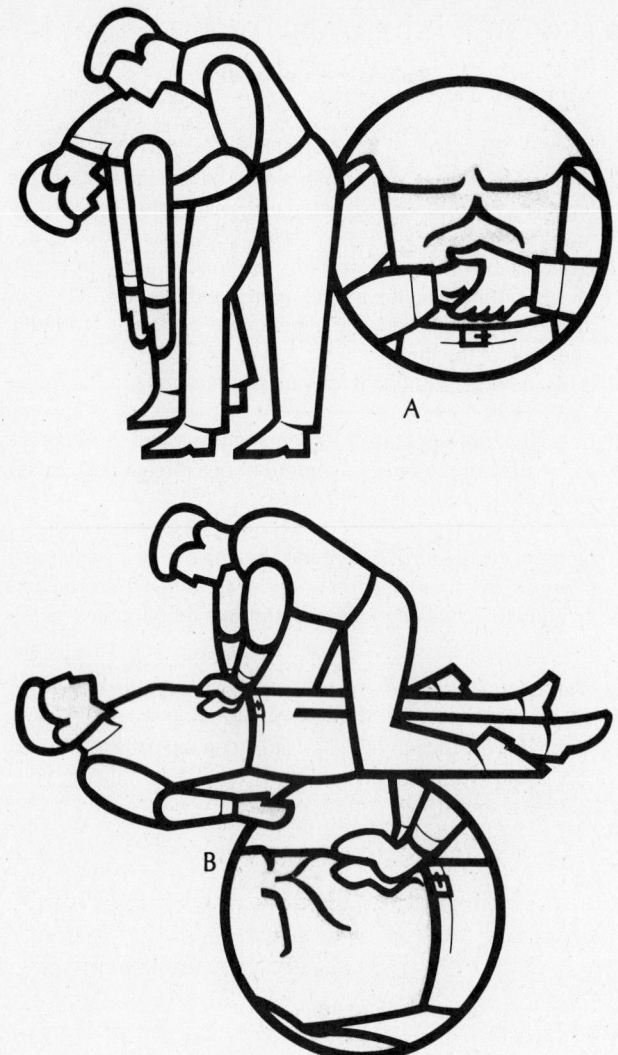

Figure 61-2. Heimlich maneuver. (© Edumed, Inc., 1976. Reprinted with permission. Posters, teaching slides, and wallet cards of the Heimlich Maneuver are now available. For information, send a stamped, self-addressed envelope to: Edumed, Box 52, Cincinnati, Ohio 45201.)

HEIMLICH MANEUVER FOR UPPER AIRWAY OBSTRUCTION BY A FOREIGN BODY

The Heimlich maneuver is a procedure designed to dislodge a food bolus or other obstructing object occluding the airway. It consists of external compression of the air in the lungs so that air is forced from the larynx expelling the obstructing object.

Choking is the sixth leading cause of accidental death in the United States. In adults, a piece of meat is the most common cause of obstruction. Other factors associated with choking on food include excessive alcohol intake, dislodgement of upper/lower dentures, and laughing and talking while chewing and swallowing. If the airway is only partially obstructed, the person may be able to spontaneously cough out the foreign body.

EMERGENCY MANAGEMENT*

If the person is standing: (Fig. 61-2A)
1. Stand behind the patient and wrap your arms around his waist. The rescuer's arms should be just above the belt line. The patient's head, arms, and upper torso are allowed to hang forward.
2. Make a fist with one hand and grasp the fist with your other hand. Place the thumb side of your fist against the patient's abdomen slightly above the navel and below the rib cage.
3. Grasp your fist with other hand and press fist into patient's abdomen with a quick upward thrust. This action produces a sudden sharp rise in intrathoracic pressure which will eject the bolus or foreign object that is occluding the airway.
4. Have a second person prepared to remove the foreign body from the mouth if necessary.

If the person is sitting:
1. Stand behind the patient's chair and perform the maneuver in the same manner.

If the person is lying on his back: (Fig. 61-2B)
1. Sit astride the patient's hips, facing his head, and with one of your hands on top of the other, place the heel of the bottom hand on the patient's abdomen slightly above the navel and below the rib cage.
2. Press into the patient's abdomen with a quick upward thrust. Repeat several times if necessary.
3. Place the patient on his side, if he begins to vomit, to prevent aspiration.
4. The patient should be examined by a physician after the emergency maneuver is performed.

Insertion of Oropharyngeal Airway

An oropharyngeal airway is a plastic or metal airway device inserted into the pharynx above the tongue in a spontaneously breathing patient in order to keep the tongue clear of the airway and permit suctioning of secretions.

EMERGENCY MANAGEMENT
1. Extend patient's head by placing one hand beneath the neck close to the occiput and gently lifting the neck while tilting the head backward by pressure on the forehead with the other hand.
2. Insert the airway upside down and rotate through 180 degrees as airway is introduced over the tongue to the pharynx.

OR

3. Insert from side of mouth and rotate into position.

Insertion of Esophageal Obturator Airway (EOA)

The esophageal obturator airway (Fig. 61-3) is a device consisting of three parts: (1) a mask—to seal off the nose and mouth and anchor the airway; (2) a flexible tube with openings at the level of the pharynx—to permit ventilation of the lungs; and (3) a balloon on the distal end of the tube—to prevent aspiration of gastric contents.

The tube is inserted through the mouth and advanced

*From Heimlich, H. J.: A life-saving maneuver to prevent food choking. JAMA, *234*:398-401, Oct. 27, 1975.

into the esophagus just below the bifurcation of the trachea. The proximal part of the tube has airholes at the level of the pharynx through which air or oxygen is blown into the lungs.

The purpose is to ventilate the apneic unconscious patient; it is an alternative to endotracheal intubation when skilled personnel and special facilities are not available.

Equipment

> Esophageal obturator airway
> 50 ml. syringe
> Lubricant jelly

EMERGENCY MANAGEMENT

1. Lubricate the tube and attach the mask to the tube.
2. Grasp the patient's tongue and lower jaw between the thumb and index finger and lift upward and forward.
3. Insert the esophageal obturator airway into the mouth, carefully guiding the tube over the tongue and past the pharynx; rotate the tube 180 degrees into the esophagus.
4. Stop advancing the tube when the mask reaches the face; press the mask firmly against the face.
5. Ventilate the patient by blowing a few breaths through the tube or by attaching a bag mask to it. IF THE TUBE IS IN THE ESOPHAGUS THE CHEST WILL RISE.
6. If the tube is in the trachea, take it out immediately and make another attempt at insertion.
7. Auscultate over both lung fields to check that *both* lungs are receiving adequate ventilation and that the airway is in the esophagus and *not* in the trachea.
8. Inflate the cuff (balloon) with approximately 30 ml. of air. Inflating the cuff results in occlusion of the esophagus and minimizes the incidence of regurgitation.

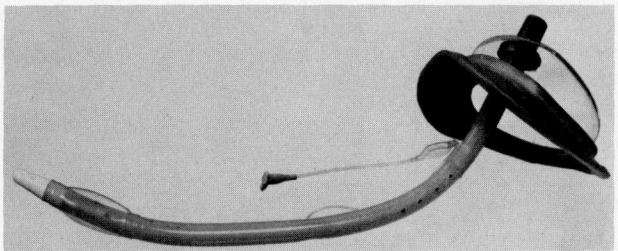

Figure 61-3. Esophageal obturator airway. (From Cosgriff, J. H., Jr.: Atlas of Diagnostic and Therapeutic Procedures for Emergency Personnel. Philadelphia, J. B. Lippincott, 1978)

9. Connect the end of the esophageal obturator to a bag-mask or mechanical ventilator, or continue mouth-to-tube ventilation.
10. Do not remove EOA until the patient regains consciousness or has a gag reflex *OR* until endotracheal intubation has been accomplished. If the tube is taken out prematurely, regurgitation and aspiration are almost inevitable.
11. This procedure is contraindicated in conscious or semiconscious patients or in those with corrosive poisoning, esophageal disease, or a foreign body in the trachea.

EMERGENCY ENDOTRACHEAL PROCEDURES

Emergency Endotracheal Intubation

The purpose of endotracheal intubation is to establish and maintain the airway in patients with respiratory insufficiency or hypoxia. Endotracheal intubation is in-

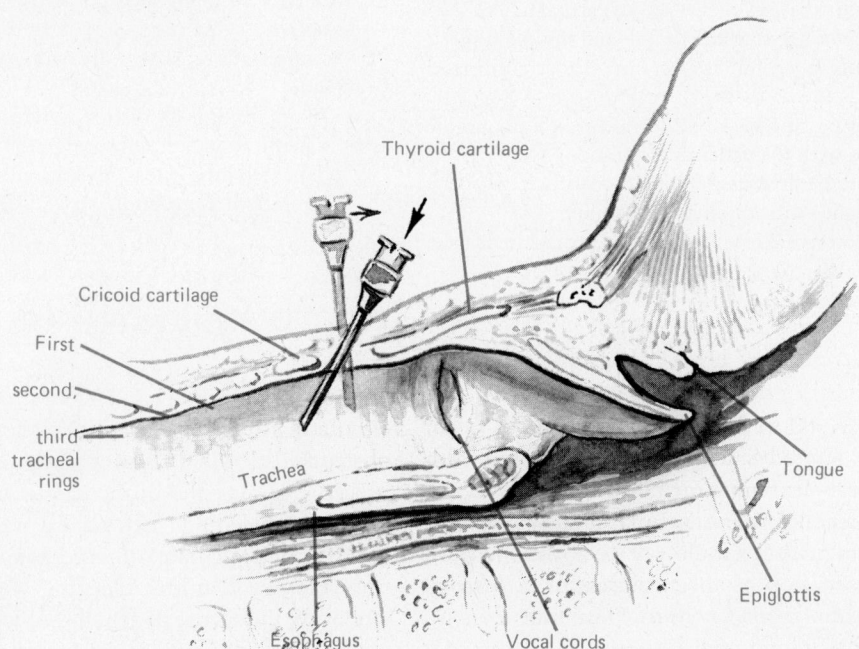

Figure 61-4. Crycothyroidotomy, or cricothyroid membrane puncture. (From Cosgriff, J. H., Jr.: Atlas of Diagnostic and Therapeutic Procedures for Emergency Personnel. Philadelphia, J. B. Lippincott, 1978, page 23.)

dicated for the following reasons: (1) to establish an airway for patients who cannot be adequately ventilated with an oropharyngeal airway, (2) to bypass an upper airway obstruction, (3) to prevent aspiration, (4) to permit connection of the patient to a resuscitation bag or mechanical ventilator, and (5) to facilitate the removal of tracheobronchial secretions.

Because the procedure requires skill, endotracheal intubation should be done after intensive training in which the technique is practiced on a manikin. It should be done under expert clinical supervision.

Details for emergency endotracheal intubation are outlined in the chart beginning on page 1418.

Crycothyroidotomy, or Cricothyroid Membrane Puncture

Crycothyroidotomy is the puncture of the cricothyroid membrane of the larynx with a large bore needle or a specially designed blade (Fig. 61-4). It is used during acute airway obstruction caused by laryngospasm, laryngeal edema (allergic reaction), hemorrhage into neck tissue, or obstruction of the larynx. It is usually done as a last resort after attempts at ventilation or removal of a foreign body are not successful or when personnel or equipment are not available for endotracheal intubation or tracheostomy.

EMERGENCY MANAGEMENT

1. Extend the neck.
2. Identify the thyroid notch and allow finger to descend in the midline to the prominence of the cricoid cartilage, which is above the superior margin of the cricoid cartilage.
3. Stabilize the larynx between the thumb and middle finger.
4. Insert the needle perpendicularly into the cricothyroid membrane.
   a. Listen for air passing back and forth through the needle synchronous with the patient's respiration.
   b. Direct the needle downward and posteriorly.
   c. Tape the needle with adhesive for stability.
5. Prepare for endotracheal intubation. This procedure is usually followed by elective tracheostomy (page 451).

NEAR DROWNING

An estimated 7,000 to 8,000 drowning deaths occur each year in the United States. Factors associated with drowning and near-drowning include inability to swim, diving injuries, alcohol, hypothermia, and exhaustion. Efforts to save the victim should not be abandoned too soon, since resuscitation has been successful in persons who have been submerged for 10 to 40 minutes.

Following resuscitation, the primary problems of a victim who has nearly drowned are hypoxia and acidosis, which will require immediate intervention in the emergency department. The resultant pathophysiological changes and pulmonary injury following this experience depend on the type of fluid (fresh water or salt water) and the volume of aspiration. When water has been aspirated, alterations of pulmonary function may be anticipated. After a person has survived immersion, secondary drowning (acute adult respiratory distress syndrome) with hypoxia, hypercarbia, and respiratory and/or metabolic acidosis can occur.

EMERGENCY MANAGEMENT IN EMERGENCY DEPARTMENT

The objectives are to treat for ventilatory insufficiency, hypoxia, and resultant acidosis.

1. Assess for airway, breathing, circulation, vital signs, level of responsiveness.

   Use rectal probe to determine true temperature if patient has been submerged in cold water.
2. Start IV line; draw arterial blood—to evaluate oxygen and carbon dioxide tensions, pH, and bicarbonate levels; these parameters will determine the type of ventilatory support required and subsequent dosage of sodium bicarbonate to be given.
3. Initiate endotracheal intubation and use volume controlled ventilator with PEEP if needed to improve oxygenation and prevent pulmonary injury as indicated by patient's condition.
4. Continue with 100 percent oxygen via mask (if patient is breathing spontaneously) or via endotracheal tube (if patient is not breathing spontaneously).
5. Assist with nasogastric intubation to prevent patient from regurgitating gastric contents.
6. Continue to monitor patient closely—vital signs, serial arterial blood gas tensions, pH, ECG, urinary output, serum electrolytes, chest x-ray.
7. Admit to hospital; the appearance of the patient may be deceptive.

   Complications of near drowning which can lead to death include:
   a. Acute respiratory distress syndrome (page 446).
   b. Chemical pneumonitis, which may be superimposed on damaged lung due to aspiration of gastric contents. (See aspiration, page 466.)

CONTROL OF HEMORRHAGE DUE TO TRAUMA

One of the primary causes of shock is the reduction in circulating blood volume. Only a few conditions, such as obstructed airway or a sucking wound of the chest, take precedence over the immediate control of hemorrhage. "Stop the bleeding" is fundamental to the care and the survival of patients in an emergency or a disaster situation. However, minor bleeding will usually stop spontaneously unless the patient has a bleeding disorder. Most of this type of blood loss will be venous. The objectives of emergency management are to control the bleeding, maintain an adequately circulating blood volume for tissue oxygenation, and prevent shock.

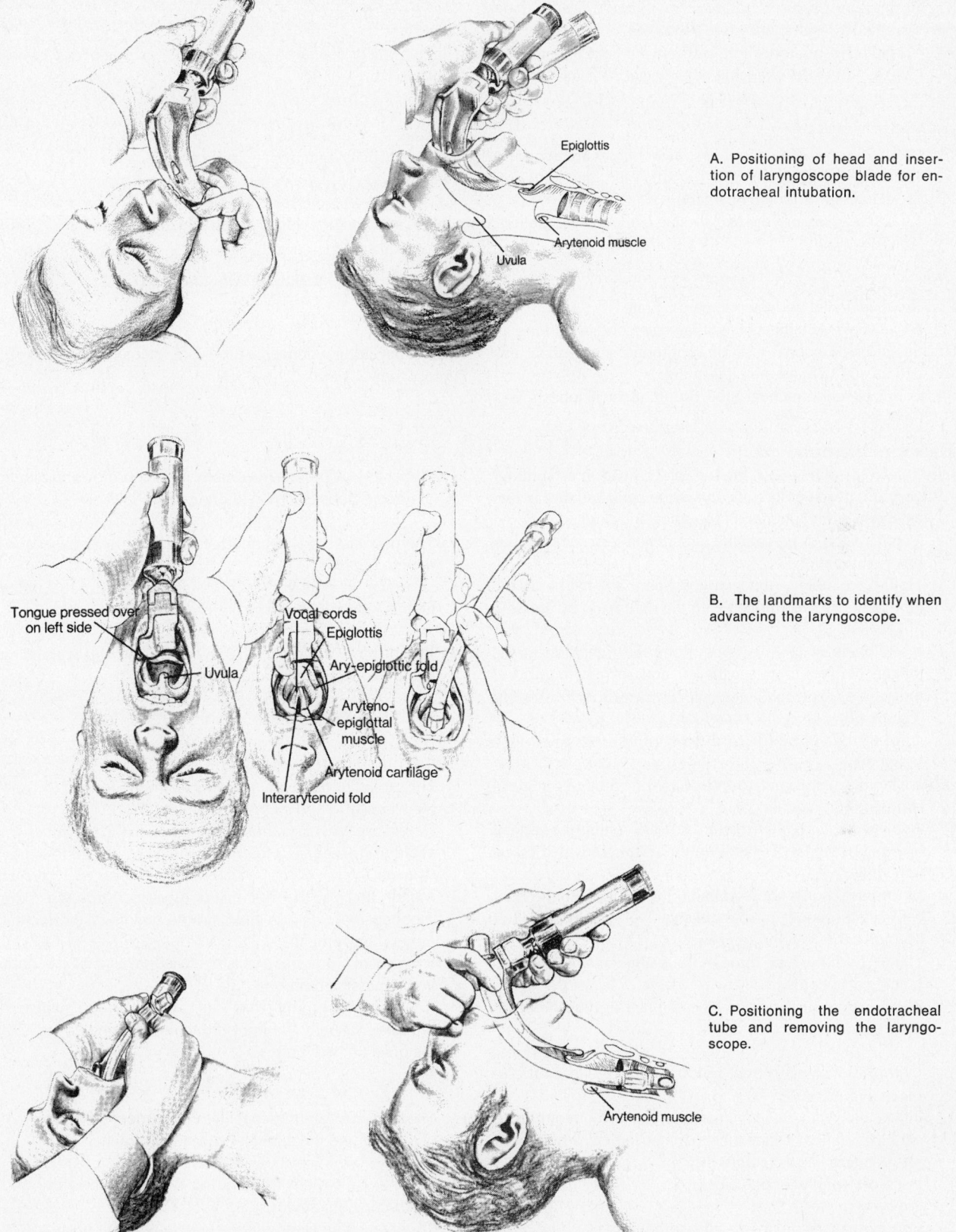

A. Positioning of head and insertion of laryngoscope blade for endotracheal intubation.

Epiglottis

Arytenoid muscle

Uvula

B. The landmarks to identify when advancing the laryngoscope.

Tongue pressed over on left side

Uvula

Vocal cords

Epiglottis

Ary-epiglottic fold

Aryteno-epiglottal muscle

Arytenoid cartilage

Interarytenoid fold

C. Positioning the endotracheal tube and removing the laryngoscope.

Arytenoid muscle

Figure 61-5.   Sequence of steps for endotracheal intubation. (Reprinted with permission of Nursing Update, May 1972. Copyright © Miller and Fink Publishing Corporation, Darien, Conn. All rights reserved)

CLINICAL SIGNS FOR INTUBATION
1. Respiratory arrest
2. Respiratory insufficiency (see page 446)

    Marked respiratory effort, substernal retraction, nostril flaring, increasing or decreasing pulse rate, increasing or decreasing respiratory rate, changing color (*cyanosis is a late sign*)
3. Airway obstruction (asphyxia)

EQUIPMENT
1. Laryngoscope with curved or straight blades and working light source. (Check batteries and bulb periodically.)
2. Endotracheal tubes with low-pressure cuffs and adaptor to connect tube to ventilator or bag
3. Stylet to guide endotracheal tube
4. Oral airway (assorted sizes), tongue blade to keep patient from biting into and occluding endotracheal tube
5. Adhesive tape   6. Lubricant jelly   7. Syringe

Action	Rationale/Amplification
1. Remove dental bridgework, partial plate.	
2. Make sure that light source of laryngoscope is working.	
3. Select endotracheal tube of appropriate size. Inflate and deflate cuff to make sure it is intact.	The average adult will need a tube with an internal diameter of 7.5 to 9 mm.
4. Lubricate endotracheal tube. Insert stylet if tube is very flexible.	

ASSIST WITH THE FOLLOWING:

Action	Rationale/Amplification
1. If cervical spine is not injured, place head in a "sniffing" position, flexed at the junction of the neck and thorax and extended at the junction of the spine and skull.	1. Upper airway is open maximally in this position and mouth of unconscious patient will often open.
2. Ventilate and oxygenate the patient with resuscitation bag before intubation.	2. This decreases the likelihood of cardiac arrhythmias secondary to hypoxia.
3. Hold the handle of the laryngoscope in the left hand and hold patient's mouth open with the right hand by crossing fingers (Fig. 61-5A).	3. Leverage is improved by crossing the thumb and index fingers when opening the patient's mouth.
4. Insert blade of laryngoscope along the right side of the tongue, pointing tongue to the left, and use right thumb and index finger to pull patient's lower lip away from lower teeth (Fig. 61-5B).	4. Rolling lip away from teeth prevents injury of lip by its being caught between teeth and blade.
5. Lift laryngoscope forward (toward ceiling) to expose epiglottis.	
6. Lift laryngoscope upward and forward at 45-degree angle to expose glottis (vocal cords).	6. This stretches the hypoepiglottis ligament, folding the epiglottis upward and exposing the glottis.
7. As the epiglottis is lifted forward (toward ceiling) the vertical opening of the larynx between the vocal cords will come into view.	7. Do not use wrist; use shoulder and arm to lift epiglottis—to avoid using teeth as a fulcrum, which could lead to dental damage.
8. Once vocal cords are visualized, insert tube into the right corner of the mouth and pass the tube—guided by blade but keeping cords in constant view.	8. Make sure you do not insert tube in esophagus; the esophageal mucosa is pink and the opening is horizontal rather than vertical.
9. Gently push the tube through the triangular space formed by the vocal cords.	9. If the vocal cords are in spasm (closed), wait a few seconds before passing tube.
10. Stop insertion just after the tube cuff has disappeared from view beyond the cords.	10. Advancing tube further may lead to its entry into a mainstem bronchus (usually the right bronchus) causing collapse of the unventilated lung.
11. Withdraw laryngoscope, holding endotracheal tube in place (Fig. 61-5C).	
12. Inflate cuff with the minimal amount of air required to occlude trachea. Attach tube to a mechanical ventilator or resuscitation bag as required.	12. The amount of air used for cuff inflation depends on the size of the cuff and the diameter of patient's trachea.
13. Insert oral airway or bite block.	13. This keeps patient from biting down on the tube and obstructing the airway.
14. Observe expansion of both sides of the chest by observation and auscultation of breath sounds.	14. Observation and auscultation help in determining that tube remains in position and has not slipped into right mainstem bronchus and that both lungs are being aerated.
15. Mark proximal end of tube with marking pen or tape.	15. This will allow for detection of any later change in position.
16. Secure tube with adhesive tape to the patient's face.	16. Taping the tube prevents expulsion.
17. Take chest x-ray to verify tube position.	

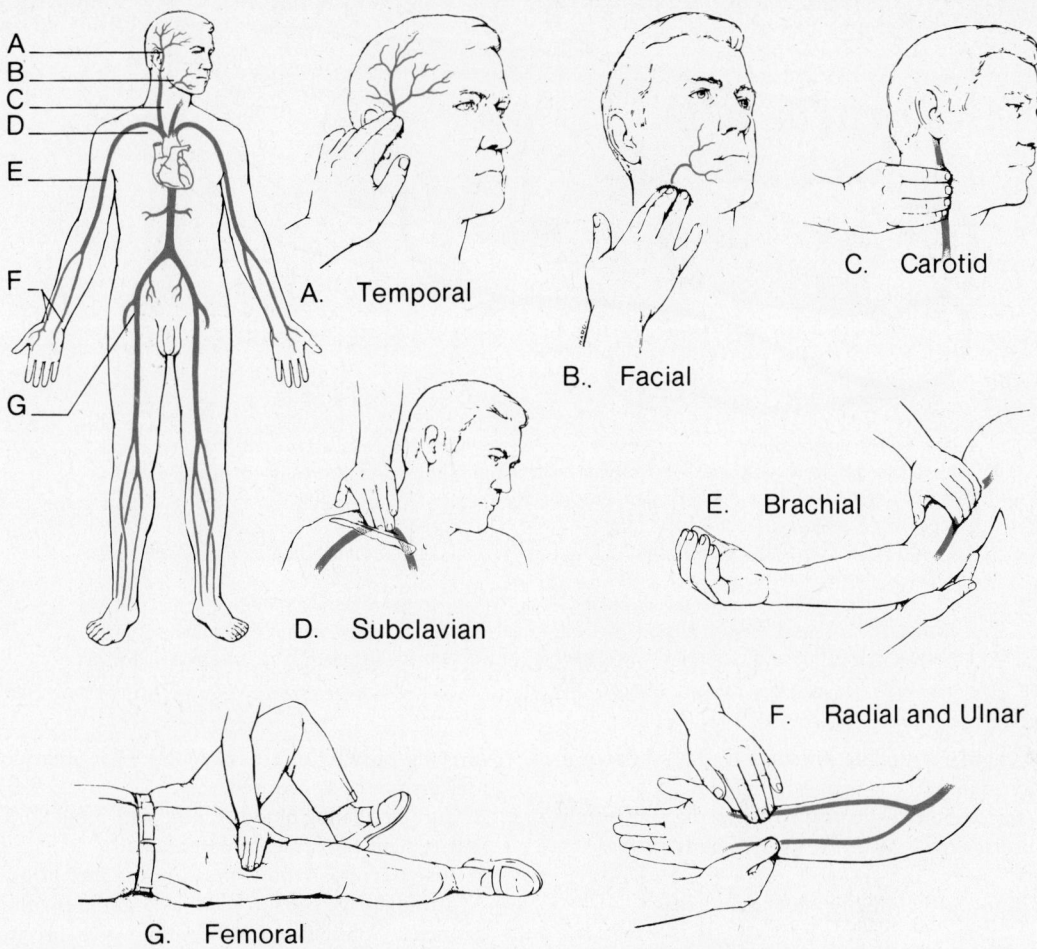

A. Temporal

B. Facial

C. Carotid

D. Subclavian

E. Brachial

F. Radial and Ulnar

G. Femoral

Figure 61-6. Pressure points for control of hemorrhage.

EMERGENCY MANAGEMENT

1. Cut the patient's clothing away quickly to identify area of hemorrhage and carry out a rapid physical assessment.

2. Apply direct, firm pressure over the bleeding area or the artery involved (Fig. 61-6). Almost all bleeding can be stopped by direct pressure (except when a major artery has been severed). Unchecked arterial bleeding produces death.

3. Apply a firm pressure dressing. Elevate the injured part to stop venous and capillary bleeding. Immobilize an injured extremity to control blood loss.

4. Insert intravenous cannula to provide means of blood replacement.
   a. Withdraw blood samples for analysis, typing, and cross-matching.
   b. Give replacement fluids including plasma, plasma protein fractions, blood, isotonic electrolyte solutions — depending on clinical estimates of type and volume of fluids lost.
      (1) Additional platelets and clotting factors (in form of fresh frozen plasma) are given when large amounts of blood are needed, since replacement blood is deficient in clotting factors.
      (2) Warm the blood (commercial warmer or basin of warm water) — massive blood replacement has a cooling effect that can cause cardiac arrest.
   c. Rate of infusion depends on severity of blood loss and clinical evidence of hypovolemia.

5. Take the following steps for internal bleeding:
   a. Suspect internal bleeding in patients with hypovolemic shock with no external signs of bleeding: rising pulse rate, falling blood pressure, thirst, apprehension, cool moist skin.
   b. Give whole blood or plasma expanders at the rate of blood loss.
   c. Prepare patient immediately for surgical intervention.
   d. Apply wraparound inflatable counterpressure suit ("G" suit, compression suit), if available, to control bleeding (Fig. 61-7).
   e. Obtain blood gas determination; establish central venous pressure monitoring as an index of the amount of fluid the patient can tolerate.

6. Apply a tourniquet only as a *last resort,* when the hemorrhage cannot be controlled by any other method. Anticipate loss of an extremity if tourniquet is applied.
   a. Apply the tourniquet just proximal to the wound; tie it tightly enough to control arterial blood flow.
   b. Tag the patient with a skin-marking pencil or on adhesive tape on his forehead with a "T" stating the location of the tourniquet and the time applied.
   c. Loosen the tourniquet as directed to prevent irreparable vascular or neurologic damage if patient is in emergency facility. If there is no arterial bleeding, remove the tourniquet and again try pressure dressing.

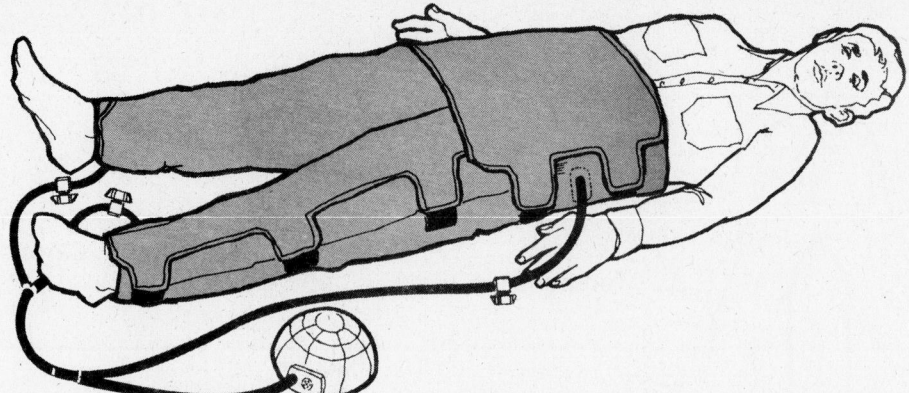

Figure 61-7. The Medical Anti-Shock Trouser (MAST) is a garment designed to correct and counteract internal bleeding conditions and hypovolemia by developing an encircling pressure of up to 2 psi or 104 mm. Hg around both legs and abdomen, thus effectively
  a. slowing or stopping arterial bleeding
  b. forcing any available blood from the lower body to the heart, brain and other vital organs in the upper body, and
  c. preventing return of available circulating blood volume to the lower extremities.
It should be applied as soon as possible after injury, preferably before patient is transferred to the Emergency Department. (Courtesy David Clark Co., Inc., 373 Franklin Street, Worcester, Mass. 01604)

  d. In the event of a traumatic amputation, leave the tourniquet applied until the patient is in the O.R.
7. Watch for cardiac arrest; patients who hemorrhage are candidates for cardiac arrest caused by hypovolemia with secondary anoxia.
8. See page 370 for further discussion of hemorrhage.

CONTROL OF HYPOVOLEMIC SHOCK*

Shock is a condition in which there is loss of effective circulating blood volume; inadequate organ and tissue perfusion results, leading to derangements of cellular function. In any emergency situation it is wise to anticipate shock before it develops. Any injured person should be assessed immediately to determine the presence of shock. Its underlying cause must be discovered (hypovolemic, cardiogenic, neurogenic, septic shock). Hypovolemia is the most common cause of shock.

The following signs and symptoms, in varying combinations, indicate that the patient is in some degree of shock: decreasing arterial pressure, increasing pulse rate, cold moist skin, circumoral pallor, thirst, alteration of mental status, and suppression of kidney function. Of these, the most dependable criterion is the level of arterial blood pressure. Start treatment at the first signs of shock.

EMERGENCY MANAGEMENT

The objectives of treatment are to restore and maintain tissue perfusion and to correct physiologic abnormalities.
1. Establish and maintain an airway; start resuscitation procedures if necessary. Give oxygen to augment the oxygen-

*See also pages 364–370.

carrying capacity of arterial blood. Give additional ventilatory assistance as required.
2. Restore circulating blood volume with rapid fluid and blood replacement to correct hypotension.
   a. Insert central venous pressure catheter in or near right atrium (page 516) to serve as a guide for fluid replacement. Continuing CVP readings give direction and degree of change from baseline readings; catheter also is a vehicle for emergency fluid volume replacement.
   b. Insert intravenous catheter or needles; two or more catheters may be necessary for rapid replacement in profound shock; the emphasis is on volume replacement.
      (1) Establish IV lines in both upper and lower extremities if there is suspicion that a major vessel in the chest or abdomen has been disrupted.
      (2) Withdraw blood for specimens; arterial blood gases (arterial blood); chemistry studies, typing and cross-matching, and hematocrit.
3. Start intravenous infusion at a rapid rate until CVP rises to a satisfactory level above baseline measurement or until there is improvement in clinical condition.
   a. Infusion of lactated Ringer's solution is useful initially to allow time for whole blood typing and cross-matching and to restore circulation and serve as an adjunct to whole blood.
   b. Start transfusion of blood component therapy, especially when blood loss has been severe or when patient continues to hemorrhage.
   c. Control hemorrhage; hemorrhage will compound the shock state. Carry out serial hematocrit examinations if continued bleeding is suspected.
   d. Maintain the systolic blood pressure at 90–110 mm. Hg via fluid and blood.
4. Insert a urinary catheter. Urinary volume reveals adequacy of kidney perfusion.

5. Carry out a rapid physical assessment to determine cause of shock.
6. Maintain ongoing nursing surveillance of *total patient*; blood pressure, heart, and respiratory rates, skin temperature, color, CVP, and urinary output to assess patient response to treatment. Keep a flow sheet of these parameters—trend analysis reveals improvement or deterioration of patient.
7. Elevate the feet slightly to improve cerebral circulation and promote return of venous blood to the heart. (*This position is contraindicated in patients with head injuries.*)
8. Give specific pharmacologic agents (sodium bicarbonate, dopamine, etc.) when indicated by the patient's condition.
9. Support the defense mechanisms of the body.
   a. Reassure and comfort the patient; sedation may be necessary to relieve apprehension.
   b. Relieve pain by *cautious* use of analgesics or narcotics.
   c. Maintain the body temperature.
      (1) Too much heat produces vasodilatation, which counteracts the body's compensatory mechanism of vasoconstriction and also increases fluid loss by perspiration.
      (2) A patient who is in septic shock should be kept cool, since high fever will increase the cellular metabolic effects of shock.

INTRA-ABDOMINAL INJURIES

PENETRATING ABDOMINAL INJURIES

Penetrating abdominal injuries (gunshot wounds, stab wounds) are serious and usually require surgery. In penetrating injuries, the most important factor is the velocity with which the missile entered the body. High velocity missiles (bullets) create extensive tissue damage. Almost all gunshot wounds require surgical exploration. Stab wounds may be managed more conservatively.

The objectives of emergency management are to control the bleeding and maintain the blood volume.
- Assess the patient for progression of distention, involuntary guarding, tenderness, pain, muscular rigidity or rebound tenderness, diminished bowel sounds, hypotension and shock.
- Auscultate for bowel sounds as the absence of bowel sounds is an early sign of intraperitoneal involvement. If signs of peritoneal irritation are present, an immediate exploratory celiotomy (surgical incision into abdominal cavity) is usually performed.
- Record all physical signs as the patient is examined.
- Look for chest injuries which frequently accompany intra-abdominal injuries.

EMERGENCY MANAGEMENT
1. Keep the patient on the stretcher, since movement may cause fragmentation of a clot in a large vessel and produce massive hemorrhage.
   a. Ensure patency of airway, adequacy of respirations and circulatory competence.
   b. Cut the clothing away from the wound.
   c. Tabulate the number of wounds.
   d. Look for entrance and exit wounds.
2. Assess for signs and symptoms of hemorrhage. *Hemorrhage frequently accompanies abdominal injury,* especially if the liver and spleen have been traumatized.
3. Control the bleeding and maintain the blood volume until surgery can be performed.
   a. Apply compression to external bleeding wounds and occlusion of chest wounds.
   b. Insert indwelling intravenous catheter(s) for rapid fluid replacement to restore circulatory dynamics.
   c. Watch for occurrence of shock after an initial response to transfusion therapy; this is often the first sign of internal hemorrhage.
4. Aspirate the stomach contents with nasogastric tube. This procedure also helps detect gastric wounds and prevents lung complications due to aspiration.
5. Cover protruding abdominal viscera with sterile saline dressings to prevent viscera from drying.
   a. Flex patient's knees as this position will prevent further protrusion.
   b. Withhold oral fluids to prevent increased peristalsis and vomiting.
6. Insert indwelling urethral catheter to ascertain the presence of hematuria and to monitor the urinary output.
7. Keep an ongoing flow sheet of the patient's vital signs, urinary output, central venous pressure readings (when indicated) and neurological status.
8. Prepare for paracentesis or peritoneal lavage (see chart, page 1422) when there is uncertainty about intraperitoneal bleeding.
9. For stab wounds, prepare for sinography to determine whether there is peritoneal penetration.
10. Carry out tetanus prophylaxis as directed.
11. Give broad-spectrum antibiotic to prevent infection, since bacterial contamination is a frequent complication.
12. Prepare for surgery if patient shows continuing evidence of shock, blood loss, free air, evisceration, hematuria, etc.

BLUNT ABDOMINAL TRAUMA

Blunt trauma to the abdomen may result from automobile accidents, falls, and blows to the abdomen. These patients are a challenge because of potential hidden injuries that may be difficult to detect. The incidence of delayed trauma-related complications is greater than that associated with penetrating injuries. This is especially true of blunt injuries involving the liver, kidneys, spleen, and pancreas. Blunt abdominal trauma is frequently associated with extra-abdominal injuries to the chest, head, extremities, etc.

The clinical manifestations of blunt abdominal trauma include pain (especially on movement), rebound and maximal point tenderness (may indicate peritoneal irritation from blood or gastrointestinal fluid), muscle guarding, and diminishing or absent bowel sounds.

(*Text continues, page 1423*)

Peritoneal lavage is the introduction of solution into the peritoneum in order to evaluate the effects of trauma to the abdomen.

PURPOSES
1. To detect blood in the peritoneal cavity following trauma.
2. To look for injuries requiring surgical treatment.
3. To test patients with equivocal abdominal findings.
4. To avoid unnecessary operation, especially in patients with altered states of consciousness (from head injuries, drugs, alcohol) and when physical findings are unreliable (spinal cord injuries).

CONTRAINDICATIONS
1. Multiple abdominal scars
2. Pregnancy

EQUIPMENT
Peritoneal dialysis tray
Sterile solution (lactated Ringer's solution; normal saline)
IV tubing; IV pole
Peritoneal dialysis catheter (multiple perforations)
Local skin anesthetic; sterile gloves

PROCEDURE

Nursing Action	Rationale/Amplification
Preparatory Phase	
1. Explain the procedure to the patient; see that the consent form has been signed.	
2. Empty the bladder (by catheter if necessary).	2. To prevent puncture of urinary bladder.
3. Shave the lower abdomen from umbilicus to pubic area. Prepare the abdomen as for surgery.	3. To minimize or eliminate surface bacteria and decrease the possibility of wound contamination and infection.
4. Fill the IV tubing with solution using aseptic technique.	
Performance Phase (by the physician)	
1. The skin is infiltrated 2-3 cm. (.7-1.2") below the umbilicus in the midline with local anesthetic.	1. The midline area is relatively avascular.
2. A 2-3 cm. (.7-1.2") vertical incision is made down to the linea alba.	
3. Bleeding vessels are carefully ligated.	3. Ligation of vessels helps avoid a false positive lavage.
4. The peritoneum is brought upward between 2 hemostats and is punctured under direct vision. The peritoneum is opened and a peritoneal dialysis catheter is directed into the incision and advanced toward the pelvis.	
5. A gauze sponge is packed into the subcutaneous tissue.	5. To absorb minor bleeding.
6. A syringe is attached to the catheter and the peritoneal cavity is aspirated.	6. If nonclotted blood is obtained (or bile or intestinal contents) the tap shows positive findings and the patient is prepared for immediate celiotomy (incision into abdominal cavity).
7. If no blood is present, the catheter is attached to the IV tubing; 500-1,000 ml. of solution is infused into the peritoneal cavity through the intravenous tubing attached to the dialysis catheter.	7. If not contraindicated by the patient's condition, he may be turned from side to side to ensure that the solution reaches all parts of the abdominal cavity.
8. Clamp off the IV tubing. Remove the empty IV bottle from the pole and lower the bottle to the floor.	8. Lowering the bottle creates a siphon effect to drain the excess fluid. As much of the fluid as possible is siphoned out of the peritoneal cavity by gravity.
9. Dislodge the air vent from the rubber stopper by removing the IV tubing. Reinsert the IV tubing into the vent hole itself. Unclamp the tubing and allow the fluid to be siphoned from the abdominal cavity.	
10. The fluid recovered from the peritoneal cavity is examined visually and is usually sent to the laboratory for cell counts and microscopic inspection of a spun down sediment.	

(Continued)

PERITONEAL LAVAGE (CONTINUED)

Interpretation of lavage fluid

1. *Gross examination (visual)*

   Inability to read newsprint through the intravenous tubing usually means that the amount of blood is sufficient to indicate a laparotomy.

2. *Laboratory evaluation (positive tests)*

   RBC greater than 100,000/cu. mm.

   WBC greater than 500/cu. mm.

   Bacteria—pathologic when present

   Bile—pathologic when present

   Amylase level—greater than 100 Somogyi units/100 ml.

If the test is positive, a laparotomy is usually done.

If the test is negative, the catheter is removed and the wound closed.

If the test is questionable, the catheter may be left in place and the lavage repeated.

If the test is weakly positive, the patient may have echography and arteriography if his condition is stable.

Follow-up Phase

1. Assess patient for complications.

2. Watch the patient closely for any type of deterioration.

1. Complications include visceral perforation, wound hematoma, perforated bowel, puncture of bladder, laceration of major vessels, lack of fluid return.

2. *Repeated physical examinations* of the abdomen should be carried out when intra-abdominal injury is suspected.

(Continued from page 1421)

EMERGENCY MANAGEMENT

1. Take a detailed history (although this is frequently unobtainable, inaccurate, and misleading). Obtain all possible data about the following:
   a. Method of injury.
   b. Time of onset of symptoms.
   c. Passenger location; driver frequently sustains rupture of spleen/liver.
   d. Time of last food/fluid intake.
   e. Bleeding tendencies.
   f. Concurrent disease/medications.
   g. Immunization history, with attention to tetanus.
   h. Allergies.
2. Carry out ongoing physical assessment: inspection, palpation, auscultation, and percussion of the abdomen.
   a. Avoid moving the patient until initial assessment is done.
   b. Look for chest injuries, especially for fractures of the lower ribs.
   c. Inspect front, flanks, and back for bluish discoloration, asymmetry, abrasion, and contusion.
   d. Evaluate for signs and symptoms of hemorrhage which frequently accompanies abdominal injury, especially if liver and spleen have been traumatized.
   e. Note tenderness, rebound tenderness, guarding, rigidity, and spasm.
      (1) Press the area of maximal tenderness (let patient point to the area).
      (2) Remove the fingers quickly; pain at suspected point indicates peritoneal irritation.
   f. Look for increasing abdominal distention. Measure abdominal girth at umbilical level upon admission; this serves as a baseline from which changes can be determined.
   g. Auscultate for bowel sounds; silent abdomen accompanies peritoneal irritation.
   h. Note loss of dullness over solid organs (liver/spleen); indicates presence of free air. Dullness over regions normally containing gas indicates presence of blood.
3. Assist with rectal or vaginal examination for diagnosis of injury to pelvis, bladder and intestinal wall.
4. Avoid giving narcotics during observation period, since this may mask clinical picture.
5. Monitor vital signs frequently and carefully. This may be the only clue to intra-abdominal bleeding.
6. Obtain baseline laboratory studies.
   a. Urinalysis—as a guide to possible urinary tract injury (hematuria) and to monitor urinary output.
   b. Serial hemoglobin and hematocrit levels—their trend reflects presence or absence of bleeding.
   c. CBC—white blood cell count may be elevated with rupture of spleen.
   d. Serum amylase—rising level may indicate pancreatic injury.
7. Obtain abdominal and chest x-rays—may reveal free air beneath diaphragm, indicating ruptured hollow viscus.
8. Prepare for peritoneal lavage (page 1422); organ laceration or bleeding may be diagnosed by gross and microscopic examination of fluid returned after peritoneal lavage.
9. Assist with insertion of nasogastric tube to prevent vomiting and subsequent aspiration. It is also helpful in decompressing (removing fluid/air from) gastrointestinal tract.
10. Patient may be admitted for observation or exploratory laparotomy.

CRUSH INJURIES

Crush injuries occur when a person is crushed beneath debris, run over, or compressed by machinery.

The first step is to assess the patient for oligemic shock resulting from the extravasation of blood and plasma into the injured tissues after the compression has been released. The extremity may be paralyzed, erythematous, swollen, tense, and hard, and the skin blistered. If the shock persists, prolonged hypotension can cause kidney damage and acute renal insufficiency.

EMERGENCY MANAGEMENT

1. Control shock.
2. Observe carefully for acute renal insufficiency. Injury to the back may cause severe kidney damage.
3. Splint major soft tissue injuries to control bleeding and pain early.
4. Elevate the extremity. Incise fascia if the blood supply is blocked to relieve the pressure of extravasated fluid.
5. Administer medication for pain and anxiety.

MULTIPLE INJURIES

The patient with multiple injuries requires a team approach, with one person responsible for coordinating the treatment. Following trauma, there may be general depression of body functions leading to such complications as reduced blood pressure, oxygen deficiency in the blood stream and primary organ systems, arrhythmias, and respiratory and heart failure. The patient may ultimately die of a combination of malfunctions. It is thought that the defense mechanism of the body becomes depressed, contributing to total organ failure.

The objectives of treatment are to determine the extent of injuries and to establish priorities of treatment. Obtaining a patent airway and support of respiration and circulation are key priorities. Imperative lifesaving procedures are performed simultaneously by the emergency team. As soon as the patient is resuscitated, the clothes are usually cut off and a rapid physical assessment is done. Critically traumatized patients should not be moved.

EMERGENCY MANAGEMENT (FIG. 61-8)

Carry out a *rapid* physical examination to determine if patient is breathing, bleeding, or in shock; determine the status of his responsiveness and if he has severe wounds or fracture deformities.

1. Establish an open airway.*
   a. Ask conscious patient if he is having difficulty in breathing. Ask if he has chest pain.
   b. Apply suction to clear the trachea and bronchial tree.

   c. Hold hand above patient's nose to determine adequacy of ventilation. (Not always reliable.)
   d. Insert oropharyngeal airway—to prevent occlusion by tongue.
   e. Ventilate the patient (bag-mask system).
   f. Prepare for endotracheal intubation (page 450) if adequate airway cannot be maintained.
   g. Suspect serious intrathoracic injuries if respiratory distress continues after adequate airway has been established. See pages 497-501 for management of chest injuries.
2. Assess cardiac function and treat cardiac arrest—hypoxia, metabolic acidosis, and chest trauma may precipitate cardiac arrest.*
   a. For cardiac arrest, start closed chest compression and ventilation (page 548).
   b. If chest wall is unstable (flail chest), emergency thoracotomy and manual compression may be necessary.
   c. Give sodium bicarbonate (IV) to compensate for acidosis if indicated—severely traumatized patients with respiratory and circulatory embarrassment will have some degree of metabolic acidosis.
3. Control hemorrhage.*
   a. Apply pressure over bleeding points if hemorrhage is overt (page 1419).
   b. Expect significant blood loss in patient with fracture of shaft of femur, with multiple fractures, or with major pelvic trauma.
   c. Use tourniquet(s) for massive arterial bleeding from extremities which cannot be halted with pressure.
   d. Prepare for immediate surgical intervention if patient is bleeding internally.
4. Prevent and treat hypovolemic shock.
   a. Insert at least two (sometimes 4) IV lines; one above the diaphragm and one below. Use venous cutdown if necessary.
   b. Draw blood for laboratory studies as directed (typing and cross-matching, baseline CBC, electrolytes, blood urea nitrogen, glucose, prothrombin time).
   c. Introduce central venous catheter to monitor patient's response to fluid infusion and to prevent fluid overload.
   d. Start intravenous infusions.
      (1) Balanced saline solution, plasma or plasma protein fraction is given in sufficient quantity to maintain blood pressure until blood is available.
      (2) Give blood as directed—massive transfusions have a cooling effect which can cause cardiac irritability and arrest; blood should be warmed.
   e. Give intravenous infusions rapidly enough to keep central venous pressure readings at 5-15 cm. H_2O; monitor rate and direction of change (important parameters).
   f. Monitor ECG.
   g. Carry out ongoing clinical evaluation to observe for improvement or deterioration; improvement in level of responsiveness, skin warmth, speed of capillary filling, etc., shows reversal of shock state.
   h. Prepare for immediate surgical intervention if patient does not respond to fluids or blood. Inability to restore blood pressure and circulatory volume in patient usually indicates major internal bleeding.

---

*Imperative lifesaving procedures are performed simultaneously by the emergency team.

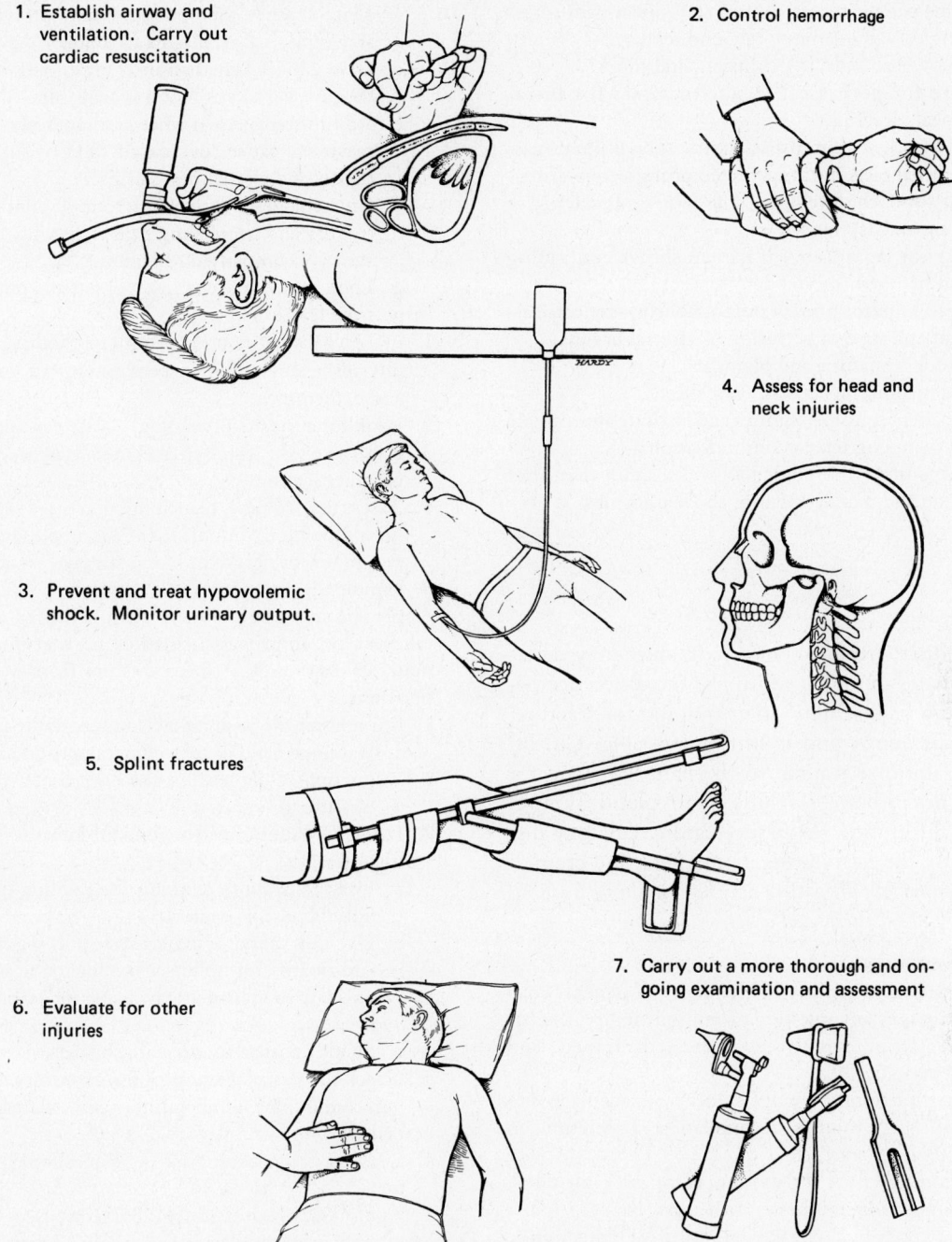

1. Establish airway and ventilation. Carry out cardiac resuscitation

2. Control hemorrhage

3. Prevent and treat hypovolemic shock. Monitor urinary output.

4. Assess for head and neck injuries

5. Splint fractures

6. Evaluate for other injuries

7. Carry out a more thorough and on-going examination and assessment

Figure 61-8.   The patient with multiple injuries.

5. Insert indwelling urethral catheter and monitor urinary output. Do not force the catheter; the patient may have a ruptured urethra.
6. Assess for head and neck injuries.
   a. Make definite statements concerning baseline neurologic status of patient: level of responsiveness, size and reactivity of pupils, motor power, reflexes.
   b. Neck (and chest) films may be taken; apply rigid cervical collar before x-ray examinations if there is any suspicion of cervical neck injury.
   c. Catheter may be inserted into ventricle of brain (page 1186) to measure intracranial pressure if patient does not show signs of cerebral improvement.
7. Administer dexamethasone as directed—corticosteroids appear to protect pulmonary function in patients with multiple injuries and to help prevent posttraumatic pulmonary insufficiency. (However, this is considered a controversial issue.)
8. Splint fractures to prevent further trauma to soft tissues and blood vessels and to relieve pain; note presence or absence of pulses in fractured extremities.
9. Assess patient for gastrointestinal injuries.

a. Examine patient repeatedly for abdominal pain, muscular rigidity, tenderness, rebound tenderness, diminished bowel sounds, hypotension, and shock.

b. Prepare for peritoneal lavage to assess for intraperitoneal bleeding.

c. Assist with insertion of nasogastric tube if upper gastrointestinal bleeding is suspected or if gaseous distension of stomach develops — will decrease incidence of vomiting and aspiration.

d. Prepare for laparotomy if patient shows continuing signs of hemorrhage and deterioration.

10. Continue to monitor urinary output hourly — reflects cardiac output and state of perfusion of visceral organs.
    a. Assess for hematuria and oliguria.
    b. Record measurements on a flow sheet.

11. Evaluate patient for other injuries and institute appropriate treatment including tetanus immunization.

12. Carry out a more thorough physical examination after resuscitation and management of above priorities.

FRACTURES

The immediate management of a fracture may determine the patient's outcome and make the difference between recovery or disability. In examining for fracture, handle the part gently and as little as possible. Cut off clothing to minimize trauma to the part. Evaluate for pain over or near a bone, swelling (from blood, lymph, and exudate infiltrating the tissue), and circulatory disturbance. Look for ecchymosis, tenderness, and crepitation. *Keep in mind that the patient may have multiple fractures accompanied by head, chest, and other serious injuries.*

EMERGENCY MANAGEMENT

A. Give immediate attention to the patient's general condition. If there is any question of multiple injury, the patient needs to be completely undressed, draped, and examined periodically.
   1. Evaluate for respiratory difficulties from edema due to facial and neck injuries, accumulation of secretions in the respiratory tract, etc.
      a. Examine chest for evidences of sucking chest wounds, pneumothorax, flail chest, etc.
      b. Prepare for tracheal intubation or emergency tracheostomy.
   2. Control hemorrhage.
      a. Control venous bleeding by applying direct pressure along with digital pressure over the artery nearest to the bleeding area.
      b. Suspect internal hemorrhage (pleural, pericardial, or abdominal) in the event of continuing shock and in the presence of injuries to the chest and abdomen.
   3. Treat for shock which is usually the result of blood loss in patients with fractures.
      a. Assess for falling blood pressure, cold and clammy skin, and rapid thready pulse.
      b. Keep in mind that a large amount of blood loss may accompany fractures of the femur and pelvis.

c. Maintain the blood pressure with intravenous infusions, plasma, or plasma expanders.

d. Give blood transfusion(s) or blood component therapy as soon as blood is available.

e. Administer oxygen since cardiopulmonary embarrassment causes decreased oxygen supply to the tissues and circulatory collapse.

f. Give analgesic to control pain. (Splinting the extremity and controlling pain are essential in treating shock accompanying fractures.)

g. Look for evidence of head, chest, and other injuries.

B. Inspect the fractured part(s).
   1. Observe the entire body using a methodical head to toe physical examination; inspect for lacerations, swelling, and deformities.
   2. Look for *angulation* (bending), *shortening*, and *rotation*.
   3. Feel the pulse distal to the limb fracture. Check all peripheral pulses.
   4. Assess for coolness, blanching, decreased sensation and motor function, diminished or absent pulses; these indicate injury to nerves or blood supply.
   5. Handle the part gently and as little as possible.

C. Apply the splint before the patient is moved as splinting relieves pain, improves circulation, prevents further tissue injury and prevents a closed fracture from becoming an open one.
   1. Immobilize the joint above and below the fracture.
      a. Place one hand distal to the fracture and apply some traction while placing the other hand beneath the fracture for support.
   2. Extend the splints well beyond the joints adjacent to the fracture.
      a. Use the patient's clothing for padding (shirt, tie) if nothing else is available.
      b. Use newspapers, magazines, pillows, tree limbs, and boards for splints if nothing else is available. Specialized splints are available on ambulances and in hospital.
      c. Splint joints in functional positions.
   3. Check the vascular status of the extremity after splinting; check color, temperature, pulse, blanching of nail bed.
   4. Evaluate for neurological deficits caused by the fracture.
   5. Apply a sterile dressing if the fracture is an open one.

D. Investigate any complaint of pain or pressure.

E. Transport the patient carefully and gently.

F. See pages 1299-1313 for a complete discussion of the treatment of fractures at specific sites.

Emergency Splinting and Transporting

The act of improperly moving an accident victim from one position to another may make a closed fracture an open one, may puncture a lung, or may sever a spinal cord or major blood vessel. A suspected fracture should be splinted before the patient is moved. In general, splints should be rigid but well padded and wrapped with nonconstricting material. A splint is applied so that the joints above and below the fracture are immobilized.

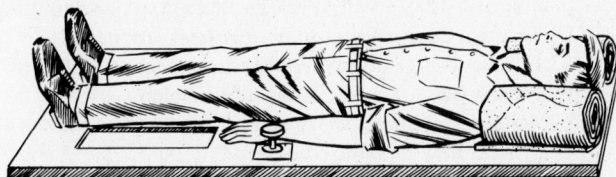

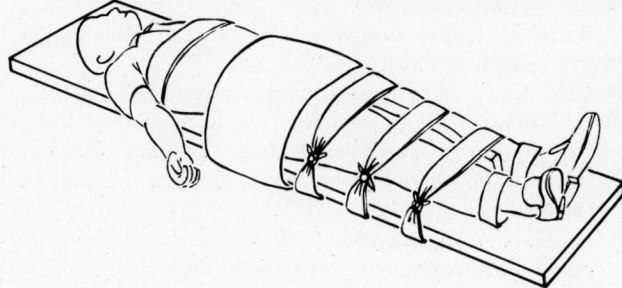

Figure 61-9. Transporting a patient with a cervical injury of the spine. While transporting patient, assign someone to stabilize the patient's head.

Figure 61-10. Emergency splinting of a pelvic fracture. Immobilize the pelvis as much as possible.

1. **Skull**
   a. If there is no cervical spine injury, elevate the head slightly on the stretcher, but do not place a pillow under the head.
   b. Maintain adequate respiration. Transport patient with head to one side to promote drainage of mucus, blood, or vomitus if level of responsiveness does not permit patient to do so himself.
2. **Jaw**
   a. Hold the jaw up and in by tying with a bandage, if there is no spinal cord injury.
   b. Transport the patient in a sitting position, with the head slightly bent forward.
   c. Be alert for possible vomiting; cut bandages immediately to prevent aspiration of vomitus.
3. **Cervical spine**
   a. Place your hands on each side of the head so that the ears are cupped in the hands. (The thumb should be in the temporal region, the second finger just below the zygoma, the third finger along the zygoma, and the fourth finger beneath the mandible and extending traction.)
   b. Hold the patient's head, keeping it in line with the body. Slide him on a rigid surface *flat on his back, face up*. The entire body is moved as a unit. Avoid twisting, turning, or pulling the spine (Fig. 61-9).
   c. Watch for inadequate respiratory exchange due to paralysis of chest muscles and for neurogenic shock.
4. **Lumbar spine** — Straighten patient carefully and place him on a rigid surface such as a long spinal board. Avoid flexion, extension, or rotation of the spine.
5. **Pelvis** — Turn the patient carefully on his back. Place padding between the legs and splint them together to prevent unnecessary motion. Immobilize the pelvis by binding a folded blanket around the pelvis. Transport on a firm stretcher (Fig. 61-10).
6. **Shoulder, Arm, and Elbow** — Place elbow at right angle and apply sling. Bind arm and sling to body with a circular bandage or binder. Check radial pulse in an elbow injury. Do not compromise circulation with bandage in antecubital area. Check radial pulse. If injured elbow is in extension, bandage the extremity to the body in the position in which it is found.
7. **Forearm, Wrist, and Hand** — Immobilize with newspaper splint or with commercial or inflatable air splint. Place arm in sling with elbow at right angle (Fig. 61-11).
8. **Hip** — Splint from axilla to ankle with board. If board is not available, bind the legs together. Use a half-ring trac-

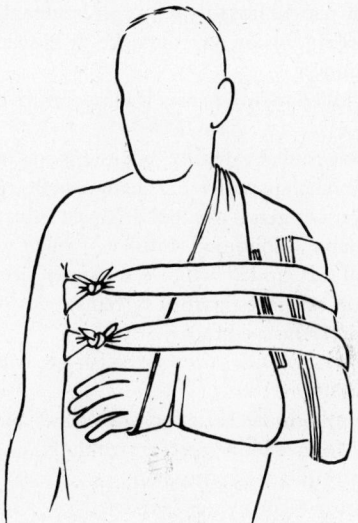

Figure 61-11. Splinting for a broken arm.

tion if available; traction is obtained by means of a hitch around the foot and ankle. Transport patient on a stretcher.
9. **Lower extremity** — Apply steady, even traction and splint fracture from hip to ankle. Transport patient on stretcher.
10. **Ankle** — Wrap pillow around lower leg, ankle, and foot. Transport patient on a stretcher.

HEAT STROKE

Heat stroke is a medical emergency caused by failure of the heat-regulating mechanisms of the body when the temperature-humidity index is high. Persons who are not acclimatized to heat exposure, the elderly, and those with cardiovascular problems are particularly vulnerable. Young persons exercising strenuously in a hot environment and persons on certain medications are at risk.

When assessing the patient, note the following: (1) headache and visual disturbances, (2) dizziness and nausea, (3) hot dry flushed skin, later becoming ashen, (4) weak, rapid, or irregular pulse, (5) sudden loss of consciousness, (6) high fever (41-43° C. [105-109° F.]) or cessation of sweating, (7) muscle cramping, and (8) convulsions.

EMERGENCY MANAGEMENT

The objective of management is to reduce the high temperature as quickly as possible.

1. Reduce the core (internal) temperature to 39° C. (102° F. rectally) as rapidly as possible. If available, monitor the rectal temperature by a rectal thermistor probe left in place. One or more of the following temperature-lowering methods may be used.
   a. Place patient in a tub of cold water with ice cubes added.
      (1) Rub extremities continuously during immersion—promotes circulation and maintains cutaneous vasodilation.
   b. Place patient on a hypothermia blanket if available.
   c. Sponge patient liberally with cool water; place electric fan so that it blows on patient, since air movement increases evaporation.
   d. Give chilled saline enemas if temperature does not come down.
   e. Monitor patient carefully; vital signs and level of responsiveness change with rapid changes in body temperature.
2. Administer oxygen—to supply tissue needs exaggerated by hypermetabolic condition. Intubate patient with cuffed endotracheal tube and attach to ventilator if necessary to support failing cardiorespiratory systems.
3. Give medications as directed.
   a. Small doses of chlorpromazine IV—to control shivering and agitation.
   b. Mannitol—to decrease cerebral edema and ensure urine flow. Monitor blood pressure carefully, since these agents may precipitate hypotension.
   c. Potassium—for hypokalemia.
   d. Sodium bicarbonate—to correct metabolic acidosis.
4. Start intravenous infusions as directed; give slowly because of danger of acute pulmonary edema.
5. Measure urinary output—acute tubular necrosis is a complication of heat stroke.
6. Admit to intensive care unit—permanent liver, cardiac, and central nervous system damage may occur.
7. Advise patient to avoid immediate re-exposure to high temperatures (after condition has stabilized); patient may remain hypersensitive to high temperatures for considerable length of time.

COLD INJURIES

The extent of injury from exposure to cold is not always known when the patient is seen initially. A frozen extremity may be hard, cold and insensitive to touch and appear white or mottled blue-white. Color changes (purple; cyanosis) after rewarming may be transient or they may indicate pressure within the fascial compartment.

EMERGENCY MANAGEMENT

The objective of management is to restore normal body temperature.

1. Do not allow the patient to walk if lower extremities are involved.
2. Remove all constricting clothing.
3. Rewarm extremity gently and rapidly in warm water bath, 37.8–42° C. (100–108° F.)—early thawing appears to give better chance for maximum tissue preservation.
   a. Handle part gently to avoid further mechanical injury.
   b. Protect thawed part; do not rupture blebs.
   c. Administer analgesic for pain if necesary—thawing process may be quite painful.
4. Carry out physical assessment—to look for concomitant injury (soft tissue injury, fracture, dehydration, alcohol coma, fat embolism).
5. Restore electrolyte balance; check for acidosis.
6. Give tetanus prophylaxis if indicated by associated trauma.
7. Use bedside isolation with sterile technique during bleb stage to protect patient from contamination.
8. Encourage hourly active motion of affected digits to promote maximum restoration of function.
9. The following measures may be carried out when appropriate:
   a. Whirlpool bath for affected extremity
   b. Escharotomy to permit joint motion
   c. Fasciotomy and sympathectomy if there is distal ischemia
10. Prohibit use of tobacco because of vasoconstrictive effect.

Accidental Hypothermia

Accidental hypothermia is a condition in which the core (internal) temperature is less than 35° C. (95° F.) as a result of exposure to cold.

There is progressive deterioration with apathy, poor judgment, ataxia, dysarthria, drowsiness, and, eventually coma. Shivering may be suppressed below a temperature of 32.2° C. (90° F.). Below this temperature the body's self-warming mechanisms become ineffective. The heartbeat and the blood pressure may be so weak that the peripheral pulsation becomes undetectable. Cardiac irregularities also may occur. Other physiologic abnormalities include hypoxemia and acidosis.

EMERGENCY MANAGEMENT

Management consists of continuing monitoring, rewarming, and supportive care.

1. Monitor patient—vital signs, CVP, urinary output, arterial blood gases, electrolytes, glucose, BUN.
   a. Monitor body temperature with esophageal or rectal thermistor probe.
   b. Employ continuous ECG monitoring.
   c. Maintain arterial line for recording blood pressure and to facilitate blood sampling.
2. Rewarm patient: rewarming methods include active core (internal) rewarming, active external rewarming, and passive or spontaneous rewarming. The optimal method is controversial.
3. Supportive care during rewarming includes:
   a. External cardiac massage if indicated.
   b. Mechanical ventilation with PEEP and heated oxygen—to maintain tissue oxygenation.
   c. IV fluids (warmed)—to correct hypotension, maintain urinary output.
   d. Sodium bicarbonate—to correct metabolic acidosis.
   e. Electrical cardioversion of ventricular fibrillation.

ANAPHYLACTIC REACTION

An anaphylactic reaction is a generalized systemic and frequently fatal reaction occurring with seconds to minutes after exposure to the causative agent, namely, foreign sera, drugs, or insect venoms. Repeated administration of parenteral or oral therapeutic agents also may precipitate an anaphylactic reaction.

An anaphylactic reaction is the result of an antigen-antibody interaction in a sensitized individual who, as a consequence of previous exposure, has developed a special type of antibody (immunoglobin) that is specific for this particular allergen. The antibody immunoglobulin IgE is responsible for the great majority of immediate type of human allergic responses—the individual becomes sensitive to a particular antigen after production of IgE to this antigen.

Anaphylactic reaction produces a wide range of clinical manifestations.

- *Respiratory signs* include (1) possible respiratory distress which progresses rapidly and is caused by bronchospasm or edema of the larynx, (2) sneezing and coughing, (3) tightness of the chest, and (4) other respiratory difficulties such as wheezing, dyspnea, and cyanosis.
- *Skin manifestations* appear in the form of flushing with a sense of warmth and diffuse erythema. *Generalized itching over the entire body indicates that a general systemic reaction is developing.* Urticaria (hives) may also appear. When massive facial angioedema develops, upper respiratory edema may occur.
- *Cardiovascular manifestations* include tachycardia or bradycardia and peripheral vascular collapse as indicated by pallor, imperceptible pulse, falling blood pressure, and circulatory failure leading to coma and death.
- *Gastrointestinal discomforts* such as nausea, vomiting, and colicky abdominal pains or diarrhea, may contribute to the general sense of malaise.

EMERGENCY MANAGEMENT

1. Establish an airway while another person administers epinephrine.
   a. Turn face to one side; support angles of mandible.
   b. Insert oropharyngeal or endotracheal tube; apply oropharyngeal suction for excessive secretions.
   c. Employ resuscitative measures (especially for patients with stridor and progressive pulmonary edema).
   d. If glottic edema is present, an incision through the cricothyroid ligament will provide an airway.
   e. Use positive pressure oxygen therapy by mask and compression bag.
   f. Use closed chest cardiac massage if necessary.
2. Give epinephrine as directed—to provide rapid relief of hypersensitivity reaction. This should be done while another person is establishing the airway.

   Use judgment in choosing route of administration for epinephrine.
   a. Subcutaneous injection for mild, generalized symptoms.
   b. Intramuscular or sublingual injection when reaction is more severe and progressive and when there is concern that vascular collapse will inhibit absorption.
   c. Intravenous route (aqueous epinephrine diluted in saline and given *slowly*) for profound hypotension: this method may precipitate cardiac arrhythmias.
3. Start an intravenous infusion of saline for emergency route.
4. Apply tourniquet above injection site if anaphylactic reaction followed injection or insect sting—to retard absorption.

   Infiltrate injection site with epinephrine as directed.
5. Give antihistamine drugs, e.g., diphenhydramine hydrochloride (Benadryl) (IM)—to block further histamine binding at target cells.
6. Give aminophylline IV *slowly* over a period of time for patients with severe bronchospasm and asthmatic symptoms. This is usually not given if patient is responding to epinephrine.
7. Treat prolonged hypotension with plasma or colloids (dextran), vasoconstrictors (metaraminol bitartrate (Aramine), or levarterenol bitartrate (Levophed); patient with reduced cardiac output may respond to an infusion of isoproterenol or dopamine.
8. Watch for arrhythmias and cardiorespiratory arrest.
9. If the patient is convulsing, give IV injection of short-acting barbiturate or diazepam over a period of several minutes.
10. Administer corticosteroids if the patient is having a prolonged reaction and persistent hypotension or bronchospasm.

Preventive Measures

1. Be aware of the danger of anaphylactic reactions.
2. Ask about the patient's previous allergies to medications; if positive, do not give medication or injection.
3. Question the patient before giving a foreign serum or other types of antigenic agents to determine whether he has had it at some earlier time.
4. Question the patient concerning previous allergic reactions to food or pollen.
5. Avoid giving drugs to patients with hay fever, asthma, and other allergic disorders unless absolutely necessary.
6. Do skin testing before administering foreign serum. Skin testing can precipitate anaphylaxis in highly sensitive individuals.

   A negative skin test does not always indicate safety. Have epinephrine on hand to control acute untoward reactions.
7. If patient is being treated as an outpatient, keep him in the office, hospital, or clinic at least 30 minutes after injection of any agent.
8. Caution patients who are sensitive to insect bites to carry kits equipped to treat insect stings (tourniquet, epinephrine).
9. Avoid giving parenteral medications unless absolutely indicated.

   Anaphylactic reactions are more likely to occur when agent is given parenterally.
10. Encourage allergic individuals to wear identification tags.

POISONING

Poison is any substance which when ingested, inhaled, absorbed, applied to the skin, or produced within the body in relatively small amounts, causes injury to the body by its chemical action. Poisoning from inhalation and ingestion of toxic materials, both accidental and by design, constitutes a major health hazard. The problem is one of real magnitude, as is reflected in the high number of such patients — more than 1 million cases of poisoning occur in the United States annually.

The objectives of emergency treatment are (1) to remove or inactivate the poison before it is absorbed, (2) to give supportive care to maintain vital organ systems, (3) to use the specific antidote to neutralize the poison, and (4) to give treatment to hasten the elimination of the absorbed poison.

SWALLOWED POISONS

GENERAL MANAGEMENT

1. Try to discover the nature of the poison. Call the poison control center in the area if an unknown toxic agent has been taken, or if it is necessary to identify an antidote for a known toxic agent.
2. Maintain the airway; in the absence of cerebral or renal damage the patient's prognosis largely depends upon successful management of respiratory and circulatory systems.
   a. Administer oxygen for respiratory depression, unconsciousness, cyanosis, shock.
   b. Give artificial respiration if respiration is depressed. Positive expiratory pressure applied to airway may help keep alveoli inflated.
   c. Take arterial blood samples to measure pH and blood gas tensions.
   d. Insert indwelling urinary catheter to monitor kidney function.
   e. Assess for central nervous system depression.
3. Consider gastric lavage or induce emesis as the clinical situation dictates.
4. Treat shock appropriately.
5. Support the patient having convulsions; many poisons excite the central nervous system, or else the patient may convulse from oxygen deprivation.
6. Give specific therapy. Administer special chemical antidote or specific pharmacologic antagonists as early as possible (if indicated).
7. Monitor central venous pressure as indicated.
8. Monitor for fluid and electrolyte imbalance.
9. Reduce elevated temperature.
10. Give analgesics for pain cautiously; severe pain causes vasomotor collapse and reflex inhibition of normal physiologic functions.
11. Provide constant nursing surveillance and attention to the patient in a coma; coma from poisoning results from interference with brain cell function or metabolism.
12. Assist with forced diuresis, hemodialysis, or peritoneal dialysis to shorten period of unconsciousness in the event of barbiturate and other hypnotic or tranquilizer poisoning.
13. Assist in securing specimens of blood, urine, stomach contents, and vomitus.

Corrosive Poisons

Corrosive poisons include *acid and acidlike substances* such as sodium acid sulfate (toilet bowl cleaners), acetic acid, sulfuric acid, nitric acid, oxalic acid, hydrofluoric acid (rust removers), iodine, or silver nitrate, and *alkali corrosives,* such as sodium hydroxide (lye, drain cleaners), dish washer detergents, sodium carbonate (washing soda), ammonia water, and sodium hypochlorite (household bleach).

Patients suspected of swallowing corrosive poisons should be assessed for severe pain and burning sensations in the mouth and throat, pain in swallowing or an inability to swallow, destruction of oral mucosa, vomiting, and drooling (in children).

EMERGENCY MANAGEMENT

- If the patient can swallow after ingestion of a *corrosive poison,* offer milk as an emollient agent.
- *Do not induce vomiting if person has consumed a strong acid, alkali, or other corrosive substance.*

Noncorrosive Poisons

EMERGENCY MANAGEMENT

1. Remove poison from the patient's stomach immediately by inducing vomiting. *Do not induce vomiting if person has consumed a strong acid, alkali, or other corrosive or hydrocarbon solvent. Do not induce vomiting if patient is in a coma, is unconscious, or having convulsions.*
   a. Give 3 to 4 glassfuls of milk or water to dilute poison.
   b. Induce vomiting by giving syrup of ipecac or inserting the index finger or blunt end of a spoon at the back of the patient's throat.
2. Carry out gastric lavage to remove any unabsorbed poison (see procedure on page 1431). This is *not* done if corrosives or hydrocarbon solvents have been ingested (turpentine, kerosene, gasoline, liquid wax, charcoal lighter fluid, etc.). Persons ingesting hydrocarbons should have a chest film to evaluate for chemical pneumonia.
3. Instruct the family to bring the unused poison to the hospital for identification.
4. Know the poison control center in the area; call the center if an unknown toxic agent has been taken or if it is necessary to identify an antidote for a known toxic agent.

INHALED POISONS

GENERAL MANAGEMENT

1. Carry the patient to fresh air immediately; open all doors and windows.
2. Loosen all tight clothing.
3. Apply artificial respiration if required.

ASSISTING WITH GASTRIC LAVAGE

Gastric lavage is the aspiration of the stomach contents and washing out of the stomach by means of a gastric tube.

Gastric lavage may be dangerous after acid or alkali ingestion, in the presence of convulsions, or after ingestion of hydrocarbons or petroleum distillates. It is dangerous after ingestion of strong corrosive agents.

PURPOSES

1. To remove unabsorbed poison after ingestion of poison.
2. To diagnose gastric hemorrhage and to arrest hemorrhage.
3. To cleanse the stomach before endoscopic procedures.
4. To remove liquid or small particles of material from the stomach.

EQUIPMENT

Stomach tubes (large lumen)
Large irrigating syringe with adapter
Large plastic funnel with adapter to fit stomach tube
Water soluble lubricant
Tap water or appropriate antidote (milk, saline solution, sodium bicarbonate solution, fruit juice, activated charcoal*)
Bucket for aspirate
Mouth gag; nasotracheal or endotracheal tubes with inflatable cuffs
Containers for specimens

PROCEDURE

Action	Rationale/Amplification
1. Remove dental appliances and inspect oral cavity for loose teeth.	1. This will prevent accidental aspiration.
2. Measure the distance between the bridge of the nose and the xiphoid process. Mark tube with indelible pencil or tape.	2. This distance is a rule of thumb measurement of the distance the tube is passed to reach the stomach.
3. Lubricate the tube with water soluble lubricant.	
4. If the patient is comatose he is intubated with a cuffed nasotracheal or endotracheal tube.	4. A cuffed endotracheal tube prevents aspiration of gastric contents.
5. Place the patient in a left lateral position with the head, neck, and trunk forming a straight line. After the lavage tube is passed, the head of the table is lowered. Have standby suction available.	5. This position prevents fluid from running into the trachea and keeps reflux vomitus from being aspirated.
6. Pass the tube via the oral (or nasal) route while keeping the head in a neutral position. Pass the tube to the adhesive marking or about 50 cm. (20 inches).	6. The depth of insertion of the tube will vary with the height of the patient. If the tube enters the larynx instead of the esophagus the patient will experience coughing and dyspnea.
7. Submerge free end of tube below water level at the moment of patient's exhalation.	7. If tube is inadvertently in the lungs, the water will bubble with each exhalation.
8. Aspirate the stomach contents with syringe attached to the tube before instilling water or antidote. Save the specimen for analysis.	8. Aspiration is carried out to remove the stomach contents.
9. Remove syringe. Attach funnel to the stomach tube or use 50-ml. syringe to put lavage solution in gastric tube. Volume of fluid placed in the stomach should be small.	9. Overfilling of the stomach may cause regurgitation and aspiration or force the stomach contents through the pylorus.
10. Elevate funnel above the patient's head and pour approximately 120-300 ml. of solution into funnel.	10. If the syringe method is used, the turbulence from the pressure of the syringe will cause the fluid to mix with the stomach contents and assist in washing all of the mucosal surface. It is possible for poison/drugs to be trapped in the rugae of stomach.
11. Lower the funnel and siphon the gastric contents into the bucket.	
12. Save samples of first 2 washings.	12. Keep first washings isolated from other washings for possible analysis.
13. Repeat lavage procedure until the returns are relatively clear.	

(Continued)

---

*Activated charcoal will absorb significant quantities of many drugs and chemicals and thus retards absorption from the gastrointestinal tract.

14. At the completion of lavage:
    a. Stomach may be left empty.
    b. Antidote may be instilled in tube and allowed to remain in stomach.
    c. Cathartic may be put down tube.
15. Pinch off tube during removal or maintain suction while tube is being withdrawn.

16. Give the patient a cathartic if prescribed.

15. Pinching off the tube prevents aspiration and the initiation of the gag reflex. Keeping the patient's head lower than the body also gives this protection.
16. A cathartic may be given if the poison has no corrosive action on the bowel. The cathartic will help remove unabsorbed material from the intestine.

---

4. Prevent chilling; wrap patient in blankets.
5. Keep patient as quiet as possible.
6. Do not give alcohol in any form.

Carbon Monoxide Poisoning

Carbon monoxide poisoning may occur as an industrial or household accident or as an attempted suicide. It causes more deaths than any other toxic agent except alcohol. Carbon monoxide exerts its toxic effect by binding to circulating hemoglobin to reduce the oxygen-carrying capacity of the blood. The affinity between carbon monoxide and hemoglobin is 200 to 300 times that between oxygen and hemoglobin. (Carbon monoxide combines with hemoglobin to form carboxyhemoglobin). As a result there is tissue anoxia.

The central nervous system has a critical need of oxygen and will show signs of carbon monoxide toxicity. A person suffering from carbon monoxide poisoning will appear intoxicated (from cerebral hypoxia). Other symptoms and signs include headache, muscular weakness, palpitation, dizziness, and mental confusion which can progress rapidly to coma. The skin color is not a reliable sign. Skin color may be pink, cherry red, or cyanotic and pale. History of exposure to carbon monoxide should justify immediate treatment.

EMERGENCY MANAGEMENT

The objectives of management are to reverse cerebral and myocardial hypoxia and to hasten carbon monoxide elimination.
1. Give 100% oxygen at atmospheric or hyperbaric pressures to reverse hypoxia and accelerate elimination of carbon monoxide.
2. Oberve the patient constantly. Psychoses, spastic paralysis, ataxia, visual disturbances, and deterioration of personality may persist following resuscitation and may be symptoms of permanent central nervous system damage.

SKIN CONTAMINATION POISONS

EMERGENCY MANAGEMENT
1. Drench skin with water (shower, hose, faucet).
2. Apply stream of water to skin while removing clothing.
3. Cleanse skin thoroughly with water; rapidity in washing is most important in reducing extent of injury.

INJECTED POISONS

Stinging Insects (bee, yellow jacket, hornet, wasp)

A person may have an extreme sensitivity to the stings of bees, yellow jackets, hornets, and wasps. This constitutes an acute emergency. Stings of the head and neck are especially serious, although stings in any area of the body can result in anaphylaxis.

The clinical response may range from generalized urticaria, itching, malaise, and anxiety to constriction in the throat, difficulty in breathing, respiratory obstruction, collapse, and death. In general, the shorter the time between the sting and the onset of severe symptoms, the worse the prognosis.

EMERGENCY MANAGEMENT
1. Give epinephrine as directed. Massage the site to hasten absorption.
2. See page 1429 for treatment of anaphylactic shock.
3. Counsel all persons known to be sensitive to hymenoptera venom to carry an emergency insect sting kit (kit with tourniquet, epinephrine, syringe and needles, aerosol inhalator containing epinephrine bitartrate, and oral antihistamine tablets).
    a. Instruct the patient to take epinephrine immediately if he is stung.
    b. Flick stinger off with fingernail, or scrape away with knife.
    c. Do not squeeze venom sac; may cause additional venom to be injected.
4. A person with this allergy should be encouraged to undergo hyposensitization injections and to wear a medical warning bracelet.

5. Instruct the patient to avoid the following:
   a. Locales with stinging insects (camp and picnic sites, orchards, clover patches)
   b. Going barefoot outdoors—yellow jackets may nest on ground.
   c. Perfumes, scented soaps, and bright colors—attract bees.
   d. Eating sweets outdoors.

Snakebite

Only about 10 percent of the snakes in the United States are poisonous. The majority of these belong to the *Crotalidae* (pit vipers) which includes rattlesnakes, ground rattlers, moccasins (cotton mouth or water moccasins, copperhead or highland moccasin). The remainder (less than 2 percent) belong to the *Elapidae* family (coral snakes) which includes the Eastern coral snake and the Arizona coral snake.

Immediately following a poisonous snakebite there is usually burning pain and rapidly spreading edema at the site of the bite. The toxic effects of snake venom affect the hematologic, cardiovascular, respiratory, and nervous systems. There is local tissue destruction that often results in loss of function.

IMMEDIATE FIRST AID TO SNAKEBITE VICTIMS

Snakebites are considered a medical emergency. The treatment of poisonous snakebites is controversial.

1. Try to identify the offending snake; kill the snake and bring it in for identification.
2. Apply a mildly constricting tourniquet above the bite area; one should be able to pass a finger under the tourniquet—to retard spread of venom.
   a. Obstruct only lymphatic and superficial venous flow.
   b. Release every 30 minutes for 60-90 seconds; some authorities disagree, since they feel that this causes additional venom to be propelled from the limb.
3. Wash the skin over the fang marks. Make an incision 4 to 6 mm. long (¼ inch) through the fang marks, cutting only through the skin; this is only effective if done within the first few minutes.
4. Apply suction by suction cup (provided in snakebite kits)—preferable to oral suction since there are wound contaminating organisms in the mouth.
5. Immobilize the extremity below the heart level.
6. In the event of severe envenomation when no other treatment is available for many hours, a tight occlusive tourniquet may have to be applied as a lifesaving measure; this may result in loss of the extremity.
7. *Do not use any form of cooling.*
8. Transport the patient to the medical facility on a stretcher if available.
9. Splint the extremity in a functional position.
10. Notify police to telephone ahead to Emergency Department.

TREATMENT IN EMERGENCY DEPARTMENT

1. Reassure the patient—victims of snakebite are extremely frightened.
2. Perform skin or eye test for hypersensitivity to horse serum; antivenin is prepared from horse serum.
   a. Testing is described in detail in the brochure enclosed with each unit of antivenin.
   b. Obtain history of previous illnesses and allergies, especially allergy to horse serum.
3. Start an intravenous infusion.
4. Give prescribed antivenin IV as soon as possible (the mainstay of treatment).
   a. Have epinephrine drawn up in syringe available for immediate use in the event of an unfavorable reaction.
   b. Give antivenin slowly, according to package brochure directions.
5. Cleanse the bite site; cover with sterile dressing. Immobilize affected extremity in position of function.
6. If tight tourniquet has been in place for less than 1 hour prior to patient's admission, apply a looser one closer to the bite site and remove the first tourniquet.
   a. Do not suddenly release a tourniquet that has been left in place for several hours; rapid systemic absorption of unneutralized venom may ensue.
   b. Release tourniquet gradually, as directed, after antivenin therapy is started.
7. Give broad-spectrum antimicrobial as required—pathogenic bacteria in snake's mouth and venoms are predominantly gram-negative.
8. Give tetanus toxoid and, if necessary, human tetanus immune globulin.
9. Use supportive measures—blood transfusion, pressor agents, etc., as required by patient's symptoms and condition.
10. Carry out careful ongoing patient assessment and monitoring.
    a. Note blood pressure, pulse, level of consciousness.
    b. Measure circumference of involved extremity.
11. Assist with fasciotomy, which is done occasionally.

FOOD POISONING

Food poisoning is a sudden, explosive illness which may occur after ingestion of contaminated food or drink. Botulism, a serious form of food poisoning, is discussed on page 1389 since the treatment differs and the patient requires continuing surveillance.

EMERGENCY MANAGEMENT

1. Determine the source and type of food poisoning.
   a. Have family bring suspected food to medical facility.
   b. Take the history:
      (1) How soon after eating did the symptoms occur? Immediate onset suggests chemical, plant, or animal poisoning.
      (2) What was eaten in the previous meal? Did the food have any unusual odor or taste. Most foods causing bacterial poisoning do not have unusual odor or taste.

(3) Did vomiting occur? What was the appearance of the vomitus?

(4) Did diarrhea occur? Diarrhea is usually absent with botulism, shell-fish, or other fish poisoning.

(5) Are any neurologic symptoms present? These occur in botulism, chemical, plant, and animal poisoning.

(6) Does the patient have fever? Fever is seen in salmonella, favism (ingestion of fava beans), and some fish poisoning.

(7) What is the patient's appearance?

2. Monitor vital signs on a continuing basis.
   a. Assess respiration, blood pressure, sensorium, central venous pressure (if indicated), and muscular activity.
   b. Weigh the patient for future comparisons.

3. Support the respiratory system. Death from respiratory paralysis can occur with botulism, fish poisoning, etc.

4. Maintain fluid and electrolyte balance; severe vomiting produces alkalosis and severe diarrhea produces acidosis; large amounts of electrolytes and water are lost by vomiting and diarrhea.
   a. Watch for oligemic shock from severe fluid and electrolyte losses.
   b. Evaluate for apathy, rapid pulse, fever, oliguria, anuria, hypotension, delirium.
   c. Carry out blood electrolyte studies.
   d. Obtain stool specimen for culture and sensitivity.

5. Correct and control hypoglycemia.

6. Control the nausea.
   a. Give antiemetic drug parenterally if patient cannot tolerate fluids or medications by mouth.
   b. Give sips of weak tea, carbonated drinks, tap water for mild nausea.
   c. Give clear liquids 12 to 24 hours after nausea and vomiting subside.
   d. Graduate to a low residue bland diet.

DRUG ABUSE

Drug abuse is the use of drugs for other than legitimate medical purposes. The clinical manifestations may vary with the drug used, but the underlying principles of management are essentially the same. Table 61-1 notes the most commonly abused drugs, listing their clinical manifestations and therapeutic management.

There is a growing tendency among drug users to take a variety of drugs simultaneously, including alcohol, barbiturates, tranquilizers, and sedatives which may have additive effects. The immediate management of a patient suffering from drug intoxication is to support the respiratory and cardiovascular functions and then to give definitive treatment for the drug overdose. In addition, if the patient is unconscious and drug abuse is suspected, he should be undressed and examined for needle marks and antecubital scarring.

Acute Drug Reaction

EMERGENCY MANAGEMENT

1. Provide a patent airway. Maintain the patient's respirations.
   a. Use a cuffed endotracheal tube and provide assisted ventilation in a severely depressed patient with absent gag or cough reflexes.
   b. Measure arterial blood gases for hypoxia due to hypoventilation and acid-base derangements.
   c. Administer oxygen.

2. Start intravenous fluids and stabilize the cardiovascular system. (This is done simultaneously with airway management.)
   a. Begin external cardiac compression and ventilation in the absence of heartbeat.
   b. Start ECG monitoring.

3. Give specific drug antagonist if drug is known; naloxone hydrochloride (Narcan) is frequently used.

4. Remove the drug from the stomach as soon as possible.
   a. Induce vomiting if patient is seen early after ingestion.
   b. Use gastric lavage if the patient is unconscious or if there is no way to determine when the drug was ingested.
      In patients with absent gag or cough reflexes, carry out this procedure only after intubation with cuffed endotracheal tube to prevent aspiration of the stomach contents.
   c. Activated charcoal may be a useful adjunct to therapy and is used after emesis or lavage.
   d. Save gastric contents for toxicologic analysis.

5. Consider hemodialysis or peritoneal dialysis for potentially lethal poisoning.

6. Try to maintain a free urine flow since the drug or metabolites are excreted by the kidneys.

7. Do a thorough physical examination to rule out insulin shock, meningitis, subdural hematoma, stroke, etc.
   a. Look for needle marks.
   b. There is a high incidence of infectious hepatitis among drug users which is thought to be the result of communal use of nonsterile needles and syringes.
   c. Keep in mind that many drug users take multiple drugs at the same time.
   d. Examine breath for characteristic odor of alcohol, acetone, etc.

8. Try to obtain a history of the drug experience (from the person accompanying the patient or the patient himself).
   a. Adapt a supportive, empathetic, and realistic relationship with the patient.
   b. Do not leave the patient alone.

9. Make every effort to enroll the patient in a drug treatment program (detoxication and rehabilitation) to intervene in a life style that fosters addiction.

ALCOHOLISM

Acute Alcohol Intoxication

According to the AMA Manual on Alcoholism, "Alcoholism is an illness characterized by preoccupation with alcohol and loss of control over its consumption such as

(Text continues, page 1438)

TABLE 61-1. EMERGENCY MANAGEMENT OF DRUG ABUSES

DRUG	CLINICAL MANIFESTATIONS	THERAPEUTIC MANAGEMENT
Narcotics Heroin (most frequently involved) Opium or paregoric Morphine, codeine, synthetic narcotics (methadone)	*Acute Intoxication* Pinpoint pupils Depressed vital signs Apnea or slow respirations (2-6/minute) Fresh needle marks along course of any superficial vein Thrombophlebitis Healed skin abscesses	Support respiratory and cardiovascular functions. Give narcotic antagonist to counteract respiratory depression (naloxone hydrochloride [Narcan]). Patient may slip back into severe respiratory depression once antagonist wears off. Do not leave patient unattended until fully responsive. Send urine for analysis; opiates can be detected in urine. Secure blood for chemical and toxicologic analysis for baseline studies. Establish an IV line; patient may be given a bolus of glucose to eliminate possibility of hypoglycemia. Secure an ECG. Gastric lavage may be necessary to obtain sample of drug for analysis and for treatment. Hemodialysis may be indicated for severe drug intoxication.
	Heroin Withdrawal Syndrome Lethargy, yawning Perspiration, lacrimation, runny nose Dilated pupils, poorly reactive to light Gooseflesh, muscular aches Twitching, anorexia, nausea, vomiting, abdominal pain Chills and fever	Methadone may be prescribed if patient is receiving treatment at a methadone center, or substitution therapy should be given in hospital setting. Give intravenous fluids since patient is dehydrated from vomiting; may progress to toxic delirium. Assess for concomitant medical problems (hepatitis, pneumonia, severe diarrhea). Place patient in a protected environment under proper medical supervision. Make every effort to enroll patient in narcotics treatment program.

Barbiturates
Pentobarbital (Nembutal)
Secobarbital (Seconal)
Amobarbital (Amytal)
	Acute Intoxication
	Flushed face
	Decreased pulse rate
	Increasing nystagmus
	Depressed tendon reflexes
	Decreasing mental alertness
	Difficulty in speaking
	Poor motor coordination
	Coma; death
		Maintain airway and stimulate depressed respirations.
		Consider endotracheal intubation or tracheostomy if there is any doubt about the adequacy of airway exchange.
		  a. Check airway frequently.
		  b. Perform *regular* suctioning.
		Support cardiovascular and respiratory functions—most deaths result from depression of these systems.
		Start intravenous infusion through large gauge needle or intravenous catheter to support blood pressure—coma and dehydration result in hypotension and respond to infusion of intravenous fluids with elevation of blood pressure.
		Carry out physical and neurological examinations.
		Maintain neurological and vital sign flow sheet.
		Patient awakening from overdose may demonstrate hostility; this can stimulate automatic angry response by health personnel.

(Continued)

TABLE 61-1. (Continued)

DRUG	CLINICAL MANIFESTATIONS	THERAPEUTIC MANAGEMENT
Barbiturates (Continued)	*Withdrawal Syndrome* Shakiness, anxiety, muscular irritability, orthostatic hypotension Tachycardia Seizures Withdrawal psychosis Hyperpyrexia Death	*Symptoms of barbiturate withdrawal are serious because of life-threatening nature of abrupt abstinence.* Maintain airway; stimulate depressed respiration. Administer phenobarbital according to patient's tolerance. Carry out gastric lavage to evacuate stomach. Give oxygen, antibiotics, intravenous fluids as required. Gradually reduce dosage of barbiturates. Watch for excessive agitation, confusion, and convulsions. Consider treatment in residential treatment center.

Amphetamine Type Drugs
(Pep pills, "uppers," "speed")
Amphetamine (Benzedrine)
Dextroamphetamine (Dexedrine)
Methamphetamine (Desoxyn)
	Aggressive type of behavior
	Irritability; insomnia
	Visual misperceptions; auditory hallucinations
	Hyperactivity, rapid speech, euphoria
	Dilated pupils
	Increasing pulse rate and blood pressure
	Paranoid suspiciousness
	Hallucinosis; high temperature
	Convulsions—coma—death
		1. Try to communicate with patient—amphetamine paranoid psychosis is frequently seen.
		   Patient may have delusions of persecution, ideas of reference, visual and auditory hallucinations, changes in body image, hyperactivity, excitation.
		2. Use specific drug therapy to alleviate agitative state.
		   a. Usually within 24 hours after last dose of amphetamine patient will begin to spend increasing amounts of time sleeping.
		   b. Keep patient relatively quiet and reassured; patient may become aggressive/assaultive and reach a state of panic.
		3. Carry out urine checks for amphetamines.
		4. Place patient in protective environment—observe for suicidal attempts.
		   a. Use techniques of dealing with acutely paranoid individuals; do not move close to patient or behind him.
		   b. Avoid confined spaces; refer to psychiatric nursing textbook.

Hallucinogens or Psychedelic Type Drugs
1. Lysergic acid diethylamide (LSD)
2. Phencyclidine HCl (PCP; "angel dust," "crystal," "sheets," "hog," "peace pill," "PeaCe pill")
3. Mescaline, Psilocybin
4. Jimson weed seeds
	Marked confusion bordering on panic
	Confusion, incoherence, hyperactivity
	Hazardous behavior—delirium, mania, self-injury
	Hallucinations
	Flashback—recurrence of LSD-like state without having taken the drug; may occur weeks or months after drug was taken.
	Convulsions, coma, circulatory collapse, death
		Emergency Management
		1. Determine whether patient has ingested hallucinogenic drug or has a toxic psychosis.
		2. Try to communicate with the patient—use "vocal anesthesia" to reassure him.
		   a. "Talking down" involves understanding the process through which the patient is proceeding and helping him overcome his fears while establishing contact with reality.
		   b. Remind the patient that fear is common with this problem.
		   c. Reassure the patient that he is not losing his mind; that he is experiencing effect of drugs and that this will wear off.
		   d. Instruct the patient to keep his eyes open—reduces intensity of reaction.
		   e. *Reduce sensory stimuli*—minimize noise, lights, movement, tactile stimulation.

TABLE 61-1. (Continued)

DRUG	CLINICAL MANIFESTATIONS	THERAPEUTIC MANAGEMENT

Hallucinogens or Psychedelic Type Drugs *(Continued)*		f. Do not leave the patient alone.
		3. Sedate the patient if his hyperactivity cannot be controlled—diazepam (Valium), or a barbiturate may be given.
		4. Search for evidences of trauma—hallucinogen users have a tendency to "act out" their hallucinations.
		5. Manage convulsions; place patient in Intensive Care Unit.
		6. Watch patient closely—his behavior may become hazardous.
		7. Monitor for hypertensive crisis if patient has prolonged psychosis due to drug ingestion.
		8. Place patient in a protected environment under proper medical supervision to prevent self-inflicted bodily harm.
		9. *For phencyclidine abusers:*
		  a. Drug effects are unpredictable and prolonged.
		  b. Symptoms likely to exacerbate; patient becomes out of control.

Drugs producing sedation, intoxication,
  psychologic and physical dependence
  (nonbarbiturate sedatives)
Glutethimide (Doriden)
Methyprylon (Noludar)
Ethchlorvynol (Placidyl)
Ethinamate (Valmid)
Meprobamate (Miltown, Equanil)
Chlordiazepoxide (Librium)
Diazepam (Valium)
Bromides
	Acute Intoxication
	Decreasing mental alertness
	Confusion
	Slurred speech
	Ataxia
	Pulmonary edema
	Coma—death
		Management
		1. Insert endotracheal tube as a precaution; utilize assisted ventilation.
		  Watch for sudden apnea and laryngeal spasm (especially in patients habituated to Doriden).
		2. Start ECG monitoring.
		  Watch for cardiovascular instability with arrhythmia.
		3. Assess for hypotension.
		  a. Insert indwelling catheter for comatose patient—decreased urinary volume is an index of reduced renal flow associated with reduced intravascular volume or vascular collapse.
		  b. Start volume expansion with saline, plasma, or dextrose as required.
		4. Assist with gastric lavage.
		5. Use hemodialysis therapy if needed.

Salicylate Poisoning
Aspirin (present in all compound analgesic tablets)
	Abdominal pain, hematemesis (early)
	Late signs and symptoms:
	  Hyperpnea
	  Disturbed acid-base balance
	  Tinnitus and vertigo
	  Mental aberrations
	  Hyperventilation
	  Convulsions; coma
		1. Treat respiratory depression.
		2. Carry out gastric lavage; will remove significant amounts of salicylates up to 10 hours, or give Ipecac.
		3. Give water, milk, or activated charcoal to delay absorption of ingested poison.
		4. Support patient with intravenous infusions to correct electrolyte imbalance and maintain hydration.
		5. Correct acid-base disturbances.
		  Give blood transfusion as indicated.
		6. Prepare for peritoneal dialysis (page 916) or hemodialysis for patients with severe intoxication.
		7. Give vitamin K for bleeding; salicylates lower the plasma prothrombin by interfering with vitamin K utilization in the liver.
		8. Monitor electrolytes.

(Continued from page 1434)

to lead usually to intoxication if drinking is begun; by chronicity; by progresssion; and by tendency toward relapse. It is typically associated with physical disability and impaired emotional, occupational, and/or social adjustments as a direct consequence of persistent and excessive use."

Because alcoholic patients are frequent return visitors to the emergency department, they are infamous and exasperating, taxing the endurance of the health professionals caring for them. Thus, their management requires thoughtful and correct treatment.

Ethanol (alcohol) is a direct multisystem toxin and central nervous system depressant that causes drowsiness, incoordination, slurring of speech or belligerency, grandiosity, and uninhibited behavior. It can cause stupor and coma and even death if taken in excessive amounts.

EMERGENCY MANAGEMENT

The treatment of alcoholism involves (1) detoxication of the acute poisoning, (2) recovery, or "drying out," and (3) rehabilitation.

1. Approach the patient in a nonjudgmental manner, without condemnation or reproach.
   a. Expect him to use mechanisms of denial and defensiveness.
   b. Adapt a firm, consistent, accepting, and reasonable attitude.
   c. Speak calmly.
   d. If he appears drunk, he is probably drunk even though he denies alcohol intake.
2. Take a blood alcohol test as directed.
3. Allow the drowsy patient to "sleep off" the state of alcoholic intoxication. Acute alcoholic intoxication usually resolves spontaneously within several hours.
   a. Keep the patient under observation.
   b. Undress the patient and cover with a blanket.
   c. Observe for symptoms of respiratory depression.
   d. Protect the airway.
4. Sedate the noisy, belligerent patient as directed.
   a. *Monitor the patient carefully.*
   b. Check vital signs and monitor heart rate and blood pressure.
5. Examine the patient for injuries and organic disease which can easily be masked by alcoholic intoxication. (Alcoholics suffer more injuries than the general population.)
   a. Look for symptoms of head injury.
   b. Evaluate for pulmonary infection.
      (1) Pulmonary infections are more common in alcoholic individuals due to impaired defense system and tendency toward gastric aspiration.
      (2) Patient may show little increase in temperature or white blood count.
   c. Assess the neurologic status of the patient. (See page 83.)
   d. Watch for hypoglycemia.
6. Hospitalize if necessary.

For the severely intoxicated patient
   a. Provide respiratory support if necessary.
   b. Place patient in semiprone position with mouth down to avoid aspiration of vomitus and pharyngeal secretions.
   c. Start intravenous drip.

Delirium Tremens (Alcoholic Hallucinosis)

Delirium tremens is an acute toxic state that follows a prolonged bout of steady drinking or diminution or withdrawal of alcoholic intake. It may be precipitated by acute injury or infection. Delirium tremens is a serious complication and is considered a medical emergency.

Patients suspected of delirium tremens will show signs of anxiety, uncontrollable fear, tremulousness, irritability, agitation, and insomnia. They will be talkative and preoccupied, and will experience visual, tactile, olfactory, and auditory hallucinations that are frequently terrifying. Autonomic overactivity will occur and is evidenced by tachycardia, dilated pupils, and profuse perspiration. Usually all vital signs are elevated in the alcoholic toxic state.

EMERGENCY MANAGEMENT

The objective of management is to give proper sedation and support to enable the patient to rest and recover without danger of injury or exhaustion.

1. Take the blood pressure, since the patient's subsequent medication may depend on blood pressure readings.
2. Carry out a physical examination to identify preexisting or contributing illnesses or injuries (head injury, pneumonia, etc.).
3. Sedate the patient with a sufficient dosage of medication to produce adequate sedation—to reduce agitation, prevent exhaustion, and promote sleep.
   a. A variety of drugs and combinations of drugs are used—chloral hydrate, diazepam (Valium), hydroxyzine (Vistaril), etc.
   b. The dosage is adjusted according to the patient's symptoms (agitation, anxiety) and blood pressure response.
4. Place the patient in a private room and observe closely.
   a. Keep room lighted—to reduce incidence of visual hallucinations.
   b. Close closet and bathroom doors to eliminate shadows.
   c. Keep the environment calm and nonstressful.
   d. Observe the patient closely—homicidal or suicidal responses may result from hallucinations.
   e. Have someone stay with the patient as much as possible—the presence of another person has a reassuring and quieting effect and helps maintain contact with reality.
   f. Explain visual misrepresentations (illusions)—to strengthen link with reality.
   g. Explain in detail every procedure being done to the patient.
   h. Shut out loud noises; call patient by name.
   i. Take patient to the bathroom if permitted.
   j. Use restraints if necessary, if the patient is not under direct and constant observation.
5. Maintain electrolyte balance and hydration via oral or intravenous route—fluid losses may be extreme because of profuse perspiration and agitation.

6. Record temperature, pulse, respiration, and blood pressure frequently (every 30 minutes in severe forms of delirium)—in anticipation of peripheral circulatory collapse and/or hyperthermia (the 2 most lethal complications).

7. Administer phenytoin (Dilantin) or other anticonvulsant drugs as prescribed to prevent or control alcoholic or epileptic convulsions.

8. Assess respiratory, hepatic, and cardiovascular status of patient—pneumonia, liver disease, and cardiac failure are complications.

   a. Hypoglycemia may accompany alcoholic withdrawal, because alcohol depletes liver glycogen stores and impairs gluconeogenesis; also many alcoholic patients suffer from malnutrition.

   b. Administer parenteral dextrose if liver glycogen is depleted.

      Give orange juice, Gatorade, or other carbohydrates to stabilize blood sugar and to counteract tremulousness.

9. Give supplemental vitamin therapy and a high protein diet; these patients are usually vitamin deficient.

10. Refer to alcoholic treatment center for subsequent follow-up and rehabilitation.

PSYCHIATRIC EMERGENCY

A psychiatric emergency is an urgent, serious disturbance of behavior, affect, or thought which makes the patient unable to cope with life situations and interpersonal relationships. A patient presenting with a psychiatric emergency may be (1) overactive (or violent), (2) underactive or depressed, or (3) suicidal.

The most important concern of the Emergency Department personnel is whether the patient is likely to cause personal harm or injury to others. In general, the aim is to try to maintain the patient's self-esteem (and life, if necessary) while carrying out assessment and management. The patient is asked if he is under psychiatric treatment at the current time.

Overactive Patients

Patients in the overactive category will display disturbed, uncooperative, and paranoid behavior, as well as anxiety and paniclike feelings. They may be prone to assaultive and destructive impulses and abnormal social behavior. Intense nervousness, depression, and crying are also evident in some patients. Their disturbed and noisy behavior may be compounded by alcohol and/or drug intoxication.

EMERGENCY MANAGEMENT

1. Determine from the family or another reliable source, whether the patient has had past mental illness, hospitalizations, injuries, or serious illnesses, uses alcohol or drugs, or has experienced crises in interpersonal relationships or intrapsychic conflicts.

2. Be aware that abnormal thought and behavior may be a manifestation of an underlying physical disorder such as hypoglycemia, cerebrovascular accident, epilepsy, and drug toxicity, including alcohol.

3. Try to gain control of the situation.

   a. Approach the patient with a calm, confident, and firm manner—this attitude is therapeutic and will have a calming effect.

   b. Introduce yourself by name.

   c. Tell him, "I am here to help you."

   d. Repeat patient's name from time to time.

   e. Speak in one-thought sentences. Be consistent.

   f. Give the patient space. Let him slow down by himself and allow him to become compliant.

   g. Be interested in and listen to the patient—encourage him to talk of his thoughts and *feelings*.

   h. Offer appropriate explanations. Tell the truth.

4. Give tranquilizer or psychotropic agent for emergency management of functional psychosis. Chlorpromazine (Thorazine) or haloperidol (Haldol) act specifically against psychotic symptoms of thought fragmentation and perceptual and behavioral aberrations.

   a. Initial dosage depends on body weight and severity of symptoms.

   b. Observe patient for 1 hour after initial dose to determine degree of change in psychotic behavior.

   c. Subsequent dosages depend on patient's reaction.

   d. If behavior is caused by hallucinogens (LSD, etc.), psychotropic drugs (exerting an effect on the mind) are not used.

5. Use restraints only as a last resort.

6. Admit to psychiatric unit or arrange for psychiatric outpatient treatment.

The Violent Patient

Violent and aggressive behavior is usually episodic and is a means of expressing feelings of anger, fear, or hopelessness about a situation. Usually the patient has a history of outbursts of rage, temper tantrums, or generally impulsive behavior. Persons with a tendency to violence frequently lose control when intoxicated with alcohol or drugs. Family members are the most frequent victims of their aggression. Patients with violent behavior usually fall into one of four diagnostic categories: (1) functional (usually psychotic), (2) organic brain syndrome, (3) toxic psychosis, and (4) drug withdrawal.

The goal is to protect the patient and staff from harm and to control the violent or disturbed episode. If possible, two persons should see the patient initially and a specially designated room should be used. Objects that could be used as weapons should not be in sight.

EMERGENCY MANAGEMENT

1. Keep the door of the room open and be in clear view of the staff. Do not block the patient's exit to the door; patient may feel closed in and threatened.

2. Give the patient space. Do not make any sudden movement. If the patient is carrying a weapon ask him to place it in a neutral area.

3. Adapt a calm, noncritical approach and remain in control of the situation. External calm and structure may help patient to gain control.
4. Talk and listen to the patient.
    a. Crisis intervention is best done with an attitude of interest in the patient's well-being and with an attempt to "tune in" to the patient while at the same time remaining firm.
    b. Acknowledge the patient's state of agitation. "I want to work with you to relieve your distress, etc."
    c. Give the patient the opportunity to ventilate his anger verbally.
    d. Try to hear what the patient is saying.
    e. Convey to the patient that help is available for him to gain control.
        (1) Let patient know that his behavior is frightening to those around him.
        (2) Describe the help available in crisis situations — clinic, emergency department, mental health facility.
5. Allow the security personnel/police to intervene if the patient does not become calm.
    a. Offer protection of hospitalization — usually welcomed by the patient who fears his loss of control.
    b. Use restraints when necessary but with minimum of force.
        (1) Use restraints with verbal intervention.
        (2) Have enough personnel available when applying restraints.
    c. Administer intramuscular medication (haloperidol, diazepam, chlorpromazine) as directed.
    d. Refer patient for further mental health treatment after combativeness, agitation, and fear have cooled.

Underactive or Depressed Patients

During any given year, 125,000 persons are hospitalized in the United States for depressive symptoms. Another 200,000 depressed people are treated as outpatients. Fifteen percent of all American adults between 18 and 74 will experience some type of depressive episode at some time in their lives. Seventy-five percent of those who attempt suicide suffer from a depressive illness.

The underactive or depressed patient will be fearful, depressed, slow to respond, plagued by feelings of worthlessness, guilt, ambivalence, and indecision, and prone to insomnia, a worsening mood in the morning, sad facial expression, and feelings of isolation.

EMERGENCY MANAGEMENT

1. Listen to the patient in a calm, unhurried manner.
    a. Patient will benefit from ventilation of feelings.
    b. Give patient an opportunity to talk about his problems.
    c. Anticipate that the patient may be suicidal.
    d. Attempt to find out if the patient has thought about or attempted suicide.
        (1) "Have you ever thought about taking your own life?"
        (2) The patient is generally relieved because of the opportunity to discuss his feelings.
    e. Notify relatives about a seriously depressed patient. Do not leave the patient alone, since suicide is usually an act committed in solitude.

f. Find out if there is an illness, perceived or real.
    g. Assess whether there has been sudden worsening of depression.
2. Give antidepressant and antianxiety agents as prescribed.
3. Point out to the patient that depression is treatable.
4. Refer patient for psychiatric consultation or to psychiatric unit.

Suicidal Patients

Suicide ranks as the eleventh cause of death in the United States and is actually an act that stems from depression. Many people who are suicidal have suffered the recent loss of a loved one, of body integrity, or status. The high-risk patient for suicide is male, over 45, unemployed, divorced, living alone, and showing significant depression (weight loss, sleep disturbances, somatic complaints, and suicidal preoccupation).

Others at risk are persons with a history of previous suicidal attempts, those with psychiatric illness and lack of resources, and those who express hopelessness.

EMERGENCY MANAGEMENT

1. Treat the emergency condition brought about by the suicidal attempt. The patient may need respiratory or circulatory support, gastric lavage, or surgery. (The majority arriving alive at the emergency department have ingested some type of drug.)
2. Prevent further self-injury; a patient who has made a suicidal gesture may do so again.
3. Admit to intensive care unit or psychiatric unit.

Prevention

1. Have an awareness of persons at risk.
2. Determine whether person has communicated *suicidal intent*
    "tired of living"   "put my affairs in order"
    "better off dead"   preoccupied with death
    "burden to my family"   talking of someone else's suicide
3. Determine whether he has ever attempted suicide; risk is much greater.
4. Is there a family history of suicide?
5. Was there loss of a parent at an early age?

SEXUAL ASSAULT

Legally, rape is defined as carnal knowledge of a female by force or the threat of force. It is one of the fastest growing crimes of violence. The feminist movement has focused on the rights and care of rape victims, and law enforcement agencies are becoming increasingly sensitive and aggressive in the management of these crimes. Rape crisis centers offer extensive support and education of victims and help them through the subsequent courtroom experience.

The manner in which the patient is received and treated in the Emergency Department is important to her future psychological well-being. Crisis intervention should begin when the patient enters the health facility. She should be seen immediately upon entrance into the Emergency Department. Most hospitals have a written protocol that reflects consideration for the victim's physical and emotional needs as well as concern for meeting requirements for subsequent legal proceedings.

EMERGENCY MANAGEMENT

The objectives of management are to give sympathetic support and to reduce the emotional trauma of the patient.

1. Respect the privacy and sensitivity of the patient; be kind and supportive.
   a. Emotional trauma may be present for weeks, months, or years. The patient may go through phases of psychologic reactions:
      (1) Phase of disorganization—fear, guilt, humiliation, anger, self-blame.
      (2) Phase of resolution (putting incident into perspective); patient may have sleep disturbances, phobias, sexual fears.
   b. Reassure patient that anxiety is natural and that appropriate support is available from professional and community resources.
   c. Accept the emotional reactions of the patient (hysteria, stoicism, overwhelmed feeling, etc.).
   d. Do not leave the patient alone.
2. Assist with the physical assessment.
   a. Take history *only* if patient has not already talked to police officer, crisis intervention worker, etc. Do not ask patient to repeat the history.
   b. Secure informed consent from patient (or parent/guardian if patient is a minor) for conducting the examination and for taking photographs which are used as legal evidence.
   c. Ask if patient has bathed, douched, brushed teeth, changed clothes, or defecated since attack—may alter interpretation of subsequent findings.
   d. Record time of admission, time of examination, and the general appearance of the patient.
      (1) Document any evidence of trauma—discoloration, bruises, lacerations, secretions, torn and bloody clothing.
      (2) Record emotional state.
   e. Assist patient to undress; drape properly.
      (1) Save clothing; label.
      (2) Give to appropriate law enforcement authorities.
3. Assist with pelvic and rectal examination.
   a. Advise the patient of the nature and necessity of each procedure; give the rationale for each question asked.
      (1) Use water-moistened vaginal speculum for examination; do not use lubricant.
      (2) Note color and consistency of any discharge present.
   b. Assist with securing laboratory specimens.
      (1) Collect vaginal aspirate, which is examined for presence or absence of motile/nonmotile sperm.
      (2) Sterile swab from vaginal pool for acid phosphatase, blood group antigen of semen, and precipitin test against human sperm and blood.
      (3) Obtain separate smears from vulva.
      (4) Obtain culture of body orifices for gonorrhea (page 1373).
      (5) Conduct test for pregnancy if there is question that patient may be pregnant.
      (6) Collect foreign material (leaves, grass, dirt) and place in a clean envelope.
      (7) Comb the pubic hairs with prepackaged clean comb; place in separate container.
      (8) Inspect fingers for broken nails and tissue and foreign materials under nails.
      (9) Label all specimens with name of patient, date, and initials of personnel handling specimens to preserve chain of evidence; give to pathologist or designated person (forensic laboratory, etc.)
      (10) Photographs are taken by designated person; film is usually given to police for development and printing.
4. Treat associated injuries as indicated.
5. Give patient option of prophylaxis against venereal disease.
   a. Probenecid orally, followed in 30 minutes by IM penicillin.
   b. Patient with allergy to penicillin may receive alternate therapy (page 1375) which may not be effective in treatment of incubating syphilis; patient should have a serology check in 6 weeks.
6. Antipregnancy measures may be considered if patient is of childbearing age, is using no contraceptives, and is at high risk in menstrual cycle.
   a. Hormonal therapy—oral diethylstilbestrol, etc., for 5 days renders endometrium inhospitable for implantation; usually effective in preventing pregnancy following unprotected intercourse.
   b. Give prescription of antiemetic; the side effects of diethylstilbestrol are nausea and vomiting.
   c. Inform patient that if she misses a menstrual period she has the option of having menstrual extraction or abortion.
7. Offer cleansing douche if patient desires.
8. Provide for follow-up services:
   a. Make appointment for follow-up surveillance for pregnancy and venereal disease.
   b. Encourage patient to return to previous level of functioning as soon as possible.
   c. Inform patient of counseling services to prevent long-term psychologic effects.
      (1) Most patients benefit from this type of service.
      (2) Counseling services to parents, husband, etc., of victim can be beneficial.
   d. Patient should be accompanied by family/friend when leaving health facility.

BIBLIOGRAPHY

BOOKS

American Academy of Orthopaedic Surgeons: Emergency Care and Transportation of the Sick and Injured, 2nd ed. Menasha, Wis., George Banta Co., 1977.

American Nurses Association Division on Medical-Surgical Nursing Practice and Emergency Department Nurses' Association: Standards of Emergency Nursing Practice. Kansas City, ANA, 1975.

Barry, J., ed.: Emergency Nursing. New York, McGraw-Hill, 1978.

Bourne, P. G.: Acute Drug Abuse Emergencies. New York, Academic Press, 1976.

Cohen, A. S., Freidin, R. B., and Samuels, M. A.: Medical Emergencies: Diagnosis and Management Procedures from Boston City Hospital. Boston, Little, Brown, 1977.

Condon, R. E., and Nyhus, L. M.: Manual of Surgical Therapeutics. Boston, Little, Brown, 1978.

Cosgriff, J. H.: Atlas of Diagnostic and Therapeutic Procedures for Emergency Personnel. Philadelphia, J. B. Lippincott, 1978.

Dreisbach, R. H.: Handbook of Poisoning: Diagnosis and Treatment, 9th ed. Los Altos, Lange Medical Pub., 1977.

Eisenberg, M. S., and Copass, M. K.: Manual of Emergency Medical Therapeutics. Philadelphia, W. B. Saunders, 1978.

Frey, C. F., ed.: Initial Management of the Trauma Patient. Philadelphia, Lea and Febiger, 1976.

Garfield, C. A., ed.: Stress and Survival. St. Louis, C. V. Mosby, 1979.

Halpern, S., Hicks, D. J., and Crenshaw, T. L.: Rape. Helping the Victim. Oradell: Medical Economics Co., 1978.

Lion, J. R., and Madden, D.: Management of the violent patient. *In* Balis, G. U., Wurmser, L., and McDaniel, E., eds.: Psychiatric Problems in Medical Practice. Boston, Butterworth Pub., 1978, pages 265-273.

Klippel, A. P., and Anderson, C. B.: Manual of Emergency and Outpatient Techniques. Boston, Little, Brown, 1979.

Mott, T., Jr.: Management of the Suicidal Patient. *In* Balis, G. U., Wurmser, L., and McDaniel, E., eds.: Psychiatric Problems in Medical Practice. Boston, Butterworth Pub., 1978, pages 251-263.

Najarian, J. S., and Delaney, J. P., eds.: Critical Surgical Care. New York, Stratton Intercontinental Medical Book Corp., 1977.

O'Doherty, D. S.: Handbook of Neurologic Emergencies. Garden City, Medical Examination Pub. Co., 1977.

Parcel, G. S.: First Aid in Emergency Care. St. Louis, C. V. Mosby, 1977.

Robbins, A. S., and Tamkin, J. A.: Manual of Ambulatory Medicine. Philadelphia, W. B. Saunders, 1979.

Robinson, J., ed.: Giving Emergency Care Competently. Horsham, Intermed Communications, 1978.

Rosen, P., and Sternbach, G. L.: Atlas of Emergency Medicine. Baltimore, Williams and Wilkins, 1979.

Rumack, B. H., and Temple, A. R.: Management of the Poisoned Patient. Princeton, Science Press, 1977.

Sanders, J. H., and Gardner, L. B.: Handbook of Medical Emergencies. Garden City, Medical Examination Pub. Co., 1978.

Schwartz, G. R., et al.: Principles and Practice of Emergency Medicine. Vols. 1 and 2. Philadelphia, W. B. Saunders, 1978.

Sharp, E. G.: Handbook of General Surgical Emergencies. Flushing, Medical Examination Pub. Co., 1977.

Stephenson, H. E., Jr.: Immediate Care of the Acutely Ill and Injured, 2nd ed. St. Louis, C. V. Mosby, 1978.

Warner, C. G., ed.: Emergency Care, 2nd ed. St. Louis, C. V. Mosby, 1978.

Weil, M. H., and DaLuz, P. L.: Critical Care Medicine Manual. New York, Springer-Verlag, 1978.

Westermeyer, J.: A Primer on Chemical Dependency. A Clinical Guide to Alcohol and Drug Problems. Baltimore, Williams and Wilkins, 1976.

Wilkins, E. W., et al.: MGH Textbook of Emergency Medicine. Baltimore, Williams and Wilkins, 1978.

ARTICLES

General

August-Miler, S.: Dealing with sudden death: The survivors. Crit. Care Quart., *1*:71-77, May 1978.

Carden, T. S.: "Emergency": — A redefinition. JAMA, *240*:377, July 28, 1978.

Creighton, H.: Your legal risks in emergency care. Nursing '78, *8*:52-55, Feb. 1978.

Miller, M.: Patient teaching in the emergency department. JEN, *4*:21-23, Jan.-Feb. 1978.

Sharer, P. S.: Helping survivors cope with the shock of sudden death. Nursing '79, *9*:20-23, Jan. 1979.

Heat/Cold Injuries

Mills, W. J.: Out in the cold. Emerg. Med., *8*:134-147, Jan. 1976.

Stine, R. J.: Accidental hypothermia. JACEP, *6*:413-416, Sept. 1977.

Sturzenberger, A. J.: Differentiating among heat syndromes. JEN, *4*:25-28, July-Aug. 1978.

Poisoning/Drug Abuse

Haracz, N. L.: Emergency management of mushroom poisoning. JEN, *4*:12-16, May-June 1978.

Hardin, K.: Treating intoxicated patients in the emergency department. JEN, *5*:11-14, Jan.-Feb. 1979.

Hooper, R. G., et al.: Acute poisoning from over-the-counter sleep preparations. JACEP, *8*:98-100, Mar. 1979.

Jozwiak, J. S.: Acetaminophen overdose. RN, *41*:56-62, Dec. 1978.

Mennear, J. H.: The poisoning emergency. AJN, 77:842-844, May 1977.

Pisarcik, G.: Management of phencyclidine toxicity. JEN, *4*:35-37, Sept.-Oct. 1978.

Rothstein, R. J.: Emergency management of poisoning and overdose. Compr. Ther., *5*:7-14, Jan. 1979.

Vourakis, C., and Bennett, G.: Angel dust—not heaven sent. AJN, 79:649-653, Apr. 1979.

Yowell, S., and Brose, C.: Working with drug abuse patients in the ER. AJN, 77:82-85, Jan. 1977.

Psychiatric Emergencies

Edelman, S. E.: Managing the violent patient in the community mental health center. Hosp. Community Psychiatry, *29*:460-462, July 1978.

Guirguis, E.: Management of disturbed patients: An alternative to the use of mechanical restraints. J. Clin. Psychiatry, *39*:295-299, 303, Apr. 1978.

Imboden, J. M., and Urbaitis, J. C.: Practical Psychiatry in Medicine. Part 7. Suicidal behavior and other psychiatric emergencies. J. Fam. Pract., *6*:415-432, Feb. 1978.

Murphy, G. E.: Suicide and attempted suicide. Hosp. Pract., *12*:73-81, Nov. 1977.

Reubin, R.: Spotting and stopping the suicide patient. Nursing '79, *9*:82-85, Apr. 1979.

Shevitz, S.: Emergency management of the agitated patient. Primary Care, *5*:625-634, Dec. 1978.

Skodol, A. E., and Karastu, T. B.: Emergency psychiatry and the assaultive patient. Am. J. Psychiatry, *135*:202-205, Feb. 1978.

Weissenberg, M. P., and Dubovsky, S. L.: Assessment of psychiatric emergencies in medical practice. Primary Care, *4*:651-660, Dec. 1977.

Resuscitation

DeLaurentis, D. A.: Resuscitation in the injured patient. Hosp. Med., *14*:82-88, June 1978.

Donaldson, J. C., and Royall, J. D.: Drowning and near-drowning. Pathophysiology and therapy. Postgrad. Med., *64*:71-73 passim, July 1978.

Hart, R.: What to do when you're number 1.: A review of CPR for adults. Nursing '79, *9*:54-59, Feb. 1979.

Hartong, J. M., and Dixon, R. S.: Monitoring resuscitation of the injured patient. JAMA, *237*:242-244, Jan. 17, 1977.

Heimlich, H. J.: Heimlich defends his maneuver (letter). New Eng. J. Med., *299*:1415, Dec. 21, 1978.

———: The Heimlich maneuver: Prevention of death from choking on foreign bodies. J. Occ. Med., *19*:208-210, Mar. 1977.

Jackson, D. L., and Beraducci, A.: Carbon monoxide poisoning — A growing hazard. Med. Times, *106*:28-37, Feb. 1978.

Knopp, R.: Near drowning. JACEP, 7:249-254, June 1978.

LeFort, S.: Cardiopulmonary resuscitation (CPR): Step-by-step. Can. Nurse, *74*:38-47, Feb. 1978.

McElroy, C. R.: The esophageal obturator airway. JEN, *4*:35-38, Mar.-Apr. 1978.

Modell, J. H.: Biology of drowning. Annu. Rev. Med., *29*:1-8, 1978.

Near-drowning (editorial). Lancet, *2*, No. 8082:194-195, July 23, 1978.

To ventilate, obturate. Emerg. Med., *9*:75-78, July 1977.

Sexual Assault

Enos, W. F., and Beyer, J. C.: Management of the rape victim. Am. Fam. Phys., *18*:97-102, Sept. 1978.

Burgess, A., and Laszlo, A. T.: Courtroom use of hospital records in sexual assault cases. AJN, 77:64-68, Jan. 1977.

Evans, H. I.: Psychotherapy for the rape victim: Some treatment models. Hosp. Community Psychiatry, *29*:309-312, May 1978.

Halbert, D. R., and Jones, D. E.: Medical management of the sexually assaulted woman. J. Reprod. Med., *20*:265-274, May 1978.

Hicks, D. J.: Rape: Sexual assault. Obstet. Gyn. Annu., 7:447-465, 1978.

Moynihan, B., and Coughlin, P.: Sexual assault: A comprehensive response to a complex problem. JEN, *4*:22-26, Nov.-Dec. 1978.

Pepitone-Rockwell, F.: Patterns of rape and approaches to care. J. Fam. Pract., *6*:521-529, Mar. 1978.

Schaefer, J. L., Sullivan, R. A., and Goldstein, F. L.: Counseling sexual abuse victims. Am. Fam. Phys., *18*:85-91, Nov. 1978.

Silverman, D. C.: Sharing the crisis of rape: Counseling the males and families of victims. Am. J. Orthopsychiatry, *48*:166-173, Jan. 1978.

Snakebites, Stings

Clement, J. F., and Pietrusko, R.: Pit viper snakebite in the United States. J. Fam. Pract., *6*:269-279, Feb. 1978.

Frazier, C. A.: The hazards of hymenoptera. Am. Fam. Phys., *15*:91-96, Apr. 1977.

Hutchinson, R.: What to do — and what to worry about — when treating stings and bites. Nursing '77, 7:69-71, June 1977.

Van Mierop, L. H. S.: Poisonous snakebite: A review. 2. Symptomatology and treatment. J. Fla. Med. Assoc., *63*:201-210, Mar. 1976.

Watt, C. H.: Poisonous snakebite treatment in the United States. JAMA, *240*:654-656, Aug. 18, 1978.

Wingert, W. A., and Wainschel, J.: A quick handbook on snakebites. Med. Times, *105*:68-75, Apr. 1977.

Trauma

Allen, R. E., et al.: The organization of emergency medical services. Western. J. Med., *130*:83-89, Jan. 1979.

Berg, E.: Management of acute orthopedic injuries. Compr. Ther., *5*:38-44, Jan. 1979.

Bietz, D. S.: Algorithm for critically injured patients. J. Trauma, *17*:55-60, Jan. 1977.

Canizaro, P. C.: Trauma to the abdomen: II. Management, Bull. N.Y. Acad. Med., *55*:212-226, Feb. 1979.

Cayten, C. G., and Evans, W.: Severity indices and their implications for emergency medical services research and evaluation. J. Trauma, *19*:98-102, Feb. 1979.

Danzl, D. F., and Berg, B. C.: Peritoneal lavage and scintigraphic evaluation of blunt abdominal trauma. JACEP, *6*:397-404, Sept. 1977.

Dillman, P. A.: The bio-physical response to shock trousers. JEN, *3*:21-25, Nov.-Dec. 1977.

Edlich, R. F., et al.: Emergency department treatment. Triage and transfer. JACEP, 7:152-158, Apr. 1978.

Geelhoed, G. W.: Blunt and penetrating abdominal trauma. Am. Fam. Phys., *17*:96-104, Mar. 1978.

Harley, R. D.: Blunt trauma to the eye. Compr. Ther., *3*:29-32, Mar. 1977.

Jergens, M. E.: Peritoneal lavage. Am. J. Surg., *133*:365-369, Mar. 1977.

Jones, C. A., and Feller, I.: Burns: What to do the first crucial hours. Nursing '77, 7:22-31, Mar. 1977.

Kelly, C. A.: Ocular trauma. JEN, *4*:23-28, Mar.-Apr. 1978.

Meyd, C. J.: Acute brain trauma. AJN, *78*:40-44, Jan. 1978.

Miller, J. D., et al.: Early insults to the injured brain. JAMA, *240*:439-442, Aug. 4, 1978.

Minar, V.: Fluid resuscitation of the burn patient. JEN, *4*:39-43, Sept.-Oct. 1978.

Molyneux-Luick, M., and Knecht, J.: Hypovolemic shock. Nursing '77, 7:32-37, Nov. 1977.

Molyneux-Luick, M.: The ABCs of multiple trauma. Nursing '77, 7:30-36, Oct. 1977.

Notes from a trauma team. Emerg. Med., 8:153-179, Mar. 1976.

Podgorny, G.: Priorities in the management of severe trauma. Med. Times, 106:2d-6d, Feb. 1978.

Podgorny, G., and Stanley, L.: Dealing with the special dangers of gunshot wounds. RN, 40:62-71, Oct. 1977.

Schutz, M. K.: What must be done when all else fails. RN, 42:52-54, May 1979.

Shires, G. T.: Management of hypovolemic shock. Bull. N.Y. Acad. Med., 55:139-149, Feb. 1979.

Stone, W. S.: Trauma: A continuing U.S. health problem. J. Trauma, 17:89-92, Feb. 1977.

Symposium on trauma. Nurs. Clin. N. Am., 13:175-265, June 1978.

Thai, E. R.: Trauma to the abdomen: I. Diagnosis. Bull. N.Y. Acad. Med., 55:201-211, Feb. 1979.

Walraven, G., and Romano, T.: Anti-shock trousers. JEN, 3:31, Nov.-Dec. 1977.

Yarington, C. T.: Managing soft tissue injuries. Am. Fam. Phys., 16:108-114, Oct. 1977.

AGENCIES

Governmental

Alcohol, Drug Abuse, and Mental Health Administration; National Institute on Drug Abuse; National Institute of Mental Health; National Institute on Alcohol Abuse and Alcoholism; 5600 Fishers Lane, Rockville, Md. 20857

Voluntary

American National Red Cross, 17th and D Sts., N.W., Washington, D.C. 20006

National Council on Alcoholism, Inc., 733 Third Ave., Suite 1405, New York, N.Y. 10017

National Safety Council, 444 North Michigan Ave., Chicago, Ill. 60611

APPENDIX

DIAGNOSTIC STUDIES AND THEIR MEANING

TABLE OF ABBREVIATIONS

kg. = kilogram	L. = liter	mm. = millimeter
gm. = gram	dl. = 100 milliliters	μ. = micron or micrometer
mg. = milligram	ml. = milliliter	mm. Hg = millimeters of mercury
μg. = microgram	cu. mm. = cubic millimeter	mU = milliunit
$\mu\mu$g. = micromicrogram	nM. = nanomolar	μU = microunit
ng. = nanogram		mEq. = milliequivalent
pg. = picogram		IU = International Unit
		mIU = milliInternational Unit

NORMAL VALUES—HEMATOLOGY*

DETERMINATION	NORMAL VALUE	CLINICAL SIGNIFICANCE
A$_2$ hemoglobin	1.90-3.86%	Increased in certain types of thalassemia
Bleeding time	30 sec.-6 min.	Prolonged in purpura hemorrhagica, in which platelets are reduced, and in chloroform and phosphorus poisoning
Clotting time	5-10 min.	Prolonged in hemorrhagic disease and in various coagulation factor deficiencies
Factor V assay	75-125%	Pro-accelerin factor
Factor VIII assay (antihemophiliac factor)	50-150%	Deficient in classical hemophilia
Factor IX assay (plasma thromboplastin component)	75-125%	Deficient in Christmas disease (pseudohemophilia)
Factor X (Stuart factor)	75-125%	Stuart clotting defect
Fibrinogen	200-400 mg./dl.	Increased in pregnancy, pneumonia, infections accompanied by leukocytosis, and nephrosis. Decreased in acute yellow atrophy of liver, cirrhosis, typhoid fever, chloroform poisoning, abruptio placentae
Fibrinolysins (whole blood clot lysis time)	No lysis in 24 hrs.	Increased activity associated with massive hemorrhage, extensive surgery, and transfusion reactions
Partial thromboplastin time (activated)	20-45 sec.	Prolonged in Factor VIII, IX, and X deficiency
Prothrombin consumption	Over 20 sec.	Impaired in factor VIII, IX, and X deficiency
Prothrombin time	60-100% of control	Prolonged in factor X deficiency and other hemorrhagic diseases, and in cirrhosis, hepatitis, and acute toxic necrosis of the liver

*Laboratory values vary according to the techniques used in different laboratories.

NORMAL VALUES—HEMATOLOGY (CONTINUED)

DETERMINATION	NORMAL VALUES	CLINICAL SIGNIFICANCE
Erythrocyte count	Males: 4,600,000-6,200,000 per cu. mm. Females: 4,200,000-5,400,000 per cu. mm.	Increased in severe diarrhea and dehydration, polycythemia, secondary polycythemia, acute poisoning, pulmonary fibrosis, and Ayerza disease. Decreased in all anemias, in leukemia, and after hemorrhage, when blood volume has been restored.
Erythrocyte indices		
Mean corpuscular volume (MCV)	80-94 (cu. microns)	Increased in macrocytic anemias, decreased in microcytic anemia
Mean corpuscular hemoglobin (MCH)	27-32 $\mu\mu$g. per cell	Increased in macrocytic anemias, decreased in microcytic anemia
Mean corpuscular hemoglobin concentration (MCHC)	33-38%	Decreased in severe hypochromic anemia
Reticulocytes	0.5-1.5% of red cells	Increased with any condition stimulating increase in bone marrow activity, i.e., infection, blood loss (acute and chronic); following iron therapy in iron deficiency anemia, polycythemia rubra vera. Decreased with any condition depressing bone marrow activity, acute leukemia, late stage of severe anemias
Erythrocyte sedimentation rate	Males: 0-9 mm./hr. Females: 0-20 mm./hr.	Increased in tissue destruction, whether inflammatory or degenerative, and during menstruation, pregnancy, and in acute febrile diseases
Hematocrit	Males: 42-50% Females: 40-48%	Decreased in severe anemias, anemia of pregnancy, acute massive blood loss. Increased in erythrocytosis of any cause, and in dehydration or hemoconcentration associated with shock
Hemoglobin	Males: 13-16 gm./dl. Females: 12-14 gm./dl.	Decreased in various anemias, pregnancy, severe or prolonged hemorrhage, and with excessive fluid intake. Increased in polycythemia, chronic obstructive pulmonary diseases, failure of oxygenation because of congestive heart failure, and normally, in people living at high altitudes
Hemoglobin F	Less than 2%	Increased in infants and children, in thalassemia and many anemias
Leukocyte alkaline phosphatase	Score of 40-100	Decreased in chronic myelocytic leukemia and chronic lymphocytic leukemia. Increased in nonleukemic leukocytosis and myeloproliferative diseases
Leukocyte count Neutrophils Eosinophils Basophils Lymphocytes Monocytes	Total: 5,000-10,000 cu. mm. 60-70% 1-4% 0-0.5% 20-30% 2-6%	Elevated in acute infectious diseases—predominantly in the neutrophilic fraction with bacterial diseases, and in the lymphocytic and monocytic fractions in viral diseases. Eosinophils elevated in collagen diseases, allergy, intestinal parasitosis. Elevated in acute leukemia, following menstruation, and following surgery or trauma. Depressed in aplastic anemia, agranulocytosis, and by toxic agents, such as chemotherapeutic agents used in treating malignancy
Osmotic fragility of red cells	Increase if hemolysis occurs in over 0.5% NaCl Decrease if hemolysis is incomplete in 0.3% NaCl	Increased in congenital spherocytosis, idiopathic acquired hemolytic anemia, isoimmune hemolytic disease, ABO hemolytic disease of newborn. Decreased in sickle-cell anemia, thalassemia
Platelet count	200,000-350,000 per cu. mm.	Increased with chronic granulocytic leukemia, hemoconcentration. Decreased in thrombocytopenic purpura, acute leukemia, aplastic anemia, and during cancer chemotherapy

NORMAL CHEMISTRIES—SERUM, PLASMA, WHOLE BLOOD

DETERMINATION	NORMAL ADULT VALUES	CLINICAL SIGNIFICANCE	
		(Increased)	(Decreased)
Acetoacetate and acetone	0.3-2.0 mg./dl.	Diabetic acidosis Fasting Toxemia of pregnancy Carbohydrate-free diet High-fat diet	
Adrenocorticotropic hormone (ACTH) (plasma), RIA*	Less than 100 pg./ml.	Pituitary-dependent Cushing's syndrome Ectopic ACTH syndrome Primary adrenal atrophy	Adrenocortical tumor Adrenal insufficiency secondary to hypopituitarism
Aldolase	0.5-3.1 mU/ml.	Hepatic necrosis Granulocytic leukemia Myocardial infarction Skeletal muscle disease	
Aldosterone (plasma), RIA	Supine: 3-10 ng./dl. Upright: 5-30 ng./dl. Adrenal vein: 200-800 ng./dl.	Primary (Conn's syndrome) Secondary aldosteronism	Addison's disease
Alpha amino nitrogen	3.0-5.5 mg./dl.	Phosphorus, arsenic, chloroform, carbon tetrachloride poisoning Infectious hepatitis Eclampsia	Bacterial pneumonia Administration of anterior pituitary extracts Administration of insulin
Alpha-1-antitrypsin	200-400 mg./dl.	Early inflammatory processes Pneumonia Abscess formations Arthritis	Chronic lung disease
Alpha-1-fetoprotein	None detected	Hepatocarcinoma Metastatic carcinoma of liver Germinal cell carcinoma of the testis or ovary	
Alpha-hydroxybutyric dehydrogenase	up to 140 mU/ml.	Myocardial infarction Granulocytic leukemia Hemolytic anemias Muscular dystrophy	
Ammonia (plasma)	5-70 μg./dl.	Severe liver disease Hepatic decompensation	
Amylase	15-200 units/dl.	Acute pancreatitis Mumps Duodenal ulcer Carcinoma of head of pancreas Prolonged elevation with pseudocyst of pancreas	Chronic pancreatitis Pancreatic fibrosis and atrophy Cirrhosis of liver Acute alcoholism Toxemias of pregnancy
Androstenedione, RIA	Females: 0.6-3.0 ng./ml.	Increases in many cases of hirsutism and virilization	
Arsenic	6-20 μg./dl.	Accidental or intentional poisoning Excessive occupational exposure	
Ascorbic acid (vitamin C)	0.4-1.5 mg./dl.	Large doses of ascorbic acid as a prophylactic against the common cold	Rheumatic fever Collagen diseases Deficient vitamin C intake Renal and hepatic disease Congestive heart failure
Bilirubin	Total: 0.1-1.0 mg./dl. Direct: 0.1-0.2 mg./dl. Indirect: 0.1-0.8 mg./dl.	Hemolytic anemia (indirect) Biliary obstruction Hepatocellular damage Pernicious anemia Hemolytic disease of newborn Eclampsia	*(Continued)*

* By radioimmunoassay

NORMAL CHEMISTRIES—SERUM, PLASMA, WHOLE BLOOD (CONTINUED)

DETERMINATION	NORMAL ADULT VALUES	CLINICAL SIGNIFICANCE	
		(Increased)	(Decreased)
Bromsulphalein (BSP)	Less than 5% retention in 45 minutes	Acute hepatic diseases	
Calcitonin	Basal: Nondetectable (below 400 pg./ml.)	Medullary carcinoma of the thyroid Some nonthyroid tumors Zollinger-Ellison syndrome Pernicious anemia Chronic renal failure	
Calcium	8.5-10.5 mg./dl.	Tumor or hyperplasia of parathyroid Hyperparathyroidism Hypervitaminosis D Multiple myeloma Nephritis with uremia	Hypoparathyroidism Diarrhea Celiac disease Rickets Osteomalacia Malnutrition Nephrosis After parathyroidectomy
CO_2 content	Adults: 24-32 mEq./L. Infants: 18-24 mEq./L.	Tentany Respiratory disease Intestinal obstruction Vomiting	Acidosis Nephritis Eclampsia Diarrhea Anesthesia
Carcinoembryonic antigen (CEA), RIA	0-2.5 ng./ml.	The repeatedly high incidence of this antigen in cancers of the colon, rectum, pancreas, and stomach suggest that CEA levels may be a useful adjunct in the diagnosis of these conditions	
Carotene, beta	70-250 μg./dl.	Carotenemia Hypothyroidism Diabetes Hyperlipemia	Malabsorption syndromes Hepatic disease Dietary deficiencies
Catecholamines, plasma, RIA	Recumbent: 200-600 ng./L. Upright: 300-1000 ng./L.	Pheochromocytoma	
Cephalin flocculation	Negative to 1+	Severe liver disease Atypical viral pneumonia Malaria Syphilis Infectious mononucleosis Congestive heart failure	
Ceruloplasmin	Males: 29-80 mg./dl. Females: 32-156 mg./dl.	Pregnancy Myocardial infarction Hepatic cirrhosis	Wilson's disease (hepatolenticular degeneration)
C_1 Esterase inhibitor	50-100% of normal control		Hereditary angioneurotic edema Lymphoproliferative disorders
Chloride	95-105 mEq./L.	Nephritis Urinary obstruction Cardiac decompensation Anemia Ether anesthesia	Diabetes Diarrhea Vomiting Pneumonia Heavy metal poisoning Cushing's syndrome Burns Intestinal obstruction Febrile conditions
Cholesterol	150-300 mg./dl.	Lipemia Obstructive jaundice Diabetes Hypothyroidism	Pernicious anemia Hemolytic anemia Hyperthyroidism Severe infection Terminal states of debilitating disease

NORMAL CHEMISTRIES—SERUM, PLASMA, WHOLE BLOOD (CONTINUED)

DETERMINATION	NORMAL ADULT VALUES	CLINICAL SIGNIFICANCE	
		(Increased)	(Decreased)
Cholesterol esters	60-70% of total		The esterified fraction decreases in liver disease
Cholinesterase	Serum: 0.61-1.50 delta pH Red cells: 0.60-1.00 delta pH	Nephrosis Exercise	Nerve gas intoxication (greater effect on red cell activity) Insecticides, organic phosphates (greater effect on plasma activity)
Chorionic gonadotrophin, beta subunit, RIA	0-5 IU/L.	Pregnancy Hydatidiform mole Choriocarcinoma	
Chorionic somatomammotrophin	None detectable	Pregnancy	
Complement, Human C₃	Males: 88-252 mg./dl. Females: 88-206 mg./dl.	Some inflammatory diseases	Acute glomerulonephritis Disseminated lupus erythematosus with renal involvement
Complement, C₄	14-51 mg./dl.	Some inflammatory diseases	Often decreased in immunlogical diseases, especially with active SLE Hereditary angioneurotic edema
Complement, total (hemolytic)	90-94% complement	Some inflammatory diseases	Acute glomerulonephritis Epidemic meningitis Subacute bacterial endocarditis
Congo red	60-100% retained in bloodstream		Deposits of amyloid in tissue absorb congo red. In amyloid disease, less than 40% of the dye will remain in the plasma. In severe cases, less than 10% is retained.
Copper	70-165 μg./dl.	Cirrhosis of liver Pregnancy	Wilson's disease
Cortisol, RIA	8 A.M.: 7-25 μg./dl. 4 P.M.: 2-9 μg./dl.	Stress: infectious disease, surgery, burns, etc. Pregnancy Cushing's syndrome Pancreatitis Eclampsia	Addison's disease Anterior pituitary hypofunction
C-peptide Reactivity	1.5-10 ng./ml.	Insulinoma	Diabetes
Creatine	0.2-0.8 mg./dl.	Biliary obstruction Pregnancy Nephritis Renal destruction Trauma to muscle Pseudohypertrophic muscular dystrophy	
Creatine phosphokinase (CPK)	Males: 50-325 mU/ml. Females: 50-250 mU/ml.	Myocardial infarction Skeletal muscle diseases Intramuscular injections Crush syndrome Hypothyroidism Delirium tremens Cerebrovascular disease	
Creatine phosphokinase isoenzymes	MM band present (skeletal muscle): MB band absent (heart muscle)	MB band increased in myocardial infarction	
Creatinine	0.7-1.4 mg./dl.	Nephritis Chronic renal disease	
Creatinine clearance	100-150 mls. of blood cleared of creatinine/min.		Kidney diseases

(Continued)

NORMAL CHEMISTRIES—SERUM, PLASMA, WHOLE BLOOD (CONTINUED)

DETERMINATION	NORMAL ADULT VALUES	CLINICAL SIGNIFICANCE	
		(Increased)	(Decreased)
Cryofibrinogen, qualitative (plasma)	Negative	Neoplasms Acute rheumatic fever Acute glomerulonephritis Ulcerative colitis Thromboembolic states	
Cryoglobulins, qualitative	Negative	Multiple myeloma Chronic lymphocytic leukemia Lymphosarcoma Systemic lupus erythematosus Rheumatoid arthritis Subacute bacterial endocarditis Some malignancies	
Cyclic AMP (plasma), RIA	Males: 17-33 nM./L. Females: 11-27 nM./L.	Has proved valuable in differentiating nephrogenic diabetes insipidus from that of primary hypothalamic diabetes insipidus. Administration of ADH appears to be incapable of eliciting an increase of cyclic AMP in nephrogenic diabetes insipidus.	
11-Desoxycortisol	0-2 μg./dl.	Hypertensive form of virilizing adrenal hyperplasia due to an 11-beta hydroxylase defect.	
Dibucaine number	Normal: 70-85% inhibition Heterozygote: 50-65% inhibition Homozygote: 16-25% inhibition		Important in detecting carriers of abnormal cholinesterase activity who are susceptible to succinyldicholine anesthetic shock
Dihydrotestosterone	Males: 50-210 ng./dl. Females: None detectable		Testicular feminization syndrome
Erythropoietin	7-36 milli-immuno-chemical units/ml.	Many red blood cell anemias Some cases of "secondary" polycythemia Possible as an early manifestation of kidney transplant rejection	Polycythemia vera Some types of renal disease
Estradiol, RIA	Males: 0.5-5.0 ng./dl. Females: Menstruation: 1.5-7.5 ng./dl. Follicular phase: 2.0-20 ng./dl. Midcycle: 12-40 ng./dl. Luteal phase: 10-30 ng./dl. Postmenopausal: 1.0-5.0 ng./dl.	Pregnancy	Depressed or failure to peak—ovarian failure
Estriol, RIA	Males: less than 0.5 ng./ml. Nonpregnant females: less than 0.5 ng./ml. Pregnant females: 1st trimester— up to 1.0 ng./ml. 2nd trimester— 0.8 to 7.0 ng./ml. 3rd trimester— 5.0 to 25.0 ng./ml.	Pregnancy	Depressed or failure to peak—ovarian failure
Estrogens, total, RIA	Males: 47-74 ng./dl. Females: Menstrual flow: 43-67 ng./dl.	Pregnancy Measured on a daily basis can be used to evaluate response of hypogonadotrophic,	Fetal distress Ovarian failure

NORMAL CHEMISTRIES—SERUM, PLASMA, WHOLE BLOOD (CONTINUED)

DETERMINATION	NORMAL ADULT VALUES	CLINICAL SIGNIFICANCE	
		(Increased)	(Decreased)
Estrogens, total, RIA (*Continued*)	Follicular phase: 40-103 ng./dl. Ovulation peak: 75-139 ng./dl. Luteal phase: 47-113 ng./dl.	hypoestrogenic women to human menopausal or pituitary gonadotropin	
Estrone, RIA	Females: Day 1-10: 4.3-18.0 ng./dl. Day 11-20: 7.5-19.6 ng./dl. Day 21-30: 13.0-20.0 ng./dl. Males: 2.5-7.5 ng./dl.	Pregnancy	Depressed or failure to peak— ovarian failure
Fatty acids	Total: 250-300 mg./dl.	Diabetes Anemia Nephrosis Hypothyroidism Nephritis	Hyperthyroidism
Ferritin, RIA	Males: 10-270 ng./ml. Females: 5-100 ng./ml.	Hemochromatosis Certain neoplastic diseases Acute myelogenous leukemia Multiple myeloma	Iron deficiency
Fibrinogen degradation products (FDP)	Less than 10 μg./ml. (negative in the 1:5 dilution)	Thrombotic episodes of any kind, including myocardial infarction, postoperative deep vein thrombosis, and certain pregnancy disorders	
Folic acid, RIA	4-16 ng./ml.		Megaloblastic anemias of infancy and pregnancy Inadequate diets Liver disease Malabsorption syndrome Severe hemolytic anemia
Follicle stimulating hormone (FSH), RIA	Normal Males: 5-25 mIU/ml. Normal Females: Follicular phase: 5-20 mIU/ml. Peak of middle cycle: 12-30 mIU/ml. Luteinic phase: 5-15 mIU/ml. Menopausal Females: 40-200 mIU/ml.	Menopause and primary ovarian failure	Pituitary failure
Galactose-1-phosphate uridyl transferase	Above 18 units of activity per gram of hemoglobin 0.05-1.5: Possibly galactosemic 0-0.05: Galactosemic		Galactosemia
Gamma glutamyl transpeptidase	Males: less than 45 IU/L. Females: less than 30 IU/L.	Hepatobiliary disease Anicteric alcoholics Drug therapy damage	
Gastrin, RIA	Fasting: 50-155 pg./ml. Postprandial: 80-170 pg./ml. Zollinger-Ellison syndrome: 200- over 2000 pg./ml. Pernicious anemia: 130-2260 (mean 912) pg./ml.	Zollinger-Ellison syndrome Peptic ulceration of the duodenum Pernicious anemia	
Glucose	Fasting: 60-110 mg./dl. Postprandial (2 hour): 65-140 mg./dl.	Diabetes Nephritis Hyperthyroidism	Hyperinsulinism Hypothyroidism Late hyperpituitarism

(Continued)

NORMAL CHEMISTRIES—SERUM, PLASMA, WHOLE BLOOD (CONTINUED)

DETERMINATION	NORMAL ADULT VALUES	CLINICAL SIGNIFICANCE	
		(Increased)	(Decreased)
Glucose (*Continued*)		Early hyperpituitarism Cerebral lesions Infections Pregnancy Uremia	Pernicious vomiting Addison's disease Extensive hepatic damage

Glucose tolerance (oral)	Features of a normal response:
	1. Normal fasting between 60-125 mg./dl.
	2. No sugar in urine
	3. The upper limits of normal are:
	    fasting—125
	    1 hour—190
	    2 hours—140
	    3 hours—125
		(Flat or inverted curve)
		Hyperinsulinism
		Adrenal cortical insufficiency (Addison's disease)
		Anterior pituitary hypofunction
		Hypothyroidism
		Sprue and celiac disease
			(High or prolonged curve)
			Diabetes
			Hyperthyroidism
			Primary adrenal cortical tumor or hyperplasia
			Severe anemia
			Certain central nervous system disorders

Glucose-6-phosphate dehydrogenase (red cells)	Screening: Decolorization in 20-100 minutes Quantitative: 1.86-2.50 IU/ml. RBC		Drug induced hemolytic anemia Hemolytic disease of newborn
Glycoprotein	110-140 mg./dl.	Neoplasm Tuberculosis Diabetes complicated by degenerative vascular disease Pregnancy Rheumatoid arthritis Rheumatic fever Infectious liver disease Lupus erythematosus	
Growth hormone, RIA	Males: up to 3 ng./ml. Females: up to 5 ng./ml.	Acromegaly	Failure to stimulate with arginine or insulin—hypopituitarism
Haptoglobin	50-200 mg./dl.	Pregnancy Estrogen therapy Chronic infections Various inflammatory conditions Tissue destruction or necrosis	Hemolytic anemia Hemolytic blood transfusion reaction
Hemoglobin (plasma)	2-7 mg./dl.	Transfusion reactions Paroxysmal nocturnal hemoglobinuria Intravascular hemolysis	
Hexosaminidase, total	Controls: 333-375 nM./ml./hr. Heterozygotes: 288-644 nM./ml./hr. Tay-Sachs disease: 284-1232 nM./ml./hr. Diabetics: 567-3560 nM./ml./hr.	Diabetes Tay-Sachs disease	
Hexosaminidase A	Controls: 49-68% of total Heterozygotes: 26-45% of total Tay-Sachs disease: 0-4% of total Diabetics: 39-59% of total		Tay-Sachs disease and heterozygotes

NORMAL CHEMISTRIES—SERUM, PLASMA, WHOLE BLOOD (CONTINUED)

DETERMINATION	NORMAL ADULT VALUES	CLINICAL SIGNIFICANCE	
		(Increased)	(Decreased)
High density lipoprotein Cholesterol (HDL cholesterol)	Males / Females Age (years) — Males (mg./dl.) — Females (mg./dl.) 0-19 — 30-65 — 30-70 20-29 — 35-70 — 35-75 30-39 — 30-65 — 35-80 40-49 — 30-65 — 40-85 50-59 — 30-65 — 35-85 60-69 — 30-65 — 35-85		HDL cholesterol is lower in patients with increased risk for coronary heart disease
17-Hydroxyprogesterone, RIA	Males: 0.4-4.0 ng./ml. Females: 0.1-3.3 ng./ml. Children: 0.1-0.5 ng./ml.	Congenital adrenal hyperplasia Pregnancy Some cases of adrenal or ovarian adenomas	
Icterus index	1-6 units	Biliary obstruction Hemolytic anemias	Secondary anemias
Immunoglobulin A	Adult Males: 60-297 mg./dl. Adult Females: 48-295 mg./dl. (In children the normals are lower and vary with age.)	Gamma A myeloma Wiscott-Aldrich syndrome Autoimmune disease Hepatic cirrhosis	Ataxia telangiectasis Agammaglobulinemia Hypogammaglobulinemia, transient Dysgammaglobulinemia Protein-losing enteropathies
Immunoglobulin D	0-30 mg./dl.	IgD multiple myeloma Some patients with chronic infectious diseases	
Immunoglobulin E	20-740 ng./ml.	Allergic patients and those with parasitic infestations	
Immunoglobulin G	Adult Males: 635-1400 mg./dl. Adult Females: 645-1300 mg./dl. (In children the normals are lower and vary with age.)	IgG myeloma Following hyperimmunization Autoimmune disease states Chronic infections	Congenital and acquired hypogammaglobulinemia IgA myelomas, Waldenstrom's (IgM) macroglobulinemia Some malabsorption syndromes Extensive protein loss
Immunoglobulin M	Adult Males: 41-248 mg./dl. Adult Females: 59-280 mg./dl. (In children the normals are lower and vary with age.)	Waldenstrom's macroglobulinemia Parasitic infections Hepatitis	Agammaglobulinemias Some IgG and IgA myelomas Chronic lymphatic leukemia
Insulin, RIA	5-25 μU/ml.	Insulinoma Acromegaly	Diabetes mellitus
Iodine, protein-bound	4.0-8.0 μg./dl.	Hyperthyroidism	Hypothyroidism
Ionized calcium	2.04-2.44 mEq./L.	Ionized calcium is a much more sensitive indicator of disease states than the total calcium. Useful in diagnosing hyperparathyroidism in patients with normal and near normal total calcium levels. Also a necessary protocol in management of hemodialysis patients.	Hypothyroidism
Iron	65-170 μg./dl.	Pernicious anemia Aplastic anemia Hemolytic anemia Hepatitis Hemochromatosis	Iron deficiency anemia

(Continued)

NORMAL CHEMISTRIES—SERUM, PLASMA, WHOLE BLOOD (CONTINUED)

DETERMINATION	NORMAL ADULT VALUES	CLINICAL SIGNIFICANCE	
		(Increased)	(Decreased)
Iron binding capacity	IBC: 150-235 μg./dl. TIBC: 250-420 μg./dl. % Saturation: 20-50	Iron deficiency anemia	Chronic infectious diseases
Isocitric dehydrogenase	50-180 units	Hepatitis, cirrhosis Obstructive jaundice Metastatic carcinoma of the liver Megaloblastic anemia	

Lactic acid
(whole blood)
	9-16 mg./dl.	Increased muscular activity
		Congestive heart failure
		Hemorrhage
		Shock
		Some varieties of metabolic
		  acidosis
		Some febrile infections
		May be increased in severe liver
		  disease	

Lactic dehydrogenase (LDH)	100-225 mU/ml.	Untreated pernicious anemia Myocardial infarction Pulmonary infarction Liver disease	
Lactic dehydrogenase isoenzymes			

Total lactic dehydrogenase
LDH-1
LDH-2
LDH-3
LDH-4
LDH-5
	100-225 mU/ml.
	20-35%
	25-40%
	20-30%
	0-20%
	0-25%
		LDH-1 and LDH-2 are increased
		  in myocardial infarction,
		  megaloblastic anemia, and
		  hemolytic anemia
		LDH-4 and LDH-5 are increased
		  in pulmonary infarction,
		  congestive heart failure, and
		  liver disease	

Lead (whole blood)	up to 40 μg./dl.	Lead poisoning	
Leucine aminopeptidase	1-3 micromoles/hr./ml.	Liver or biliary tract diseases Pancreatic disease Metastatic carcinoma of liver and pancreas Biliary obstruction	
Lipase	0.2-1.5 units/ml.	Acute and chronic pancreatitis Biliary obstruction Cirrhosis Hepatitis Peptic ulcer	
Lipids, total	400-1000 mg./dl.	Hypothyroidism Diabetes Nephrosis Glomerulonephritis	Hyperthyroidism

NORMAL CHEMISTRIES—SERUM, PLASMA, WHOLE BLOOD (CONTINUED)

DETERMINATION	NORMAL ADULT VALUES	CLINICAL SIGNIFICANCE	
		(Increased)	(Decreased)
Lipoprotein phenotype			

SUMMARY OF FINDINGS IN THE PRIMARY HYPERLIPOPROTEINEMIAS

TYPE	APPEAR-ANCE	TRIGLYC-ERIDE	CHOLES-TEROL	LIPOPROTEIN STAINING				SECONDARY CAUSES
				Beta	Pre-Beta	Alpha	Chylomi-crons	
Normal	Clear	Normal	Normal	Moderate	Zero to moderate	Moderate	Weak	
I	Creamy	Markedly increased	Normal to moderately increased	Weak	Weak	Weak	Markedly increased	Dysglobulinemia
II	Clear	Normal to slightly increased	Slightly to markedly increased	Strong	Zero to strong	Moderate	Weak	Hypothyroidism, myeloma, hepatic disease, nephrotic syndrome, macroglobulinemia, and high dietary cholesterol
III	Clear, cloudy or milky	Increased	Increased	Broad in-tense band	Extends into beta	Moderate	Weak	
IV	Clear, cloudy or milky	Slightly to markedly increased	Normal to slightly increased	Weak to moderate	Moderate to strong	Weak to moderate	Weak	Hypothyroidism, diabetes mellitus, pancreatitis, glycogen storage diseases, nephrotic syndrome, myeloma, pregnancy, and oral contraceptives
V	Cloudy to creamy	Markedly increased	Increased	Weak	Moderate	Weak	Strong	Diabetes mellitus, pancreatitis, and alcoholism

Types I and II are fat induced; III and IV are carbohydrate induced; type V is fat and carbohydrate induced.

DETERMINATION	NORMAL ADULT VALUES	(Increased)	(Decreased)
Lithium	Usual maintenance level: 0.5-1.0 mEq./L.		
Low density lipoprotein cholesterol (LDL cholesterol)	Age (years) mg./dl. 0-19 50-170 20-29 60-170 30-39 70-190 40-49 80-190 50-59 80-210	LDL cholesterol is higher in patients with increased risk for coronary heart disease.	
Luteinizing hormone, RIA	Males: 6-30 mIU/ml. Children: 4-20 mIU/ml. Females: Follicular Phase: 2-30 mIU/ml. Ovulatory Peak: 40-200 mIU/ml. Luteal Phase: 0-20 mIU/ml. Postmenopausal: 35-120 mIU/ml.	Pituitary tumor Ovarian failure	Depressed or failure to peak— pituitary failure
Lysozyme (muramidase)	2.8-8.0 μg./ml.	Certain types of leukemia (acute monocytic leukemia) Inflammatory states and infections	Acute lymphocytic leukemia
Magnesium	1.3-2.4 mEq./L.	Ingestion of Epsom salts Parathyroidectomy	Chronic alcoholism Toxemia of pregnancy Severe renal disease
Manganese	0.08-0.26 μg./dl.		Defective growth

(Continued)

NORMAL CHEMISTRIES—SERUM, PLASMA, WHOLE BLOOD (CONTINUED)

DETERMINATION	NORMAL ADULT VALUES	CLINICAL SIGNIFICANCE	
		(Increased)	(Decreased)
Mercury	up to 10 μg./dl.	Mercury poisoning	
Myoglobin, RIA	up to 85 ng./ml.	Myocardial infarction	
Nonprotein nitrogen	20-35 mg./dl.	Acute nephritis Polycystic kidneys Obstructive uropathy Peritonitis Congestive heart failure Pregnancy	
5' Nucleotidase	3.2-11.6 IU/L.	Hepatobiliary disease	
Osmolality	280-300 milliosmoles/kg.	Useful in the study of electrolyte and water balance	Inappropriate secretion of antidiuretic hormone
Oxygen saturation arterial (whole blood)	96-100%	Polycythemia Anhydremia	Anemia Cardiac decompensation Chronic obstructive pulmonary disease
pCO_2 (whole blood) arterial	35-45 mm. Hg	Respiratory acidosis Metabolic alkalosis	Respiratory alkalosis Metabolic acidosis
pH (whole blood) arterial	7.35-7.45	Vomiting Hyperpnea Fever Intestinal obstruction	Uremia Diabetic acidosis Hemorrhage Nephritis
pO_2 (whole blood) arterial	95-100 mm. Hg	Directly related to oxygen saturation	
Parathyroid hormone	163-347 pg./ml.	Hyperparathyroidism	
Pepsinogen	200-425 units/ml.		Conditions which decrease gastric acidity Pernicious anemia Achlorhydria
Phenylalanine	0-6 mg./dl. first week 0.7-3.5 mg./dl. thereafter	Phenylketonuria Oasthouse urine disease	
Phosphatase, acid, total	0-11 IU/L.	Carcinoma of prostate Advanced Paget's disease Hyperparathyroidism	
Phosphatase, acid, prostatic, RIA	0-10 ng./ml. Borderline: 2.5-3.3 IU/L.	Carcinoma of prostate	
Phosphatase, alkaline	Adults: 30-115 mU/ml. Children: 60-300 mU/ml.	Conditions reflecting increased osteoblastic activity of bone Rickets Hyperparathyroidism Liver disease	
Phosphatase, alkaline, thermostable fraction	Thermostable fraction greater than 35%: hepatic disease and combined disease with predominant hepatic component. Thermostable fraction between 25-35%: combined hepatic and skeletal disease. Thermostable fraction less than 25%: skeletal disease with increased osteoblastic activity.	Hepatic disease	
Phosphohexose isomerase	20-90 IU/L.	Malignancy Diseases of heart, liver, and skeletal muscles	

NORMAL CHEMISTRIES—SERUM, PLASMA, WHOLE BLOOD (CONTINUED)

DETERMINATION	NORMAL ADULT VALUES	CLINICAL SIGNIFICANCE	
		(Increased)	(Decreased)
Phospholipids	125-300 mg./dl.	Diabetes Nephritis	
Phosphorus, inorganic	2.5-4.5 mg./dl.	Chronic nephritis Hypoparathyroidism	Hyperparathyroidism
Potassium	3.5-5.0 mEq./L.	Addison's disease Oliguria Anuria Tissue breakdown or hemolysis	Diabetic acidosis Diarrhea Vomiting
Progesterone, RIA	Follicular phase: up to 0.8 ng./ml. Luteal phase: 10-20 ng./ml. End of cycle: less than 1 ng./ml. Pregnant: up to 50 ng./ml. in 20th week	Useful in evaluation of menstrual disorders and infertility and the evaluation of placental function during pregnancies complicated by toxemia, diabetes mellitus, or threatened miscarriage.	
Prolactin, RIA	Males: 7-18 ng./ml. Females: 6-24 ng./ml.	Pregnancy Functional or structural disorders of the hypothalamus Pituitary stalk section Pituitary tumors Primary hypothyroidism	
Protein, total Albumin Globulin	6.0-8.0 gm./dl. 3.5-5.0 gm./dl. 1.5-3.0 gm./dl.	Hemoconcentration Shock Multiple myeloma (globulin fraction) Chronic infections (globulin fraction) Liver disease (globulin)	Malnutrition Hemorrhage Loss of plasma from burns Proteinuria
Electrophoresis (Cellulose acetate) Albumin Alpha$_1$ globulin Alpha$_2$ globulin Beta globulin Gamma globulin	 3.3-5.0 gm./dl. 0.2-0.4 gm./dl. 0.6-1.0 gm./dl. 0.6-1.2 gm./dl. 0.7-1.5 gm./dl.		
Protoporphyrin, erythrocyte (whole blood)	15-100 μg./dl.	Lead toxicity Erythropoietic porphyria	
Pyridoxine	3.6-18 ng./ml.		A wide spectrum of clinical conditions such as mental depression, peripheral neuropathy, anemia, neonatal seizures, and reactions to certain drug therapy
Pyruvic acid (whole blood)	0.3-0.7 mg./dl.	Diabetes Severe thiamine deficiency Acute phase of some infections, possibly secondary to increased glycogenolysis and glycolysis	
Renin (plasma), RIA	*Normal Diet:* Supine: 0.3-1.9 ng./ml./hr. Upright: 0.6-3.6 ng./ml./hr. *Low Salt Diet:* Supine: 0.9-4.5 ng./ml./hr. Upright: 4.1-9.1 ng./ml./hr.	Renovascular hypertension Malignant hypertension Untreated Addison's disease Primary salt-losing nephropathy Low-salt diet Diuretic therapy Hemorrhage	Frank primary aldosteronism Increased salt intake Salt-retaining steroid therapy Antidiuretic hormone therapy Blood transfusion
Riboflavin (whole blood)	0.9-1.31 (activity coefficient)		Riboflavin deficiency

(Continued)

NORMAL CHEMISTRIES—SERUM, PLASMA, WHOLE BLOOD (CONTINUED)

DETERMINATION	NORMAL ADULT VALUES	CLINICAL SIGNIFICANCE	
		(Increased)	(Decreased)
Sodium	135-145 mEq./L.	Hemoconcentration Nephritis Pyloric obstruction	Alkali deficit Addison's disease Myxedema
Sulfate	0.5-1.5 mg./dl.	Nephritis Nitrogen retention	

Testosterone, RIA	Females: 25-100 ng./dl.
	Males: 300-800 ng./dl.
		Females:
		  Polycystic ovary
		  Virilizing tumors
			Males:
			Orchidectomy for neoplastic
			  disease of the prostate or breast
			Estrogen therapy
			Klinefelter's syndrome
			Hypopituitarism
			Hypogonadism
			Hepatic cirrhosis

Thymol turbidity	1-4.5 units/ml.	Liver disease Infectious diseases with antibody production	
T_3 uptake	25-35%	Hyperthyroidism TBG deficiency Androgens and anabolic steroids	Hypothyroidism Pregnancy TBG excess Estrogens and antiovulatory drugs
T_3, Triiodothyronine (total circulating), RIA	75-200 ng./dl.	Pregnancy Hyperthyroidism	Hypothyroidism

T_4, Thyroxine, RIA	4.5-11.5 μg./dl.	Hyperthyroidism
		Thyroiditis
		Cases of elevated thyroxine-
		  binding proteins caused by oral
		  contraceptives
		Pregnancy
			Primary and pituitary
			  hypothyroidism
			Idiopathic involvement
			Cases of diminished thyroxine-
			  binding proteins caused by
			  androgenic and anabolic
			  steroids
			Hypoproteinemia
			Nephrotic syndrome

T_4, Thyroxine, free	1.0-2.2 ng./dl.	Euthyroid patients with normal
		  free thyroxine levels may have
		  abnormal T_3 and T_4 levels
		  caused by drug preparations	

Thyroid stimulating hormone (TSH), RIA	0-10 μIU/ml.	Primary hypothyroidism	
Thyroid binding globulin	10-26 μg./dl.	Hypothyroidism Pregnancy Estrogen therapy Oral contraceptives Genetic and idiopathic	Androgens and anabolic steroids Nephroic syndromes Marked hypoproteinemia Hepatic disease
Transaminase (SGOT) (Aspartate aminotransferase)	7-40 mU/ml.	Myocardial infarction Skeletal muscle disease Liver disease	

Transaminase (SGPT)
(Alanine aminotransferase)
	10-40 mU/ml.	Same conditions as SGOT, but
		  increase is more marked in liver
		  disease than SGOT	

Transferrin	230-320 mg./dl.	Pregnancy
		Iron-deficiency anemia due to
		  hemorrhaging
		Acute hepatitis
		Polycythemia
		Oral contraceptives
			Pernicious anemia in relapse
			Thalassemic and sickle cell
			  anemia
			Chromatosis
			Neoplastic and hepatic diseases

Transketolase (whole blood)	Pentose utilization: 9.66-15.50 micromoles/hr./ml. or 1.70-3.04 micromoles/hr./10^9 red blood cells		Thiamine deficiency

NORMAL CHEMISTRIES—SERUM, PLASMA, WHOLE BLOOD (CONTINUED)

DETERMINATION	NORMAL ADULT VALUES	CLINICAL SIGNIFICANCE	
		(Increased)	(Decreased)
Triglycerides	10-150 mg./dl.	See lipoprotein phenotype	
Tryptophan	1.4-3.0 mg./dl.		Tryptophan-specific malabsorption syndrome
Tyrosine	0.5-4.0 mg./dl.	Hyperthyroidism Tyrosinosis	
Urea nitrogen (BUN)	10-20 mg./dl.	Acute glomerulonephritis Obstructive uropathy Mercury poisoning Nephrotic syndrome	Severe hepatic failure Pregnancy
Uric acid	2.5-8.0 mg./dl.	Gouty arthritis Acute leukemia Lymphomas treated by chemotherapy Toxemia of pregnancy	Xanthinuria Defective tubular reabsorption
Viscosity	1.4-1.8 relative to water at 37° C. (98.6° F.)	Patients with marked increases of the gamma globulins	
Vitamin A	50-220 μg./dl.	Hypervitaminosis A	Vitamin A deficiency Celiac disease Sprue Obstructive jaundice Cystic fibrosis Giardiasis Parenchymal hepatic disease
Vitamin B_1 (thiamine)	1.6-4.0 μg./dl.		Anorexia Beriberi Polyneuropathy Cardiomyopathies
Vitamin B_6 (pyridoxal phosphate)	3.6-18.0 ng./ml.		Chronic alcoholism Malnutrition Uremia Neonatal seizures Malabsorption, such as celiac syndrome
Vitamin B_{12} RIA	130-785 pg./ml.	Hepatic cell damage and in association with the myeloproliferative disorders (the highest levels are encountered in myeloid leukemia)	Strict vegetarianism Alcoholism Pernicious anemia Total or partial gastrectomy Ileal resection Sprue and celiac disease Fish tapeworm infestation
Vitamin E	0.5-2.0 mg./dl.		Vitamin E deficiency
Water content	92.6-94.3 gm./dl.	Useful in the study of electrolyte and water balance	
Xylose absorption test	2 hr. 30-50 mg./dl.		Malabsorption syndrome
Zinc	55-150 μg./dl.	Zinc is essential for the growth and propagation of cell cultures and the functioning of several enzymes	
Zinc turbidity	2-12 units/ml.	Same clinical significance as thymol turbidity	

NORMAL VALUES—URINE CHEMISTRY

DETERMINATION	NORMAL VALUE	CLINICAL SIGNIFICANCE	
		(Increased)	(Decreased)
Acetone and acetoacetate	Zero	Uncontrolled diabetes Starvation	
Acid mucopolysaccharides	Negative	Hurler's syndrome Marfan's syndrome Morquio-Ulrich disease	
Aldosterone	*Normal salt:* Normal: 4-20 μg./24 hr. Renovascular: 10-40 μg./24 hr. Tumor: 20-100 μg./24 hr. *Low salt:* Normal: 10-40 μg./24 hr. Renovascular: 20-100 μg./24 hr. Tumor: 20-100 μg./24 hr.	Primary aldosteronism (adrenocortical tumor) Secondary aldosteronism Salt depletion Potassium loading ACTH in large doses Cardiac failure Cirrhosis with ascites formation Nephrosis Pregnancy	
Alpha amino nitrogen	64-199 mg./24 hr.	Leukemia Diabetes Phenylketonuria Other metabolic diseases	
Amylase	35-260 units excreted/hr.	Acute pancreatitis	
Arylsulfatase A	Greater than 2.4 units/ml.		Metachromatic leukodystrophy
Bence-Jones protein	None detected	Myeloma	
Bile melanin	Zero	Advanced melanoma Ochronosis	
Calcium	Less than 150 mg./24 hr.	Hyperparathyroidism Vitamin D intoxication Fanconi syndrome	Hypoparathyroidism Vitamin D deficiency
Catecholamines	Total: 0-275 μg./24 hr. Epinephrine: 10-40% Norepinephrine: 60-90%	Pheochromocytoma Neuroblastoma	
Chloride	70-250 mEq./24 hr.	Urine chloride levels vary with excretion of sodium, potassium, ammonia, and bicarbonate	
Chorionic gonadotrophin, qualitative (pregnancy test)	Negative	Pregnancy Chorionepithelioma Hydatidiform mole	
Copper	20-70 μg./24 hr.	Wilson's disease Cirrhosis Nephrosis	
Coproporphyrin	50-300 μg./24 hr.	Poliomyelitis Lead poisoning Porphyria hepatica Porphyria erythropoietica Porphyria cutanea tarda	
Cortisol, free	20-90 μg./24 hr.	Cushing's syndrome	
Creatine	0-200 mg./24 hr.	Muscular dystrophy Fever Carcinoma of liver Pregnancy Hyperthyroidism Myositis	
Creatinine	0.8-2.0 gm./24 hr.	Typhoid fever Salmonella infections Tetanus	Muscular atrophy Anemia Advanced degeneration of kidneys Leukemia

NORMAL VALUES—URINE CHEMISTRY (CONTINUED)

DETERMINATION	NORMAL ADULT VALUES	CLINICAL SIGNIFICANCE	
		(Increased)	(Decreased)
Creatinine clearance	100-150 mls. of blood cleared of creatinine/min.		Measures glomerular filtration rate Renal diseases
Cystine	10-100 mg./24 hr.	Cystinuria	
Delta amino-levulinic acid	0.00-0.54 mg./dl.	Lead poisoning Porphyria hepatica Hepatitis Hepatic carcinoma	
11-Desoxycortisol	20-100 μg./24 hr.	Hypertensive form of virilizing adrenal hyperplasia due to an 11-beta hydroxylase defect	
Diagnex blue	Greater than 0.6 mg. Presumptive evidence for hypochlorhydria: 0.3-0.6 mg. Presumptive evidence for achlorhydria: less than 0.3 mg.		Hypochlorhydria Achlorhydria
Estriol (placental)	*Weeks of pregnancy mg./24 hr.* 12 — less than 1 16 — 2-7 20 — 4-9 24 — 6-13 28 — 8-22 32 — 12-43 36 — 14-45 40 — 19-46		Decreased values occur with fetal distress of many conditions, including preeclampsia, placental insufficiency, and poorly controlled diabetes mellitus
Estrogens, total (fluorimetric)	Females: Onset of menstruation: 4-25 μg./24 hr. Ovulation peak: 28-99 μg./24 hr. Luteal peak: 22-105 μg./24 hr. Menopausal: 1.4-19.6 μg./24 hr. Males: 5-18 μg./24 hr.	Hyperestrogenism due to gonadal or adrenal neoplasm	Primary or secondary amenorrhea
Etiocholanolone	Males: 1.9-6.0 mg./24 hr. Females: 0.5-4.0 mg./24 hr.	Adrenogenital syndrome Idiopathic hirsutism	
Follicle stimulating hormone, RIA	Males: 5-25 IU/24 hr. Females: Follicular: 5-20 IU/24 hr. Luteal: 5-15 IU/24 hr. Midcycle: 15-60 IU/24 hr. Menopausal: 50-100 IU/24 hr.	Menopause and primary ovarian failure	Pituitary failure
Glucose	Negative	Diabetes mellitus Pituitary disorders Intracranial pressure Lesion in floor of 4th ventricle	
Hemoglobin and myoglobin	Negative	Extensive burns Transfusion of incompatible blood Myoglobin increased in severe crushing injuries to muscle	
Homogentisic acid, qualitative	Negative	Alkaptonuria Ochronosis	

NORMAL VALUES—URINE CHEMISTRY (CONTINUED)

DETERMINATION	NORMAL ADULT VALUES	CLINICAL SIGNIFICANCE	
		(Increased)	(Decreased)
Homovanillic acid	Up to 15 mg./24 hrs.	Neuroblastoma	
17-hydroxycorticosteroids	2-10 mg./24 hr.	Cushing's syndrome	Addison's disease Anterior pituitary hypofunction
5-hydroxyindoleacetic acid, qualitative	Negative	Malignant carcinoid tumors	
Hydroxyproline	25-77 mg./24 hr.	Paget's disease Fibrous dysplasia Osteomalacia Neoplastic bone disease Hyperparathyroidism	
17-ketosteroids, alpha-beta fractionation	Alpha concentration 85% or more	Adrenal carcinomas (in beta fraction)	

17-ketosteroids, total	Males: 10-22 mg./24 hr.
	Females: 6-16 mg./24 hr.
	Children:
	  Up to 1 yr.:
	    less than 1 mg./24 hr.
	  1-4 yrs.:
	    less than 2 mg./24 hr.
	  5-8 yrs.:
	    less than 3 mg./24 hr.
	  9-12 yrs.: 3-10 mg./24 hr.
	  13-16 yrs.: 5-12 mg./24 hr.
		Interstitial cell tumor of testes
		Simple hirsutism, occasionally
		Adrenal hyperplasia
		Cushing's syndrome
		Adrenal cancer, virilism
		Arrhenoblastoma
			Thyrotoxicosis
			Female hypogonadism
			Diabetes mellitus
			Hypertension
			Debilitating disease of mild to
			  moderate severity
			Eunuchoidism
			Addison's disease
			Panhypopituitarism
			Myxedema
			Nephrosis

Kynurenic and xanthurenic acids	Kynurenic acid:
	  up to 18.0 mg./24 hr.
	Xanthurenic acid:
	  up to 4.0 mg./24 hr.
		Vitamin B_6 deficiency
		Acute typhoid fever
		Sandfly fever
		Tularemia	

Lead	up to 150 μg./24 hr.	Lead poisoning	
Lipase	0.1-0.75 units/ml.	Pancreatitis	

Luteinizing hormone	Males: 5-18 IU/24 hr.
	Females:
	  Follicular phase:
	    2-25 IU/24 hr.
	  Ovulatory peak:
	    30-95 IU/24 hr.
	  Luteal phase: 2-20 IU/24 hr.
	  Postmenopausal:
	    40-110 IU/24 hr.
		Pituitary tumor
		Ovarian failure
			Depressed or failure to peak—
			  pituitary failure

Metanephrines, total	Less than 1.3 mg./24 hr.	Pheochromocytoma, a few patients with pheochromocytoma may have elevated urinary metanephrines but normal catecholamines and VMA	

Osmolality	Males:
	  390-1090 milliosmoles/kg.
	Females:
	  300-1090 milliosmoles/kg.
		Useful in the study of electrolyte and water balance	

Oxalate	up to 40 mg./24 hrs.	Primary hyperoxaluria	
Phenolphthalein (PSP)	At least 25% excreted in 15 min., 40% by 30 min., and 60% by 120 min.	Primarily measures renal tubular function	Delayed in renal diseases Low in nephritis, cystitis, pyelonephritis, congestive heart failure
Phenylpyruvic acid, qualitative	Negative	Phenylketonuria	

NORMAL VALUES—URINE CHEMISTRY (CONTINUED)

DETERMINATION	NORMAL ADULT VALUES	CLINICAL SIGNIFICANCE	
		(Increased)	(Decreased)
Phosphorus, inorganic	0.8-1.3 gm./24 hr.	Fever Nervous exhaustion Tuberculosis Rickets Chronic lead poisoning	Acute infections Nephritis Chlorosis Pregnancy
Porphobilinogen, qualitative	Negative	Acute porphyria Liver disease	
Porphobilinogen, quantitative	0.00-0.03 mg./dl.	Acute porphyria Liver disease	
Porphyrins, qualitative	Negative	See porphyrins, quantitative	
Porphyrins, quantitative (Coproporphyrin and Uroporphyrin)	Coproporphyrin: 50-300 μg./24 hr. Uroporphyrin: up to 50 μg./24 hr.	Porphyria hepatica Porphyria erythropoietica Porphyria cutanea tarda Lead poisoning (only coproporphyrin increased)	
Potassium	40-65 mEq./24 hr.	Hemolysis	
Pregnanediol	Males: 0.1-2.0 mg./24 hr. Females: Proliferative phase: 0.5-1.5 mg./24 hr. Luteal phase: 2-7 mg./24 hr. Menopause: 0.2-1.0 mg./24 hr. Pregnancy: *(Weeks of* *gestation)* *mg./24 hr.* 10-12 5-15 12-18 5-25 18-24 15-33 24-28 20-42 28-32 27-47	Corpus luteum cysts When placental tissue remains in the uterus following parturition Some cases of adrenocortical tumors Pregnancy	Placental dysfunction Threatened abortion Intrauterine death
Pregnanetriol	0.4 mg./24 hr.	Congenital adrenal androgenic hyperplasia	
Protein	up to 100 mg./24 hr.	Nephritis Cardiac failure Mercury poisoning Bence-Jones protein in multiple myeloma Febrile states Hematuria Amyloidosis	
Sodium	130-200 mEq./24 hr.	Useful in detecting gross changes in water and salt balance	
Titratable acidity	20-40 mEq./24 hr.	Metabolic acidosis	Metabolic alkalosis
Urea nitrogen	9-16 gm./24 hr.	Excessive protein catabolism	Impaired kidney function
Uric acid	250-750 mg./24 hr.	Gout	Nephritis
Urobilinogen	Random urine: less than 0.25 mg./dl. 24 hr. urine: up to 4 mg./24 hr.	Liver and biliary tract disease Hemolytic anemias	Complete or nearly complete biliary obstruction Diarrhea Renal insufficiency
Uroporphyrins	up to 50 μg./24 hr.	Porphyria	
Vanillymandelic acid (VMA)	0.7-6.8 mg./24 hr.	Pheochromocytoma Neuroblastoma Coffee, tea, aspirin, bananas, and several different drugs	
Xylose absorption test (5 hour)	16-33% of ingested xylose		Malabsorption syndromes
Zinc	0.15-1.2 mg./24 hr.	Zinc is an essential nutritional element	

NORMAL VALUES—CEREBROSPINAL FLUID

DETERMINATION	NORMAL VALUE	CLINICAL SIGNIFICANCE	
		(Increased)	(Decreased)
Albumin	15.5-32.0 mg./dl.	Certain neurological disorders Lesion in the choroid plexus or blockage of the flow of CSF Damage to the blood-CNS barrier	
Cell count	0-5 mononuclear cells/cu. mm.	Bacterial meningitis Neurosyphilis Anterior poliomyelitis Encephalitis lethargica	
Chloride	100-130 mEq./L.	Uremia	Acute generalized meningitis Tubercular meningitis
Colloidal gold	0000000000	Acute meningitis Neurosyphilis	
Glucose	50-75 mg./dl.	Diabetes mellitus Diabetic coma Epidemic encephalitis Uremia	Acute meningitides Tuberculous meningitis Insulin shock
Glutamine	6-15 mg./dl.	Hepatic encephalopathies, including Reye's syndrome Hepatic coma Cirrhosis	
IgG	0-6.6 mg./dl.	Damage to the blood-CNS barrier Multiple sclerosis Neurosyphilis Subacute sclerosing panencephalitis Chronic phases of CNS infections	
Lactic acid	Less than 24 mg./dl.	Bacterial meningitis Hypocapnia Hydrocephalus Brain abscesses Cerebral ischemia	
Lactic dehydrogenase	One tenth that of serum	CNS disease	

Protein
  Lumbar
  Cisternal
  Ventricular
	
	15-45 mg./dl.
	15-25 mg./dl.
	5-15 mg./dl.
		Acute meningitides
		Tubercular meningitis
		Neurosyphilis
		Poliomyelitis
		Guillain-Barré syndrome	

Protein Electrophoresis
  (Cellulose acetate)
  Prealbumin
  Albumin
  Alpha$_1$ globulin
  Alpha$_2$ globulin
  Beta globulin
  Gamma globulin
	% of total
	
	3.0-7.0
	56.0-74.0
	2.0-6.5
	3.0-12.0
	8.0-18.5
	4.0-14.0
		An increase in the level of
		  albumin alone can be the result
		  of a lesion in the choroid plexus
		  or a blockage of the flow of CSF.
		  An elevated gamma globulin
		  value with a normal albumin
		  level has been reported in
		  multiple sclerosis, neurosyphilis,
		  subacute sclerosing
		  panencephalitis, and the
		  chronic phase of CNS
		  infections. If the blood-CNS
		  barrier has been severely
		  damaged during the course of
		  these diseases, the CSF albumin
		  level may also be elevated.	

MISCELLANEOUS VALUES

DETERMINATIONS	NORMAL VALUE	CLINICAL SIGNIFICANCE	
Acetaminophen	Zero	Therapeutic level = 10-20 μg./ml.	
Aminophylline (theophylline)	Zero	Therapeutic level = 10-20 μg./ml.	
Bromide	Zero	Therapeutic level = 5-50 mg./dl.	
Carbon monoxide	0-2%	Symptoms with over 20% saturation	
Digitoxin	Zero	Therapeutic level = 5-30 ng./ml.	
Digoxin	Zero	Therapeutic level = 0.5-2.0 ng./ml.	
Dilantin (phenytoin)	Zero	Therapeutic level = 10-20 μg./ml.	
Ethanol	0-0.01%	Legal intoxication level = 0.10% or above 0.3-0.4% = marked intoxication 0.4-0.5% = alcoholic stupor	
Gentamicin	Zero	Therapeutic level = 4-10 μg./ml.	
Librium (chlordiazepoxide)	Zero	Therapeutic level = 1-3 μg./ml.	
Methanol	Zero	May be fatal in concentrations as low as 10 mg./dl.	
Mysoline (primidone)	Zero	Therapeutic level = 5-12 μg./ml.	
Phenobarbital	Zero	Therapeutic level = 15-40 μg./ml.	
Quinidine	Zero	Therapeutic level = 0.2-0.5 mg./dl.	
Salicylate	Zero	Therapeutic level = 2-25 mg./dl. Toxic level = over 30 mg./dl.	

Sulfonamide	Zero	Therapeutic levels:
		    Sulfadiazine 8-15 mg./dl.
		    Sulfaguanidine 3-5 mg./dl.
		    Sulfamerazine 10-15 mg./dl.
		    Sulfanilamide 10-15 mg./dl.	

Valium (diazepam)	Zero	Therapeutic level: 0.5-2.5 μg./dl.	
Gastric Analysis		(Increased)	(Decreased)
Free HCl	0-30 mEq./L.	Neuroses	Pernicious anemia
Total acidity	15-45 mEq./L.	Peptic ulcer	Gastric carcinoma
Combined acid	10-15 mEq./L.	Zollinger-Ellison syndrome	Chronic atrophic gastritis Decreases normally with age

INDEX

Page numbers in *italics* refer to figures; page numbers followed by (t) refer to tables.

Abdomen, incisions of, 714, *715*
  as an indicator of nutritional status, 142(t)
  injuries to, emergency nursing in, 1421
  pain, assessment of, 76
  physical examination of, 75-79
  postoperative distention of, 356, *356*
  radiologic examination of, 287, *288*
  size of internal organs of, 77
  topography of, 75, *75,* 713, *715*
Abduction, definition of, 184
Abortion, habitual, 974
  management following, 975
  patient education following, 975
  septic, 975
  spontaneous, types of, 973
  therapeutic, management of, 974
    types of, 974
Abscess(es), anorectal, 792, *792*
  brain, clinical manifestations of, 1229
  dentoalveolar, chronic, 685
  liver, 826
    amebic, 1403
  lung, 478-479
  mammary, lactational, 1008
  periapical, 685
  perinephric, 940
  peritonsillar, clinical manifestations of, 392
  rectal, 792
  renal, 940
Acceptance, as a stage of dying, 175
Accidents, as a cause of death, 12(t)
  motor vehicle, as a cause of death, 12(t)
  prevention of, in the elderly, 215
Accommodation, visual, 1125
Acetohexamide, pharmacology of, 843(t)
  in the treatment of diabetes, 843
Acetone, urine testing for, 835
Acetylcysteine, for bronchial asthma, 1115
  for pulmonary emphysema, 486(t)
Achalasia, esophageal, management of, 701
Achlorhydria, altered drug responses in, 223(t)
Acid-base balance, *121*
  disturbances in, 125-127
    diagnosis of, 126-127
    therapy of, 127, 129-131
  regulation of acid excretion in, 896
Acidemia, *121*
Acidosis, definition of, *121,* 125
  metabolic, 125-126, *127*
  respiratory, 126, *127*

Acne vulgaris, 1050-1051
  dermabrasion for, 1078
Acoustic nerve, assessment of, 84
  neuroma of, clinical manifestations of, 1225
Acromegaly, changes in head size in, 51
ACTH, in cancer therapy, 264
  role in regulation of homeostasis, 111
Actinomycin, site of action in the cell cycle, *254*
  toxicity of, 255(t)
Actinomycosis, clinical manifestations of, 1391
  management of, 1392
Active transport, definition of, 119
  role in internal exchange of electrolytes, 120
Activities of daily living, adaptive equipment as aids to, 196
  sample chart, *195*
  following stroke, 1202
  teaching of, 194, 196
Addison's disease, assessment of, 872
  clinical manifestations of, 872
  management of, 872
  pathophysiology of, 114, *115,* 872
Adduction, definition of, 184
Adenoid(s), anatomy of, 384, *384*
  infection of, management of, 391
Adenoidectomy, nursing management following, 391
  patient education following, 392
Adenomyosis, clinical manifestations and treatment of, 999
Adenosine triphosphate (ATP), as an energy source for active transport, 120
ADH, role in the regulation of water elimination, 120
Adhesions, postoperative, as a cause of intestinal obstruction, 789
Adrenal gland, cancer of, chemotherapy response rates in, 266(t)
  cortex, activity of, 111
    function of, 859
    hormone secretion by, 872
  glucocorticoid secretion by, 859
  hormones secreted by, site and function of, 857(t)
  medulla, activity of, 111
    function of, 859
  mineralocorticoid secretion by, 859
  pheochromocytoma of, 870
  sex hormones of, 860
  tumors of, adrenalectomy for, 874

Adrenalectomy, for adrenal tumors, 874
  for malignancy of breasts or prostate, 874, 1017(t)
Adrenocortical insufficiency, chronic primary, assessment of, 872
  clinical manifestations and pathophysiology of, 872
  management of, 872
  pathophysiology of, 114-115, *115*
Adrenocorticotrophin. See *ACTH.*
Adriamycin, site of action in the cell cycle, *254*
  toxicity of, 255(t), 267(t)
Adult, recommended daily requirements of vitamins and minerals, 144(t)
Adulthood, mature, developmental concepts of, 206-207
Aerotitis media, causes and prevention of, 1155
Affection, need for, by patients, 165-166
Aging. See also *Elderly people.*
  American, profile of, 209, *209*
  biological, 208
  developmental theories and themes of, 207-208
  and disease, 215-216
  impact and implications for health care of, 209-210
  physiologic changes of, 210-213
  psychological, 208
  sociogenic, 208-209
Agranulocytosis, management of, 666
Air embolism, as a complication of intravenous therapy, 138
Airway, esophageal obturator, insertion of, 1414, *1415*
  maintenance of, during anesthesia, 348
    following head injuries, 1249
    in patient with maxillofacial problems, 1076
    in the postoperative period, 347-350, *348, 350*
    in shock, 369
  oropharyngeal, insertion of, 1414
Albumin, serum, interpretation of laboratory findings, 150(t)
  in the treatment of shock, 677
Alcoholism, acute intoxication, emergency management of, 1438
  in the clinical interview, 40
  delirium tremens, emergency management of, 1438
  and surgery, 310